MW00563498

DIAGNOSTIC AND SURGICAL

IMAGING ANATOMY

BRAIN • HEAD & NECK • SPINE

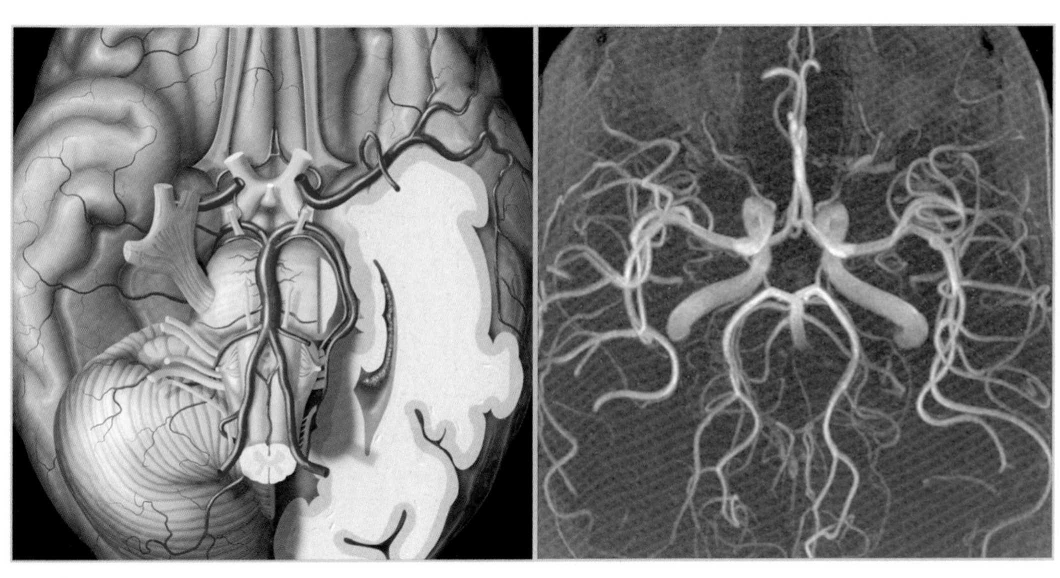

DIAGNOSTIC AND SURGICAL IMAGING ANATOMY
BRAIN • HEAD & NECK • SPINE

H. Ric Harnsberger, MD
Professor of Radiology
R.C. Willey Chair in Neuroradiology
University of Utah School of Medicine

Anne G. Osborn, MD, FACR
Distinguished Professor of Radiology
William H. and Patricia W. Child
Presidential Endowed Chair in Radiology
University of Utah School of Medicine
GE Healthcare Visiting Professor in Diagnostic Imaging
Armed Forces Institute of Pathology

Jeffrey S. Ross, MD
Staff Neuroradiologist
Head, Radiology Research
Cleveland Clinic Foundation

Kevin R. Moore, MD
Pediatric Neuroradiologist
Primary Children's Medical Center
Adjunct Assistant Professor of Radiology
University of Utah School of Medicine

Karen L. Salzman, MD
Associate Professor of Radiology
Division of Neuroradiology
University of Utah School of Medicine

Charles R. Carrasco, MD
Assistant Professor of Radiology
University of Utah School of Medicine

Bronwyn E. Hamilton, MD
Assistant Professor of Radiology
Oregon Health Sciences University

H. Christian Davidson, MD
Assistant Professor of Radiology
Vice Chairman, Department of Radiology
University of Utah School of Medicine

Richard H. Wiggins, MD
Associate Professor of Radiology
Division of Neuroradiology
Head and Neck Imaging
University of Utah School of Medicine

Managing Editor
André J. Macdonald, MBChB
Attending Radiologist, VA Salt Lake City Healthcare System
Adjunct Assistant Professor, Radiology
University of Utah School of Medicine

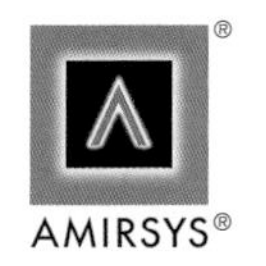

AMIRSYS®
Names you know, content you trust

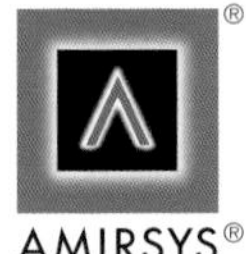

AMIRSYS®

Names you know, content you trust®

First Edition

Second Printing - October 2006
Third Printing - December 2007

Composition by Amirsys Inc, Salt Lake City, Utah

Printed in Canada by Friesens, Altona, Manitoba, Canada

ISBN-13: 978-1-9318-8429-7
ISBN-10: 1-9318-8429-3
ISBN-13: 978-1-9318-8430-3 (International English Edition)
ISBN-10: 1-9318-8430-7 (International English Edition)

Notice and Disclaimer

The information in this product ("Product") is provided as a reference for use by licensed medical professionals and no others. It does not and should not be construed as any form of medical diagnosis or professional medical advice on any matter. Receipt or use of this Product, in whole or in part, does not constitute or create a doctor-patient, therapist-patient, or other healthcare professional relationship between Amirsys Inc. ("Amirsys") and any recipient. This Product may not reflect the most current medical developments, and Amirsys makes no claims, promises, or guarantees about accuracy, completeness, or adequacy of the information contained in or linked to the Product. The Product is not a substitute for or replacement of professional medical judgment. Amirsys and its affiliates, authors, contributors, partners, and sponsors disclaim all liability or responsibility for any injury and/or damage to persons or property in respect to actions taken or not taken based on any and all Product information.

In the cases where drugs or other chemicals are prescribed, readers are advised to check the Product information currently provided by the manufacturer of each drug to be administered to verify the recommended dose, the method and duration of administration, and contraindications. It is the responsibility of the treating physician relying on experience and knowledge of the patient to determine dosages and the best treatment for the patient.

To the maximum extent permitted by applicable law, Amirsys provides the Product AS IS AND WITH ALL FAULTS, AND HEREBY DISCLAIMS ALL WARRANTIES AND CONDITIONS, WHETHER EXPRESS, IMPLIED OR STATUTORY, INCLUDING BUT NOT LIMITED TO, ANY (IF ANY) IMPLIED WARRANTIES OR CONDITIONS OF MERCHANTABILITY, OF FITNESS FOR A PARTICULAR PURPOSE, OF LACK OF VIRUSES, OR ACCURACY OR COMPLETENESS OF RESPONSES, OR RESULTS, AND OF LACK OF NEGLIGENCE OR LACK OF WORKMANLIKE EFFORT. ALSO, THERE IS NO WARRANTY OR CONDITION OF TITLE, QUIET ENJOYMENT, QUIET POSSESSION, CORRESPONDENCE TO DESCRIPTION OR NON-INFRINGEMENT, WITH REGARD TO THE PRODUCT. THE ENTIRE RISK AS TO THE QUALITY OF OR ARISING OUT OF USE OR PERFORMANCE OF THE PRODUCT REMAINS WITH THE READER.

Amirsys disclaims all warranties of any kind if the Product was customized, repackaged or altered in any way by any third party.

Library of Congress Cataloging-in-Publication Data

Diagnostic and surgical imaging anatomy. Brain, head & neck, spine /
H. Ric Harnsberger ... [et al.] ; managing editor, André Macdonald.
-- 1st ed.
p. ; cm.
Includes index.
ISBN 1-931884-29-3 (alk. paper) -- ISBN 1-931884-30-7 (International ed. : alk. paper)
1. Brain--Anatomy--Atlases. 2. Head--Anatomy--Atlases. 3. Neck--Anatomy--Atlases. 4. Spine--Anatomy--Atlases. 5. Brain--Imaging--Atlases. 6. Head--Imaging--Atlases. 7. Neck--Imaging--Atlases. 8. Spine--Imaging--Atlases. I. Harnsberger, H. Ric. II. Macdonald, André. III. Title: Imaging anatomy. Brain, head & neck, spine. IV. Title: Brain, head & neck, spine.
[DNLM: 1. Brain--anatomy & histology--Atlases. 2. Head--anatomy & histology--Atlases. 3. Magnetic Resonance Spectroscopy--Atlases. 4. Neck--anatomy & histology--Atlases. 5. Spine--anatomy & histology--Atlases. 6. Tomography, X-Ray Computed--Atlases.
WL 17 D536 2006]
QM455.D486 2006
611'.91--dc22

2006040720

This book is dedicated to the busy physician who desires to be anatomically correct in their work but often lacks ready access to key imaging anatomy reference material. To this intrepid physician group we offer the Diagnostic and Surgical Imaging Anatomy series as an in depth critical imaging anatomy reference book to assist in your daily work. We hope that easy access to anatomically precise reporting will take some of the load off your increasingly challenging work days. Enjoy!

H. Ric Harnsberger, MD

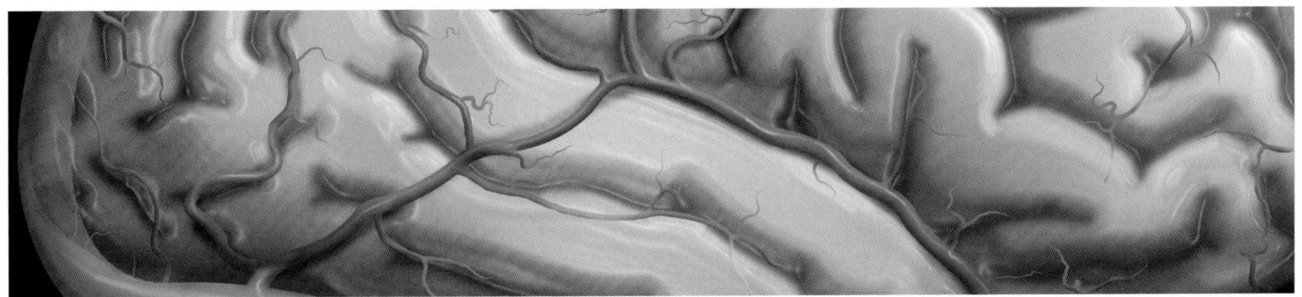

DIAGNOSTIC AND SURGICAL IMAGING ANATOMY: BRAIN, HEAD & NECK, SPINE

We at Amirsys, together with our distribution colleagues at LWW, are proud to present *Diagnostic and Surgical Imaging Anatomy: Brain, Head & Neck, Spine*, the first in a brand-new 3 volume series of anatomy reference titles. All books in the series are designed specifically to serve clinicians in both medical imaging and the related subspecialty surgeons. We focus on anatomy that is generally visible on imaging studies, crossing modalities and presenting bulleted single page anatomy descriptions along with a rich offering of color normal anatomy graphics and in-depth multimodality, multiplanar high-resolution imaging.

Each imaging anatomy textbook contains over 2,500 labeled color graphics and radiologic images, with heavy emphasis on 3 Tesla MR and state-of-the-art multi-detector CT. It is designed to give the medical professional rapid answers to imaging anatomy questions with each normal anatomy sequence providing views of anatomic structures never before seen and discussed in an anatomy reference textbook. *Brain, Head & Neck, Spine* is organized into 3 major parts, then further subdivided to reflect the normal anatomy topics inherent to each major part.

In summary, *Diagnostic and Surgical Imaging Anatomy: Brain, Head & Neck, Spine* is a product designed with you, the reader, in mind. Today's typical radiologic or surgical practice settings demand both accuracy and efficiency in image interpretation for clinical decision-making. We think you'll find this new approach to anatomy a highly efficient and wonderfully rich resource that will be the core of your reference collection in Brain, Head & Neck and Spine anatomy. Future volumes arriving later in 2006 and 2007 will cover musculoskeletal, chest, abdomen, and pelvis imaging, among other relevant topics.

We hope that you will sit back, dig in, and enjoy seeing anatomy and imaging with a whole different eye.

Anne G. Osborn, MD
Executive Vice President and Editor-in-Chief, Amirsys Inc.

H. Ric Harnsberger, MD
CEO & Chairman, Amirsys Inc.

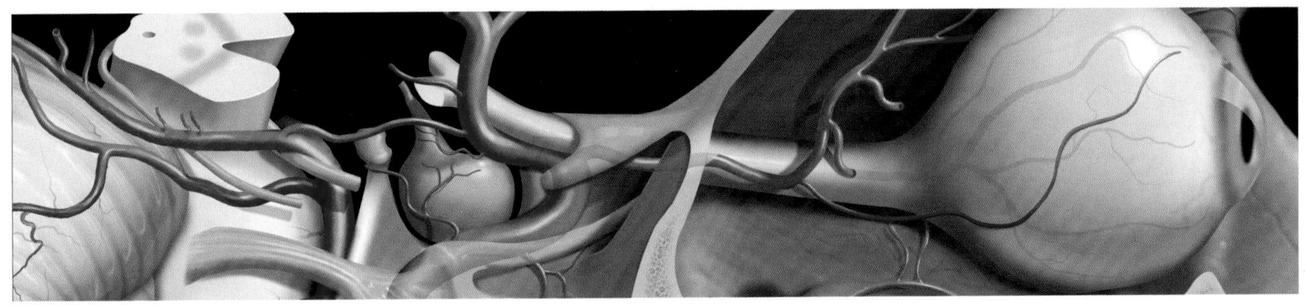

FOREWORD

As freshman medical students in the late 1950's we studied anatomy in the traditional manner with manuals of dissection, cadavers, and no idea of the importance of what we were learning. As radiologists into the 1960's and early 70's, our anatomic universe was still two-dimensional, and texts of radiographic anatomy consisted of line drawings highlighting the larger structures seen on film. Structures were separated into a few categories of density from air to bone with fat and water in between and contrast material to provide silhouettes.

Sectional imaging changed all of that and has revealed anatomic structures that no one would have dreamed could be visualized in vivo without a scalpel, let alone in three dimensions. Early on, a few anatomic-radiographic manuals appeared, but labeling was gross, images were of varying quality, and anatomic comparisons were usually used "with permission" from a variety of classical anatomic textbooks.

In this volume, which deals with the anatomy of the brain, head and neck, and spine, the Amirsys team, led again by H. Ric Harnsberger, Anne G. Osborn and Jeff S. Ross, has built on its tradition of brevity of verbiage, uniformity of anatomic drawings and high quality medical images. The reference anatomic images that accompany CT and MR scans are created to look at human anatomy *in the projections radiologists use*, vistas that Gray, Cunningham, Willis, Galen, Hunter et al. could never have imagined. What is most unique is the accompanying text organization, which includes the clinical and pathological entities to consider in a given anatomic area.

As in their previous texts, radiological images are superb and discreetly labeled so as not to intrude on the anatomic lesson. Images in different planes are often juxtaposed in the manner in which they might be viewed on a PACS station. Correlative anatomic images are in color, and were created by a team of superb medical illustrators, and often include three dimensional surface rendered CT images that are almost indistinguishable from a photograph of the anatomic specimen. In fact this book raises the question of where the boundaries between classical anatomy and medical imaging lie.

With the bulk of diagnoses today being made in the radiology department, this is anatomy for 21st century medicine. This textbook not only teaches what the radiologist needs to know, but this should become a "bible" for the teaching of anatomy to medical students. Its title appropriately eliminates reference to "radiological anatomy." It is anatomy for the entire universe of medical and allied professionals and, as a bonus, will help them understand why they see what they see on those increasingly important diagnostic images. The only thing missing is the formaldehyde.

Michael S. Huckman, MD
Professor of Radiology
Rush Medical College
Director of Neuroradiology
Rush University Medical Center

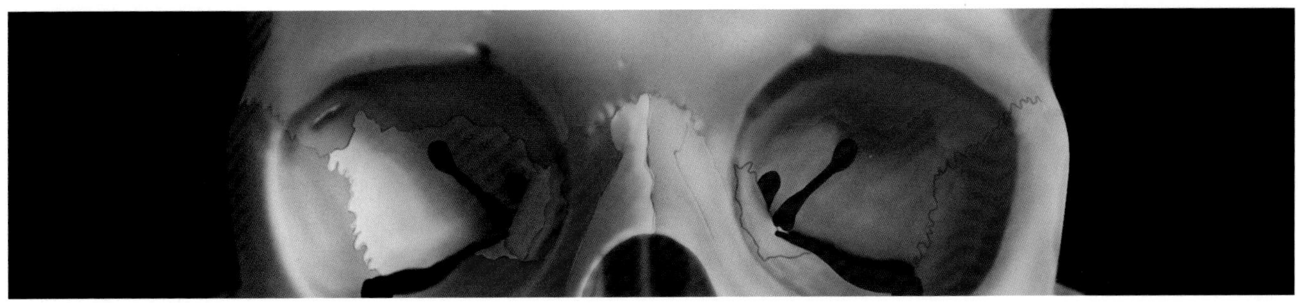

PREFACE

When I began my radiology career as a resident at Stanford University, CT was in its infancy and MR wasn't even in our vocabulary. Neuroimaging was primarily plain film radiographs, cerebral angiography, and (ugh) pneumoencephalography. In my attempt to relearn neuroanatomy I discovered a real treasure: a small book, scarcely larger than one of today's paperbacks, by McClure Wilson that was titled something like "Anatomic Foundations of Neuroradiology." It was prose, mostly text, with relatively few images and line drawings but it did something no other book did, viz., it put the anatomic foundation firmly under our crude neuroimaging procedures and taught me a principle that still holds true today: at least half of learning neuroradiology is understanding neuroanatomy.

As CT and then MR became part of our standard neuroimaging armamentarium, I longed for a new book that would do for today's radiologists what Dr. Wilson's book did for me. While a number of atlases and other volumes have been published, nothing has ever come close to the impact his book had on us. Until now. H. Ric Harnsberger came up with the idea of building on our enormously successful Diagnostic Imaging series, using succinct, bulleted text combined with our signature graphics, 3T MR imaging and MDR CT to create a new series, Diagnostic and Surgical Imaging Anatomy. Jeff S. Ross and several of our favorite co-authors have joined Ric and me in writing the first book in this innovative new series. Brain, Head & Neck, Spine are combined into a single volume that we believe will help radiologists understand the detailed anatomy that underlies neuroimaging. Each topic is lavishly illustrated, not only with gorgeous graphics but many series of high-resolution images that portray the relevant anatomy in many planes.

We hope that this, the first in our series, will do for you what Dr. Wilson's book accomplished for an earlier generation of radiologists. Sit down, put your feet up, and dig into what we hope will be a veritable imaging feast! You might even keep the book on your coffee table—the graphics/imaging correlates are so clear that your family, friends and neighbors can tell at a glance what it is that you do all day long. Enjoy!

Anne G. Osborn, MD, FACR
Distinguished Professor of Radiology
William H. and Patricia W. Child
Presidential Endowed Chair in Radiology
University of Utah School of Medicine

GE Healthcare Visiting Professor in Diagnostic Imaging
Armed Forces Institute of Pathology
Washington, D.C.

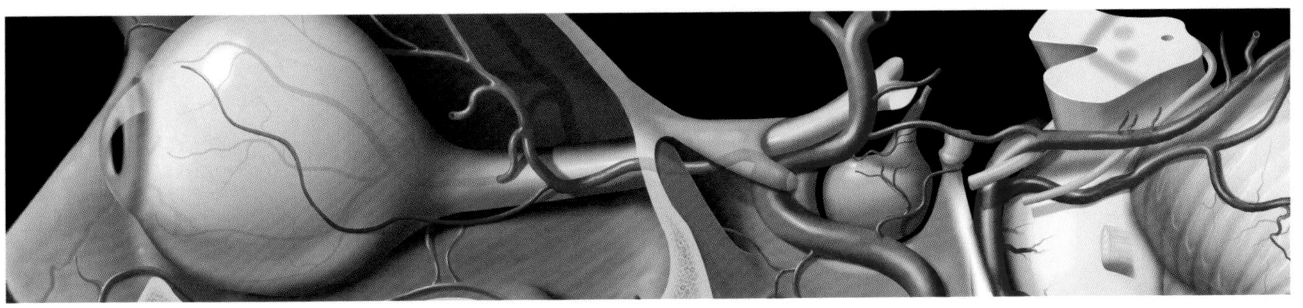

ACKNOWLEDGMENTS

Illustrations

Lane R. Bennion, MS
Richard Coombs, MS
James A. Cooper, MD

Image/Text Editing

Melissa A. Hoopes
Kaerli Main

Medical Text Editing

André J. Macdonald, MD
Richard H. Wiggins, MD
Karen L. Salzman, MD
R. Kent Sanders, MD
H. Christian Davidson, MD

Case Management

Roth LaFleur
Christopher Odekirk

Project Lead

Angie D. Mascarenaz

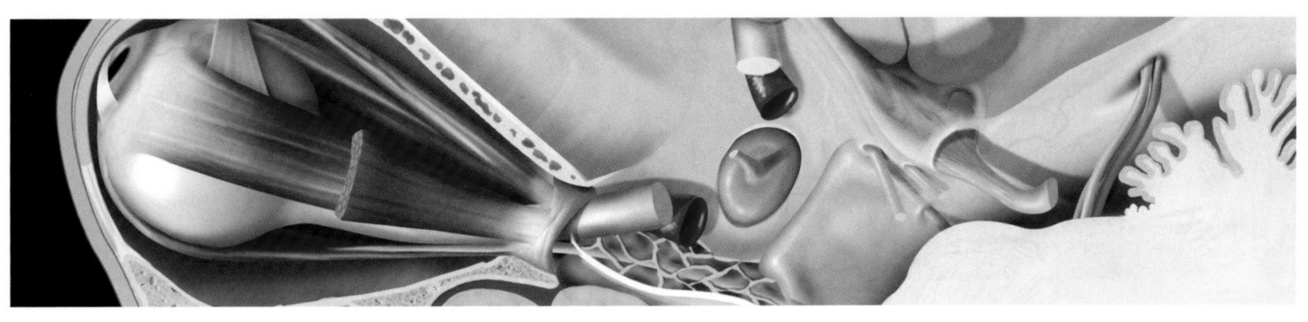

SECTIONS

PART I
Brain

PART II
Head & Neck

PART III
Spine

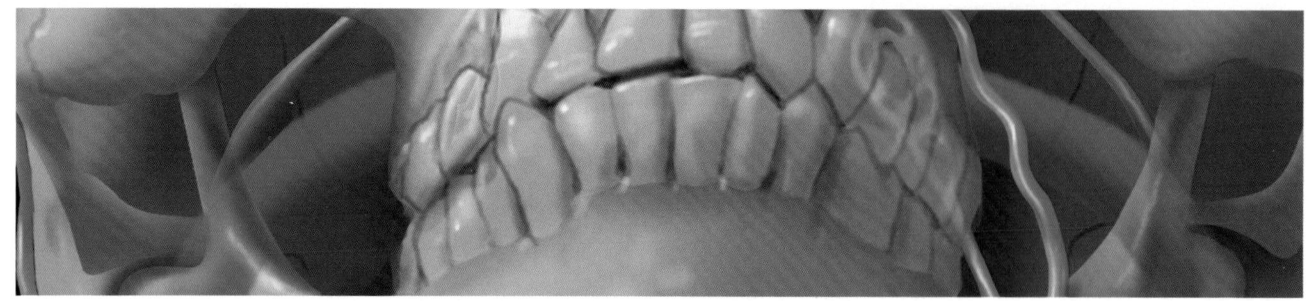

TABLE OF CONTENTS

PART I
Brain

Section 1
Scalp, Skull and Meninges

Section 2
Supratentorial Brain

Section 3
Infratentorial Brain

Section 4
CSF Spaces

Section 5
Cranial Nerves

Section 6
Extracranial Arteries

Section 7
Intracranial Arteries

Section 8
Veins and Venous Sinuses

PART II
Head & Neck

Section 1
Temporal Bone and Skull Base

Section 2
Orbit, Nose and Sinuses

Section 3
Suprahyoid and Infrahyoid Neck

Section 4
Oral Cavity

PART III
Spine

Section 1
Vertebral Column, Discs & Paraspinal Muscle

Section 2
Cord, Meninges and Spaces

Section 3
Vascular

Section 4
Plexus

Section 5
Peripheral Nerves

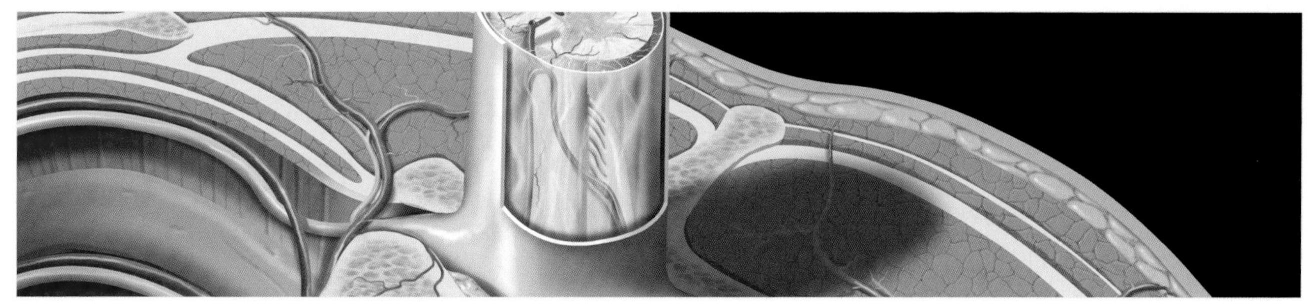

ABBREVIATIONS

Brain

AA: Aortic arch

ACA: Anterior cerebral artery

AChoA: Anterior choroidal artery

ACoA: Anterior communicating artery

AH: Adenohypophysis

aICA: Aberrant ICA

AICA: Anterior inferior cerebellar artery

APMV: Anterior pontomesencephalic vein/venous plexus

BA: Basilar artery

BCT: Brachiocephalic trunk

BG: Basal ganglia

BVR: Basal vein of Rosenthal

CCA: Common carotid artery

CC: Corpus callosum

CHD: Congenital heart disease

CN: Cranial nerve

CN1: Olfactory nerve

CN2: Optic nerve

CN3: Oculomotor nerve

CN4: Trochlear nerve

CN5: Trigeminal nerve

CN6: Abducens nerve

CN7: Facial nerve

CN8: Vestibulocochlear nerve

CN9: Glossopharyngeal nerve

CN10: Vagus nerve

CN11: Accessory nerve

CN12: Hypoglossal nerve

COW: Circle of Willis

CPA: Cerebellopontine angle

CS: Cavernous sinus

CSF: Cerebrospinal fluid

dAVF: Dural arteriovenous fistula

DMCV: Deep middle cerebral vein

ECA: External carotid artery

EDS: Extradural space

GP: Globus pallidus

IAC: Internal auditory canal

ICA: Internal carotid artery

ICV: Internal cerebral vein

IJV: Internal jugular vein

IPS: Inferior petrosal sinuses

ISF: Interstitial fluid

ISS: Inferior sagittal sinus

IVN: Inferior vestibular nerve

IVV: Inferior vermian vein

LAO: Left anterior oblique

LCCA: Left common carotid artery

LSCA: Left subclavian artery

MCA: Middle cerebral artery

MHT: Meningohypophyseal trunk

MLF: Medial longitudinal fasciculus

MMA: Middle meningeal artery

NH: Neurohypophysis

OA: Ophthalmic artery

PCA: Posterior cerebral artery

PCoA: Posterior communicating artery

PCV: Precentral cerebellar vein

PICA: Posterior inferior cerebellar artery

PVS: Perivascular space

RCCA: Right common carotid artery

RAH: Recurrent artery of Heubner

RSCA: Right subclavian artery

SAS: Subarachnoid space

SCA: Superior cerebellar artery

SDS: Subdural space

SHN: Suprahyoid neck

SMCV: Superficial middle cerebral vein

SNHL: Sensorineural hearing loss

SOF: Superior orbital fissure

SPS: Superior petrosal sinuses

SS: Straight sinus

SSS: Superior sagittal sinus

SV: Septal vein

SVN: Superior vestibular nerve

SVV: Superior vermian vein

TS: Transverse sinus

TSV: Thalamostriate vein

VA: Vertebral artery

VB: Vertebrobasilar

VofG: Vein of Galen

VofT: Vein of Trolard

VRS: Virchow-Robin spaces

Head & Neck

ACS: Anterior cervical space

ASB: Anterior skull base

BS: Buccal space

CCA: Common carotid artery

CG: Crista galli

CN: Cranial nerve

CP: Cribriform plate

CPA: Cerebellopontine angle

CS: Carotid space

CSB: Central skull base

CSF: Cerebrospinal fluid

DL-DCF: Deep layer, deep cervical fascia

DS: Danger space

EAC: External auditory canal

ECA: External carotid artery

EOM: Extra-ocular muscles

FOM: Floor of mouth

FL: Frontal lobe

FO: Foramen ovale

FR: Foramen rotundum

FS: Foramen spinosum

FVC: False vocal cord

GWS: Greater wing of sphenoid

IAC: Internal auditory canal

ICA: Internal carotid artery

IE: Inner ear

IHN: Infrahyoid neck

IJC: Internal jugular (nodal) chain

IJV: Internal jugular vein

IOF: Inferior orbital fissure

IOV: Inferior ophthalmic vein

JF: Jugular foramen

LWS: Lesser wing of sphenoid

Md: Mandible

ME: Middle ear

ME-M: Middle ear-mastoid

ML-DCF: Middle layer, deep cervical fascia

MS: Masticator space

MSG: Minor salivary glands

Mx: Maxilla

OA: Ophthalmic artery

OMC: Ostiomeatal complex

OMS: Oral mucosal space/surface

OMU: Ostiomeatal unit

ONSC: Optic nerve-sheath complex

OphA: Ophthalmic artery

OC: Oral cavity

OpC: Optic canal

PA: Petrous apex

PCA: Posterior cerebral artery

PCS: Posterior cervical space

PNT: Perineural tumor

PMR: Pterygomandibular raphe

PMS: Pharyngeal mucosal space

PPF: Pterygopalatine fossa

PPS: Parapharyngeal space

PS: Parotid space

PSB: Posterior skull base

PTG: Parathyroid gland

PTH: Parathormone

PVS: Perivertebral space

REZ: Root entry zone

RMT: Retromolar trigone

ROT: Root of tongue

RPS: Retropharyngeal space

SAC: Spinal accessory (nodal) chain

SAN: Spinal accessory nodes

SAS: Subarachnoid space

SB: Skull base

SCA: Superior cerebral artery

SCCa: Squamous cell carcinoma

SER: Sphenoethmoidal recess

SHN: Suprahyoid neck

SL-DCF: Superficial layer, deep cervical fascia

SLS: Sublingual space

SMS: Submandibular space

SN: Sinonasal

SNHL: Sensorineural hearing loss

SOF: Superior orbital fissure

SOV: Superior ophthalmic vein

TEG: Tracheoesophageal groove

TG: Trigeminal ganglion

TMJ: Temporomandibular joint

TVC: True vocal cord

VC: Vidian canal

VS: Visceral space

Spine

AA: Atlanto-axial

ADI: Atlanto-dental interval

AIN: Anterior interosseous nerve

ALL: Anterior longitudinal ligament

AM: Arachnoid matter

AO: Atlanto-occipital

ASA: Anterior spinal artery

ATP: Adenosine triphosphate

BA: Basilar artery

BP: Brachial plexus

CCJ: Craniocervical junction

CE: Cauda equina

CTS: Carpal tunnel syndrome

CSF: Cerebrospinal fluid

CN: Cranial nerve

CPN: Common peroneal nerve

CV: Costovertebral

DL: Denticulate ligament

DM: Dura matter

DPR: Dorsal primary ramus

DRG: Dorsal root ganglion

EDNAC: Extradural neural axis compartment

EOP: External occipital protuberance

FCU: Flexor carpi ulnaris

FN: Femoral nerve

IJV: Internal jugular vein

IVC: Inferior vena cava

LN: Ligamentum nuchae

LP: Lumbar plexus

LS: Lumbosacral

LSP: Lumbosacral plexus

LST: Lumbosacral trunk

mm: Muscles

MCP: Metacarpal phalangeal joint

MN: Median nerve

OC: Occipital condyle

PIN: Posterior interosseous nerve

PLL: Posterior longitudinal ligament

PM: Pia matter

PNS: Peripheral nervous system

PSP: Posterior spinal arteries

RN: Radial nerve

RTS: Radial tunnel syndrome

SAS: Subarachnoid spaces

SC: Spinal cord

SI: Sacroiliac

SN: Sciatic nerve

SP: Spinous process

SVC: Superior vena cava

TN: Tibial nerve

TP: Transverse process

UN: Ulnar nerve

VA: Vertebral artery

VPR: Ventral primary ramus

VVP: Vertebral venous plexus

VVS: Vertebral venous system

DIAGNOSTIC AND SURGICAL

IMAGING ANATOMY

BRAIN • HEAD & NECK • SPINE

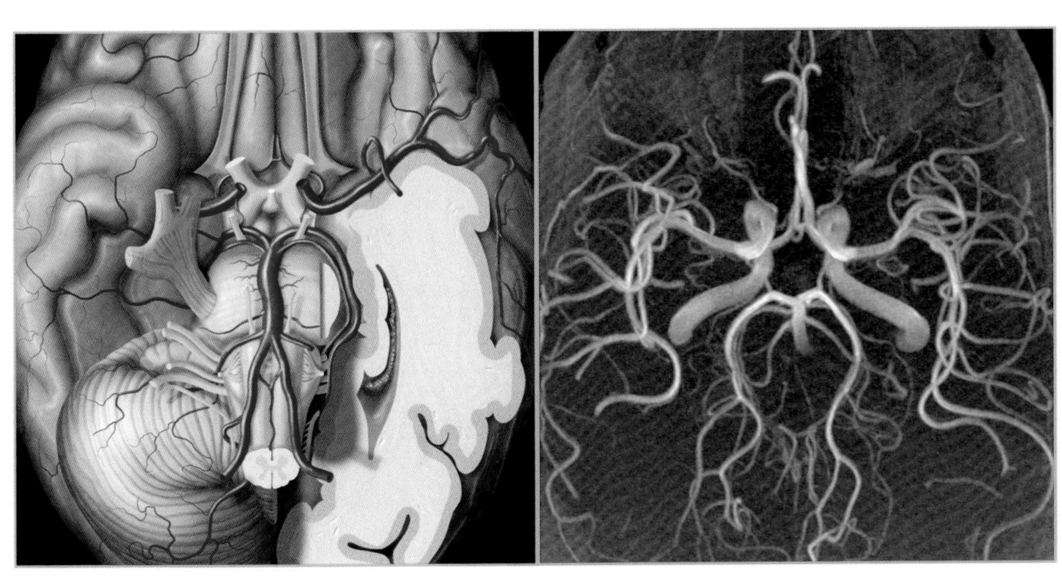

PART I

Brain

Scalp, Skull and Meninges

Supratentorial Brain

Infratentorial Brain

CSF Spaces

Cranial Nerves

Extracranial Arteries

Intracranial Arteries

Veins and Venous Sinuses

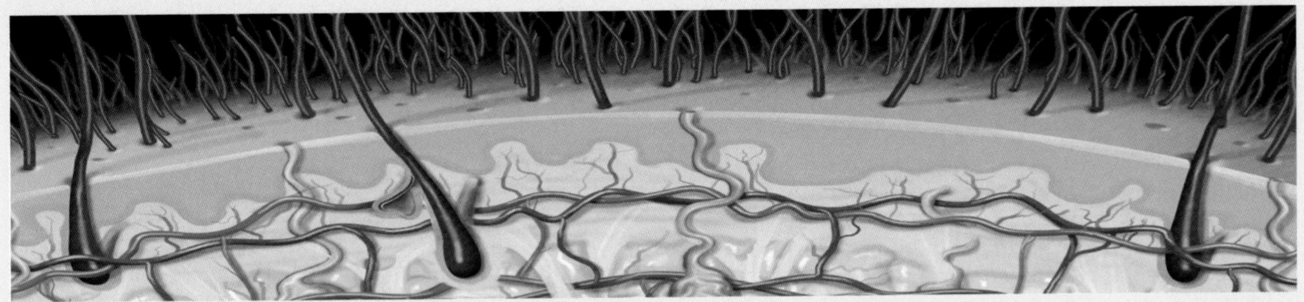

SECTION 1: Scalp, Skull and Meninges

SCALP AND CALVARIAL VAULT

Terminology

Definitions

- Bregma: Meeting of sagittal, coronal sutures (anterior fontanelle in neonates)
- Lambda: Meeting of sagittal, lambdoid sutures (site of posterior fontanelle in neonates)
- Pterion
  - "H-shaped" junction between frontal, parietal bones plus greater sphenoid wing, squamous temporal bone
  - Site of anterolateral, i.e., sphenoidal, fontanelle

Gross Anatomy

Overview

- **Scalp**
  - Scalp has five layers
    - **Skin** (epidermis, dermis, hair, sebaceous glands)
    - **Subcutaneous tissue** (very vascular fibro-adipose tissue)
    - **Epicranial tissue** (scalp muscles, galea aponeurotica)
    - **Subaponeurotic tissue** (loose areolar connective tissue)
    - **Pericranium** (periosteum of skull)
- **Skull** (28 separate bones, mostly connected by fibrous sutures)
  - **Cranium** has several parts
    - Calvarial vault
    - Cranial base
    - Facial skeleton
  - **Calvarial vault** composed of several bones
    - Frontal bone
    - Paired parietal bones
    - Squamous occipital bone
    - Paired squamous temporal bones
  - Three major serrated fibrous joints (**sutures**) connect bones of vault
    - Coronal suture
    - Sagittal suture
    - Lambdoid suture
  - **Outer, inner tables**
    - Two thin plates of compact cortical bone
    - Separated by diploic space (cancellous bone containing marrow)
  - **Endocranial surface**
    - Lined by outer (periosteal) layer of dura
    - Grooved by vascular furrows
    - May have areas of focal thinning (arachnoid granulations), foramina (emissary veins)

Imaging Anatomy

Overview

- **Scalp** largely high signal (fat) on T1WI
- **Calvarium** low signal outer/inner tables; diploic space filled with fatty marrow, usually high signal on T1WI
  - **Frontal bones**
    - Frontal sinuses show wide variation in aeration
    - Frontal bones often appear thickened, hyperostotic (especially in older females)
  - **Parietal bones**
    - Areas of parietal thinning, granular foveolae (for arachnoid granulations) common adjacent to sagittal suture
    - Inner tables often slightly irregular (convolutional markings caused by gyri), grooved by paired middle meningeal arteries + vein
  - **Occipital bone**
    - Deeply grooved by superior sagittal, transverse sinuses
    - Internal occipital protuberance marks sinus confluence (torcular Herophili)
  - **Temporal bones**
    - Thin, inner surface grooved by middle meningeal vessels
    - Outer surface grooved by superficial temporal artery

Anatomy-Based Imaging Issues

Imaging Recommendations

- Skull radiographs limited utility for evaluating calvarium, skull base
- Bone algorithm (not just soft tissue algorithm with bone windows) recommended, should be routine on all head CT scans
- 3D volume-rendered NECT excellent for overall calvarial anatomy, suspected craniosynostosis
- Contrast-enhanced fat suppressed MR excellent for suspected calvarial, dural lesions

Imaging Pitfalls

- Most common cause of "thick skull" is normal variant
- Striking hyperostosis, especially of frontal bone, common in older females
- Areas of calvarial thinning, lucencies (foramina, vascular grooves, diploic venous lakes) are normal (should not be mistaken for osteolytic metastases)
- Vascular grooves are corticated, usually less distinct than acute linear skull fracture

Embryology

Embryologic Events

- Skull base formed from endochondral ossification
- Calvarial vault forms via membranous ossification
  - Curved mesenchymal plates appear at day 30
  - Extend towards each other, skull base
  - As paired bones meet in midline, metopic and sagittal sutures are induced (coronal suture is present from onset of ossification)
  - Unossified centers at edges of parietal bone form fontanelles
  - Vault grows rapidly in first postnatal year
    - If separate ossification center develops, "sutural" bone forms

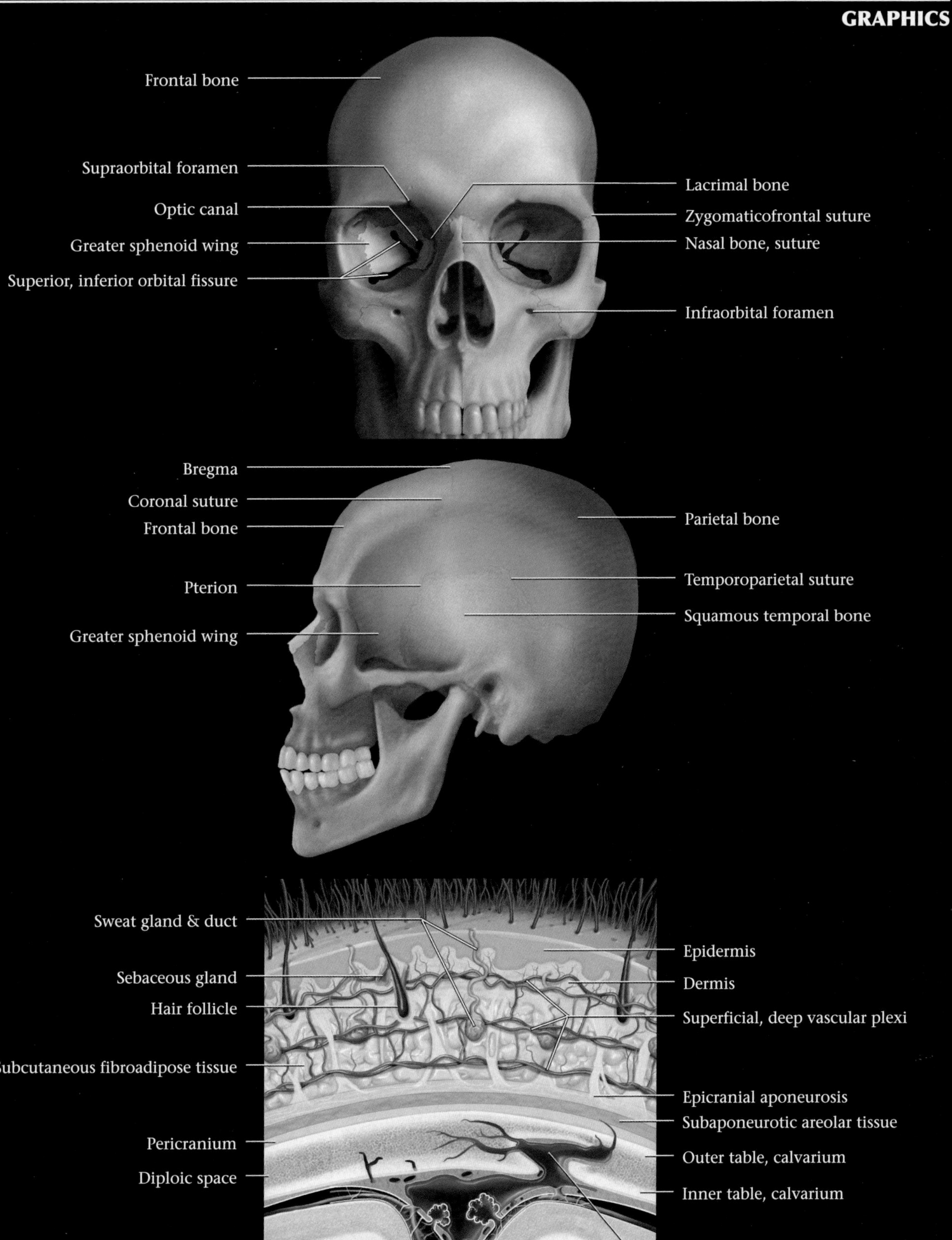
Frontal bone
Supraorbital foramen
Optic canal
Greater sphenoid wing
Superior, inferior orbital fissure
Lacrimal bone
Zygomaticofrontal suture
Nasal bone, suture
Infraorbital foramen
Bregma
Coronal suture
Frontal bone
Pterion
Greater sphenoid wing
Parietal bone
Temporoparietal suture
Squamous temporal bone
Sweat gland & duct
Sebaceous gland
Hair follicle
Subcutaneous fibroadipose tissue
Pericranium
Diploic space
Epidermis
Dermis
Superficial, deep vascular plexi
Epicranial aponeurosis
Subaponeurotic areolar tissue
Outer table, calvarium
Inner table, calvarium
Venous "lake"

(Top) Graphic depiction of cranium, frontal view. Frontal bone is rendered in purple. Two parts of the sphenoid bone are shown here: The greater and lesser wings, separated by the superior orbital fissure (SOF). The optic canal lies just above the SOF and is separated from it by a bony optic strut. **(Middle)** Lateral view of the calvarial vault. The pterion is a small area on the lateral skull at the intersection of the frontal, sphenoid, parietal and temporal squama. It is an important landmark for surgical approach to the sylvian fissure and middle cranial fossa. **(Bottom)** Scalp and calvarium are depicted in cross section. The five scalp layers are depicted. Skin consists of epidermis and dermis. Hair follicles and a sebaceous gland, the subcutaneous fibro-adipose tissue, sweat glands and ducts, as well as superficial and deep cutaneous vascular plexi are shown.

SCALP AND CALVARIAL VAULT

AXIAL NECT

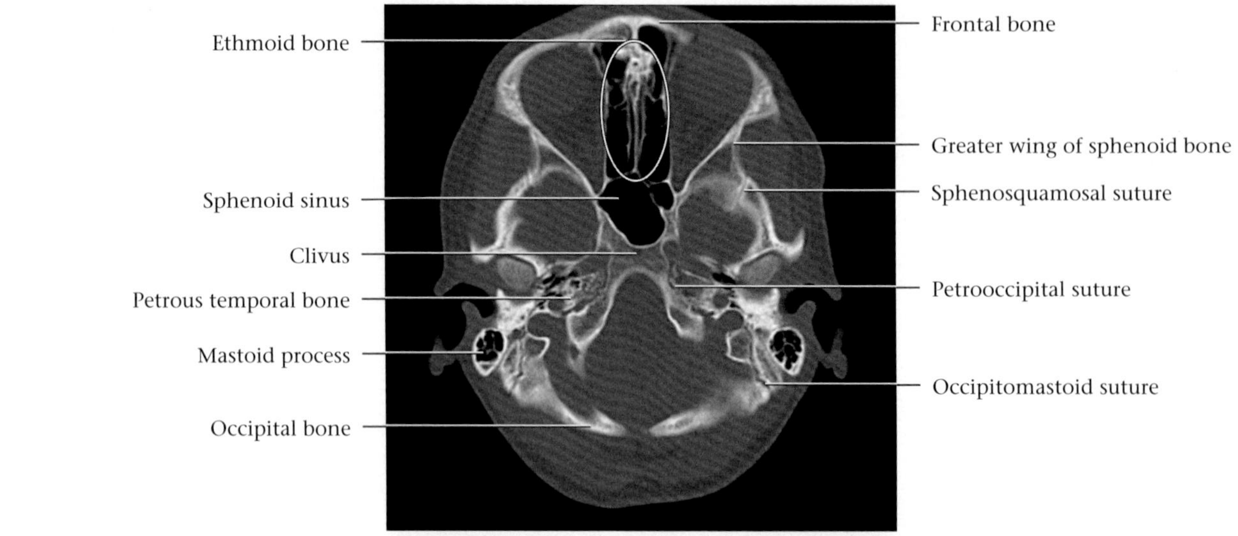

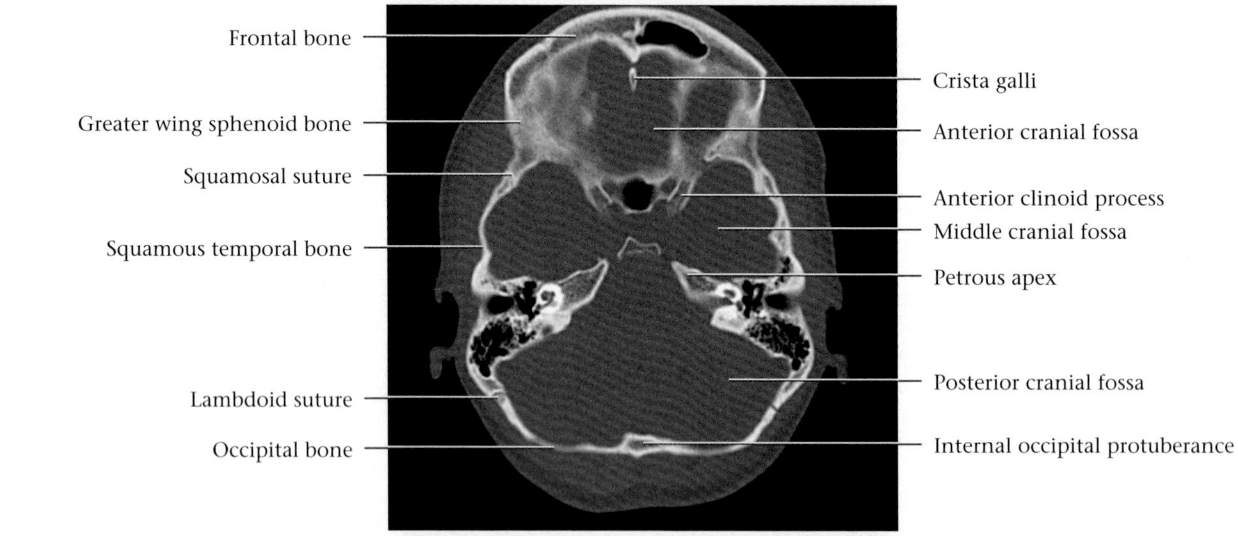

Ethmoid bone
Frontal bone
Greater wing of sphenoid bone
Sphenosquamosal suture
Sphenoid sinus
Clivus
Petrous temporal bone
Petrooccipital suture
Mastoid process
Occipitomastoid suture
Occipital bone

Frontal bone
Crista galli
Greater wing sphenoid bone
Anterior cranial fossa
Squamosal suture
Anterior clinoid process
Middle cranial fossa
Squamous temporal bone
Petrous apex
Posterior cranial fossa
Lambdoid suture
Occipital bone
Internal occipital protuberance

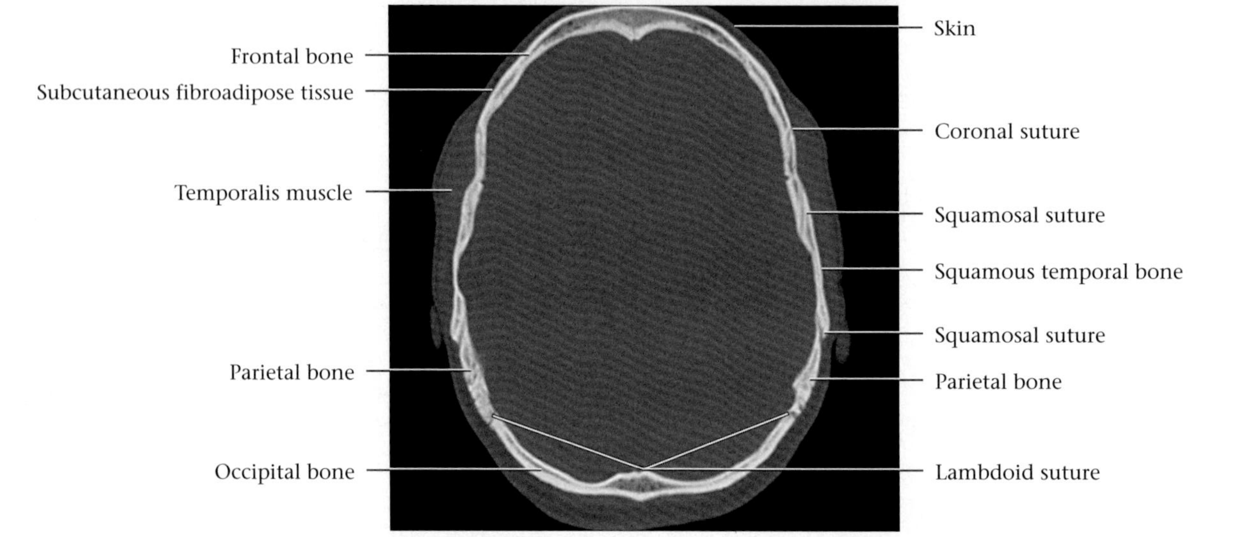

Skin
Frontal bone
Subcutaneous fibroadipose tissue
Coronal suture
Temporalis muscle
Squamosal suture
Squamous temporal bone
Squamosal suture
Parietal bone
Parietal bone
Occipital bone
Lambdoid suture

(Top) Five sequential axial NECT images from presented inferior to superior through skull base, calvarium, are depicted. Section through skull base shows major bones, sutures forming skull base. Sphenosquamosal, petrooccipital, occipitomastoid sutures are normally well seen and should not be confused with fractures. **(Middle)** Section through upper skull base shows anterior, middle and posterior cranial fossae as well as formation of lower vault by frontal, greater wing sphenoid, squamous temporal and occipital bones. **(Bottom)** Section through lower calvarial vault showing antero-posterior linear configuration of squamosal suture, not to be confused with a fracture. Major bones forming vault are frontal, parietal, and occipital bones which are now all visible.

AXIAL NECT & SAGITTAL T1 MR

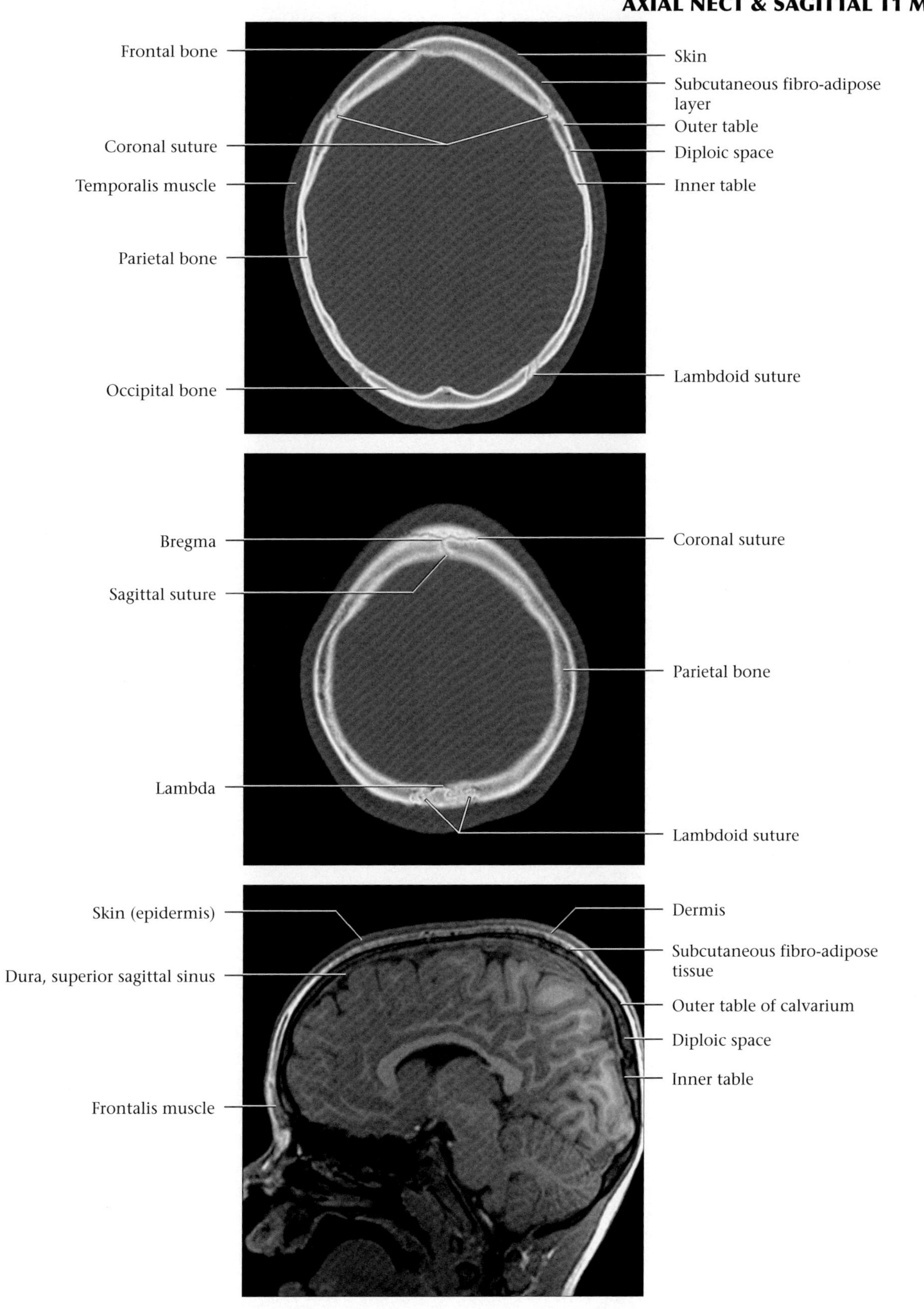
Frontal bone
Coronal suture
Temporalis muscle
Parietal bone
Occipital bone
Skin
Subcutaneous fibro-adipose layer
Outer table
Diploic space
Inner table
Lambdoid suture
Bregma
Sagittal suture
Lambda
Coronal suture
Parietal bone
Lambdoid suture
Skin (epidermis)
Dura, superior sagittal sinus
Frontalis muscle
Dermis
Subcutaneous fibro-adipose tissue
Outer table of calvarium
Diploic space
Inner table

(Top) Section through vault shows the frontal, parietal and occipital bones separated by coronal and lambdoid sutures. The calvarium consists of compact bone forming the external and inner tables with interposed diploic space. **(Middle)** Section through upper vault shows coronal, sagittal and lambdoid sutures separating frontal, parietal and occipital bones. The junction between the coronal and sagittal sutures is the bregma. Sagittal and lambdoid sutures meet at the lambda. **(Bottom)** Sagittal T1 MR volume acquisition with 1 mm sections shows details of the scalp and calvarial vault. The skin (epidermis, dermis) and subcutaneous fatty tissue can be distinguished. Marrow-bearing diploic space is contained between the hypointense outer/inner tables. The image is of an eight year old child and the hemopoietic marrow is hypointense. In adults it is hyperintense on T1.

SCALP AND CALVARIAL VAULT

3D-VRT NECT

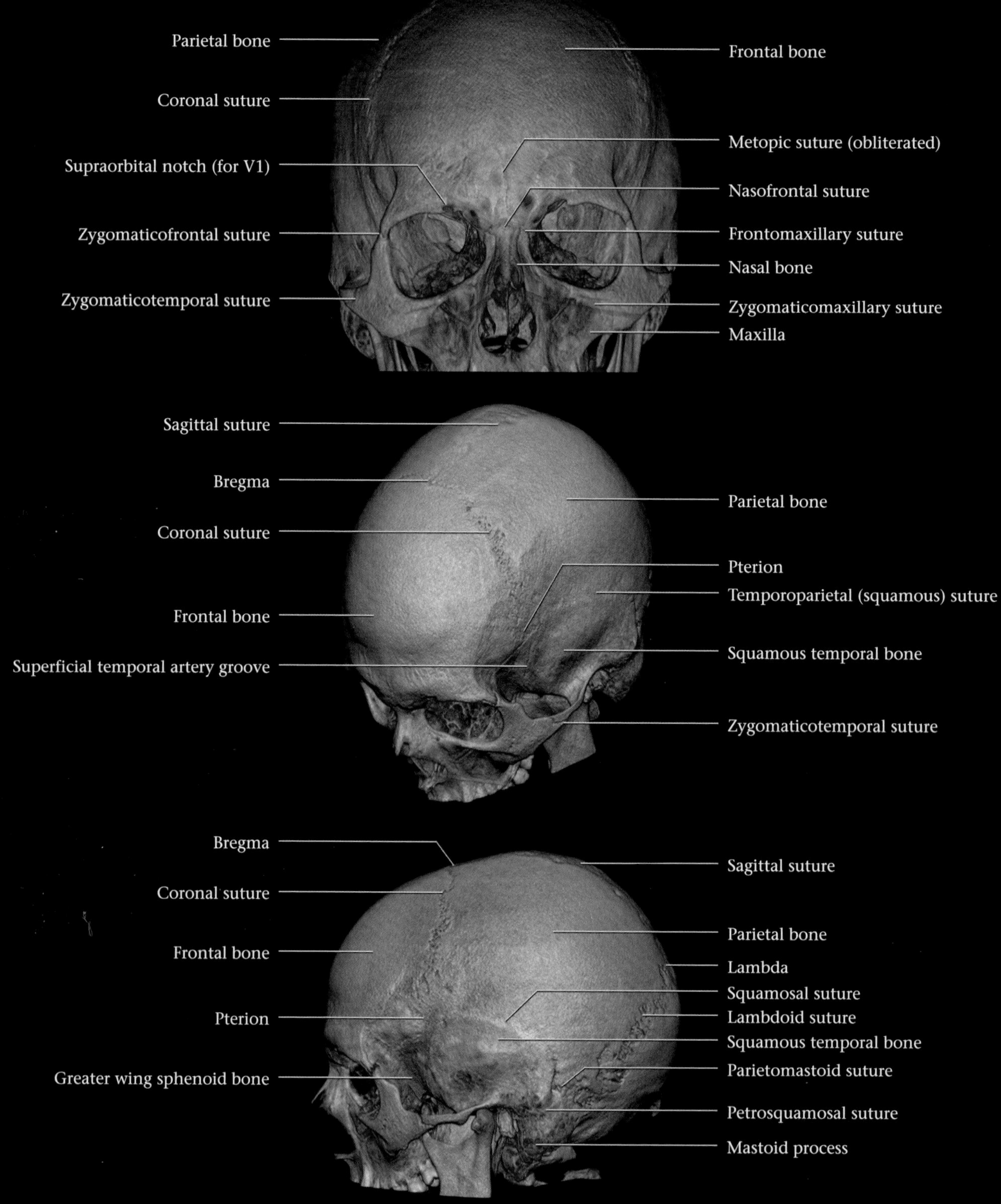
Parietal bone
Coronal suture
Supraorbital notch (for V1)
Zygomaticofrontal suture
Zygomaticotemporal suture
Frontal bone
Metopic suture (obliterated)
Nasofrontal suture
Frontomaxillary suture
Nasal bone
Zygomaticomaxillary suture
Maxilla
Sagittal suture
Bregma
Coronal suture
Frontal bone
Superficial temporal artery groove
Parietal bone
Pterion
Temporoparietal (squamous) suture
Squamous temporal bone
Zygomaticotemporal suture
Bregma
Coronal suture
Frontal bone
Pterion
Greater wing sphenoid bone
Sagittal suture
Parietal bone
Lambda
Squamosal suture
Lambdoid suture
Squamous temporal bone
Parietomastoid suture
Petrosquamosal suture
Mastoid process

(Top) First of six 3D reconstruction images using volume rendering technique (VRT) of data acquired from multislice NECT shows anterior skull. Anterior calvarial vault is dominated by frontal bone, which also forms floor of anterior cranial fossa (roof of orbit). **(Middle)** Antero-superior view shows coronal suture separating frontal & parietal bones. Sagittal suture separates paired parietal bones. Zygomatic arch is formed by zygomatic process of temporal bone & temporal process of zygomatic bone. **(Bottom)** The lateral calvarial vault is formed by parietal bone, with lesser portions formed by frontal, greater wing sphenoid, squamous temporal & occipital bones with intervening sutures.

SCALP AND CALVARIAL VAULT

3D-VRT NECT

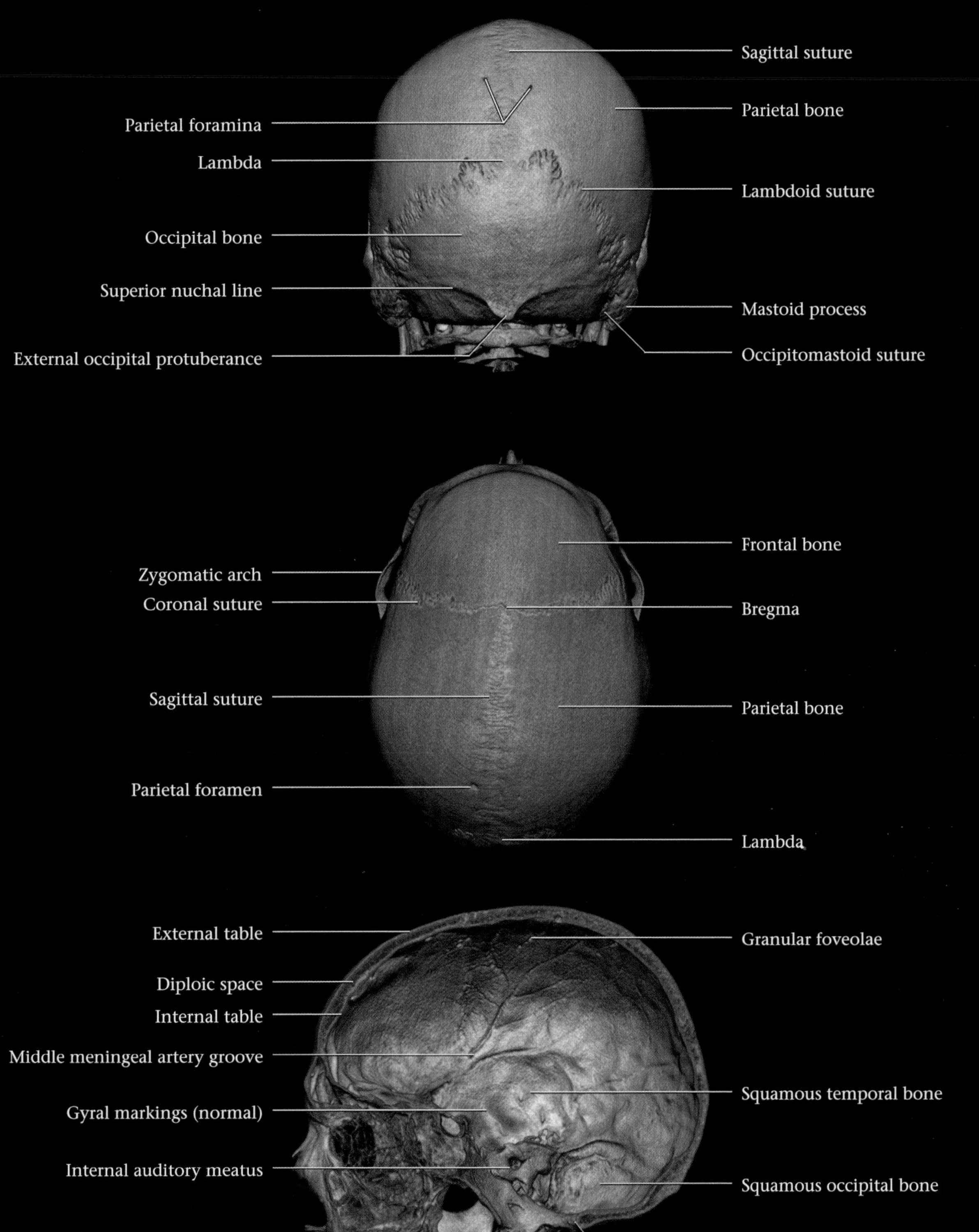

Parietal foramina
Lambda
Occipital bone
Superior nuchal line
External occipital protuberance
Sagittal suture
Parietal bone
Lambdoid suture
Mastoid process
Occipitomastoid suture
Zygomatic arch
Coronal suture
Sagittal suture
Parietal foramen
Frontal bone
Bregma
Parietal bone
Lambda
External table
Diploic space
Internal table
Middle meningeal artery groove
Gyral markings (normal)
Internal auditory meatus
Granular foveolae
Squamous temporal bone
Squamous occipital bone
Foramen magnum

(Top) Reconstruction of posterior skull formed by posterior parietal and squamous portion of occipital bones. Parietal foramina are present which transmit emissary veins and may occasionally be particularly large. **(Middle)** View of superior skull shows coronal & sagittal sutures. Coronal suture separates frontal & parietal bones. Sagittal suture separates paired parietal bones & extends from bregma anteriorly to lambda posteriorly. **(Bottom)** The inner surface of lateral calvarium shows prominent groove for middle meningeal artery. Sectioned vault demonstrates compact external & inner table with interposed diploic space. Numerous indentations of variable size called granular foveolae occur in parasagittal parietal bone into which arachnoid granulations extend.

CRANIAL MENINGES

Terminology

Abbreviations

- Extradural space (EDS)
- Subdural space (SDS)
- Subarachnoid space (SAS)
- Subpial space (SPS)
- Perivascular space (PVS)
- Interstitial fluid (ISF)
- Cerebrospinal fluid (CSF)
- Internal carotid artery (ICA)
- External carotid artery (ECA)

Definitions

- Pachymeninges: Dura
- Leptomeninges: Arachnoid, pia
- EDS: Potential space between dura, skull; seen only in pathologic conditions (infection, hematoma, etc.)
- SDS: Potential space between inner dura, arachnoid; seen only in pathologic conditions
- SAS: Normal CSF-filled space between arachnoid, pial-covered brain
- SPS: Potential space between pia, glia limitans of cortex
- PVS: Pial-lined, ISF-filled invagination along penetrating arteries

Gross Anatomy

Overview

- Brain encased by three meninges
  - **Dura**
    - Dense fibrocollagenous sheet
    - Two layers (outer/periosteal, inner/meningeal)
    - Closely adherent except where separate to enclose venous sinus
    - Outer layer forms periosteum of inner calvarium
    - Inner layer folds inward (forming falx cerebri, tentorium cerebelli, etc.), also continues extracranially (into orbit, through foramen magnum into spinal canal)
    - At other foramina, meningeal dura fuses with epineurium of cranial/peripheral nerves, adventitia of carotid/vertebral arteries
    - Blood supply from numerous dural vessels (middle, accessory meningeal arteries; cavernous/tentorial branches of ICA; posterior meningeal branches of vertebral artery; transosseous meningeal branches of ECA, etc.), many with extensive extra/intracranial anastomoses
    - Dura tightly adherent to skull at sutural attachments
  - **Arachnoid**
    - Thin, nearly transparent
    - Outer surface loosely adherent to dura, easily separated
    - Arachnoid follows dura, does **not** invaginate into sulci
    - SAS lies between arachnoid, pia and is traversed by sheet-like bridging trabeculae
    - Arachnoid villi/granulations = endothelial-lined extensions of arachnoid + SAS into dural sinus
  - **Pia**
    - Innermost layer of leptomeninges
    - Covers brain, invaginates into sulci
    - Follows penetrating cortical arteries into brain, forming **PVSs (Virchow-Robin spaces)**

Imaging Anatomy

Overview

- **Dura**
  - Capillaries lack endothelial tight junctions so macromolecules (e.g., contrast agents) easily leak into dura
  - Dura enhances normally on CECT, T1 C+ scans
    - Should be smooth, 1-2 mm thick
    - Most prominent near vertex, least prominent under temporal lobes
    - Enhancing segments appear discontinuous on 1.5T but typically well seen on 3T as continuous curvilinear enhancement that hugs inner calvarium
- **Arachnoid**
  - Normally not seen
  - Pathologic processes typically affect both dura, arachnoid which become involved/thickened together and are indistinguishable on imaging
  - Arachnoid granulations seen as round/ovoid areas of CSF density/signal intensity that project into dural venous sinus (most typically in transverse/sigmoid sinuses)
  - Trabeculae/vessels that bridge SAS occasionally seen on 3T T2WI or if they become pathologically enlarged (e.g., in Sturge-Weber syndrome)
- Pia normally not seen on imaging **but** perivascular spaces often normally seen as linear/ovoid CSF areas in basal ganglia around anterior commissure, basal ganglia, midbrain, deep cerebral white matter

Anatomy-Based Imaging Issues

Imaging Recommendations

- T1 C+ scans in both axial, coronal planes

Imaging Pitfalls

- "Giant" arachnoid granulations (up to 1-2 cm) may occur as normal variant in dural venous sinuses; should not be mistaken for thrombus
- Veins in, around tentorium may appear quite prominent on CECT, T1 C+ scans; should not be mistaken for dAVF

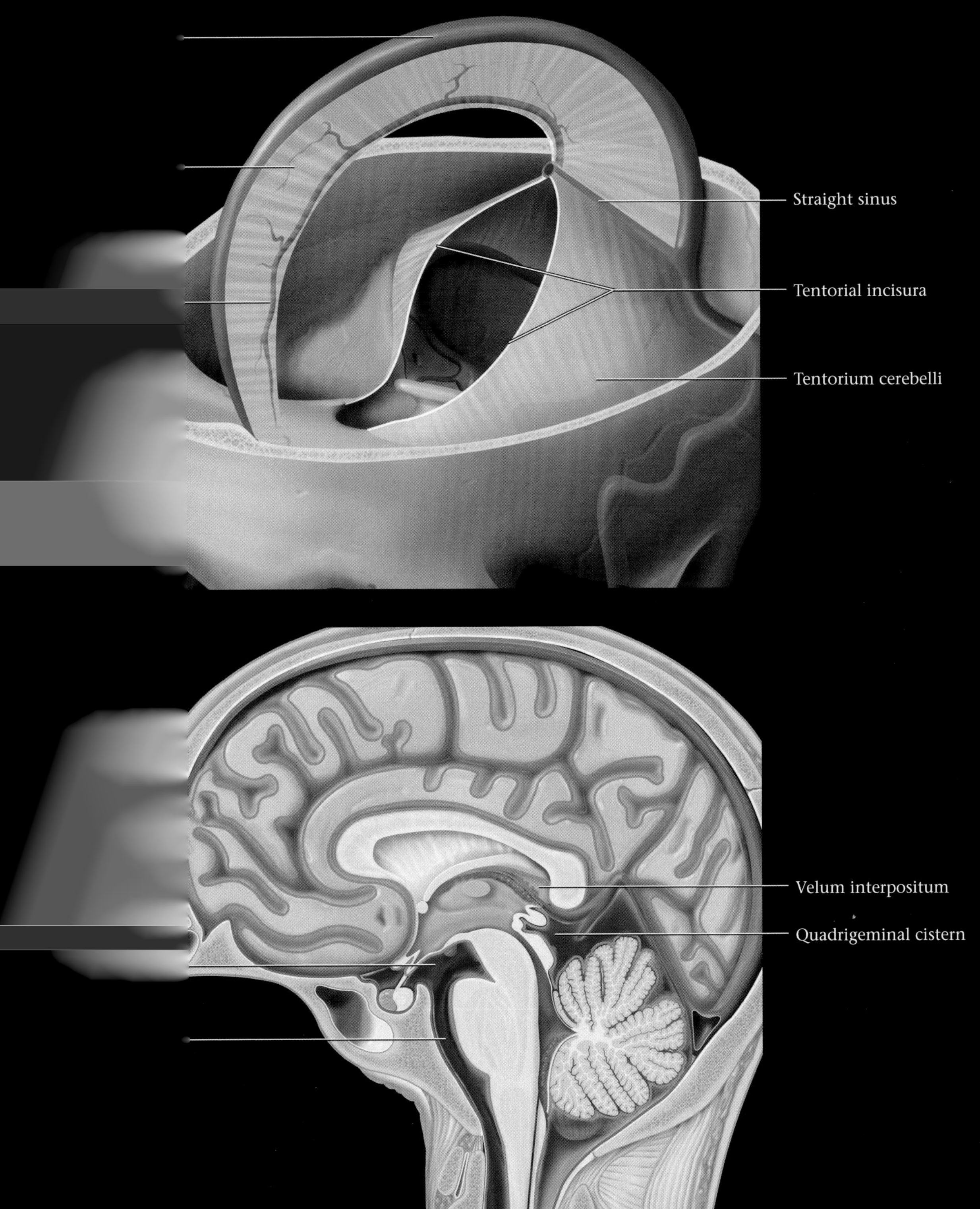
Straight sinus
Tentorial incisura
Tentorium cerebelli
Velum interpositum
Quadrigeminal cistern

phic shows relationship of the major dural sinuses to the falx cerebri and tentorium
on the crista galli anteriorly and sweeps backwards in the midline to the straight sinus,
s posteriorly between the cerebral hemispheres. The tentorium cerebelli meets the falx
ex and curves downwards to contain the transverse sinuses. The leaves of the tentorium
trous apex and fibers extend forward to the anterior clinoid processes. The tentorial
ewhat U-shaped. **(Bottom)** Sagittal graphic depicts cranial leptomeninges enclosing CSF
noid follows the dura around the inner calvarium and is shown in purple; the pia (orange)

GRAPHICS

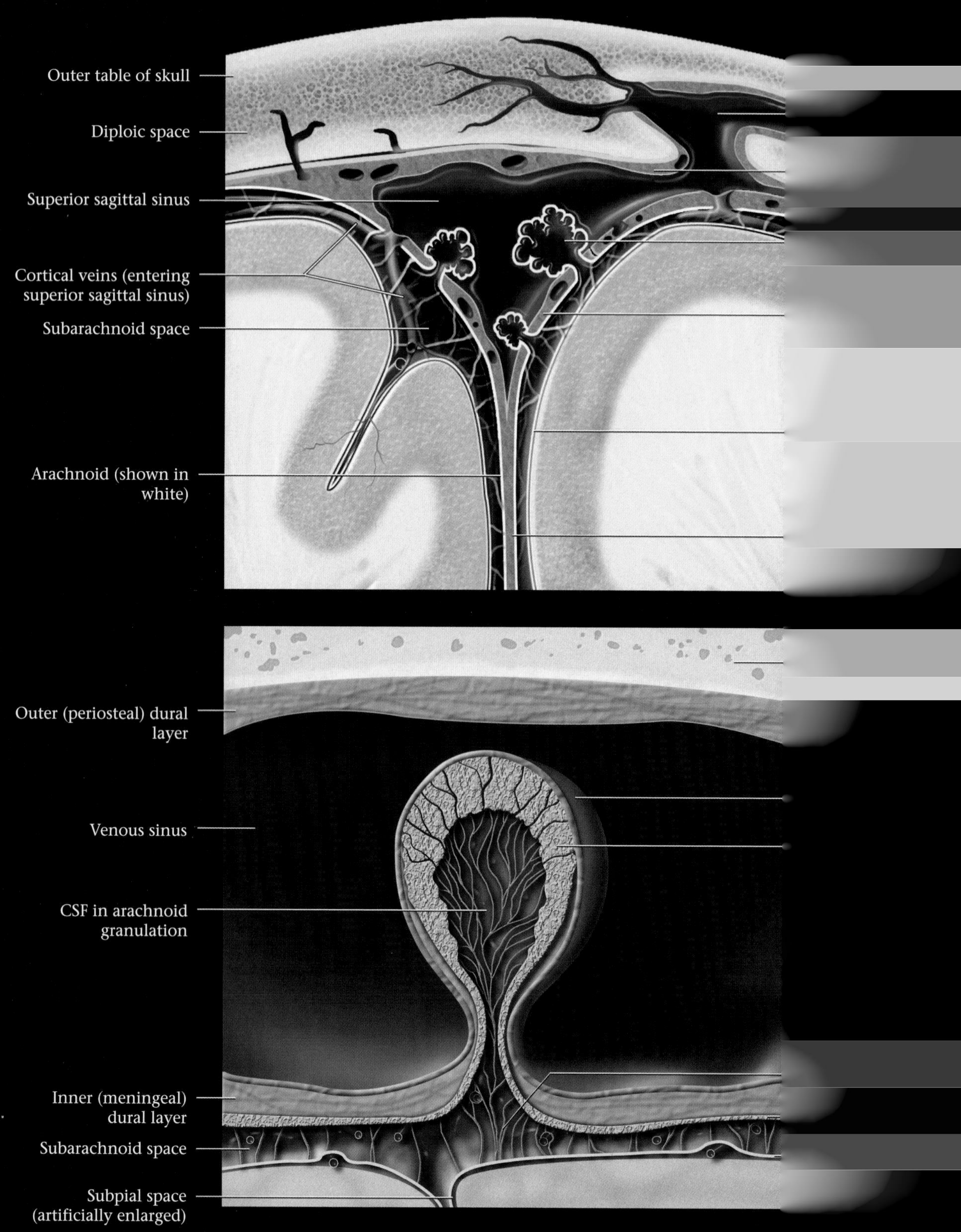
Outer table of skull
Diploic space
Superior sagittal sinus
Cortical veins (entering superior sagittal sinus)
Subarachnoid space
Arachnoid (shown in white)
Outer (periosteal) dural layer
Venous sinus
CSF in arachnoid granulation
Inner (meningeal) dural layer
Subarachnoid space
Subpial space (artificially enlarged)

(Top) Close-up coronal view shows the superior sagittal sinus as it is enclosed between the c
layers. Note CSF-containing projections (arachnoid granulations) that extend from the suba
superior sagittal sinuses. **(Bottom)** Graphic depiction of an arachnoid granulation projecting
sinus. A core of CSF extends from the SAS into the granulation and is covered by an apical c
Channels extend through the cap to the sinus endothelium and drain CSF into the venous c
numerous trabeculae as well as small arteries and veins within the SAS over the brain.

AXIAL T1 C+ MR

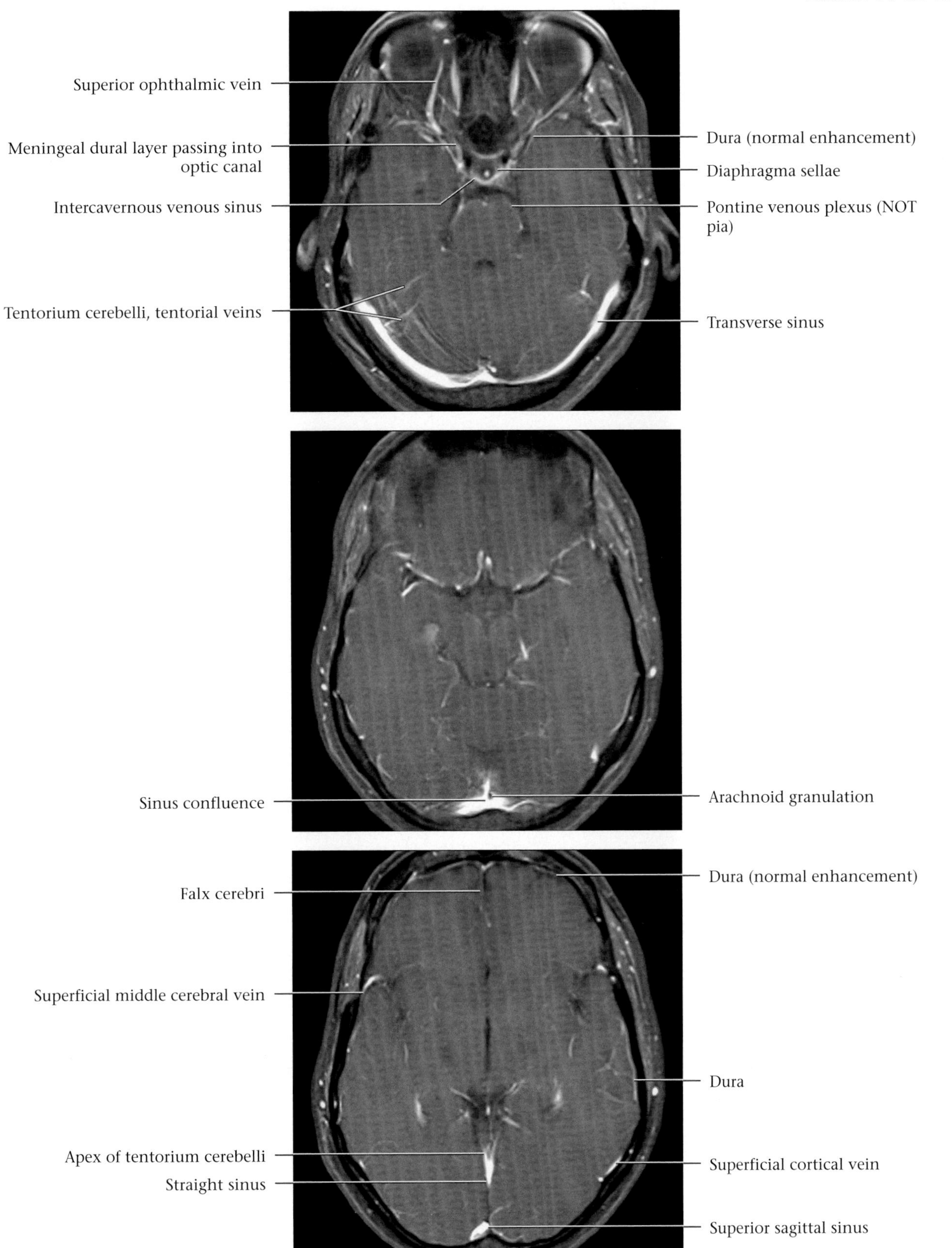
Superior ophthalmic vein
Meningeal dural layer passing into optic canal
Intercavernous venous sinus
Tentorium cerebelli, tentorial veins
Dura (normal enhancement)
Diaphragma sellae
Pontine venous plexus (NOT pia)
Transverse sinus
Sinus confluence
Arachnoid granulation
Falx cerebri
Superficial middle cerebral vein
Apex of tentorium cerebelli
Straight sinus
Dura (normal enhancement)
Dura
Superficial cortical vein
Superior sagittal sinus

(Top) A series of six selected axial T1 C+ MR images through brain from inferior to superior shows normal meningeal enhancement at 1.5T. Unlike arachnoid microvessels, dural microvessels lack capillary endothelial tight junctions. Dural enhancement is therefore normal following contrast administration. **(Middle)** The outer and inner dural layers adhere to each other, except where encase dural venous sinuses. Venous flow in sinuses is relatively slow so strong enhancement is normal. A small arachnoid granulation is present, seen here as a CSF-intensity filling defect within the strongly enhancing sinus confluence. **(Bottom)** The falx cerebri encases the superior and inferior sagittal sinuses at its upper and lower margins respectively. The Y-shaped tentorial apex is seen very well on this image. Note inhomogeneous signal within the superior sagittal sinus, a normal finding.

AXIAL T1 C+ MR

Frontal cortical vein
Dura (normal enhancement)
Dura

Superior sagittal sinus
Falx cerebri
Inferior sagittal sinus
Dura (normal enhancement)

Falx cerebri
Superficial cortical veins
Vein of Trolard
Superior sagittal sinus

(Top) Normal dural enhancement is thin, smooth, discontinuous and symmetric (best appreciated on coronal sections). Enhancing superficial cortical veins travel within subarachnoid space before traversing potential subdural space to drain into dural sinuses. Superficial cortical veins are typically seen as thicker, more strongly enhancing structures that branch and communicate with draining tributaries extending into sulci. **(Middle)** Section through the centrum semiovale shows the falx cerebri with a prominent inferior sagittal sinus arcing above the corpus callosum. **(Bottom)** Scan through the vertex shows the triangular-shaped superior sagittal sinus, which is larger posteriorly than anteriorly. The anastomotic vein of Trolard is seen here as it courses superiorly from the sylvian fissure towards the superior sagittal sinus.

CRANIAL MENINGES

CORONAL T1 C+ MR

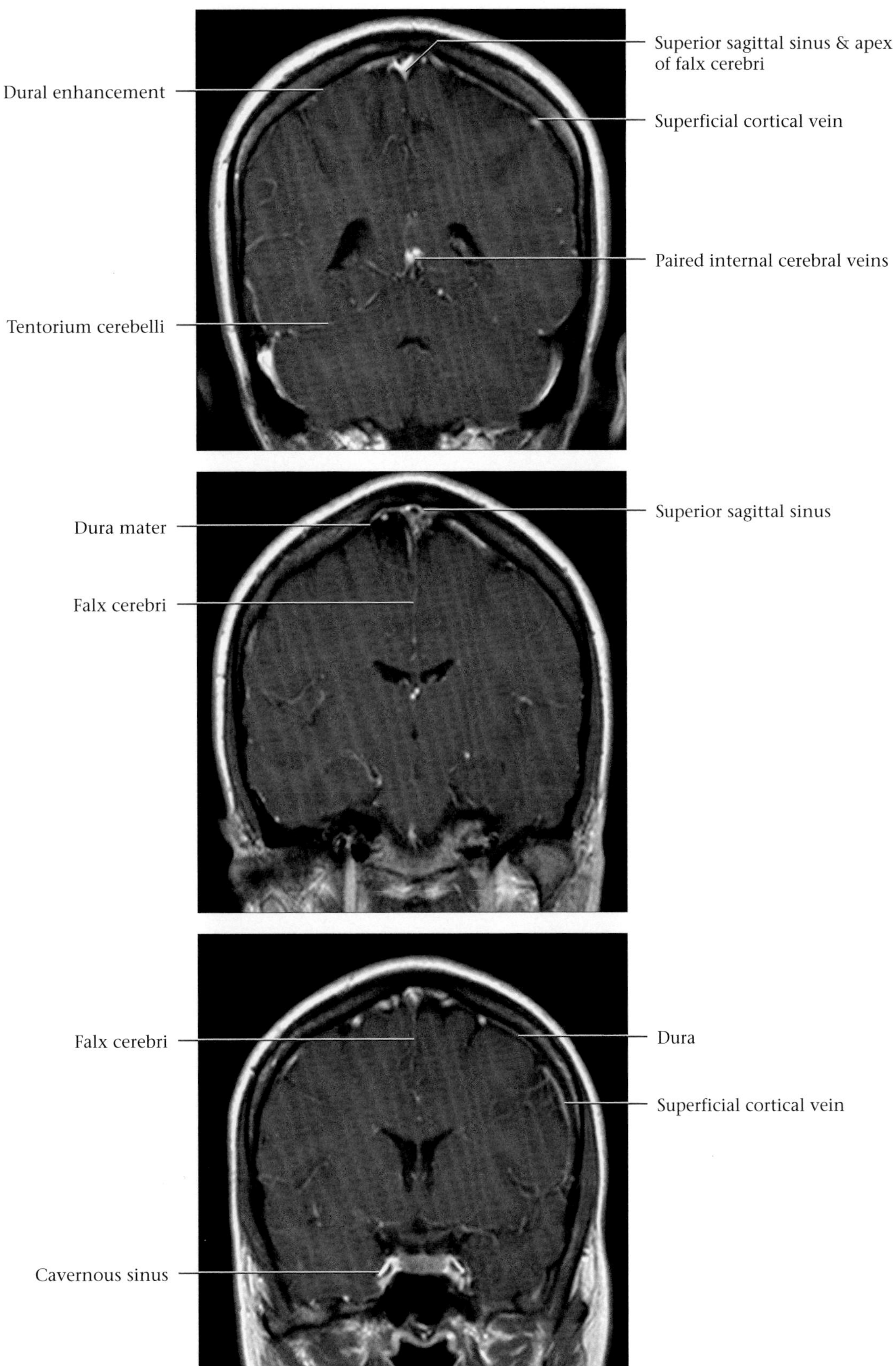

Superior sagittal sinus & apex of falx cerebri
Dural enhancement
Superficial cortical vein
Paired internal cerebral veins
Tentorium cerebelli
Superior sagittal sinus
Dura mater
Falx cerebri
Falx cerebri
Dura
Superficial cortical vein
Cavernous sinus

(Top) First of three coronal T1 C+ MR images from posterior to anterior shows normal dural enhancement at 1.5T following contrast administration. At this field strength, dura is thickest near the superior sagittal sinus and typically appears discontinuous as it sweeps inferiorly. Arachnoid microvessels have tight junctions and are part of blood-brain barrier which normally does not enhance. **(Middle)** Normal dural enhancement is thin, smooth, and discontinuous. Enhancement is less intense than adjacent dural venous sinuses. The falx cerebri and tentorium cerebelli are dural reflections and therefore also normally enhance. **(Bottom)** Dural enhancement is most prominent near vertex, least striking around and under the temporal lobes. Note that dural enhancement is less intense than the cavernous sinus.

CORONAL T2 MR

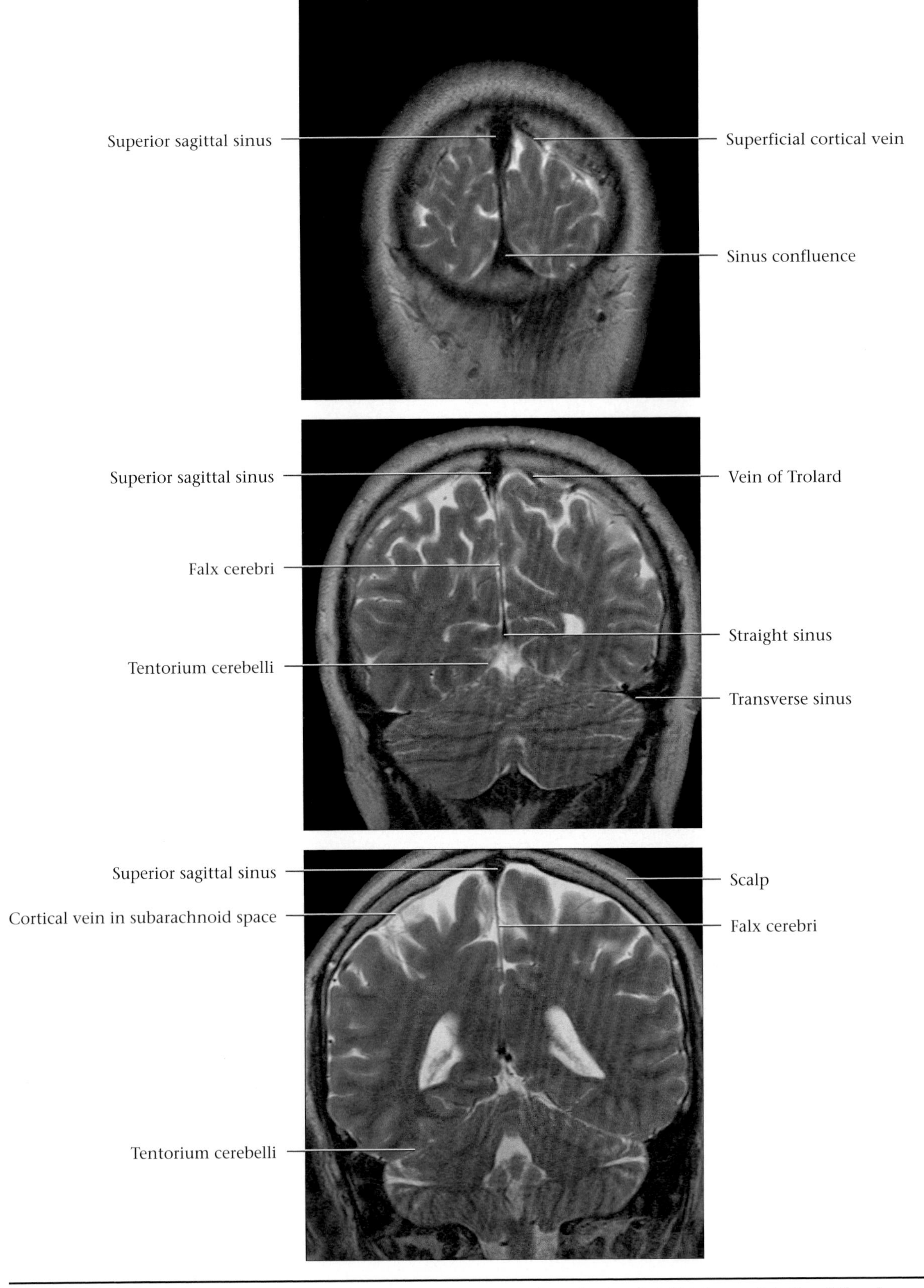

Superior sagittal sinus
Superficial cortical vein
Sinus confluence
Superior sagittal sinus
Vein of Trolard
Falx cerebri
Straight sinus
Tentorium cerebelli
Transverse sinus
Superior sagittal sinus
Scalp
Cortical vein in subarachnoid space
Falx cerebri
Tentorium cerebelli

(Top) First of six coronal T2 MR images from posterior to anterior obtained at 3T shows details of the dura and cortical veins as they drain into the superior sagittal sinus. **(Middle)** Section through the straight sinus shows its enclosure by leaves of the falx and tentorium cerebelli. The tentorium sweeps superiorly from the tops of the petrous ridges and transverse sinuses to meet the falx cerebri in the midline and form the straight sinus. **(Bottom)** The hypointense outer dura and inner table of the skull are indistinguishable but reflections of the inner (meningeal) dural layer as it forms the falx cerebri and tentorium cerebelli are easily seen here.

CRANIAL MENINGES

CORONAL T2 MR

Superior sagittal sinus
Falx cerebri
Trabeculae in subarachnoid space
Sylvian (lateral cerebral) fissure
Tentorium cerebelli

Falx cerebri
Perivascular spaces
Lateral wall, cavernous sinus
Dura

Superior sagittal sinus
Falx cerebri
Crista galli

(Top) The tentorial incisura is seen here between the two leaves of the tentorium and transmits the midbrain and basilar artery. **(Middle)** Several perivascular spaces are seen here as linear areas of high signal intensity within the centrum semiovale. Pia invaginates along penetrating vessels, forming the PVSs which contain interstitial fluid. **(Bottom)** Section through the frontal lobes demonstrates attachment of the falx cerebri to the crista galli. The superior sagittal sinus is seen here and appears much smaller than on more posterior sections. The pia covering the cortex is not distinguishable, even on these high-resolution 3T images.

PIA AND PERIVASCULAR SPACES

Terminology

Abbreviations

- Perivascular spaces (PVSs)
- Subarachnoid space (SAS)
- Cerebrospinal fluid (CSF)
- Interstitial fluid (ISF)

Synonyms

- Virchow-Robin spaces (VRSs)

Definitions

- Pial-lined, ISF-filled structures that accompany vessels entering (penetrating arteries) or leaving (draining veins) cerebral cortex

Gross Anatomy

Overview

- **Leptomeninges**: "Thin" meninges (arachnoid, pia)
  - **Arachnoid**: Translucent sheet of tissue loosely adherent to inner surface of meningeal layer of dura
  - **Pia**: Innermost layer of meninges consisting of thin sheet (one or two cells thick) covering brain surface
    - Pial cells form anatomic barrier between SAS, brain
    - Pia functions as regulatory interface between SAS, brain (exhibit pinocytosis, enzymatic activity)
- **SAS**
  - CSF-filled space contained between arachnoid (outer wall), pia (inner wall)
  - Contains traversing arteries, veins
  - Numerous sheet-like filiform trabeculae extend across SAS from arachnoid to pia, forming bridging chordae coated by leptomeningeal cells that are continuous with pia, inner arachnoid
- **PVSs**
  - Accompany small, medium-sized arteries as they penetrate brain parenchyma
  - Flattened layer of pial cells invaginates along penetrating arteries
    - Basal ganglia, midbrain PVSs contain double layer of pia so PVSs are "interpial" space
    - Cortex, white matter PVSs lined by single pial layer so PVS is between adventitia, pia
    - PVSs inapparent as pass through cortex, become larger in subcortical white matter
    - Pia becomes fenestrated, then disappears at capillary level
  - PVSs are filled with ISF, not CSF
    - PVSs may drain ISF along periarterial compartments, functionally bypassing SAS
  - Most PVSs are 1-2 mm but can become very large
  - Immunocompetent lymphocytes, monocytes enter brain through postcapillary venule walls into perivenular spaces
    - Perivenular spaces have discontinuous groups of pial cells, not complete pial sheath

Imaging Anatomy

Overview

- PVSs found in all parts of the brain
  - Most common locations
    - Around anterior commissure
    - Inferior 1/3 of basal ganglia
    - Anterior perforated substance
    - Hemispheric white matter (centrum semiovale)
    - Midbrain (around substantia nigra)
  - Other locations
    - Extreme capsule
    - Subinsular white matter
    - Dentate nuclei
- PVSs occur at all ages, although prominence/prevalence ↑ with age
- Seen commonly at 1.5T, almost universally on 3T MR
  - Usually 5 mm or less in size but can be up to 2-3 cm as normal variant
  - Appear as round, ovoid or linear (depending on orientation of PVSs to plane of section)
    - Usually suppress completely on FLAIR (25% have small hyperintense rim)
    - Do not enhance (sometimes linear enhancement of central vessel can be seen)
    - Typically not seen as pass through cortex, only become visible as enter subcortical white matter
    - Isointense with CSF on all sequences

Anatomy Relationships

- Pia invaginates along small/medium-sized arteries as they penetrate brain and creates the PVSs
- Pia separates SAS from brain parenchyma

Internal Structures-Critical Contents

- PVSs are filled with interstitial fluid (not CSF)

Normal Variants, Anomalies

- **Giant ("tumefactive") PVSs** may cause mass effect, obstructive hydrocephalus, mimic neoplasm
  - Typically occur as clusters of variable-sized CSF-like cysts
  - Suppress on FLAIR, don't enhance
- **Widespread enlarged PVSs** in cerebral white matter may appear bizarre but is extreme normal variant, usually asymptomatic

Anatomy-Based Imaging Issues

Imaging Recommendations

- FLAIR sequence helpful in distinguishing PVS from lacunar infarct

Imaging Pitfalls

- Prominent PVSs in subinsular white matter, temporal lobes common; should not be mistaken for demyelinating/dysmyelinating disorders
- PVSs **do not** communicate with SAS (even when extensive, subarachnoid hemorrhage does not enter PVSs)

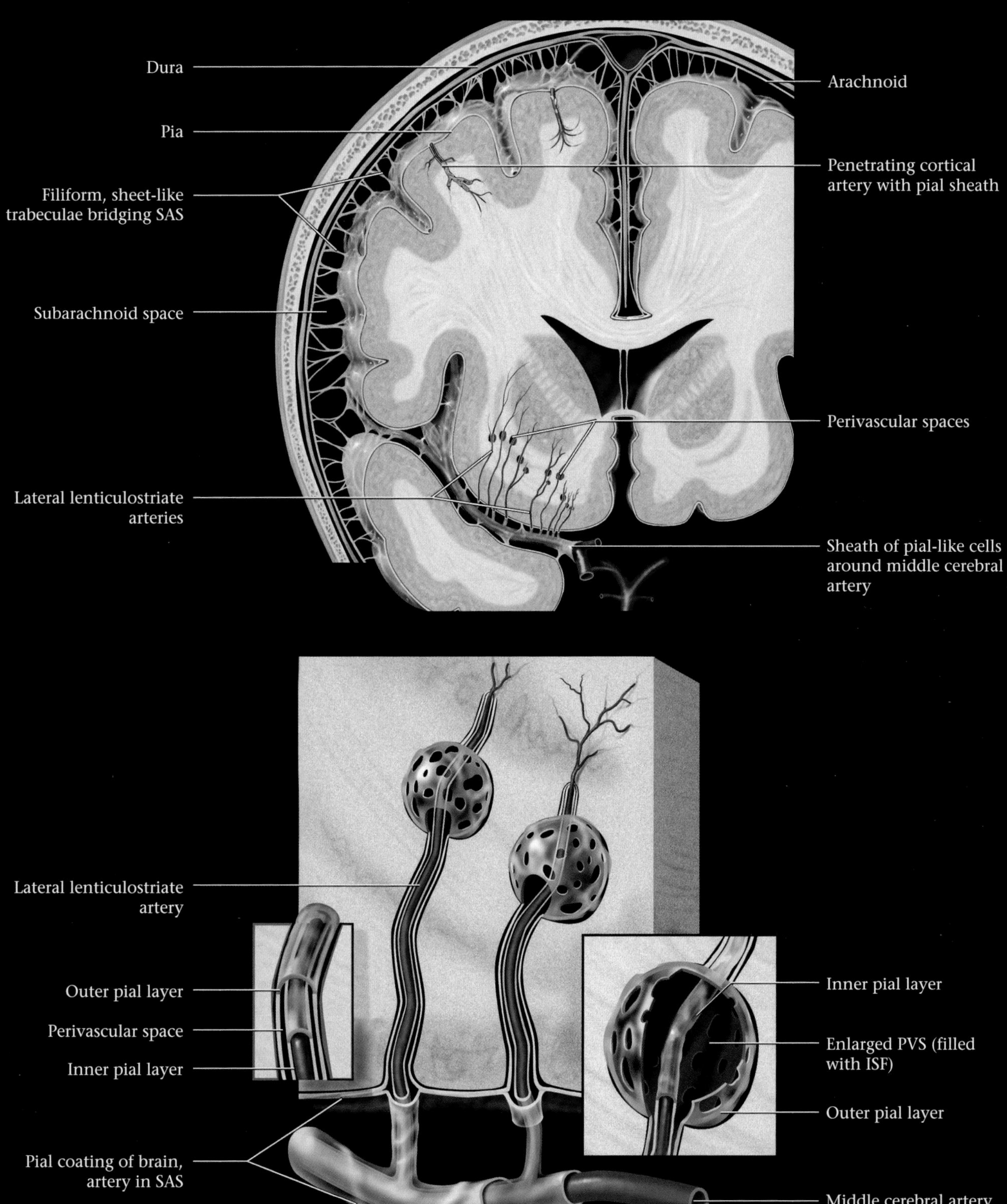

Dura
Pia
Filiform, sheet-like trabeculae bridging SAS
Subarachnoid space
Lateral lenticulostriate arteries
Arachnoid
Penetrating cortical artery with pial sheath
Perivascular spaces
Sheath of pial-like cells around middle cerebral artery
Lateral lenticulostriate artery
Outer pial layer
Perivascular space
Inner pial layer
Pial coating of brain, artery in SAS
Inner pial layer
Enlarged PVS (filled with ISF)
Outer pial layer
Middle cerebral artery

(Top) Coronal overview shows relationship of the cranial meninges to brain and subarachnoid space. Inner (meningeal) dural layer and arachnoid are closely but loosely adherent to each other. Pia (not arachnoid) covers the cortical surface and accompanies penetrating arteries through the cortex. CSF-filled subarachnoid space is filled with bridging trabeculae and vessels, all of which are coated with a thin layer of pial-like cells. Small but numerous dilated perivascular spaces are seen in the basal ganglia surrounding lateral lenticulostriate arteries as they pass cephalad through the anterior perforated substance. **(Bottom)** Close-up view shows prominent PVSs clustered in inferior 1/3 of basal ganglia. PVSs here are composed of two pial layers and are thus an "interpial" compartment. Focal enlargement at the ends of these PVSs is common in the basal ganglia.

PIA AND PERIVASCULAR SPACES

GRAPHICS

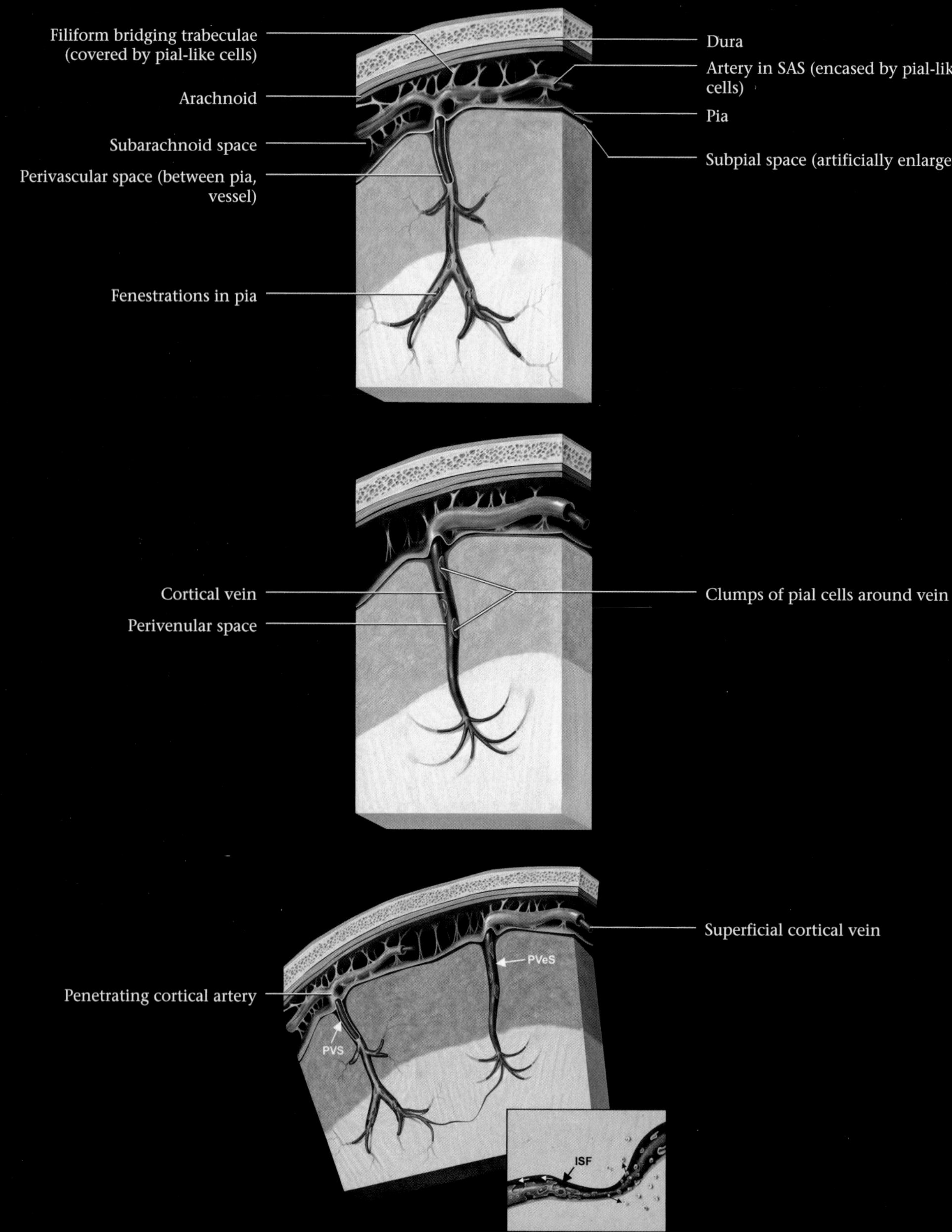

Filiform bridging trabeculae (covered by pial-like cells)
Arachnoid
Subarachnoid space
Perivascular space (between pia, vessel)
Fenestrations in pia
Dura
Artery in SAS (encased by pial-like cells)
Pia
Subpial space (artificially enlarged)
Cortical vein
Perivenular space
Clumps of pial cells around vein
Superficial cortical vein
PVeS
Penetrating cortical artery
PVS
ISF

(Top) Close-up view of cranial meninges and a penetrating cortical artery. Note pia coats vessels, trabeculae within the SAS and covers brain surface, accompanying artery as it penetrates through cortex. Pia covering excludes the PVSs from the SAS so these two spaces do not communicate with each other. **(Middle)** A cortical vein is depicted. While a thin sheet of pial-like cells encases all vessels and trabeculae within the SAS, only isolated groups of pial cells surround draining cortical veins. The perivenular spaces are thus in direct contact with the brain parenchyma. **(Bottom)** Interrelationship between arterial (PVS) and venous (PVeS) perivascular spaces. Fenestrated pial sheath disappears at capillary level. PVSs are filled with interstitial fluid. Activated lymphocytes (insert, small arrows) escape from post-capillary venule into surrounding parenchyma.

PIA AND PERIVASCULAR SPACES

AXIAL T2 MR

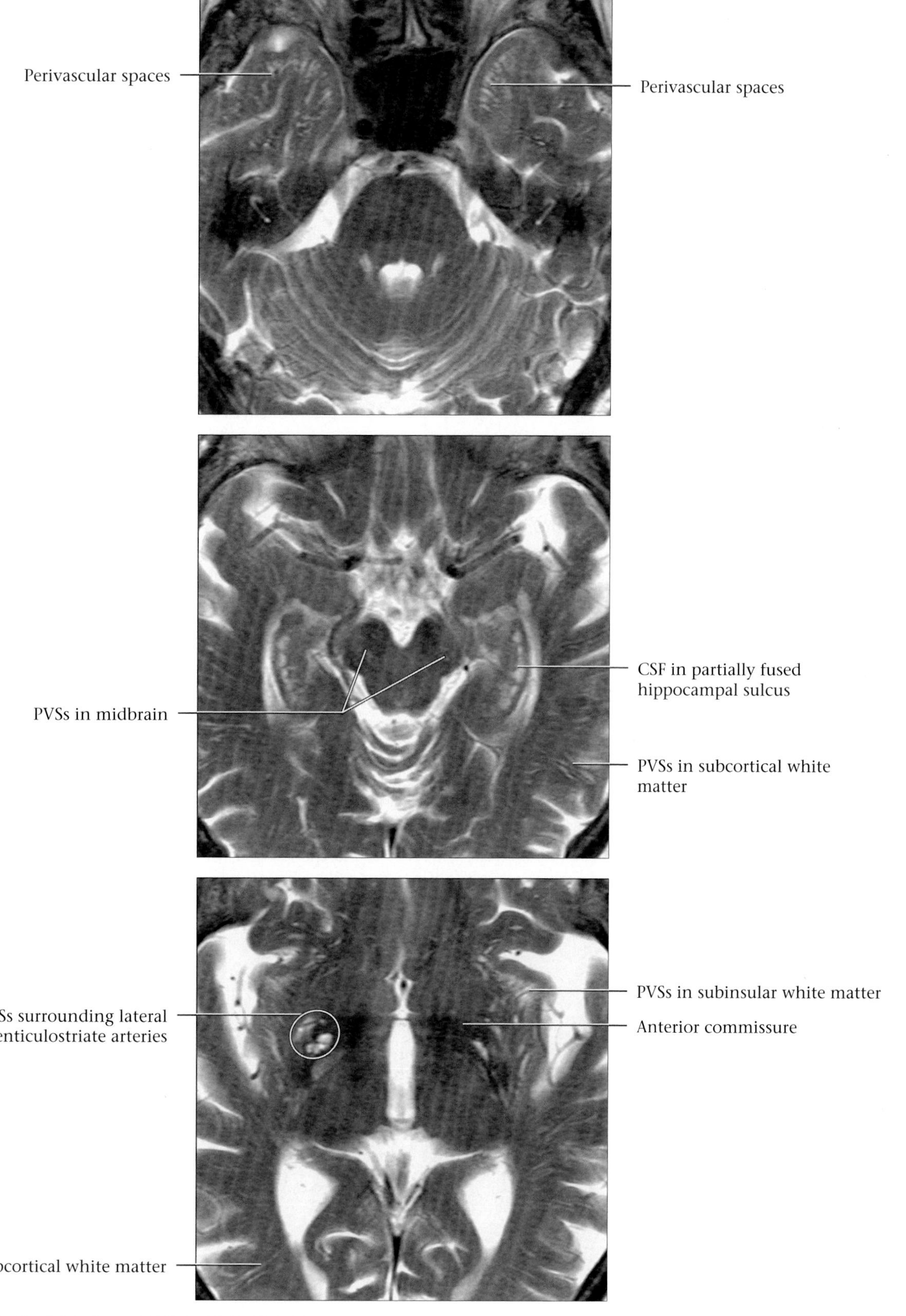
Perivascular spaces
Perivascular spaces
CSF in partially fused hippocampal sulcus
PVSs in midbrain
PVSs in subcortical white matter
PVSs in subinsular white matter
PVSs surrounding lateral lenticulostriate arteries
Anterior commissure
PVSs in subcortical white matter

(Top) First of six 3T axial T2 MR images from inferior to superior demonstrate normal appearance of perivascular spaces (PVS) in a middle-aged patient. This section shows prominent PVSs in the subcortical white matter of both temporal lobes, a common location. Note that even at 3T, the PVSs are not seen as they pass through the cortex and only become apparent once they reach the subcortical white matter. **(Middle)** PVSs are seen here in the midbrain and white matter of the temporal lobes. The larger high signal collections just medial to the temporal lobes represent CSF in a partially fused hippocampal sulcus, a normal congenital variant, and should not be mistaken for PVSs or lacunar infarcts. **(Bottom)** PVSs are most common along the anterior commissure, clustered in the inferior third of the basal ganglia. The subinsular region is another common normal site.

PIA AND PERIVASCULAR SPACES

AXIAL T2 MR

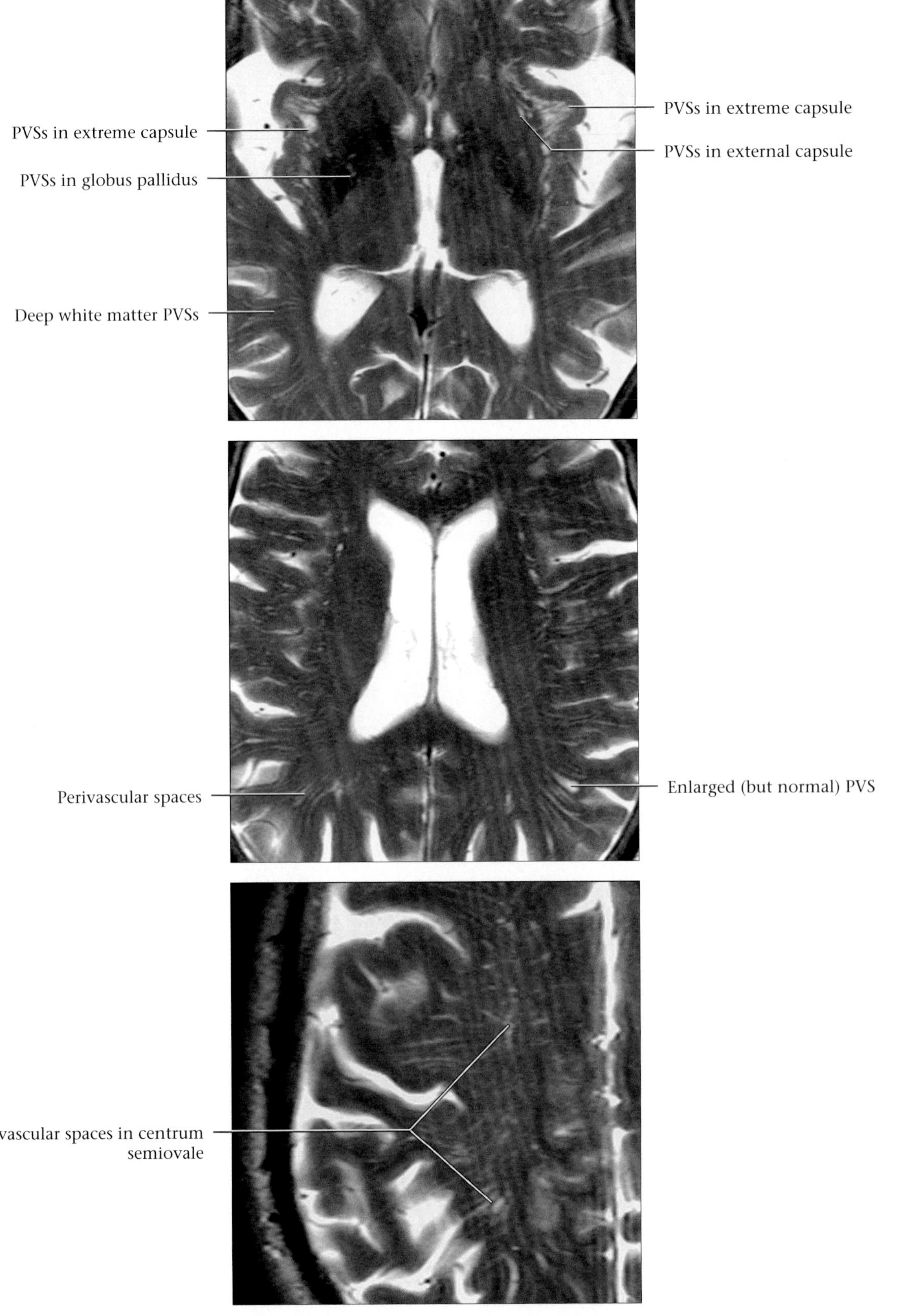
PVSs in extreme capsule
PVSs in globus pallidus
Deep white matter PVSs
PVSs in extreme capsule
PVSs in external capsule
Perivascular spaces
Enlarged (but normal) PVS
Perivascular spaces in centrum semiovale

(Top) Section through the third ventricle and insular regions shows unusually prominent but normal PVSs in the subinsular white matter (extreme capsule). A few "dot-like" PVSs are seen end-on here in the globi pallidi. PVSs in the deep white matter of the posterior temporal and occipital lobes appear mostly linear at this level. **(Middle)** PVSs are commonly seen in the corona radiata and centrum semiovale and may normally be quite prominent, as in this patient. At the midventricular level, most are seen as linear streaks of CSF signal intensity (although they are filled with interstitial fluid, not CSF). On FLAIR (not shown), these would suppress completely. Some PVSs may appear larger but are still normal. **(Bottom)** Close-up view shows PVSs in the deep white matter are seen as either linear or dot-like or ovoid, depending on orientation within the plane of section.

CORONAL T2 MR

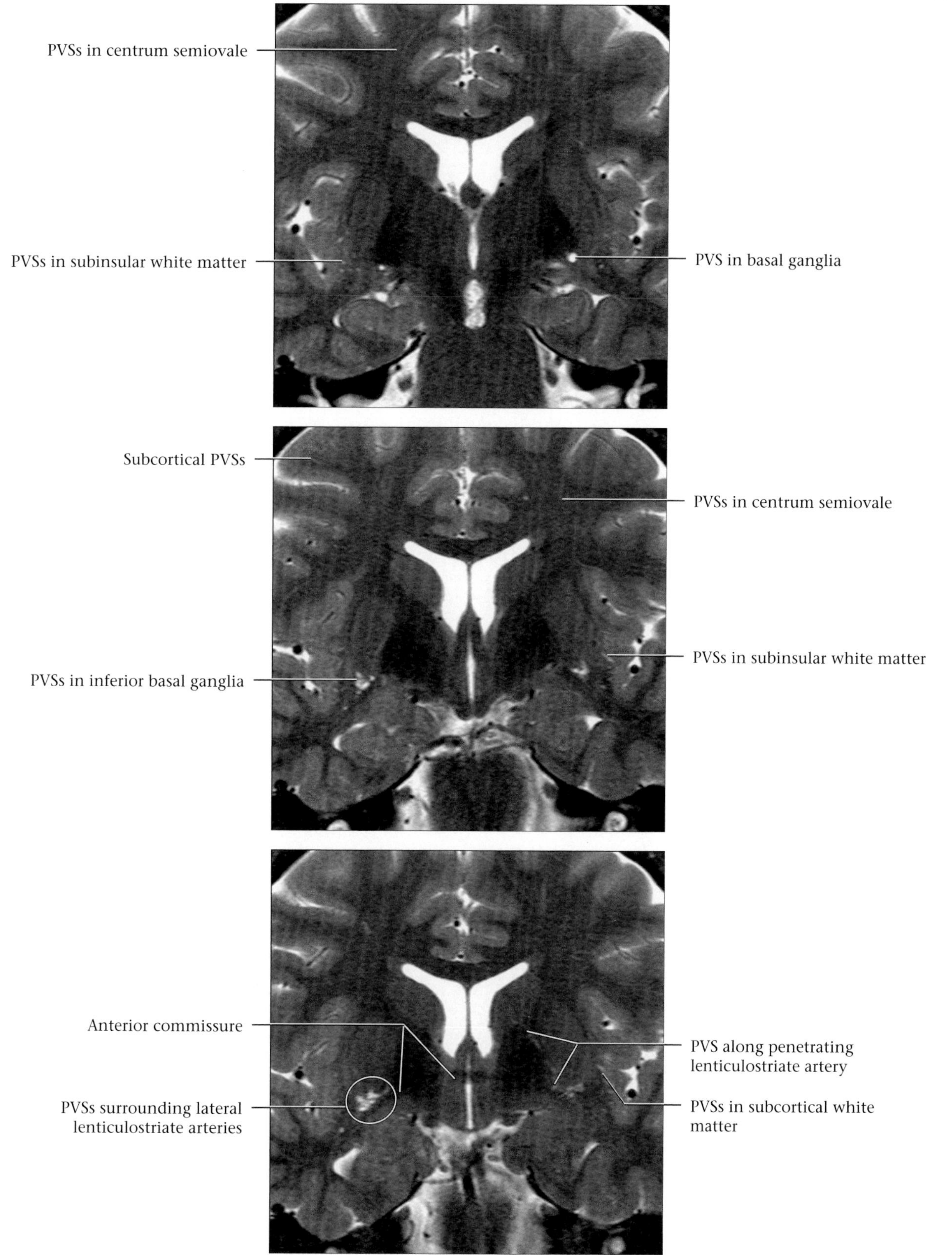

PVSs in centrum semiovale
PVSs in subinsular white matter
PVS in basal ganglia
Subcortical PVSs
PVSs in centrum semiovale
PVSs in subinsular white matter
PVSs in inferior basal ganglia
Anterior commissure
PVS along penetrating lenticulostriate artery
PVSs surrounding lateral lenticulostriate arteries
PVSs in subcortical white matter

(Top) First of six 3T coronal T2 MR images from posterior to anterior demonstrate normal appearance of PVS in a young patient. **(Middle)** Relatively few linear-appearing PVSs are seen in the subcortical and deep white matter here but can be detected on careful examination. More prominent PVSs are seen in the inferior basal ganglia and infralenticular internal capsule. **(Bottom)** PVSs often occur in clusters, especially in the inferior basal ganglia and around the anterior commissure. Sometimes they can be seen following a penetrating artery along nearly its entire course.

CORONAL T2 MR

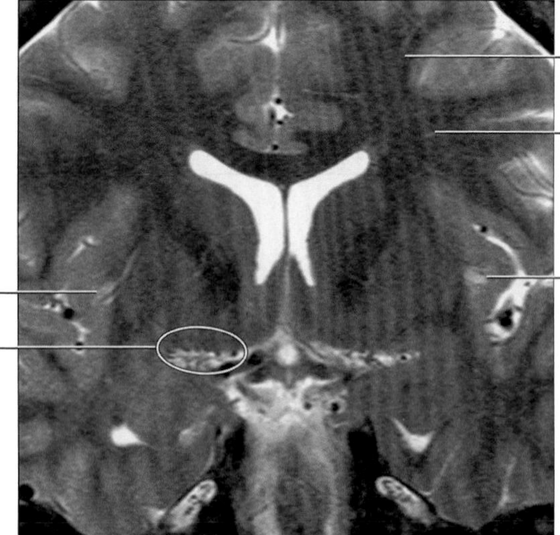
PVSs in subcortical white matter
PVS in centrum semiovale
PVSs in extreme capsule (subinsular white matter)
PVSs in subinsular region
PVSs, lateral lenticulostriate arteries in anterior perforated substance

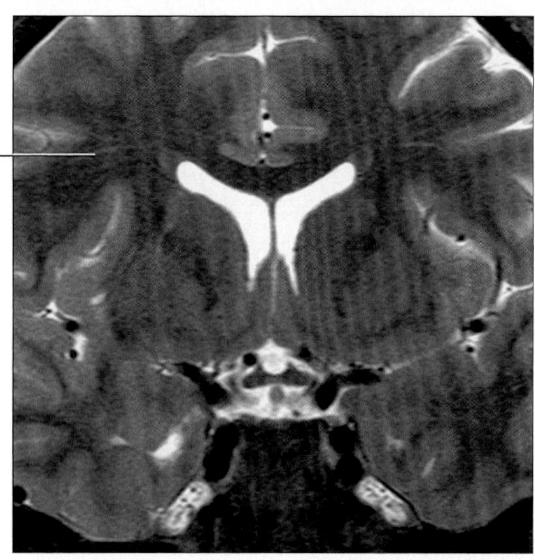
PVSs in centrum semiovale

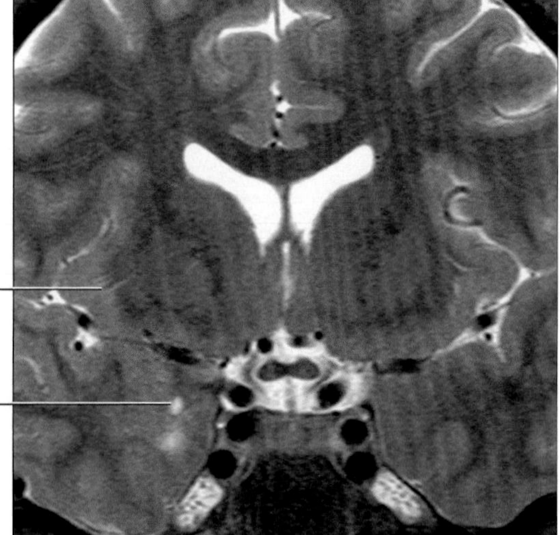
PVSs in subinsular white matter
Choroid fissure cyst

(Top) A double layer of pia accompanies penetrating arteries (here the lateral lenticulostriate arteries) as they pass cephalad through the anterior perforated substance into the basal ganglia, seen especially well in this section. PVSs in the basal ganglia and midbrain are contained within the two pial layers. **(Middle)** Relatively fewer PVSs are seen as sections include basal ganglia in front of the anterior commissure. PVSs are still seen in the centrum semiovale in this image. **(Bottom)** A single, somewhat prominent collection of CSF is seen above the temporal horn, possibly a small choroid fissure cyst. Numerous smaller PVSs are seen as dots and linear streaks of high signal intensity in white matter of the deep temporal lobe and in the subinsular regions.

SAGITTAL T1, AXIAL T2, AXIAL FLAIR MR

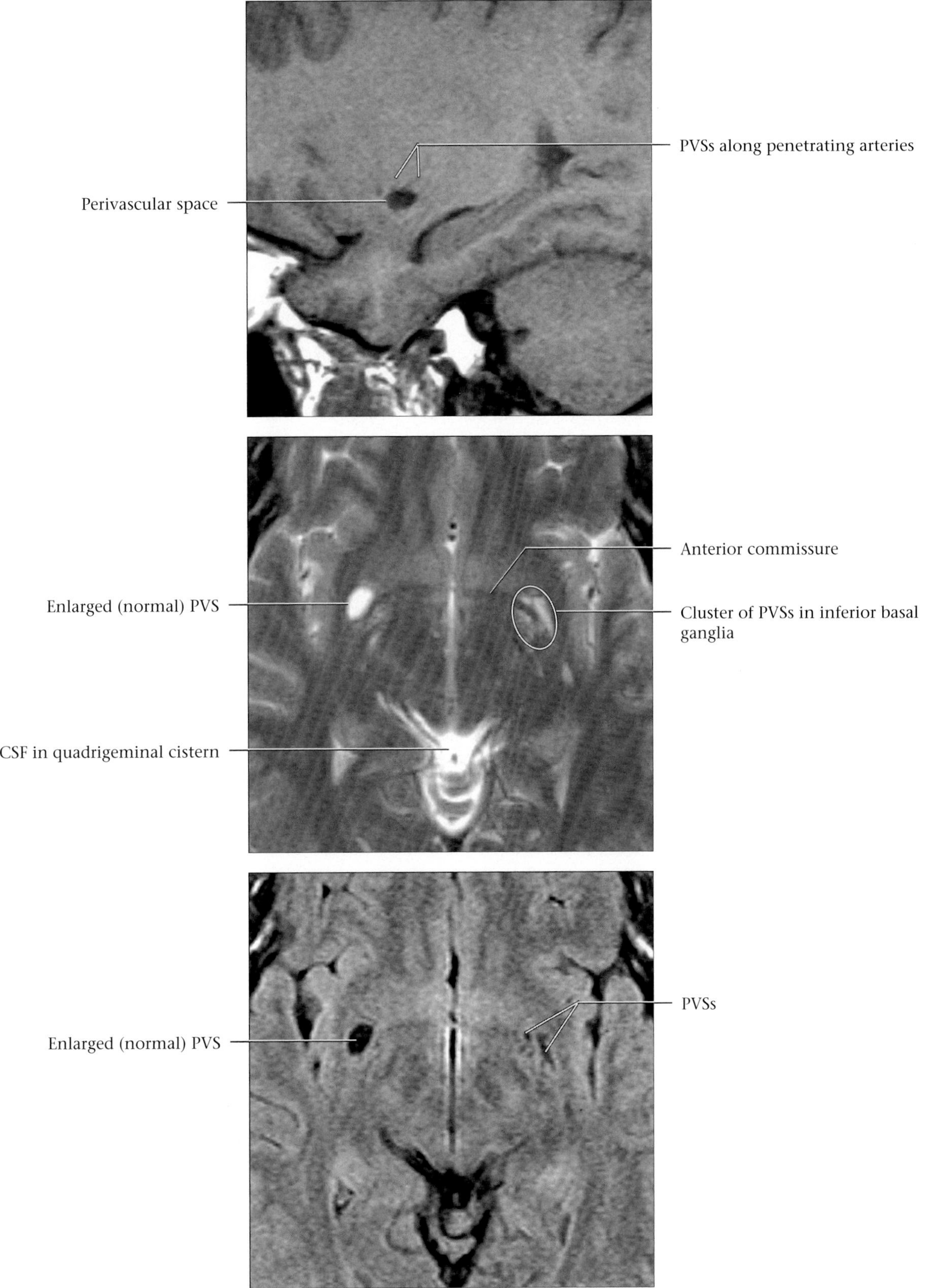

PVSs along penetrating arteries
Perivascular space
Anterior commissure
Enlarged (normal) PVS
Cluster of PVSs in inferior basal ganglia
CSF in quadrigeminal cistern
PVSs
Enlarged (normal) PVS

(Top) These three images compare normal signal intensity of PVSs on MR. Sagittal T1 MR image through an enlarged perivascular space demonstrates hypointense fluid signal that is virtually identical to CSF even though it is interstitial fluid. Also note linear penetrating arteries radiating from superior margin of perivascular space. **(Middle)** Axial T2 MR image shows the enlarged PVS has hyperintense signal similar to CSF in the quadrigeminal cistern and third ventricle. Multiple other smaller perivascular spaces are seen in in the inferior basal ganglia around the anterior commissure and in the subinsular white matter. **(Bottom)** Axial FLAIR image shows suppression of fluid signal within perivascular spaces with normal signal in surrounding brain parenchyma. A thin hyperintense rim can sometimes be seen around the PVSs and is a normal finding.

CORONAL T2, AXIAL T2, AXIAL FLAIR MR

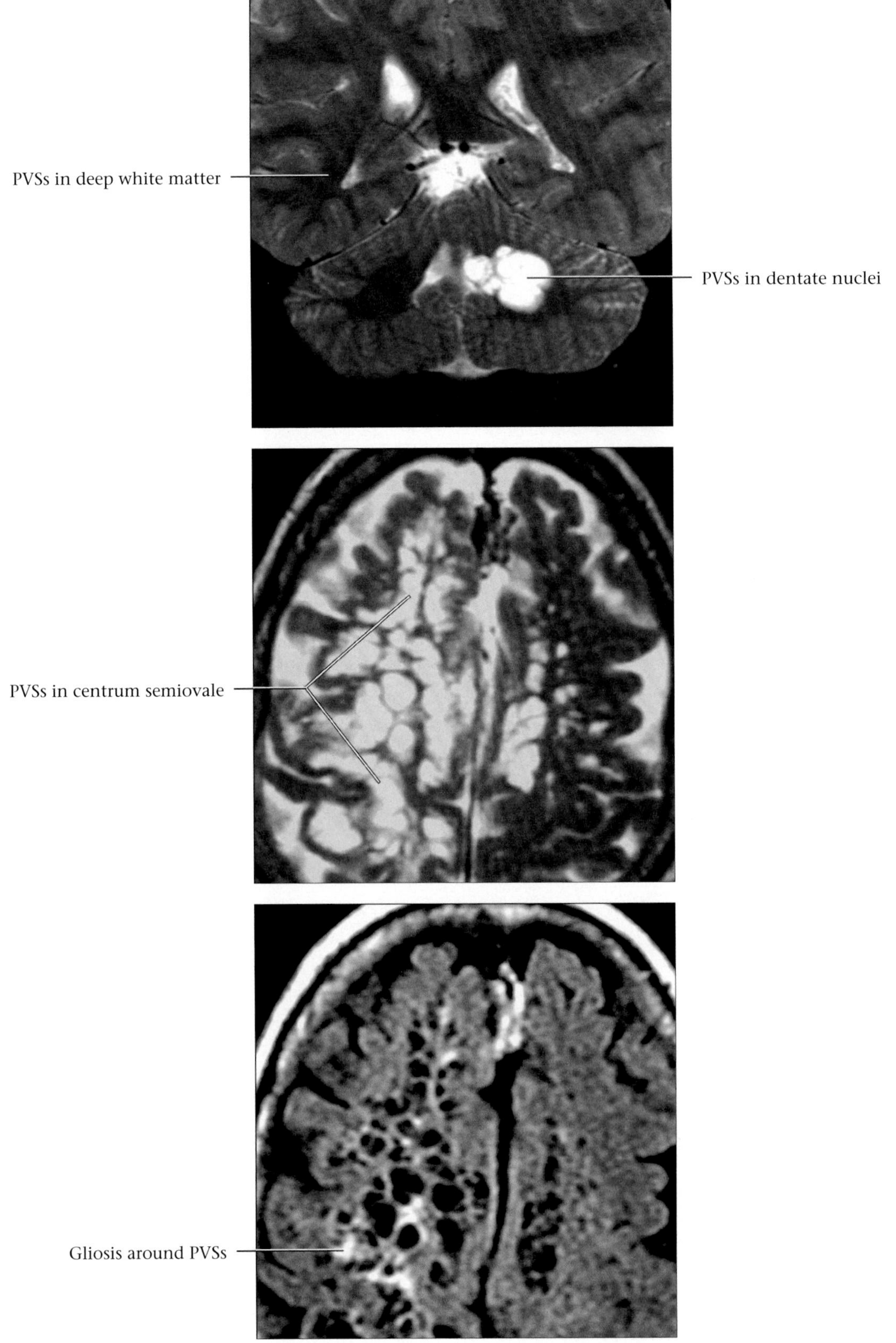

PVSs in deep white matter
PVSs in dentate nuclei
PVSs in centrum semiovale
Gliosis around PVSs

(Top) MR scans of variant perivascular spaces are illustrated in this and the following images. Coronal T2WI in an 8 year old male shows a cluster of CSF-like cysts in the left dentate nucleus. Originally called a low grade cystic neoplasm, these are simply prominent PVSs. They suppressed completely on FLAIR and did not enhance. **(Middle)** Axial T2 MR shows bilateral subcortical and deep white matter cysts with CSF-like signal intensity. Note focal expansion of cortex over the more superficial cysts. Patient was middle-aged, asymptomatic. **(Bottom)** FLAIR MR scan in same case shows fluid in cysts suppresses completely. A few areas of increased signal intensity surround some of the enlarged PVSs, a finding seen in approximately 25% of cases that may represent mild adjacent spongiosis. This is an example of unusually enlarged PVSs that are extreme variants of normal.

CORONAL T1, AXIAL T2, AXIAL T1 C+ MR

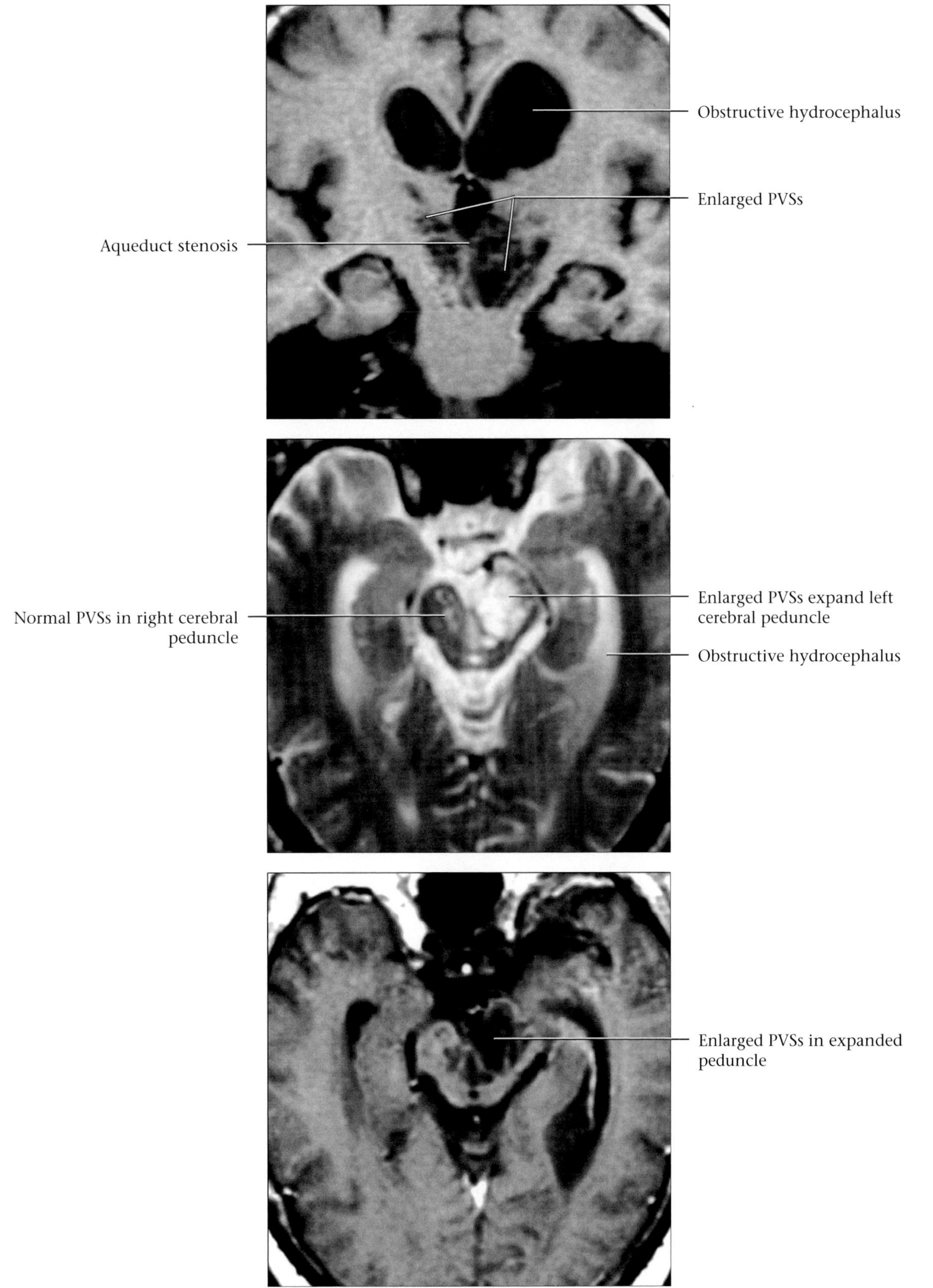
Obstructive hydrocephalus
Enlarged PVSs
Aqueduct stenosis
Enlarged PVSs expand left cerebral peduncle
Normal PVSs in right cerebral peduncle
Obstructive hydrocephalus
Enlarged PVSs in expanded peduncle

(Top) Coronal T1 MR of a middle-aged patient with headaches demonstrates numerous CSF-like cysts in the midbrain and thalami causing local mass effect, aqueduct obstruction, and hydrocephalus. This image shows that the cysts are variable in size. **(Middle)** Axial T2 MR shows the cysts, enlarged PVSs, expand the left cerebral peduncle. Prominent midbrain PVSs occur in many patients but this degree of enlargement and mass effect is atypical. The PVSs in the right cerebral peduncle are more normal-sized. **(Bottom)** Axial T1 C+ MR shows the cystic midbrain lesions do not enhance. Initially diagnosed as cystic neoplasm, these are enlarged PVSs. When they occur in the midbrain, expanded PVSs may cause obstructive hydrocephalus but should not be mistaken for tumor.

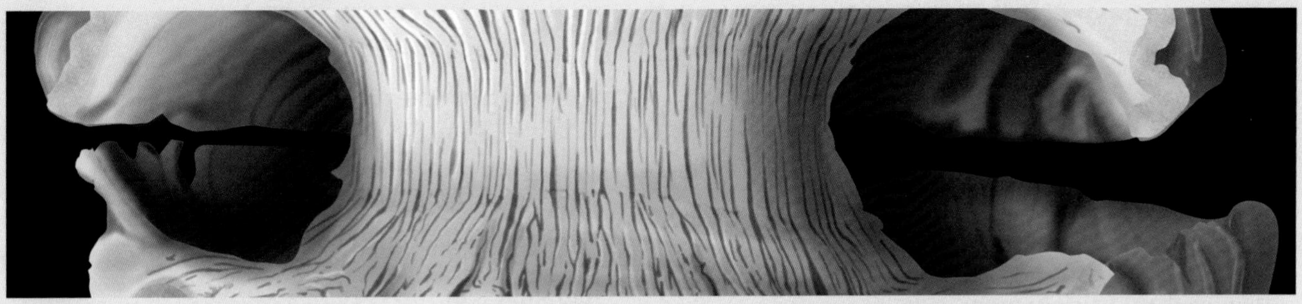

SECTION 2: Supratentorial Brain

CEREBRAL HEMISPHERES OVERVIEW

Terminology

Definitions

- Gyri: Complex convolutions of brain cortex
- Sulci (fissure): CSF-filled grooves or clefts that separate gyri
- Operculae: Parts of frontal, temporal, parietal lobes that overhang/enclose insula

Gross Anatomy

Cerebral Hemispheres

- Two hemispheres, typically of nearly equal size, linked by commissural fibers
  - Separated by a deep median cleft, the great longitudinal (interhemispheric) fissure
  - Falx cerebri lies within interhemispheric fissure
- External highly convoluted mantle of cortical gray matter overlies white matter
- Central sulcus separates frontal, parietal lobes
- Sylvian fissure separates frontal, parietal lobes above from temporal lobe below
- Deep gray nuclei (basal ganglia, thalami), ventricles centrally

Lobes

- Frontal lobe: Anterior region of hemisphere; anterior to central sulcus, superior to sylvian fissure
- Parietal lobe: Posterior region of hemisphere; posterior to central sulcus, anterior to parietooccipital sulcus
- Occipital lobe: Posterior to parietooccipital sulcus
- Temporal lobe: Inferior to sylvian fissure, anterior to angular gyrus
- Insula: Cortical region hidden within depths of lateral (sylvian) fissure; covered by frontal, temporal, parietal opercula

Imaging Anatomy

Overview

- **Frontal lobe**
  - Central sulcus separates frontal, parietal lobes
  - Precentral gyrus contains primary motor cortex
    - Detailed topographically-organized map ("motor homunculus") of contralateral body
    - Head/face lateral, legs/feet along medial surface
  - Premotor cortex: Within gyrus just anterior to precentral gyrus (motor cortex)
  - Three additional major gyri: Superior frontal gyrus, middle frontal gyrus & inferior frontal gyrus separated by superior & inferior frontal sulci
- **Parietal lobe**
  - Posterior to central sulcus
  - Separated from occipital lobe by parietooccipital sulcus (medial surface)
  - Postcentral gyrus: Primary somatosensory cortex
    - Contains topographical map of contralateral body
    - Face, tongue, lips are inferior; trunk, upper limb superolateral; lower limb on medial aspect
  - Superior & inferior parietal lobules lie posterior to postcentral gyrus
  - Supramarginal gyrus lies at end of sylvian fissure
  - Angular gyrus lies ventral to supramarginal gyrus
  - Medial surface of parietal lobe is precuneus
- **Occipital lobe**
  - Posterior to parietooccipital sulcus
  - Primary visual cortex on medial occipital lobe
  - Cuneus on medial surface
- **Temporal lobe**
  - Inferior to sylvian fissure
  - Superior temporal gyrus: Contains primary auditory cortex
  - Middle temporal gyrus: Connects with auditory, somatosensory, visual association pathways
  - Inferior temporal gyrus: Higher visual association area
  - Includes major subdivisions of limbic system
    - Parahippocampal gyrus on medial surface, merges into uncus
- **Insula**
  - Lies deep in floor of sylvian fissure, overlapped by frontal, temporal, parietal operculae
  - Somatosensory function
- **Limbic system**
  - Subcallosal, cingulate, parahippocampal gyri
  - Cingulate gyrus extends around corpus callosum; tapers rostrally (anteriorly) into paraterminal gyrus, subcallosal area
  - Hippocampus including dentate gyrus, Ammon horn (cornu ammonis)
- **Base of brain**
  - Orbital gyri cover base of frontal lobe: Gyrus rectus medially
  - Olfactory bulb/tract lie within olfactory sulcus
- **White matter tracts**: Three major types of fibers
  - Association fibers: Interconnect different cortical regions in same hemisphere
    - Cingulum is a long association fiber which lies beneath cingulate gyrus
  - Commissural fibers: Interconnect similar cortical regions of opposite hemispheres
    - Corpus callosum is largest commissural fiber, links cerebral hemispheres
  - Projection fibers: Connect cerebral cortex with deep nuclei, brainstem, cerebellum, spinal cord
    - Internal capsule is a major projection fiber
- **Basal ganglia**
  - Paired deep bray nuclei
  - Caudate nucleus, putamen, globus pallidus
- **Thalamus**: Paired nuclear complexes, serve as relay station for most sensory pathways

Anatomy-Based Imaging Issues

Imaging Recommendations

- Multiplanar MR best evaluates cerebral hemispheres
- White matter best evaluated by diffusion tensor imaging (DTI) on 1.5 or 3 Tesla MR
- Limbic system best evaluated with high-resolution coronal T2 MR, T1 volume images & FLAIR
- Multiplanar MR best evaluates basal ganglia, thalami
- Diffusion imaging often very helpful for evaluation of supratentorial disease processes

CEREBRAL HEMISPHERES OVERVIEW

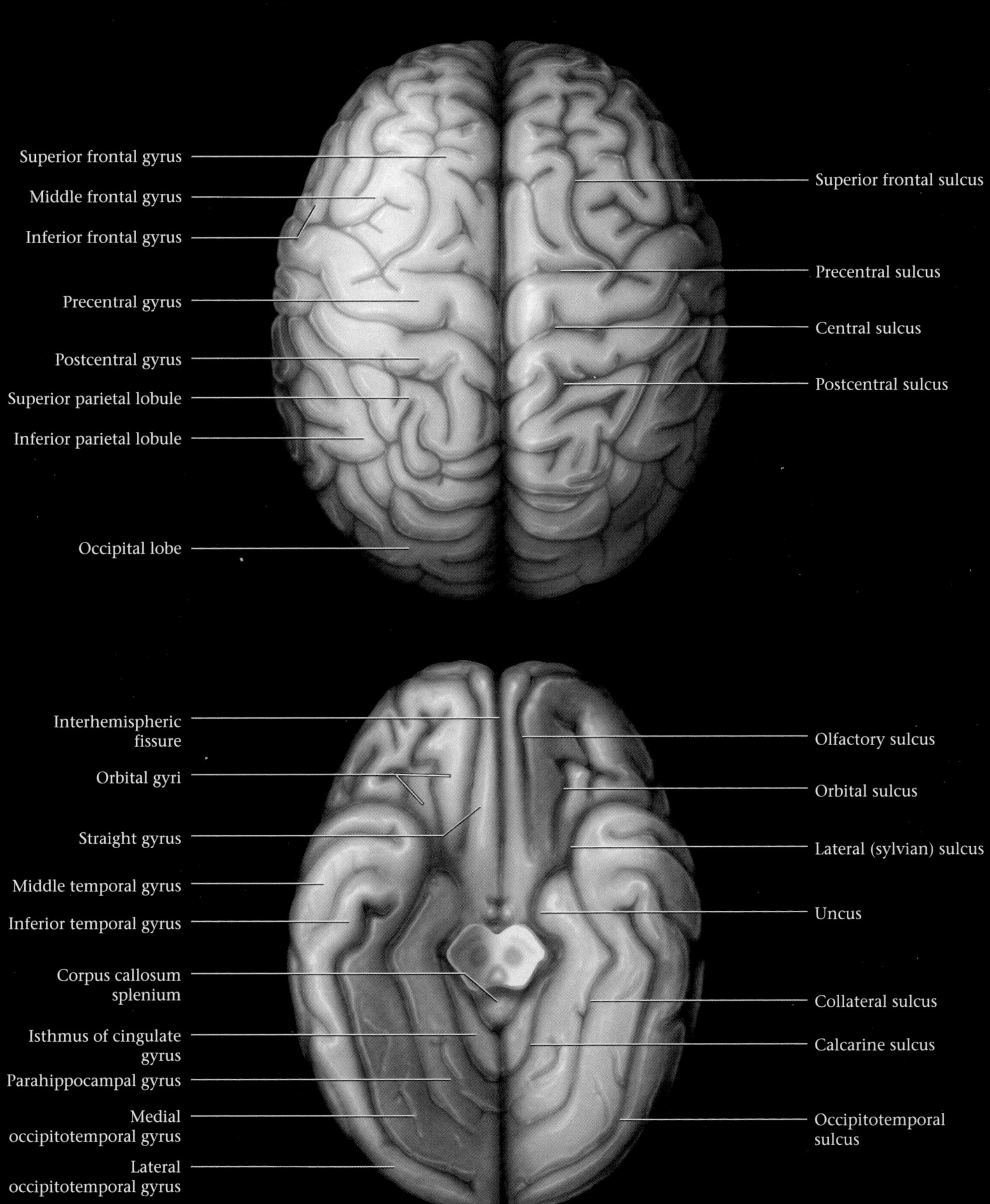
Superior frontal gyrus
Middle frontal gyrus
Inferior frontal gyrus
Precentral gyrus
Postcentral gyrus
Superior parietal lobule
Inferior parietal lobule
Occipital lobe
Superior frontal sulcus
Precentral sulcus
Central sulcus
Postcentral sulcus
Interhemispheric fissure
Orbital gyri
Straight gyrus
Middle temporal gyrus
Inferior temporal gyrus
Corpus callosum splenium
Isthmus of cingulate gyrus
Parahippocampal gyrus
Medial occipitotemporal gyrus
Lateral occipitotemporal gyrus
Olfactory sulcus
Orbital sulcus
Lateral (sylvian) sulcus
Uncus
Collateral sulcus
Calcarine sulcus
Occipitotemporal sulcus

(Top) Surface anatomy of cerebral hemisphere, seen from above. Gyri and lobules shown on left; sulci on right. Central (Rolandic) sulcus separates anterior frontal lobe from posterior parietal lobe. Precentral gyrus of frontal lobe is primary motor cortex while postcentral gyrus of parietal lobe is primary sensory cortex. Central sulcus can be reliably identified on CT & MR imaging. **(Bottom)** Inferior view with major sulci, gyri depicted. Orbital gyri cover base of frontal lobe. Gyrus rectus (straight gyrus) is most medial. Olfactory bulb/tract (not shown) lie within olfactory sulcus. Sylvian (lateral) fissure separates frontal lobe from inferior temporal lobe. Uncus forms medial border of temporal lobe, merges with parahippocampal gyrus. Collateral sulcus separates parahippocampal gyrus from medial occipitotemporal (fusiform or lingual) gyrus.

CEREBRAL HEMISPHERES OVERVIEW

GRAPHICS

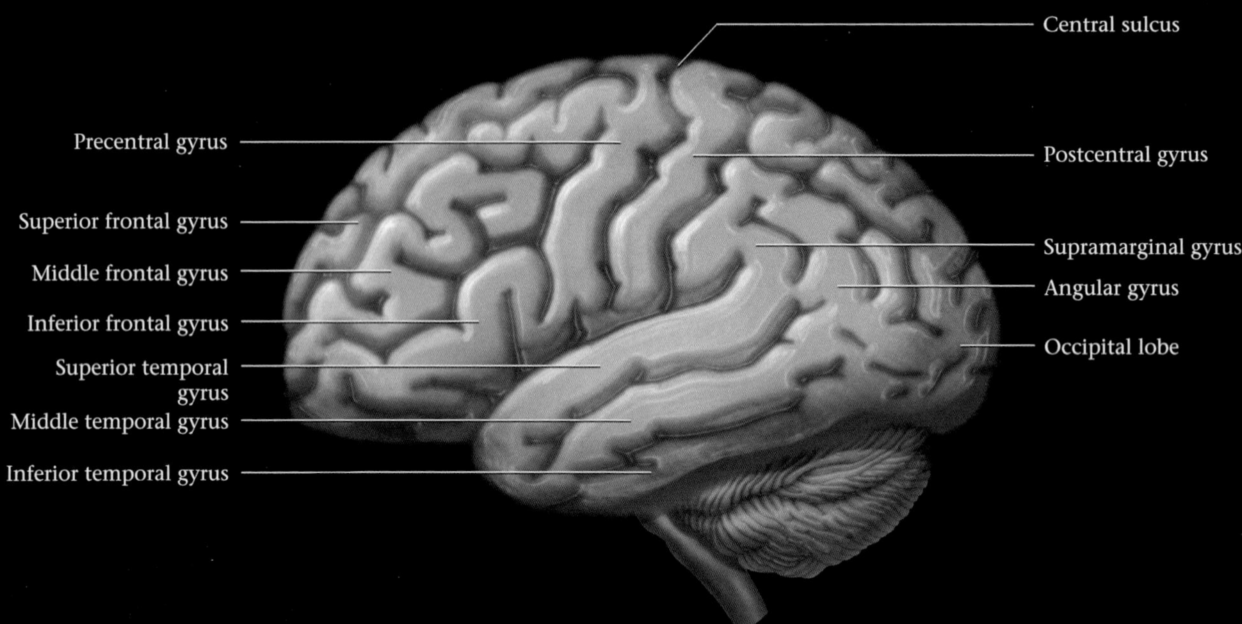
Central sulcus
Precentral gyrus
Postcentral gyrus
Superior frontal gyrus
Middle frontal gyrus
Supramarginal gyrus
Angular gyrus
Inferior frontal gyrus
Occipital lobe
Superior temporal gyrus
Middle temporal gyrus
Inferior temporal gyrus

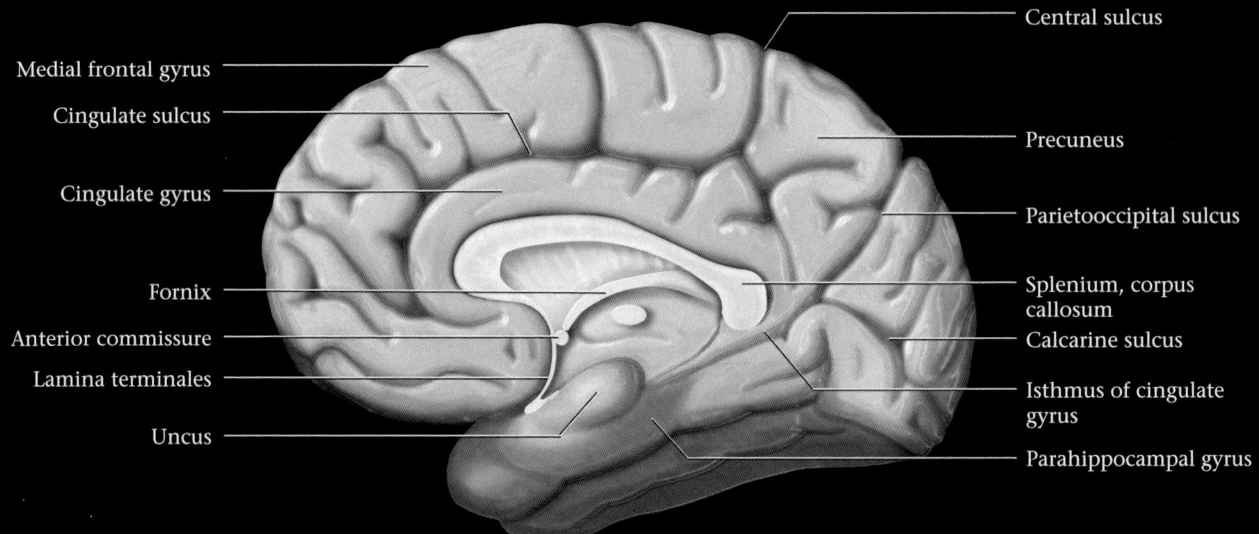
Central sulcus
Medial frontal gyrus
Cingulate sulcus
Precuneus
Cingulate gyrus
Parietooccipital sulcus
Fornix
Splenium, corpus callosum
Anterior commissure
Calcarine sulcus
Lamina terminales
Isthmus of cingulate gyrus
Uncus
Parahippocampal gyrus

(Top) Lateral surface of brain depicts major gyri, sulci. Frontal lobe extends from frontal pole to central sulcus. Supramarginal & angular gyri are part of parietal lobe. Supramarginal gyrus has somatosensory function while angular gyrus is important in auditory & visual input, language comprehension. Superior temporal gyrus contains primary auditory cortex, also forms temporal operculum. Insular cortex lies within sylvian fissure beneath frontal, temporal & parietal opercula. **(Bottom)** Sagittal graphic shows medial view of cerebral hemisphere. Corpus callosum represents major commissural fiber. Fornix & cingulate gyrus are important in limbic system. Fornix extends from fimbria of hippocampus posteriorly to anterior thalamus, mamillary body & septal region. Cingulate gyrus is involved with emotion formation & processing, learning & memory.

AXIAL CECT

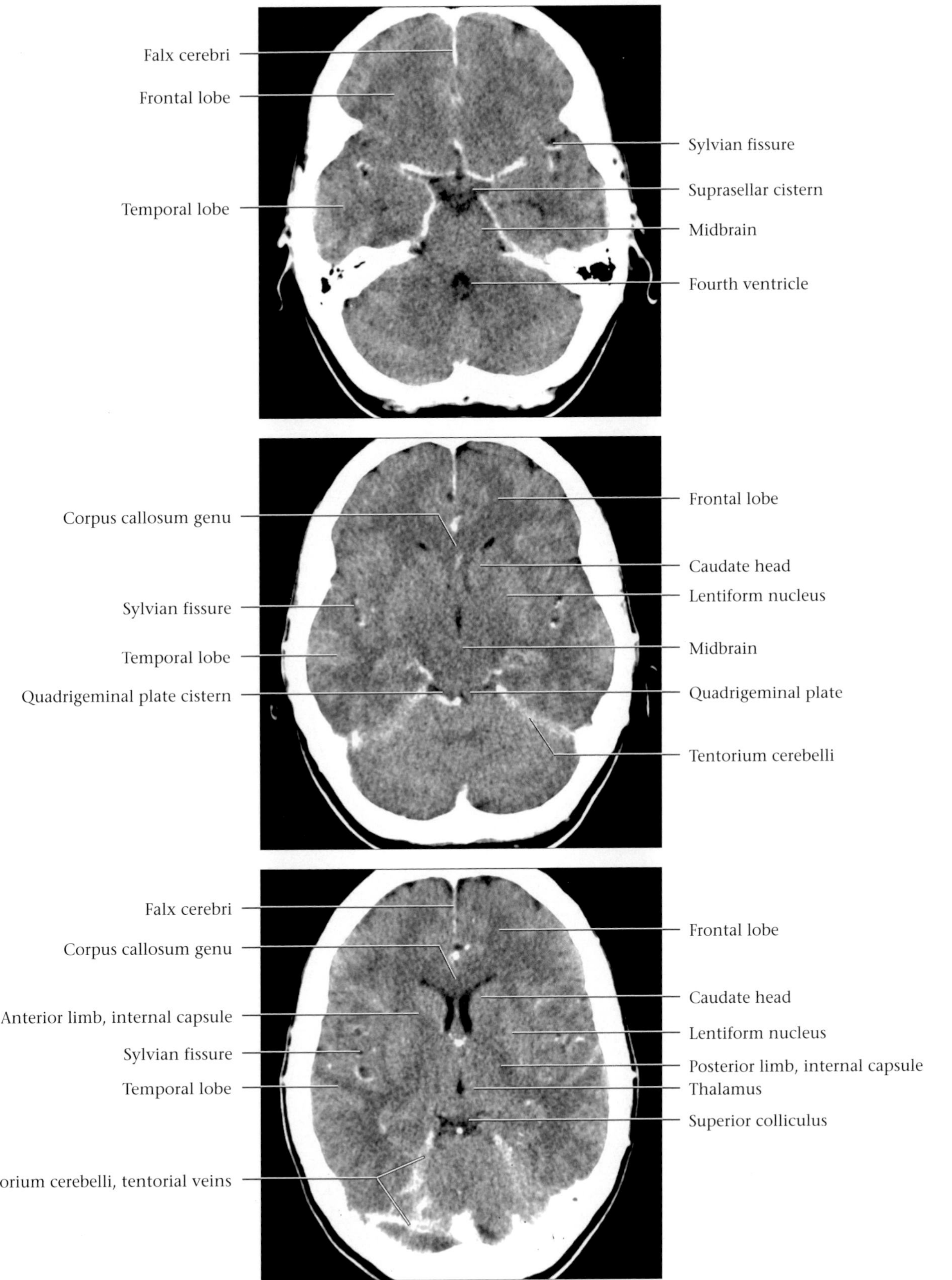

Falx cerebri
Frontal lobe
Temporal lobe
Sylvian fissure
Suprasellar cistern
Midbrain
Fourth ventricle
Corpus callosum genu
Sylvian fissure
Temporal lobe
Quadrigeminal plate cistern
Frontal lobe
Caudate head
Lentiform nucleus
Midbrain
Quadrigeminal plate
Tentorium cerebelli
Falx cerebri
Corpus callosum genu
Anterior limb, internal capsule
Sylvian fissure
Temporal lobe
Tentorium cerebelli, tentorial veins
Frontal lobe
Caudate head
Lentiform nucleus
Posterior limb, internal capsule
Thalamus
Superior colliculus

(Top) First of six axial CECT images of cerebral hemispheres from inferior to superior shows interhemispheric fissure containing falx cerebri. Sylvian (lateral) fissure is seen separating frontal & temporal lobes. **(Middle)** This image shows frontal & temporal lobes & basal ganglia. Anterior limb of internal capsule separates caudate head from lentiform nucleus (putamen & globus pallidus). Posterior limb contains corticospinal tract & separates thalamus from lentiform nucleus. **(Bottom)** More superior image shows parts of basal ganglia including caudate, putamen & globus pallidus. Anterior limb, genu & posterior limb of internal capsule are seen. Internal capsule is major projection fiber to & from cerebral cortex & it fans out to form the corona radiata. Thalamus borders third ventricle & is separated from basal ganglia by internal capsule.

CEREBRAL HEMISPHERES OVERVIEW

AXIAL CECT

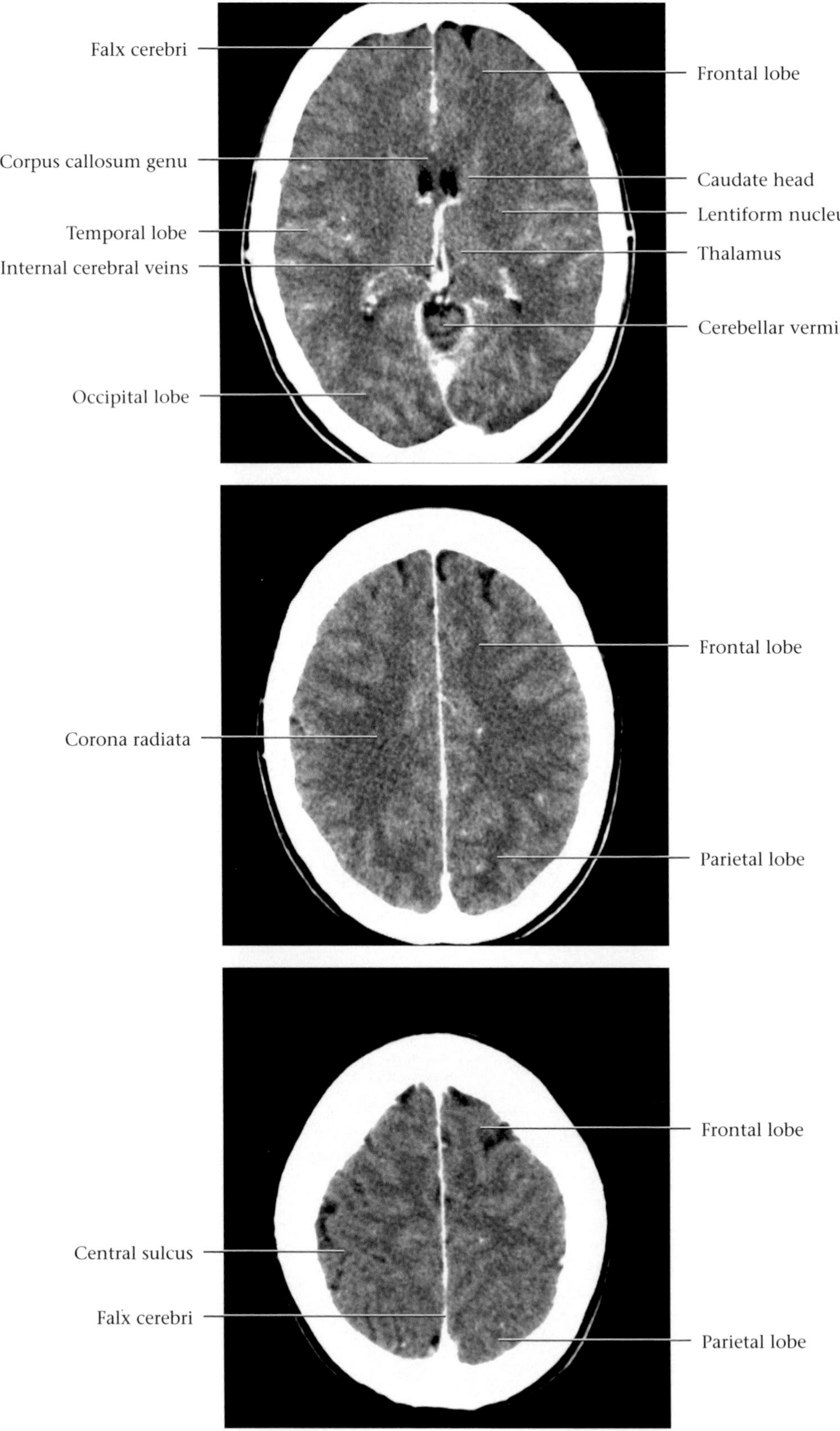

Falx cerebri
Frontal lobe
Corpus callosum genu
Caudate head
Lentiform nucleus
Temporal lobe
Internal cerebral veins
Thalamus
Cerebellar vermis
Occipital lobe
Frontal lobe
Corona radiata
Parietal lobe
Frontal lobe
Central sulcus
Falx cerebri
Parietal lobe

(Top) Image more superior shows thalamus & internal cerebral veins at level of lateral ventricles. Falx cerebri is present within interhemispheric (great longitudinal) fissure. Occipital lobe is present posteriorly, just above tentorium cerebelli & contains primary visual cortex. **(Middle)** The corona radiata (centrum semiovale) is comprised of radial projection fibers from cortex to brainstem. Corona radiata is continuous with internal capsule inferiorly. Occipital lobe is not seen on this and higher scans. **(Bottom)** Image at cerebral vertex shows central sulcus separating frontal from parietal lobes. Primary motor cortex is within frontal lobe precentral gyrus while primary somatosensory cortex is within parietal postcentral gyrus. Specific sulci & gyri are better resolved on MR imaging, although sylvian fissure & central sulcus are reliably found on CT imaging.

AXIAL T1 MR

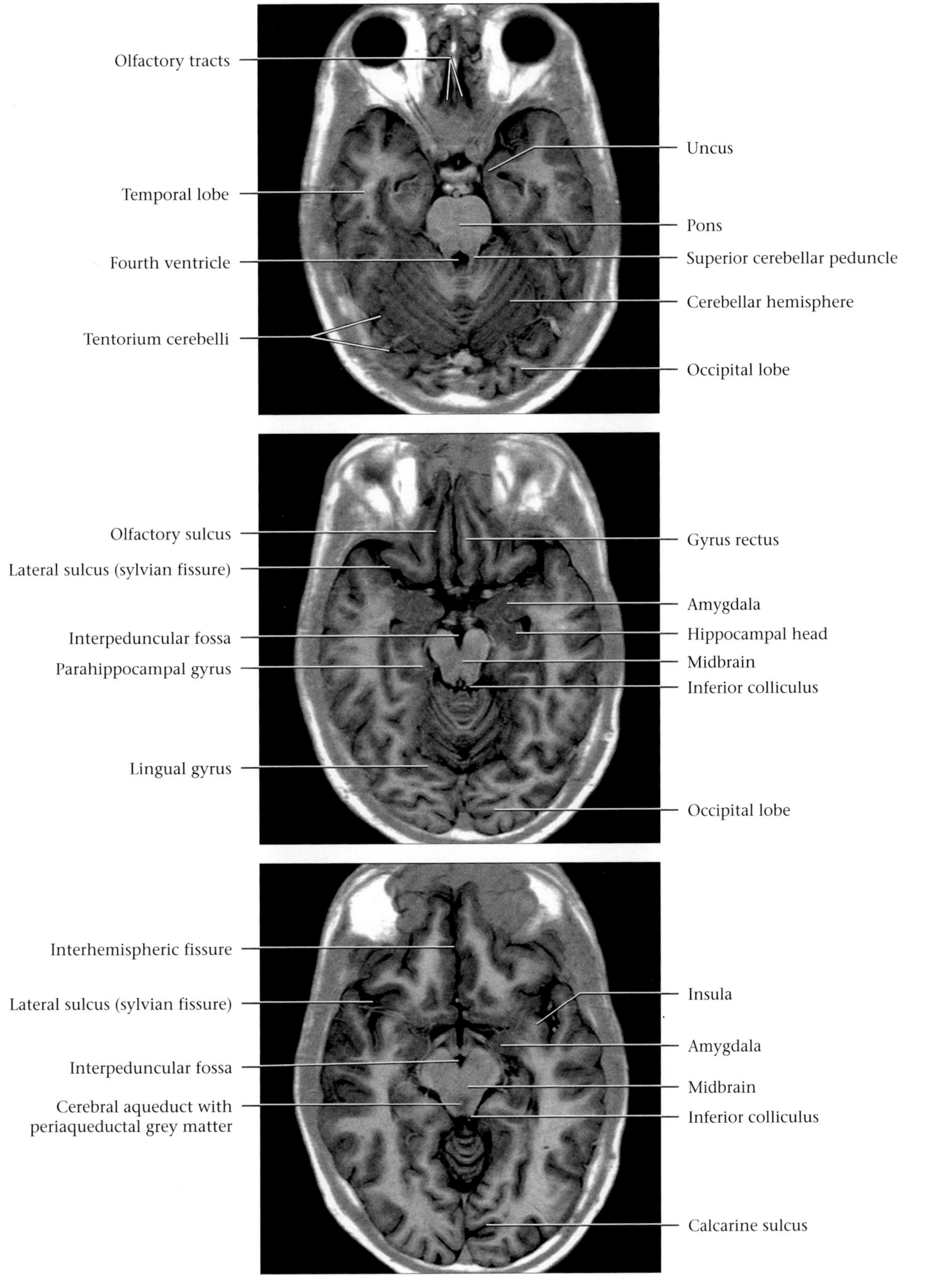
Olfactory tracts
Temporal lobe
Fourth ventricle
Tentorium cerebelli
Uncus
Pons
Superior cerebellar peduncle
Cerebellar hemisphere
Occipital lobe
Olfactory sulcus
Lateral sulcus (sylvian fissure)
Interpeduncular fossa
Parahippocampal gyrus
Lingual gyrus
Gyrus rectus
Amygdala
Hippocampal head
Midbrain
Inferior colliculus
Occipital lobe
Interhemispheric fissure
Lateral sulcus (sylvian fissure)
Interpeduncular fossa
Cerebral aqueduct with periaqueductal grey matter
Insula
Amygdala
Midbrain
Inferior colliculus
Calcarine sulcus

(Top) First of nine axial T1 MR images through cerebral hemispheres from inferior to superior shows inferior aspect of hemispheres. Occipital lobe is partially seen, superior to the sloping tentorium cerebelli. Uncus forms medial border of temporal lobe, merges posteriorly with parahippocampal gyrus. **(Middle)** Basal aspect of frontal lobes is formed by orbital gyri. Olfactory bulb/tract lies in/below olfactory sulcus. Hippocampus lies posterior & inferior to amygdala. Parahippocampal gyrus is separated from medial occipitotemporal (lingual or fusiform) gyrus by collateral sulcus. **(Bottom)** Axial image at level of midbrain shows sylvian fissure separating frontal & temporal lobes. Insula lies deep to sylvian fissure covered by surrounding frontal, temporal & parietal operculae. Calcarine sulcus is surrounded by primary motor cortex in posterior occipital lobe.

CEREBRAL HEMISPHERES OVERVIEW

AXIAL T1 MR

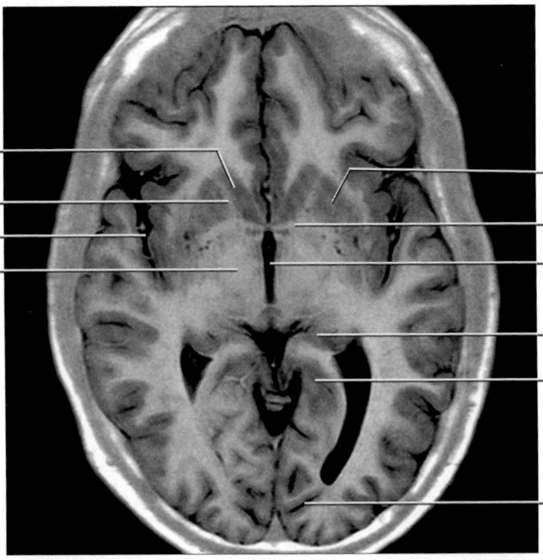

Caudate head
Anterior limb, internal capsule
Sylvian fissure
Thalamus
Putamen
Anterior commissure
Third ventricle
Hippocampus tail
Parietooccipital sulcus
Calcarine sulcus

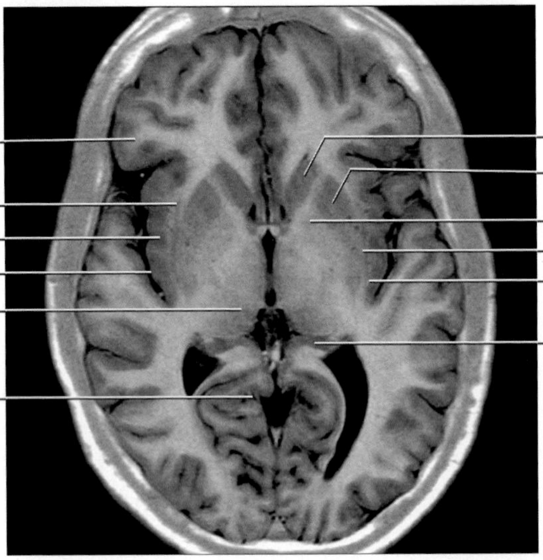

Frontal operculum
Claustrum
Insula
Sylvian fissure
Thalamus
Parietooccipital sulcus
Caudate head
Putamen
Globus pallidus
External capsule
Extreme capsule
Hippocampus tail

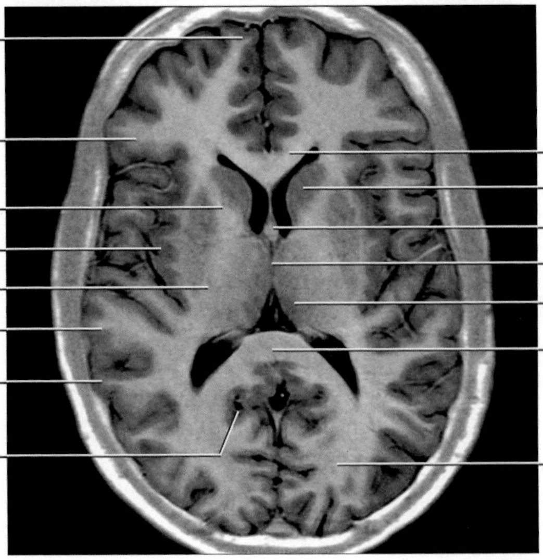

Superior frontal gyrus
Frontal operculum
Anterior limb, internal capsule
Cortex of insula
Posterior limb, internal capsule
Supramarginal gyrus
Angular gyrus
Parietooccipital sulcus
Genu, corpus callosum
Caudate head
Pillars of fornix
Third ventricle
Thalamus
Splenium, corpus callosum
Occipital lobe

(Top) More superior image at level of inferior basal ganglia shows anterior limb of internal capsule separating caudate head from lentiform nucleus. Anterior commissure is a major commissural fiber which is seen anterior to fornix in lamina terminales in anterior third ventricle. Anterior commissure connects anterior perforated substance & olfactory tracts anteriorly & temporal lobe, amygdala & stria terminales posteriorly. **(Middle)** This image shows basal ganglia & thalamus. Globus pallidus is hyperintense relative to putamen. Parietooccipital sulcus separates parietal & occipital lobes. Hippocampal tail is seen wrapping around midbrain & thalamus. External capsule lies between putamen & claustrum. Extreme capsule lies between claustrum & insula. **(Bottom)** Image through superior basal ganglia shows supramarginal gyrus & angular gyrus of parietal lobe.

CEREBRAL HEMISPHERES OVERVIEW

AXIAL T1 MR

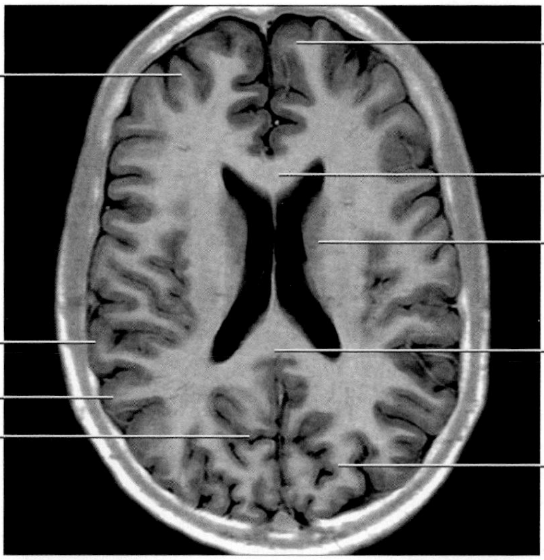

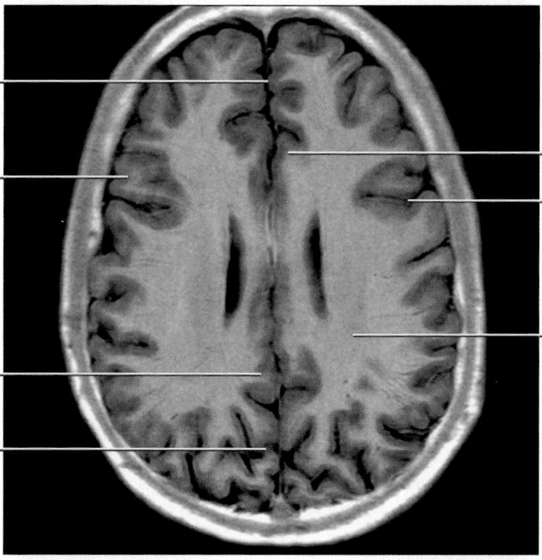

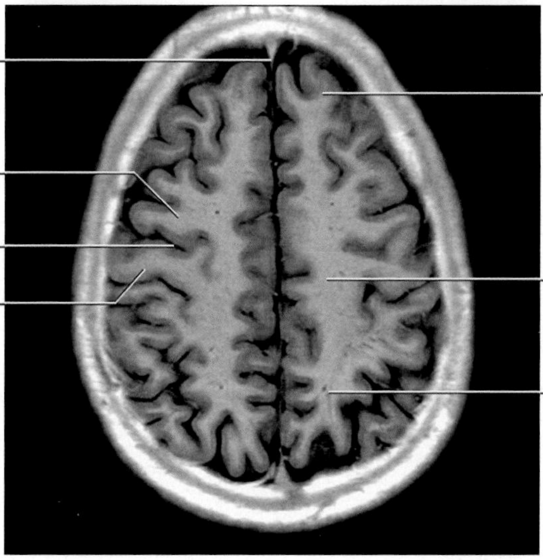

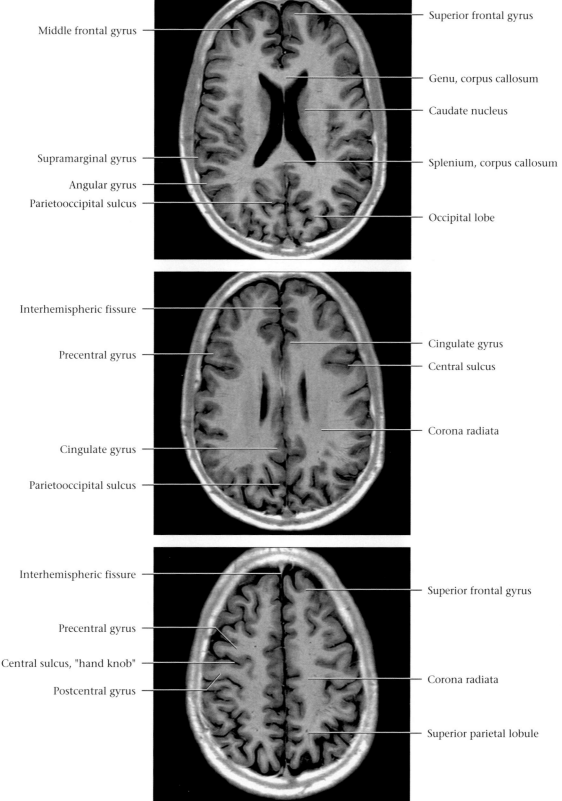

Middle frontal gyrus
Superior frontal gyrus
Genu, corpus callosum
Caudate nucleus
Supramarginal gyrus
Splenium, corpus callosum
Angular gyrus
Parietooccipital sulcus
Occipital lobe

Interhemispheric fissure
Cingulate gyrus
Precentral gyrus
Central sulcus
Corona radiata
Cingulate gyrus
Parietooccipital sulcus

Interhemispheric fissure
Superior frontal gyrus
Precentral gyrus
Central sulcus, "hand knob"
Corona radiata
Postcentral gyrus
Superior parietal lobule

(Top) More superior image shows top of caudate nucleus body as it wraps around lateral ventricle. Parietooccipital sulcus on medial aspect of hemispheres separates parietal & occipital lobes. **(Middle)** Cerebral hemispheres are separated by interhemispheric (longitudinal) fissure which contains falx cerebri. Central sulcus separates frontal & parietal lobes. Corona radiata (centrum semiovale) is formed by fibers from all cortical areas in internal capsule fanning out into superior hemispheres. **(Bottom)** Image more superior shows falx cerebri within interhemispheric fissure. Falx cerebri is a dural fold which contains superior sagittal sinus. Central sulcus separates frontal & parietal lobes & is typically identified on MR imaging. Often, the "hand knob" representing hand motor area of precentral gyrus can be identified.

CORONAL T1 MR

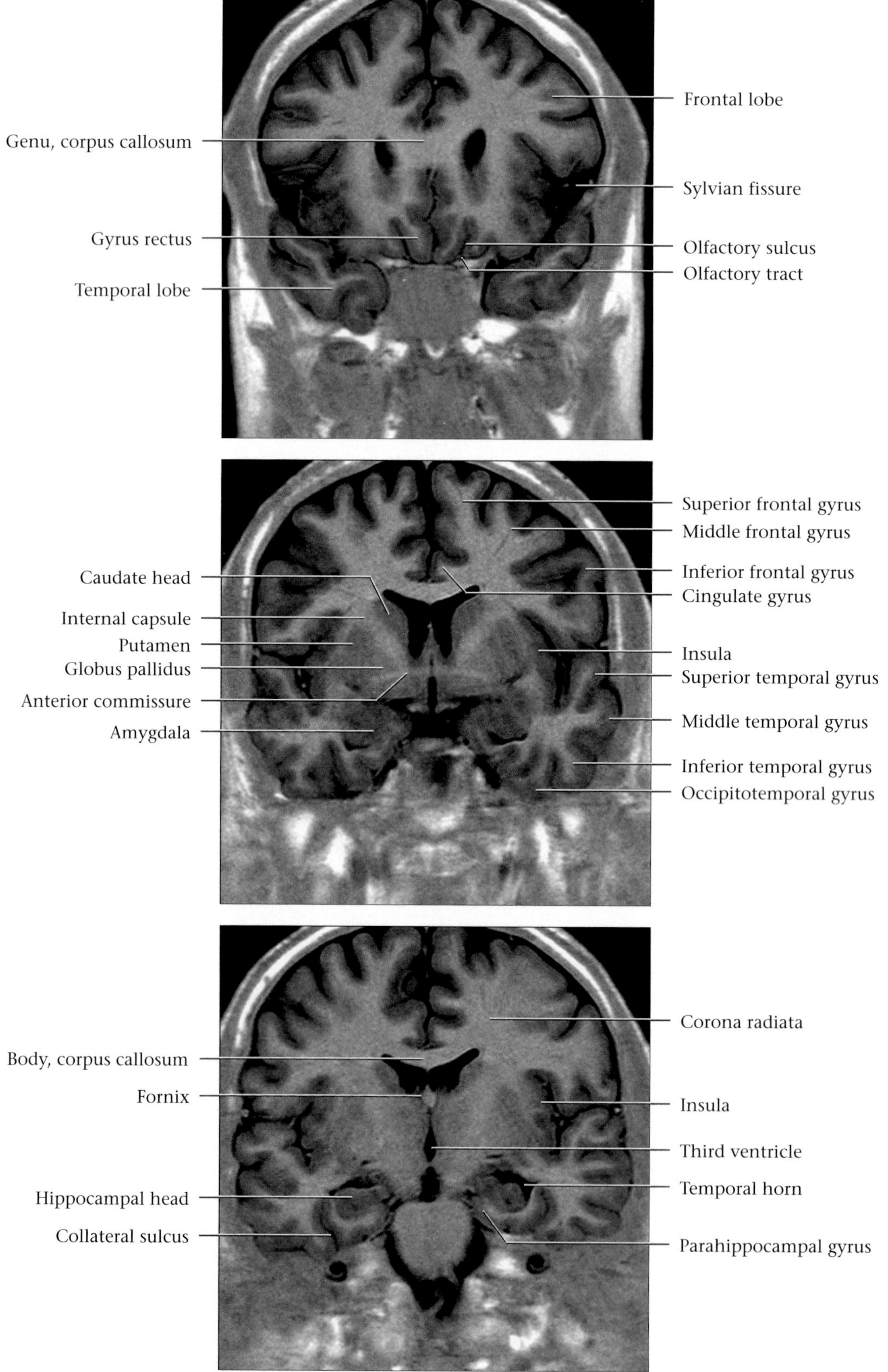
Genu, corpus callosum
Frontal lobe
Sylvian fissure
Gyrus rectus
Olfactory sulcus
Olfactory tract
Temporal lobe
Superior frontal gyrus
Middle frontal gyrus
Caudate head
Inferior frontal gyrus
Cingulate gyrus
Internal capsule
Putamen
Globus pallidus
Insula
Superior temporal gyrus
Anterior commissure
Amygdala
Middle temporal gyrus
Inferior temporal gyrus
Occipitotemporal gyrus
Corona radiata
Body, corpus callosum
Fornix
Insula
Third ventricle
Hippocampal head
Temporal horn
Collateral sulcus
Parahippocampal gyrus

(Top) First of six coronal T1 MR images through cerebral hemispheres from anterior to posterior shows genu of corpus callosum. Olfactory tract is embedded in olfactory sulcus. Olfactory sulcus defines lateral margin of gyrus rectus at base of brain. **(Middle)** More posterior image shows anterior limb of internal capsule & anterior commissure. Anteriorly, caudate head & putamen are connected. Central regions of frontal & temporal lobes are seen. Insula is covered by frontal & temporal opercula. Superior, middle & inferior gyri of temporal lobe are well seen on coronal imaging as are superior, middle & inferior frontal gyri. **(Bottom)** This image shows lobulated superior surface of hippocampal head. Body of fornix runs below corpus callosum. Collateral sulcus separates parahippocampal & medial occipitotemporal (fusiform) gyri.

CORONAL T1 MR

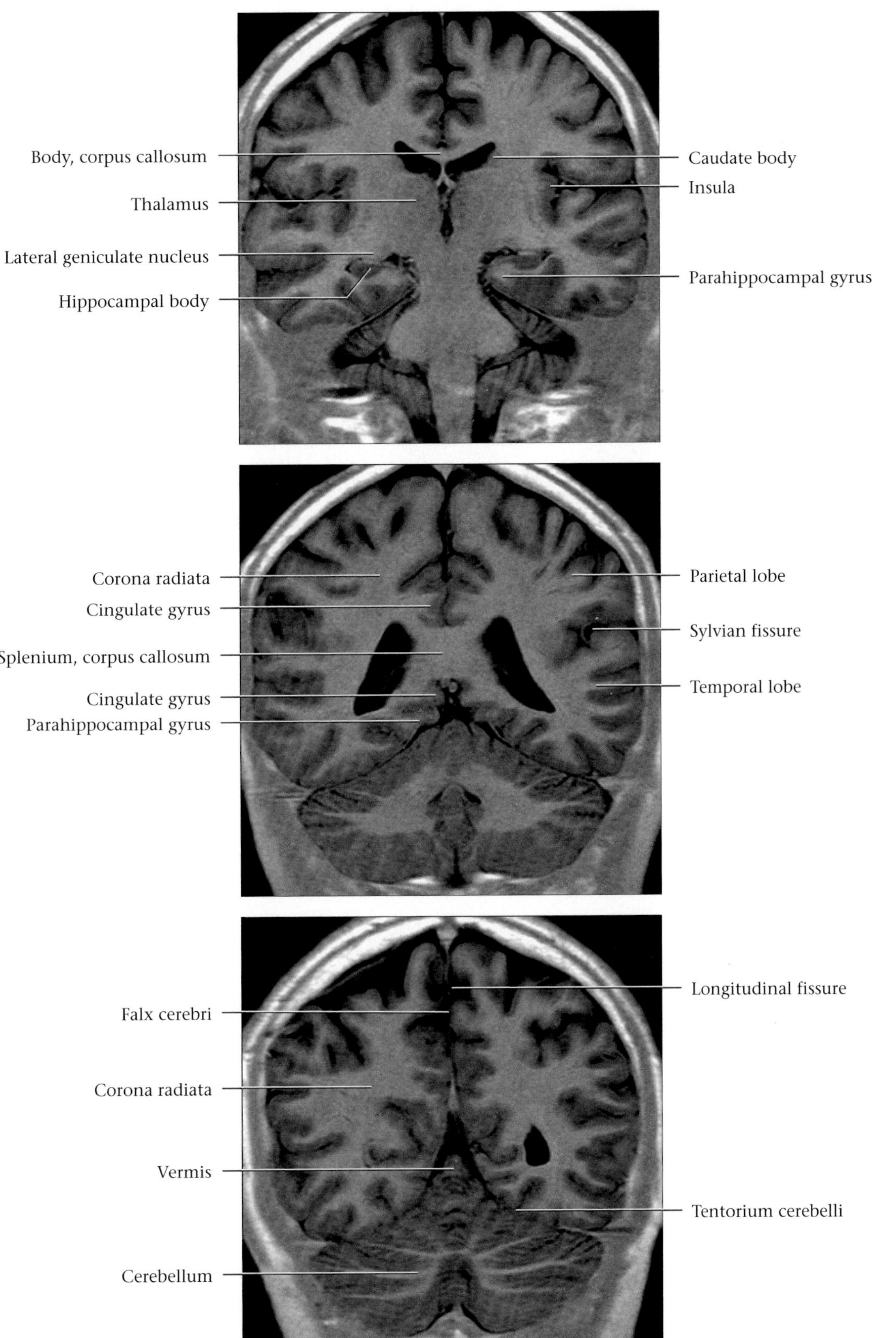
Body, corpus callosum
Thalamus
Lateral geniculate nucleus
Hippocampal body
Caudate body
Insula
Parahippocampal gyrus
Corona radiata
Cingulate gyrus
Splenium, corpus callosum
Cingulate gyrus
Parahippocampal gyrus
Parietal lobe
Sylvian fissure
Temporal lobe
Falx cerebri
Corona radiata
Vermis
Cerebellum
Longitudinal fissure
Tentorium cerebelli

(Top) More posterior image shows body of hippocampus & parahippocampal gyrus forming medial surface of posterior temporal lobe. Lateral geniculate nucleus, a thalamic nucleus involved in visual pathway, is seen at this level. Optic radiations course posteriorly from lateral geniculate nucleus to occipital lobe. **(Middle)** Image at corpus callosum splenium. Cingulate gyrus encircles splenium in an arch to lie superior & inferior to it. Posterior parahippocampal gyrus merges with cingulate gyrus. Posterior sylvian fissure is visible separating parietal lobe above from temporal lobe below. **(Bottom)** Image more posterior shows interhemispheric fissure, falx cerebri & tentorium cerebelli. Tentorium cerebelli is a dural fold in horizontal plane separating supratentorial & infratentorial compartments & is continuous superiorly with falx cerebri.

SAGITTAL T1 MR

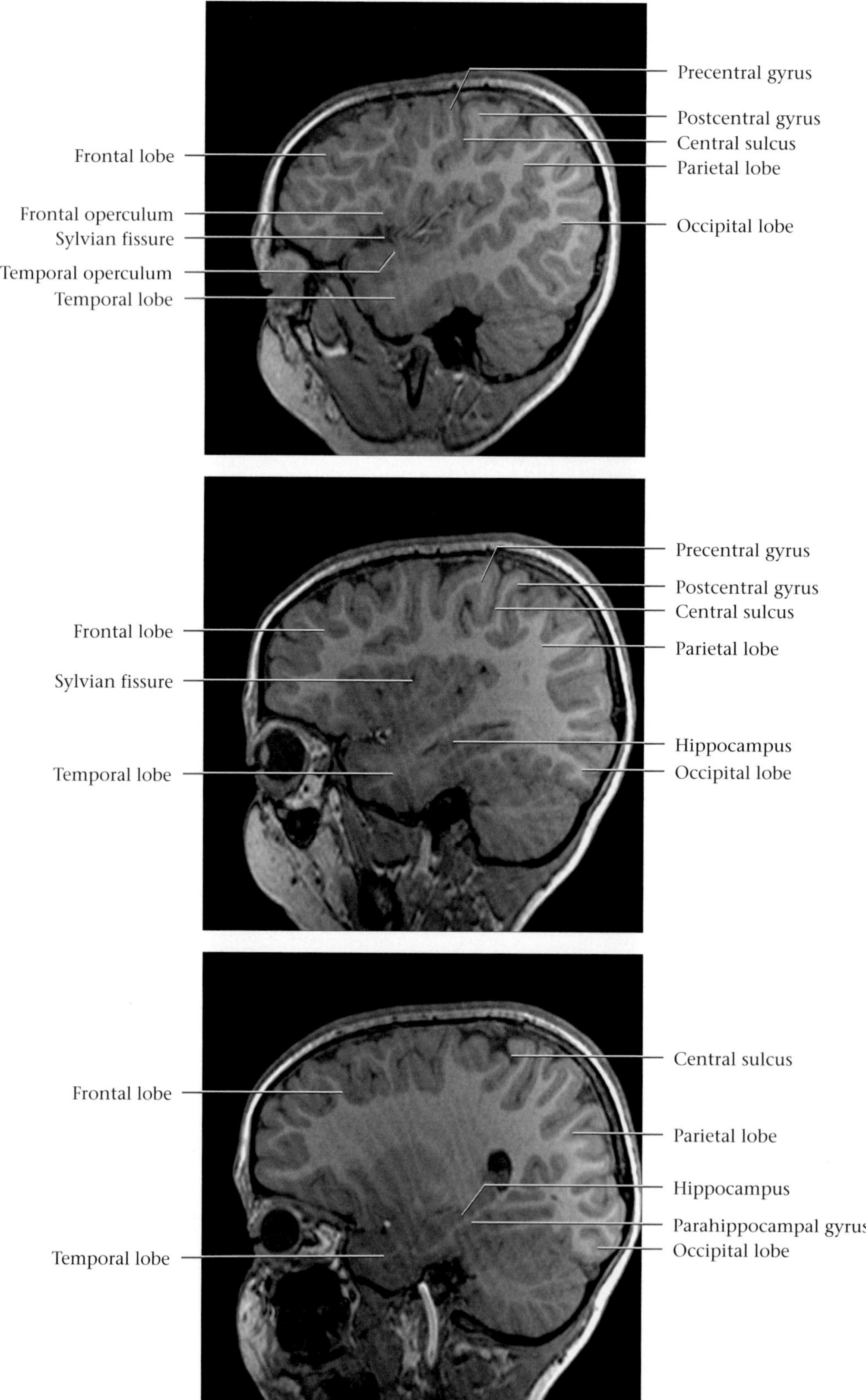
Precentral gyrus
Postcentral gyrus
Central sulcus
Parietal lobe
Occipital lobe
Frontal lobe
Frontal operculum
Sylvian fissure
Temporal operculum
Temporal lobe
Precentral gyrus
Postcentral gyrus
Central sulcus
Parietal lobe
Hippocampus
Occipital lobe
Frontal lobe
Sylvian fissure
Temporal lobe
Central sulcus
Parietal lobe
Hippocampus
Parahippocampal gyrus
Occipital lobe
Frontal lobe
Temporal lobe

(Top) First of six sagittal T1 MR images from lateral to medial shows lateral aspect of sylvian fissure bounded superiorly by frontal operculum & inferiorly by temporal operculum. Sylvian fissure contains insular (M2) and opercular (M3) segments of middle cerebral artery. **(Middle)** This image shows central sulcus bordered by precentral & postcentral gyri. Location of central sulcus & precentral gyrus (primary motor cortex) is extremely important in pre-surgical planning. Hippocampus is seen along temporal horn. **(Bottom)** Image through medial temporal lobe demonstrates hippocampus & parahippocampal gyrus. White matter along superior margin of hippocampus represents fimbria which curves superiorly & anteriorly beneath corpus callosum as fornix, terminating in mamillary body. Lateral sulcus (sylvian fissure) separates temporal lobe from frontal & parietal lobes.

CEREBRAL HEMISPHERES OVERVIEW

SAGITTAL T1 MR

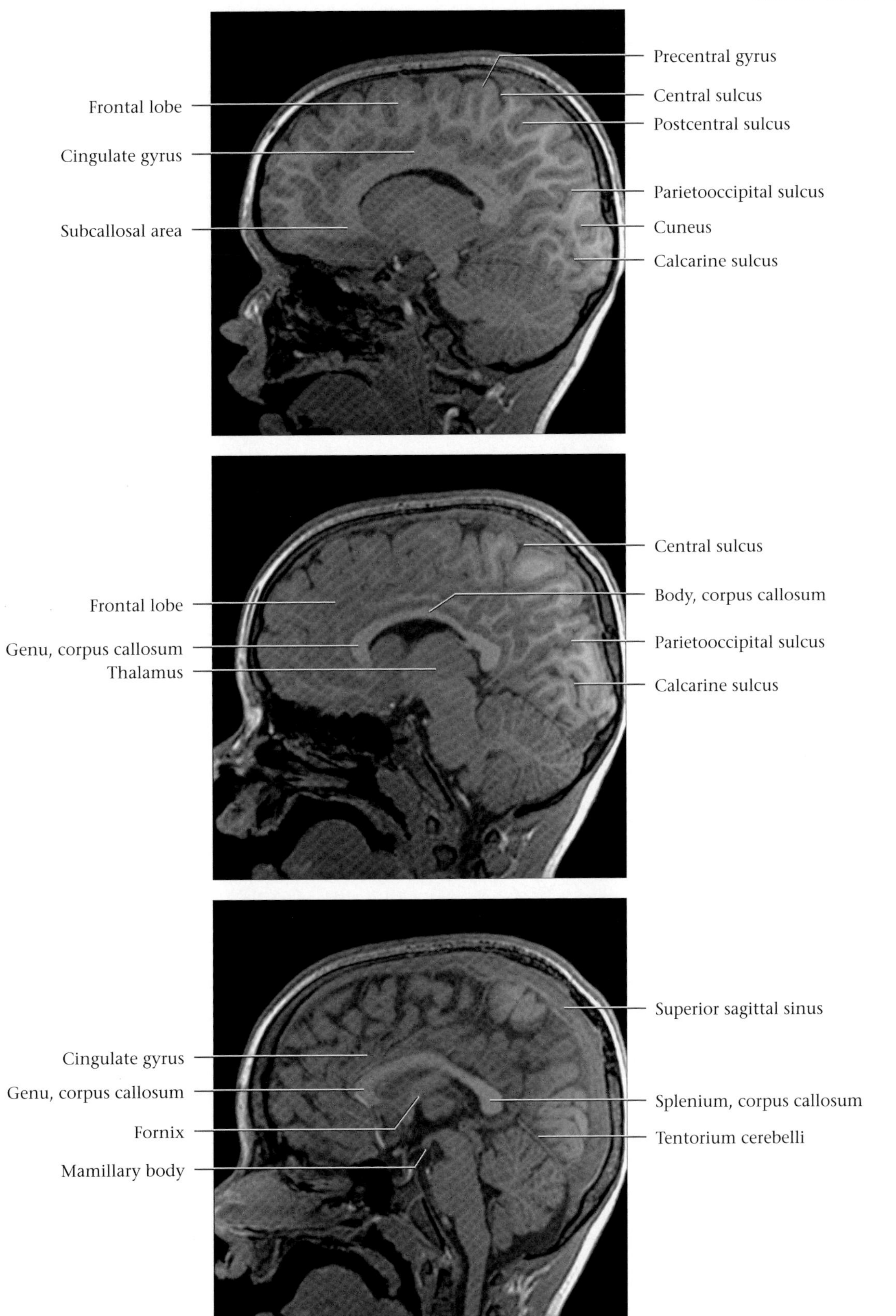
Frontal lobe
Cingulate gyrus
Subcallosal area
Precentral gyrus
Central sulcus
Postcentral sulcus
Parietooccipital sulcus
Cuneus
Calcarine sulcus
Frontal lobe
Genu, corpus callosum
Thalamus
Central sulcus
Body, corpus callosum
Parietooccipital sulcus
Calcarine sulcus
Cingulate gyrus
Genu, corpus callosum
Fornix
Mamillary body
Superior sagittal sinus
Splenium, corpus callosum
Tentorium cerebelli

(Top) More medial image shows central sulcus, bordered anteriorly by precentral gyrus (motor cortex) & posteriorly by postcentral gyrus (sensory cortex). Calcarine sulcus & parietooccipital sulcus define cuneus of occipital lobe. Cingulate gyrus extends around corpus callosum from paraterminal gyrus & subcallosal area rostrally to parahippocampal gyrus of temporal lobe. **(Middle)** Central sulcus separates frontal & parietal lobes. Parietooccipital sulcus, located on medial side of hemispheres, separates parietal & occipital lobes. **(Bottom)** Midline sagittal image shows fornix arching towards mamillary body. Cerebral hemispheres are above tentorium cerebelli, a dural fold separating brain into supratentorial & infratentorial compartments. Cerebral hemispheres are connected via corpus callosum, largest commissural fiber.

AXIAL T2 MR

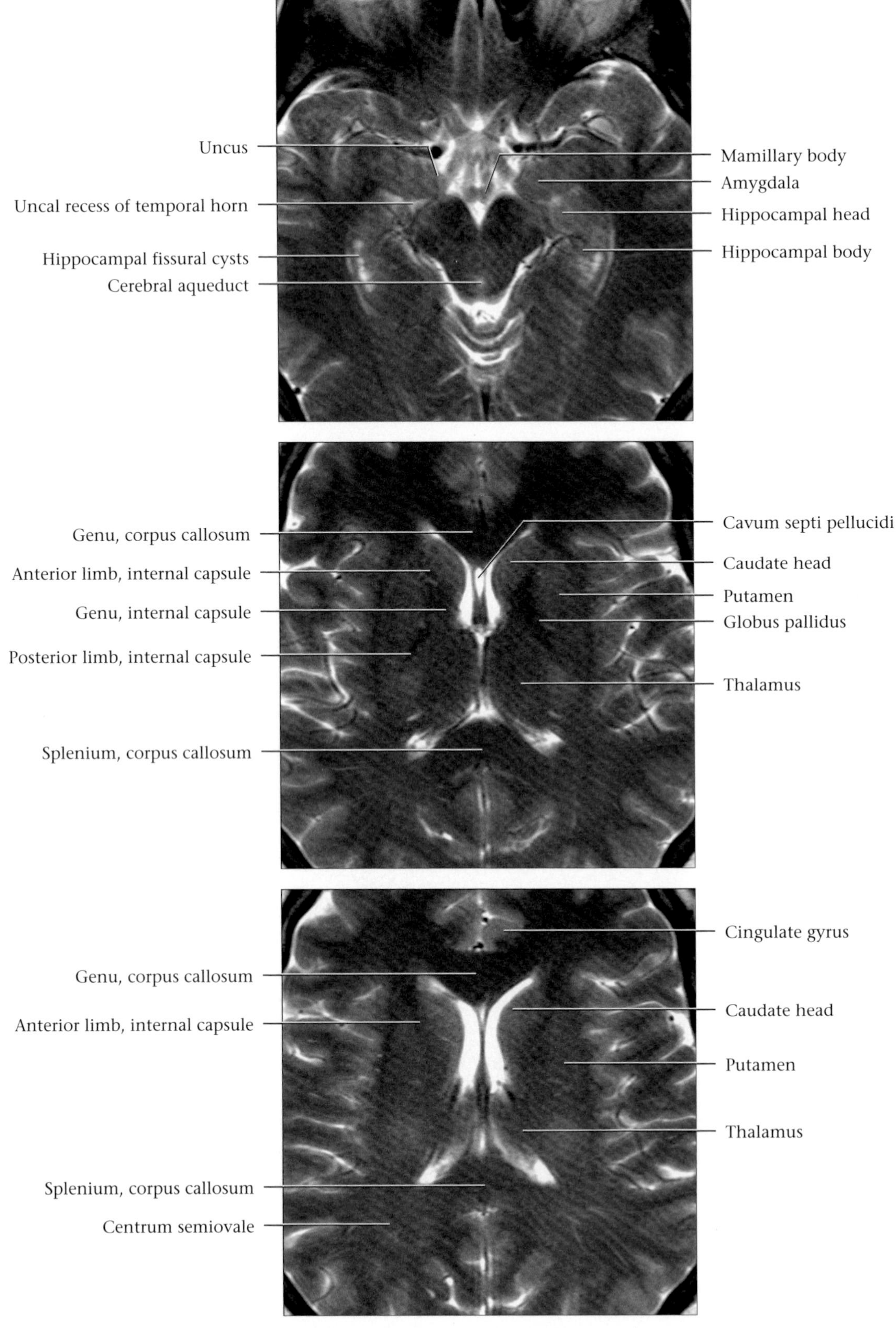
Uncus
Uncal recess of temporal horn
Hippocampal fissural cysts
Cerebral aqueduct
Mamillary body
Amygdala
Hippocampal head
Hippocampal body
Genu, corpus callosum
Anterior limb, internal capsule
Genu, internal capsule
Posterior limb, internal capsule
Splenium, corpus callosum
Cavum septi pellucidi
Caudate head
Putamen
Globus pallidus
Thalamus
Genu, corpus callosum
Anterior limb, internal capsule
Splenium, corpus callosum
Centrum semiovale
Cingulate gyrus
Caudate head
Putamen
Thalamus

(Top) First of three axial T2 MR images from inferior to superior shows hippocampus & amygdala. Hippocampal fissural cysts (hippocampal sulcus remnants), a normal variant, are noted. Temporal horn separates amygdala anteriorly & superiorly from hippocampus. **(Middle)** More superior image shows basal ganglia & thalamus. Putamen is hypointense relative to other deep gray nuclei related to increased myelin content & iron deposition in older patients. Globus pallidus is same signal intensity as internal capsule. Anterior limb, genu & posterior limbs of internal capsule are seen. Anterior limb contains frontopontine fibers & thalamocortical projections. Genu contains corticobulbar fibers & posterior limb contains corticospinal tracts. **(Bottom)** Image at level of superior thalamus. Nerve fibers of corpus callosum radiate into centrum semiovale (white matter core) of hemispheres.

CORONAL T2 MR

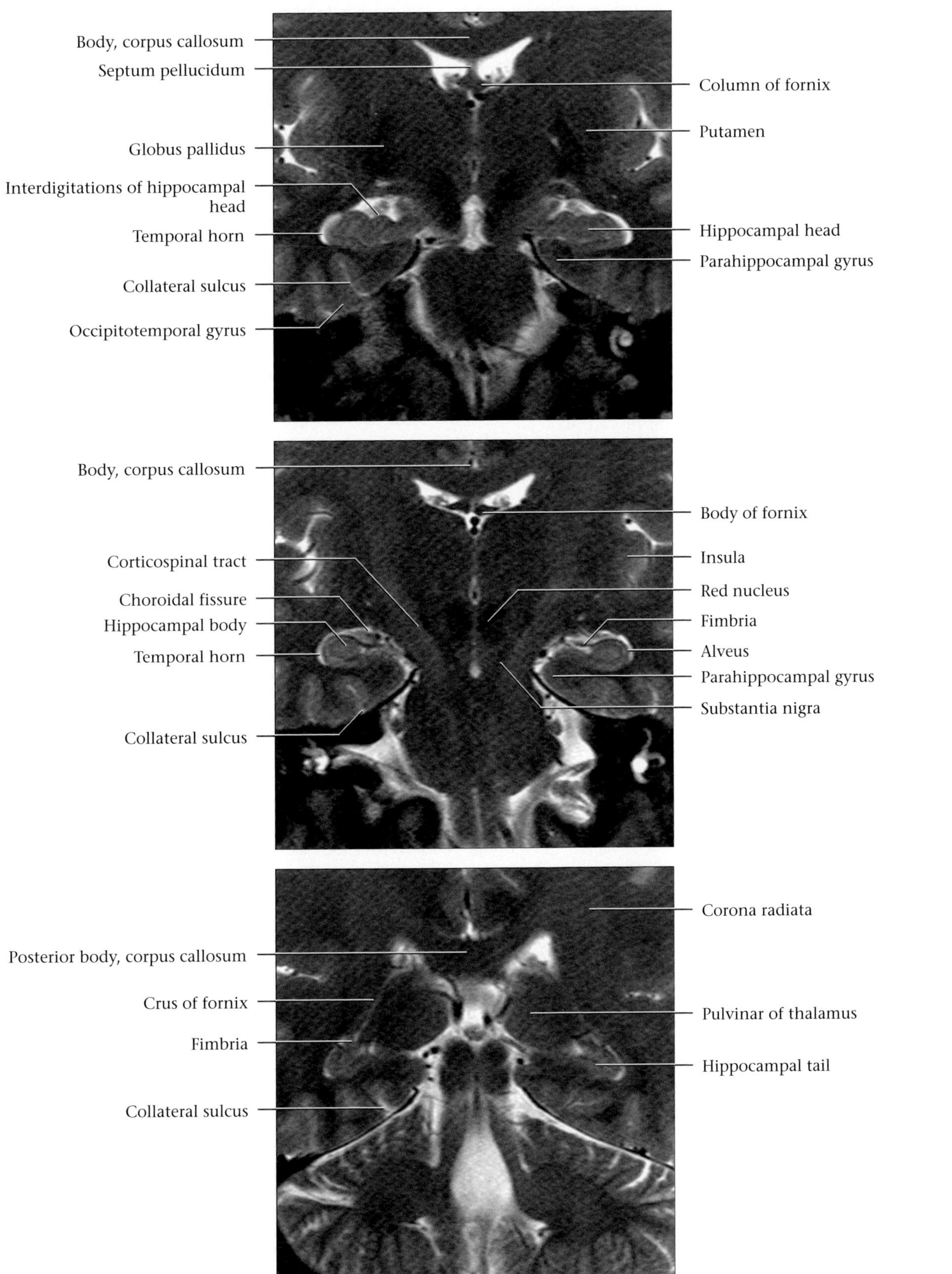
Body, corpus callosum
Septum pellucidum
Column of fornix
Putamen
Globus pallidus
Interdigitations of hippocampal head
Temporal horn
Hippocampal head
Parahippocampal gyrus
Collateral sulcus
Occipitotemporal gyrus
Body, corpus callosum
Body of fornix
Corticospinal tract
Insula
Choroidal fissure
Red nucleus
Hippocampal body
Fimbria
Temporal horn
Alveus
Parahippocampal gyrus
Substantia nigra
Collateral sulcus
Corona radiata
Posterior body, corpus callosum
Crus of fornix
Pulvinar of thalamus
Fimbria
Hippocampal tail
Collateral sulcus

(Top) First of three coronal T2 MR images through limbic system from anterior to posterior shows amygdala separated from hippocampus by uncal recess of temporal horn. Hippocampal head is recognized by digitations on its superior surface. Collateral sulcus separates parahippocampal gyrus from occipitotemporal (fusiform) gyrus. **(Middle)** More posterior image shows body of hippocampus with normal architecture. Body of fornix arcs over thalamus to split into two anterior columns which curve anteriorly to foramen of Monro & send fibers to mamillary body, anterior thalamus & septal region. White matter tracts from internal capsule are seen coursing through cerebral peduncles to pons. **(Bottom)** Image at posterior thalamus (pulvinar) shows hippocampal tail, smallest portion of hippocampus. Fimbria arise from hippocampus & become crus of fornix which attaches to splenium.

WHITE MATTER TRACTS

Gross Anatomy

Overview

- Hemispheric white matter tracts divided by course, connections into **association, commissural, projection fibers**
- **Association fibers** (may be short or long)
  - Short (arcuate or "U" fibers) link adjacent gyri, course parallel to long axis of sulci
  - Long fibers form fasciculi connecting widely spaced gyri
    - **Cingulum**: Long, curved fasciculus deep to cingulate gyrus; interconnects parts of frontal/parietal/temporal lobes
    - **Uncinate fasciculus:** Connects motor speech area & orbital gyri of frontal lobe with temporal lobe cortex
    - **Superior longitudinal (arcuate) fasciculus**: Connects frontal to parietal, temporal and occipital cortex
    - **Inferior longitudinal fasciculus**: Connects temporal and occipital cortex, contributes to sagittal stratum
    - **Superior occipitofrontal fasciculus**: Connects occipital & frontal lobes, lies beneath corpus callosum (CC)
    - **Inferior occipitofrontal fasciculus**: Connects occipital & frontal lobes, inferiorly; posteriorly forms sagittal stratum which connects occipital lobe to rest of brain
- **Commissural fibers**
  - **Corpus callosum**
    - Largest commissure; links hemispheres
    - Four parts: Rostrum, genu, body, splenium
    - Rostral fibers extend laterally connecting orbital surfaces of frontal lobes
    - Genu fibers curve forward as forceps minor, connect lateral/medial frontal lobes
    - Body fibers pass laterally, intersect with projection fibers of corona radiata to connect wide areas of hemispheres
    - Tapetum: Formed by body, some splenium fibers; course around posterior & inferior lateral ventricles
    - Most fibers from splenium curve into occipital lobes as forceps major
  - **Anterior commissure**
    - Transversely oriented bundle of compact myelinated fibers
    - Crosses anterior to fornix, embedded in anterior wall of third ventricle
    - Splits into two bundles laterally
    - Anterior bundle to anterior perforated substance, olfactory tract
    - Larger posterior fans out into temporal lobe
  - **Posterior commissure**: Small; courses transversely in posterior pineal lamina to connect midbrain, thalamus/hypothalamus
- **Projection fibers**
  - **Corona radiata:** Fibers from internal capsule fan out to form corona radiata, represent all cortical areas
  - **Internal capsule**: Major conduit of fibers to/from cerebral cortex
    - Anterior limb: Frontopontine fibers, thalamocortical projections
    - Genu: Corticobulbar fibers
    - Posterior limb: Corticospinal tracts, upper limb-anterior, trunk & lower limbs-posterior
  - **Corticospinal tract**: Major efferent projection fibers connect motor cortex to brainstem, spinal cord
    - Converge into corona radiata, continue through posterior limb of internal capsule to cerebral peduncle and lateral funiculus
  - **Corticobulbar tract**: Major efferent projection fibers connect motor cortex to brainstem and spinal cord
    - Converge into corona radiata to genu of internal capsule to cerebral peduncle, terminate in motor cranial nerve nuclei
  - **Corticopontine tract**: Motor information to pons
  - **Corticothalamic tract**: Connects entire cerebral cortex with isotopic location in thalamus

Imaging Anatomy

Overview

- Myelination generally proceeds inferior to superior; central to peripheral; posterior to anterior
- MR signal depends on maturation
- Fully myelinated white matter hyperintense on T1-, hypointense on T2WI

White Matter Maturation

- Occurs at different rates, times on T1/T2 imaging
  - Up to six months, T1WI most useful
  - After six months, T2 is most useful
- Newborn
  - T1WI: Newborn brain resembles T2 image in an adult
    - White matter has lower signal than gray matter
    - With maturation, intensity of white matter increases
  - T2WI: Newborn brain resembles T1 image in an adult
    - White matter has higher signal than gray matter
    - T2 superior for evaluating cerebellum and brainstem maturation
- First six months
  - T1WI
    - Three months: High signal in anterior limb, internal capsule ans cerebellar folia
    - Four months: High signal in CC splenium
    - Six months: High signal in CC genu
    - Eight months: Near adult appearance, except most peripheral fibers
- Six to eighteen months
  - T2WI
    - Six months: Low signal in CC splenium
    - Eight months: Low signal in CC genu
    - Eleven months: Low signal in anterior limb, internal capsule
    - Fourteen months: Low signal in deep frontal white matter
    - Eighteen months: Near adult appearance, except most peripheral fibers

WHITE MATTER TRACTS

GRAPHICS

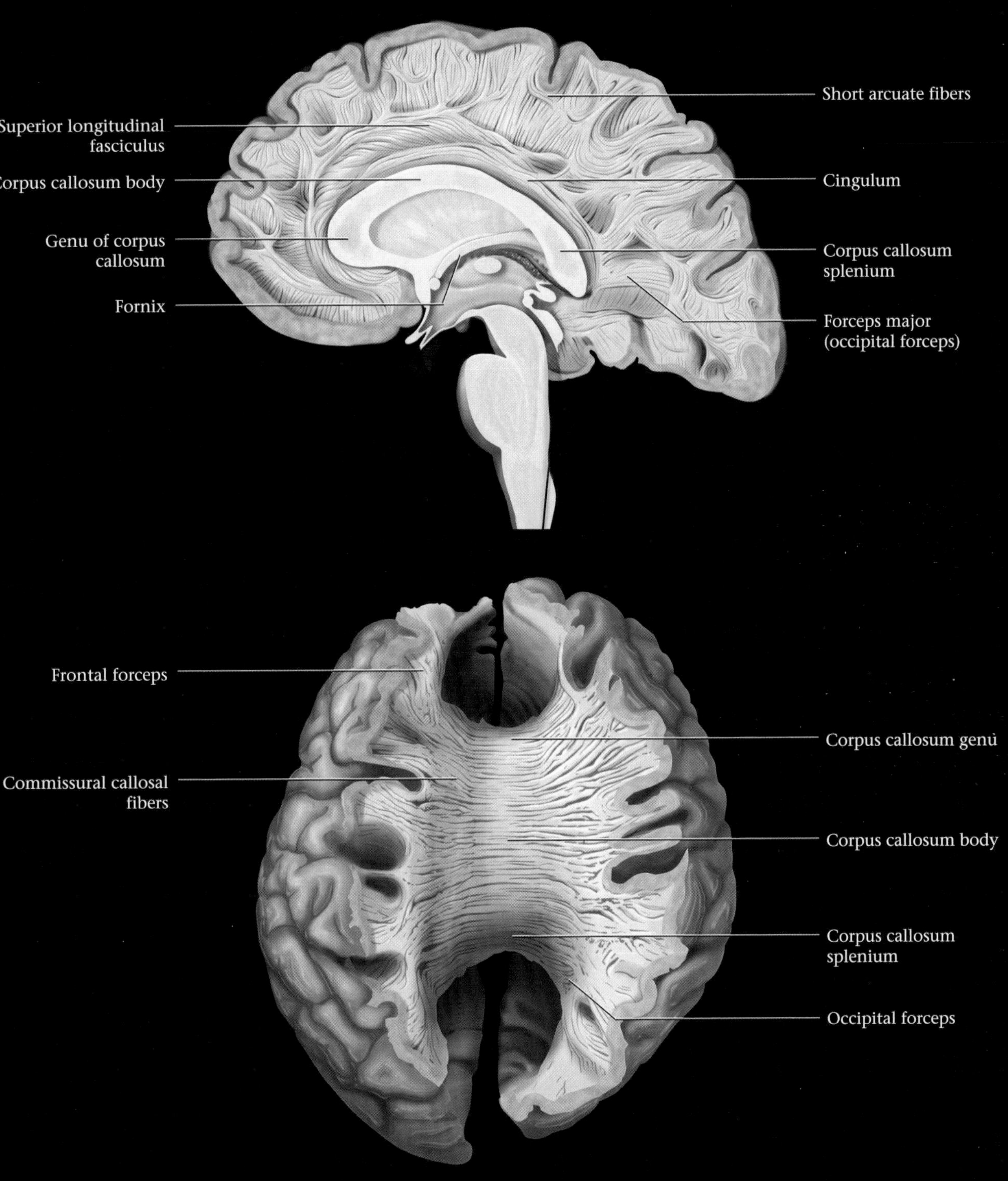
Superior longitudinal fasciculus
Corpus callosum body
Genu of corpus callosum
Fornix
Short arcuate fibers
Cingulum
Corpus callosum splenium
Forceps major (occipital forceps)
Frontal forceps
Commissural callosal fibers
Corpus callosum genu
Corpus callosum body
Corpus callosum splenium
Occipital forceps

(Top) Sagittal graphic shows midline white matter tracts. Corpus callosum, the largest commissure, connects corresponding areas of cortex between hemispheres. Fibers traversing corpus callosum body are transversely oriented, while those traversing CC genu & splenium arch anteriorly & posteriorly to reach anterior & posterior poles of hemispheres. Cingulum, an association fiber, starts in medial cortex below CC rostrum, courses within cingulate gyrus, arches around CC & extends forward to parahippocampal gyrus & uncus. **(Bottom)** Graphic shows superior view of largest white matter fiber bundle, corpus callosum which connects corresponding areas of cortex between hemispheres. Close to midline, CC fibers are primarily left-right oriented. More laterally, CC fibers fan out & intermingle with projection & association tracts.

WHITE MATTER TRACTS

GRAPHICS

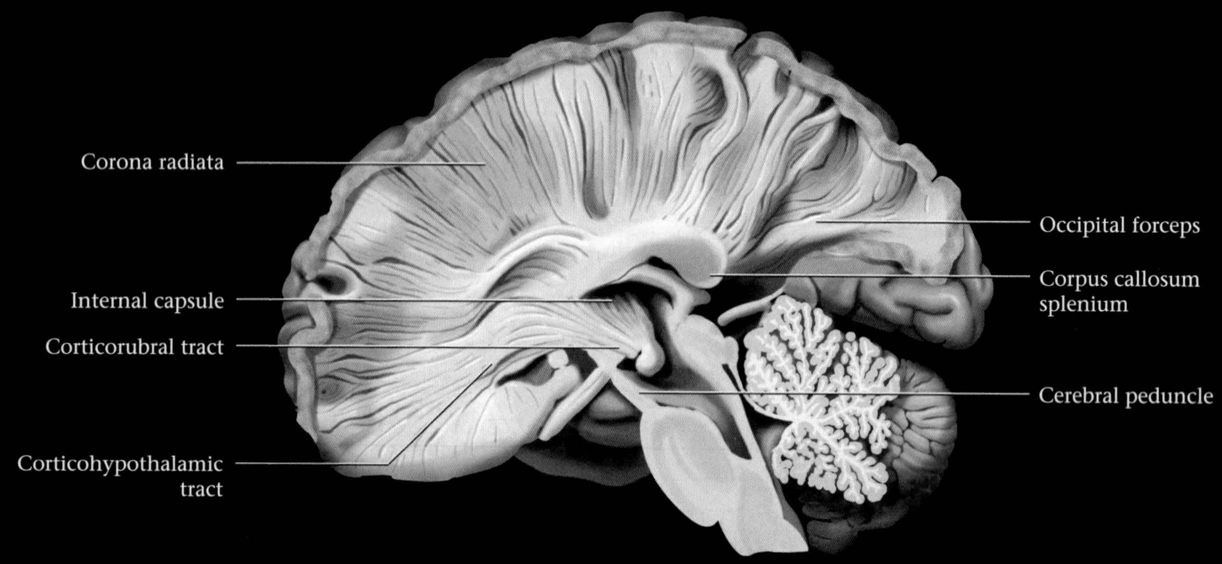
Corona radiata
Internal capsule
Corticorubral tract
Corticohypothalamic tract
Occipital forceps
Corpus callosum splenium
Cerebral peduncle

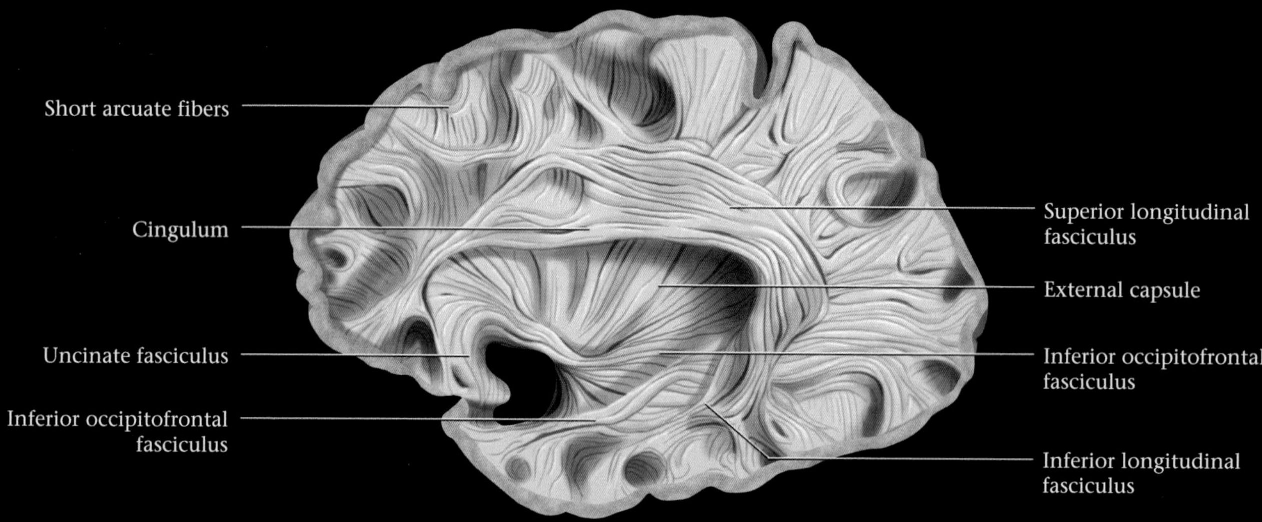
Short arcuate fibers
Cingulum
Uncinate fasciculus
Inferior occipitofrontal fasciculus
Superior longitudinal fasciculus
External capsule
Inferior occipitofrontal fasciculus
Inferior longitudinal fasciculus

(Top) Sagittal graphic shows major projection fibers, which interconnect cortical areas with deep nuclei, brainstem, cerebellum & spinal cord. There are both efferent (corticofugal) & afferent (corticopetal) projection fibers. Efferent fibers converge from all directions to form dense subcortical white matter mass of corona radiata. Corona radiata is continuous with internal capsule which contains majority of cortical projection fibers. Major projection fibers of internal capsule include corticospinal, corticobulbar & corticopontine tracts. Optic radiations extend from lateral geniculate nucleus to occipital lobe. **(Bottom)** Sagittal graphic laterally shows association fibers which interconnect cortical areas in each hemisphere. Superior longitudinal fasciculus is largest association bundle & connects frontal lobe to parietal, temporal & occipital lobe cortices.

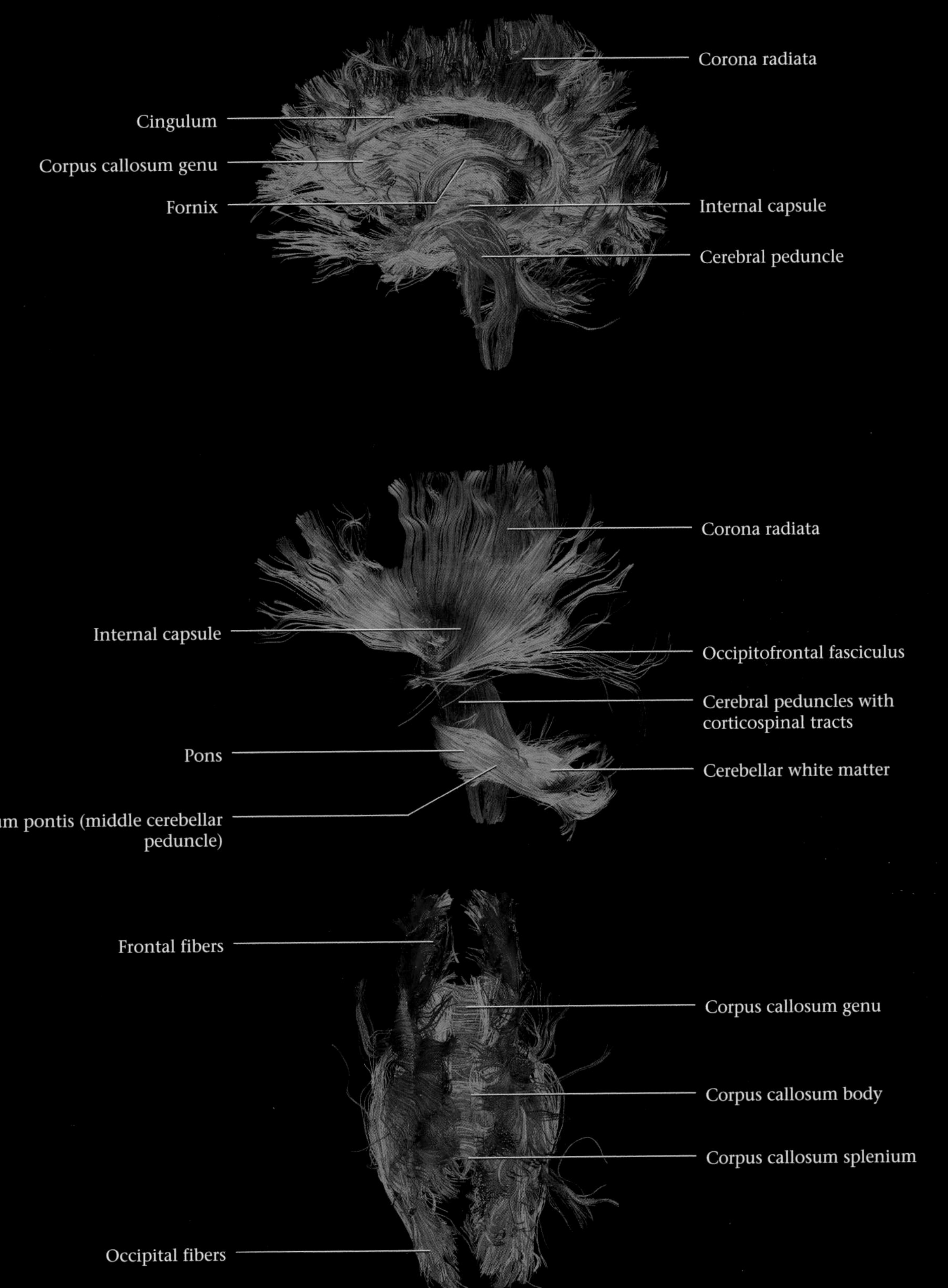

Corona radiata
Cingulum
Corpus callosum genu
Fornix
Internal capsule
Cerebral peduncle
Corona radiata
Internal capsule
Occipitofrontal fasciculus
Cerebral peduncles with corticospinal tracts
Pons
Cerebellar white matter
Brachium pontis (middle cerebellar peduncle)
Frontal fibers
Corpus callosum genu
Corpus callosum body
Corpus callosum splenium
Occipital fibers

(Top) Sagittal 3T diffusion tensor imaging (DTI) color map shows midline white matter tracts. Standard directional encoding is shown: Red is left-right, blue is superior-inferior, green is anterior-posterior. Mixtures of colors reflect changing angle of fibers along their course. **(Middle)** Sagittal DTI color map showing corona radiata, major projection fibers, which are continuous with internal capsule. **(Bottom)** DTI color map shows axial view of largest white matter bundle fiber, corpus callosum which is a commissural fiber. Close to midline, fibers are primarily left-right oriented so show primarily red, but as they fan out laterally & intermingle with projection & association tracts, more complex color patterns are seen. Images courtesy of A. Gregory Sorensen MD & Ruopeng Wang, MGH-HST Martinos Center, Massachusetts General Hospital, Boston, MA.

WHITE MATTER TRACTS

3T DTI

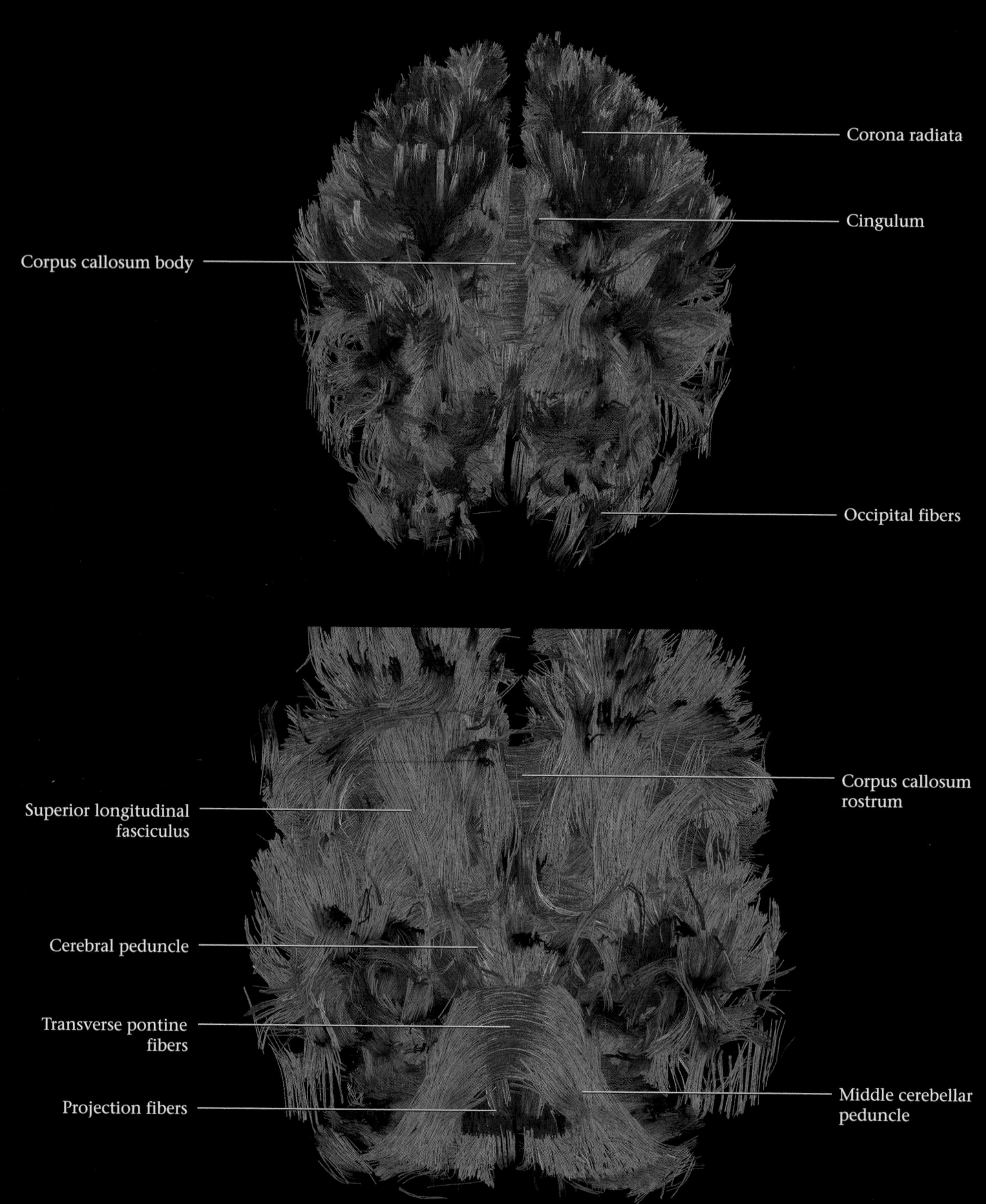
Corona radiata
Cingulum
Corpus callosum body
Occipital fibers
Corpus callosum rostrum
Superior longitudinal fasciculus
Cerebral peduncle
Transverse pontine fibers
Projection fibers
Middle cerebellar peduncle

(Top) First of two axial DTI color mapping shows level of superior corpus callosum. The colors have standard directional encoding: Red is left-right, blue is superior-inferior & green is anterior-posterior. Note central callosal red fibers related to primarily left-right orientation. Cingulum is an association fiber that connects portions of frontal, parietal & temporal lobes. Corona radiata is major projection fiber & is contiguous with internal capsule. **(Bottom)** Axial DTI color map shows inferior corpus callosum & surrounding white matter tracts. Pons has red, left-right fibers, centrally related to transverse pontine fibers, green fibers related to middle cerebellar peduncle & blue projection fibers related to corticospinal tracts. Images courtesy of A. Gregory Sorensen MD & Ruopeng Wang, MGH-HST Martinos Center, Massachusetts General Hospital, Boston, MA.

WHITE MATTER TRACTS

AXIAL T1 MR 32 WEEKS PREMATURE

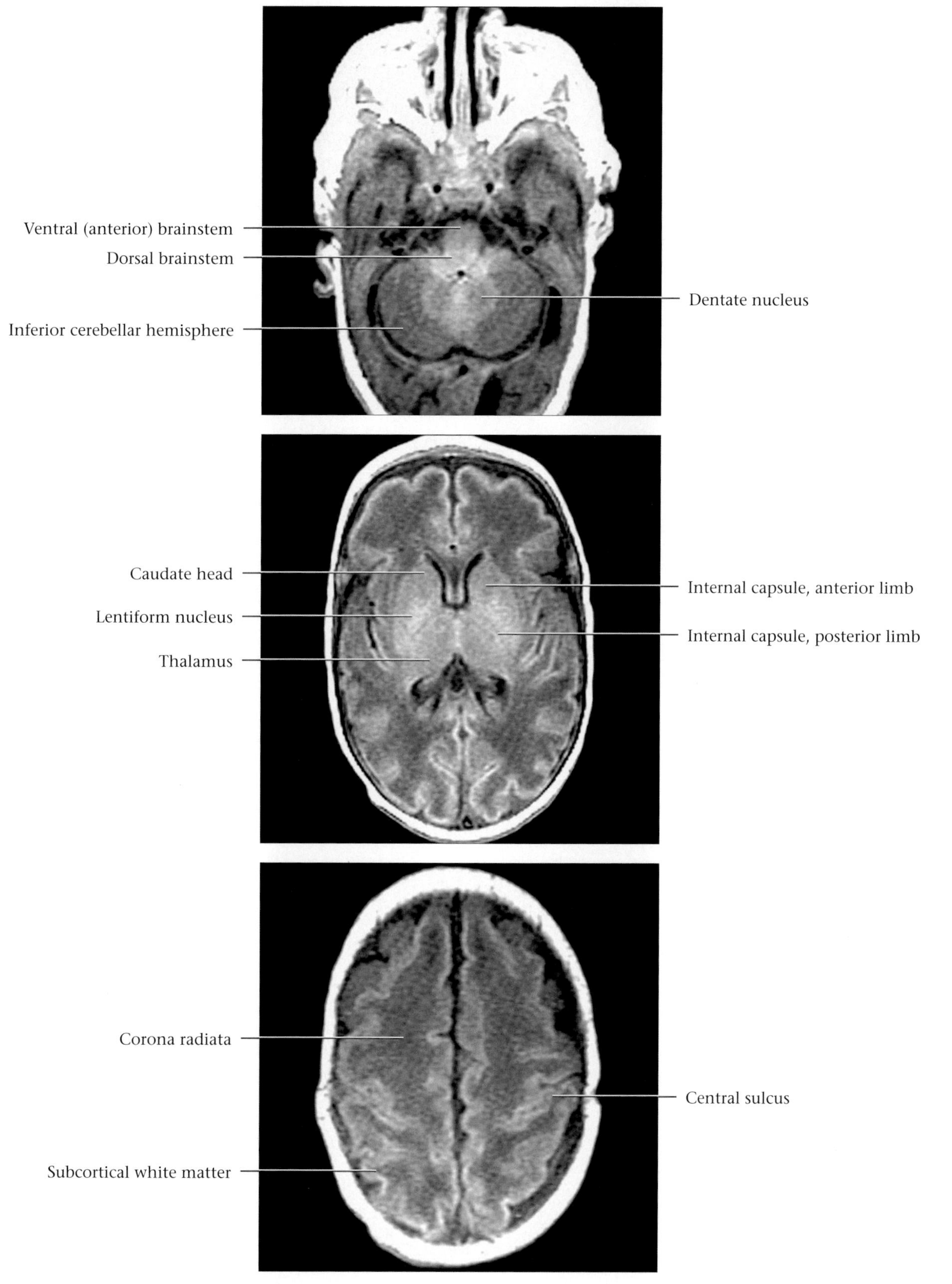

Ventral (anterior) brainstem
Dorsal brainstem
Inferior cerebellar hemisphere
Dentate nucleus
Caudate head
Lentiform nucleus
Thalamus
Internal capsule, anterior limb
Internal capsule, posterior limb
Corona radiata
Subcortical white matter
Central sulcus

(Top) First of three axial T1 MR images from inferior to superior of a normal 32 week premature infant shows posterior fossa structures. Superior & inferior cerebellar peduncles are bright on T1 images, but middle cerebellar peduncles remain unmyelinated, isointense to cerebral white matter & dark on T1 images. Dorsal brainstem is relatively hyperintense on T1 images compared with ventral pons. **(Middle)** Image at level of internal capsule shows internal capsule is hypointense compared with lentiform nucleus. Sylvian fissures remain prominent. White matter is hypointense related to lack of myelination. **(Bottom)** Image at level of corona radiata shows white matter as completely unmyelinated, showing a T1 hypointense appearance. Sulci are prominent related to immaturity. Signal intensity of entire cerebral cortex is uniform on T1 & T2 weighted images.

WHITE MATTER TRACTS

AXIAL T2 MR 32 WEEKS PREMATURE

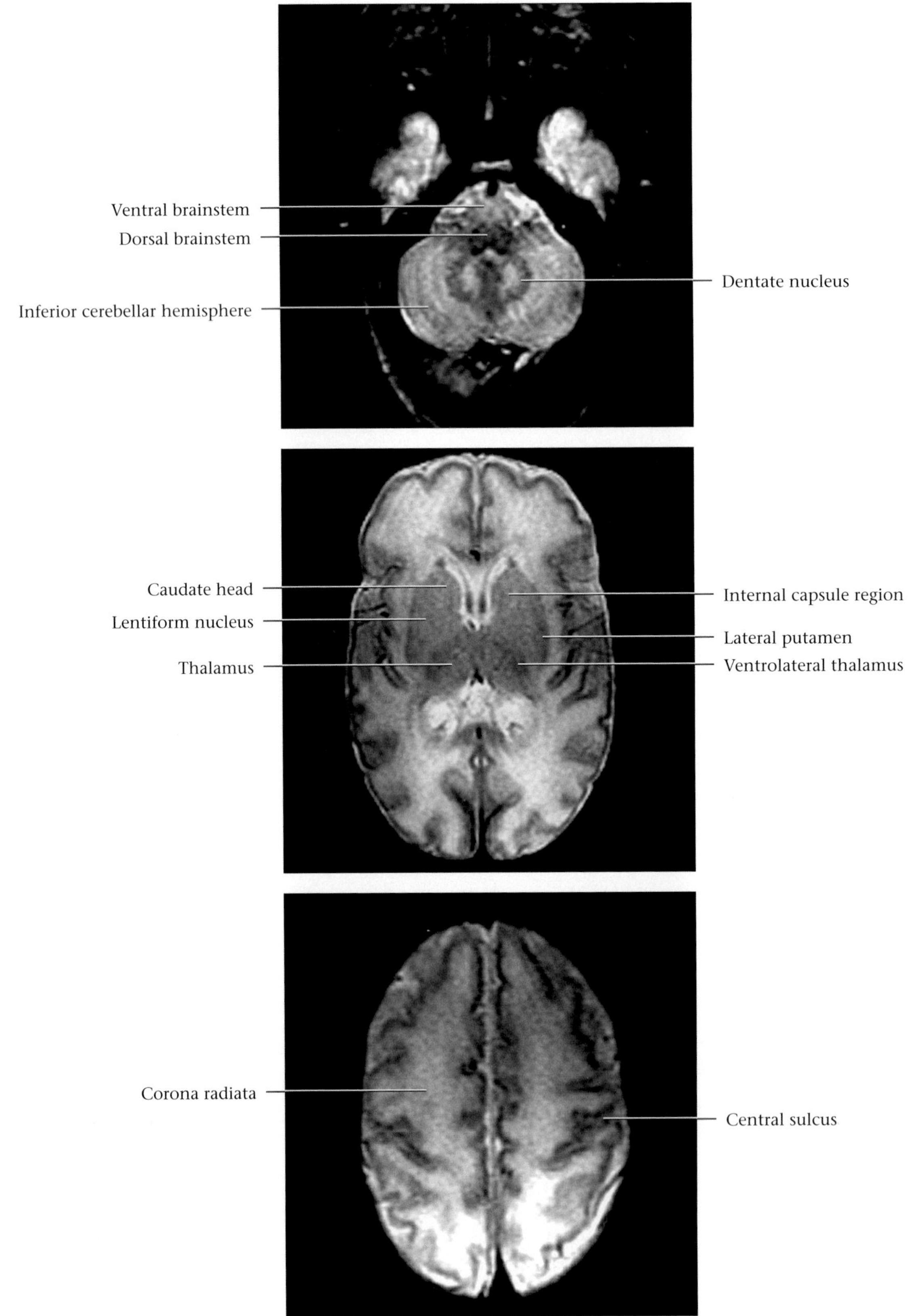
Ventral brainstem
Dorsal brainstem
Inferior cerebellar hemisphere
Dentate nucleus
Caudate head
Lentiform nucleus
Thalamus
Internal capsule region
Lateral putamen
Ventrolateral thalamus
Corona radiata
Central sulcus

(Top) First of three axial T2 MR images from inferior to superior of a normal 32 week premature infant shows posterior fossa structures. Dorsal (posterior) brainstem is relatively hypointense (dark) on T2 images compared with unmyelinated ventral (anterior) pons. Superior & inferior peduncles are hypointense on T2 images. Middle cerebellar peduncle is hyperintense on T2 images, similar to cerebral white matter. **(Middle)** Image at level of internal capsule shows the thalamus & basal ganglia are hypointense (dark). Internal capsule is typically hyperintense at this age, although is difficult to differentiate in this case. T2 also shows hypointensity in far lateral putamen & ventrolateral thalamus at this 32 week premature age. **(Bottom)** Image through corona radiata shows unmyelinated white matter, hyperintense compared with gray matter.

AXIAL T1 MR BIRTH

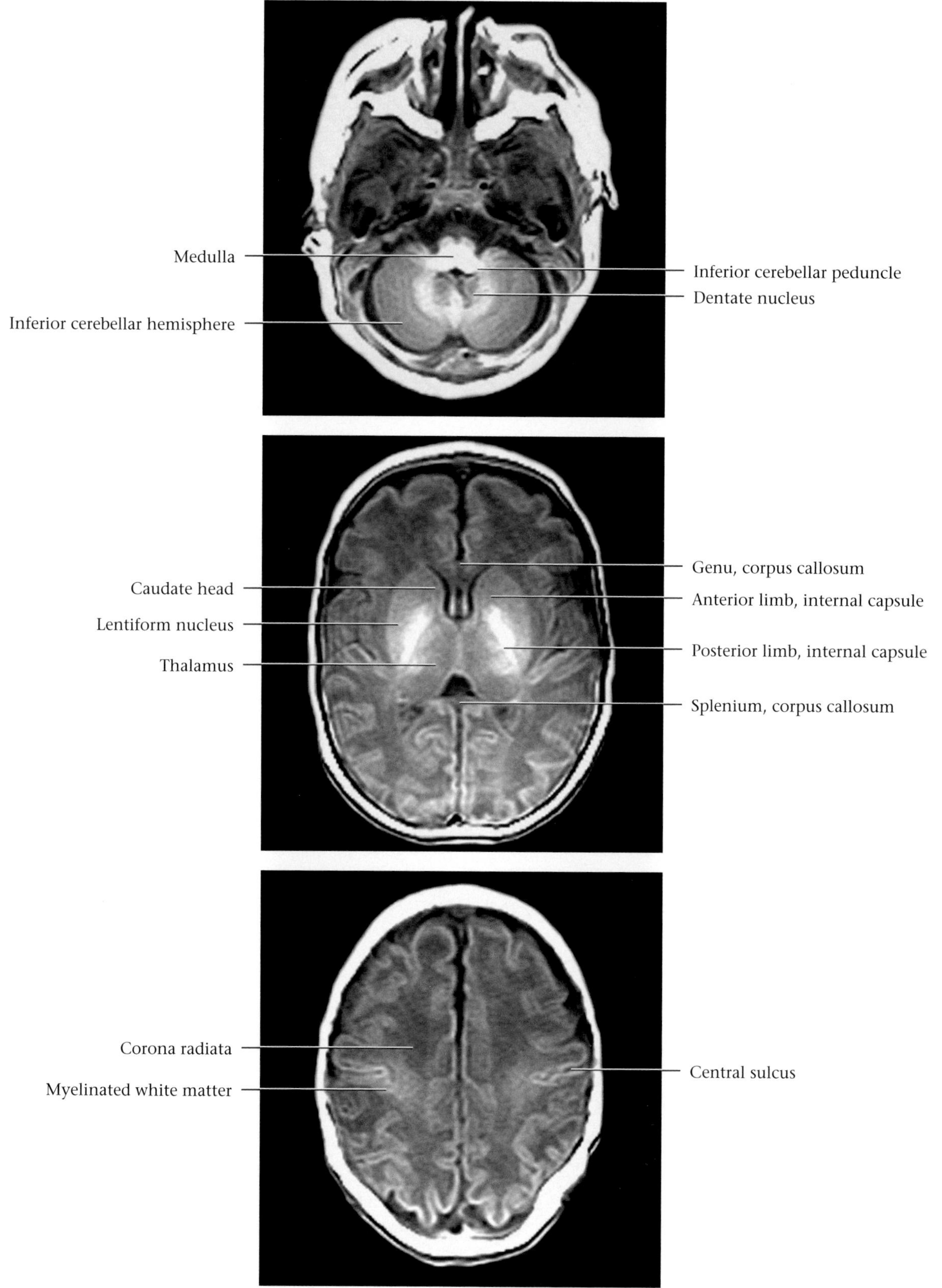
Medulla
Inferior cerebellar hemisphere
Inferior cerebellar peduncle
Dentate nucleus
Caudate head
Lentiform nucleus
Thalamus
Genu, corpus callosum
Anterior limb, internal capsule
Posterior limb, internal capsule
Splenium, corpus callosum
Corona radiata
Myelinated white matter
Central sulcus

(Top) First of three axial T1 MR images from inferior to superior of a normal full-term infant at birth shows posterior fossa structures. Superior & inferior cerebellar peduncles are bright on T1 images, but middle cerebellar peduncles remain unmyelinated, isointense to cerebral white matter & dark on T1 images. Dorsal brainstem is relatively hyperintense on T1 images compared with ventral brainstem. **(Middle)** Image at level of internal capsule shows hyperintensity of posterior limb compared with anterior limb. Lateral thalamus is also bright compared with remainder of thalamus. **(Bottom)** Image through corona radiata shows increased signal intensity in rolandic (precentral) & perirolandic gyri corresponding to known myelination within these gyri at or shortly after birth. Reminder of cerebral white matter remains hypointense, related to lack of myelination.

WHITE MATTER TRACTS

AXIAL T2 MR BIRTH

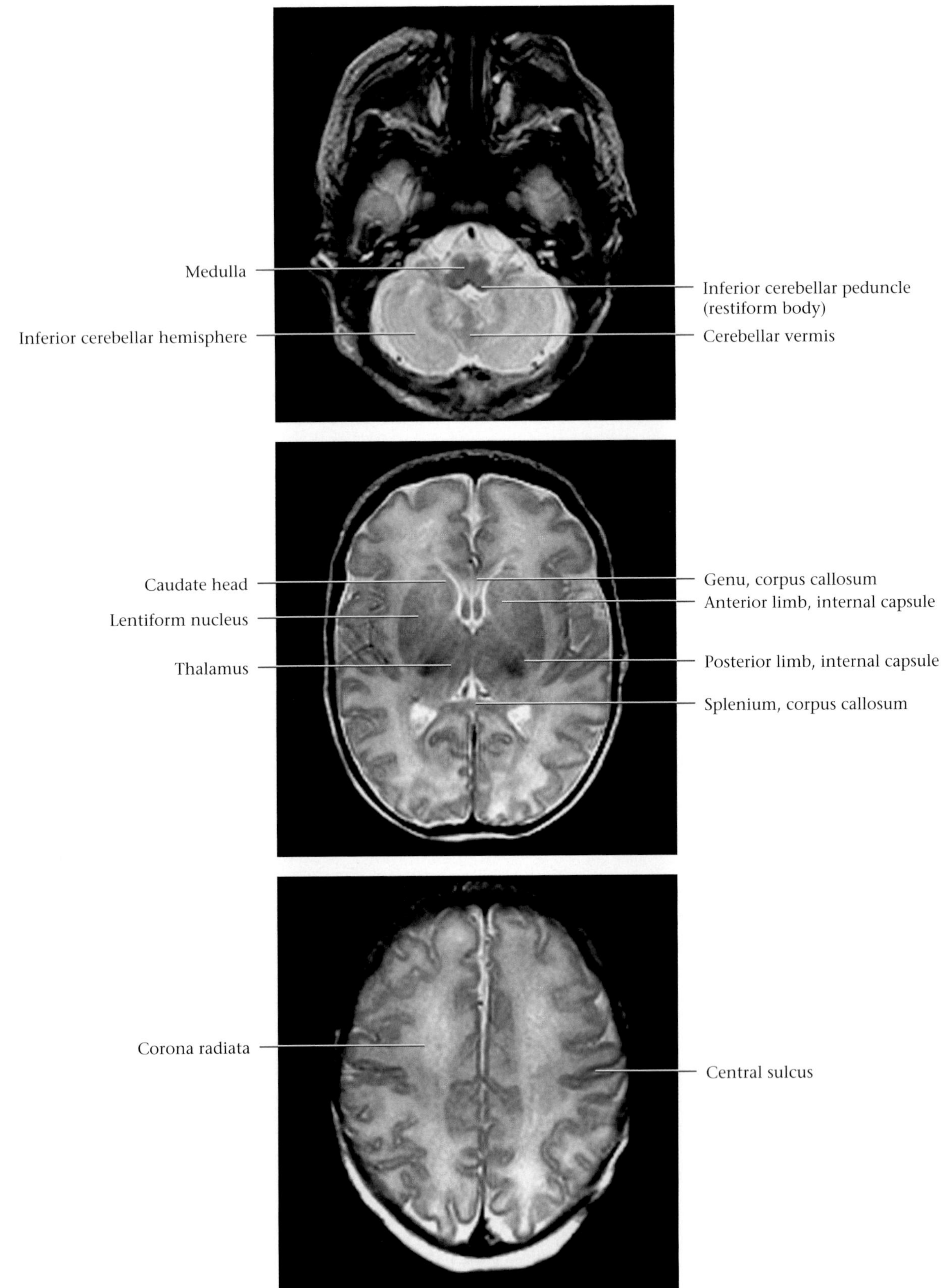
Medulla
Inferior cerebellar peduncle (restiform body)
Inferior cerebellar hemisphere
Cerebellar vermis
Caudate head
Genu, corpus callosum
Anterior limb, internal capsule
Lentiform nucleus
Thalamus
Posterior limb, internal capsule
Splenium, corpus callosum
Corona radiata
Central sulcus

(Top) First of three axial T2 MR images from inferior to superior of a normal infant at birth shows posterior fossa structures. At birth, low signal is present in inferior & superior cerebellar peduncles. Cerebellar vermis is also low signal compared with rest of cerebellum. T2 imaging is more sensitive for evaluation of posterior fossa structure maturation. **(Middle)** Image at level of internal capsule shows a small patch of hypointensity within posterior limb of internal capsule & within lateral putamen. Ventral lateral region of thalamus is also hypointense (dark) at birth. Corpus callosum is unmyelinated at birth & matures in a posterior to anterior fashion. **(Bottom)** Image at corona radiata shows predominantly unmyelinated white matter, hyperintense compared with gray matter. Subtle hypointensity in cortex of pre- & postcentral gyri can be seen and is normal.

WHITE MATTER TRACTS

AXIAL T1 MR 3 MONTHS

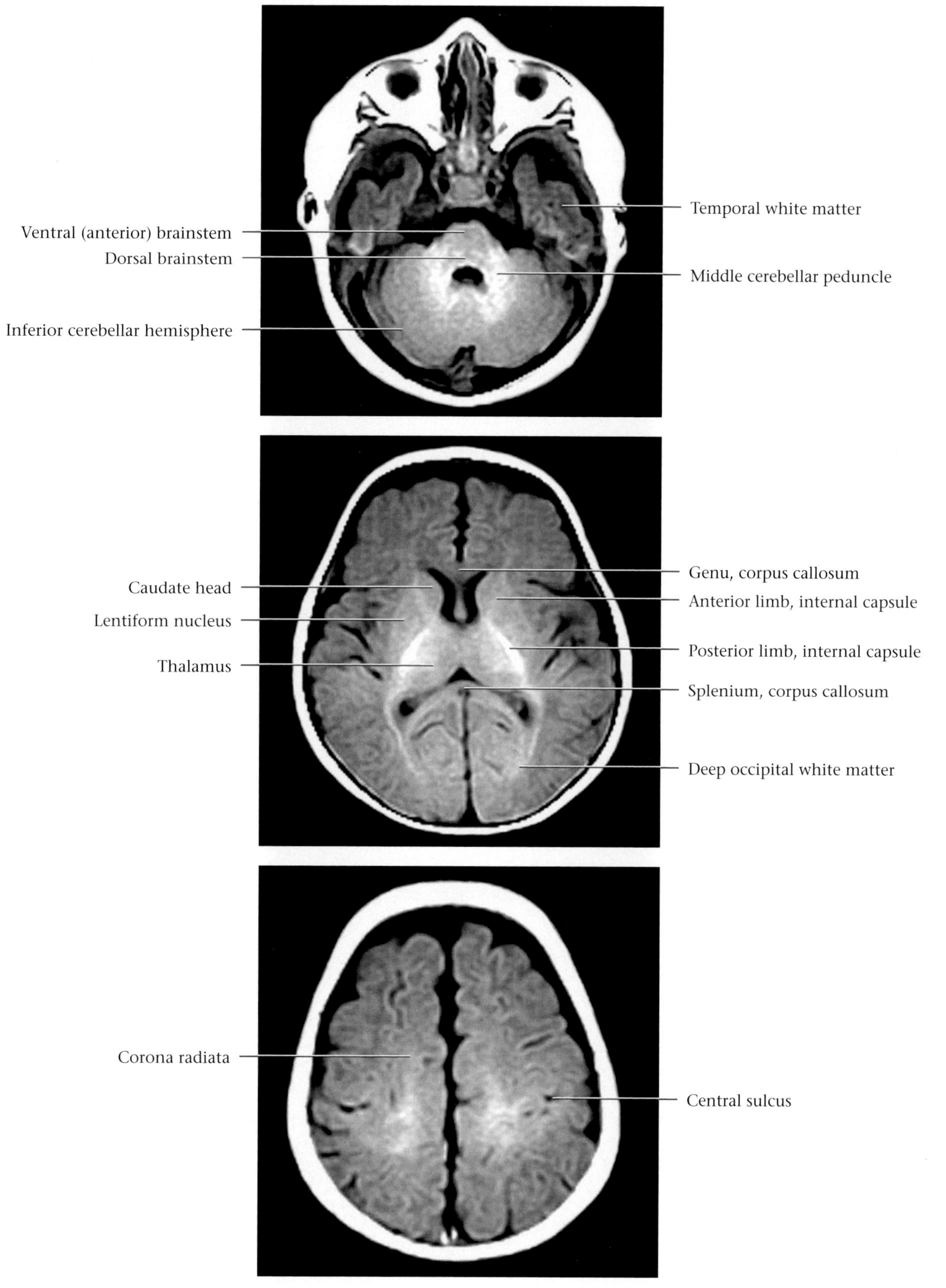
Ventral (anterior) brainstem
Dorsal brainstem
Inferior cerebellar hemisphere
Temporal white matter
Middle cerebellar peduncle
Caudate head
Lentiform nucleus
Thalamus
Genu, corpus callosum
Anterior limb, internal capsule
Posterior limb, internal capsule
Splenium, corpus callosum
Deep occipital white matter
Corona radiata
Central sulcus

(Top) First of three axial T1 MR images from inferior to superior of a normal infant at three months shows posterior fossa structures. Cerebellum has a nearly adult appearance by three months. Dorsal brainstem remains slightly hyperintense compared with ventral brainstem. **(Middle)** Image at level of internal capsule shows high signal in posterior limb & early, subtle high signal in anterior limb of internal capsule. Corpus callosum remains unmyelinated, but splenium will show high signal by approximately four months. Deep white matter begins myelinating around three months, appearing first in deep occipital white matter. **(Bottom)** Image through corona radiata shows predominantly unmyelinated white matter, hypointense compared with gray matter. Deep white matter matures in a posterior to anterior direction & early maturation in seen posteriorly.

WHITE MATTER TRACTS

AXIAL T2 MR 3 MONTHS

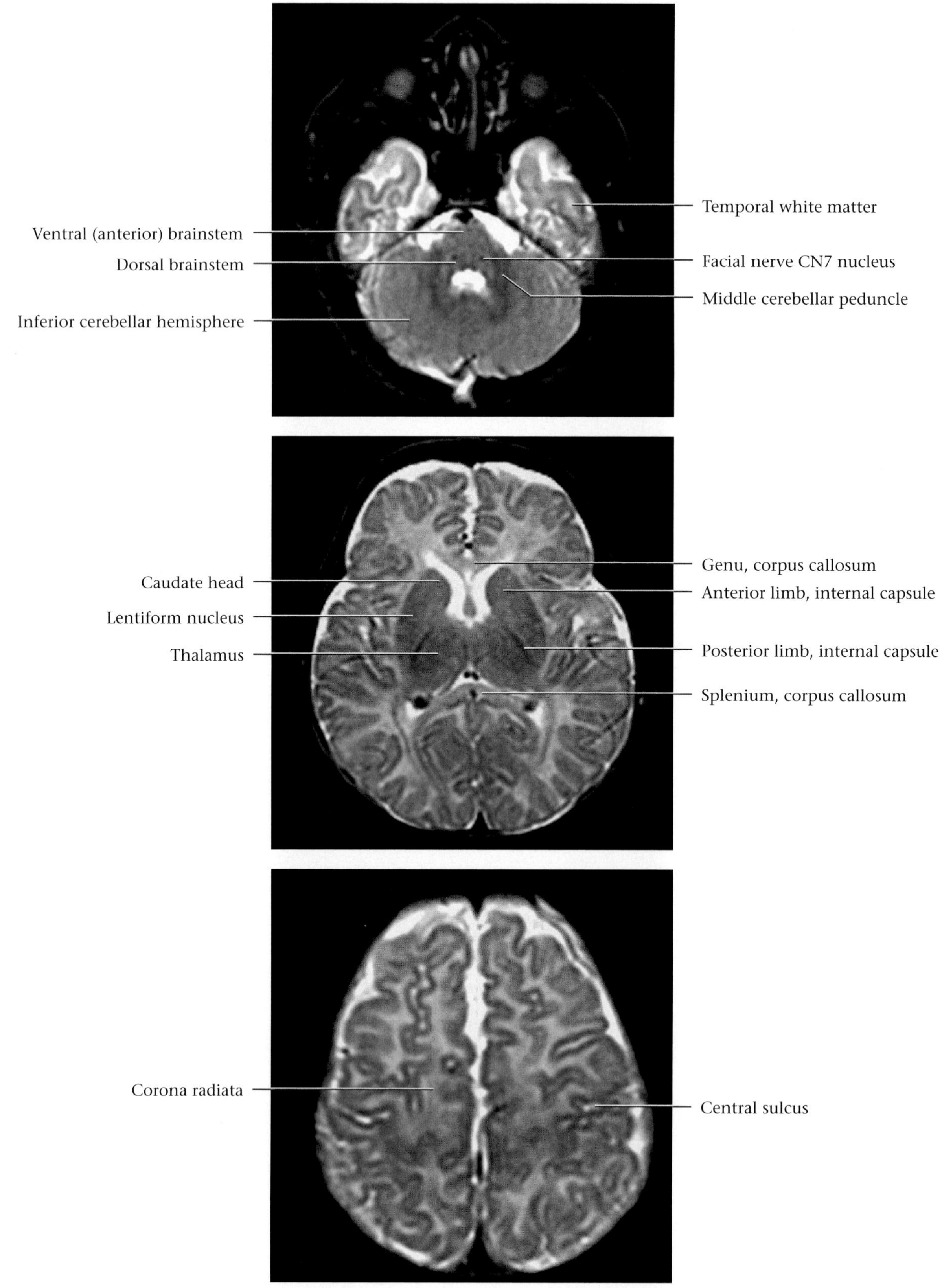
Temporal white matter
Ventral (anterior) brainstem
Dorsal brainstem
Facial nerve CN7 nucleus
Middle cerebellar peduncle
Inferior cerebellar hemisphere
Genu, corpus callosum
Caudate head
Anterior limb, internal capsule
Lentiform nucleus
Thalamus
Posterior limb, internal capsule
Splenium, corpus callosum
Corona radiata
Central sulcus

(Top) First of three axial T2 MR images from inferior to superior of a normal infant at three months shows posterior fossa structures. Low signal intensity is noted in cranial nerve nuclei including: Abducens CN6, facial CN7, & vestibulocochlear CN8 nerves. Dorsal brainstem is mildly hypointense compared with ventral brainstem & becomes isointense at about five months. Middle cerebellar peduncles are low signal by three months. **(Middle)** Image at level of internal capsule shows hypointense (dark) signal in posterior limb of internal capsule. Internal capsule matures in a posterior to anterior fashion. Corpus callosum, deep & subcortical white matter remains unmyelinated. **(Bottom)** Image through corona radiata shows predominantly unmyelinated white matter, hyperintense compared with gray matter. Newborn white matter on T2 resembles adult on T1 images.

WHITE MATTER TRACTS

AXIAL T1 MR 6 MONTHS

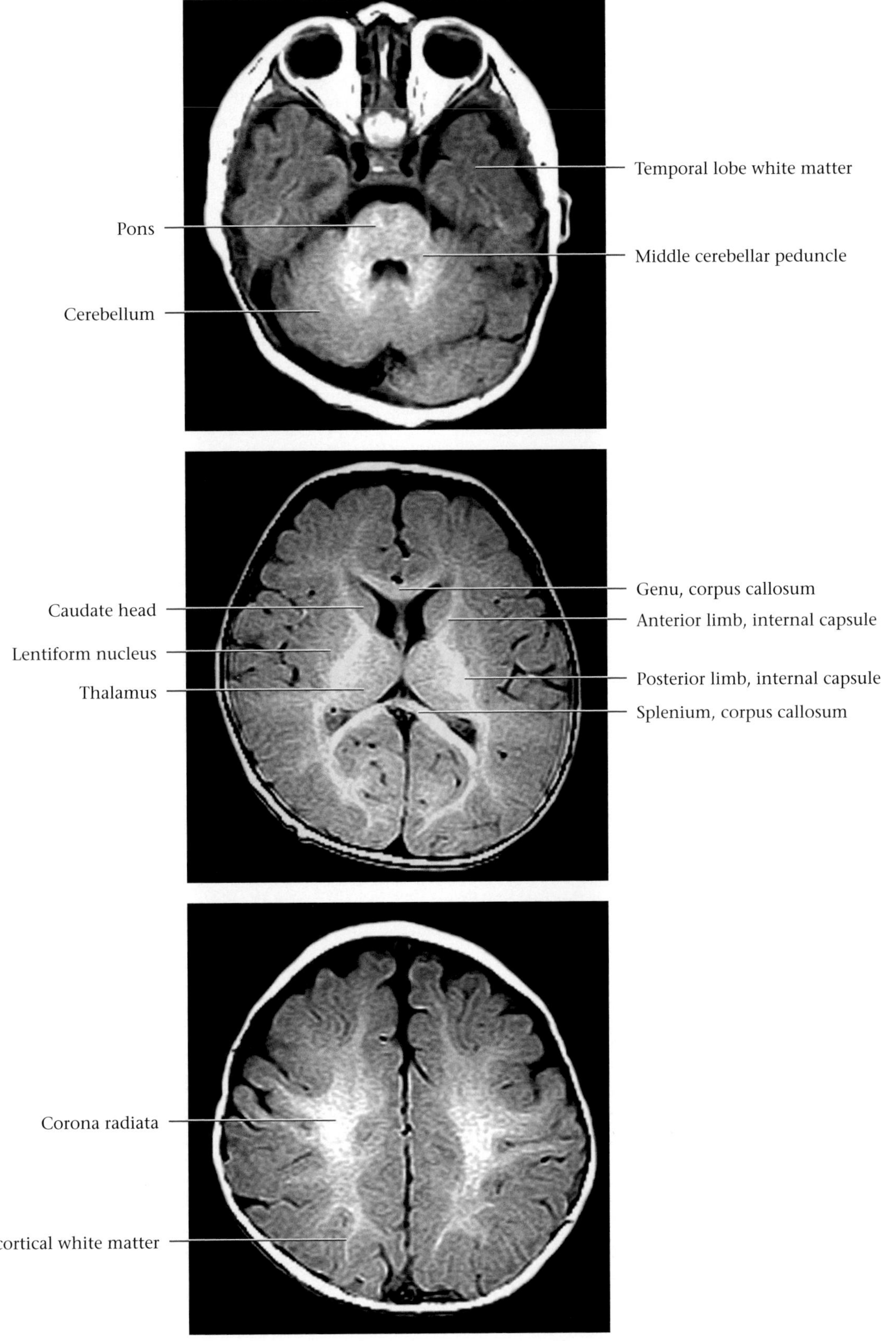
Temporal lobe white matter
Pons
Middle cerebellar peduncle
Cerebellum
Genu, corpus callosum
Caudate head
Anterior limb, internal capsule
Lentiform nucleus
Posterior limb, internal capsule
Thalamus
Splenium, corpus callosum
Corona radiata
Subcortical white matter

(Top) First of three axial T1 MR images from inferior to superior of a normal six month old shows posterior fossa structures. Cerebellum has an adult appearance by three months. Signal intensity in ventral (anterior) pons is bright with an adult appearance at this age. **(Middle)** Image at level of internal capsule shows hyperintensity (bright) in genu & splenium of corpus callosum. Internal capsule is hyperintense throughout. At birth, only posterior limb is bright, but by three months, anterior limb is also bright. **(Bottom)** Image through corona radiata shows progressive maturation of white matter with increasing hyperintensity of subcortical white matter, notably in occipital & parietal regions. Deep white matter matures in a posterior to anterior direction with deep occipital white matter maturing first, frontal & temporal white matter last.

WHITE MATTER TRACTS

AXIAL T2 MR 6 MONTHS

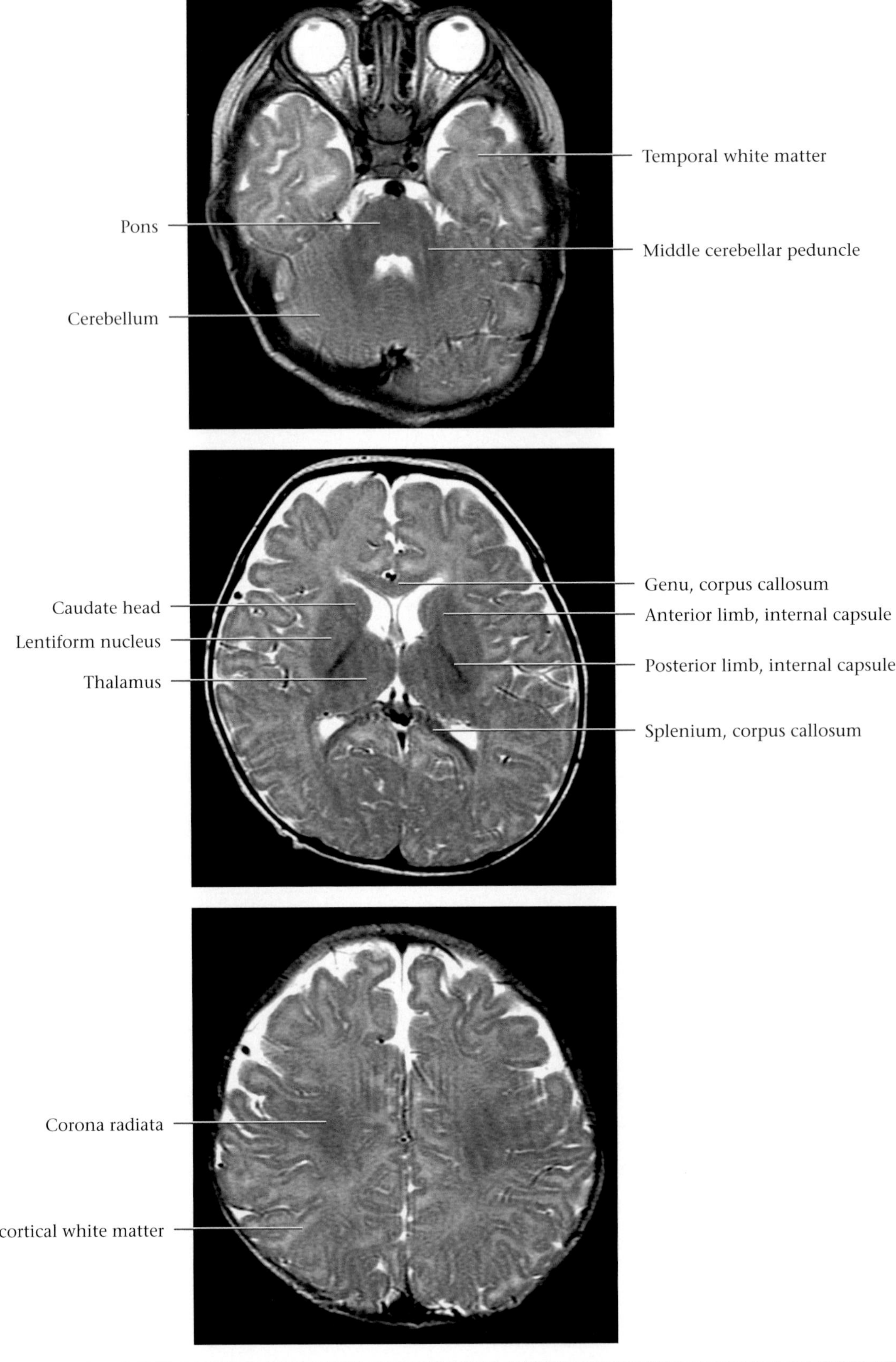
Temporal white matter
Pons
Middle cerebellar peduncle
Cerebellum
Genu, corpus callosum
Caudate head
Anterior limb, internal capsule
Lentiform nucleus
Posterior limb, internal capsule
Thalamus
Splenium, corpus callosum
Corona radiata
Subcortical white matter

(Top) First of three axial T2 MR images from inferior to superior of a normal six month old shows posterior fossa structures. Ventral brainstem becomes similar to dorsal brainstem at about five months, & is similar throughout pons in this case. Cerebellar peduncles are hypointense, similar to adult patient, by about four months. **(Middle)** Image at level of internal capsule shows dark posterior limb relative to anterior limb. Internal capsule matures in a posterior to anterior fashion. Corpus callosum also matures in posterior to anterior fashion. Splenium is hypointense (dark) compared with genu of corpus callosum. **(Bottom)** Image at level of corona radiata shows a relative decrease of signal in deep white matter. Subcortical white matter matures last, beginning in posterior occipital lobes & extending anteriorly to frontal & temporal lobes.

WHITE MATTER TRACTS

AXIAL T1 MR 9 MONTHS

Temporal lobe white matter
Ventral (anterior) pons
Dorsal pons
Middle cerebellar peduncle
Inferior cerebellar hemisphere

Genu, corpus callosum
Caudate head
Anterior limb, internal capsule
Lentiform nucleus
Posterior limb, internal capsule
Thalamus
Splenium, corpus callosum

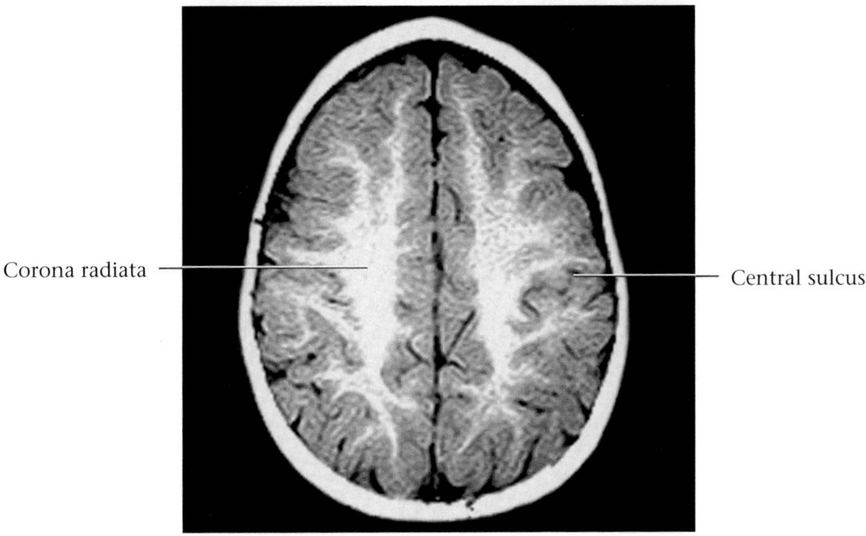
Corona radiata
Central sulcus

(Top) First of three axial T1 MR images from inferior to superior of a normal nine month old shows posterior fossa structures. Brainstem & cerebellum have an adult appearance. Temporal lobe white matter remains unmyelinated. **(Middle)** Image at level of internal capsule shows near adult appearance on T1 images. White matter of internal capsule & corpus callosum is hyperintense compared with basal ganglia & thalamus, similar to an adult. Deep & subcortical white matter of frontal lobes appears unmyelinated compared with occipital lobes. **(Bottom)** Image through corona radiata shows further myelination of deep & subcortical white matter. Frontal & temporal lobe white matter is last to completely myelinate & appear slightly hypointense compared with parietal lobe white matter. Only minimal changes are seen in white matter after eight months on T1 images.

WHITE MATTER TRACTS

AXIAL T2 MR 9 MONTHS

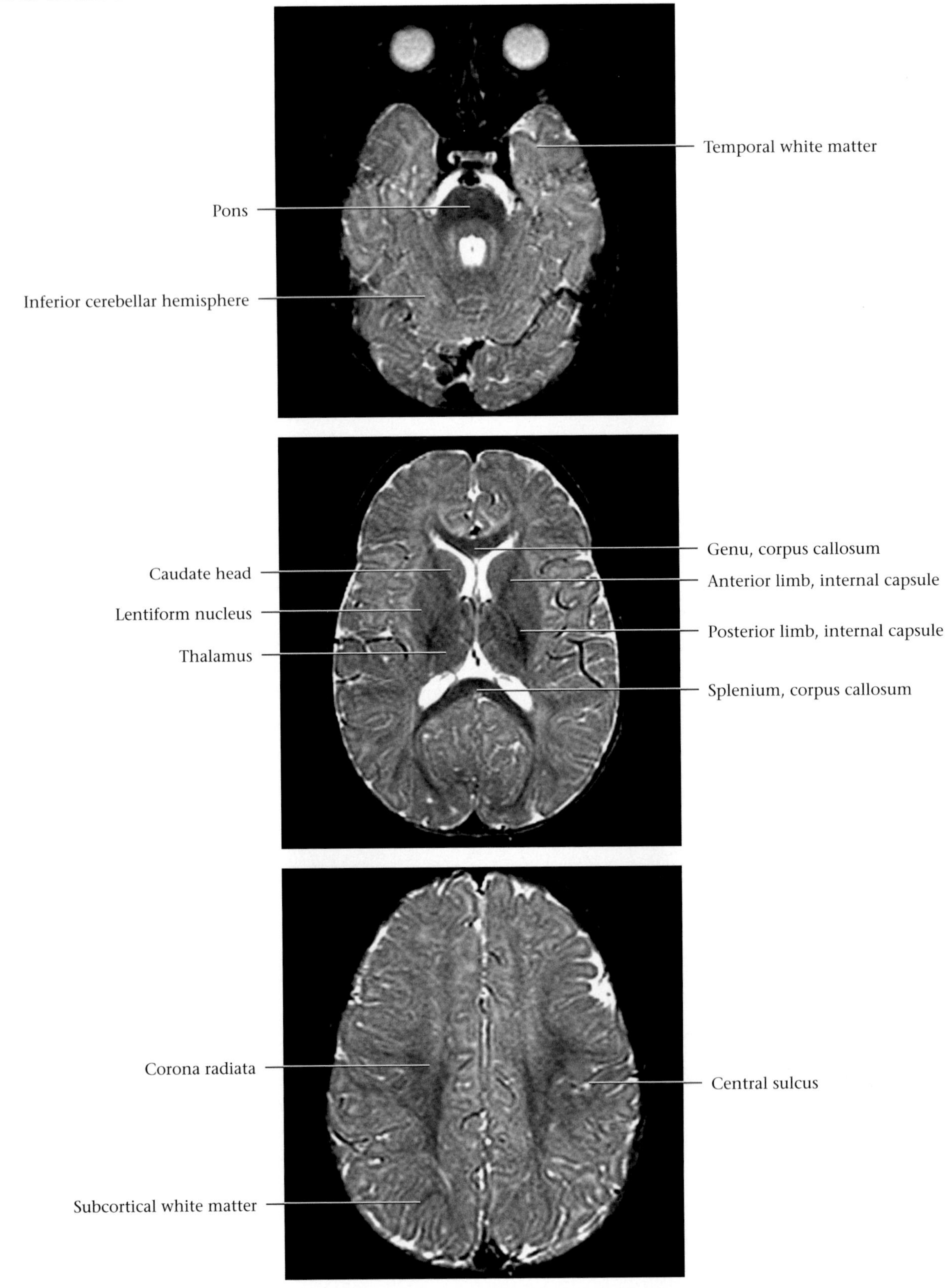
Temporal white matter
Pons
Inferior cerebellar hemisphere
Genu, corpus callosum
Caudate head
Anterior limb, internal capsule
Lentiform nucleus
Posterior limb, internal capsule
Thalamus
Splenium, corpus callosum
Corona radiata
Central sulcus
Subcortical white matter

(Top) First of three axial T2 MR images from inferior to superior of a normal nine month old shows posterior fossa structures. Cerebellum begins to develop low signal in white matter of cerebellar folia (arborization) by eight months, but does not reach an adult appearance until approximately eighteen months. **(Middle)** Image at level of internal capsule shows hypointensity in anterior & posterior limbs. Anterior limb continues to thicken until approximately ten months. Corpus callosum is myelinated by approximately eight months. **(Bottom)** Image through corona radiata shows partial myelination of deep & subcortical white matter, proceeding from occipital region anteriorly to frontal & temporal lobes. Myelination of subcortical white matter begins at approximately nine to twelve months in occipital lobes. Temporal lobe white matter matures last.

AXIAL T1 MR 12 MONTHS

Temporal lobe white matter
Pons
Middle cerebellar peduncle
Cerebellum

Caudate head
Genu, corpus callosum
Anterior limb, internal capsule
Lentiform nucleus
Thalamus
Posterior limb, internal capsule
Splenium, corpus callosum

Corona radiata
Subcortical white matter

(Top) First of three axial T1 MR images from inferior to superior of a normal twelve month old shows posterior fossa structures. Cerebellum has an adult appearance. Signal intensity in ventral (anterior) pons is bright as in an adult. Only temporal lobe white matter remains immature. **(Middle)** Image at level of internal capsule shows adult appearance on T1 images. White matter of internal capsule & corpus callosum is hyperintense compared with basal ganglia & thalamus. Globus pallidus is distinguishable as slightly hyperintense compared with putamen located laterally. **(Bottom)** Image at level of corona radiata shows an adult appearance of deep white matter & near adult appearance of subcortical white matter. Subcortical white matter matures last, beginning in posterior occipital lobes & extending anteriorly to frontal & temporal lobes.

WHITE MATTER TRACTS

AXIAL T2 MR 12 MONTHS

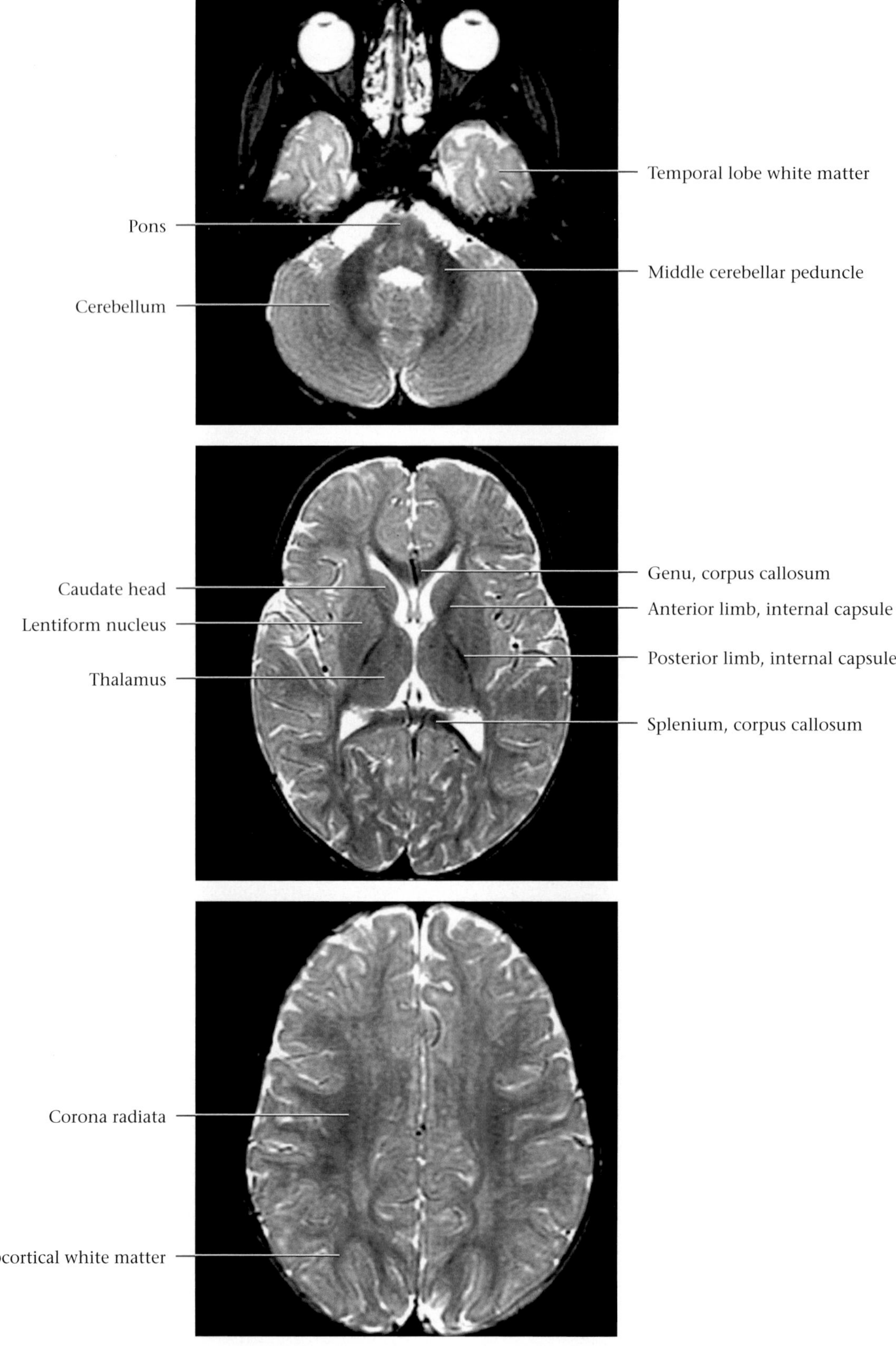
Temporal lobe white matter
Pons
Middle cerebellar peduncle
Cerebellum
Genu, corpus callosum
Caudate head
Anterior limb, internal capsule
Lentiform nucleus
Posterior limb, internal capsule
Thalamus
Splenium, corpus callosum
Corona radiata
Subcortical white matter

(Top) First of three axial T2 MR images from inferior to superior of a normal twelve month old shows posterior fossa structures. Arborization of cerebellum, low signal in cerebellar folia subcortical white matter, begins at six to eight months, but is not complete until eighteen months. Temporal white matter remains immature. **(Middle)** Image at level of internal capsule shows dark anterior & posterior limbs by twelve months. Basal ganglia & thalamus appears dark relative to white matter. Cortex & underlying white matter are essentially isointense throughout most of brain at this age, making T1 images better for identifying structural abnormalities. **(Bottom)** Image at level of corona radiata shows increased dark signal in white matter of paracentral & occipital regions. White matter maturation occurs in occipital regions first & moves anteriorly.

AXIAL T1 MR 18 MONTHS

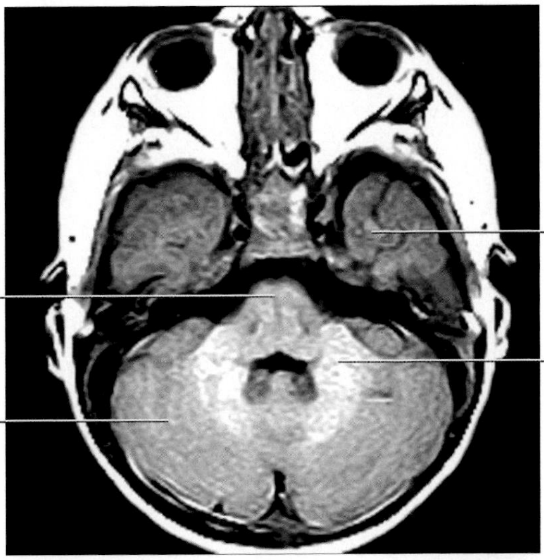

Temporal lobe white matter
Pons
Middle cerebellar peduncle
Cerebellum

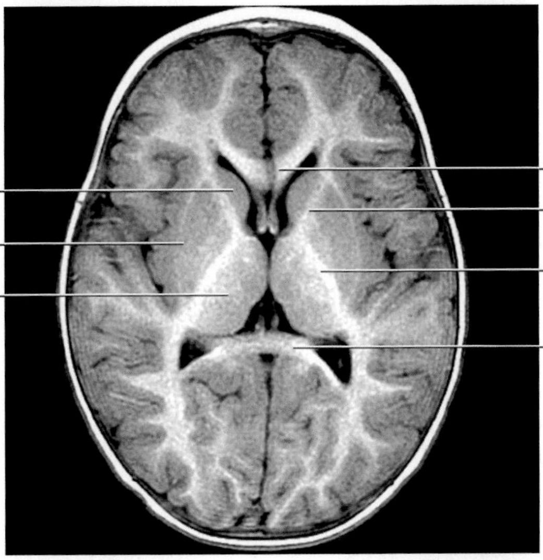

Caudate head
Genu, corpus callosum
Anterior limb, internal capsule
Lentiform nucleus
Posterior limb, internal capsule
Thalamus
Splenium, corpus callosum

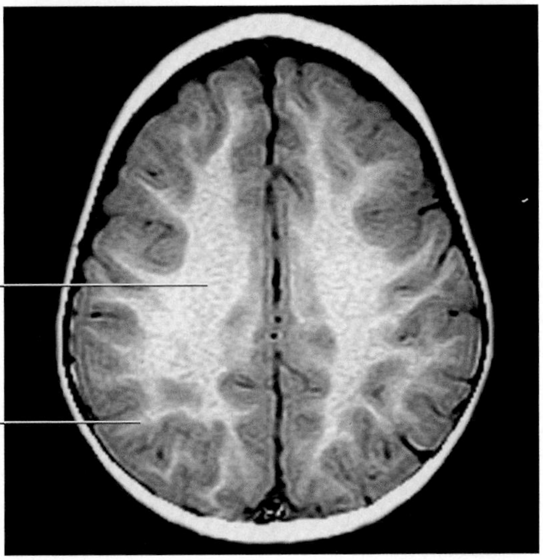

Corona radiata
Subcortical white matter

(Top) First of three axial T1 MR images from inferior to superior of a normal eighteen month old shows posterior fossa structures. Posterior fossa structures have an adult appearance on T1 images. Temporal & frontal lobe white matter is last to myelinate, but has an adult appearance on T1 images by eleven to twelve months. **(Middle)** Image at level of internal capsule shows adult appearance of basal ganglia, thalamus & white matter. Corpus callosum has an adult appearance on T1 images by six months while internal capsule has adult appearance by three months. **(Bottom)** Image at level of corona radiata shows adult appearance with hyperintensity seen in deep white matter & subcortical white matter. Myelination has adult appearance in white matter T1 images by eleven to twelve months & an adult appearance on T2 images by eighteen months.

WHITE MATTER TRACTS

AXIAL T2 MR 18 MONTHS

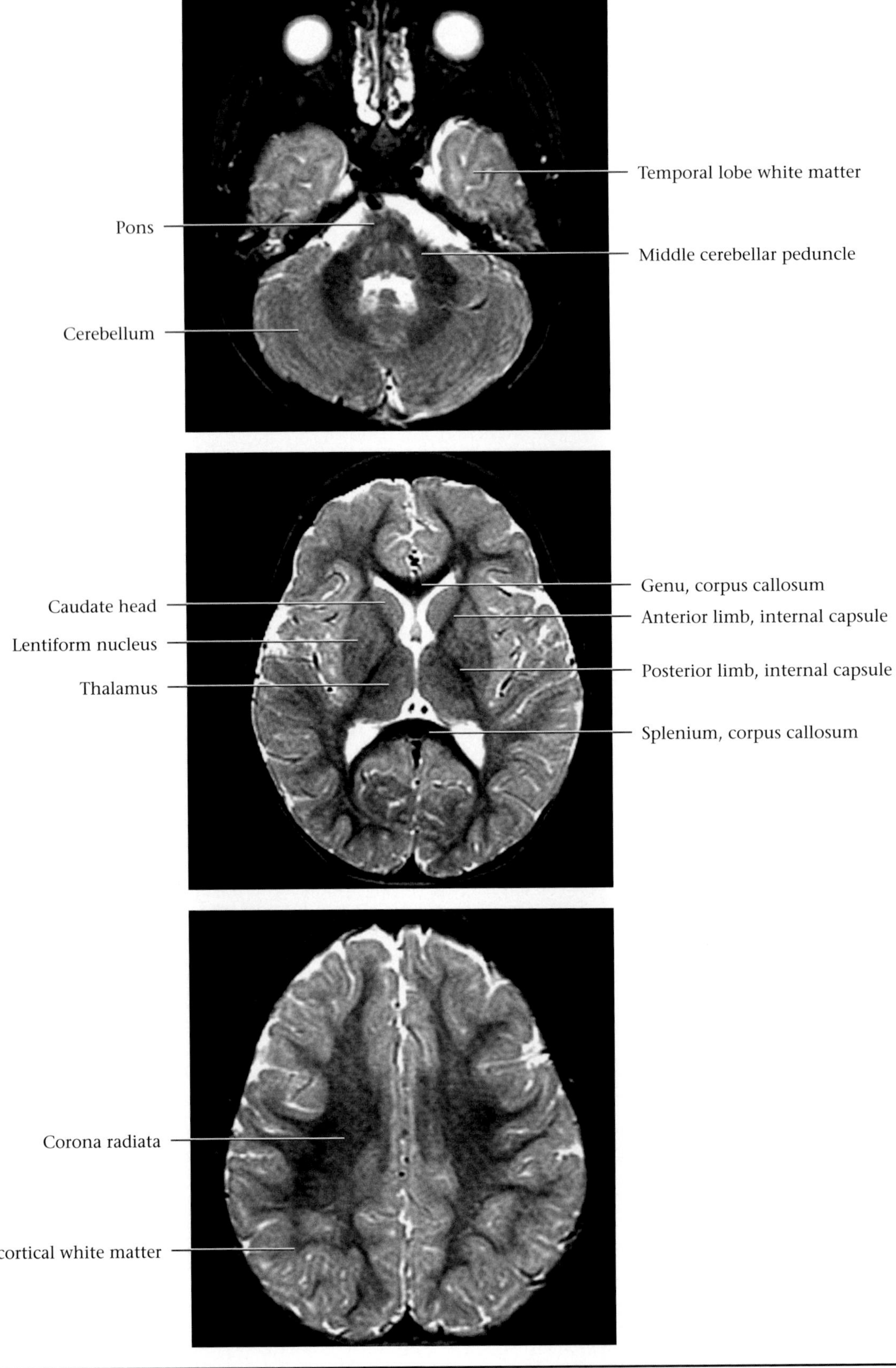
Temporal lobe white matter
Pons
Middle cerebellar peduncle
Cerebellum
Genu, corpus callosum
Caudate head
Anterior limb, internal capsule
Lentiform nucleus
Posterior limb, internal capsule
Thalamus
Splenium, corpus callosum
Corona radiata
Subcortical white matter

(Top) First of three axial T2 MR images from inferior to superior of a normal eighteen month old shows posterior fossa structures. Posterior fossa structures including brainstem & cerebellum have an adult appearance. Cerebellum reaches adult appearance on T2 images by eighteen months. Temporal lobe subcortical white matter is last to mature & reaches full maturity by 22-24 months. **(Middle)** Image at level of internal capsule shows adult appearance of corpus callosum & internal capsule. White matter of frontal & temporal lobes is last to appear mature on T2 images & remains relatively hyperintense, particularly in temporal lobes. **(Bottom)** Image at level of corona radiata shows further hypointensity in the deep & subcortical white matter. Although somewhat patchy, subcortical white matter is hypointense in majority of brain.

AXIAL T1 MR 3 YEARS

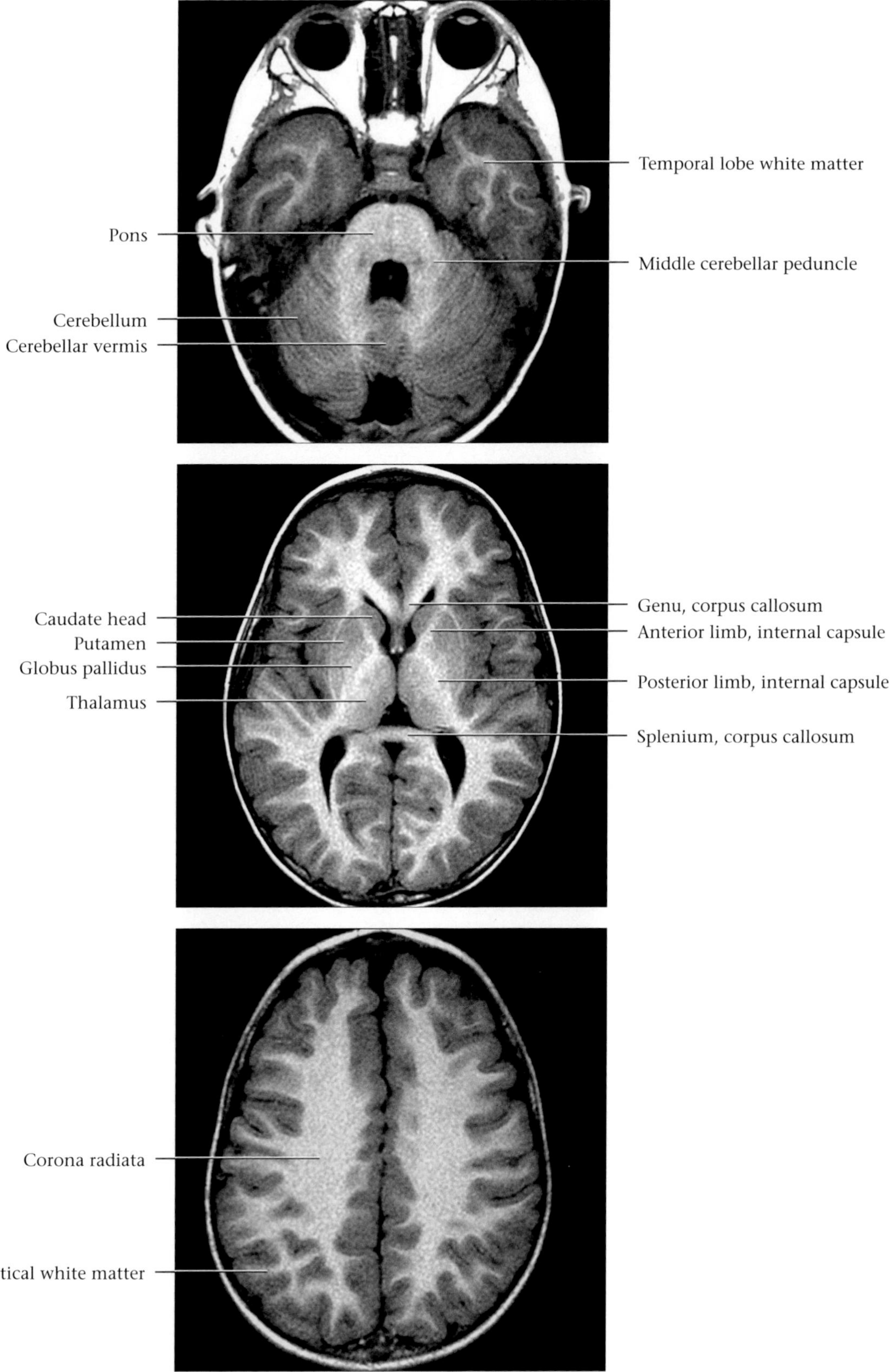
Temporal lobe white matter
Pons
Middle cerebellar peduncle
Cerebellum
Cerebellar vermis
Caudate head
Genu, corpus callosum
Putamen
Anterior limb, internal capsule
Globus pallidus
Posterior limb, internal capsule
Thalamus
Splenium, corpus callosum
Corona radiata
Subcortical white matter

(Top) First of three axial T1 MR images from inferior to superior of a normal three year old shows adult appearance. Cerebellar folia maturation, arborization, occurs much earlier on T1 than T2 images. Cerebellum appears mature on T1 images by approximately three months. However, maturation of brainstem & cerebellum is more sensitively assessed on T2 MR images. **(Middle)** Image at level of internal capsule shows adult appearance of internal capsule, corpus callosum & deep gray nuclei including basal ganglia & thalamus. Temporal lobe subcortical white matter is last to appear mature at approximately eleven to twelve months on T1 images. **(Bottom)** Image at corona radiata shows adult appearance of deep & subcortical white matter. Although conventional MR imaging suggests an adult appearance by two years, functional studies suggest complete myelination is not achieved until adolescence.

WHITE MATTER TRACTS

AXIAL T2 MR 3 YEARS

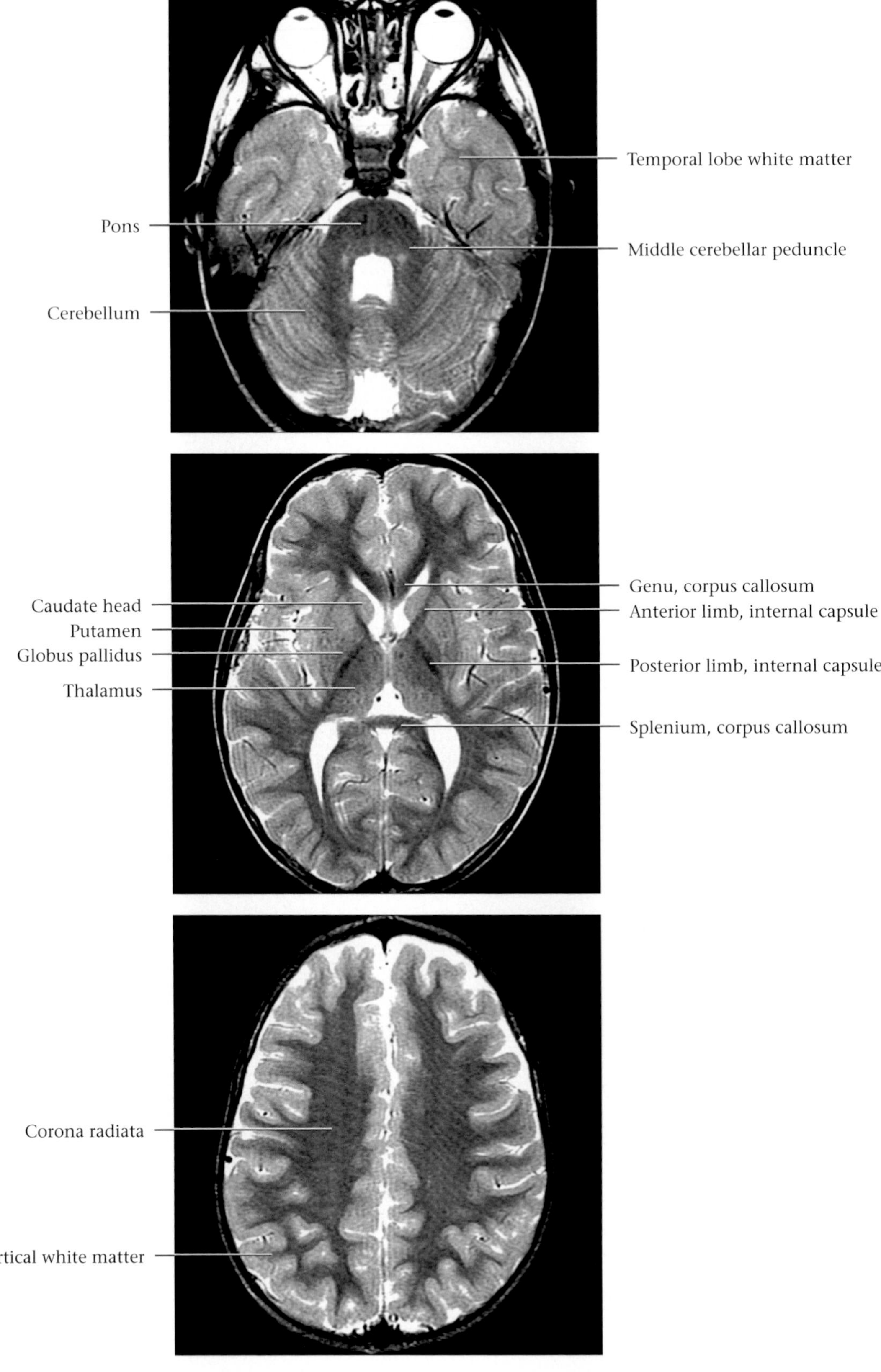
Temporal lobe white matter
Pons
Middle cerebellar peduncle
Cerebellum
Genu, corpus callosum
Caudate head
Anterior limb, internal capsule
Putamen
Globus pallidus
Posterior limb, internal capsule
Thalamus
Splenium, corpus callosum
Corona radiata
Subcortical white matter

(Top) First of three axial T2 MR images in a normal, mature three year old. Adult appearance of posterior fossa structures is noted. Temporal lobe subcortical white matter is also mature. **(Middle)** Image at level of internal capsule shows a near adult appearance in this three year old patient. Globus pallidus becomes more hypointense at around ten years related to normal iron deposition. **(Bottom)** Image at level of corona radiata shows normal adult appearance of deep & subcortical white matter. Corona radiata is formed by fibers from all cortical areas which fan out from internal capsule. T2 MR imaging is superior for evaluating brain maturation after six months of age. Normal adult appearance is usually obtained by eighteen months, except for most peripheral fibers.

CORONAL STIR MR

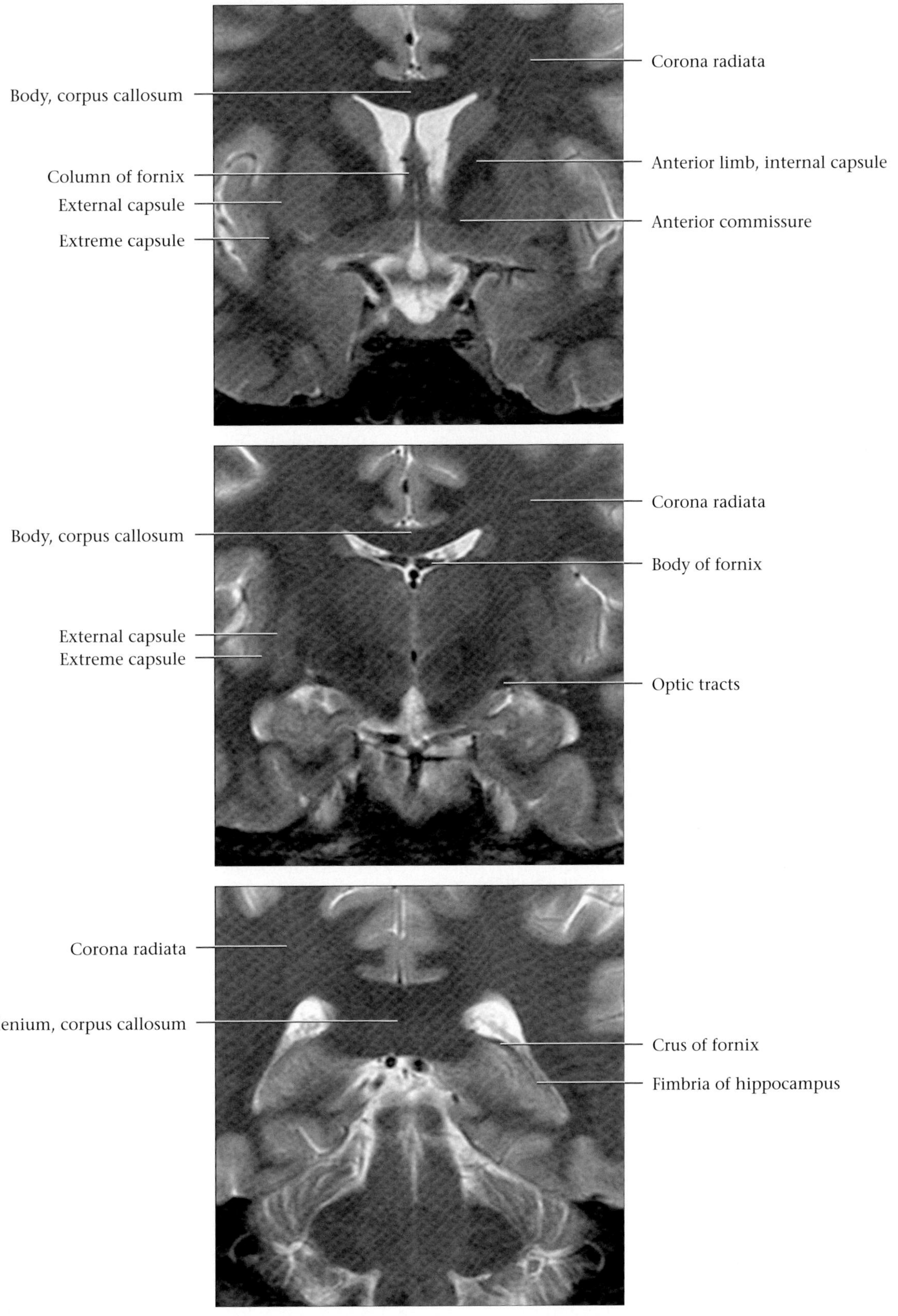

Corona radiata
Body, corpus callosum
Anterior limb, internal capsule
Column of fornix
External capsule
Anterior commissure
Extreme capsule
Corona radiata
Body, corpus callosum
Body of fornix
External capsule
Extreme capsule
Optic tracts
Corona radiata
Splenium, corpus callosum
Crus of fornix
Fimbria of hippocampus

(Top) First of three coronal STIR MR images through white matter tracts from anterior to posterior. Anterior commissure crosses through lamina terminalis. Anterior fibers of anterior commissure connect olfactory bulbs & nuclei while posterior fibers connect middle & inferior temporal gyri. Anterior limb of internal capsule lies between head of caudate & lentiform nucleus & passes projection fibers to & from thalamus (thalamocortical projections) & frontopontine tracts. **(Middle)** Image more posterior shows body of fornix. Fornix is major white matter tract associated with hippocampus & limbic system. **(Bottom)** Image posteriorly shows splenium of corpus callosum & crus of fornix. Hippocampal fimbria continue along undersurface of splenium to form crus of fornix which extend under body of corpus callosum to form commissure which becomes body anteriorly.

BASAL GANGLIA AND THALAMUS

Terminology

Definitions

- Basal ganglia (BG): Subcortical nuclear masses in inferior hemispheres
  - Involved in motivation, controlling movement
  - Lentiform nucleus: Putamen + globus pallidus (GP)
  - Corpus striatum: Caudate nucleus + putamen + GP; neostriatum = putamen, caudate
  - Definition recently narrowed to exclude claustrum, amygdala
- Thalamus: Paired ovoid nuclear complexes; relay stations for most sensory pathways
- Subthalamus: Complex region of nuclear masses, fiber tracts that plays major role in normal BG function

Gross Anatomy

Overview

- **Basal ganglia**: Caudate nucleus, putamen, GP
  - Anterior limb of internal capsule separates caudate head from putamen, GP
  - Posterior limb separates thalamus from BG
- **Caudate nucleus**: "C-shaped" curved nucleus with large head, tapered body, down-curving tail
  - Head forms floor/lateral wall of anterior horn of lateral ventricle
  - Body borders, parallels lateral ventricle
  - Tail follows curve of inferior horn, lies in ventricular roof
  - Deep groove (sulcus terminalis) separates caudate from thalamus; its stria terminalis lies deep to ependyma, helps form choroid fissure
  - Caudate continuous anteriorly with inferior putamen above anterior perforated substance; with posteroinferior putamen at caudate tail
- **Putamen**: Located lateral to GP, separated by lateral (external) medullary lamina
- **GP**: Two segments
  - Lateral (external), medial (internal) segments separated by internal medullary lamina
  - Higher myelin content than putamen (darker on T2)
- **Thalamus**: Ovoid nucleus, extends from foramen of Monro to quadrigeminal plate of midbrain
  - Medially forms lateral walls of third ventricle
  - Laterally bordered by internal capsule
  - Subdivided into nuclear groups (anterior, medial, lateral), geniculate nuclei (lateral, medial), pulvinar
    - Nuclear groups further subdivided into 10 additional nuclei
    - Internal medullary lamina separates medial, lateral, anterior nuclear groups
    - External medullary lamina separates lateral nuclear group, reticular nucleus
  - Geniculate nuclei
    - Lateral geniculate nucleus: Ovoid ventral projection from posterior thalamus (part of visual system)
    - Medial geniculate nucleus: Medial to lateral geniculate nucleus along posterior thalamus (part of auditory system)
  - Pulvinar: Occupies caudal third of thalamus & overhangs superior colliculus
  - Massa intermedia (interthalamic adhesion): Connects thalami across third ventricle
- **Subthalamus**
  - Associated with Parkinson disease, ballism
  - Subthalamic, reticular nuclei included
  - Subthalamic nucleus is lens-shaped, lies superolateral to red nucleus
  - Reticular nucleus: Lamella that wraps around lateral thalamus, separated from it by external medullary lamina

Vascular Supply

- BG: Mostly lenticulostriate arteries
- Thalamus: Mostly thalamoperforators from posterior communicating, basilar, P1 posterior cerebral arteries
  - Large thalamoperforator (artery of Percheron or paramedian thalamic artery) may supply bilateral medial thalami

Imaging Anatomy

Overview

- CT: Deep gray nuclei hyperdense to white matter; isodense with cortex
  - Punctate or dense globular Ca++ common
  - Usually symmetric, in medial GP
  - Common in middle-aged, older patients
- MR
  - Iron deposition in BG occurs with normal aging
    - No Fe in brain at birth
    - Progressive ↑ with aging, ↓ signal intensity on T2WI
    - GP hypointensity begins to ↑ in 2nd decade, plateaus after age 30
    - Putamen = GP hypointensity at 80 years

Anatomy-Based Imaging Issues

Imaging Recommendations

- MR (axial, coronal) best general imaging; NECT for Ca++
- DWI, T2* helpful additions

Clinical Implications

Clinical Importance

- Disorders of the BG are characterized by abnormalities of movement, muscle tone & posture
- Putamen is most common location affected by hypertensive hemorrhage
- GP is most sensitive area of brain to hypoxia (in addition to hippocampus)
- BG is common location for strokes, particularly lacunar infarcts & hypertensive hemorrhages

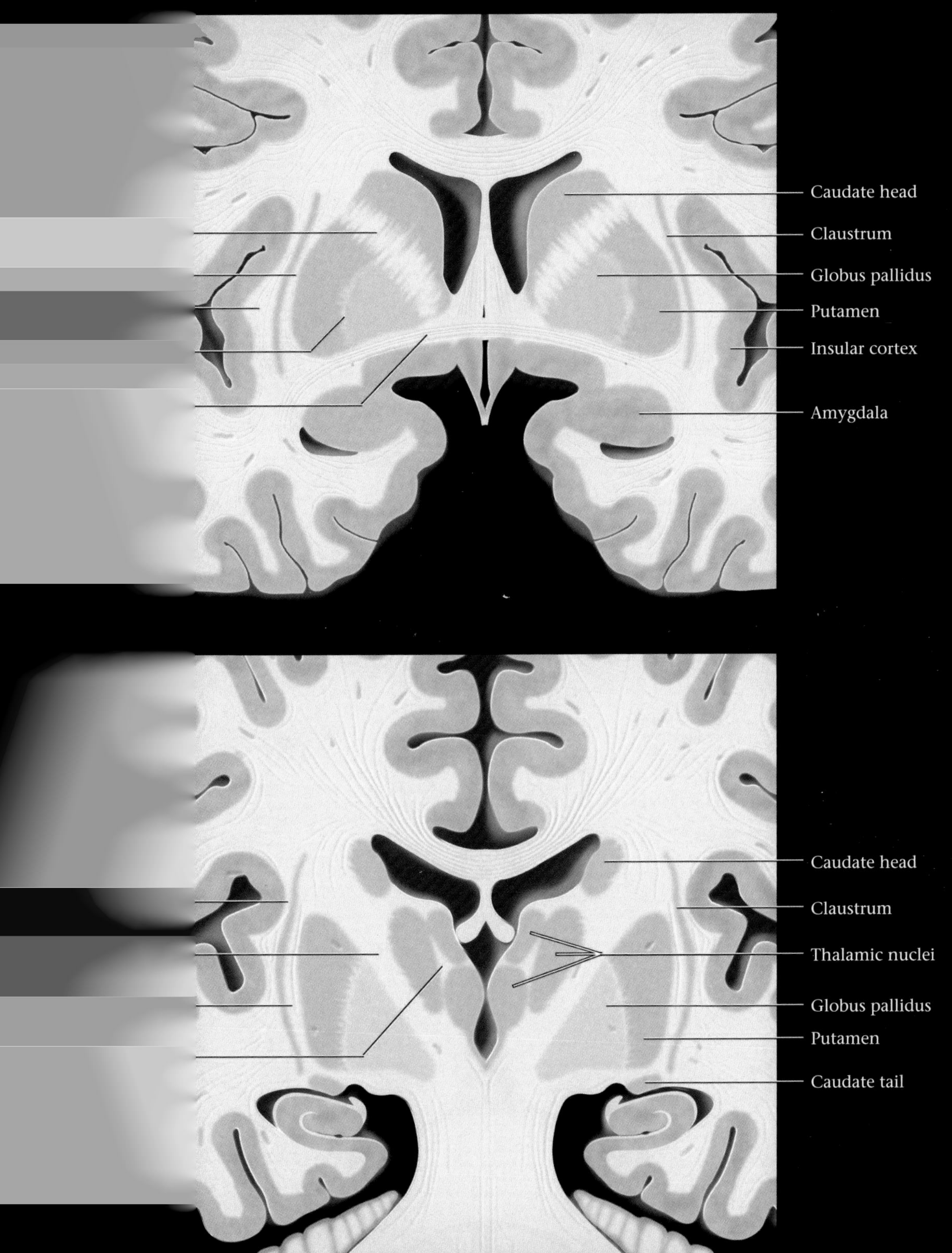

Caudate head
Claustrum
Globus pallidus
Putamen
Insular cortex
Amygdala
Caudate head
Claustrum
Thalamic nuclei
Globus pallidus
Putamen
Caudate tail

basal ganglia at level of anterior commissure & frontal horns of lateral ventricles. Caudate l of frontal horn & is separated from globus pallidus & putamen by anterior limb of nal medullary lamina separates putamen from globus pallidus. The GP has two segments, a t, separated by an internal medullary lamina (not shown). **(Bottom)** Coronal graphic of through anterior third ventricle shows division of thalamic nuclei into 3 main groups: lei & anterior nuclei. Anterior nuclei border lateral & third ventricle while medial nuclei are ricle. Internal medullary lamina separates these main thalamic groups. These main

GRAPHICS

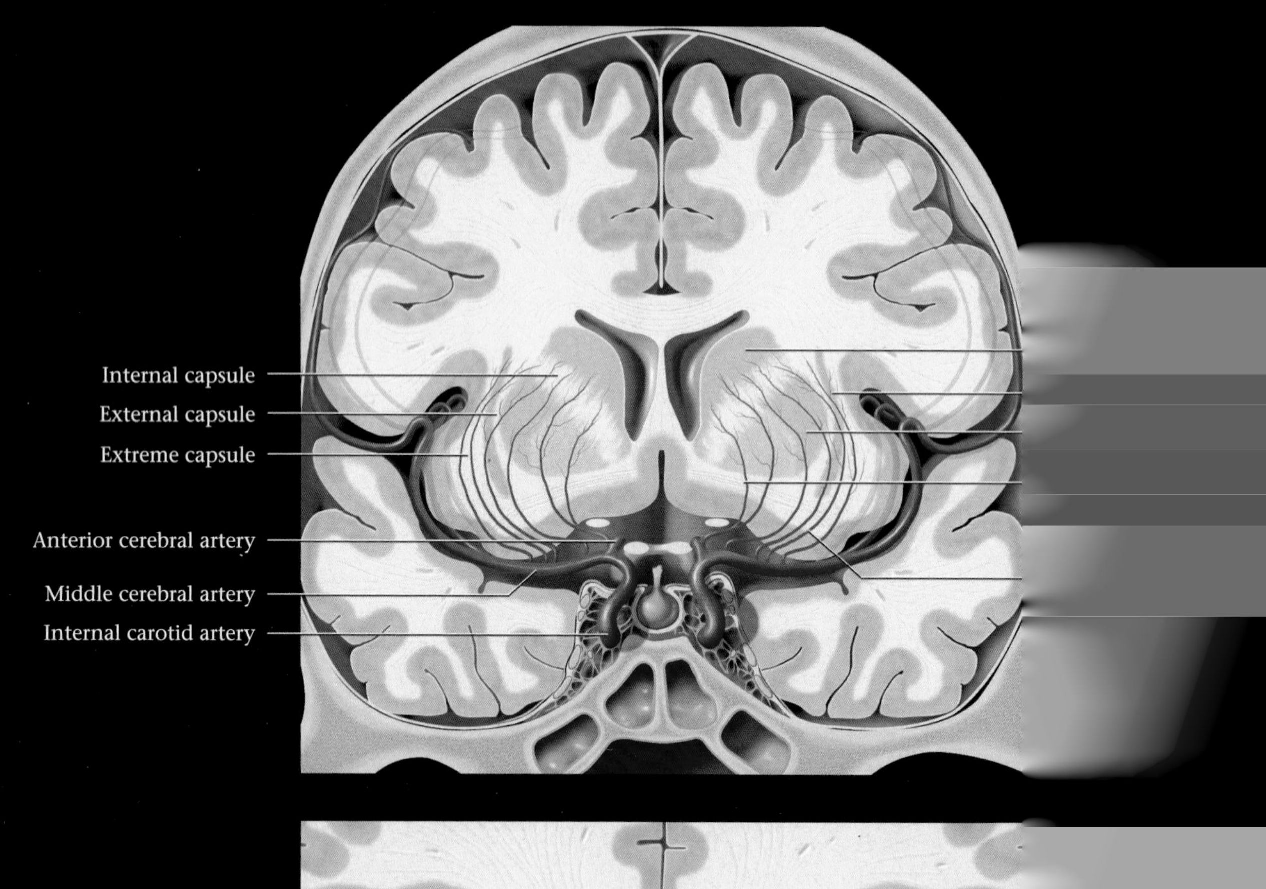
Internal capsule
External capsule
Extreme capsule
Anterior cerebral artery
Middle cerebral artery
Internal carotid artery
Anterior limb, internal capsule
External capsule
Genu, internal capsule
Extreme capsule
Posterior limb, internal capsule

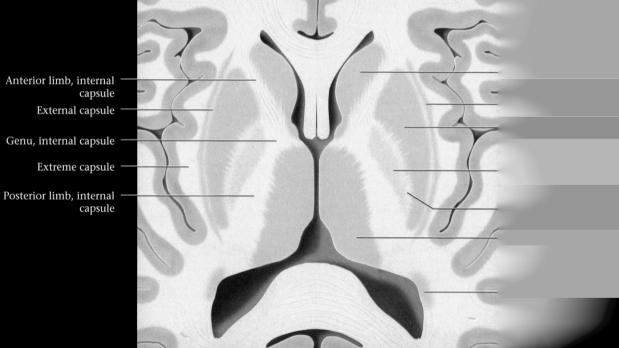

(Top) Coronal graphic of basal ganglia at level of frontal horns of lateral ventricles showing anterior circulation. Note medial lenticulostriate arteries supply head of caudate, anterior pc globus pallidus & anterior limb of internal capsule while lateral lenticulostriate arteries supp pallidus, putamen & internal capsule. Note lack of collateral supply to basal ganglia. **(Bottor** ganglia & thalamus shows internal capsule separating caudate & thalamus from putamen & limb primarily contains fibers from frontal lobes. Genu of internal capsule contains corticob fibers while posterior limb contains corticospinal tracts & thalamic fibers. Fibers from upper within posterior limb while lower extremity fibers are posterior.

AXIAL CECT

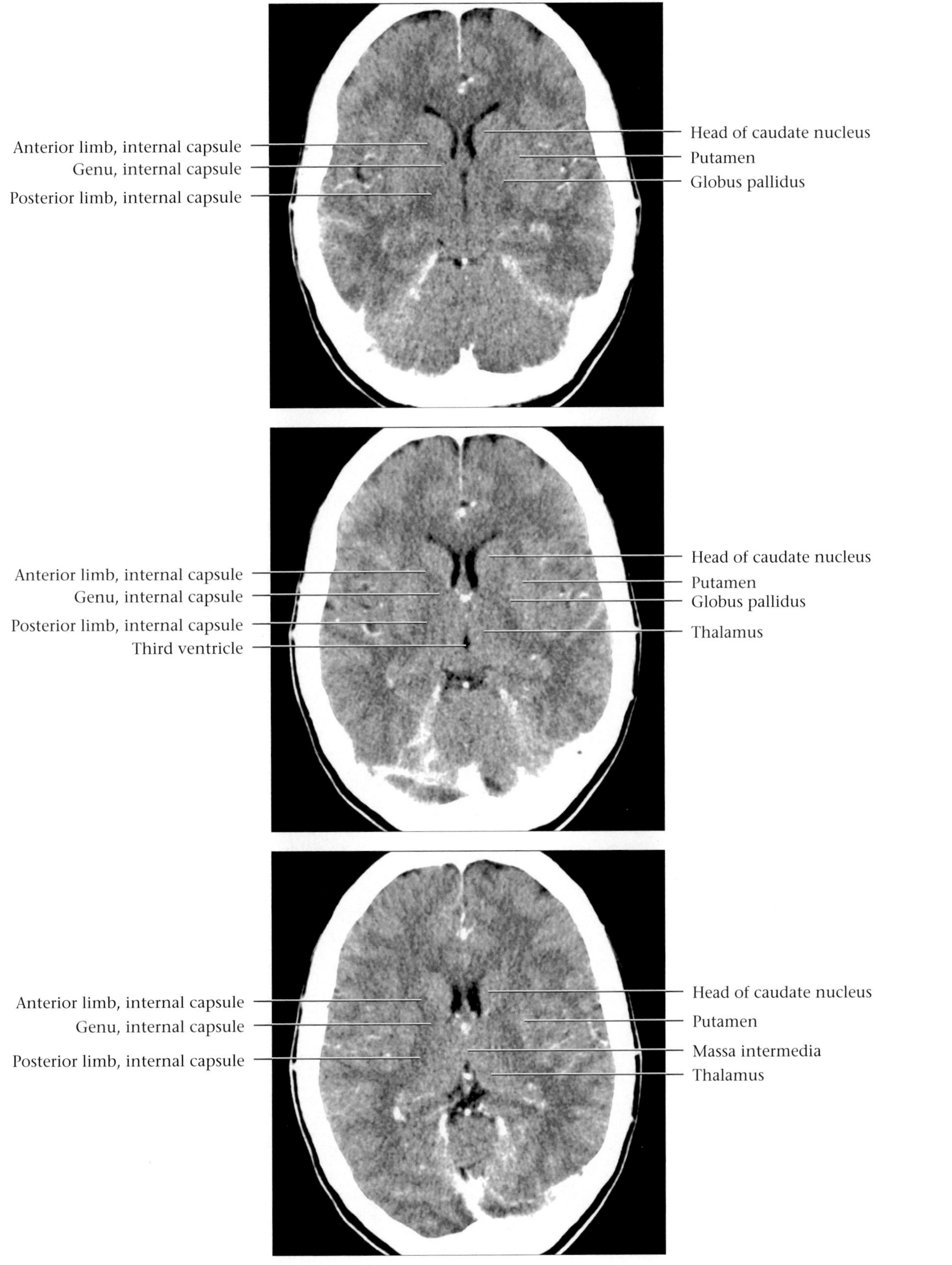
Anterior limb, internal capsule
Genu, internal capsule
Posterior limb, internal capsule
Head of caudate nucleus
Putamen
Globus pallidus
Anterior limb, internal capsule
Genu, internal capsule
Posterior limb, internal capsule
Third ventricle
Head of caudate nucleus
Putamen
Globus pallidus
Thalamus
Anterior limb, internal capsule
Genu, internal capsule
Posterior limb, internal capsule
Head of caudate nucleus
Putamen
Massa intermedia
Thalamus

(Top) First of three CECT images of basal ganglia & thalamus from inferior to superior. Note internal capsule appears hypodense & helps separate caudate head from putamen & globus pallidus. External capsule, claustrum & extreme capsule cannot be resolved on CT imaging. Unenhanced CT is an excellent choice for initial evaluation of possible basal ganglia stroke as hypertensive hemorrhages & lacunar infarcts are common in basal ganglia & thalami & are well seen by CT. **(Middle)** This image shows large anterior caudate head lying in floor & lateral wall of frontal horn of lateral ventricle. Putamen, globus pallidus are separated on CT by location & subtle differences in density. GP is often slightly less dense than putamen. **(Bottom)** Image more superior shows thalamus as it extends posteriorly. Massa intermedia (interthalamic adhesion) connects thalami across third ventricle.

BASAL GANGLIA AND THALAMUS

AXIAL T1 MR

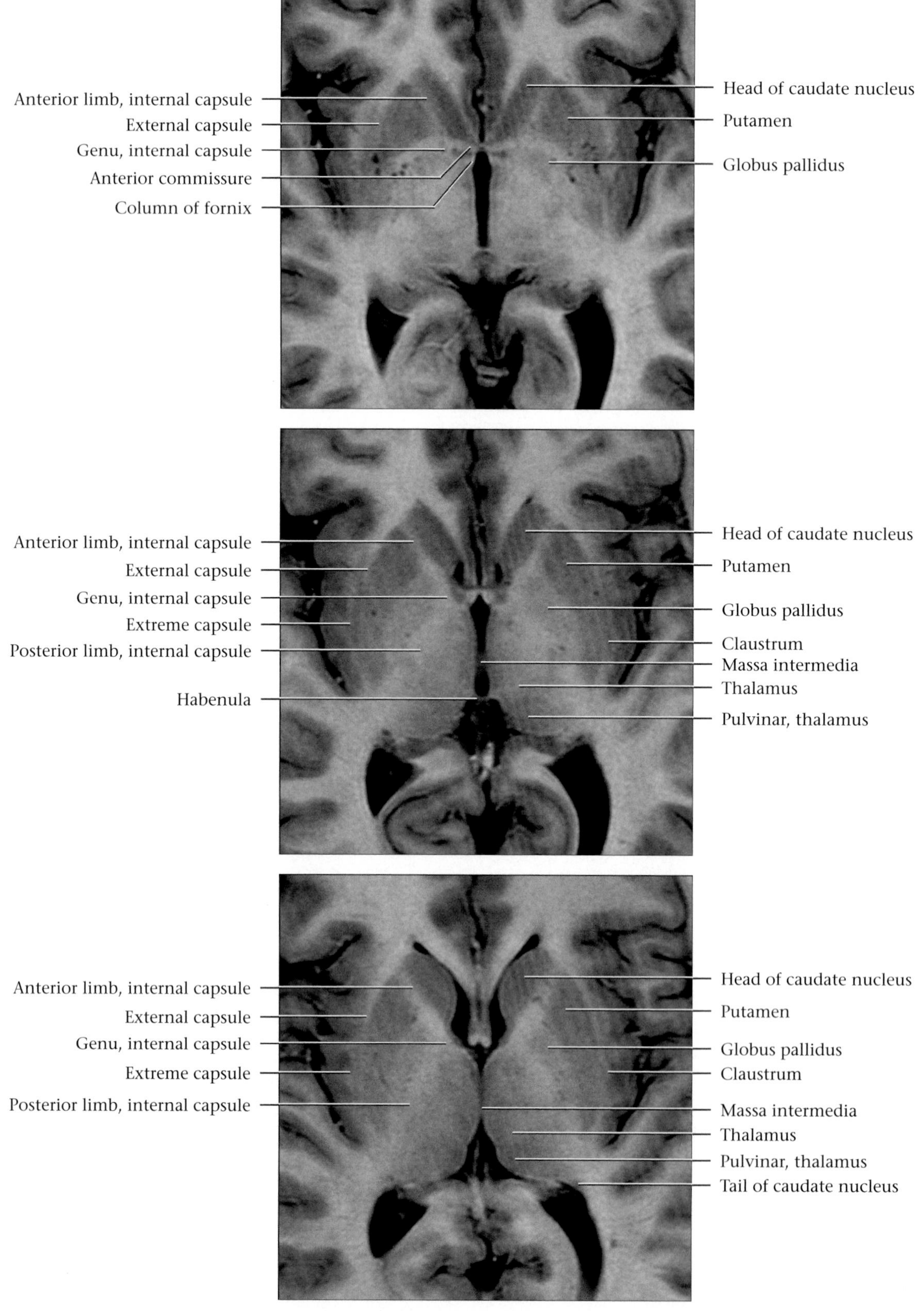
Anterior limb, internal capsule
External capsule
Genu, internal capsule
Anterior commissure
Column of fornix
Head of caudate nucleus
Putamen
Globus pallidus
Anterior limb, internal capsule
External capsule
Genu, internal capsule
Extreme capsule
Posterior limb, internal capsule
Habenula
Head of caudate nucleus
Putamen
Globus pallidus
Claustrum
Massa intermedia
Thalamus
Pulvinar, thalamus
Anterior limb, internal capsule
External capsule
Genu, internal capsule
Extreme capsule
Posterior limb, internal capsule
Head of caudate nucleus
Putamen
Globus pallidus
Claustrum
Massa intermedia
Thalamus
Pulvinar, thalamus
Tail of caudate nucleus

(Top) First of six axial T1 MR images from inferior to superior shows inferior aspect of basal ganglia & thalamus. Note caudate head lies inferior to frontal horns of lateral ventricles at this level. **(Middle)** Image thorough basal ganglia & thalamus shows distinct nuclei of caudate, putamen & globus pallidus. Note massa intermedia (interthalamic adhesion) across the third ventricle. The habenula (which connects olfactory impulses to brain stem nuclei) is seen at this level. Lateral to putamen, external capsule, claustrum, extreme capsule & insular cortex are present. **(Bottom)** This image shows internal capsule in its entirety with anterior limb, genu & posterior limb. Genu of internal capsule contains corticobulbar fibers & thalamic fibers while posterior limb contains corticospinal tracts & thalamic fibers. Lenticulostriate arteries supply internal capsule.

BASAL GANGLIA AND THALAMUS

AXIAL T1 MR

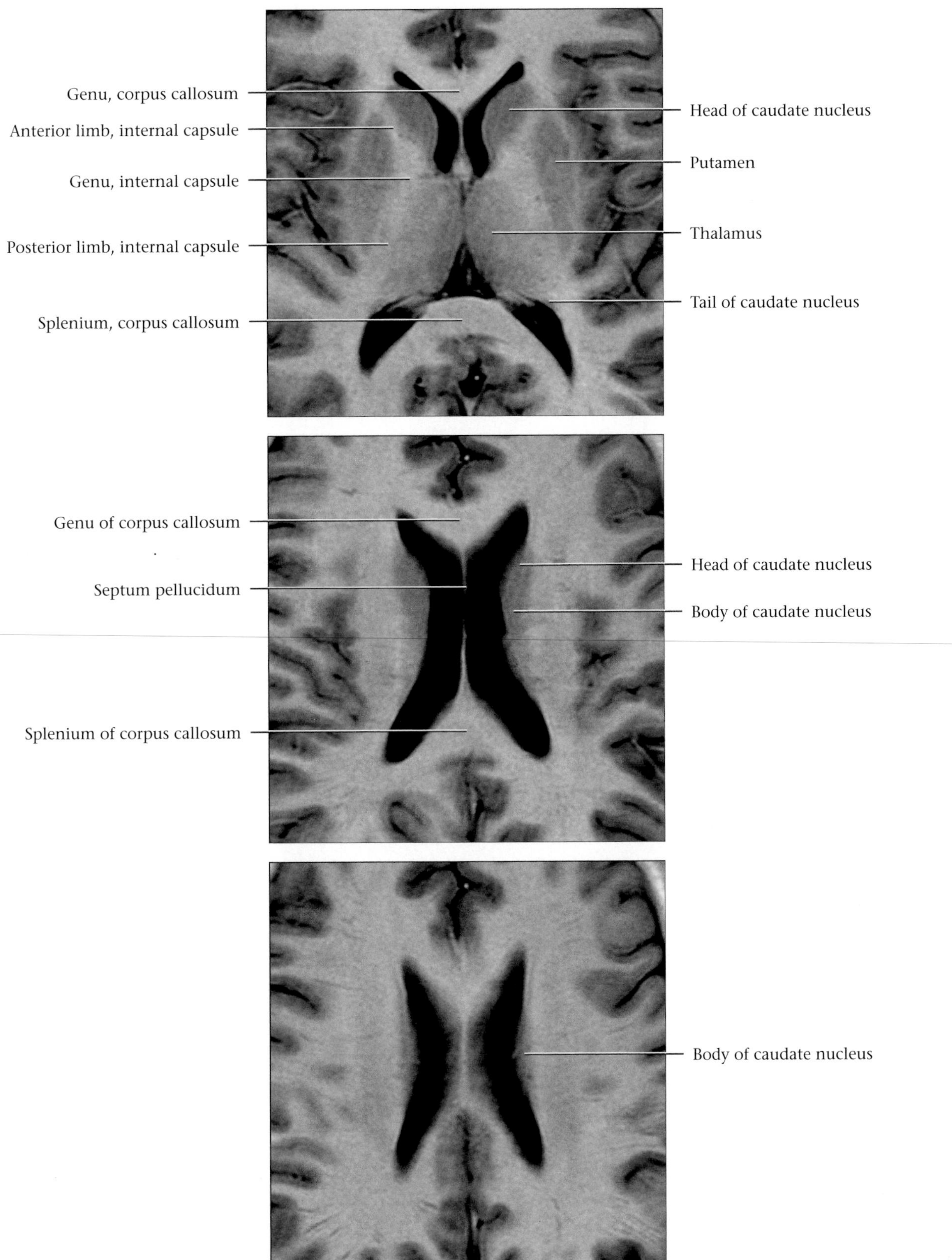
Genu, corpus callosum
Anterior limb, internal capsule
Genu, internal capsule
Posterior limb, internal capsule
Splenium, corpus callosum
Head of caudate nucleus
Putamen
Thalamus
Tail of caudate nucleus
Genu of corpus callosum
Septum pellucidum
Splenium of corpus callosum
Head of caudate nucleus
Body of caudate nucleus
Body of caudate nucleus

(Top) Image more superior through basal ganglia at level of genu & splenium of corpus callosum. Head & tail of caudate nucleus are seen as caudate curves around lateral ventricle. Tail of caudate lies in ventricular roof in temporal lobe. Caudate is separated from thalamus by sulcus terminalis which contains stria terminalis & thalamostriate veins anteriorly. Putamen is larger than globus pallidus & continues more superiorly. **(Middle)** Image at level of centrum semiovale shows head & body of caudate as it wraps around lateral ventricle. Caudate nucleus lies in frontal lobe & wraps around ventricle to end in temporal lobe at the amygdala. **(Bottom)** Image more superior shows body of caudate head as it parallels the lateral ventricles.

BASAL GANGLIA AND THALAMUS

CORONAL T1 MR

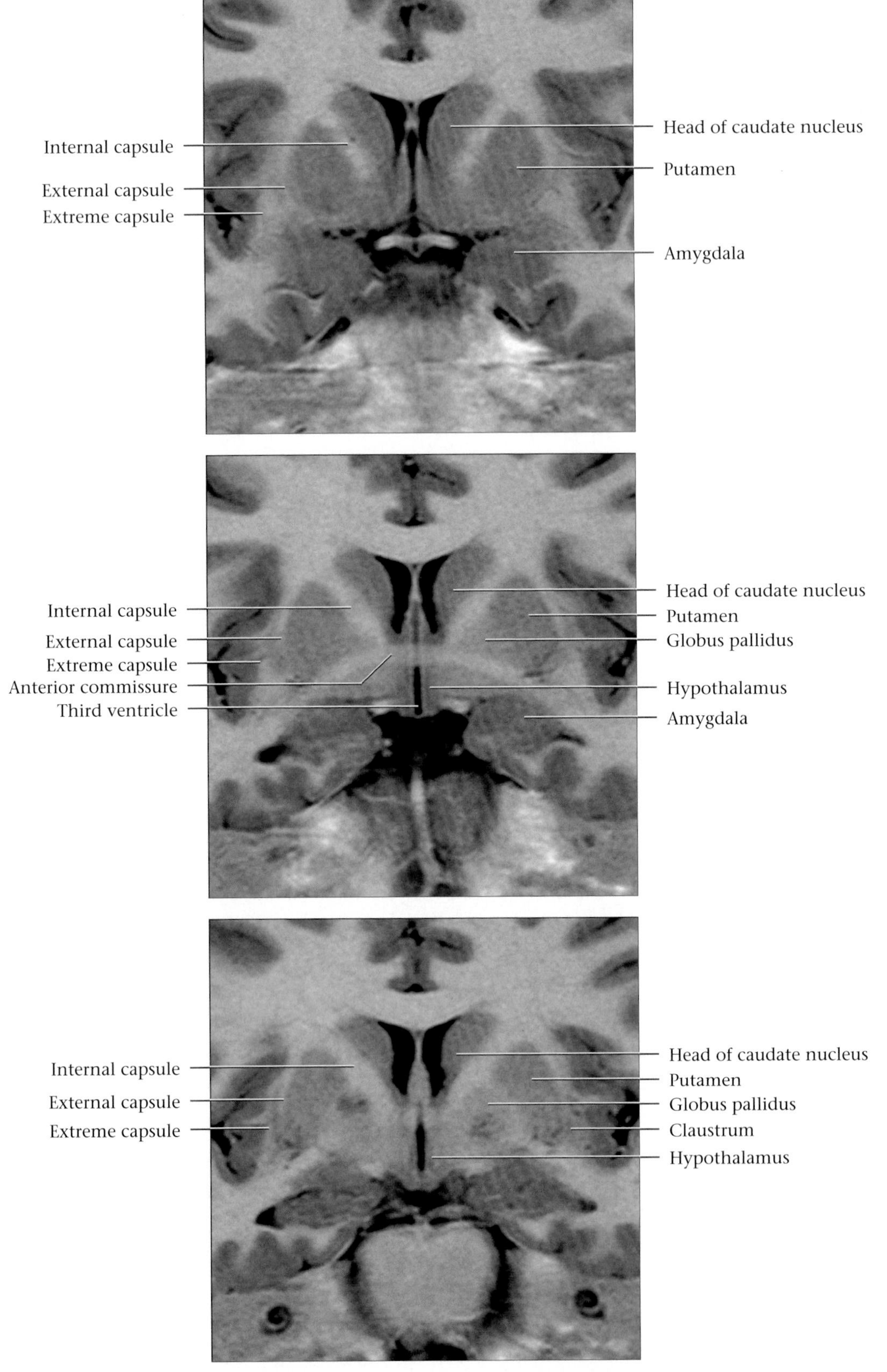
Internal capsule
External capsule
Extreme capsule
Head of caudate nucleus
Putamen
Amygdala
Internal capsule
External capsule
Extreme capsule
Anterior commissure
Third ventricle
Head of caudate nucleus
Putamen
Globus pallidus
Hypothalamus
Amygdala
Internal capsule
External capsule
Extreme capsule
Head of caudate nucleus
Putamen
Globus pallidus
Claustrum
Hypothalamus

(Top) First of six coronal T1 MR images from anterior to posterior through basal ganglia & thalamus. Note inferior part of caudate head becomes continuous with most inferior part of putamen just above anterior perforated substance. **(Middle)** Image at level of anterior commissure shows anterior limb of internal capsule as it separates caudate head from putamen & globus pallidus. Globus pallidus & putamen have different signal intensity related to increased myelin in globus pallidus. Lateral & medial segments of globus pallidus cannot be distinguished on conventional imaging. **(Bottom)** Image more posterior through third ventricle shows components of basal ganglia: Caudate, putamen & globus pallidus. Typical pathologic conditions of basal ganglia include hypoxic-ischemic insults & toxic-metabolic processes. Imaging with T1 & T2 as well as DWI sequences are useful.

BASAL GANGLIA AND THALAMUS

CORONAL T1 MR

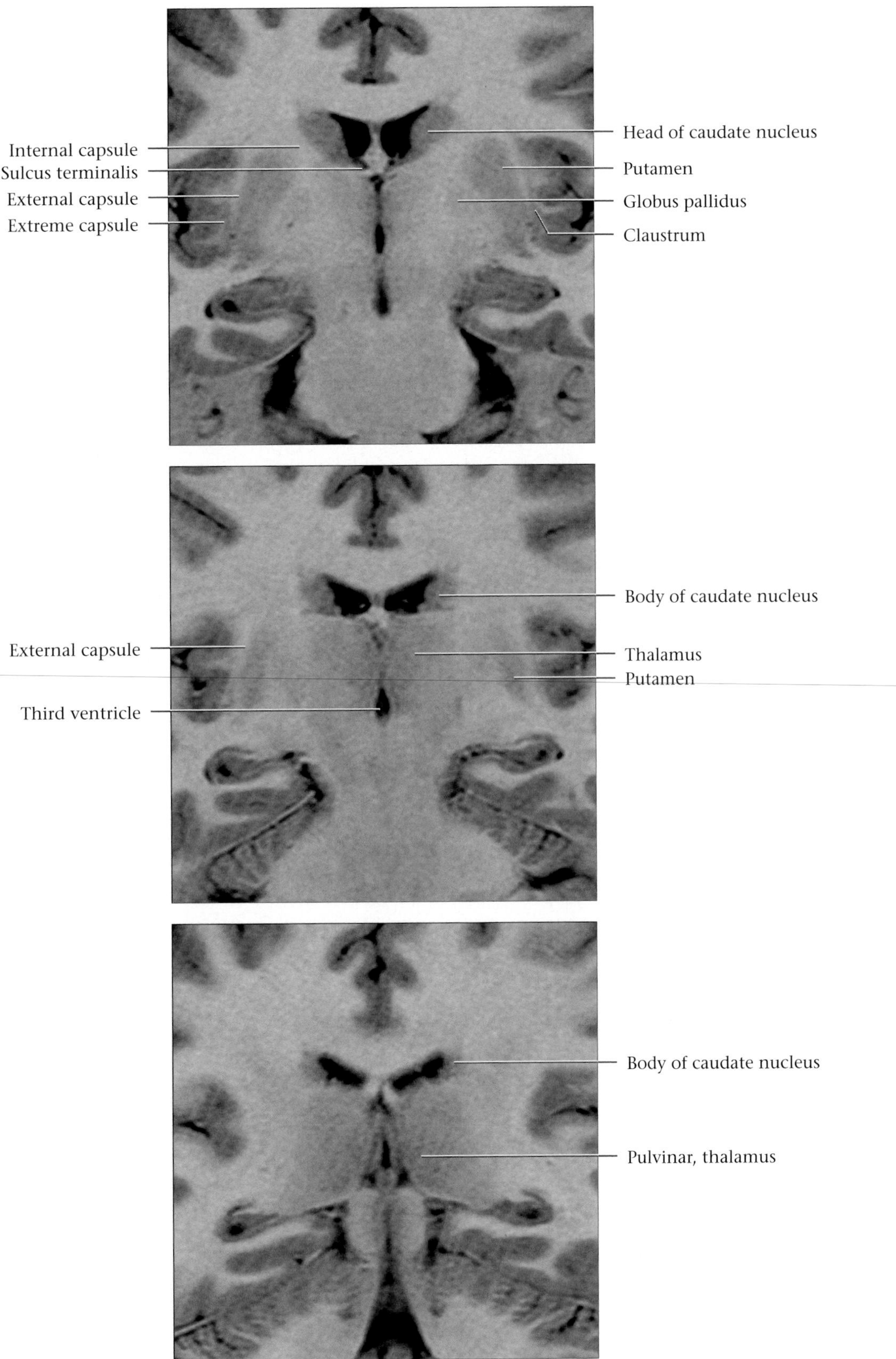
Internal capsule
Sulcus terminalis
External capsule
Extreme capsule
Head of caudate nucleus
Putamen
Globus pallidus
Claustrum
External capsule
Third ventricle
Body of caudate nucleus
Thalamus
Putamen
Body of caudate nucleus
Pulvinar, thalamus

(Top) Image more posterior shows basal ganglia & thalamus. The sulcus terminalis which separates caudate head from thalamus contains thalamostriate vein & stria terminalis. Stria terminalis is most important efferent fiber system of amygdala, runs below thalamostriate vein, but is not seen on conventional imaging. **(Middle)** Image more posterior shows thalamus bordering third ventricle. Thalamus contains three major nuclear groups (anterior, medial, lateral) which are not resolved on conventional imaging. Other thalamic nuclei include lateral & medial geniculate nuclei which may be seen on high-resolution images. Subthalamic nuclei are located superolateral to red nucleus & are important in movement disorders. **(Bottom)** Image more posterior shows caudate body as it parallels lateral ventricle. Pulvinar occupies posterior third of thalamus.

BASAL GANGLIA AND THALAMUS

AXIAL T2 MR

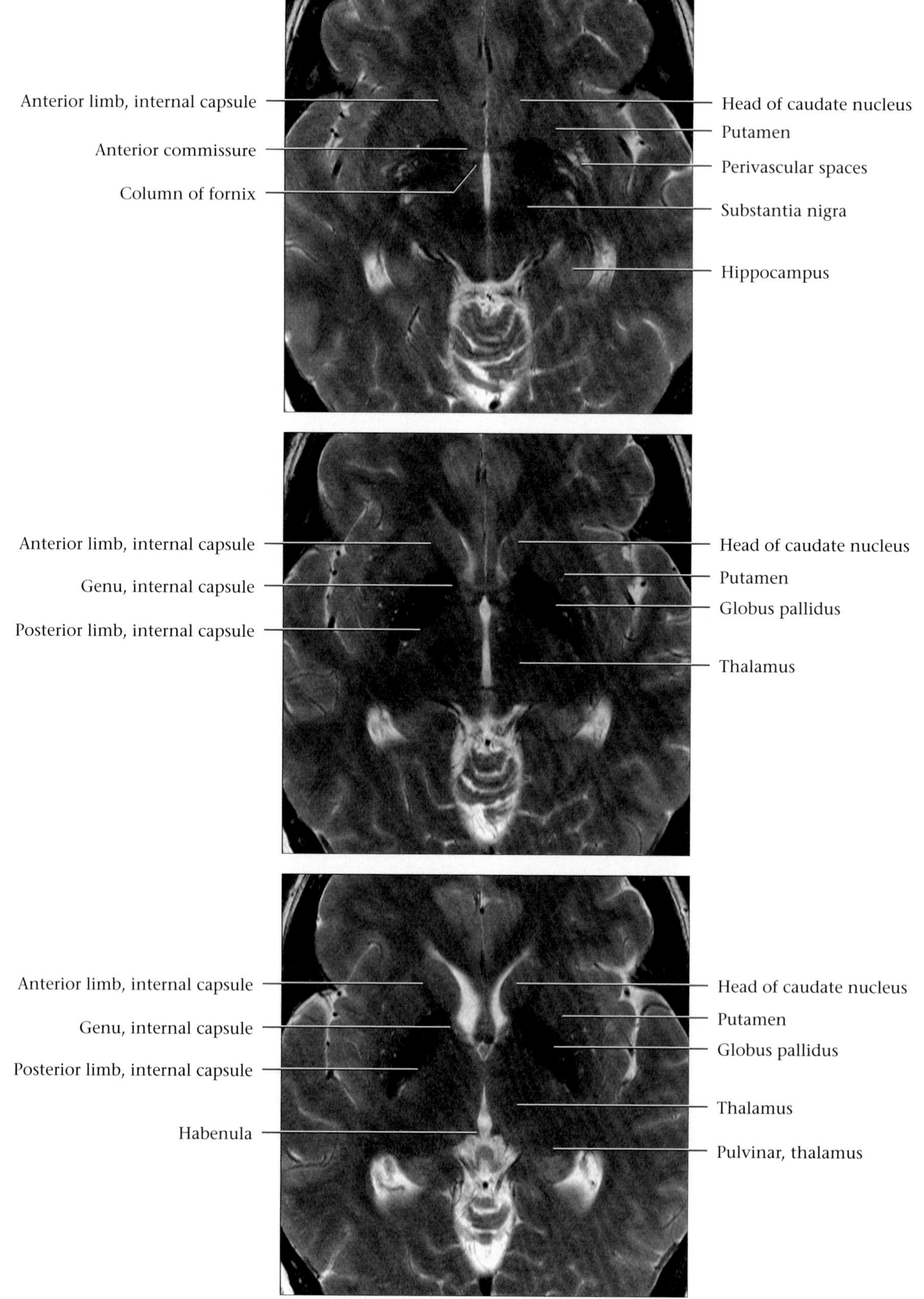
Anterior limb, internal capsule
Anterior commissure
Column of fornix
Head of caudate nucleus
Putamen
Perivascular spaces
Substantia nigra
Hippocampus
Anterior limb, internal capsule
Genu, internal capsule
Posterior limb, internal capsule
Head of caudate nucleus
Putamen
Globus pallidus
Thalamus
Anterior limb, internal capsule
Genu, internal capsule
Posterior limb, internal capsule
Habenula
Head of caudate nucleus
Putamen
Globus pallidus
Thalamus
Pulvinar, thalamus

(Top) First of six axial T2 MR images from inferior to superior shows caudate head as it lies along floor of lateral ventricle. Perivascular spaces, a normal variant, are seen in a typical location along lateral aspect of anterior commissure. Perivascular spaces follow CSF on all pulse sequence & have no surrounding gliosis or edema & no enhancement. Substantia nigra is within midbrain cerebral peduncles. **(Middle)** Image through basal ganglia shows GP is hypointense compared with other deep gray nuclei because of normal age-related iron deposition. **(Bottom)** Image more superior through basal ganglia & thalamus shows internal capsule components including anterior limb, genu & posterior limb. Habenula, part of epithalamus, transmits olfactory impulses to brainstem. Habenula also attaches to pineal gland.

AXIAL T2 MR

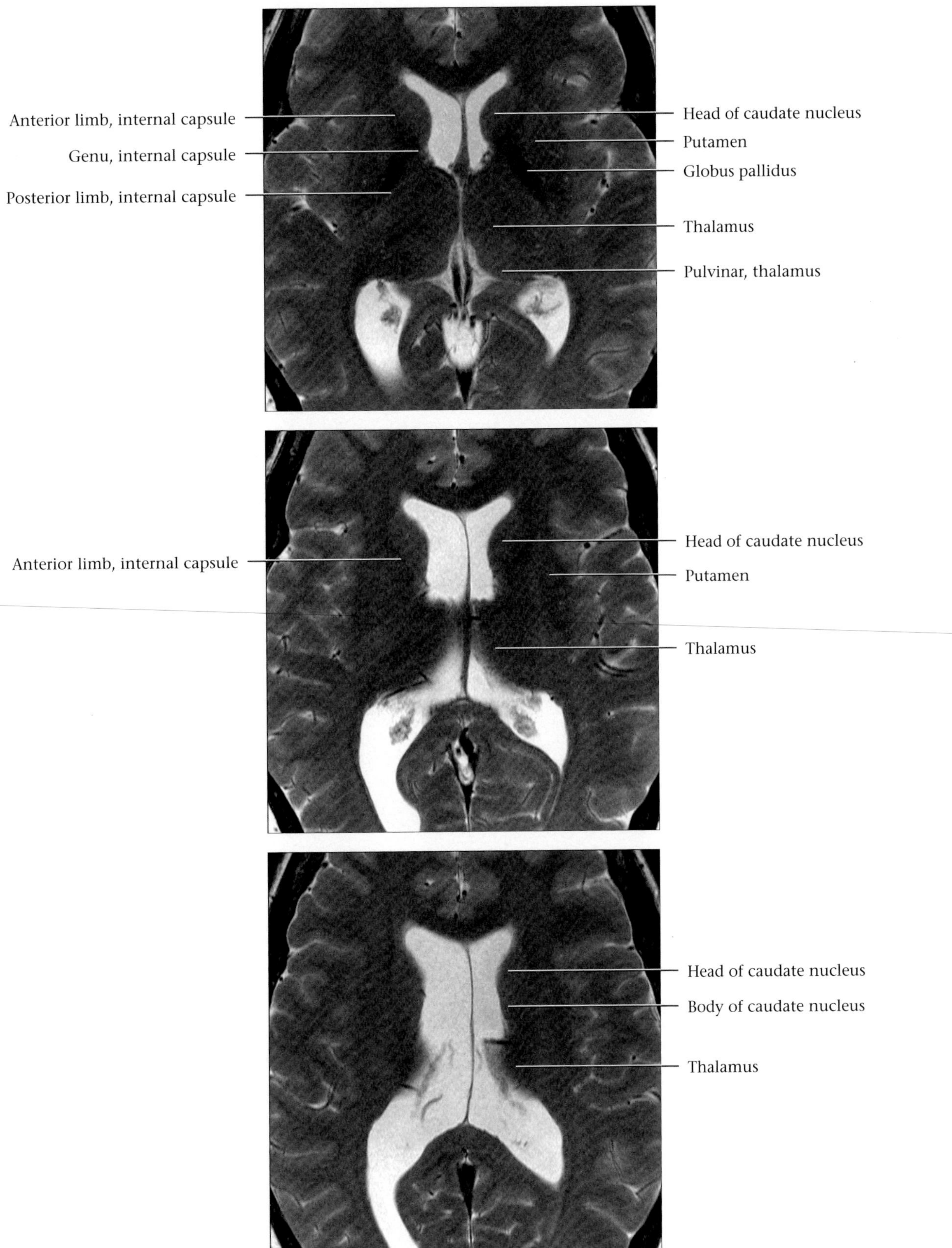
Anterior limb, internal capsule
Genu, internal capsule
Posterior limb, internal capsule
Head of caudate nucleus
Putamen
Globus pallidus
Thalamus
Pulvinar, thalamus
Anterior limb, internal capsule
Head of caudate nucleus
Putamen
Thalamus
Head of caudate nucleus
Body of caudate nucleus
Thalamus

(Top) Image more superior shows basal ganglia & thalamus. Occasionally, a single large thalamoperforator artery, called artery of Percheron or paramedian thalamic artery, supplies both medial thalami & can result in bilateral medial thalamic infarcts. This condition may mimic neoplasm such as lymphoma or glioma on imaging. **(Middle)** This image shows superior thalamus & superior aspects of caudate head & putamen. Anterior limb of internal capsule separates caudate head from putamen, while posterior limb separates thalamus from globus pallidus & putamen. **(Bottom)** Image at level of centrum semiovale shows caudate nucleus as it wraps around lateral ventricles. Huntington disease is characterized by an inability to prevent unwanted movement. Caudate head becomes atrophied in this disease making a "box-car" appearance of frontal horns of lateral ventricles.

BASAL GANGLIA AND THALAMUS

CORONAL STIR MR

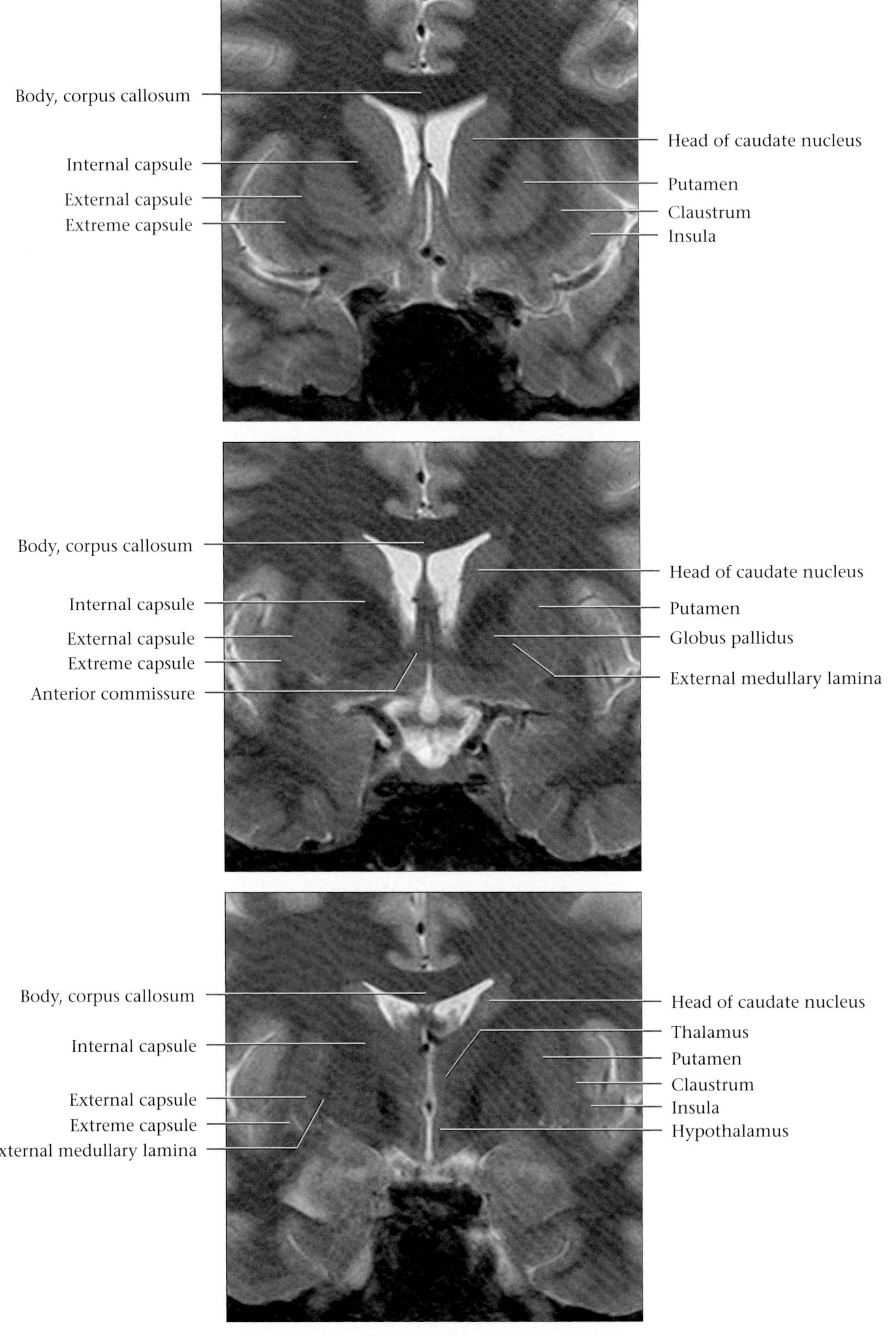
Body, corpus callosum
Internal capsule
External capsule
Extreme capsule
Head of caudate nucleus
Putamen
Claustrum
Insula
Body, corpus callosum
Internal capsule
External capsule
Extreme capsule
Anterior commissure
Head of caudate nucleus
Putamen
Globus pallidus
External medullary lamina
Body, corpus callosum
Internal capsule
External capsule
Extreme capsule
External medullary lamina
Head of caudate nucleus
Thalamus
Putamen
Claustrum
Insula
Hypothalamus

(Top) First of six coronal STIR MR images from anterior to posterior shows caudate head continuous with inferior putamen immediately above anterior perforated substance. Other connections between caudate & putamen can be seen along course of anterior limb of internal capsule. **(Middle)** Image through anterior commissure shows decreased signal of globus pallidus relative to putamen related to increased iron deposition in globus pallidus. Putamen is separated from globus pallidus by external medullary lamina. Globus pallidus contains two segments, lateral & medial, which are not resolved on conventional imaging. **(Bottom)** Image through anterior limb internal capsule. The insula lies deep in floor of sylvian fissure & is overlapped by the operculum. Insula has many connections with thalamus & amygdala, as well as with olfactory & limbic systems.

CORONAL STIR MR

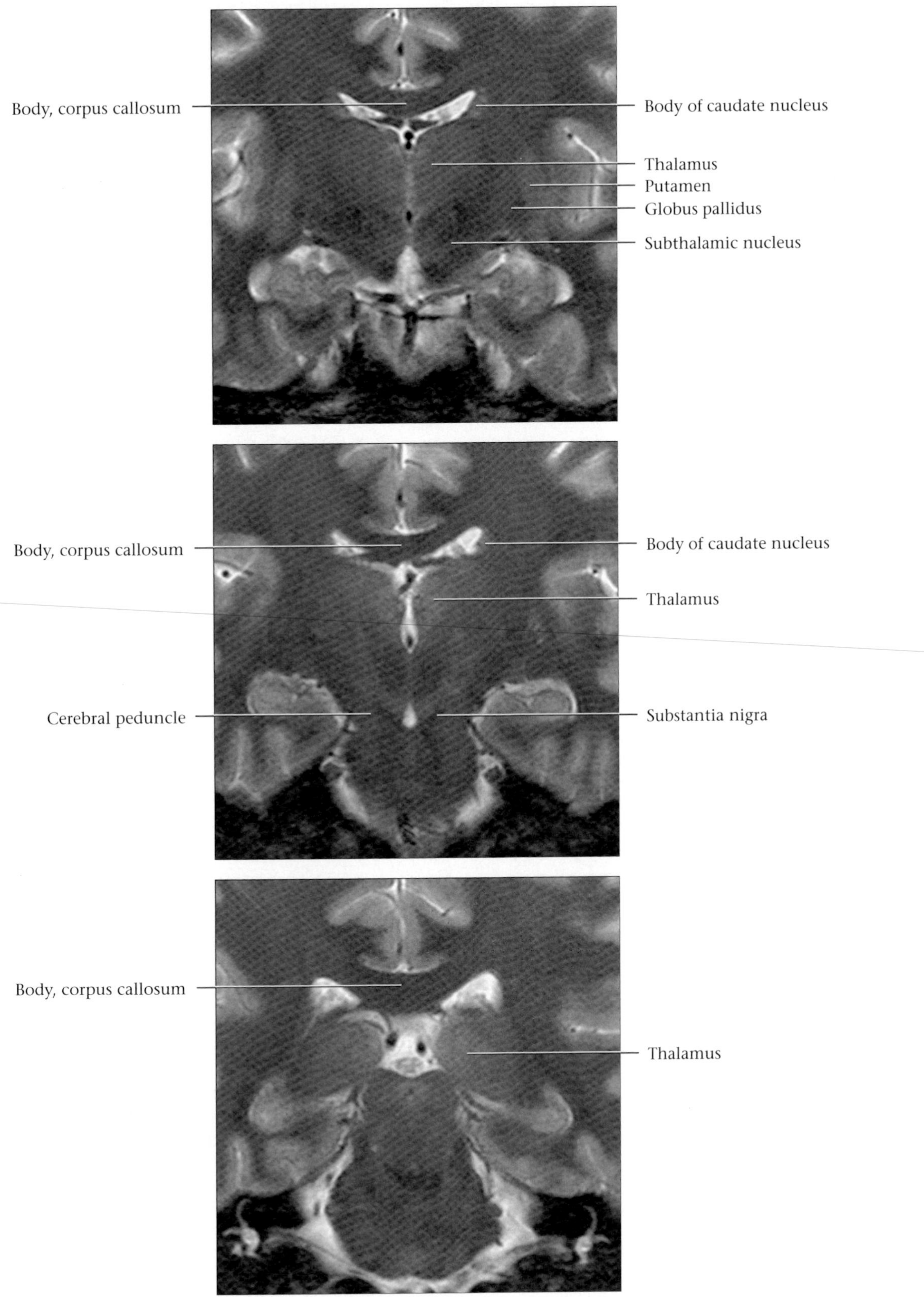
Body, corpus callosum
Body of caudate nucleus
Thalamus
Putamen
Globus pallidus
Subthalamic nucleus
Body, corpus callosum
Body of caudate nucleus
Thalamus
Cerebral peduncle
Substantia nigra
Body, corpus callosum
Thalamus

(Top) Image more posterior through thalamus shows approximate location of subthalamic nucleus which is a biconvex, lens-shaped nucleus medial to internal capsule & superolateral to red nucleus. Subthalamic nucleus plays major role in normal function of basal ganglia. Pathologically, subthalamic nucleus is associated with Parkinson disease & ballism. **(Middle)** Image through thalamus shows pigmented, dopaminergic neurons of substantia nigra. Parkinson disease is most common pathologic condition of basal ganglia, related to degeneration of dopaminergic neurons of substantia nigra & secondary depletion of dopamine in putamen & caudate. **(Bottom)** Image through thalamus shows pulvinar which occupies posterior third of thalamus. Pulvinar function is poorly understood, but it is thought to be an integration nucleus.

LIMBIC SYSTEM

Terminology

Definitions

- Limbic lobe
  - Phylogenetically older cortex
  - Fewer layers than neocortex
  - Major role in memory, olfaction, emotion
  - Composed of subcallosal, cingulate, parahippocampal gyri + hippocampus, dentate gyrus, subiculum, entorhinal cortex
- Limbic system
  - Limbic lobe
  - Plus some subcortical structures (e.g., amygdala, mammillary bodies, septal nuclei, etc.)

Gross Anatomy

Overview

- **Limbic lobe** formed by nested "C-shaped" arches of tissues surrounding diencephalon, basal ganglia
- **Outer arch**
  - Largest of the three arches
  - Extends from temporal to frontal lobes, comprised of
    - Uncus (anterior end of parahippocampal gyrus)
    - Parahippocampal gyrus (swings medially at posterior temporal lobe, becomes isthmus of cingulate gyrus)
    - Cingulate gyrus (anterosuperior continuation of parahippocampal gyrus)
    - Subcallosal (paraolfactory area) is anteroinferior continuation of cingulate gyrus
  - Curves above callosal sulcus (continuous with hippocampal sulcus of temporal lobe)
- **Middle arch**
  - Extends from temporal to frontal lobes, comprised of
    - Hippocampus proper (Ammon horn)
    - Dentate gyrus
    - Supracallosal gyrus (indusium griseum, a thin strip of gray matter that extends from dentate/hippocampus all the way around corpus callosum to paraterminal gyrus)
    - Paraterminal gyrus (below corpus callosum rostrum)
  - Curves over corpus callosum, below callosal sulcus
- **Inner arch**
  - Smallest arch
  - Extends from temporal lobe to mamillary bodies
  - Comprised of fornix, fimbria

Imaging Anatomy

Overview

- **Hippocampus**
  - Curved structure on medial aspect of temporal lobe that bulges into floor of temporal horn
  - Consists of two interlocking "U-shaped" gray matter structures
    - Hippocampus proper (Ammon horn) forms more superolateral, upside-down **U**
    - Dentate gyrus forms inferomedial **U**
  - Has three anatomic subdivisions
    - Head (pes hippocampus): Most anterior part, oriented transversely; has 3-4 digitations on superior surface
    - Body: Cylindrical, oriented parasagittally
    - Tail: Most posterior portion; narrows then curves around splenium to form indusium griseum above corpus callosum (CC)
- **Ammon horn** (hippocampus proper)
  - Subdivided into four zones (based on histology of main cell layers)
    - CA1 (Sommer sector): Small pyramidal cells (most vulnerable; commonly affected by anoxia, mesial temporal sclerosis)
    - CA2: Narrow, dense band of large pyramidal cells ("resistant sector")
    - CA3: Wide loose band of large pyramidal cells
    - CA4 (end-folium): Loosely structured inner zone, enveloped by dentate gyrus
  - Blends laterally into subiculum
    - Subiculum forms transition to neocortex of parahippocampal gyrus (entorhinal cortex)
  - Covered by layer of efferent fibers, the alveus
    - Alveus borders temporal horn of lateral ventricle ventricle
    - Forms fimbria → crus of fornix
- **Fornix**
  - Primary efferent system from hippocampus
  - Four parts
    - Crura (arch under CC splenium, form part of medial wall of lateral ventricles)
    - Commissure (connects crura)
    - Body (formed by convergence of crura, attached to inferior surface of septum pellucidum)
    - Columns (curve inferiorly to mammillary bodies, anterior thalamus, mamillary bodies, septal nuclei)
- **Amygdala**
  - Large complex of gray nuclei medial to uncus, just in front of temporal horn of lateral ventricle
  - Tail of caudate nucleus ends in amygdala
  - Major efferent is stria terminalis
    - Stria terminalis arches in sulcus between caudate nucleus, thalamus
    - Forms one margin of choroid fissure (other is fornix)

Anatomy-Based Imaging Issues

Imaging Recommendations

- MR is best performed in a slightly oblique plane, perpendicular to long axis of hippocampus
  - Coronal T1 volume images (SPGR): 1-3 mm
  - Coronal T2 high-resolution: 2.5-3 mm
  - Coronal FLAIR whole brain: 4-5 mm

Imaging Pitfalls

- Normal variant is incomplete fusion of hippocampal sulcus → CSF-containing "cysts" along medial hippocampus

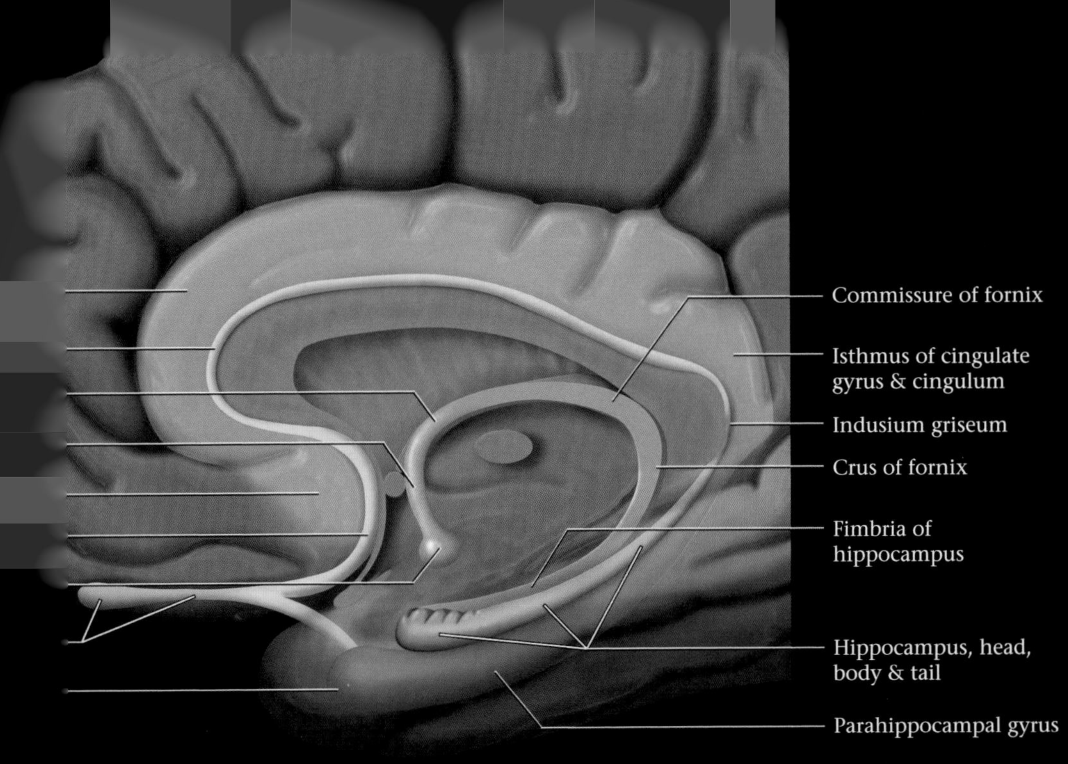

Commissure of fornix
Isthmus of cingulate gyrus & cingulum
Indusium griseum
Crus of fornix
Fimbria of hippocampus
Hippocampus, head, body & tail
Parahippocampal gyrus

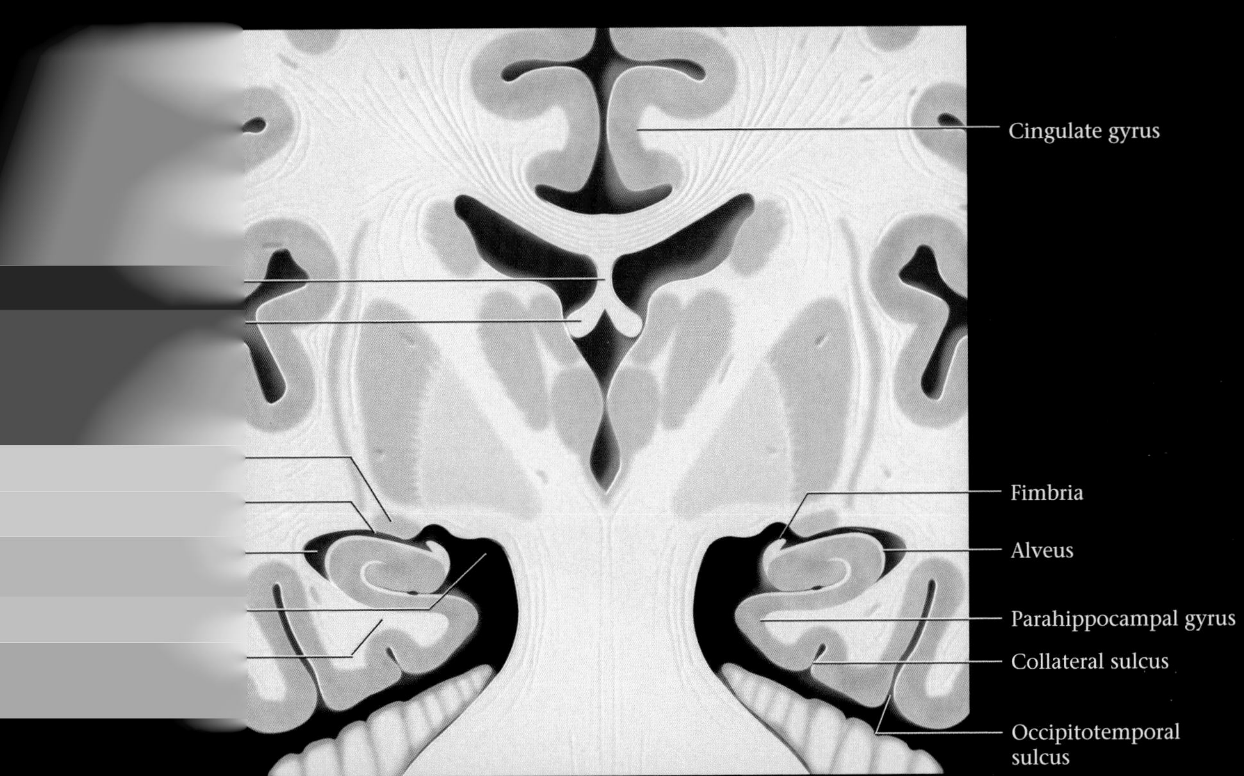
Cingulate gyrus
Fimbria
Alveus
Parahippocampal gyrus
Collateral sulcus
Occipitotemporal sulcus

ws 3 arches of limbic system. Outer arch (blue) is parahippocampal gyrus-cingulate gyrus. ppocampus-indusium griseum & inner arch (purple) is fimbria-fornix. Hippocampus lies at largely covered by parahippocampal gyrus. Hippocampus extends to corpus callosum es a thin layer of gray matter, indusium griseum. Indusium griseum continues along to end near anterior commissure. Fimbria on dorsal hippocampus continue as fornix which body. **(Bottom)** Coronal graphic at level of anterior third ventricle & columns of fornix. ociation fibers which lie deep to cingulate gyrus cannot be separated from cingulate gyrus. atter which extends along superior corpus callosum is also not seen on imaging.

GRAPHIC & HISTOLOGY

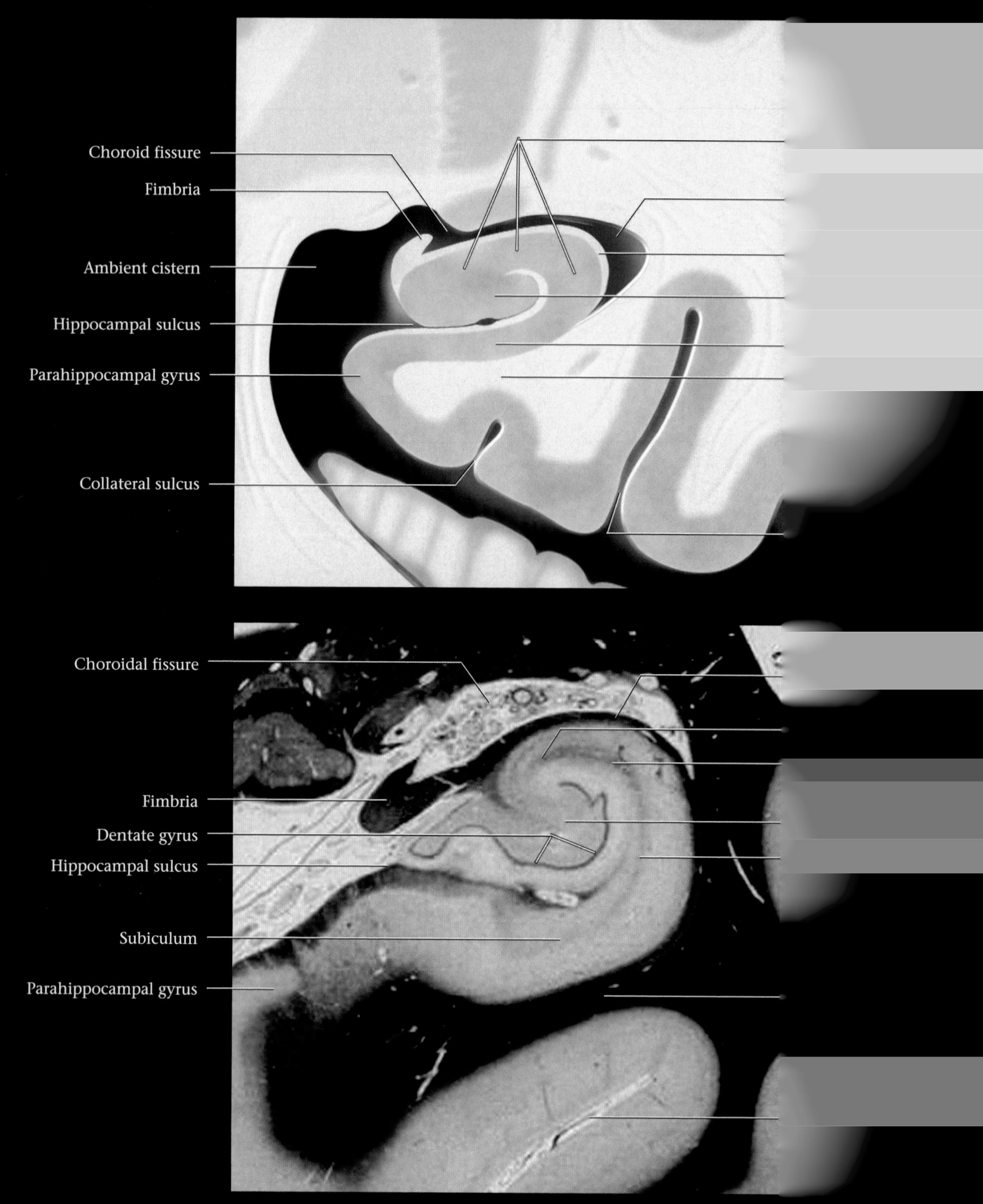
Choroid fissure
Fimbria
Ambient cistern
Hippocampal sulcus
Parahippocampal gyrus
Collateral sulcus
Choroidal fissure
Fimbria
Dentate gyrus
Hippocampal sulcus
Subiculum
Parahippocampal gyrus

(Top) Coronal graphic shows hippocampus & surrounding structures. Hippocampus is a cur aspect of temporal lobe. It is composed of two "U-shaped" gray matter structures, dentate gy (cornu ammonis) which are interlocked. Ammon horn is further subdivided into 4 parts bas cell density. Ammon horn blends into the subiculum, transitional area between Ammon ho entorhinal cortex, the parahippocampal gyrus. White matter tracts extend from Ammon ho converge to form fimbria. **(Bottom)** Coronal histology section of hippocampus shows interl Ammon horn & dentate gyrus. Ammon horn is divided into fields CA1, CA2, CA3 and CA4. dentate gyrus. Alveus contains efferent fibers from Ammon horn which continue along as fi

LIMBIC SYSTEM

CORONAL T1 MR

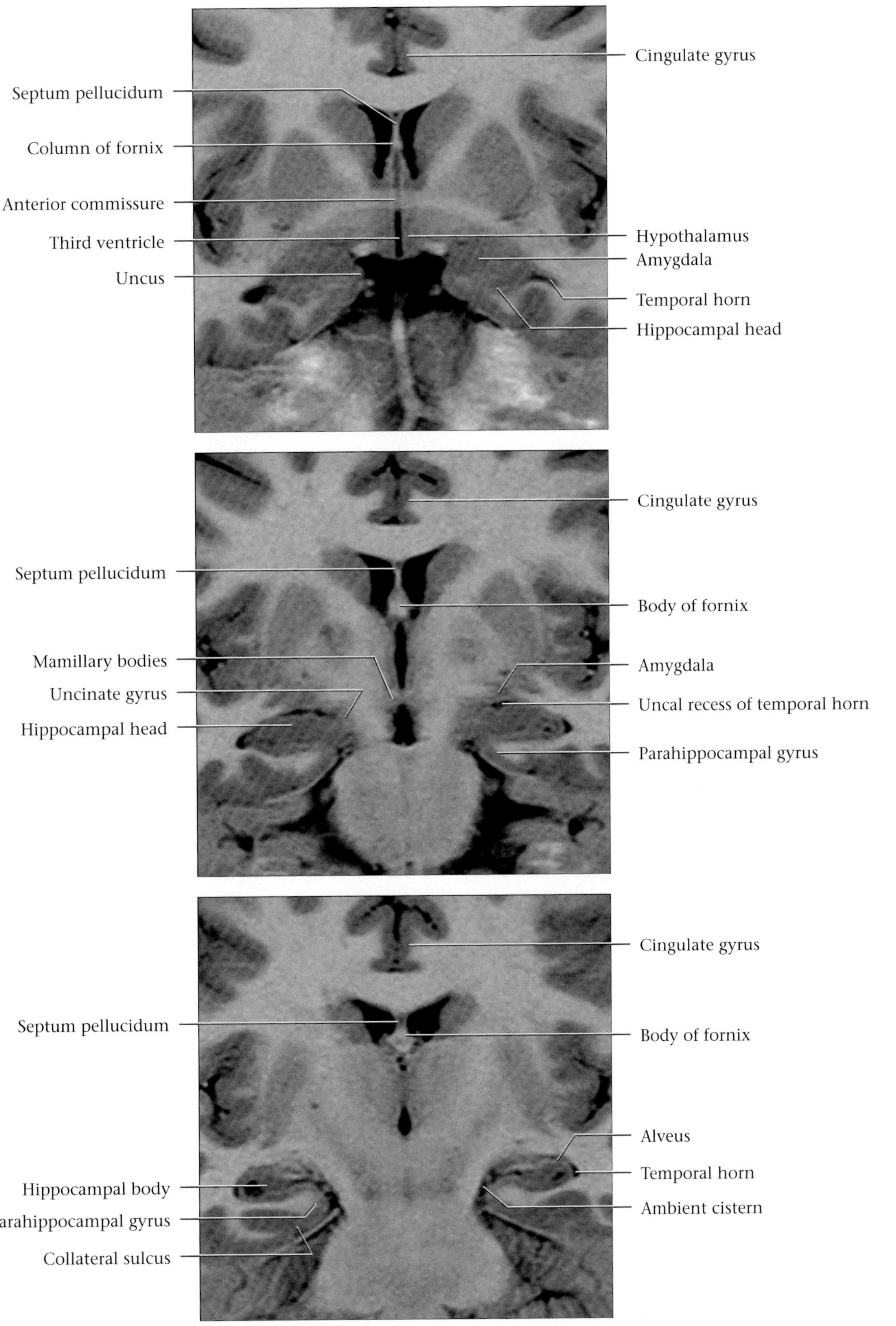
Cingulate gyrus
Septum pellucidum
Column of fornix
Anterior commissure
Third ventricle
Uncus
Hypothalamus
Amygdala
Temporal horn
Hippocampal head
Cingulate gyrus
Septum pellucidum
Body of fornix
Mamillary bodies
Uncinate gyrus
Hippocampal head
Amygdala
Uncal recess of temporal horn
Parahippocampal gyrus
Cingulate gyrus
Septum pellucidum
Body of fornix
Alveus
Temporal horn
Ambient cistern
Hippocampal body
Parahippocampal gyrus
Collateral sulcus

(Top) First of six coronal T1 MR images through limbic system from anterior to posterior. Note amygdala lies anterior & superior to hippocampus, at medial aspect of temporal lobe, just lateral to the uncus. Tail of caudate nucleus ends in amygdala. Pes hippocampus (hippocampal head) lies just posterior to amygdala. Anterior commissure contains crossing fibers of temporal cortex, amygdala & stria terminales. **(Middle)** A more posterior image through third ventricle shows digitations of the hippocampal head (pes hippocampus). The hippocampus is separated from amygdala by uncal recess of temporal horn. The uncinate gyrus connects medial hippocampus with amygdala. **(Bottom)** More posterior image shows hippocampal body with loss of hippocampal head digitations. Hippocampal body is bordered medially by ambient cistern & laterally by temporal horn of lateral ventricle.

LIMBIC SYSTEM

CORONAL T1 MR

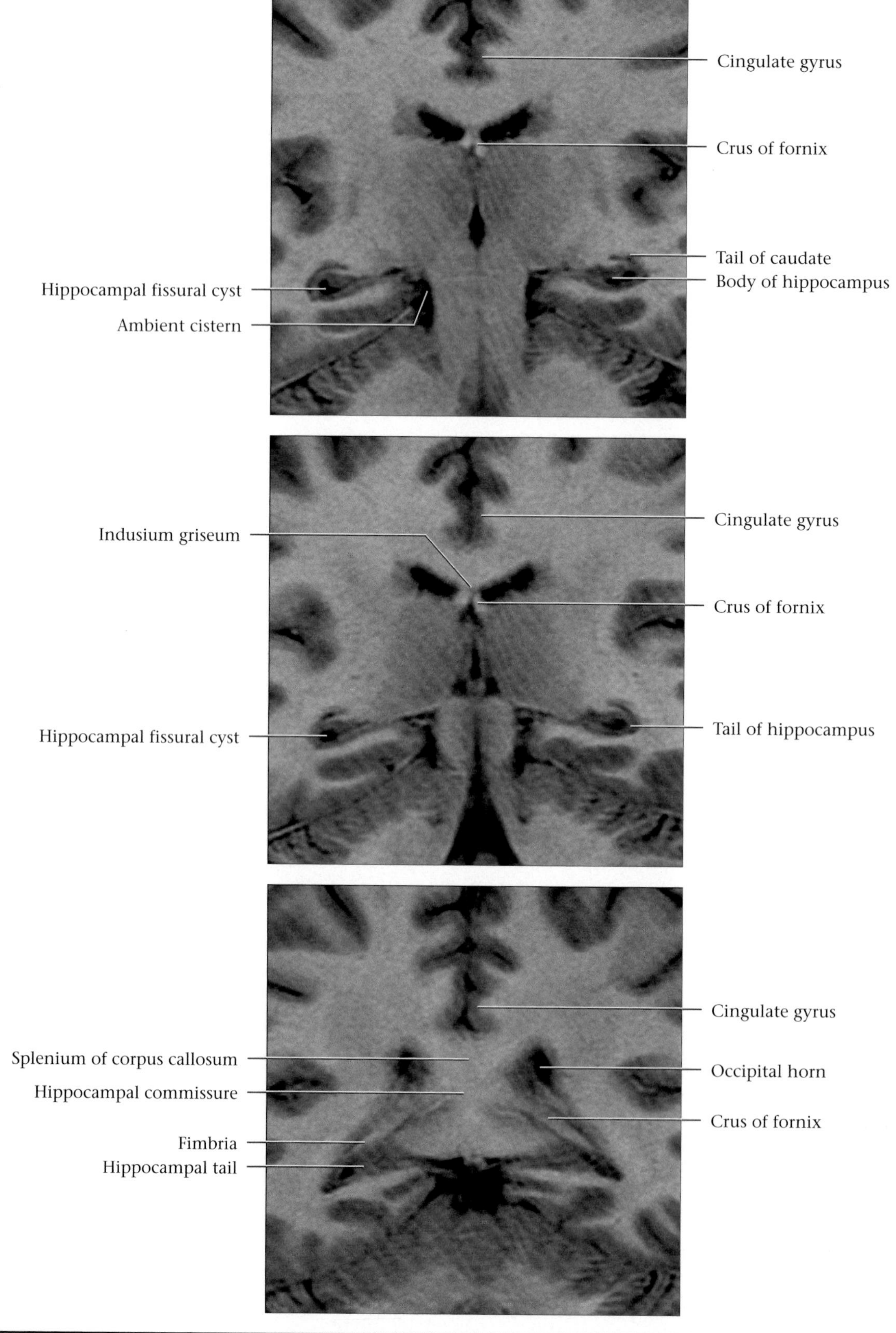
Cingulate gyrus
Crus of fornix
Tail of caudate
Body of hippocampus
Hippocampal fissural cyst
Ambient cistern
Indusium griseum
Cingulate gyrus
Crus of fornix
Hippocampal fissural cyst
Tail of hippocampus
Cingulate gyrus
Splenium of corpus callosum
Occipital horn
Hippocampal commissure
Crus of fornix
Fimbria
Hippocampal tail

(Top) A more posterior image through mid thalamus shows crura of fornices which join anteriorly to form body of fornix. The body of hippocampus typically shows the normal internal architecture of hippocampus. In this case, there are hippocampal fissural cysts bilaterally which mildly distort the typical architecture. These cysts are benign & represent partially unfused hippocampal sulcus. **(Middle)** Image at posterior thalamus shows tail of hippocampus. Tail is narrowest portion of hippocampus as it extends posteriorly. Indusium griseum may be the tiny area of gray matter above corpus callosum. **(Bottom)** Image through splenium of corpus callosum shows fimbria as it becomes crus of fornix. The crus attaches to anterior surface of splenium of corpus callosum. At inferior corpus callosum, the two crus of fornix unite to form commissure of fornix (hippocampal commissure).

CORONAL T2 MR

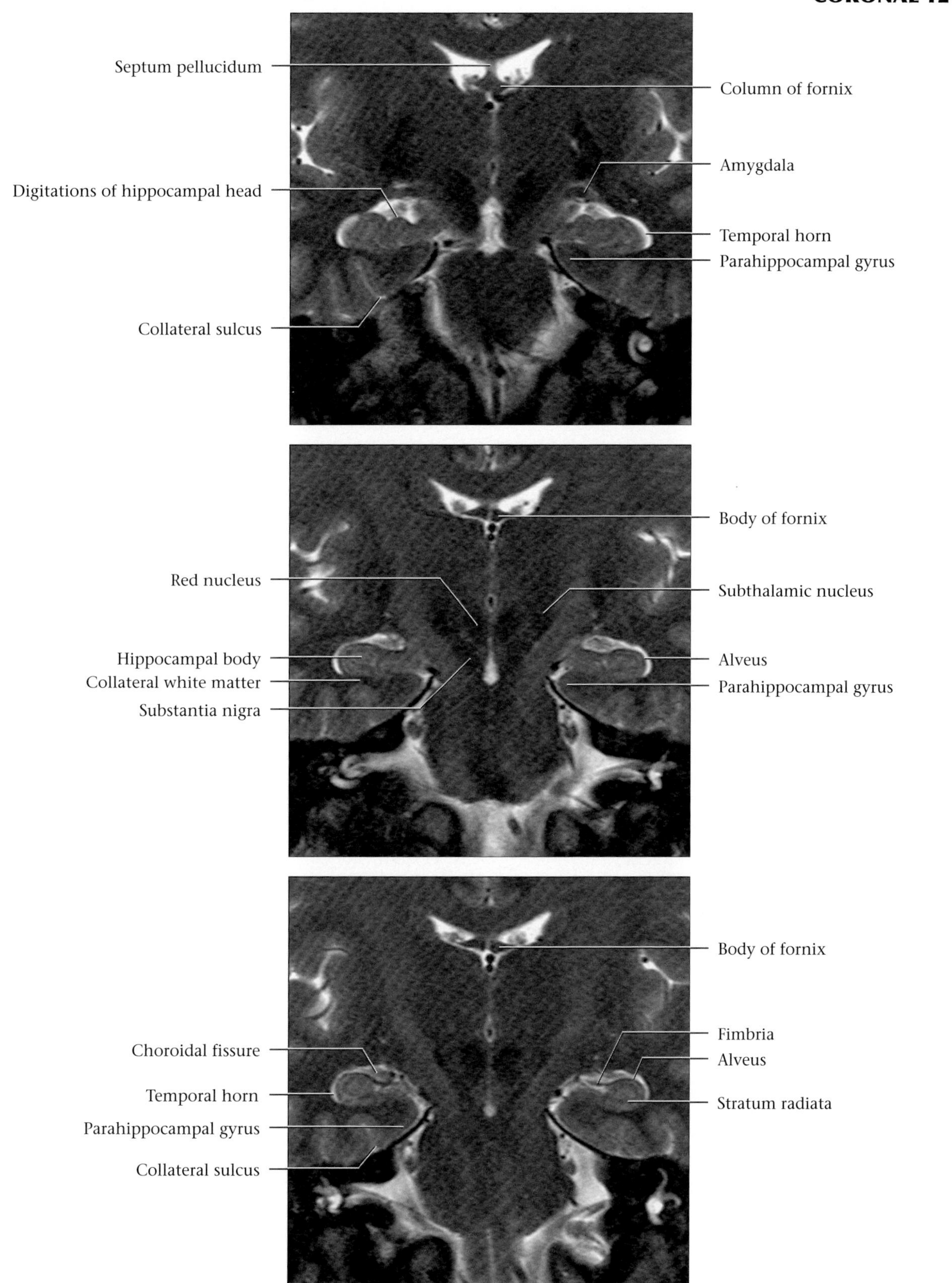
Septum pellucidum
Column of fornix
Amygdala
Digitations of hippocampal head
Temporal horn
Parahippocampal gyrus
Collateral sulcus
Body of fornix
Red nucleus
Subthalamic nucleus
Hippocampal body
Alveus
Collateral white matter
Parahippocampal gyrus
Substantia nigra
Body of fornix
Fimbria
Choroidal fissure
Alveus
Temporal horn
Stratum radiata
Parahippocampal gyrus
Collateral sulcus

(Top) First of six coronal T2 MR images through limbic system from anterior to posterior. Hippocampal head (pes hippocampus) is recognized by digitations on its superior surface. Amygdala is separated from hippocampus by uncal recess of temporal horn or alveus of hippocampus. **(Middle)** Image more posterior shows body of hippocampus which loses digitations seen in head. Body of fornix arcs over thalamus to split into two anterior columns which curve anterior to foramen of Monro & send fibers to mamillary bodies, anterior thalamus & septal region. **(Bottom)** More posteriorly, hippocampal body is seen with its normal architecture. The stratum radiata primarily makes up white matter between Ammon horn & dentate gyrus. Loss of this normal architecture is one of major features of mesial temporal sclerosis. Other major features are bright T2 signal & atrophy.

LIMBIC SYSTEM

CORONAL T2 MR

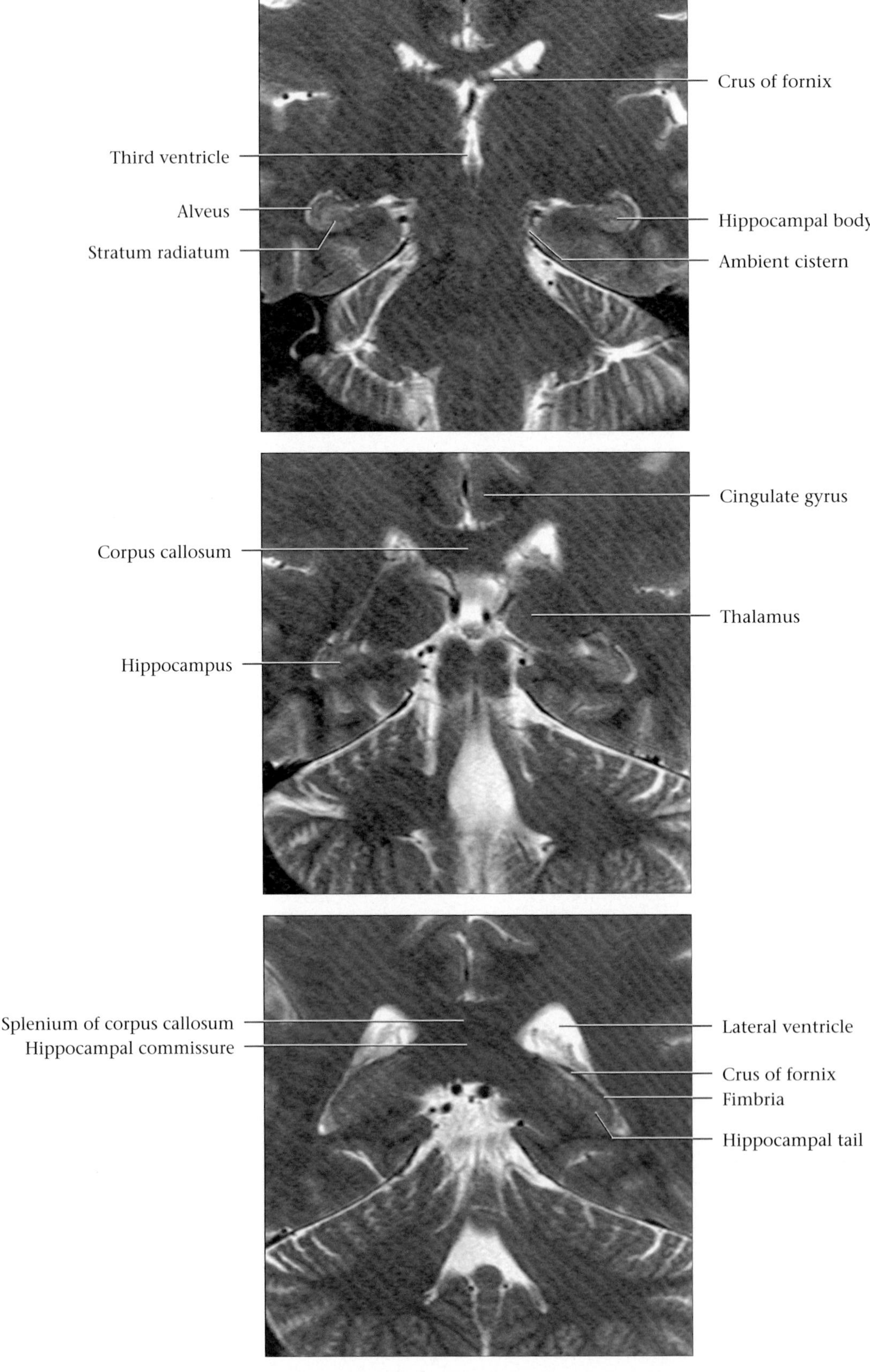
Crus of fornix
Third ventricle
Alveus
Hippocampal body
Stratum radiatum
Ambient cistern
Cingulate gyrus
Corpus callosum
Thalamus
Hippocampus
Splenium of corpus callosum
Hippocampal commissure
Lateral ventricle
Crus of fornix
Fimbria
Hippocampal tail

(Top) Image more posteriorly through thalamus shows crus of fornix. Hippocampal body is seen with its normal architecture, bordered laterally by temporal horn of lateral ventricle & medially by ambient cistern. In mesial temporal sclerosis, the hippocampal body is affected in approximately 90% of patients. Typically CA1 & CA4 regions are most affected by mesial temporal sclerosis, although the entire Ammon horn & dentate gyrus may be involved. **(Middle)** Image at posterior thalamus (pulvinar) shows transition of hippocampal body to hippocampal tail, the most narrow portion of hippocampus. **(Bottom)** Image through splenium of corpus callosum shows fimbria arising from hippocampus & becoming crus of fornix. Crus attach to anterior splenium. At inferior corpus callosum, two crus of fornix unite to form hippocampal commissure (commissure of fornix).

CORONAL T2 MR

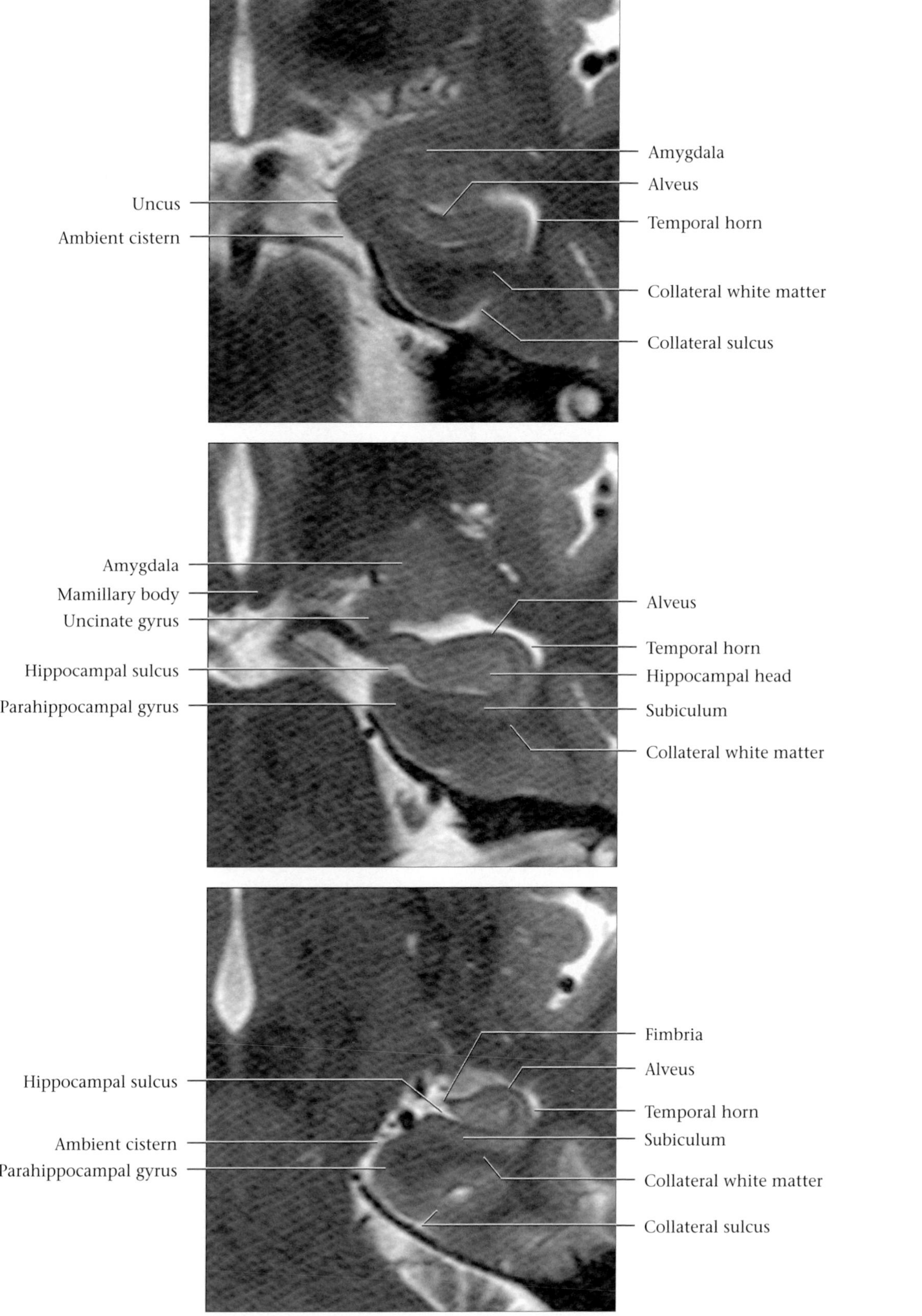
Amygdala
Alveus
Uncus
Temporal horn
Ambient cistern
Collateral white matter
Collateral sulcus
Amygdala
Mamillary body
Alveus
Uncinate gyrus
Temporal horn
Hippocampal sulcus
Hippocampal head
Parahippocampal gyrus
Subiculum
Collateral white matter
Fimbria
Alveus
Hippocampal sulcus
Temporal horn
Subiculum
Ambient cistern
Parahippocampal gyrus
Collateral white matter
Collateral sulcus

(Top) First of three high-resolution coronal T2 MR images through anterior aspect of limbic system. Amygdala is anterior & superior to head of hippocampus. Amygdala is separated from hippocampus by alveus or uncal recess of temporal horn. **(Middle)** Image at hippocampal head shows typical digitations at superior margin. Note uncinate gyrus which connects medial hippocampus with amygdala. Mamillary body is well seen along the inferior third ventricle. Mamillary body may be atrophied in severe cases of mesial temporal sclerosis as can the fornix. **(Bottom)** Image at hippocampal body shows normal hippocampal architecture. Hippocampal sulcus is typically closed in adult patients, as seen here. Parahippocampal gyrus (entorhinal cortex) continues as cingulate gyrus under splenium of corpus callosum & above body of corpus callosum as part of the limbic lobe.

LIMBIC SYSTEM

AXIAL T2 MR

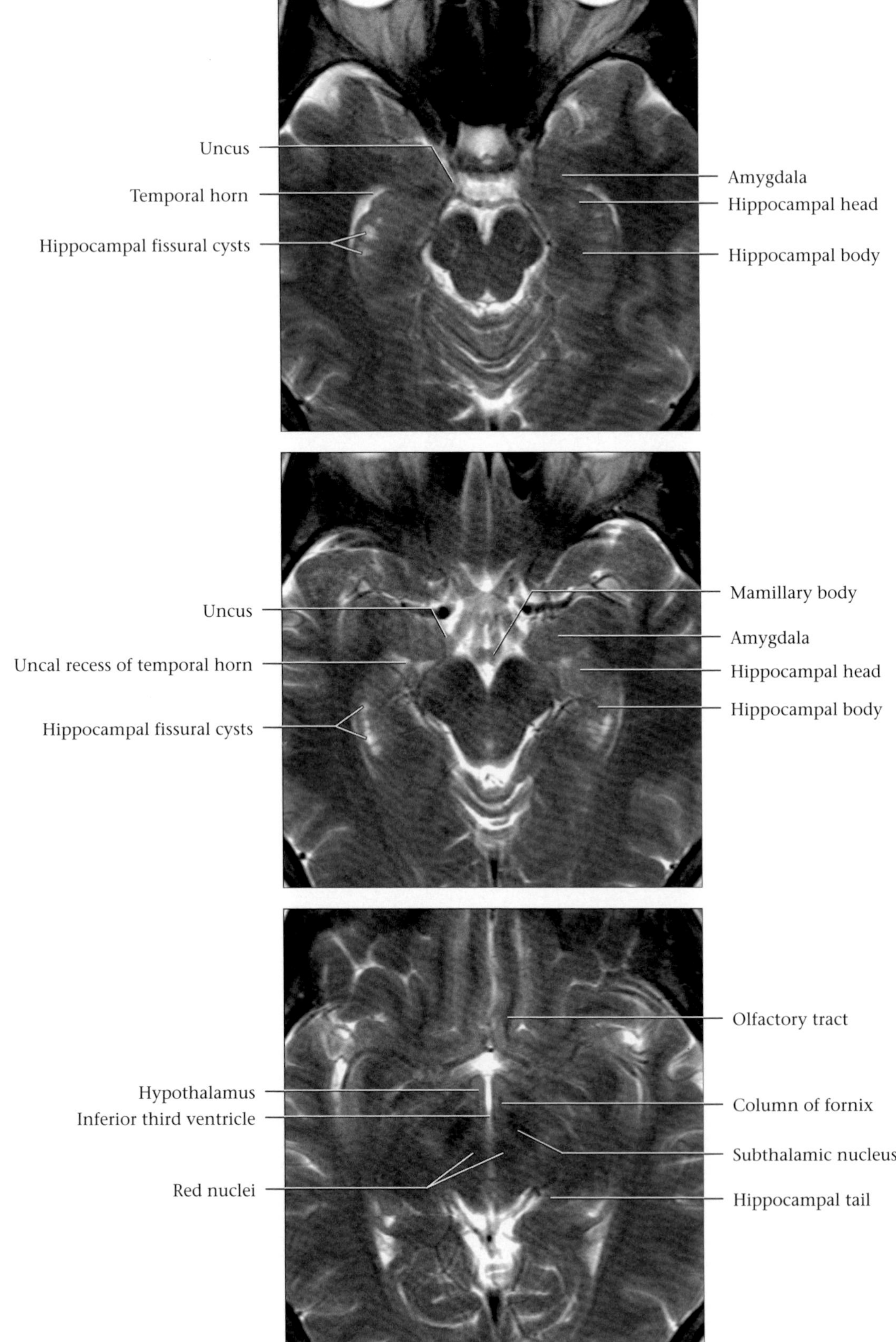
Uncus
Temporal horn
Hippocampal fissural cysts
Amygdala
Hippocampal head
Hippocampal body
Uncus
Uncal recess of temporal horn
Hippocampal fissural cysts
Mamillary body
Amygdala
Hippocampal head
Hippocampal body
Olfactory tract
Hypothalamus
Inferior third ventricle
Red nuclei
Column of fornix
Subthalamic nucleus
Hippocampal tail

(Top) First of three axial T2 MR images from inferior to superior at level of cerebral peduncles shows hippocampus & amygdala. Note failure of normal involution of hippocampal sulcus resulting in hippocampal fissural cysts (hippocampal sulcus remnants). These cysts are usually bilateral & occur between dentate gyrus & Ammon horn. This normal variant occurs in 10-15% of patients. **(Middle)** More superior image shows hippocampal head, body. Uncal recess of temporal horn separates amygdala from hippocampus. Mamillary bodies lie in interpeduncular cistern. Uncus forms lateral border of suprasellar cistern. **(Bottom)** Image through superior aspect of midbrain/inferior third ventricle shows hypothalamus, fornix, olfactory tract. Hippocampal tail is seen curving posteriorly around midbrain. Subthalamic nucleus is almond-shaped, lies anterolateral to red nucleus.

LIMBIC SYSTEM

SAGITTAL T1 MR

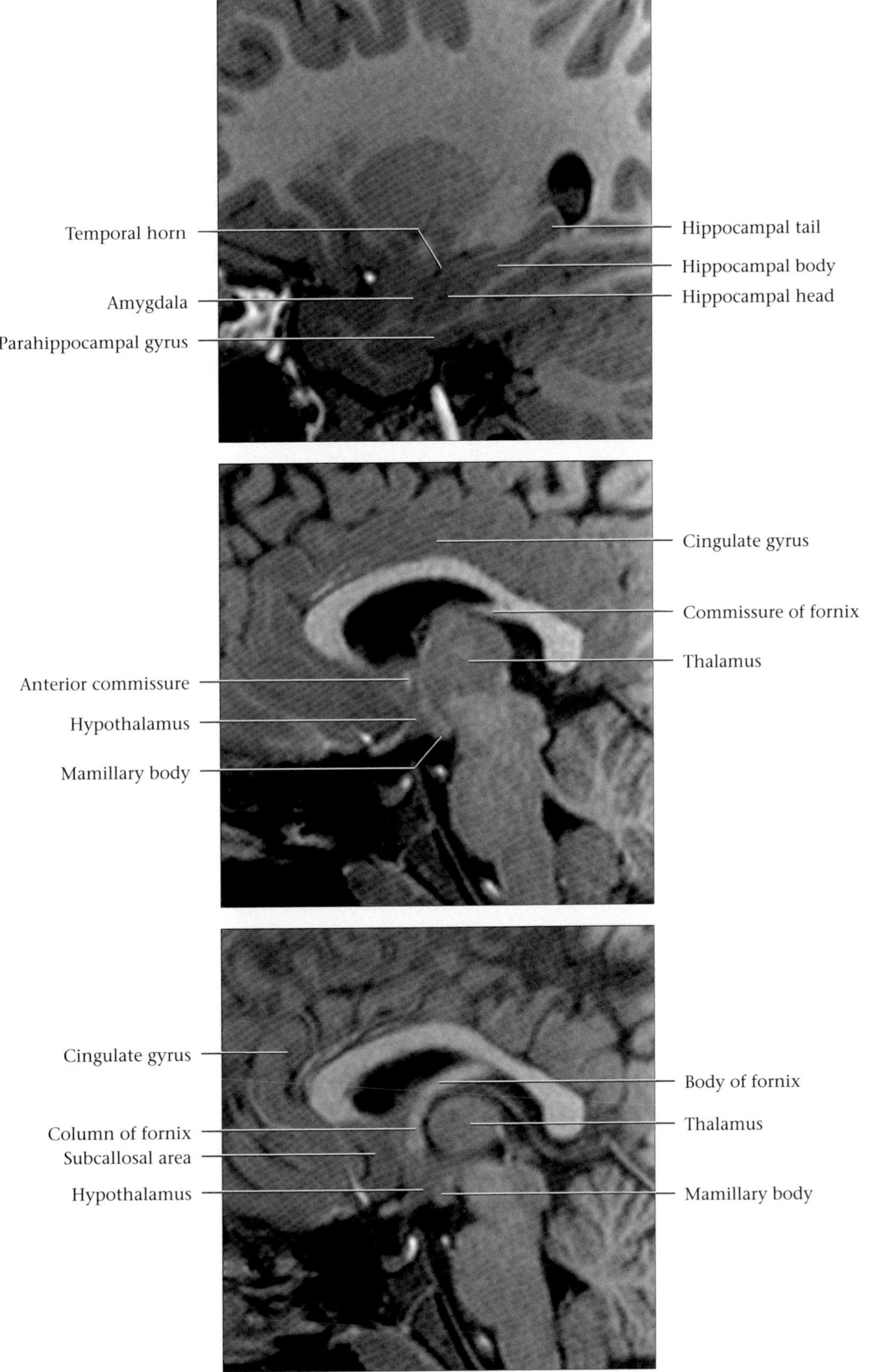
Temporal horn
Amygdala
Parahippocampal gyrus
Hippocampal tail
Hippocampal body
Hippocampal head
Cingulate gyrus
Commissure of fornix
Thalamus
Anterior commissure
Hypothalamus
Mamillary body
Cingulate gyrus
Column of fornix
Subcallosal area
Hypothalamus
Body of fornix
Thalamus
Mamillary body

(Top) First of three sagittal T1 MR images from lateral to medial shows hippocampus & amygdala. Note thin temporal horn which separates amygdala anteriorly from hippocampal head posteriorly. **(Middle)** A more medial image shows commissure of fornix as it extends under body of corpus callosum. Anterior commissure is seen in cross section as it crosses anterior to columns of fornix within anterior third ventricle. Anterior commissure divides into small anterior bundle which connects anterior perforated substance & olfactory tracts, while larger posterior bundle connects medial temporal gyrus, amygdala & stria terminalis. **(Bottom)** Midline sagittal image shows body of fornix which divides at anterior thalamus to become columns of fornix. Fornix ends in anterior thalamus, mamillary body & septal region. Cingulate gyrus continues anteriorly to become subcallosal area.

SELLA, PITUITARY AND CAVERNOUS SINUS

Terminology

Abbreviations

- Adenohypophysis (AH); neurohypophysis (NH)

Synonyms

- Pituitary gland = hypophysis

Gross Anatomy

Overview

- **Sella** (concave midline depression in basisphenoid)
  - Anterior borders: Tuberculum sellae, anterior clinoid processes of lesser sphenoid wing
  - Posterior borders: Dorsum sellae, posterior clinoid processes
  - Dural reflections
    - Diaphragma sellae covers sella
    - Variable-sized central opening transmits infundibulum
    - Dura lines floor of hypophyseal fossa
- **Hypophysis** (pituitary gland)
  - **Adenohypophysis**
    - 80% of gland; wraps anterolaterally around NH
    - Includes pars anterior (pars distalis or glandularis), pars intermedia, pars tuberalis
    - Function: Cells secrete somato-, lactogenic, other hormones
    - Vascular supply: Venous (portal venous via hypothalamus)
  - **Pars intermedia**
    - < 5% of pituitary, located between AH/NH
    - Contains axons from hypothalamus, infundibulum
    - Function: Carries releasing hormones to AH, NH
  - **Neurohypophysis**
    - 20% of pituitary
    - Includes pars posterior (nervosa), infundibular stem, median eminence of tuber cinereum
    - Contains pituicytes, hypothalamohypophysial tract
    - Function: Stores vasopressin, oxytocin from hypothalamus
    - Vascular supply: Arterial (superior and inferior hypophyseal arteries)
- **Cavernous sinuses** (CS)
  - Paired septated, dural-lined venous sinuses that lack valves
    - Communicate with each other, clival plexus via intercavernous, basal venous sinuses; posteriorly to transverse sinuses via superior petrosal sinuses
    - Drain inferiorly to pterygoid venous plexi via emissary veins, to IJV via inferior petrosal sinuses
    - Thicker lateral, thinner medial dural walls enclose CS, separate it from pituitary
    - Posteriorly dural walls enclose Meckel cave (arachnoid-lined, CSF-filled extension of prepontine cistern; contains fascicles of CN5, trigeminal ganglion)
  - Venous tributaries
    - Superior, inferior ophthalmic veins
    - Sphenoparietal sinus
  - Contents (venous blood, cranial nerves, ICAs + sympathetic plexus)
    - **CN3** lies within superior lateral dural wall
    - **CN4** just below CN3
    - **V1** (ophthalmic division of CN5) in lateral wall below CN4
    - **V2** (maxillary division of CN5) is most inferior CN in lateral CS wall
    - **V3** (mandibular division of CN5) does NOT enter CS proper (passes from Meckel cave inferiorly into foramen ovale)
    - **CN6** lies within CS proper, next to ICA

Imaging Anatomy

Overview

- Hypophysis
  - NH usually has short T1 (posterior pituitary "bright spot") caused by vasopressin/oxytocin (NOT fat!)
  - Gland enhances strongly, uniformly, somewhat < CS
    - 15-20% of normal patients have incidental finding of "filling defects" on T1 C+ MR (cyst, nonfunctioning microadenoma)
- CS (inconstantly visualized at DSA)
  - Strong, uniform enhancement on CT, T1 C+ MR
  - Lateral dural walls should be flat or concave
  - Medial dural walls difficult to image even at 3T

Anatomy-Based Imaging Issues

Imaging Recommendations

- MR for pituitary, hypothalamic imaging
  - Coronal/sagittal, 2 mm, small FOV
    - Pre-contrast T1-, T2WI
    - T1 C+ with fat-saturated helpful in differentiating post-operative fat packing from enhancing tissue
  - "Dynamic" scan with rapid bolus of contrast, sequential scans sorted by slice q10-12 secs

Normal Variants

- Normal size, configuration of pituitary varies with age, gender
  - ≤ 6 mm children; 8 mm males, post-menopausal females; physiologic hypertrophy with 10 mm upper limit in young females (can bulge upwards); 12 mm pregnant/lactating females
- "Empty" sella
  - Protrusion of arachnoid, CSF into sella
  - Normal pituitary becomes flatted, displaced posteroinferiorly against sellar floor
  - Rarely symptomatic (may be associated with pseudotumor cerebri)

Imaging Pitfalls

- Paramedian ICAs ("kissing carotids") can mimic intrasellar aneurysm, compress pituitary
- Anterior clinoid pneumatization may mimic ICA aneurysms
- Asymmetric skull base marrow (short T1) can mimic pathology: Fat-saturated MR or CT resolves
- Suprasellar "bright spot" usually ectopic NH, less often lipoma, etc.

GRAPHICS

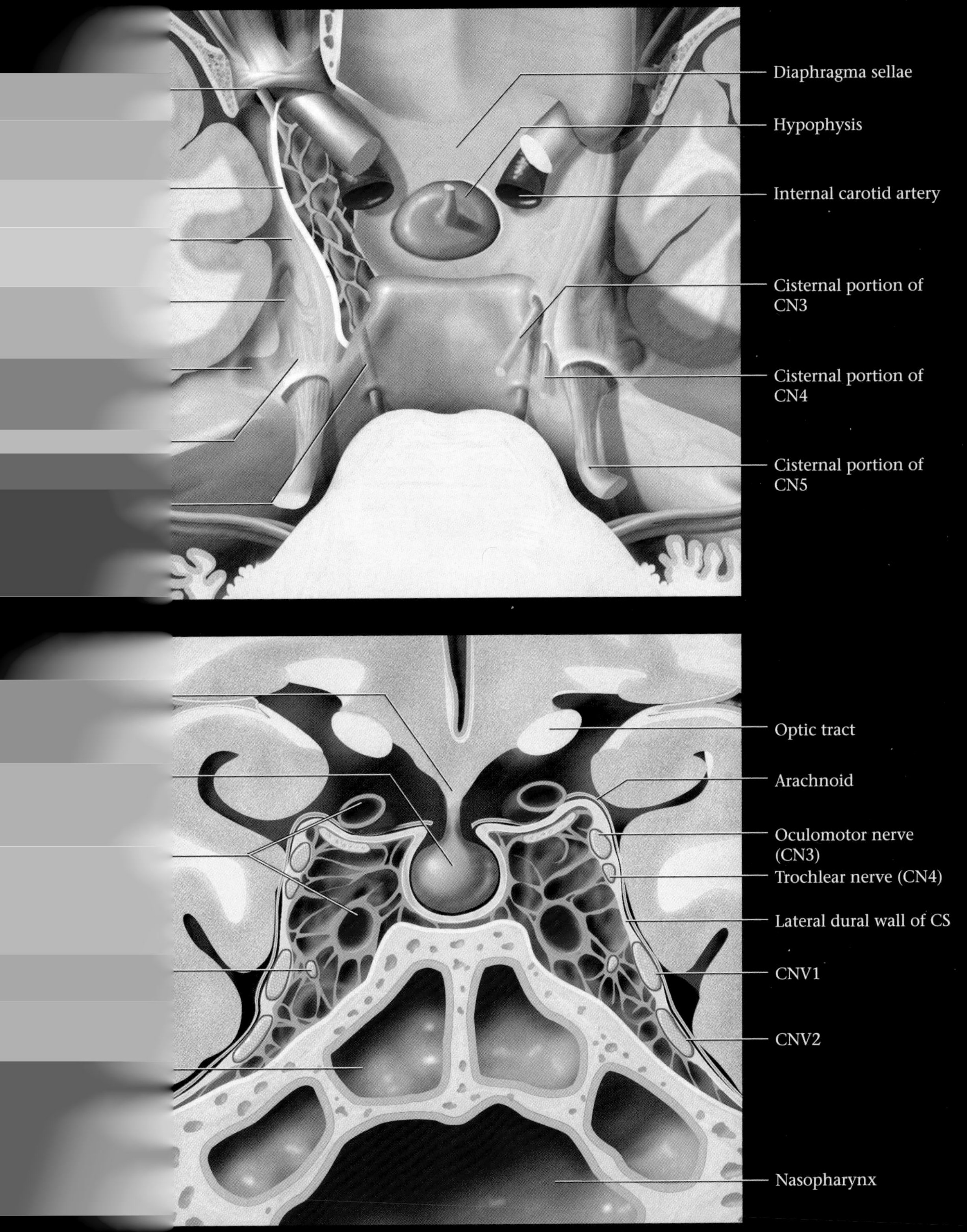
Diaphragma sellae
Hypophysis
Internal carotid artery
Cisternal portion of CN3
Cisternal portion of CN4
Cisternal portion of CN5
Optic tract
Arachnoid
Oculomotor nerve (CN3)
Trochlear nerve (CN4)
Lateral dural wall of CS
CNV1
CNV2
Nasopharynx

... sella turcica, as viewed from above, depicts normal sellar and parasellar anatomy. Dura ...ous sinus is removed to show CN5 & 6. All CNs are shown in the left CS. The mandibular ... run through the CS but exits from Meckel cave inferiorly to enter foramen ovale. Note the ... channel but is extensively septated. **(Bottom)** Coronal graphic depicting contents of the ... llowing cranial nerves traverse the cavernous sinus within the lateral wall of the cavernous ... ferior: Oculomotor (CN3), trochlear (CN4), first (ophthalmic or V1) and second (maxillary ... inal (CN5) nerves. The only cranial nerve actually within the venous sinusoids of the

GRAPHICS

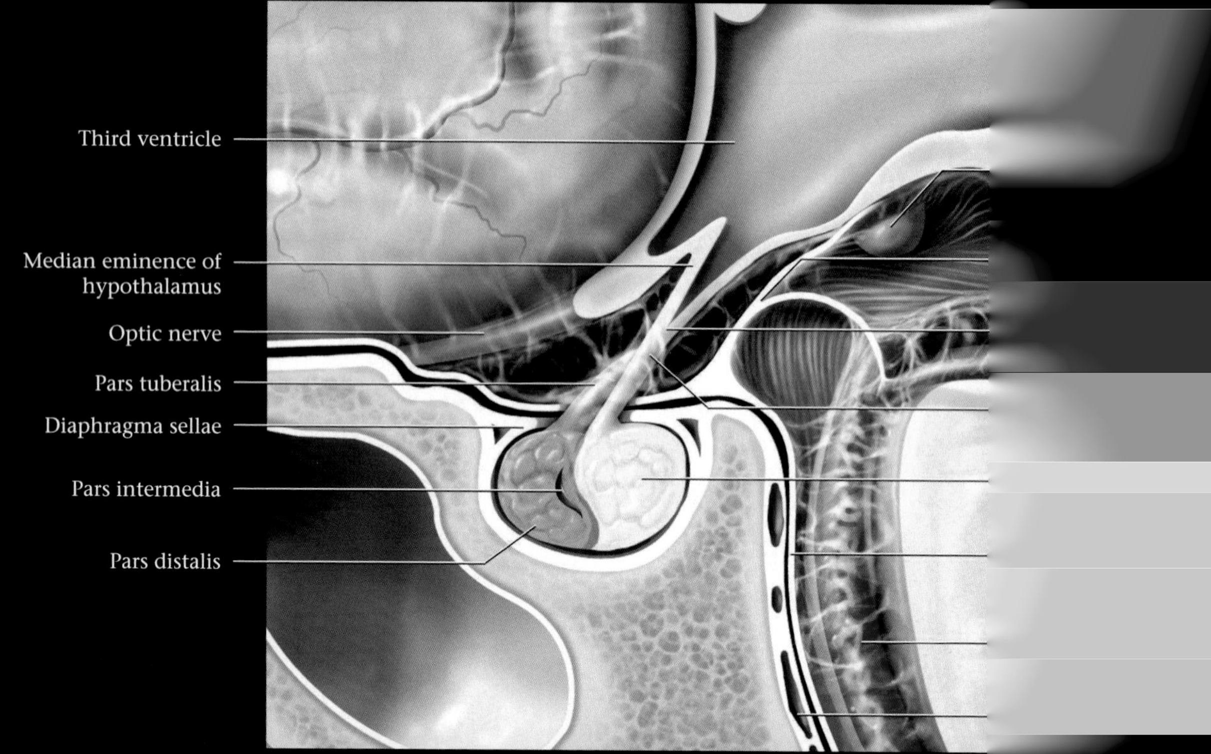
Third ventricle
Median eminence of hypothalamus
Optic nerve
Pars tuberalis
Diaphragma sellae
Pars intermedia
Pars distalis

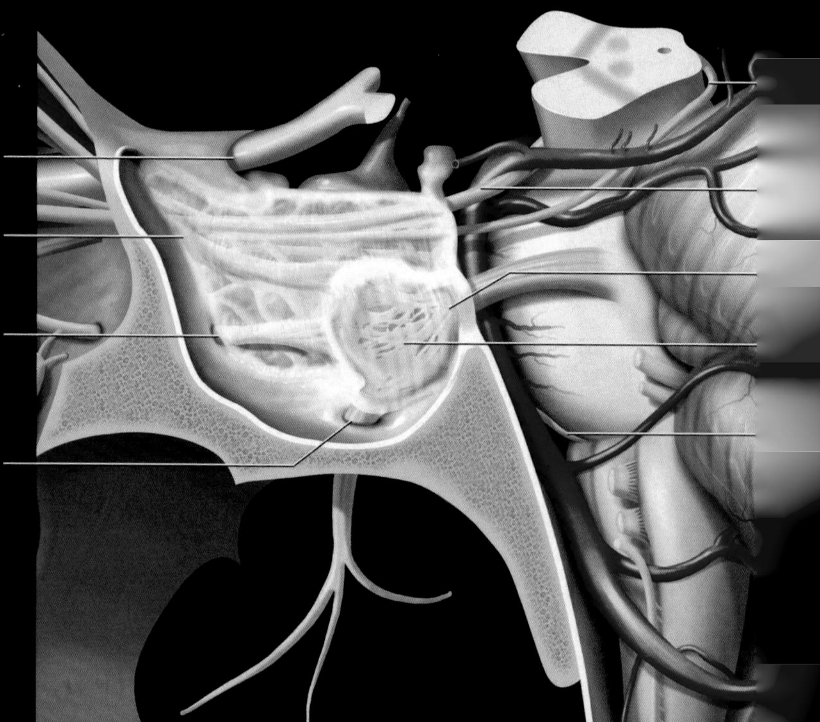
Optic nerve (CN2) entering optic canal
Ophthalmic (V1) division of CN5 (trigeminal)
Maxillary nerve (CNV2) entering foramen rotundum
Mandibular nerve (CNV3) entering foramen ovale

(Top) Lateral graphic of normal pituitary: The adenohypophysis is comprised of the pars tub and pars distalis. The neurohypophysis is comprised of the median eminence of hypothalam pars nervosa. Periosteal dural layer covers the sellar floor. **(Bottom)** Lateral graphic demonst detail in the sellar region. CN3, 4, V1 and V2 are in the lateral dural wall of the cavernous si the venous sinusoids of the CS, adjacent to the internal carotid artery (not shown). Meckel c and arachnoid-lined invagination that communicates freely with the prepontine cistern. It c

AXIAL T1 C+ MR

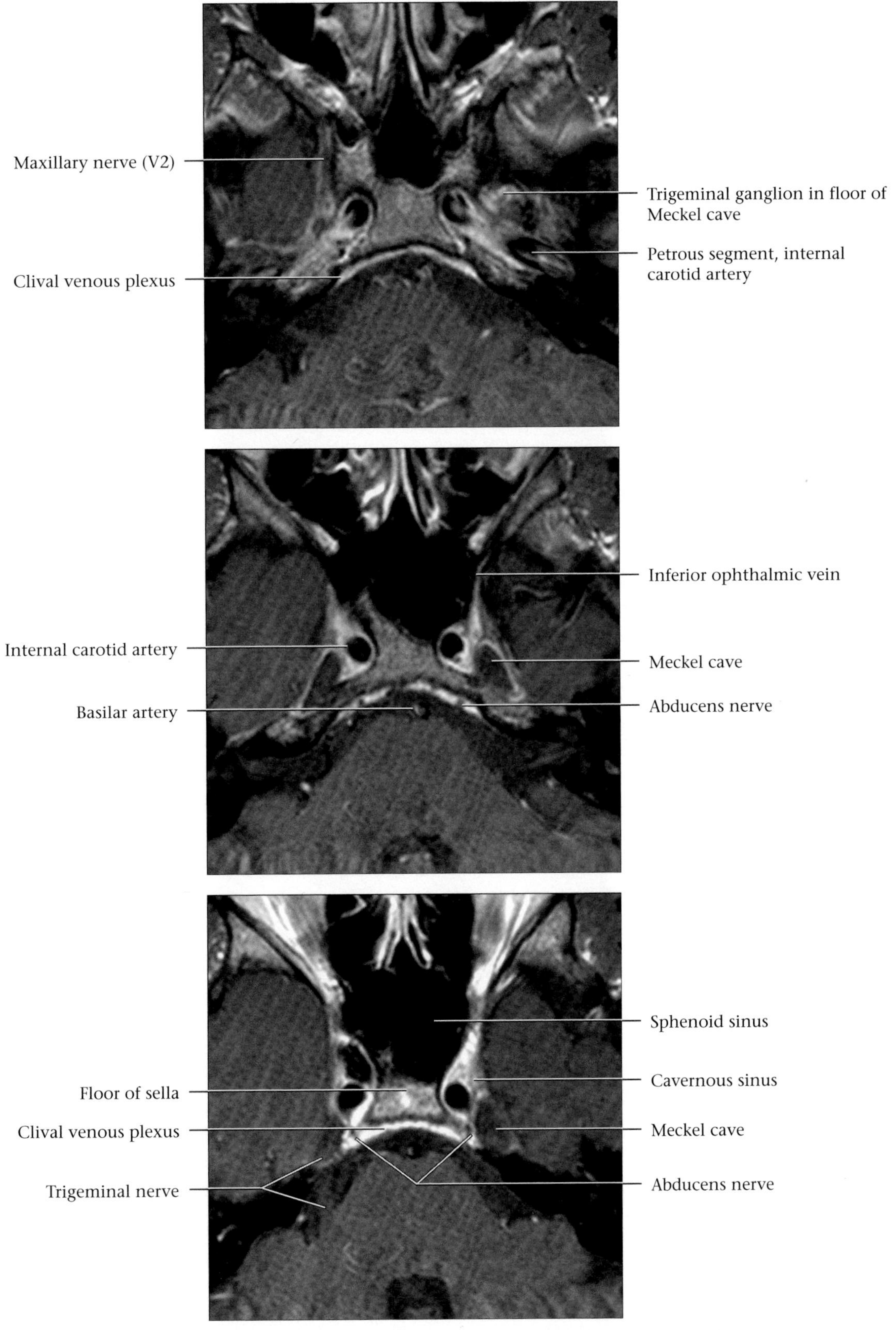
Maxillary nerve (V2)
Trigeminal ganglion in floor of Meckel cave
Petrous segment, internal carotid artery
Clival venous plexus
Inferior ophthalmic vein
Internal carotid artery
Meckel cave
Basilar artery
Abducens nerve
Sphenoid sinus
Cavernous sinus
Floor of sella
Clival venous plexus
Meckel cave
Trigeminal nerve
Abducens nerve

(Top) Series of six axial contrast-enhanced T1 MR images presented from inferior to superior through skull base and cavernous sinus demonstrate right maxillary nerve (V2) passing anteriorly into foramen rotundum and the left trigeminal ganglion. The mandibular nerve (V3) will exit inferiorly through foramen ovale (not shown). **(Middle)** Meckel cave is located posterior, inferior and lateral relative to cavernous sinus. Dura forming posterior part of lateral wall of cavernous sinus also forms upper medial third of Meckel cave, separating the two structures. Note the abducens nerve (CN6), seen here as a filling defect within the clival venous plexus, just before entering Dorello canal. **(Bottom)** Both abducens nerves are seen coursing through Dorello canal to enter the posterior cavernous sinus. The right trigeminal nerve is seen entering Meckel cave.

SELLA, PITUITARY AND CAVERNOUS SINUS

AXIAL T1 C+ MR

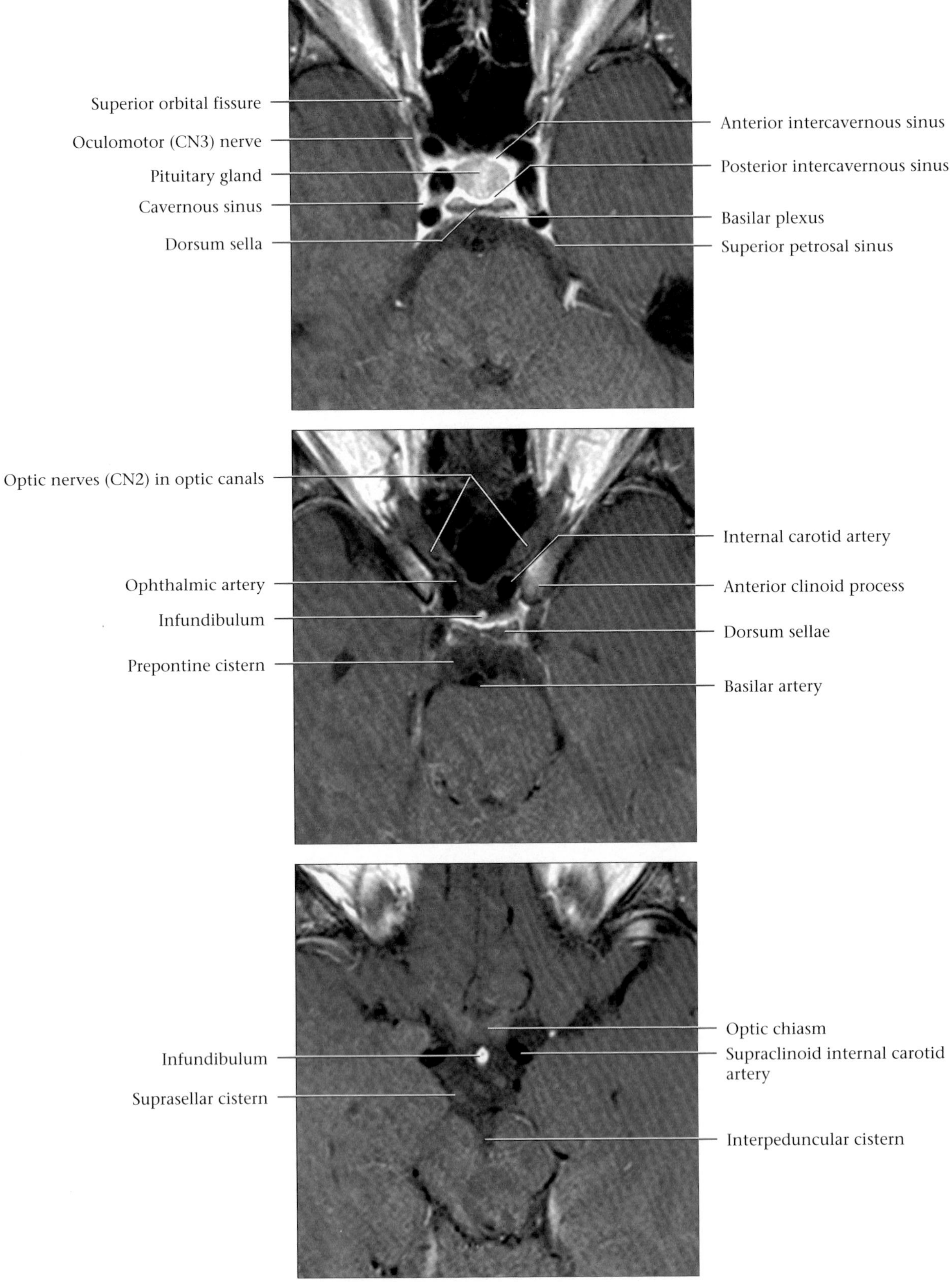
Superior orbital fissure
Oculomotor (CN3) nerve
Pituitary gland
Cavernous sinus
Dorsum sella
Anterior intercavernous sinus
Posterior intercavernous sinus
Basilar plexus
Superior petrosal sinus
Optic nerves (CN2) in optic canals
Ophthalmic artery
Infundibulum
Prepontine cistern
Internal carotid artery
Anterior clinoid process
Dorsum sellae
Basilar artery
Infundibulum
Suprasellar cistern
Optic chiasm
Supraclinoid internal carotid artery
Interpeduncular cistern

(Top) Cranial nerves exiting the cavernous sinus through the superior orbital fissure are: CN3, 4, 6, and the first (ophthalmic or V1) division of CN5. **(Middle)** The optic nerve in the optic canal is located anteromedial to the anterior clinoid and superomedial to the superior orbital fissure (SOF). It is separated from the SOF by a thin bony strut, the "optic strut." The cavernous carotid is posteromedial to the anterior clinoid. Note origin of the ophthalmic artery from the internal carotid artery, just above the transition from intracavernous carotid (below) to intradural carotid (above) segments. **(Bottom)** Pituitary infundibulum is seen within the suprasellar cistern posterior to the optic chiasm; avid enhancement seen here is typical. The supraclinoid internal carotid artery (or terminal segment) is seen laterally.

SELLA, PITUITARY AND CAVERNOUS SINUS

CORONAL T2 MR

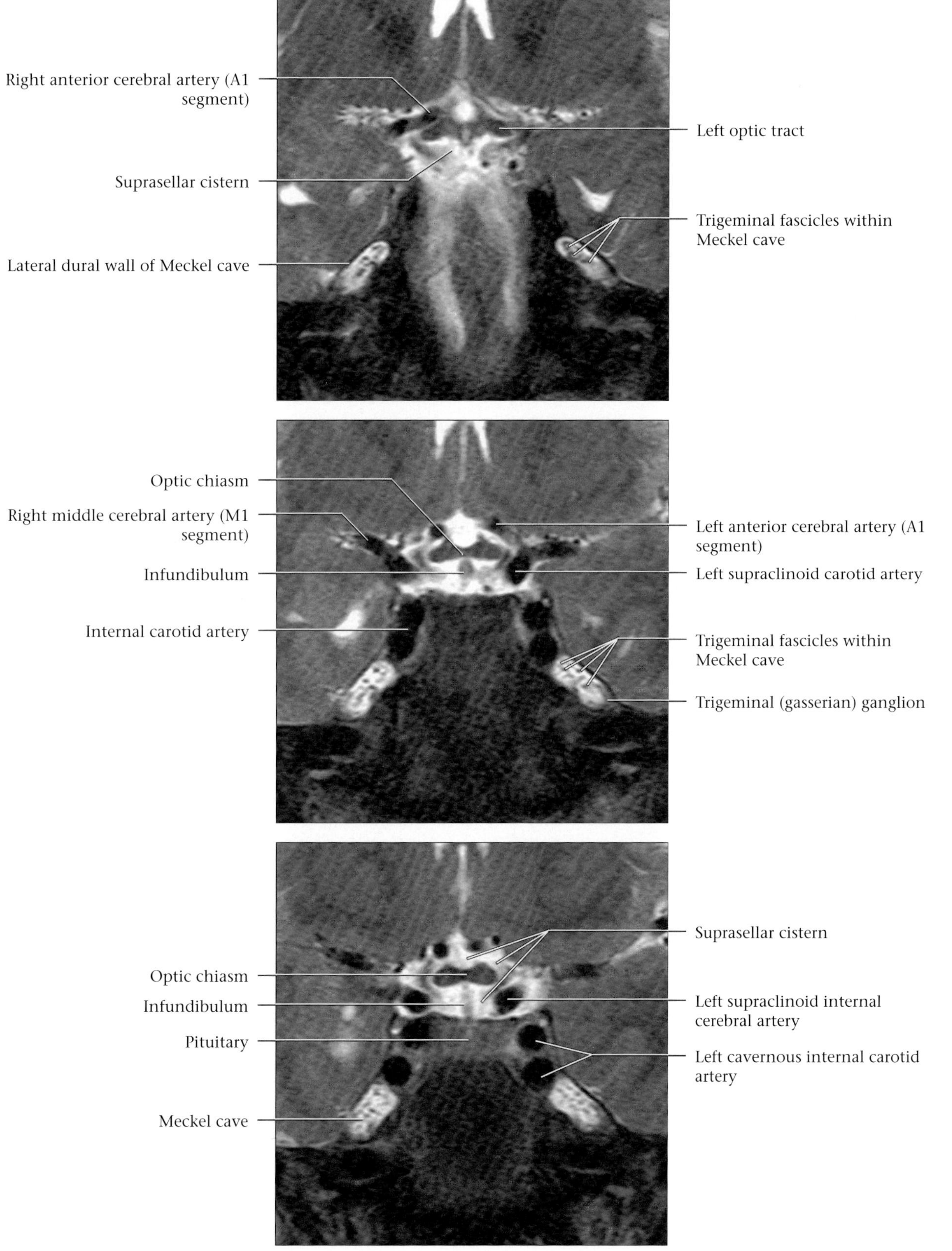
Right anterior cerebral artery (A1 segment)
Suprasellar cistern
Lateral dural wall of Meckel cave
Left optic tract
Trigeminal fascicles within Meckel cave
Optic chiasm
Right middle cerebral artery (M1 segment)
Infundibulum
Internal carotid artery
Left anterior cerebral artery (A1 segment)
Left supraclinoid carotid artery
Trigeminal fascicles within Meckel cave
Trigeminal (gasserian) ganglion
Optic chiasm
Infundibulum
Pituitary
Meckel cave
Suprasellar cistern
Left supraclinoid internal cerebral artery
Left cavernous internal carotid artery

(Top) First of six sequential coronal T2 MR images presented from posterior to anterior demonstrate the optic tracts within the posterior aspect of the suprasellar cistern, and anterior cerebral and supraclinoid internal carotid arteries. **(Middle)** The posterior optic chiasm and part of the pituitary infundibulum are seen here. Note the internal carotid, middle cerebral, and anterior cerebral arteries. Individual trigeminal nerve rootlets are well demonstrated within Meckel cave on thin-section imaging. **(Bottom)** Image at the level of the optic chiasm within the suprasellar cistern demonstrates normal pituitary gland and regional vascular anatomy. Note the normal location and appearance of Meckel cave, seen inferior and lateral. The pituitary gland and venous blood within the cavernous sinus are nearly isointense with each other on T2WIs.

SELLA, PITUITARY AND CAVERNOUS SINUS

CORONAL T2 MR

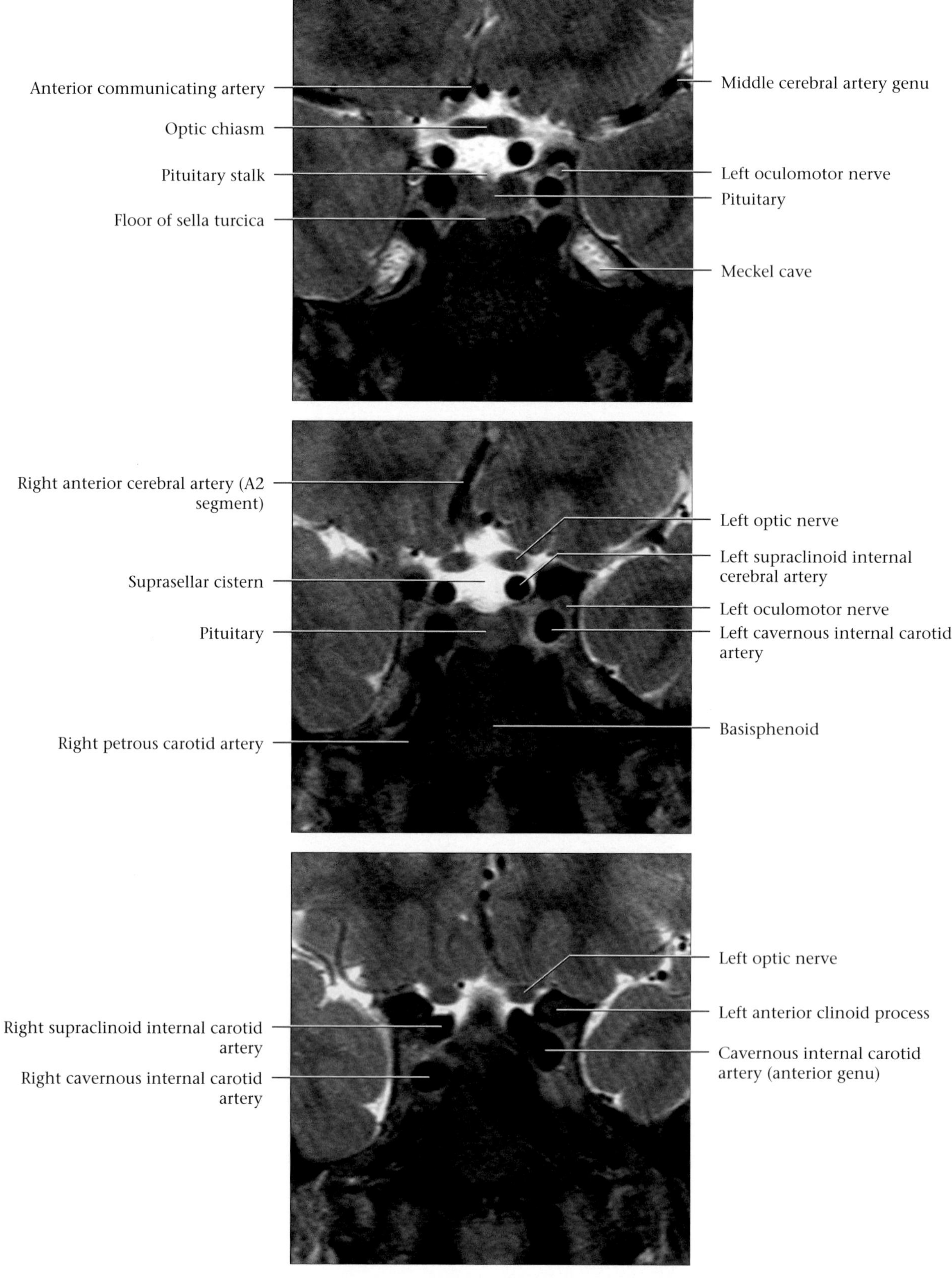
Anterior communicating artery
Optic chiasm
Pituitary stalk
Floor of sella turcica
Middle cerebral artery genu
Left oculomotor nerve
Pituitary
Meckel cave
Right anterior cerebral artery (A2 segment)
Suprasellar cistern
Pituitary
Right petrous carotid artery
Left optic nerve
Left supraclinoid internal cerebral artery
Left oculomotor nerve
Left cavernous internal carotid artery
Basisphenoid
Right supraclinoid internal carotid artery
Right cavernous internal carotid artery
Left optic nerve
Left anterior clinoid process
Cavernous internal carotid artery (anterior genu)

(Top) Normal appearance of the anterior pituitary gland, cavernous sinus, Meckel cave, and suprasellar cistern are seen here. The oculomotor nerves (CN3), and optic nerves (CN2) are well seen. The anterior communicating artery, which connects the two anterior cerebral arteries, and the left middle cerebral artery genu, are visible here. **(Middle)** The most anterior aspect of the suprasellar cistern demonstrates normal optic nerves (CN2), oculomotor nerves (CN3), cavernous internal carotid arteries, and anterior cerebral artery within the anterior interhemispheric fissure. **(Bottom)** The anterior clinoid processes seen here form the anterolateral boundaries of the sella turcica. Note normal optic nerves, located medial to the anterior clinoids, and the anterior genu of the cavernous internal carotid artery on the left.

CORONAL T1 C+ MR

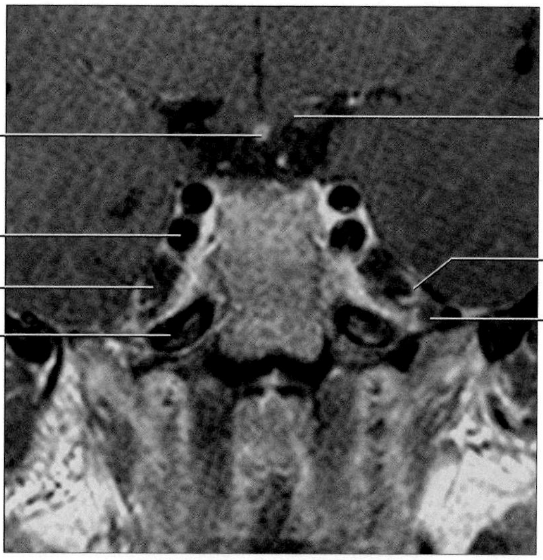

Infundibulum (pituitary stalk) upper aspect
Posterior cavernous internal carotid artery
Meckel cave
Petrous internal carotid artery
Optic chiasm
Gasserian ganglion
Mandibular nerve (V3)

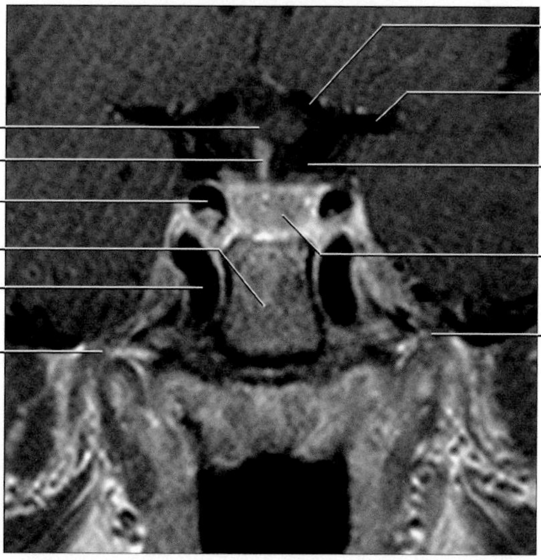

Optic chiasm
Infundibulum (pituitary stalk)
Cavernous internal carotid artery
Basisphenoid
Petrous internal carotid artery
Mandibular nerve (V3) exiting foramen ovale
Left anterior cerebral artery (A1 segment)
Left middle cerebral artery (M1 segment)
Supraclinoid left internal carotid artery
Pituitary gland
Left foramen ovale

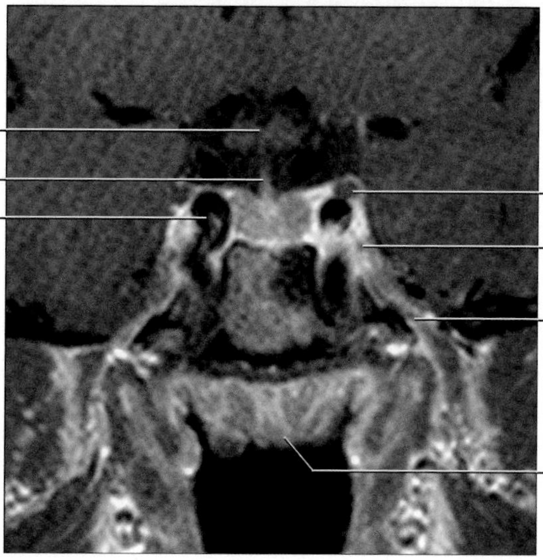

Optic chiasm
Infundibulum (pituitary stalk)
Cavernous internal carotid artery
Oculomotor nerve (CN3)
Abducens nerve within cavernous sinus sinusoids
Mandibular nerve (V3)
Nasopharyngeal/adenoidal tissue

(Top) First of six sequential contrast-enhanced T1 MR images through the sella, presented from posterior to anterior, demonstrates detail of Meckel cave. The mandibular (V3) division of the trigeminal nerve is seen inferior to the normally enhancing gasserian ganglion. **(Middle)** The pituitary infundibulum insertion into the gland is well seen here. Note the mandibular nerve (3rd division of trigeminal nerve, or V3), best seen on the right, as it exits through foramen ovale, entering the high masticator space. It is easy to see how extracranial tumors may gain access to the intracranial compartment without destroying the skull base, either through direct extension or via perineural spread. **(Bottom)** The left foramen ovale is well seen here. Note the third and sixth cranial nerves within the cavernous sinus. All of the cranial nerves are not well seen on this image.

SELLA, PITUITARY AND CAVERNOUS SINUS

CORONAL T1 C+ MR

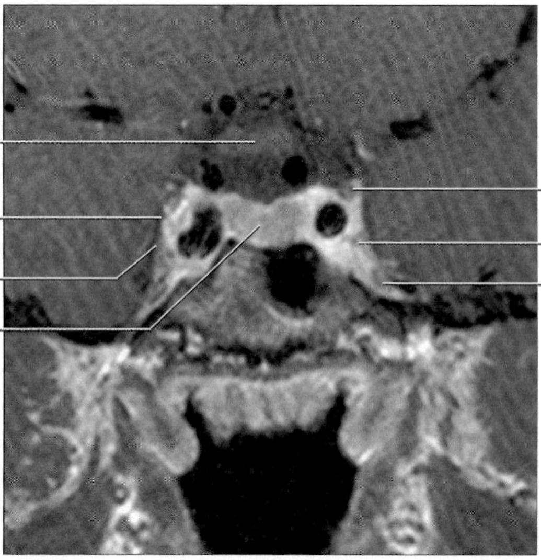

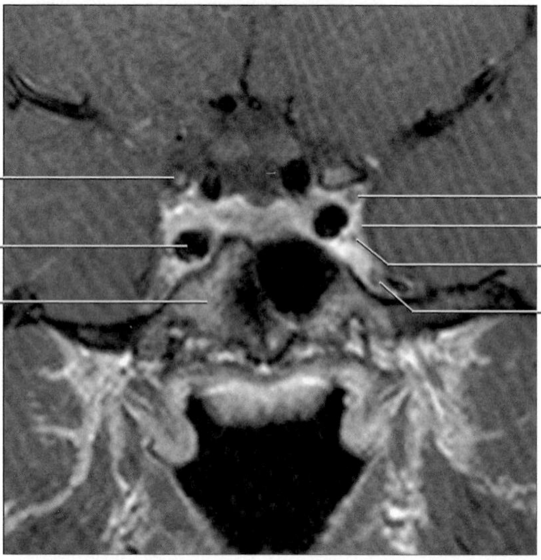

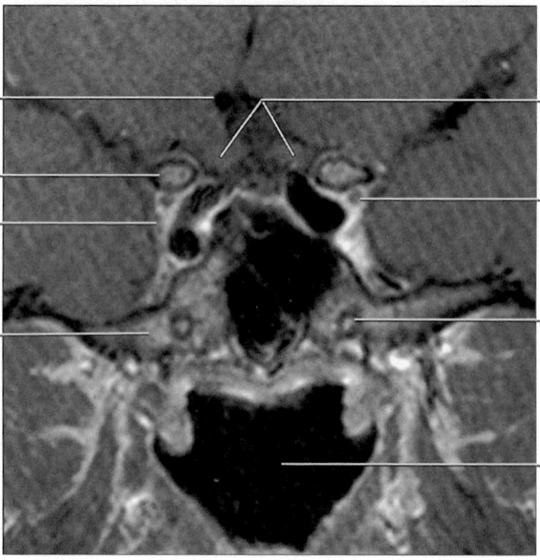

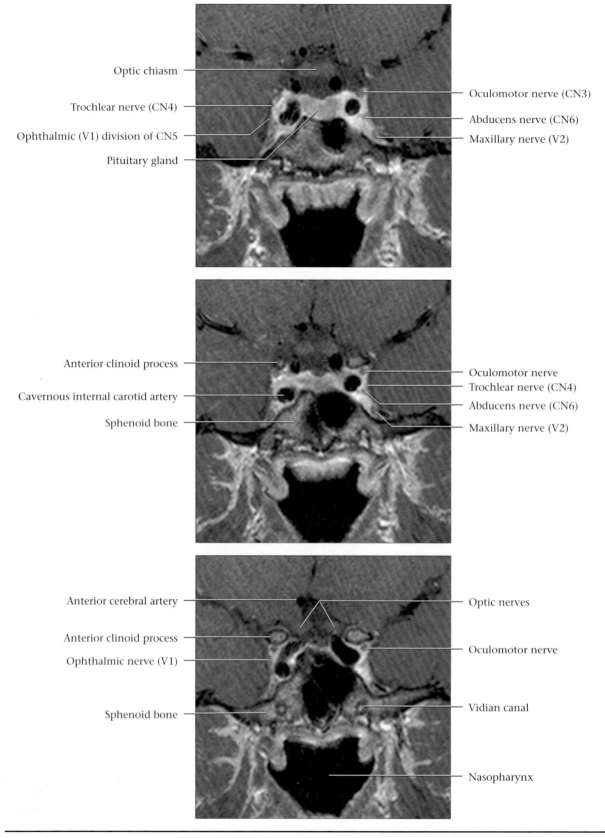

Optic chiasm
Trochlear nerve (CN4)
Ophthalmic (V1) division of CN5
Pituitary gland
Oculomotor nerve (CN3)
Abducens nerve (CN6)
Maxillary nerve (V2)

Anterior clinoid process
Cavernous internal carotid artery
Sphenoid bone
Oculomotor nerve
Trochlear nerve (CN4)
Abducens nerve (CN6)
Maxillary nerve (V2)

Anterior cerebral artery
Anterior clinoid process
Ophthalmic nerve (V1)
Sphenoid bone
Optic nerves
Oculomotor nerve
Vidian canal
Nasopharynx

(Top) This image demonstrates the oculomotor, abducens, and maxillary nerves. The pituitary gland enhances less strongly than venous blood in the cavernous sinus. **(Middle)** Normal cranial nerves traversing the cavernous sinus from superior to inferior include: Oculomotor nerve, trochlear nerve, abducens nerve, ophthalmic nerve (V1), and maxillary nerve (V2). The fourth cranial nerve (trochlear) is small and difficult to visualize, but is normally located in the lateral cavernous sinus, between the oculomotor and trigeminal nerves, lateral to the abducens. **(Bottom)** The oculomotor nerve is again well seen in the anterior cavernous sinus, before it traverses the superior orbital fissure. The vidian canal, which contains the vidian artery and nerve, is seen in the sphenoid bone. Note the optic nerves medial to the anterior clinoids before entering the optic canals.

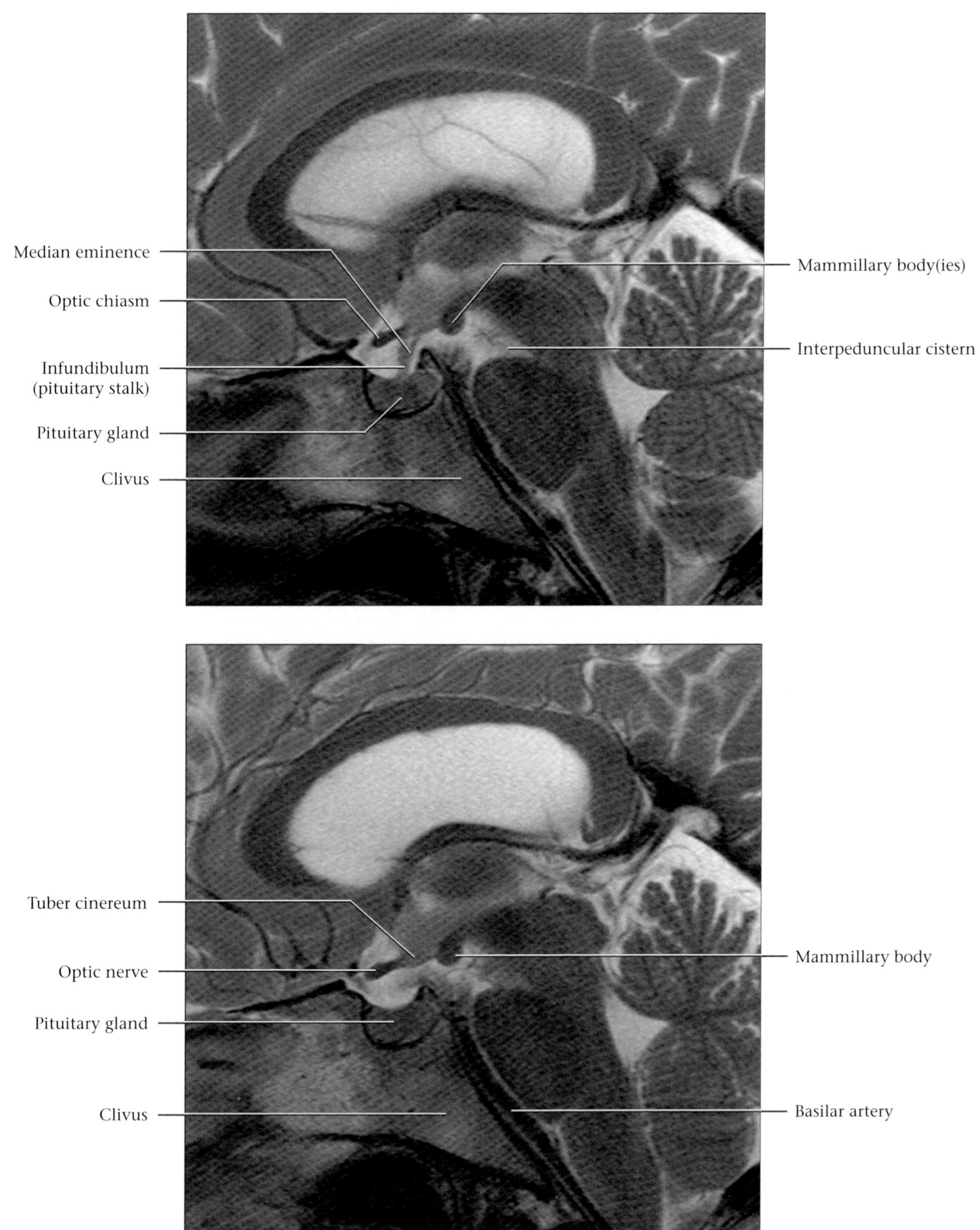
Median eminence
Optic chiasm
Infundibulum (pituitary stalk)
Pituitary gland
Clivus
Mammillary body(ies)
Interpeduncular cistern
Tuber cinereum
Optic nerve
Pituitary gland
Clivus
Mammillary body
Basilar artery

(Top) First of four sequential fat-saturated sagittal T2 MR images, presented midline to lateral, depicts normal sellar osseous boundaries: Sphenoid and clivus (floor), anterior clinoids anterolaterally, tuberculum sella anteriorly, dorsum sella and posterior clinoids posteriorly. The pituitary sits in the sella, connected superiorly to the hypothalamus via the pituitary infundibulum. Note the median eminence of hypothalamus, which forms part of the neurohypophysis. **(Bottom)** The tuber cinereum of hypothalamus is located between the optic chiasm anteriorly and mammillary bodies posteriorly. Its ventral aspect has small grooves and eminences but on imaging it should be smooth, flat, and slightly convex inferiorly. Thickening or nodularity should raise suspicion for pathology. The infundibulum courses inferiorly from the tuber cinereum to the hypophysis.

SAGITTAL T2 MR

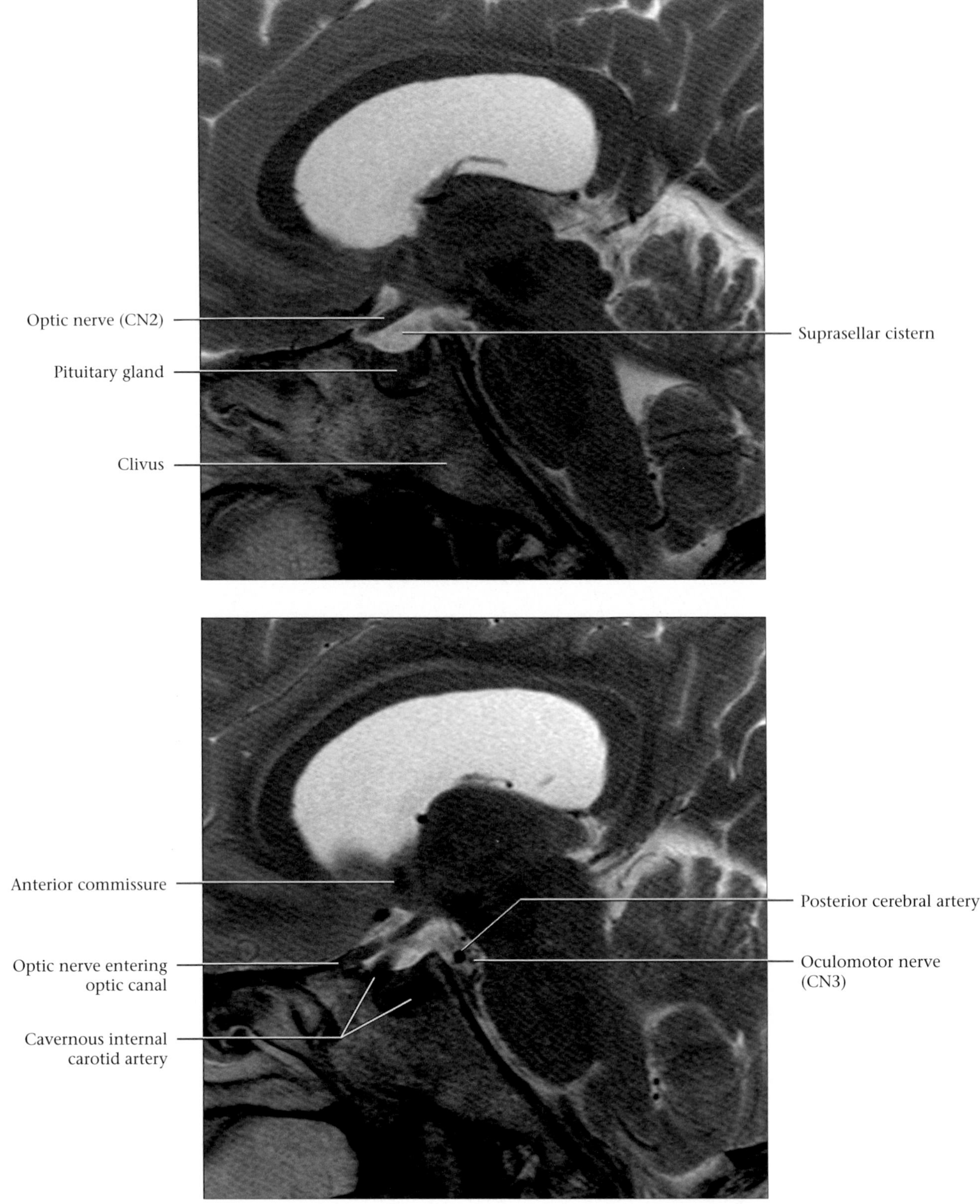
Optic nerve (CN2)
Pituitary gland
Clivus
Suprasellar cistern
Anterior commissure
Optic nerve entering optic canal
Cavernous internal carotid artery
Posterior cerebral artery
Oculomotor nerve (CN3)

(Top) The optic nerve traverses the suprasellar cistern. Note lack of sphenoid sinus pneumatization in this case, a normal anatomical variant that may make transsphenoidal surgery more difficult. **(Bottom)** The optic nerve is seen here entering the posterior aspect of the optic canal. The suprasellar and interpeduncular cisterns are normally in communication, are appreciated here. Volume averaging of the cavernous internal carotid artery together with part of the pituitary gland on off-midline images, as seen here, is common and should not be mistaken for abnormality. The oculomotor nerve courses anteriorly between the posterior cerebral artery above and the superior cerebellar artery below.

SAGITTAL FAT-SATURATED T1 MR

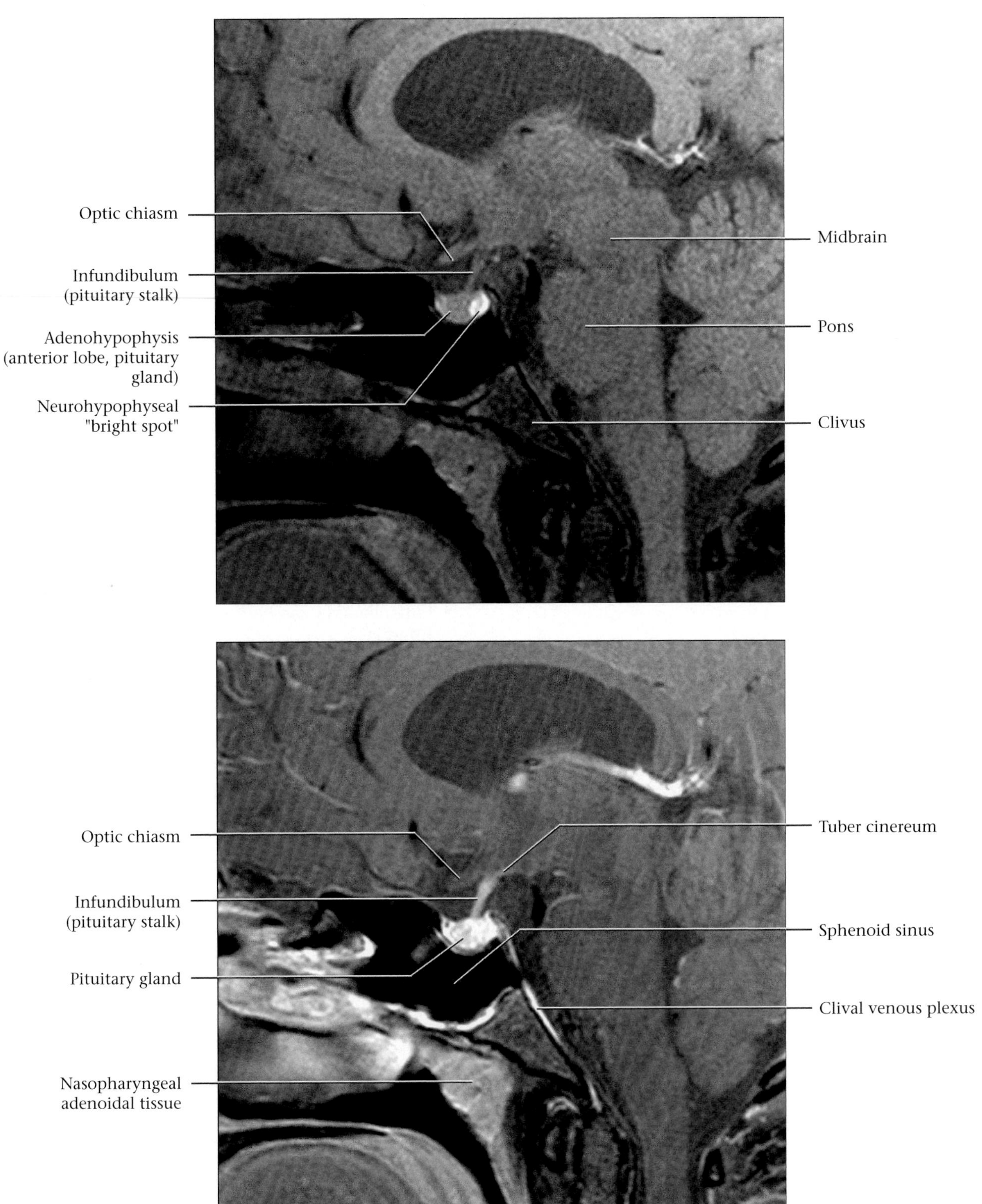
Optic chiasm
Infundibulum (pituitary stalk)
Adenohypophysis (anterior lobe, pituitary gland)
Neurohypophyseal "bright spot"
Midbrain
Pons
Clivus
Optic chiasm
Infundibulum (pituitary stalk)
Pituitary gland
Nasopharyngeal adenoidal tissue
Tuber cinereum
Sphenoid sinus
Clival venous plexus

(Top) Unenhanced sagittal T1 fat-saturated MR image through the midline sella turcica demonstrates T1 shortening in the neurohypophysis (posterior pituitary "bright spot" or PPBS). The PPBS is caused by vasopressin and oxytocin, not fat, and therefore does not suppress. Note prominent developmental sphenoid pneumatization in this case. **(Bottom)** Enhanced sagittal T1 fat-saturated MR image through the midline in the same case shows normal pituitary gland and stalk enhancement. The tuber cinereum and hypothalamus between the infundibulum and mammillary bodies lacks a blood-brain barrier and also enhances. Note normal enhancement of the nasopharyngeal tissue and its proximity to the central skull base.

PINEAL REGION

Terminology

Synonyms
- Pineal gland, pineal body, epiphysis cerebri
- Posterior commissure: Epithalamic commissure

Definitions
- Epithalamus: Dorsal nuclei of diencephalon

Gross Anatomy

Overview
- Major components of pineal region
  - Pineal gland
  - Posterior recesses of third ventricle
  - Internal cerebral veins, vein of Galen; medial posterior choroidal artery
  - Epithalamus, quadrigeminal plate (tectum), corpus callosum
  - Dura, arachnoid
- Pineal gland
  - Unpaired midline endocrine organ located within quadrigeminal cistern
  - Structure
    - Attached to diencephalon & posterior wall of third ventricle by pineal stalk
    - Pineal stalk consists of superior/inferior lamina (form superior & inferior borders of pineal recess of third ventricle)
    - Superior/inferior lamina connect habenular/posterior commissures, respectively, to pineal gland
  - Vascular supply: Primarily medial posterior choroidal artery (lacks blood-brain barrier)
  - Contents: Pineal parenchymal cells, germ cells, some neuroglial cells (predominately astrocytes)
  - Functions: Incompletely understood but include
    - Secretion of melatonin, thought to regulate sleep/wake cycle in humans
    - Regulation of reproductive function, such as onset of puberty in humans
- Pineal gland connections
  - Habenular commissure: Connects habenular, amygdaloid nuclei and hippocampi
  - Posterior commissure: Connections with dorsal thalamus, superior colliculi, pretectal nuclei and others; medial longitudinal fasciculus fibers also cross here
  - Stria medullaris thalami: Fibers connecting both habenular nuclei
  - Habenular nuclei: Relay station for olfactory centers, brain stem, and pineal
  - Paraventricular nuclei: Connections with hypothalamus, hippocampus, amygdala, brain stem, septal nuclei and stria terminalis
  - Superior cervical ganglia sympathetic fibers
  - Dorsal tegmentum nonadrenergic tract

Anatomy Relationships
- Pineal gland boundaries
  - Superior: Cistern of velum interpositum and internal cerebral veins
  - Inferior: Superior colliculi of midbrain tectum
  - Anterior: Pineal and suprapineal recesses, third ventricle
  - Posterior and superior: Vein of Galen
  - Posterior and inferior: Superior cerebellar cistern

Imaging Anatomy

Overview
- Pineal gland lacks blood-brain barrier, enhances after contrast administration
- CT
  - Pineal gland calcifications common, increase with age
    - Globular or concentric lamellar patterns common
    - Incidence increases with age (< 3% at 1 year, 7% by 10 years, 33% by 18 years, > 50% of older patients)
    - Central calcifications normal, generally ≤ 10 mm
    - Larger, peripheral or "exploded" calcifications abnormal, may signify underlying neoplasm
  - Habenular commissure sometimes calcifies ("C-shaped" on lateral projections)
- MR
  - Homogeneous enhancement is typical
  - Incidental, nonneoplastic intrapineal cysts common
    - Usually proteinaceous (FLAIR bright)
    - Enhancement can be nodular, crescentic or ring-like

Anatomy-Based Imaging Issues

Imaging Recommendations
- MR: Thin-section enhanced sagittal images (1 mm) and smaller field of view (16 cm) best

Imaging Pitfalls
- Benign, nonneoplastic pineal cysts are common
  - Most appropriate management and follow-up recommendations are controversial
  - Unilocular small simple cysts most common (on routine imaging), usually do not require follow-up
  - Suggested follow-up if > 1 cm or atypical enhancement pattern; some authors suggest follow-up based on clinical indications
  - Large cysts can become symptomatic (cause hydrocephalus or Parinaud syndrome)
- Pineal cysts may mimic tumors (pineocytoma) and vice versa
- Exophytic midbrain tectal masses may mimic primary pineal region tumors (pineal tumors usually compress tectum and displace it inferiorly)

Clinical Implications
- Parinaud syndrome
  - Dorsal midbrain or collicular syndrome caused by mass in pineal region compressing tectal plate
  - Loss of vertical gaze; nystagmus on attempted convergence; pseudo-Argyll-Robertson pupil
- "Pineal apoplexy"
  - Sudden onset severe headache, visual problems
  - Hemorrhage into pineal cyst or neoplasm

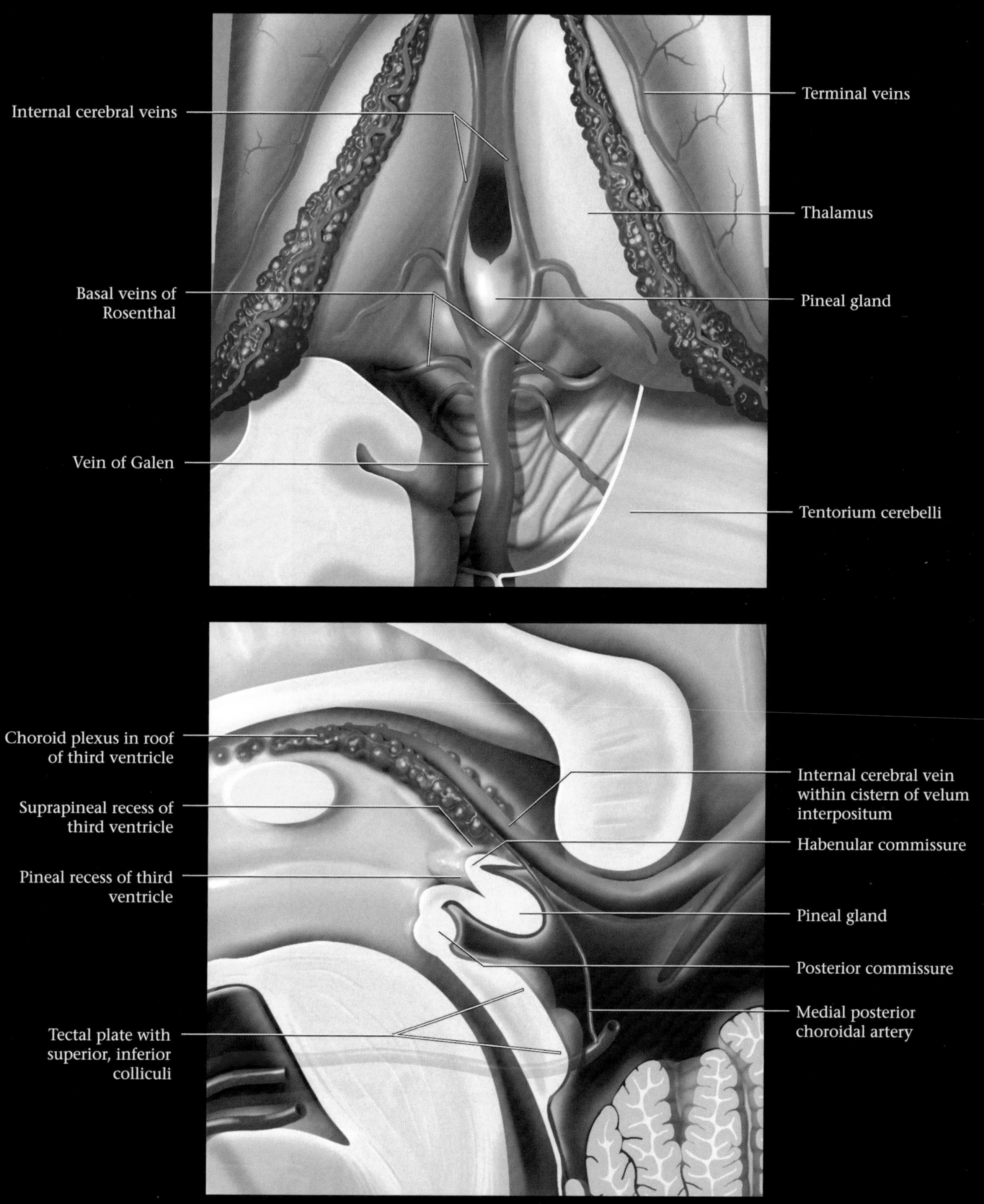
Internal cerebral veins
Terminal veins
Thalamus
Basal veins of Rosenthal
Pineal gland
Vein of Galen
Tentorium cerebelli
Choroid plexus in roof of third ventricle
Suprapineal recess of third ventricle
Pineal recess of third ventricle
Tectal plate with superior, inferior colliculi
Internal cerebral vein within cistern of velum interpositum
Habenular commissure
Pineal gland
Posterior commissure
Medial posterior choroidal artery

(Top) Midline graphic demonstrating detail of the pineal region. The pineal gland is viewed from above, with the corpus callosum and fornices removed. The internal cerebral veins extend posteriorly from foramen of Monro, traversing the cistern of velum interpositum just superior to the pineal, and unite posteriorly to form the vein of Galen. **(Bottom)** Sagittal midline graphic demonstrates normal anatomy of the pineal region. The pineal stalk has 2 lamina; these attach the pineal gland superiorly to the habenular commissure, with connections to the amygdala and hippocampus. The inferior lamina attaches the pineal gland to the posterior commissure, allowing communication with numerous nuclei of the thalamus, superior colliculi, tectal and habenular nuclei and also contains crossing fibers of the medial longitudinal fasciculus.

PINEAL REGION

CORONAL T2 MR

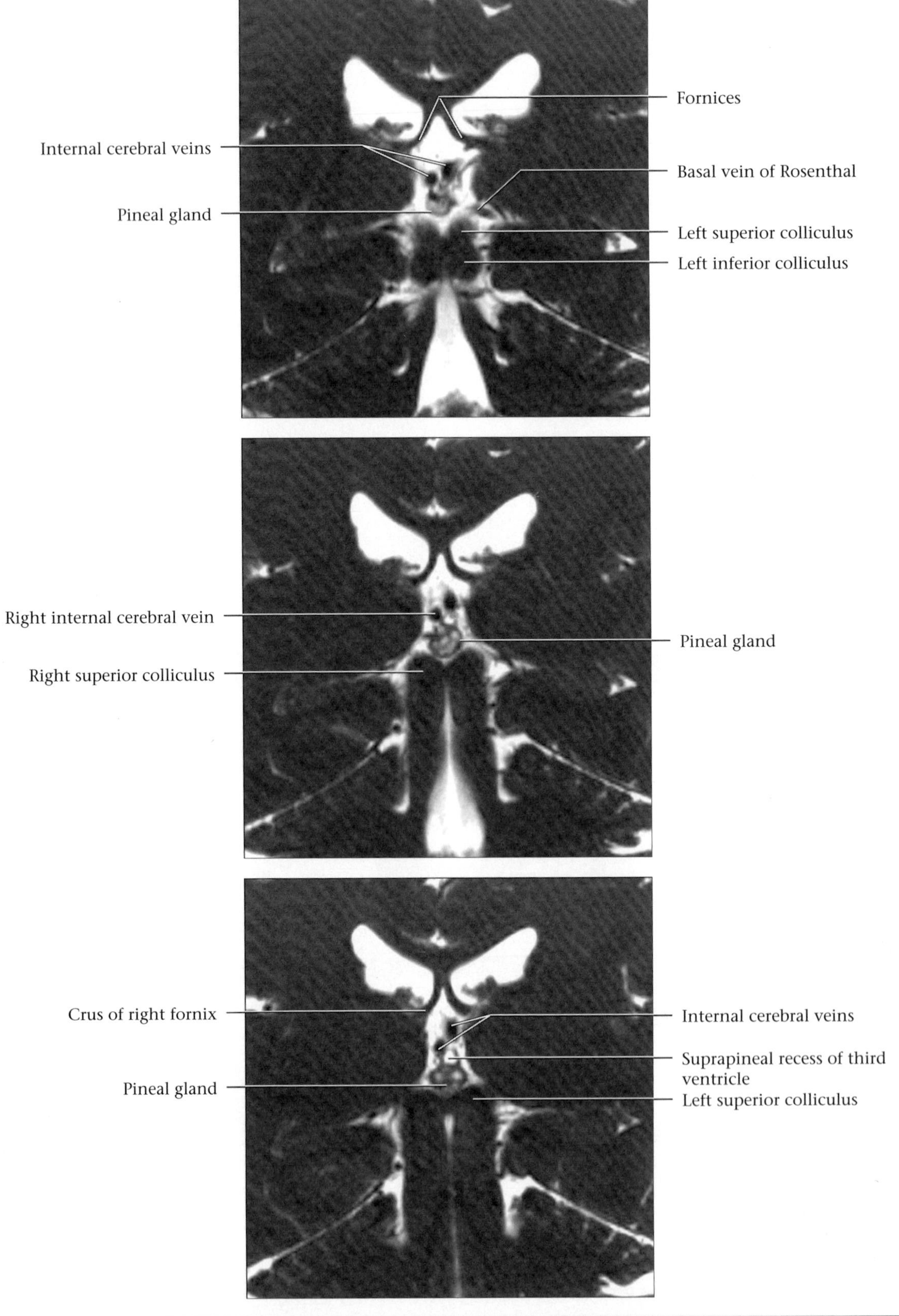
Fornices
Internal cerebral veins
Basal vein of Rosenthal
Pineal gland
Left superior colliculus
Left inferior colliculus
Right internal cerebral vein
Pineal gland
Right superior colliculus
Crus of right fornix
Internal cerebral veins
Suprapineal recess of third ventricle
Pineal gland
Left superior colliculus

(Top) First of three coronal T2 MR images, presented sequentially from posterior to anterior, is seen at the level of the superior and inferior colliculi and posterior pineal gland. **(Middle)** Image through body of pineal gland demonstrating multiple small cysts within the gland, a common finding on high-resolution scans. The pineal is located just above the superior colliculi of the midbrain tectum. Exophytic tectal masses can be difficult to distinguish from pineal origin masses because of this proximity; thin slice sagittal and/or coronal imaging best evaluates this area in this situation. **(Bottom)** The suprapineal recess of third ventricle is seen here as a small fluid-filled space located between the pineal gland inferiorly and internal cerebral veins superiorly. The internal cerebral veins traverse the cistern of the velum interpositum.

PINEAL REGION

SAGITTAL T2 MR

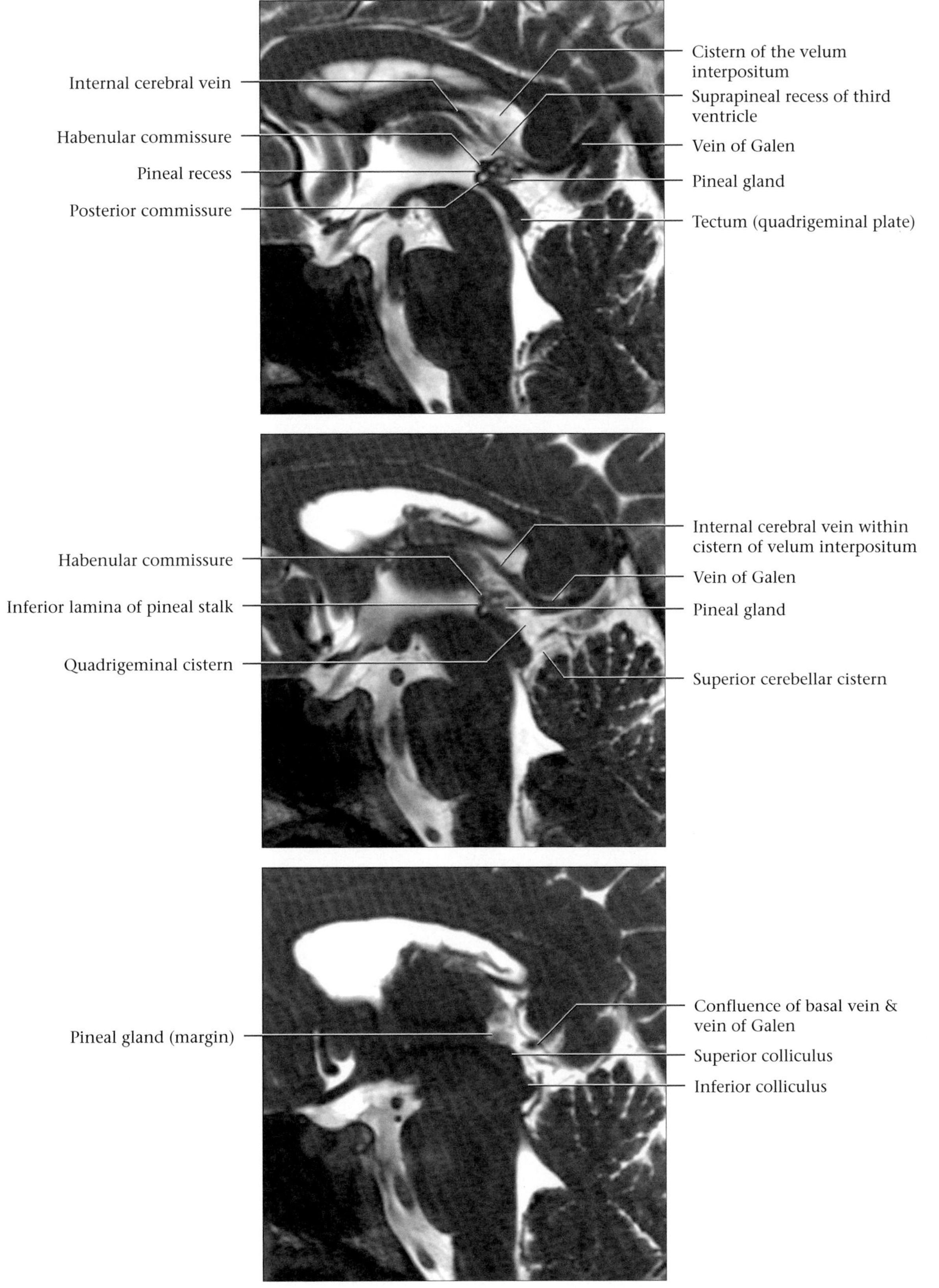
Internal cerebral vein
Habenular commissure
Pineal recess
Posterior commissure
Cistern of the velum interpositum
Suprapineal recess of third ventricle
Vein of Galen
Pineal gland
Tectum (quadrigeminal plate)
Habenular commissure
Inferior lamina of pineal stalk
Quadrigeminal cistern
Internal cerebral vein within cistern of velum interpositum
Vein of Galen
Pineal gland
Superior cerebellar cistern
Pineal gland (margin)
Confluence of basal vein & vein of Galen
Superior colliculus
Inferior colliculus

(Top) Series of three sagittal T2 MR images presented from medial to lateral. Midline section through the pineal gland demonstrates multiple small cysts, commonly seen with high-resolution imaging. Note the habenular and posterior commissures, which are connected to the pineal by the superior and inferior lamina, respectively. The posterior recesses of the third ventricle are well seen here: The suprapineal recess just above the pineal gland, and the pineal recess immediately anterior to the gland. **(Middle)** Note the normal pineal location just superior to the tectum. The inferior lamina is seen here, connecting the pineal gland and posterior commissure. Internal cerebral veins drain into the posteriorly located vein of Galen. **(Bottom)** The lateral aspect of the pineal gland is demonstrated here. Note the superior and inferior colliculi of the midbrain tectum.

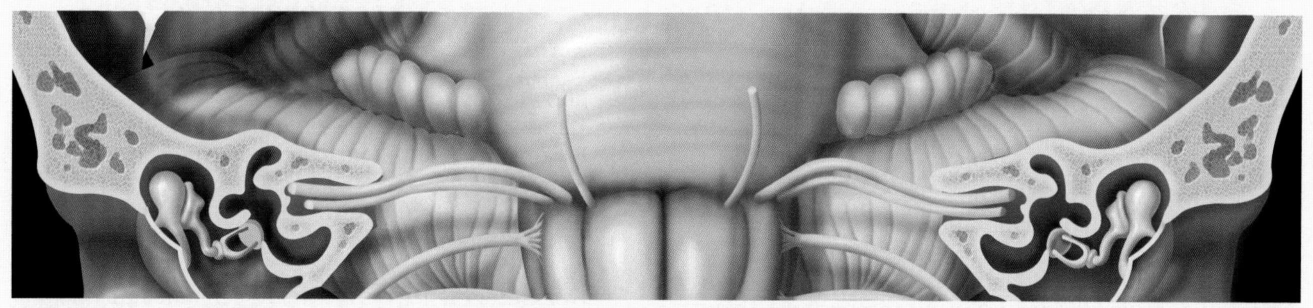

SECTION 3: Infratentorial Brain

BRAINSTEM AND CEREBELLUM OVERVIEW

Terminology

Abbreviations

- Cerebrospinal fluid (CSF)
- Cranial nerves (CN): Oculomotor nerve (CN3), trochlear nerve (CN4), trigeminal nerve (CN5), abducens nerve (CN6), facial nerve (CN7), vestibulocochlear nerve (CN8), glossopharyngeal nerve (CN9), vagus nerve (CN10), accessory nerve (CN11), hypoglossal nerve (CN12)

Synonyms

- Classical nomenclature (simplified nomenclature)
  - Superior (tentorial), inferior (suboccipital), anterior (petrosal) cerebellar surfaces
  - Primary (tentorial), horizontal (petrosal), prebiventral/prepyramidal (suboccipital) cerebellar fissures

Definitions

- Posterior fossa: Houses brainstem and cerebellum, below tentorium cerebelli (infratentorial)
- Brainstem: Composed of midbrain (mesencephalon), pons and medulla oblongata
- Cerebellum: Largest part of hindbrain, integrates coordinations & fine-tuning of movement & regulation of muscle tone

Gross Anatomy

Overview

- **Posterior fossa**: Infratentorial contents
  - Protected space surrounded by calvarium, contains:
    - Brainstem anteriorly, cerebellum posteriorly
    - Cerebral aqueduct and fourth ventricle
    - CSF cisterns containing CNs, vertebrobasilar arterial system and veins
  - CSF cisterns suspend & cushion brainstem and cerebellum
- **Brainstem**
  - Anatomic divisions
    - **Midbrain (mesencephalon)**: Upper brainstem, connects pons and cerebellum with forebrain
    - **Pons**: Mid portion of brainstem, relays information from brain to cerebellum
    - **Medulla**: Caudal (inferior) brainstem, relays information from spinal cord to brain
  - Functional divisions
    - Ventral part: Contains large descending white matter tracts: Midbrain cerebral peduncles, pontine bulb, medullary pyramids
    - Dorsal part: Tegmentum, common to midbrain, pons and medulla; contains CN nuclei and reticular formation
- **Cerebellum**
  - Two hemispheres & midline vermis, three surfaces
  - Connected to brainstem by three paired peduncles
  - Cortical gray matter, central white matter & four paired deep gray nuclei

Anatomy Relationships

- **Posterior fossa** boundaries
  - Tentorium cerebelli superiorly
  - Bony clivus anteriorly
  - Temporal bones and calvarium laterally
  - Foramen magnum and calvarium inferiorly
- **Midbrain**
  - Ventral: **Cerebral peduncles** (crus cerebri) containing corticospinal, corticobulbar and corticopontine tracts
  - **Dorsal tegmentum**: Ventral to cerebral aqueduct
    - White matter tracts: Medial longitudinal fasciculus, medial lemniscus, lateral lemniscus, spinothalamic tract, central tegmental tract
    - Gray matter: Substantia nigra and red nucleus
    - Upper midbrain: Contains CN3 nucleus, at superior colliculus level
    - Lower midbrain: Contains CN4 nucleus, at inferior colliculus level
  - **Tectum (quadrigeminal plate)**: Dorsal to cerebral aqueduct
    - Superior & inferior colliculi
    - Periaqueductal gray matter
- **Pons**
  - Ventral: Longitudinal fibers primarily from corticospinal, corticobulbar & corticopontine tracts
  - Dorsal tegmentum: White matter tracts & CN nuclei
    - White matter tracts: Medial longitudinal fasiculus, medial lemniscus, lateral lemniscus, trapezoid body, spinothalamic tract, central tegmental tract
    - Upper pons: Contains main nuclei of CN5
    - Lower pons: Contains nuclei of CN6, 7 & 8
- **Medulla**
  - Ventral: **Olives & pyramids**
  - **Dorsal tegmentum**: White matter tracts & CN nuclei
    - White matter tracts: Medial longitudinal fasiculus, medial lemniscus, spinothalamic tract, central tegmental tract, spinocerebellar tract
    - CN nuclei: CN9, 10 & 11 (bulbar portion) in upper & mid medulla; CN12 nuclei in mid medulla
- **Cerebellum**
  - Three surfaces: Superior (tentorial), inferior (suboccipital), anterior (petrosal)
  - Two **hemispheres** and a midline **vermis**
    - Divided into lobes & lobules by transverse **fissures**
    - Major fissures: Primary (tentorial), horizontal (petrosal), prebiventral/prepyramidal (suboccipital) cerebellar fissures
  - Three paired **peduncles**
    - **Superior cerebellar peduncle** (brachium conjunctivum) connects to cerebrum via midbrain
    - **Middle cerebellar peduncle** (brachium pontis) connects to pons
    - **Inferior cerebellar peduncle** (restiform body) connects to medulla
- **Vertebrobasilar system**
  - Midbrain: Perforating branches from basilar, superior cerebellar & posterior cerebral arteries
  - Pons: Superior cerebellar artery, perforating branches of basilar artery
  - Medulla: Anterior spinal artery, vertebral artery penetrating branches, posterior inferior cerebellar artery
  - Cerebellum: Superior cerebellar, posterior inferior cerebellar & anterior inferior cerebellar arteries

GRAPHICS

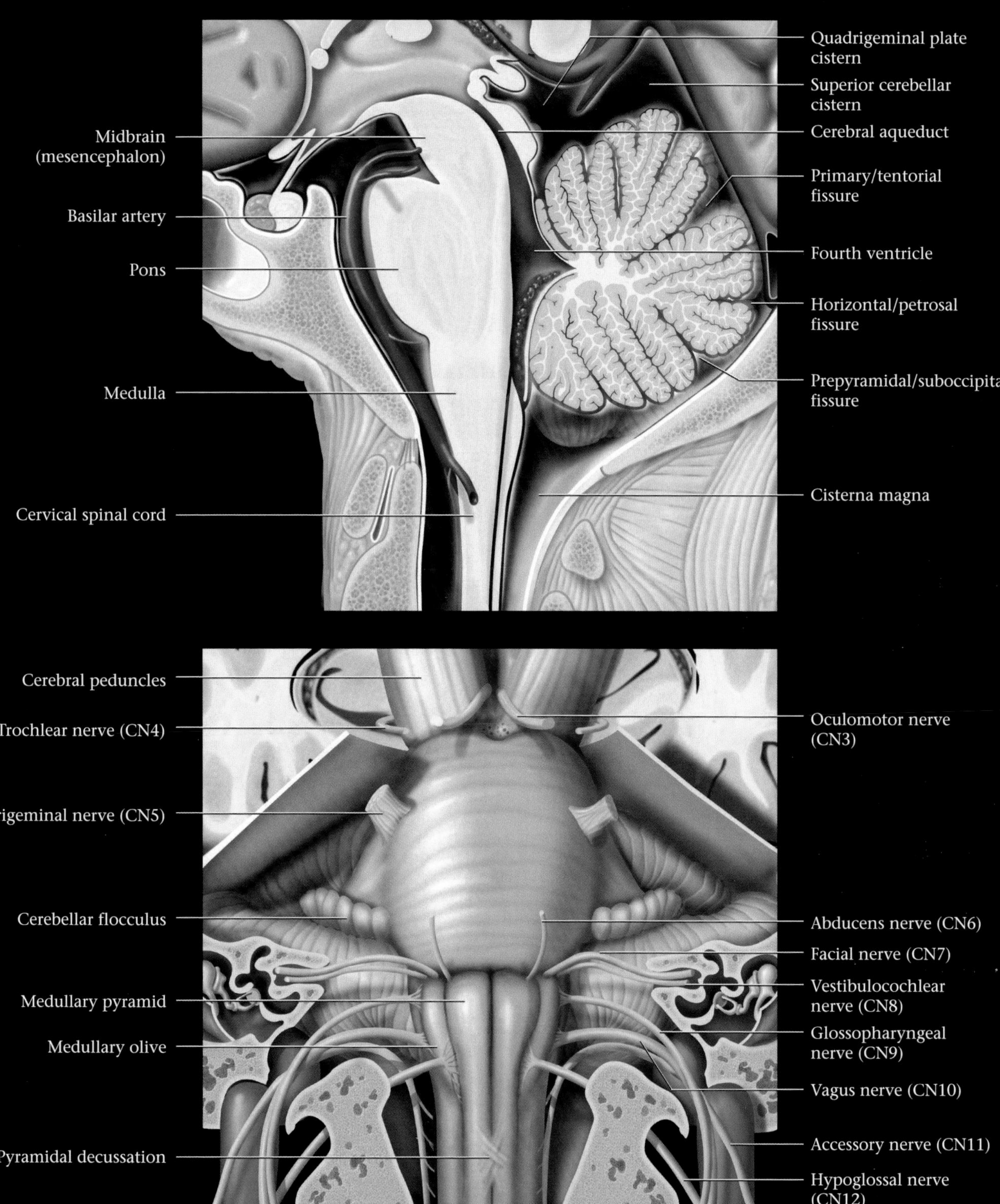
Midbrain (mesencephalon)
Basilar artery
Pons
Medulla
Cervical spinal cord
Quadrigeminal plate cistern
Superior cerebellar cistern
Cerebral aqueduct
Primary/tentorial fissure
Fourth ventricle
Horizontal/petrosal fissure
Prepyramidal/suboccipital fissure
Cisterna magna
Cerebral peduncles
Trochlear nerve (CN4)
Trigeminal nerve (CN5)
Cerebellar flocculus
Medullary pyramid
Medullary olive
Pyramidal decussation
Oculomotor nerve (CN3)
Abducens nerve (CN6)
Facial nerve (CN7)
Vestibulocochlear nerve (CN8)
Glossopharyngeal nerve (CN9)
Vagus nerve (CN10)
Accessory nerve (CN11)
Hypoglossal nerve (CN12)

(Top) Sagittal midline graphic of posterior fossa demonstrates anterior brainstem & posterior cerebellum, separated by fourth ventricle. Brainstem consists of midbrain (mesencephalon), pons & medulla. Cerebellum has superior (tentorial), inferior (suboccipital) & anterior (petrosal) surfaces. Primary (tentorial) fissure & horizontal (petrosal) fissures divide vermis & cerebellar hemispheres into lobules. Horizontal (petrosal) fissure is most prominent fissure on anterior (petrosal) surface & curves posteriorly onto inferior (suboccipital) surface. **(Bottom)** Coronal graphic of anterior brainstem & exiting cranial nerves. CN3 through CN12 nuclei are located within brainstem. CN3 & 4 nuclei are within midbrain, CN5 through CN8 nuclei are within pons, CN9 through CN12 nuclei are within medulla. CN4 is only dorsally exiting CN & wraps around lateral midbrain in tentorial margin.

AXIAL T2 MR

Clivus
Junction of cervical spinal cord & medulla
Inferior cerebellar hemisphere
Vertebral artery
Cerebellar tonsil

Clivus
Medullary pyramid
Medullary olive
Dorsal median sulcus
Inferior cerebellar hemisphere
Vertebral artery
Cerebellar tonsil

Medullary pyramid
Medullary olive
Inferior fourth ventricle
Inferior cerebellar hemisphere
Medullary cistern
Pre-olivary sulcus
Postolivary sulcus
Hypoglossal eminence
Cerebellar tonsil

(Top) First of nine axial T2 MR images from inferior to superior shows inferior posterior fossa at junction of cervical spinal cord & medulla. Cerebellar tonsils are seen at foramen magnum. **(Middle)** Image at level of inferior "closed" medulla shows ventral (anterior) medullary pyramids & olives which include white matter fibers from corticospinal & corticobulbar tracts which continue through ventral pons & ventral midbrain. Dorsal median sulcus continues superiorly to divide floor of fourth ventricle. **(Bottom)** Image of mid medulla shows hypoglossal eminence, formed by hypoglossal nerve CN12 nucleus as a bulge in fourth ventricular floor. CN12 exits anterolateral medulla in pre-olivary sulcus while glossopharyngeal CN9, vagus CN10, & cranial roots of accessory CN11 nerves exit lateral medulla in postolivary sulcus, posterior to medullary olive.

BRAINSTEM AND CEREBELLUM OVERVIEW

AXIAL T2 MR

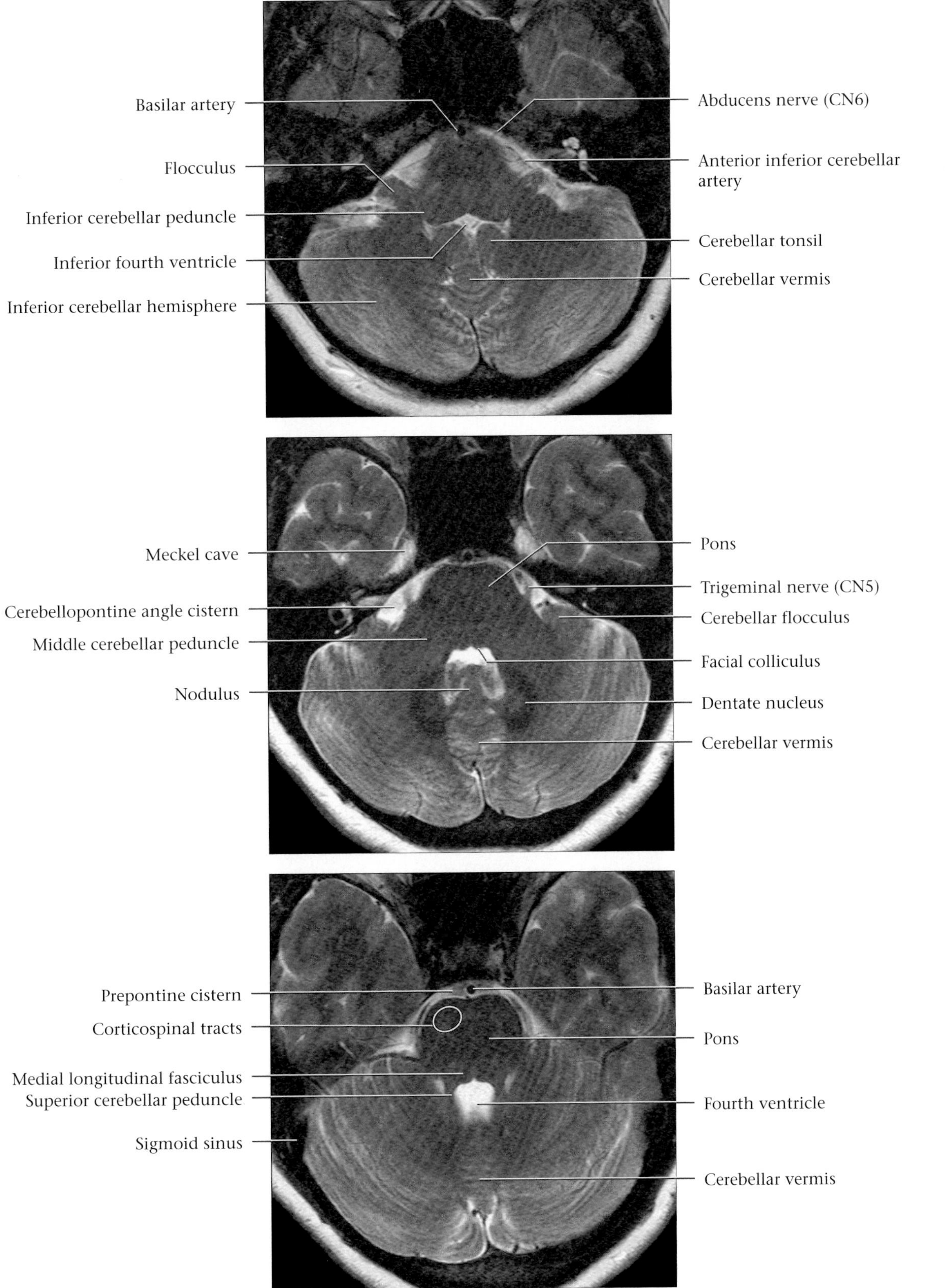

Basilar artery
Flocculus
Inferior cerebellar peduncle
Inferior fourth ventricle
Inferior cerebellar hemisphere
Abducens nerve (CN6)
Anterior inferior cerebellar artery
Cerebellar tonsil
Cerebellar vermis
Meckel cave
Cerebellopontine angle cistern
Middle cerebellar peduncle
Nodulus
Pons
Trigeminal nerve (CN5)
Cerebellar flocculus
Facial colliculus
Dentate nucleus
Cerebellar vermis
Prepontine cistern
Corticospinal tracts
Medial longitudinal fasciculus
Superior cerebellar peduncle
Sigmoid sinus
Basilar artery
Pons
Fourth ventricle
Cerebellar vermis

(Top) Image more superiorly at pontomedullary junction shows inferior cerebellar peduncles (restiform body) where cochlear nuclei of vestibulocochlear nerve CN8 are found. Abducens nerve (CN6) exits anteriorly at pontomedullary junction. Anterior inferior cerebellar artery, which arises from basilar artery, is seen looping in region of internal auditory canal. **(Middle)** Image at mid pons shows middle cerebellar peduncles (brachium pontis), major cerebellar peduncle. Facial colliculus, formed by axons of facial nerve CN7 looping around abducens nucleus CN6, creating bulge in floor of fourth ventricle. Trigeminal nerve CN5 is seen as it courses toward Meckel cave. Dentate nucleus is only cerebellar nucleus that is seen on imaging. **(Bottom)** Image at superior pons shows superior cerebellar peduncles (brachium conjunctivum). Corticospinal tracts are present in ventral pons.

BRAINSTEM AND CEREBELLUM OVERVIEW

AXIAL T2 MR

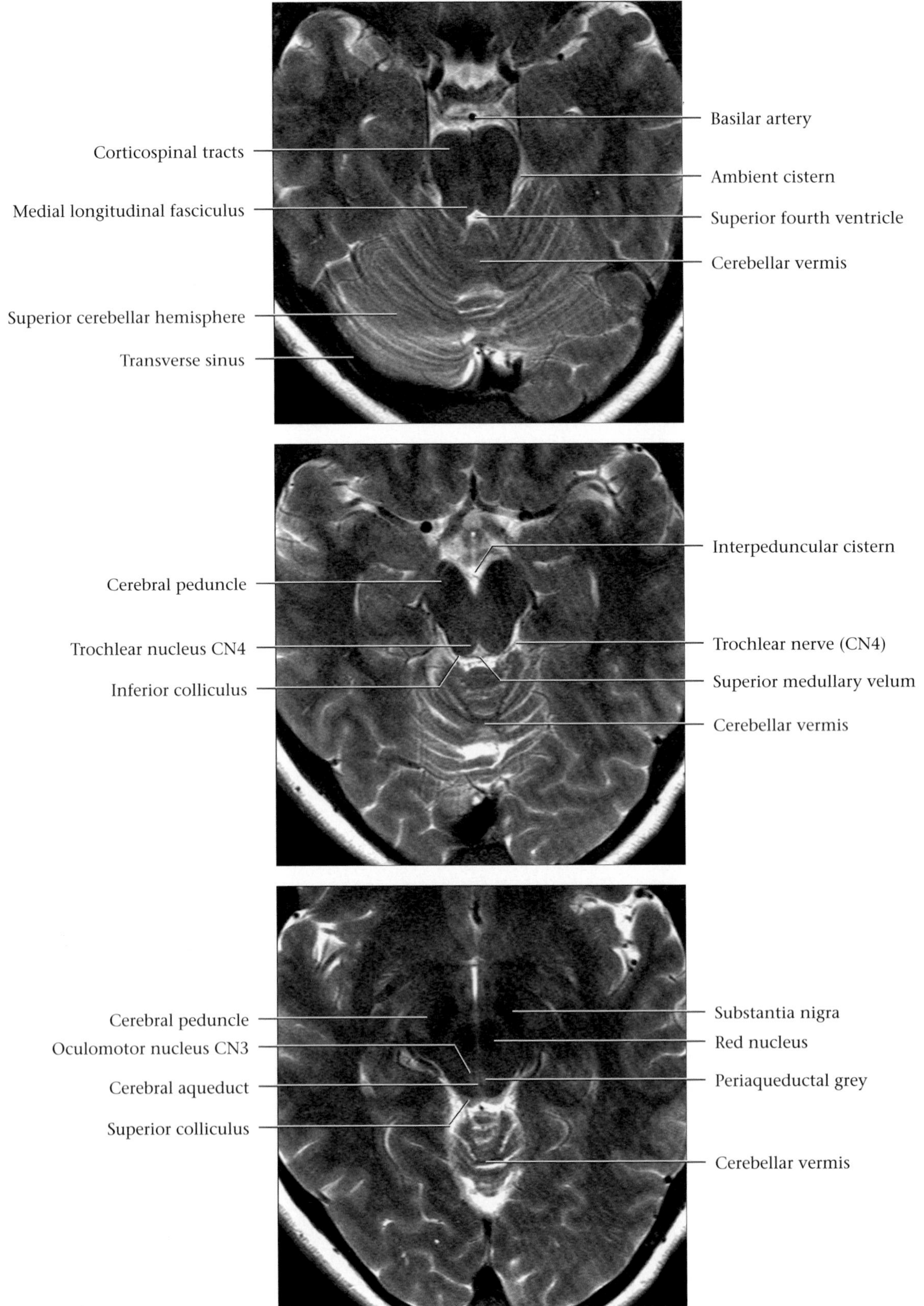
Basilar artery
Corticospinal tracts
Ambient cistern
Medial longitudinal fasciculus
Superior fourth ventricle
Cerebellar vermis
Superior cerebellar hemisphere
Transverse sinus
Interpeduncular cistern
Cerebral peduncle
Trochlear nucleus CN4
Trochlear nerve (CN4)
Superior medullary velum
Inferior colliculus
Cerebellar vermis
Cerebral peduncle
Substantia nigra
Red nucleus
Oculomotor nucleus CN3
Cerebral aqueduct
Periaqueductal grey
Superior colliculus
Cerebellar vermis

(Top) Image more superiorly shows junction of pons & midbrain. Major white matter tracts including corticospinal tracts & medial longitudinal fasciculus are known by typical location, but are not directly seen. **(Middle)** Image at inferior midbrain shows interpeduncular fossa where oculomotor nerve CN3 exits. Trochlear nucleus CN4 is present in paramedian gray matter, just dorsal to medial longitudinal fasciculus, approximate location shown. CN4 decussates in superior medullary velum & is seen exiting dorsally & wrapping around midbrain in ambient cistern. **(Bottom)** Image of superior midbrain shows cerebral peduncles where major white matter tracts including corticospinal tracts travel. Major pigmented gray nuclei, substantia nigra & red nucleus are seen. Oculomotor nerve CN3 nucleus is present at level of superior colliculus, approximate location shown.

AXIAL T1 MR

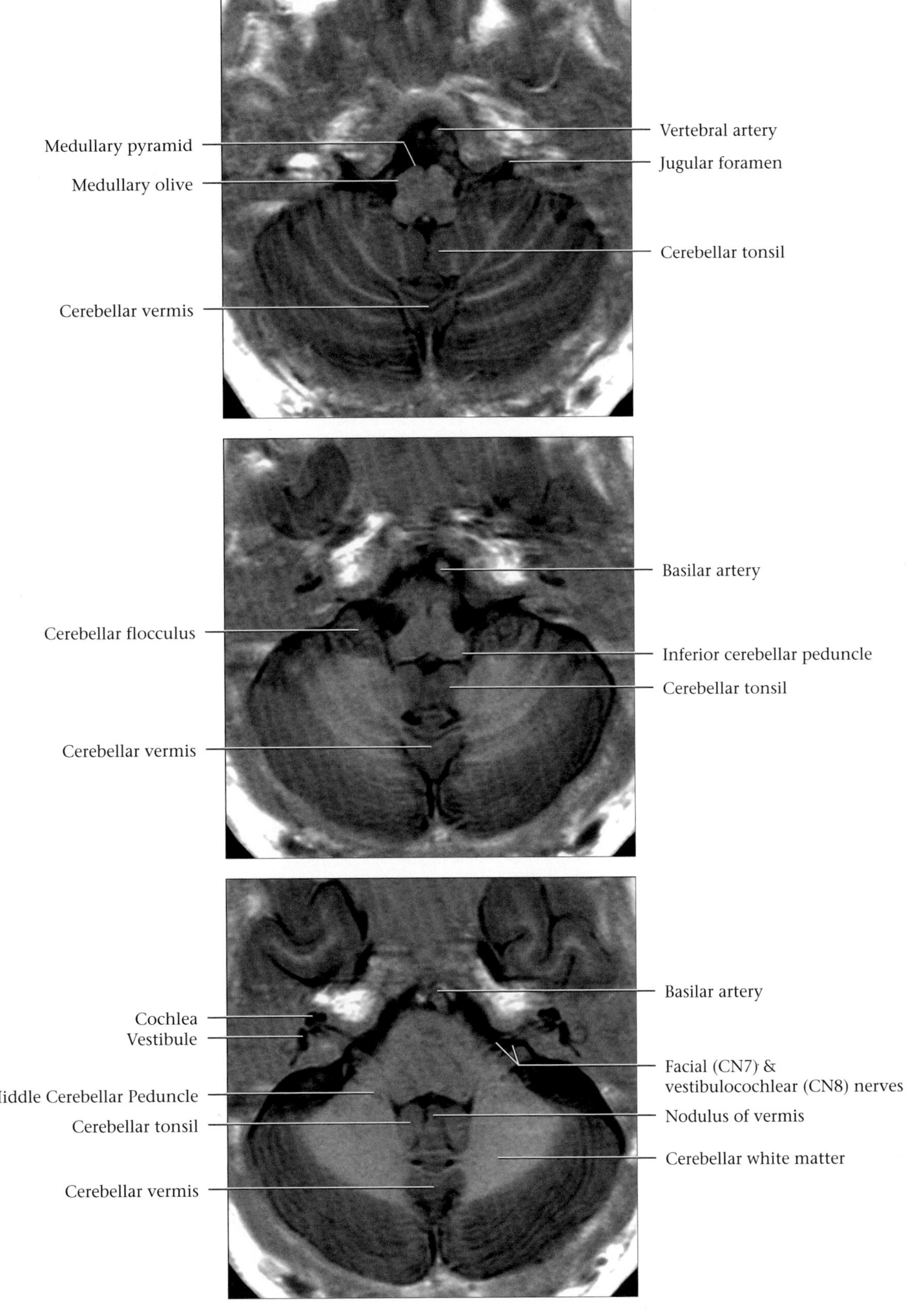

Medullary pyramid
Medullary olive
Cerebellar vermis
Vertebral artery
Jugular foramen
Cerebellar tonsil
Cerebellar flocculus
Cerebellar vermis
Basilar artery
Inferior cerebellar peduncle
Cerebellar tonsil
Cochlea
Vestibule
Middle Cerebellar Peduncle
Cerebellar tonsil
Cerebellar vermis
Basilar artery
Facial (CN7) &
vestibulocochlear (CN8) nerves
Nodulus of vermis
Cerebellar white matter

(Top) First of six axial T1 MR images from inferior to superior through posterior fossa at level of medulla. Dorsal medulla (tegmentum) contains cranial nerve nuclei & white matter tracts which can be identified by typical location, but are not directly visualized. **(Middle)** Image at level of superior medulla/pontomedullary junction shows inferior cerebellar peduncles (restiform body) where cochlear nuclei arise. Cerebellar flocculus is a common pseudolesion. **(Bottom)** Image at level of lower pons shows facial nerve CN7 & vestibulocochlear nerve CN8 coursing towards interior auditory canal. Nodulus of vermis may protrude into fourth ventricle & cause a pseudolesion. Middle cerebellar peduncle (brachium pontis) is major cerebellar peduncle & contains fibers from pontine nuclei.

AXIAL T1 MR

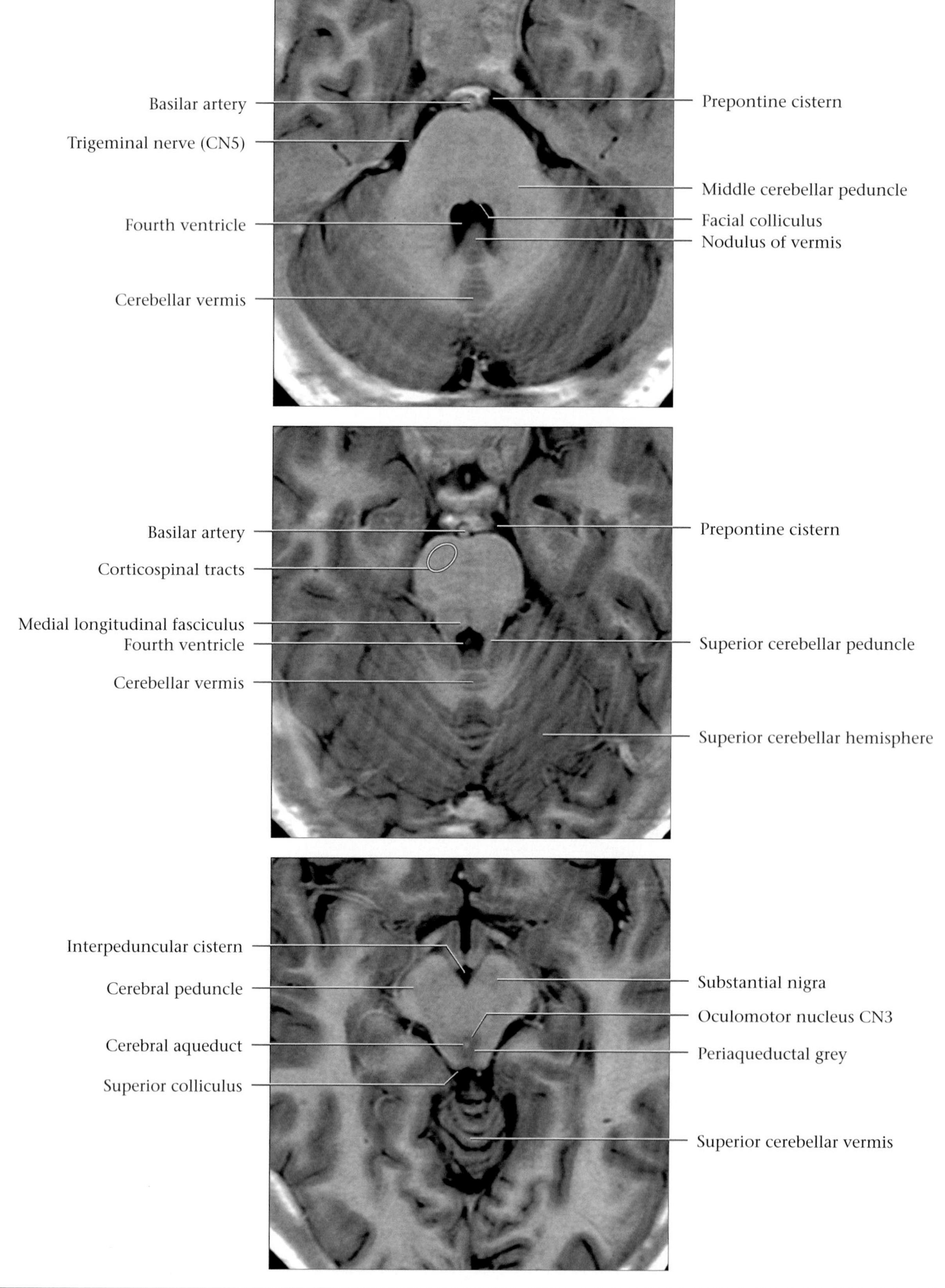

Basilar artery
Trigeminal nerve (CN5)
Fourth ventricle
Cerebellar vermis
Prepontine cistern
Middle cerebellar peduncle
Facial colliculus
Nodulus of vermis
Basilar artery
Corticospinal tracts
Medial longitudinal fasciculus
Fourth ventricle
Cerebellar vermis
Prepontine cistern
Superior cerebellar peduncle
Superior cerebellar hemisphere
Interpeduncular cistern
Cerebral peduncle
Cerebral aqueduct
Superior colliculus
Substantial nigra
Oculomotor nucleus CN3
Periaqueductal grey
Superior cerebellar vermis

(Top) Image more superiorly through mid pons shows middle cerebellar peduncles & trigeminal nerve CN5. Facial colliculus represents axons of facial nerve CN7 wrapping around nucleus of abducens nerve CN6. **(Middle)** Image at superior pons shows superior cerebellar peduncle (brachium conjunctivum). Approximate location of medial longitudinal fasciculus is shown, just lateral to midline, which is important in extraocular muscle movement & head location. **(Bottom)** Image through midbrain at superior colliculus shows approximate location of oculomotor nerve CN3 nucleus. Cerebral peduncles (crus cerebri) contain descending white matter tracts from cerebral hemispheres including corticospinal, corticobulbar & corticopontine tracts. Periaqueductal grey surrounds cerebral aqueduct.

CORONAL T2 MR

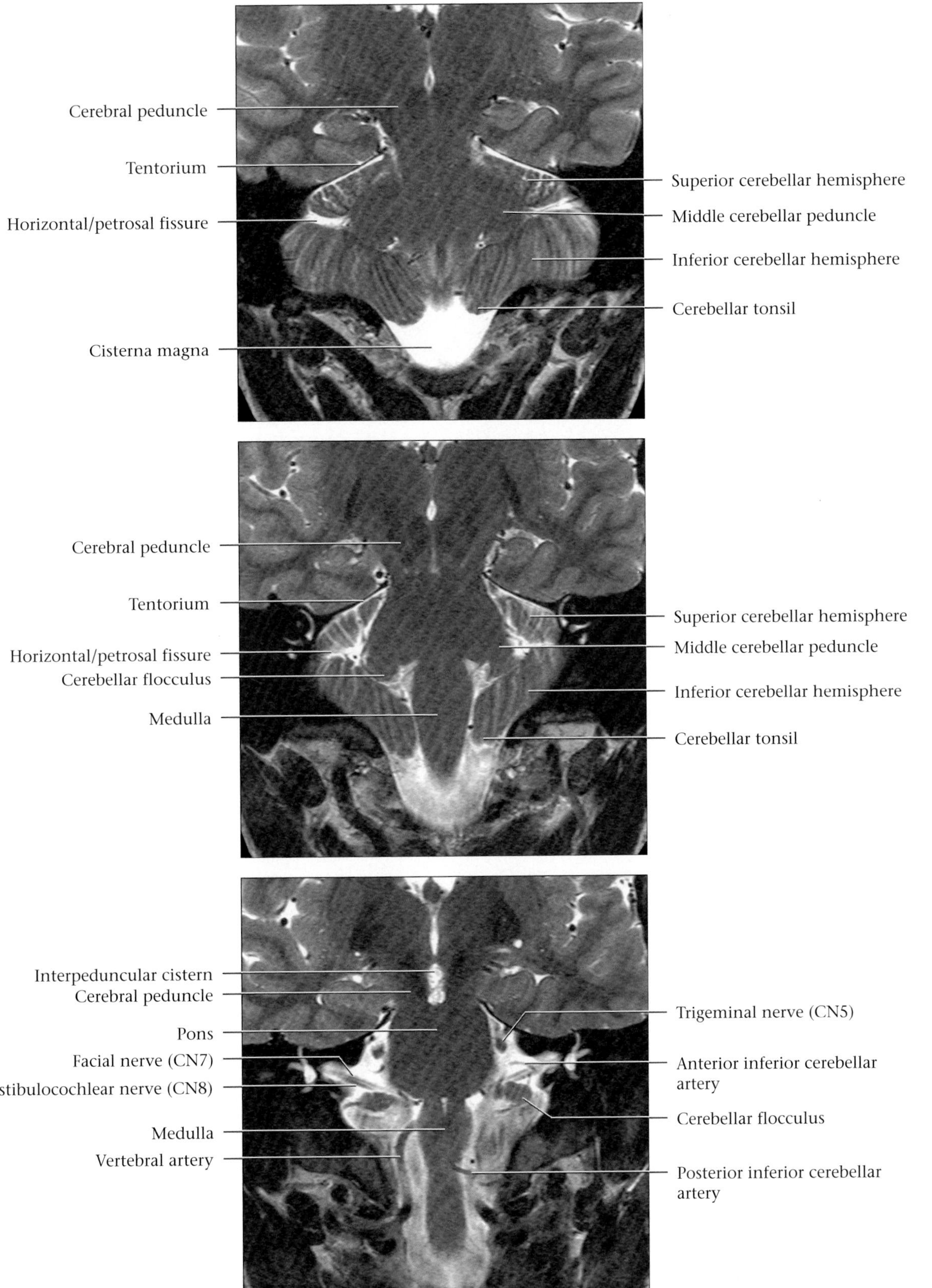
Cerebral peduncle
Tentorium
Horizontal/petrosal fissure
Cisterna magna
Superior cerebellar hemisphere
Middle cerebellar peduncle
Inferior cerebellar hemisphere
Cerebellar tonsil
Cerebral peduncle
Tentorium
Horizontal/petrosal fissure
Cerebellar flocculus
Medulla
Superior cerebellar hemisphere
Middle cerebellar peduncle
Inferior cerebellar hemisphere
Cerebellar tonsil
Interpeduncular cistern
Cerebral peduncle
Pons
Facial nerve (CN7)
Vestibulocochlear nerve (CN8)
Medulla
Vertebral artery
Trigeminal nerve (CN5)
Anterior inferior cerebellar artery
Cerebellar flocculus
Posterior inferior cerebellar artery

(Top) First of six coronal T2 MR images through posterior fossa from posterior to anterior shows prominent horizontal (petrosal) fissure of cerebellum which extends from middle cerebellar peduncle onto inferior (suboccipital) surface of cerebellum. **(Middle)** This image shows continuation of midbrain, pons & medulla. Cerebral peduncles contain corticospinal & other white matter tracts which are continuous with anterior (ventral) pons white matter tracts & continue to extend to medullary pyramids in ventral medulla. **(Bottom)** Image through brainstem at level of internal auditory canals. Trigeminal nerve is seen arising from lateral pons. Facial CN7 & vestibulocochlear CN8 nerves are seen coursing in cerebellopontine angle to internal auditory canal. Vertebrobasilar system is seen which supplies vast majority of brainstem & cerebellum.

BRAINSTEM AND CEREBELLUM OVERVIEW

CORONAL T2 MR

Oculomotor nerve (CN3)
Cerebral peduncle
Trigeminal nerve (CN5)
Pons
Internal auditory canal
Anterior inferior cerebellar artery
Cerebellopontine angle cistern
Medulla
Vertebral artery
Posterior inferior cerebellar artery

Posterior cerebral artery
Oculomotor nerve (CN3)
Superior cerebellar artery
Pons
Trigeminal nerve (CN5)
Cochlea
Cerebellopontine angle cistern
Vertebral artery

Posterior cerebral artery
Oculomotor nerve (CN3)
Superior cerebellar artery
Pons
Trigeminal nerve (CN5)
Cerebellopontine angle cistern
Basilar artery
Vertebral artery

(Top) Image more anteriorly shows anterior aspect of pons, pons belly or bulb, which contains multiple transverse pontine fibers & descending tracts. Vertebral arteries form basilar artery in region of pontomedullary junction. Posterior inferior cerebellar artery arises from vertebral artery & has a reciprocal relationship with anterior inferior cerebellar artery which arises from basilar artery. **(Middle)** This image shows oculomotor nerve CN3 coursing between posterior cerebral artery above & superior cerebellar artery below. **(Bottom)** Image through anterior pons shows trigeminal nerve CN5 entering porus trigeminus of Meckel cave. Basilar artery is seen coursing along anterior surface of pons giving rise to superior cerebellar & posterior cerebral arteries. Pons is supplied by perforating branches from basilar artery & superior cerebellar artery branches.

BRAINSTEM AND CEREBELLUM OVERVIEW

SAGITTAL T2 MR

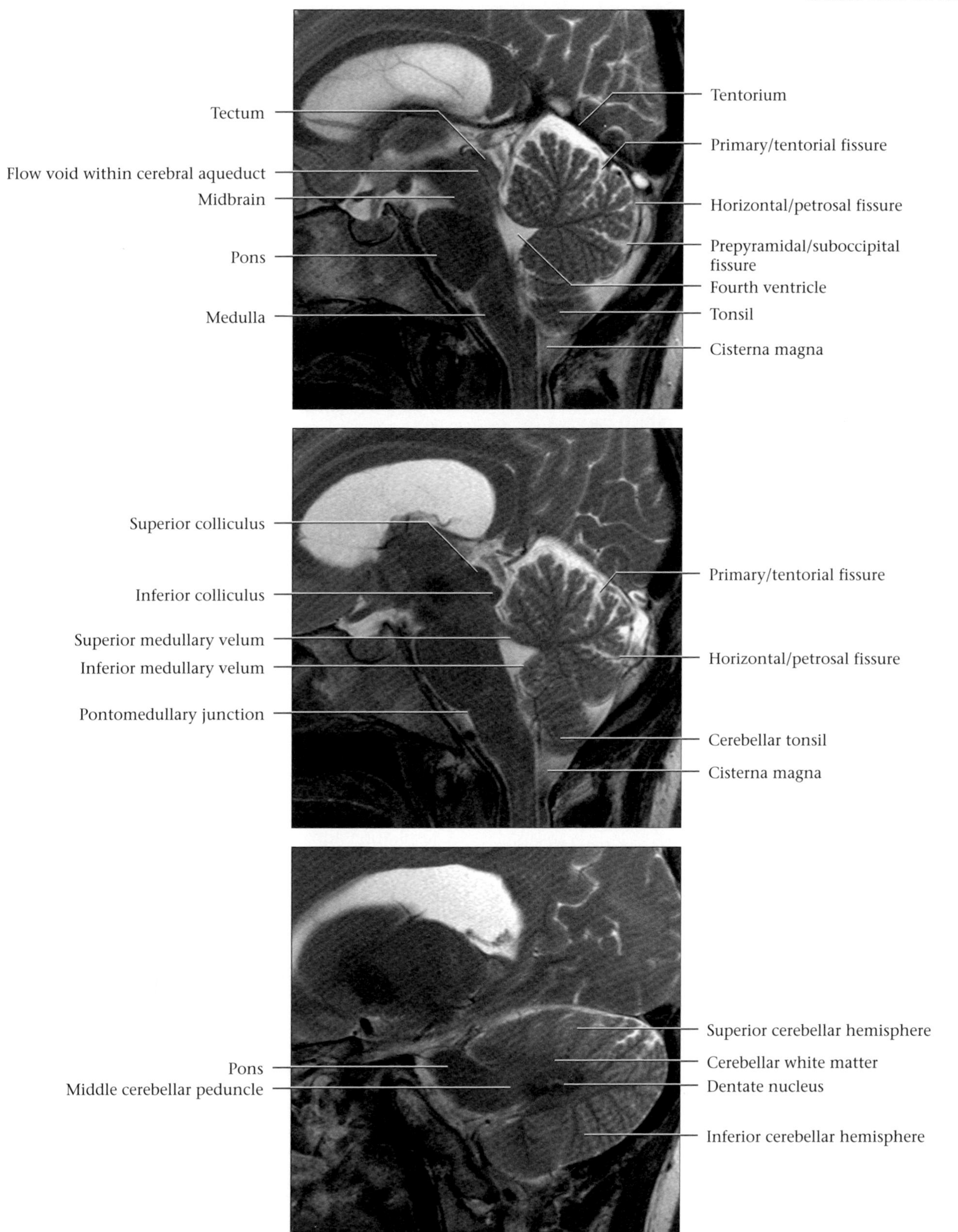

Tectum
Flow void within cerebral aqueduct
Midbrain
Pons
Medulla
Tentorium
Primary/tentorial fissure
Horizontal/petrosal fissure
Prepyramidal/suboccipital fissure
Fourth ventricle
Tonsil
Cisterna magna
Superior colliculus
Inferior colliculus
Superior medullary velum
Inferior medullary velum
Pontomedullary junction
Primary/tentorial fissure
Horizontal/petrosal fissure
Cerebellar tonsil
Cisterna magna
Pons
Middle cerebellar peduncle
Superior cerebellar hemisphere
Cerebellar white matter
Dentate nucleus
Inferior cerebellar hemisphere

(Top) First of three sagittal T2 MR images from medial to lateral shows midline posterior fossa structures situated below tentorium cerebelli. Brainstem is anterior & separated from cerebellum by cerebral aqueduct & fourth ventricle. Brainstem consists of midbrain (mesencephalon), pons & medulla. Major fissures of cerebellum separate cerebellum & vermis into lobules. **(Middle)** Image just lateral of midline shows continuation of primary (tentorial) & horizontal (petrosal) fissures dividing cerebellar hemisphere into lobules. Superior & inferior medullary velum makes up roof of fourth ventricle. Superior & inferior colliculi of tectum are seen. **(Bottom)** Image more lateral shows white matter core of cerebellum, arbor vitae (tree of life). Largest gray nucleus of cerebellum, dentate nucleus is visible.

MIDBRAIN

Terminology

Abbreviations

- Cerebrospinal fluid (CSF)
- Cranial nerves (CN): Oculomotor nerve (CN3), trochlear nerve (CN4)

Synonyms

- Midbrain, mesencephalon

Definitions

- Midbrain: Portion of brainstem which connects pons and cerebellum with forebrain

Gross Anatomy

Overview

- "Butterfly-shaped" upper brainstem which passes through hiatus in tentorium cerebelli
- Composed of **gray matter formations, CN nuclei** (CN3-4) and **white matter tracts**
- Three main parts
  - **Cerebral peduncles**: White matter tracts
    - Continuous with pontine bulb and medullary pyramids
  - **Tegmentum**: CN nuclei, gray matter nuclei, white matter tracts
    - Continuous with pontine tegmentum
    - Ventral to cerebral aqueduct
  - **Tectum (quadrigeminal plate)**: Superior and inferior colliculi
    - Dorsal to cerebral aqueduct
- Midbrain **connections**
  - Rostral (superior): Cerebral hemispheres, basal ganglia and thalami
  - Dorsal (posterior): Cerebellum
  - Caudal (inferior): Pons
- **Cerebral aqueduct** passes through dorsal midbrain between tectum posteriorly and tegmentum anteriorly, connecting third and fourth ventricles
- Adjacent CSF cisterns
  - Interpeduncular: Anterior, contains CN3
  - Ambient (perimesencephalic): Lateral, contains CN4
  - Quadrigeminal plate: Posterior, contains CN4
- Blood supply by vertebrobasilar circulation
  - Small perforating branches from basilar, superior cerebellar and posterior cerebral arteries

Cerebral Peduncles (Crus Cerebri)

- **Corticospinal, corticobulbar & corticopontine fibers**
- Cerebral peduncles separated in midline by interpeduncular fossa

Mesencephalic Tegmentum

- Directly continuous with pontine tegmentum, contains same tracts
- Multiple **white matter tracts** (not resolved on conventional imaging)
  - **Medial longitudinal fasciculus**: Oculomotor-vestibular
  - **Medial lemniscus**: Somatosensory
  - **Lateral lemniscus**: Auditory
  - **Spinothalamic tract**: Somatosensory
  - **Central tegmental tract**: Motor
- **Gray matter formations**
  - **Substantia nigra**: Pigmented nucleus, extends through midbrain from pons to subthalamic region, important in movement
    - Pars compacta: Contains dopaminergic cells (atrophied in Parkinson disease)
    - Pars reticularis: Contains GABAergic cells
  - **Red nucleus**: Relay and control station for cerebellar, globus pallidus and corticomotor impulses
    - Important for muscle tone, posture, locomotion
  - **Periaqueductal grey**: Surrounds cerebral aqueduct
    - Important in modulation of pain and defensive behavior
- **Cranial nerve nuclei**
  - **CN3** nuclei at superior colliculus level
    - Paramedian, anterior to cerebral aqueduct
    - Motor nuclei consists of five individual motor subnuclei that supply individual extraocular muscles
    - Edinger-Westphal parasympathetic nuclei: Dorsal to CN3 nucleus in periaquaductal grey
    - CN3 fibers course anteriorly through midbrain to exit at interpeduncular fossa
  - **CN4** nuclei at inferior colliculus level
    - Paramedian, anterior to cerebral aqueduct
    - Dorsal to medial longitudinal fasciculus
    - CN4 fibers course posteriorly around cerebral aqueduct, decussate in superior medullary velum
    - CN4 exits dorsal midbrain just inferior to inferior colliculus
- **Reticular formation**: Expands from medulla to rostral midbrain
  - Occupies central tegmentum
  - Afferent and efferent connections
  - Important in consciousness, motor function, respiration and cardiovascular control

Tectum (Quadrigeminal Plate)

- **Superior colliculi**: Visual pathway
- **Inferior colliculi**: Auditory pathway

Imaging Anatomy

Overview

- CN3 & 4 seen as they exit midbrain
  - CN3 at level of superior colliculus, seen in interpeduncular fossa
  - CN4 at level of inferior colliculus, seen dorsally and in ambient cistern as wraps around midbrain
- Cerebral aqueduct: Signal varies due to flow artifact
- CN nuclei and white matter tracts can be identified by typical location, but are not resolved on imaging
- Substantia nigra and red nucleus well seen

Anatomy-Based Imaging Issues

Imaging Recommendations

- MR for cranial neuropathy or acute ischemia
- CT may be helpful in acute setting
- CTA and MRA for vertebrobasilar circulation

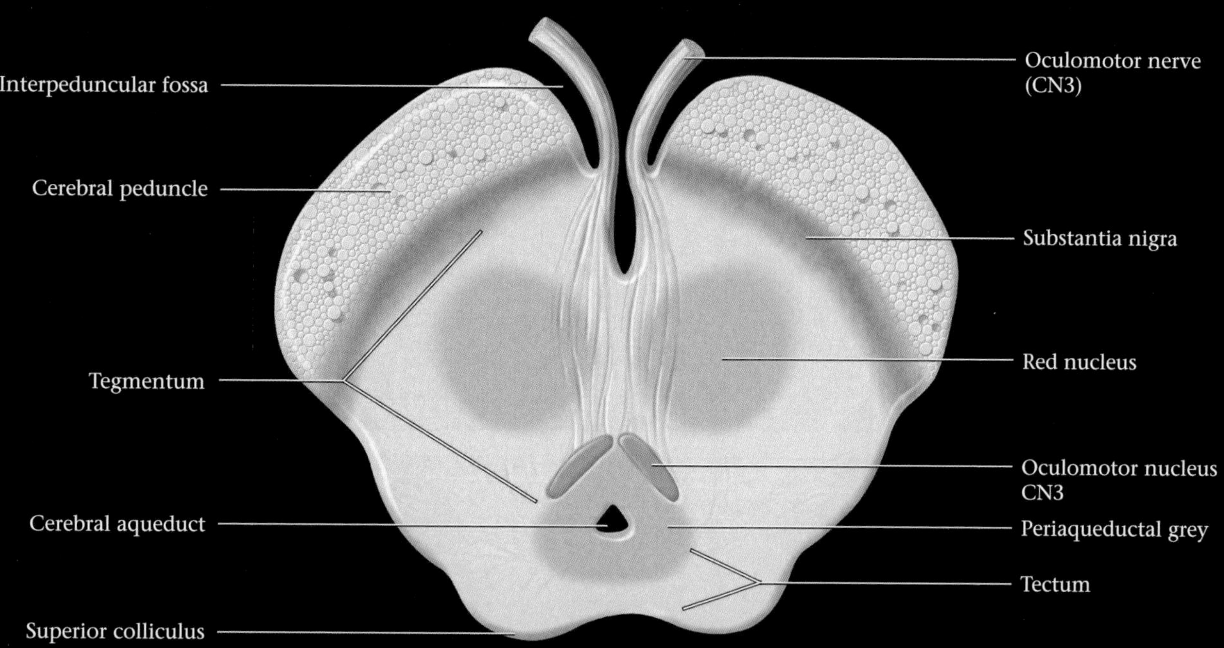
Interpeduncular fossa
Cerebral peduncle
Tegmentum
Cerebral aqueduct
Superior colliculus
Oculomotor nerve (CN3)
Substantia nigra
Red nucleus
Oculomotor nucleus CN3
Periaqueductal grey
Tectum

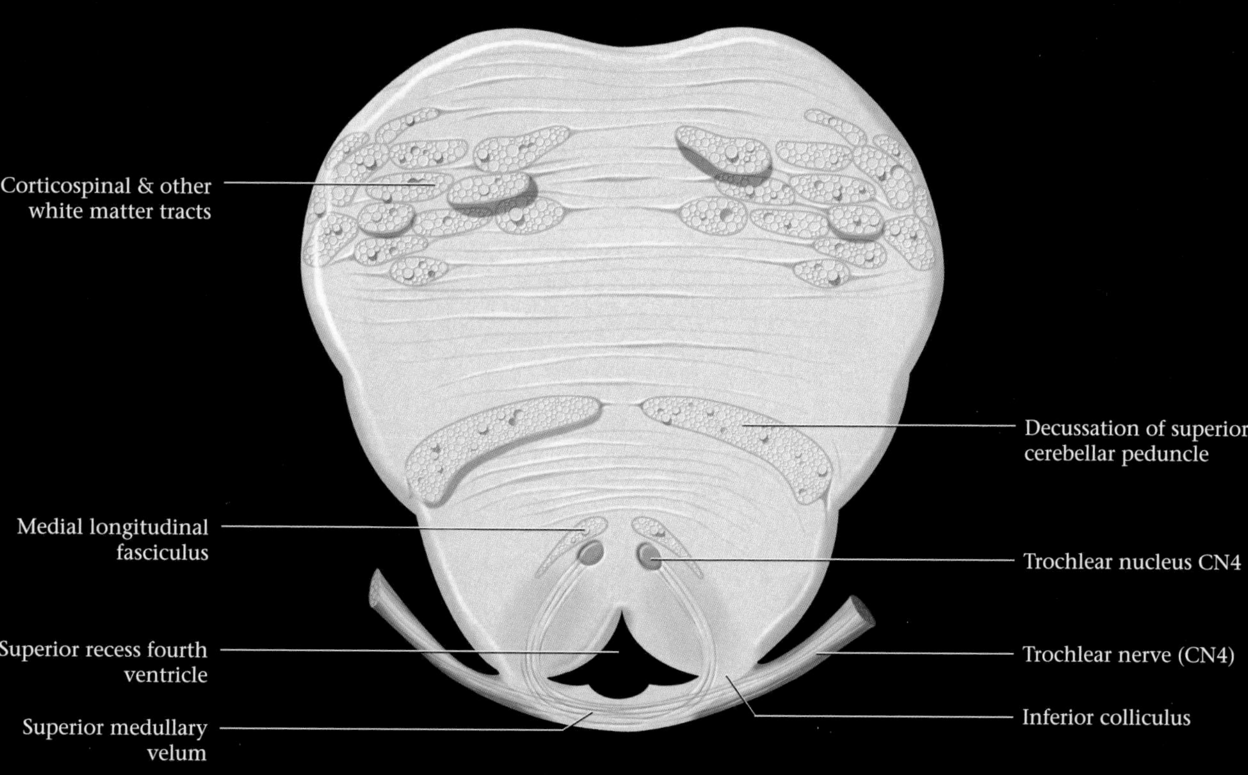
Corticospinal & other white matter tracts
Medial longitudinal fasciculus
Superior recess fourth ventricle
Superior medullary velum
Decussation of superior cerebellar peduncle
Trochlear nucleus CN4
Trochlear nerve (CN4)
Inferior colliculus

(Top) Axial graphic through level of superior colliculus shows oculomotor nucleus (CN3) just anterior to cerebral aqueduct. CN3 exits into interpeduncular fossa. Cerebral peduncles are anterior & contain corticospinal & other white matter tracts. Tegmentum is anterior & tectum is posterior to cerebral aqueduct. Substantia nigra consists of two layers of cells: Pars compacta posteriorly & pars reticulata anteriorly & plays a vital role in Parkinson disease. **(Bottom)** Axial graphic of midbrain at level of inferior colliculi shows trochlear nucleus (CN4) & nerve fibers as they decussate in superior medullary velum which forms roof of fourth ventricle. Each superior oblique muscle is innervated by contralateral trochlear nucleus. CN4 exits dorsally, just inferior to inferior colliculus & is the only cranial nerve to exit dorsal brainstem.

AXIAL T1 MR

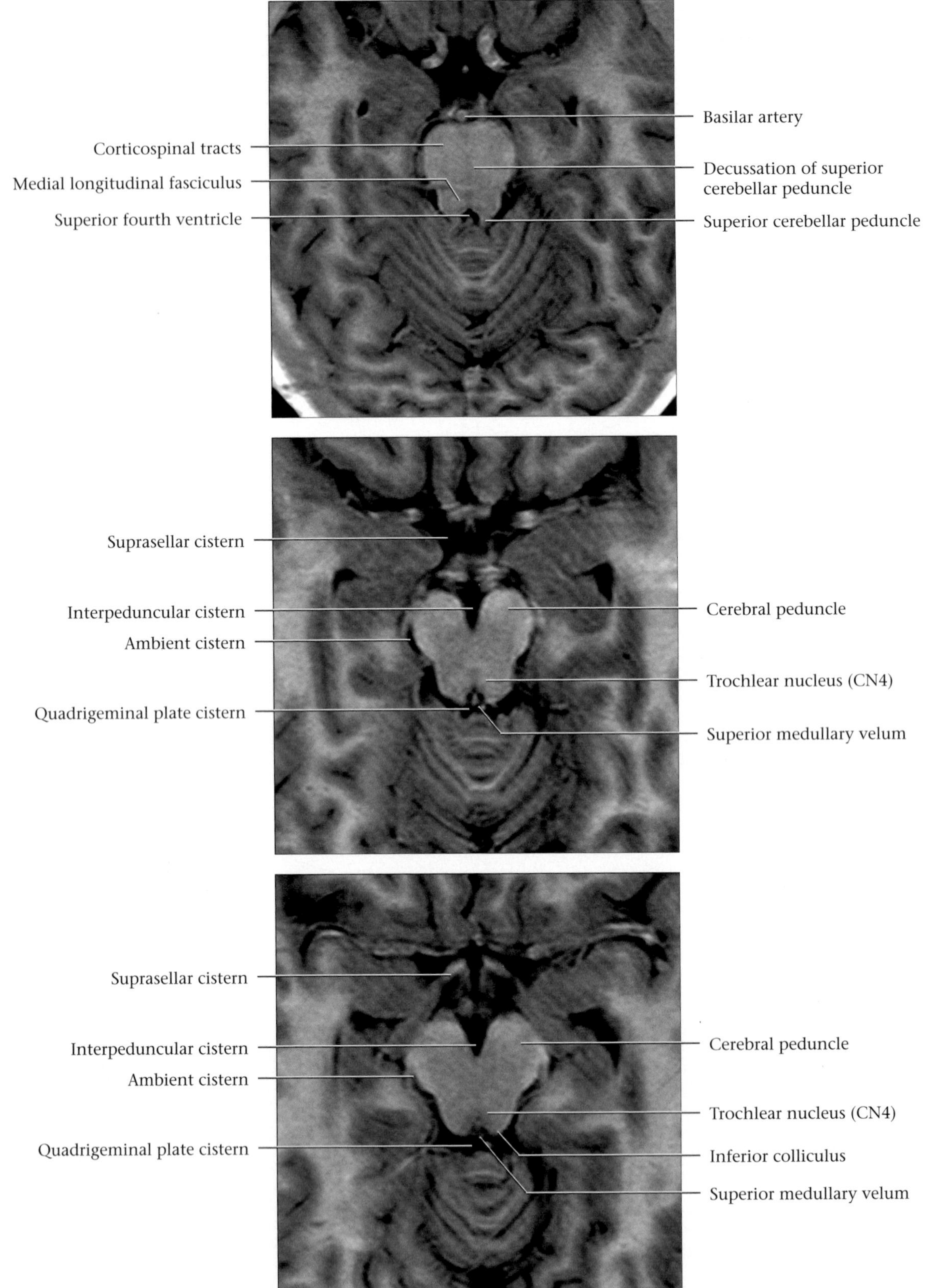
Corticospinal tracts
Medial longitudinal fasciculus
Superior fourth ventricle
Basilar artery
Decussation of superior cerebellar peduncle
Superior cerebellar peduncle
Suprasellar cistern
Interpeduncular cistern
Ambient cistern
Quadrigeminal plate cistern
Cerebral peduncle
Trochlear nucleus (CN4)
Superior medullary velum
Suprasellar cistern
Interpeduncular cistern
Ambient cistern
Quadrigeminal plate cistern
Cerebral peduncle
Trochlear nucleus (CN4)
Inferior colliculus
Superior medullary velum

(Top) First of six axial T1 MR images of midbrain from inferior to superior shows junction of pons with inferior midbrain. The brainstem tegmentum is dorsal & is common to all three parts of the brainstem: Medulla, pons & midbrain. At pons level, tegmentum is covered by cerebellum, while at midbrain level, tectal plate (superior & inferior colliculi) covers tegmentum. **(Middle)** Image through inferior midbrain shows location of trochlear nucleus CN4, in paramedian midbrain anterior to cerebral peduncle at level of inferior colliculus. Although not seen, medial longitudinal fasciculus is just ventral (anterior) to CN4 nucleus. **(Bottom)** Image through inferior midbrain & inferior colliculus shows superior medullary velum which contains decussation of CN4. CN4 exits dorsally & wraps around midbrain in ambient cistern.

AXIAL T1 MR

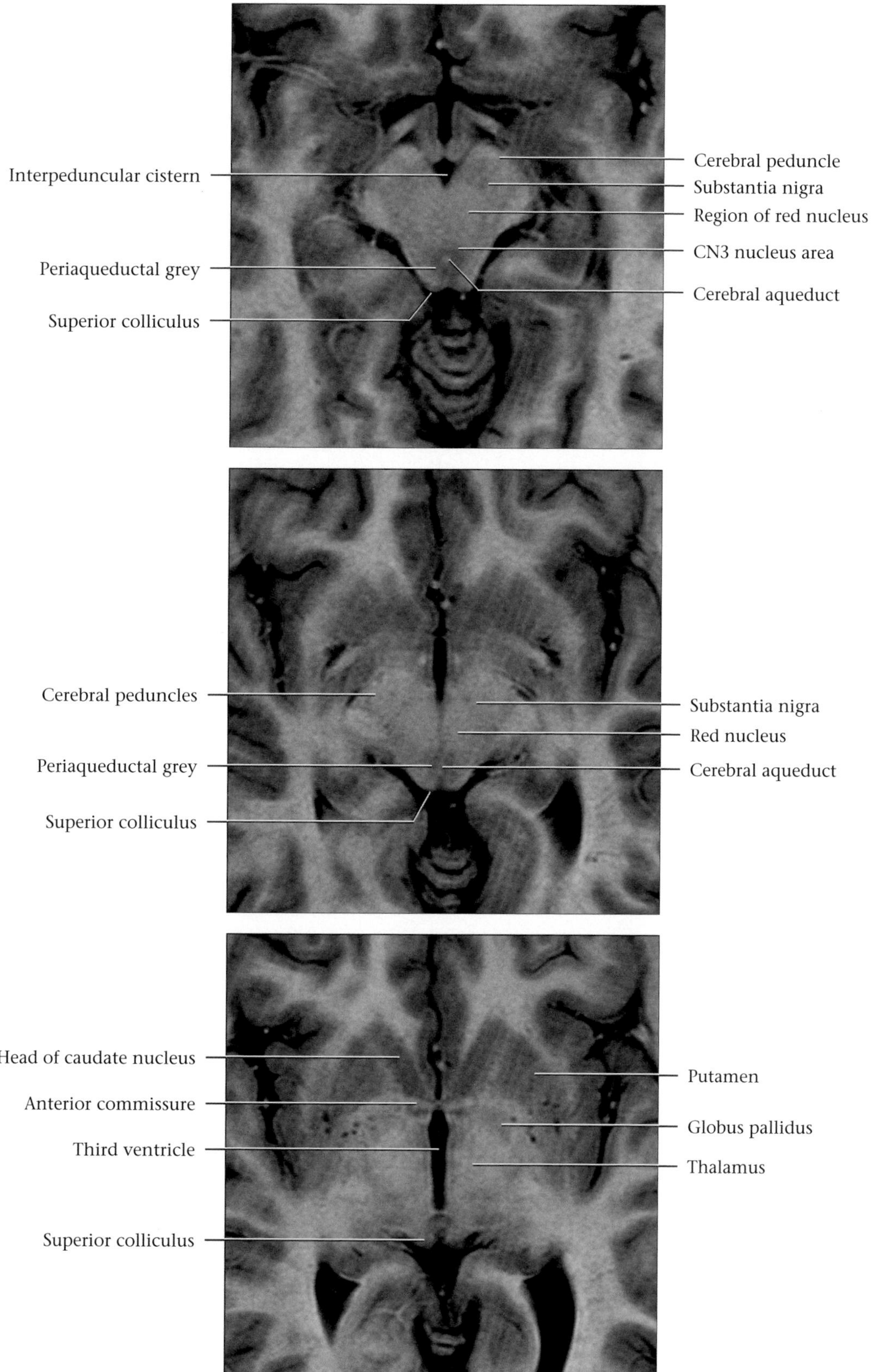
Interpeduncular cistern
Periaqueductal grey
Superior colliculus
Cerebral peduncle
Substantia nigra
Region of red nucleus
CN3 nucleus area
Cerebral aqueduct
Cerebral peduncles
Periaqueductal grey
Superior colliculus
Substantia nigra
Red nucleus
Cerebral aqueduct
Head of caudate nucleus
Anterior commissure
Third ventricle
Superior colliculus
Putamen
Globus pallidus
Thalamus

(Top) Image through superior midbrain at level of superior colliculus shows approximate location of oculomotor nerve CN3 nucleus along anterolateral periaqueductal grey. CN3 exits midbrain in interpeduncular fossa. Pigmented nuclei, substantia nigra & red nucleus are seen at this level, although are better seen on T2 images. **(Middle)** Image through superior midbrain shows cerebral peduncles as they descend from cerebral hemispheres. Cerebral peduncles (crus cerebri) contain descending white matter tracts from cerebral hemispheres including corticospinal, corticobulbar & corticopontine tracts. Periaqueductal grey surrounds cerebral aqueduct & is important in modulation of pain & defensive behavior. **(Bottom)** Image through junction of midbrain with inferior basal ganglia. White matter tracts extend from midbrain to basal ganglia & thalamus.

MIDBRAIN

AXIAL T2 MR

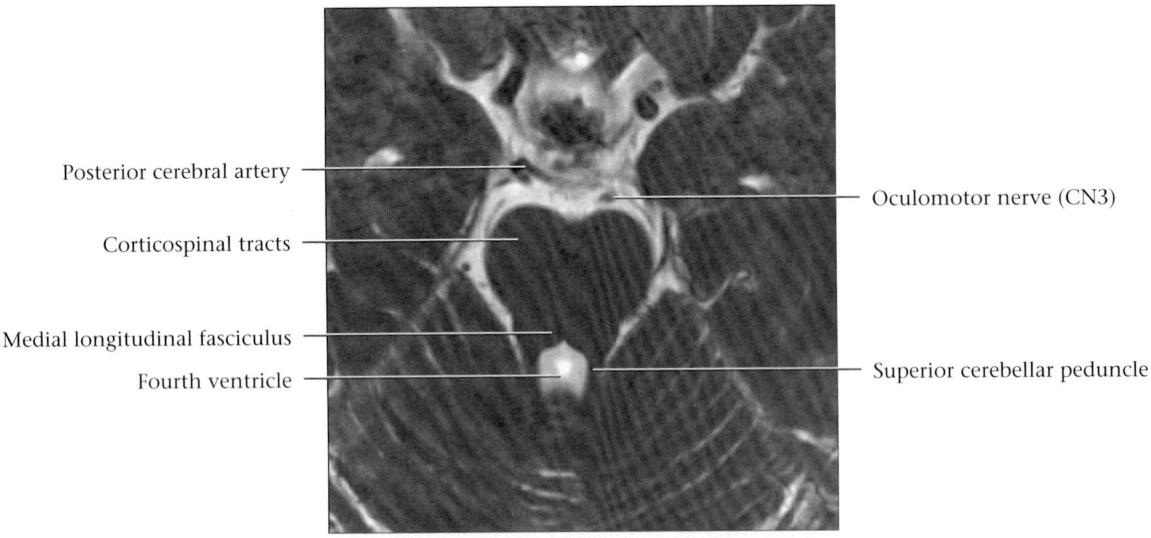

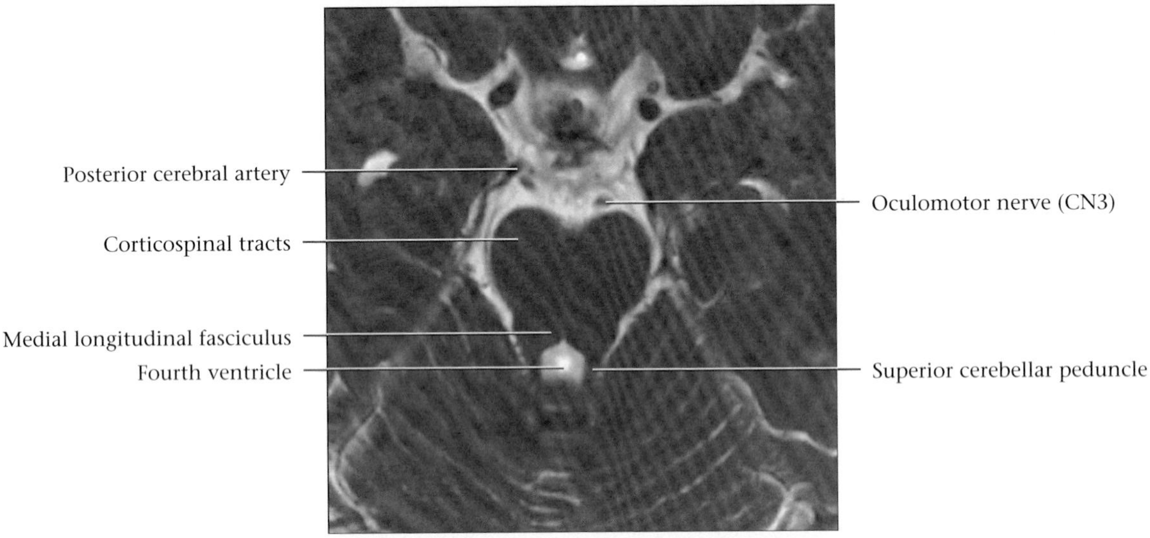

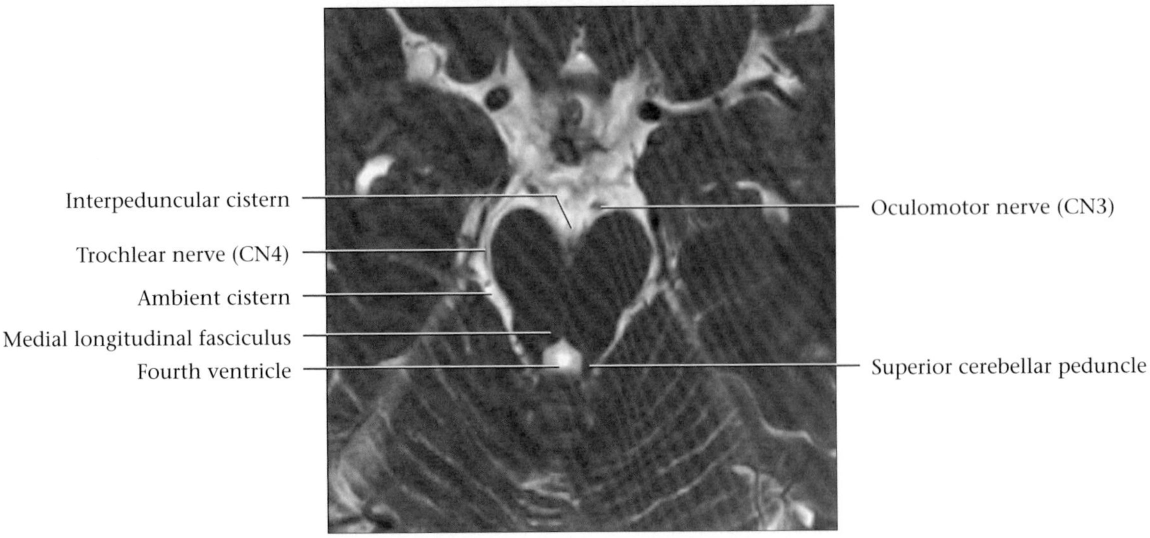

Posterior cerebral artery
Corticospinal tracts
Medial longitudinal fasciculus
Fourth ventricle
Oculomotor nerve (CN3)
Superior cerebellar peduncle

Posterior cerebral artery
Corticospinal tracts
Medial longitudinal fasciculus
Fourth ventricle
Oculomotor nerve (CN3)
Superior cerebellar peduncle

Interpeduncular cistern
Trochlear nerve (CN4)
Ambient cistern
Medial longitudinal fasciculus
Fourth ventricle
Oculomotor nerve (CN3)
Superior cerebellar peduncle

(Top) First of six axial T2 MR images (balanced steady state free precession technique) from inferior to superior through midbrain shows junction of pons & midbrain. White matter tracts including corticospinal tracts & medial longitudinal fasciculus continue into midbrain in approximately same location as they are seen in pons. **(Middle)** This image shows oculomotor nerves CN3 bilaterally, anterior to midbrain. Posterior cerebral artery is noted just anterior to CN3. CN3 passes between posterior cerebral artery & superior cerebellar artery. A posterior communicating artery aneurysm may result in a CN3 palsy. **(Bottom)** Image at inferior midbrain shows trochlear nerve CN4 as it wraps around midbrain in ambient cistern. It is only cranial nerve to exit dorsally from brainstem. Oculomotor nerves CN3 exit midbrain at interpeduncular fossa.

MIDBRAIN

AXIAL T2 MR

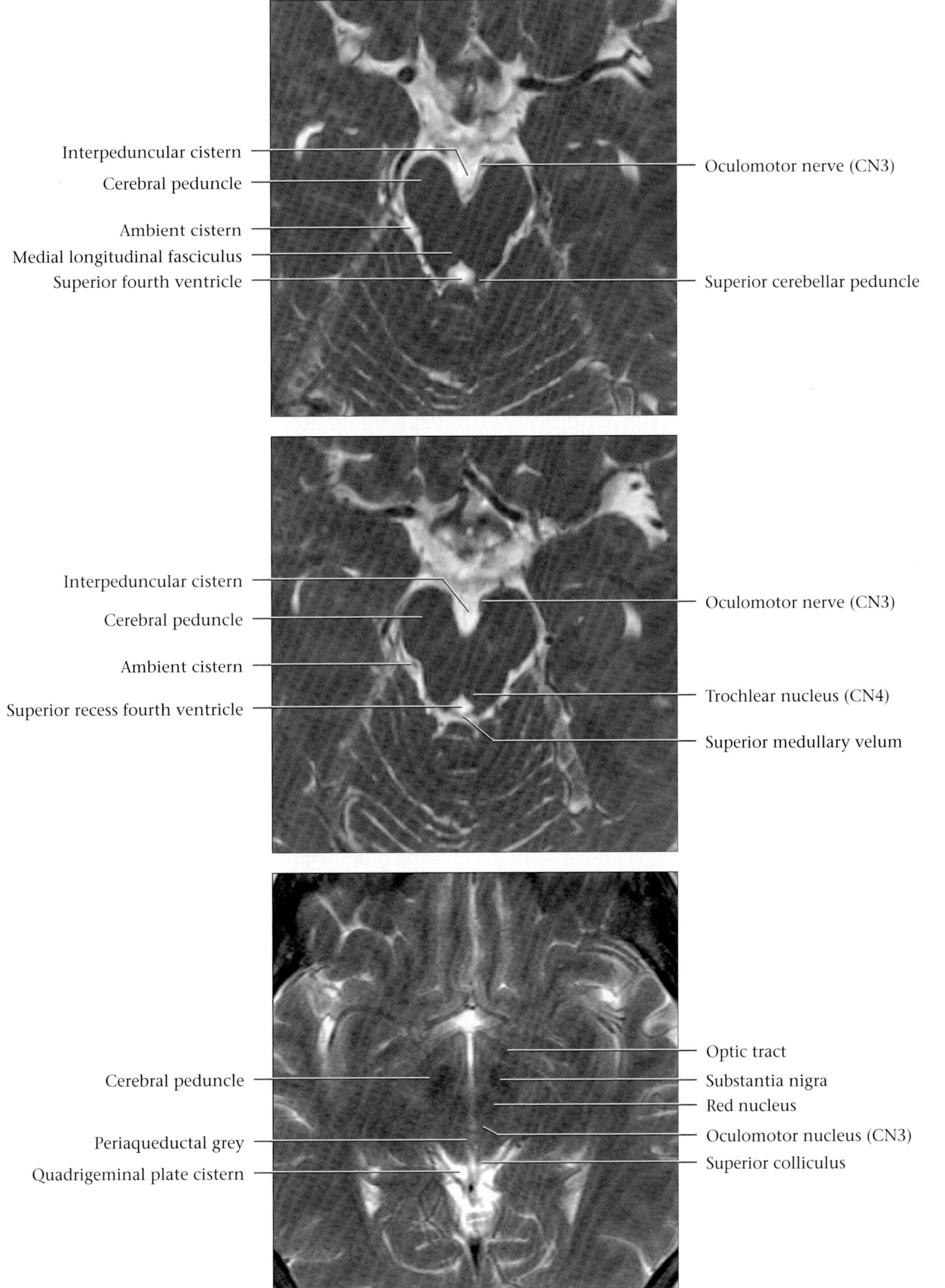

Interpeduncular cistern
Cerebral peduncle
Ambient cistern
Medial longitudinal fasciculus
Superior fourth ventricle
Oculomotor nerve (CN3)
Superior cerebellar peduncle
Interpeduncular cistern
Cerebral peduncle
Ambient cistern
Superior recess fourth ventricle
Oculomotor nerve (CN3)
Trochlear nucleus (CN4)
Superior medullary velum
Cerebral peduncle
Periaqueductal grey
Quadrigeminal plate cistern
Optic tract
Substantia nigra
Red nucleus
Oculomotor nucleus (CN3)
Superior colliculus

(Top) A more superior image shows midbrain at level of superior fourth ventricle. Oculomotor nerve is seen in interpeduncular fossa as it heads towards cavernous sinus. **(Middle)** Image more superiorly shows midbrain at level of superior recess of fourth ventricle. Trochlear nucleus CN4 is located in paramedial gray matter, just dorsal to medial longitudinal fasciculus, approximate location shown. CN4 decussates in superior medullary velum. **(Bottom)** Image more superiorly in a different patient shows superior midbrain at level of superior colliculi. The pigmented nuclei, substantia nigra & red nucleus are well seen. Substantia nigra contains two parts, pars compacta & pars reticularis. Pars compacta becomes atrophied in Parkinson's disease where there is a loss of dopaminergic cells. Oculomotor nucleus CN3 is present at this level, approximate location shown.

PONS

Terminology

Abbreviations

- Cerebellopontine angle (CPA)
- Cranial nerves (CN): Trigeminal nerve (CN5), abducens nerve (CN6), facial nerve (CN7), vestibulocochlear nerve (CN8)

Definitions

- Pons: Portion of brain stem which relays information from brain to cerebellum

Gross Anatomy

Overview

- Bulbous mid portion of brainstem located between midbrain (superiorly) & medulla oblongata (inferiorly)
- Composed of gray matter formations, CN nuclei (CN5-8) and white matter tracts
- Two main parts
  - Ventral (anterior) pons: White matter tracts
    - Continuous with cerebral peduncles superiorly and medullary pyramids inferiorly
  - Dorsal tegmentum: CN nuclei, gray matter nuclei, white matter tracts
    - Continuation of midbrain tegmentum superiorly and medullary tegmentum inferiorly
- Dorsal surface of pons forms rostral half of rhomboid fossa of fourth ventricle
- Adjacent CSF cisterns
  - Prepontine cistern: Anterior to pons; contains CN5 & 6
  - CPA cistern: Lateral to pons; contains CN7 & 8
- Blood supply by vertebrobasilar circulation
  - Medial branches of superior cerebellar arteries
  - Perforating branches of basilar artery, thalamoperforator arteries

Ventral (Anterior) Pons

- Contains longitudinal fibers primarily from **corticospinal, corticobulbar & corticopontine tracts**
- Multiple **transverse pontine fibers** make up bulk
- May be referred to as pontine bulb or belly

Dorsal Tegmentum

- Continuation of medulla except medullary pyramids
- Multiple **white matter tracts of tegmentum** (not resolved on conventional imaging)
  - Medial lemniscus: Somatosensory
  - Medial longitudinal fasciculus: Oculomotor-vestibular
  - Lateral lemniscus: Auditory
  - Trapezoid body: Auditory
  - Spinothalamic tract: Somatosensory
  - Central tegmental tract: Motor
- **Cranial nerve nuclei**
  - **CN5** nuclei located throughout brainstem and upper cord
    - Bulk of motor, main sensory and mesencephalic nuclei located in pons
  - **CN6** nucleus
    - Nucleus located in pontine tegmentum near midline, anterior to fourth ventricle
    - Axons of facial nerve (CN7) loop around abducens nucleus creating a bulge in floor of fourth ventricle, the facial colliculus
  - **CN7** nucleus
    - CN7 has three main nuclei within pons: Motor, superior salivatory, solitary tract
    - Located in ventrolateral aspect of tegmentum of lower pons
  - **CN8** nuclei
    - CN8 has cochlear and vestibular nuclei
    - Vestibular nuclei beneath lateral recess along floor of fourth ventricle (rhomboid fossa)
    - Dorsal and ventral cochlear nuclei on lateral surface of inferior cerebellar peduncle (restiform body)

Imaging Anatomy

Overview

- CN root entry & exit zones visualized
  - CN5 root entry zone at mid lateral pons
  - CN6 exit brainstem anteriorly at pontomedullary junction
  - CN7 exit lateral brainstem at root exit zone in pontomedullary junction
  - CN8 enters brainstem, posterior to CN7 at pontomedullary junction
- CN nuclei not resolved on conventional imaging
- Specific white matter tracts can be identified by typical location, but are not resolved on imaging
- CPA: Junction between pons and cerebellum

Anatomy-Based Imaging Issues

Imaging Recommendations

- CT may be useful for acute setting
  - Pontine hemorrhage, ischemia
- MR for cranial neuropathy
- Diffusion imaging for acute ischemia
- CTA and MRA for vertebrobasilar circulation

Clinical Issues

- White matter lesions affecting middle cerebellar peduncle (brachium pontis) or location of medial longitudinal fasciculus, think multiple sclerosis
- Hypertensive hemorrhages and lacunar infarcts are common pontine lesions
- Acute pontine ischemia often not seen on routine CT or MR
  - Use diffusion weighted imaging (DWI) sequence when acute ischemia suspected
- Osmotic demyelination (central pontine myelinolysis) is characterized by central T1 hypointensity and T2 hyperintensity in ventral pons
- Cerebellopontine angle lesions are common
  - Enhancing mass: Vestibulocochlear schwannoma (most common) or meningioma
  - Nonenhancing: Epidermoid or arachnoid cyst
  - Don't forget posterior circulation aneurysm for fusiform or unusual masses

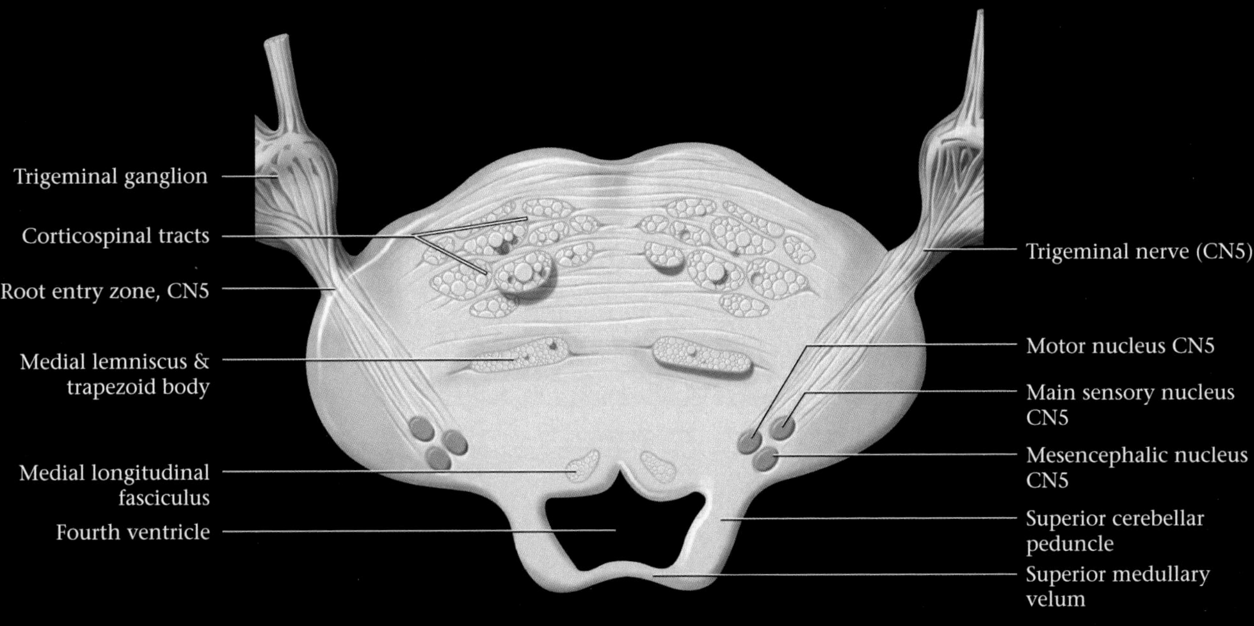

Trigeminal ganglion
Corticospinal tracts
Root entry zone, CN5
Medial lemniscus & trapezoid body
Medial longitudinal fasciculus
Fourth ventricle
Trigeminal nerve (CN5)
Motor nucleus CN5
Main sensory nucleus CN5
Mesencephalic nucleus CN5
Superior cerebellar peduncle
Superior medullary velum

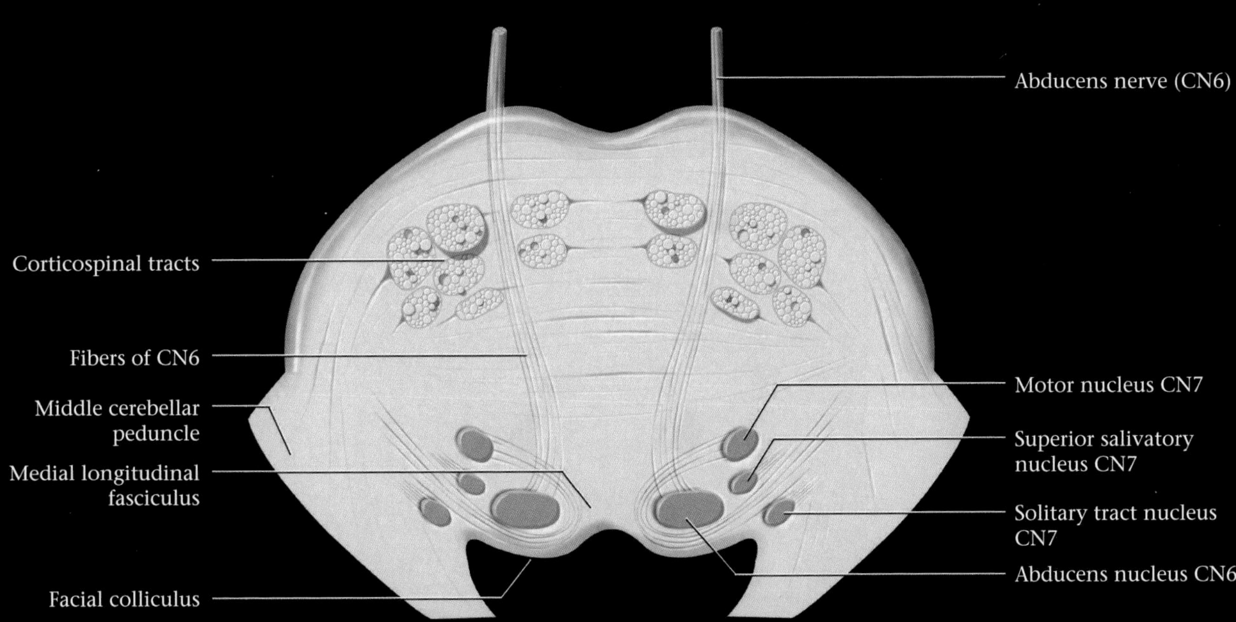

Abducens nerve (CN6)
Corticospinal tracts
Fibers of CN6
Middle cerebellar peduncle
Medial longitudinal fasciculus
Facial colliculus
Motor nucleus CN7
Superior salivatory nucleus CN7
Solitary tract nucleus CN7
Abducens nucleus CN6

(Top) Axial graphic of pons at level of trigeminal nerve shows main trigeminal nuclei: Main sensory nucleus, motor nucleus & mesencephalic nucleus. Root entry zone of CN5 is seen as preganglionic segment of CN5. Corticospinal tracts are seen as transversely cut fiber bundles which continue as pyramidal tract into medulla. Medial longitudinal fasciculus (MLF) is noted just anterior to fourth ventricle & is important in extraocular muscle movement. A lesion involving the MLF may result in internuclear ophthalmoplegia, which is often associated with multiple sclerosis. **(Bottom)** Axial graphic of pons at level of CN6 & 7. Axons of CN7 loop around CN6 nucleus creating bulge in fourth ventricle, facial colliculus. CN7 has three main nuclei: Motor, superior salivatory & solitarius tract nuclei. Middle cerebellar peduncle is a common location for multiple sclerosis plaques.

AXIAL T1 MR

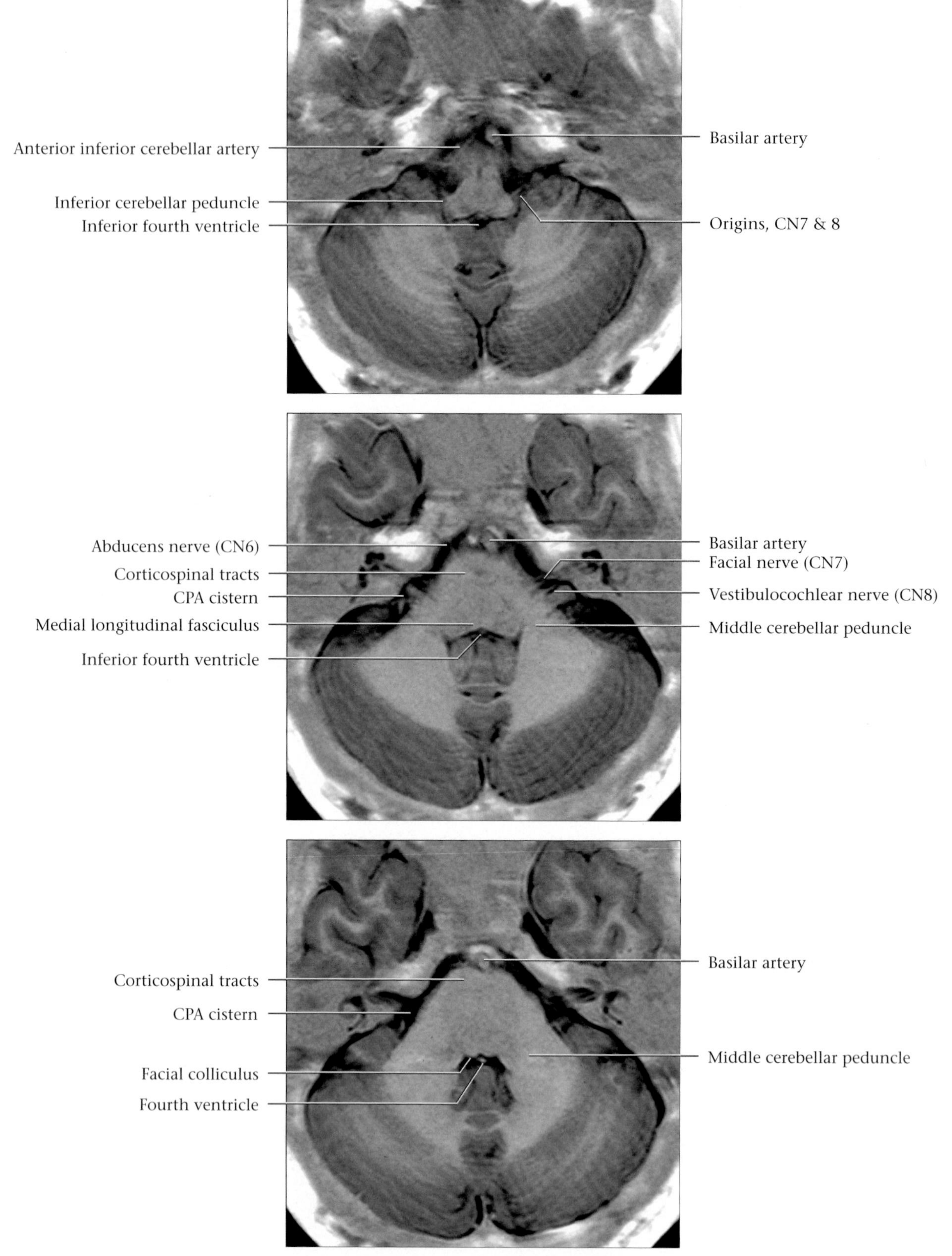
Anterior inferior cerebellar artery
Inferior cerebellar peduncle
Inferior fourth ventricle
Basilar artery
Origins, CN7 & 8
Abducens nerve (CN6)
Corticospinal tracts
CPA cistern
Medial longitudinal fasciculus
Inferior fourth ventricle
Basilar artery
Facial nerve (CN7)
Vestibulocochlear nerve (CN8)
Middle cerebellar peduncle
Corticospinal tracts
CPA cistern
Facial colliculus
Fourth ventricle
Basilar artery
Middle cerebellar peduncle

(Top) First of six axial T1 MR images of pons from inferior to superior shows pontomedullary junction & inferior aspect of inferior cerebellar peduncle (restiform body). Cochlear nerve nuclei are found on lateral surface of inferior cerebellar peduncle. **(Middle)** Image through inferior pons shows cisternal segment of CN6 as it ascends anterosuperiorly in prepontine cistern. Basilar artery is seen anteriorly along belly of pons as it sits in shallow median sulcus. CN7 & 8 exit laterally in pontomedullary junction to enter cerebellopontine angle (CPA) cistern. **(Bottom)** Image through pons at level of facial colliculus which is formed by axons of CN7 as they wrap around nucleus of CN6 just anterior to fourth ventricle. A lesion in this location would result in both CN6 & 7 palsies.

AXIAL T1 MR

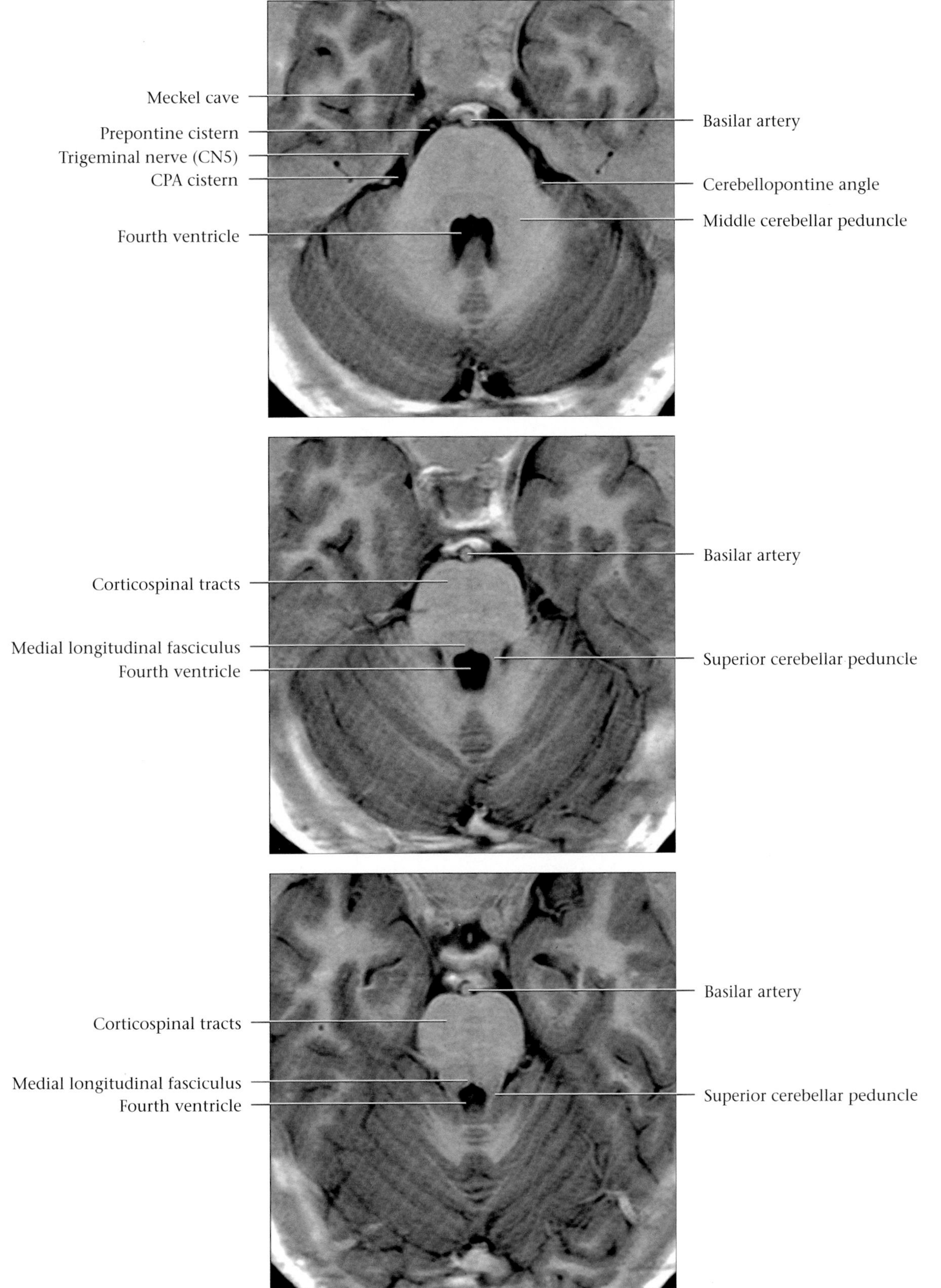
Meckel cave
Preponti ne cistern
Trigeminal nerve (CN5)
CPA cistern
Fourth ventricle
Basilar artery
Cerebellopontine angle
Middle cerebellar peduncle
Corticospinal tracts
Medial longitudinal fasciculus
Fourth ventricle
Basilar artery
Superior cerebellar peduncle
Corticospinal tracts
Medial longitudinal fasciculus
Fourth ventricle
Basilar artery
Superior cerebellar peduncle

(Top) A more superior image through pons at level of CN5 root entry zone, where CN5 exits lateral pons. From here, CN5 courses anteriorly through prepontine cistern, passes over petrous ridge & enters middle cranial fossa passing through porus trigeminus to enter Meckel cave. Meckel cave is an arachnoid lined, dural diverticulum filled with CSF & houses trigeminal ganglion. **(Middle)** Image through superior pons shows approximate location of corticospinal tracts which continue as pyramidal tracts into medulla. The anterior aspect of pons which contains corticospinal tracts will become atrophied in cortical strokes that affect motor cortex, related to Wallerian degeneration. **(Bottom)** Image through superior pons shows approximate location of medial longitudinal fasciculus, just lateral to midline. MLF is important in extraocular muscle movement.

AXIAL T2 MR

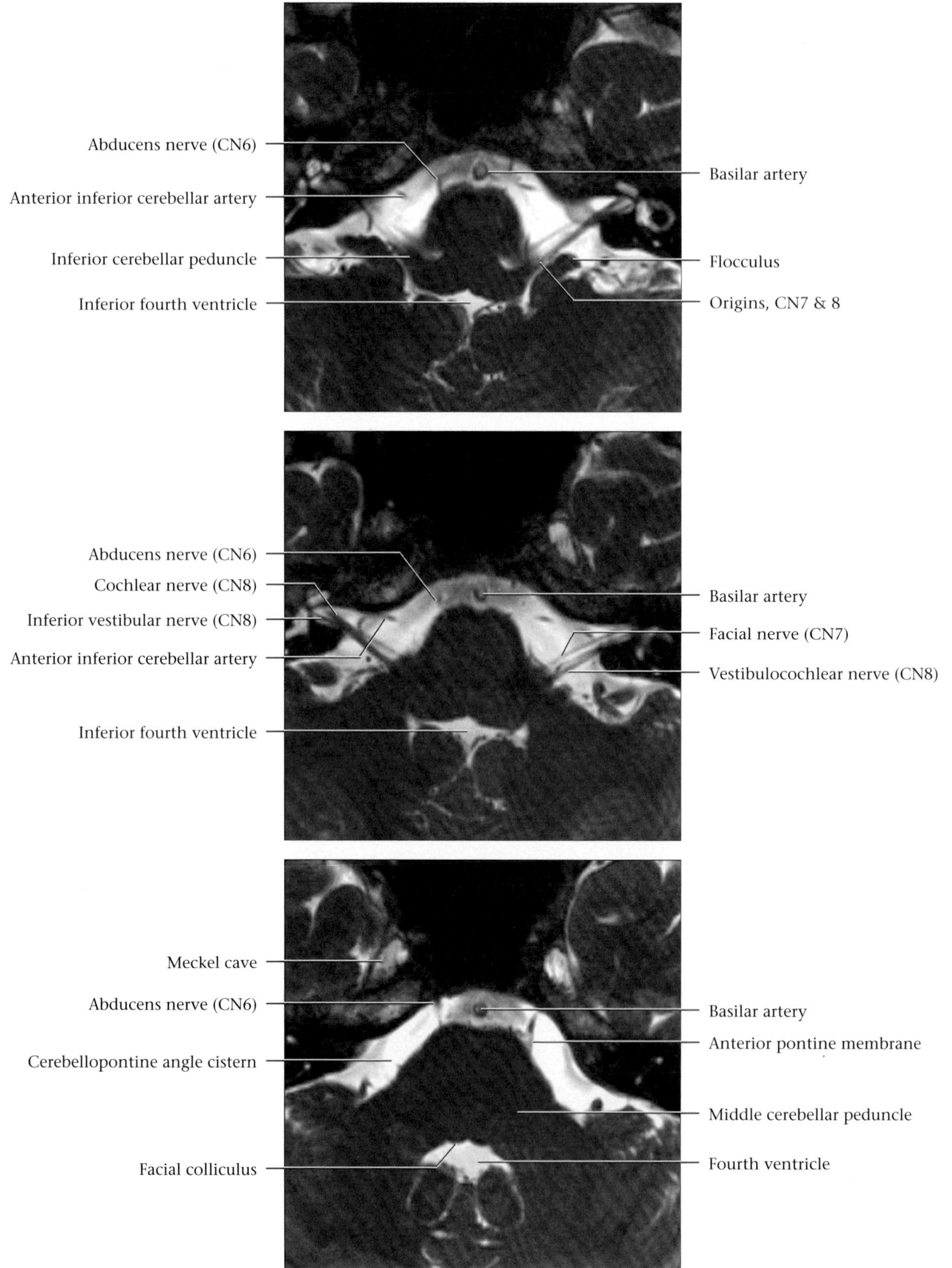
Abducens nerve (CN6)
Anterior inferior cerebellar artery
Inferior cerebellar peduncle
Inferior fourth ventricle
Basilar artery
Flocculus
Origins, CN7 & 8
Abducens nerve (CN6)
Cochlear nerve (CN8)
Inferior vestibular nerve (CN8)
Anterior inferior cerebellar artery
Inferior fourth ventricle
Basilar artery
Facial nerve (CN7)
Vestibulocochlear nerve (CN8)
Meckel cave
Abducens nerve (CN6)
Cerebellopontine angle cistern
Facial colliculus
Basilar artery
Anterior pontine membrane
Middle cerebellar peduncle
Fourth ventricle

(Top) First of six axial T2 MR images of pons from inferior to superior shows pontomedullary junction & inferior aspect of inferior cerebellar peduncle (restiform body). CN6 exits brainstem anteriorly at pontomedullary junction just above medullary pyramid. Inferior cerebellar peduncle (restiform body) lateral surface is where dorsal & ventral cochlear nuclei are found. **(Middle)** Image through inferior pons shows cisternal segment of CN6 as it ascends in prepontine cistern. Basilar artery is seen anteriorly. It gives rise to thalamoperforator arteries which supply majority of pons & anterior inferior cerebellar arteries which loop in region of internal auditory canals. CN7 and 8 exit laterally at pontomedullary junction. **(Bottom)** Image through mid pons shows middle cerebellar peduncle (brachium pontis), a common location for multiple sclerosis plaques.

AXIAL T2 MR

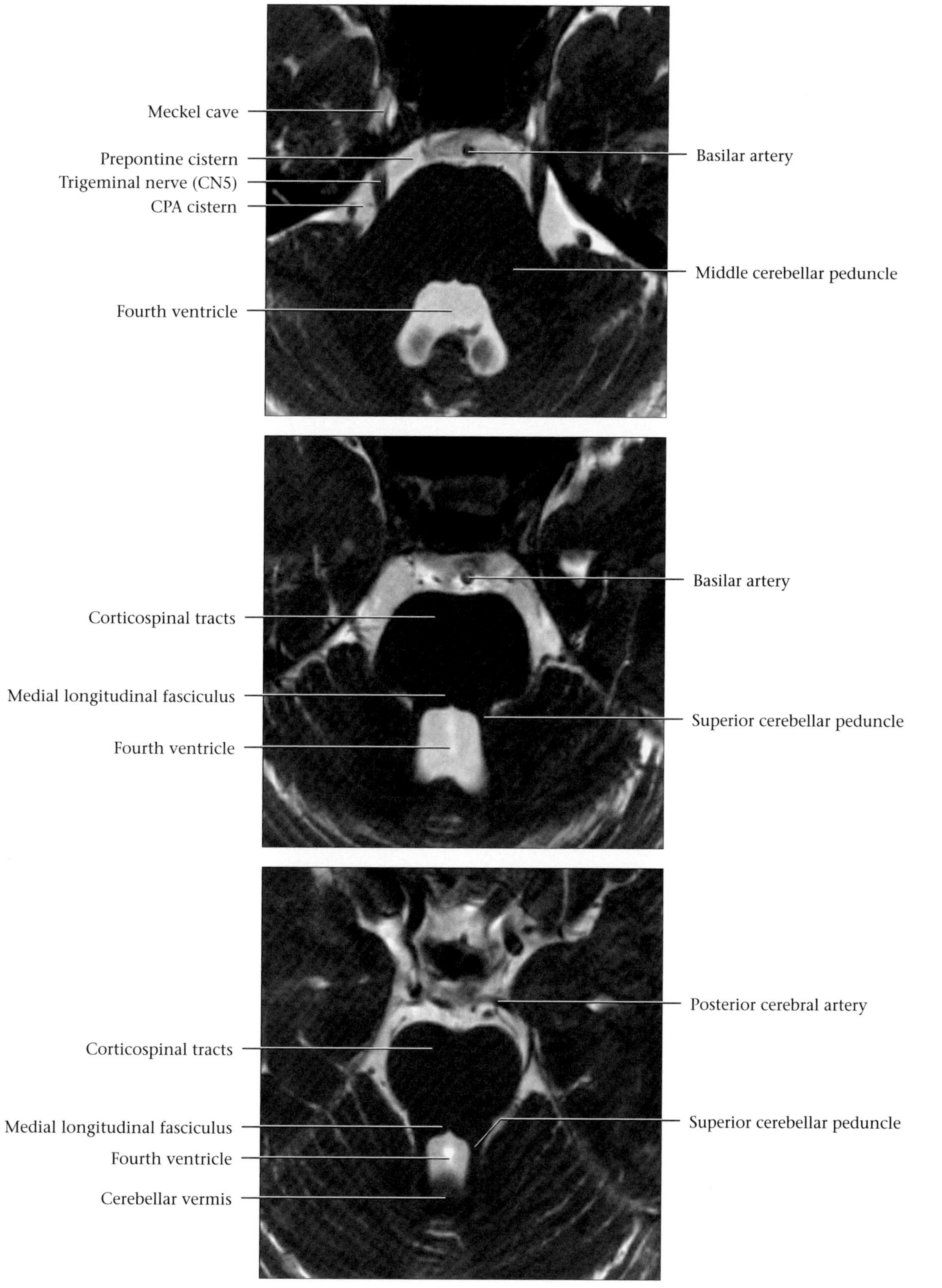

Meckel cave
Prepontine cistern
Trigeminal nerve (CN5)
CPA cistern
Fourth ventricle
Basilar artery
Middle cerebellar peduncle
Corticospinal tracts
Medial longitudinal fasciculus
Fourth ventricle
Basilar artery
Superior cerebellar peduncle
Corticospinal tracts
Medial longitudinal fasciculus
Fourth ventricle
Cerebellar vermis
Posterior cerebral artery
Superior cerebellar peduncle

(Top) A more superior image through pons at level of CN5 root entry zone, where CN5 exits lateral pons. From here, CN5 courses through prepontine cistern, enters middle cranial fossa & passes through opening in dura to enter Meckel cave which houses trigeminal ganglion. **(Middle)** Image through superior pons shows approximate location of corticospinal tracts & medial longitudinal fasciculus. These specific fibers cannot be resolved on conventional imaging, but knowledge of their location is useful when evaluating patients with weakness or cranial neuropathies. **(Bottom)** Image through superior pons shows superior cerebellar peduncles. The superior medullary velum, a thin sheet of tissue that covers dorsal fourth ventricle attaches laterally to superior cerebellar peduncles. The lingula of cerebellar vermis overlies superior medullary velum.

CORONAL T2 MR

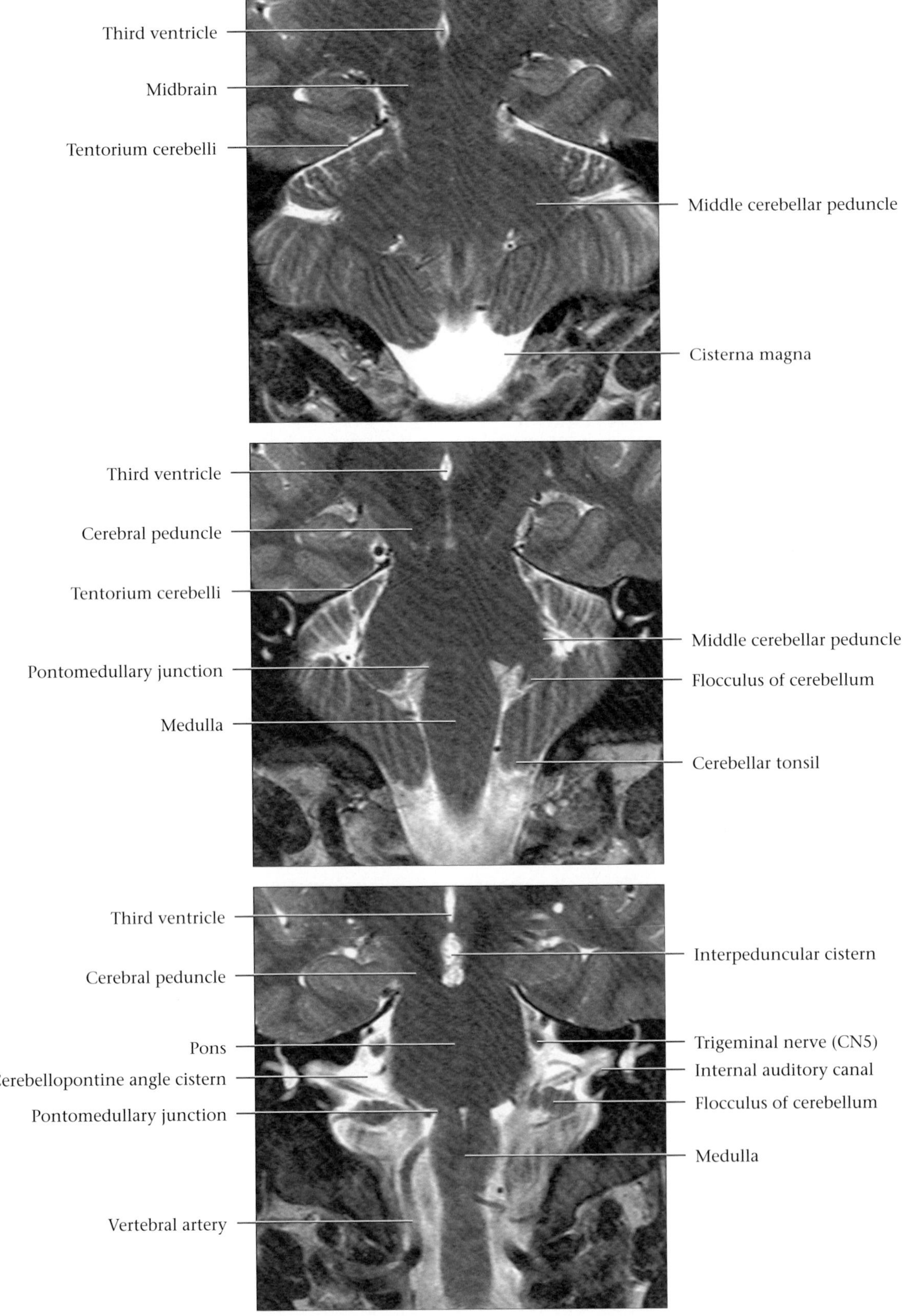
Third ventricle
Midbrain
Tentorium cerebelli
Middle cerebellar peduncle
Cisterna magna
Third ventricle
Cerebral peduncle
Tentorium cerebelli
Middle cerebellar peduncle
Pontomedullary junction
Flocculus of cerebellum
Medulla
Cerebellar tonsil
Third ventricle
Interpeduncular cistern
Cerebral peduncle
Pons
Trigeminal nerve (CN5)
Cerebellopontine angle cistern
Internal auditory canal
Pontomedullary junction
Flocculus of cerebellum
Medulla
Vertebral artery

(Top) First of six coronal T2 MR images of pons from posterior to anterior shows dorsal pons & middle cerebellar peduncles, largest of cerebellar peduncles. Superior & inferior cerebellar peduncles are small. Dorsal surface of pons is hidden by cerebellum which covers posterior aspect of fourth ventricle (rhomboid fossa). **(Middle)** This image shows pontomedullary junction at inferior border of pons where pons & medulla meet. Cerebral peduncles which contain corticospinal tracts are continuous with anterior pons where corticospinal tracts continue inferiorly to medullary pyramids. **(Bottom)** A more anterior image shows preganglionic segment of CN5 arising from lateral pons. CN7 and 8 exit brainstem laterally at pontomedullary junction & traverse the cerebellopontine angle cistern before entering internal auditory canal.

CORONAL T2 MR

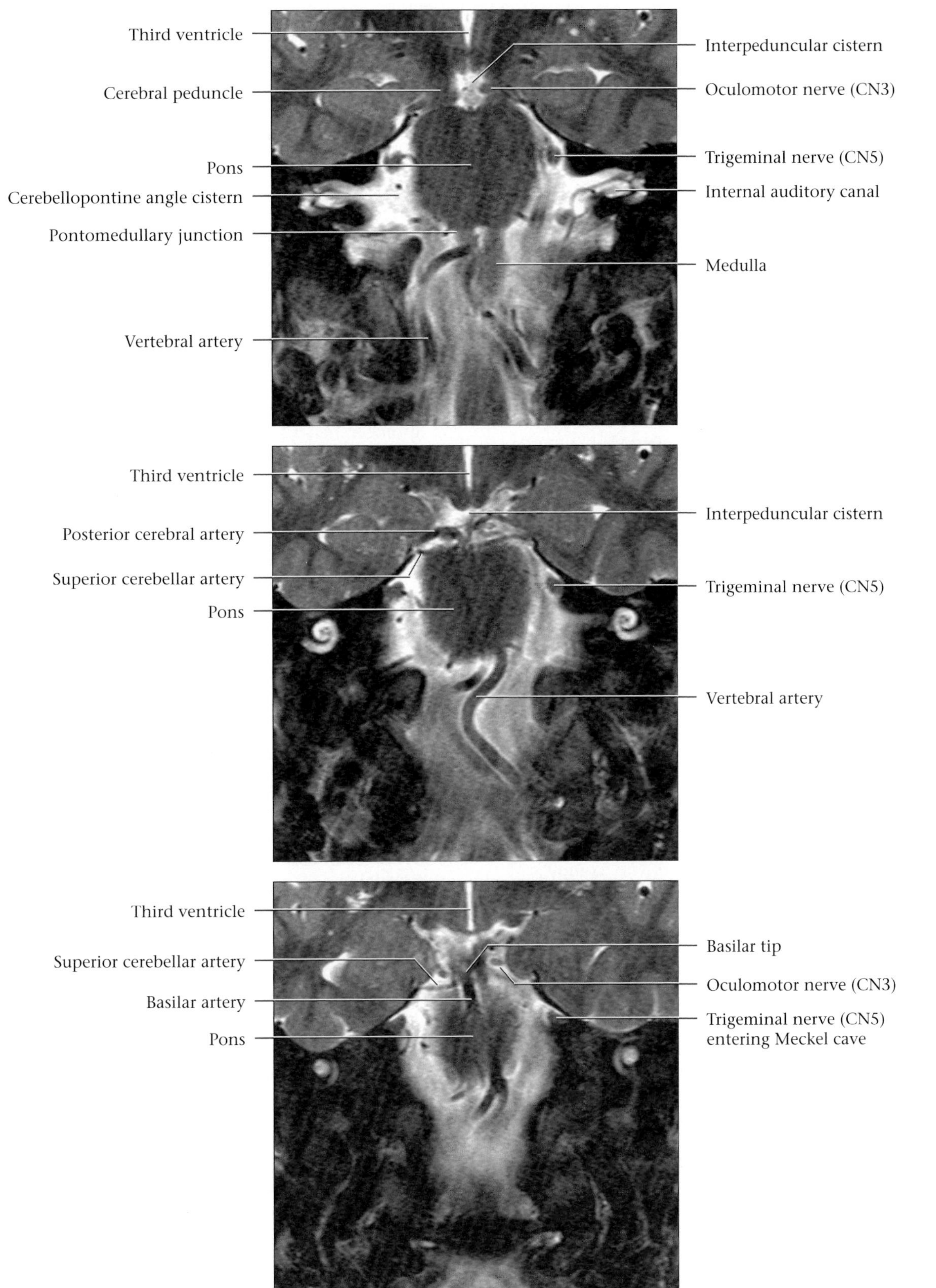
Third ventricle
Cerebral peduncle
Pons
Cerebellopontine angle cistern
Pontomedullary junction
Vertebral artery
Interpeduncular cistern
Oculomotor nerve (CN3)
Trigeminal nerve (CN5)
Internal auditory canal
Medulla
Third ventricle
Posterior cerebral artery
Superior cerebellar artery
Pons
Interpeduncular cistern
Trigeminal nerve (CN5)
Vertebral artery
Third ventricle
Superior cerebellar artery
Basilar artery
Pons
Basilar tip
Oculomotor nerve (CN3)
Trigeminal nerve (CN5)
entering Meckel cave

(Top) A more anterior image shows anterior aspect of pons which contains multiple transverse pontine fibers & descending corticospinal, corticobulbar & corticopontine tracts. Vertebral arteries unite to form basilar artery in region of pontomedullary junction. Ectasia & tortuosity of the vertebrobasilar system (dolichoectasia) is often seen in elderly adults, particularly those with atherosclerotic disease. **(Middle)** A more anterior image shows preganglionic segment of CN5, largest of cranial nerves. Pons is a common location for lacunar infarcts related to small thalamoperforator arteries that supply it. **(Bottom)** This image shows most anterior aspect of pons with basilar artery coursing along surface. The basilar tip is the most cephalad aspect of basilar artery & a location for posterior circulation aneurysms.

MEDULLA

Terminology

Abbreviations

- Cranial nerves (CN): Trigeminal nerve (CN5), vestibulocochlear nerve (CN8), glossopharyngeal nerve (CN9), vagus nerve (CN10), accessory nerve (CN11), hypoglossal nerve (CN12)

Definitions

- Medulla: Caudal brainstem, transition from spinal cord to brain

Gross Anatomy

Overview

- Caudal part of brainstem composed of gray matter formations, CN nuclei (CN9-12) & white matter tracts
  - Located between pons (superiorly) and spinal cord
  - Fourth ventricle and cerebellum dorsal to medulla
  - Caudal border: First cervical nerves
- Medulla subdivided into two main parts
  - Ventral (anterior) medulla: Olive & pyramidal tract
  - Tegmentum (dorsal): CN nuclei and white matter tracts
- Medulla may also be divided into rostral (superior) defined by fourth ventricle (open) and caudal (inferior) defined by central canal (closed portion)
- **Medulla** external features
  - **Pyramid**
    - Paired structure on anterior surface, separated in midline by ventral median fissure
    - Contains ipsilateral corticospinal tracts prior to decussation more inferiorly
  - **Olive**
    - Medullary olives are lateral to pyramids, separated by ventrolateral sulcus (pre-olivary sulcus)
    - Formed by underlying inferior olivary complex of nuclei
    - Posterolateral sulcus (postolivary sulcus) is lateral to olives
  - **Inferior cerebellar peduncle** (restiform body)
    - Arise from superior aspect of dorsal medulla; peduncles diverge and incline to enter cerebellar hemispheres
    - Nuclei of CN8 located along dorsal surface
  - **Gracile and cuneate tubercles**
    - Form lower aspect of dorsal medulla
    - Produced by paired nuclei gracilis (medial) and cuneatus (lateral)
    - Dorsal median sulcus separates gracile tubercles
- **Fourth ventricle**
  - Dorsal median sulcus divides ventricular floor longitudinally
  - Terminates in caudal medulla
  - Roof formed by superior and inferior medullary velum
- Blood supply from vertebrobasilar circulation
  - Distal vertebral arteries
  - Posterior inferior cerebellar arteries
  - Anterior spinal artery

Ventral (Anterior) Medulla

- Medullary pyramids
  - Corticospinal tracts (pyramidal tracts) make up bulk
- Medullary olives
  - Consists of inferior olivary nucleus, dorsal & medial accessory olivary nuclei & superior olivary nucleus
  - Inferior olivary nucleus is largest and forms bulge on surface of medulla, "medullary olive"

Dorsal Tegmentum

- Multiple **white matter tracts of tegmentum** (not resolved on conventional imaging)
  - Medial longitudinal fasciculus: Oculomotor-vestibular
  - Medial lemniscus: Auditory
  - Spinothalamic tract: Somatosensory
  - Central tegmental tract: Motor
  - Spinocerebellar tract: Somatosensory
- **Cranial nerve nuclei**
  - **CN9** nuclei in upper and mid medulla: Nucleus ambiguus, solitary tract nucleus, inferior salivatory nucleus
    - Sensory fibers terminate in spinal nucleus CN5
    - CN9 exits medulla in postolivary sulcus above CN10
  - **CN10** nuclei in upper and mid medulla: Nucleus ambiguus, solitary tract nucleus, dorsal vagal nucleus
    - Sensory fibers terminate in spinal nucleus CN5
    - CN10 exits medulla in postolivary sulcus between CN9 and 11
  - **CN11** bulbar nuclei in lower nucleus ambiguus in upper and mid medulla
    - CN11 exits medulla in postolivary sulcus below CN10
  - **CN12** nuclei in mid medulla, dorsally results in hypoglossal eminence or trigone (bulge in fourth ventricle)
    - CN12 exits anterior medulla in pre-olivary sulcus
- **Reticular formation**
  - Occupies central tegmentum, afferent and efferent connections
  - Important in consciousness, motor function, respiration and cardiovascular control

Imaging Anatomy

Overview

- Medullary olives and pyramids well seen on imaging
- CN9-12 seen as they exit medulla
  - CN9-11 exit medulla in postolivary sulcus
  - CN12 exits anterior medulla in pre-olivary sulcus
- CN nuclei and white matter tracts can be identified by typical location, but are not resolved on imaging

Anatomy-Based Imaging Issues

Imaging Recommendations

- MR for cranial neuropathy or acute ischemia
- CTA and MRA for vertebrobasilar circulation

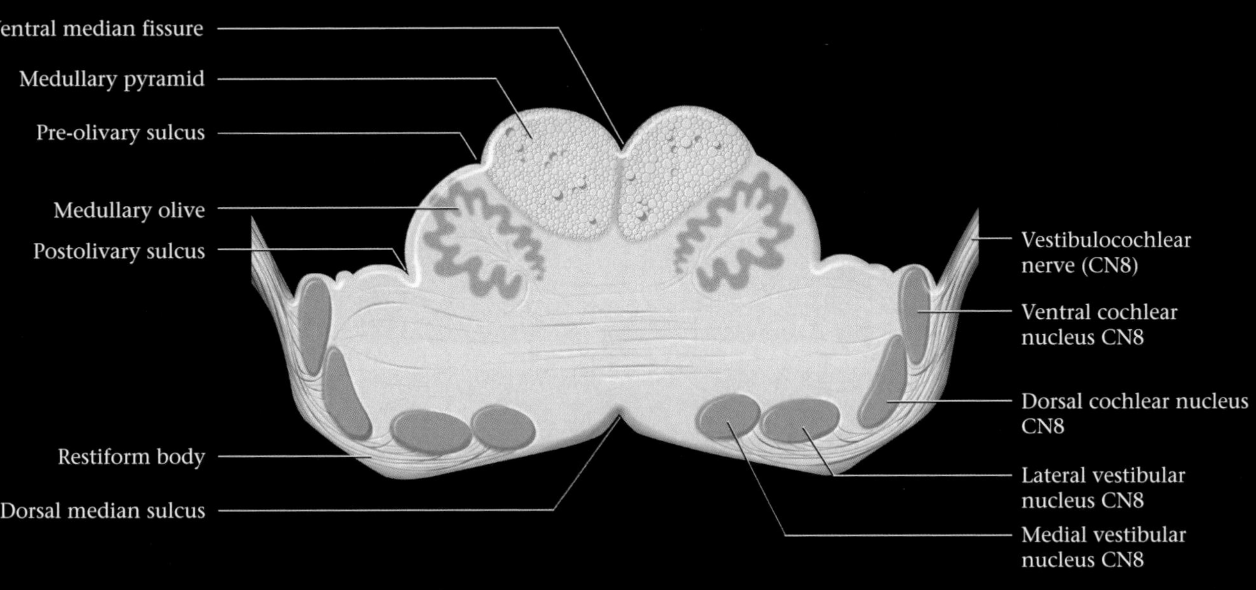
Ventral median fissure
Medullary pyramid
Pre-olivary sulcus
Medullary olive
Postolivary sulcus
Restiform body
Dorsal median sulcus
Vestibulocochlear nerve (CN8)
Ventral cochlear nucleus CN8
Dorsal cochlear nucleus CN8
Lateral vestibular nucleus CN8
Medial vestibular nucleus CN8

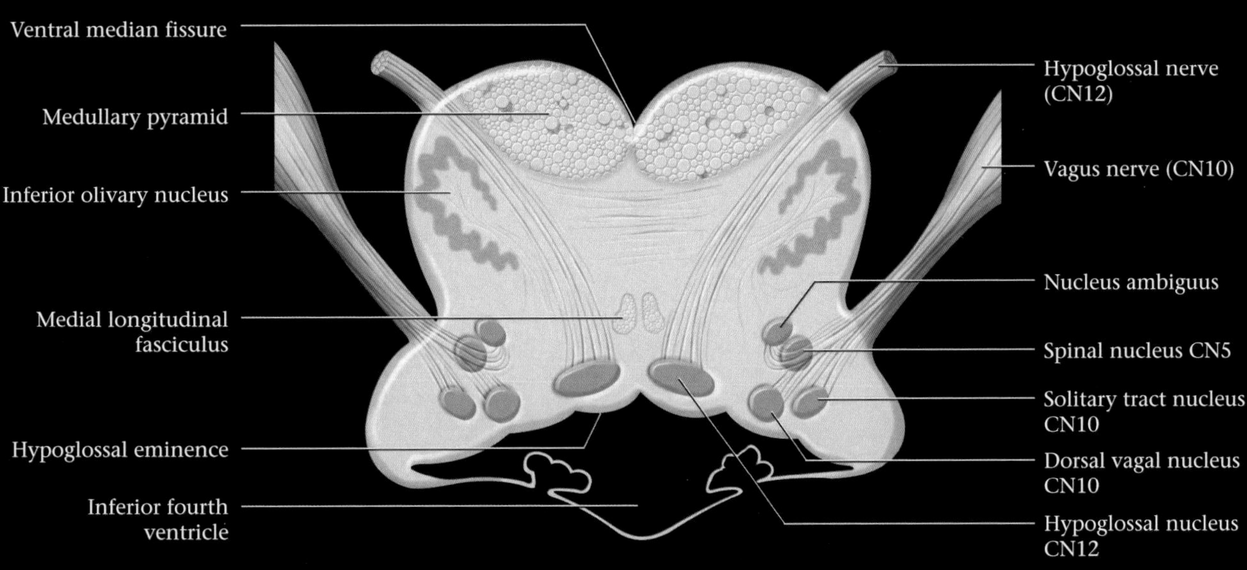
Ventral median fissure
Medullary pyramid
Inferior olivary nucleus
Medial longitudinal fasciculus
Hypoglossal eminence
Inferior fourth ventricle
Hypoglossal nerve (CN12)
Vagus nerve (CN10)
Nucleus ambiguus
Spinal nucleus CN5
Solitary tract nucleus CN10
Dorsal vagal nucleus CN10
Hypoglossal nucleus CN12

(Top) Axial graphic of superior medulla at level of pontomedullary junction showing vestibulocochlear CN8 nuclei. Both cochlear nuclei & two of four vestibular nuclei are are seen. Each medullary pyramid contains descending corticospinal tracts from ipsilateral cerebral cortex which have traversed internal capsule, midbrain & pons. CN9-11 exit postolivary sulcus & CN12 exits at pre-olivary sulcus. **(Bottom)** Axial graphic of mid medulla at level of CN12 nucleus & CN10 nuclei. CN12 nucleus forms bulge on floor of fourth ventricle, hypoglossal eminence. Fibers of CN12 cross medulla to exit between pyramid & olive in pre-olivary sulcus. CN10 nuclei are in upper & middle medulla & include nucleus ambiguus, solitary tract nucleus & dorsal vagal nucleus. CN10 exits lateral medulla in postolivary sulcus inferior to CN9 & superior to bulbar portion of CN11.

AXIAL T2 MR

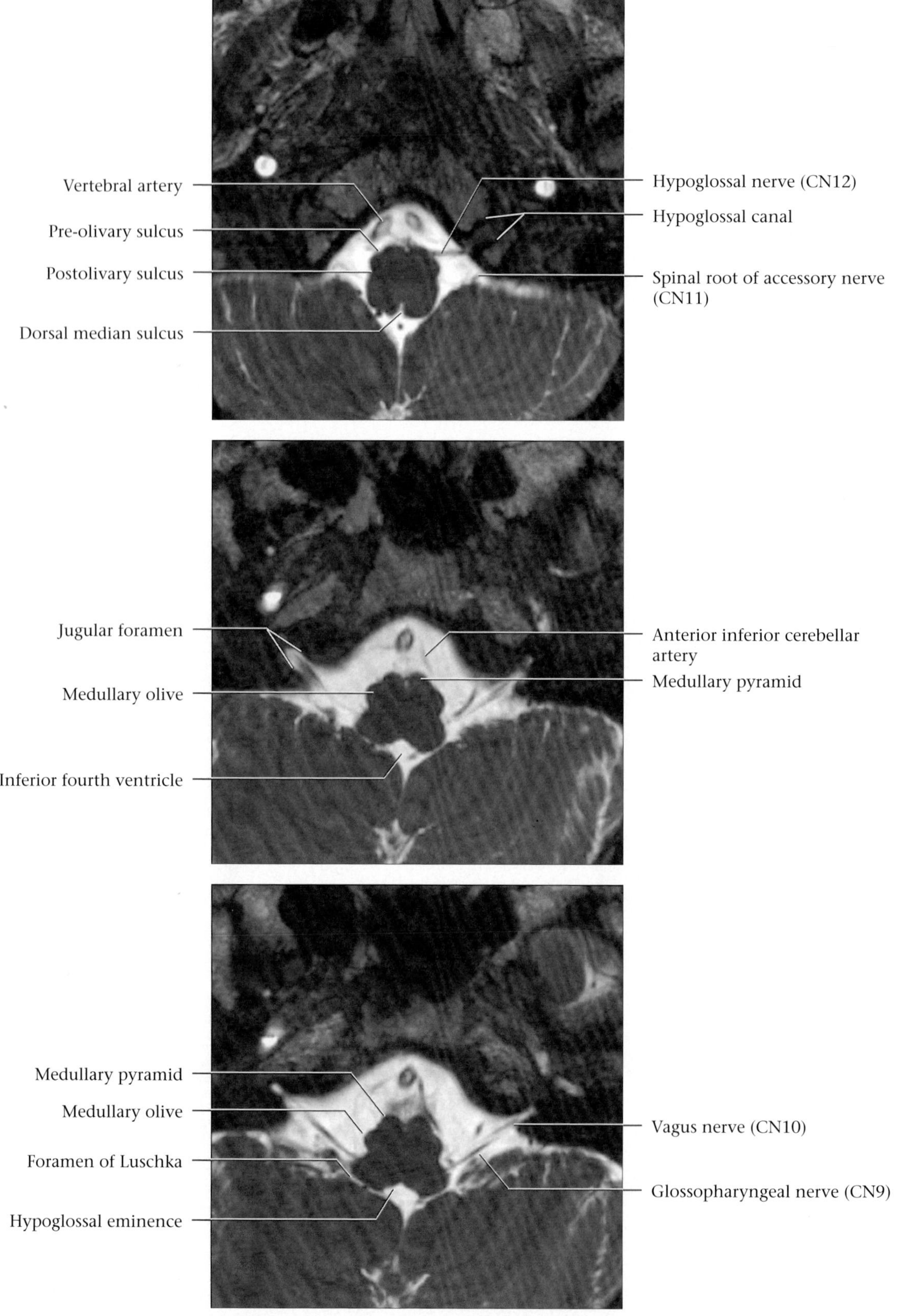

Vertebral artery
Pre-olivary sulcus
Postolivary sulcus
Dorsal median sulcus
Hypoglossal nerve (CN12)
Hypoglossal canal
Spinal root of accessory nerve (CN11)
Jugular foramen
Medullary olive
Inferior fourth ventricle
Anterior inferior cerebellar artery
Medullary pyramid
Medullary pyramid
Medullary olive
Foramen of Luschka
Hypoglossal eminence
Vagus nerve (CN10)
Glossopharyngeal nerve (CN9)

(Top) First of six axial T2 MR images through medulla from inferior to superior shows hypoglossal nerve CN12 exiting medulla at pre-olivary sulcus. Spinal root of accessory nerve CN11 is seen laterally as it ascends through foramen magnum to unite with cranial roots of CN11 before exiting via jugular foramen. Dorsal median sulcus continues superiorly to divide floor of fourth ventricle longitudinally. **(Middle)** Image at level of jugular foramen shows medullary olives & pyramids. **(Bottom)** This image shows hypoglossal eminence (trigone), formed by CN12 nucleus as bulge in fourth ventricular floor. Glossopharyngeal CN9, vagus CN10, & cranial roots of accessory CN11 nerves exit lateral medulla in postolivary sulcus, posterior to olive. These nerves exit skull base via jugular foramen. Thin-section, high-resolution imaging allows identification of CN9-11.

AXIAL T2 MR

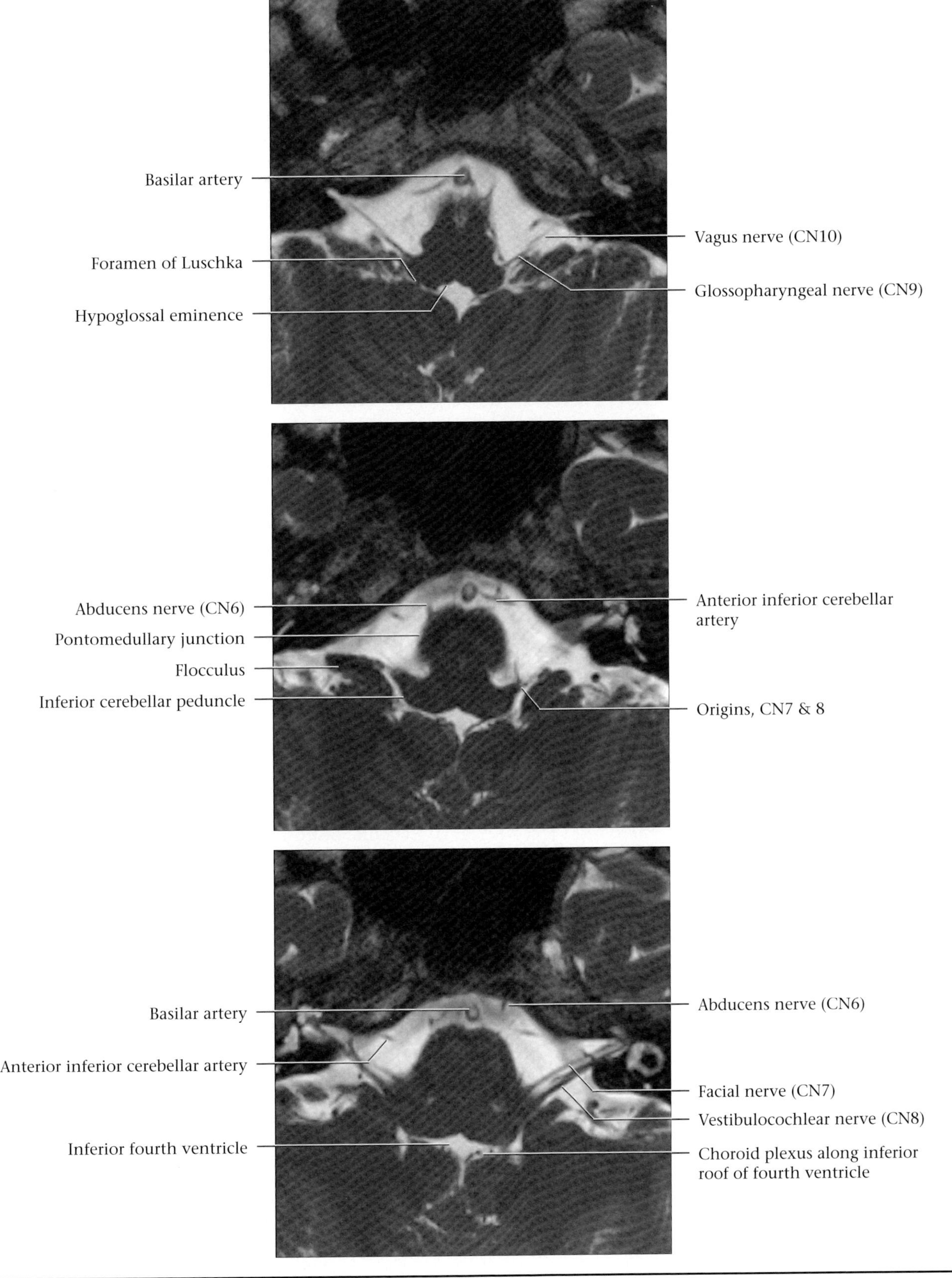
Basilar artery
Foramen of Luschka
Hypoglossal eminence
Vagus nerve (CN10)
Glossopharyngeal nerve (CN9)
Abducens nerve (CN6)
Pontomedullary junction
Flocculus
Inferior cerebellar peduncle
Anterior inferior cerebellar artery
Origins, CN7 & 8
Basilar artery
Anterior inferior cerebellar artery
Inferior fourth ventricle
Abducens nerve (CN6)
Facial nerve (CN7)
Vestibulocochlear nerve (CN8)
Choroid plexus along inferior roof of fourth ventricle

(Top) Image more superiorly shows medullary olives bilaterally. Olives become atrophied in the degenerative disease, olivopontocerebellar atrophy. Wallenberg syndrome is a neurological condition caused by ischemia of lateral medulla related to vertebral or posterior inferior cerebellar artery disease. **(Middle)** Image more superiorly at level of pontomedullary junction. Inferior cerebellar peduncle (restiform body) is where cochlear nuclei of vestibulocochlear nerve CN8 are found. Abducens nerve CN6 exits anteriorly at pontomedullary junction, just above medullary pyramid. Important to remember that anterior inferior cerebellar artery is seen about brainstem in order to not mistake it for a cranial nerve. **(Bottom)** Image at inferior pons junction with upper medulla. Facial nerve CN7 & vestibulocochlear nerve CN8 exit laterally at pontomedullary junction.

CEREBELLUM

Terminology

Abbreviations

- Cerebrospinal fluid (CSF)

Synonyms

- Classical nomenclature (simplified nomenclature): Superior (tentorial), inferior (suboccipital), anterior (petrosal) cerebellar surfaces
- Primary (tentorial), horizontal (petrosal), prebiventral/prepyramidal (suboccipital) cerebellar fissures

Definitions

- Cerebellum: Integrative organ for coordination & fine-tuning of movement & regulation of muscle tone

Gross Anatomy

Overview

- Bilobed posterior fossa structure located posterior to brainstem and fourth ventricle
  - Two hemispheres & midline vermis
  - Three surfaces
  - Divided into lobes & lobules by transverse fissures
  - Connected to brainstem by three paired peduncles
  - Cortical gray matter, central white matter & four paired deep gray nuclei

Anatomy Relationships

- **Surfaces**
  - **Superior (tentorial) surface**
    - Faces & conforms to inferior surface of tentorium
    - Transition between vermis & hemispheres is smooth
    - Primary (tentorial) fissure divides superior (tentorial) surface into anterior & posterior parts
  - **Inferior (suboccipital) surface**
    - Located below, between lateral & sigmoid sinuses
    - Vermis is contained within a deep vertical depression, the posterior cerebellar incisura which separates the cerebellar hemispheres
    - Prebiventral/prepyramidal (suboccipital) fissure divides inferior (suboccipital) surface into superior & inferior parts
    - Tonsil is part of hemisphere, located on inferomedial part of inferior (suboccipital) surface
  - **Anterior (petrosal) surface**
    - Faces the posterior surface of petrous bone, brainstem & fourth ventricle
    - Vermis lies dorsal to fourth ventricle
    - Horizontal (petrosal) fissure divides anterior (petrosal) surface into superior & inferior parts
    - Horizontal (petrosal) fissure continues posterolaterally onto inferior (suboccipital) surface
- **Peduncles**: 3 paired peduncles attach cerebellum to brainstem
  - **Superior cerebellar peduncle (brachium conjunctivum)**
    - Connects to cerebrum via midbrain
    - Contains efferent fiber systems extending to red nucleus & thalamus
  - **Middle cerebellar peduncle (brachium pontis)**
    - Connects to pons
    - Contains fiber mass originating from pontine nuclei & represent continuation of corticopontine tracts
  - **Inferior cerebellar peduncle (restiform body)**
    - Connects to medulla
    - Contains spinocerebellar tracts & connections to vestibular nuclei
- Adjacent CSF cisterns
  - Cerebellopontine angle cistern: Lateral to pons
  - Cisterna magna: Inferior to cerebellum
  - Quadrigeminal plate cistern: Posterior to midbrain, above cerebellum
  - Superior cerebellar cistern: Above cerebellum, below tentorium
- Blood supply from vertebrobasilar circulation
  - Superior cerebellar artery, anterior inferior cerebellar artery & posterior inferior cerebellar artery

Cerebellar Lobes and Lobules

- **Vermis**: Superior & inferior, separated by horizontal (petrosal) fissure
  - Superior vermis: Lingula (anterior), central lobule, culmen, declive, folium (posterior) lobules
  - Inferior vermis: Tuber (posterior), pyramid, uvula, nodule (anterior) lobules
- **Lobules of vermis** are associated with pair of **hemispheric lobules**
  - Lingula: Wing of lingula
  - Central lobule: Wing of central lobule
  - Culmen: Quadrangular lobule
    - Primary (tentorial) fissure
  - Declive: Simple lobule
  - Folium: Superior semilunar lobule
    - Horizontal (petrosal) fissure
  - Tuber: Inferior semilunar lobule
    - Prebiventral/prepyramidal (suboccipital) fissure
  - Pyramid: Biventral lobule
  - Uvula: Tonsils
  - Nodule: Flocculus

Cerebellar Nuclei

- Located deep in cerebellar white matter
- Nuclei project fibers to coordinate goal directed movement
- Fastigial nucleus: Medial group (vermis)
  - Fibers from vermis cortex, vestibular nuclei and other medulla nuclei
- Globose (posterior) nucleus: Intermediate group
  - Fibers from vermis cortex, sends fibers to medulla nuclei
- Emboliform (anterior) nucleus: Intermediate group
  - Fibers from cerebellar cortex between vermis and hemispheres, sends fibers to thalamus
- Dentate nucleus: Lateral group
  - Fibers from hemispheric cortex, sends fibers to red nucleus and thalamus
  - Largest nucleus, shaped as a heavily folded band with medial opening (hilum)

GRAPHICS

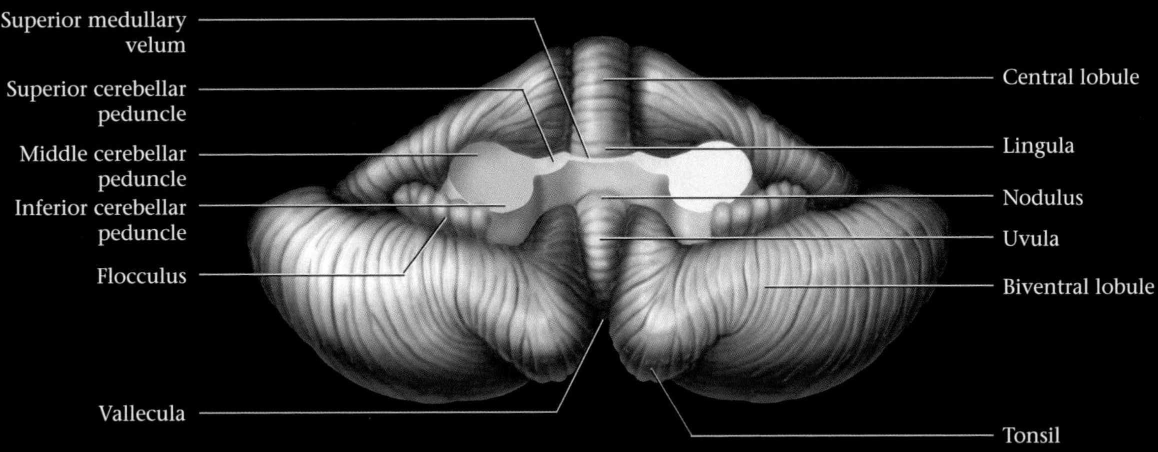
Superior medullary velum
Superior cerebellar peduncle
Middle cerebellar peduncle
Inferior cerebellar peduncle
Flocculus
Vallecula
Central lobule
Lingula
Nodulus
Uvula
Biventral lobule
Tonsil

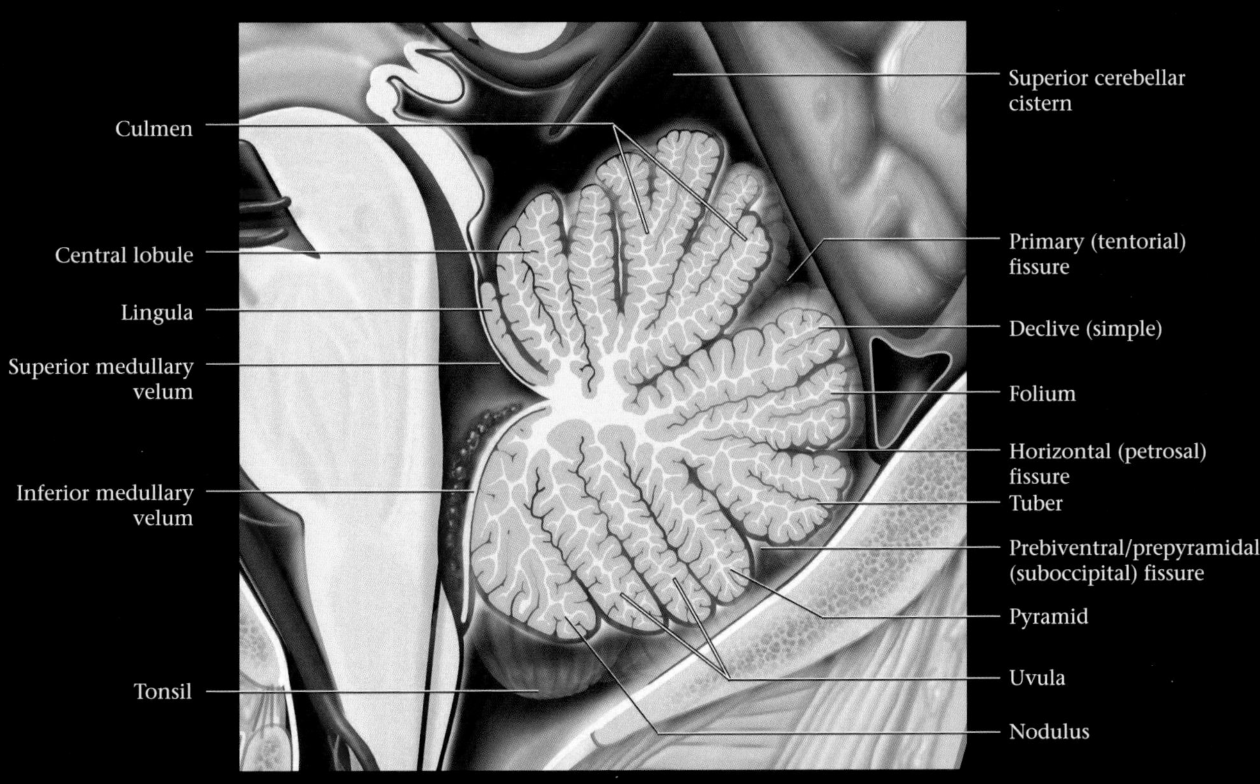
Culmen
Central lobule
Lingula
Superior medullary velum
Inferior medullary velum
Tonsil
Superior cerebellar cistern
Primary (tentorial) fissure
Declive (simple)
Folium
Horizontal (petrosal) fissure
Tuber
Prebiventral/prepyramidal (suboccipital) fissure
Pyramid
Uvula
Nodulus

(Top) Graphic of anterior (petrosal) surface of cerebellum shows cut surfaces of cerebellar peduncles. Middle cerebellar peduncle is largest & contains corticopontine tracts from pons. Superior cerebellar peduncle contains fibers from red nucleus & thalamus. Inferior cerebellar peduncle contains spinocerebellar tracts & connections to vestibular nuclei. Cerebellum is divided into two large lateral hemispheres united by a midline vermis. **(Bottom)** Sagittal graphic of midline cerebellum shows parts of cerebellar vermis: Lingula, central, culmen, declive, folium, tuber, pyramid, uvula & nodulus. Primary (tentorial) fissure separates culmen from declive (simple). Horizontal (petrosal) fissure separates folium from tuber dividing vermis into superior & inferior parts. Prebiventral/prepyramidal (suboccipital) fissure separates tuber from pyramid.

AXIAL T1 MR

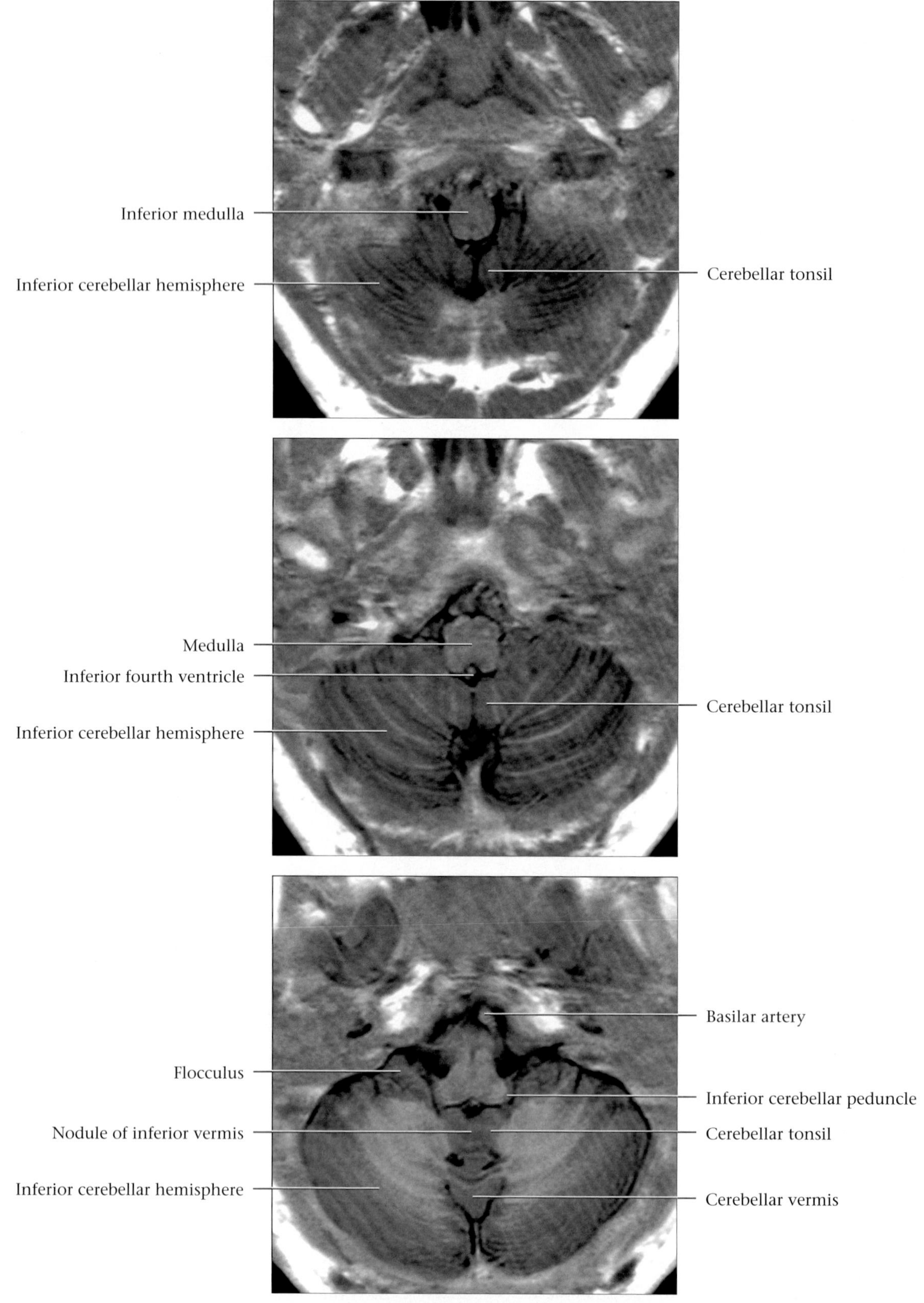
Inferior medulla
Inferior cerebellar hemisphere
Cerebellar tonsil
Medulla
Inferior fourth ventricle
Inferior cerebellar hemisphere
Cerebellar tonsil
Basilar artery
Flocculus
Inferior cerebellar peduncle
Nodule of inferior vermis
Cerebellar tonsil
Inferior cerebellar hemisphere
Cerebellar vermis

(Top) First of six axial T1 MR images through cerebellum from inferior to superior shows junction of medulla with cervical spinal cord. Cerebellar tonsils are most inferior extension of cerebellum & may herniate inferiorly in patients with cerebellar edema or mass resulting in descending tonsillar herniation. **(Middle)** Image shows inferior cerebellar hemispheres which are supplied primarily by posterior inferior cerebellar artery (PICA). Anterior inferior cerebellar artery (AICA) supplies anterolateral aspect of cerebellar hemispheres. Ischemia in a PICA distribution is most common cerebellar stroke. **(Bottom)** Image more superiorly shows inferior cerebellar peduncle (restiform body) which ascends from lower medulla to cerebellum & contains spinocerebellar tracts & connections to vestibular nuclei. It is also location of cochlear nerve CN8 nuclei.

AXIAL T1 MR

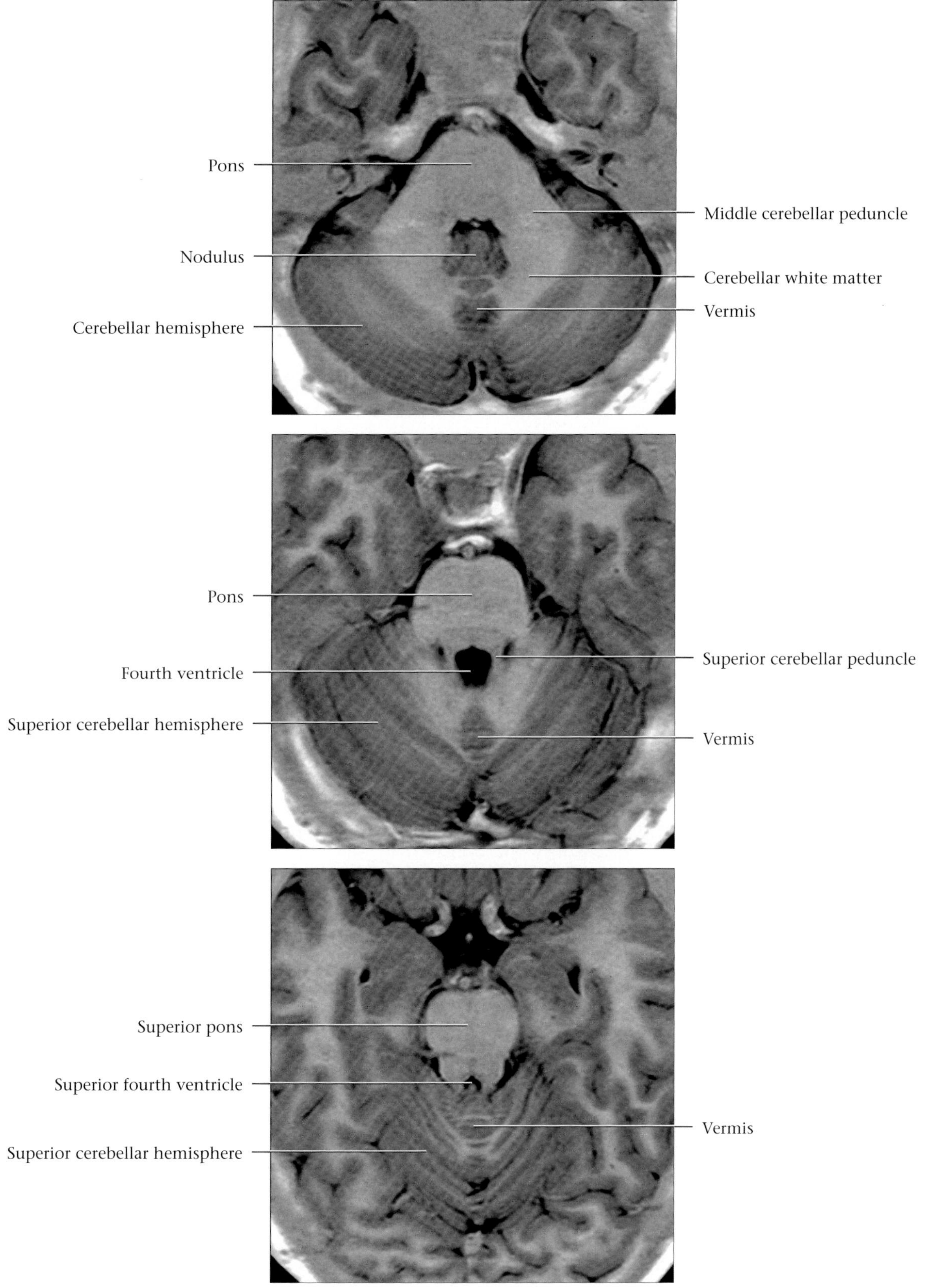
Pons
Nodulus
Cerebellar hemisphere
Middle cerebellar peduncle
Cerebellar white matter
Vermis
Pons
Fourth ventricle
Superior cerebellar hemisphere
Superior cerebellar peduncle
Vermis
Superior pons
Superior fourth ventricle
Superior cerebellar hemisphere
Vermis

(Top) Image more superiorly at level of middle cerebellar peduncles shows midline vermis & nodulus. Nodulus, just posterior to fourth ventricle, is occasionally mistaken for a lesion in fourth ventricle. Middle cerebellar peduncle (brachium pontis) connect pons with cerebellum & contains corticopontine tracts. It is a common location for multiple sclerosis plaques. **(Middle)** This image shows superior cerebellar peduncles (brachium conjunctivum) which connects cerebellum with red nucleus & thalamus. Superior cerebellar hemisphere is supplied primarily by superior cerebellar arteries which arise from basilar artery just before posterior cerebral arteries, which are terminal branches. Superior cerebellar arteries also supply superior cerebellar peduncle, dentate nucleus, & part of middle cerebellar peduncle. **(Bottom)** Image more superiorly shows midline vermis.

CORONAL T2 MR

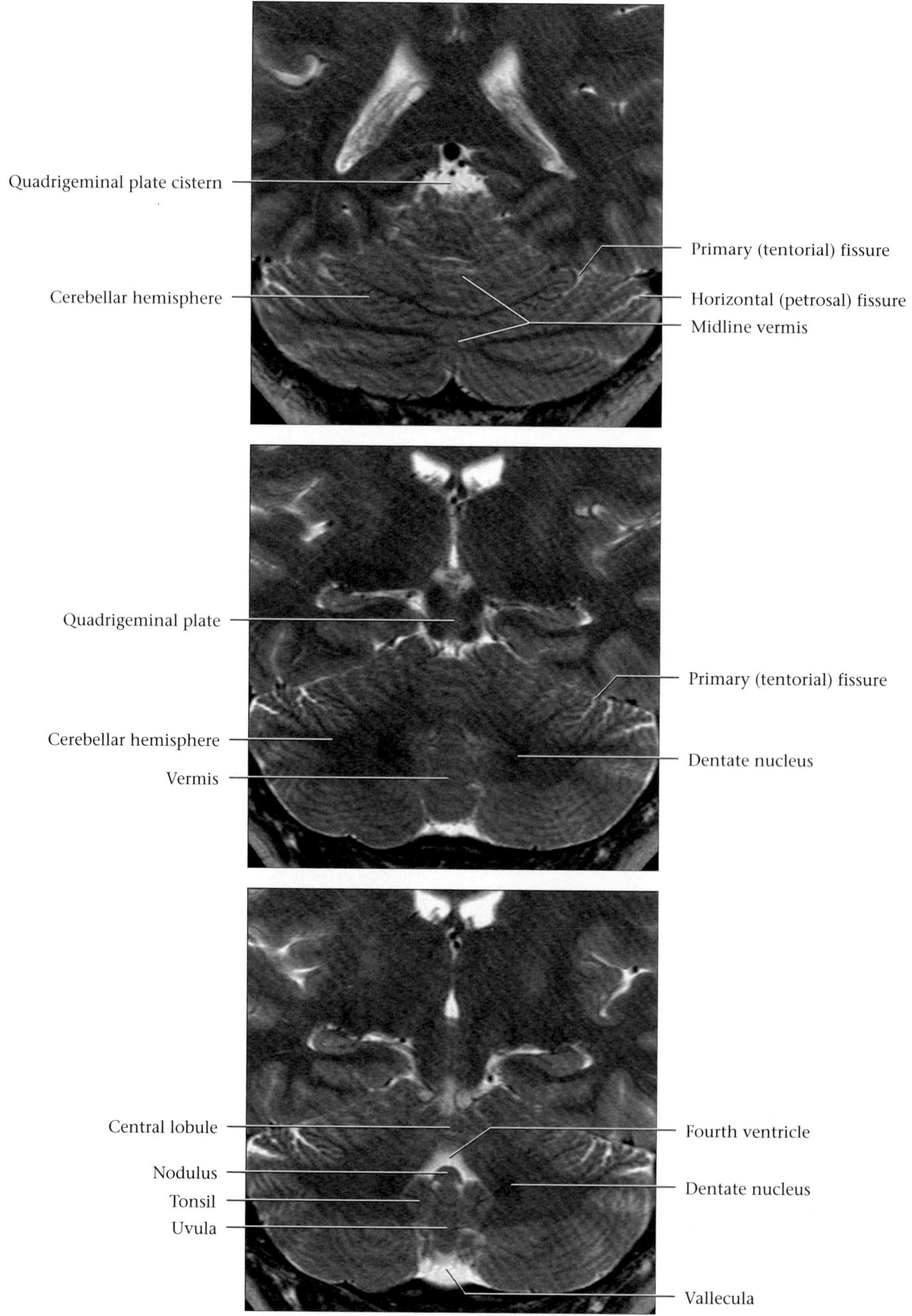

Quadrigeminal plate cistern
Cerebellar hemisphere
Primary (tentorial) fissure
Horizontal (petrosal) fissure
Midline vermis
Quadrigeminal plate
Primary (tentorial) fissure
Cerebellar hemisphere
Dentate nucleus
Vermis
Central lobule
Fourth ventricle
Nodulus
Dentate nucleus
Tonsil
Uvula
Vallecula

(Top) First of six coronal T2 MR images from posterior to anterior shows primary (tentorial) fissure which is deepest fissure on superior (tentorial) surface of cerebellum. Other main fissure is horizontal (petrosal) fissure which extends from middle cerebellar peduncle on anterior (petrosal) surface posterolaterally onto inferior (suboccipital) surface of cerebellum. **(Middle)** Image more anteriorly shows dentate nucleus which receives cortical fibers of cerebellar hemispheres & sends fibers through superior cerebellar peduncles to red nucleus & thalamus. Other cerebellar nuclei are midline & paramedian & are not resolved on conventional imaging. **(Bottom)** This image shows some of vermian lobules including central lobule, uvula & nodulus. Typically, vermis is discussed as single entity on imaging, with exception of nodulus.

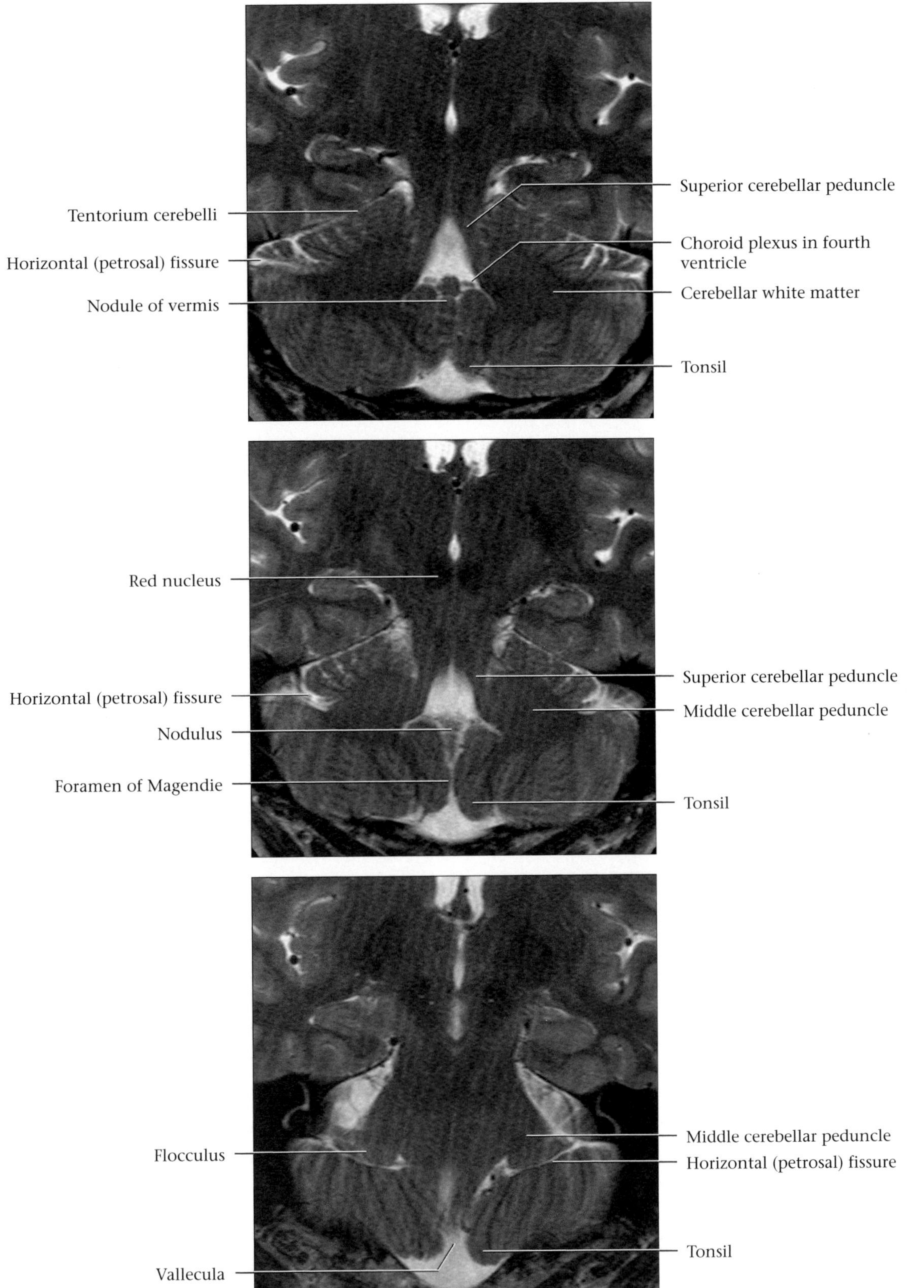

Tentorium cerebelli
Horizontal (petrosal) fissure
Nodule of vermis
Superior cerebellar peduncle
Choroid plexus in fourth ventricle
Cerebellar white matter
Tonsil
Red nucleus
Horizontal (petrosal) fissure
Nodulus
Foramen of Magendie
Superior cerebellar peduncle
Middle cerebellar peduncle
Tonsil
Flocculus
Vallecula
Middle cerebellar peduncle
Horizontal (petrosal) fissure
Tonsil

(Top) Image more anteriorly shows nodulus projecting into fourth ventricle. Superior cerebellar peduncle is seen along superior fourth ventricle as it extends to superior pons & midbrain to send fibers to red nucleus & thalamus. **(Middle)** This image shows horizontal (petrosal) fissure curving anteriorly onto anterior (petrosal) surface of cerebellum. Surface of cerebellum exhibits numerous narrow, almost parallel convolutions called folia. Cerebellar hemispheres contain lobules or wings that are paired with vermis lobules. **(Bottom)** Image more anteriorly shows middle cerebellar peduncles & cerebellar tonsils. Flocculus & nodulus make up flocculonodular lobe of cerebellum. Flocculus is a common pseudolesion in CPA cistern. Inferiorly, cerebellar hemispheres are separated by a deep vallecula which contains falx cerebelli. Vallecula is bounded by tonsils bilaterally.

CEREBELLUM

SAGITTAL T2 MR

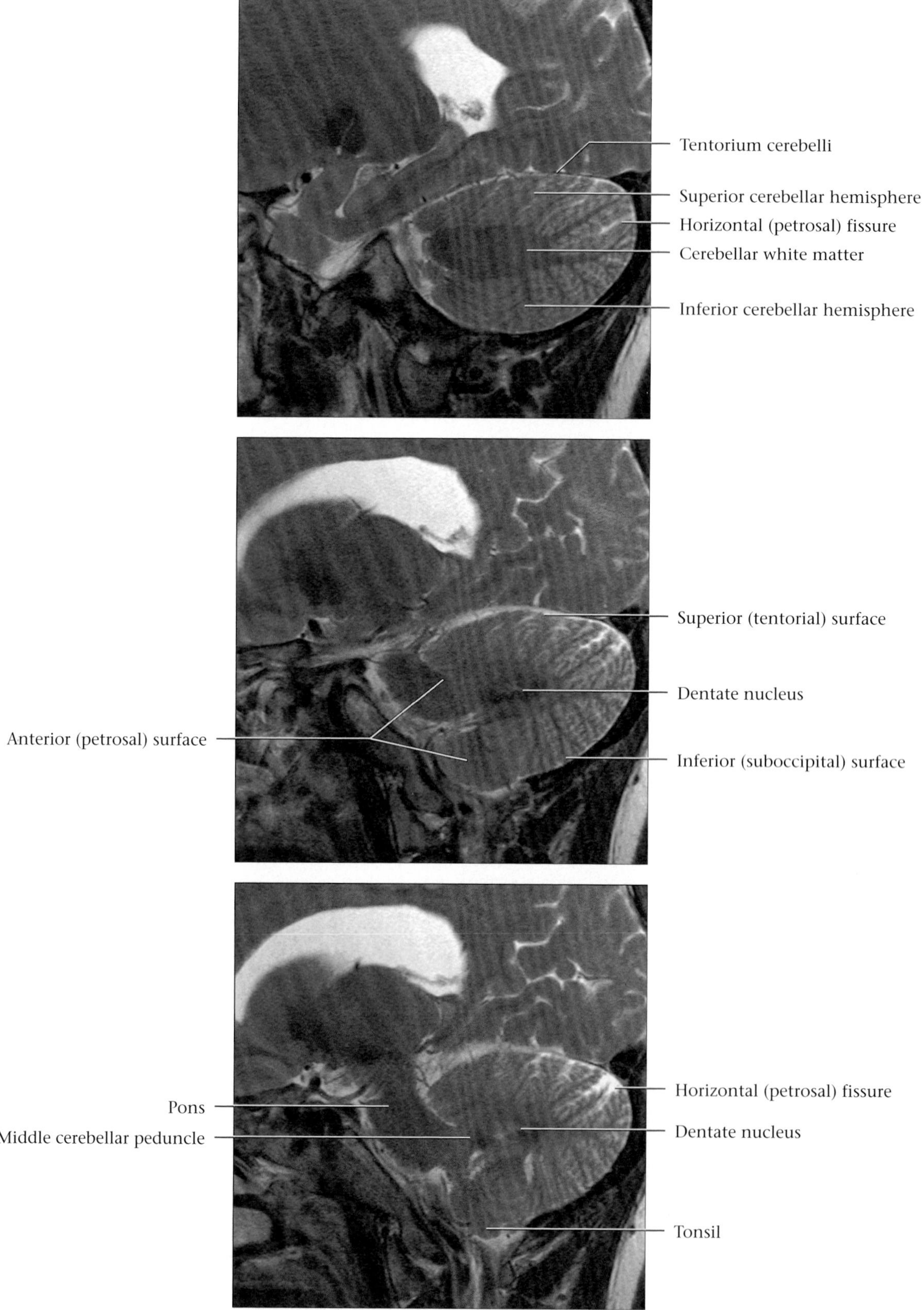
Tentorium cerebelli
Superior cerebellar hemisphere
Horizontal (petrosal) fissure
Cerebellar white matter
Inferior cerebellar hemisphere
Superior (tentorial) surface
Dentate nucleus
Anterior (petrosal) surface
Inferior (suboccipital) surface
Horizontal (petrosal) fissure
Pons
Dentate nucleus
Middle cerebellar peduncle
Tonsil

(Top) First of six sagittal T2 MR images form lateral to medial show white matter core of cerebellum which branches into medullary laminae, which occupy central lobules & are covered by cerebellar cortex. In sagittal section, the highly branched pattern of medullary laminae is known as arbor vitae (tree of life). Cerebellar nuclei are located deep in white matter, but only dentate nucleus is resolved on imaging. **(Middle)** Image through lateral cerebellar hemisphere showing superior (tentorial), inferior (suboccipital) & anterior (petrosal) surfaces. Dentate nucleus has a folded band appearance with medial part remaining open (hilum of dentate nucleus). **(Bottom)** Image more medially shows relationship of cerebellum to brainstem. Note middle cerebellar peduncle connects cerebellum to pons.

SAGITTAL T2 MR

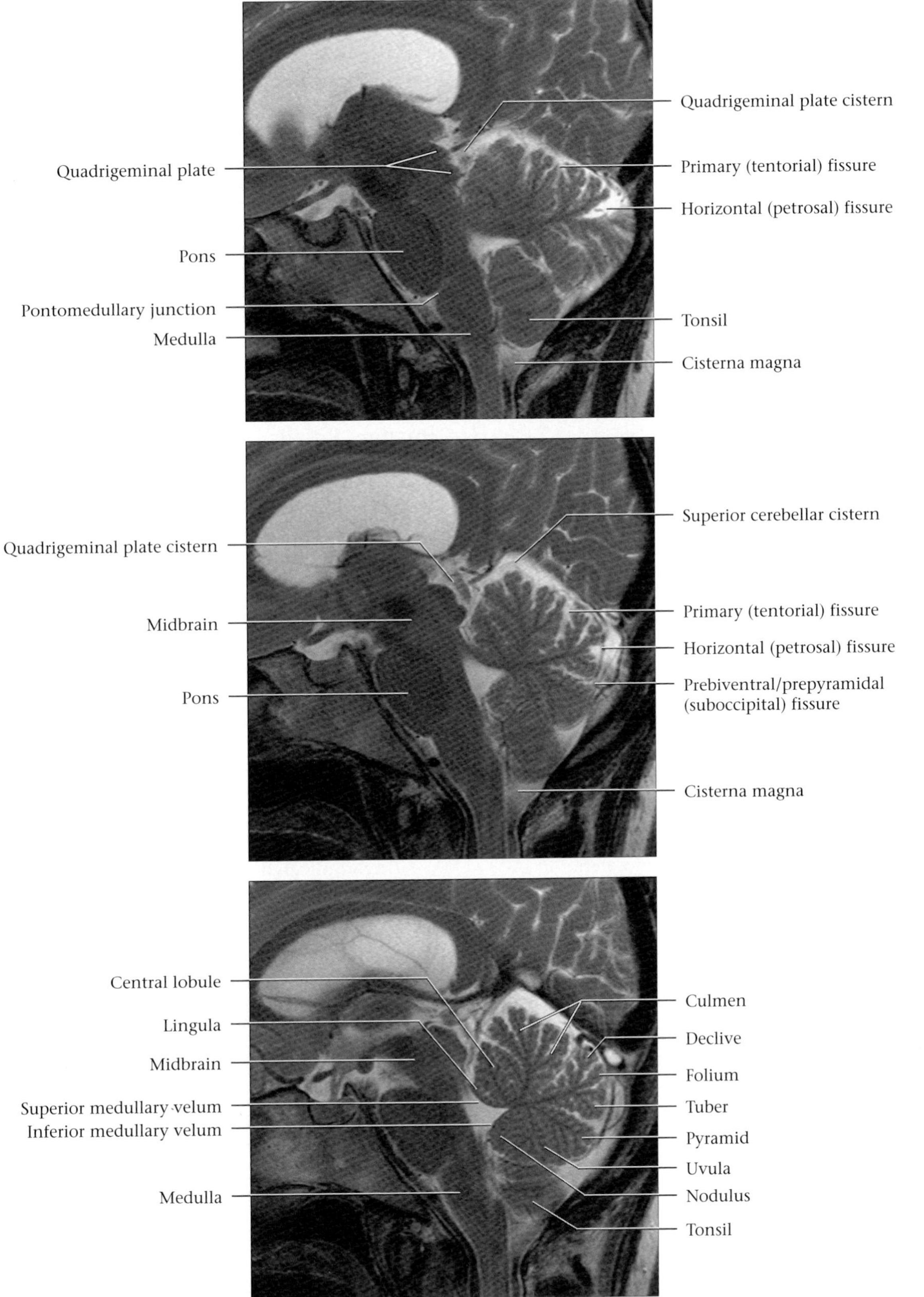

Quadrigeminal plate cistern
Quadrigeminal plate
Primary (tentorial) fissure
Horizontal (petrosal) fissure
Pons
Pontomedullary junction
Tonsil
Medulla
Cisterna magna
Superior cerebellar cistern
Quadrigeminal plate cistern
Primary (tentorial) fissure
Midbrain
Horizontal (petrosal) fissure
Prebiventral/prepyramidal (suboccipital) fissure
Pons
Cisterna magna
Central lobule
Culmen
Lingula
Declive
Midbrain
Folium
Superior medullary velum
Tuber
Inferior medullary velum
Pyramid
Uvula
Medulla
Nodulus
Tonsil

(Top) This image shows quadrigeminal plate cistern, anterior & superior to cerebellum. **(Middle)** Slightly off-midline image shows major fissures. Primary (tentorial) fissure separates anterior culmen from posterior declive. Horizontal (petrosal) fissure separates folium above from tuber below. Prebiventral/prepyramidal (suboccipital) fissure separates posterior tuber from anterior pyramid. Superior cerebellar cistern is above cerebellum, below tentorium. **(Bottom)** Midline image shows components of vermis. Superior vermis includes lingula, central lobule, culmen, declive & folium from anterior to posterior. Horizontal (petrosal) fissure separates superior from inferior vermis. Inferior vermis includes tuber, pyramid, uvula & nodulus from superior to inferior. Cerebellum forms roof of fourth ventricle with superior & inferior medullary velum.

CEREBELLOPONTINE ANGLE/IAC

Terminology

Abbreviations

- Cerebellopontine angle (CPA) & internal auditory canal (IAC)
- Superior vestibular nerve (SVN) & inferior vestibular nerve (IVN)
- Anterior inferior cerebellar artery (AICA)

Definitions

- **CPA-IAC cistern**: Cerebrospinal fluid (CSF) space in CPA & IAC containing CN7 & CN8 and AICA loop
- **IAC fundus**: Lateral CSF-filled cap of IAC cistern containing distal CN7, SVN, IVN & cochlear nerve
- **Cochlear aperture**: Bony opening connecting IAC fundus to cochlea

Imaging Anatomy

Internal Structures-Critical Contents

- **Vestibulocochlear nerve (CN8)**: CPA-IAC cistern
  - Components
    - Vestibular (balance) & cochlear portions (hearing)
  - **Cochlear nerve portion, CN8 course**
    - Leaves **spiral ganglion** as auditory axons
    - Travels as **cochlear nerve** in anterior-inferior quadrant of IAC
    - Joins SVN & IVN at porus acusticus to become CN8 bundle in CPA cistern
    - Crosses CPA cistern as posterior nerve bundle to enter brainstem at pontomedullary junction
    - Enters brainstem, bifurcates to synapse with both dorsal & ventral cochlear nuclei
  - **CN7 & CN8 orientation in IAC cistern**
    - **"Seven-up, coke down"** useful pneumonic
    - CN7 anterosuperior; cochlear nerve anteroinferior
    - SVN posterosuperior; IVN posteroinferior in IAC
- **Facial nerve (CN7): CPA-IAC cistern**
  - Root exit zone in pontomedullary junction
  - Travels anterior to CN8 in CPA cistern
  - Anterosuperior in IAC cistern
- **Anterior inferior cerebellar artery** (AICA loop)
  - Arises from basilar artery then rises into IAC
  - Continues in IAC as **internal auditory artery** (IAA)
  - May mimic cranial nerve on high-resolution T2
  - IAA supplies 3 branches to inner ear
- **Other structures in CPA cistern**
  - **Flocculus** of cerebellum in posteromedial CPA
  - **Choroid plexus** may pass from fourth ventricle though foramen of Luschka into CPA cistern
- **Other structures in IAC cistern**
  - **Crista falciformis** (horizontal crest): Horizontal bony projection from IAC fundus
  - **Vertical crest** (Bill bar): Vertical bony ridge in superior portion IAC fundus (not visible on CT or MR)
  - **Cochlear aperture**: IAC outlet for cochlear nerve to cochlea
  - **Macula cribrosa**: Perforated bone between IAC & vestibule of inner ear

Anatomy-Based Imaging Issues

Imaging Approaches

- Cochlear portion of CN8
  - Principal impetus for imaging CN8
  - Bone CT used in trauma, otosclerosis & Paget disease
  - MR used for all other indications
- MR imaging approach to **uncomplicated** unilateral sensorineural hearing loss (SNHL)
  - Screening MR involves high-resolution thin-section T2 MR imaging through CPA-IAC
- MR imaging approach to **complex** SNHL (unilateral SNHL + other symptoms)
  - Whole brain & posterior fossa sequences
  - Begin with whole brain axial T2 & FLAIR sequences
  - Conclude with axial & coronal T1 thin-section C+ MR of posterior fossa & CPA-IAC

Imaging Pitfalls

- Normal variants in CPA-IAC
  - Normal structures, when unusually prominent, trouble radiologist evaluating CPA-IAC
  - **AICA loop** flow void on high-resolution T2 MR
    - Will not prominently enhance on T1 C+ MR
    - Subtle enhancement in IAC on T1 C+ MR may be mistaken for small acoustic schwannoma
  - **Marrow space foci** in walls of IAC can mimic IAC tumor on T1 C+ MR images
    - Correlate location of foci with IAC cistern
    - Bone CT of T-bone may be necessary to identify this normal variant

Clinical Implications

Function-Dysfunction

- CPA-IAC lesions most commonly present with SNHL
  - **Uncomplicated unilateral SNHL**: Patient otherwise healthy & presents with unilateral SNHL
  - **Complicated SNHL**: Patient has other symptoms in addition to unilateral SNHL
    - Symptoms include other cranial neuropathy, long tract signs & headache
- Cochlear nerve injury
  - SNHL & tinnitus primary symptoms
- Facial nerve injury, CPA-IAC portion
  - Peripheral facial neuropathy
    - Lacrimation, stapedial reflex, anterior 2/3 tongue taste loss & complete loss of muscles of facial expression on side of lesion
    - CN7 rarely injured by lesion in CPA-IAC
    - If lesion in CPA-IAC and CN7 is out, consider non-acoustic schwannoma causes such as facial nerve schwannoma or metastatic disease

Embryology

Embryologic Events

- IAC forms separately from inner ear & external ear
- Forms in response to migration of CN7 & CN8 through this area

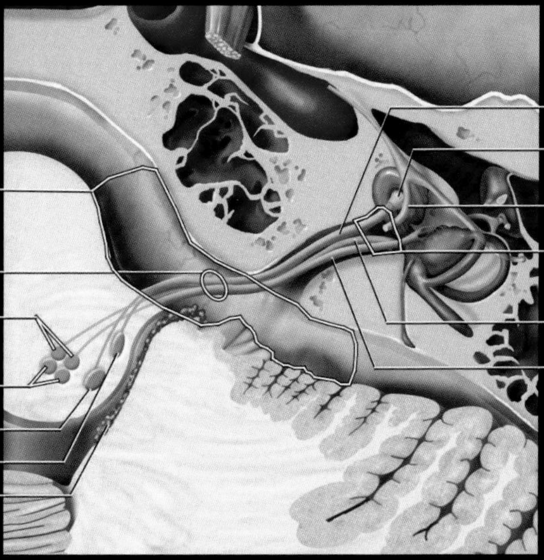

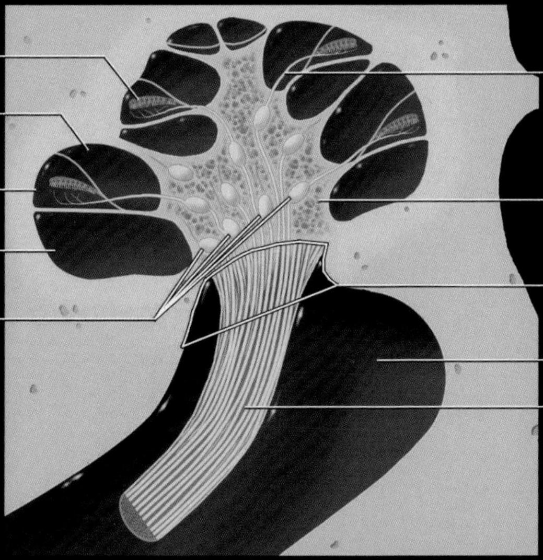

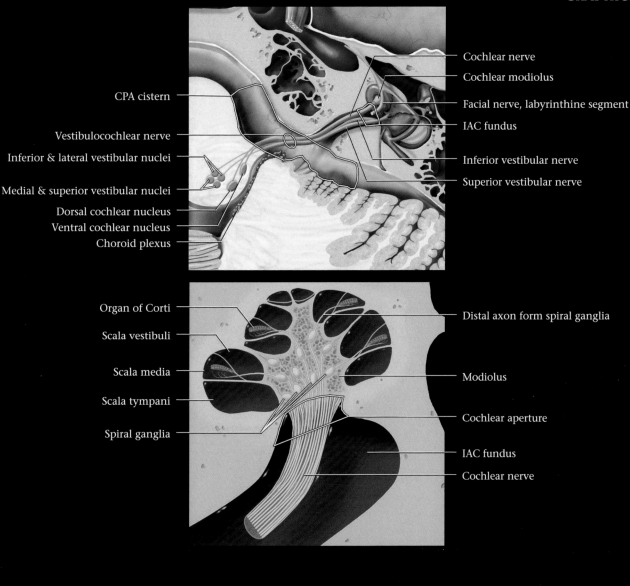

CPA cistern
Vestibulocochlear nerve
Inferior & lateral vestibular nuclei
Medial & superior vestibular nuclei
Dorsal cochlear nucleus
Ventral cochlear nucleus
Choroid plexus
Cochlear nerve
Cochlear modiolus
Facial nerve, labyrinthine segment
IAC fundus
Inferior vestibular nerve
Superior vestibular nerve

Organ of Corti
Scala vestibuli
Scala media
Scala tympani
Spiral ganglia
Distal axon form spiral ganglia
Modiolus
Cochlear aperture
IAC fundus
Cochlear nerve

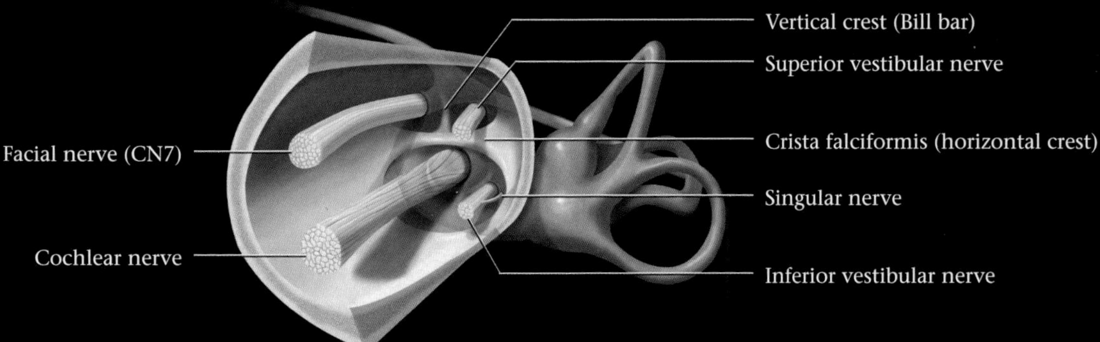
Vertical crest (Bill bar)
Superior vestibular nerve
Crista falciformis (horizontal crest)
Singular nerve
Inferior vestibular nerve
Facial nerve (CN7)
Cochlear nerve

(Top) Graphic of CPA-IAC cisterns & inner ear. The inferior & superior vestibular nerves begin in cell bodies in the vestibular ganglion, from there coursing centrally to 4 vestibular nuclei. Cochlear component of CN8 begins in bipolar cell bodies in spiral ganglion of the modiolus. Central fibers run in cochlear nerve to dorsal & ventral cochlear nuclei in inferior cerebellar peduncle. **(Middle)** Axial graphic of magnified cochlea shows the modiolus & cochlear nerve in IAC fundus. Note cells in spiral ganglion are bipolar contributing proximal axons that constitute the cochlear nerve & distal fibers to organ of Corti. **(Bottom)** Graphic depicting fundus of IAC. Notice the crista falciformis separates cochlear nerve & inferior vestibular nerve below from CN7 & superior vestibular nerve above. Also note vertical crest separating CN7 from the superior vestibular nerve.

AXIAL BONE CT

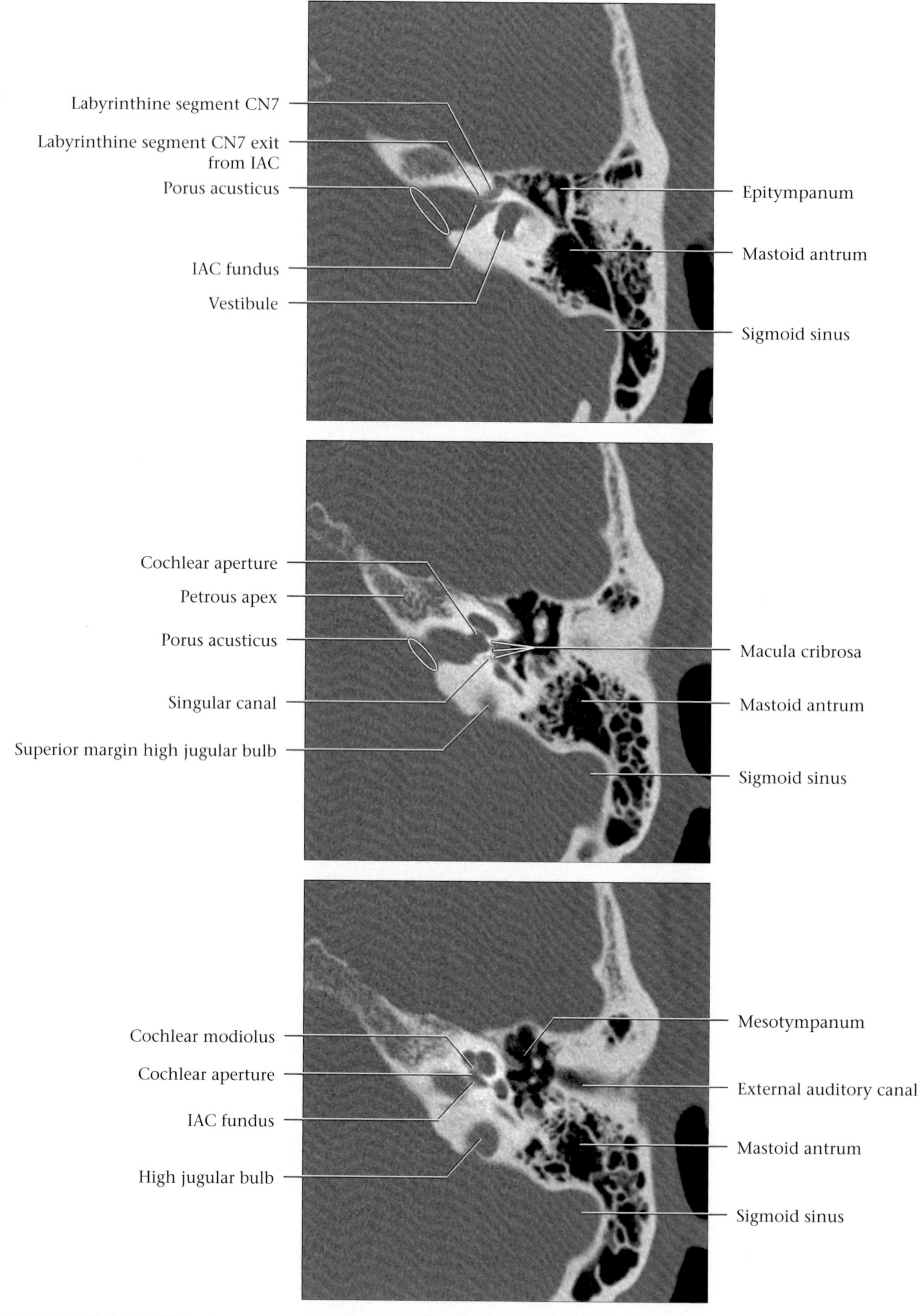
Labyrinthine segment CN7
Labyrinthine segment CN7 exit from IAC
Porus acusticus
IAC fundus
Vestibule
Epitympanum
Mastoid antrum
Sigmoid sinus
Cochlear aperture
Petrous apex
Porus acusticus
Singular canal
Superior margin high jugular bulb
Macula cribrosa
Mastoid antrum
Sigmoid sinus
Cochlear modiolus
Cochlear aperture
IAC fundus
High jugular bulb
Mesotympanum
External auditory canal
Mastoid antrum
Sigmoid sinus

(Top) First of three axial bone CT images of the left ear through the internal auditory canal presented from superior to inferior. In this CT image the labyrinthine segment of the facial nerve is seen exiting the anterosuperior fundus of the IAC. **(Middle)** In this image the cochlear aperture is seen connecting the anteroinferior fundus of the IAC to the cochlea. The cochlear nerve accesses the modiolus of the cochlea through this aperture. Note the posterolateral fundal bony wall abutting the medial vestibule. Multiple branches of the vestibular nerves pass to the vestibule and semicircular canals through this wall called the macula cribrosa. **(Bottom)** The cochlear modiolus is visible as a high density structure at the cochlear base directly inside the cochlea from the cochlear aperture. The high jugular bulb projects cephalad behind the internal auditory canal.

SAGITTAL T2 MR

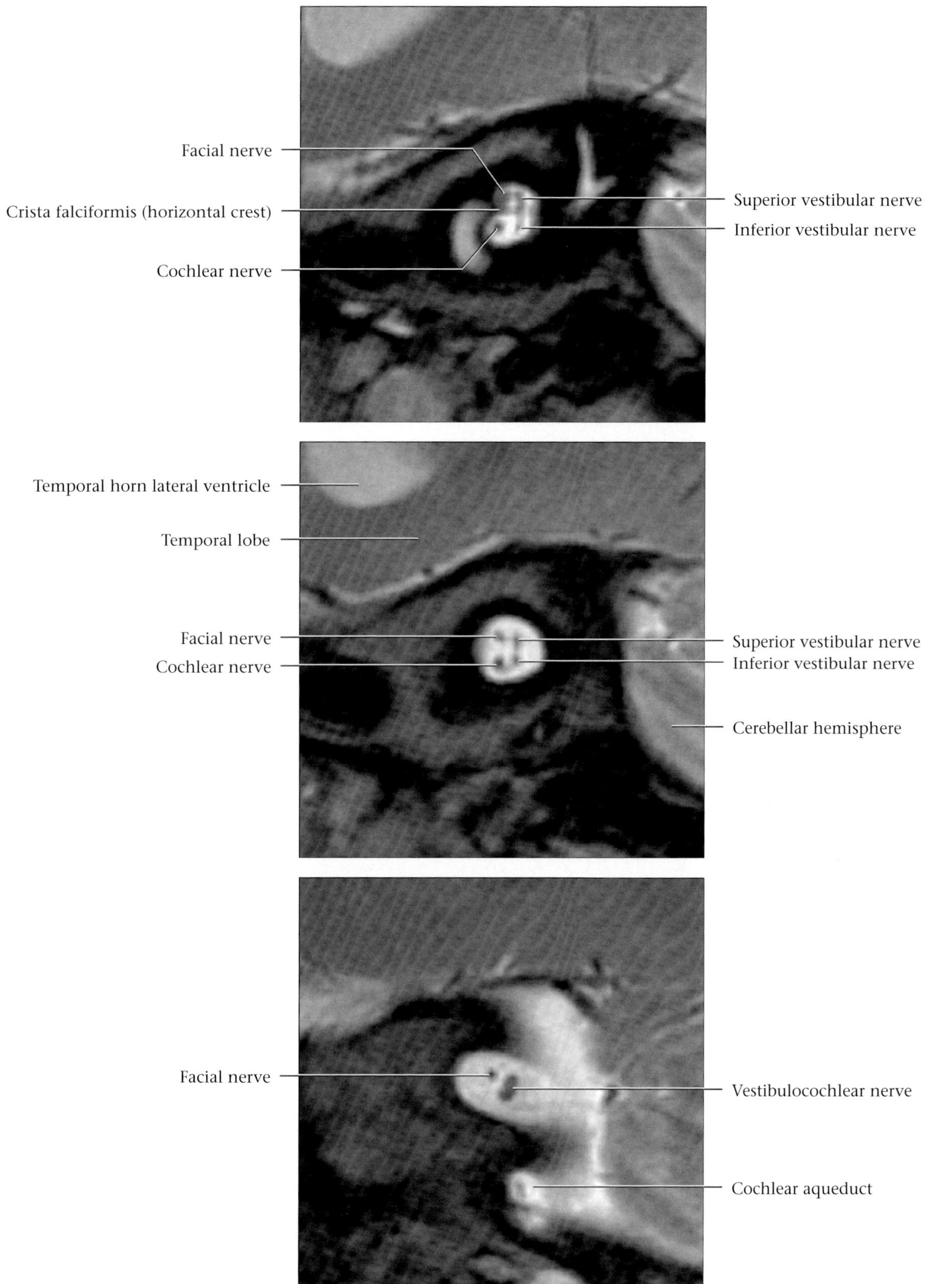

Facial nerve
Crista falciformis (horizontal crest)
Cochlear nerve
Superior vestibular nerve
Inferior vestibular nerve
Temporal horn lateral ventricle
Temporal lobe
Facial nerve
Cochlear nerve
Superior vestibular nerve
Inferior vestibular nerve
Cerebellar hemisphere
Facial nerve
Vestibulocochlear nerve
Cochlear aqueduct

(Top) First of 3 oblique sagittal high-resolution T2 MR images presented from lateral to medial shows the fundus of the internal auditory canal (IAC) filled with high signal cerebrospinal fluid. The horizontal low signal line in the fundus is the crista falciformis. The facial nerve is anterosuperior while the cochlear nerve is anteroinferior. **(Middle)** In this image through the mid-IAC the 4 discrete nerves are well seen. Notice that the anteroinferior cochlear nerve is normally slightly larger than the other three nerves in the IAC. **(Bottom)** At the level of the porus acusticus the facial nerve is visible just anterior to the vestibulocochlear nerve. The overall appearance of these two nerves is that of a "ball" (facial nerve) in a "catcher's mitt" (vestibulocochlear nerve). The vestibulocochlear nerve contains the cochlear, inferior & superior vestibular nerves.

CEREBELLOPONTINE ANGLE/IAC

AXIAL T2 MR

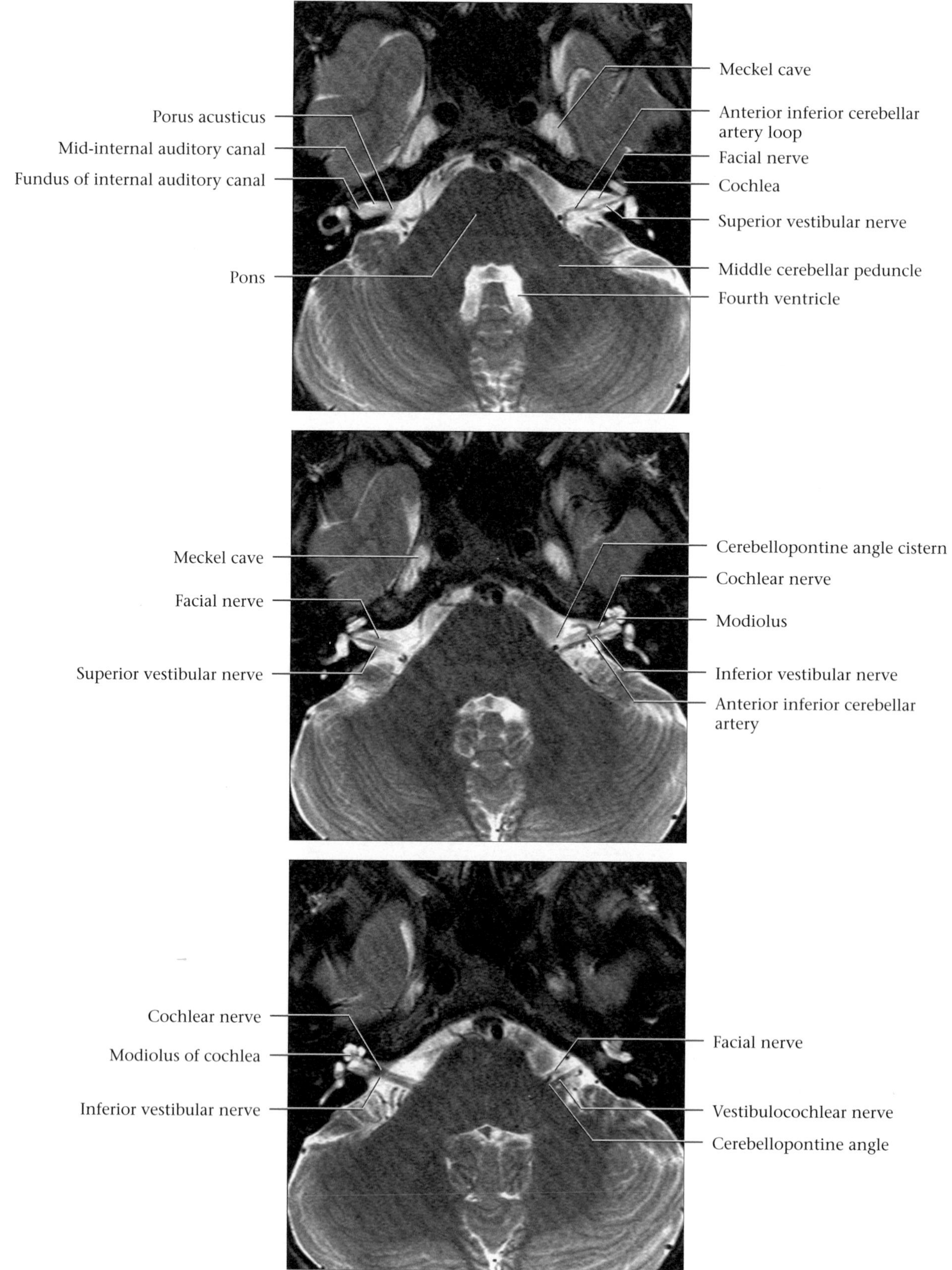
Porus acusticus
Mid-internal auditory canal
Fundus of internal auditory canal
Pons
Meckel cave
Anterior inferior cerebellar artery loop
Facial nerve
Cochlea
Superior vestibular nerve
Middle cerebellar peduncle
Fourth ventricle
Meckel cave
Facial nerve
Superior vestibular nerve
Cerebellopontine angle cistern
Cochlear nerve
Modiolus
Inferior vestibular nerve
Anterior inferior cerebellar artery
Cochlear nerve
Modiolus of cochlea
Inferior vestibular nerve
Facial nerve
Vestibulocochlear nerve
Cerebellopontine angle

(Top) First of three axial T2 MR images presented from superior to inferior reveals the porus acusticus, mid-portion and fundus of the internal auditory canal (IAC) on the right. On the left the anterior inferior cerebellar artery is seen looping through the cerebellopontine angle cistern. Also note the facial nerve and superior vestibular nerve on the left within the IAC. **(Middle)** In this image the facial nerve and superior vestibular nerve are seen in the right internal auditory canal while the cochlear nerve and inferior vestibular are visible on the left. **(Bottom)** In this image the cochlear nerve is seen in the right internal auditory canal exiting through the cochlear aperture to reach the modiolus of the cochlea. On the left the cerebellopontine angle is seen with the vestibulocochlear nerve emerging from the brainstem at this point.

CORONAL T2 MR

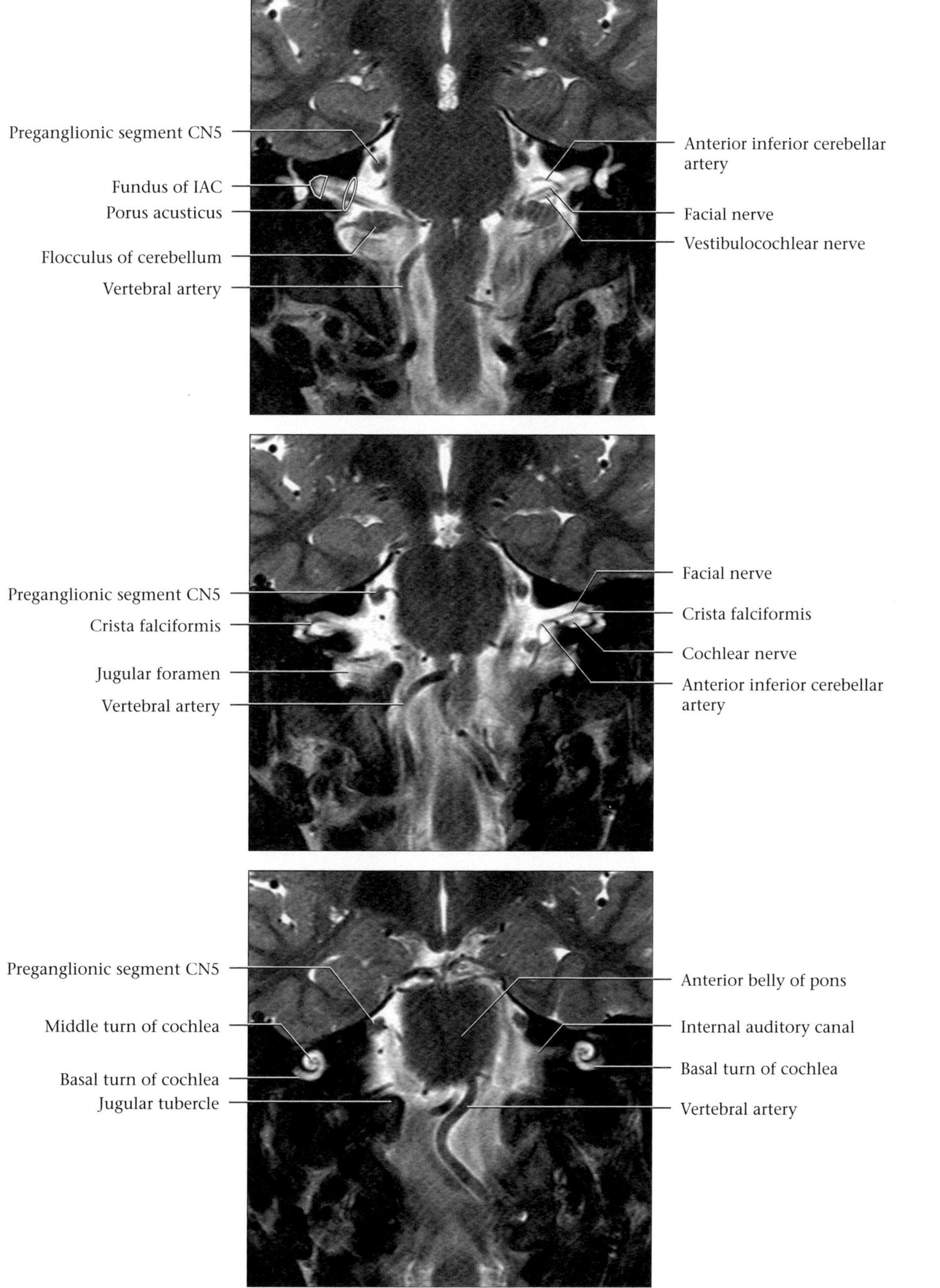
Preganglionic segment CN5
Fundus of IAC
Porus acusticus
Flocculus of cerebellum
Vertebral artery
Anterior inferior cerebellar artery
Facial nerve
Vestibulocochlear nerve
Preganglionic segment CN5
Crista falciformis
Jugular foramen
Vertebral artery
Facial nerve
Crista falciformis
Cochlear nerve
Anterior inferior cerebellar artery
Preganglionic segment CN5
Middle turn of cochlea
Basal turn of cochlea
Jugular tubercle
Anterior belly of pons
Internal auditory canal
Basal turn of cochlea
Vertebral artery

(Top) First of three coronal T2 MR images presented from posterior to anterior through the cerebellopontine angle and internal auditory canal cisterns shows important regional structures including the preganglionic segment of CN5, anterior inferior cerebellar artery loop, flocculus of cerebellum and vertebral artery. **(Middle)** In this image the crista falciformis in the fundus of the internal auditory canal is seen. The facial nerve & superior vestibular nerve are above and the cochlear nerve & inferior vestibular nerve are below the crista falciformis. **(Bottom)** At the level of the cochlea the anterior belly of the pons is visible. The preganglionic segment of the trigeminal nerve is in the anterosuperior portion of the cerebellopontine angle cistern while the jugular tubercle is in the anteroinferior portion.

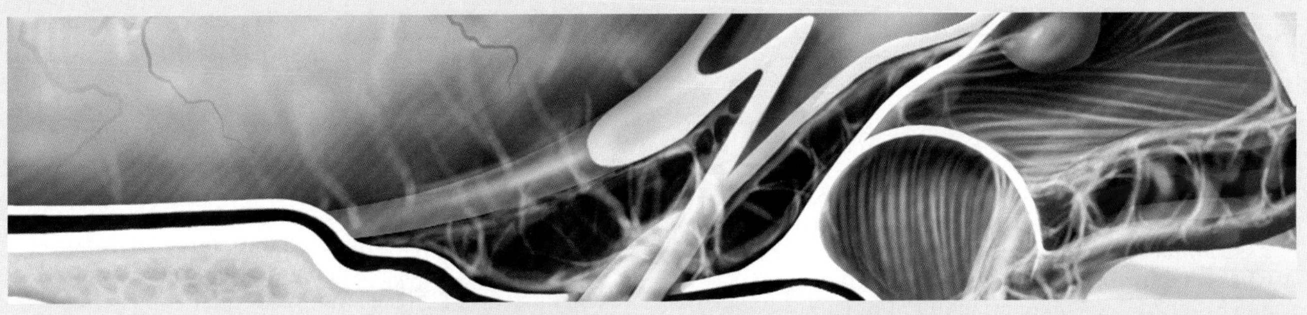

SECTION 4: CSF Spaces

VENTRICLES AND CHOROID PLEXUS

Terminology

Definitions

- Tela choroidea: Double layer of pia, formed during folding of brain where hemispheres overgrow diencephalon & cerebellum apposes dorsal brainstem
- Choroidal fissure: Narrow, pial-lined channel between SAS & ventricles; Site of attachment of choroid plexus in lateral ventricles

Gross Anatomy

Overview

- **Cerebral ventricles**
  - Four cerebrospinal fluid-filled, ependymal lined cavities deep within brain
  - Paired lateral, midline third and fourth ventricles
  - Communicate with each other as well as central canal of spinal cord, subarachnoid space (SAS)
- **Choroid plexus**
  - Secretory epithelium that produces cerebrospinal fluid (CSF)
  - Choroid plexus forms where tela choroidea contacts ependymal lining of ventricles: Roof of third ventricle, body & temporal horn of lateral ventricle via choroidal fissure, inferior roof of fourth ventricle
  - CSF flows from lateral ventricles through foramen of Monro into third ventricle, through cerebral aqueduct into fourthventricle; exits through foramina of Luschka & Magendie to SAS
  - Bulk of CSF resorption through arachnoid granulations in region of superior sagittal sinus

Anatomy Relationships

- **Lateral ventricles**
  - Each has body, atrium, three horns
  - **Frontal horn** formed by
    - Roof: Corpus callosum
    - Lateral wall, floor: Caudate nucleus
    - Medial wall: Septum pellucidum (thin midline structure that separates right, left frontal horns)
  - **Body** formed by
    - Roof: Corpus callosum
    - Floor: Dorsal surface of thalamus
    - Medial wall, floor: Fornix
    - Lateral wall, floor: Body, tail of caudate nucleus
  - **Temporal horn** formed by
    - Roof: Tail of caudate nucleus
    - Medial wall, floor: Hippocampus
    - Lateral wall: Geniculocalcarine tract, arcuate fasciculus
  - **Occipital horn**: Surrounded by white matter (forceps major of corpus callosum, geniculocalcarine tract)
  - **Atrium**: Confluence of horns; contains glomi of choroid plexus
  - Lateral ventricles communicate with each other, third ventricle via "Y-shaped" **foramen of Monro**
- **Third ventricle**
  - Midline, slit-like vertical cavity between right, left diencephalon that contains interthalamic adhesion (not a true commissure)
  - Borders
    - Anterior: Lamina terminalis, anterior commissure
    - Lateral: Thalami
    - Roof: Tela choroidea, choroid plexus
    - Floor: Optic chiasm, infundibulum & tuber cinereum, mammillary bodies, posterior perforated substance, tegmentum of midbrain
    - Posterior: Pineal gland, habenular & posterior commissures
  - Recesses
    - Inferior: Optic, infundibular
    - Posterior: Suprapineal, pineal
  - Communicates with fourth ventricle via cerebral aqueduct
- **Fourth ventricle**
  - Diamond-shaped cavity (rhomboid fossa) along dorsal pons & upper medulla
  - Borders
    - Roof: Tent-shaped, covered by anterior (superior) medullary velum above & inferior medullary velum below
    - Walls: Dorsal surface of pons & medulla, cerebral peduncles (superior/middle/inferior)
  - Five recesses
    - Paired posterior superior: Thin, flat pouch capping tonsils
    - Paired lateral: Curve anteriorly under brachium pontis, contain choroid plexus, communicate with SAS via foramina of Luschka
    - Fastigium: Blind-ending, dorsally pointed midline outpouching from body of fourth ventricle
  - Communicates with SAS via **foramina of Magendie and Luschka**, with central canal of cord via obex

Imaging Anatomy

Overview

- Lateral ventricles: Paired, "C-shaped", curve posteriorly from temporal horns, arch around/above thalami
- Third ventricle: Thin, usually slit-like; 80% have central adhesion between thalami (massa intermedia)
  - Recesses: Optic is rounded, superior to optic chiasm; infundibular is pointed, extends inferiorly into infundibular stalk; suprapineal is thin, extends over pineal; pineal is pointed projecting into pineal stalk
- Fourth ventricle: Diamond-shaped midline infratentorial ventricle
  - Terminates inferiorly at obex, which communicates with central canal of spinal cord (dorsal "bump" covering obex is nucleus gracilis)

Normal Variants

- Ventricles: Cavum septi pellucidi, cavum vergae, cavum veli interpositi
- Choroid plexus: Calcification, xanthogranulomas (glomi appear lobulated, cystic)

Anatomy-Based Imaging Issues

Imaging Pitfalls

- Spin dephasing with pulsatile CSF flow can mimic intraventricular mass (e.g., colloid cyst)!

VENTRICLES AND CHOROID PLEXUS

GRAPHICS

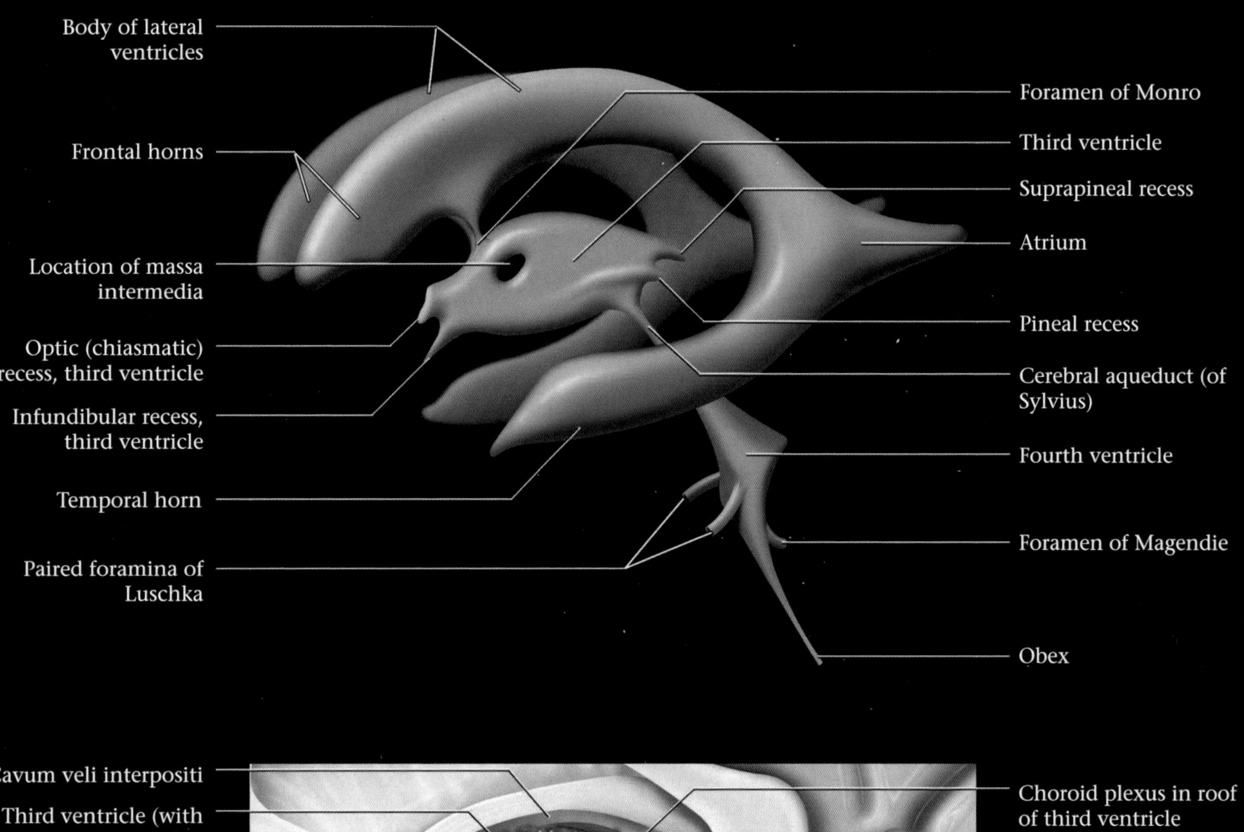

Body of lateral ventricles
Frontal horns
Location of massa intermedia
Optic (chiasmatic) recess, third ventricle
Infundibular recess, third ventricle
Temporal horn
Paired foramina of Luschka
Foramen of Monro
Third ventricle
Suprapineal recess
Atrium
Pineal recess
Cerebral aqueduct (of Sylvius)
Fourth ventricle
Foramen of Magendie
Obex

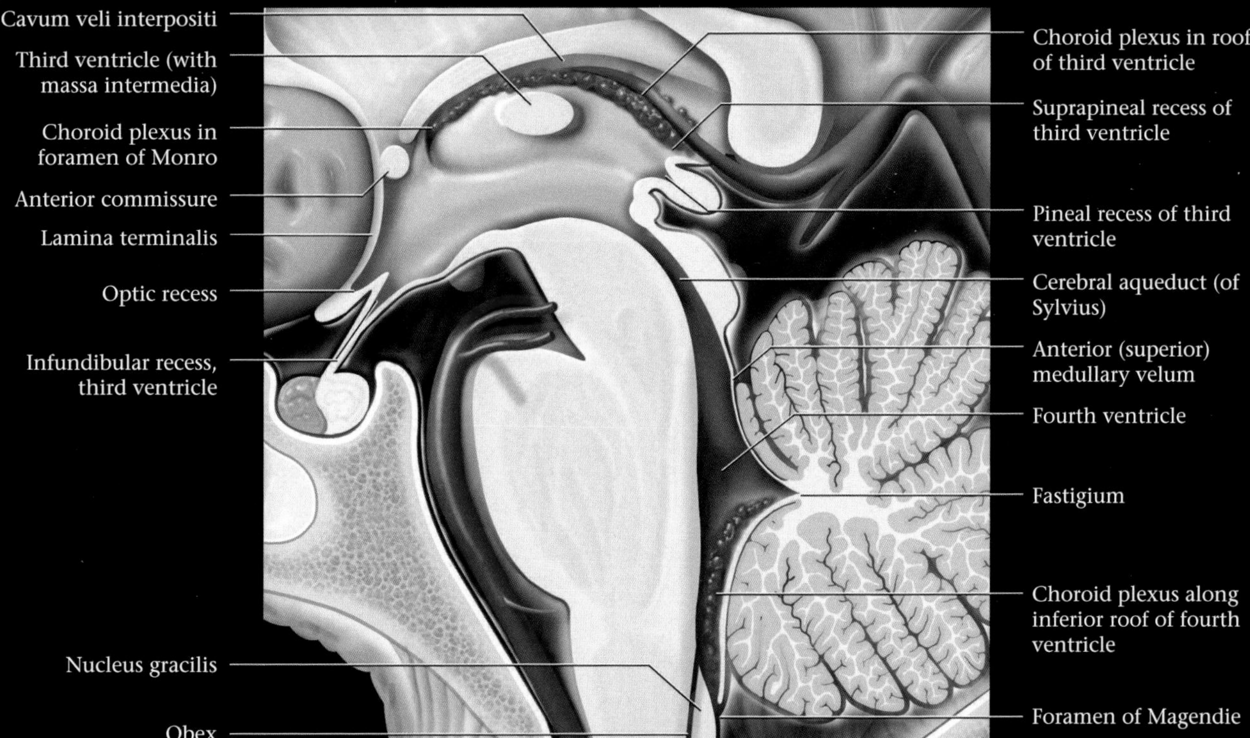

Cavum veli interpositi
Third ventricle (with massa intermedia)
Choroid plexus in foramen of Monro
Anterior commissure
Lamina terminalis
Optic recess
Infundibular recess, third ventricle
Nucleus gracilis
Obex
Choroid plexus in roof of third ventricle
Suprapineal recess of third ventricle
Pineal recess of third ventricle
Cerebral aqueduct (of Sylvius)
Anterior (superior) medullary velum
Fourth ventricle
Fastigium
Choroid plexus along inferior roof of fourth ventricle
Foramen of Magendie

(Top) Schematic 3D representation of the ventricular system, viewed in the sagittal plane, demonstrates the normal appearance and communicating pathways of the cerebral ventricles. **(Bottom)** Sagittal midline graphic of normal midline ventricular anatomy. Choroid plexus from the lateral ventricles (not shown) extends through the foramina of Monro and curves dorsally and posteriorly along the roof of the third ventricle. Choroid plexus is not found in the frontal or occipital horns of the lateral ventricles, the cerebral aqueduct or foramen of Magendie. The foramen of Magendie is a slit-like median aperture which allows posterior communication of the fourth ventricle with the cisterna magna. The obex is the inferior terminus of the fourth ventricle in the upper cord.

VENTRICLES AND CHOROID PLEXUS

AXIAL T2 MR

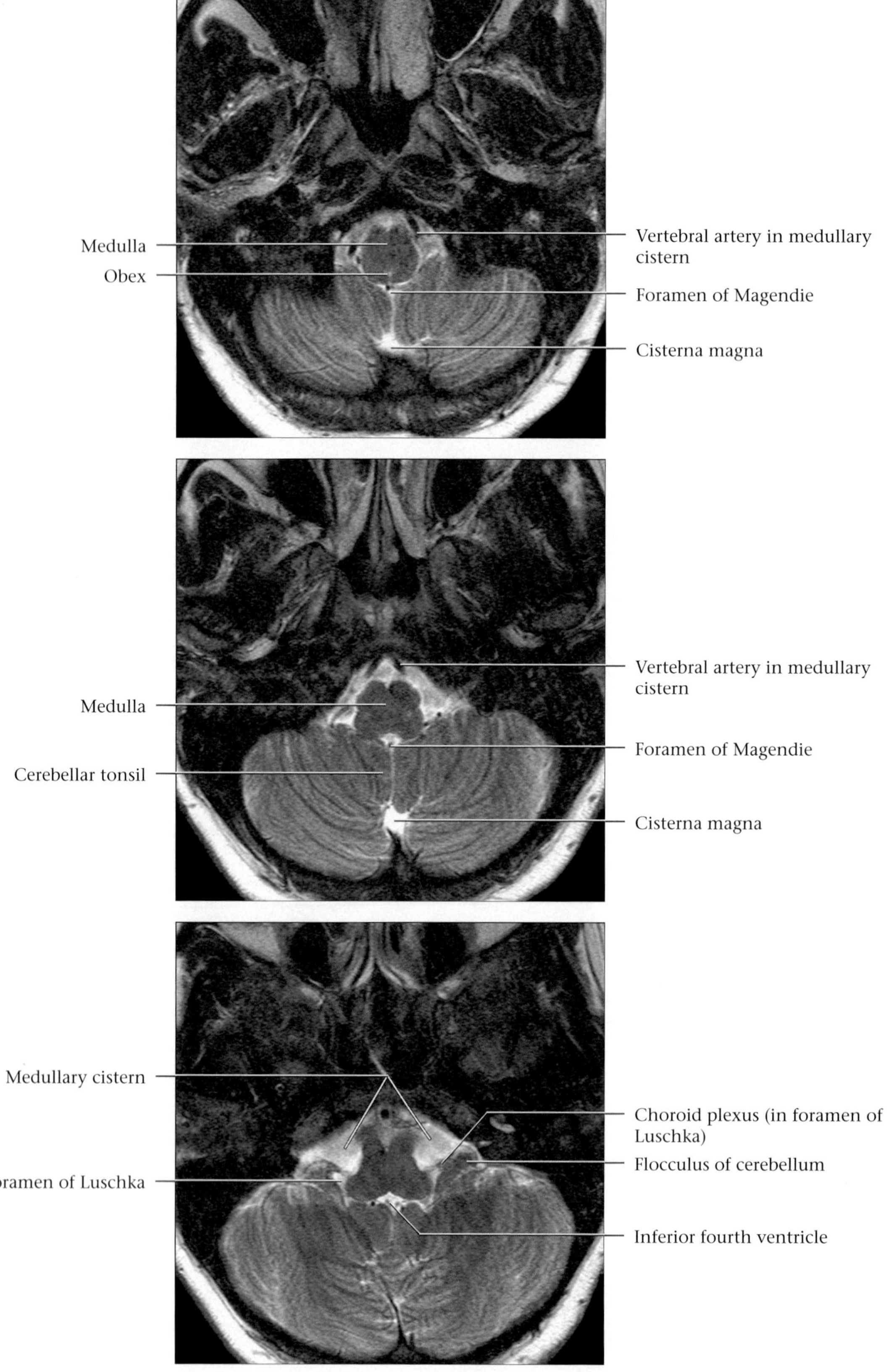
Medulla
Obex
Vertebral artery in medullary cistern
Foramen of Magendie
Cisterna magna
Medulla
Cerebellar tonsil
Vertebral artery in medullary cistern
Foramen of Magendie
Cisterna magna
Medullary cistern
Foramen of Luschka
Choroid plexus (in foramen of Luschka)
Flocculus of cerebellum
Inferior fourth ventricle

(Top) First of 12 sequential axial T2 MR images from inferior to superior demonstrates the obex, which is the inferior termination of the fourth ventricle in the upper cord. The obex separates the central canal of the spinal cord from the intracranial ventricular system. **(Middle)** Scan at lower medulla demonstrates foramen of Magendie (median aperture), which allows communication between the fourth ventricle and cisterna magna. In contrast to the foramina of Luschka, the foramen of Magendie contains no choroid plexus. **(Bottom)** Image at the level of the medulla. The fourth ventricle communicates laterally with the medullary cisterns via the foramina of Luschka as demonstrated here. Choroid plexus in the foramina of Luschka normally protrudes through the lateral recess into the medullary cisterns and should not be mistaken for an enhancing mass.

AXIAL T2 MR

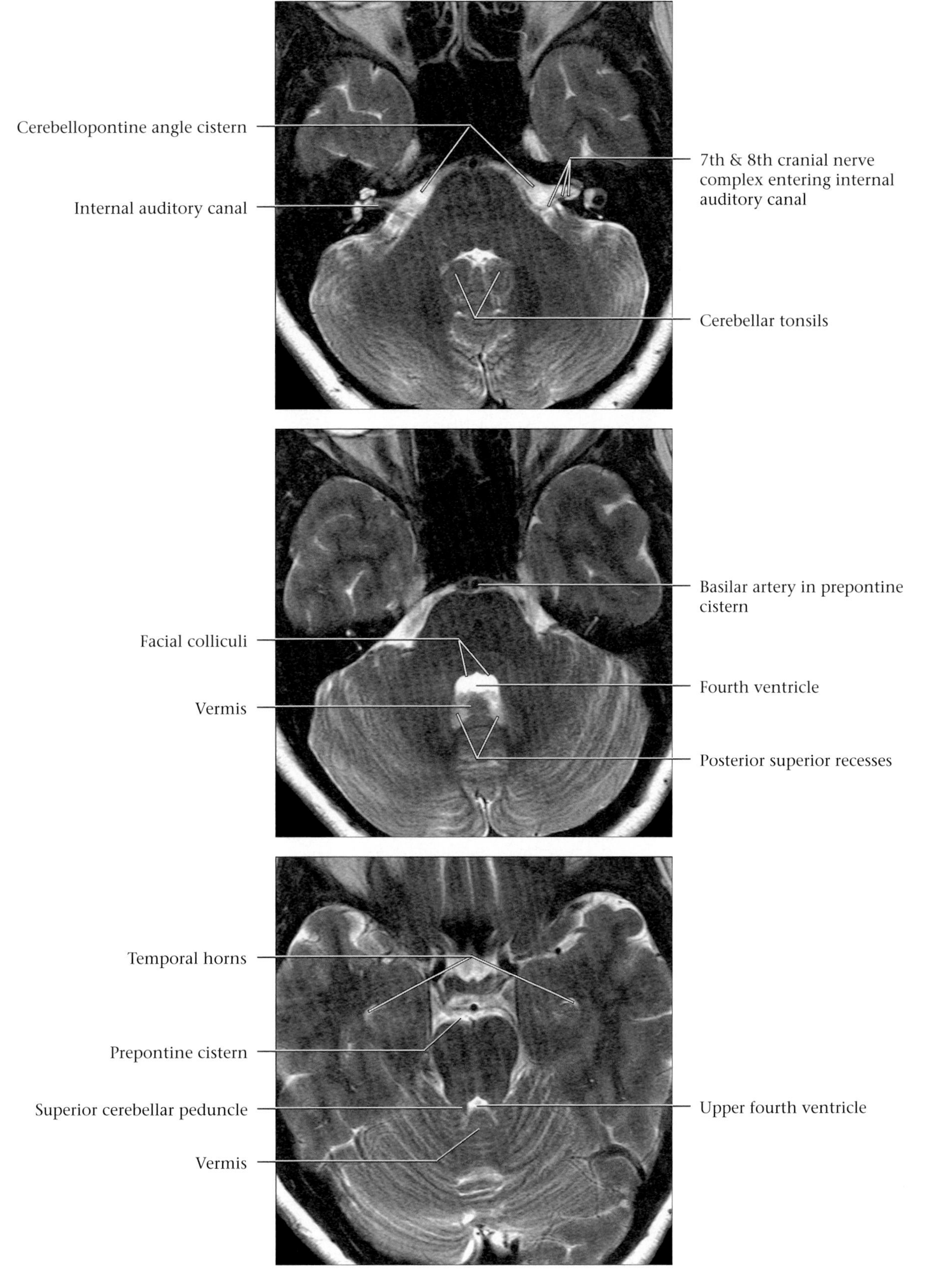
Cerebellopontine angle cistern
Internal auditory canal
7th & 8th cranial nerve complex entering internal auditory canal
Cerebellar tonsils
Basilar artery in prepontine cistern
Facial colliculi
Vermis
Fourth ventricle
Posterior superior recesses
Temporal horns
Preportine cistern
Superior cerebellar peduncle
Vermis
Upper fourth ventricle

(Top) Image at the level of lower pons demonstrates the seventh & eighth cranial nerves as they traverse the cerebellopontine angle cistern towards the internal auditory canals. The anterior inferior cerebellar artery loop usually extends into the proximal internal auditory canal. **(Middle)** Image through the body of the fourth ventricle shows the thin, CSF-filled blind-ending posterior superior recesses capping the tonsils. **(Bottom)** Image at the level of the superior cerebellar peduncles shows the normal appearing upper fourth ventricle, which begins at the inferior aspect of the cerebral aqueduct (of Sylvius). Note the normally crescentic appearance of the temporal horns also seen here, which are bounded medially by the hippocampi. Rounding of the temporal horns should raise suspicion for obstruction.

VENTRICLES AND CHOROID PLEXUS

AXIAL T2 MR

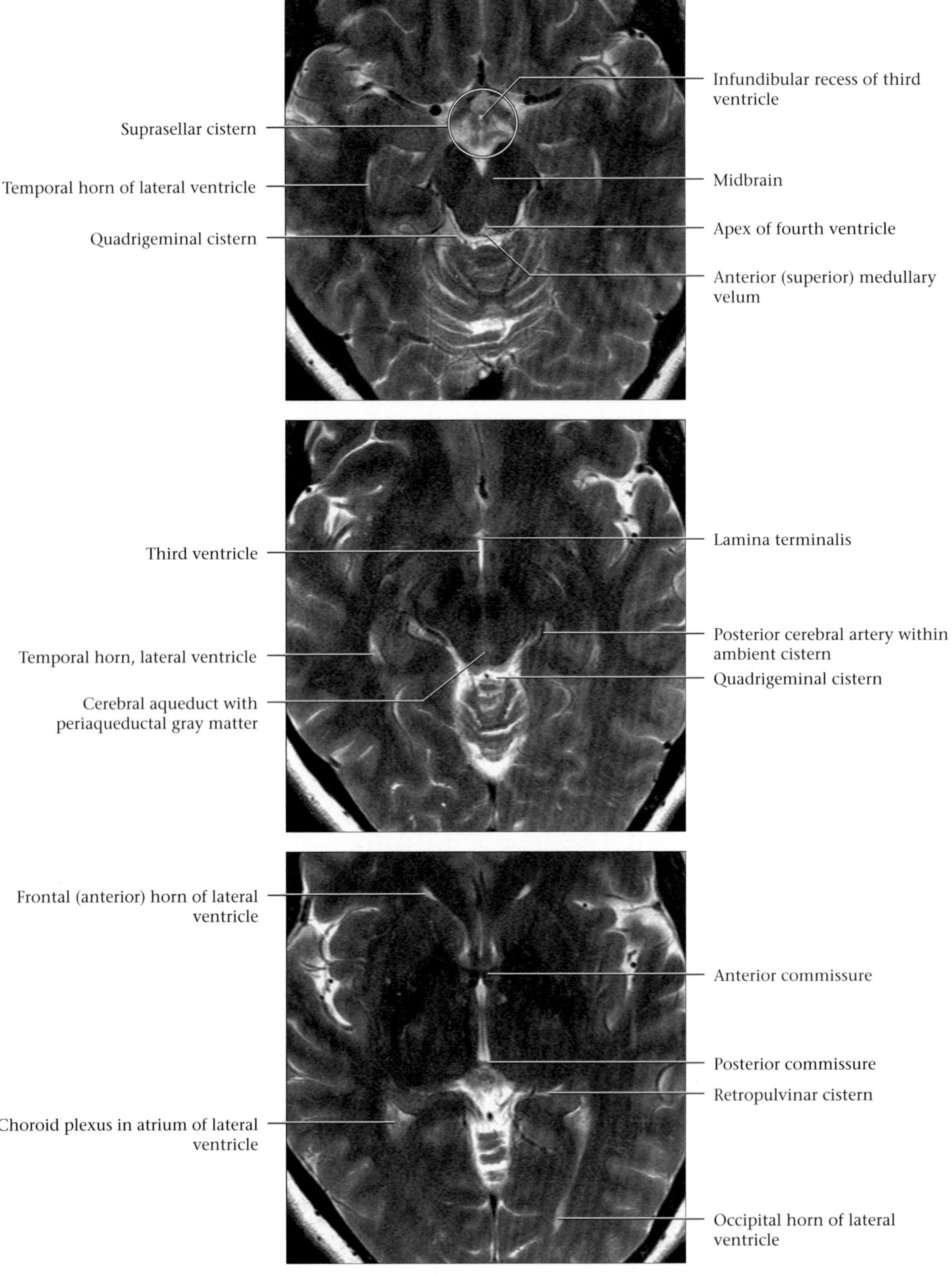

Suprasellar cistern
Temporal horn of lateral ventricle
Quadrigeminal cistern
Infundibular recess of third ventricle
Midbrain
Apex of fourth ventricle
Anterior (superior) medullary velum
Third ventricle
Temporal horn, lateral ventricle
Cerebral aqueduct with periaqueductal gray matter
Lamina terminalis
Posterior cerebral artery within ambient cistern
Quadrigeminal cistern
Frontal (anterior) horn of lateral ventricle
Choroid plexus in atrium of lateral ventricle
Anterior commissure
Posterior commissure
Retropulvinar cistern
Occipital horn of lateral ventricle

(Top) The suprasellar cistern and infundibular recess of the third ventricle are seen at this level. Note the normal thin crescentic appearance to the temporal horns. The hippocampi line the inner margins of the temporal horns. **(Middle)** Image at the midbrain level shows the lamina terminalis as a thin tract of white matter crossing midline at the anterior margin of the third ventricle. The cerebral aqueduct, barely visible in this case, may have increased T2 signal (due to CSF) or decreased signal (from high flow). **(Bottom)** Image at the level of the anterior commissure, which forms part of the anterior boundary of the third ventricle. Choroid plexus is normally present within the trigone (atrium) of the lateral ventricle. Choroid plexus in roof of the third ventricle is often hypoplastic or inapparent, even on contrast-enhanced T1 weighted MR scans.

VENTRICLES AND CHOROID PLEXUS

AXIAL T2 MR

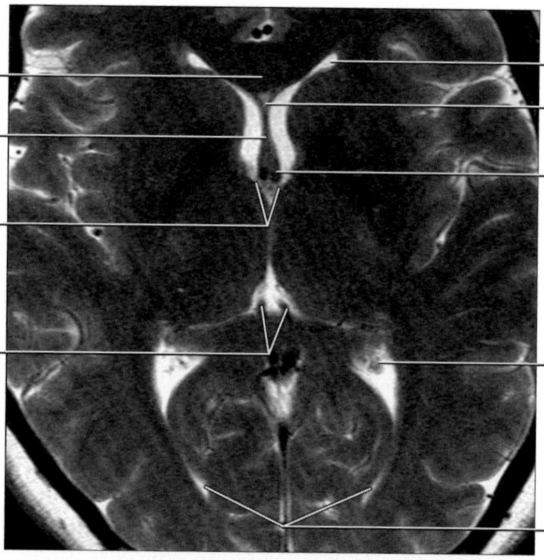

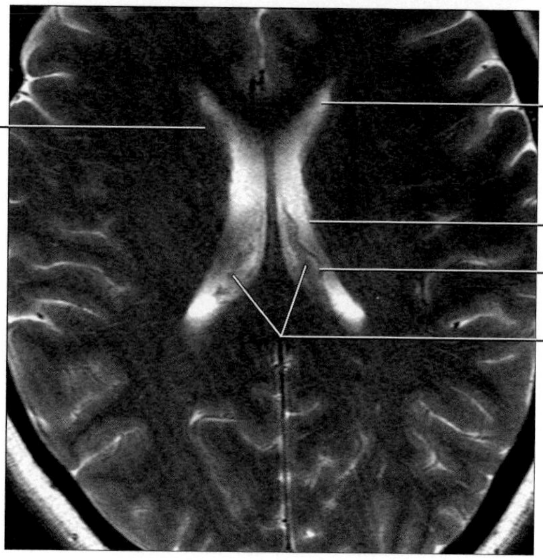

Genu of corpus callosum
Septum pellucidum
Foramina of Monro
Internal cerebral veins in cistern of velum interpositum
Frontal horn
Cavum septi pellucidi
Columns of fornix
Choroid plexus glomus in atrium of lateral ventricle
Occipital horns of lateral ventricles

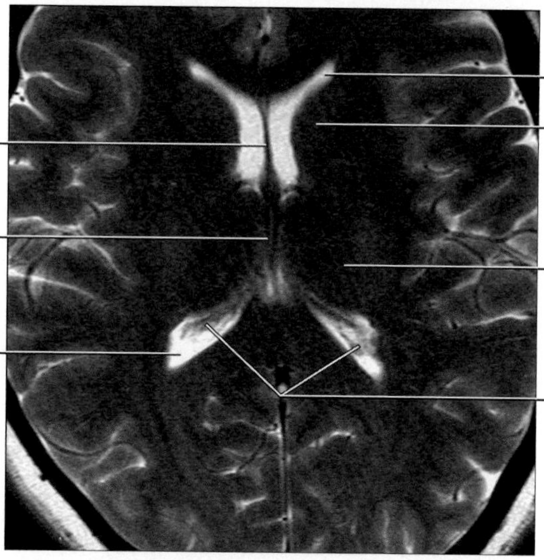

Septum pellucidum
Internal cerebral vein
Atrium of lateral ventricle
Frontal horn of lateral ventricle
Caudate head
Thalamus
Choroid plexus within lateral ventricular atria

Caudate head
Frontal horn of lateral ventricle
Body of lateral ventricle
Choroidal arteries, veins
Choroid plexus in lateral ventricles

(Top) Image at the foramina of Monro level shows connection between the lateral and third ventricles. Choroid plexus is seen in the lateral ventricular atria. The occipital horns contain no choroid plexus, and are a common place for subtle intraventricular blood to collect dependently. **(Middle)** Image at the level of the lateral ventricular atria. Note the septum pellucidum which separates the lateral ventricles. Choroid plexus is normally seen in the anteromedial body and atria of the lateral ventricles. The caudate head impresses upon the floor and lateral wall of the frontal horn, and the thalamus forms the lateral boundary of the lateral ventricle body. **(Bottom)** This image demonstrates normal choroid plexus in the anteromedial body of the lateral ventricles. Note the normal concavity along the lateral margins of the lateral ventricles from the caudate nuclei.

CORONAL T2 MR

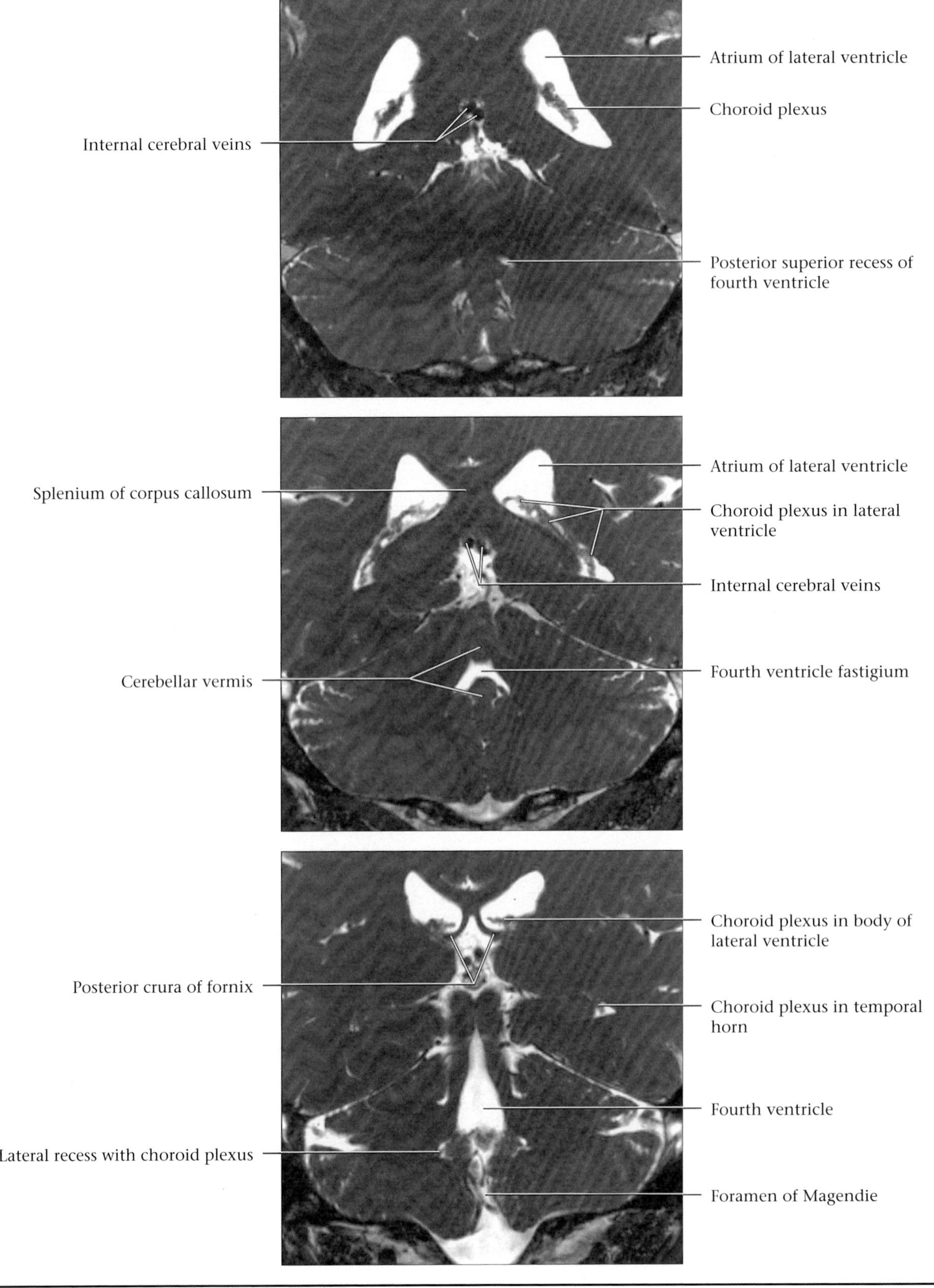

Atrium of lateral ventricle
Choroid plexus
Internal cerebral veins
Posterior superior recess of fourth ventricle
Atrium of lateral ventricle
Splenium of corpus callosum
Choroid plexus in lateral ventricle
Internal cerebral veins
Cerebellar vermis
Fourth ventricle fastigium
Choroid plexus in body of lateral ventricle
Posterior crura of fornix
Choroid plexus in temporal horn
Fourth ventricle
Lateral recess with choroid plexus
Foramen of Magendie

(Top) First of 12 sequential coronal T2 MR images from posterior to anterior, through the ventricles. Here normal choroid plexus is seen in the trigone (atria) of the lateral ventricles. The posterior superior recesses of the fourth ventricle are partly imaged here. **(Middle)** Normal choroid plexus is seen in the lateral ventricular atria. **(Bottom)** The fornices, seen here, are thin white matter tracts with complex communications with the hippocampus, thalamus, hypothalamus, septal nuclei and entorhinal cortex. Anatomically, the fornix separates posteriorly into two posterior crura along the inferior surface of the corpus callosum as seen here, then unites in the mid portion (body) and separates again anteriorly into the anterior columns (pillars) that descend towards the mammillary bodies and form the anterior border of the foramen of Monro.

VENTRICLES AND CHOROID PLEXUS

CORONAL T2 MR

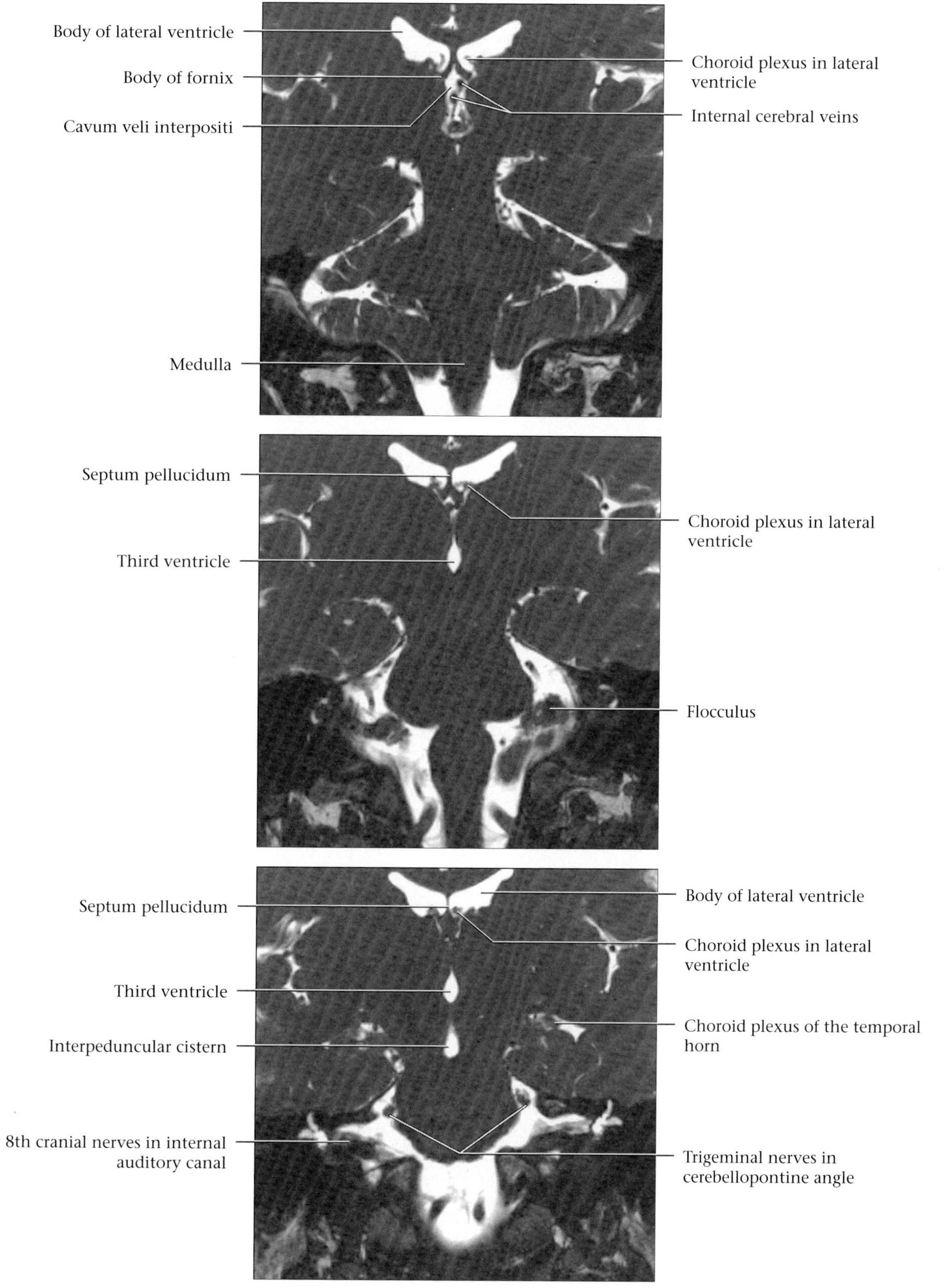
Body of lateral ventricle
Body of fornix
Cavum veli interpositi
Choroid plexus in lateral ventricle
Internal cerebral veins
Medulla
Septum pellucidum
Third ventricle
Choroid plexus in lateral ventricle
Flocculus
Septum pellucidum
Third ventricle
Interpeduncular cistern
7th & 8th cranial nerves in internal auditory canal
Body of lateral ventricle
Choroid plexus in lateral ventricle
Choroid plexus of the temporal horn
Trigeminal nerves in cerebellopontine angle

(Top) Choroid plexus is seen here within the lateral ventricles. The internal cerebral veins traverse normally within the cistern of the velum interpositum, located superior to the pineal gland. **(Middle)** The lateral ventricles are separated in the midline by a thin membrane(s), the septum pellucidum. Choroid plexus is normally present in the lateral ventricle body, as again is appreciated here. The caudate nuclei are located along the lateral margins of the lateral ventricles, and form an outwardly concave appearance. **(Bottom)** Choroid plexus is normally seen within the temporal horn and body of the lateral ventricle as appreciated here. Note also the interpeduncular cistern, which should not be confused with the third ventricle on coronal scans. The cisternal portions of the trigeminal nerves are well demonstrated within the prepontine cisterns.

VENTRICLES AND CHOROID PLEXUS

CORONAL T2 MR

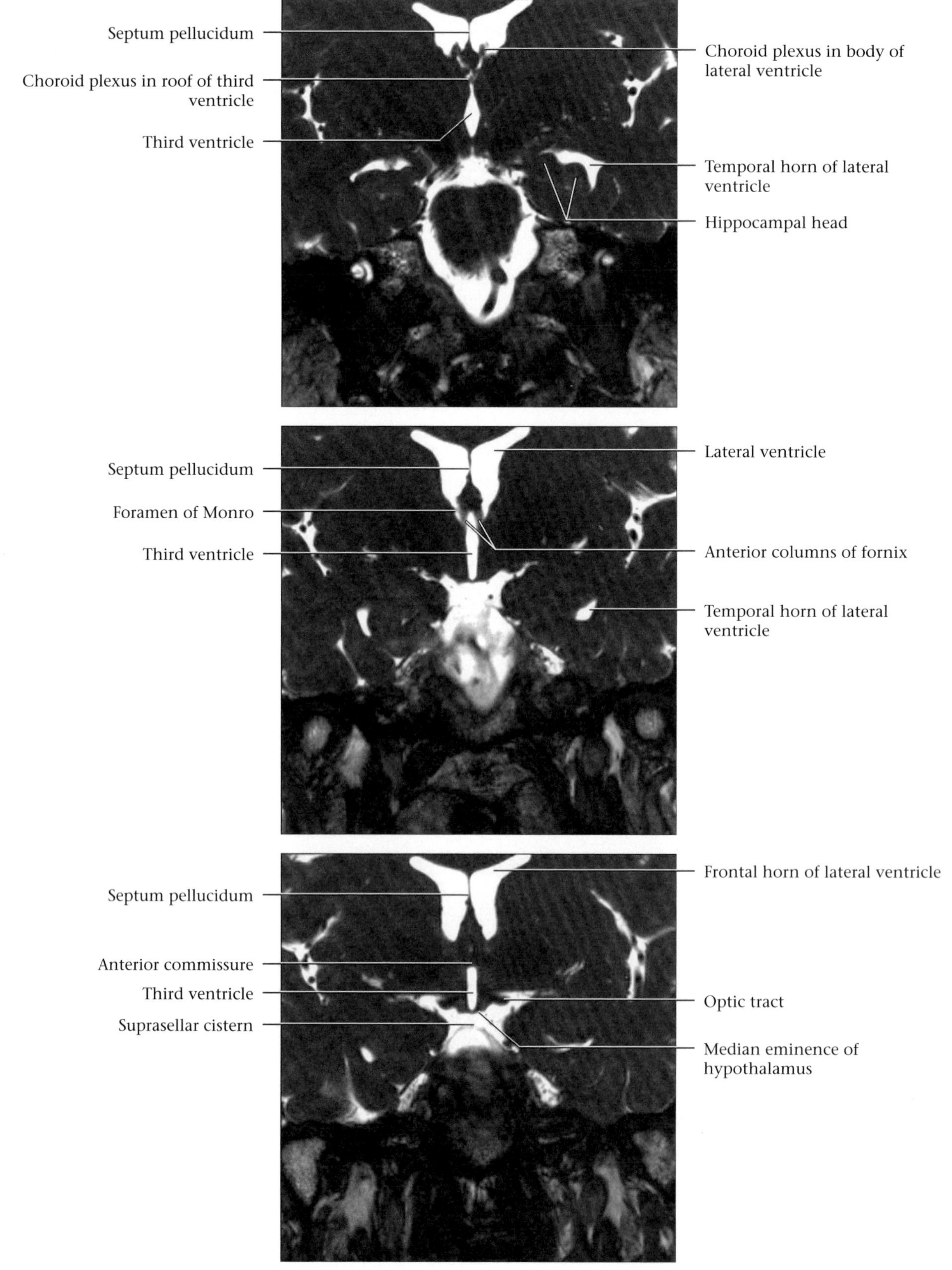
Septum pellucidum
Choroid plexus in roof of third ventricle
Third ventricle
Choroid plexus in body of lateral ventricle
Temporal horn of lateral ventricle
Hippocampal head
Septum pellucidum
Foramen of Monro
Third ventricle
Lateral ventricle
Anterior columns of fornix
Temporal horn of lateral ventricle
Septum pellucidum
Anterior commissure
Third ventricle
Suprasellar cistern
Frontal horn of lateral ventricle
Optic tract
Median eminence of hypothalamus

(Top) This image demonstrates normal choroid plexus in the roof of the third ventricle and body of the lateral ventricle. Note the normal undulations along the superior aspect of the hippocampal head which are in contact with the temporal horn. **(Middle)** The anterior temporal horns are well seen here. Note the normally narrow transverse dimension of the third ventricle; when this configuration widens, or is outwardly convex, concern for obstruction should be considered. Note also the fornix again divides into two anterior columns at this level, anterior to the foramina of Monro. **(Bottom)** Image through the anterior third ventricle through the level of the anterior commissure, which forms part of the anterior boundary of the third ventricle. The median eminence of the hypothalamus forms part of the anterior floor of third ventricle. The optic tracts are also well demonstrated.

VENTRICLES AND CHOROID PLEXUS

CORONAL T2 MR

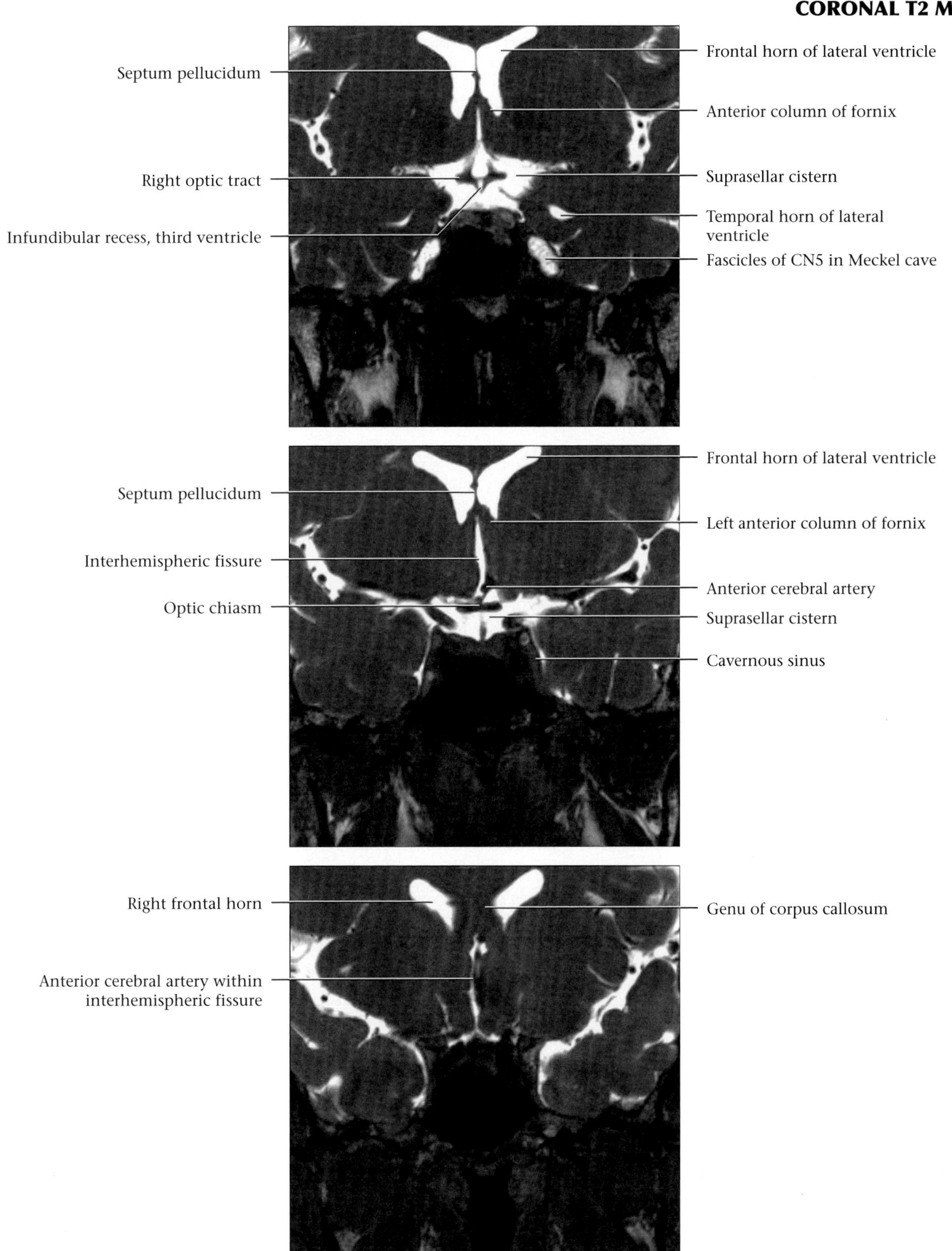
Septum pellucidum
Frontal horn of lateral ventricle
Anterior column of fornix
Right optic tract
Suprasellar cistern
Infundibular recess, third ventricle
Temporal horn of lateral ventricle
Fascicles of CN5 in Meckel cave
Frontal horn of lateral ventricle
Septum pellucidum
Left anterior column of fornix
Interhemispheric fissure
Anterior cerebral artery
Optic chiasm
Suprasellar cistern
Cavernous sinus
Right frontal horn
Genu of corpus callosum
Anterior cerebral artery within interhemispheric fissure

(Top) Image through the frontal horns of the lateral ventricles. The suprasellar cistern has the appearance of a five pointed star at this level. **(Middle)** Image through the optic chiasm and frontal horns of lateral ventricles is shown here. The thin linear fluid collection inferior to the frontal horns is the interhemispheric fissure, not the third ventricle. Note the presence of the anterior cerebral arteries inferiorly within the interhemispheric fissure. This part of the interhemispheric fissure is sometimes called the "cistern of the lamina terminalis." **(Bottom)** The frontal horns of the lateral ventricles normally show concave lateral margins. Note slice is anterior to the septum pellucidum; the midline white matter tract is the genu of the corpus callosum. Choroid plexus is not present in the frontal horns.

VENTRICLES AND CHOROID PLEXUS

SAGITTAL T2 MR

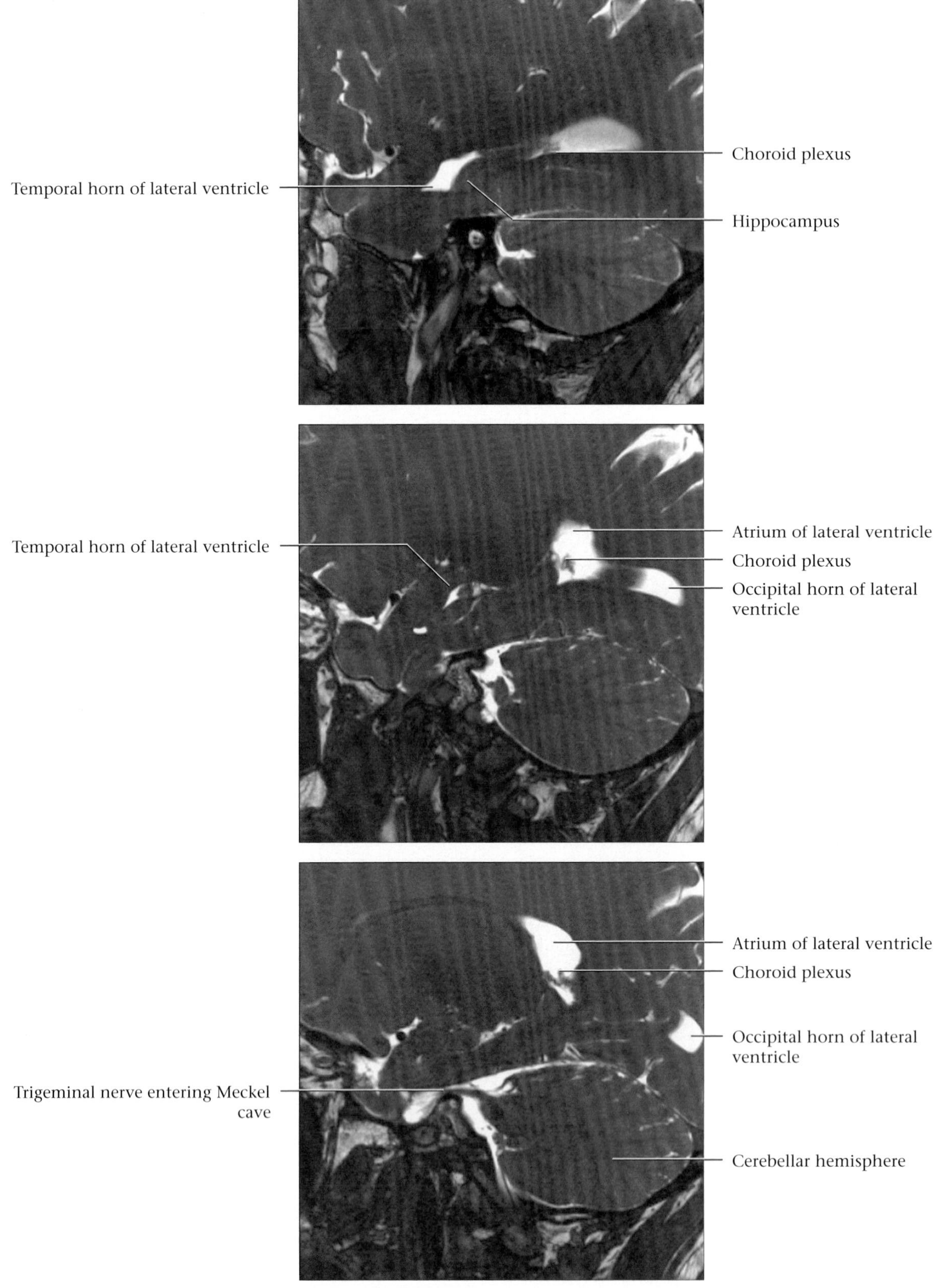

Choroid plexus
Temporal horn of lateral ventricle
Hippocampus
Temporal horn of lateral ventricle
Atrium of lateral ventricle
Choroid plexus
Occipital horn of lateral ventricle
Atrium of lateral ventricle
Choroid plexus
Occipital horn of lateral ventricle
Trigeminal nerve entering Meckel cave
Cerebellar hemisphere

(Top) First of 6 sagittal T2 MR images from lateral to medial, through the temporal horn and atrium of the lateral ventricle demonstrating normal choroid plexus within the atrium. Note also normal appearing hippocampus along the inferior margin of the temporal horn. **(Middle)** Image showing normal choroid plexus within the atrium (collateral trigone) of the lateral ventricle. Choroid plexus is not normally located within the occipital horns of the lateral ventricle. **(Bottom)** This image demonstrates normal choroid plexus within the atrium (collateral trigone) of the lateral ventricle. Note the normal cisternal portion the trigeminal nerve as it passes anteriorly over the petrous ridge to enter Meckel cave.

VENTRICLES AND CHOROID PLEXUS

SAGITTAL T2 MR

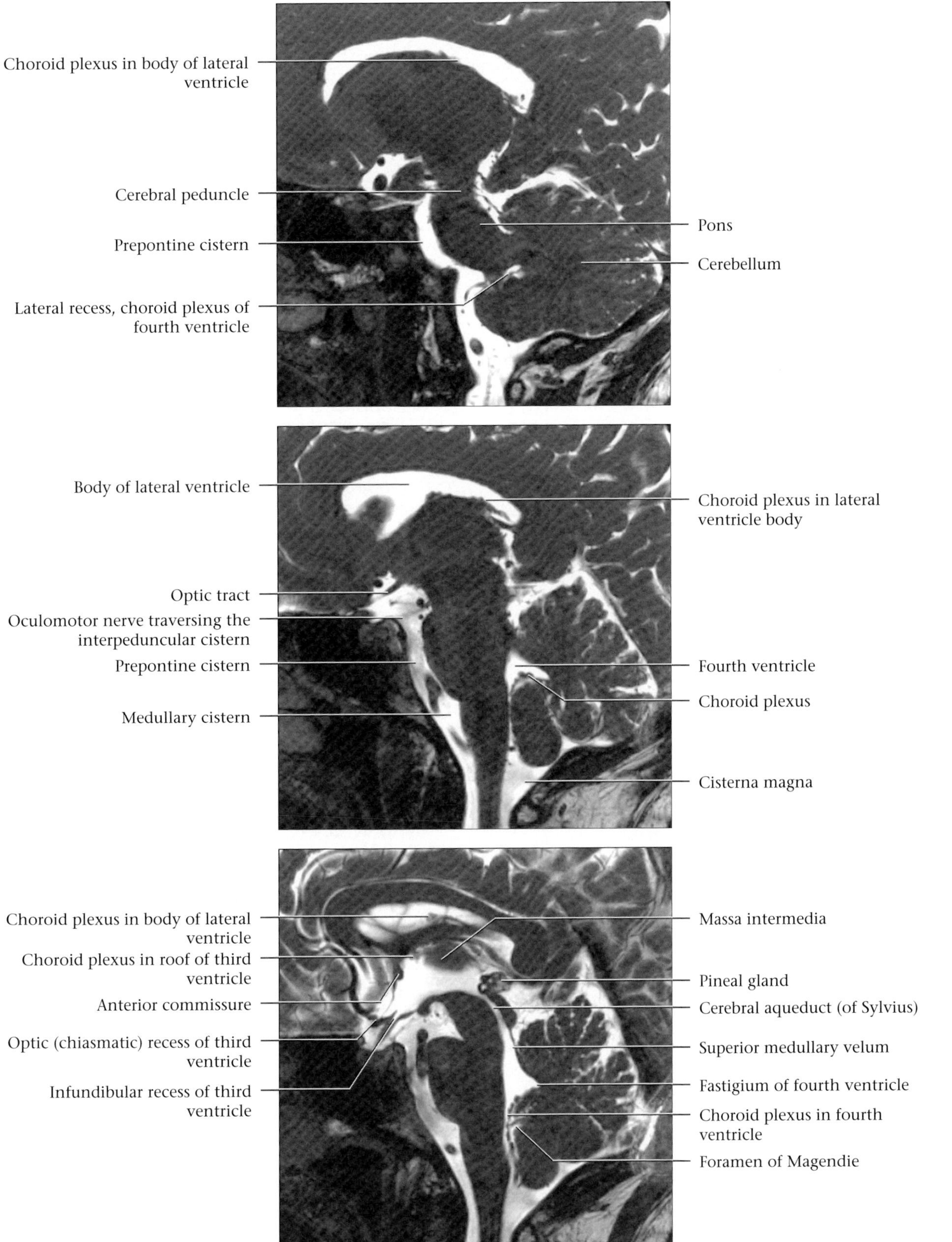
Choroid plexus in body of lateral ventricle
Cerebral peduncle
Prepontine cistern
Lateral recess, choroid plexus of fourth ventricle
Pons
Cerebellum
Body of lateral ventricle
Optic tract
Oculomotor nerve traversing the interpeduncular cistern
Prepontine cistern
Medullary cistern
Choroid plexus in lateral ventricle body
Fourth ventricle
Choroid plexus
Cisterna magna
Choroid plexus in body of lateral ventricle
Choroid plexus in roof of third ventricle
Anterior commissure
Optic (chiasmatic) recess of third ventricle
Infundibular recess of third ventricle
Massa intermedia
Pineal gland
Cerebral aqueduct (of Sylvius)
Superior medullary velum
Fastigium of fourth ventricle
Choroid plexus in fourth ventricle
Foramen of Magendie

(Top) Image at the level of the cerebral peduncle demonstrates choroid plexus within the body of the lateral ventricle. The lateral wing of the fourth ventricle is seen here. **(Middle)** Choroid plexus is seen within the body of the lateral ventricle and inferior roof of fourth ventricle. Note also the oculomotor nerve traversing the interpeduncular cistern. **(Bottom)** This image demonstrates normal choroid plexus in the roof of third ventricle, body of lateral ventricle, and posterior roof of fourth ventricle. The posterior choroidal artery is seen passing forward into the third ventricle. The superior medullary velum and pons, which form part of the fourth ventricle boundaries, are well seen here. The anteriorly located optic and infundibular recesses of the third ventricle are also well demonstrated. The lamina terminalis forms the anterior border of third ventricle.

SUBARACHNOID SPACES/CISTERNS

Terminology

Abbreviations

- SASs: Subarachnoid spaces

Definitions

- SASs: Cerebrospinal fluid-filled spaces between pia, arachnoid; expand at base of brain, around brainstem, tentorial incisura
- Liliequist membrane: Thin arachnoid membrane separates suprasellar, interpeduncular & prepontine cisterns
- Velum interpositum: Double layer of pia (tela choroidea), the result of folding of brain where hemispheres overgrow diencephalon, forms velum interpositum which may remain open & communicate posteriorly with quadrigeminal cistern (cavum veli interpositi)
- Choroidal fissure: Narrow, pial-lined channel between SAS & ventricles; site of attachment of choroid plexus in lateral ventricles

Gross Anatomy

Overview

- Numerous trabeculae, septae, membranes cross SAS → create smaller compartments termed cisterns
  - **Liliequist membrane** separates suprasellar, interpeduncular & prepontine cisterns
  - Anterior/lateral pontine, medial/lateral pontomedullary membranes separate posterior fossa cisterns
- All cranial nerves, major arteries/veins traverse cisterns
- All structures within cisterns invested with thin pial-like layer of cells
- All SAS cisterns communicate with each other and with ventricular system (through foramina of Magendie and Luschka)
- Cisterns provide natural pathways for disease spread as well as surgical approaches
- SAS cisterns divided into supra- and peritentorial, infratentorial groups
- Sulci separate gyri, fissures separate hemispheres/lobes

Imaging Anatomy

Overview

- **Supratentorial/peritentorial cisterns**
  - **Suprasellar cistern**: Superior to pituitary gland
  - **Interpeduncular cistern**: Between cerebral peduncles, Liliequist membrane
  - **Ambient (perimesencephalic) cisterns**: Wrap around midbrain, connect suprasellar, quadrigeminal cisterns
  - **Quadrigeminal cistern**: Under corpus callosum splenium, behind pineal gland, tectum; continuous anteriorly with velum interpositum
  - **Cistern of velum interpositum**: Formed by double layers of tela choroidea (pia), lies above third ventricle; communicates posteriorly with quadrigeminal cistern
- **Infratentorial (posterior fossa) cisterns**
  - Midline (unpaired)
    - **Prepontine cistern**: Between upper clivus, anterior pons
    - **Premedullary cistern**: From pontomedullary junction above to foramen magnum below; between lower clivus and medulla
    - **Superior cerebellar cistern**: Between upper vermis, straight sinus
    - **Cisterna magna**: Between medulla (anterior) and occiput (posterior), below/behind inferior vermis
  - **Lateral** (paired)
    - **Cerebellopontine cistern**: Between anterolateral pons/cerebellum, petrous temporal bone
    - **Cerebellomedullary cistern** (sometimes included as lower cerebellopontine cistern): From dorsal margin of inferior olive laterally around medulla
- **Fissures**
  - **Interhemispheric fissure**: Longitudinal cerebral fissure separates hemispheres
    - Inferior part contains cistern of the lamina terminalis; upper part contains pericallosal cistern
  - **Sylvian (lateral) fissure**: Separates frontal, temporal lobes anteriorly, courses laterally to cover insula

Internal Structures-Critical Contents

- **Supratentorial/peritentorial cisterns**
  - **Suprasellar cistern**: Infundibulum, optic chiasm, circle of Willis
  - **Interpeduncular cistern**: Oculomotor nerves (CN3), basilar artery (BA) bifurcation, posterior thalamoperforating arteries
  - **Ambient cisterns**: Trochlear nerves (CN4), P2 posterior cerebral artery (PCA) segments and branches, superior cerebellar arteries (SCAs), basal veins of Rosenthal
  - **Quadrigeminal cistern**: Pineal gland, trochlear nerves (CN4), P3 PCA segments, medial & lateral posterior choroidal arteries, vein of Galen (VofG) + tributaries
  - **Cistern of velum interpositum**: Internal cerebral veins (ICVs), MPChAs
- **Infratentorial cisterns**
  - **Prepontine cistern**: BA, anterior inferior cerebellar artery (AICA), CN5 and 6
  - **Premedullary cistern**: Vertebral arteries (VAs), anterior spinal artery, posterior inferior cerebellar artery (PICAs), CN12
  - **Superior cerebellar cistern**: SCA branches, superior vermian and precentral cerebellar veins
  - **Cisterna magna**: Cerebellar tonsils (often have dense trabecular attachments), tonsillohemispheric PICA branches
  - **Cerebellopontine cistern**: CN5, 7 & 8; AICA; petrosal vein
  - **Cerebellomedullary cistern**: CN9, 10 & 11
- **Fissures**
  - **Interhemispheric fissure**: Falx cerebri with inferior sagittal sinus, anterior cerebral artery (ACA) and branches
  - **Lateral fissure**: Middle cerebral artery (M1-3 segments) & vein

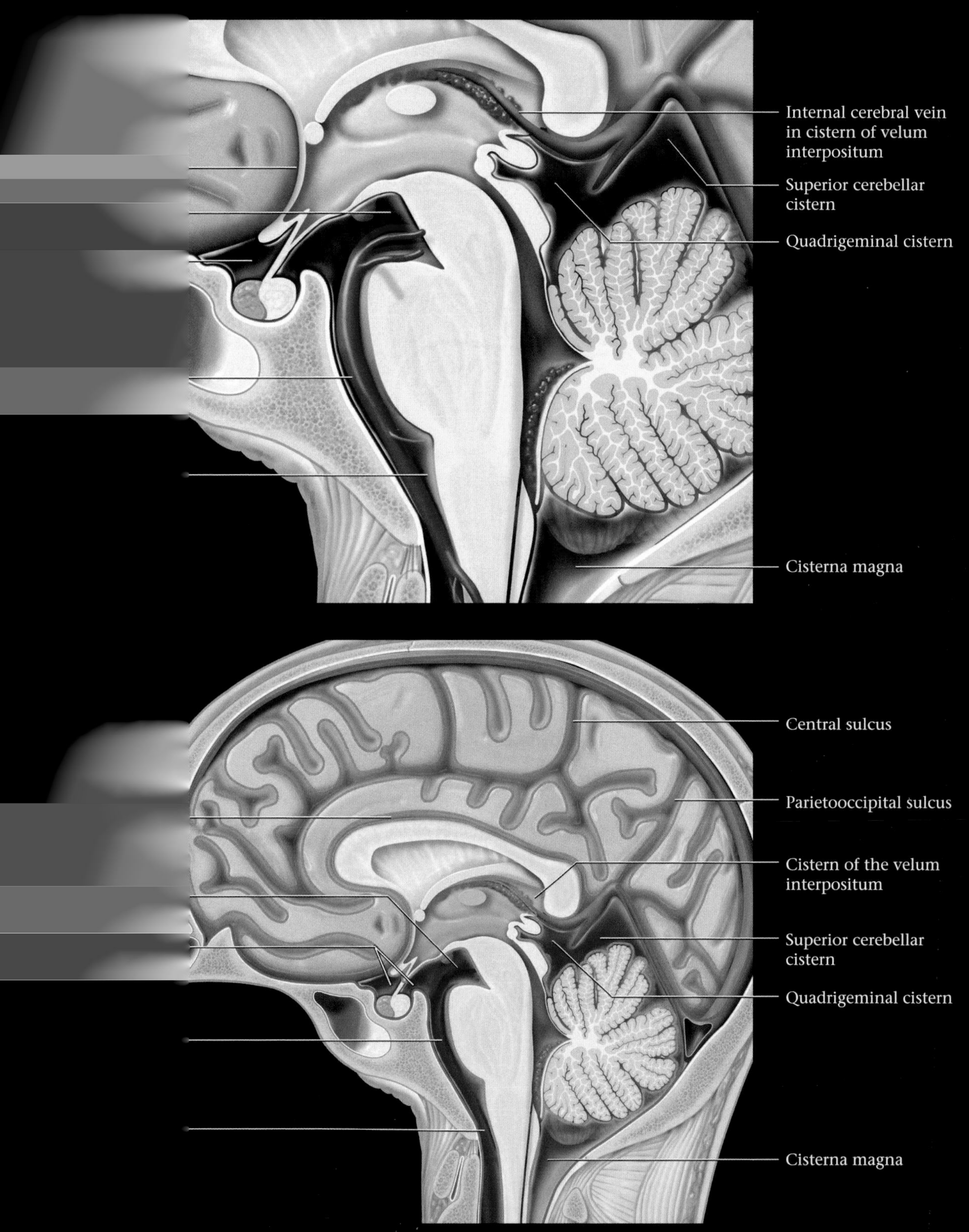
Internal cerebral vein in cistern of velum interpositum
Superior cerebellar cistern
Quadrigeminal cistern
Cisterna magna
Central sulcus
Parietooccipital sulcus
Cistern of the velum interpositum
Superior cerebellar cistern
Quadrigeminal cistern
Cisterna magna

phic demonstrates normal cisternal, regional anatomy. The anterior circulation (anterior communicating arteries) have been removed to illustrate some of the major structures in **ottom)** Sagittal midline graphic through interhemispheric fissure depicts SASs with CSF (purple) and pia (orange). The central sulcus separates frontal lobe (anterior) from parietal nater is closely applied to the brain surface whereas the arachnoid is adherent to the dura. ate with the cisterns and subarachnoid space via the foramina of Luschka and Magendie.

GRAPHICS

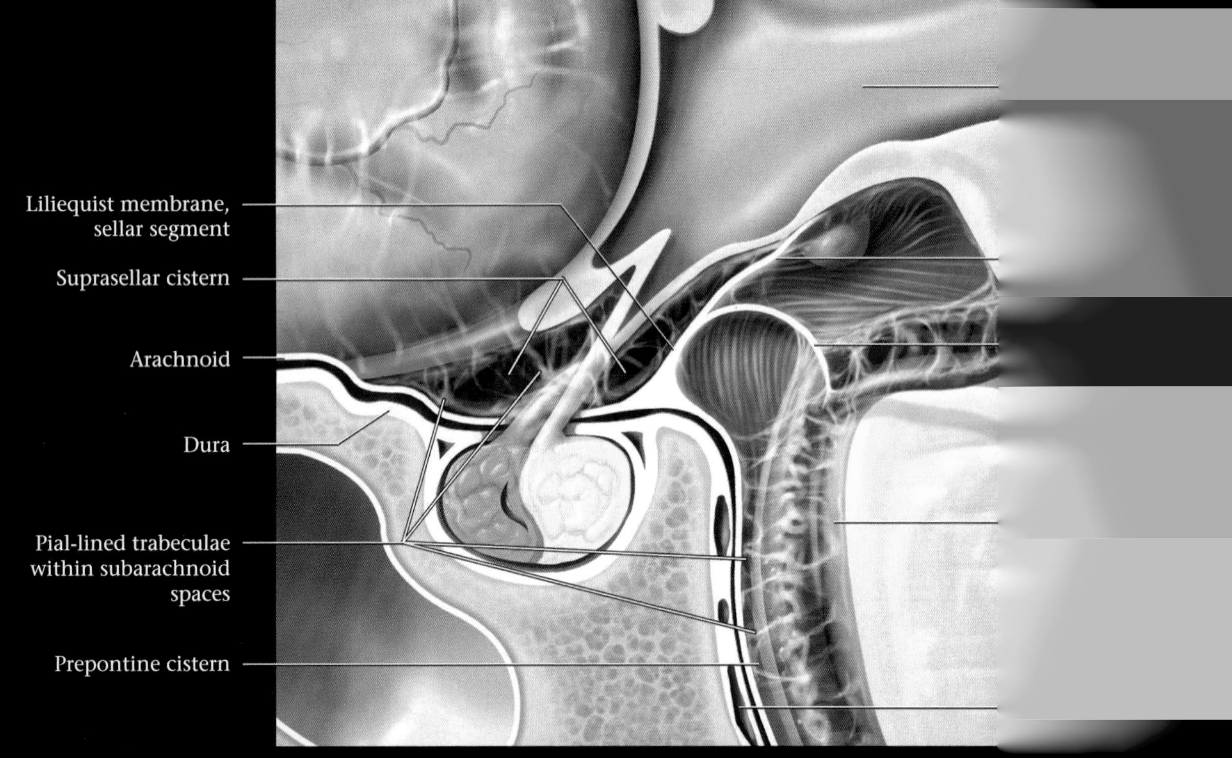
Liliequist membrane, sellar segment
Suprasellar cistern
Arachnoid
Dura
Pial-lined trabeculae within subarachnoid spaces
Prepontine cistern

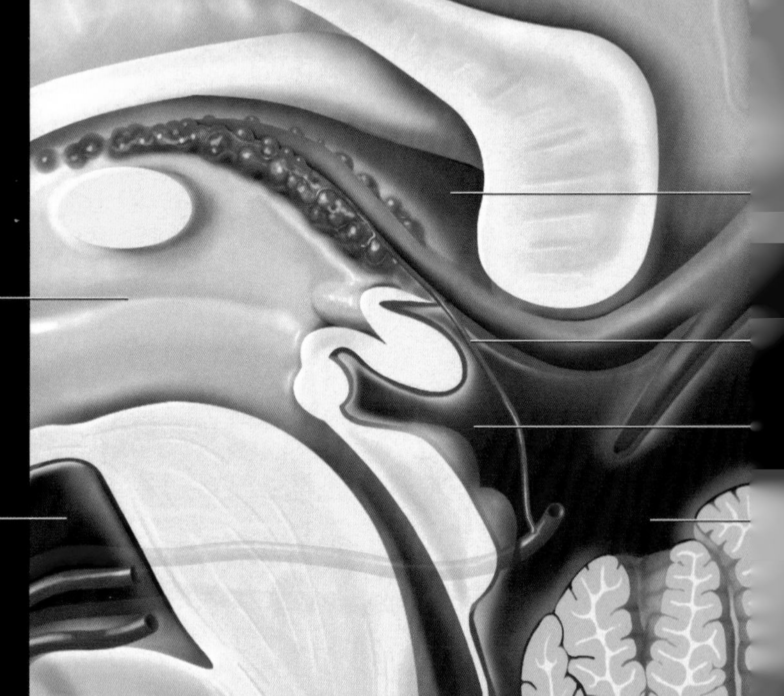
Third ventricle
Interpeduncular cistern

(Top) The membrane of Liliequist is a thin arachnoid membrane which can potentially obst suprasellar cistern; the sellar segment detailed here attaches inferiorly along the dorsum sell membrane divides into less constant segments: A superior diencephalic membrane (attaches and a posterior mesencephalic membrane. Numerous small pial-lined trabeculae are present subarachnoid space. **(Bottom)** Detail midline graphic of the pineal region demonstrates the interpositum which lies between double layers of the tela choroidea and contains the intern its inferolateral margins. The quadrigeminal cistern is posterior to the pineal gland; it comm the superior cerebellar cistern and anteriorly with the cistern of the velum interpositum.

SUBARACHNOID SPACES/CISTERNS

AXIAL T2 MR

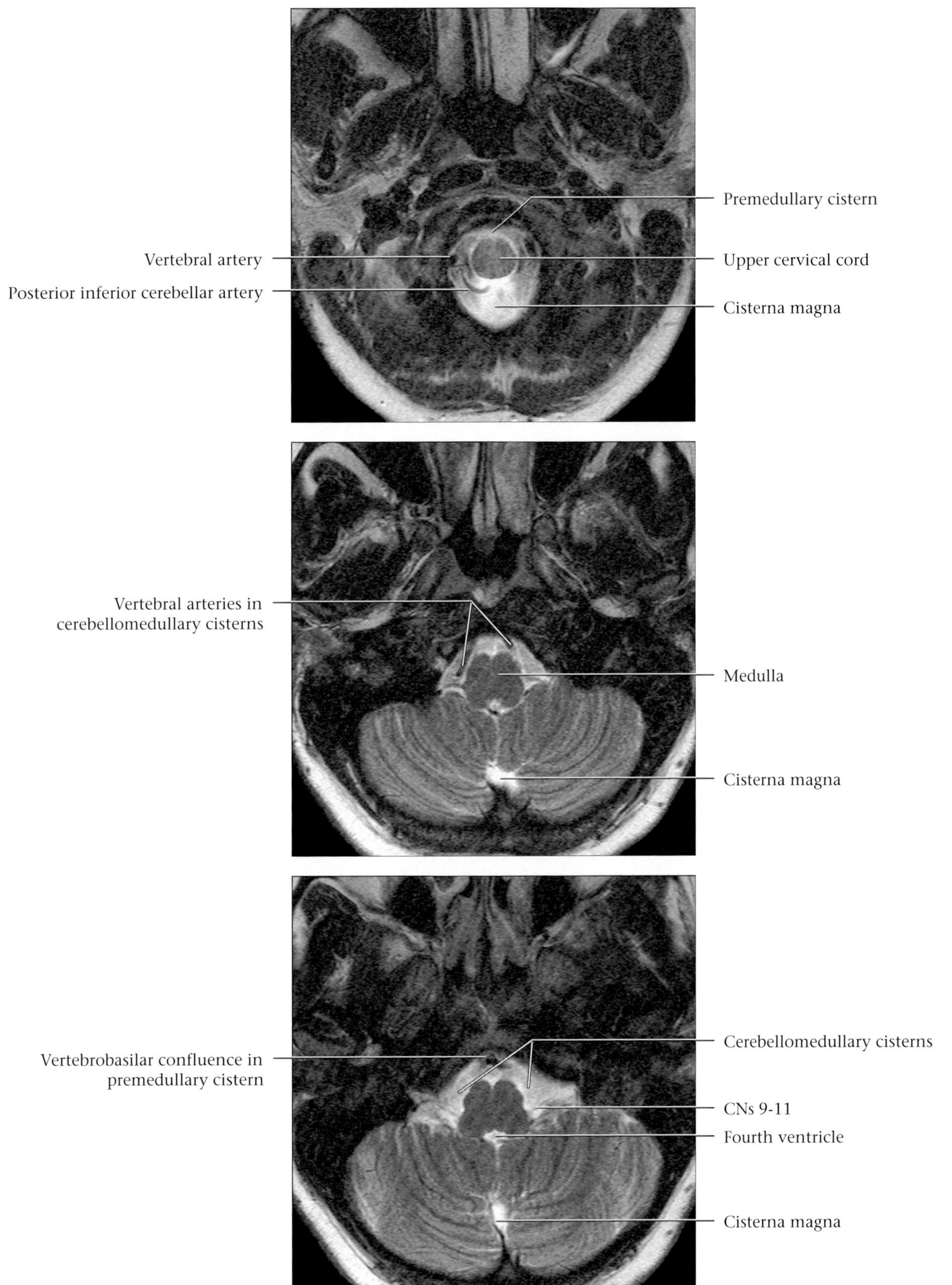
Premedullary cistern
Vertebral artery
Upper cervical cord
Posterior inferior cerebellar artery
Cisterna magna
Vertebral arteries in cerebellomedullary cisterns
Medulla
Cisterna magna
Cerebellomedullary cisterns
Vertebrobasilar confluence in premedullary cistern
CNs 9-11
Fourth ventricle
Cisterna magna

(Top) First of nine sequential axial T2 MR images presented from inferior to superior demonstrates the subarachnoid spaces and cisterns. The cisterna magna is located behind the upper cervical cord and lower medulla, and below the cerebellar hemispheres. It is continuous with the subarachnoid space of the spinal cord. The vertebral arteries and posterior inferior cerebellar arteries normally traverse the cisterna magna, as seen here. **(Middle)** The cisterna magna is seen here as a small CSF-filled space posterior to the cerebellum in the midline. The vertebral arteries travel within the medullary cisterns. **(Bottom)** The vertebral arteries are seen in the medullary cistern at their confluence with the basilar artery.

AXIAL T2 MR

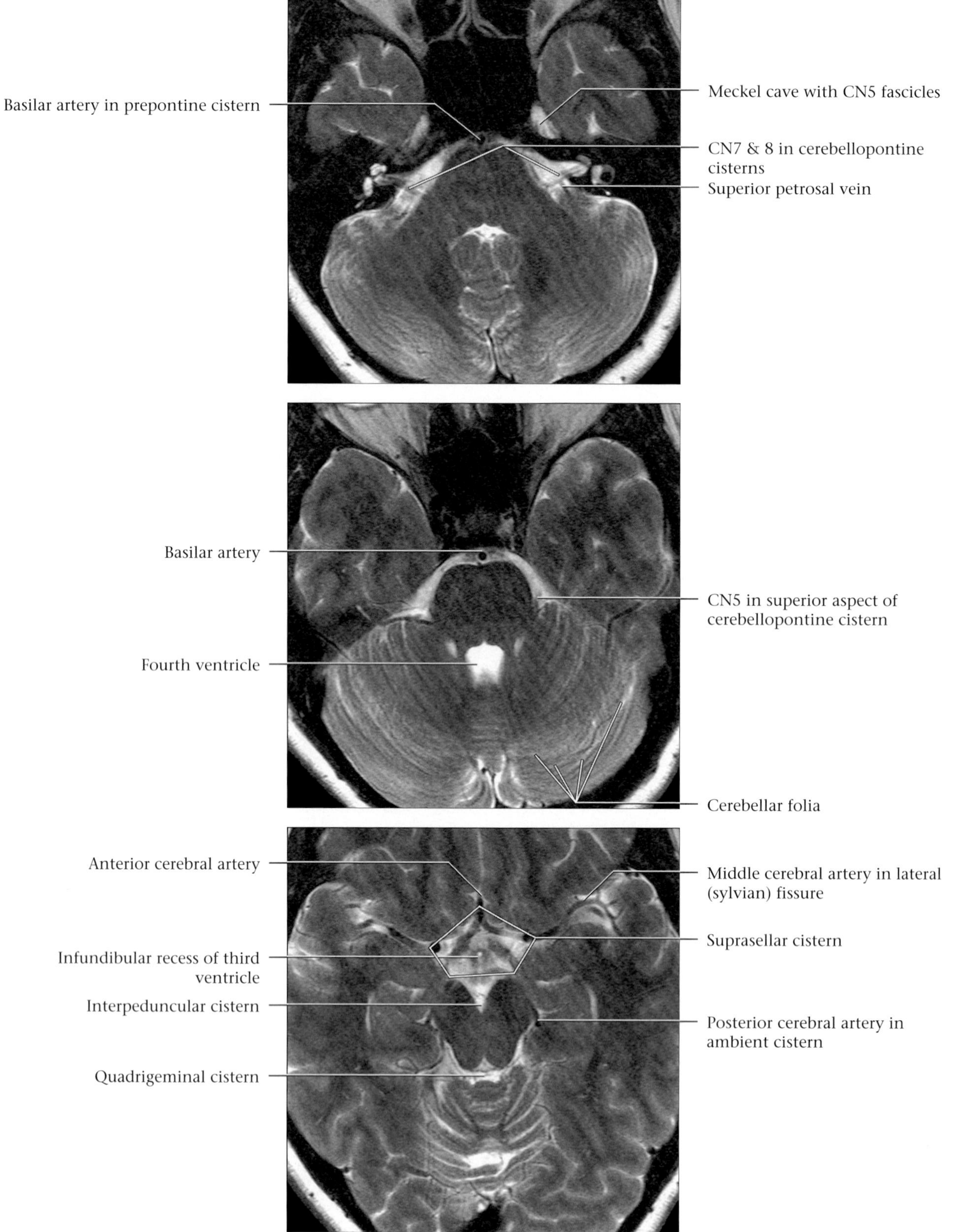

Basilar artery in prepontine cistern
Meckel cave with CN5 fascicles
CN7 & 8 in cerebellopontine cisterns
Superior petrosal vein
Basilar artery
CN5 in superior aspect of cerebellopontine cistern
Fourth ventricle
Cerebellar folia
Anterior cerebral artery
Middle cerebral artery in lateral (sylvian) fissure
Suprasellar cistern
Infundibular recess of third ventricle
Interpeduncular cistern
Posterior cerebral artery in ambient cistern
Quadrigeminal cistern

(Top) Cranial nerves 7 & 8 are demonstrated traversing the cerebellopontine cisterns. The anterior inferior cerebellar arteries and posterior inferior cerebellar arteries also course through this cistern. CSF in Meckel cave communicates freely with the prepontine and cerebellopontine angle cisterns. **(Middle)** The basilar artery is seen in the prepontine cistern. Cerebellar folia are seen here as the numerous curvilinear fluid-filled subarachnoid spaces over the cerebellum. **(Bottom)** The pituitary infundibulum lies in the center of the suprasellar cistern; the small fluid-filled structure centrally is the variably hollow portion of the infundibulum which is contiguous with the infundibular recess. The ambient cisterns surround the midbrain and connect the suprasellar and quadrigeminal cisterns.

SUBARACHNOID SPACES/CISTERNS

AXIAL T2 MR

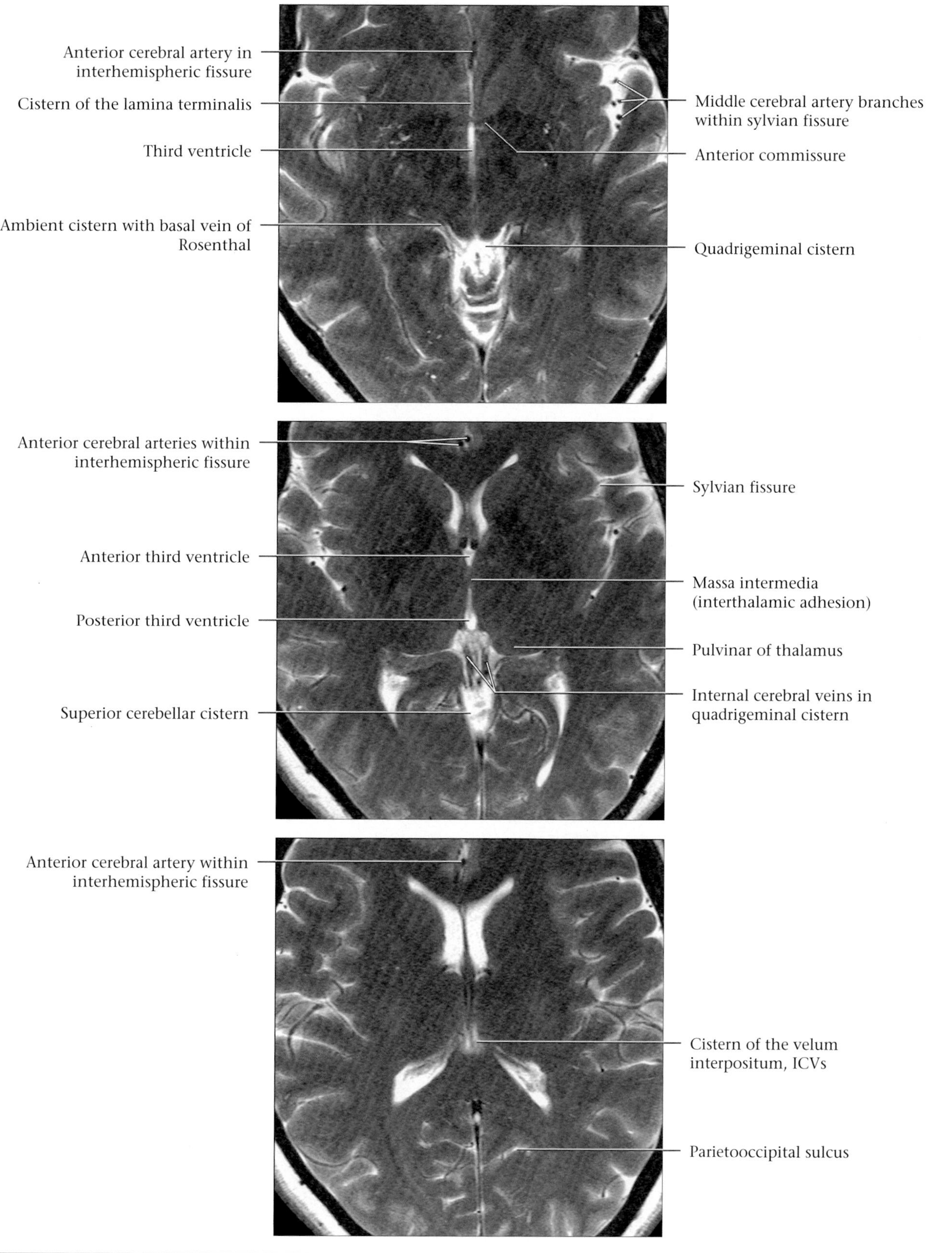

Anterior cerebral artery in interhemispheric fissure
Cistern of the lamina terminalis
Third ventricle
Ambient cistern with basal vein of Rosenthal
Middle cerebral artery branches within sylvian fissure
Anterior commissure
Quadrigeminal cistern
Anterior cerebral arteries within interhemispheric fissure
Anterior third ventricle
Posterior third ventricle
Superior cerebellar cistern
Sylvian fissure
Massa intermedia (interthalamic adhesion)
Pulvinar of thalamus
Internal cerebral veins in quadrigeminal cistern
Anterior cerebral artery within interhemispheric fissure
Cistern of the velum interpositum, ICVs
Parietooccipital sulcus

(Top) The quadrigeminal plate cistern is located between the cerebellar vermis and the colliculi. Middle cerebral artery branches are well demonstrated within the sylvian fissure. The anterior commissure is only partly visualized on this image, but demarcates the anterior aspect of the third ventricle. The interhemispheric fissure is visualized anteriorly. **(Middle)** The sylvian and interhemispheric fissures are demonstrated here. The retropulvinar cisterns are the lateral extensions of the ambient cisterns, located posterior to the thalami. The internal cerebral veins are located within the cistern of the velum interpositum. **(Bottom)** The parietooccipital sulci and interhemispheric sulci are demonstrated here. The superior aspect of the cistern of the velum interpositum is also visible.

CORONAL T2 MR

Third ventricle
Oculomotor nerve (CN3)
Interpeduncular cistern
Posterior cerebral artery (in ambient cistern)
Vertebral artery within premedullary cistern
Posterior perforated substance
Ambient cistern
Cerebellopontine angle cistern

Third ventricle
Cerebellopontine angle cistern
Oculomotor nerves traversing interpeduncular cistern
Vertebrobasilar junction at prepontine & medullary cistern junction

Right posterior cerebral artery
Oculomotor nerve (CN3)
Right superior cerebellar arteries
Interpeduncular cistern
Ambient cistern
Basilar artery within prepontine cistern

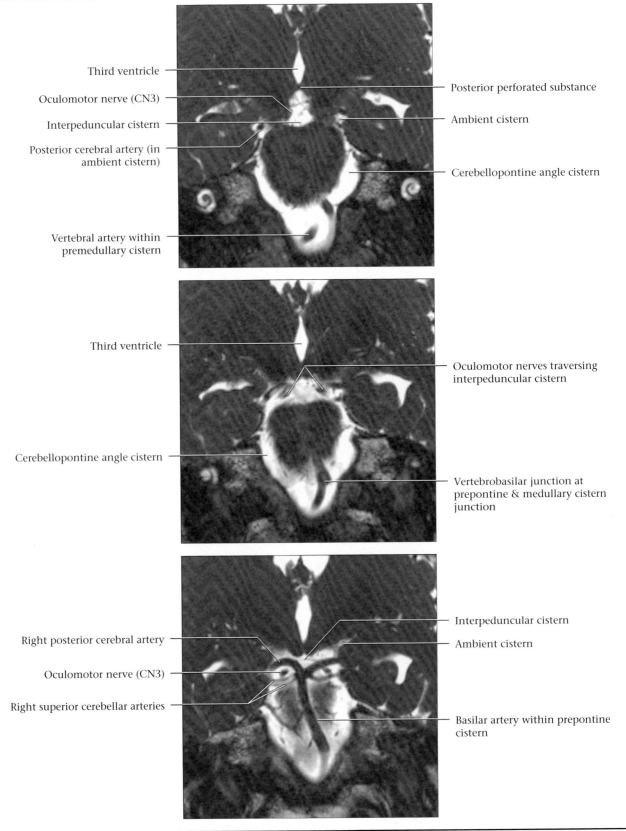

(Top) First of 12 coronal T2 MR images through the central cisterns presented from posterior to anterior demonstrates the posterior third ventricle, interpeduncular and cerebellopontine cisterns. The vertebral arteries run within the premedullary cisterns. **(Middle)** The oculomotor nerves traverse in the interpeduncular cistern. Note the vertebrobasilar junction, at the junction of the prepontine and medullary cisterns. **(Bottom)** The anterior vasculature within the prepontine cistern is well seen here: Top of basilar artery, which divides into the posterior cerebral arteries, and the superior cerebellar arteries. Duplication of the superior cerebellar artery, as seen here, is a common anatomical variant. Note the position of the oculomotor nerves which travel between the posterior cerebral and superior cerebellar arteries in the interpeduncular cistern.

CORONAL T2 MR

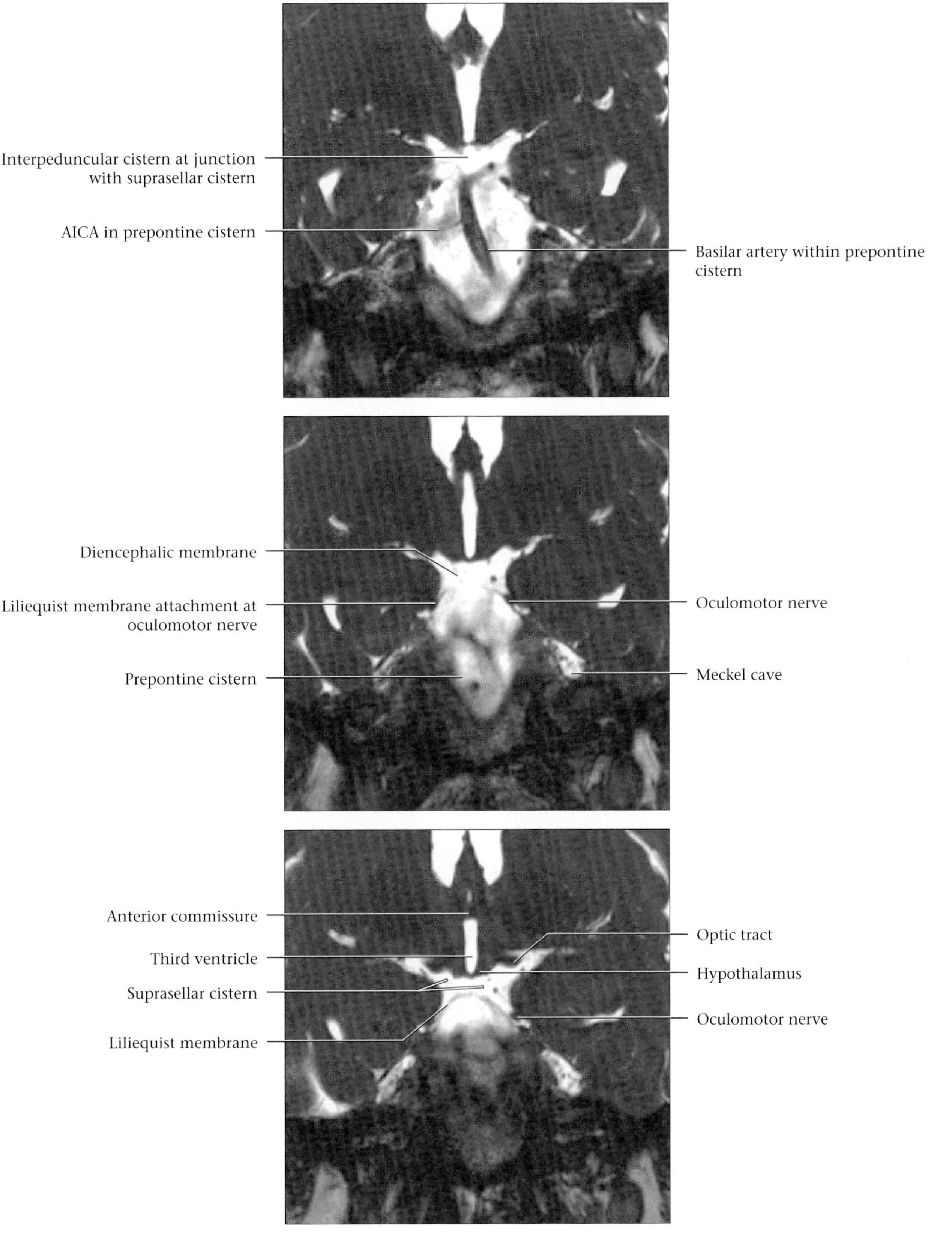
Interpeduncular cistern at junction with suprasellar cistern
AICA in prepontine cistern
Basilar artery within prepontine cistern
Diencephalic membrane
Liliequist membrane attachment at oculomotor nerve
Preponitine cistern
Oculomotor nerve
Meckel cave
Anterior commissure
Third ventricle
Suprasellar cistern
Liliequist membrane
Optic tract
Hypothalamus
Oculomotor nerve

(Top) Scan just anterior to basilar bifurcation shows confluence of suprasellar, interpeduncular, mesencephalic, prepontine cisterns. **(Middle)** The Liliequist membrane is seen at its lateral attachments to/around the oculomotor nerves. Suprasellar cistern is anterosuperior; interpeduncular is posterosuperior; prepontine is posteroinferior. **(Bottom)** The normal transverse appearance of the Liliequist membrane is appreciated here; it is normally about half the width of the third ventricular floor. Laterally, the Liliequist membrane attaches to the oculomotor nerves or the arachnoid membranes around them. The interpeduncular and suprasellar cisterns are thus separated anatomically when this membrane is completely intact. Note also how the hypothalamus forms part of the anterior floor of the third ventricle. Note also the midline crossing fibers of the anterior commissure.

CORONAL T2 MR

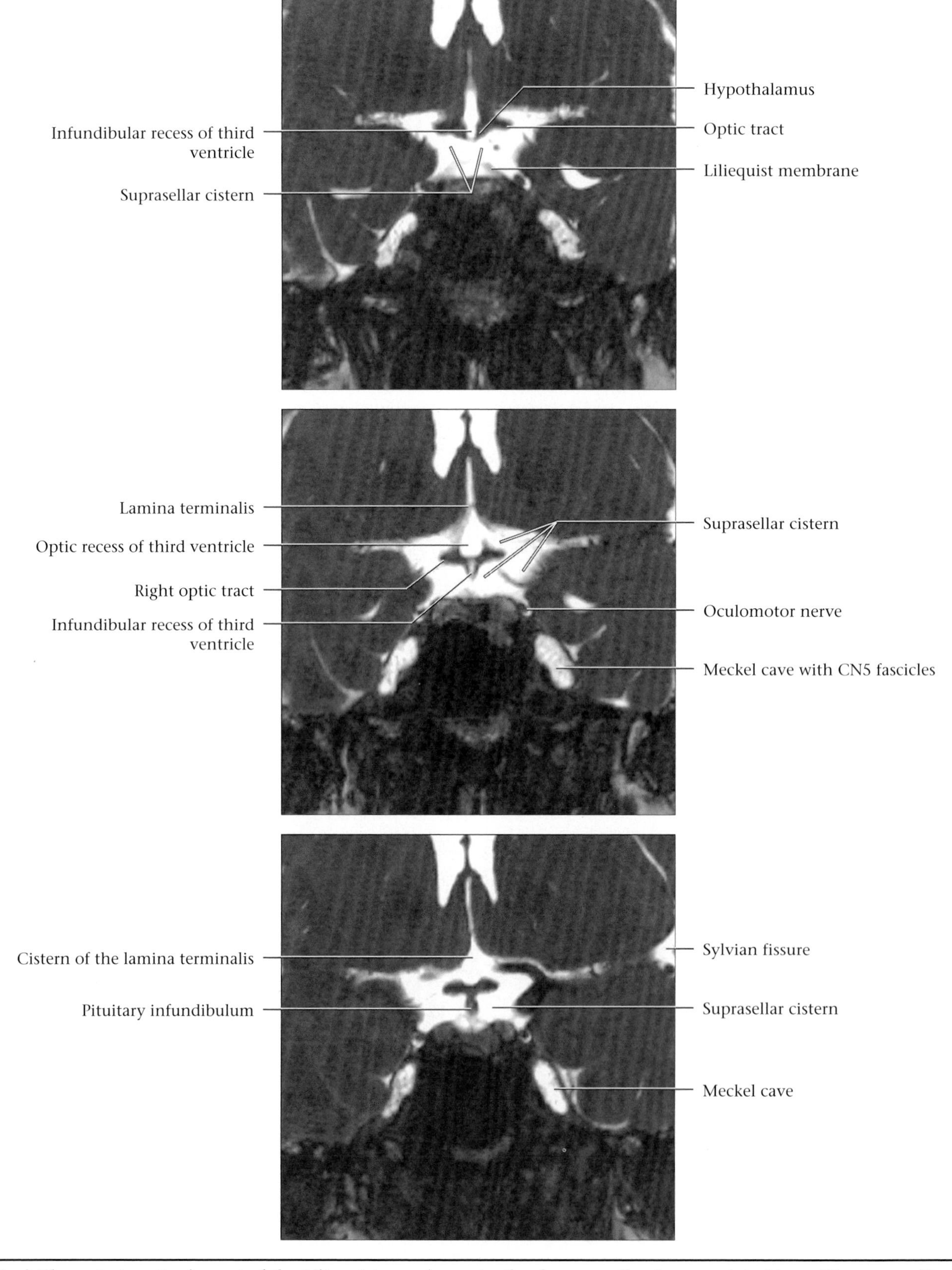

Hypothalamus
Infundibular recess of third ventricle
Optic tract
Liliequist membrane
Suprasellar cistern
Lamina terminalis
Suprasellar cistern
Optic recess of third ventricle
Right optic tract
Oculomotor nerve
Infundibular recess of third ventricle
Meckel cave with CN5 fascicles
Sylvian fissure
Cistern of the lamina terminalis
Pituitary infundibulum
Suprasellar cistern
Meckel cave

(Top) The anterior attachment of the Liliequist membrane to the dorsum sellae is appreciated here. The suprasellar cistern is seen above and surrounding the pituitary infundibulum. **(Middle)** The anterior recesses of the third ventricle are seen here in the midline: Optic and infundibular recesses. The lamina terminalis, which forms part of the third ventricle, is seen here. A small CSF-filled extension of the suprasellar and interpeduncular cisterns surrounds the third cranial (oculomotor) nerve. CSF in Meckel cave contains fascicles of the trigeminal nerve (CN5) and communicates freely with the prepontine cistern. **(Bottom)** The suprasellar cistern is visualized here, above the pituitary gland, surrounding the pituitary infundibulum and optic chiasm.

CORONAL T2 MR

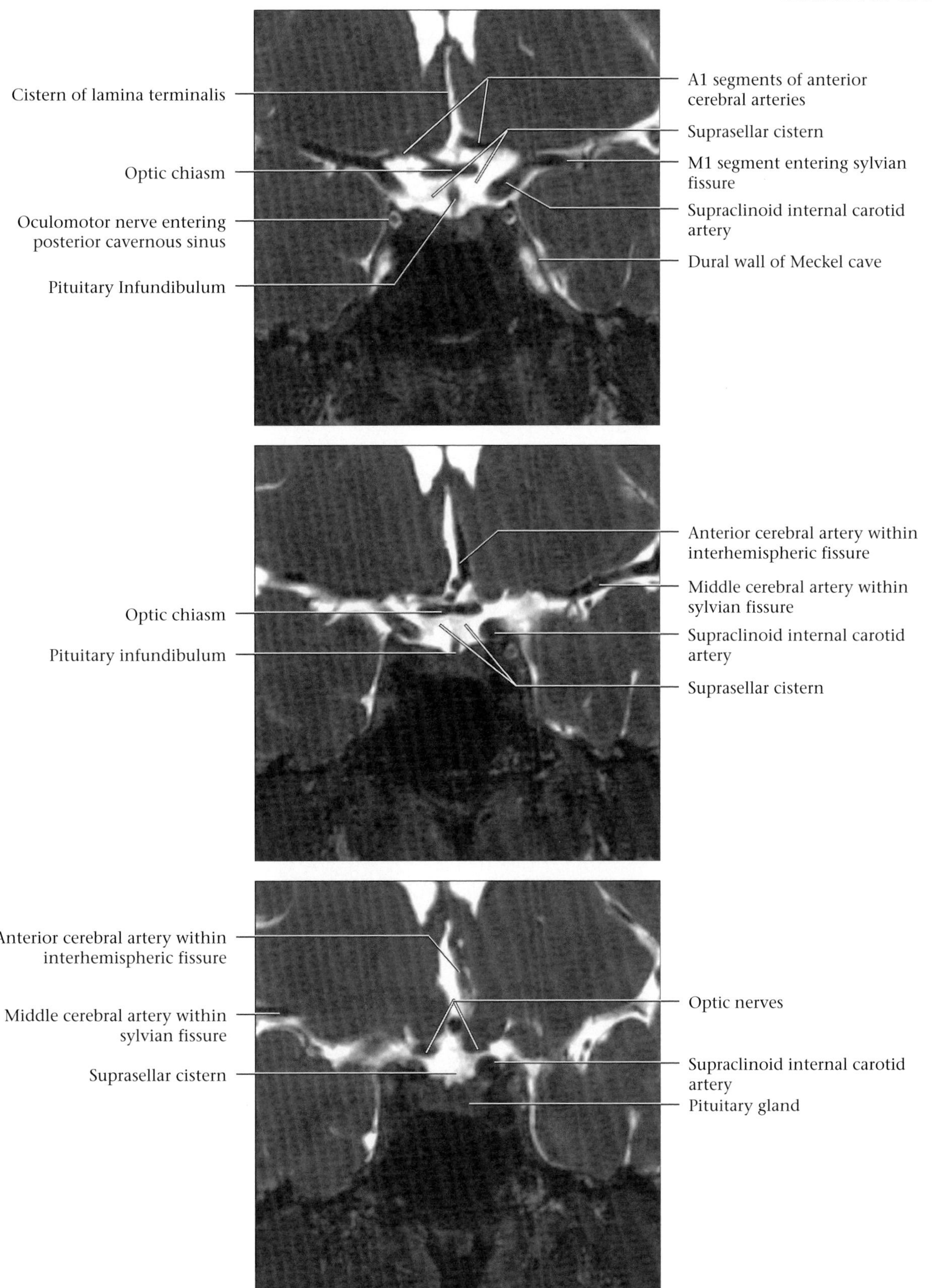

Cistern of lamina terminalis
A1 segments of anterior cerebral arteries
Suprasellar cistern
Optic chiasm
M1 segment entering sylvian fissure
Oculomotor nerve entering posterior cavernous sinus
Supraclinoid internal carotid artery
Dural wall of Meckel cave
Pituitary Infundibulum
Anterior cerebral artery within interhemispheric fissure
Middle cerebral artery within sylvian fissure
Optic chiasm
Supraclinoid internal carotid artery
Pituitary infundibulum
Suprasellar cistern
Anterior cerebral artery within interhemispheric fissure
Optic nerves
Middle cerebral artery within sylvian fissure
Suprasellar cistern
Supraclinoid internal carotid artery
Pituitary gland

(Top) The anterior circle of Willis vasculature is well seen in the suprasellar cistern at this level with A1 and M1 segments arising from the supraclinoid internal carotid arteries. The proximal M1 segments are seen entering the sylvian fissures. **(Middle)** The pituitary infundibulum is seen at the anterior inferior insertion into the pituitary gland. The optic chiasm is seen in the suprasellar cistern. The anterior cerebral arteries are identified within the anterior interhemispheric fissure, and the proximal middle cerebral arteries within the sylvian fissures. **(Bottom)** The optic nerves are seen separately in the anterior aspect of the suprasellar cistern. The anterior curvature of the anterior cerebral arteries is visualized in the interhemispheric fissure, and middle cerebral artery within the sylvian fissure.

SUBARACHNOID SPACES/CISTERNS

SAGITTAL T2 MR

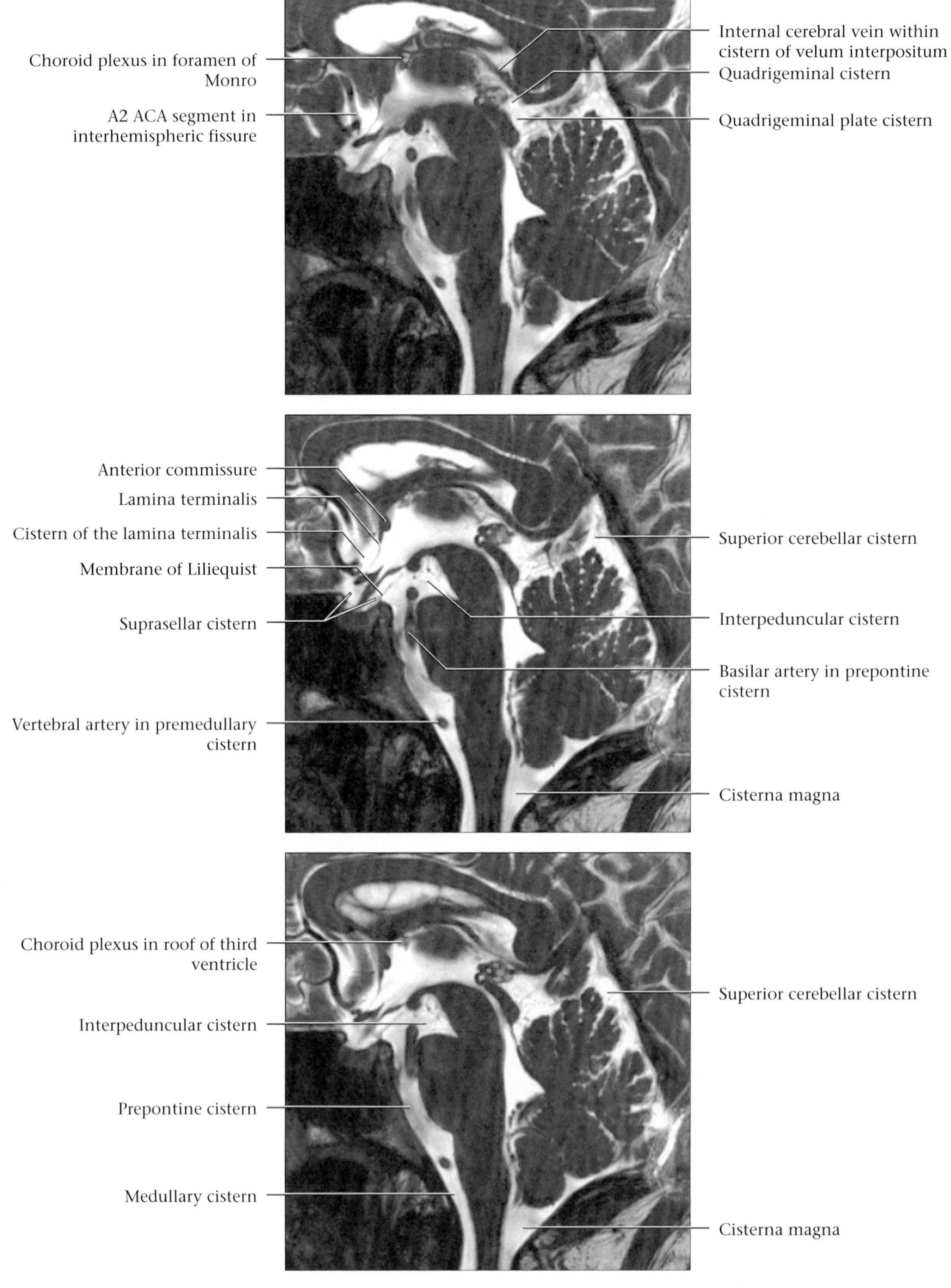
Choroid plexus in foramen of Monro
A2 ACA segment in interhemispheric fissure
Internal cerebral vein within cistern of velum interpositum
Quadrigeminal cistern
Quadrigeminal plate cistern
Anterior commissure
Lamina terminalis
Cistern of the lamina terminalis
Membrane of Liliequist
Suprasellar cistern
Vertebral artery in premedullary cistern
Superior cerebellar cistern
Interpeduncular cistern
Basilar artery in prepontine cistern
Cisterna magna
Choroid plexus in roof of third ventricle
Interpeduncular cistern
Prepontine cistern
Medullary cistern
Superior cerebellar cistern
Cisterna magna

(Top) First of 6 sequential sagittal T2 MR images shown from left to right demonstrates the internal cerebral veins traversing the cistern of the velum interpositum. The quadrigeminal cistern is posterior to the pineal gland and the collicular plate. **(Middle)** This image demonstrates the membrane of Liliequist, a delicate arachnoid membrane between the dorsum sella and mamillary bodies, separating the prepontine, interpeduncular & suprasellar cisterns. Note how the thin lamina terminalis and the anterior commissure form part of the anterior third ventricular margin The cistern of the lamina terminalis is seen anterior to the lamina terminalis. **(Bottom)** Cisterns anterior to the brainstem, and the superior cerebellar cistern are well demonstrated here. Note course of the basilar artery, which travels in the prepontine cistern.

SAGITTAL T2 MR

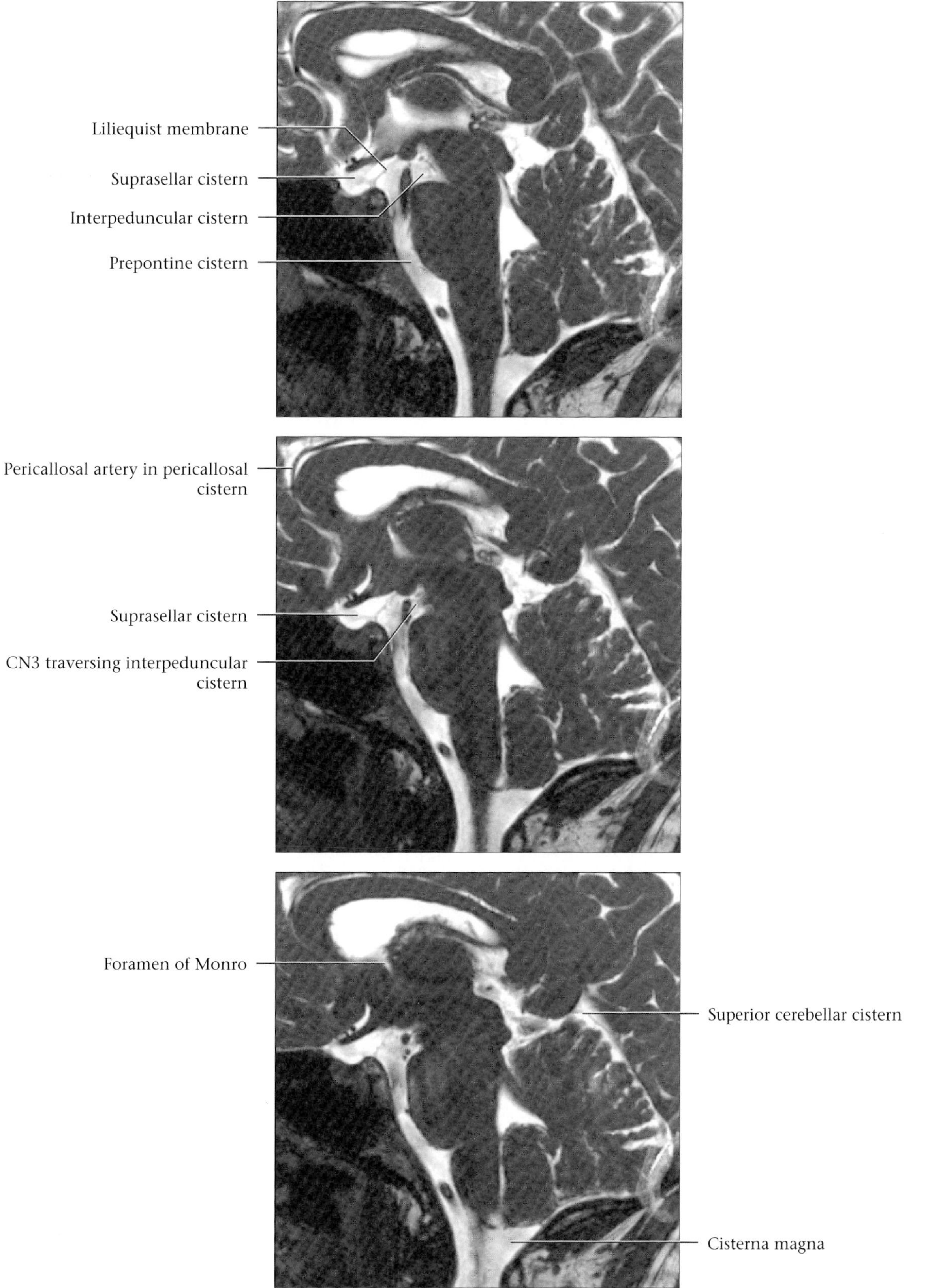
Liliequist membrane
Suprasellar cistern
Interpeduncular cistern
Prepontine cistern
Pericallosal artery in pericallosal cistern
Suprasellar cistern
CN3 traversing interpeduncular cistern
Foramen of Monro
Superior cerebellar cistern
Cisterna magna

(Top) The Liliequist membrane is again seen attaching posterosuperiorly to the mammillary bodies and anteroinferiorly to the dorsum sella. This small arachnoid membrane may also require perforation when third ventriculostomies are performed to relieve obstruction when anatomically complete. **(Middle)** The pericallosal artery, an A2 branch of the anterior cerebral artery, is seen in the pericallosal cistern above the corpus callosum. The oculomotor nerve is seen as it emerges from the midbrain in the interpeduncular cistern. **(Bottom)** The superior cerebellar cistern lies above the vermis and cerebellar hemispheres and connects to the ambient and quadrigeminal cisterns. The right stem of the foramen of Monro is seen here. The cisterna magna is dorsal to the cervicomedullary junction.

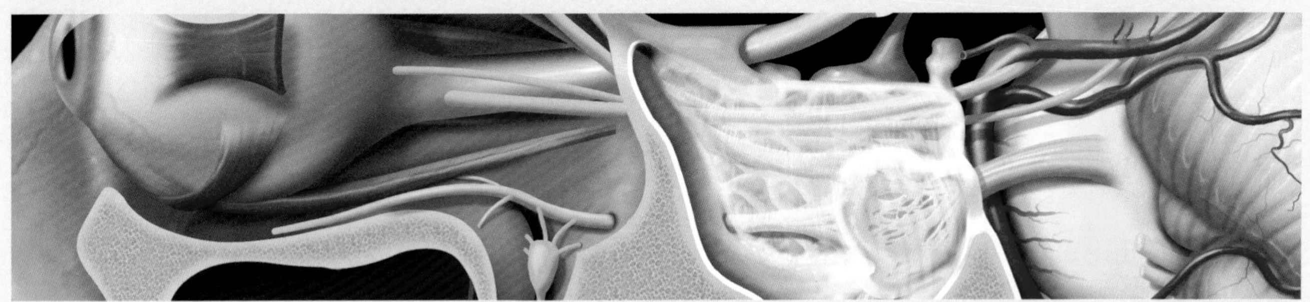

SECTION 5: Cranial Nerves

CRANIAL NERVES OVERVIEW

Terminology

Abbreviations

- Olfactory nerve: CN1
- Optic nerve: CN2
- Oculomotor nerve: CN3
- Trochlear nerve: CN4
- Trigeminal nerve: CN5
- Abducens nerve: CN6
- Facial nerve: CN7
- Vestibulocochlear nerve: CN8
- Glossopharyngeal nerve: CN9
- Vagus nerve: CN10
- Accessory nerve: CN11
- Hypoglossal nerve: CN12

Imaging Anatomy

Overview

- Cranial nerve groupings based on area of brainstem origin
  - Diencephalon: CN2
  - Mesencephalon (midbrain): CN3 and CN4
  - Pons: CN5, CN6, CN7, and CN8
  - Medulla: CN9, CN10, CN11 and CN12

Anatomy-Based Imaging Issues

Imaging Recommendations

- Best imaging modality for any simple or complex cranial neuropathy is **MR**
  - Single exception to this directive is distal vagal neuropathy where it is necessary to image to aortopulmonic window on left
    - Contrast-enhanced CT better here as less affected by breathing, swallowing and coughing movements
- If a lesion is located in bony area such as skull base, sinuses or mandible, bone CT is highly recommended to provide complimentary bone anatomy and lesion-related information
  - Contrast-enhancement of CT is not necessary if full T1, T2 and T1 C+ MR is available

Imaging Approaches

- Remember cranial nerves do **not** stop at skull base!
- Radiologist must image to "functional endplate" of affected cranial nerve
  - **CN1, 2, 3, 4 and 6**: Include focused **orbital sequences**
  - **CN5**: Include entire **face to inferior mandible if V3** affected
  - **CN7**: Include **CPA, temporal bone and parotid space**
  - **CN8**: Include **CPA-IAC and inner ear**
  - **CN9-12**: Include **basal cistern, skull base, nasopharyngeal carotid space**
    - **CN10**: Follow carotid space to aortopulmonic window on left, cervicothoracic junction on right
    - **CN12**: Remember to reach hyoid bone to include distal loop as it rises into sublingual space

Imaging Pitfalls

- Radiologist forgets to image the extracranial structures associated with cranial nerve affected

Clinical Implications

Clinical Importance

- Cranial nerves and their functions
  - Olfactory nerve
    - Sense of **smell**
  - Optic nerve
    - Sense of **vision**
  - Oculomotor nerve
    - **Motor** to all **extraocular muscles** except lateral rectus and superior oblique
    - **Parasympathetic** supply to ciliary and pupillary constrictor muscles
  - Trochlear nerve
    - **Motor** to **superior oblique**
  - Trigeminal nerve
    - **Motor** (V3) to **muscles of mastication**, anterior belly digastric, mylohyoid, tensor tympani and palatini
    - **Sensory** to surface of **forehead and nose** (V1), **cheek** (V2) and **jaw** (V3)
    - **Sensory** to surfaces of nose, sinuses, meninges and external surface of tympanic membrane (auriculotemporal nerve)
  - Abducens nerve
    - **Motor** to **lateral rectus** muscle
  - Facial nerve
    - **Motor** to **muscles of facial expression**
    - **Motor** to **stapedius muscle**
    - **Parasympathetic** to lacrimal, submandibular and sublingual glands
    - Anterior 2/3 tongue taste (chorda tympanic nerve)
    - General sensation for periauricular skin, external surface of tympanic membrane
  - Vestibulocochlear nerve
    - Senses of **hearing and balance**
  - Glossopharyngeal nerve
    - **Motor** to **stylopharyngeus** muscle
    - **Parasympathetic** to parotid gland
    - Visceral sensory to carotid body
    - Posterior 1/3 tongue **taste**
    - General sensation to posterior 1/3 of tongue and internal surface of tympanic membrane
  - Vagus nerve
    - **Motor** to **pharynx-larynx**
    - Parasympathetic to pharynx, larynx, thoracic and abdominal viscera
    - Visceral sensory from pharynx, larynx and viscera
    - General sensation from small area around external ear
  - Accessory nerve
    - **Motor** to **sternocleidomastoid and trapezius** muscles
  - Hypoglossal nerve
    - **Motor** to intrinsic and extrinsic **tongue muscles** except palatoglossus

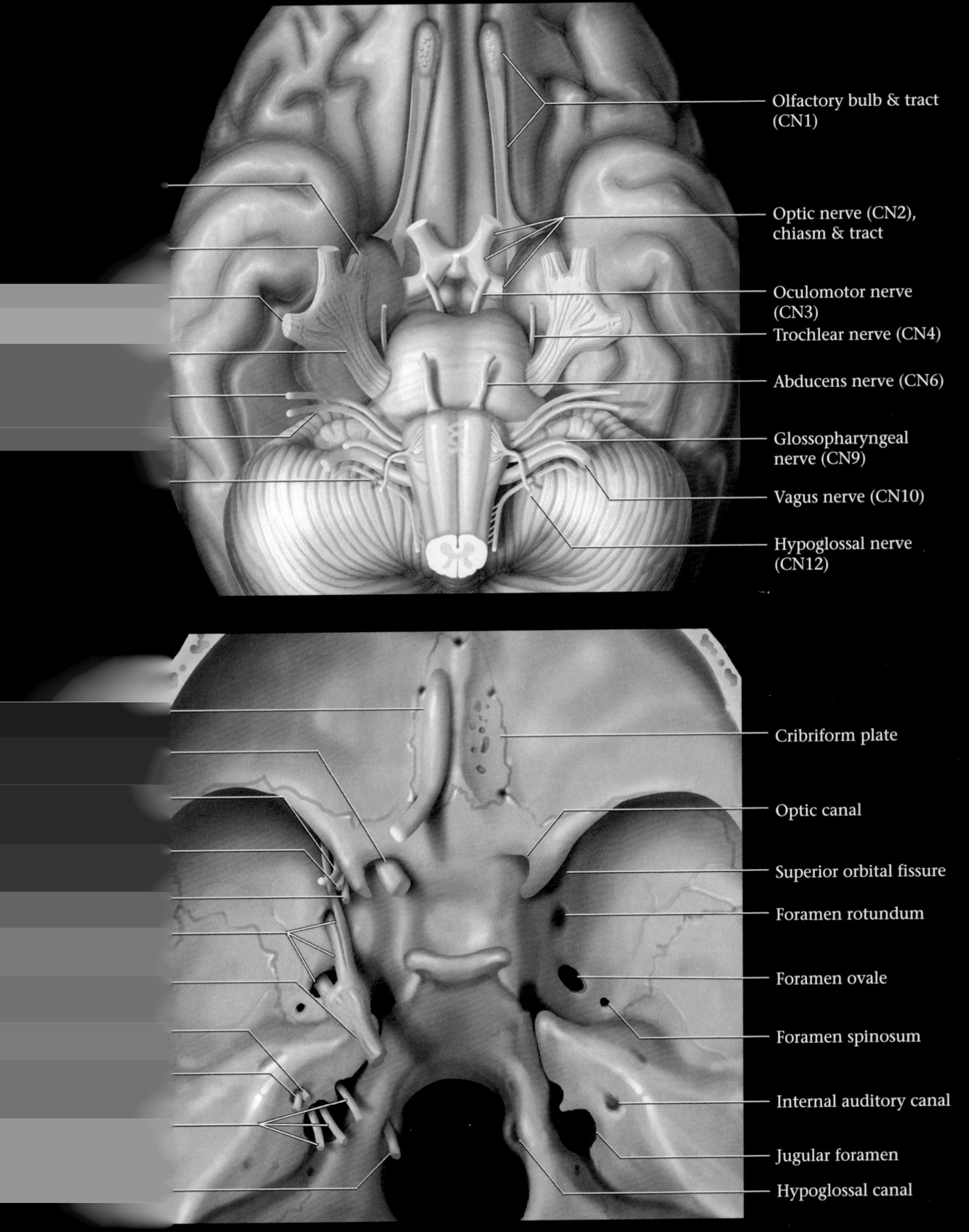
Olfactory bulb & tract (CN1)
Optic nerve (CN2), chiasm & tract
Oculomotor nerve (CN3)
Trochlear nerve (CN4)
Abducens nerve (CN6)
Glossopharyngeal nerve (CN9)
Vagus nerve (CN10)
Hypoglossal nerve (CN12)
Cribriform plate
Optic canal
Superior orbital fissure
Foramen rotundum
Foramen ovale
Foramen spinosum
Internal auditory canal
Jugular foramen
Hypoglossal canal

es graphic with all cranial nerves visible when viewing the brainstem from below. CN4 are associated with the midbrain (mesencephalon) while CN5-8 are affiliated with the n various aspects of the medulla. **(Bottom)** In this graphic of the skull base viewed from selves are on the patient's right while the nerves with the foramen are on the left. CN1 exits ny openings in the cribriform plate. CN2 exits via the optic canal while CN3, 4, 6 and V1 r orbital fissure. V2 traverses foramen rotundum with V3 seen exiting the foramen ovale. internal auditory canal with CN9-11 found in jugular foramen. Finally, CN12 uses its own

GRAPHICS, UPPER CRANIAL NERVES

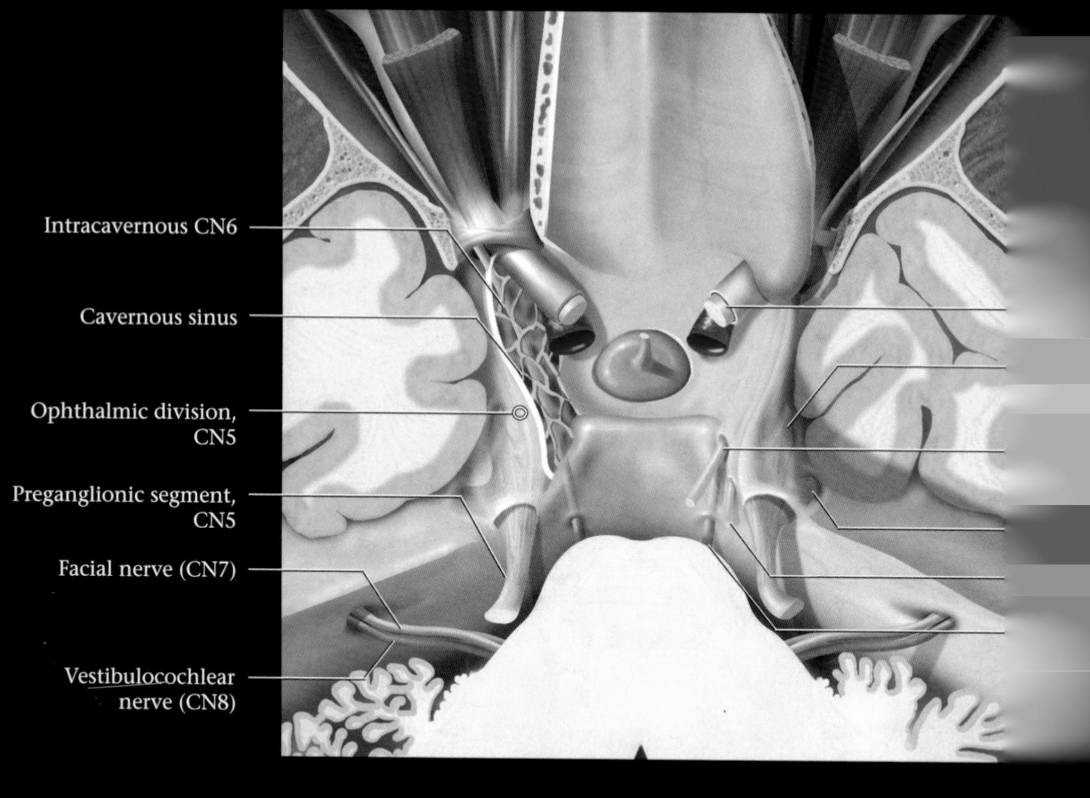
Intracavernous CN6
Cavernous sinus
Ophthalmic division, CN5
Preganglionic segment, CN5
Facial nerve (CN7)
Vestibulocochlear nerve (CN8)

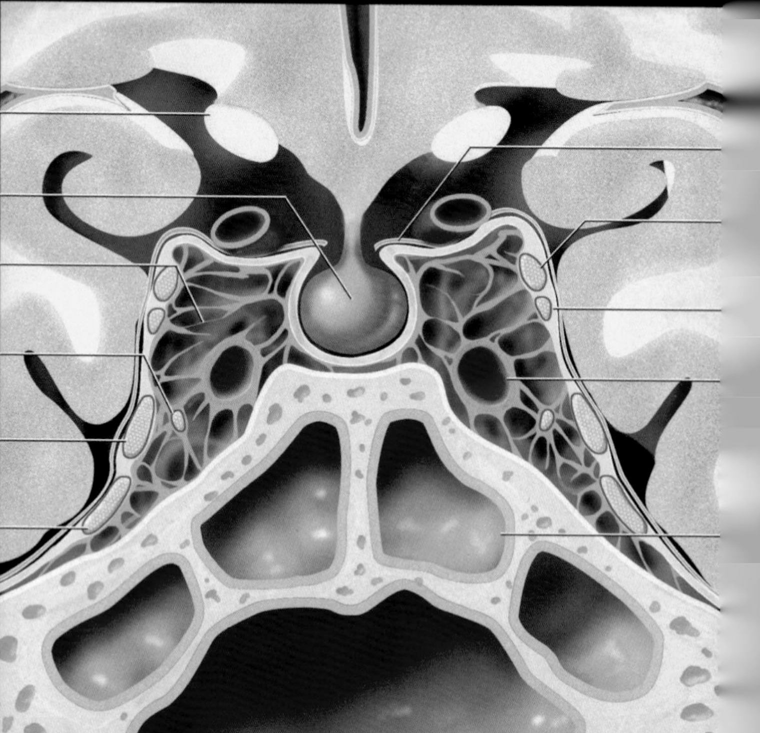
Optic tract (CN2)
Pituitary gland
Cavernous sinus
Abducens nerve (CN6)
Ophthalmic division, CN5 (V1)
Maxillary division, CN5 (V2)

(Top) Axial graphic of the prepontine cistern and cavernous sinus areas seen from above. Th of CN5 can be seen in the lateral prepontine cistern. It enters Meckel cave through the poru 6 are seen piercing the dura to enter the cavernous sinus. Only CN6 is within the venous sin sinus while CN3 and 4 remain in its wall. **(Bottom)** Coronal graphic through cavernous sinu located intracavernous cranial nerve to be the abducens nerve (CN6). CN3 and 4 are all also cavernous sinus, just laterally positioned. V1 and V2 are in the lateral wall of the cavernous

GRAPHICS, LOWER CRANIAL NERVES

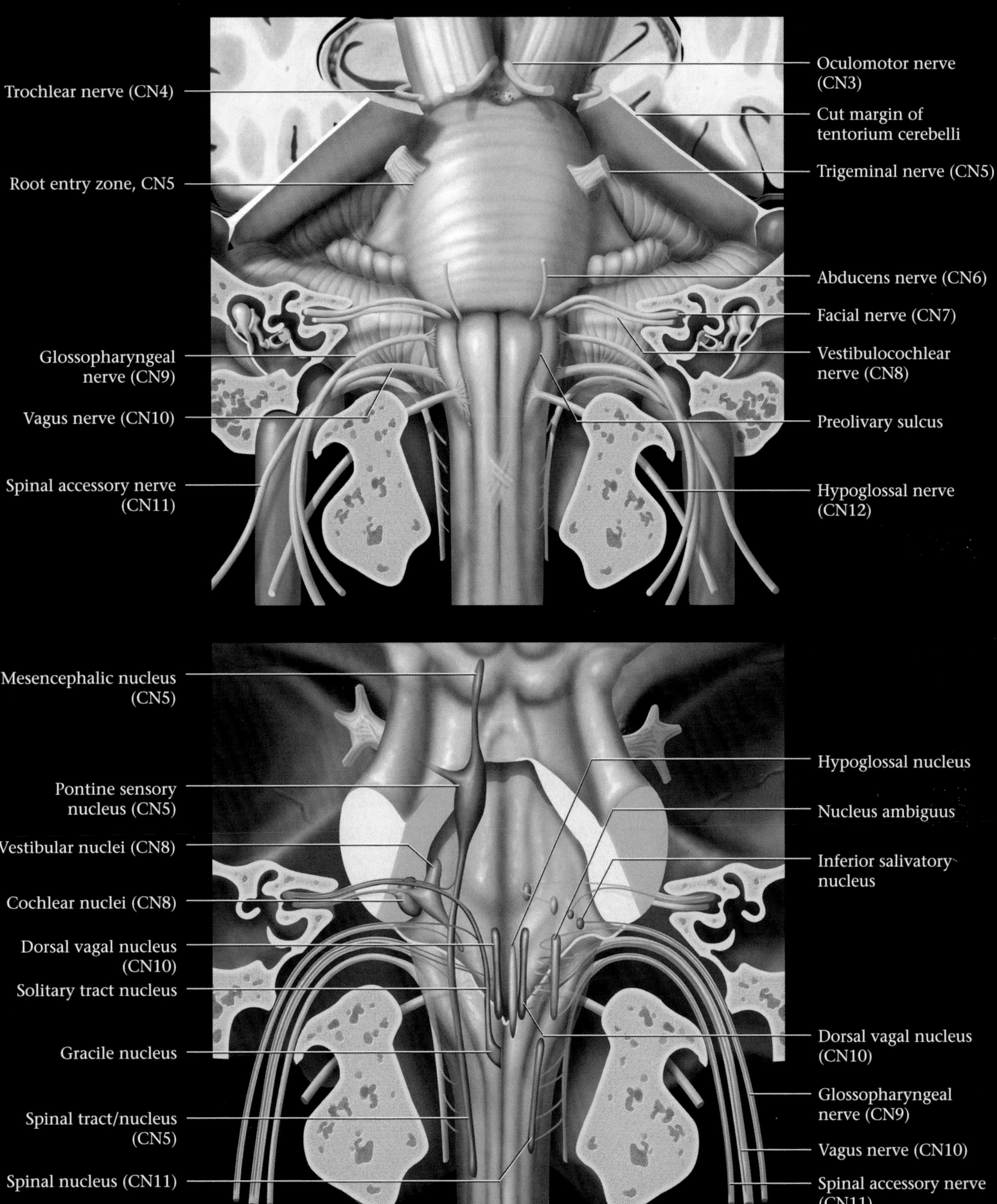

Trochlear nerve (CN4)
Root entry zone, CN5
Glossopharyngeal nerve (CN9)
Vagus nerve (CN10)
Spinal accessory nerve (CN11)
Oculomotor nerve (CN3)
Cut margin of tentorium cerebelli
Trigeminal nerve (CN5)
Abducens nerve (CN6)
Facial nerve (CN7)
Vestibulocochlear nerve (CN8)
Preolivary sulcus
Hypoglossal nerve (CN12)
Mesencephalic nucleus (CN5)
Pontine sensory nucleus (CN5)
Vestibular nuclei (CN8)
Cochlear nuclei (CN8)
Dorsal vagal nucleus (CN10)
Solitary tract nucleus
Gracile nucleus
Spinal tract/nucleus (CN5)
Spinal nucleus (CN11)
Hypoglossal nucleus
Nucleus ambiguus
Inferior salivatory nucleus
Dorsal vagal nucleus (CN10)
Glossopharyngeal nerve (CN9)
Vagus nerve (CN10)
Spinal accessory nerve (CN11)

(Top) Graphic of frontal view of brainstem & exiting cranial nerves. CN3 is seen exiting midbrain into interpeduncular cistern. CN4 wraps around lateral midbrain in tentorial margin. CN6 exits at pontomedullary junction. CN7 and CN8 exit brainstem at cerebellopontine angle. Inferiorly CN9-11 leave lateral medulla in post-olivary sulcus. CN12 on the other hand exits via pre-olivary sulcus. **(Bottom)** Graphic of brainstem from behind emphasizes lower cranial nerve nuclei. On patient's right are efferent fibers, on left are afferent fibers connecting to brainstem nuclei. Highlights of this drawing include nucleus ambiguus providing voluntary motor fibers for CN9 and CN10. Inferior salivatory nucleus provides secretomotor fibers to the parotid via CN9. Dorsal motor nucleus provides involuntary motor and sensory fibers to CN10. Solitary tract receives taste from CN7 and CN9.

AXIAL BONE CT

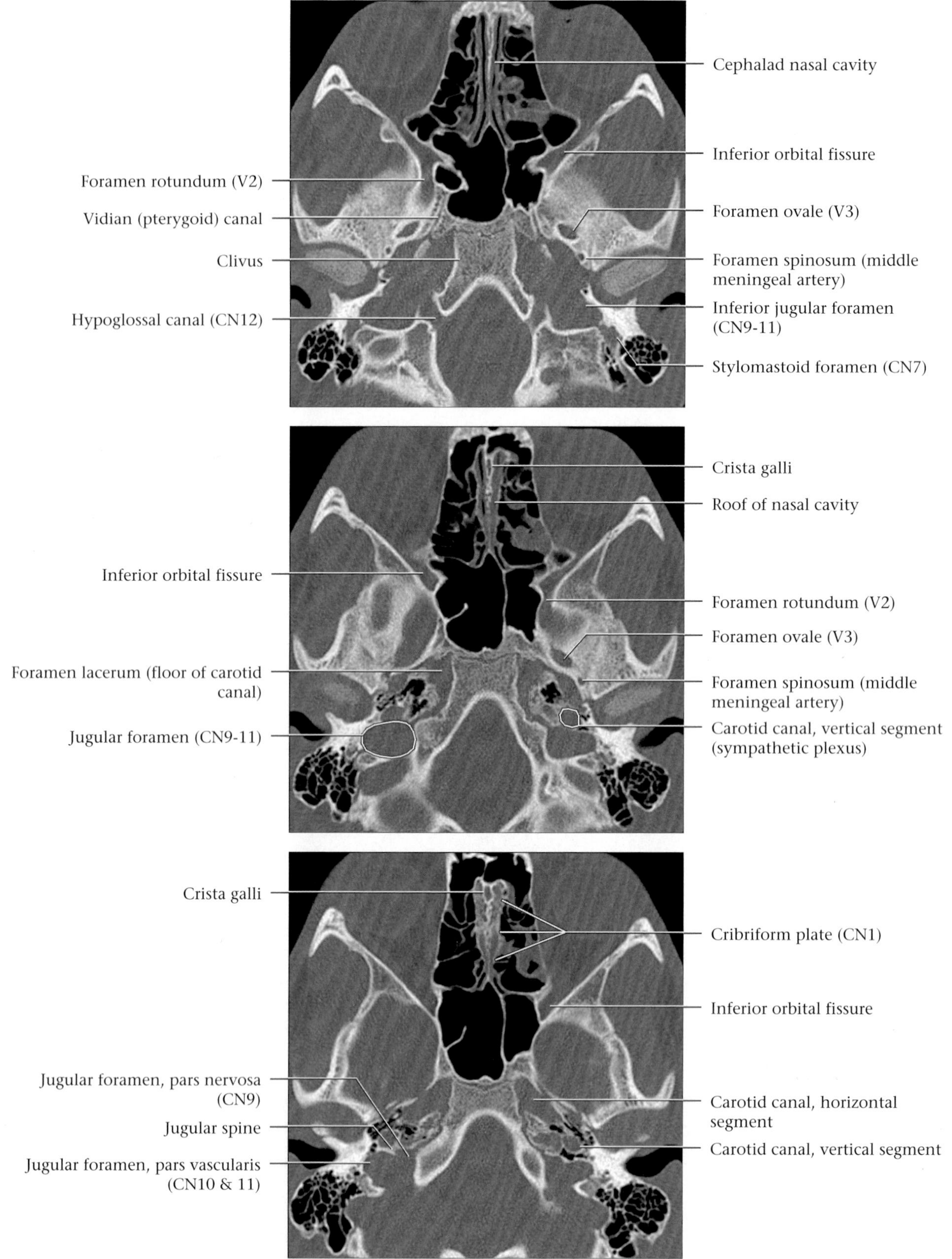

Cephalad nasal cavity
Inferior orbital fissure
Foramen rotundum (V2)
Vidian (pterygoid) canal
Foramen ovale (V3)
Clivus
Foramen spinosum (middle meningeal artery)
Hypoglossal canal (CN12)
Inferior jugular foramen (CN9-11)
Stylomastoid foramen (CN7)
Crista galli
Roof of nasal cavity
Inferior orbital fissure
Foramen rotundum (V2)
Foramen ovale (V3)
Foramen lacerum (floor of carotid canal)
Foramen spinosum (middle meningeal artery)
Jugular foramen (CN9-11)
Carotid canal, vertical segment (sympathetic plexus)
Crista galli
Cribriform plate (CN1)
Inferior orbital fissure
Jugular foramen, pars nervosa (CN9)
Carotid canal, horizontal segment
Jugular spine
Carotid canal, vertical segment
Jugular foramen, pars vascularis (CN10 & 11)

(Top) First of six sequential axial bone CT images through skull base presented from inferior to superior shows foramina of sphenoid bone including foramen rotundum (CNV2) & foramen ovale (CNV3). More posteriorly oblique hypoglossal canal is visible bilaterally in the occipital bone. **(Middle)** At the level of the inferior jugular foramen the entry to the vertical segment of the carotid canal is also seen just anterior to jugular foramen. Notice the ovoid shape of the jugular foramen at this level. The floor of the anteromedial aspect of the horizontal segment of petrous ICA is called the foramen lacerum. **(Bottom)** At the level of the cribriform plate the jugular foramen is now divided by the jugular spine into more anterior pars nervosa (CN9, Jacobsen nerve and inferior petrosal sinus) and more posterolateral pars vascularis (CN10, 11, Arnold nerve and jugular bulb).

AXIAL BONE CT

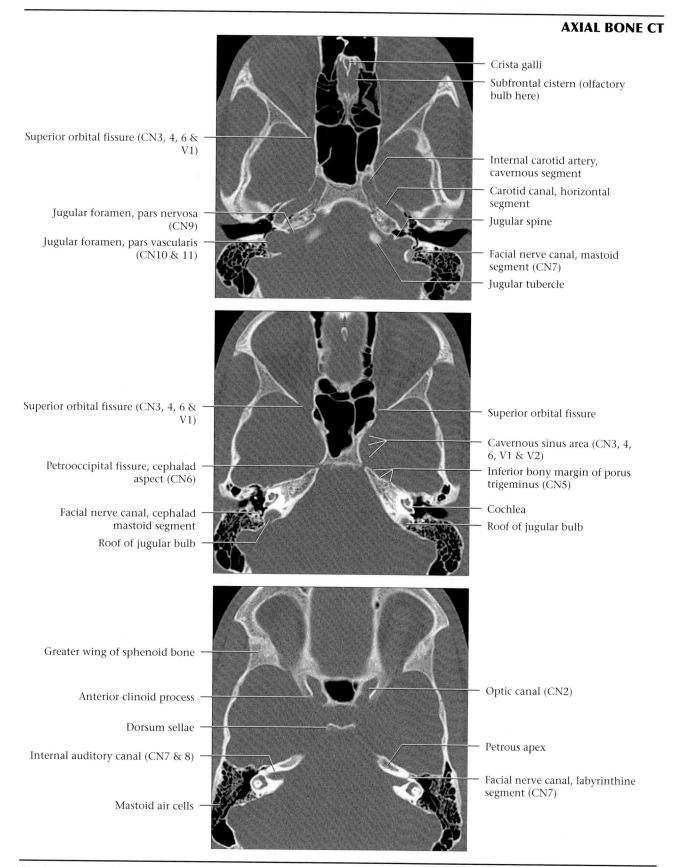

Crista galli
Subfrontal cistern (olfactory bulb here)
Superior orbital fissure (CN3, 4, 6 & V1)
Internal carotid artery, cavernous segment
Carotid canal, horizontal segment
Jugular foramen, pars nervosa (CN9)
Jugular spine
Jugular foramen, pars vascularis (CN10 & 11)
Facial nerve canal, mastoid segment (CN7)
Jugular tubercle

Superior orbital fissure (CN3, 4, 6 & V1)
Superior orbital fissure
Cavernous sinus area (CN3, 4, 6, V1 & V2)
Petrooccipital fissure, cephalad aspect (CN6)
Inferior bony margin of porus trigeminus (CN5)
Cochlea
Facial nerve canal, cephalad mastoid segment
Roof of jugular bulb
Roof of jugular bulb

Greater wing of sphenoid bone
Anterior clinoid process
Optic canal (CN2)
Dorsum sellae
Petrous apex
Internal auditory canal (CN7 & 8)
Facial nerve canal, labyrinthine segment (CN7)
Mastoid air cells

(Top) At the level of the mid-horizontal portion of the petrous ICA the superior orbital fissure is seen. Remember that CN3, 4 and 6 as well as the ophthalmic division of CN5 and the superior ophthalmic vein all enter the orbit through this structure. **(Middle)** At the level of the cochlea and upper petrous apex, the petrooccipital fissure is seen. This is approximately the location of CN6 after it pierces the dura to leave the prepontine cistern on its way to the cavernous sinus. On bone CT the area of the cavernous sinus can only be approximated. Notice also the inferior margin of the porus trigeminus. **(Bottom)** The internal auditory canal is visible on this most cephalad CT image. The facial (CN7) and vestibulocochlear (CN8) nerves pass through the IAC. The optic nerve (CN2) enters orbit via the optic canal which lies medial to the anterior clinoid process.

CRANIAL NERVES OVERVIEW

AXIAL T2 MR

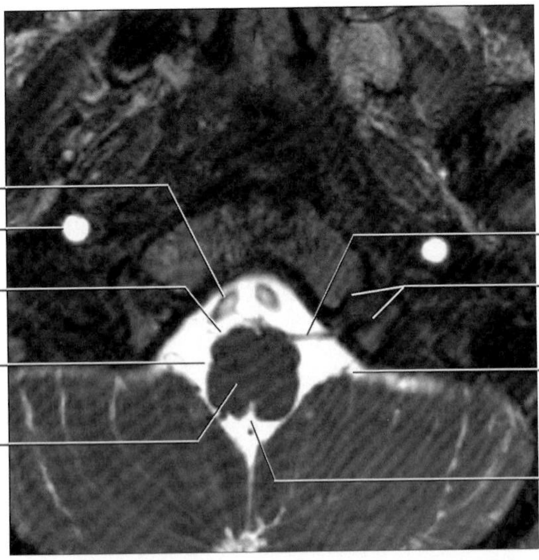

Vertebral artery
Nasopharyngeal internal carotid artery
Preolivary sulcus
Postolivary sulcus
Medulla
Hypoglossal nerve (CN12)
Hypoglossal canal
Spinal root of accessory nerve (CN11)
Dorsal median sulcus

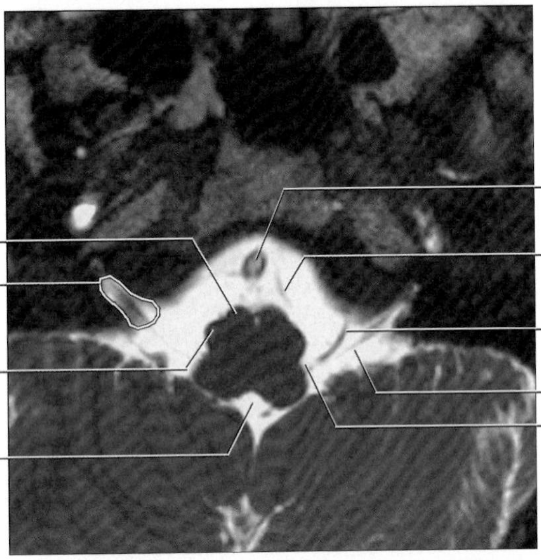

Pyramid
Jugular foramen
Olive
Inferior fourth ventricle
Basilar artery
Anterior inferior cerebellar artery
Posterior inferior cerebellar artery
CN9-11
Postolivary sulcus

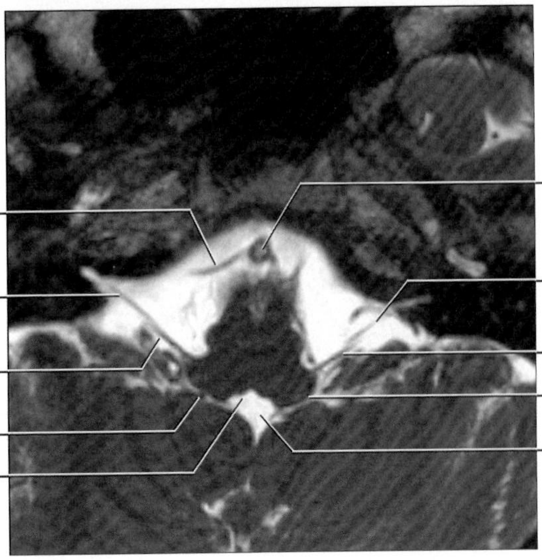

Anterior inferior cerebellar artery
Glossopharyngeal nerve (CN9)
Vagus nerve (CN10)
Foramen of Luschka
Hypoglossal trigone
Basilar artery
Glossopharyngeal nerve (CN9)
Vagus nerve (CN10)
Inferior cerebellar peduncle
Fourth ventricle

(Top) First of twelve axial T2 MR image sequence presented from inferior to superior shows the left hypoglossal nerve leaving the preolivary sulcus of the medulla. Spinal root of accessory nerve (CN11) ascends through foramen magnum, lateral to brainstem to unite with cranial roots of accessory nerve before exiting via jugular foramen. **(Middle)** Glossopharyngeal (CN9), vagus (CN10) and cranial (bulbar) roots of spinal accessory (CN11) nerves emerge from lateral brainstem posterior to olive in the postolivary sulcus and exit the skull base via jugular foramen. Do not confuse the posterior or anterior inferior cerebellar arteries for cranial nerves. **(Bottom)** Nucleus of hypoglossal nerve (CN12) forms a characteristic bulge on floor of fourth ventricle called the hypoglossal trigone. It is often difficult to separate CN9 from CN10 in the basal cistern.

AXIAL T2 MR

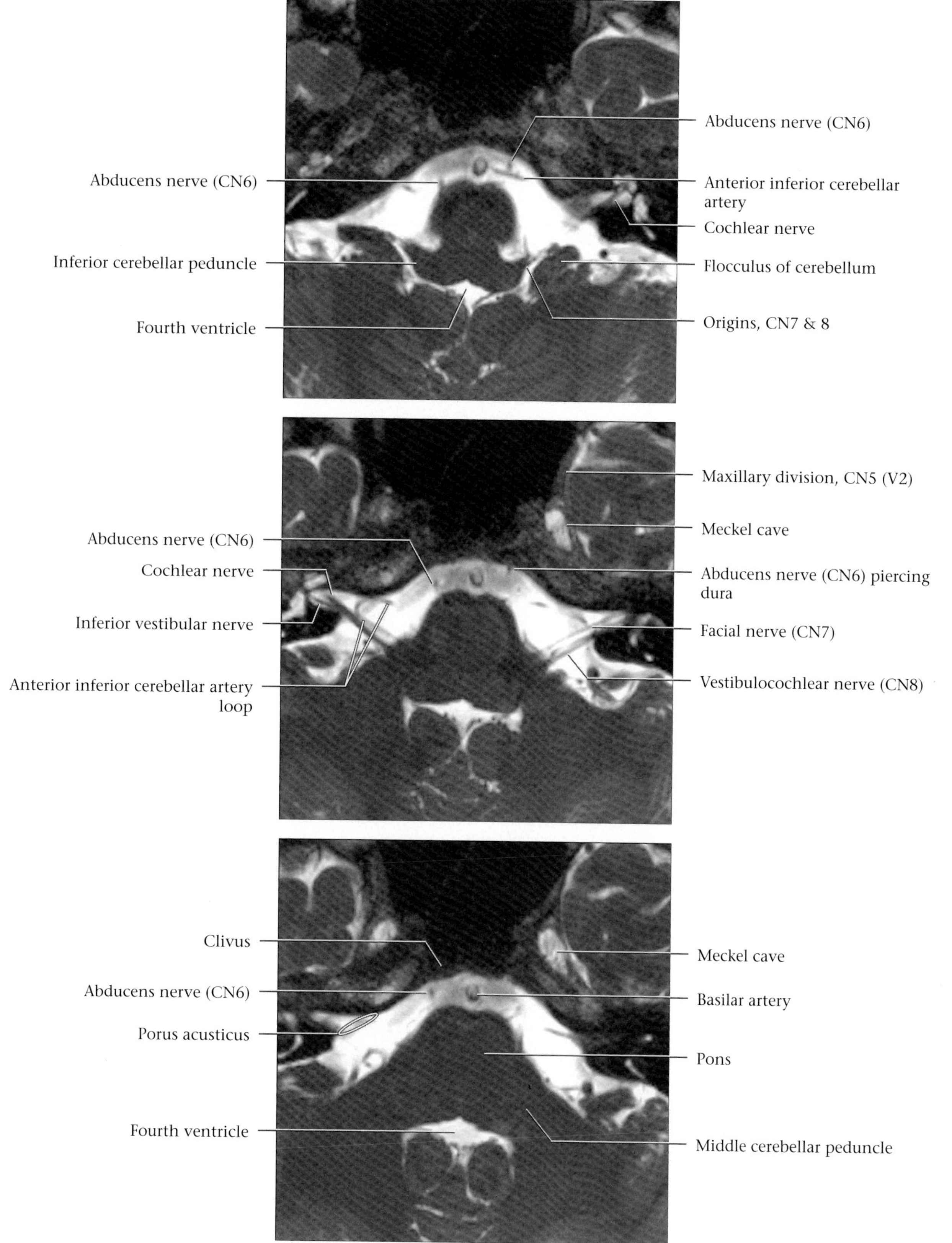
Abducens nerve (CN6)
Abducens nerve (CN6)
Anterior inferior cerebellar artery
Cochlear nerve
Inferior cerebellar peduncle
Flocculus of cerebellum
Fourth ventricle
Origins, CN7 & 8
Maxillary division, CN5 (V2)
Meckel cave
Abducens nerve (CN6)
Cochlear nerve
Abducens nerve (CN6) piercing dura
Inferior vestibular nerve
Facial nerve (CN7)
Anterior inferior cerebellar artery loop
Vestibulocochlear nerve (CN8)
Clivus
Meckel cave
Abducens nerve (CN6)
Basilar artery
Porus acusticus
Pons
Fourth ventricle
Middle cerebellar peduncle

(Top) Abducens (CN6) nerves exit brainstem anteriorly at pontomedullary junction just above pyramid, ascending from there through prepontine cistern towards clivus. Cochlear nerve nuclei are found on lateral surface of inferior cerebellar peduncle (restiform body). **(Middle)** CN7 and CN8 exit brainstem laterally at pontomedullary junction to enter cerebellopontine angle cistern. CN7 lies anterior to CN8 in cerebellopontine angle cistern. Notice CN6 piecing dura on patient's left to enter Dorello canal an interdural channel passing along dorsal surface of clivus within basilar venous plexus towards cavernous sinus. **(Bottom)** Meckel cave is formed by a dural reflection, lined with arachnoid and containing cerebrospinal fluid. The Gasserian ganglion (trigeminal ganglion) is semi-lunar in shape and lies antero-inferiorly in Meckel cave.

AXIAL T2 MR

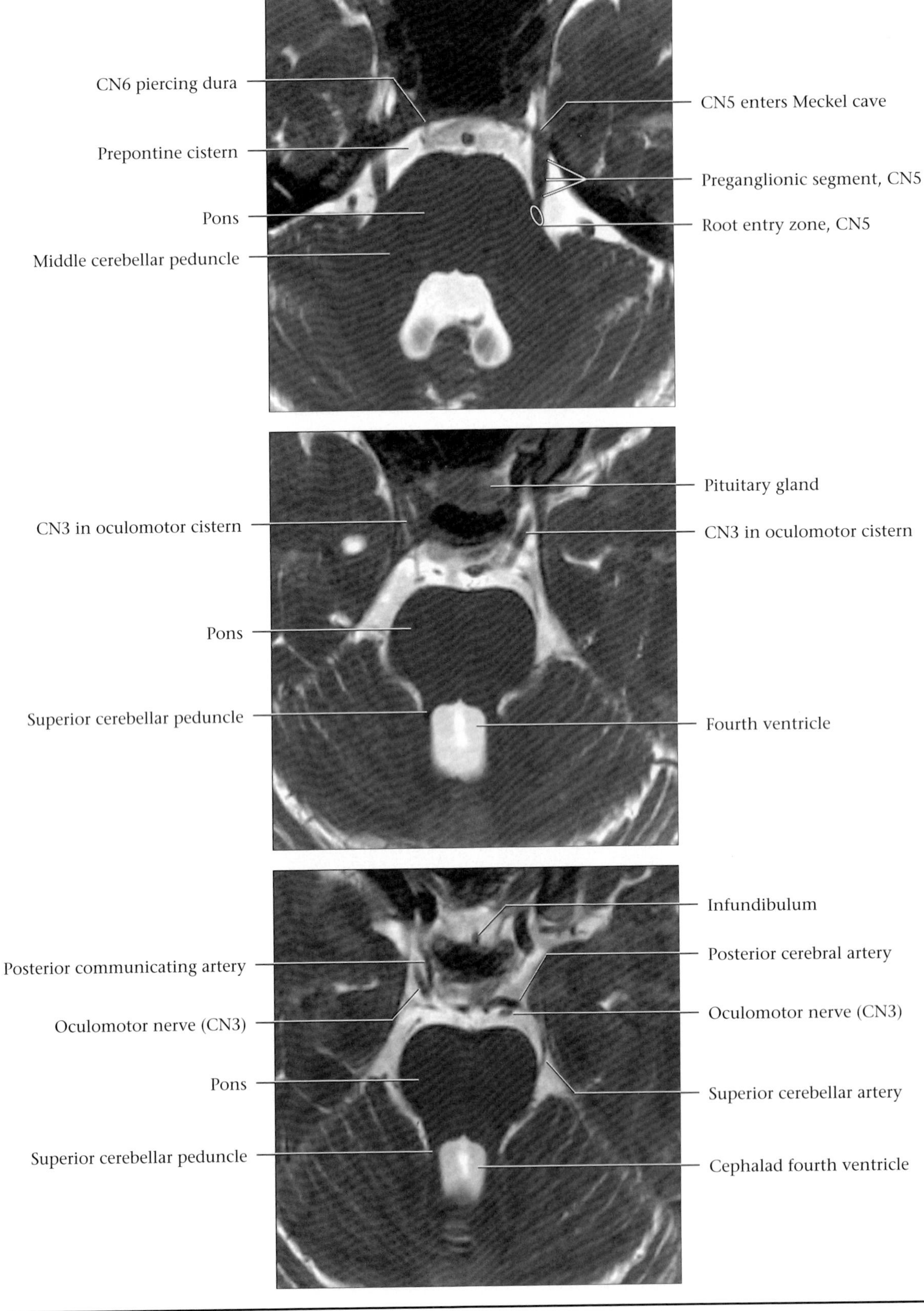

CN6 piercing dura
Preportine cistern
Pons
Middle cerebellar peduncle
CN5 enters Meckel cave
Preganglionic segment, CN5
Root entry zone, CN5
Pituitary gland
CN3 in oculomotor cistern
CN3 in oculomotor cistern
Pons
Superior cerebellar peduncle
Fourth ventricle
Infundibulum
Posterior cerebral artery
Posterior communicating artery
Oculomotor nerve (CN3)
Oculomotor nerve (CN3)
Pons
Superior cerebellar artery
Superior cerebellar peduncle
Cephalad fourth ventricle

(Top) CN5 exits lateral pons at point referred to as the root entry zone. Preganglionic segment courses anteriorly through prepontine cistern and passes over petrous apex to enter Meckel cave via porus trigeminus (entrance to Meckel cave). **(Middle)** In this image the oculomotor nerve (CN3) can be seen surrounded by high signal cerebrospinal fluid as it enters the roof of the cavernous sinus. This area is referred to as the oculomotor cistern **(Bottom)** At level of upper pons important vascular relationships of CN3 passing between posterior cerebral and superior cerebellar arteries visible. Notice CN3 coursing anteriorly within suprasellar cistern adjacent to posterior communicating artery. An aneurysm of posterior communicating artery will result in compression of CN3.

CRANIAL NERVES OVERVIEW

AXIAL T2 MR

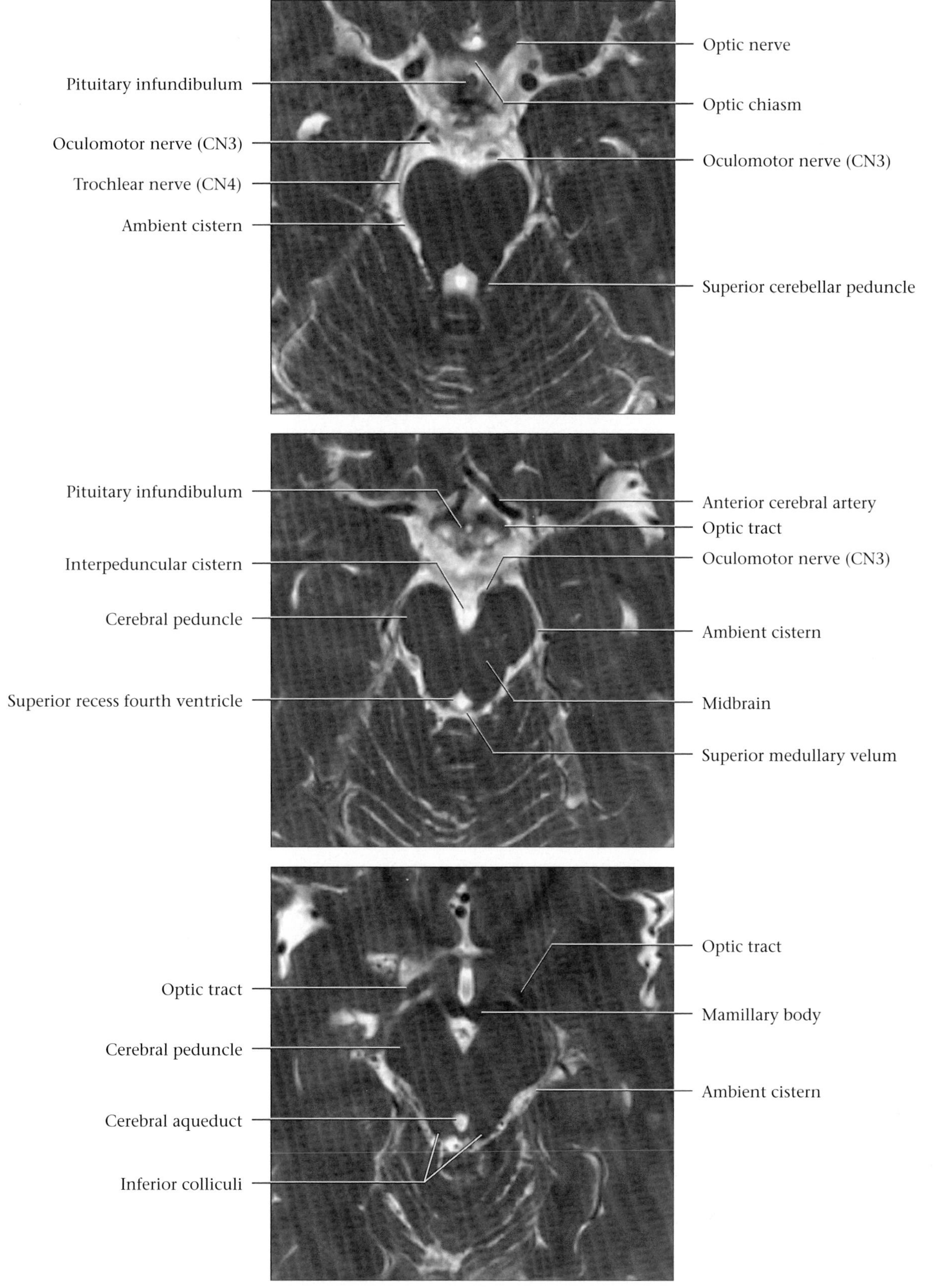
Pituitary infundibulum
Oculomotor nerve (CN3)
Trochlear nerve (CN4)
Ambient cistern
Optic nerve
Optic chiasm
Oculomotor nerve (CN3)
Superior cerebellar peduncle
Pituitary infundibulum
Interpeduncular cistern
Cerebral peduncle
Superior recess fourth ventricle
Anterior cerebral artery
Optic tract
Oculomotor nerve (CN3)
Ambient cistern
Midbrain
Superior medullary velum
Optic tract
Cerebral peduncle
Cerebral aqueduct
Inferior colliculi
Optic tract
Mamillary body
Ambient cistern

(Top) Anteriorly note the optic nerves (CN2) form optic chiasm in suprasellar cistern. Fibers originating from nasal halves of retina cross within optic chiasm. CN3 course anteriorly within suprasellar cistern towards cavernous sinus. **(Middle)** Note CN3 is seen on the patient's left exiting the brainstem along medial aspect of cerebral peduncle where it enters the interpeduncular cistern. The trochlear nerve decussates in the superior medullary velum, then exits dorsal surface of the midbrain below the inferior colliculus to enter quadrigeminal plate cistern. From there CN4 courses around brainstem below tentorium cerebelli in ambient cistern passing between posterior cerebral and superior cerebellar arteries. **(Bottom)** Optic tracts connect the lateral geniculate body to the optic chiasm. Only a portion of the optic tracts are visible here.

CRANIAL NERVES OVERVIEW

CORONAL T2 MR

Third ventricle
Tentorium cerebelli
Proximal preganglionic segment, CN5
Vestibulocochlear nerve (CN8)
Facial nerve (CN7)
Cerebellopontine angle cistern
Vertebral artery
Interpeduncular cistern
Cerebral peduncle
Superior cerebellar artery
Anterior inferior cerebellar artery
Flocculus of cerebellum
Medulla

Oculomotor nerve (CN3)
Prepontine segment, CN5
Porus acusticus
Interpeduncular cistern
Oculomotor nerve (CN3)
Pons
Crista falciformis
Pontomedullary junction
Vertebral artery

Posterior cerebral artery
Oculomotor nerve (CN3)
Tentorium cerebelli
Preganglionic segment, CN5
Vertebral artery
Posterior cerebral artery
Oculomotor nerve (CN3)
Superior cerebellar artery
Cochlea
Ventral belly of pons

(Top) First of six coronal T2 MR images of brainstem, cisterns and cranial nerves presented from posterior to anterior. Preganglionic segment of trigeminal nerve is seen arising from lateral pons. Also seen are facial and vestibulocochlear nerves traversing cerebellopontine angle cistern into internal auditory canal. **(Middle)** Oculomotor nerves are seen emerging from medial aspect of cerebral peduncle into interpeduncular cistern. Basal cistern cranial nerves are not visible. The abrupt transition between the pons and the medulla is termed the pontomedullary junction. **(Bottom)** In this image notice the oculomotor nerves passing between posterior cerebral artery above and superior cerebellar artery below. The distal preganglionic segment of CN5 is poised to enter the porus trigeminus on its way into Meckel cave.

CRANIAL NERVES OVERVIEW

CORONAL T2 MR

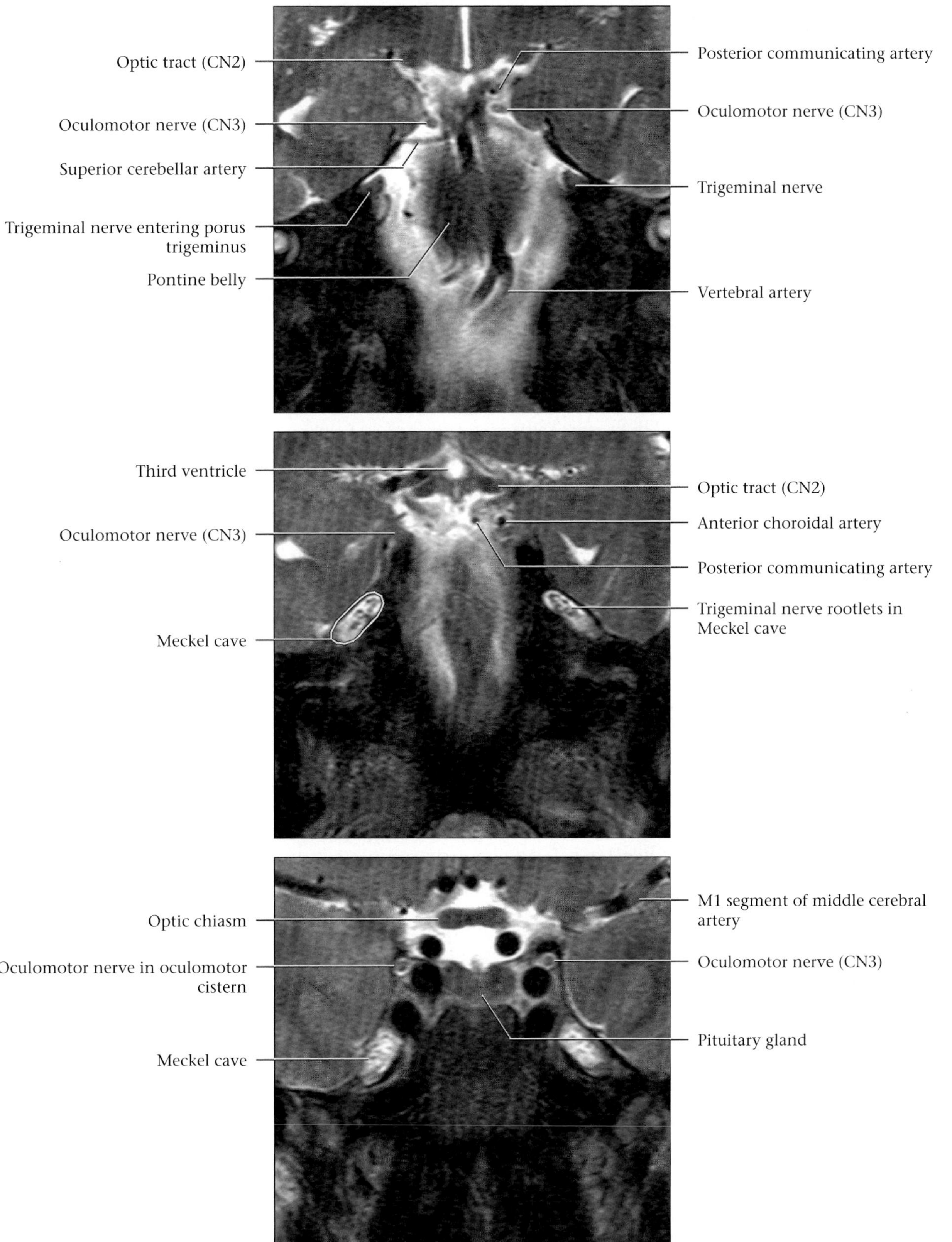
Optic tract (CN2)
Oculomotor nerve (CN3)
Superior cerebellar artery
Trigeminal nerve entering porus trigeminus
Pontine belly
Posterior communicating artery
Oculomotor nerve (CN3)
Trigeminal nerve
Vertebral artery
Third ventricle
Oculomotor nerve (CN3)
Meckel cave
Optic tract (CN2)
Anterior choroidal artery
Posterior communicating artery
Trigeminal nerve rootlets in Meckel cave
Optic chiasm
Oculomotor nerve in oculomotor cistern
Meckel cave
M1 segment of middle cerebral artery
Oculomotor nerve (CN3)
Pituitary gland

(Top) This image shows the oculomotor nerve between the posterior communicating artery above and the superior cerebellar artery below. The trigeminal nerve is visible entering the porus trigeminus of Meckel cave. **(Middle)** Here the optic tracts are seen converging toward optic chiasm. Note a large left anterior choroidal artery coursing posterolaterally within suprasellar cistern. Preganglionic fibers of trigeminal nerve are seen within Meckel cave. Meckel cave is formed by a reflection of dura which is lined with arachnoid and contains cerebrospinal fluid which communicates freely with prepontine cistern. **(Bottom)** In this most anterior coronal T2 image the pituitary is seen below optic chiasm. Notice the oculomotor nerve is entering the cavernous sinus in the oculomotor cistern. The high signal ring around CN3 is cerebrospinal fluid.

CN1 (OLFACTORY NERVE)

Terminology

Abbreviations
- Olfactory nerve: CN1, CN I

Synonyms
- First cranial nerve

Definitions
- CN1: Special visceral afferent cranial nerve for olfaction (sense of smell)

Imaging Anatomy

Overview
- Visceral afferent system providing sense of smell
- Olfactory nerve segments
  - End receptor in olfactory epithelium in nasal vault
  - Transethmoidal segment through cribriform plate
  - Intracranial olfactory bulb, tract and cortex

Nasal Epithelium
- Approximately 2 cm² nasal epithelium in roof of each nasal cavity
  - Extends onto nasal septum and lateral wall of nasal cavity including superior turbinates
- **Bipolar olfactory receptor cells** (neurosensory cells) located in nasal pseudostratified columnar epithelium
  - Peripheral processes of receptor cells in olfactory epithelium act as sensory receptors for smell
- Olfactory glands (of Bowman) secrete mucous which solubilizes inhaled scents (aromatic molecules)

Transethmoidal Segment
- Central processes of bipolar receptor cells traverse **cribriform plate** to synapse with olfactory bulb
- Hundreds of central processes traverse cribriform plate as unmyelinated fascicles (fila olfactoria)
  - **Fila olfactoria** are actual **olfactory nerves**
  - Each side of nasal cavity has ~ 20 fila olfactoria

Intracranial, Olfactory Bulb and Tract
- Olfactory bulb and tracts are extensions of the brain, not nerves
  - Historically bulb and tract are called "**olfactory nerve**"
- **Olfactory bulb** closely apposed to cribriform plate at ventral surface of medial frontal lobe
  - Rostral enlargement of olfactory tract
  - Bipolar cells synapse in olfactory bulb with secondary neuronal cells (mitral and tufted cells)
  - Mitral cell axons project posteriorly in olfactory tract
  - Granule cells modulate mitral cells
- **Olfactory tract** divides into medial, intermediate and lateral stria at **anterior perforated substance**
  - This trifurcation creates **olfactory trigone**
  - Anterior perforated substance is perforated by multiple small vascular structures
  - Olfactory tract is made up of **secondary sensory axons**, not primary sensory axons
  - Majority of fibers project through lateral olfactory stria and intermediate stria

Intracranial, Central Pathways
- Complex pattern of central connections
- **Lateral olfactory striae**
  - Formed by majority of fibers of olfactory tracts
  - Course over insula to prepiriform area (anterior to uncus) and amygdala
  - On way to prepiriform area collaterals are given to subfrontal or frontal olfactory cortex
  - Fibers to subthalamic nuclei with collaterals/terminal fibers to thalamus and stria medullaris
- **Medial olfactory striae**
  - Majority terminate in parolfactory area of Broca (medial surface in front of the subcallosal gyrus)
  - Some fibers end in subcallosal gyrus and in anterior perforated substance
  - Few fibers cross in anterior commissure to opposite olfactory tract
- **Intermediate olfactory striae**
  - Intermediate olfactory stria terminate in anterior perforated substance
  - Intermediate olfactory area contains anterior olfactory nucleus and nucleus of diagonal band
- **Medial forebrain bundle**
  - Formed by fibers from basal olfactory region, periamygdaloid area and septal nuclei
  - Some fibers terminate in hypothalamic nuclei
  - Majority of fibers extend to brainstem to autonomic areas in reticular formation, salivatory nuclei and dorsal vagus nucleus

Anatomy-Based Imaging Issues

Imaging Recommendations
- Coronal sinus CT is best study for isolated anosmia
  - Identifies nasal vault and cribriform plate lesions
- MR of brain, anterior cranial fossa and sinonasal region used in complex anosmia cases
  - Identifies intracranial dural and parenchymal lesions

Imaging "Sweet Spots"
- Intracranial: Include anterior cranial fossa floor and medial temporal lobes
- Extracranial: Include nasal vault and cribriform plate

Imaging Pitfalls
- Coronal sinus CT insensitive to intracranial pathology

Clinical Implications

Clinical Importance
- CN1 dysfunction produces unilateral **anosmia**
  - Each side of nose must be tested individually
- **Esthesioneuroblastoma** arises from olfactory epithelium in nasal vault
- Head trauma may cause anosmia: Cribriform plate fracture or shear forces; anterior temporal lobe injury
- Seizure activity in lateral olfactory area may produce "uncinate fits", imaginary odor, oroglossal automatisms and impaired awareness

CN1 (OLFACTORY NERVE)

GRAPHICS

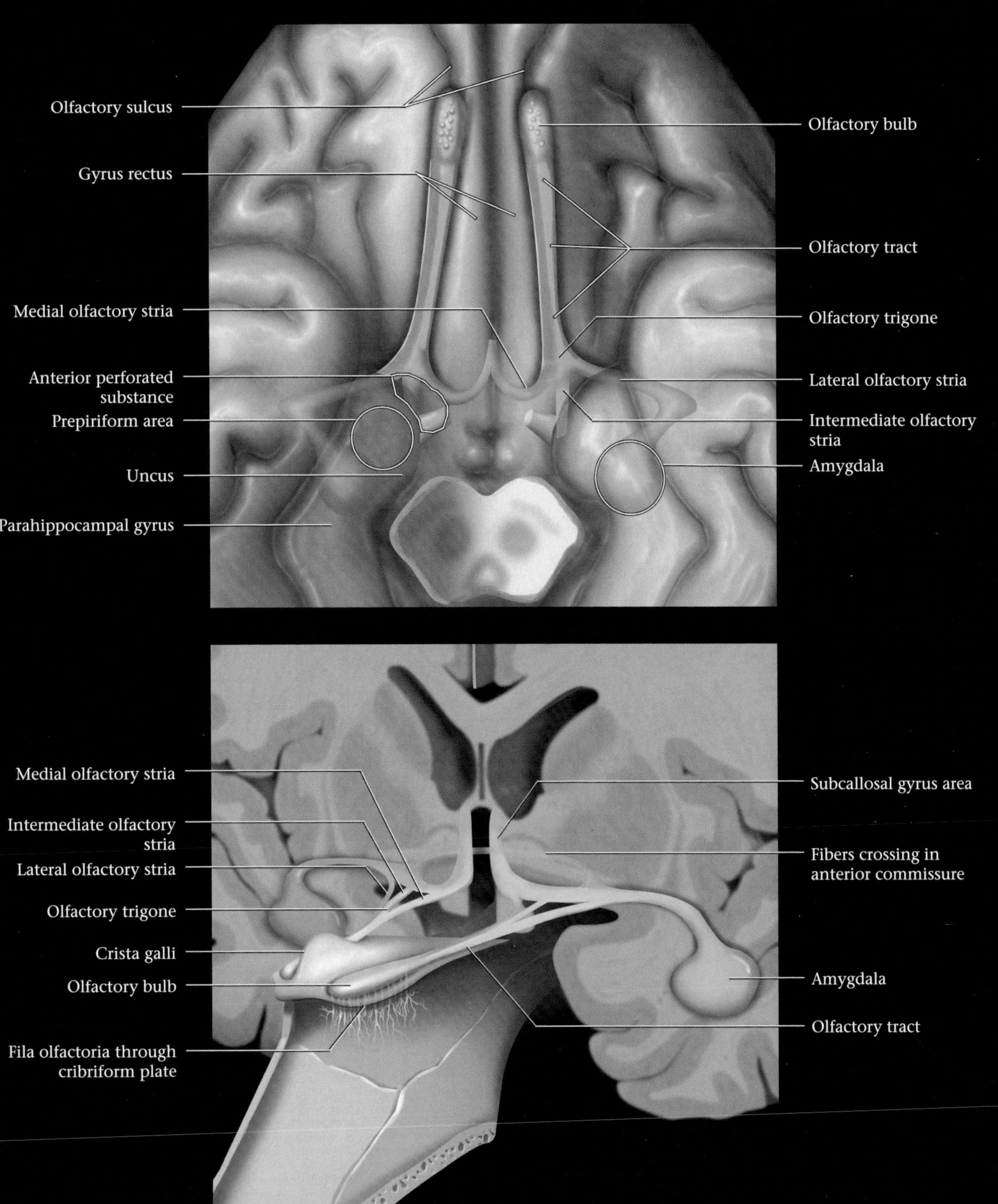
Olfactory sulcus
Gyrus rectus
Medial olfactory stria
Anterior perforated substance
Prepiriform area
Uncus
Parahippocampal gyrus
Olfactory bulb
Olfactory tract
Olfactory trigone
Lateral olfactory stria
Intermediate olfactory stria
Amygdala
Medial olfactory stria
Intermediate olfactory stria
Lateral olfactory stria
Olfactory trigone
Crista galli
Olfactory bulb
Fila olfactoria through cribriform plate
Subcallosal gyrus area
Fibers crossing in anterior commissure
Amygdala
Olfactory tract

(Top) Graphic of olfactory system viewed from below shows olfactory tracts coursing from olfactory bulbs to the olfactory trigone. In the olfactory trigone fibers split up into lateral, intermediate and medial striae. The majority of fibers course through lateral stria to prepiriform area and amygdala. Some fibers in medial stria course through anterior commissure to connect to opposite tract. Majority of intermediate stria fibers terminate in anterior perforated substance. **(Bottom)** Graphic of olfactory system seen from an anterolateral oblique perspective shows central processes from bipolar olfactory cells in olfactory epithelium crossing cribriform plate bundled as fila olfactoria (about 20 per side) and connecting with secondary neurons in olfactory bulbs. The olfactory trigone is visible dividing into the lateral, intermediate and medial stria.

CN1 (OLFACTORY NERVE)

CORONAL NECT

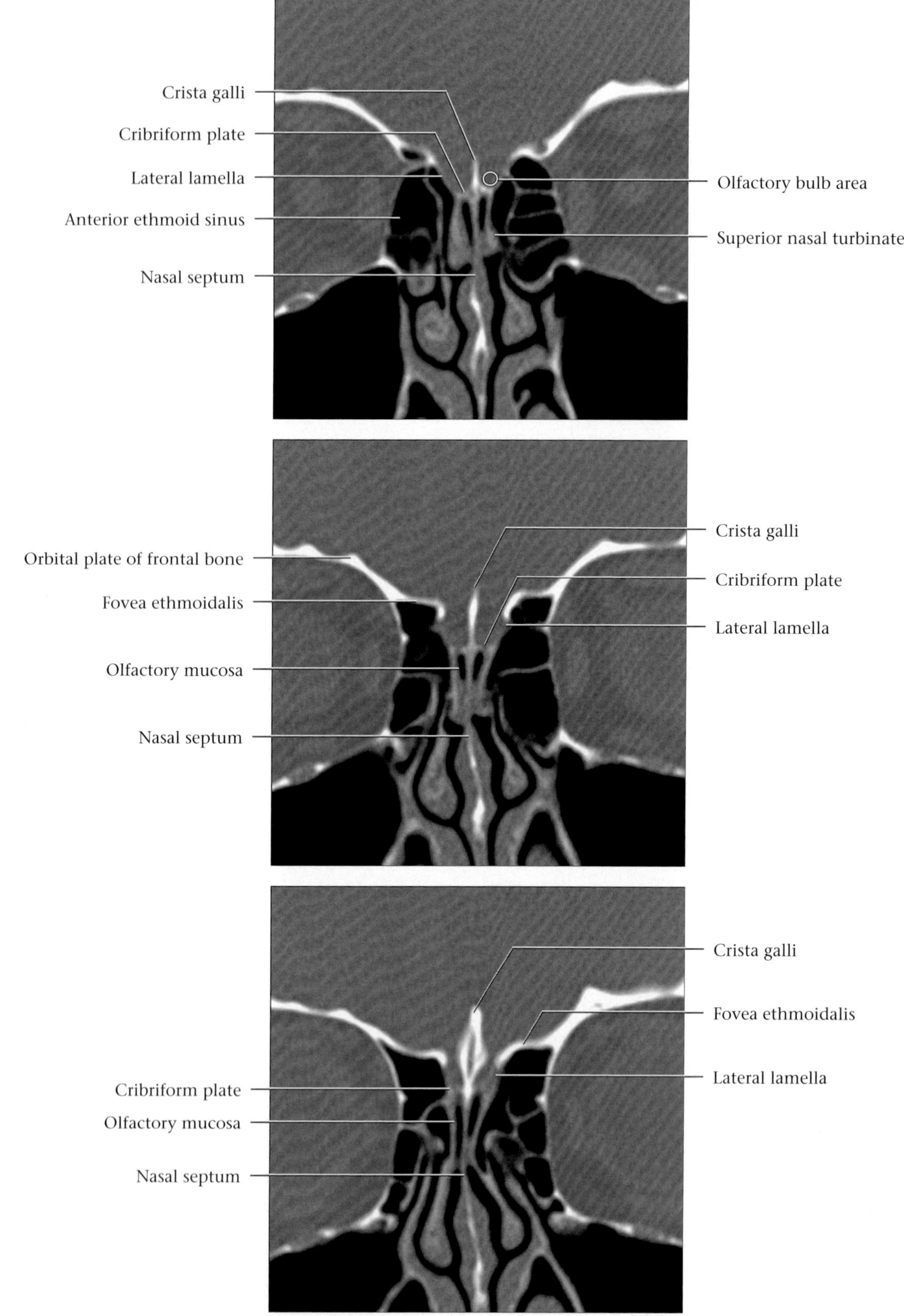
Crista galli
Cribriform plate
Lateral lamella
Anterior ethmoid sinus
Nasal septum
Olfactory bulb area
Superior nasal turbinate
Orbital plate of frontal bone
Fovea ethmoidalis
Olfactory mucosa
Nasal septum
Crista galli
Cribriform plate
Lateral lamella
Crista galli
Fovea ethmoidalis
Lateral lamella
Cribriform plate
Olfactory mucosa
Nasal septum

(Top) First of three coronal bone CTs through anterior cranial fossa presented from posterior to anterior. Olfactory epithelium is found on roof of nasal cavity, extending inferolaterally on superior turbinate and inferomedially on nasal septum. Olfactory nerves pass through perforations in cribriform plate. The olfactory bulbs sit just above the cribriform plates. **(Middle)** In this CT image ethmoid bone forms medial floor of anterior cranial fossa and consists of cribriform plate and crista galli. Fenestrated cribriform plate is depressed relative to orbital plate of frontal bone. Fovea ethmoidalis is most medial portion of orbital plate of frontal bone and separates ethmoid labyrinth from anterior cranial fossa. **(Bottom)** Anterior cribriform plate is seen at the base of the larger anterior crista galli.

CORONAL T2 MR

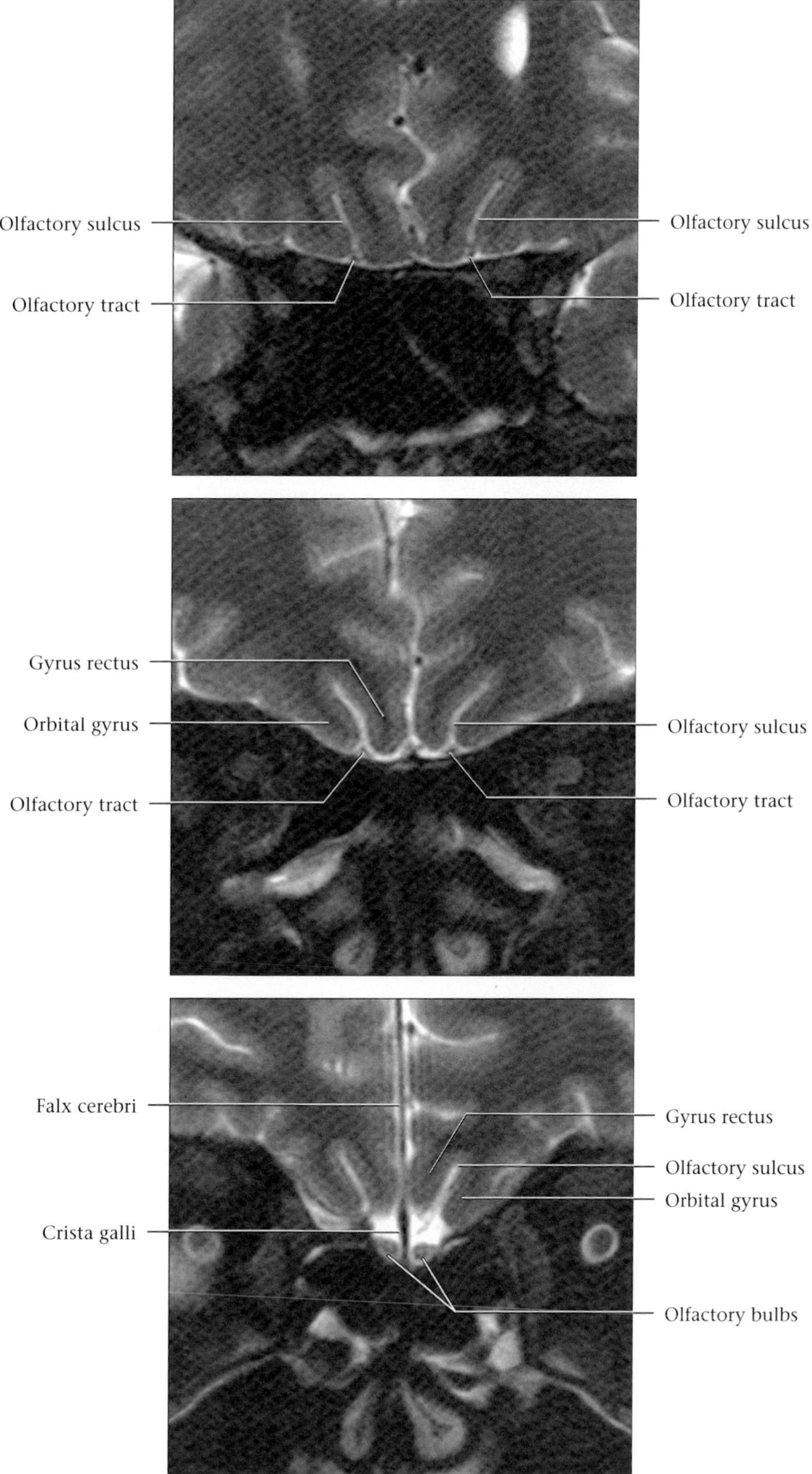
Olfactory sulcus
Olfactory sulcus
Olfactory tract
Olfactory tract
Gyrus rectus
Orbital gyrus
Olfactory sulcus
Olfactory tract
Olfactory tract
Falx cerebri
Gyrus rectus
Olfactory sulcus
Orbital gyrus
Crista galli
Olfactory bulbs

(Top) First of three sequential coronal T2 MR images presented from posterior to anterior shows triangular olfactory tracts which are comprised of centrally projecting axons, embedded within olfactory sulcus. **(Middle)** Olfactory sulcus is easily identified separating gyrus rectus medially from orbital gyrus laterally. Again note the olfactory tracts at the base of the olfactory sulcus. **(Bottom)** In this image through the anterior cribriform plate note the olfactory bulbs. The olfactory bulbs are rostral enlargement of olfactory tracts which lie on either side of midline on intracranial surface of cribriform plate. Olfactory nerves arise from olfactory epithelium located in roof nasal cavity and pass through fenestrated cribriform plate to end in olfactory bulbs.

CN2 (OPTIC NERVE)

Terminology

Abbreviations

- Optic nerve: CN2, CN II

Synonyms

- Second cranial nerve

Definitions

- CN2: Nerve of sight
- Visual pathway consists of optic nerve, optic chiasm and retrochiasmal structures

Imaging Anatomy

Overview

- Optic nerve **not** true cranial nerve but rather **extension of the brain**
  - Represents collection of retinal ganglion cell axons
  - Myelinated by **oligodendrocytes** not by Schwann cells as with true cranial nerves
  - Enclosed by meninges
  - Throughout its course to visual cortex nerve fibers are arranged in **retinotopic order**
- Optic nerve has four segments
  - Intraocular, intraorbital, intracanalicular and intracranial
- Partial decussation CN2 fibers within optic chiasm
  - Axons from medial portion of each retina cross to join those from lateral portion of opposite retina
- Retrochiasmal structures: Optic tract, lateral geniculate body, optic radiation and visual cortex

Optic Pathway

- **Optic nerve: Intraocular segment**
  - 1 mm length
  - Region of sclera termed **lamina cribrosa** where ganglion cell axons exit globe
- **Optic nerve: Intraorbital segment**
  - 20-30 mm in length
  - Extends posteromedially from back of globe to orbital apex within intraconal space of orbit
  - CN2 longer than actual distance from optic chiasm to globe allowing for movements of eye
  - Covered by same 3 meningeal layers as brain
    - Outer dura, middle arachnoid and inner pia
    - Subarachnoid space (SAS) between arachnoid and pia contains cerebrospinal fluid (CSF); continuous with SAS of suprasellar cistern
    - Fluctuations in intracranial pressure transmitted via SAS of optic nerve-sheath complex
  - Central retinal artery
    - 1st branch of ophthalmic artery
    - Enters optic nerve about 1 cm posterior to globe with accompanying vein to run to retina
- **Optic nerve: Intracanalicular segment**
  - 4-9 mm segment within bony optic canal
  - Ophthalmic artery lies inferior to CN2
  - Dura of CN2 fuses with orbit periosteum (periorbita)
- **Optic nerve: Intracranial segment**
  - About 10 mm length from optic canal to chiasm
  - Covered by pia and surrounded by CSF within suprasellar cistern
  - Ophthalmic artery runs inferolateral to nerve
- **Optic chiasm**
  - Horizontally oriented; "X-shaped" structure within suprasellar cistern
  - Forms part of floor of 3rd ventricle between optic recess anteriorly and infundibular recess posteriorly
  - Immediately anterior to infundibulum (pituitary stalk), superior to diaphragma sellae
  - Anteriorly chiasm divides into optic nerves
  - In chiasm nerve fibers from the medial half of retina cross to opposite side
  - Posteriorly chiasm divides into optic tracts
  - Medial fibers of optic tracts cross in chiasm to connect lateral geniculate bodies of both sides (commissure of Gudden)
- **Optic tracts**
  - Posterior extension of optic chiasm
  - Fibers pass posterolaterally curving around cerebral peduncle and divide into medial and lateral bands
    - Lateral band (majority of fibers) ends in **lateral geniculate body** of the thalamus
    - Medial band goes by medial geniculate body to pretectal nuclei deep to superior colliculi
- **Optic radiation and visual cortex**
  - Efferent axons from lateral geniculate body form **optic radiations** (geniculocalcarine tracts)
  - Fan out from lateral geniculate body and run as broad fiber tract to calcarine fissure
    - Initially pass laterally behind posterior limb internal capsule and basal ganglia
    - Extend posteriorly around lateral ventricle passing through posterior temporal and parietal lobes
    - Terminate in calcarine cortex (primary visual cortex) on medial surface of occipital lobes

Anatomy-Based Imaging Issues

Imaging Recommendations

- CT best for skull base and optic canal bony anatomy
- MR for CN2, optic chiasm and retrochiasmal structures
  - Axial and coronal thin-section T2, T1 and T1 C+

Imaging Pitfalls

- Orbital CT may see subtle calcified optic sheath meningioma when MR may not

Clinical Implications

Clinical Importance

- Lesion location
  - Optic nerve pathology: **Monocular visual loss**
  - Optic chiasm pathology: **Bitemporal heteronymous hemianopsia** (loss of bilateral temporal visual fields)
  - Retrochiasmal pathology: **Homonymous hemianopsia** (vision loss in contralateral eye)
- Increased intracranial pressure transmitted along SAS of optic nerve-sheath complex
  - Manifests clinically as **papilledema**
  - Imaging shows flattening of posterior sclera, tortuosity and elongation of intraorbital optic nerves and dilatation of perioptic SAS

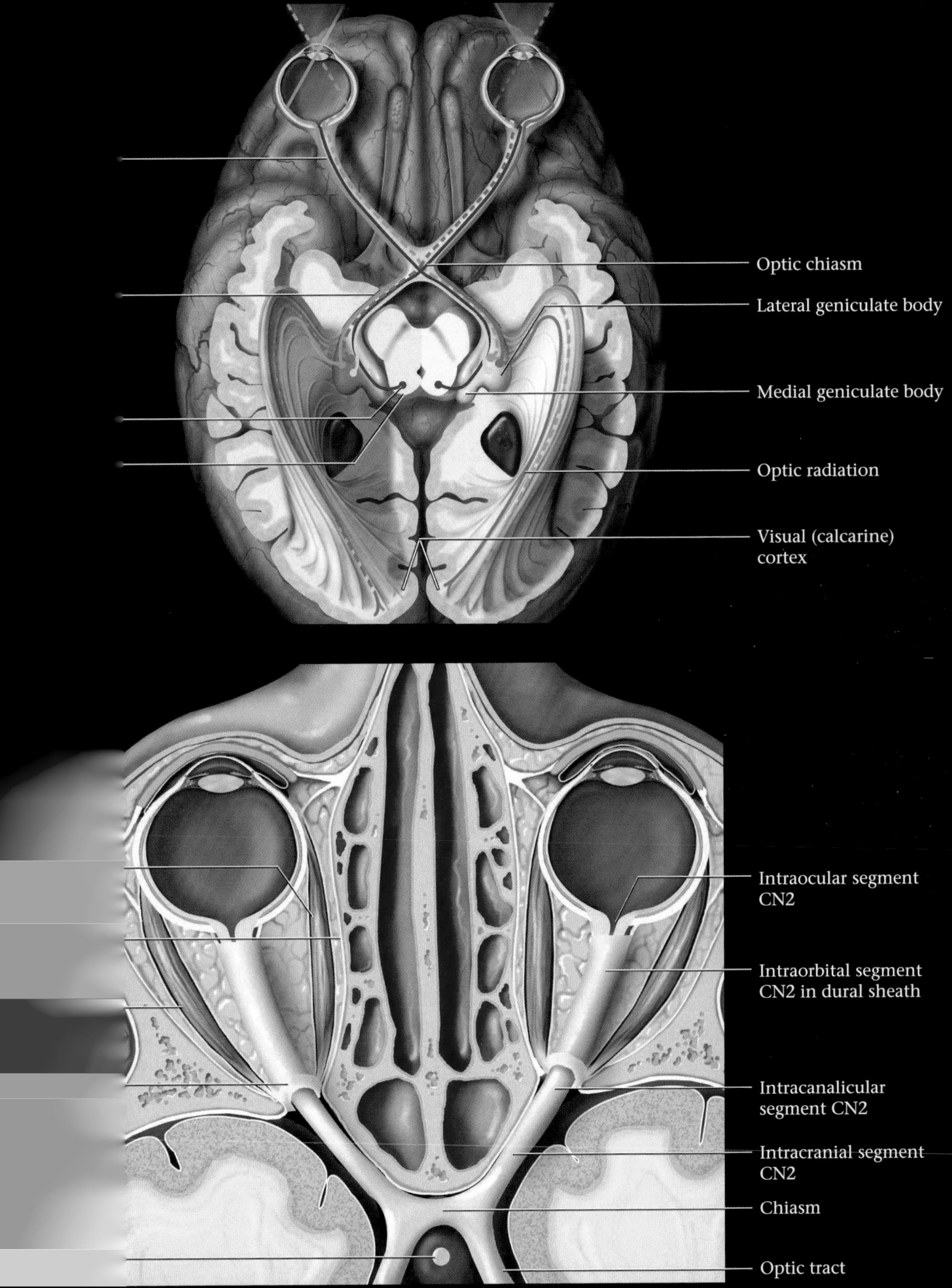
Optic chiasm
Lateral geniculate body
Medial geniculate body
Optic radiation
Visual (calcarine) cortex
Intraocular segment CN2
Intraorbital segment CN2 in dural sheath
Intracanalicular segment CN2
Intracranial segment CN2
Chiasm
Optic tract

gh visual pathway shows medial retinal fibers crossing in optic chiasm so that fibers from urse in left optic tract and fibers in right half of both retinas course in right optic tract vely). Majority of retinal nerve fibers terminate in lateral geniculate bodies, where new radiation, which extends to visual cortex. A few retinal nerve fibers (blue) involved in optic iculate bodies and terminate in pretectal nuclei. Medial fibers of optic tracts cross in chiasm ate bodies of both sides (yellow). **(Bottom)** Axial graphic of orbit shows the 4 segments of ntraorbital, intracanalicular and intracranial). At annulus of Zinn dural sheath of

GRAPHICS

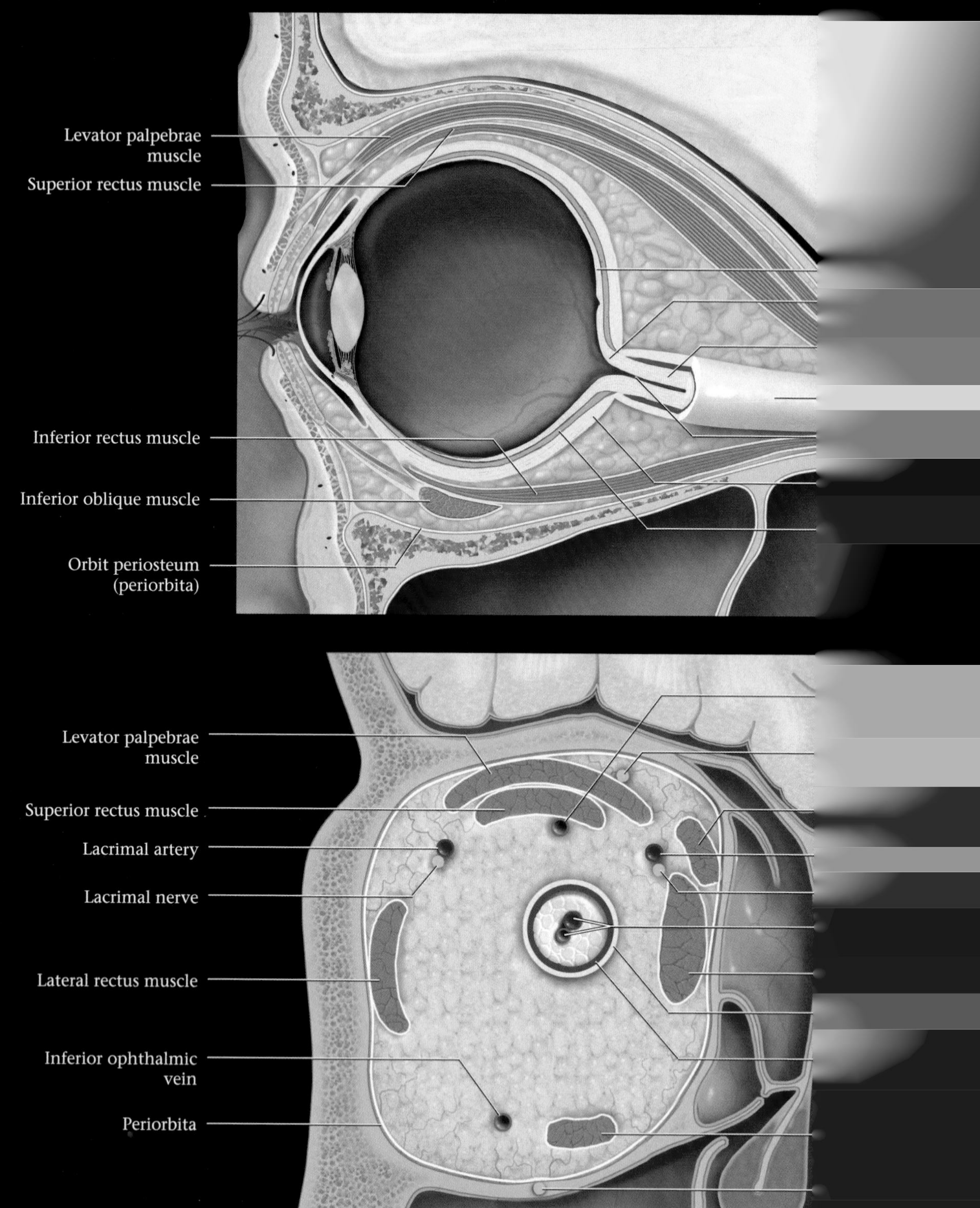
Levator palpebrae muscle
Superior rectus muscle
Inferior rectus muscle
Inferior oblique muscle
Orbit periosteum (periorbita)
Levator palpebrae muscle
Superior rectus muscle
Lacrimal artery
Lacrimal nerve
Lateral rectus muscle
Inferior ophthalmic vein
Periorbita

(Top) Sagittal graphic through the orbit shows continuity of dural sheath of intraorbital seg
At annulus of Zinn dural sheath is continuous with periorbita (not seen in this graphic). Ce
vein enter the distal intraorbital segment of CN2 to supply retina. **(Bottom)** Coronal graphi
nerve shows encasement of optic nerve by arachnoid and dura. Subarachnoid space of CN2
cerebral subarachnoid space. Central retinal artery and vein pierce dura of distal intraorbital

AXIAL STIR MR

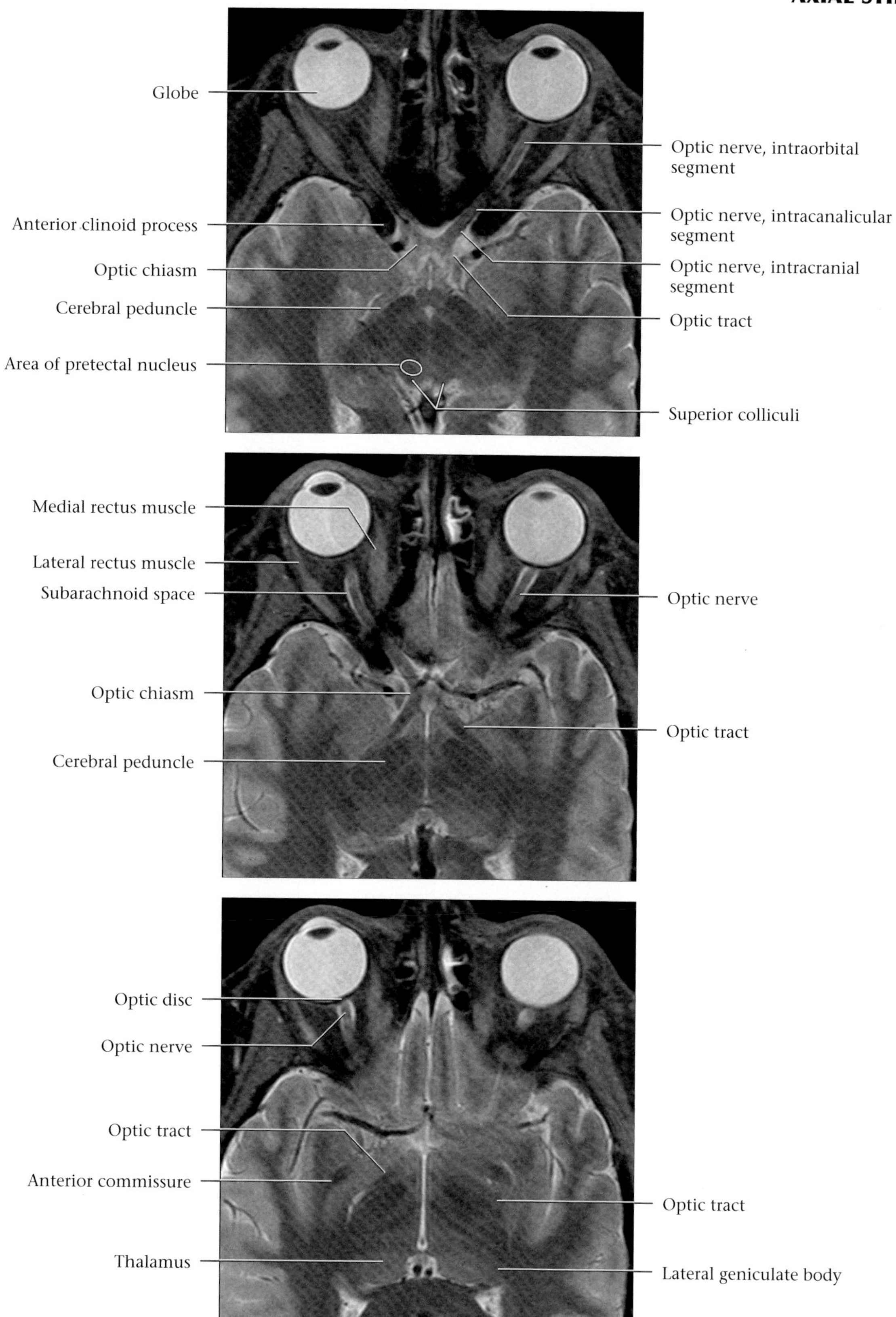
Globe
Optic nerve, intraorbital segment
Anterior clinoid process
Optic nerve, intracanalicular segment
Optic chiasm
Optic nerve, intracranial segment
Cerebral peduncle
Optic tract
Area of pretectal nucleus
Superior colliculi
Medial rectus muscle
Lateral rectus muscle
Subarachnoid space
Optic nerve
Optic chiasm
Optic tract
Cerebral peduncle
Optic disc
Optic nerve
Optic tract
Anterior commissure
Optic tract
Thalamus
Lateral geniculate body

(Top) First of three axial STIR MR images from inferior to superior demonstrate intraorbital, intracanalicular and intracranial segments of optic nerve. Intraorbital segment extends from back of globe posteromedially to orbital apex within intraconal space. Intracanalicular segment passes through bony optic canal. Intracranial segment is about 10 mm long from optic canal to chiasm. **(Middle)** Subarachnoid space with cerebrospinal fluid surrounds optic nerve and is continuous with subarachnoid space of suprasellar cistern. Optic chiasm lies within suprasellar cistern. Optic tracts extend posteriorly around cerebral peduncles to lateral geniculate body. **(Bottom)** Majority of fibers from optic tracts terminate in lateral geniculate body located at posteroinferior aspect of thalamus. Efferent axons from lateral geniculate body form optic radiation extending to calcarine cortex.

CN2 (OPTIC NERVE)

CORONAL T1 MR

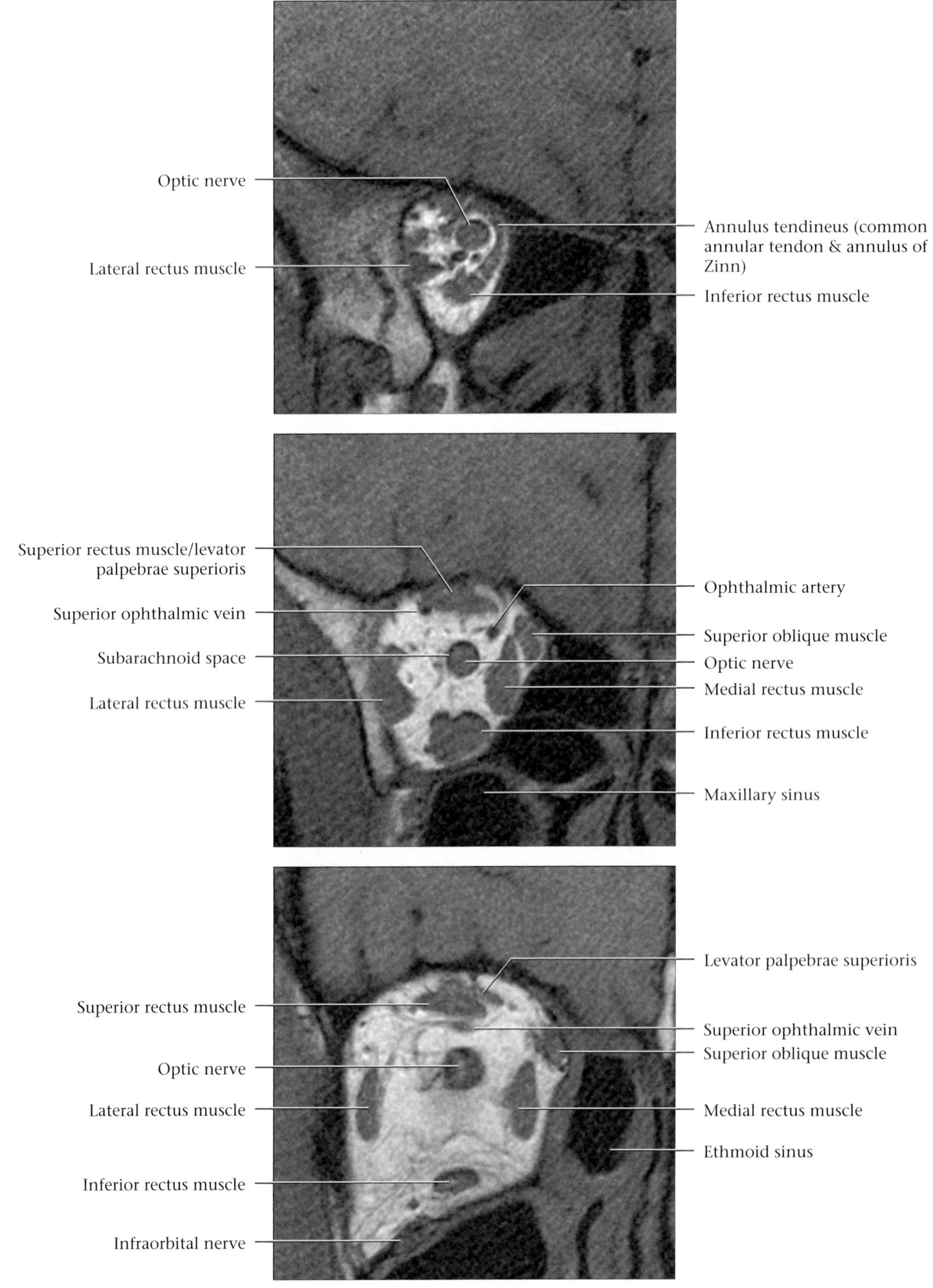
Optic nerve
Lateral rectus muscle
Annulus tendineus (common annular tendon & annulus of Zinn)
Inferior rectus muscle
Superior rectus muscle/levator palpebrae superioris
Superior ophthalmic vein
Subarachnoid space
Lateral rectus muscle
Ophthalmic artery
Superior oblique muscle
Optic nerve
Medial rectus muscle
Inferior rectus muscle
Maxillary sinus
Superior rectus muscle
Optic nerve
Lateral rectus muscle
Inferior rectus muscle
Infraorbital nerve
Levator palpebrae superioris
Superior ophthalmic vein
Superior oblique muscle
Medial rectus muscle
Ethmoid sinus

(Top) First of three coronal T1 MR images through orbit from posterior to anterior. Section through orbital apex shows optic nerve passing through common annular tendon which serves as site of origin of rectus muscles. **(Middle)** In this image both the superolateral ophthalmic vein and the superomedial ophthalmic artery are visible. Note that the subarachnoid space is visible as a thin black line surrounding the optic nerve, a finding often not seen on routine T1 imaging of the orbit. **(Bottom)** In this image just behind the globe all the extraocular muscles are clearly visible. Notice the levator palpebrae superioris muscle may be difficult to distinguish from the superior rectus muscle even with high resolution MR imaging.

CN2 (OPTIC NERVE)

CORONAL T2 MR

Optic tract
Basal vein
Oculomotor nerve (CN3)
Trigeminal nerve, preganglionic segment
Optic tract
Mamillary body
Posterior cerebral artery
Superior cerebellar artery
Trigeminal nerve
Pontine belly

Third ventricle
Optic tract
Oculomotor nerve (CN3)
Basilar artery
Basal vein
Optic tract
Uncus
Trigeminal nerve entering Meckel cave

Third ventricle
Optic tract
Tuber cinereum
Meckel cave

(Top) First of six coronal T2 MR images showing the optic tracts and chiasm from posterior to anterior. Optic tracts course posterolaterally curving around cerebral peduncle to eventually terminate in lateral geniculate body (lateral root) and pretectal nuclei at superior colliculi (medial band). **(Middle)** Optic tracts course through posterior suprasellar cistern towards ambient cistern closely related to basal vein (of Rosenthal). **(Bottom)** In this image through the back of the optic chiasm the optic tracts are shown as the posterior extension of optic chiasm carrying fibers from the ipsilateral half of both retinae. The tuber cinereum leads to infundibulum (pituitary stalk). Notice the third ventricle just above the posterior optic chiasm.

CN2 (OPTIC NERVE)

CORONAL T2 MR

Anterior cerebral artery
Optic chiasm
Suprasellar cistern
Cavernous internal carotid artery
Third ventricle
M1 segment, middle cerebral artery
Supraclinoid internal carotid artery
Infundibulum
Meckel cave

Suprasellar cistern
Oculomotor nerve (CN3)
Infundibulum
Anterior cerebral arteries
Optic chiasm
Internal carotid artery
Pituitary gland

Optic nerve, intracranial segment
Anterior clinoid process
Internal carotid artery
Cavernous internal carotid artery
Optic nerve, intracranial segment

(Top) In this image the optic chiasm is seen forming part of the floor of the third ventricle between optic recess anteriorly and infundibular recess posteriorly. It is immediately anterior to infundibulum (pituitary stalk). **(Middle)** Optic chiasm is horizontally oriented, "X-shaped" structure within suprasellar cistern. Nerve fibers from the medial halves of both retinae cross to continue to lateral geniculate bodies. Interruption of crossing chiasmatic fibers leads to bitemporal hemianopia. **(Bottom)** The intracranial segment of optic nerves are visible in this image. This segment is approximately 10 mm in length from optic canal anteriorly to optic chiasm posteriorly. Although not seen, they are covered by pia. The bright CSF within suprasellar cistern surrounds the nerves.

Lacrimal gland

Lateral rectus muscle

Retrobulbar Fat

Globe

Medial rectus muscle

Superior oblique muscle

Optic nerve, intraorbital segment

Ophthalmic artery

Optic nerve, intracanalicular segment

Lacrimal gland

Retrobulbar fat

Globe

Superior oblique muscle

Optic nerve

Superior ophthalmic vein

Levator palpebrae superioris

Globe

Superior rectus muscle

Optic nerve

Retrobulbar fat

Choroid

Sclera

Inferior rectus muscle

(Top) Axial T1 MR demonstrates intraorbital segment of optic nerve extending posteromedially from back of globe to orbital apex surrounded by fat within intraconal space. Note intracanalicular segment passing through bony optic canal. **(Middle)** Axial T1 MR image shows origin of optic nerve from globe. Nerve fibers of retina unite forming optic nerve before exiting eyeball through lamina cribrosa, a thin, perforated portion of sclera. In the superior orbit the lacrimal gland is seen in its superolateral fossa. **(Bottom)** Sagittal T1 MR image through optic nerve demonstrating intraorbital segment of optic nerve. Sclera of globe is hypointense while pigmented choroid of uvea is hyperintense due to T1 shortening effects of melanin.

CN3 (OCULOMOTOR NERVE)

Terminology

Abbreviations
- Oculomotor nerve: CN3; CN III

Synonyms
- Third cranial nerve

Definitions
- CN3: Motor nerve to extraocular muscles except lateral rectus (CN6) & superior oblique muscles (CN4); parasympathetic to pupillary sphincter & ciliary muscle

Imaging Anatomy

Overview
- Mixed cranial nerve (motor and parasympathetic)
- Four anatomic segments: Intra-axial, cisternal, cavernous and extracranial

Intra-Axial Segment
- **Oculomotor nuclear complex**
  - Paired paramedian nuclear complex
    - Located in midbrain anterior (ventral) to cerebral aqueduct at level of superior colliculus
    - Partially embedded in periaqueductal gray matter
    - Bounded laterally and inferiorly by medial longitudinal fasciculus
  - Consists of five individual motor subnuclei that supply individual extraocular muscles
- **Edinger-Westphal parasympathetic nuclei**
  - Located dorsal to oculomotor nuclear complex in poorly myelinated periaqueductal gray matter
  - Preganglionic parasympathetic fibers exit nucleus, course ventrally with motor CN3 fibers
  - Innervation of internal eye muscles (sphincter pupillae and ciliary muscles)
- Oculomotor fascicles course anteriorly through medial longitudinal fasciculus, red nucleus, substantia nigra and medial cerebral peduncle
  - Exit midbrain into **interpeduncular cistern**
- Parasympathetic Perlia nuclei
  - Located between the Edinger-Westphal nuclei
  - Thought to be involved in ocular convergence

Cisternal Segment
- Courses anterolaterally through interpeduncular and prepontine cisterns
- Passes between posterior cerebral (PCA) and superior cerebellar arteries (SCA)
- Courses inferior to posterior communicating artery and medial to free edge of tentorium cerebelli
- Crosses the petroclinoid ligament and penetrates dura to enter roof of cavernous sinus

Cavernous Segment
- Enters roof of cavernous sinus surrounded by narrow **oculomotor CSF cistern**
- Courses anteriorly through lateral dural wall of cavernous sinus
- CN3 remains most cephalad of all cranial nerves within cavernous sinus
- CN3 superolateral to cavernous internal carotid artery

Extracranial Segment
- CN3 enters orbit through **superior orbital fissure** and passes through annulus tendineus (annulus of Zinn)
- Divides into superior and inferior branches
  - Superior branch supplies levator palpebrae superioris and superior rectus muscles
  - Inferior branch supplies inferior rectus, medial rectus and inferior oblique muscles
- Preganglionic parasympathetic fibers follow inferior branch to ciliary ganglion of orbit
  - Postganglionic parasympathetic fibers continue as short ciliary nerves to enter globe with optic nerve
  - In globe short ciliary nerves to ciliary body and iris
  - Control papillary sphincter function and accommodation via ciliary muscle

Anatomy-Based Imaging Issues

Imaging Recommendations
- Bone CT best for skull base, bony foramina
- MR for intra-axial, cisternal, cavernous segments
  - Thin-section high-resolution T2 MR sequences in axial and coronal planes
    - Depicts cisternal CN3 surrounded by CSF with high contrast and high spatial resolution

Imaging "Sweet Spots"
- CN3 nuclear complex and intra-axial segment not directly visualized
  - Find periaqueductal gray matter to localize

Imaging Pitfalls
- Negative MR and MRA does **not** completely exclude posterior communicating artery aneurysm
  - Cerebral angiography still represents gold standard to exclude this diagnosis

Clinical Implications

Clinical Importance
- Uncal herniation pushes CN3 on petroclinoid ligament
- During trauma downward shift of brainstem upon impact can stretch CN3 over petroclinoid ligament
- CN3 susceptible to compression by PCA aneurysms
- CN3 neuropathy divided into **simple** if isolated and **complex** if with other CN involvement (CN4 & CN6)
  - **Simple** CN3 with pupillary involvement
    - Must exclude PCA **aneurysm** as cause
    - Explanation: Parasympathetic fibers are peripherally distributed
  - Simple CN3 with pupillary sparing
    - Presumed microvascular infarction involves vessels supplying core of nerve with relative sparing of peripheral pupillary fibers

Clinical Findings
- **Oculomotor ophthalmoplegia**
  - Strabismus, ptosis, pupillary dilatation, downward abducted globe and paralysis of accommodation

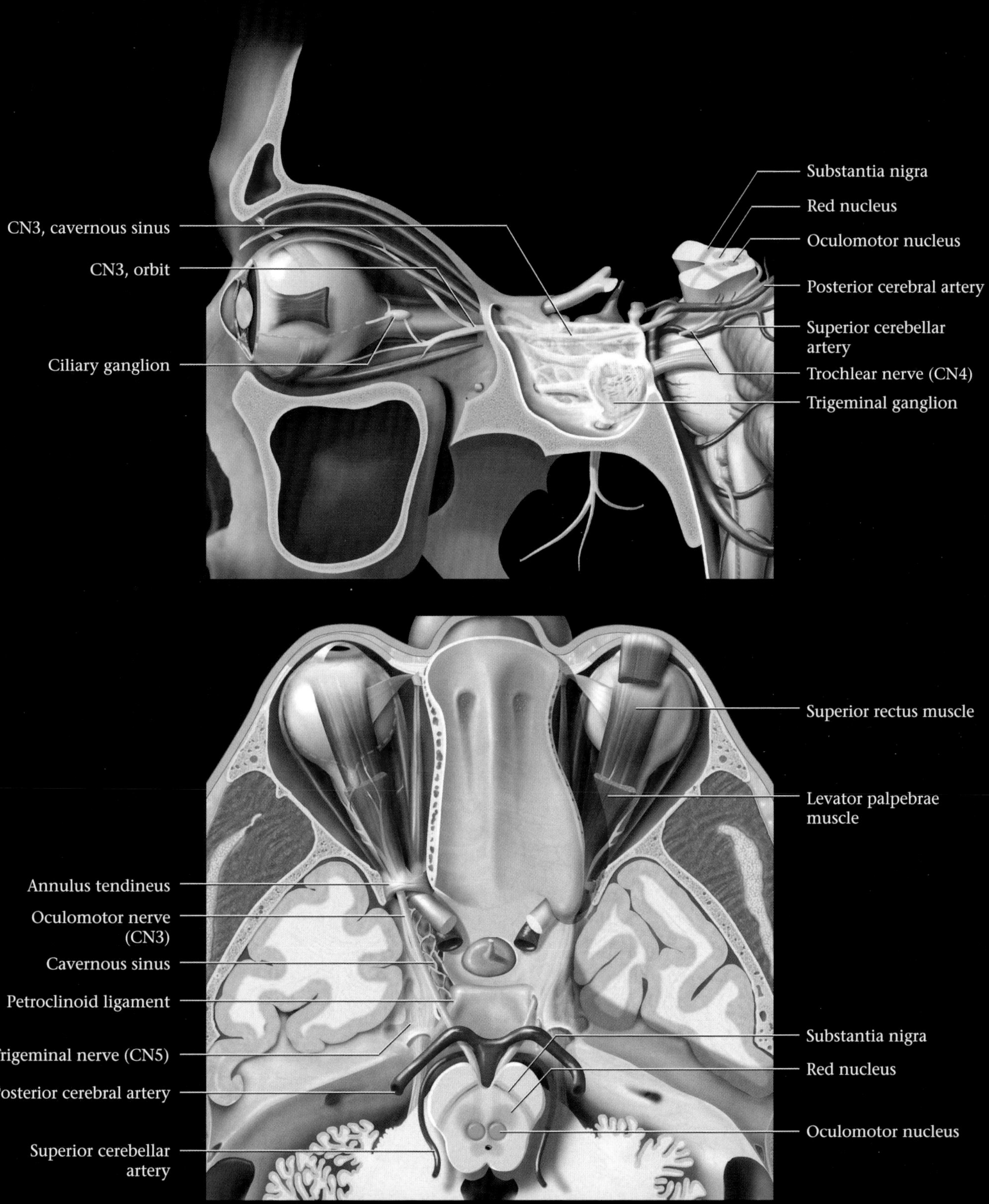

CN3, cavernous sinus
CN3, orbit
Ciliary ganglion
Substantia nigra
Red nucleus
Oculomotor nucleus
Posterior cerebral artery
Superior cerebellar artery
Trochlear nerve (CN4)
Trigeminal ganglion
Superior rectus muscle
Levator palpebrae muscle
Annulus tendineus
Oculomotor nerve (CN3)
Cavernous sinus
Petroclinoid ligament
Trigeminal nerve (CN5)
Posterior cerebral artery
Superior cerebellar artery
Substantia nigra
Red nucleus
Oculomotor nucleus

(Top) Sagittal graphic shows occulomotor nerve exiting from anterior brainstem. After passing medially to trochlear nerve (CN4) between superior cerebellar artery and posterior cerebral artery it enters cavernous sinus. CN3 is the most superior nerve coursing through cavernous sinus. Once in orbit it divides into superior and inferior divisions. Preganglionic parasympathetic fibers travel with inferior division to join ciliary ganglion. **(Bottom)** Axial graphic clearly depicts CN3 originating from the oculomotor nuclei complex to travel through medial aspect of red nucleus and substantia nigra before exiting into prepontine cistern. After traversing the cavernous sinus it enters the orbit through the superior orbital fissure through annulus tendineus (annulus of Zinn) to divide into superior and inferior branches.

CN3 (OCULOMOTOR NERVE)

AXIAL T2 MR

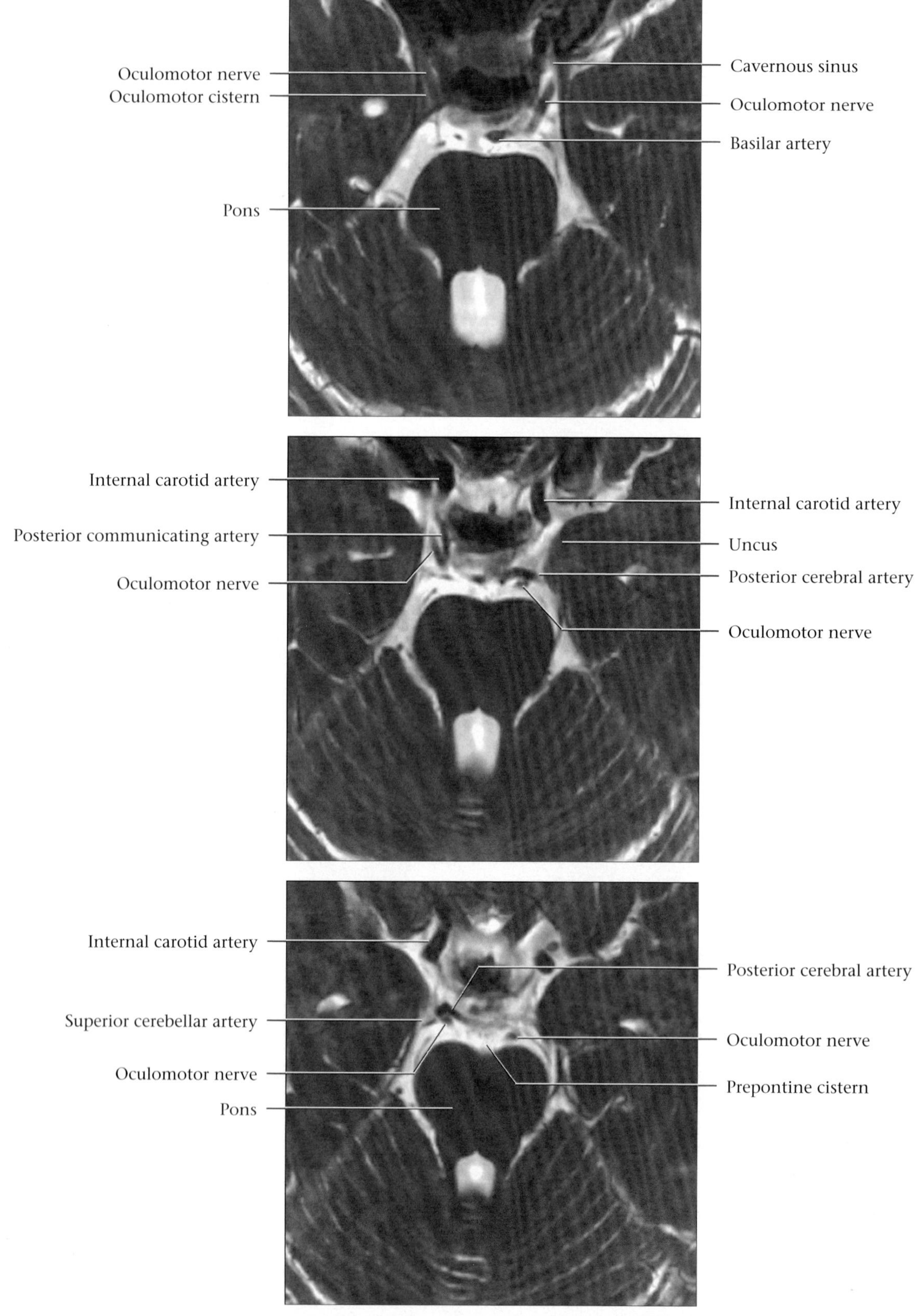
Oculomotor nerve
Oculomotor cistern
Cavernous sinus
Oculomotor nerve
Basilar artery
Pons
Internal carotid artery
Posterior communicating artery
Oculomotor nerve
Internal carotid artery
Uncus
Posterior cerebral artery
Oculomotor nerve
Internal carotid artery
Superior cerebellar artery
Oculomotor nerve
Pons
Posterior cerebral artery
Oculomotor nerve
Prepontine cistern

(Top) First of five axial T2 MR images presented from inferior to superior demonstrates the oculomotor nerves entering the oculomotor cisterns in the posterior roof of cavernous sinus. Notice the nerves are surrounded by high signal cerebrospinal fluid. From here the oculomotor nerves course anteriorly in the wall of the cavernous sinus above trochlear nerve and enters orbit via superior orbital fissure. **(Middle)** Oculomotor nerves course anteriorly through prepontine cistern inferolateral to posterior communicating artery and medial to uncus of temporal lobe. Left oculomotor nerve is seen passing below posterior cerebral artery. **(Bottom)** After exiting brainstem, oculomotor nerves course anteriorly through interpeduncular and prepontine cisterns towards cavernous sinus, passing between posterior cerebral and superior cerebellar arteries.

AXIAL T2 & T1 MR

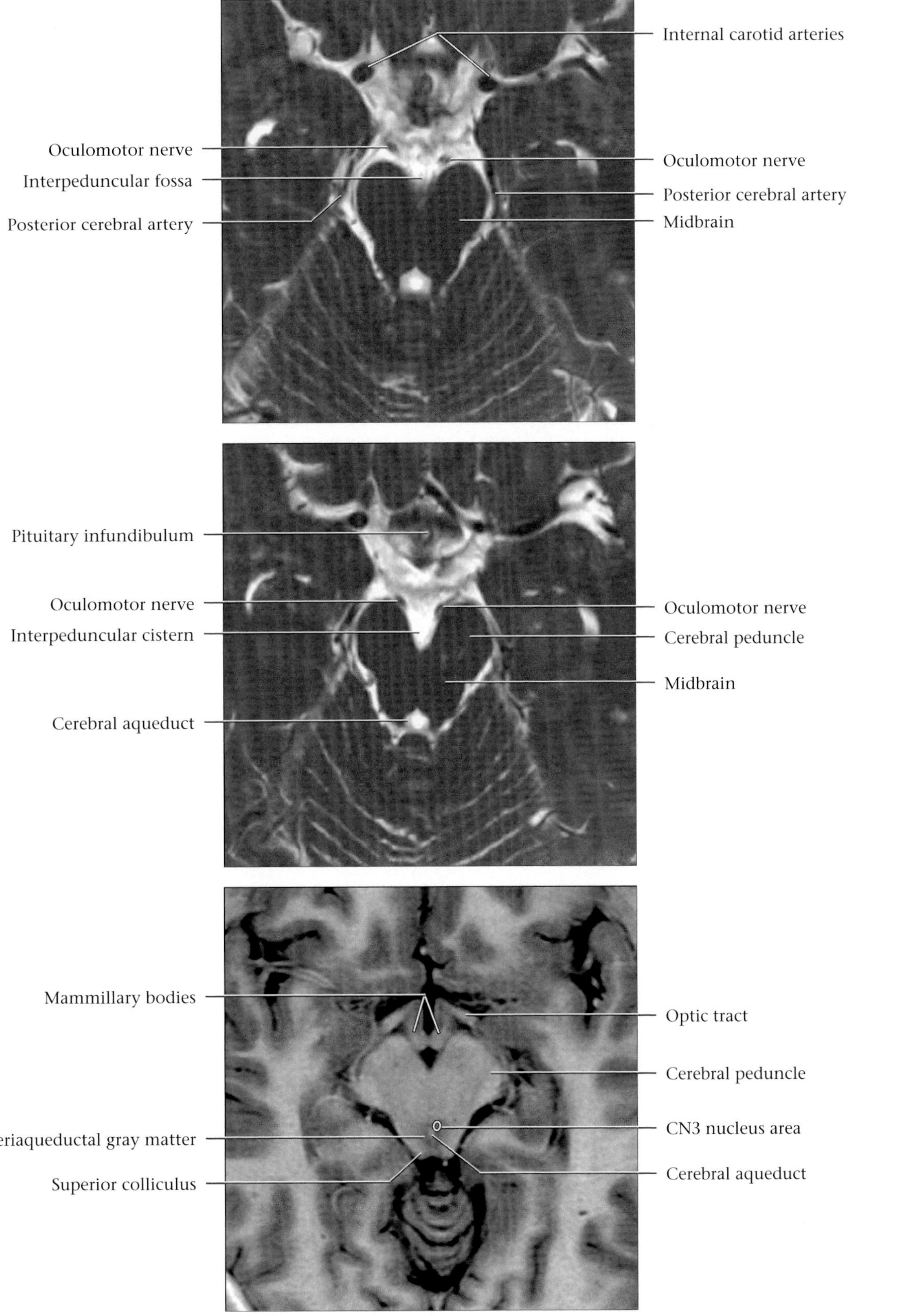

Internal carotid arteries
Oculomotor nerve
Interpeduncular fossa
Posterior cerebral artery
Oculomotor nerve
Posterior cerebral artery
Midbrain
Pituitary infundibulum
Oculomotor nerve
Interpeduncular cistern
Cerebral aqueduct
Oculomotor nerve
Cerebral peduncle
Midbrain
Mammillary bodies
Periaqueductal gray matter
Superior colliculus
Optic tract
Cerebral peduncle
CN3 nucleus area
Cerebral aqueduct

(Top) This image shows both oculomotor nerves coursing through the interpeduncular cistern. **(Middle)** Oculomotor nerves exit midbrain from medial surface of cerebral peduncle to enter interpeduncular cistern and continue anteriorly underneath the posterior cerebral arteries. **(Bottom)** Axial inversion recovery prepared T1 weighted MR image through brainstem at level of superior colliculus. Paired oculomotor nuclear complex is not directly visualized. However, since it is partially embedded in periaqueductal gray matter anterior to cerebral aqueduct at level of superior colliculus, its position can be inferred by these landmarks. Approximate location of oculomotor nucleus in marked on left.

CN3 (OCULOMOTOR NERVE)

CORONAL T2 MR

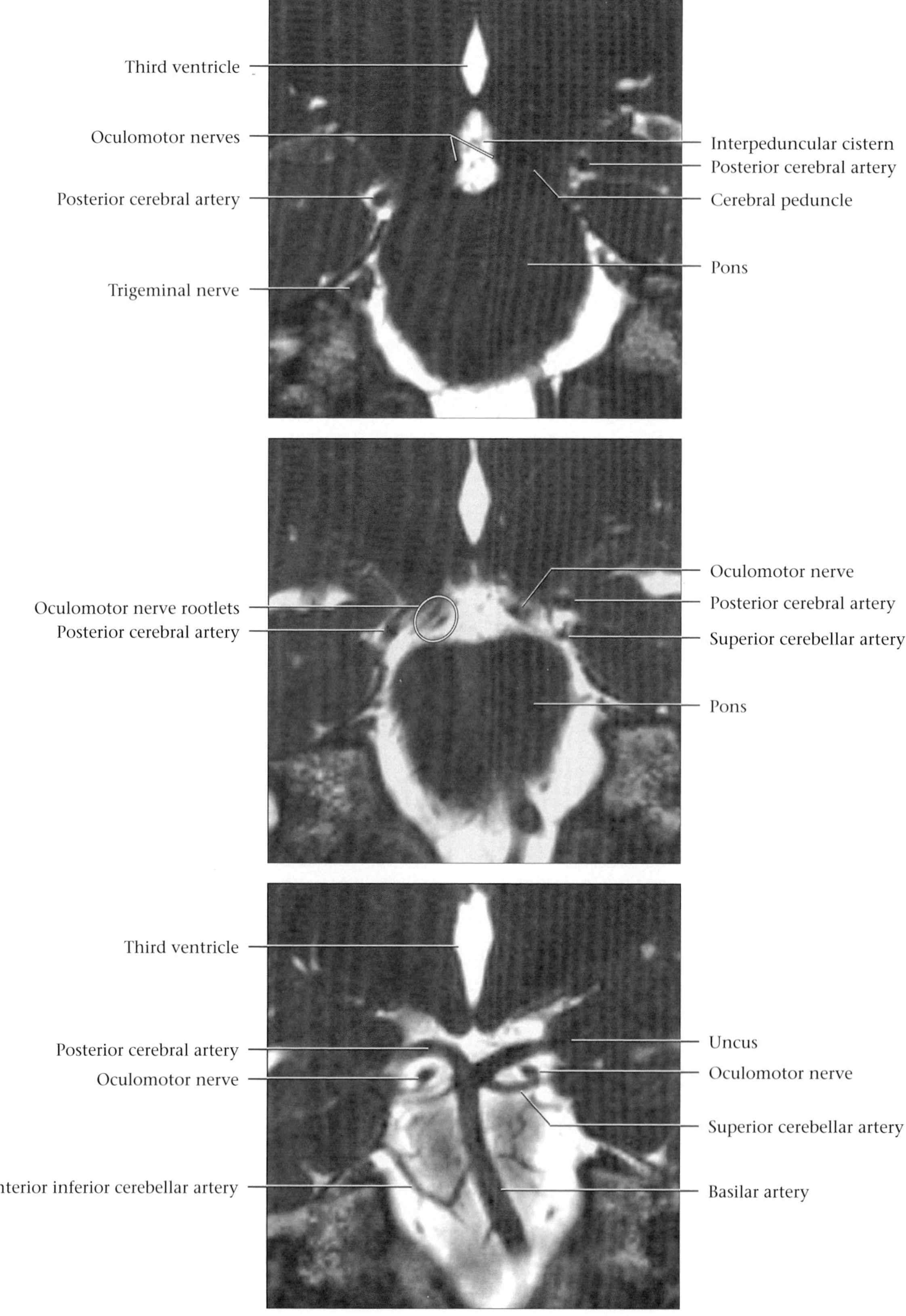

Third ventricle
Oculomotor nerves
Posterior cerebral artery
Trigeminal nerve
Interpeduncular cistern
Posterior cerebral artery
Cerebral peduncle
Pons
Oculomotor nerve rootlets
Posterior cerebral artery
Oculomotor nerve
Posterior cerebral artery
Superior cerebellar artery
Pons
Third ventricle
Posterior cerebral artery
Oculomotor nerve
Anterior inferior cerebellar artery
Uncus
Oculomotor nerve
Superior cerebellar artery
Basilar artery

(Top) First of six coronal T2 MR images presented from posterior to anterior reveals the most proximal aspects of both oculomotor nerves exiting the midbrain from the medial surface of cerebral peduncle to enter interpeduncular cistern. **(Middle)** Oculomotor nerves often emerge from midbrain by several rootlets as seen in this T2 coronal image (circle), which subsequently fuse to form a single trunk. **(Bottom)** Oculomotor nerves pass between posterior cerebral artery above and superior cerebellar artery below. Proximity of the oculomotor nerve to the uncus makes the nerve vulnerable to injury through uncal herniation. Its nearness to the posterior communicating, posterior cerebral and superior cerebellar arteries makes it easily injured by aneurysm.

CN3 (OCULOMOTOR NERVE)

CORONAL T2 MR

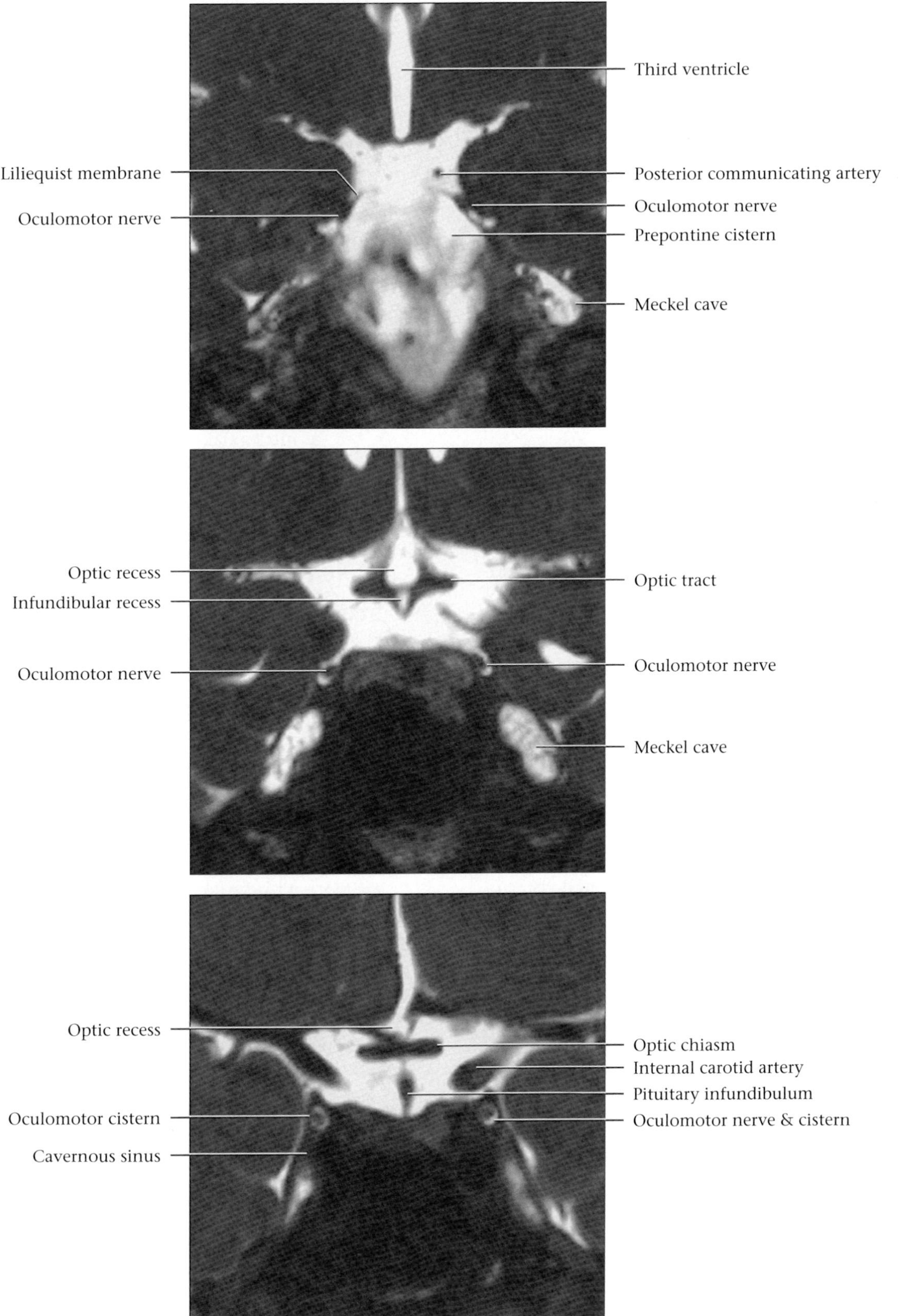

Third ventricle
Liliequist membrane
Posterior communicating artery
Oculomotor nerve
Oculomotor nerve
Prepontine cistern
Meckel cave
Optic recess
Optic tract
Infundibular recess
Oculomotor nerve
Oculomotor nerve
Meckel cave
Optic recess
Optic chiasm
Internal carotid artery
Pituitary infundibulum
Oculomotor cistern
Oculomotor nerve & cistern
Cavernous sinus

(Top) Oculomotor nerves are seen coursing through interpeduncular cistern towards cavernous sinus closely related to posterior communicating artery. An aneurysm of posterior communicating artery can result in compression of oculomotor nerve. Lateral margin of Liliequist membrane attaches to arachnoidal sheath surrounding oculomotor nerves. **(Middle)** The oculomotor nerve crosses petroclinoid ligament and is situated medial to and slightly beneath level of free edge of tentorium at point of entry into roof of cavernous sinus. **(Bottom)** A short length of oculomotor nerve is surrounded by a dural and arachnoid cuff to create the oculomotor cistern within roof and lateral wall of cavernous sinus. Oculomotor nerve courses anteriorly above trochlear nerve within lateral wall of cavernous sinus and enters orbit via superior orbital fissure.

CN4 (TROCHLEAR NERVE)

Terminology

Abbreviations

- Trochlear nerve: CN4, CN IV

Synonyms

- Fourth cranial nerve

Definitions

- CN4: Motor nerve to superior oblique muscle

Imaging Anatomy

Overview

- CN4 is a pure motor nerve
- Four segments: Intra-axial, cisternal, cavernous and extracranial

Intra-Axial Segment

- **Trochlear nuclei**
  - Paired nuclei located in paramedian midbrain
    - Anterior to cerebral aqueduct
    - Dorsal to medial longitudinal fasciculus
    - Caudal to oculomotor nuclear complex at level of inferior colliculus
- Trochlear nerve fascicles course posteriorly & inferiorly around cerebral aqueduct
  - Fibers then decussate within **superior medullary velum**
  - Key concept: Each superior oblique muscle is innervated by **contralateral** trochlear nucleus
- CN4 exists dorsal midbrain just inferior to inferior colliculus
  - Key concept: CN4 is the only cranial nerve to exit dorsal brainstem

Cisternal Segment

- CN4 courses anterolaterally in ambient cistern
  - Runs underneath the margin of the tentorium
  - Passes between free edge of tentorium cerebelli and midbrain just superolateral to pons
- Passes between posterior cerebral artery above and superior cerebellar artery below
  - Oculomotor nerve travels this gap as well
  - CN4 is just inferolateral to oculomotor nerve
- Penetrates dura to enter lateral wall of cavernous sinus just inferior to oculomotor nerve

Cavernous Segment

- Courses anteriorly through **lateral dural wall** of cavernous sinus
- Intracavernous relationships of CN4
  - Remains inferior to CN3
  - Superior to ophthalmic division of trigeminal nerve (CNV1)
  - Lateral to cavernous internal carotid artery

Extracranial Segment

- CN4 enters orbit through **superior orbital fissure** together with CN3 and CN6
- Crosses over CN3 and courses medially
- Passes **above** annulus of Zinn (CN3 and CN6 go through annulus)
- Supplies motor innervation to superior oblique muscle

Anatomy-Based Imaging Issues

Imaging Recommendations

- CT best for skull base, bony foramina
- MR best for brainstem, cisternal, cavernous and intra-orbital imaging
- Intra-orbital segment not visualized by any imaging modality or sequence

Imaging "Sweet Spots"

- CN4 nucleus and intra-axial segment not directly visualized
  - Nuclei position inferred by identifying periaqueductal gray matter and cerebral aqueduct at level of inferior colliculi on high-resolution MR
- MR for intra-axial, cisternal and cavernous segments
  - Thin-section high-resolution T2 and T1 C+ MR in axial and coronal planes
    - Coronal imaging margins: Fourth ventricle to anterior globe
    - Axial imaging margins: Orbital roof-diencephalon to maxillary sinus roof-medulla

Imaging Pitfalls

- Difficult to visualize CN4 despite best MR imaging efforts
- During image interrogation by radiologist, view known landmarks along its course
  - Midbrain → tentorial margin → cavernous sinus → superior orbital fissure → extraconal orbit

Normal Measurements

- CN4 is smallest cranial nerve
- CN4 has longest intracranial course (~ 7.5 cm)

Clinical Implications

Clinical Importance

- CN4 neuropathy divided into **simple and complex**
  - **Simple** CN4 neuropathy (isolated)
    - Most common form; usually secondary to trauma
    - Cisternal segment injury by free edge of tentorium cerebelli or from posterior cerebral or superior cerebellar artery aneurysm
    - Contusion of superior medullary velum
  - **Complex** CN4 neuropathy (associated with other CN injury, CN3 ± CN6)
    - Brainstem stoke or tumor
    - Cavernous sinus thrombosis, tumor
    - Orbital tumor

Clinical Findings

- Paralysis of superior oblique muscle results in **extorsion** (outward rotation) of affected eye
- Extorsion is secondary to unopposed action of inferior oblique muscle
- Patient complaints: Diplopia, weakness of downward gaze, neck pain from head tilting
- Physical exam: Compensatory head tilt usually away from affected side

CN4 (TROCHLEAR NERVE)

GRAPHICS

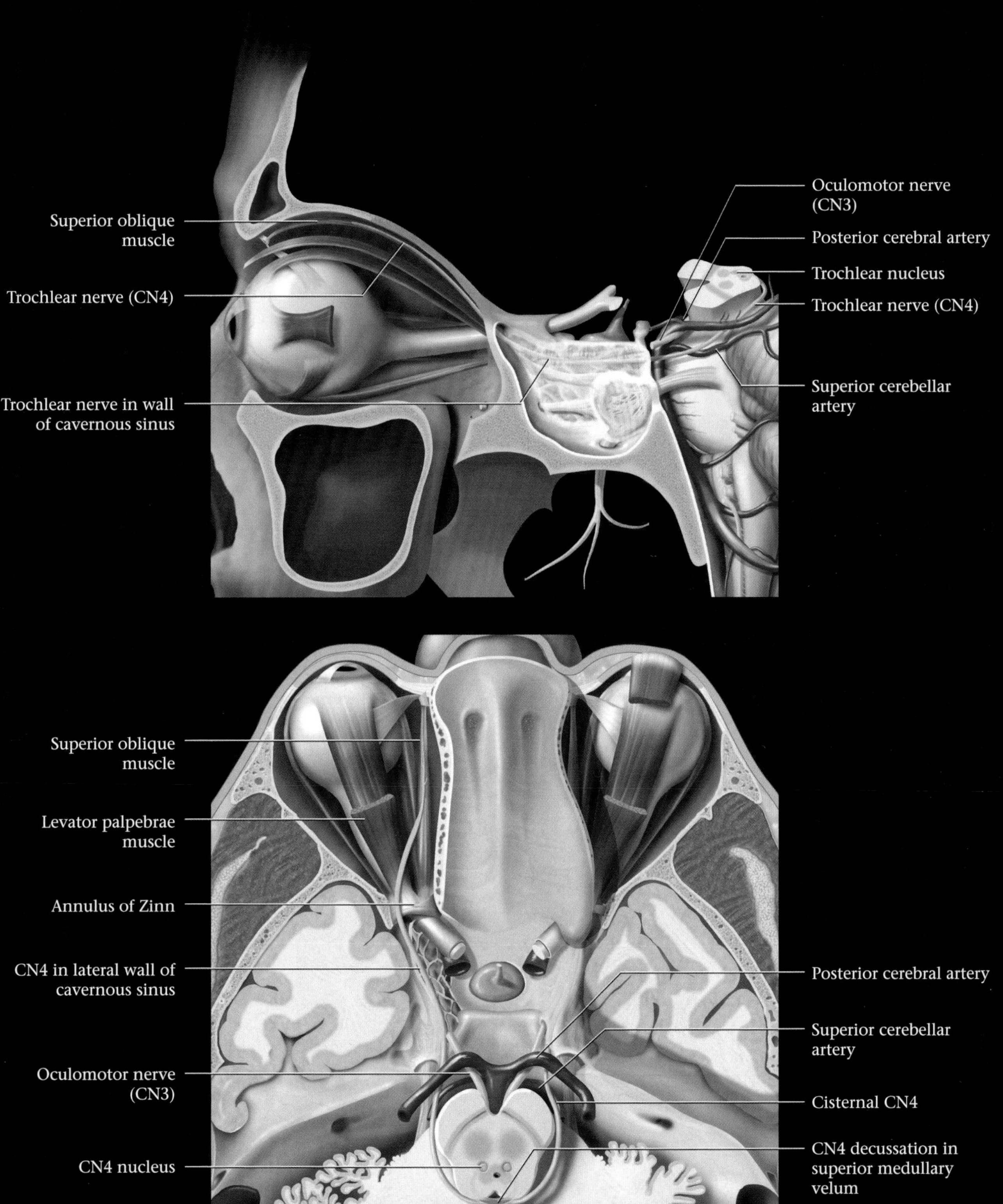

Superior oblique muscle
Trochlear nerve (CN4)
Trochlear nerve in wall of cavernous sinus
Oculomotor nerve (CN3)
Posterior cerebral artery
Trochlear nucleus
Trochlear nerve (CN4)
Superior cerebellar artery
Superior oblique muscle
Levator palpebrae muscle
Annulus of Zinn
CN4 in lateral wall of cavernous sinus
Oculomotor nerve (CN3)
CN4 nucleus
Posterior cerebral artery
Superior cerebellar artery
Cisternal CN4
CN4 decussation in superior medullary velum

(Top) Sagittal graphic shows trochlear nucleus gives rise to fibers that form contralateral trochlear nerve. After exiting dorsal brainstem, CN4 courses lateral to oculomotor nerve between posterior cerebral artery & superior cerebellar artery. After its long cisternal course CN4 enters cavernous sinus & runs inferolateral to CN3 and superior to ophthalmic division of trigeminal nerve (CNV1). **(Bottom)** Axial graphic shows trochlear nerves originating from the trochlear nuclei & decussating in the superior medullary velum. CN4 runs lateral to the oculomotor nerve between posterior cerebral artery and superior cerebellar artery to continue inferolateral with CN3 through cavernous sinus. It crosses over CN3 to enter orbit above annulus of Zinn, then courses medially over levator palpebrae muscle to innervate superior oblique muscle.

CN4 (TROCHLEAR NERVE)

AXIAL T2 MR

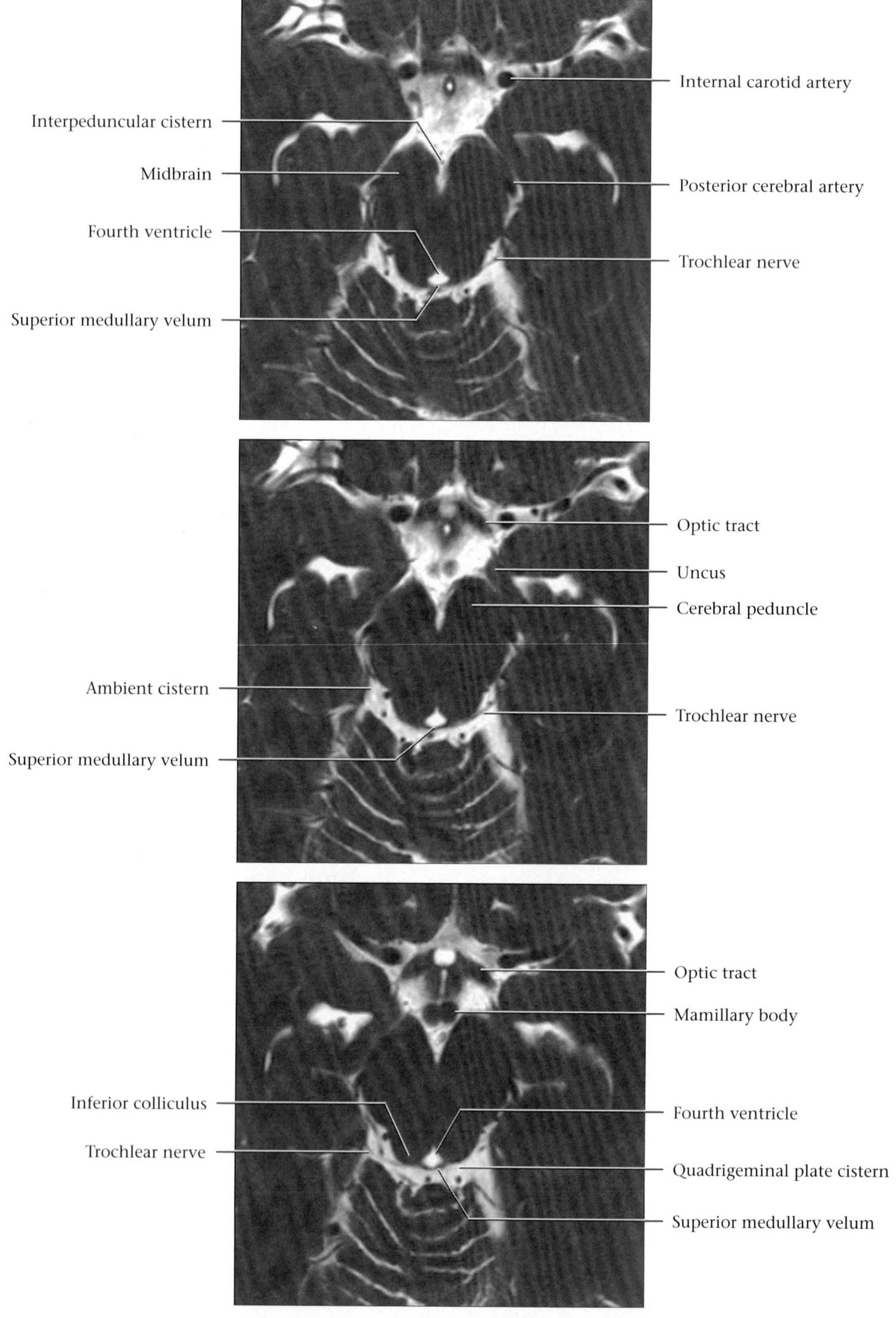
Internal carotid artery
Interpeduncular cistern
Midbrain
Posterior cerebral artery
Fourth ventricle
Trochlear nerve
Superior medullary velum
Optic tract
Uncus
Cerebral peduncle
Ambient cistern
Trochlear nerve
Superior medullary velum
Optic tract
Mamillary body
Inferior colliculus
Fourth ventricle
Trochlear nerve
Quadrigeminal plate cistern
Superior medullary velum

(Top) First of three axial T2 MR images presented from inferior to superior through midbrain. The left trochlear nerve passes around the brainstem within ambient cistern where it courses anteriorly below tentorium cerebelli. The trochlear nerves decussate in the superior medullary velum with fibers from the nucleus passing to the contralateral CN4. **(Middle)** Trochlear nerve (CN4) is smallest cranial nerve (0.75-1.00 mm diameter) and is not routinely visualized. In addition trochlear nerve may easily be confused with numerous small arteries and veins in the ambient cistern. **(Bottom)** After decussating in superior medullary velum, trochlear nerve exits dorsal surface of brainstem below the inferior colliculus to enter quadrigeminal plate cistern. Trochlear nerve is only cranial nerve to exit dorsal brainstem.

CN4 (TROCHLEAR NERVE)

CORONAL T2 MR

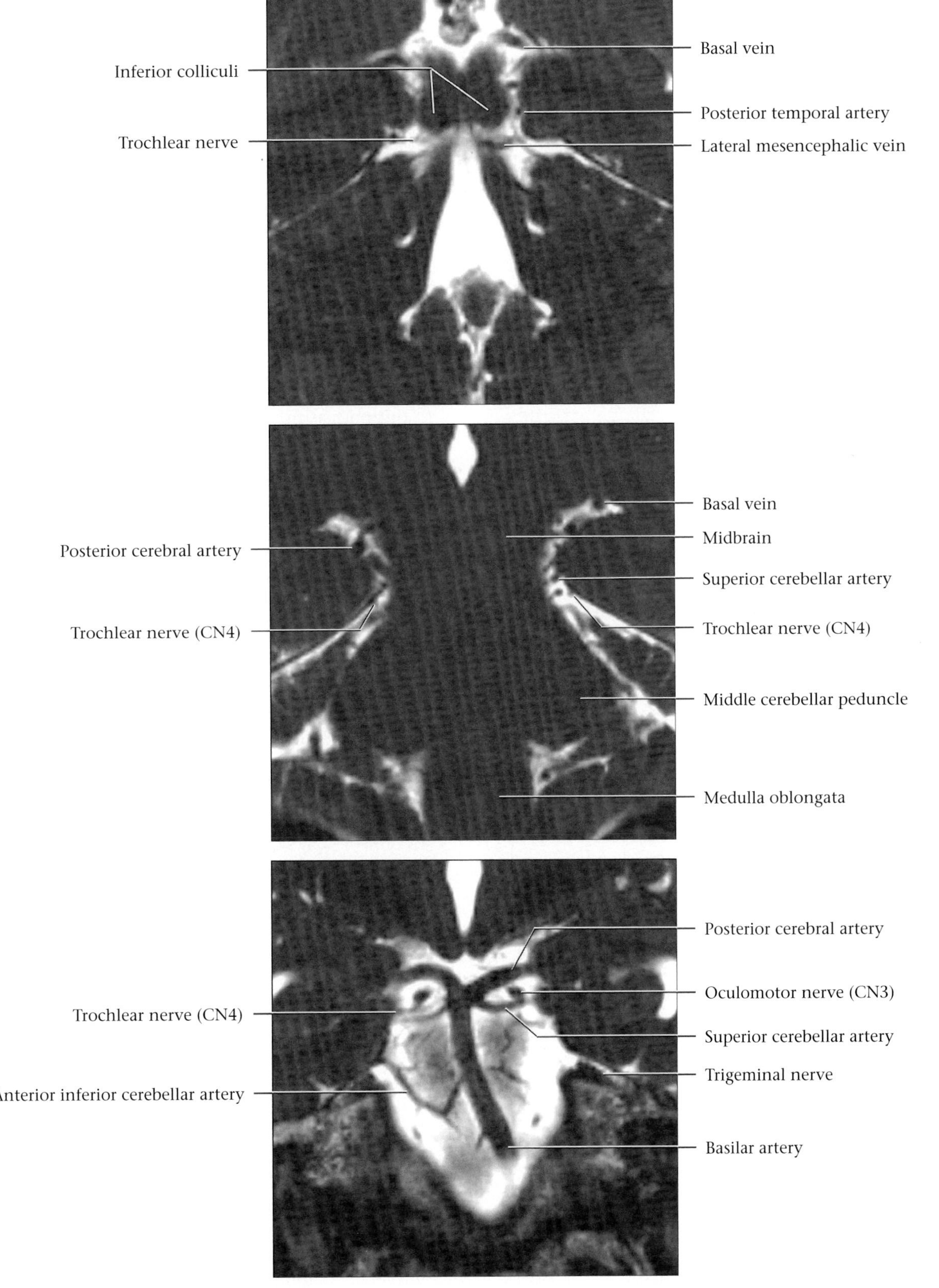
Inferior colliculi
Trochlear nerve
Basal vein
Posterior temporal artery
Lateral mesencephalic vein
Posterior cerebral artery
Trochlear nerve (CN4)
Basal vein
Midbrain
Superior cerebellar artery
Trochlear nerve (CN4)
Middle cerebellar peduncle
Medulla oblongata
Trochlear nerve (CN4)
Anterior inferior cerebellar artery
Posterior cerebral artery
Oculomotor nerve (CN3)
Superior cerebellar artery
Trigeminal nerve
Basilar artery

(Top) First of three coronal T2 MR images from posterior to anterior through brainstem demonstrates right the trochlear nerve exiting from dorsal brainstem below inferior colliculus as multiple discrete rootlets to enter quadrigeminal plate cistern. Left trochlear nerve is obscured by lateral mesencephalic vein. **(Middle)** Trochlear nerves can be visualized bilaterally coursing anteriorly within the ambient cistern below free margin of tentorium cerebelli. Only very focused thin-section high-resolution T2 MR imaging has any chance of seeing CN4 in this location. **(Bottom)** At the level of the basilar artery the trochlear nerve is hidden on the left but visible on the right inferolateral to the oculomotor nerve. Both nerves pass between the posterior cerebral artery and the superior cerebellar artery.

CN5 (TRIGEMINAL NERVE)

Terminology

Abbreviations

- Trigeminal nerve: CN5, CNV
- Ophthalmic division, trigeminal nerve: CNV1
- Maxillary division, trigeminal nerve: CNV2
- Mandibular division, trigeminal nerve: CNV3

Synonyms

- Fifth cranial nerve, nervus trigeminus

Definitions

- CN5: Great sensory cranial nerve of head and face; motor nerve for muscles of mastication

Imaging Anatomy

Overview

- Mixed nerve (both sensory, motor components)
- Four segments: Intra-axial, cisternal, interdural and extracranial

Intra-Axial Segment

- Four nuclei (3 sensory, 1 motor)
- Located in brainstem, upper cervical cord
  - **Mesencephalic nucleus CN5**
    - Slender column of cells projecting cephalad from pons to level of inferior colliculus
    - Found anterior to upper fourth ventricle/aqueduct near lateral margin of central gray
    - Afferent fibers for **facial proprioception** (teeth, hard palate and temporomandibular joint)
    - Sickle-shaped mesencephalic tract descends to motor nucleus, conveys impulses that **control mastication and bite force**
  - **Main sensory nucleus CN5**
    - Nucleus lies lateral to entering trigeminal root
    - Provides **facial tactile sensation**
  - **Motor nucleus CN5**
    - Ovoid column of cells anteromedial to principal sensory nucleus
    - Supplies **muscles of mastication** (medial/lateral pterygoids, masseter, temporalis), tensor palatine/tensor tympani, mylohyoid and anterior belly of digastric
  - **Spinal nucleus CN5**
    - Extends from principal sensory root in pons into upper cervical cord (between C2 to C4 level)
    - Conveys **facial pain, temperature**

Cisternal (Preganglionic) Segment

- Two roots: Smaller motor, larger sensory
- Emerges from lateral pons at **root entry zone** (REZ)
- Courses anterosuperiorly through prepontine cistern
- Enters middle cranial fossa by passing beneath tentorium at apex of petrous temporal bone
- Passes through an opening in dura matter called **porus trigeminus** to enter Meckel cave

Interdural Segment

- **Meckel cave** formed by meningeal layer of dura lined by arachnoid
  - Cave is filled with cerebrospinal fluid (CSF) (90%) and continuous with prepontine subarachnoid space
- Pia covers CN5 in trigeminal cave
- Preganglionic CN5 ends at **trigeminal ganglion** (TG)
  - TG located in inferior aspect of Meckel cave
  - TG synonyms: Gasserian or semilunar ganglion

Divisions (Post-Ganglionic) of CN5

- **Ophthalmic nerve**
  - Courses in lateral cavernous sinus wall below CN4
  - Exits skull through superior orbital fissure
  - Enters orbit, divides into lacrimal, frontal and nasociliary nerves
    - **Sensory** innervation **scalp, forehead, nose, globe**
- **Maxillary nerve**
  - Courses in cavernous sinus lateral wall below CNV1
  - Exits skull through **foramen rotundum**
  - Traverses roof of pterygopalatine fossa
  - Continues as **infraorbital nerve** in floor of orbit
  - Exits orbit through infraorbital foramen
    - **Sensory** to **cheek and upper teeth**
- **Mandibular nerve**
  - Does **not** pass through cavernous sinus
  - Exits directly from Meckel cave, passing inferiorly through foramen ovale into masticator space
  - Carries both motor and sensory fibers
    - Motor root bypasses TG, joins V3 as it exits through **foramen ovale**
    - Divides into masticator (muscles of mastication) and mylohyoid nerves (mylohyoid and anterior belly of digastric muscles)
    - **Masticator nerve** takeoff just below skull base
    - **Mylohyoid nerve** takeoff at mandibular foramen
  - Main sensory branches include inferior alveolar, lingual and auriculotemporal nerves

Anatomy-Based Imaging Issues

Imaging Recommendations

- CT best for skull base and bony foramina
- MR for intra-axial, cisternal and intradural segments
  - Thin-section T2 in axial and coronal planes
- T1 C+ fat-saturated MR of entire extracranial course

Imaging Pitfalls

- Trigeminal ganglion is small crescent of tissue found in the anteroinferior Meckel cave
  - Trigeminal ganglion lacks blood-nerve barrier therefore normally enhances with contrast

Clinical Implications

Clinical Importance

- Sensory complaints: Pain, burning, numbness in face
- Motor (V3 only): Weakness in chewing
  - Proximal V3 injury causes motor atrophy of masticator muscles within 6 weeks to 3 months
  - Distal V3 injury (above mylohyoid nerve takeoff) affects only anterior belly of digastric & mylohyoid
- Tic douloureux (trigeminal neuralgia)
  - Sharp, excruciating pain in V2-3 distributions
  - Look for vascular compression at REZ (on MR)

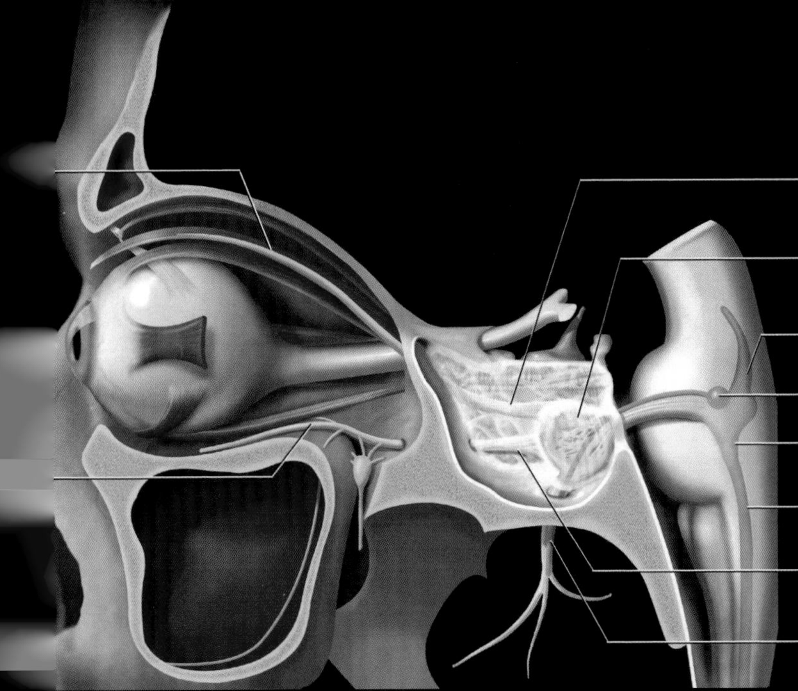
Ophthalmic division, CN5 (CNV1)
Meckel cave with trigeminal ganglion
Mesencephalic nucleus CN5
Motor nucleus CN5
Main sensory nucleus CN5
Spinal nucleus CN5
Maxillary division, CN5 (CNV2)
Mandibular division, CN5 (CNV3)

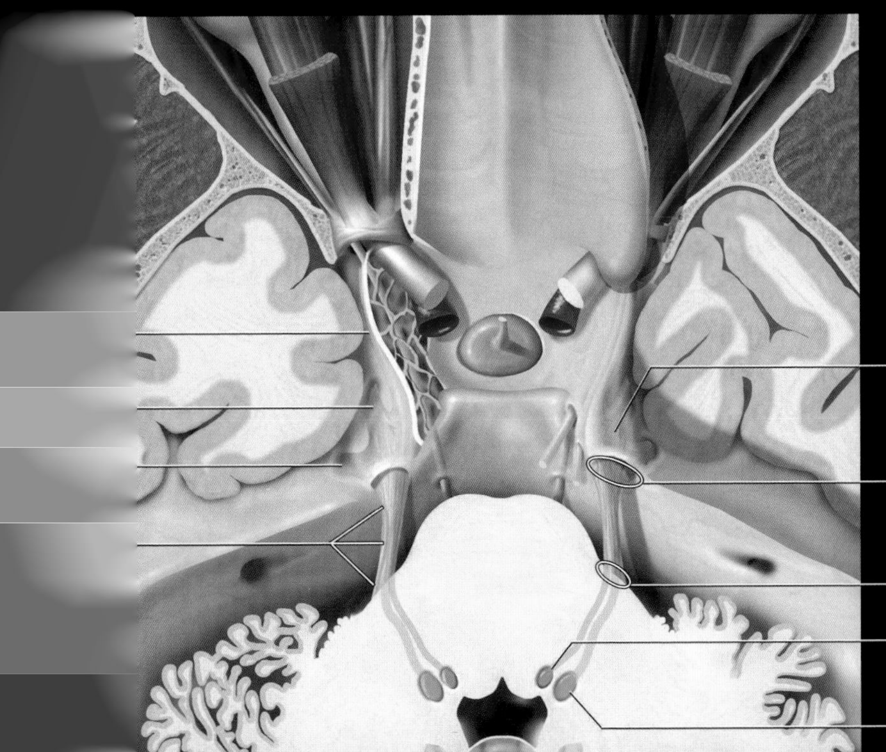
Trigeminal ganglion
Porus trigeminus
Root entry zone
Main motor nucleus CN5
Main sensory nucleus CN5

used on the four nuclei of the trigeminal nerve. From superior to inferior note the the midbrain, the motor nucleus and main sensory nucleus in the pons and the spinal he lower pons into the upper cervical spinal cord. The motor root of CN5 sends fibers along nly. **(Bottom)** Axial graphic depicting the course of the trigeminal nerve from its pontine motor nuclei) to its main three branches (CNV1, CNV2, CNV3). Notice the large iting the lateral pons at the root entry zone. It then enters Meckel cave through the porus trigeminal ganglion. Vascular loop irritation of the root entry zone is the most common

GRAPHICS

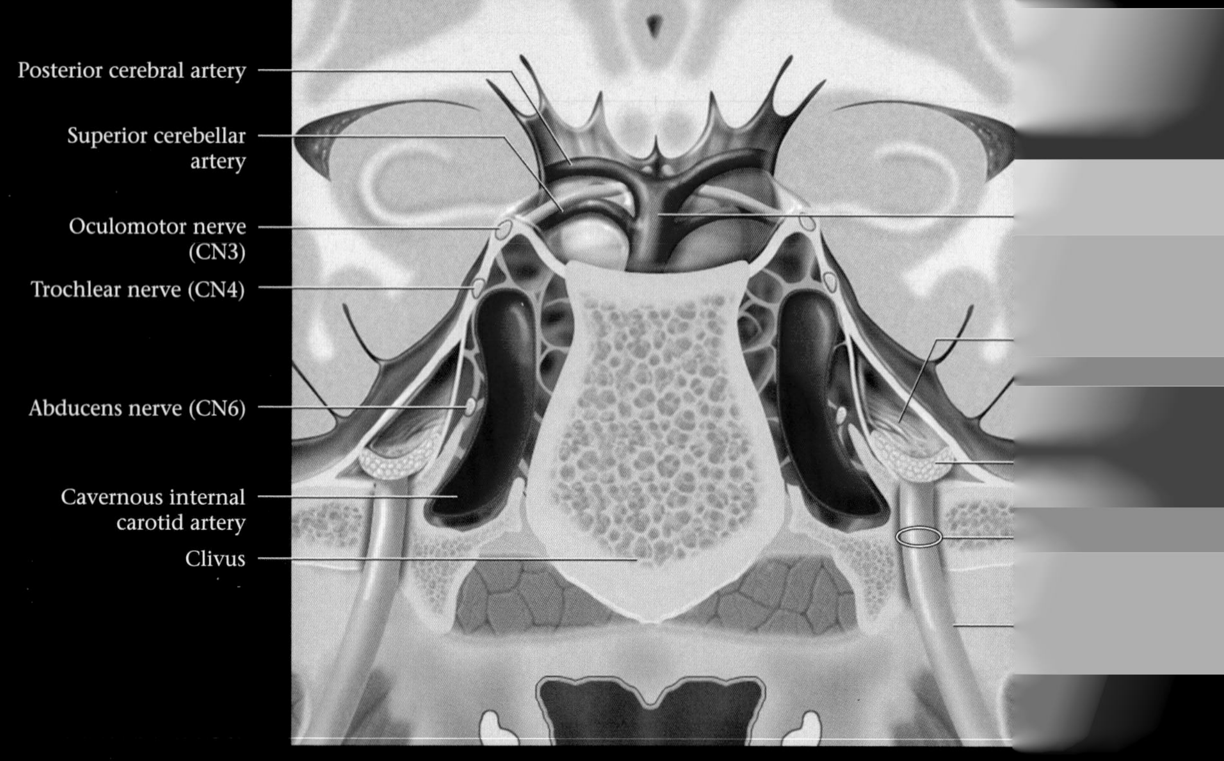
Posterior cerebral artery
Superior cerebellar artery
Oculomotor nerve (CN3)
Trochlear nerve (CN4)
Abducens nerve (CN6)
Cavernous internal carotid artery
Clivus

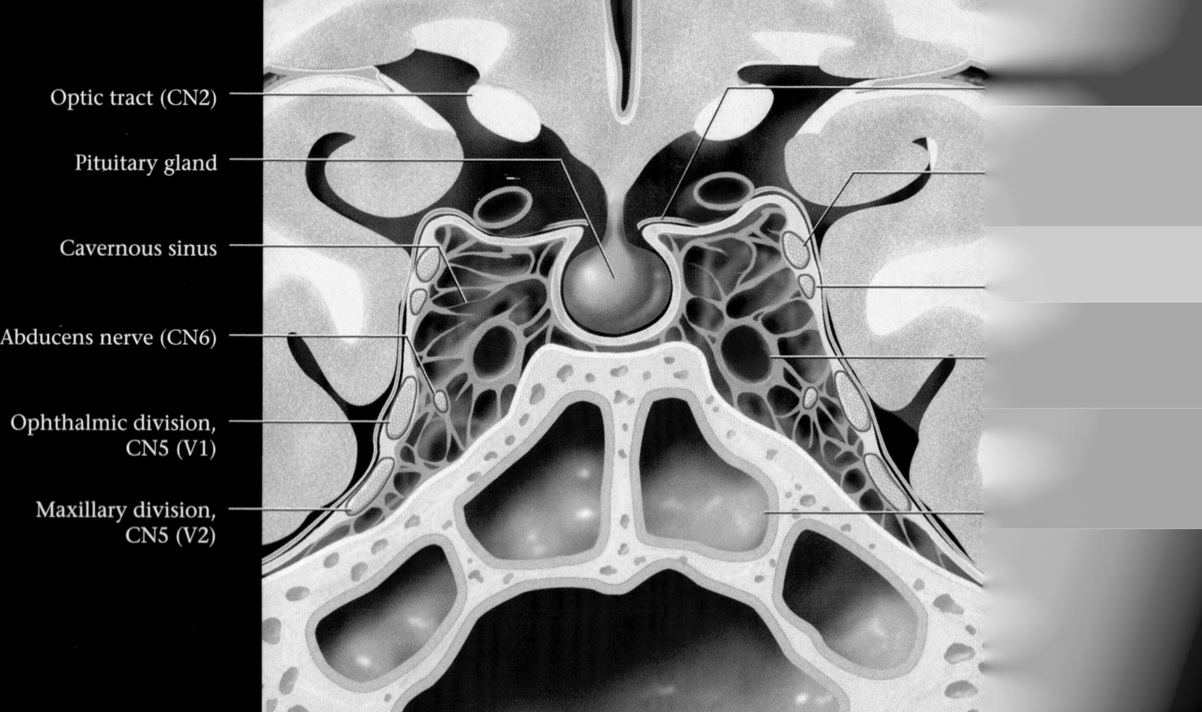
Optic tract (CN2)
Pituitary gland
Cavernous sinus
Abducens nerve (CN6)
Ophthalmic division, CN5 (V1)
Maxillary division, CN5 (V2)

(Top) Coronal graphic aimed at depicting the fact that the mandibular division of the triger
enters the cavernous sinus. Instead CNV3 exits directly from Meckel cave, passing inferiorly
into the nasopharyngeal masticator space. Meckel cave is actually a "pseudopod" of the later
containing both the trigeminal nerve rootlets and the trigeminal ganglion. Remember it is C
motor fibers of the trigeminal nerve. **(Bottom)** Coronal graphic through cavernous sinus sh
lateral wall of the cavernous sinus just inferior to CNV1. CNV1 is embedded in the lateral w
as are CN3 and CN4. The only centrally located intracavernous cranial nerve to be the abdu

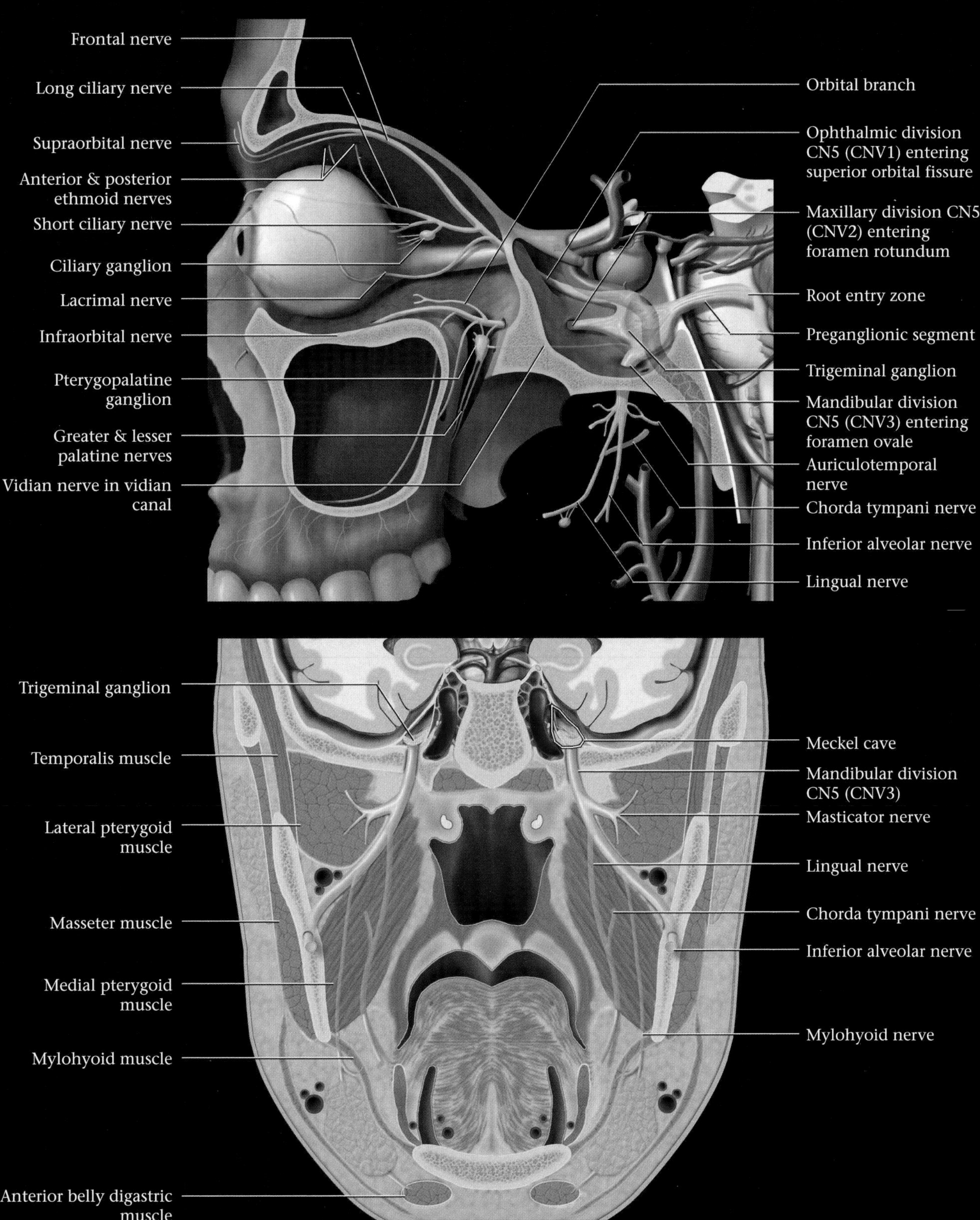

Frontal nerve
Long ciliary nerve
Supraorbital nerve
Anterior & posterior ethmoid nerves
Short ciliary nerve
Ciliary ganglion
Lacrimal nerve
Infraorbital nerve
Pterygopalatine ganglion
Greater & lesser palatine nerves
Vidian nerve in vidian canal
Orbital branch
Ophthalmic division CN5 (CNV1) entering superior orbital fissure
Maxillary division CN5 (CNV2) entering foramen rotundum
Root entry zone
Preganglionic segment
Trigeminal ganglion
Mandibular division CN5 (CNV3) entering foramen ovale
Auriculotemporal nerve
Chorda tympani nerve
Inferior alveolar nerve
Lingual nerve
Trigeminal ganglion
Temporalis muscle
Lateral pterygoid muscle
Masseter muscle
Medial pterygoid muscle
Mylohyoid muscle
Anterior belly digastric muscle
Meckel cave
Mandibular division CN5 (CNV3)
Masticator nerve
Lingual nerve
Chorda tympani nerve
Inferior alveolar nerve
Mylohyoid nerve

(Top) Sagittal graphic of trigeminal nerve showing the major branches and exiting foramina. The ophthalmic division of CN5 enters into the orbit via superior orbital fissure where it divides into frontal, ciliary and lacrimal branches. The maxillary division of CN5 exits via the foramen rotundum to become the infraorbital nerve as well as drop the greater and lesser palatine nerves inferiorly to provide sensation for the hard and soft palates. The mandibular division exits through foramen ovale, then divides into 2 main trunks, lingual and inferior alveolar nerves. **(Bottom)** Coronal graphic of the mandibular division of CN5. Notice CNV3 exits the skull base through the foramen ovale without entering the cavernous sinus. The two motor branches from CNV3 are the masticator nerve (to muscles of mastication) and the mylohyoid nerve (to mylohyoid and anterior belly of digastric muscle).

CN5 (TRIGEMINAL NERVE)

AXIAL BONE CT

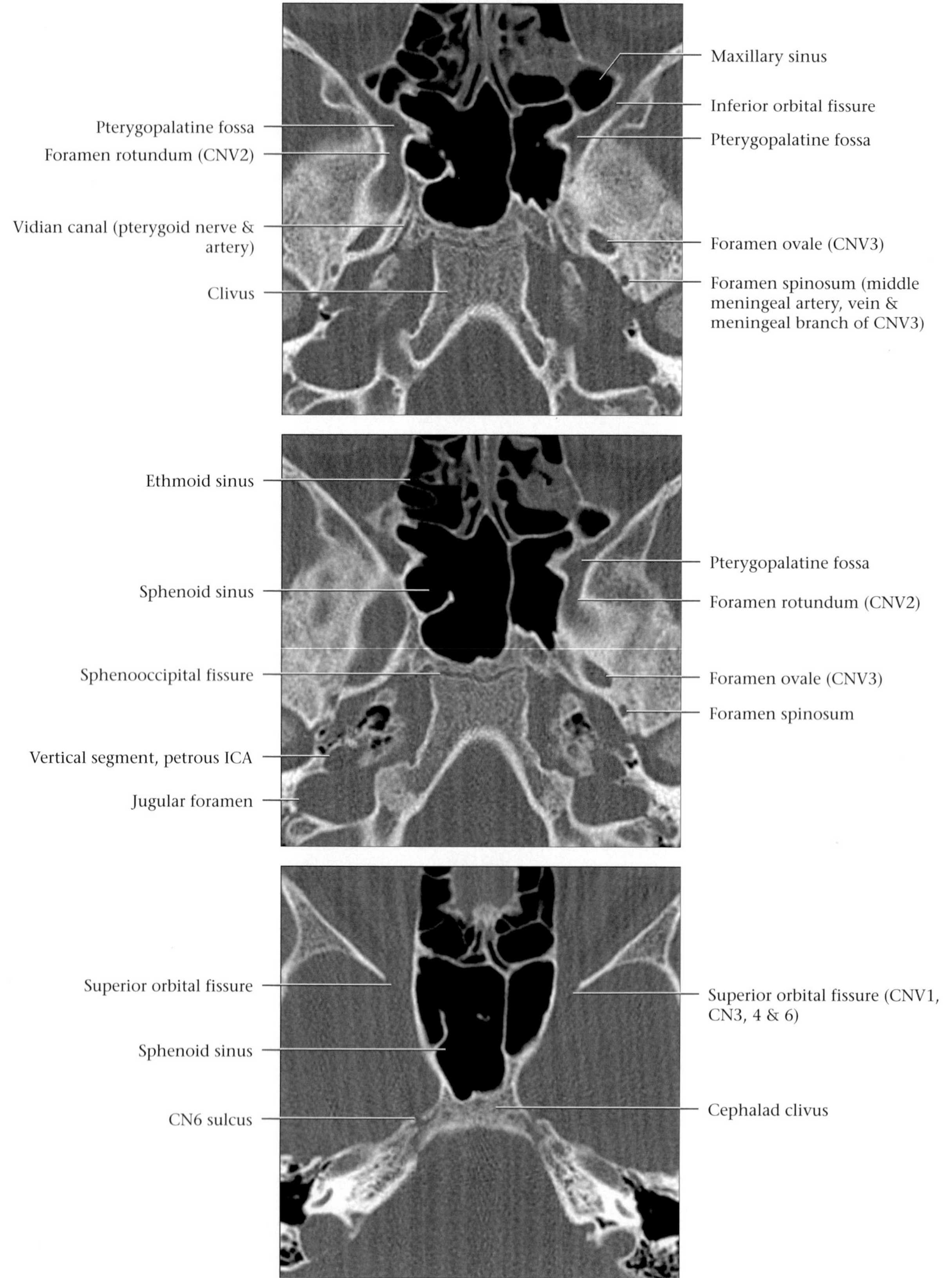
Maxillary sinus
Inferior orbital fissure
Pterygopalatine fossa
Foramen rotundum (CNV2)
Pterygopalatine fossa
Vidian canal (pterygoid nerve & artery)
Foramen ovale (CNV3)
Clivus
Foramen spinosum (middle meningeal artery, vein & meningeal branch of CNV3)
Ethmoid sinus
Pterygopalatine fossa
Sphenoid sinus
Foramen rotundum (CNV2)
Sphenooccipital fissure
Foramen ovale (CNV3)
Foramen spinosum
Vertical segment, petrous ICA
Jugular foramen
Superior orbital fissure
Superior orbital fissure (CNV1, CN3, 4 & 6)
Sphenoid sinus
Cephalad clivus
CN6 sulcus

(Top) First of three axial bone CT images presented from inferior to superior through central skull base. CNV2 exits skull base through foramen rotundum to enter superior margin of pterygopalatine fossa. CNV3 exits via foramen ovale to enter masticator space where it supplies motor innervation to muscles of mastication and sensory branches inferior alveolar, lingual and auriculotemporal nerves. **(Middle)** In this image the foramen ovale (CNV3) and foramen rotundum (CNV2) are now best seen on the patient's left. Notice left foramen rotundum is seen opening into then superior pterygopalatine fossa. **(Bottom)** The superior orbital fissure transmits ophthalmic division of trigeminal nerve from cranium to orbit. Other structures which pass through superior orbital fissure include oculomotor nerve (CN3), trochlear nerve (CN4) and abducens nerve (CN6) and the superior ophthalmic vein.

CN5 (TRIGEMINAL NERVE)

AXIAL T2 MR

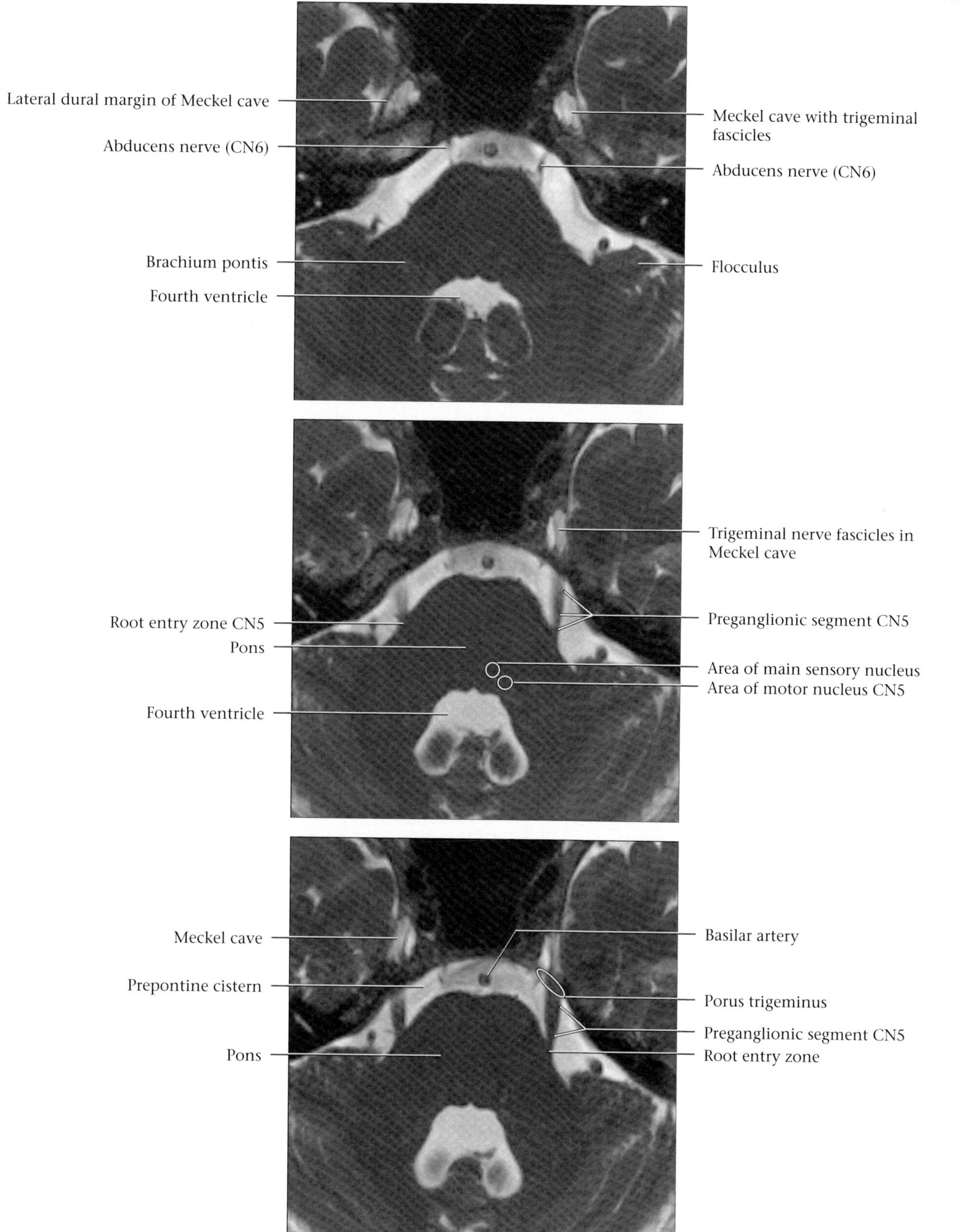
Lateral dural margin of Meckel cave
Abducens nerve (CN6)
Brachium pontis
Fourth ventricle
Meckel cave with trigeminal fascicles
Abducens nerve (CN6)
Flocculus
Root entry zone CN5
Pons
Fourth ventricle
Trigeminal nerve fascicles in Meckel cave
Preganglionic segment CN5
Area of main sensory nucleus
Area of motor nucleus CN5
Meckel cave
Prepontine cistern
Pons
Basilar artery
Porus trigeminus
Preganglionic segment CN5
Root entry zone

(Top) First of three axial T2 MR images through the trigeminal nerve and Meckel cave presented from inferior to superior demonstrates a layer of hypointense dura mater forming lateral wall and roof of Meckel cave. Right abducens nerve is seen penetrating dura to enter Dorello canal. Trigeminal nerve fascicles can be seen with the cerebrospinal fluid of Meckel cave. **(Middle)** Preganglionic fascicles of CN5 are seen within Meckel cave. Meckel cave is an arachnoid lined, dural diverticulum protruding from the lateral aspect of the prepontine cistern. It contains cerebrospinal fluid, trigeminal fascicles and trigeminal ganglion. Note approximate location of the main sensory and motor nuclei of CN5. **(Bottom)** In this image the preganglionic segment of CN5 is seen spanning the distance between the root entry zone on the lateral pons and the porus trigeminus of Meckel cave.

CN5 (TRIGEMINAL NERVE)

AXIAL T1 C+ MR

Foramen rotundum
Maxillary nerve (CNV2)
Petrous ICA turning cephalad into cavernous sinus
Sphenoid sinus
Mandibular nerve (CNV3)
Middle meningeal artery in foramen spinosum
Clivus

Trigeminal ganglion
Clivus
Abducens nerve in Dorello canal
Sphenoid sinus
Cavernous ICA
Meckel cave
Abducens nerve in Dorello canal

Superior orbital fissure
Cavernous sinus
Cavernous ICA
Pons
CN5 in porus trigeminus
Preganglionic segment CN5
Root entry zone CN5

(Top) First of three axial T1 C+ fat-saturated MR images presented from inferior to superior through central skull base demonstrates right maxillary nerve (CNV2) passing anteriorly into foramen rotundum and left mandibular nerve (CNV3) passing inferiorly through foramen ovale. Both nerves are surrounded by enhancing veins communicating with extracranial venous system. **(Middle)** This more superior image demonstrates the ovoid shape of the cerebrospinal fluid-filled Meckel cave. The trigeminal ganglion is the linear anteroinferior structure in Meckel cave. It lacks a blood-nerve barrier and therefore normally enhances with contrast. **(Bottom)** Preganglionic segment of trigeminal nerve arises from lateral pons at root entry zone. Right internal carotid artery is tortuous within cavernous sinus.

CORONAL T2 MR

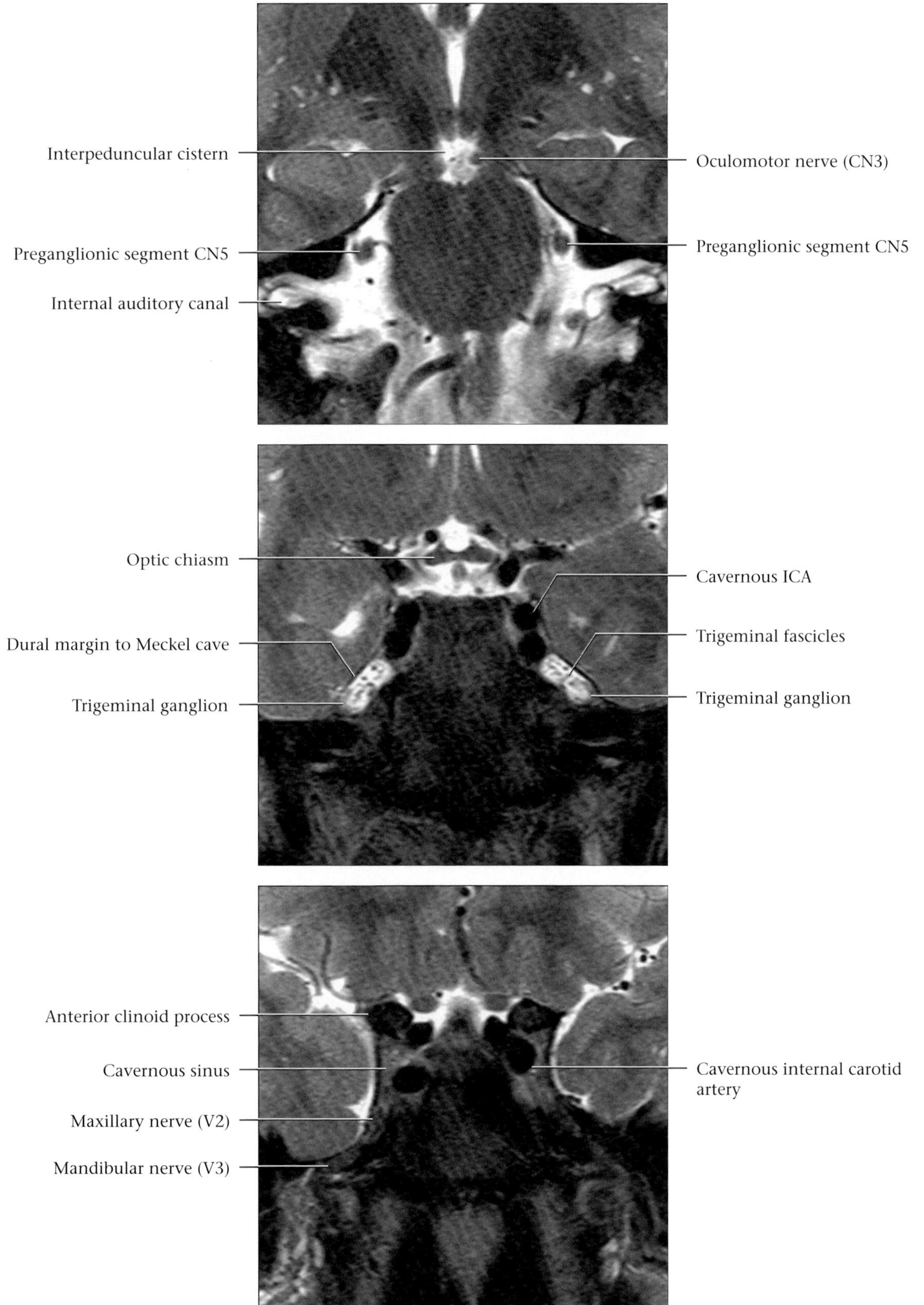
Interpeduncular cistern
Oculomotor nerve (CN3)
Preganglionic segment CN5
Preganglionic segment CN5
Internal auditory canal
Optic chiasm
Cavernous ICA
Dural margin to Meckel cave
Trigeminal fascicles
Trigeminal ganglion
Trigeminal ganglion
Anterior clinoid process
Cavernous sinus
Cavernous internal carotid artery
Maxillary nerve (V2)
Mandibular nerve (V3)

(Top) First of three coronal T2 MR images presented from posterior to anterior demonstrates the ovoid preganglionic segment of the trigeminal nerve surrounded by high signal cerebrospinal fluid. The preganglionic segment has just exited the lateral pons root entry zone area. **(Middle)** This more anterior image through Meckel cave delineates the trigeminal fascicles of preganglionic trigeminal nerve. The trigeminal ganglion is visible as a semilunar structure in the floor of Meckel cave bilaterally. **(Bottom)** This image through the anterior cavernous sinus shows the maxillary nerve (CNV2) passing anteriorly within lateral wall of cavernous sinus and the mandibular nerve (CNV3) passing inferiorly to its exit point in the skull base (foramen ovale).

CN5 (TRIGEMINAL NERVE)

CORONAL T1 C+ MR

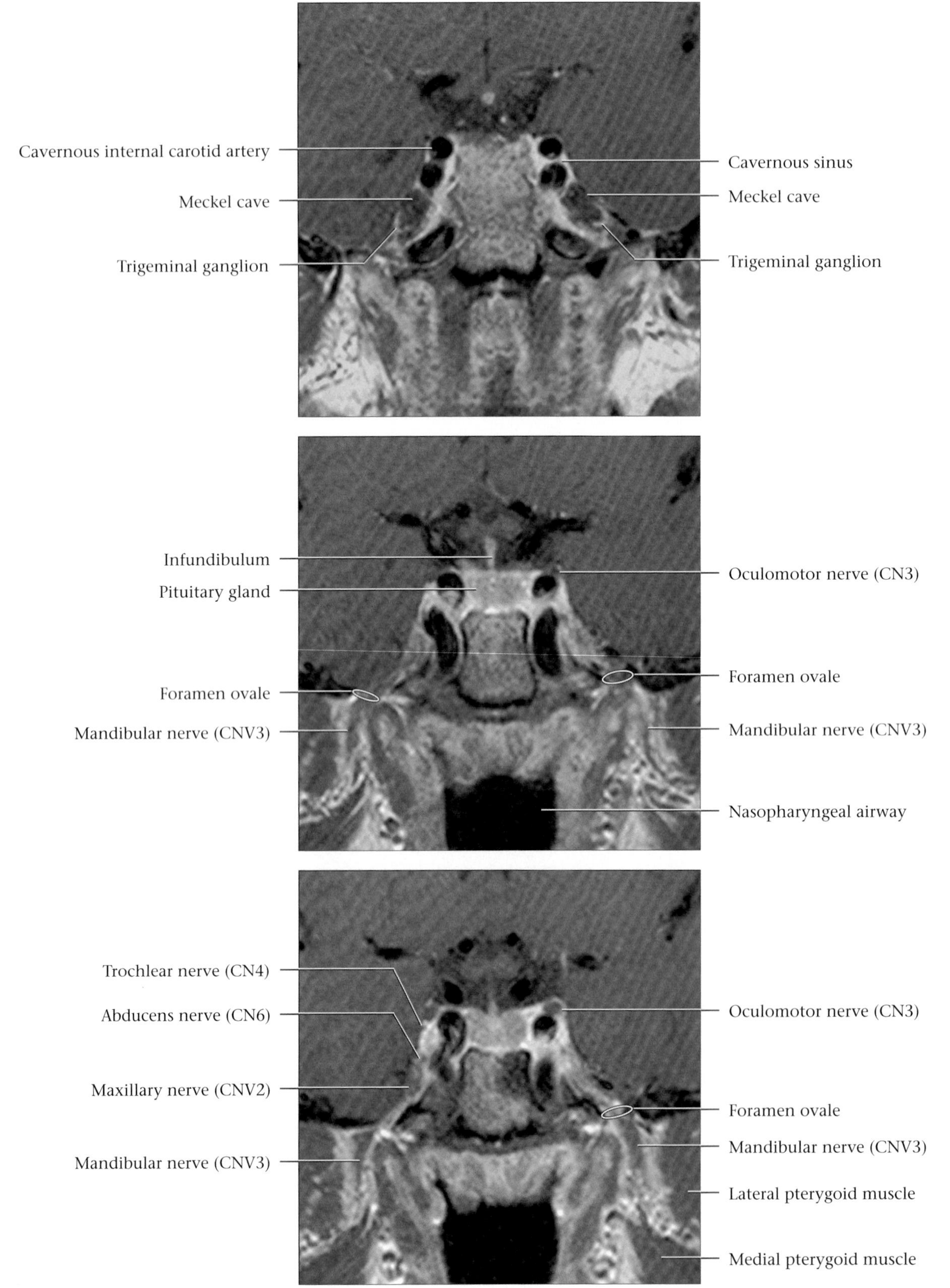
Cavernous internal carotid artery
Meckel cave
Trigeminal ganglion
Cavernous sinus
Meckel cave
Trigeminal ganglion
Infundibulum
Pituitary gland
Foramen ovale
Mandibular nerve (CNV3)
Oculomotor nerve (CN3)
Foramen ovale
Mandibular nerve (CNV3)
Nasopharyngeal airway
Trochlear nerve (CN4)
Abducens nerve (CN6)
Maxillary nerve (CNV2)
Mandibular nerve (CNV3)
Oculomotor nerve (CN3)
Foramen ovale
Mandibular nerve (CNV3)
Lateral pterygoid muscle
Medial pterygoid muscle

(Top) First of six coronal T1 C+ MR images through cavernous sinus presented from posterior to anterior. The trigeminal ganglion is seen as a crescentic area of enhancement in floor of Meckel cave. Trigeminal ganglion enhances because it lacks a blood-nerve barrier. **(Middle)** In this image through foramen ovale mandibular nerve (CNV3) is visible exiting inferiorly into masticator space. The 1st branch of CNV3, masticator nerve, supplies motor innervation to all 4 muscles of mastication (masseter, medial and lateral pterygoid and temporalis muscles). **(Bottom)** In this image the patient's left foramen ovale and mandibular nerve are seen. Mandibular nerve plunges directly into masticator space where it gives of its main motor branch (masticator nerve) to innervate muscles of mastication. It also give off sensory branches including inferior alveolar, lingual and auriculotemporal branches.

CORONAL T1 C+ MR

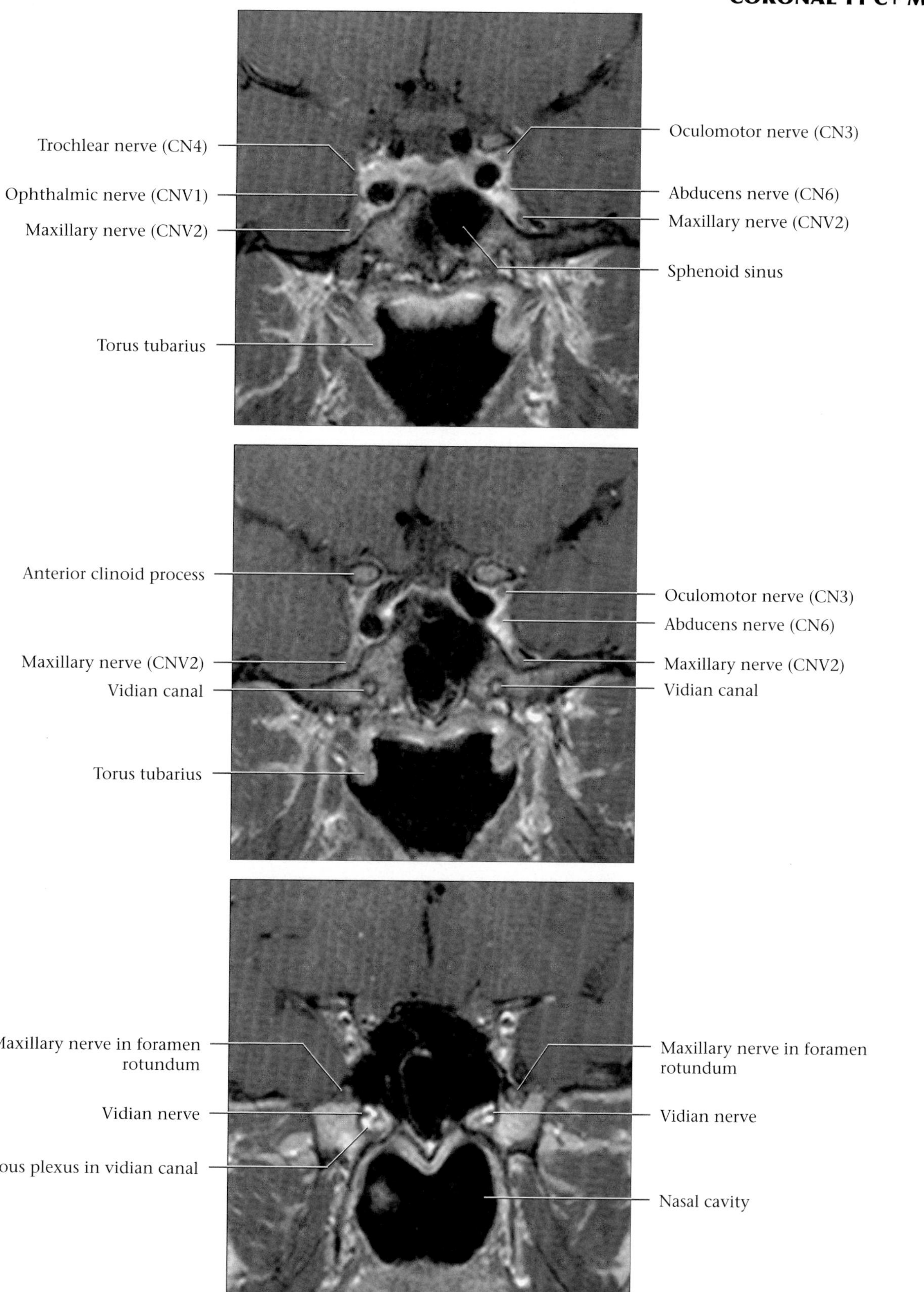
Trochlear nerve (CN4)
Ophthalmic nerve (CNV1)
Maxillary nerve (CNV2)
Torus tubarius
Oculomotor nerve (CN3)
Abducens nerve (CN6)
Maxillary nerve (CNV2)
Sphenoid sinus
Anterior clinoid process
Maxillary nerve (CNV2)
Vidian canal
Torus tubarius
Oculomotor nerve (CN3)
Abducens nerve (CN6)
Maxillary nerve (CNV2)
Vidian canal
Maxillary nerve in foramen rotundum
Vidian nerve
Venous plexus in vidian canal
Maxillary nerve in foramen rotundum
Vidian nerve
Nasal cavity

(Top) In this image through the anterior margin of the pituitary gland, the maxillary nerve (CNV2) is well seen bilaterally in the inferolateral wall of the cavernous sinus. **(Middle)** In this more anterior image the maxillary nerves are seen in the inferolateral wall of the cavernous sinus just prior to its entry into the foramen rotundum. Inferomedially note the vidian canals. **(Bottom)** In this image the maxillary nerve can be seen in the foramen rotundum. Notice also the vidian canal widening on its extracranial side with the vidian nerve visible surrounded by a venous plexus. The vidian nerve carries secretomotor fibers originally in the facial nerve which are responsible for lacrimation.

CN5 (TRIGEMINAL NERVE)

SAGITTAL T2 & AXIAL T1 MR

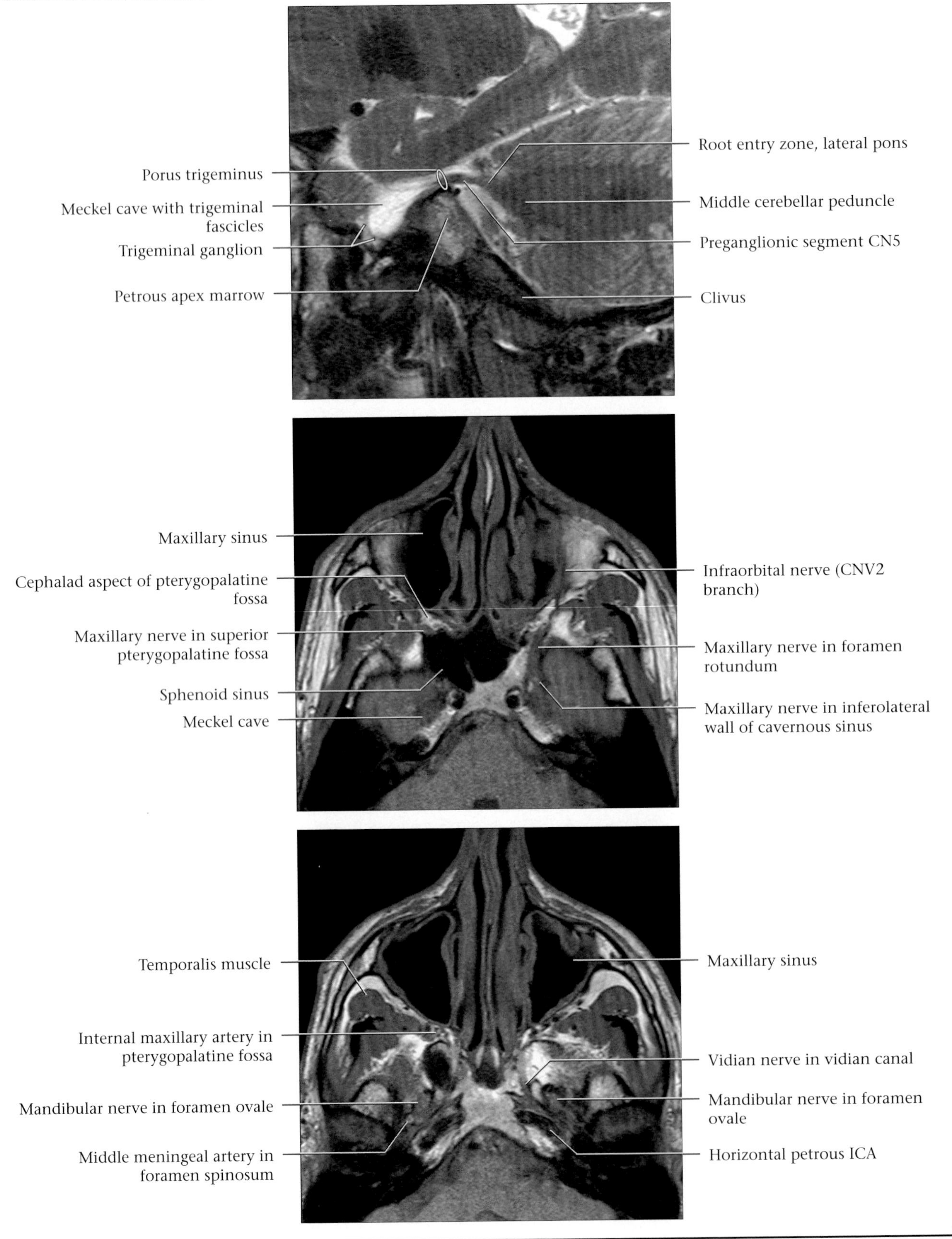
Porus trigeminus
Meckel cave with trigeminal fascicles
Trigeminal ganglion
Petrous apex marrow
Root entry zone, lateral pons
Middle cerebellar peduncle
Preganglionic segment CN5
Clivus
Maxillary sinus
Cephalad aspect of pterygopalatine fossa
Maxillary nerve in superior pterygopalatine fossa
Sphenoid sinus
Meckel cave
Infraorbital nerve (CNV2 branch)
Maxillary nerve in foramen rotundum
Maxillary nerve in inferolateral wall of cavernous sinus
Temporalis muscle
Internal maxillary artery in pterygopalatine fossa
Mandibular nerve in foramen ovale
Middle meningeal artery in foramen spinosum
Maxillary sinus
Vidian nerve in vidian canal
Mandibular nerve in foramen ovale
Horizontal petrous ICA

(Top) Sagittal T2 MR along line of proximal trigeminal nerve shows the preganglionic segment between the root entry zone in the lateral pons and the trigeminal ganglion in the anteroinferior Meckel cave. The cerebrospinal fluid within Meckel cave communicates with prepontine cistern through the porus trigeminus. **(Middle)** First of five axial T1 unenhanced MR images extending from the skull base to the mandibular body presented from superior to inferior. Notice the left maxillary nerve in the foramen rotundum. Distally it give rise to the infraorbital nerve. **(Bottom)** Image through foramen ovale of skull base. Notice the mandibular nerves exiting skull base. The vidian canal and nerve are also visible connecting the foramen lacerum to pterygopalatine fossa. The many black dots within pterygopalatine fossa are from the normal terminal internal maxillary artery.

CN5 (TRIGEMINAL NERVE)

AXIAL T1 MR

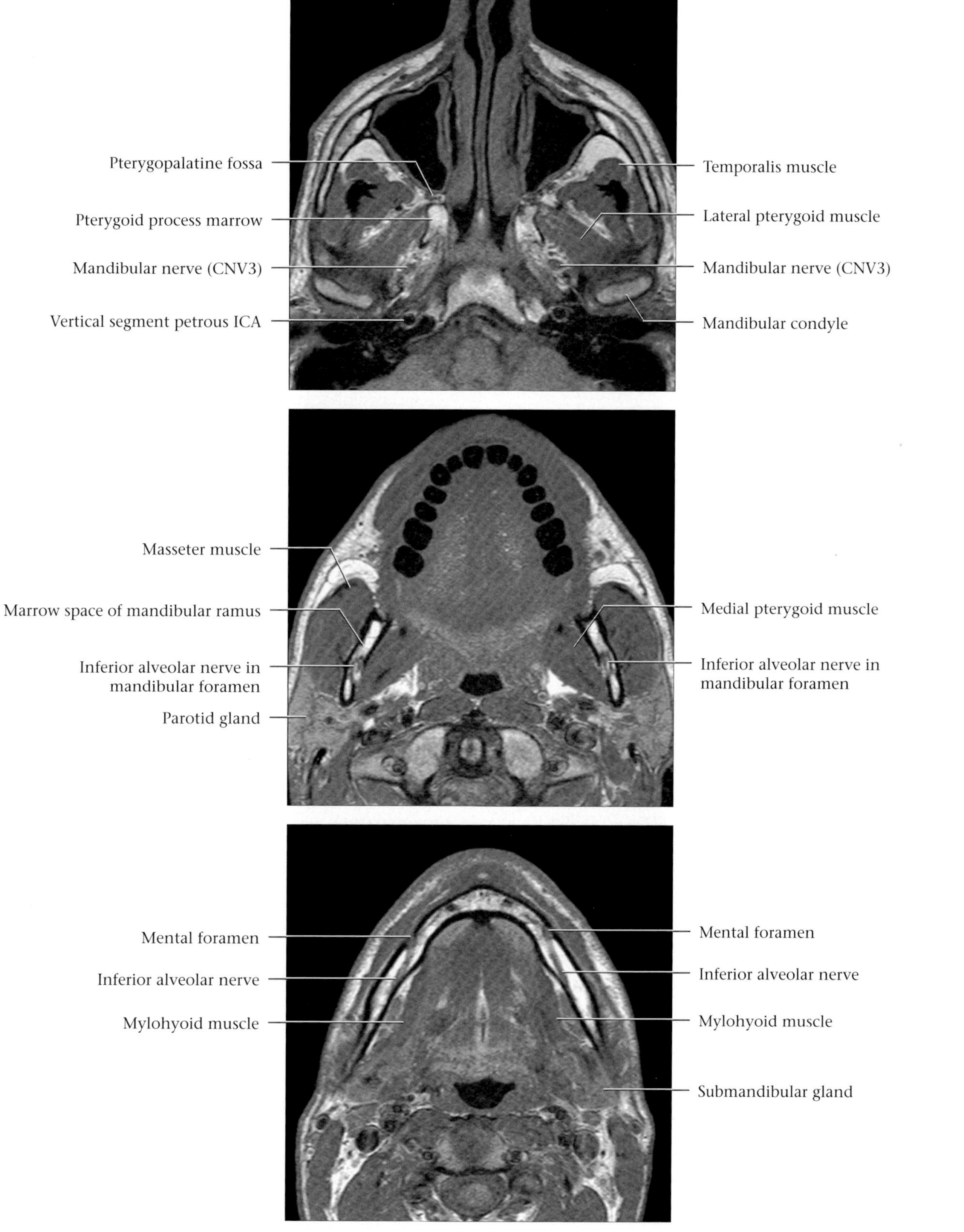
Pterygopalatine fossa
Pterygoid process marrow
Mandibular nerve (CNV3)
Vertical segment petrous ICA
Temporalis muscle
Lateral pterygoid muscle
Mandibular nerve (CNV3)
Mandibular condyle
Masseter muscle
Marrow space of mandibular ramus
Inferior alveolar nerve in mandibular foramen
Parotid gland
Medial pterygoid muscle
Inferior alveolar nerve in mandibular foramen
Mental foramen
Inferior alveolar nerve
Mylohyoid muscle
Mental foramen
Inferior alveolar nerve
Mylohyoid muscle
Submandibular gland

(Top) Image just under skull base shows both mandibular nerves are entering medial portion of upper masticator space. At this level that mandibular nerve gives off masticator nerve, motor branch to muscles of mastication. Auriculotemporal nerve branches posterolaterally at this level. **(Middle)** Image at level of mandibular foramina. Inferior alveolar nerve is seen bilaterally in the mandibular foramina. Mylohyoid nerve branches off inferior alveolar nerve just prior to mandibular foramen. It is the motor nerve to the mylohyoid and anterior belly of digastric muscles. Lingual nerve also branches anteromedially off inferior alveolar nerve at this level. **(Bottom)** In this image at level of the body of mandible the inferior alveolar nerve is seen within the high intensity marrow fat. The inferior alveolar nerve exits mandible via the mental foramen.

CN6 (ABDUCENS NERVE)

Terminology

Abbreviations

- Abducens nerve: CN6, CN VI

Synonyms

- Abducens nerve: Sixth cranial nerve

Definitions

- CN6: Motor nerve to lateral rectus muscle only

Imaging Anatomy

Overview

- CN6 is a pure motor nerve
- Five segments can be defined: Intra-axial, cisternal, interdural, cavernous and extracranial (intra-orbital)

Intra-Axial Segment

- **Abducens nucleus**
  - Paired CN6 nuclei located in pontine tegmentum near midline
    - Found just anterior to fourth ventricle
  - **Facial colliculus**: Axons of facial nerve (CN7) loop around abducens nucleus creating this bulge in floor of fourth ventricle
- Abducens nerve axons course anteroinferiorly through pontine tegmentum
- Emerges from anterior brainstem near midline through groove between pons and pyramid of medulla oblongata (bulbopontine sulcus)

Cisternal Segment

- CN6 ascends anterosuperiorly in prepontine cistern toward site where it penetrates dura
- May be posterior or anterior to anterior inferior cerebellar artery
- Penetrates dura of basisphenoid to enter Dorello canal

Interdural Segment

- **Dorello canal** represents channel within basilar venous plexus (petroclival venous confluence)
  - Channel is located **between** two layers of dura
  - Basilar venous plexus is continuous with cavernous sinus anteriorly
  - Basilar venous plexus drains into inferior petrosal sinus
- Extends from point where CN6 pierces inner (cerebral) layer dura mater to its entrance into cavernous sinus
- Within Dorello canal, abducens nerve is surrounded by layer of arachnoid mater & occasionally dura mater
- After penetrating dura, CN6 passes superiorly through basilar venous plexus
  - It then arches over petrous apex below petrosphenoidal ligament into upper posterior region of cavernous sinus
  - Bony sulcus of CN6 as it passes over top of petrous apex usually present

Cavernous Segment

- CN6 courses anteriorly within cavernous sinus
  - Abducens nerve is **only cranial nerve to lie within cavernous sinus**
  - Cranial nerves 3, 4, V1 and V2 are all embedded within lateral wall of cavernous sinus
- Within cavernous sinus CN6 runs along inferolateral aspect of cavernous internal carotid artery

Extracranial (Intra-Orbital) Segment

- CN6 enters orbit through **superior orbital fissure** together with CN3 and CN4
- Passes through annulus of Zinn
- Supplies **motor innervation** to **lateral rectus muscle**

Anatomy-Based Imaging Issues

Imaging Recommendations

- MR for intra-axial, cisternal, interdural & cavernous segments
  - Thin-section high-resolution T2 and contrast-enhanced T1 in axial and coronal planes
    - Depicts small structures including cranial nerves surrounded by CSF with high contrast & high spatial resolution
- Bone CT best for skull base and its bony foramina
- Dorello canal, cavernous sinus and orbital CN6 not visualized on routine MR imaging

Imaging "Sweet Spots"

- Axial and coronal MR sequences should include brainstem, fourth ventricle, cavernous sinus and orbit
- CN6 nucleus and intra-axial segment not directly visualized
  - Position of CN6 inferred by identifying facial colliculus in floor of fourth ventricle on high-resolution thin-section T2 MR
- Cisternal segment routinely visualized on high-resolution T2
- CN6 entrance into Dorello canal may be visualized due to invagination of cerebrospinal fluid into proximal canal

Imaging Pitfalls

- Use of fat-saturation on post-contrast T1 MR sequences can amplify blooming (susceptibility) artifact around a well aerated sphenoid sinus
  - Cavernous sinus & orbital apex subtle lesions may be obscured by this artifact
  - Remove fat-saturation and repeat T1 post-contrast MR if this artifact obscures key areas of interest

Clinical Implications

Clinical Importance

- In abducens neuropathy, affected eye will not **abduct** (rotate laterally)
- CN6 neuropathy divided into **simple** if isolated & **complex** if associated with other CN involvement (CN3, 4 and 7)
  - Simple CN6 neuropathy most common ocular motor nerve palsy
  - Usually presents as complex cranial neuropathy
    - Pontine lesions affect CN6 with CN7
    - Cavernous sinus, superior orbital fissure lesions affect CN6 with CN3, 4 and CNV1

CN6 (ABDUCENS NERVE)

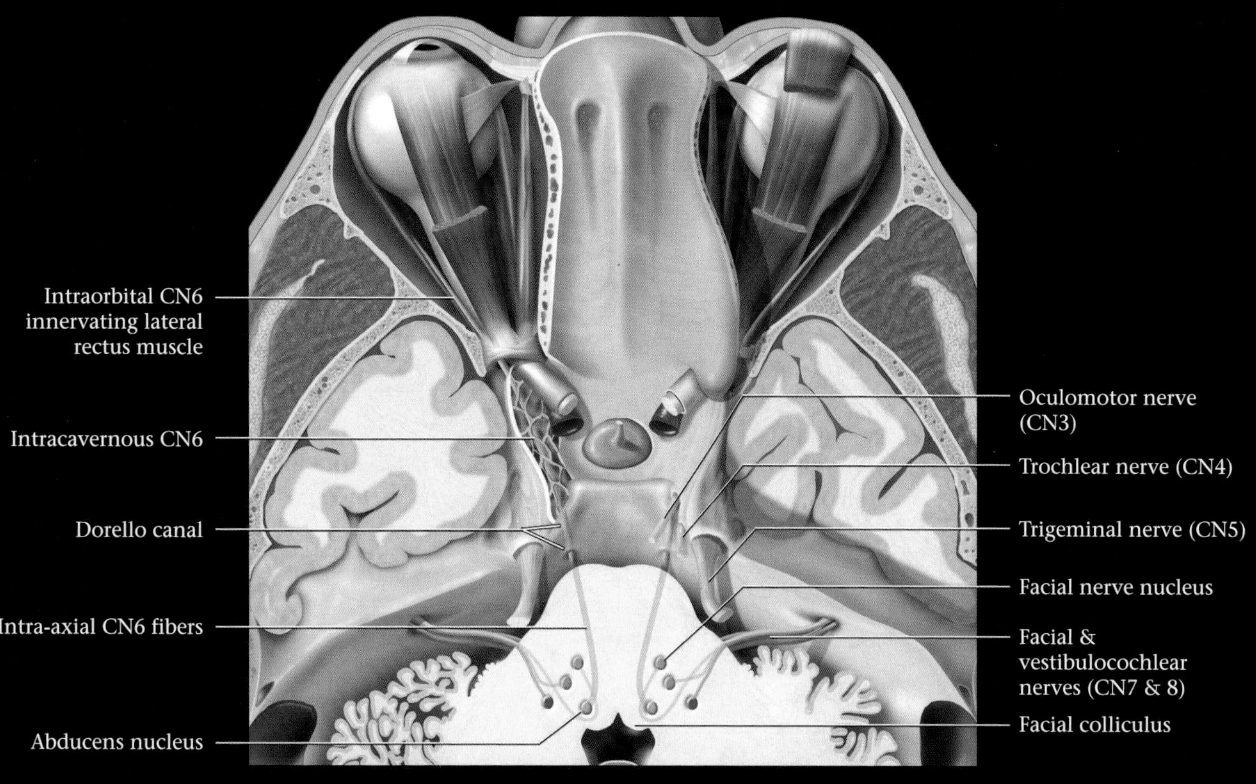
Intraorbital CN6 innervating lateral rectus muscle
Intracavernous CN6
Dorello canal
Intra-axial CN6 fibers
Abducens nucleus
Oculomotor nerve (CN3)
Trochlear nerve (CN4)
Trigeminal nerve (CN5)
Facial nerve nucleus
Facial & vestibulocochlear nerves (CN7 & 8)
Facial colliculus

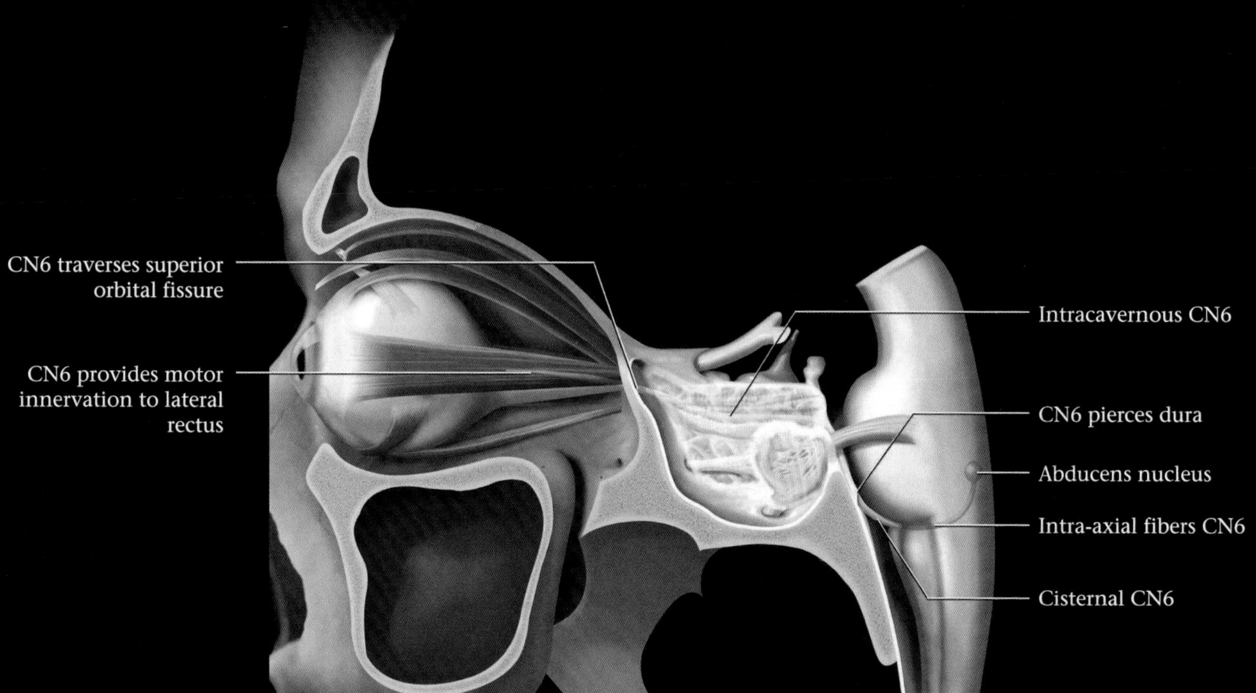
CN6 traverses superior orbital fissure
CN6 provides motor innervation to lateral rectus
Intracavernous CN6
CN6 pierces dura
Abducens nucleus
Intra-axial fibers CN6
Cisternal CN6

(Top) Axial graphic showing entire length of abducens nerve from its pontine tegmentum nuclear origin to its motor endplate in the lateral rectus muscle. Follow its progress from nucleus to its exit at anteromedial bulbopontine sulcus. From there note the dural penetration into Dorello canal leading to its intracavernous portion. Finally it passes through the superior orbital fissure and the ring of Zinn into the orbit. **(Bottom)** Sagittal graphic of abducens nerve depicted from its origin in pontine tegmentum to its motor endplate in lateral rectus muscle. Notice intra-axial CN6 fibers descend before exiting bulbopontine sulcus anteriorly. Prepontine cistern CN6 then ascends to pierce dura into Dorello canal. Intracavernous CN6 proceeds anteriorly to pass through superior orbital fissure and ring of Zinn before innervating lateral rectus muscle in orbit.

CN6 (ABDUCENS NERVE)

AXIAL T2 & T1 C+ MR

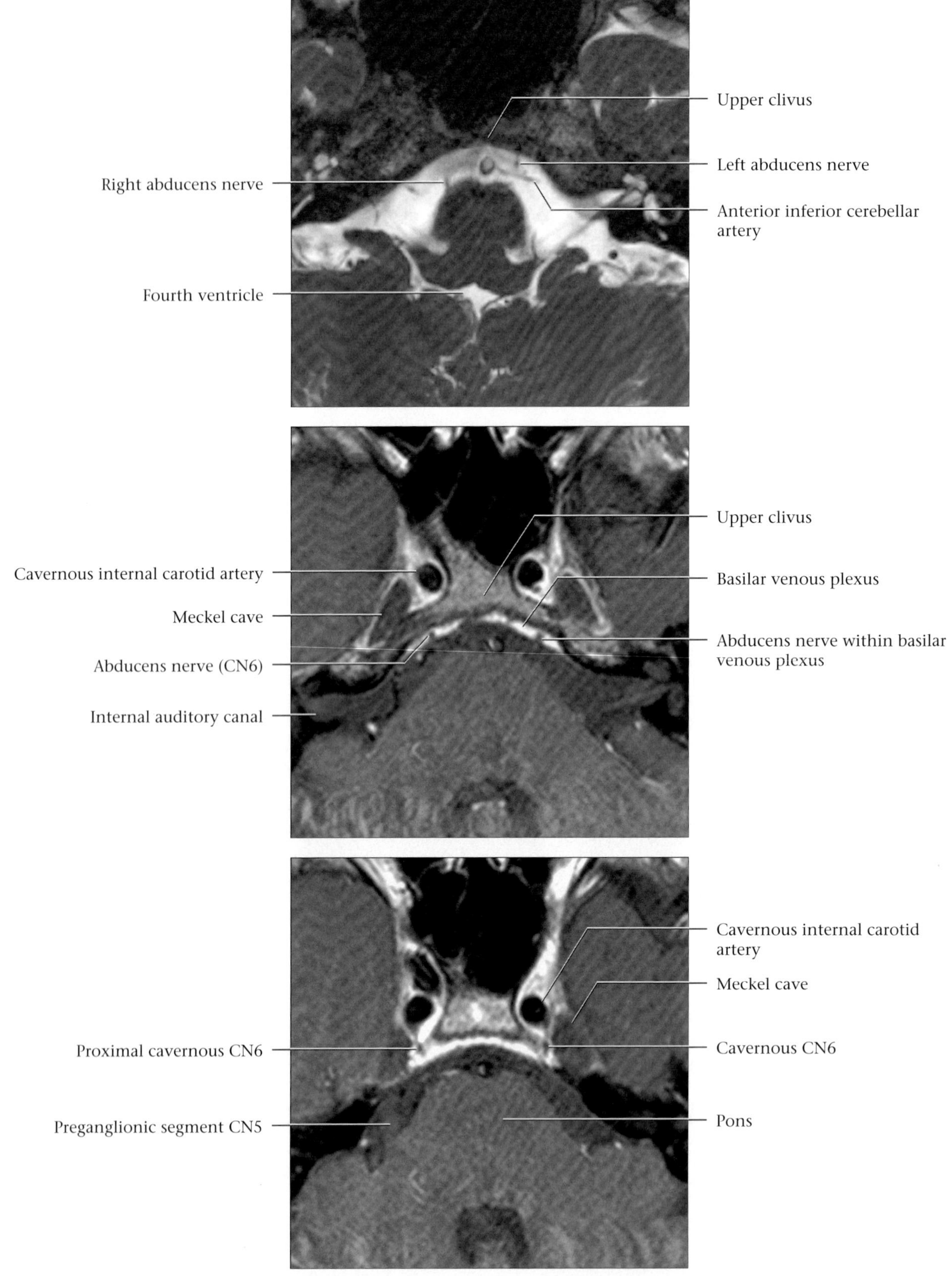
Upper clivus
Left abducens nerve
Right abducens nerve
Anterior inferior cerebellar artery
Fourth ventricle
Upper clivus
Cavernous internal carotid artery
Basilar venous plexus
Meckel cave
Abducens nerve within basilar venous plexus
Abducens nerve (CN6)
Internal auditory canal
Cavernous internal carotid artery
Meckel cave
Proximal cavernous CN6
Cavernous CN6
Preganglionic segment CN5
Pons

(Top) Axial T2 MR image near level of IAC presented to show the appearance of the abducens nerve in the prepontine cistern. On the person's right CN6 is just exiting the bulbopontine sulcus while on the left it is poised to penetrate the dura. Both nerves are rising in the prepontine cistern. **(Middle)** Axial T1 enhanced MR image demonstrates the interdural segment of abducens nerve within Dorello canal surrounded by brightly enhancing basilar venous plexus. **(Bottom)** Axial T1 enhanced MR image just above the internal auditory canal shows the abducens nerves passing through the superior basilar venous plexus to enter the posterior margin of the cavernous sinus. At this point CN6 is arching over the petrous apex below the petrosphenoidal ligament into upper posterior region of cavernous sinus.

CN6 (ABDUCENS NERVE)

SAGITTAL T2 MR

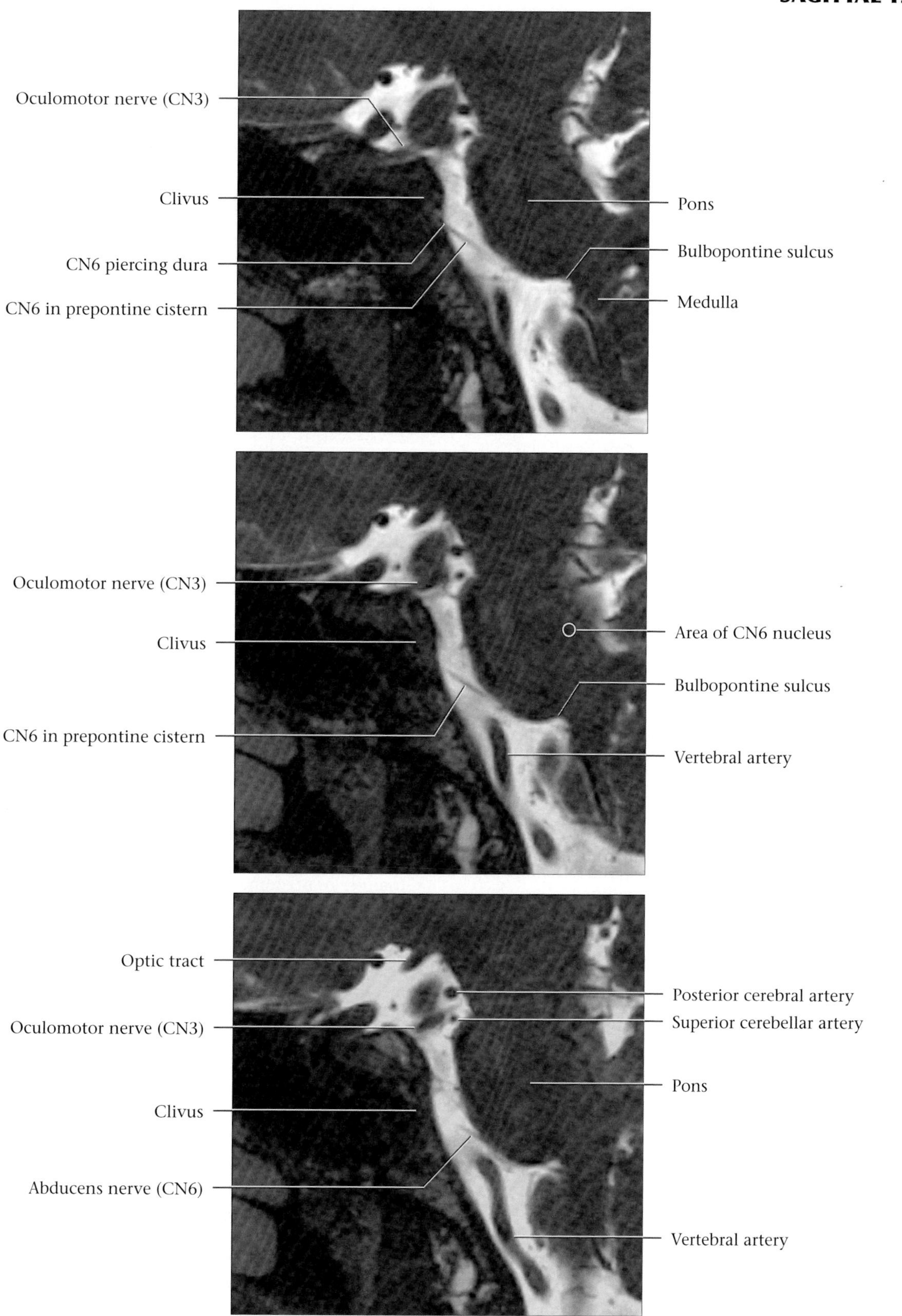

Oculomotor nerve (CN3)
Clivus
CN6 piercing dura
CN6 in prepontine cistern
Pons
Bulbopontine sulcus
Medulla
Oculomotor nerve (CN3)
Clivus
CN6 in prepontine cistern
Area of CN6 nucleus
Bulbopontine sulcus
Vertebral artery
Optic tract
Oculomotor nerve (CN3)
Clivus
Abducens nerve (CN6)
Posterior cerebral artery
Superior cerebellar artery
Pons
Vertebral artery

(Top) First of three sagittal T2 MR images presented from lateral to medial reveals the abducens nerve traversing prepontine cistern towards clivus. In this image the abducens nerve is visible penetrating the dura to enter Dorello canal which lies between cranial dura and periosteum surrounded by basilar venous plexus. **(Middle)** Image of brainstem area shows abducens nerve coursing anterosuperiorly from its exit point from the brainstem (bulbopontine sulcus) towards its point of dural penetration into Dorello canal. Notice the approximate location of CN6 nucleus and the steep course the intra-axial fibers take to reach the bulbopontine sulcus. **(Bottom)** Image of brainstem and prepontine cisterns shows proximal cisternal CN6 closely associated with the belly of the pons. CN3 is seen passing between posterior cerebral and superior cerebellar arteries.

CN7 (FACIAL NERVE)

Terminology

Abbreviations

- Facial nerve: CN7, CN VII

Synonyms

- Seventh cranial nerve

Definitions

- CN7: Cranial nerve that carries motor nerves to muscles of facial expression, parasympathetics to lacrimal, submandibular and sublingual glands and taste from anterior 2/3 of tongue

Imaging Anatomy

Overview

- Mixed nerve: Motor, parasympathetic and special sensory (taste)
- Two roots: Motor & sensory (nervus intermedius) roots
  - Nervus intermedius exits lateral brainstem between motor root of facial and vestibulocochlear nerves, hence its name
- Four segments: Intra-axial, cisternal, intratemporal and extracranial (parotid)

Intra-Axial Segment

- Three nuclei (one motor, two sensory)
- **Motor nucleus of facial nerve**
  - Located in ventrolateral pontine tegmentum
  - Efferent fibers loop dorsally around CN6 nucleus in floor of fourth ventricle forming **facial colliculus**
  - Fibers then course anterolaterally to exit lateral brainstem at pontomedullary junction
- **Superior salivatory nucleus**
  - Located lateral to CN7 motor nucleus in pons
  - Efferent **parasympathetic fibers** exit brainstem posterior to CN7 as nervus intermedius
    - To submandibular, sublingual and lacrimal glands
- **Solitarius tract nucleus**
  - Termination of taste sensation fibers from anterior 2/3 of tongue
  - **Cell bodies** of these fibers in **geniculate ganglion**
  - Fibers travel within nervus intermedius

Cisternal Segment

- Two roots in cisternal CN7
  - Larger motor root anteriorly
  - Smaller sensory nervus intermedius posteriorly
- Emerge from lateral brainstem at **root exit zone** in pontomedullary junction to enter cerebellopontine angle (CPA) cistern
  - CN8 exits brainstem posterior to CN7
- 2 roots join together & pass anterolaterally through CPA cistern with CN8 to internal auditory canal (IAC)

Intratemporal Segment

- CN7 further divided in T-bone into 4 segments: IAC, labyrinthine, tympanic and mastoid
- **IAC segment**: Porus acusticus to IAC fundus; anterosuperior position above crista falciformis
- **Labyrinthine segment**: Connects fundal CN7 to geniculate ganglion (anterior genu)
- **Tympanic segment**: Connects anterior to posterior genu, passing under lateral semicircular canal
- **Mastoid segment**: Inferiorly directed from posterior genu to stylomastoid foramen

Extracranial Segment

- CN7 exits skull base through **stylomastoid foramen** to enter parotid space
- Parotid CN7 passes lateral to retromandibular vein
- Ramifies within parotid, passes anteriorly to innervate muscles of facial expression

CN7 Branches

- **Greater superficial petrosal nerve**
  - Arises at geniculate ganglion, passes anteromedially, exits temporal bone via facial hiatus
  - Carries **parasympathetic** fibers to **lacrimal gland**
- **Stapedius nerve**
  - Arises from high mastoid segment of CN7
  - Provides **motor** innervation to **stapedius muscle**
- **Chorda tympani nerve**
  - Arises from lower mastoid segment
  - Courses across middle ear to exit anterior T-bone
  - Carries **taste** fibers from **anterior 2/3 tongue**
    - These fibers travel with lingual branch of mandibular division of trigeminal nerve
- **Terminal motor branches**

Anatomy-Based Imaging Issues

Imaging Recommendations

- Bone CT best for intratemporal segment of CN7
- MR for intra-axial, cisternal, IAC and extracranial segments
- Do not image routine Bell palsy!

Imaging "Sweet Spots"

- Include brainstem, CPA cistern, IAC, T-bone and **parotid** when MR completed for CN7 palsy

Imaging Pitfalls

- Mild enhancement of labyrinthine segment, geniculate ganglion and proximal tympanic segments of CN7 can be normal on post-contrast T1 MR
  - Secondary to circumneural arteriovenous plexus
- Always check parotid in peripheral CN7 paralysis

Clinical Issues

- Facial nerve paralysis can be central or peripheral
  - **Central**: Supranuclear injury resulting in paralysis of contralateral muscles of facial expression with forehead sparing
  - **Peripheral**: Injury to CN7 from brainstem nucleus peripherally, resulting in paralysis of all ipsilateral muscles of facial expression
    - If lesion proximal to geniculate ganglion, lacrimation, sound dampening and taste affected
    - If CN6 involved, check pons for lesion
    - If CN8 involved, check CPA-IAC for lesion
    - If lacrimation, sound dampening and taste are variably affected, T-bone lesion possible
    - If lacrimation, sound dampening and taste are spared, extracranial CN7 implicated

CN7 (FACIAL NERVE)

GRAPHICS

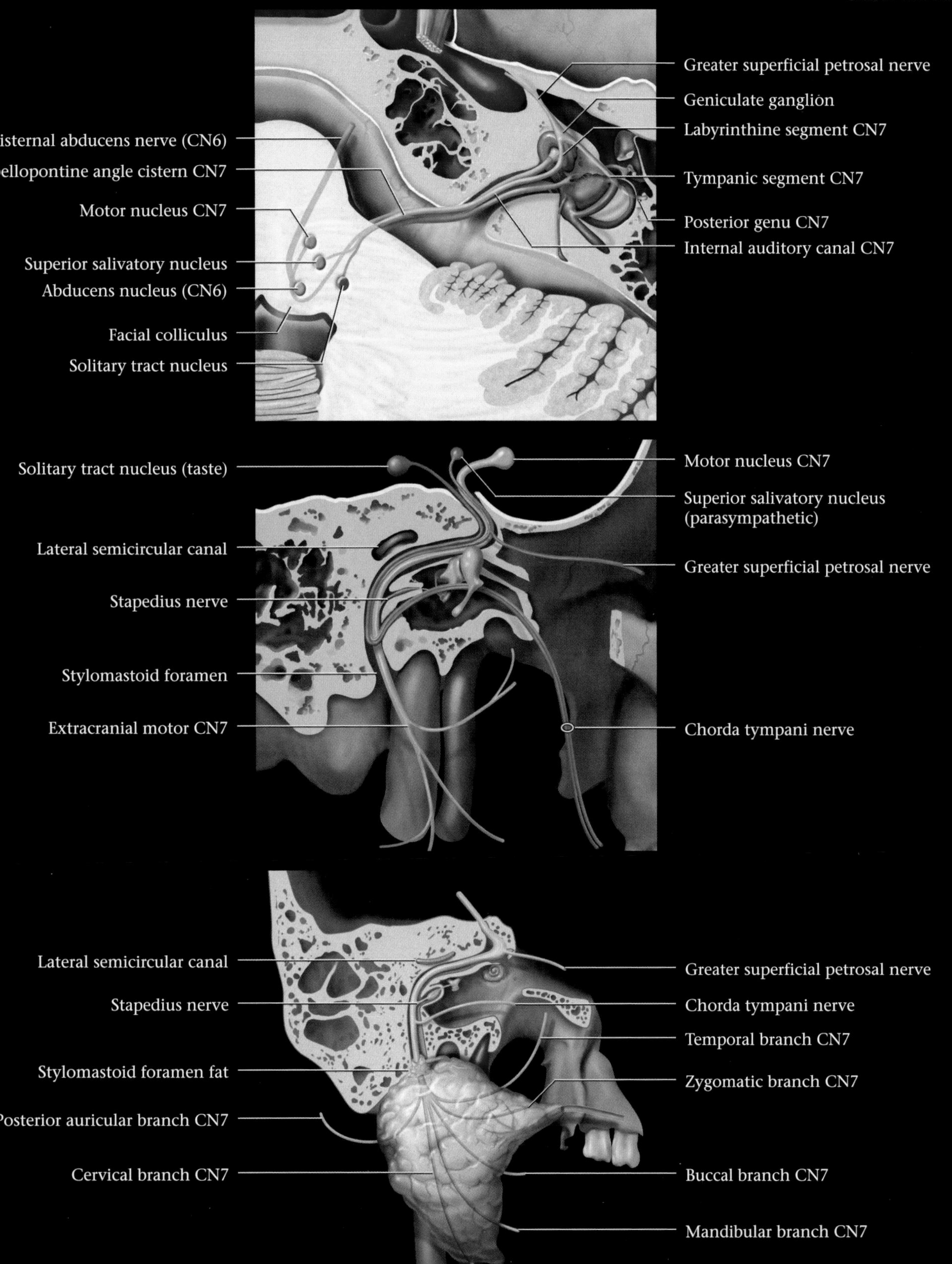

Cisternal abducens nerve (CN6)
Cerebellopontine angle cistern CN7
Motor nucleus CN7
Superior salivatory nucleus
Abducens nucleus (CN6)
Facial colliculus
Solitary tract nucleus
Greater superficial petrosal nerve
Geniculate ganglion
Labyrinthine segment CN7
Tympanic segment CN7
Posterior genu CN7
Internal auditory canal CN7
Solitary tract nucleus (taste)
Lateral semicircular canal
Stapedius nerve
Stylomastoid foramen
Extracranial motor CN7
Motor nucleus CN7
Superior salivatory nucleus (parasympathetic)
Greater superficial petrosal nerve
Chorda tympani nerve
Lateral semicircular canal
Stapedius nerve
Stylomastoid foramen fat
Posterior auricular branch CN7
Cervical branch CN7
Greater superficial petrosal nerve
Chorda tympani nerve
Temporal branch CN7
Zygomatic branch CN7
Buccal branch CN7
Mandibular branch CN7

(Top) Axial graphic of CN7 nuclei. Motor nucleus sends out its fibers to circle CN6 nucleus before reaching root exit zone at pontomedullary junction. Superior salivatory nucleus sends parasympathetic secretomotor fibers to lacrimal, submandibular and sublingual glands. Solitary tract nucleus receives anterior 2/3 tongue taste information. **(Middle)** Sagittal graphic depicts CN7 within temporal bone. Motor fibers pass through T-bone, dropping stapedius nerve to stapedius muscle, then exits via stylomastoid foramen to extracranial CN7 (entirely motor). Parasympathetic fibers from superior salivatory nucleus reach lacrimal gland via greater superficial petrosal nerve and submandibular-sublingual glands via chorda tympanic nerve. Anterior 2/3 tongue taste fibers come via chorda tympani nerve. **(Bottom)** Sagittal graphic depicting extracranial motor branches of the facial nerve.

CN7 (FACIAL NERVE)

AXIAL BONE CT

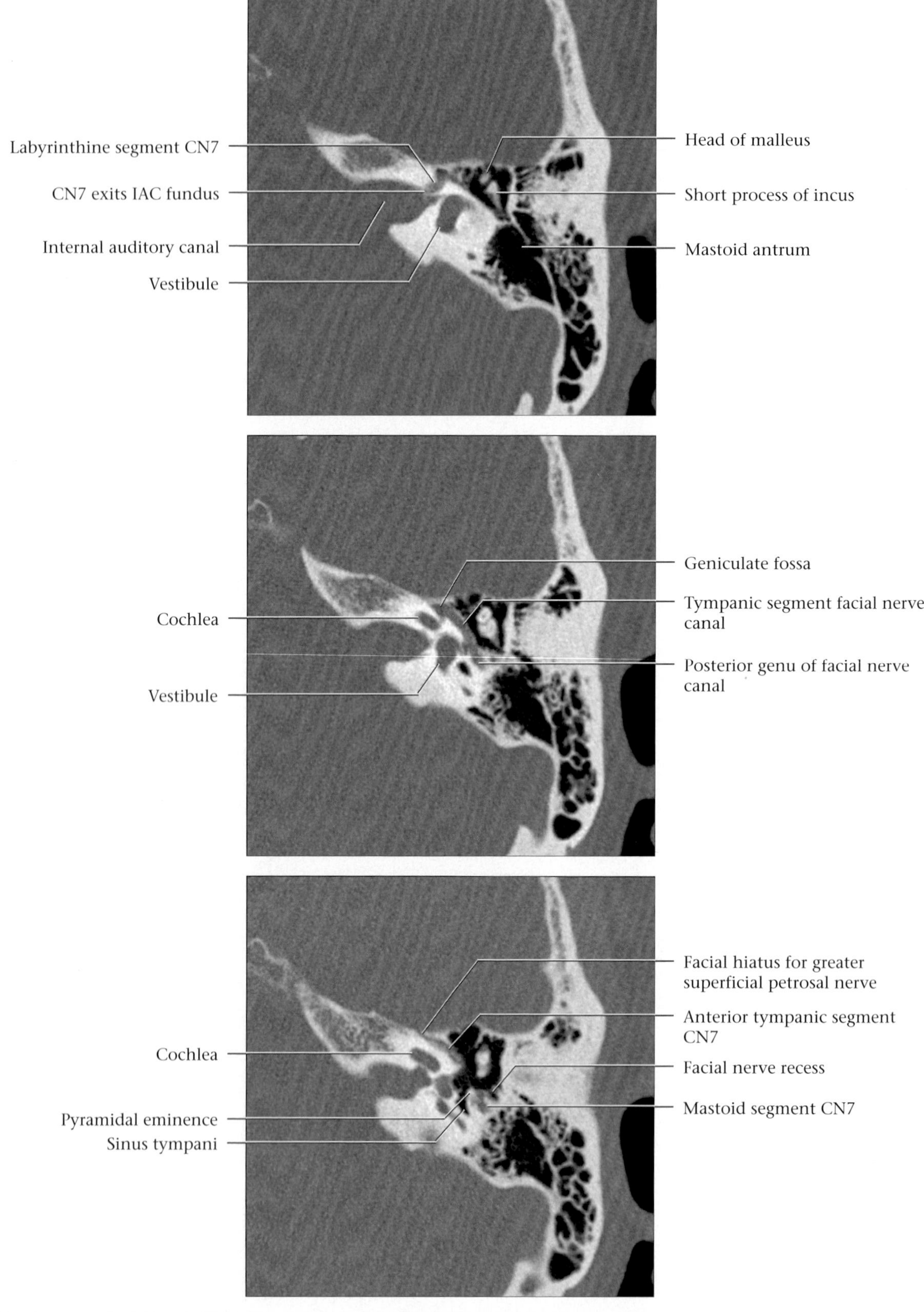
Labyrinthine segment CN7
CN7 exits IAC fundus
Internal auditory canal
Vestibule
Head of malleus
Short process of incus
Mastoid antrum
Cochlea
Vestibule
Geniculate fossa
Tympanic segment facial nerve canal
Posterior genu of facial nerve canal
Cochlea
Pyramidal eminence
Sinus tympani
Facial hiatus for greater superficial petrosal nerve
Anterior tympanic segment CN7
Facial nerve recess
Mastoid segment CN7

(Top) First of six axial bone CT images of the left temporal bone presented from superior to inferior shows the labyrinthine segment of the facial nerve canal as a C-shaped structure arching anterolaterally over the top of the cochlea. **(Middle)** In this image the labyrinthine segment CN7 canal terminates in geniculate fossa. The facial nerve canal turns abruptly at the geniculate fossa (anterior genu). The tympanic segment arises from geniculate fossa, coursing posterolaterally in axial plane, running under the lateral semicircular canal before turning 90 degrees inferiorly at posterior genu to become mastoid segment. **(Bottom)** At the level of the oval window, the mastoid segment is visible deep to the facial nerve recess. Notice the more medial pyramidal eminence and sinus tympani.

CN7 (FACIAL NERVE)

AXIAL BONE CT

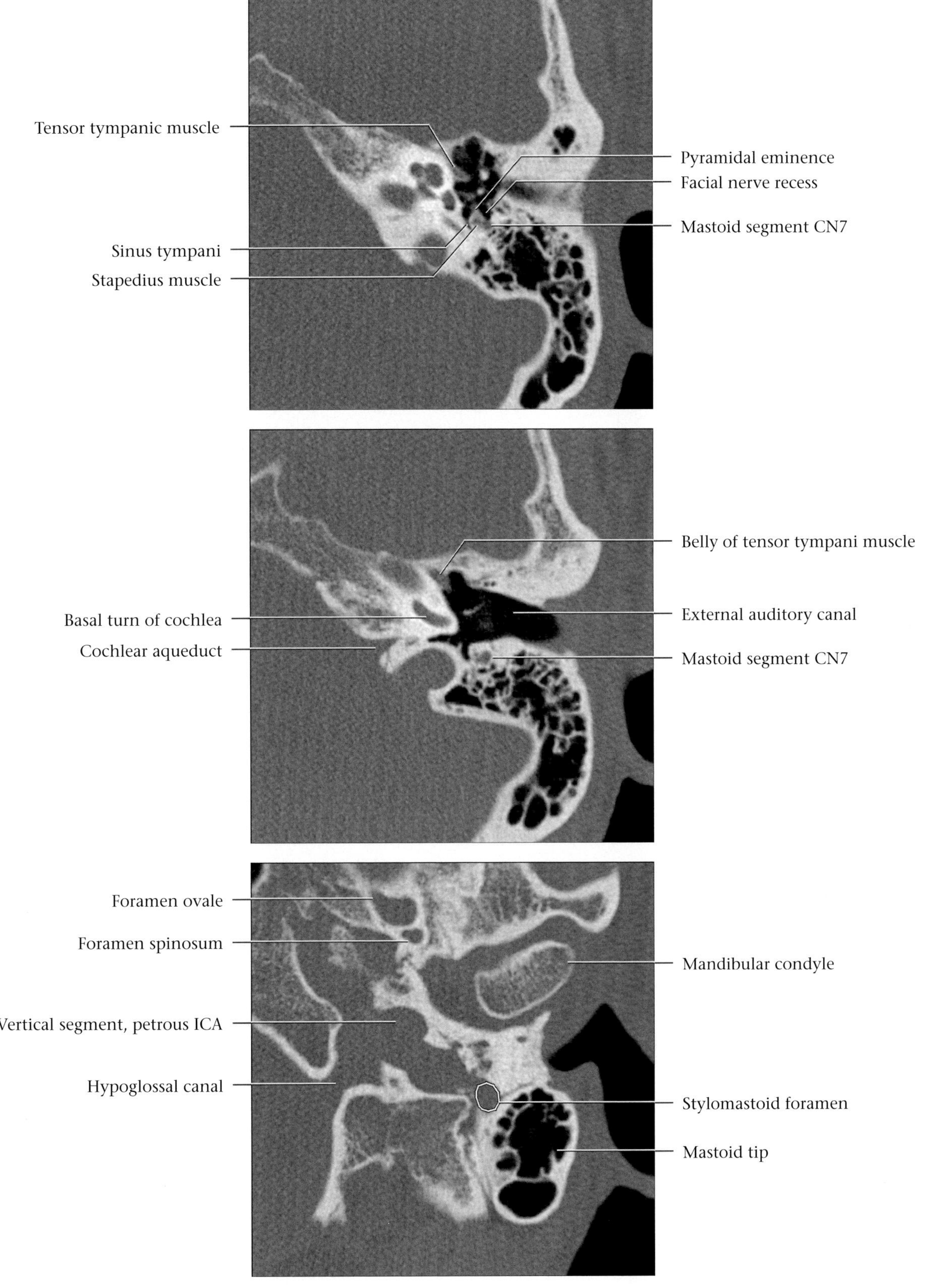
Tensor tympanic muscle
Sinus tympani
Stapedius muscle
Pyramidal eminence
Facial nerve recess
Mastoid segment CN7
Basal turn of cochlea
Cochlear aqueduct
Belly of tensor tympani muscle
External auditory canal
Mastoid segment CN7
Foramen ovale
Foramen spinosum
Vertical segment, petrous ICA
Hypoglossal canal
Mandibular condyle
Stylomastoid foramen
Mastoid tip

(Top) Mastoid segment extends approximately 13 mm from posterior genu to stylomastoid foramen coursing inferiorly within posterior wall of middle ear cavity. Mastoid segment is related anteriorly to facial nerve recess and medially to stapedius muscle within pyramidal eminence on posterior wall of middle ear cavity. **(Middle)** At the level of the basal turn of the cochlea the mastoid segment of facial nerve is still visible. Both the nerve to stapedius muscle proximally and chorda tympani distally branch off the mastoid segment CN7. **(Bottom)** Image at the level of the stylomastoid foramen. Notice the "bell" of the stylomastoid foramen is just anteromedial to the mastoid tip. The mastoid tip protects the facial nerve from traumatic injury as it exits the skull base.

CN7 (FACIAL NERVE)

CORONAL BONE CT

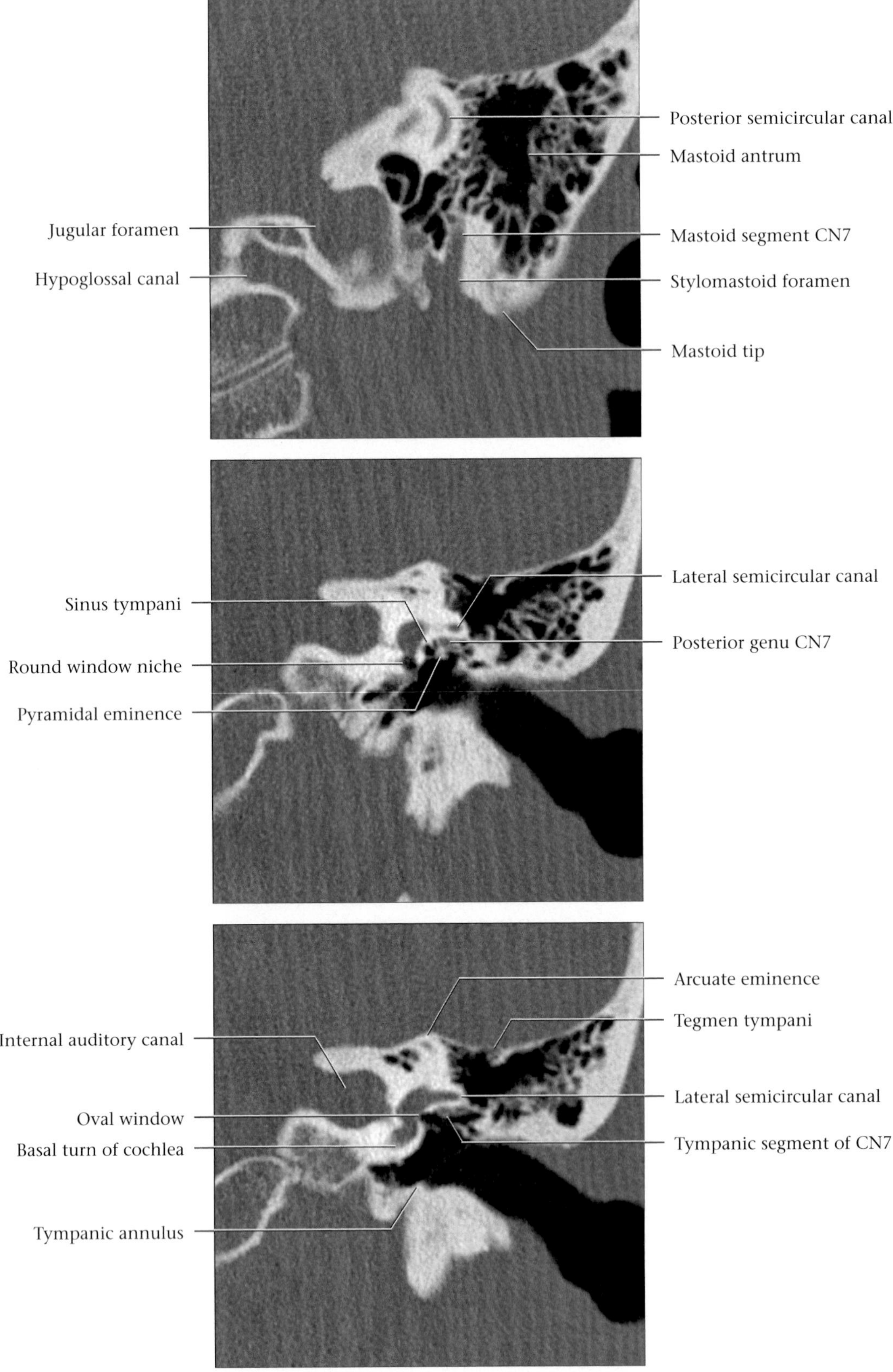
Posterior semicircular canal
Mastoid antrum
Jugular foramen
Mastoid segment CN7
Hypoglossal canal
Stylomastoid foramen
Mastoid tip
Lateral semicircular canal
Sinus tympani
Posterior genu CN7
Round window niche
Pyramidal eminence
Arcuate eminence
Tegmen tympani
Internal auditory canal
Lateral semicircular canal
Oval window
Tympanic segment of CN7
Basal turn of cochlea
Tympanic annulus

(Top) First of six coronal bone CT images of left temporal bone presented from posterior to anterior shows lower mastoid segment of the facial nerve (CN7) and stylomastoid foramen. **(Middle)** At the level of the round window the posterior genu of the facial nerve can be seen just lateral to the pyramidal eminence. Notice the sinus tympani is medial to the pyramidal eminence. **(Bottom)** At the level of the oval window the tympanic segment of the facial nerve can be seen coursing under the lateral semicircular canal. Notice the fine bony covering (thin white line) surrounding the facial nerve. Also note the location relative to the upper margin of the oval window. In patients with oval window atresia, the facial nerve is found near or within the oval window niche.

CN7 (FACIAL NERVE)

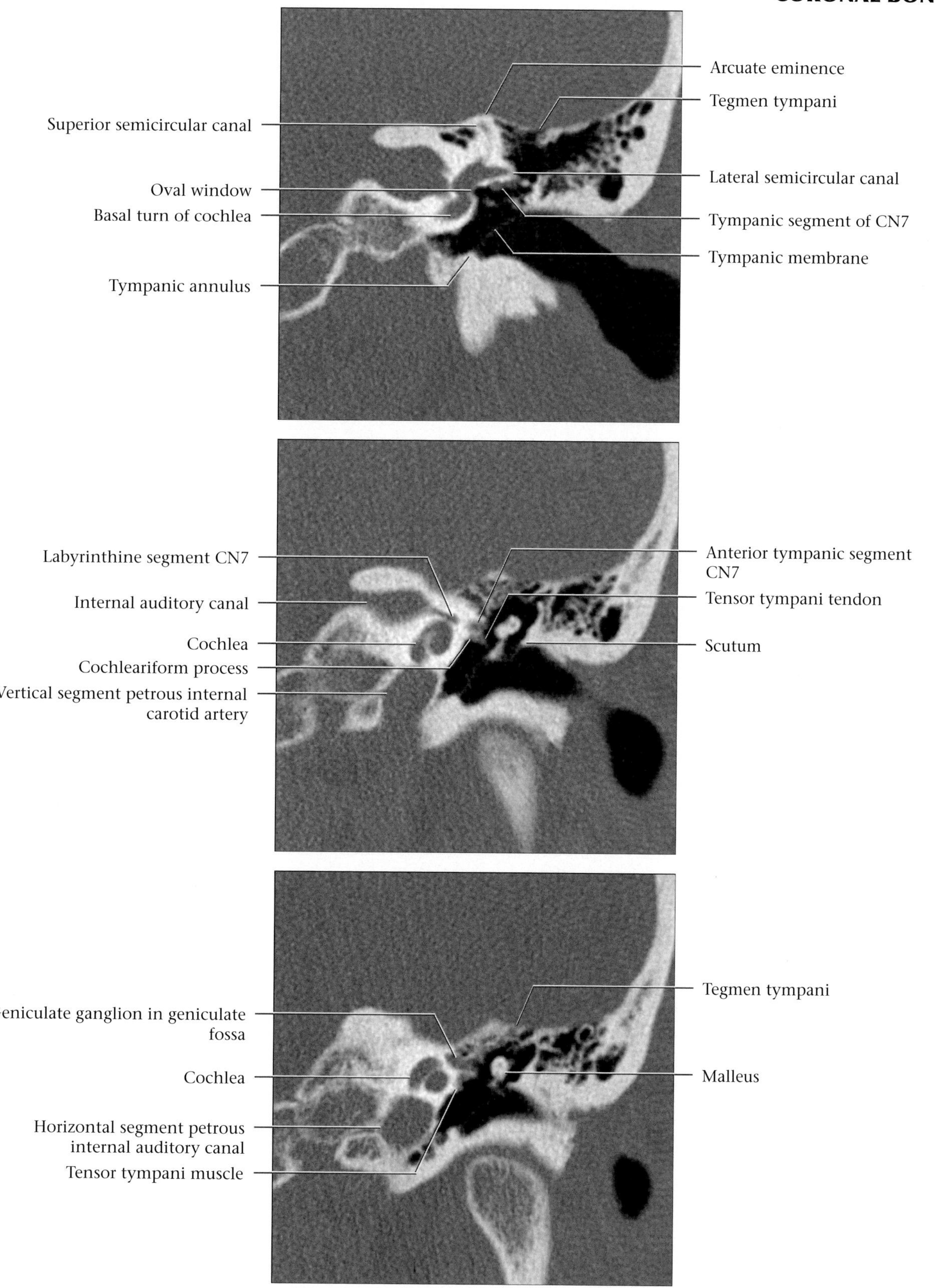
Arcuate eminence
Tegmen tympani
Superior semicircular canal
Lateral semicircular canal
Oval window
Basal turn of cochlea
Tympanic segment of CN7
Tympanic membrane
Tympanic annulus
Labyrinthine segment CN7
Anterior tympanic segment CN7
Internal auditory canal
Tensor tympani tendon
Cochlea
Scutum
Cochleariform process
Vertical segment petrous internal carotid artery
Tegmen tympani
Geniculate ganglion in geniculate fossa
Cochlea
Malleus
Horizontal segment petrous internal auditory canal
Tensor tympani muscle

(Top) At the level of the anterior margin of the oval window the tympanic segment of the facial nerve can be seen under the lateral semicircular canal. Notice the fine bony covering (thin white line) surrounding the facial nerve is now not seen. The facial nerve canal bony covering in this area is normally incomplete. **(Middle)** In the anterior middle ear cavity the labyrinthine segment of the facial nerve can be seen exiting the internal auditory canal over the top of the cochlea. The anterior tympanic segment of the facial nerve is also visible. Do not confuse the muscle-tendon of the tensor tympani in the cochleariform process with the facial nerve. **(Bottom)** In the most anterior portion of middle ear cavity (where both the carotid and the cochlea are visible), the geniculate ganglion is seen within the geniculate fossa as an ovoid structure just above the cochlea.

CN7 (FACIAL NERVE)

AXIAL T2 & T1 MR

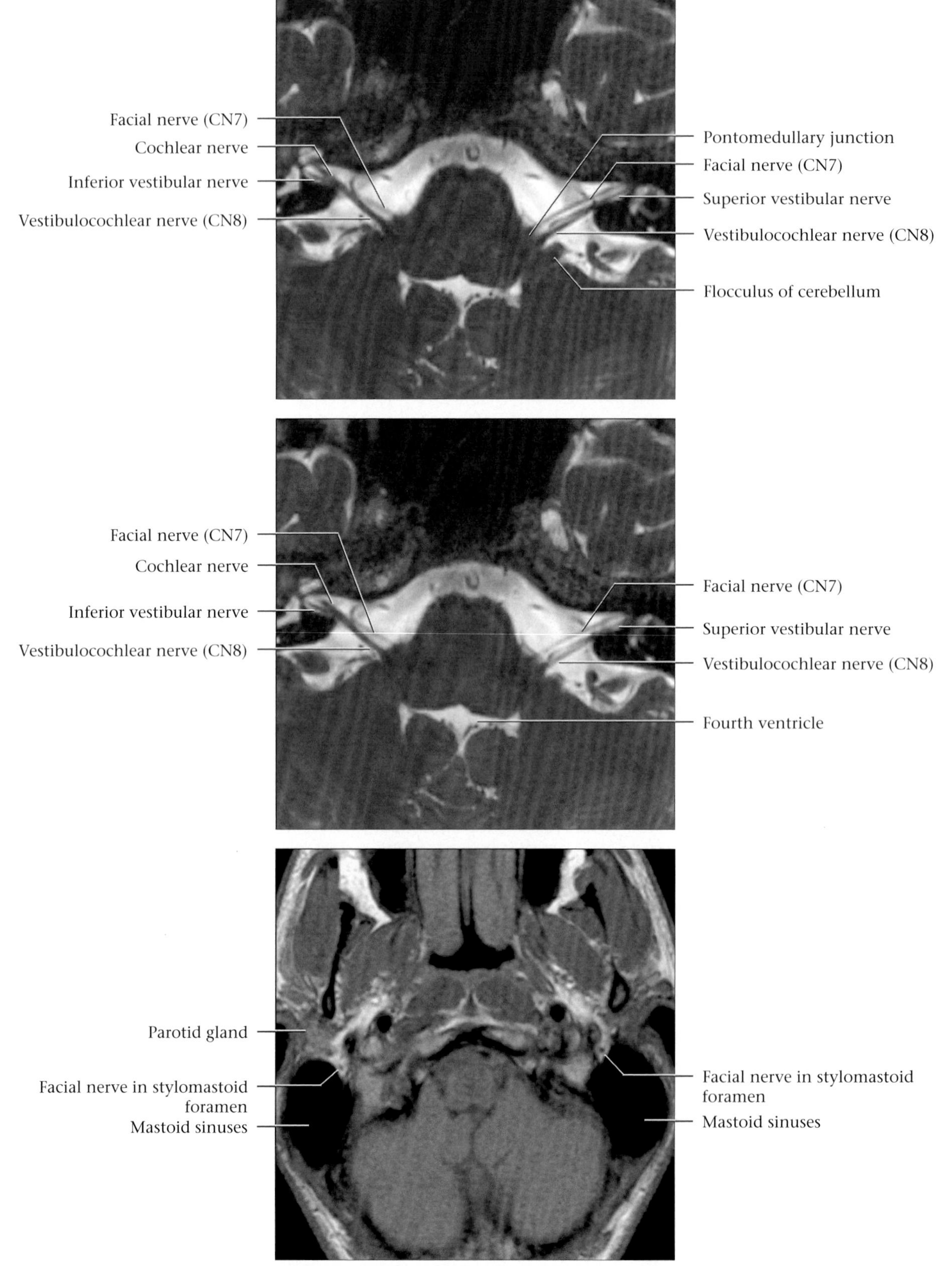
Facial nerve (CN7)
Cochlear nerve
Inferior vestibular nerve
Vestibulocochlear nerve (CN8)
Pontomedullary junction
Facial nerve (CN7)
Superior vestibular nerve
Vestibulocochlear nerve (CN8)
Flocculus of cerebellum
Facial nerve (CN7)
Cochlear nerve
Inferior vestibular nerve
Vestibulocochlear nerve (CN8)
Facial nerve (CN7)
Superior vestibular nerve
Vestibulocochlear nerve (CN8)
Fourth ventricle
Parotid gland
Facial nerve in stylomastoid foramen
Mastoid sinuses
Facial nerve in stylomastoid foramen
Mastoid sinuses

(Top) First of two axial high-resolution T2 MR images through the cerebellopontine angle cistern and internal auditory canal. The facial nerve root exit zone is seen anterior to the vestibulocochlear nerve in the pontomedullary junction bilaterally. Notice the facial nerve maintains an anterior relationship with the vestibulocochlear nerve as it crosses through the cerebellopontine angle cistern. **(Middle)** Image through cephalad internal auditory canal (IAC) on person's left shows the facial nerve anterior to the superior vestibular nerve throughout its IAC course. **(Bottom)** Axial T1 MR image at the level of the stylomastoid foramen shows the exiting low signal facial nerve surrounded by high signal fat in the "bell" of the stylomastoid foramen. If perineural parotid malignancy is present, the fat in this area is obscured.

OBLIQUE SAGITTAL T2 MR

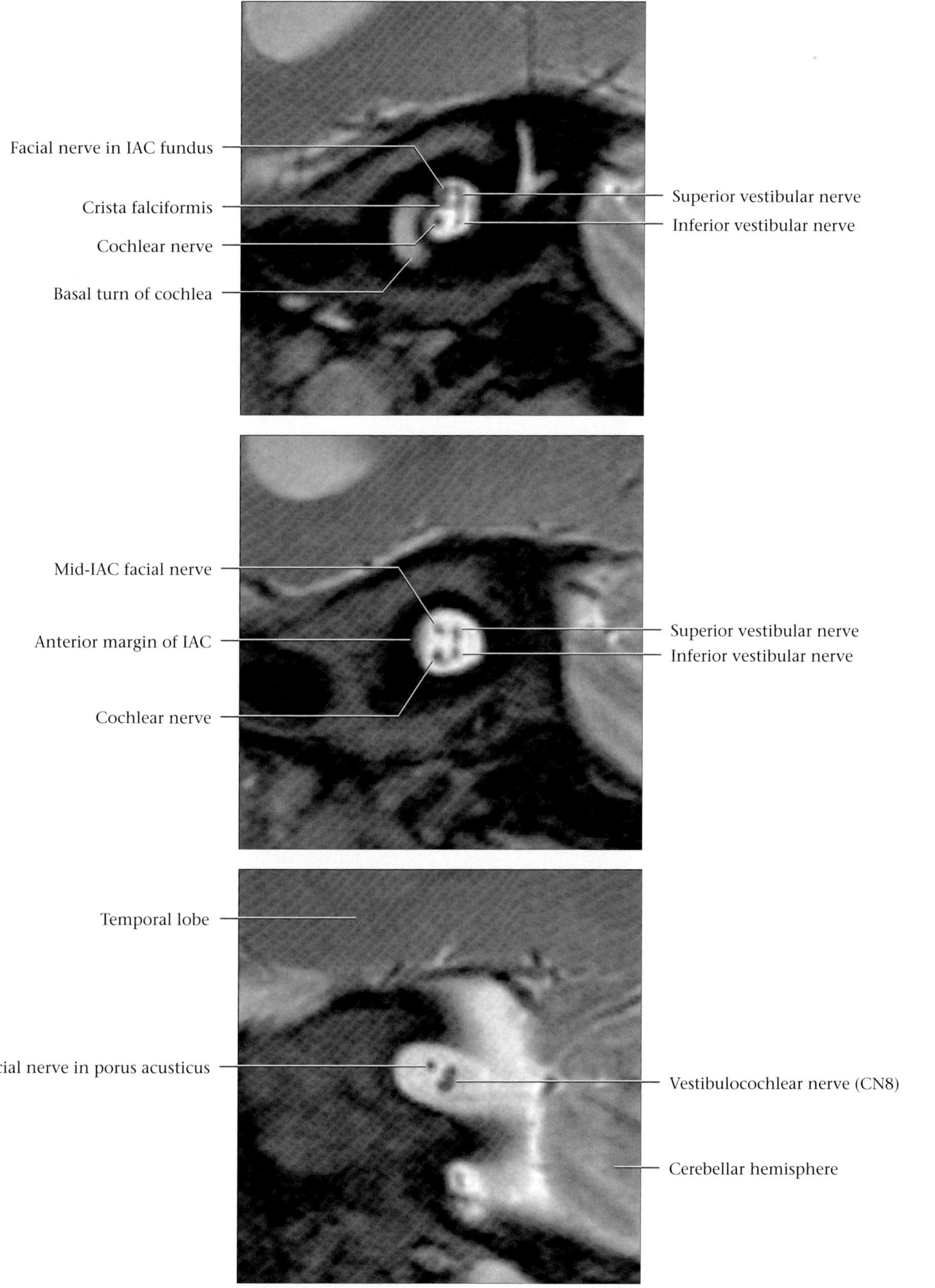
Facial nerve in IAC fundus
Crista falciformis
Cochlear nerve
Basal turn of cochlea
Superior vestibular nerve
Inferior vestibular nerve
Mid-IAC facial nerve
Anterior margin of IAC
Cochlear nerve
Superior vestibular nerve
Inferior vestibular nerve
Temporal lobe
Facial nerve in porus acusticus
Vestibulocochlear nerve (CN8)
Cerebellar hemisphere

(Top) First of three oblique sagittal T2 MR images presented from lateral to medial shows normal fundal anatomy. The horizontal crista falciformis separates the fundus into upper and lower portions. Facial nerve is anterosuperior, separated from superior vestibular nerve by a vertical bony septum called "Bill bar" which is not resolved. Below falciform crest are larger anterior cochlear nerve and posterior inferior vestibular nerve. **(Middle)** In the mid-internal auditory canal (IAC) 4 nerves are clearly identified. The facial nerve is anterosuperior. **(Bottom)** This image through the porus acusticus reveals the characteristic "ball in catcher's mitt" appearance of the facial and vestibulocochlear nerves. The facial nerve is the "ball" and the vestibulocochlear nerve is the "catcher's mitt".

CN8 (VESTIBULOCOCHLEAR NERVE)

Terminology

Abbreviations

- Vestibulocochlear nerve: CN8; CN VIII

Synonyms

- Eighth cranial nerve

Definitions

- CN8: Afferent sensory nerve of hearing & balance

Imaging Anatomy

Overview

- Sensory nerve consisting of two parts
  - Vestibular part: Balance
  - Cochlear part: Hearing
- CN8 best described from peripheral to central

Cochlear Nerve

- Arises from bipolar neurons located in **spiral ganglion** within modiolus of cochlea
  - Peripheral fibers pass to organ of Corti in cochlear duct (scala media) within cochlea
  - Central fibers coalesce & pass as auditory component of CN8 (cochlear nerve) to brainstem
- Central fibers pass from modiolus through cochlear aperture into internal auditory canal (IAC)
  - **Cochlear aperture** defined as bony opening into anteroinferior quadrant of fundus of IAC
  - Maximum diameter of cochlear aperture ~ 2 mm
- **Cochlear nerve** passes from IAC fundus to porus acusticus within **anteroinferior quadrant of IAC**
- Near porus acusticus cochlear nerve joins together with superior & inferior vestibular nerves to form vestibulocochlear nerve (CN8)
- CN8 crosses cerebellopontine angle (CPA) cistern posterior to facial nerve
- CN8 enters lateral brainstem at pontomedullary junction posterior to facial nerve
- Cochlear nerve fibers bifurcate, ending in dorsal & ventral cochlear nuclei
- **Dorsal & ventral cochlear nuclei**
  - Cochlear nuclei found on lateral surface of inferior cerebellar peduncle (restiform body)

Vestibular Nerve

- Arises from bipolar neurons located in vestibular (Scarpa) ganglion located within vestibular nerve in fundal portion of IAC
  - Vestibular ganglion not visible on imaging
  - Peripheral fibers pass to sensory epithelium of utricle, saccule & semicircular canals
    - Traverse multiple foramina in cribriform plate in lateral wall of IAC fundus
  - Central fibers coalesce to form superior & inferior vestibular nerves that pass medially to brainstem
- Fundus of IAC
  - Superior & inferior vestibular nerves are separated by **falciform crest** (transverse crest)
  - Superior vestibular nerve separated from facial nerve anteriorly by vertical bony structure called **Bill bar**
    - Bill bar not visible on imaging (CT or MR)
- Superior & inferior vestibular nerves pass medially from IAC fundus to porus acusticus within posterosuperior & posteroinferior quadrants of IAC
- Near porus acusticus superior & inferior vestibular nerves join together with cochlear nerve to form vestibulocochlear nerve (CN8)
- Vestibulocochlear nerve crosses CPA cistern posterior to facial nerve
- Enters lateral brainstem at junction pons & medulla posterior to facial nerve
- Vestibular nerve fibers divide into ascending & descending branches which mainly terminate in vestibular nuclear complex
- **Vestibular nuclear complex**
  - Four nuclei (lateral, superior, medial & inferior)
  - Located beneath lateral recess along floor of fourth ventricle (rhomboid fossa) in lower pons
  - Complex connections exist between vestibular nuclei, cerebellum, spinal cord (vestibulospinal tract) & nuclei controlling eye movement

Anatomy-Based Imaging Issues

Imaging Recommendations

- Sensorineural hearing loss (SNHL)
  - **Intracochlear lesion suspected**
    - CT & MR both useful for imaging
    - Congenital lesions of membranous labyrinth seen as abnormalities of fluid spaces on MR or in bony labyrinth shape on T-bone CT
    - T-bone CT better for otosclerosis, Paget disease, labyrinthine ossificans or if trauma suspected
    - Only MR will demonstrate labyrinthitis or intralabyrinthine tumor
  - **CN8 lesion suspected (CPA-IAC)**
    - MR imaging method of choice
    - Thin-section, high-resolution T2 sequence in axial & coronal planes may be used to screen patients with unilateral sensorineural hearing loss
    - T1 C+ MR remains gold standard

Imaging "Sweet Spots"

- Unilateral sensorineural hearing loss
  - Focus on brainstem (inferior cerebellar peduncle)-CPA-IAC-cochlea
  - Central acoustic pathway (intra-axial pathways above cochlear nuclei) rarely site of offending lesion
- Cisternal & IAC segments of CN8 routinely visualized on high-resolution T2 MR

Imaging Pitfalls

- Beware small lesions of IAC (≤ 2 mm)!
  - Follow-up imaging recommended as may be transient finding where surgery not needed

Clinical Implications

Clinical Importance

- Vestibular nerve dysfunction (dizziness, vertigo, imbalance) alone usually has negative MR
- 95% of lesions causing unilateral SNHL found by MR are **vestibulocochlear schwannoma**

CN8 (VESTIBULOCOCHLEAR NERVE)

GRAPHICS

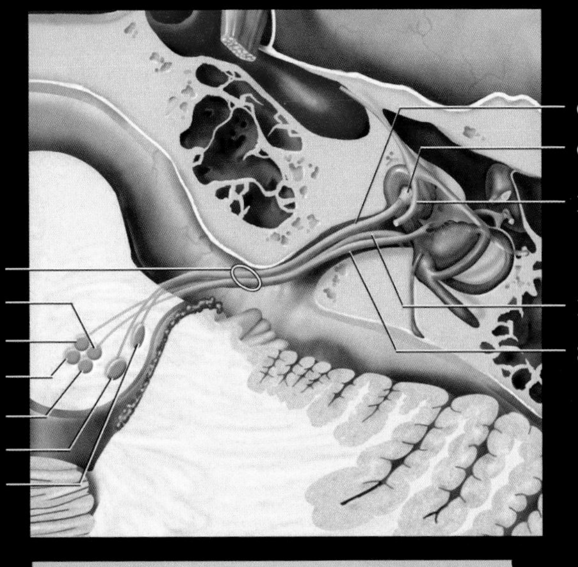
Vestibulocochlear nerve (CN8)
Inferior vestibular nucleus
Superior vestibular nucleus
Medial vestibular nucleus
Lateral vestibular nucleus
Dorsal cochlear nucleus
Ventral cochlear nucleus
Cochlear nerve
Cochlear modiolus
Facial nerve, labyrinthine segment
Inferior vestibular nerve
Superior vestibular nerve

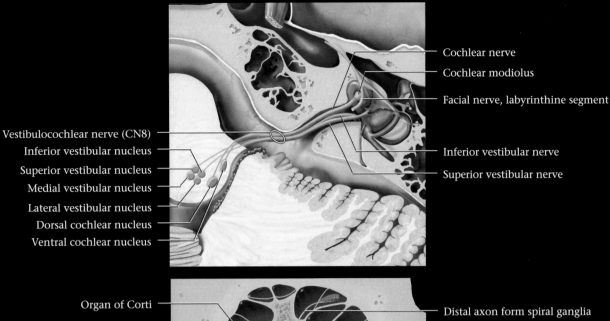

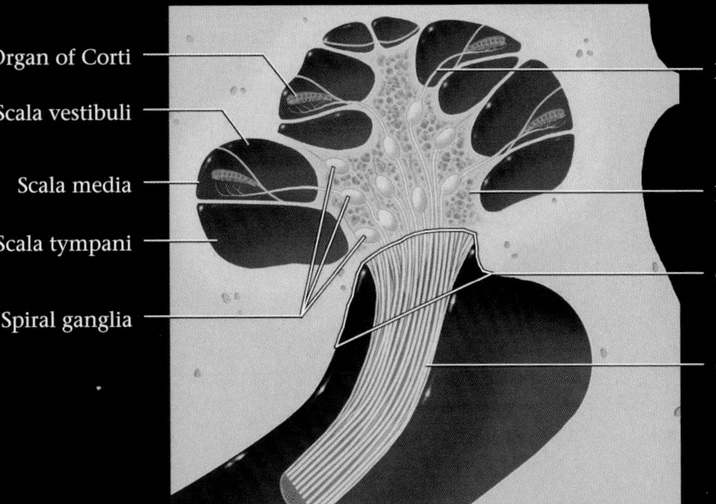
Organ of Corti
Scala vestibuli
Scala media
Scala tympani
Spiral ganglia
Distal axon form spiral ganglia
Modiolus
Cochlear aperture
Cochlear nerve

Facial nerve (CN7)
Cochlear nerve
Bill bar
Superior vestibular nerve
Crista falciformis (horizontal crest)
Singular nerve
Inferior vestibular nerve

(Top) Axial graphic of CPA, IAC & inner ear. Cochlear component of CN8 begins in bipolar cell bodies in spiral ganglion of cochlear modiolus. Central fibers run in cochlear nerve to dorsal & ventral cochlear nuclei in inferior cerebellar peduncle. The inferior & superior vestibular nerves begin in cell bodies in the vestibular ganglion, from there coursing centrally to 4 vestibular nuclei. **(Middle)** Axial graphic of magnified cochlea, modiolus & cochlear nerve. Notice the bipolar spiral ganglion cells within modiolus contribute distal fibers to organ of Corti as well as proximal axons that constitute the cochlear nerve. **(Bottom)** Graphic depicting fundus of IAC. Notice the crista falciformis separates cochlear nerve & inferior vestibular nerve below from CN7 & superior vestibular nerve above. Also note Bill bar separating CN7 from the superior vestibular nerve.

CN8 (VESTIBULOCOCHLEAR NERVE)

AXIAL & CORONAL BONE CT

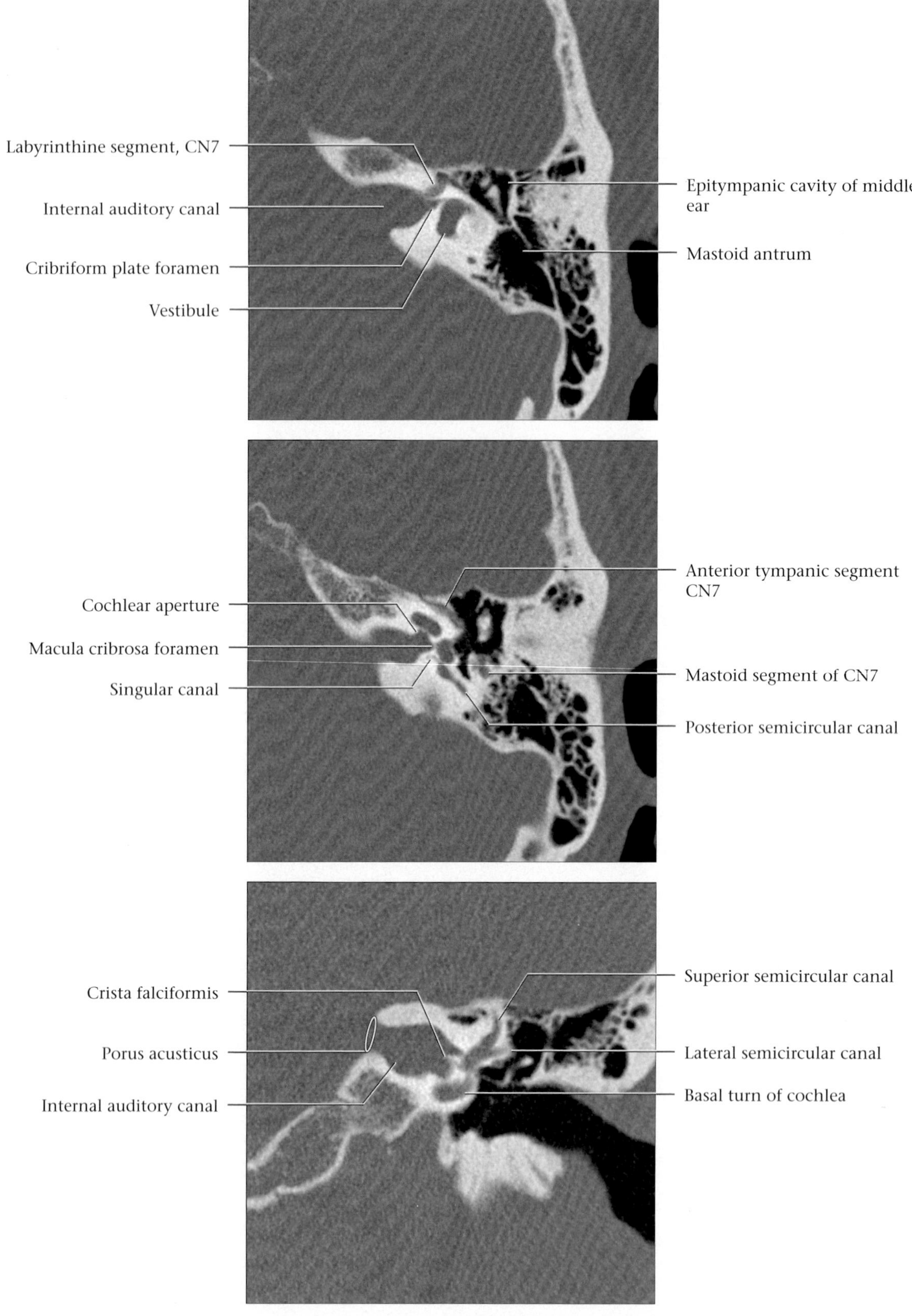
Labyrinthine segment, CN7
Internal auditory canal
Cribriform plate foramen
Vestibule
Epitympanic cavity of middle ear
Mastoid antrum
Cochlear aperture
Macula cribrosa foramen
Singular canal
Anterior tympanic segment CN7
Mastoid segment of CN7
Posterior semicircular canal
Crista falciformis
Porus acusticus
Internal auditory canal
Superior semicircular canal
Lateral semicircular canal
Basal turn of cochlea

(Top) Axial bone CT through the upper portion of the internal auditory canal shows the C-shaped labyrinthine segment of the facial nerve & a main canal of the superior vestibular nerve crossing the cribriform plate toward the vestibule. **(Middle)** Axial bone CT through the lower IAC shows anterolateral cochlear aperture through which the cochlear nerve passes on its way from the cochlear modiolus into the IAC. Also notice the cribriform plate foramen through which the inferior vestibular nerve reaches the vestibule & the smaller singular canal. **(Bottom)** Coronal bone CT image through IAC demonstrates horizontal falciform crest which divides fundus of IAC into upper & lower portions. Facial & superior vestibular nerves pass above & cochlear & inferior vestibular nerves pass below falciform crest. Porus acusticus is bony aperture of internal auditory canal.

CN8 (VESTIBULOCOCHLEAR NERVE)

AXIAL T2 MR

Cochlea
Facial nerve (CN7)
Anteroinferior cerebellar artery
Vestibulocochlear nerve (CN8)
Facial nerve
Superior vestibular nerve
Vestibulocochlear nerve (CN8)
Flocculus of cerebellum

Cochlear nerve
Cochlea
Inferior vestibular nerve
Vestibulocochlear nerve (CN8)
Facial nerve (CN7)
Abducens nerve (CN6)
Facial nerve (CN7)
Superior vestibular nerve
Vestibulocochlear nerve (CN8)

Abducens nerve (CN6)
Facial nerve (CN7)
Superior vestibular nerve
Middle cerebellar peduncle
Abducens nerve (CN6)
Anterior inferior cerebellar artery
Fourth ventricle

(Top) First of three axial T2 MR images presented from inferior to superior through cerebellopontine angle cistern & internal auditory canal. Section through superior left IAC demonstrates cochlear nerve anteriorly & inferior vestibular nerve posteriorly at fundus. **(Middle)** Vestibulocochlear nerve arises posterior to facial nerve from brainstem at pontomedullary junction & maintains a posterior position throughout its course through CPA/IAC. On patient's right the cochlear nerve is anterior to inferior vestibular nerve within fundus of IAC. On left the superior fundus of IAC is seen with the anterior facial nerve & posterior superior vestibular nerve. **(Bottom)** This MR slice through superior IAC area demonstrates the superior vestibular nerve posterior to facial nerve on the patient's right.

CN8 (VESTIBULOCOCHLEAR NERVE)

CORONAL T2 MR

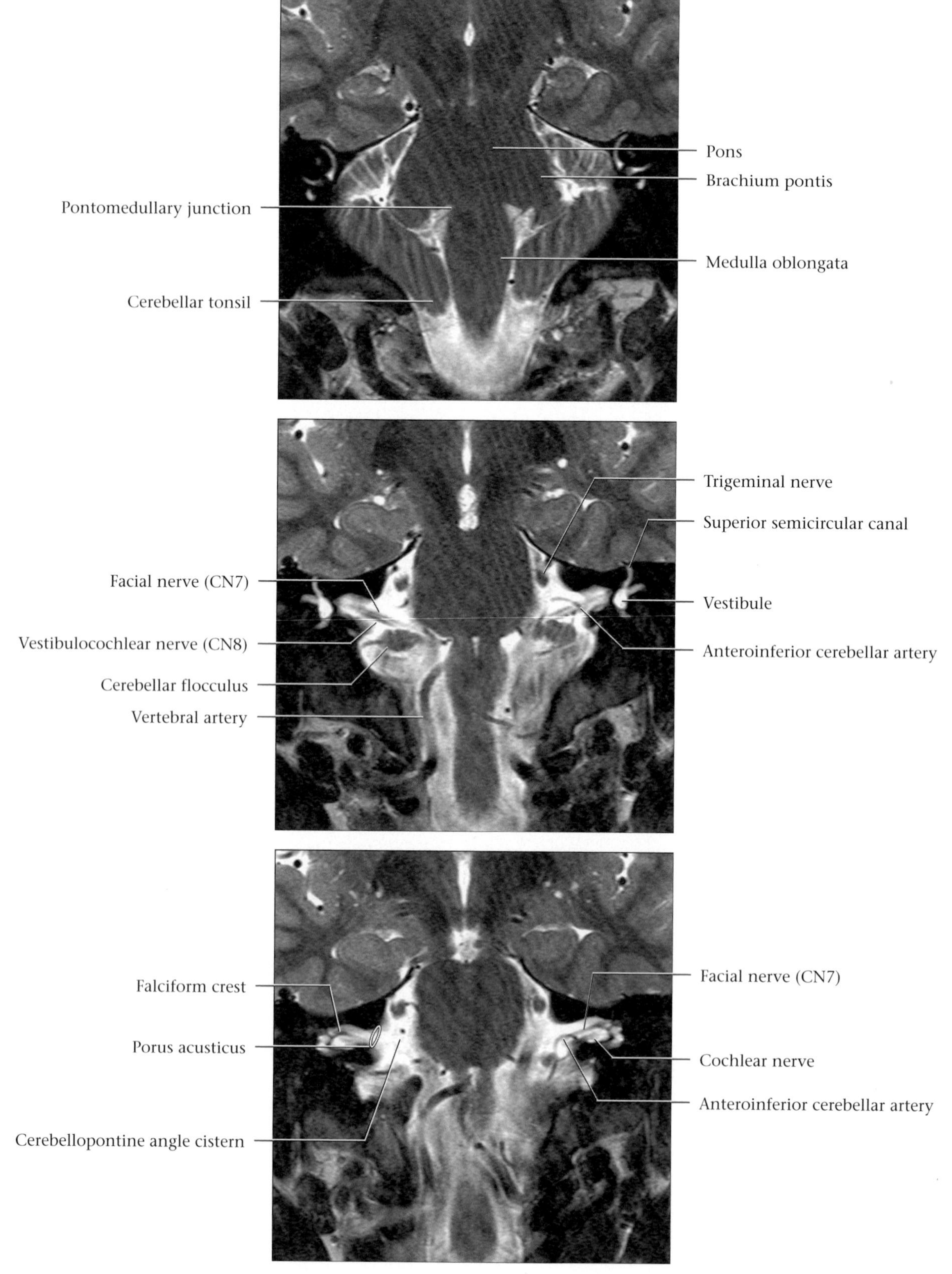
Pons
Brachium pontis
Pontomedullary junction
Medulla oblongata
Cerebellar tonsil
Trigeminal nerve
Superior semicircular canal
Facial nerve (CN7)
Vestibule
Vestibulocochlear nerve (CN8)
Anteroinferior cerebellar artery
Cerebellar flocculus
Vertebral artery
Falciform crest
Facial nerve (CN7)
Porus acusticus
Cochlear nerve
Anteroinferior cerebellar artery
Cerebellopontine angle cistern

(Top) First of three coronal T2 MR images presented from posterior to anterior. Vestibulocochlear nerve emerges from brainstem posterior to facial nerve at pontomedullary junction. **(Middle)** Facial & vestibulocochlear nerves course through CPA into IAC. Facial nerve is anterior & superior to vestibulocochlear nerve within CPA & IAC. Notice the somewhat cephalad course of CN8 as it rises into the IAC from its origin at the pontomedullary junction. **(Bottom)** Section through fundus of internal auditory canal demonstrates horizontal falciform crest separating fundus into upper & lower portions. At this level, facial nerve is above & cochlear nerve is below falciform crest. The anteroinferior cerebellar artery loop is a constant fixture in the normal anatomy of the CPA & IAC area.

OBLIQUE SAGITTAL T2 MR

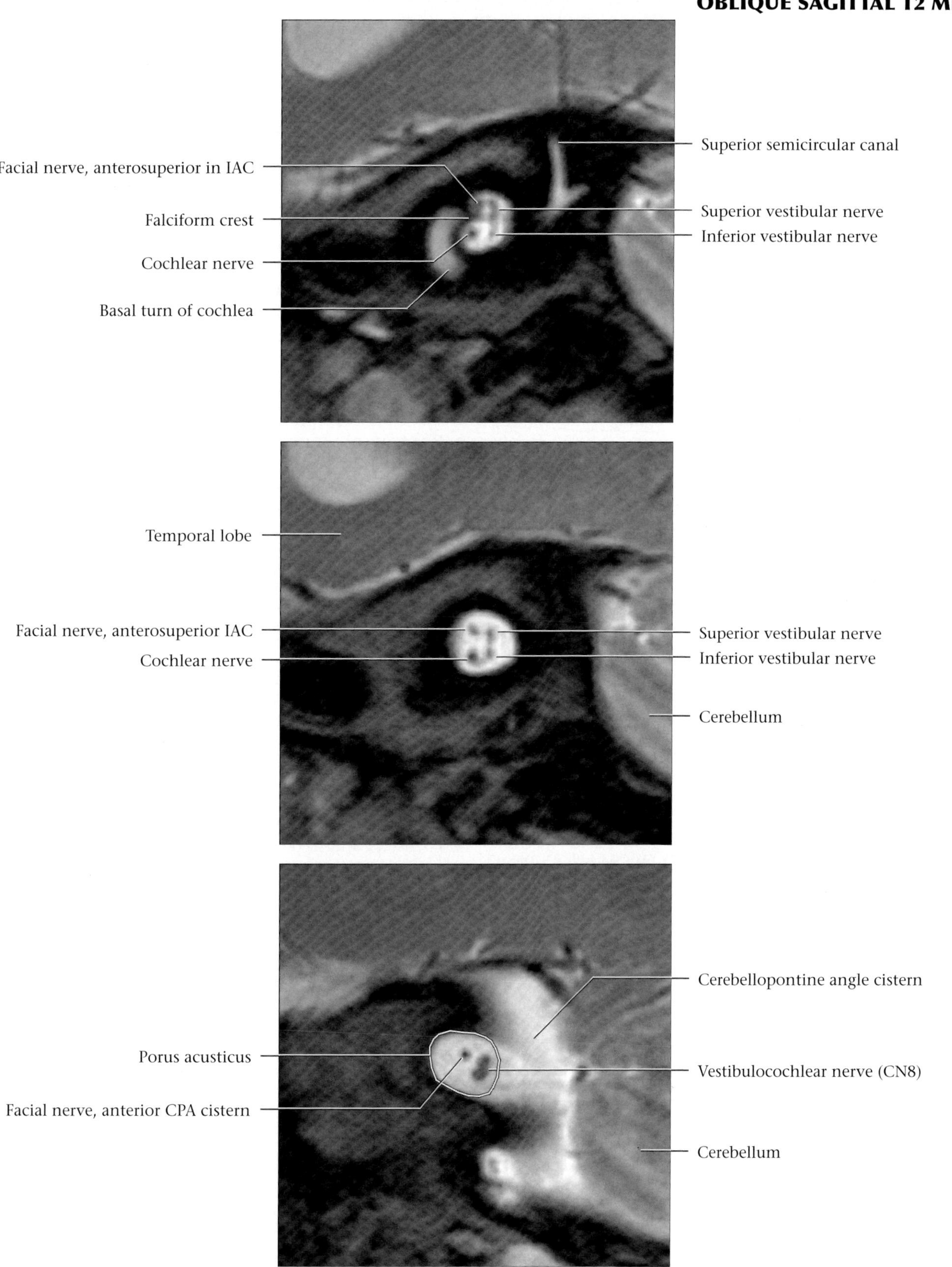
Facial nerve, anterosuperior in IAC
Falciform crest
Cochlear nerve
Basal turn of cochlea
Superior semicircular canal
Superior vestibular nerve
Inferior vestibular nerve
Temporal lobe
Facial nerve, anterosuperior IAC
Cochlear nerve
Superior vestibular nerve
Inferior vestibular nerve
Cerebellum
Porus acusticus
Facial nerve, anterior CPA cistern
Cerebellopontine angle cistern
Vestibulocochlear nerve (CN8)
Cerebellum

(Top) First of three sequential oblique sagittal T2 MR images through IAC presented from lateral to medial. Slice is through fundus of IAC showing horizontal falciform crest separating fundus into upper & lower portions. Facial nerve is anterosuperior, separated from superior vestibular nerve by a vertical bony septum called "Bill bar" which is not resolved with even focused imaging. Below falciform crest are cochlear nerve anteriorly & inferior vestibular nerve posteriorly. **(Middle)** In the mid-IAC this image shows 4 discrete nerves. **(Bottom)** At the level of porus acusticus both superior & inferior vestibular nerves join together with cochlear nerve to form a C-shaped vestibulocochlear nerve. The facial nerve remains discrete as it travels across the cerebellopontine angle cistern.

CN9 (GLOSSOPHARYNGEAL NERVE)

Terminology

Abbreviations

- Glossopharyngeal nerve: CN9, CN IX

Synonyms

- Ninth cranial nerve

Definitions

- Complex cranial nerve functions
  - Taste & sensation to posterior 1/3 tongue
  - Sensory nerve to middle ear & pharynx
  - Parasympathetic to parotid gland
  - Motor to stylopharyngeus muscle
  - Viscerosensory to carotid body & sinus

Imaging Anatomy

Overview

- Mixed nerve (sensory, taste, motor, parasympathetic)
- Four segments: Intra-axial, cisternal, skull base & extracranial

Intra-Axial Segment

- Glossopharyngeal nuclei are in upper & middle medulla
  - **Motor fibers** to stylopharyngeus muscle originate in **nucleus ambiguus**
  - **Sensory fibers** from tympanic membrane, soft palate, tongue base & pharynx terminate in **spinal nucleus CN5**
  - **Taste fibers** from posterior 1/3 tongue terminate in **solitary tract nucleus**
  - **Parasympathetic fibers** to parotid gland originate in **inferior salivatory nucleus**

Cisternal Segment

- Exits lateral medulla in **postolivary sulcus** just above vagus nerve
- Travel anterolaterally through basal cistern together with vagus nerve & bulbar portion of accessory nerve
- Passes through glossopharyngeal meatus into pars nervosa portion of jugular foramen

Skull Base Segment

- Passes through anterior **pars nervosa** portion of **jugular foramen**
  - Accompanied by inferior petrosal sinus
  - Vagus (CN10) & spinal accessory (CN11) nerves are posterior within pars vascularis portion of jugular foramen
  - Superior & inferior sensory ganglia of CN9 are found within jugular foramen

Extracranial Segment

- Exits jugular foramen into anterior **nasopharyngeal carotid space**
- Passes lateral to internal carotid artery & stylopharyngeus muscle
- Terminates in posterior sublingual space in floor of mouth (posterior 1/3 taste function)

Extracranial Branches

- **Tympanic branch (Jacobsen nerve)**
  - Sensation from middle ear & parasympathetic to parotid gland
  - Arises from inferior sensory ganglion within jugular foramen
  - Passes through **inferior tympanic canaliculus** into middle ear
    - Aberrant internal carotid artery enters middle ear via this canal
  - Forms tympanic plexus on cochlear promontory
    - Glomus bodies associated with this nerve form glomus tympanicum paraganglioma
- **Stylopharyngeus branch**
  - Motor to stylopharyngeus muscle
- **Sinus nerve**
  - Supplies viscerosensory fibers to carotid sinus & carotid body
  - Conducts impulses from mechanoreceptors of sinus & chemoreceptors of carotid body to medulla
- **Pharyngeal branches**
  - Sensory to posterior oropharynx & soft palate
- **Lingual branch**
  - Sensory & taste to posterior 1/3 of tongue

Anatomy-Based Imaging Issues

Imaging Recommendations

- MR imaging method of choice
  - Superior sensitivity to skull base, meningeal, cisternal & brainstem pathology
  - Sequences should include a combination of T2, T1 without fat-saturation & contrast-enhanced T1 with fat-saturation in axial & coronal planes
- Bone CT used to supplement MR when complex skull base pathology discovered

Imaging "Sweet Spots"

- Focused enhanced MR imaging extends from pontomedullary junction above to hyoid bone below
- CN9 nuclei & intra-axial segment not directly visualized
  - Position inferred by identifying upper medulla, posterior to postolivary sulcus
  - Cisternal segment is not always visualized on routine MR imaging
    - High-resolution thin-section T2 sequences usually demonstrate CN9, 10, 11 nerve complex passing through basal cisterns
    - Bone CT with bone algorithm clearly demonstrates bony anatomy of pars nervosa
- Extracranial segment not visualized

Imaging Pitfalls

- Remember to image entire extracranial course of CN9; do not just stop at skull base!

Clinical Implications

Clinical Importance

- Glossopharyngeal nerve dysfunction usually associated with CN10 & 11 neuropathy
  - Isolated glossopharyngeal neuropathy exceedingly rare

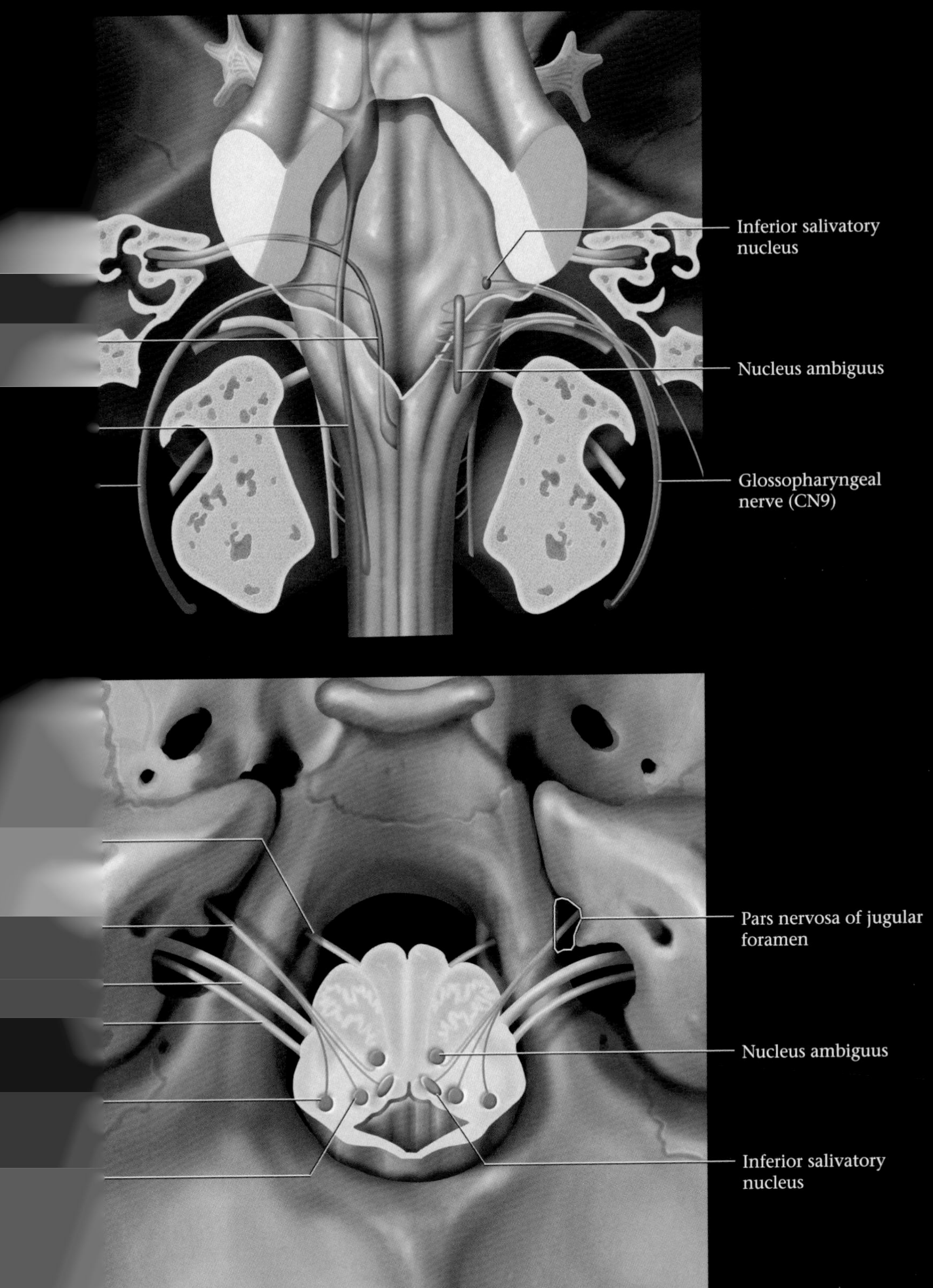
Inferior salivatory nucleus
Nucleus ambiguus
Glossopharyngeal nerve (CN9)
Pars nervosa of jugular foramen
Nucleus ambiguus
Inferior salivatory nucleus

m from behind emphasizing the four nuclei participating in the functions of the
Notice the two efferent nuclei, the nucleus ambiguus and inferior salivatory nucleus labeled
ambiguus supplies motor fibers to the stylopharyngeus muscle while the inferior salivatory
pathetic fibers to the parotid gland. On the left the afferent nuclei are the solitary tract
cleus of CN5. The solitary tract nucleus receives taste fibers from the tongue base while the
eives sensation from the soft palate, tongue base and pharynx. **(Bottom)** Axial graphic
tem from above shows the 4 nuclei of the glossopharyngeal nerve

GRAPHICS, EXTRACRANIAL

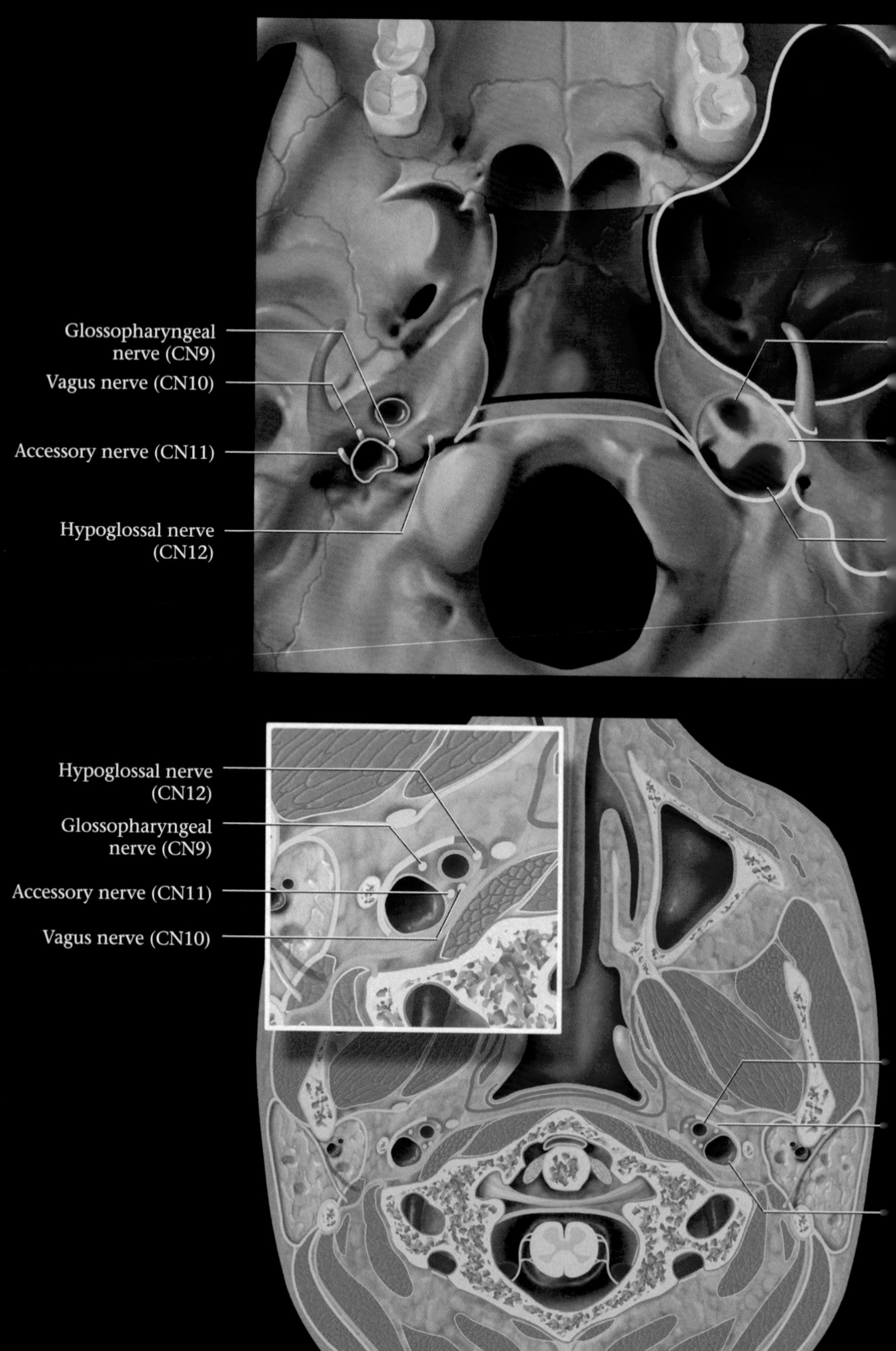

Glossopharyngeal nerve (CN9)
Vagus nerve (CN10)
Accessory nerve (CN11)
Hypoglossal nerve (CN12)
Hypoglossal nerve (CN12)
Glossopharyngeal nerve (CN9)
Accessory nerve (CN11)
Vagus nerve (CN10)

(Top) Graphic of skull base viewed from below depicting the four cranial nerves emerging ir carotid space. The glossopharyngeal nerve is just anteromedial to the internal jugular vein a of the jugular foramen. **(Bottom)** Axial graphic of nasopharyngeal carotid spaces showing tl glossopharyngeal nerve situated anteriorly in the gap between the internal carotid artery an vein. Notice that at this level, CN10, CN11 and CN12 are all still within the carotid space. T

CN9 (GLOSSOPHARYNGEAL NERVE)

GRAPHIC, EXTRACRANIAL

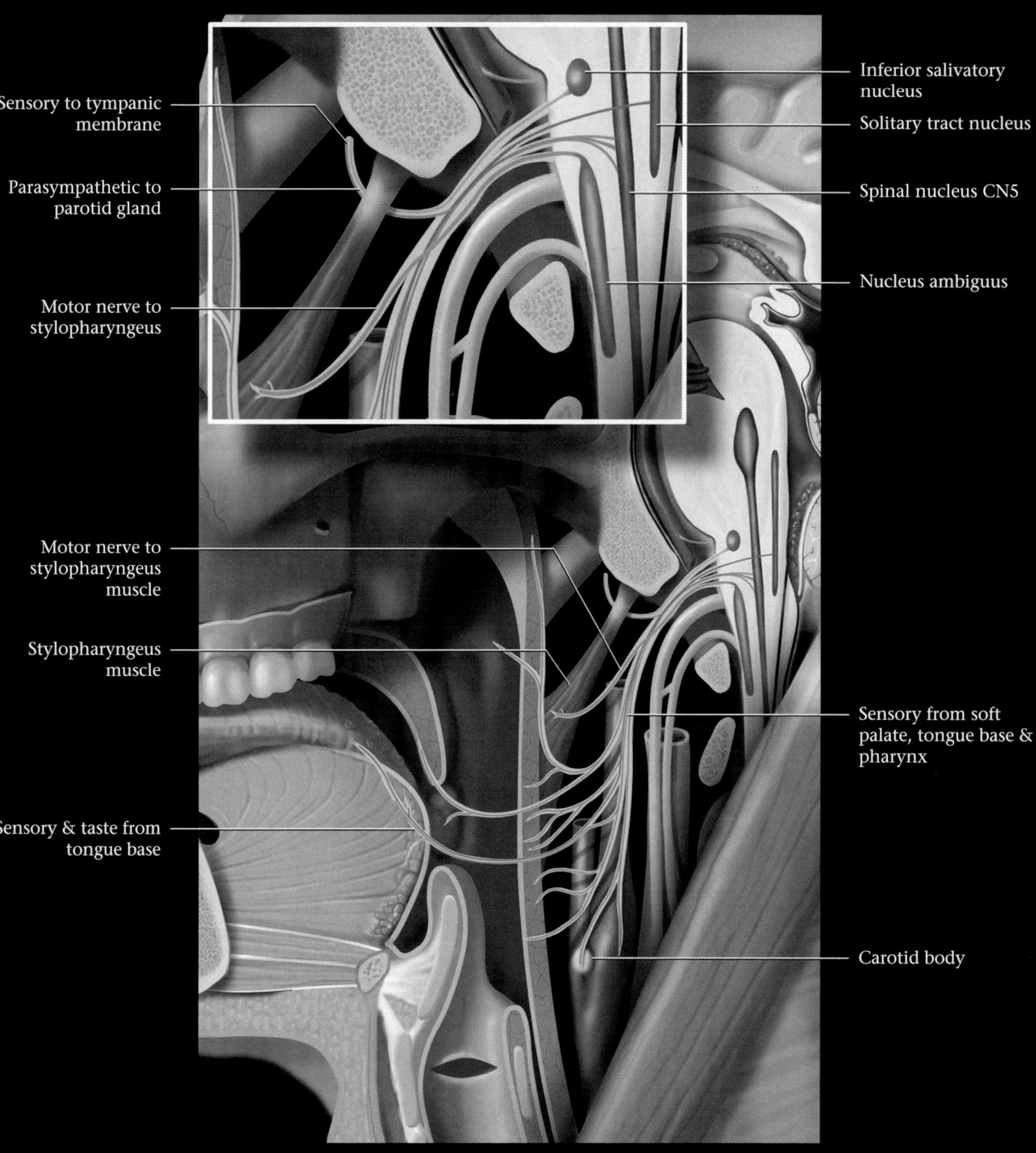
Sensory to tympanic membrane
Parasympathetic to parotid gland
Motor nerve to stylopharyngeus
Inferior salivatory nucleus
Solitary tract nucleus
Spinal nucleus CN5
Nucleus ambiguus
Motor nerve to stylopharyngeus muscle
Stylopharyngeus muscle
Sensory & taste from tongue base
Sensory from soft palate, tongue base & pharynx
Carotid body

Sagittal graphic emphasizing the extracranial component of the glossopharyngeal nerve. Only one muscle is innervated by the fibers in CN9 from the nucleus ambiguus, the stylopharyngeus. Sensory information from the tongue base, soft palate and oropharyngeal surface are transmitted via CN9 to the spinal nucleus of the trigeminal nerve. Taste sensation from the tongue base travels via CN9 to the solitary tract nucleus. Parasympathetic secretomotor fibers from the inferior salivatory nucleus bound for the parotid gland also travel in CN9.

CN9 (GLOSSOPHARYNGEAL NERVE)

AXIAL BONE CT

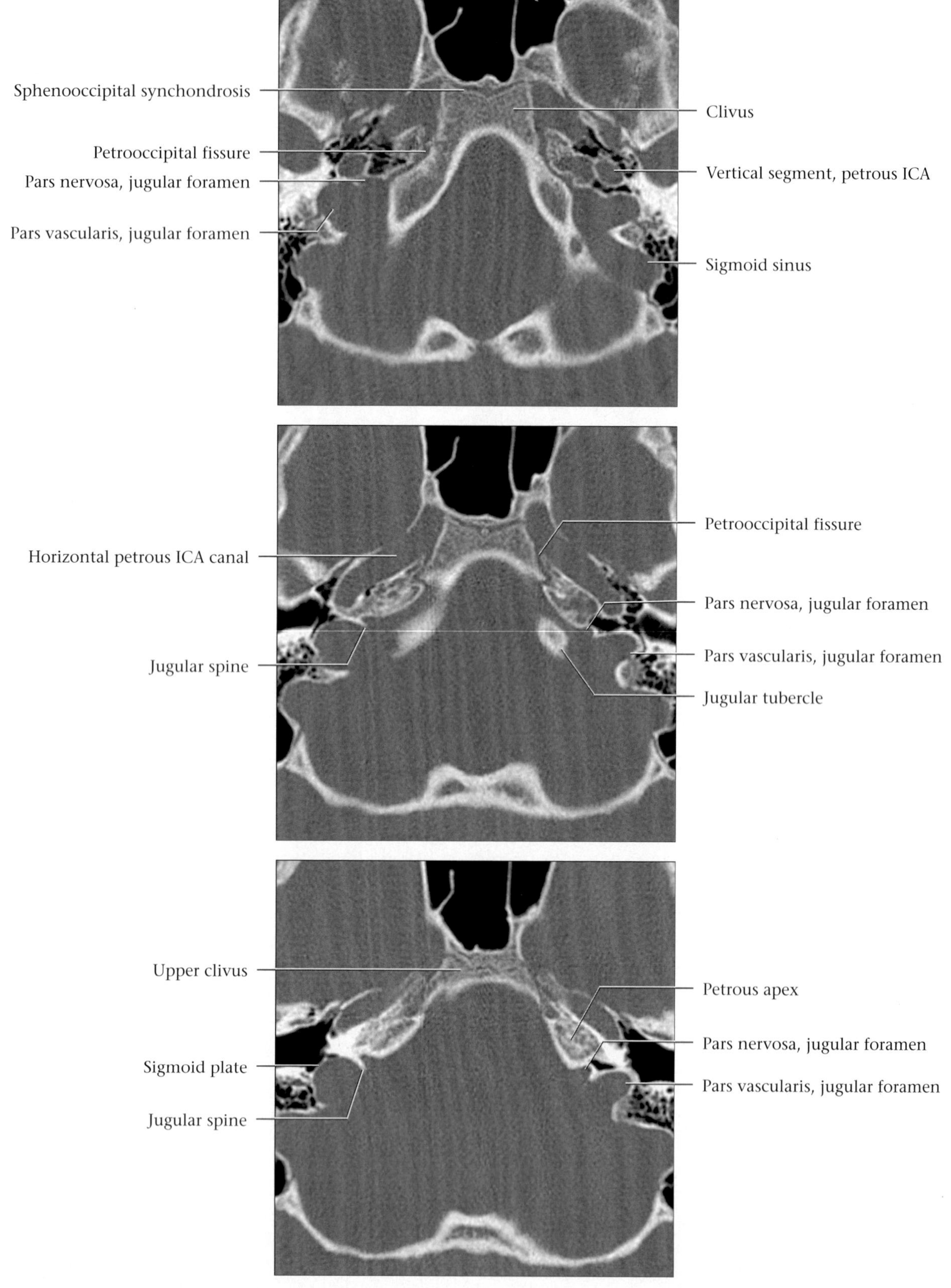
Sphenooccipital synchondrosis
Clivus
Petrooccipital fissure
Vertical segment, petrous ICA
Pars nervosa, jugular foramen
Pars vascularis, jugular foramen
Sigmoid sinus
Petrooccipital fissure
Horizontal petrous ICA canal
Pars nervosa, jugular foramen
Pars vascularis, jugular foramen
Jugular spine
Jugular tubercle
Upper clivus
Petrous apex
Pars nervosa, jugular foramen
Sigmoid plate
Pars vascularis, jugular foramen
Jugular spine

(Top) First of three axial bone CT images presented from inferior to superior through posterior skull base emphasizing the bony anatomy of the jugular foramen. The jugular foramen is located on floor of posterior cranial fossa between petrous temporal bone anterolaterally & occipital bone posteromedially. It is therefore a venous channel between these bones. **(Middle)** The jugular foramen is seen here as two discrete pieces, the smaller anteromedial pars nervosa & larger posterolateral pars vascularis, separated by jugular spine of petrous bone. **(Bottom)** The two parts of the jugular foramen are visibile. The pars nervosa transmits the glossopharyngeal nerve (CN9), Jacobsen nerve & inferior petrosal sinus. The pars vascularis transmits the vagus (CN10) & accessory (CN11) cranial nerves, Arnold nerve & sigmoid sinus which becomes the internal jugular vein.

CN9 (GLOSSOPHARYNGEAL NERVE)

AXIAL T2 MR

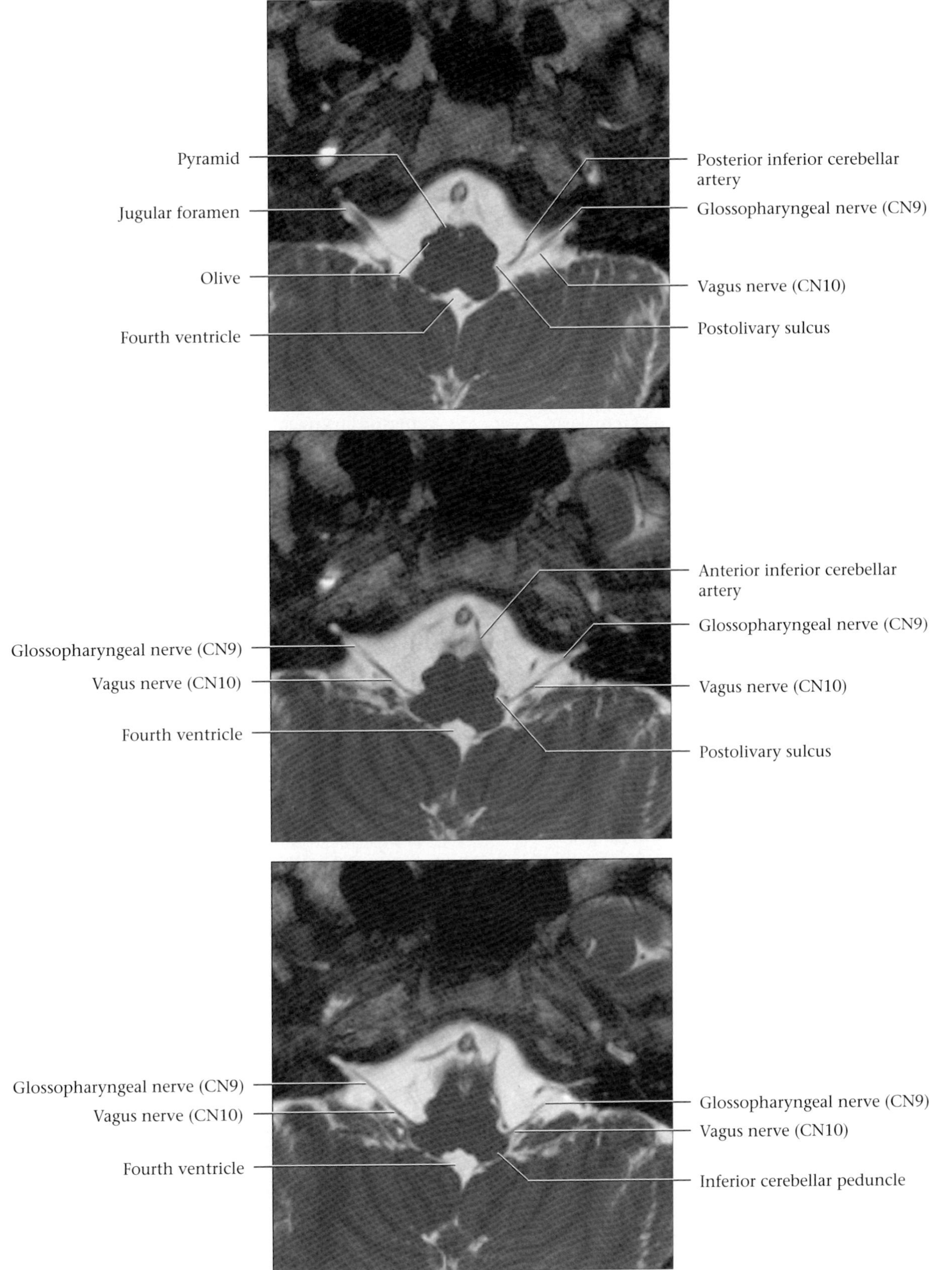
Pyramid
Jugular foramen
Olive
Fourth ventricle
Posterior inferior cerebellar artery
Glossopharyngeal nerve (CN9)
Vagus nerve (CN10)
Postolivary sulcus
Glossopharyngeal nerve (CN9)
Vagus nerve (CN10)
Fourth ventricle
Anterior inferior cerebellar artery
Glossopharyngeal nerve (CN9)
Vagus nerve (CN10)
Postolivary sulcus
Glossopharyngeal nerve (CN9)
Vagus nerve (CN10)
Fourth ventricle
Glossopharyngeal nerve (CN9)
Vagus nerve (CN10)
Inferior cerebellar peduncle

(Top) First of three axial high-resolution T2 MR images through the brainstem medulla presented from inferior to superior. Glossopharyngeal nerve is seen passing laterally into the pars nervosa of the jugular foramen. **(Middle)** The glossopharyngeal nerve (CN9), vagus nerve (CN10) and bulbar accessory nerve (CN11) all exit the medulla laterally in the postolivary sulcus. CN9 is the most cephalad of these. With routine MR imaging it is not possible to see these three cranial nerves individually. **(Bottom)** In the upper medulla the vagus nerve is well seen leaving the brainstem via the postolivary sulcus. The glossopharyngeal nerve is seen more laterally as it has already exited the brainstem above the vagus nerve.

CN10 (VAGUS NERVE)

Terminology

Abbreviations

- Vagus nerve: CN10, CN X

Synonyms

- Tenth cranial nerve

Definitions

- CN10: Parasympathetic nerve supplying regions of head and neck and thoracic and abdominal viscera
- Additional vagus nerve components
    - Motor to soft palate (except tensor veli palatini muscle), pharyngeal constrictor muscles, larynx and palatoglossus muscle of tongue
    - Visceral sensation from larynx, esophagus, trachea, thoracic and abdominal viscera
    - Sensory nerve to external tympanic membrane, external auditory canal (EAC) and external ear
    - Taste from epiglottis

Imaging Anatomy

Overview

- Mixed nerve (sensory, taste, motor, parasympathetic)
- Segments: Intra-axial, cisternal, skull base and extracranial

Intra-Axial Segment

- Vagal nuclei are in upper and middle medulla
    - **Motor fibers** originate in **nucleus ambiguus**
    - **Taste** from epiglottis goes to **solitary tract nucleus**
    - **Sensory fibers** from viscera terminate in **dorsal vagal nucleus** (afferent component)
    - **Parasympathetic fibers** project from **dorsal vagal nucleus** (efferent component)
    - Sensory from regional meninges and ear project to spinal nucleus CN5
- Fibers to and from these nuclei exit lateral medulla in postolivary sulcus inferior to CN9 and superior to bulbar portion of CN11

Cisternal Segment

- Exits lateral medulla in **postolivary sulcus** between CN9 and bulbar portion of CN11
- Travel anterolaterally through basal cistern together with CN9 and bulbar portion of CN11

Skull Base Segment

- Passes through posterior **pars vascularis** portion of jugular foramen (JF)
    - Accompanied by CN11 and jugular bulb
    - **Superior vagal ganglion** is found within JF

Extracranial Segment

- Exits JF into nasopharyngeal **carotid space**
- Inferior vagal ganglion lies just below skull base
- Descends along posterolateral aspect of internal carotid artery into thorax
    - Passes anterior to aortic arch on left and subclavian artery on right
- Forms plexus around esophagus and major blood vessels to heart and lungs
- Gastric nerves emerge from esophageal plexus and provide parasympathetic innervation to stomach
- Innervation to intestines and visceral organs follows arterial blood supply to that organ

Extracranial Branches in Head & Neck

- **Auricular branch (Arnold nerve)**
    - Sensation from external surface of tympanic membrane, EAC and external ear
    - Arises from superior vagal ganglion within JF
    - Passes through **mastoid canaliculus** extending from posterolateral JF to mastoid segment CN7 canal
    - Enters EAC via tympanomastoid fissure
- **Pharyngeal branches**
    - **Pharyngeal plexus** exits just below skull base
    - Sensory to epiglottis, trachea and esophagus
    - Motor to soft palate [except tensor veli palatini muscle (CNV3)] and pharyngeal constrictor muscles
- **Superior laryngeal nerve**
    - Motor to **cricothyroid** muscle
    - Sensory to mucosa of supraglottis
- **Recurrent laryngeal nerve**
    - On right recurs at cervicothoracic junction, passes posteriorly around subclavian artery
    - On left recurs in mediastinum by passing posteriorly under aorta at aortopulmonary window
    - Nerves recur in **tracheoesophageal grooves** (TEG)
    - Motor to all laryngeal muscles except cricothyroids
    - Sensory to mucosa of infraglottis

Anatomy-Based Imaging Issues

Imaging Recommendations

- **Proximal vagal neuropathy**
    - Image from medulla to hyoid bone
    - MR imaging method of choice
        - Superior sensitivity to skull base, meningeal, cisternal and brainstem pathology
        - Sequences should include a combination of T2, T1 without fat-saturation and contrast-enhanced T1 with fat-saturation in axial and coronal planes
        - Bone CT used to supplement MR when complex skull base pathology is present
- **Distal vagal neuropathy**
    - Image from hyoid bone to mediastinum
    - Must reach carina if **left** vagal neuropathy
    - Key areas to evaluate are carotid space and TEG
    - CECT imaging method of choice

Clinical Implications

Clinical Importance

- Vagal nerve dysfunction separated into proximal and distal symptom complexes
- **Proximal symptom complex**
    - Injury site: Between medulla and hyoid bone
    - Multiple cranial nerves involved (CN9-12) with oropharyngeal and laryngeal dysfunction
- **Distal symptom complex**
    - Injury site: Below hyoid bone
    - Isolated CN10 involvement with laryngeal dysfunction only

CN10 (VAGUS NERVE)

GRAPHICS, PROXIMAL CN10

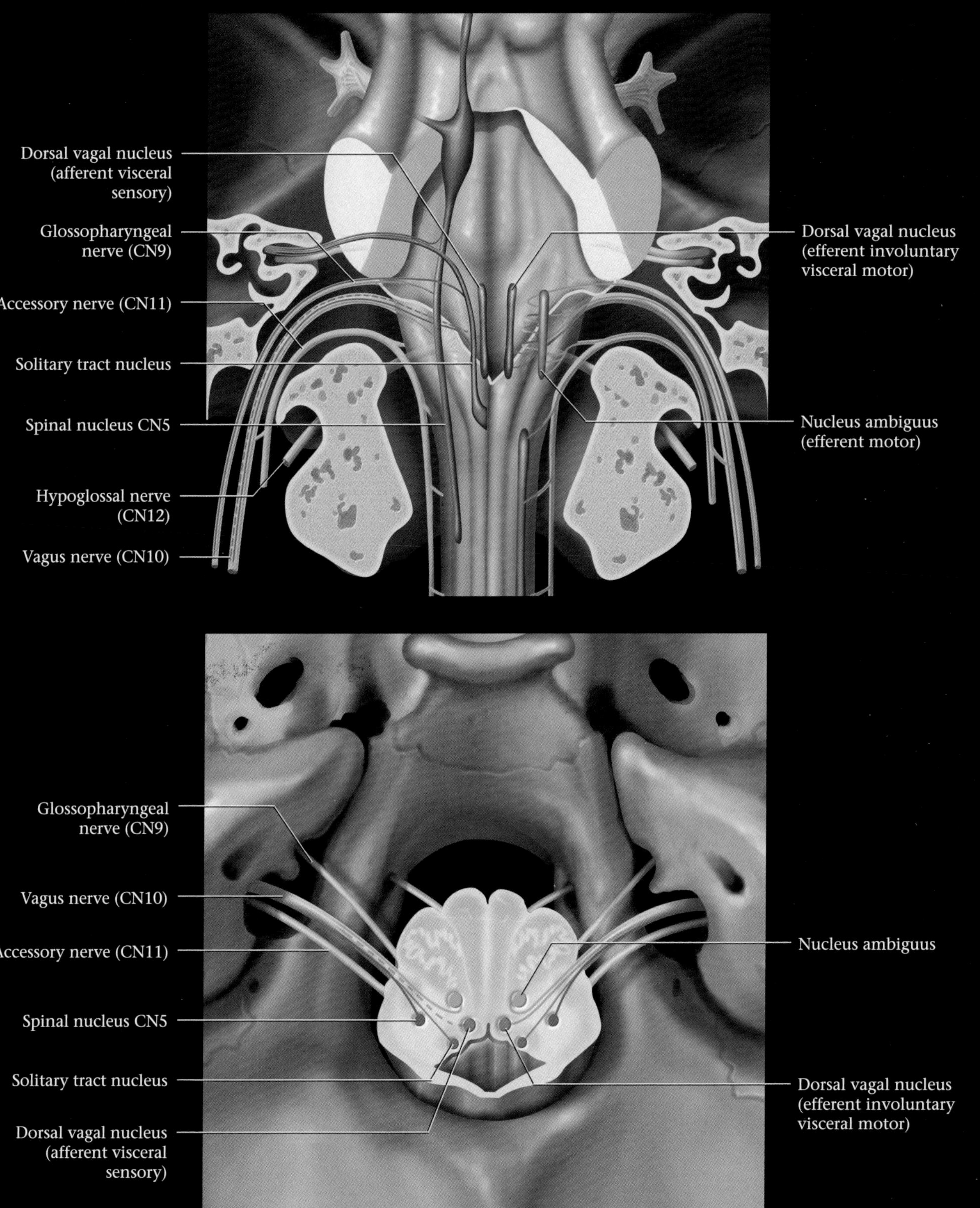

Dorsal vagal nucleus (afferent visceral sensory)
Glossopharyngeal nerve (CN9)
Accessory nerve (CN11)
Solitary tract nucleus
Spinal nucleus CN5
Hypoglossal nerve (CN12)
Vagus nerve (CN10)
Dorsal vagal nucleus (efferent involuntary visceral motor)
Nucleus ambiguus (efferent motor)
Glossopharyngeal nerve (CN9)
Vagus nerve (CN10)
Accessory nerve (CN11)
Spinal nucleus CN5
Solitary tract nucleus
Dorsal vagal nucleus (afferent visceral sensory)
Nucleus ambiguus
Dorsal vagal nucleus (efferent involuntary visceral motor)

(Top) Graphic of brainstem viewed from behind shows critical nuclear columns of CN10. Note the nucleus ambiguus supplies motor fibers to CN10. Dorsal vagal nucleus is a mixed nucleus, sending efferent parasympathetic fibers to the viscera while receiving afferent sensory fibers from these same viscera. The solitary tract nucleus receives taste information from epiglottis and vallecula via CN10. **(Bottom)** Axial graphic through medulla shows principal nuclei associated with vagus nerve function. Skeletal motor fibers to pharynx and larynx come from nucleus ambiguus. Parasympathetic fibers to the viscera are associated with the dorsal nucleus of the vagus nerve (solid pink line). Sensory information transmitted from the viscera is transmitted to the dorsal nucleus of vagus nerve (dashed pink line). The solitary tract nucleus receives taste information for the epiglottis.

CN10 (VAGUS NERVE)

GRAPHIC, EXTRACRANIAL VAGUS NERVE

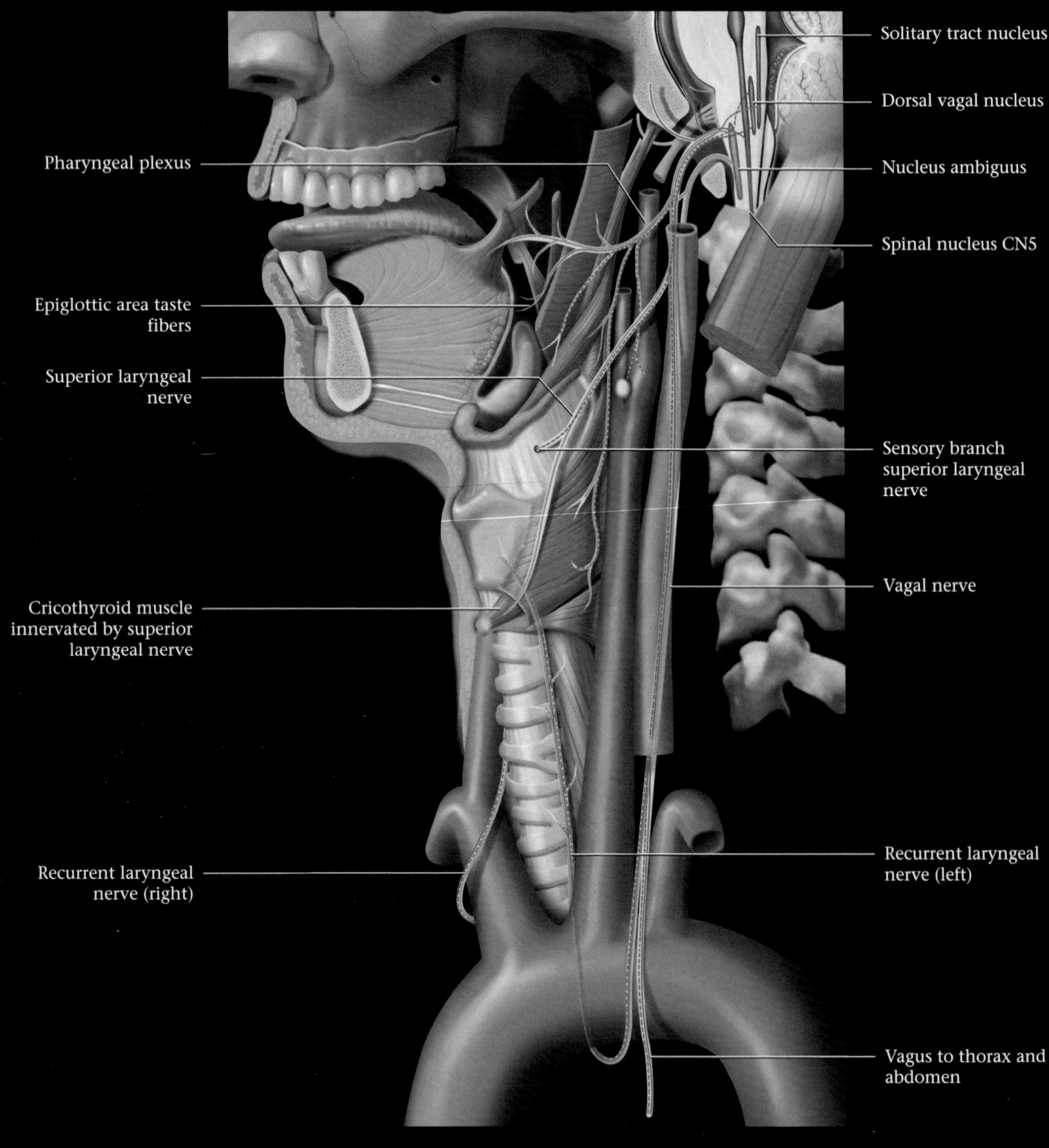
Solitary tract nucleus
Dorsal vagal nucleus
Nucleus ambiguus
Spinal nucleus CN5
Pharyngeal plexus
Epiglottic area taste fibers
Superior laryngeal nerve
Sensory branch superior laryngeal nerve
Vagal nerve
Cricothyroid muscle innervated by superior laryngeal nerve
Recurrent laryngeal nerve (right)
Recurrent laryngeal nerve (left)
Vagus to thorax and abdomen

Lateral graphic focused on neck and upper mediastinal portions CN10 including the 4 brainstem nuclei. The nucleus ambiguus supplies efferent motor innervation (green lines) via pharyngeal plexus to the soft palate and pharynx (superior, middle and inferior constrictor muscles) and via the recurrent laryngeal nerves to all laryngeal muscles except the cricothyroids. The dual functioning dorsal vagal nucleus both sends out efferent fibers for involuntary motor activity in the viscera (solid pink line) as well as receives sensations from these same viscera (dashed pink line). The solitary tract nucleus receives taste information from the region of the epiglottis and vallecula. The spinal nucleus of CN5 receives external ear and skull base-meninges sensory information. Only the visceral motor and sensory fibers from dorsal vagal nucleus continue on CN10 to rest of body.

CN10 (VAGUS NERVE)

GRAPHIC, EXTRACRANIAL CN10

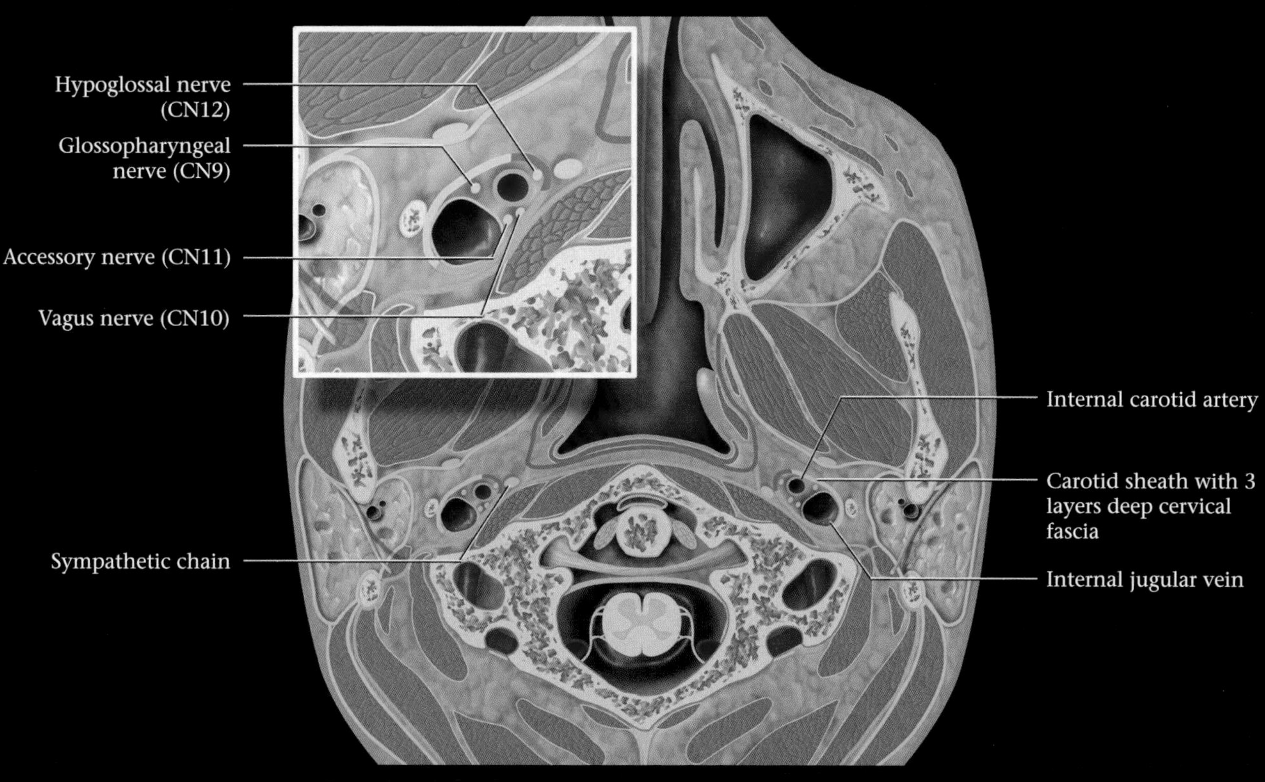
Hypoglossal nerve (CN12)
Glossopharyngeal nerve (CN9)
Accessory nerve (CN11)
Vagus nerve (CN10)
Sympathetic chain
Internal carotid artery
Carotid sheath with 3 layers deep cervical fascia
Internal jugular vein

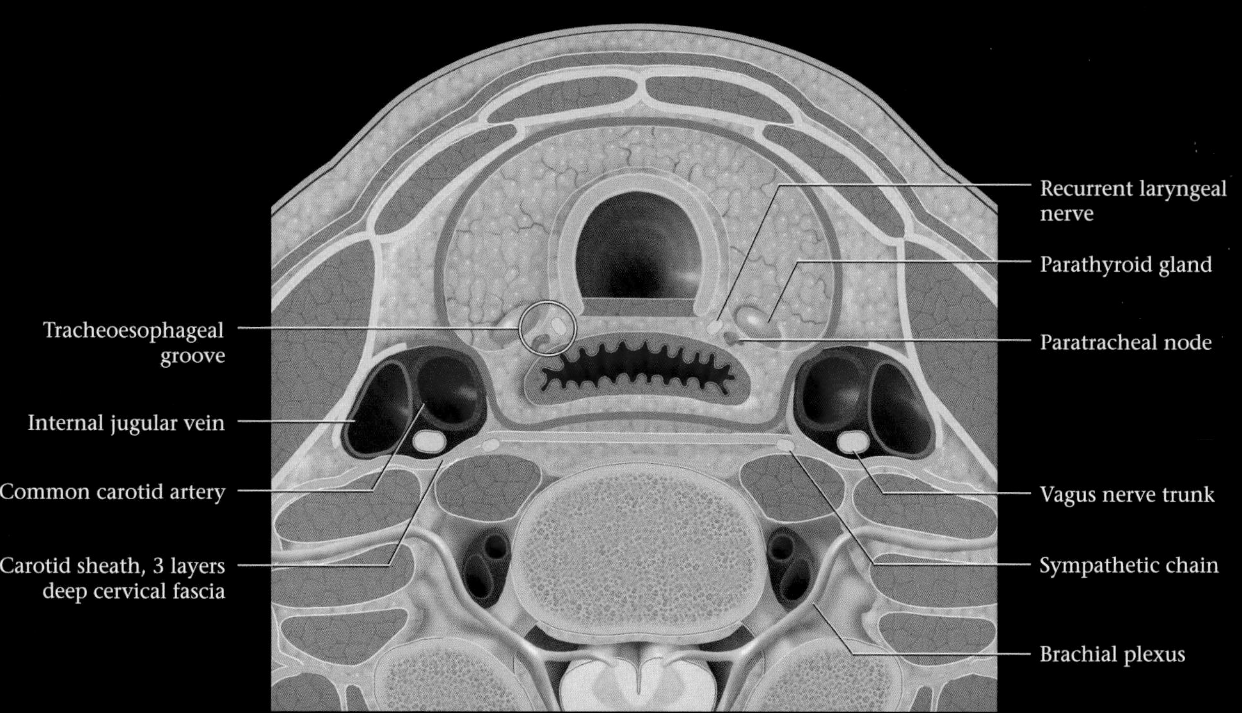
Tracheoesophageal groove
Internal jugular vein
Common carotid artery
Carotid sheath, 3 layers deep cervical fascia
Recurrent laryngeal nerve
Parathyroid gland
Paratracheal node
Vagus nerve trunk
Sympathetic chain
Brachial plexus

(Top) Axial graphic of nasopharyngeal carotid spaces shows the extracranial vagus nerve situated posteriorly in the gap between the internal carotid artery and the internal jugular vein. Notice that at this level, CN9, CN11 and CN12 are all still within the carotid space. **(Bottom)** Axial graphic through the infrahyoid carotid spaces at the level of the thyroid gland demonstrates the vagus trunk is the only remaining cranial nerve within the carotid space. It remains in the posterior gap between the common carotid artery and the internal jugular vein. Note the recurrent laryngeal nerve in the tracheoesophageal groove with the visceral space. Remember the left recurrent laryngeal nerve turns cephalad in the aortopulmonic window in the mediastinum whereas the right recurrent nerve turns at the cervicothoracic junction around the subclavian artery.

AXIAL BONE CT

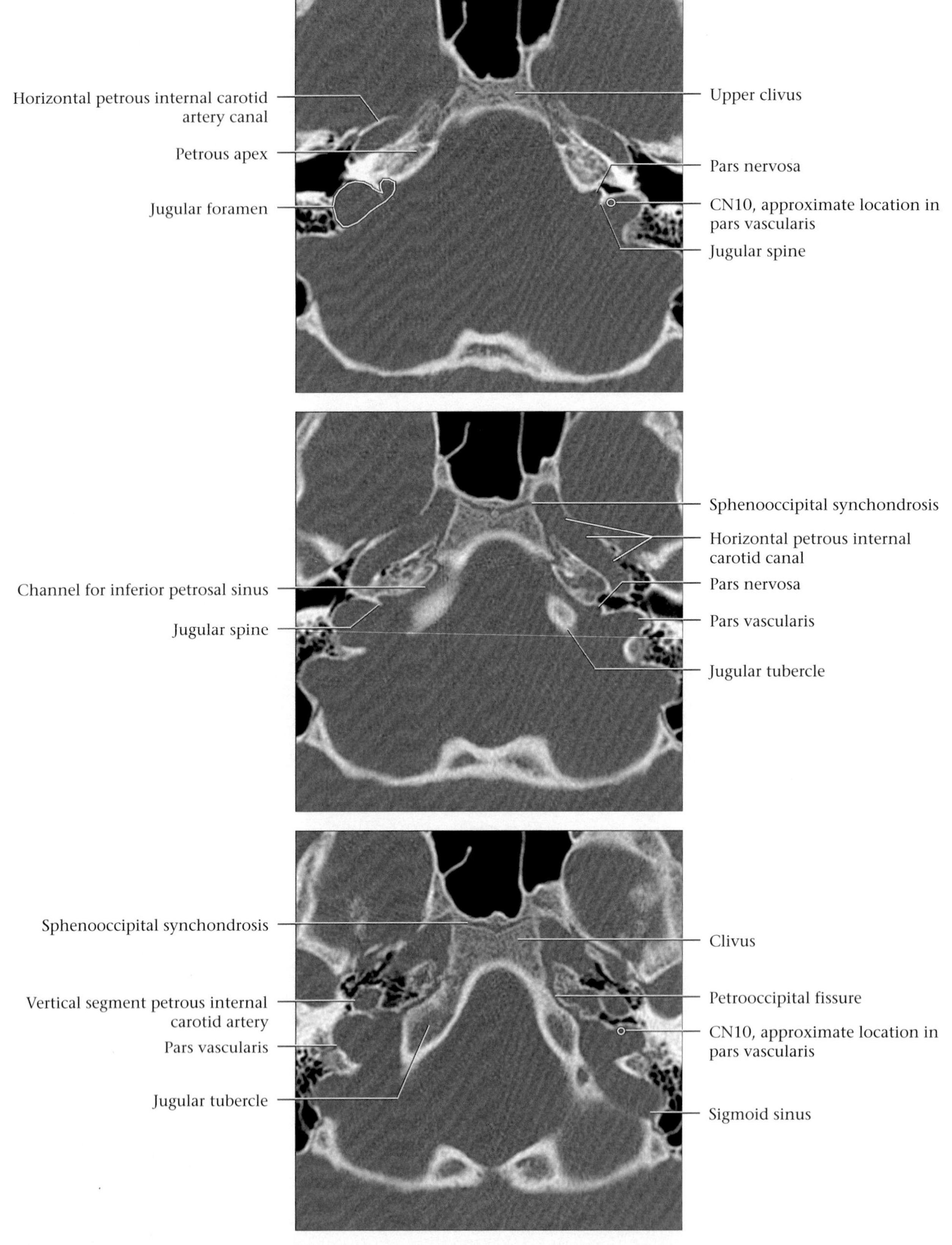

Horizontal petrous internal carotid artery canal
Petrous apex
Jugular foramen
Upper clivus
Pars nervosa
CN10, approximate location in pars vascularis
Jugular spine
Channel for inferior petrosal sinus
Jugular spine
Sphenooccipital synchondrosis
Horizontal petrous internal carotid canal
Pars nervosa
Pars vascularis
Jugular tubercle
Sphenooccipital synchondrosis
Vertical segment petrous internal carotid artery
Pars vascularis
Jugular tubercle
Clivus
Petrooccipital fissure
CN10, approximate location in pars vascularis
Sigmoid sinus

(Top) First of three axial bone CT images of the skull base presented from superior to inferior. The jugular foramen is divided by the jugular spine into the anteromedial pars nervosa and posterolateral pars vascularis. The pars vascularis transmits the vagus and accessory cranial nerves, Arnold nerve and jugular bulb which becomes internal jugular vein. **(Middle)** In this image the pars nervosa is seen to connect anteromedially to the inferior petrosal sinus. CN9, Jacobsen nerve and the inferior petrosal sinus are all found within the pars nervosa. **(Bottom)** Image through lower jugular foramen shows the sigmoid sinuses emptying into the pars vascularis of the jugular foramen. Notice the jugular foramen is located on floor of posterior cranial fossa in the seam between petrous temporal bone anterolaterally and occipital bone posteromedially.

CN10 (VAGUS NERVE)

AXIAL T2 MR

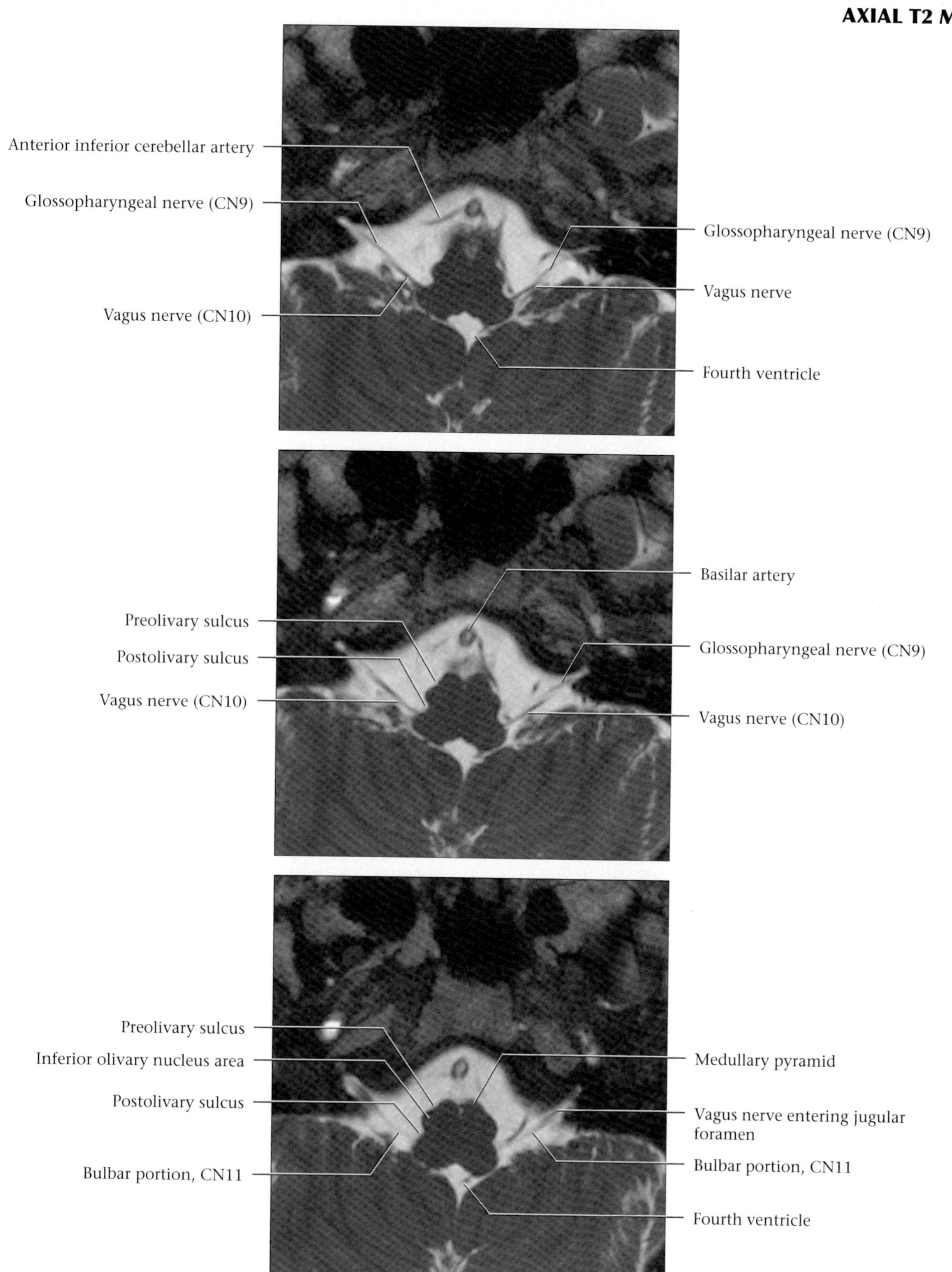
Anterior inferior cerebellar artery
Glossopharyngeal nerve (CN9)
Vagus nerve (CN10)
Glossopharyngeal nerve (CN9)
Vagus nerve
Fourth ventricle
Basilar artery
Preolivary sulcus
Postolivary sulcus
Vagus nerve (CN10)
Glossopharyngeal nerve (CN9)
Vagus nerve (CN10)
Preolivary sulcus
Inferior olivary nucleus area
Postolivary sulcus
Bulbar portion, CN11
Medullary pyramid
Vagus nerve entering jugular foramen
Bulbar portion, CN11
Fourth ventricle

(Top) First of three axial T2 MR images of low brainstem presented from superior to inferior. The vagus nerve is seen exiting the lateral medulla in postolivary sulcus inferior to glossopharyngeal nerve. **(Middle)** In this image the vagus nerve is clearly seen exiting the postolivary sulcus into the lateral basal cistern bilaterally. CN9 exits this sulcus just above the vagus nerve while the bulbar CN11 exits it just inferiorly. **(Bottom)** At the level of the cephalad margin of the jugular foramen the bulbar root of the accessory nerve is seen exiting the postolivary sulcus. The vagus nerve is entering the jugular foramen laterally. Unless thin-section focused T2 imaging is completed it is often difficulty to separate the glossopharyngeal nerve, vagus nerve and bulbar root of the accessory nerve in the basal cisterns.

CN11 (ACCESSORY NERVE)

Terminology

Abbreviations
- Accessory nerve: CN11, CN XI

Synonyms
- Eleventh cranial nerve

Definitions
- CN11: Pure motor cranial nerve supplying sternocleidomastoid & trapezius muscles

Imaging Anatomy

Overview
- Motor cranial nerve only
- Four CN11 segments are defined
  - Intra-axial, cisternal, skull base & extracranial

Intra-Axial Segment
- Two distinct nuclear origins
  - **Bulbar** (cranial) motor fibers originate in lower **nucleus ambiguus**
    - Fibers course anterolaterally to exit lateral medulla in postolivary sulcus inferior to CN9 & 10
  - **Spinal** motor fibers originate from **spinal nucleus** of accessory nerve
    - Narrow column of cells along lateral aspect of anterior horn from C1 to C5
    - Nerve fibers emerge from lateral aspect of cervical spinal cord between anterior & posterior roots
    - Fibers combine forming a bundle that ascends entering skull base via **foramen magnum**

Cisternal Segment
- Bulbar portion travels anterolaterally through basal cistern together with CN9 & 10
- Bulbar & spinal portions join together within lateral basal cistern

Skull Base Segment
- Passes through posterior **pars vascularis portion of jugular foramen**
  - Vagus nerve (CN10) & jugular bulb are also in pars vascularis
- Bulbar & spinal portions remain together in jugular foramen

Extracranial Segment
- Combined CN11 exits jugular foramen into nasopharyngeal carotid space
- Fibers from bulbar portion which arose within nucleus ambiguus transfer to vagus nerve
  - Travels via CN10 to supply muscles of pharynx & larynx
    - Larynx: Except cricothyroid muscle via recurrent laryngeal nerve
    - Pharynx: Superior constrictor & soft palate via pharyngeal plexus
- Fibers from spinal portion remain in extracranial CN11
  - Diverges posterolaterally from carotid space
  - Descend along medial aspect of sternocleidomastoid muscle
  - **Innervates sternomastoid muscle**
  - Continues across floor of posterior cervical space in cervical neck
  - Terminate in & **innervate trapezius muscle**

Anatomy-Based Imaging Issues

Imaging Recommendations
- MR imaging method of choice
  - Superior sensitivity to skull base, meningeal, cisternal & brainstem pathology
  - Sequences should include a combination of T2, T1 without fat-saturation & contrast-enhanced T1 with fat-saturation in axial & coronal planes
- Bone CT used to supplement MR when complex skull base pathology is present

Imaging "Sweet Spots"
- CN11 nuclei & intra-axial segment not directly visualized
- Cisternal segment is often not visualized on routine MR imaging
  - High-resolution thin-section T2 MR sequence usually demonstrates CN9, 10, 11 nerve complex passing through basal cisterns from post-olivary sulcus to pars vascularis of jugular foramen
- Bone CT clearly demonstrates bony anatomy of pars vascularis of jugular foramen
- Extracranial CN11 segment not directly visualized
  - Location inferred from its constant position deep to sternocleidomastoid muscle in floor of posterior cervical space

Imaging Pitfalls
- Hypertrophic levator scapulae muscle following serious CN11 injury may mimic tumor
- Don't mistake this enlarged muscle for mass!

Clinical Implications

Clinical Importance
- CN11 innervates sternocleidomastoid & trapezius muscles

Function-Dysfunction
- CN11 dysfunction: Isolated CN11 injury
  - Most common cause is radical neck dissection because spinal accessory nodal chain intimately associated CN11
  - Initial symptoms of spinal accessory neuropathy
    - Downward & lateral rotation of scapula
    - Shoulder droop resulting from loss of trapezius tone
  - Long term findings in spinal accessory neuropathy
    - Within 6 months results in **atrophy** of ipsilateral sternocleidomastoid & trapezius muscles
    - **Compensatory hypertrophy** of ipsilateral **levator scapulae muscle** occurs over months
- CN11 dysfunction: Complex CN11 dysfunction associated with CN9 & 10 neuropathy

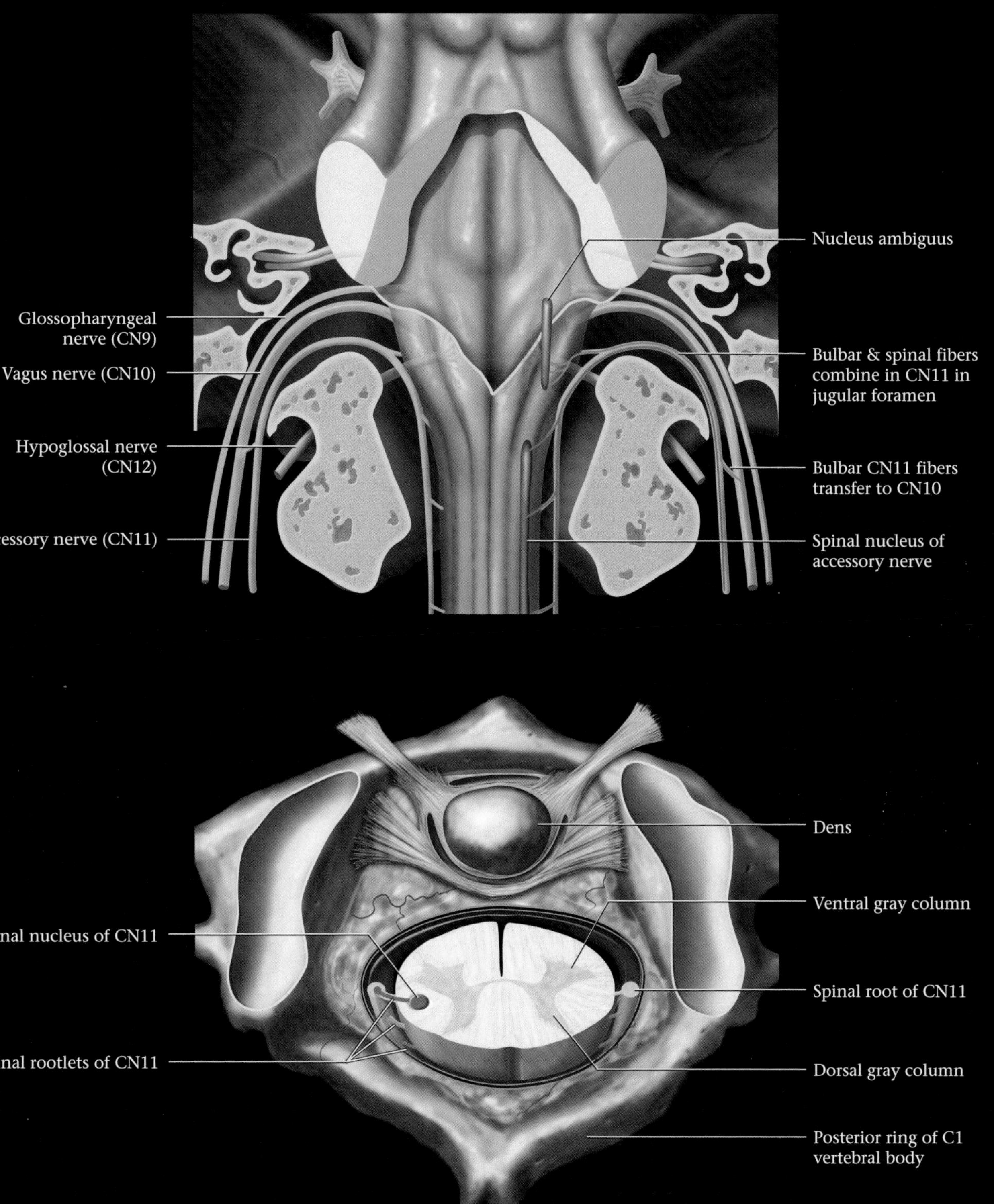
Nucleus ambiguus
Glossopharyngeal nerve (CN9)
Vagus nerve (CN10)
Bulbar & spinal fibers combine in CN11 in jugular foramen
Hypoglossal nerve (CN12)
Bulbar CN11 fibers transfer to CN10
essory nerve (CN11)
Spinal nucleus of accessory nerve
Dens
Ventral gray column
nal nucleus of CN11
Spinal root of CN11
nal rootlets of CN11
Dorsal gray column
Posterior ring of C1 vertebral body

op) Graphic of posterior brainstem reveals both the spinal & the bulbar roots of the accessory nerve (CN11). Note e lower nucleus ambiguus gives rise to multiple rootlets of bulbar root of CN11. Both the spinal & the bulbar roots mbine in lateral basal cistern & jugular foramen. The spinal root continues as extracranial CN11 to innervate the rnocleidomastoid & trapezius muscles. The bulbar root fibers cross to the vagus nerve extracranially to supply otor innervation to the pharynx (superior constrictor & soft palate) & the larynx (except the cricothyroid muscle). **ottom)** Axial graphic of the upper cervical spinal cord cut to reveal the spinal nucleus of the accessory nerve giving e to multiple rootlets that unite to form the spinal root of the accessory nerve. The rootlets exit the posterolateral cus just anterior to the posterior cervical roots.

CN11 (ACCESSORY NERVE)

GRAPHIC, INTRACRANIAL & EXTRACRANIAL

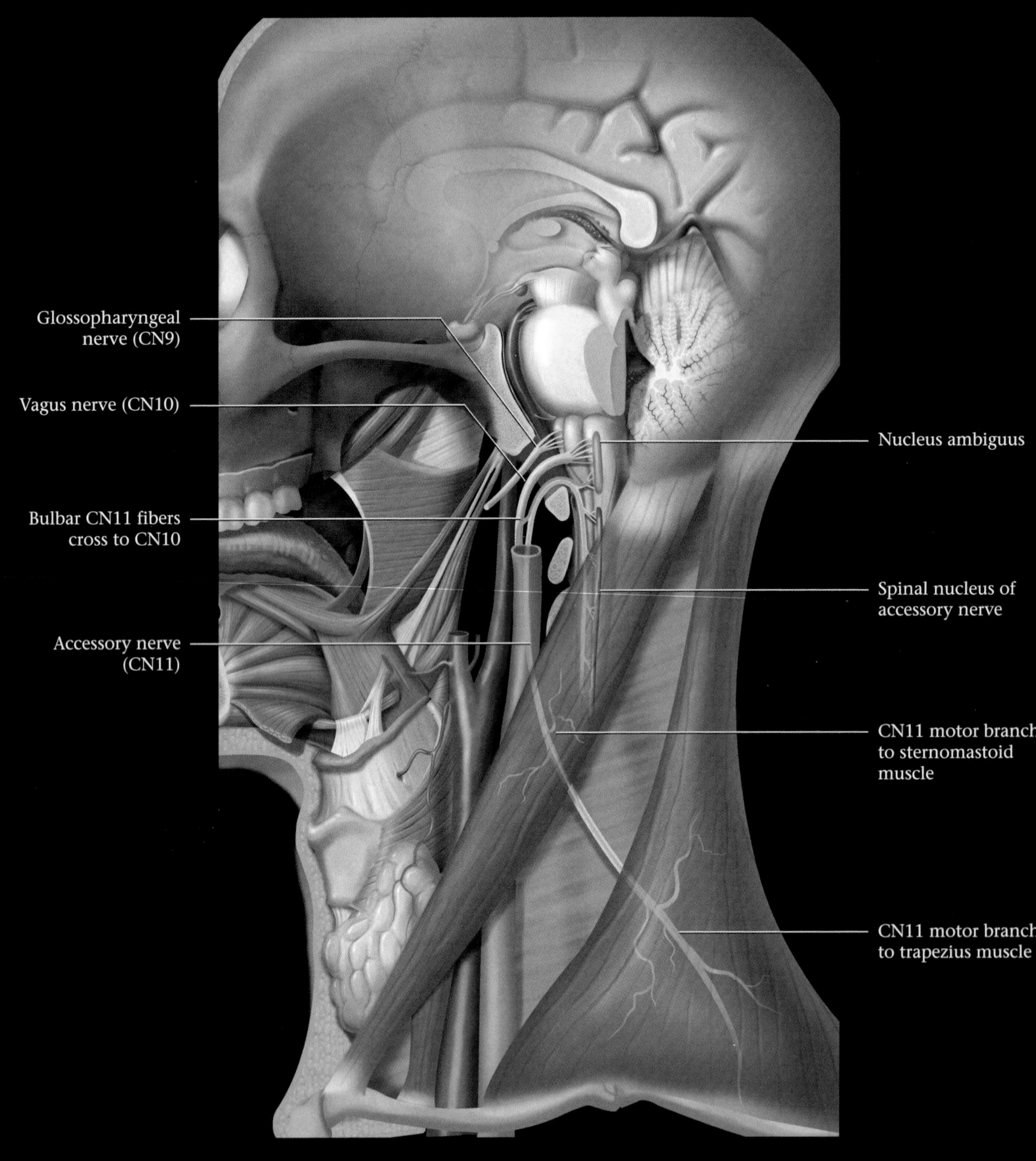
Glossopharyngeal nerve (CN9)
Vagus nerve (CN10)
Bulbar CN11 fibers cross to CN10
Accessory nerve (CN11)
Nucleus ambiguus
Spinal nucleus of accessory nerve
CN11 motor branch to sternomastoid muscle
CN11 motor branch to trapezius muscle

Overview graphic of intracranial & extracranial accessory nerve (CN11) shows the lower nucleus ambiguus at the origin of the bulbar root of CN11 while the spinal nucleus gives rise to the spinal root. Both roots combine in the jugular foramen. Extracranially the bulbar fibers cross to the vagus nerve to eventually provide motor innervation v the pharyngeal plexus to the soft palate & superior constrictor muscles & via the recurrent laryngeal nerve to the majority of the endolaryngeal muscles. The spinal fibers that remain in the accessory nerve provide motor innervation to the sternocleidomastoid & trapezius muscles. Notice the extracranial CN11 runs in the floor of the posterior cervical space.

CN11 (ACCESSORY NERVE)

AXIAL BONE CT & T2 MR

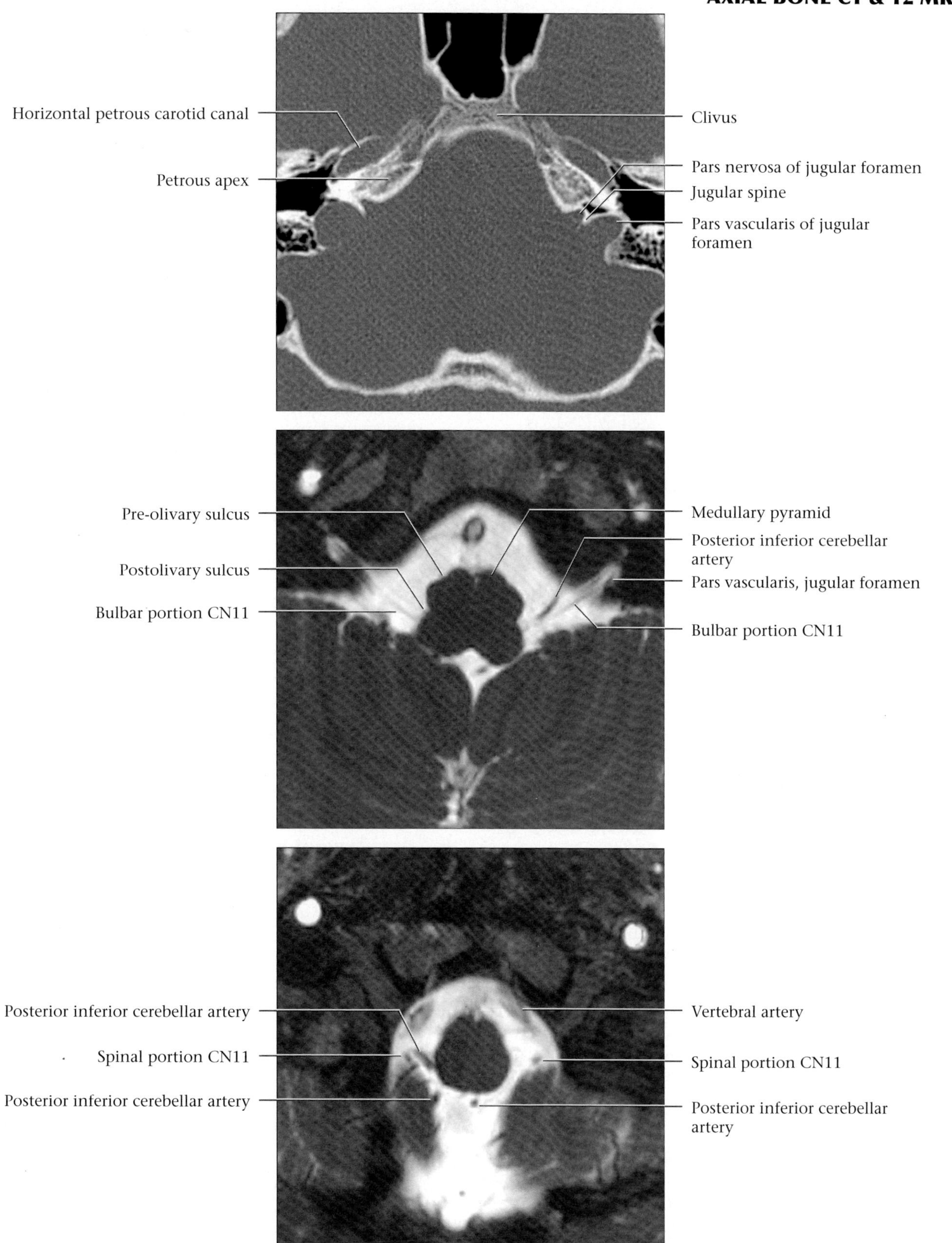

Horizontal petrous carotid canal
Petrous apex
Clivus
Pars nervosa of jugular foramen
Jugular spine
Pars vascularis of jugular foramen
Pre-olivary sulcus
Postolivary sulcus
Bulbar portion CN11
Medullary pyramid
Posterior inferior cerebellar artery
Pars vascularis, jugular foramen
Bulbar portion CN11
Posterior inferior cerebellar artery
Spinal portion CN11
Posterior inferior cerebellar artery
Vertebral artery
Spinal portion CN11
Posterior inferior cerebellar artery

(Top) Axial bone CT through the jugular foramen shows the anteromedial pars nervosa, the jugular spine & the posterolateral pars vascularis. The pars nervosa transmits CN9, Jacobsen nerve & inferior petrosal sinus. The pars vascularis transmits CN10, CN11, Arnold nerve & sigmoid sinus which becomes internal jugular vein. **(Middle)** Axial T2 MR image at level of medulla shows the bulbar portion of CN11 emerging from the postolivary sulcus just inferior to CN10. The bulbar portion travels anterolaterally through basal cistern together with CN10 & CN9. **(Bottom)** Axial T2 MR image through lower medulla reveals the spinal root of CN11 climbing cephalad through foramen magnum to join bulbar root of CN11 before they enter the pars nervosa of jugular foramen. It is spinal root that eventually becomes the extracranial CN11 with motor fibers to sternocleidomastoid & trapezius muscles.

CN12 (HYPOGLOSSAL NERVE)

Terminology

Abbreviations

- Hypoglossal nerve: CN12, CN XII

Synonyms

- Twelfth cranial nerve

Definitions

- CN12: motor cranial nerve controlling intrinsic & extrinsic muscles of tongue

Imaging Anatomy

Overview

- Motor cranial nerve to intrinsic & extrinsic muscles of tongue
  - Only extrinsic muscle **not** innervated by CN12 is **palatoglossus muscle**
    - Vagus nerve innervates palatoglossus muscle
- Hypoglossal nerve anatomic segments
  - Intra-axial segment
  - Cisternal segment
  - Skull base segment
  - Extracranial

Intra-Axial Segment

- **Hypoglossal nucleus**
  - Located in medulla between dorsal vagal nucleus & midline
  - Long, thin nucleus that is about same length as the ventrolateral olive
  - Extends from level of hypoglossal eminence in floor of fourth ventricle just inferior to stria medullares to proximal medulla
  - In axial section, hypoglossal nucleus is located in dorsal medulla, medial to dorsal vagal nucleus
- Hypoglossal intra-axial axonal course
  - Efferent fibers from hypoglossal nucleus extend ventrally through medulla, lateral to medial lemniscus
  - Efferent fibers exit between olivary nucleus & pyramid at **ventrolateral sulcus** also called **pre-olivary sulcus**

Cisternal Segment

- Efferent fibers coalesce to form multiple **rootlets**
- Rootlets fuse into hypoglossal nerve just as it exits skull base through hypoglossal canal
- Hypoglossal filaments may merge with vagal fibers

Skull Base Segment

- Hypoglossal nerve exits the occipital bone via **hypoglossal canal**
  - Hypoglossal canal is located in inferior occipital bone caudal to jugular foramen
  - Variant anatomy of hypoglossal canal
    - Osseous septa may bisect hypoglossal canal

Extracranial Segment

- **Carotid space component of CN12**
  - Hypoglossal canal "empties" into medial nasopharyngeal carotid space
  - Hypoglossal nerve immediately gives off **dural branches** after exiting hypoglossal canal
  - Hypoglossal nerve descends in posterior aspect of carotid space, closely apposed with vagus nerve
  - Exits carotid space anteriorly between jugular vein & internal carotid artery at inferior margin of posterior belly of digastric muscle
- **Trans-spatial component of CN12**
  - After leaving carotid space, runs anteroinferiorly toward hyoid bone, lateral to carotid bifurcation
  - At level of occipital artery base, hypoglossal nerve turns anterior, continuing as muscular branch below posterior belly of digastric muscle
  - Gives off superior root of ansa cervicalis from horizontal segment CN12 to anastomose with lower root of ansa cervicalis
- Distal branches of imaging importance
  - **Muscular branch** travels on lateral margin of hyoglossus muscle in posterior sublingual space
    - Muscular branch innervates extrinsic (styloglossus, hyoglossus & genioglossus) & intrinsic tongue muscles
    - **Geniohyoid** innervated by **C1** spinal nerve
  - **Ansa cervicalis**: Formed from superior and inferior (C1-C3 spinal nerves) roots
    - Innervates infrahyoid strap muscles (sternothyroid, sternohyoid, omohyoid)

Anatomy-Based Imaging Issues

Imaging Recommendations

- MR is preferred imaging study
  - Best delineates brainstem, cisterns, skull base & suprahyoid neck
- CECT with bone algorithm of skull base is excellent for skull base & suprahyoid neck

Imaging "Sweet Spots"

- Coverage of hypoglossal nerve requires CT or MR to visualize following anatomic areas
  - Brainstem, basal cistern & hypoglossal canal
  - Nasopharyngeal carotid space
  - Posterior belly digastric & carotid bifurcation
  - Hyoid bone & sublingual space

Imaging Pitfalls

- Failure to image to level of hyoid bone will result in missed diagnoses!

Clinical Implications

Clinical Importance

- Unilateral hypoglossal lesion causes tongue protrusion to "side of the lesion"
- **Acute hypoglossal injury**
  - Tongue fasciculates
  - Tongue deviates to side of injury when protruded
- **Chronic hypoglossal injury**
  - Tongue atrophy seen as fatty infiltration & volume loss on CT or MR
  - Infrahyoid strap muscles also atrophy

CN12 (HYPOGLOSSAL NERVE)

GRAPHICS, INTRACRANIAL

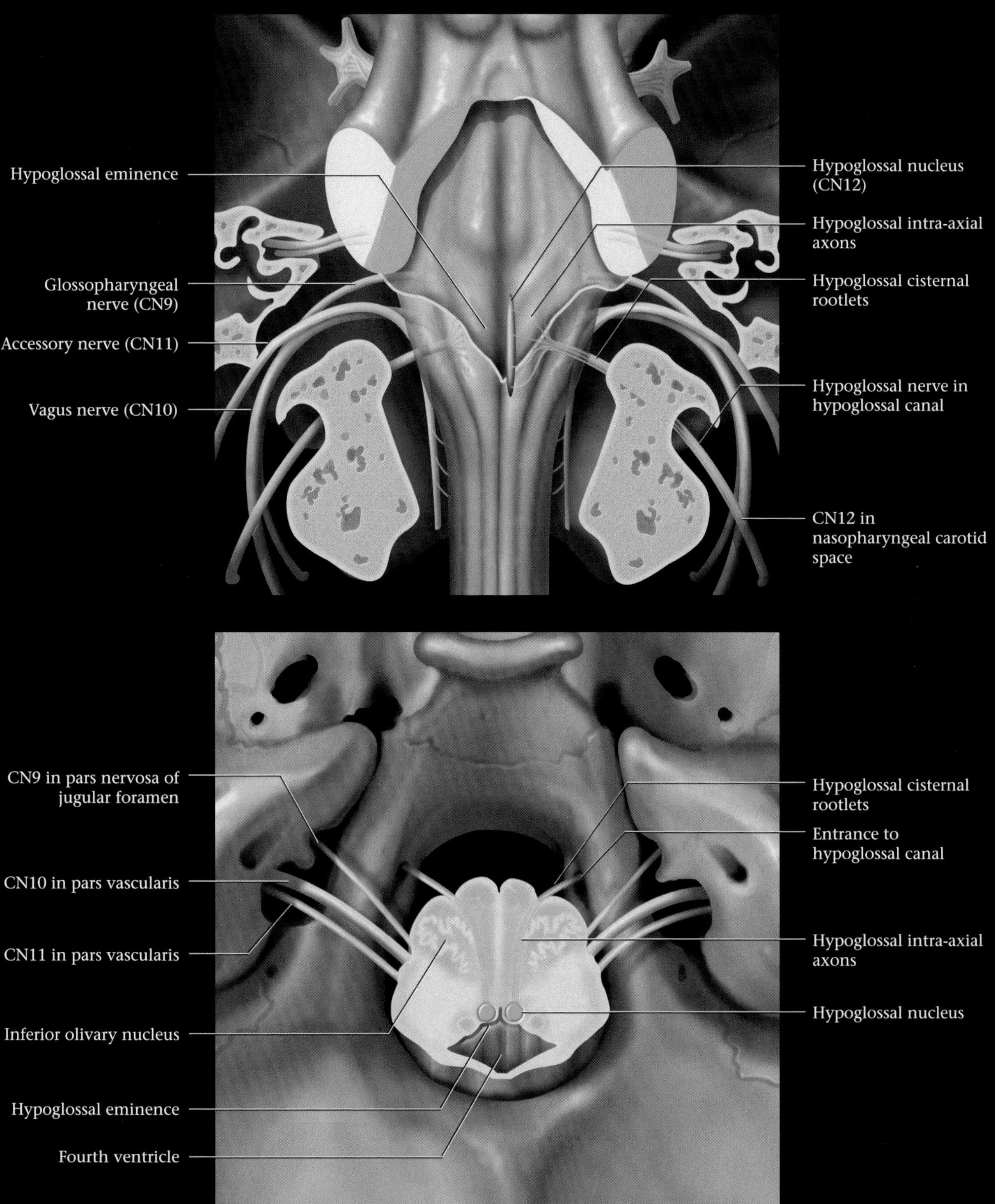
Hypoglossal eminence
Glossopharyngeal nerve (CN9)
Accessory nerve (CN11)
Vagus nerve (CN10)
Hypoglossal nucleus (CN12)
Hypoglossal intra-axial axons
Hypoglossal cisternal rootlets
Hypoglossal nerve in hypoglossal canal
CN12 in nasopharyngeal carotid space
CN9 in pars nervosa of jugular foramen
CN10 in pars vascularis
CN11 in pars vascularis
Inferior olivary nucleus
Hypoglossal eminence
Fourth ventricle
Hypoglossal cisternal rootlets
Entrance to hypoglossal canal
Hypoglossal intra-axial axons
Hypoglossal nucleus

(Top) Graphic of lower brainstem seen from behind illustrating key features of the proximal hypoglossal nerve. Notice the hypoglossal nucleus in the dorsal paramedian medulla feeding intra-axial axons that exit the pre-olivary sulcus into the anterolateral basal cistern. Cisternal rootlets fuse into the hypoglossal nerve that traverses the skull base through the hypoglossal canal. Exiting the hypoglossal canal, CN12 immediately enters the nasopharyngeal carotid space. **(Bottom)** Axial graphic through lower medulla shows the hypoglossal nucleus feeding intra-axial axons that dive ventrally to curve around the inferior olivary nucleus to exit the medulla ventrolaterally via the pre-olivary sulcus. The cisternal rootlets combine in the hypoglossal canal to become the hypoglossal nerve (CN12). Note the hypoglossal canal is anterior & inferior to the jugular foramen.

CN12 (HYPOGLOSSAL NERVE)

GRAPHIC, EXTRACRANIAL

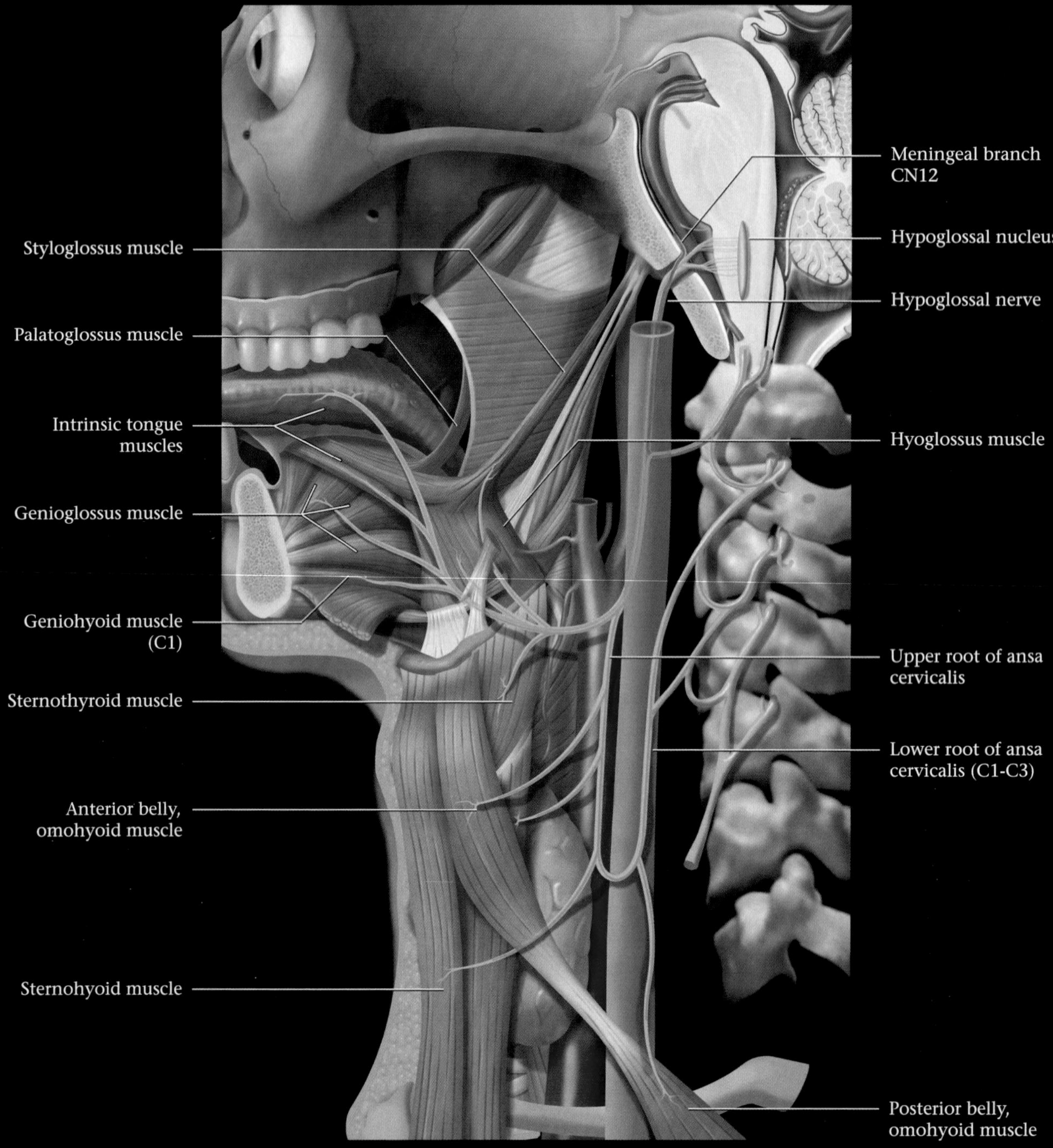
Meningeal branch CN12
Hypoglossal nucleus
Hypoglossal nerve
Hyoglossus muscle
Upper root of ansa cervicalis
Lower root of ansa cervicalis (C1-C3)
Posterior belly, omohyoid muscle
Styloglossus muscle
Palatoglossus muscle
Intrinsic tongue muscles
Genioglossus muscle
Geniohyoid muscle (C1)
Sternothyroid muscle
Anterior belly, omohyoid muscle
Sternohyoid muscle

Lateral graphic depicting entire course of hypoglossal nerve. The nerve originates in the hypoglossal nucleus in the floor of the fourth ventricle. It usually coalesces into a single trunk in the hypoglossal canal. As CN12 exits the skull base it immediately enters the nasopharyngeal carotid space just medial to the internal carotid artery. It travels inferiorly in the carotid space to exit anteriorly between the carotid artery & the internal jugular vein. CN12 supplies motor innervation to intrinsic & extrinsic (styloglossus, hyoglossus, genioglossus) tongue muscles. C1 spinal nerve supplies motor to geniohyoid muscle. Ansa cervicalis (C1-C3 spinal nerves) supplies motor innervation to infrahyoid strap muscles including sternothyroid, sternohyoid & omohyoid muscles. Also note the meningeal sensory branch from C1 following CN12 retrograde to supply clival meninges.

CN12 (HYPOGLOSSAL NERVE)

AXIAL BONE CT & T2 MR

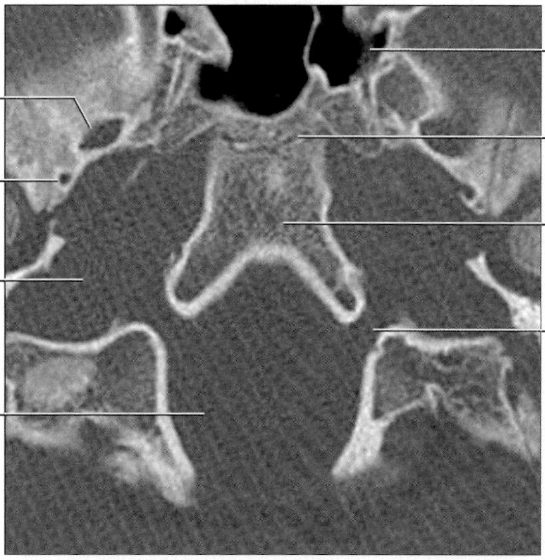

Foramen ovale
Foramen spinosum
Inferior jugular foramen
Foramen magnum
Sphenoid sinus
Sphenooccipital synchondrosis
Clivus
Hypoglossal canal

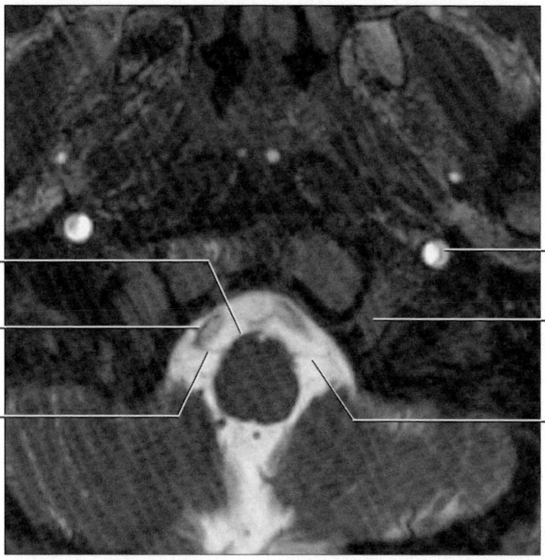

Medullary pyramid
Vertebral artery
Hypoglossal nerve
Internal carotid artery
Hypoglossal canal
Hypoglossal nerve

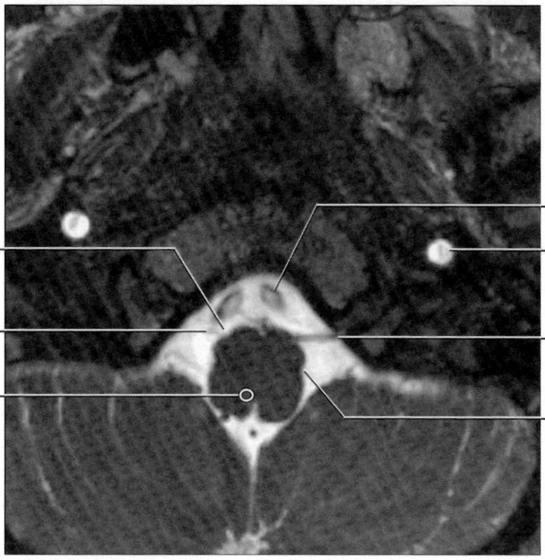

Pre-olivary sulcus
Hypoglossal rootlet
Hypoglossal nucleus location
Vertebral artery
Internal carotid artery
Hypoglossal nerve
Retro-olivary sulcus

(Top) Axial bone CT image at the level of the hypoglossal canal. Notice the margins of the hypoglossal canals are well corticated. **(Middle)** First of two axial T2 MR images through lower medulla demonstrates cisternal segment of hypoglossal nerves. Anatomy of cisternal segment is variable, but usually 12-16 rootlets emerge from pre-olivary sulcus & merge into two trunks which penetrate dura to enter hypoglossal canal. The trunks abut or pass near the vertebral arteries in the basal cisterns. **(Bottom)** Hypoglossal nerves emerge from medulla in pre-olivary sulcus between olive & pyramid. Cisternal segment of the patient's left hypoglossal nerve is seen as a thick, discrete trunk entering hypoglossal canal. Right hypoglossal nerve consists of multiple small rootlets.

CN12 (HYPOGLOSSAL NERVE)

CORONAL BONE CT

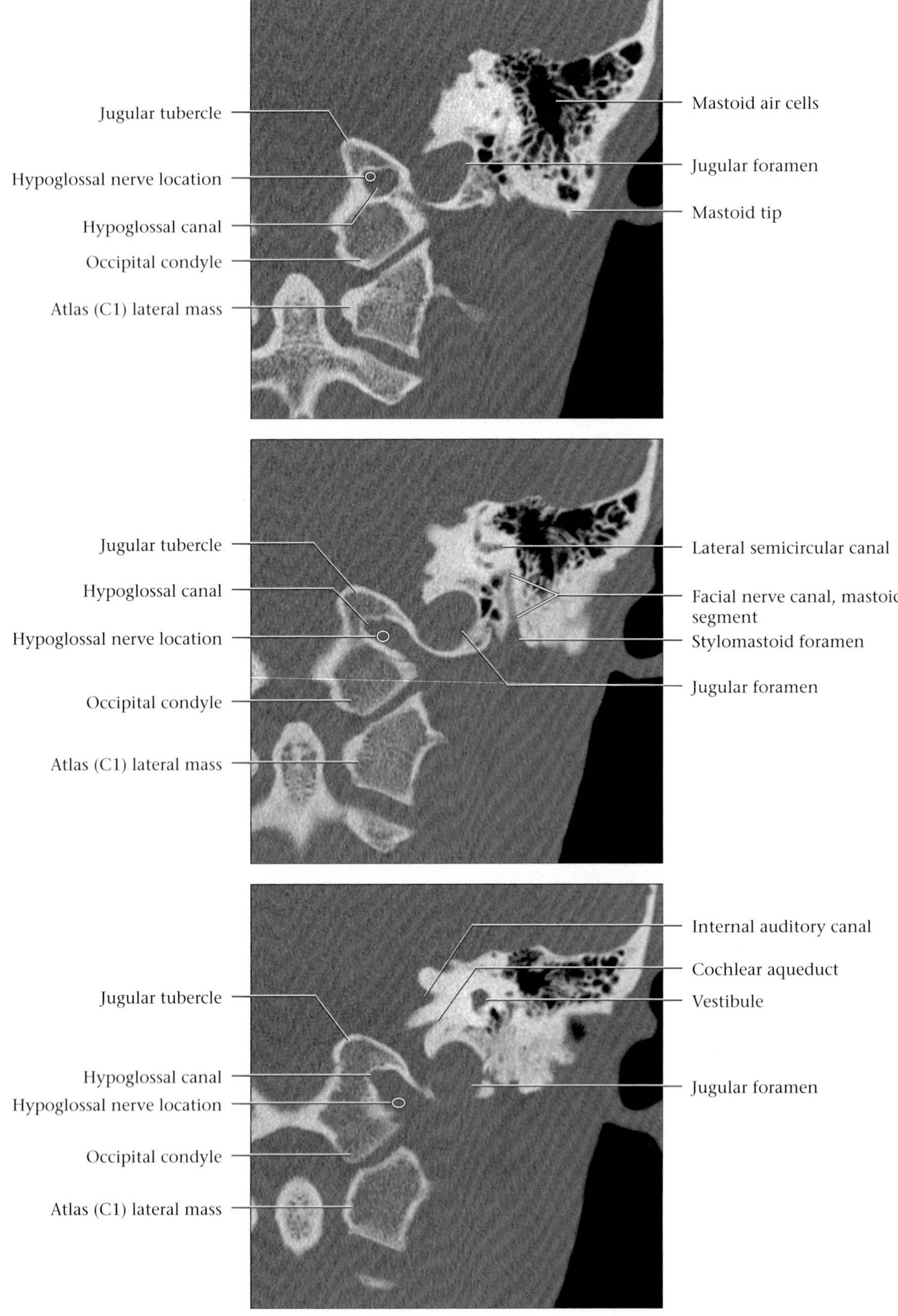
Jugular tubercle
Hypoglossal nerve location
Hypoglossal canal
Occipital condyle
Atlas (C1) lateral mass
Mastoid air cells
Jugular foramen
Mastoid tip
Jugular tubercle
Hypoglossal canal
Hypoglossal nerve location
Occipital condyle
Atlas (C1) lateral mass
Lateral semicircular canal
Facial nerve canal, mastoid segment
Stylomastoid foramen
Jugular foramen
Internal auditory canal
Cochlear aqueduct
Vestibule
Jugular tubercle
Jugular foramen
Hypoglossal canal
Hypoglossal nerve location
Occipital condyle
Atlas (C1) lateral mass

(Top) In this first of three coronal bone CT images presented from posterior to anterior shows the hypoglossal canal as a complete bony circle indicating the image is at the level of the entry into the canal. The location of CN12 is in the upper medial quadrant within the hypoglossal canal. **(Middle)** In this image of the mid-hypoglossal canal the surrounding bone appears as a "birds head & beak", with the head & beak made up of the jugular tubercle. The jugular foramen is directly lateral to the hypoglossal canal. **(Bottom)** At the level of the distal hypoglossal canal the hypoglossal nerve leaves the skull base to emerge inferiorly into the nasopharyngeal carotid space. Notice the lateral jugular foramen also empties its contents into the carotid space including the jugular vein & cranial nerves 9, 10 & 11.

CN12 (HYPOGLOSSAL NERVE)

CORONAL T1 C+ MR

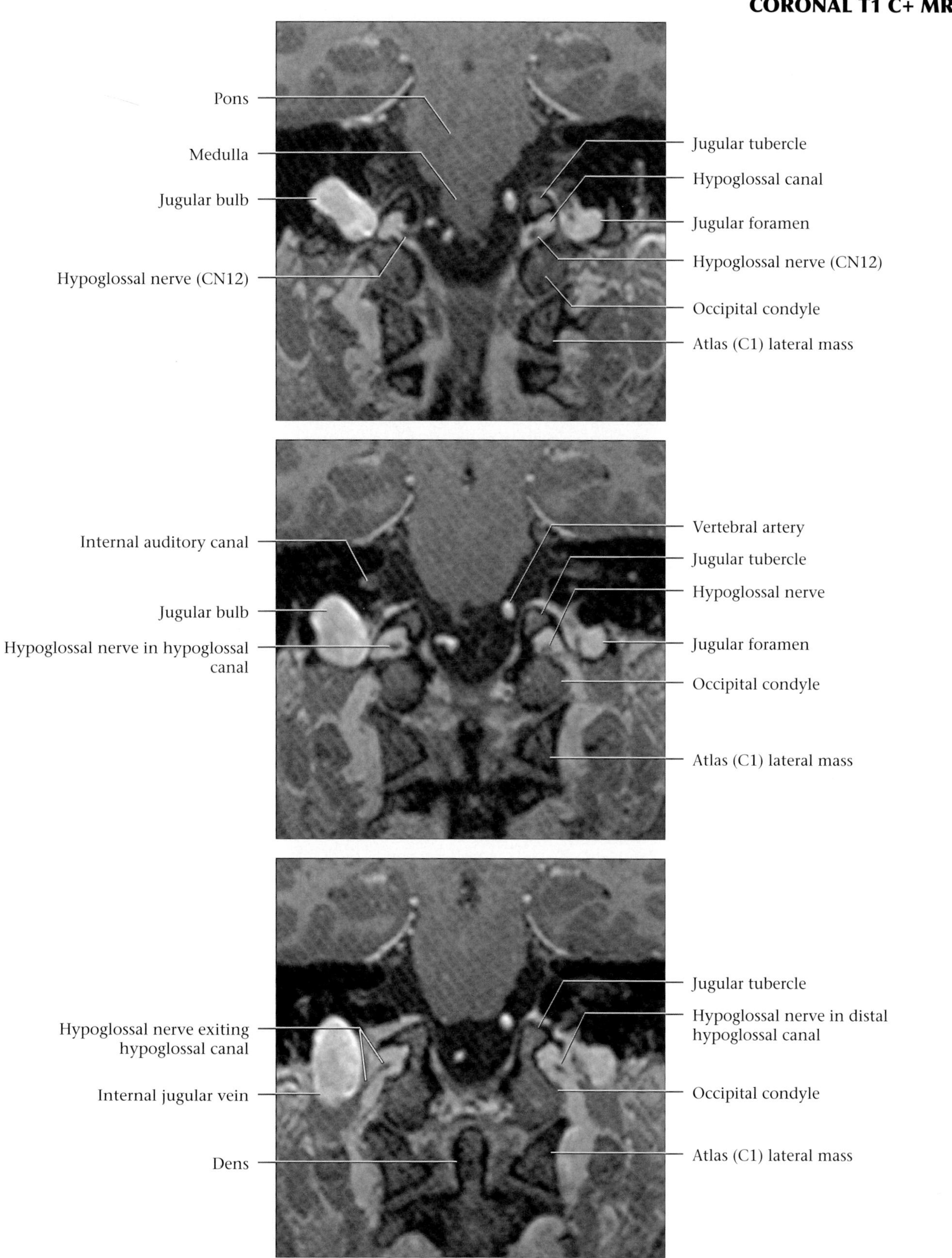
Pons
Medulla
Jugular bulb
Hypoglossal nerve (CN12)
Jugular tubercle
Hypoglossal canal
Jugular foramen
Hypoglossal nerve (CN12)
Occipital condyle
Atlas (C1) lateral mass
Internal auditory canal
Jugular bulb
Hypoglossal nerve in hypoglossal canal
Vertebral artery
Jugular tubercle
Hypoglossal nerve
Jugular foramen
Occipital condyle
Atlas (C1) lateral mass
Hypoglossal nerve exiting hypoglossal canal
Internal jugular vein
Dens
Jugular tubercle
Hypoglossal nerve in distal hypoglossal canal
Occipital condyle
Atlas (C1) lateral mass

(Top) First of three sequential coronal T1 C+ MR images presented from posterior to anterior. In this MR image the hypoglossal nerve is seen entering the proximal hypoglossal canal. The hypointense hypoglossal nerve is surrounded by strongly enhancing venous plexus & is therefore easily seen on thin-section enhanced MR. **(Middle)** In this coronal MR image of the mid-hypoglossal canal the low signal hypoglossal nerve is visible surrounded by enhancing venous plexus just beneath the "bird's beak" of the jugular tubercle. **(Bottom)** In this coronal image through the distal hypoglossal canal the hypoglossal nerves can be seen exiting inferolaterally into the nasopharyngeal carotid space. Notice also the vein of the jugular foramen exiting inferiorly on the patient's right into this same nasopharyngeal carotid space.

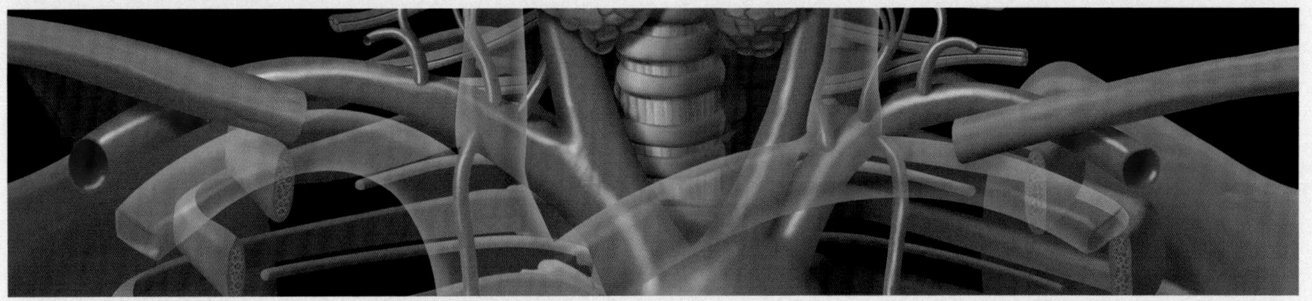

SECTION 6: Extracranial Arteries

AORTIC ARCH AND GREAT VESSELS

Terminology

Abbreviations

- Aortic arch (AA); brachiocephalic trunk (BCT)
- Right, left common carotid arteries (RCCA, LCCA)
- Right, left subclavian arteries (RSCA, LSCA)
- Congenital heart disease (CHD)

Definitions

- "Great vessels": Major vessels arising from AA (BCT, LCCA, LSCA)

Gross Anatomy

Overview

- Thoracic aorta has four major segments (ascending aorta, AA, aortic isthmus, descending aorta)
- Normal aortic arch has three major branches (BCT, LCCA, LSCA)

Imaging Anatomy

Overview

- AA curves from right to left, slightly anterior to posterior in superior mediastinum

Anatomy Relationships

- Anterior: Vagus nerve (CN10)
- Posterior
  - Trachea
  - Esophagus
  - Left recurrent laryngeal nerve
- Superior
  - Great vessels
  - Left brachiocephalic vein
- Inferior
  - Pulmonary trunk
  - Left recurrent laryngeal nerve

Branches

- **Brachiocephalic trunk** (innominate artery)
  - First (largest) AA branch
  - Arises from superior convexity of AA
  - Ascends anterior to trachea
  - At sternoclavicular level, bifurcates into RSCA, RCCA
  - RSCA branches
    - Internal thoracic (mammary) artery (courses anteroinferiorly from RSCA)
    - Right vertebral artery (courses superiorly from RSCA just distal to RCCA origin)
    - Thyrocervical trunk (gives off 2 major branches: Inferior thyroid artery and its ascending cervical, laryngeal and pharyngeal branches; suprascapular artery)
    - Costocervical trunk (gives off superior intercostal, deep cervical arteries)
  - RCCA branches
    - Bifurcates into (ICA), (ECA)
- **Left common carotid artery**
  - Arises from AA distal to BCT
  - Ascends in front of, then lateral to, trachea
  - Anteromedial to internal jugular vein
  - Branches into left ICA, ECA at level of upper thyroid cartilage
- **Left subclavian artery**
  - Arises from AA just distal to LCCA
  - Ascends into neck, passing lateral to medial border of anterior scalene
  - Crossed anteriorly by thoracic duct, left phrenic nerve
  - Branches
    - Left internal thoracic (mammary) artery
    - Left vertebral artery
    - Left thyrocervical trunk
    - Left costocervical trunk

Vascular Territory

- AA and great vessels supply neck, skull, entire brain

Normal Variants, Anomalies

- Normal variants
  - Classic pattern with three branches seen in 80% of cases
    - First branch is BCT, followed by LCCA, LSCA
  - "Bovine" configuration (misnomer)
    - Common origin of BCT, LCCA (10-25% of cases)
  - LCCA arises from BCT in 5-7%
  - "Left brachiocephalic trunk:" (LCCA, LSCA share common origin) in 1-2%
  - Left VA arises directly from AA in 0.5-1%
  - Aortic "isthmus" (circumferential bulge beyond ductus) may persist → aortic "spindle"
  - Ductus diverticulum (focal bulge along anteromedial aspect of aortic isthmus), found in 9% of adults
- Anomalies
  - Left AA with aberrant RSCA
    - Most common congenital arch anomaly (0.5-1%)
    - 70%: RCCA, LCCA, LSCA, RSCA
    - 25%: Common stem for RCCA/LCCA, LSCA, RSCA
    - 5%: Other variations with RSCA as last branch from AA
    - +/- Aneurysmal dilation of RSCA ("ductus of Kommerell")
  - Right AA with mirror image branching
    - Left brachiocephalic trunk, RCCA, RSCA
    - 98% prevalence of CHD
  - Right AA with aberrant LSCA
    - LCCA, RCCA, RSCA, LSCA
    - 10% prevalence of CHD
    - May form true vascular ring
  - Double aortic arch (multiple variations)
    - Most common vascular ring
    - Right arch typically higher, larger than left
    - Right arch usually gives origin to RSCA, RCCA; left to LCCA, LSCA
    - Rarely associated with CHD

Anatomy-Based Imaging Issues

Imaging Recommendations

- Left anterior oblique (LAO) position best visualizes AA, great vessels
- CTA, contrast-enhanced MRA rival DSA in depicting AA, great vessels

AORTIC ARCH AND GREAT VESSELS

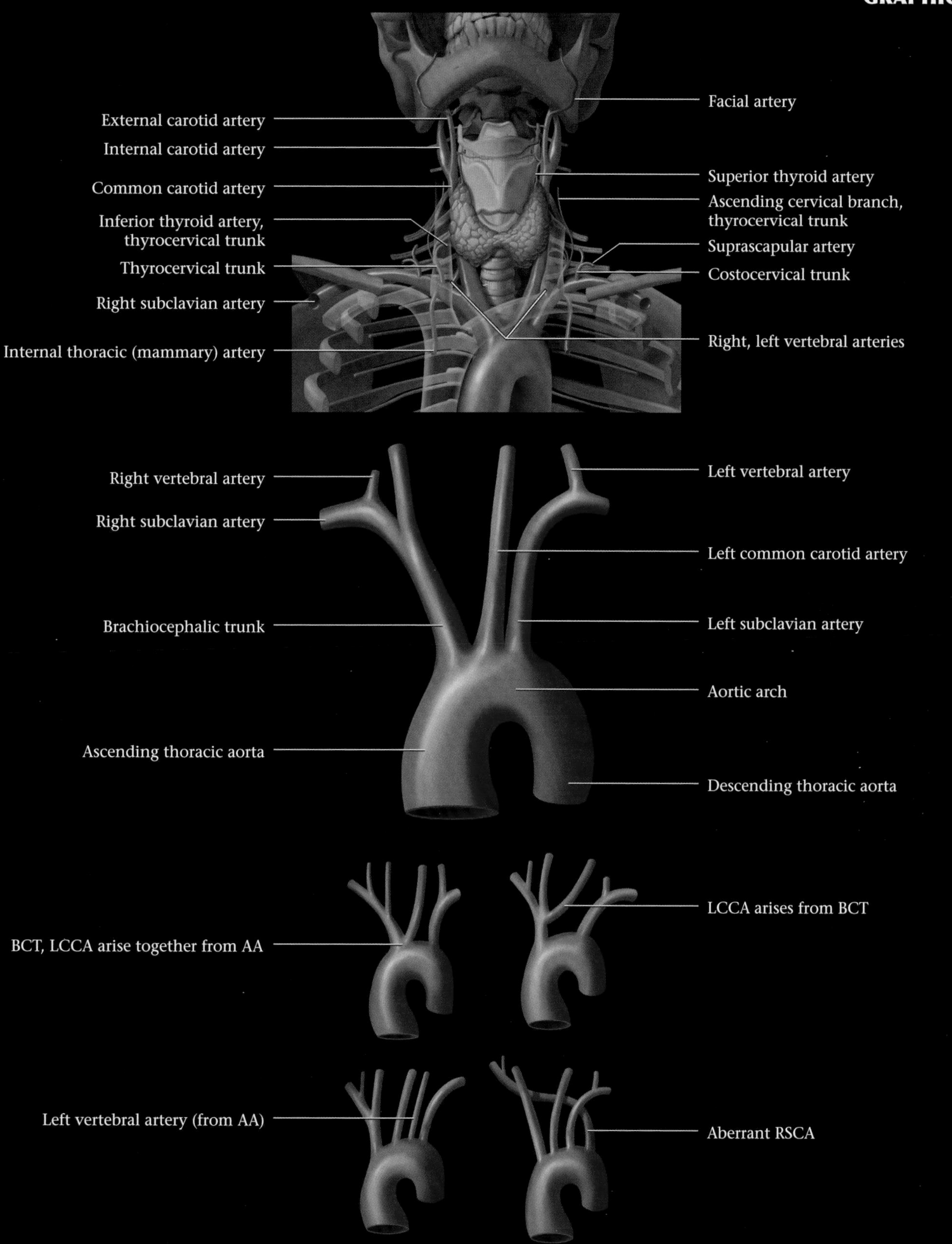
External carotid artery
Internal carotid artery
Common carotid artery
Inferior thyroid artery, thyrocervical trunk
Thyrocervical trunk
Right subclavian artery
Internal thoracic (mammary) artery
Facial artery
Superior thyroid artery
Ascending cervical branch, thyrocervical trunk
Suprascapular artery
Costocervical trunk
Right, left vertebral arteries
Right vertebral artery
Right subclavian artery
Brachiocephalic trunk
Ascending thoracic aorta
Left vertebral artery
Left common carotid artery
Left subclavian artery
Aortic arch
Descending thoracic aorta
BCT, LCCA arise together from AA
LCCA arises from BCT
Left vertebral artery (from AA)
Aberrant RSCA

(Top) AP graphic shows normal aortic arch, relationship to adjacent structures. Internal carotid artery (ICA) usually arises from the common carotid artery posterolateral to the external carotid artery (ECA). **(Middle)** Skeletonized overview of the normal aortic arch with all other structures removed. The three major "great vessels," the brachiocephalic trunk (innominate artery), left common carotid artery, and left subclavian artery are depicted. In this example we show the BCT and LCCA as having a common "V-shaped" origin together from the arch. **(Bottom)** Four common aortic arch variants and anomalies are depicted. Upper left: BCT and LCCA originate together from aortic arch. Upper right: LCCA originates from BCT; only two vessels arise from AA. Lower left: Left vertebral artery arises directly from AA. Lower right: Aberrant RSCA arises from arch as fourth "great vessel."

AORTIC ARCH AND GREAT VESSELS

LAO DSA

Right common carotid artery
Right subclavian artery
Brachiocephalic trunk
Aortic arch
Left vertebral artery
Left common carotid artery
Left subclavian artery

Inferior thyroid artery, thyrocervical trunk
Right vertebral artery
Thyrocervical trunk
Arteria thyroidea ima
Internal thoracic (mammary) artery
Ascending cervical artery, thyrocervical trunk
Costocervical trunk
Highest (superior) intercostal artery

Inferior thyroid artery
Suprascapular branch, thyrocervical trunk
Right vertebral artery
Internal thoracic (mammary) artery
Ascending cervical artery
Left vertebral artery
Thyrocervical trunk
Superior intercostal artery

(Top) Three views of DSA obtained in slight LAO projection are shown. Early arterial phase shows aortic arch, "great vessels." First branch is normally brachiocephalic trunk (innominate artery), which bifurcates into right subclavian and common carotid arteries. Left common carotid artery, second major branch, typically originates very close to (or sometimes from) brachiocephalic trunk. In this projection, origins of left common carotid and subclavian arteries slightly overlap. **(Middle)** Mid-arterial phase shows origin of the right vertebral artery (VA). A tiny inconstant branch, the thyroidea ima, arises from the BCT. **(Bottom)** Late arterial phase shows more distal branches of the "great vessels." The left vertebral artery is slightly larger than the right vertebral artery. The thyroid gland is seen as a faint blush, in between the common carotid arteries.

AORTIC ARCH AND GREAT VESSELS

3D-VRT CECT

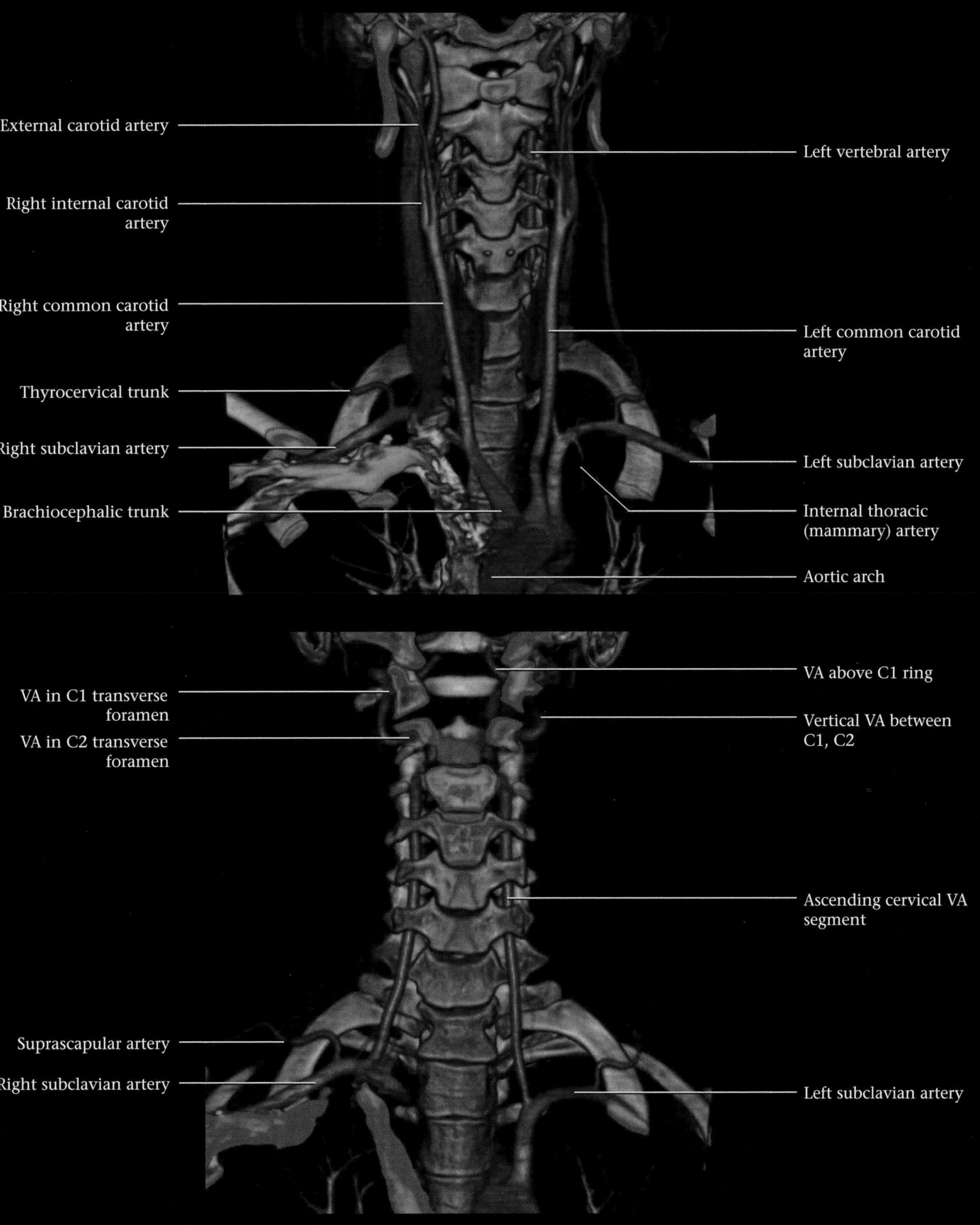
External carotid artery
Right internal carotid artery
Right common carotid artery
Thyrocervical trunk
Right subclavian artery
Brachiocephalic trunk
Left vertebral artery
Left common carotid artery
Left subclavian artery
Internal thoracic (mammary) artery
Aortic arch
VA in C1 transverse foramen
VA in C2 transverse foramen
Suprascapular artery
Right subclavian artery
VA above C1 ring
Vertical VA between C1, C2
Ascending cervical VA segment
Left subclavian artery

(Top) Two images from a 3D-VRT CT are illustrated. Here, on an AP projection, the major aortic arch branches are clearly identified. The origin of the left vertebral artery is seen. Note the two VAs as they course superiorly within the transverse foramina of the cervical spine. Both carotid bifurcations are at the C4-C5 level, the most common location. **(Bottom)** The aortic arch and carotid arteries are removed and the lateral masses of C1 and C2 are cut away to show the vertebral arteries. The VAs ascend through the transverse foramina from C6 to C3. At C2 they turn laterally in an inverted L shape, then ascend toward the transverse foramina of C1. After they exit C1 they course posteromedially around the atlantooccipital joint above the ring of C1.

CERVICAL CAROTID ARTERIES

Terminology

Abbreviations

- Aortic arch (AA); brachiocephalic trunk (BCT)
- Common (CCA), internal (ICA), external (ECA) carotid arteries
- Vertebral artery (VA), basilar artery (BA)

Gross Anatomy

Overview

- CCAs terminate by dividing into ECA, ICA
- ECA is smaller of two terminal branches
  - Supplies most of head, neck (except eye, brain)
  - Has numerous anastomoses with ICA, VA (may become important source of collateral blood flow)
- ICA has no normal extracranial branches

Imaging Anatomy

Overview

- **CCAs**
  - Right CCA originates from BCT; left CCA from AA
  - Course superiorly in carotid space, anteromedial to internal jugular vein
  - Divide into ECA, ICA at approximately C3-4 level
- **Cervical ICAs**
  - 90% arise posterolateral to ECA
  - Carotid "bulb"
    - Focal dilatation of ICA at its origin from CCA
    - Flow reversal occurs in carotid bulb
  - Ascending cervical segment
    - Courses superiorly within carotid space
    - Enters carotid canal of skull base (petrous temporal bone)
    - No named branches in neck
- **ECAs** have 8 major branches
  - **Superior thyroid artery**
    - First ECA branch (may arise from CCA bifurcation)
    - Arises anteriorly, courses inferiorly to apex of thyroid
    - Supplies superior thyroid, larynx
    - Anastomoses with inferior thyroid artery (branch of thyrocervical trunk)
  - **Ascending pharyngeal artery**
    - Arises from posterior ECA (or CCA bifurcation)
    - Courses superiorly between ECA, ICA
    - Visceral branches supply nasopharynx, oropharynx, eustachian tube
    - Muscular, tympanic branches supply middle ear, prevertebral muscles
    - Neuromeningeal branches supply dura, CNs 9-11
    - **Numerous important (potentially dangerous) anastomoses with middle/accessory meningeal, caroticotympanic and vidian arteries!**
  - **Lingual artery**
    - Second anterior ECA branch
    - Loops anteroinferiorly, then superiorly to tongue
    - Major vascular supply to tongue, oral cavity, submandibular gland
    - Common origin with facial artery in 10-20% of cases
  - **Facial artery**
    - Originates just above lingual artery
    - Curves around mandible, then passes anterosuperiorly across cheek
    - Supplies face, palate, lip, cheek
    - **Anastomoses with ophthalmic artery (ICA branch), other ECA branches**
  - **Occipital artery**
    - Originates from posterior aspect of ECA
    - Courses posterosuperiorly between occiput and C1
    - Supplies scalp, upper cervical musculature, posterior fossa meninges
    - Extensive anastomoses with muscular VA branches
  - **Posterior auricular artery**
    - Arises from posterior ECA above occipital artery
    - Courses superiorly to supply pinna, scalp, external auditory canal, chorda tympani
  - **Superficial temporal artery**
    - Smaller of two terminal ECA branches
    - Runs superiorly behind mandibular condyle, across zygoma
    - Supplies scalp, gives off transverse facial artery
  - **Maxillary artery**
    - Larger of two terminal ECA branches
    - Arises within parotid gland, behind mandibular neck
    - Gives off middle meningeal artery (supplies cranial meninges)
    - Runs anteromedially in masticator space
    - Within pterygopalatine fossa sends off terminal branches to deep face, nose
    - **Potential major source of collateral flow via inferolateral trunk of cavernous ICA, ophthalmic and recurrent meningeal arteries**
- **Cervical VAs**
  - Originate from subclavian arteries, pass upwards in transverse foramina
  - Numerous muscular branches, ECA anastomoses

Normal Variants, Anomalies

- Normal variants (common)
  - CCA bifurcation can be from T2 to C2
  - Medial (not lateral) origin of ICA from CCA in 10-15%
  - Arch origin of VA (5%)
- Anomalies (rare)
  - "Nonbifurcating" CCA
    - No ICA bulb; ECA branches arise directly from CCA
    - High association with aberrant course of ICA in middle ear!
  - Persistent hypoglossal artery
    - Second most common carotid-basilar anastomosis
    - Arises from ICA at C1-2 level, passes through hypoglossal canal to join BA
  - Proatlantal intersegmental artery
    - Arises from cervical ICA at C2-3
    - Connects cervical ICA with VA

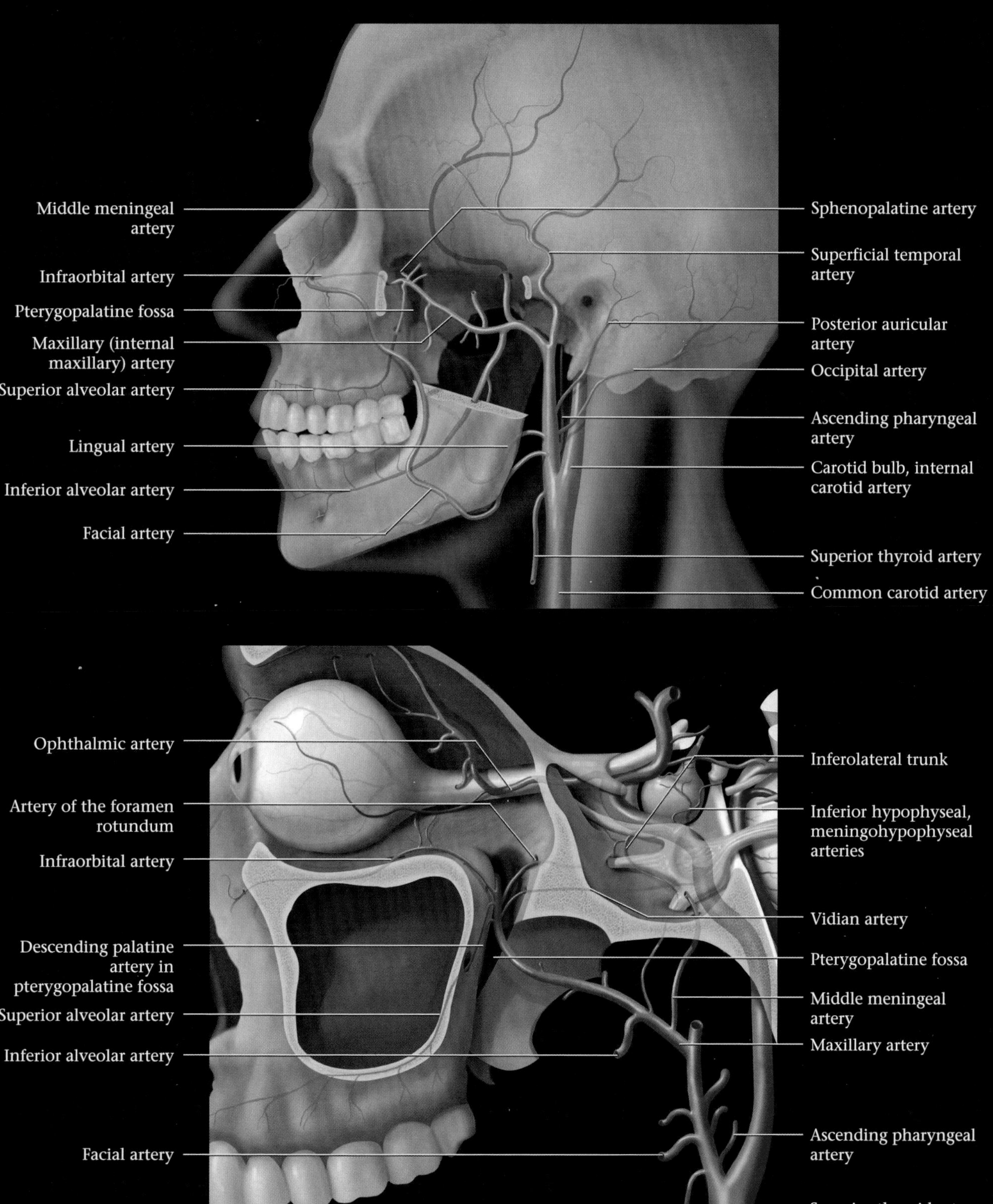
Middle meningeal artery
Infraorbital artery
Pterygopalatine fossa
Maxillary (internal maxillary) artery
Superior alveolar artery
Lingual artery
Inferior alveolar artery
Facial artery
Sphenopalatine artery
Superficial temporal artery
Posterior auricular artery
Occipital artery
Ascending pharyngeal artery
Carotid bulb, internal carotid artery
Superior thyroid artery
Common carotid artery
Ophthalmic artery
Artery of the foramen rotundum
Infraorbital artery
Descending palatine artery in pterygopalatine fossa
Superior alveolar artery
Inferior alveolar artery
Facial artery
Inferolateral trunk
Inferior hypophyseal, meningohypophyseal arteries
Vidian artery
Pterygopalatine fossa
Middle meningeal artery
Maxillary artery
Ascending pharyngeal artery
Superior thyroid artery

(Top) Lateral graphic depicts common carotid artery and its two terminal branches, external and internal carotid arteries. Scalp, superficial facial structures are removed to show deep ECA branches. ECA terminates by dividing into superficial temporal and internal maxillary arteries (IMA). Within the pterygopalatine fossa, the IMA divides into numerous deep branches. Its distal termination is the sphenopalatine artery, which passes medially into the nasal cavity. Numerous anastomoses between ECA branches (e.g., between the facial and maxillary arteries) as well as between the ECA and orbital and cavernous branches of the ICA provide potential sources for collateral blood flow. **(Bottom)** Close-up view of the deep ECA branches and their numerous anastomoses with branches from the ICA. The maxillary artery terminal branches arise deep within the pterygopalatine fossa.

CERVICAL CAROTID ARTERIES

LATERAL DSA CCA

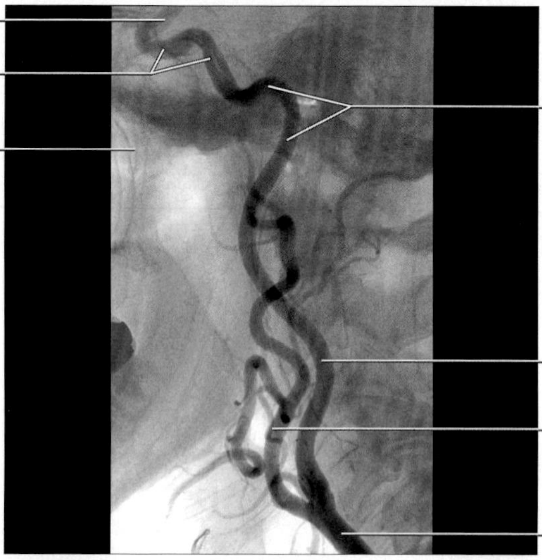

Supraclinoid internal carotid artery
Cavernous internal carotid artery
Pterygopalatine fossa
Petrous internal carotid artery
Internal carotid artery, cervical segment
External carotid artery
Common carotid artery

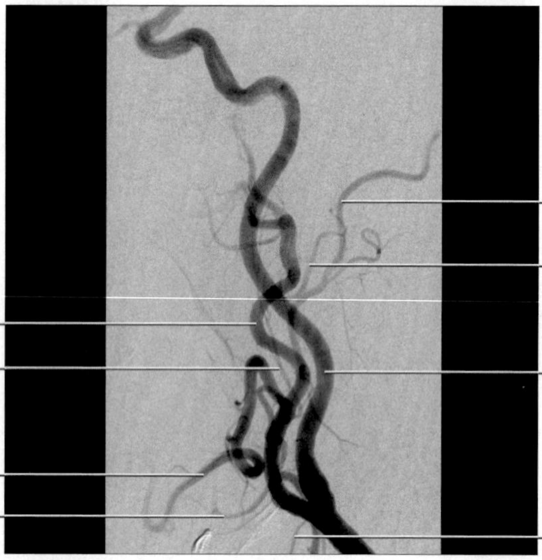

Occipital artery
Posterior auricular artery
External carotid artery
Ascending pharyngeal artery
Internal carotid artery
Facial artery
Lingual artery
Superior thyroid artery

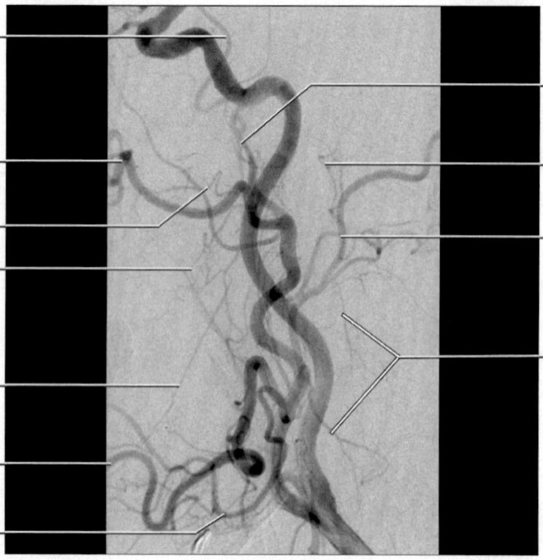

Superficial temporal artery
Superficial temporal artery
Maxillary artery branching within pterygopalatine fossa
Posterior auricular artery
Transverse facial artery
Occipital artery
Superior alveolar artery
Muscular branches of occipital artery
Inferior alveolar artery
Facial artery
Lingual artery

(Top) Lateral unsubtracted DSA of a common carotid angiogram shows the relationship of the CCA bifurcation to the cervical spine and skull base. The typical CCA bifurcation is usually around the C4-C5 level. The internal carotid artery normally arises posterior and lateral to the ECA. All branches of the carotid arteries below the skull base arise only from the ECA. The pterygopalatine fossa, seen here behind the posterior maxillary sinus wall, contains the terminal maxillary artery division into its deep facial branches. **(Middle)** Early arterial phase of the CCA angiogram is shown with bony structures subtracted. The major ECA branches are opacified. **(Bottom)** Late arterial phase shows opacification of the distal ECA branches. The main terminal ECA branch is the maxillary artery, shown here as it divides within the pterygopalatine fossa.

OBLIQUE DSA CCA

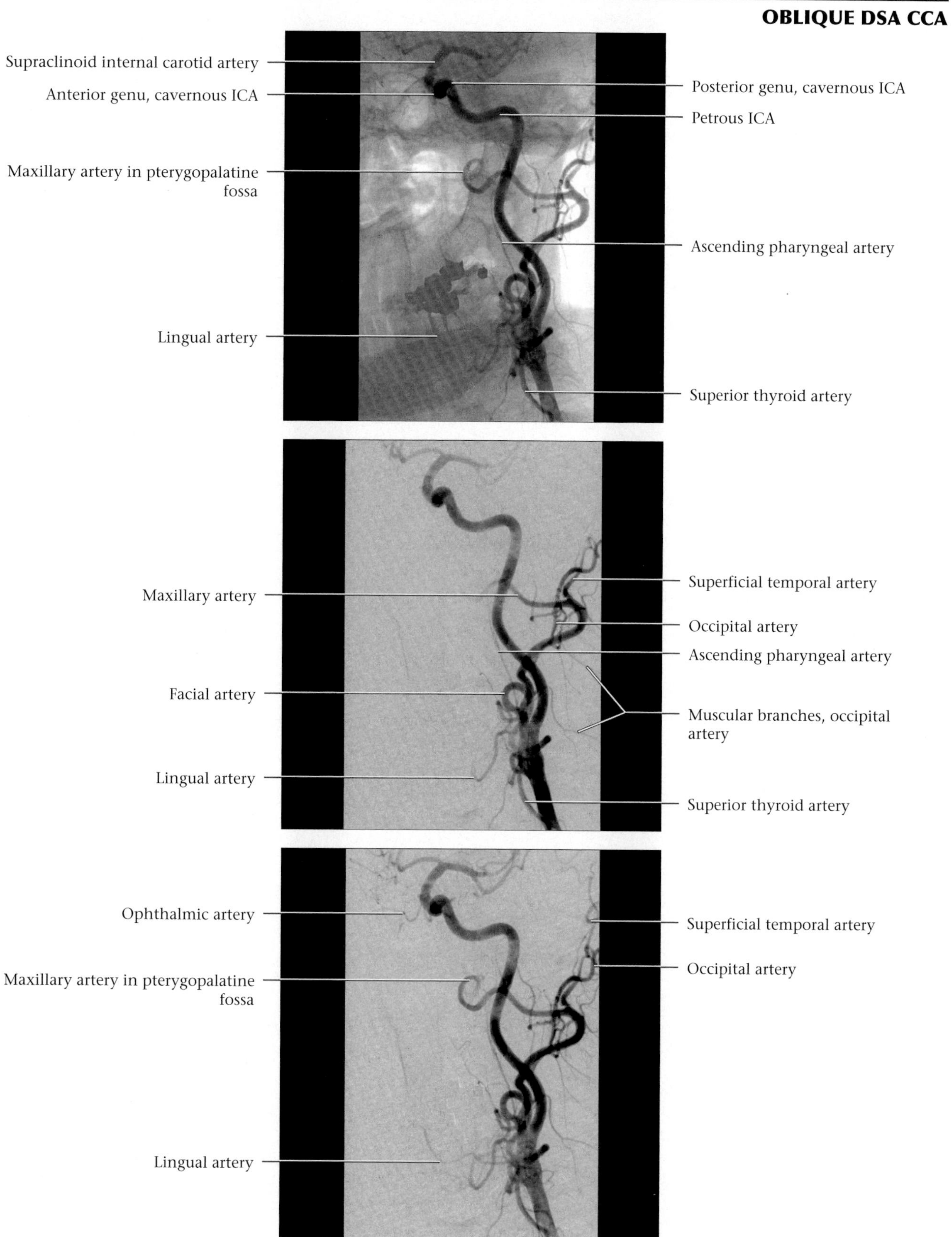
Supraclinoid internal carotid artery
Anterior genu, cavernous ICA
Maxillary artery in pterygopalatine fossa
Lingual artery
Posterior genu, cavernous ICA
Petrous ICA
Ascending pharyngeal artery
Superior thyroid artery
Maxillary artery
Facial artery
Lingual artery
Superficial temporal artery
Occipital artery
Ascending pharyngeal artery
Muscular branches, occipital artery
Superior thyroid artery
Ophthalmic artery
Maxillary artery in pterygopalatine fossa
Lingual artery
Superficial temporal artery
Occipital artery

(Top) Unsubtracted oblique view of a left common carotid DSA shows the maxillary artery coursing towards its terminal bifurcation within the pterygopalatine fossa. The ascending pharyngeal artery is a small branch that is often obscured by larger vessels on standard lateral views. **(Middle)** Subtracted view shows both proximal, distal branches of the cervical ICA. Note that the ascending pharyngeal branch, often not well seen on standard lateral or AP views, is well visualized here as it courses superiorly towards the skull base. **(Bottom)** Late arterial phase shows the terminal maxillary artery bifurcation within the pterygopalatine fossa. The superficial temporal and middle meningeal arteries typically fill late on common carotid angiograms.

CERVICAL CAROTID ARTERIES

3D-VRT CECT

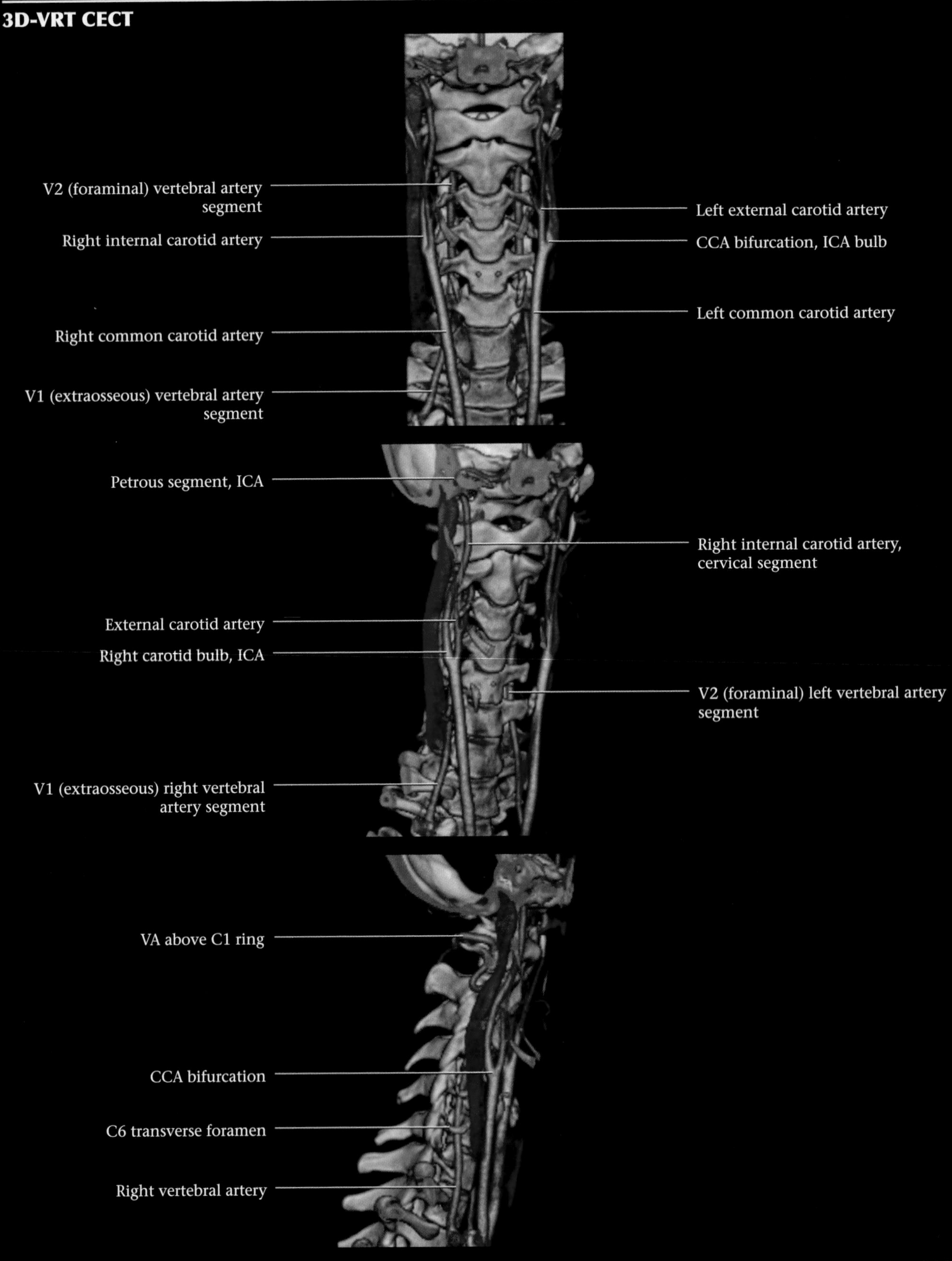
V2 (foraminal) vertebral artery segment
Right internal carotid artery
Right common carotid artery
V1 (extraosseous) vertebral artery segment
Left external carotid artery
CCA bifurcation, ICA bulb
Left common carotid artery
Petrous segment, ICA
External carotid artery
Right carotid bulb, ICA
V1 (extraosseous) right vertebral artery segment
Right internal carotid artery, cervical segment
V2 (foraminal) left vertebral artery segment
VA above C1 ring
CCA bifurcation
C6 transverse foramen
Right vertebral artery

(Top) Coned frontal 3D-VRT CECT image demonstrate the cervical carotid arteries and their relationship to the cervical spine. Here the common carotid (CCA) bifurcation is at the C4-C5 level, the most common location. The external carotid arteries arise anteromedial to the internal carotid arteries in about 90% of cases. Both the V1 (extraosseous) and V2 (foraminal) segments of both vertebral arteries can be seen ascending through the transverse foramina from C6 to C2 in this view. **(Middle)** Right oblique 3D-VRT CECT image demonstrates the right carotid bifurcation. The ICA initially ascends posterolateral to the ECA but swings anteromedially as it courses cephalad to the skull base. In this projection, the left ECA and ICA are superimposed on each other. **(Bottom)** Lateral view profiles the ICA bifurcations, right VA passing into C6 transverse foramen.

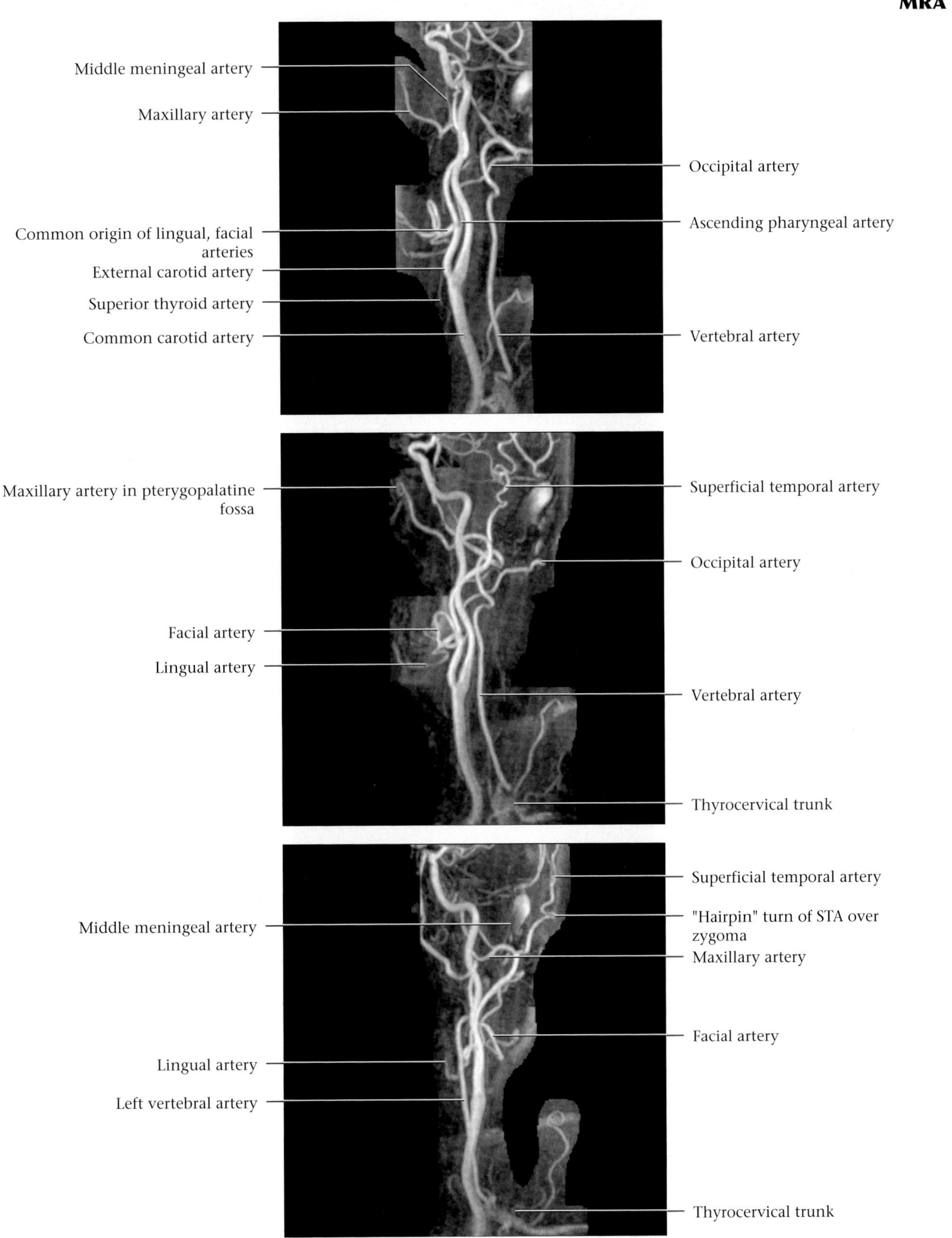

Middle meningeal artery
Maxillary artery
Occipital artery
Common origin of lingual, facial arteries
Ascending pharyngeal artery
External carotid artery
Superior thyroid artery
Common carotid artery
Vertebral artery
Maxillary artery in pterygopalatine fossa
Superficial temporal artery
Occipital artery
Facial artery
Lingual artery
Vertebral artery
Thyrocervical trunk
Superficial temporal artery
Middle meningeal artery
"Hairpin" turn of STA over zygoma
Maxillary artery
Facial artery
Lingual artery
Left vertebral artery
Thyrocervical trunk

(Top) MR angiogram of the cervical carotid and vertebral arteries profiles the carotid bifurcation. The major external carotid artery branches are well seen. **(Middle)** Oblique view shows the bifurcation. The distal loop of the maxillary artery at its termination within the pterygopalatine fossa can be seen here. **(Bottom)** On this straight AP view, the carotid bifurcation is obscured but distal ECA branches are well seen. The superficial temporal artery has a characteristic tight "hairpin" turn as it passes over the zygomatic arch.

CERVICAL CAROTID ARTERIES

LATERAL DSA DISTAL EXTERNAL CAROTID ARTERY

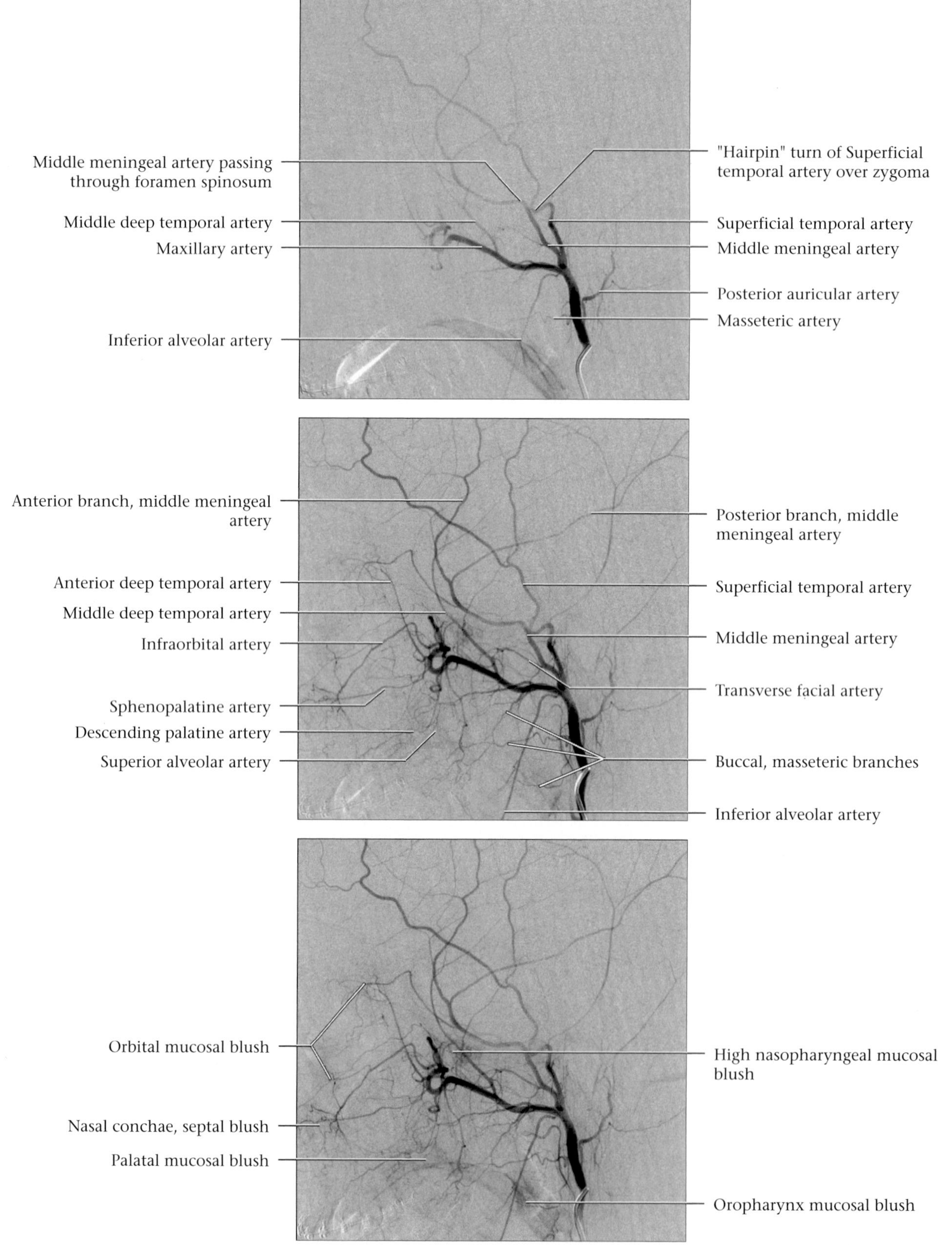

Middle meningeal artery passing through foramen spinosum
Middle deep temporal artery
Maxillary artery
Inferior alveolar artery
"Hairpin" turn of Superficial temporal artery over zygoma
Superficial temporal artery
Middle meningeal artery
Posterior auricular artery
Masseteric artery
Anterior branch, middle meningeal artery
Anterior deep temporal artery
Middle deep temporal artery
Infraorbital artery
Sphenopalatine artery
Descending palatine artery
Superior alveolar artery
Posterior branch, middle meningeal artery
Superficial temporal artery
Middle meningeal artery
Transverse facial artery
Buccal, masseteric branches
Inferior alveolar artery
Orbital mucosal blush
Nasal conchae, septal blush
Palatal mucosal blush
High nasopharyngeal mucosal blush
Oropharynx mucosal blush

(Top) Selective distal external carotid artery angiogram, early arterial phase, lateral view, shows the distal external carotid artery and its main proximal branches. The abrupt anterior angulation of the middle meningeal artery as it passes intracranially through the foramen spinosum is well demonstrated. Note "hairpin" turn of the superficial temporal artery as it courses over the zygomatic arch. **(Middle)** Mid-arterial phase shows the deep facial branches of the ECA especially well. Most arise from the termination of the maxillary artery within the pterygopalatine fossa, seen here as a distinct loop just behind the maxillary sinus wall. **(Bottom)** Late arterial phase shows very prominent vascular blushes in mucosa of the sinuses, nose, orbit and oropharynx. This is a normal finding and should not be mistaken for vascular malformation.

AP DSA INTERNAL MAXILLARY ARTERY

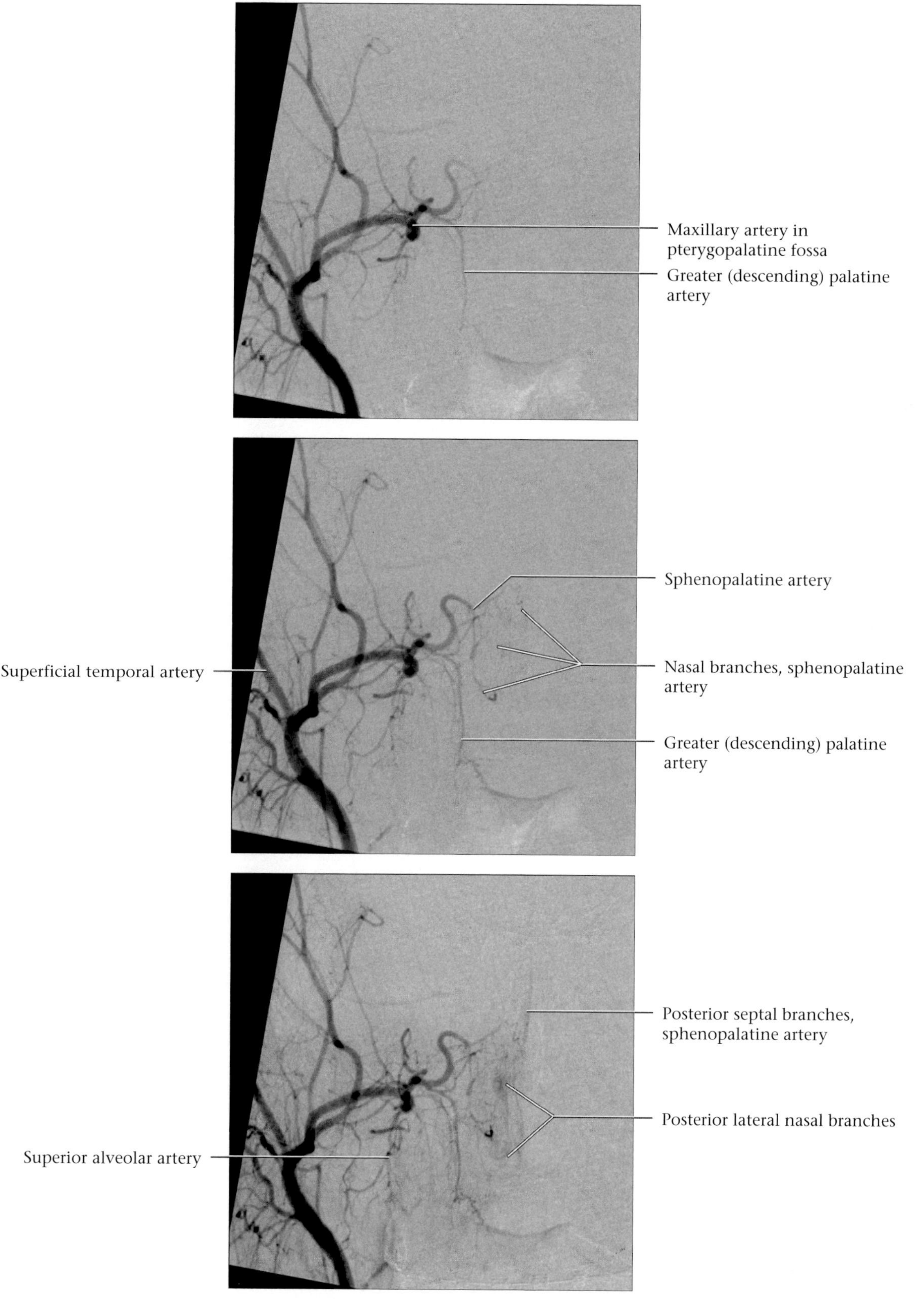
Maxillary artery in pterygopalatine fossa
Greater (descending) palatine artery
Sphenopalatine artery
Superficial temporal artery
Nasal branches, sphenopalatine artery
Greater (descending) palatine artery
Posterior septal branches, sphenopalatine artery
Posterior lateral nasal branches
Superior alveolar artery

(Top) Distal external carotid DSA, early arterial phase, AP view, shows the termination of the maxillary artery as it loops within the pterygopalatine fossa. **(Middle)** Mid-arterial phase shows the sphenopalatine artery, the distal continuation of the maxillary artery, as it passes medially through the sphenopalatine foramen into the nose. Numerous small branches supply the vascular nasal mucosa. **(Bottom)** Late arterial phase shows a prominent vascular blush along the nasal turbinates and palatal mucosa. Numerous small nasal branches of the sphenopalatine artery ramify over the conchae and meatuses and anastomose with branches of the ethmoidal arteries and nasal branches of the greater palatine artery. The sphenopalatine artery ends on the nasal septum as posterior septal branches.

CERVICAL CAROTID ARTERIES

ULTRASOUND

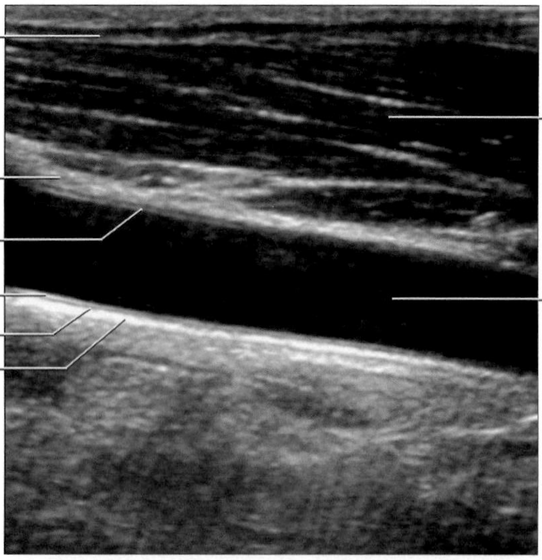

Platysma
Sternomastoid muscle
Carotid sheath
Carotid wall
Intima
Media
Adventitia
Common carotid artery (lumen)

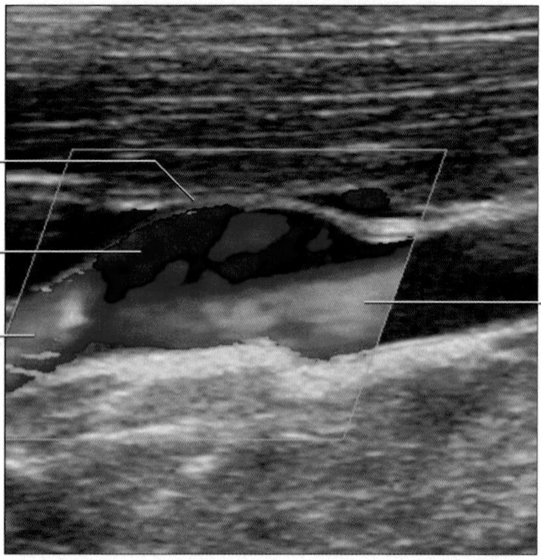

Carotid wall
Carotid bulb with slow, nonlaminar flow
Internal carotid artery lumen
Distal common carotid artery

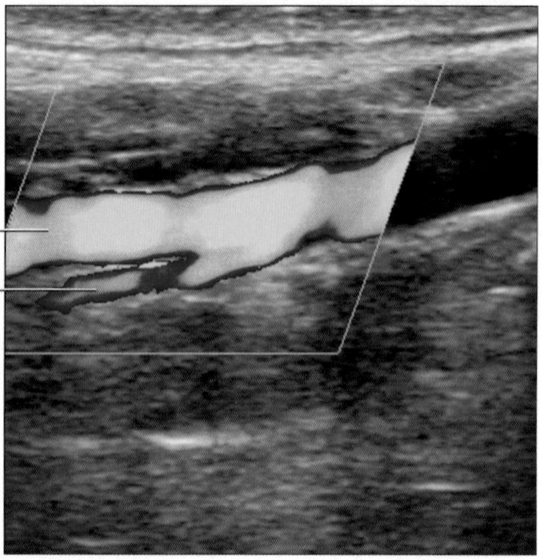

Main trunk of external carotid artery
Proximal ECA branch

(Top) M-mode ultrasound of normal carotid artery, longitudinal image, shows normal wall thickness without evidence for atherosclerosis. Three lines are seen in the carotid wall: The white endoluminal line is the intimal reflection. The darker line underneath represents the media. The thicker peripheral white line is the adventitia. **(Middle)** Color Doppler ultrasound, longitudinal image, of normal carotid bulb. Flow in the main lumen of the proximal internal carotid artery is laminar. Note the area of disturbed/reversed flow in bulbous portion of proximal ICA (mixed blue and red). **(Bottom)** Power Doppler shows normal external carotid artery with a proximal branch.

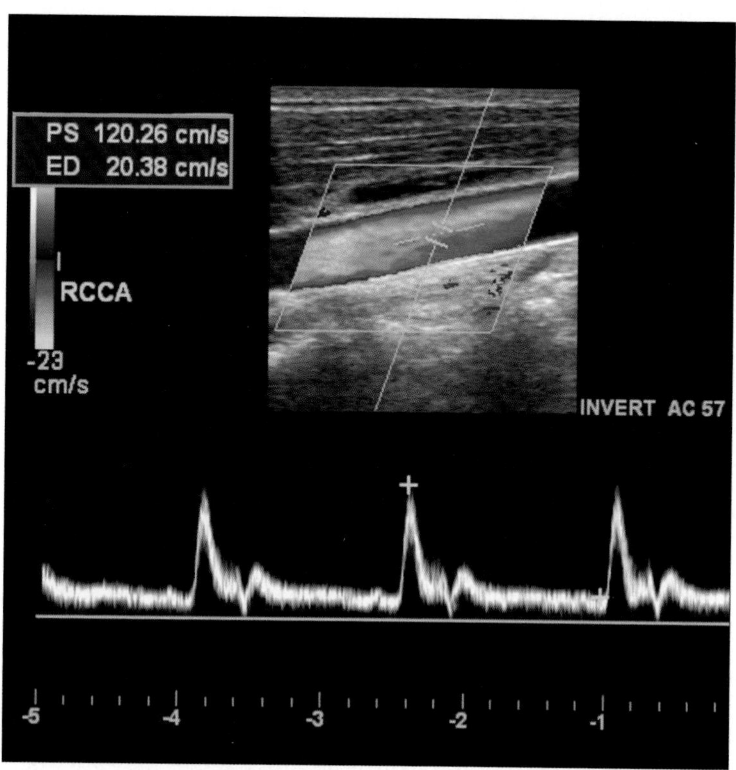
PS 120.26 cm/s
ED 20.38 cm/s
RCCA
-23
cm/s
INVERT AC 57
-5
-4
-3
-2
-1

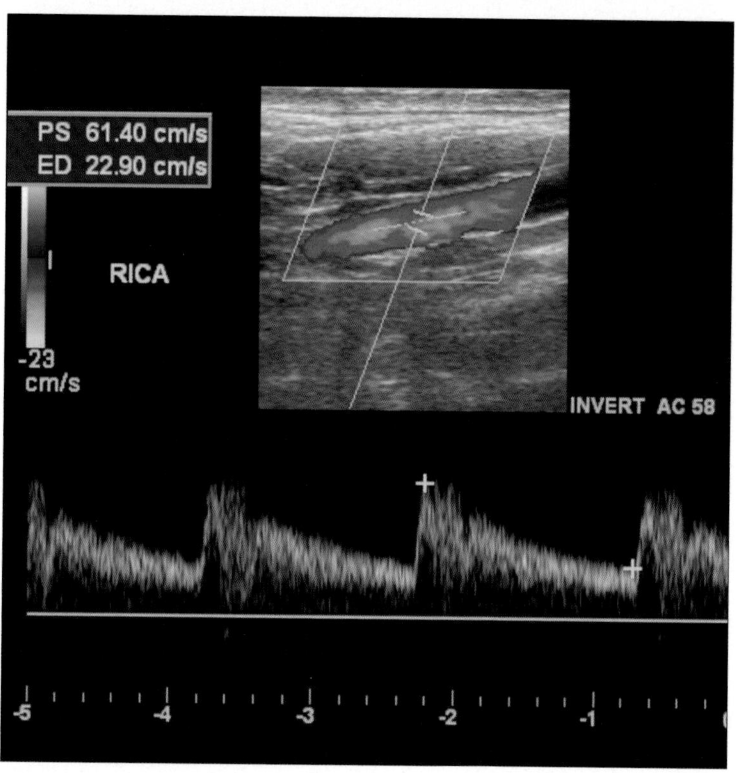
PS 61.40 cm/s
ED 22.90 cm/s
RICA
-23
cm/s
INVERT AC 58
-5
-4
-3
-2
-1

(Top) Color Doppler of right common carotid artery with normal triphasic wave form. The peak systolic velocity (PS) in this case is slightly high for physiological reasons. **(Bottom)** Color Doppler of right internal carotid artery. Notice normal low resistance waveform. The PS of 61 cm/s is normal. Note that the CCA waveform above shows higher resistance features (sharp diastolic peak and little diastolic flow) as compared with the internal carotid which has distinct low resistance features (broad systolic peaks, relatively large amount of diastolic flow).

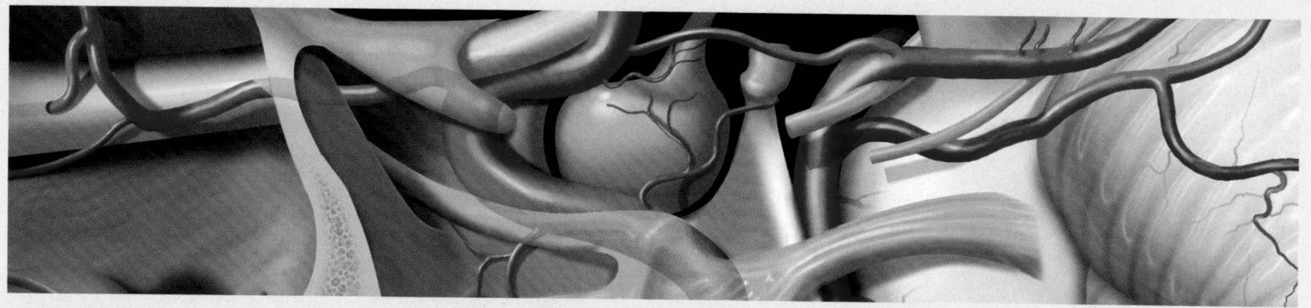

SECTION 7: Intracranial Arteries

INTRACRANIAL ARTERIES OVERVIEW

Terminology

Abbreviations

- Anterior, middle, posterior cerebral arteries (ACA, MCA, PCA)
- Anterior, posterior communicating arteries (ACoA, PCoA)
- Basilar artery (BA)
- Vertebral artery (VA)
- Anterior, posterior inferior cerebellar arteries (AICA, PICA)
- Anterior choroidal artery (AChoA)
- Recurrent artery of Heubner (RAH)

Gross Anatomy

Anterior Circulation

- ICA and its branches + ACoA, PCoA

Posterior Circulation

- BA and its branches

Imaging Anatomy

Overview

- **Internal carotid artery**
  - Proximal to termination gives off ophthalmic artery, AChoA, PCoA
  - Terminal bifurcation into ACA (smaller, medial), MCA (larger, lateral)
  - **ACA** has 4 segments
    - Horizontal or precommunicating (A1) segment courses medially above optic chiasm, joined by ACoA to contralateral A1
    - Vertical or postcommunicating (A2) segment courses superiorly in interhemispheric fissure, around corpus callosum genu
    - Distal (A3) segment courses posteriorly under inferior free margin of falx cerebri, gives off cortical branches
    - Perforating arteries arise from A1, ACoA
    - RAH arises from distal A1 or proximal A2
  - **MCA** has 4 segments
    - Horizontal (M1) segment courses laterally to sylvian fissure below anterior perforated substance, bi- or trifurcates
    - "Genu" or "knee" of MCA is gentle posterosuperior turn towards lateral cerebral (sylvian) fissure
    - Insular (M2) segments course within lateral cerebral fissure, over insula
    - Opercular (M3) segments begin at top of insula, turn laterally in sylvian fissure to reach overhanging frontal/parietal/temporal operculae
    - Cortical (M4) branches emerge from lateral cerebral fissure, course over hemispheric surface
    - Perforating arteries arise from M1
- **Basilar artery**
  - Courses cephalad in prepontine cistern to terminal bifurcation ventral to midbrain
    - Gives off **AICA**, superior cerebellar arteries (**SCAs**), pontine, midbrain perforating arteries
  - Bifurcates into **PCAs**, each of which has 4 segments
    - Mesencephalic or precommunicating (P1) segment lies within interpeduncular cistern, curves posterolaterally from BA to PCoA junction
    - Ambient (P2) segment extends from PCA-PCoA junction, curving around cerebral peduncles just above tentorium, above oculomotor nerve
    - Quadrigeminal (P3) segment extends posteromedially from level of quadrigeminal plate
    - Cortical (P4) branches arise from distal PCA at or just before reaching calcarine fissure
    - Perforating branches arise from P1
  - **Vertebral arteries**
    - Intracranial (V4) segments enter dura near foramen magnum
    - Give off anterior/posterior spinal arteries, perforating arteries to medulla, PICA

Vascular Territory

- Vascular distribution of ACA, MCA, PCA vary from individual to individual, have typical as well as maximum, minimum territories
- Two **vascular "watershed" zones** exist at confluence of territorial supply, are vulnerable to hypoperfusion
  - Cortical watershed = subpial confluence of cortical ACA/MCA/PCA branches
  - Deep white matter watershed zone = confluence of deep cortical penetrating branches, perforating branches from circle of Willis (COW)
- **ACA**
  - Perforating branches: Corpus callosum rostrum, heads of caudate nuclei, anterior commissure, anteromedial putamen/globus pallidus/anterior limb internal capsule (if RAH present)
  - Cortical branches: Inferomedial frontal lobes, anterior 2/3 of medial hemisphere surface, 1-2 cm over brain convexity
- **MCA**
  - Perforating branches: Most of putamen, globus pallidus, superior half of internal capsule, most of caudate nucleus, some deep white matter
  - Cortical branches: Most of lateral surface of cerebral hemispheres, anterior tip (pole) of temporal lobe
- **PCA**
  - Perforating branches: Much of central brain base (thalamus, hypothalamus), midbrain, choroid plexus
  - Cortical branches: Most of inferior surface of temporal lobe, occipital pole, variable amount of posterolateral surface of hemisphere
- **BA**
  - All of PCA territory (including perforating branches), most of pons, superior cerebellum/vermis
- **VA**
  - Most of medulla, cerebellar tonsils, inferior vermis/cerebellar hemispheres

Anatomy-Based Imaging Issues

Imaging Recommendations

- Late arterial (capillary) phase of DSA with "brain stain" shows vascular territory

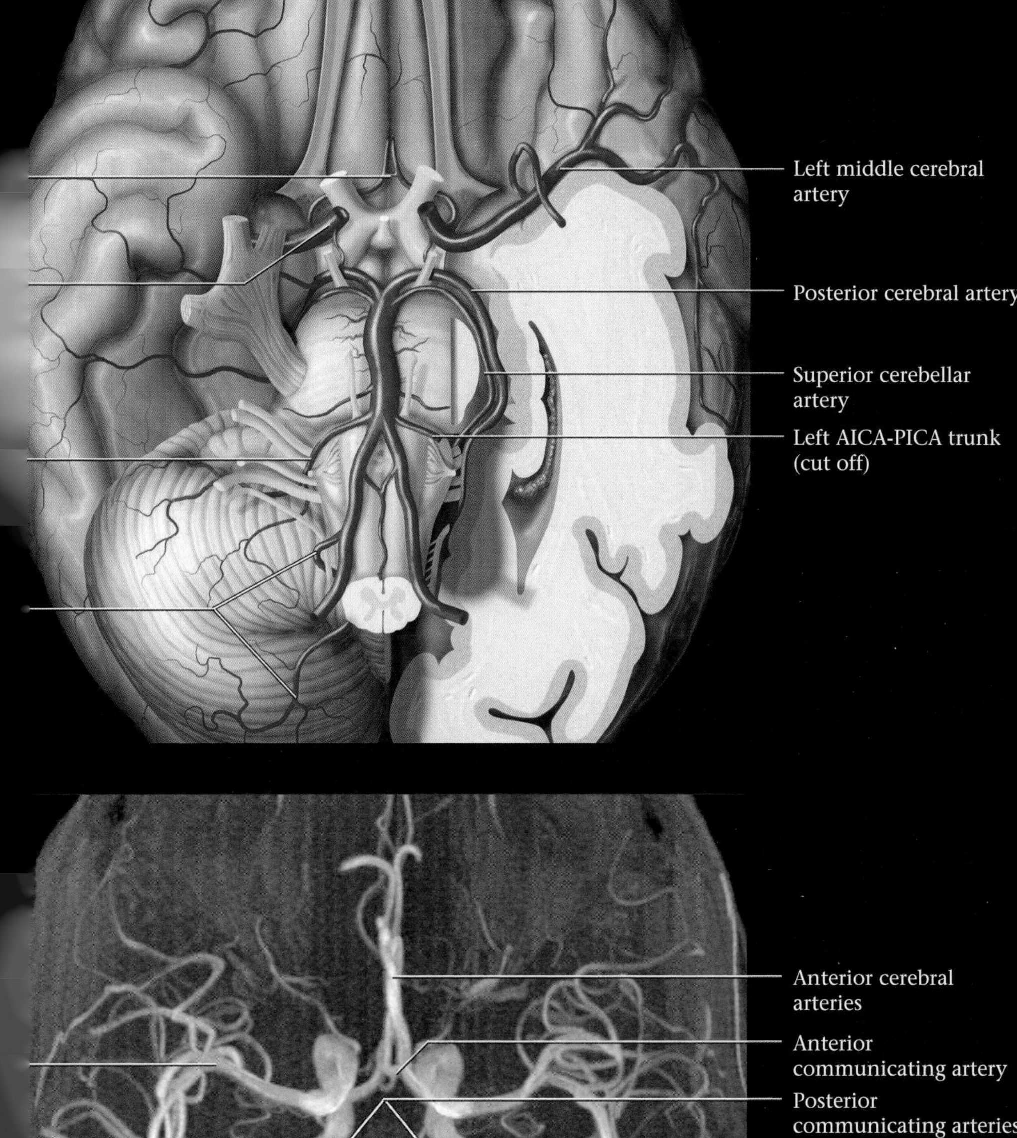

Left middle cerebral artery
Posterior cerebral artery
Superior cerebellar artery
Left AICA-PICA trunk (cut off)
Anterior cerebral arteries
Anterior communicating artery
Posterior communicating arteries
Basilar artery
Left anterior inferior cerebellar artery
Superior vermian arteries (branches of SCA)
Calcarine artery

brain vascular system and its relationship to the base of the brain. The anterior cerebral
the interhemispheric fissure from their junction at the anterior communicating artery.
medial brain surface except for the posterior third, which is supplied by the MCA. The MCA
l surface of the hemispheres. The PCA supplies most of the undersurface of the temporal
nterior tip. The right anterior and posterior inferior cerebellar arteries are shown on the
non AICA-PICA trunk is present, a frequent normal variant. **(Bottom)** Submentovertex view

INTRACRANIAL ARTERIES OVERVIEW

GRAPHICS

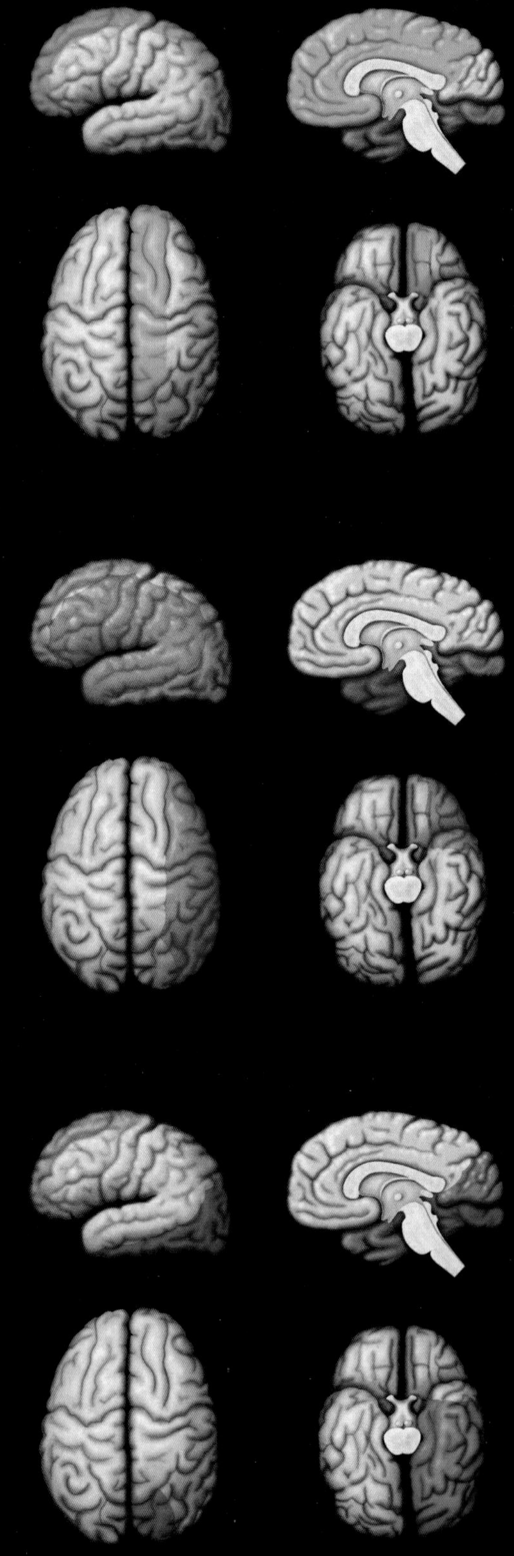

(Top) Typical vascular territories of the three major cerebral arteries are depicted. The most common distribution of the ACA is shown in green, as seen from lateral (upper left), medial (upper right), from top down (lower left) and from the submentovertex perspective (lower right). The ACA supplies most of the medial hemispheric surface except for the occipital lobe. **(Middle)** Usual vascular territory of the MCA, shown in red. MCA typically supplies most of the lateral and superior surface of the hemisphere except for a small strip over the vertex (ACA), occipital pole and inferolateral temporal lobe (PCA). **(Bottom)** Usual vascular territory of the PCA is depicted in blue. The PCA supplies the occipital poles and most of the undersurface of the temporal lobe except for its tip, which is usually supplied by the MCA.

GRAPHICS

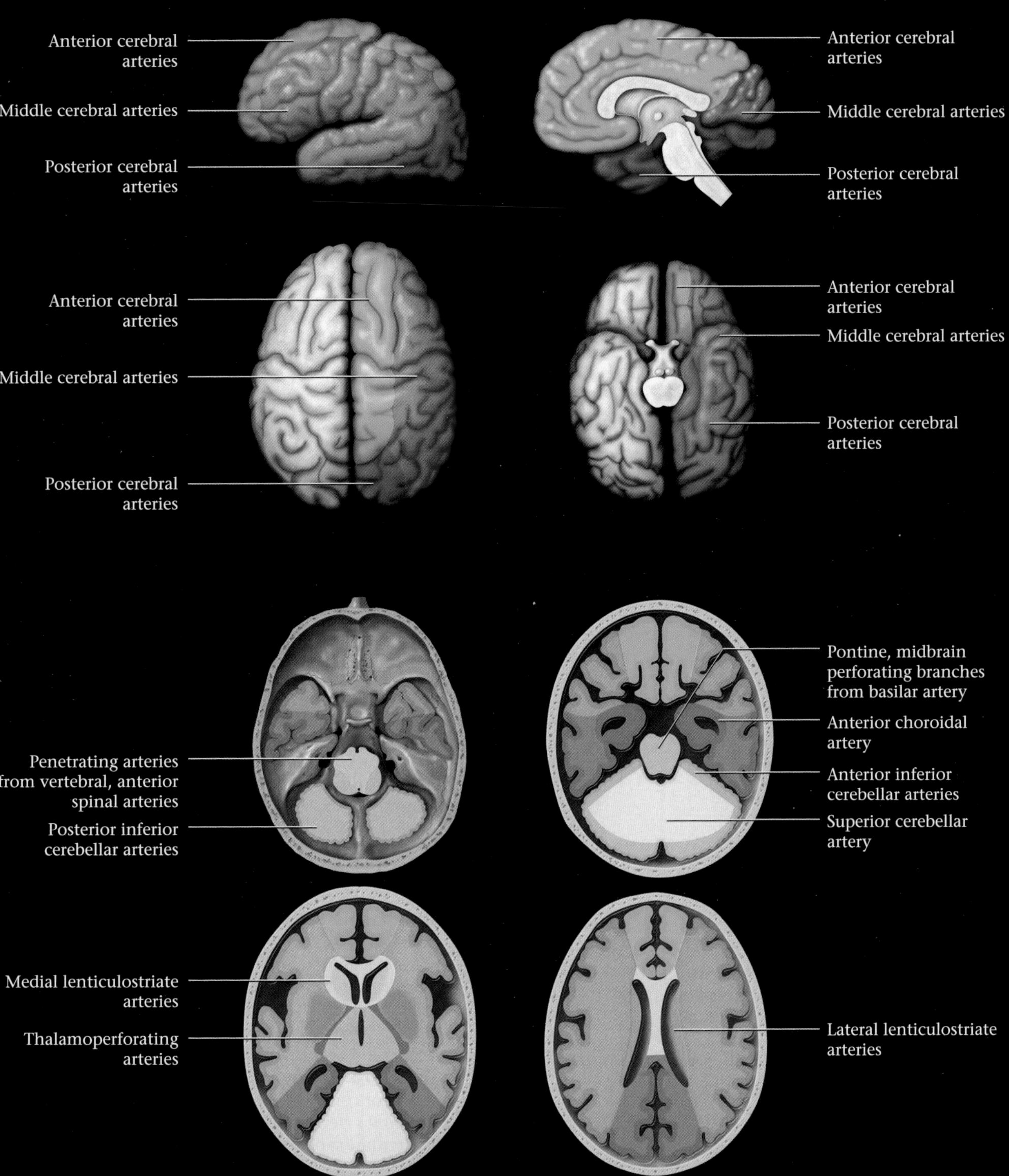

Anterior cerebral arteries
Middle cerebral arteries
Posterior cerebral arteries
Anterior cerebral arteries
Middle cerebral arteries
Posterior cerebral arteries
Anterior cerebral arteries
Middle cerebral arteries
Posterior cerebral arteries
Anterior cerebral arteries
Middle cerebral arteries
Posterior cerebral arteries
Penetrating arteries from vertebral, anterior spinal arteries
Posterior inferior cerebellar arteries
Pontine, midbrain perforating branches from basilar artery
Anterior choroidal artery
Anterior inferior cerebellar arteries
Superior cerebellar artery
Medial lenticulostriate arteries
Thalamoperforating arteries
Lateral lenticulostriate arteries

(Top) The three major cerebral artery territories fit together like a jigsaw puzzle as they supply the hemispheres. ACA is depicted in green. MCA is shown in red. The PCA is colored blue. The junction of territories forms the cortical watershed zone. The posterior confluence where all three vascular distributions meet together, seen on the lower left at the vertex, is especially vulnerable to cerebral hypoperfusion. **(Bottom)** Penetrating artery territories are shown in axial plane. PICA (tan) supplies inferior cerebellum, lateral medulla. SCA is shown in yellow, AICA in light blue. Medullary (aqua), pontine and thalamic perforating arteries (light purple) are derived from the vertebrobasilar territory. Anterior choroidal (magenta), lateral (medium blue) and medial (light green) lenticulostriate arteries supply basal ganglia, caudate, much of corpus callosum.

INTRACRANIAL INTERNAL CAROTID ARTERY

Terminology

Abbreviations

- Internal carotid, ophthalmic arteries (ICA, OA)
- Cavernous sinus (CS)

Gross Anatomy

Overview

- Complex course with several vertical/horizontal segments, 3 genus (one petrous, two cavernous)
- Six intracranial segments (cervical ICA = C1)
  - Petrous (C2), lacerum (C3), cavernous (C4)
  - Clinoid (C5), ophthalmic (C6), communicating (C7)

Imaging Anatomy

Segments, Branches

- **Petrous (C2) segment**
  - Contained within carotid canal of temporal bone
  - Surrounded by extensive sympathetic plexus
  - Two C2 subsegments joined at genu
    - Short vertical segment [anterior to internal jugular vein (IJV)]
    - "Genu" (where petrous ICA turns anteromedially in front of cochlea)
    - Longer horizontal segment
  - Exits carotid canal at petrous apex
  - Branches
    - Vidian artery (artery of pterygoid canal) anastomoses with external carotid artery (ECA)
    - Caroticotympanic artery (supplies middle ear)
- **Lacerum (C3) segment**
  - Small segment that extends from petrous apex above foramen (f.) lacerum, curving upwards toward cavernous sinus
  - Covered by trigeminal ganglion
  - No branches
- **Cavernous (C4) segment**
  - Three subsegments joined by two genus (knees)
    - Posterior vertical (ascending) portion
    - Posterior (more medial) genu
    - Horizontal segment
    - Anterior (more lateral) genu
    - Anterior vertical (subclinoid) segment
  - Covered by trigeminal ganglion posteriorly
  - Abducens nerve (CN6) is inferolateral
  - Major branches
    - Meningohypophyseal trunk (arises from posterior genu, supplies pituitary, tentorium and clival dura)
    - Inferolateral trunk arises from horizontal segment, supplies cavernous sinus (CS) dura/cranial nerves; **anastomoses with ECA branches through f. rotundum, spinosum, ovale**
- **Clinoid (C5) segment**
  - Between proximal, distal dural rings of cavernous sinus
  - Ends as ICA enters subarachnoid space near anterior clinoid process
  - No important branches unless OA arises within CS
- **Ophthalmic (C6) segment**
  - Extends from distal dural ring at superior clinoid to just below posterior communicating artery (PCoA) origin
  - Two important branches
    - OA (originates from anterosuperior ICA, passes through optic canal to orbit; gives off ocular, lacrimal, muscular branches; **extensive anastomoses with ECA**)
    - Superior hypophyseal artery (courses posteromedially; supplies anterior pituitary, infundibulum, optic nerve/chiasm)
- **Communicating (C7) segment**
  - Extends from below PCoA to terminal ICA bifurcation into anterior cerebral artery (ACA), middle cerebral artery (MCA)
  - Passes between optic (CN2), oculomotor (CN3) nerves
  - Major branches
    - Posterior communicating artery
    - Anterior choroidal artery (courses posteromedial, then turns superolateral in suprasellar cistern; enters temporal horn at choroidal fissure; supplies choroid plexus, medial temporal lobe, basal ganglia, posteroinferior internal capsule)

Normal Variants, Anomalies

- Petrous (C2) segment
  - Aberrant ICA (aICA)
    - Presents as retrotympanic pulsatile mass; should not be mistaken for glomus tympanicum tumor!
    - Absent vertical course; aICA courses more posterolaterally than normal (appears as mass in hypotympanum abutting cochlear promontory)
  - Persistent stapedial artery
    - Arises from vertical segment, crosses cochlear promontory and stapes footplate
    - Enlarges tympanic segment of facial nerve canal
    - Terminates as middle meningeal artery
    - Seen as "Y-shaped", enlarged geniculate fossa of CN7 on CT
    - F. spinosum is absent
- Cavernous (C4) segment
  - Persistent trigeminal artery
    - Most common carotid-basilar anastomosis (.02-0.5%)
    - Parallels course of CN5, passes posterolaterally around (or through) dorsum sellae
    - Connects ICA to vertebrobasilar system, forms "trident-shape" on lateral DSA, sagittal MR
    - May supply entire vertebrobasilar (VB) circulation distal to anastomosis (Saltzman type I) or fill superior cerebral arteries (SCAs) with posterior cerebral arteries (PCAs) filled via patent PCoAs (Saltzman type II)

Anatomy-Based Imaging Issues

Clinical

- Horner syndrome results from interruption of periarterial sympathetic plexus around ICA (dissection, "bruising" of plexus, etc.)

INTRACRANIAL INTERNAL CAROTID ARTERY

GRAPHICS

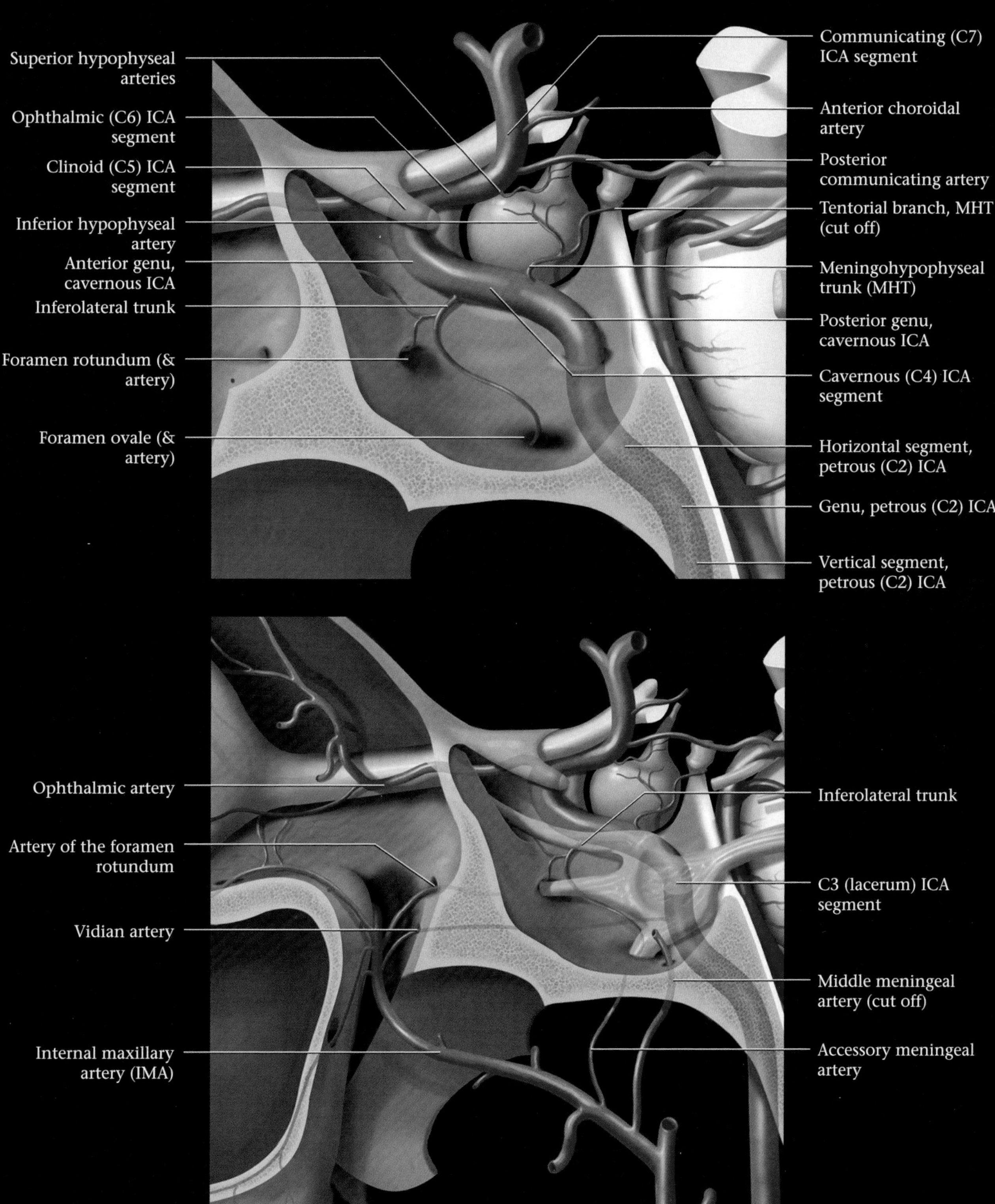
Superior hypophyseal arteries
Ophthalmic (C6) ICA segment
Clinoid (C5) ICA segment
Inferior hypophyseal artery
Anterior genu, cavernous ICA
Inferolateral trunk
Foramen rotundum (& artery)
Foramen ovale (& artery)
Communicating (C7) ICA segment
Anterior choroidal artery
Posterior communicating artery
Tentorial branch, MHT (cut off)
Meningohypophyseal trunk (MHT)
Posterior genu, cavernous ICA
Cavernous (C4) ICA segment
Horizontal segment, petrous (C2) ICA
Genu, petrous (C2) ICA
Vertical segment, petrous (C2) ICA
Ophthalmic artery
Artery of the foramen rotundum
Vidian artery
Internal maxillary artery (IMA)
Inferolateral trunk
C3 (lacerum) ICA segment
Middle meningeal artery (cut off)
Accessory meningeal artery

(Top) The C3 (lacerum) ICA segment is a short segment that begins where the petrous carotid canal ends. It passes above (not through) the foramen lacerum and is covered by the trigeminal ganglion. Major branches of the cavernous ICA (C4) segment are depicted with their numerous anastomoses with ECA branches (e.g., arteries of foramen ovale, rotundum). **(Bottom)** There are numerous ICA to ECA anastomoses through cavernous and deep facial branches of the two arteries, respectively. A small artery, the vidian artery, is an anastomosis between the IMA and the petrous ICA segment. Numerous anastomoses in and around the orbit are also present. The accessory meningeal artery is a small but important branch that enters the skull through the foramen ovale. It may supply part of the trigeminal ganglion and anastomose with the inferolateral trunk of the cavernous ICA.

AXIAL NECT

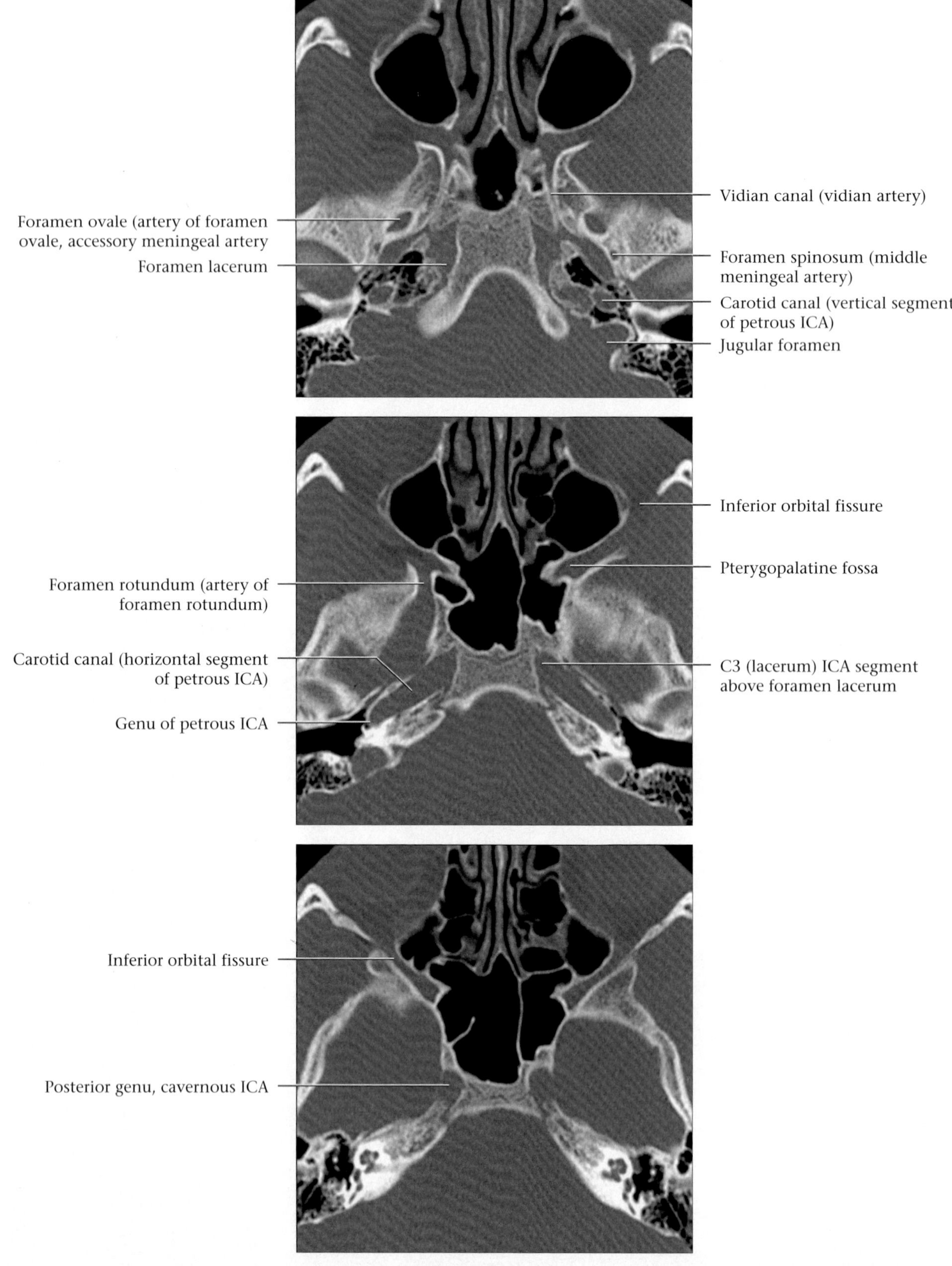

Vidian canal (vidian artery)
Foramen ovale (artery of foramen ovale, accessory meningeal artery
Foramen lacerum
Foramen spinosum (middle meningeal artery)
Carotid canal (vertical segment of petrous ICA)
Jugular foramen
Inferior orbital fissure
Pterygopalatine fossa
Foramen rotundum (artery of foramen rotundum)
Carotid canal (horizontal segment of petrous ICA)
C3 (lacerum) ICA segment above foramen lacerum
Genu of petrous ICA
Inferior orbital fissure
Posterior genu, cavernous ICA

(Top) Series of six axial NECT scans from inferior to superior with bone windows shows the major basilar foramina. The ICA follows a complex course through the petrous temporal bone. The C2 or petrous ICA enters the skull base at the exocranial opening of the carotid canal, ascending in front of the internal jugular vein. The petrous ICA has a short vertical and a longer horizontal segment. **(Middle)** Slightly more cephalad, the petrous ICA abruptly turns anteromedially and forms the posterior genu of the ICA. The posterior genu is below and slightly in front of the cochlea and middle ear cavity. The long horizontal petrous segment then courses anteromedially from the genu towards the cavernous sinus. **(Bottom)** Section just below the cavernous sinus proper shows the posterior genu of the cavernous ICA as it curves anteromedially into the cavernous sinus.

AXIAL NECT

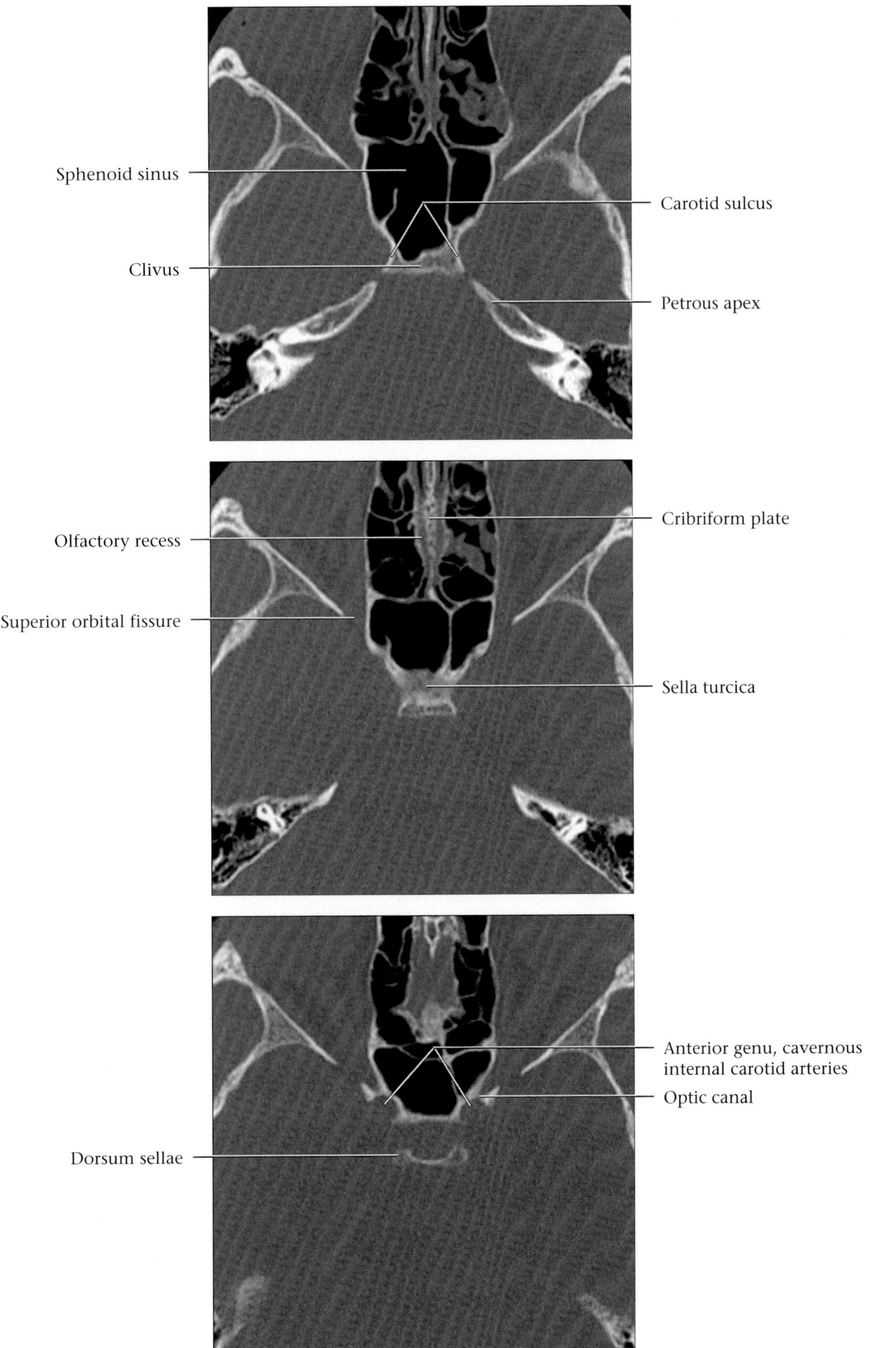

Sphenoid sinus
Carotid sulcus
Clivus
Petrous apex
Cribriform plate
Olfactory recess
Superior orbital fissure
Sella turcica
Anterior genu, cavernous internal carotid arteries
Optic canal
Dorsum sellae

(Top) Section through the middle of the cavernous sinus shows the bony grooves of the carotid sulcus along the basisphenoid bone. The cavernous (C4) ICA segment courses along the sulcus. **(Middle)** At this level, the cavernous internal carotid artery courses through the cavernous sinus proper and then turns superiorly towards the anterior clinoid process. **(Bottom)** The two cavernous carotid arteries form bony grooves just under the anterior clinoid processes as seen on this section. This represents the anterior genu of the cavernous ICAs as they curve upwards towards the dural ring where they will enter the cranial subarachnoid space. This represents the very short C5 (clinoid) ICA segment. The C6 (ophthalmic segment) begins at the distal dural ring of the cavernous sinus. The ophthalmic artery originates here and passes anteriorly through the optic canal.

INTRACRANIAL INTERNAL CAROTID ARTERY

LATERAL DSA

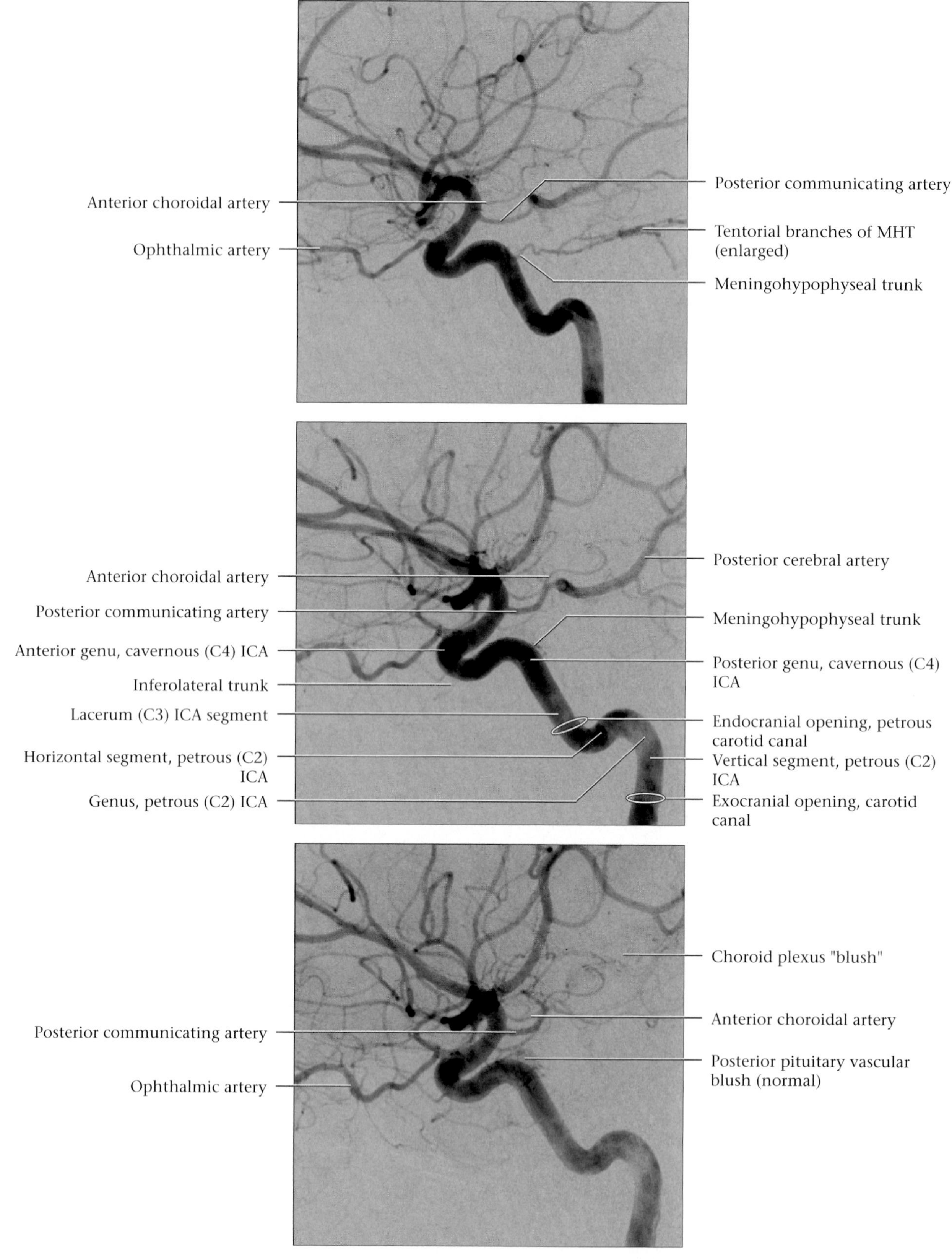

Anterior choroidal artery
Ophthalmic artery
Posterior communicating artery
Tentorial branches of MHT (enlarged)
Meningohypophyseal trunk
Anterior choroidal artery
Posterior communicating artery
Anterior genu, cavernous (C4) ICA
Inferolateral trunk
Lacerum (C3) ICA segment
Horizontal segment, petrous (C2) ICA
Genus, petrous (C2) ICA
Posterior cerebral artery
Meningohypophyseal trunk
Posterior genu, cavernous (C4) ICA
Endocranial opening, petrous carotid canal
Vertical segment, petrous (C2) ICA
Exocranial opening, carotid canal
Posterior communicating artery
Ophthalmic artery
Choroid plexus "blush"
Anterior choroidal artery
Posterior pituitary vascular blush (normal)

(Top) Lateral DSA of left internal carotid artery in a patient with a dural arteriovenous fistulas (dAVF) of left transverse sinus demonstrates an enlarged tentorial marginal branch of the meningohypophyseal trunk (MHT), also called the posterior trunk **(Middle)** Lateral DSA of right ICA of same patient shown above demonstrates normal small meningohypophyseal artery. A small inferolateral trunk is also visualized. There is transient filling of the ipsilateral posterior cerebral artery via a prominent posterior communicating artery. Approximate location of exo-, endocranial openings of petrous carotid canal are shown. **(Bottom)** Later arterial phase shows the normal vascular pituitary "blush" adjacent to the posterior genu of the cavernous ICA. The pituitary gland receives its arterial supply primarily by cavernous branches of the ICA. Note choroid plexus blush from the anterior choroidal artery.

OBL DSA

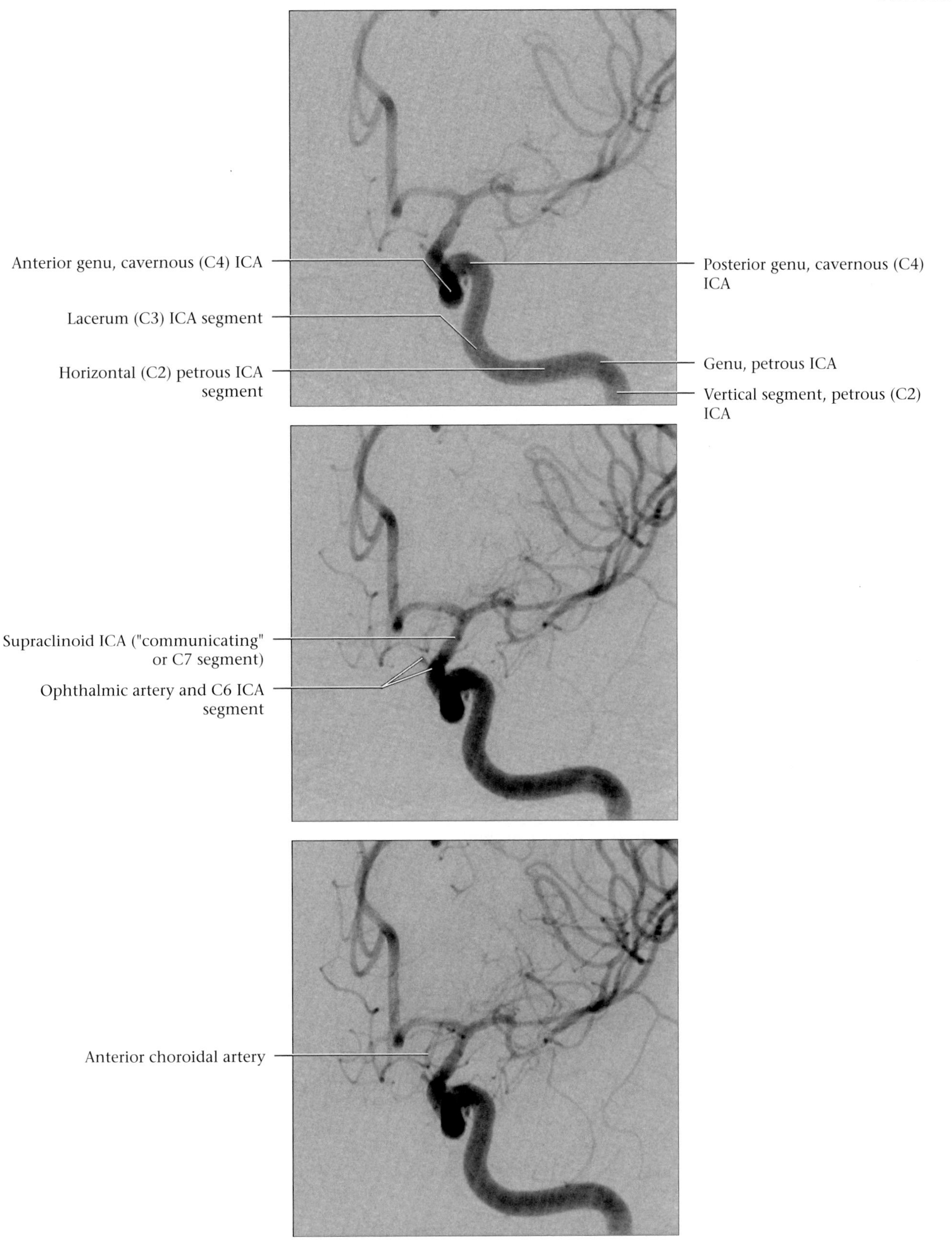
Anterior genu, cavernous (C4) ICA
Lacerum (C3) ICA segment
Horizontal (C2) petrous ICA segment
Posterior genu, cavernous (C4) ICA
Genu, petrous ICA
Vertical segment, petrous (C2) ICA
Supraclinoid ICA ("communicating" or C7 segment)
Ophthalmic artery and C6 ICA segment
Anterior choroidal artery

(Top) Series of three oblique views of a selective left internal carotid DSA are shown. The early arterial phase demonstrates the complex course of the ICA as it passes through the petrous carotid canal and enters the cavernous sinus. The vertical petrous ICA segment is much shorter than the horizontal segment. The C3 (lacerum) segment is a short portion that courses above the foramen lacerum between the endocranial opening of the petrous carotid canal and the petrolingual ligament. **(Middle)** Mid-arterial phase shows a small ophthalmic artery arising from the ophthalmic (C6) ICA segment. **(Bottom)** Late arterial phase shows the anterior choroidal artery (AChoA) arising from the C6 (communicating) ICA segment. The AChoA arises medially, coursing around the temporal lobe, before it turns posterolaterally towards the choroidal fissure.

INTRACRANIAL INTERNAL CAROTID ARTERY

AP DSA

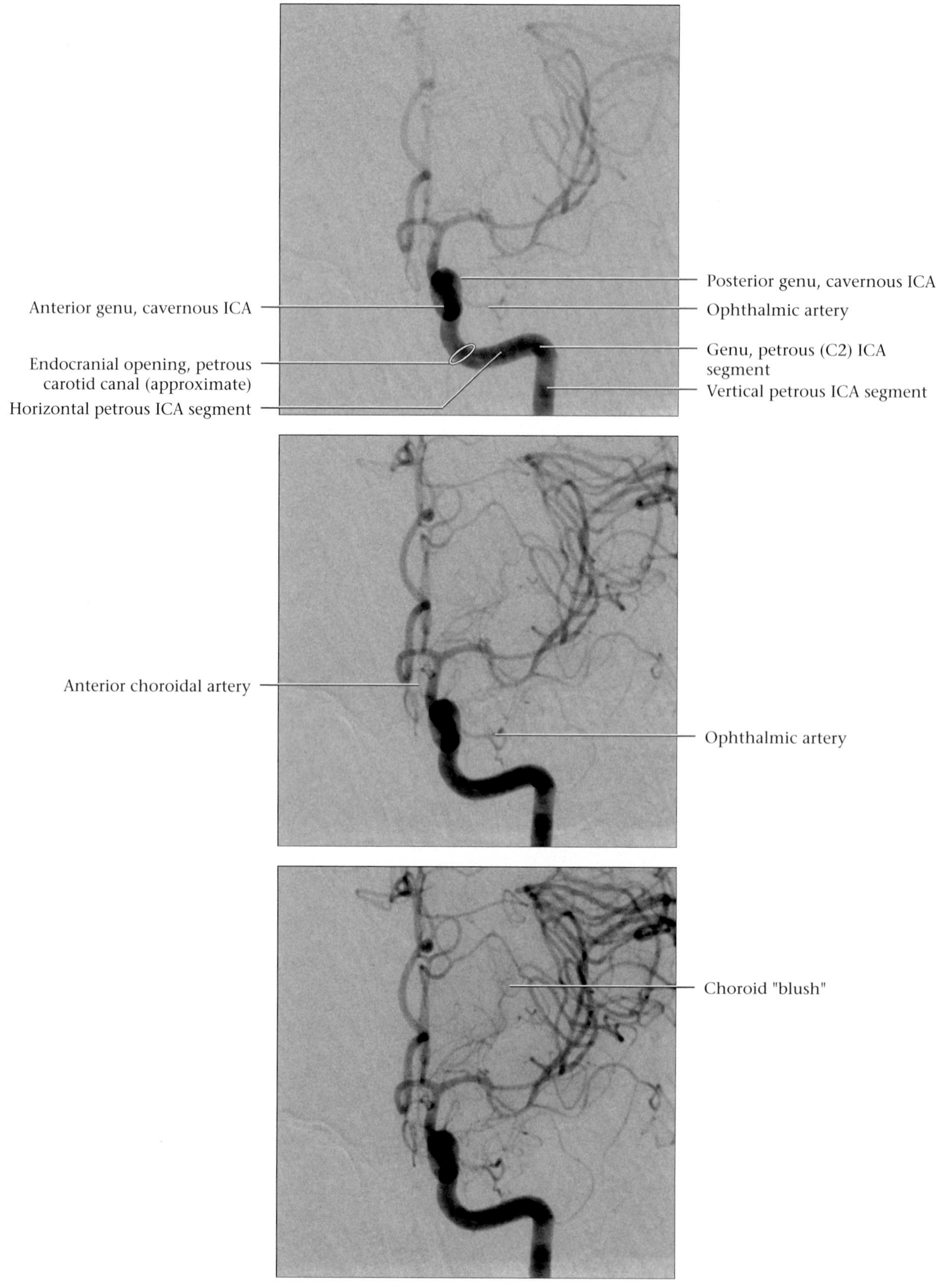
Posterior genu, cavernous ICA
Anterior genu, cavernous ICA
Ophthalmic artery
Genu, petrous (C2) ICA segment
Endocranial opening, petrous carotid canal (approximate)
Vertical petrous ICA segment
Horizontal petrous ICA segment
Anterior choroidal artery
Ophthalmic artery
Choroid "blush"

(Top) Series of three AP views, left internal carotid DSA, are illustrate. Early arterial phase shows the petrous and cavernous ICA segments. The genu between the vertical and horizontal petrous ICA segments is well seen. The approximate endocranial opening of the petrous carotid canal is indicated by the oval. The posterior and anterior genus of the cavernous ICA are superimposed on this view. The posterior ICA genu is slightly medial to the anterior genu. **(Middle)** Mid-arterial phase shows the ophthalmic and anterior choroidal arteries. **(Bottom)** Late arterial phase shows a faint "blush" of the choroid plexus within the lateral ventricle.

MRA

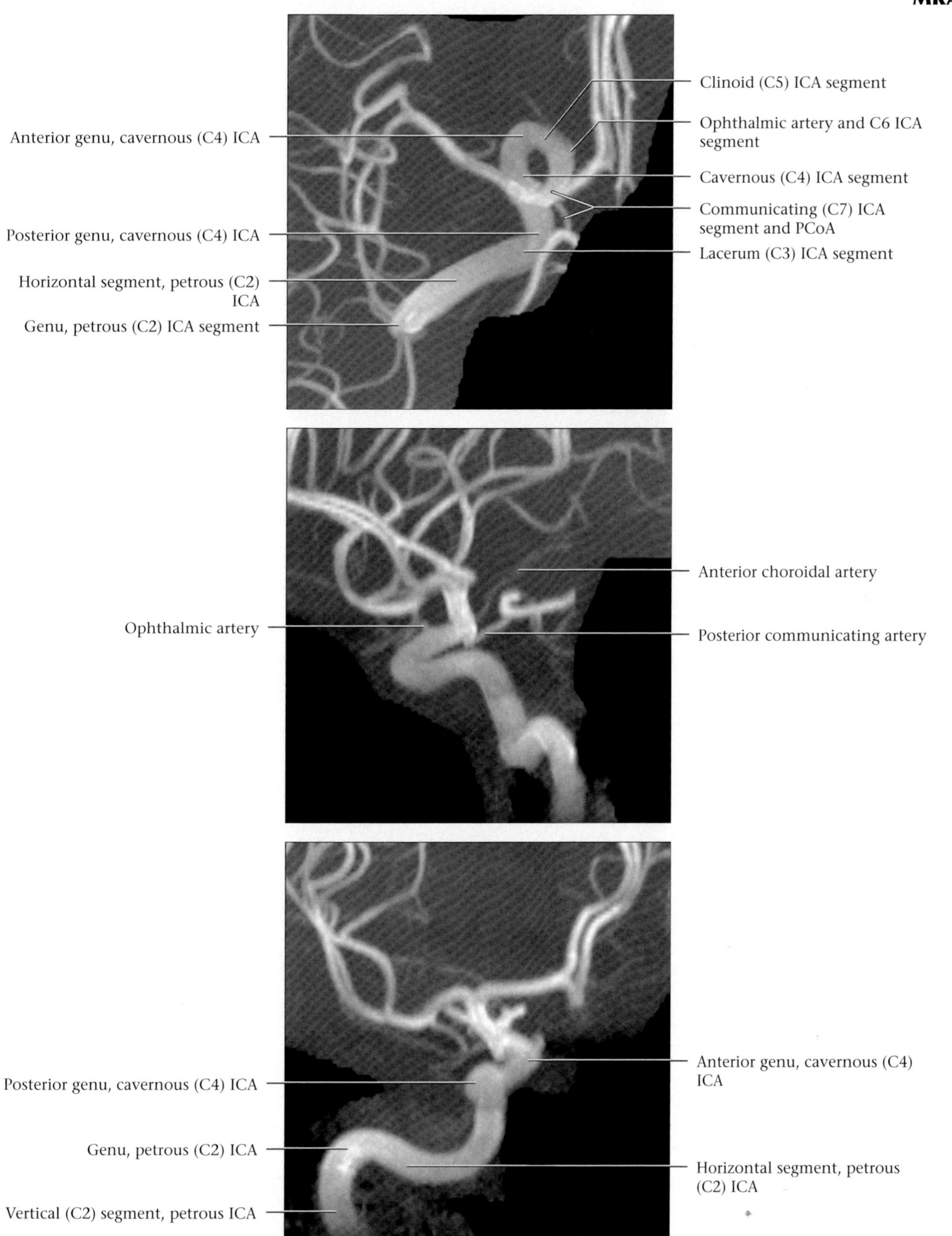
Clinoid (C5) ICA segment
Ophthalmic artery and C6 ICA segment
Anterior genu, cavernous (C4) ICA
Cavernous (C4) ICA segment
Communicating (C7) ICA segment and PCoA
Posterior genu, cavernous (C4) ICA
Lacerum (C3) ICA segment
Horizontal segment, petrous (C2) ICA
Genu, petrous (C2) ICA segment
Anterior choroidal artery
Ophthalmic artery
Posterior communicating artery
Anterior genu, cavernous (C4) ICA
Posterior genu, cavernous (C4) ICA
Genu, petrous (C2) ICA
Horizontal segment, petrous (C2) ICA
Vertical (C2) segment, petrous ICA

(Top) MRA is excellent for depicting the intracranial ICA. Note on this submentovertex reprojection that the posterior genu of the cavernous ICA is more medial than its anterior genu. The clinoid, ophthalmic, and supraclinoid (communicating) ICA segments are all medial to the cavernous ICA. **(Middle)** Lateral view shows the cavernous ICA very well. Its small branches are typically not well seen. The ophthalmic artery, seen here as it originates from the anterosuperior surface of the ICA, and the two major communicating segment branches (the posterior communicating and anterior choroidal arteries) are well visualized. **(Bottom)** Oblique view nicely shows the three knees or "genus" of the intracranial internal carotid artery: The petrous genus and the posterior and anterior genus of the internal carotid artery.

INTRACRANIAL INTERNAL CAROTID ARTERY

3D-VRT CTA

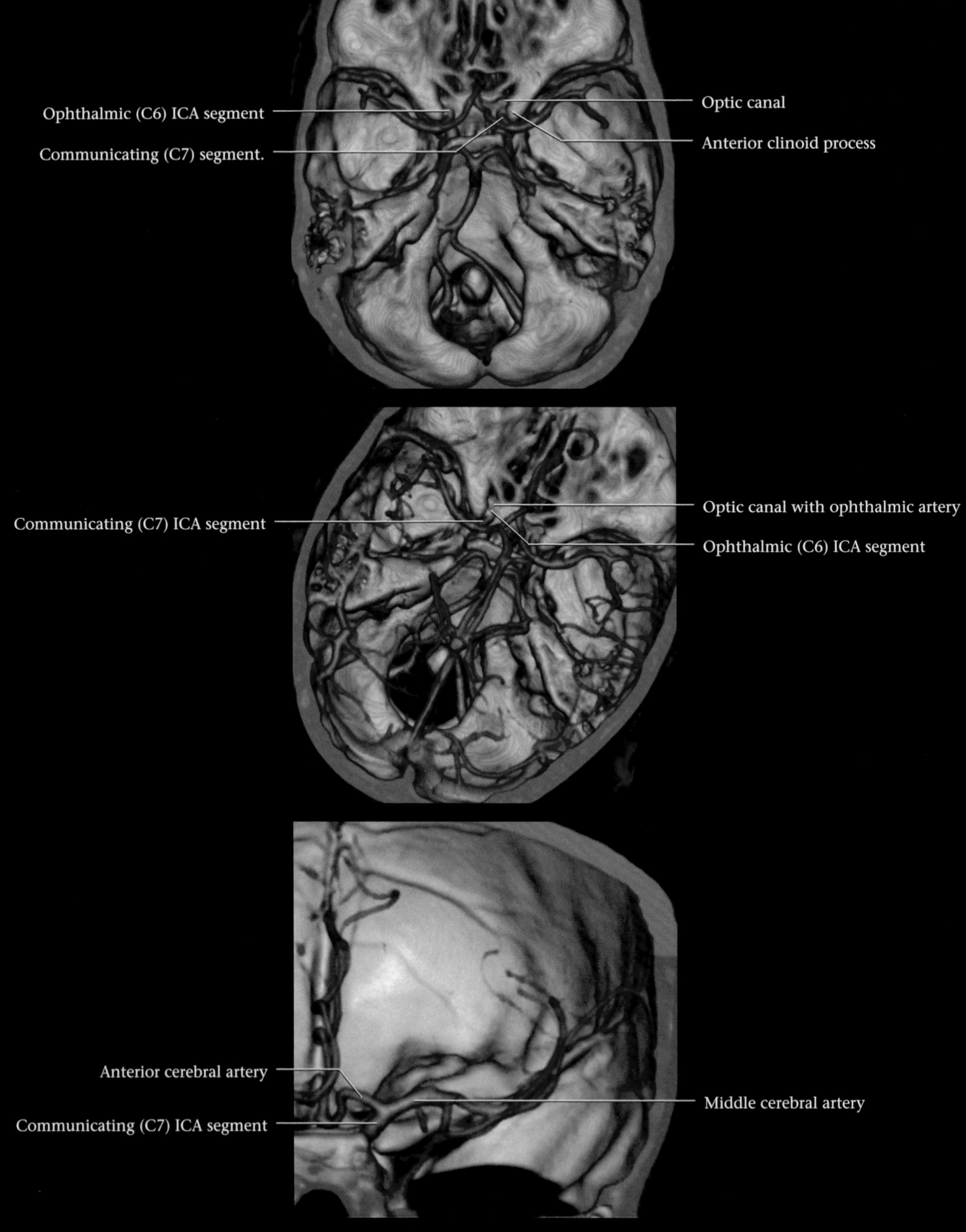
Ophthalmic (C6) ICA segment
Communicating (C7) segment.
Optic canal
Anterior clinoid process
Communicating (C7) ICA segment
Optic canal with ophthalmic artery
Ophthalmic (C6) ICA segment
Anterior cerebral artery
Communicating (C7) ICA segment
Middle cerebral artery

(Top) First of three 3D CTA volume-rendered images shows relationship between the distal ICA and the skull base. The ICA pierces the dura at approximately the level of the anterior clinoid process. The C5 (clinoid) segment lies between the inner (proximal) and outer (distal) dural rings which are not well seen. The C6 (ophthalmic) segment begins just above the optic canal, which is a good bony landmark. The supraclinoid ICA is also called the communicating (C7) segment. It gives rise to the posterior communicating and anterior choroidal arteries as well as the ICA distal bifurcation into the anterior and middle cerebral arteries (ACA, MCA). **(Middle)** Oblique view shows the optic canal very well. The ophthalmic artery is faintly seen here. **(Bottom)** AP view shows the C7 (communicating or supraclinoid) ICA segment and terminal bifurcation into the ACA and MCA.

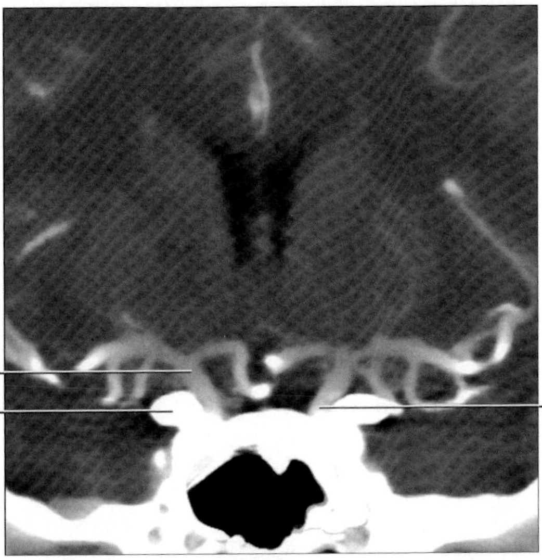

Communicating (C7) ICA segment

Anterior clinoid process

Ophthalmic (C6) ICA segment

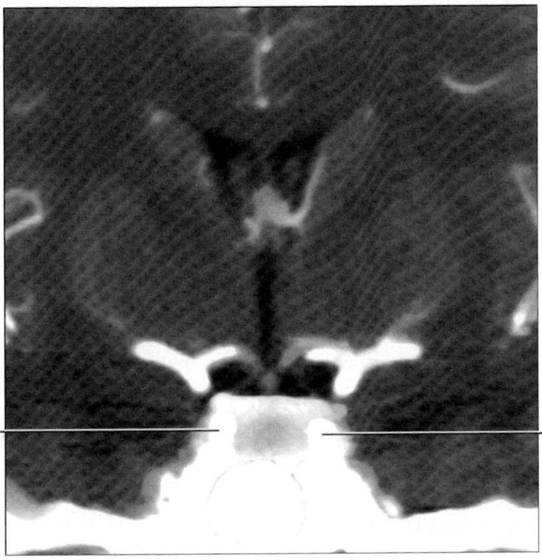

Anterior genu, cavernous (C4) ICA

Anterior genu, cavernous ICA

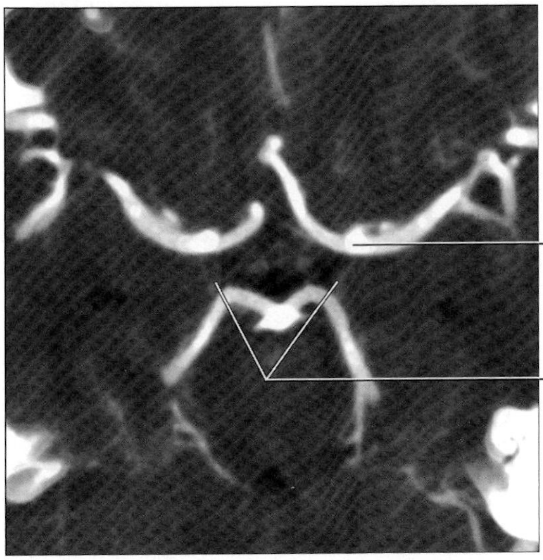

Distal ICA bifurcation

Posterior communicating arteries

(Top) Coronal MIP image from CTA shows relationship of the intracranial internal carotid artery to the anterior clinoid processes. The ICAs pierce the dural ring medial to the anterior clinoid processes. The terminal ICA bifurcation into the anterior and middle cerebral arteries is well seen. **(Middle)** Section just slightly posterior to the above level shows the anterior genus of both cavernous ICAs, seen here as contrast-enhanced rounded densities within the cavernous sinuses. **(Bottom)** Axial MIP shows the terminal ICA bifurcations. Two small posterior communicating arteries arise from the communicating (C7) ICA segment.

CIRCLE OF WILLIS

Terminology

Synonyms
- Circle of Willis (circulus arteriosus)

Definitions
- Central arterial anastomotic ring of brain

Gross Anatomy

Overview
- Circle of Willis is an arterial polygon
- Ten components
  - Two internal carotid arteries (ICAs)
  - Two proximal or horizontal (A1) anterior cerebral artery (ACA) segments
  - One anterior communicating artery (ACoA)
  - Two posterior communicating arteries (PCoAs)
  - Basilar artery
  - Two proximal or horizontal (P1) posterior cerebral artery (PCA) segments

Imaging Anatomy

Overview
- Entire COW rarely seen on single DSA but completely imaged on CTA/MRA

Anatomy Relationships
- COW lies above sella, in suprasellar cistern
- Surrounds ventral surface of diencephalon, inferolateral to hypothalamus
- Horizontal (A1) ACA segments normally course **above** optic nerves (CN2)
- PCoAs course **below** optic tracts, **above** oculomotor nerves (CN3)

Branches
- Important perforating branches arise from all parts of COW
- **ACAs**
  - Medial lenticulostriate arteries
  - Recurrent artery of Heubner
- **ACoA**
  - Unnamed perforating branches to anterior hypothalamus, optic chiasm, cingulate gyrus, corpus callosum and fornix
  - Occasionally a large vessel, median artery of corpus callosum, arises from ACoA
- **PCoA**
  - Anterior thalamoperforating arteries
- **Basilar artery (BA), PCAs**
  - Posterior thalamoperforating arteries
  - Thalamogeniculate arteries

Vascular Territory
- Entire central base of brain (including hypothalamus, internal capsule, optic tracts, thalamus, midbrain

Normal Variants, Anomalies
- Variations the rule, not exception
  - Absent/hypoplastic components (60%)
  - Hypoplastic/absent PCoA (25-33%)
  - Hypoplastic/absent A1 (10-20%)
  - "Fetal" origin of PCA from ICA (15-25%)
    - PCoA is same diameter as ipsilateral PCA
    - P1 is hypoplastic/absent
  - Absent, duplicate or multichanneled ACoA 10-15%
  - Junctional dilatation ("infundibulum") at PCoA origin from ICA in 5-15%
    - Should be 2 mm or less
    - Funnel-shaped, conical
    - PCoA arises from apex
- True anomalies rare
  - ACA-ACoA complex
    - Infraoptic origin of ACA (↑ prevalence of aneurysms)
    - Single (azygous) ACA (holoprosencephalies; ↑ prevalence of aneurysms
  - PCoA-PCA-BA complex
    - Persistent carotid-basilar anastomoses (trigeminal, hypoglossal)

Anatomy-Based Imaging Issues

Key Concepts or Questions
- COW provides major source of collateral blood flow to brain; if one (or more) segments is hypoplastic, potential for collateral flow in case of large vessel occlusion may be severely limited

Imaging Recommendations
- CTA/MRA best for imaging entire COW
- DSA requires multiple views +/- cross-compression of contralateral carotid artery to visualize ACoA

Imaging Pitfalls
- Absent COW segment usually congenital
- If PCA not visualized at vertebral angiography, anatomic variant with ICA ("fetal") origin more likely than occlusion

Embryology

Embryologic Events
- ICAs develop from third aortic arches, dorsal aortae, vascular plexus around forebrain
- Embryonic ICAs divide into cranial, caudal divisions
  - Cranial divisions give rise to
    - Primitive olfactory, anterior/middle cerebral, anterior choroidal arteries
    - Anterior communicating artery forms from coalescence of a midline plexiform network, connects developing ACAs
  - Caudal divisions
    - Become posterior communicating arteries
    - Supply stems (proximal segments) of posterior cerebral arteries
- Paired dorsal longitudinal neural arteries fuse, form basilar artery
- Developing vertebrobasilar circulation usually incorporates PCAs
- Caudal ICA divisions regress, form PCoAs

CIRCLE OF WILLIS

GRAPHICS & MRA

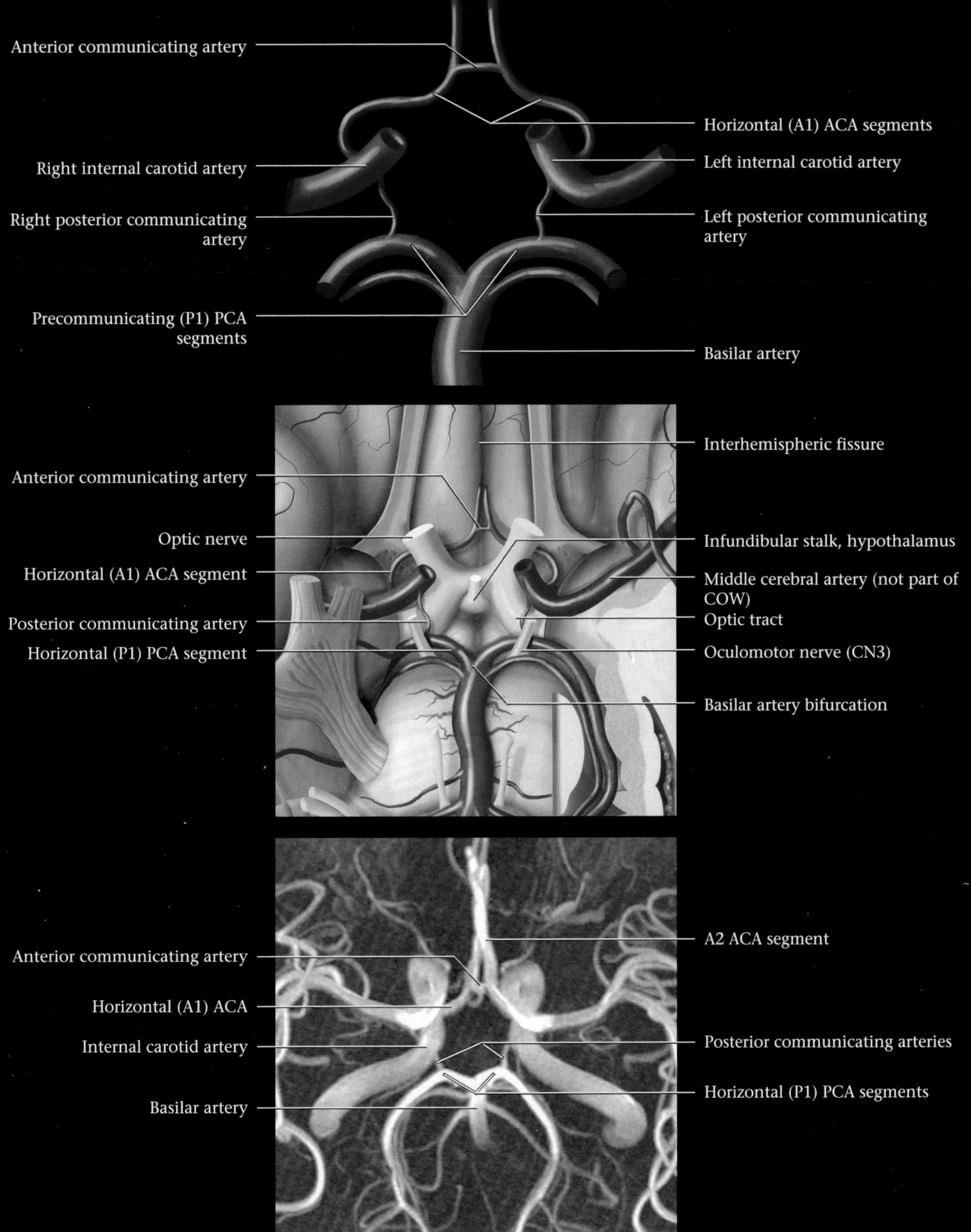
Anterior communicating artery
Horizontal (A1) ACA segments
Right internal carotid artery
Left internal carotid artery
Right posterior communicating artery
Left posterior communicating artery
Precommunicating (P1) PCA segments
Basilar artery
Interhemispheric fissure
Anterior communicating artery
Optic nerve
Infundibular stalk, hypothalamus
Horizontal (A1) ACA segment
Middle cerebral artery (not part of COW)
Posterior communicating artery
Optic tract
Horizontal (P1) PCA segment
Oculomotor nerve (CN3)
Basilar artery bifurcation
A2 ACA segment
Anterior communicating artery
Horizontal (A1) ACA
Internal carotid artery
Posterior communicating arteries
Horizontal (P1) PCA segments
Basilar artery

(Top) Schematic rendering of the circle of Willis (COW) as seen from below. All components are present but their size and configuration vary widely. Absence or hypoplasia of one or more segments is the rule, not the exception. **(Middle)** The COW and its relationship to adjacent structures is depicted. The COW is located in the suprasellar cistern just below the diencephalon. The hypothalamus, infundibular stalk and optic chiasm lie in the middle of the COW. The horizontal (A1) ACA segment passes above the optic nerves (CN2); the PCoA passes above the oculomotor nerves (CN3). The ACoA is near the midline, below the interhemispheric fissure. **(Bottom)** Submentovertex view from high resolution MR angiogram obtained at 3T is depicted for comparison with the graphic shown above. In this case all segments of the COW are present, a so-called "balanced" COW.

CIRCLE OF WILLIS

MRA

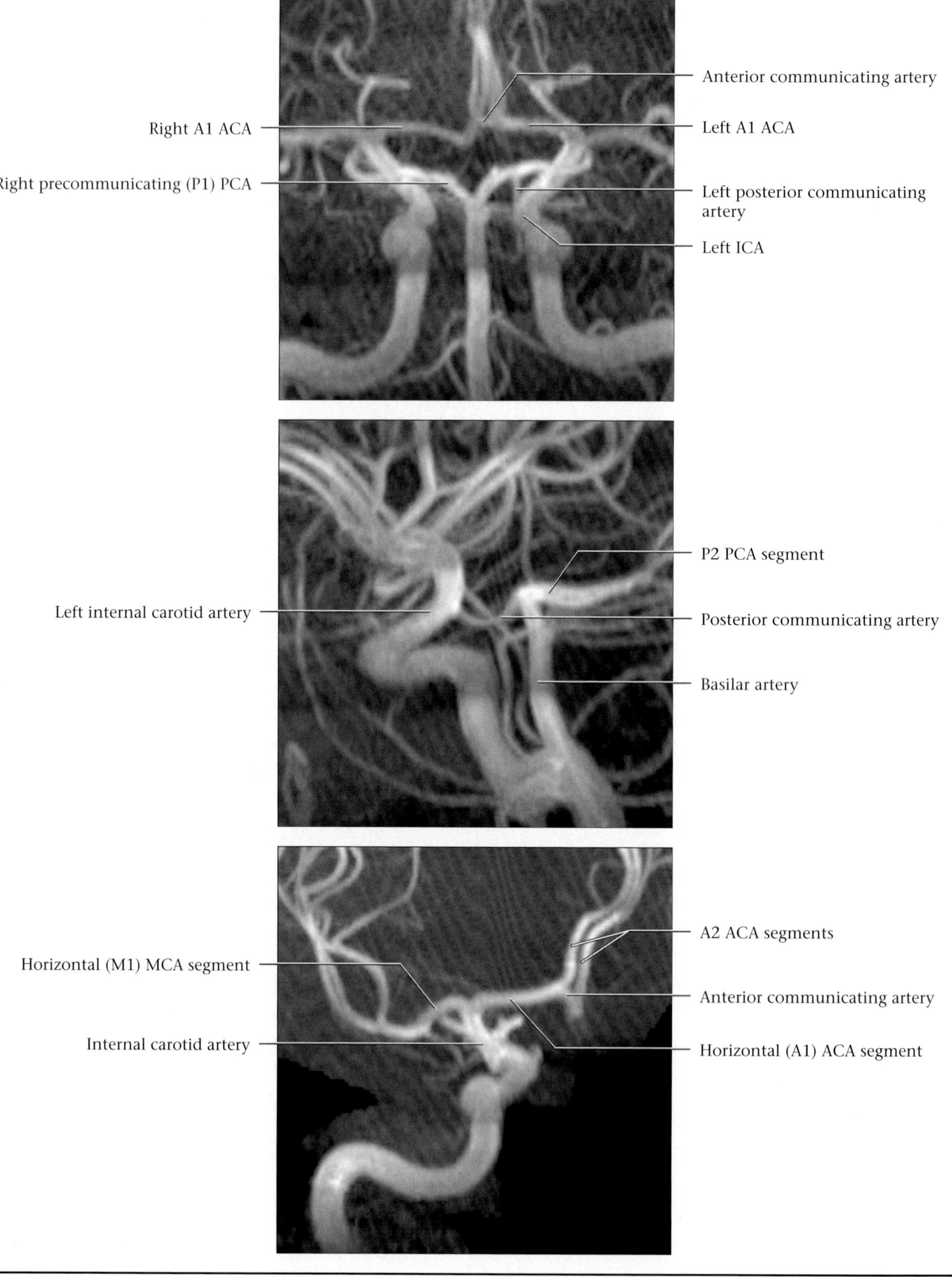
Anterior communicating artery
Right A1 ACA
Left A1 ACA
Right precommunicating (P1) PCA
Left posterior communicating artery
Left ICA
P2 PCA segment
Left internal carotid artery
Posterior communicating artery
Basilar artery
A2 ACA segments
Horizontal (M1) MCA segment
Anterior communicating artery
Internal carotid artery
Horizontal (A1) ACA segment

(Top) AP view of an MRA depicts the circle of Willis. The A1 and P1 segments of both the posterior and anterior cerebral arteries are well seen, as is the basilar bifurcation. **(Middle)** Lateral view of the MRA shows the posterior communicating arteries nicely. Neither the P1 (precommunicating) PCA segments or the A1 (horizontal) ACAs are well seen in this projection. **(Bottom)** Oblique view of a right internal carotid MRA shows the horizontal (A1) ACA segment and profiles the ACoA especially well. The vertical or post-communicating (A2) ACA segments are also well seen as is the ICA bifurcation. The MCA, which is not part of the COW, is also nicely visualized in this projection. This is an excellent projection for evaluation of the ACoA and MCA for the presence of an intracranial aneurysm.

CIRCLE OF WILLIS

3D-VRT CTA

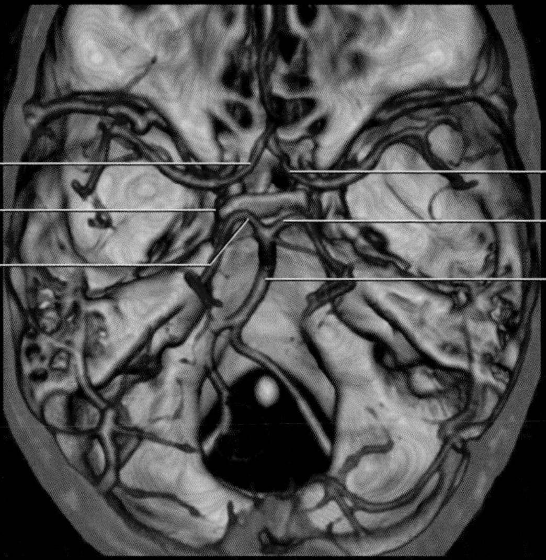

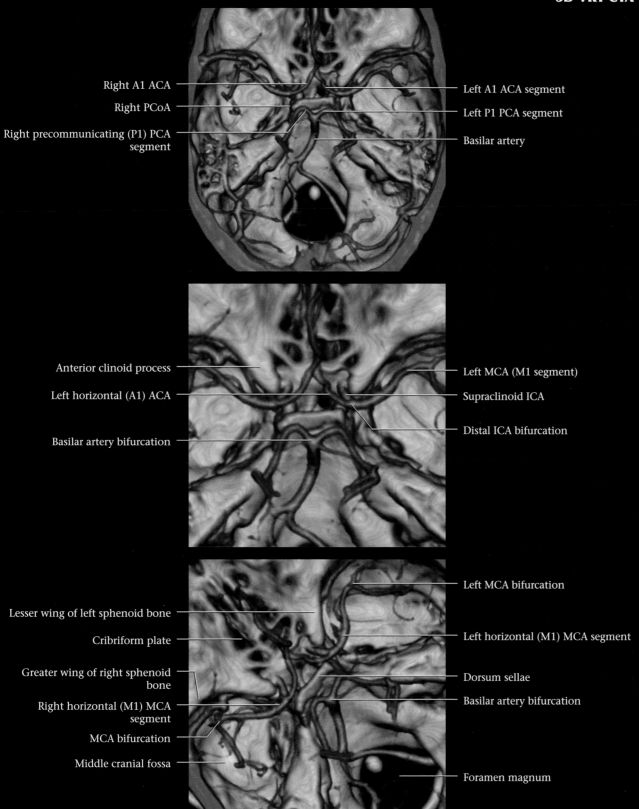

Right A1 ACA
Right PCoA
Right precommunicating (P1) PCA segment
Left A1 ACA segment
Left P1 PCA segment
Basilar artery

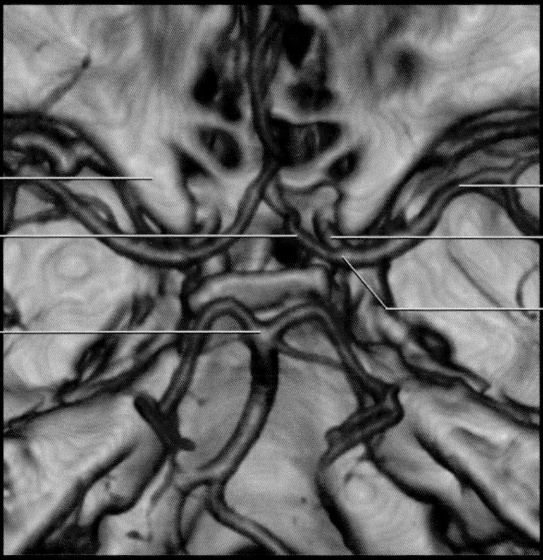

Anterior clinoid process
Left horizontal (A1) ACA
Basilar artery bifurcation
Left MCA (M1 segment)
Supraclinoid ICA
Distal ICA bifurcation

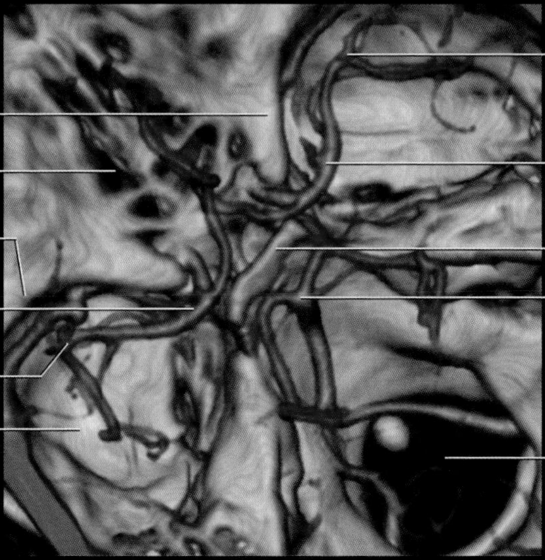

Lesser wing of left sphenoid bone
Cribriform plate
Greater wing of right sphenoid bone
Right horizontal (M1) MCA segment
MCA bifurcation
Middle cranial fossa
Left MCA bifurcation
Left horizontal (M1) MCA segment
Dorsum sellae
Basilar artery bifurcation
Foramen magnum

(Top) High-resolution CTA is shown with the brain removed. The relationship of the COW and adjacent bony structures is well seen. The COW lies above the sella turcica, within the suprasellar cistern. The ACoA is obscured in this view by overlap of the postcommunicating vertical (A2) ACA segments. **(Middle)** Close-up view delineates the distal bifurcation of the left ICA into a smaller medial branch (the horizontal or A1 ACA segment) and a larger lateral branch (the middle cerebral artery) is especially well seen here. **(Bottom)** Oblique view of the CTA as seen from above shows the relationship of the basilar artery and distal bifurcation to the clivus and dorsum sellae.

CIRCLE OF WILLIS

CTA

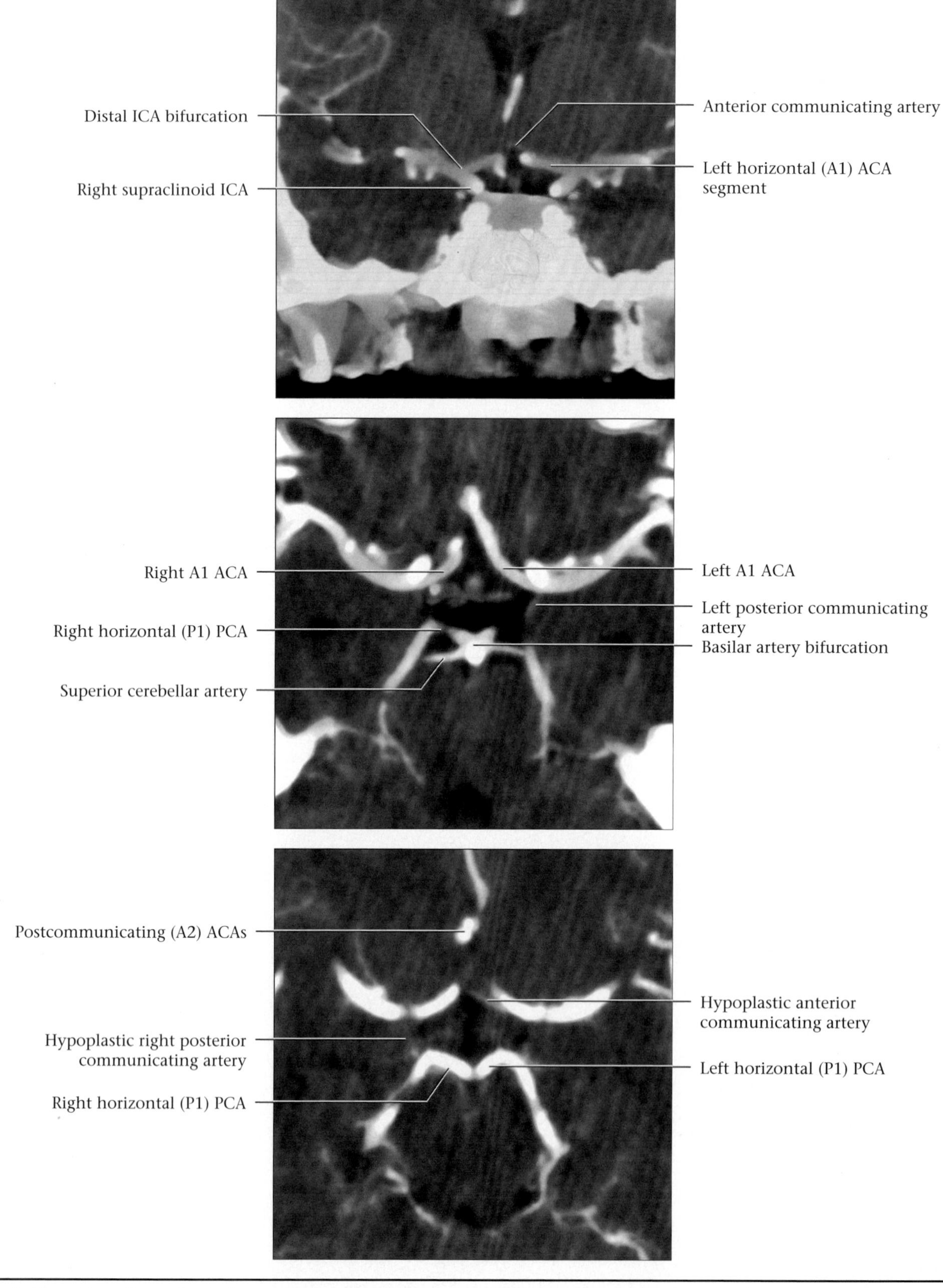
Distal ICA bifurcation
Anterior communicating artery
Left horizontal (A1) ACA segment
Right supraclinoid ICA
Right A1 ACA
Left A1 ACA
Left posterior communicating artery
Right horizontal (P1) PCA
Basilar artery bifurcation
Superior cerebellar artery
Postcommunicating (A2) ACAs
Hypoplastic anterior communicating artery
Hypoplastic right posterior communicating artery
Left horizontal (P1) PCA
Right horizontal (P1) PCA

(Top) AP section through pituitary gland, suprasellar cistern (MIP reconstruction) from high-resolution MDCT angiogram is shown. In this view the supraclinoid ICAs, their bifurcations, and horizontal (A1) ACA segments of COW are especially well seen. A very small ACoA is present connecting the two A1 segments. **(Middle)** Submentovertex view shows the right horizontal (P1) PCA and both horizontal (A1) ACA segments. The horizontal MCA segments are also well seen here. The MCA is not part of the COW. A hypoplastic left PCoA is present. **(Bottom)** Slightly higher submentovertex view shows the horizontal A1 and P1 segments. A hypoplastic ACoA can be seen on this section. The right PCoA is also hypoplastic. Hypoplasia or absence of one or more COW segments is both common and normal. These variants limit the potential for collateral blood flow in case of occlusion.

CIRCLE OF WILLIS

DSA

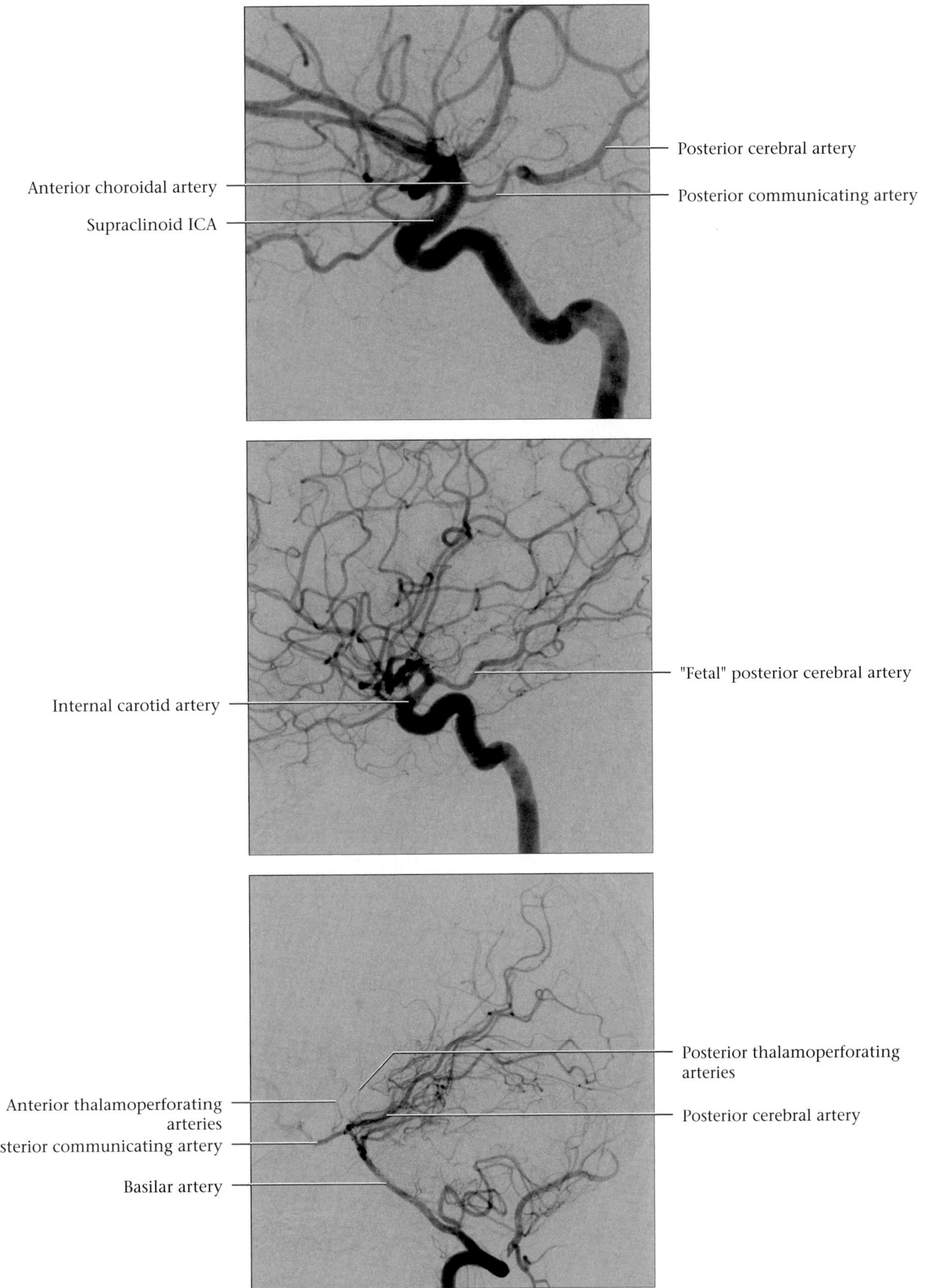
Posterior cerebral artery
Anterior choroidal artery
Posterior communicating artery
Supraclinoid ICA
"Fetal" posterior cerebral artery
Internal carotid artery
Posterior thalamoperforating arteries
Anterior thalamoperforating arteries
Posterior cerebral artery
Posterior communicating artery
Basilar artery

(Top) Lateral view of DSA from an internal carotid angiogram shows the normal relationship of the posterior communicating artery to the internal carotid and posterior cerebral arteries. Here the PCA fills transiently from the ICA injection. **(Middle)** Lateral view from another DSA of a selective internal carotid angiogram shows a so-called "fetal" origin of the posterior cerebral artery from the ICA. Here the posterior communicating artery is large and continues posteriorly as the PCA. The vertebrobasilar study in this patient (not shown) had no filling of the ipsilateral PCA as the precommunicating (P1) segment was congenitally absent. **(Bottom)** Lateral view of a vertebrobasilar DSA shows contrast refluxing into a PCoA. Perforating branches from the PCoA and proximal PCAs are especially well seen in this study.

ANTERIOR CEREBRAL ARTERY

Terminology

Abbreviations

- Anterior cerebral, anterior communicating, internal carotid arteries (ACA, ACoA, ICA)

Gross Anatomy

Overview

- Smaller, more medial terminal branch of supraclinoid ICA
- Three segments
  - Horizontal or precommunicating (**A1**) segment
  - Vertical or postcommunicating (**A2**) segment
  - Distal (**A3**) segment and cortical branches
- ACoA connects right, left A1 segments

Imaging Anatomy

Overview

- ACA excellent midline marker
- Displacement from midline common with space-occupying lesions or hemisphere atrophy

Anatomy Relationships

- **A1**: Extends medially over optic chiasm/nerves
- **A2**: Runs superiorly in interhemispheric fissure, anterior to corpus callosum rostrum
- **A3**: Curves around corpus callosum genu, divides into pericallosal, callosomarginal arteries
  - Pericallosal, callosomarginal arteries course within interhemispheric fissure, under falx cerebri

Branches

- **Cortical branches**
  - **Orbitofrontal artery**
    - Arises from proximal A2
    - Ramifies over inferior surface of frontal lobe
  - **Frontopolar artery**
    - Arises from mid-A2
    - Extends anteriorly to frontal pole
  - **Pericallosal artery**
    - Arises from A2 near corpus callosum genu
    - Larger of two major distal ACA branches
    - Courses posterosuperiorly above corpus callosum, below cingulate gyrus
  - **Callosomarginal artery**
    - Smaller of two distal ACA branches
    - Courses posterosuperiorly in cingulate sulcus, above cingulate gyrus
- **Perforating branches** (arise from A1 or ACoA)
  - **Medial lenticulostriate arteries**
    - Arise from A1, ACoA; course superiorly through anterior perforated substance
  - **Recurrent artery of Heubner**
    - Arises from distal A1 or proximal A2
    - Curves back laterally above A1 to enter anterior perforated substance

Vascular Territory

- Cortical branches supply anterior 2/3 of medial hemispheres, convexity
- Penetrating branches supply medial basal ganglia, corpus callosum genu, anterior limb of internal capsule

Normal Variants, Anomalies

- Normal variants (common)
  - Hypoplastic/absent A1
  - "Bihemispheric ACA" (distal ACA branches supply part of contralateral hemisphere)
  - ACoA can be absent, fenestrated, duplicated
- Anomalies (rare)
  - "Azygous" ACA (typically associated with holoprosencephaly)
    - Single ACA arises from junction of both A1s
    - ACoA absent
  - Infraoptic ACA
    - A1 passes under (not over) optic nerve
    - High prevalence of intracranial aneurysms

Anatomy-Based Imaging Issues

Imaging Recommendations

- Multiple views/multiplanar reconstruction required to profile ACoA
- May need to compress contralateral carotid artery during DSA to force contrast across ACoA

Imaging Pitfalls

- Lack of ACA filling on injection of ipsilateral carotid artery usually caused by absent/hypoplastic A1 (both ACA territories fill from ICA)
- Rotation of head off midline causes ACA to appear displaced on AP DSA

Clinical Implications

Clinical Importance

- ACoA is common site for aneurysm formation
- ACA occlusion much less common than middle, posterior cerebral artery involvement
- Distal ACA occlusion may occur with severe subfalcine herniation of cingulate gyrus

Embryology

Embryologic Events

- 5 weeks gestation: ACA appears as secondary branch of primitive olfactory artery (branch of primitive internal carotid artery)
- 6 weeks: Each embryonic ACA extends towards midline
  - Plexiform anastomosis forms, joining both ACAs in midline (normally regresses to form definitive ACoA)
  - Median artery of corpus callosum forms as branch from developing ACoA, then regresses (may persist, appear as "triplicate" A2s)
- 7 weeks: Definitive ACAs formed

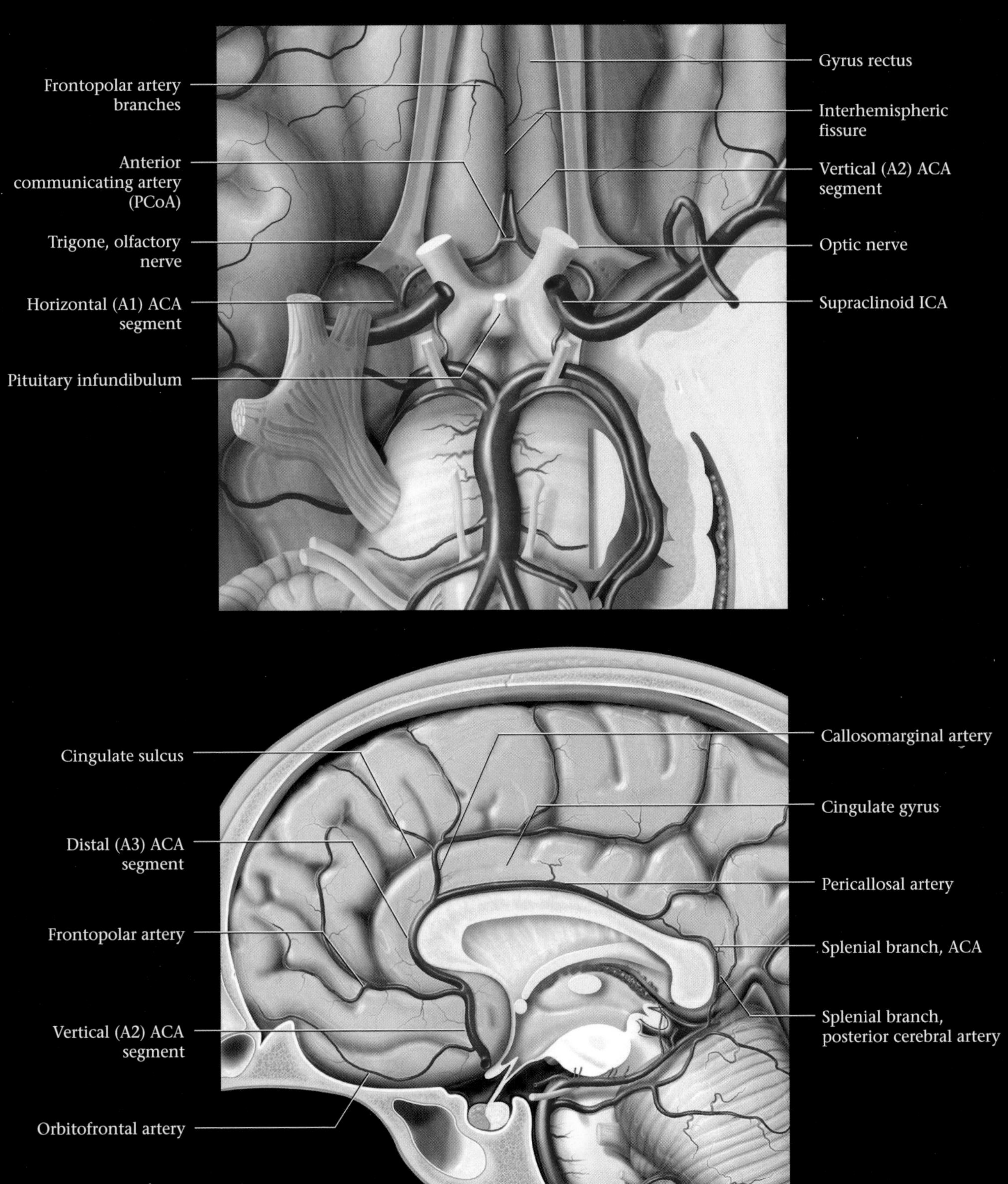
Frontopolar artery branches
Anterior communicating artery (PCoA)
Trigone, olfactory nerve
Horizontal (A1) ACA segment
Pituitary infundibulum
Gyrus rectus
Interhemispheric fissure
Vertical (A2) ACA segment
Optic nerve
Supraclinoid ICA
Cingulate sulcus
Distal (A3) ACA segment
Frontopolar artery
Vertical (A2) ACA segment
Orbitofrontal artery
Callosomarginal artery
Cingulate gyrus
Pericallosal artery
Splenial branch, ACA
Splenial branch, posterior cerebral artery

(Top) Submentovertex view shows the relationship of the circle of Willis and its components to the cranial nerves. Note that the normal course of the horizontal (A1) segment is over the optic nerves. **(Bottom)** Sagittal (midline) graphic through the interhemispheric fissure shows the relationship of the ACA and its branches to the underlying brain parenchyma. The A2 segment ascends in front of the third ventricle within the cistern of the lamina terminalis. The A3 segment curves around the corpus callosum genu. The branch point of the distal ACA into the pericallosal and callosomarginal arteries varies. Almost the entire anterior 2/3 of the medial hemisphere surface is supplied by the ACA and its branches. Branches of the posterior and anterior cerebral arteries anastomose around the corpus callosum genu.

ANTERIOR CEREBRAL ARTERY

LAT DSA

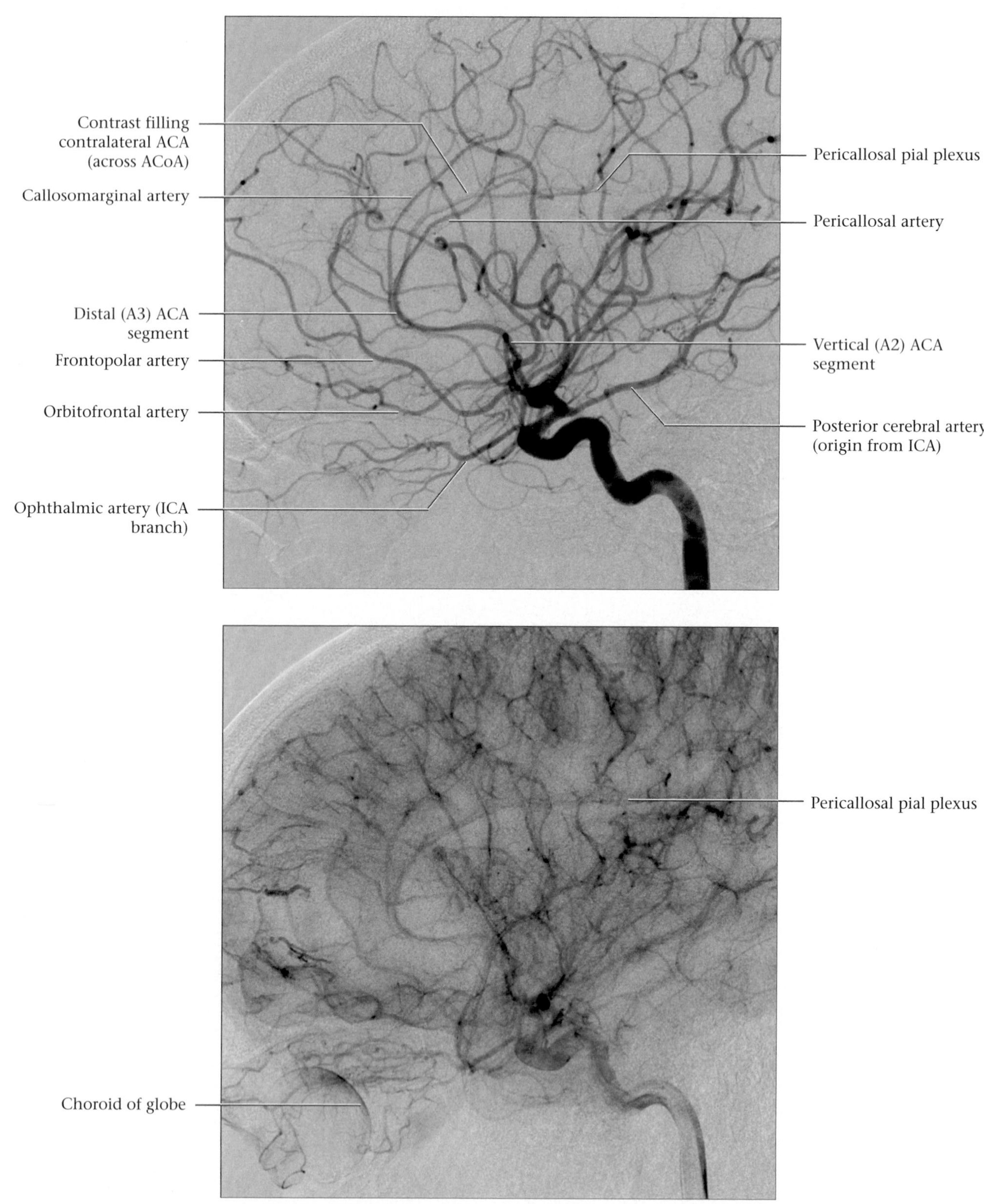
Contrast filling contralateral ACA (across ACoA)
Callosomarginal artery
Distal (A3) ACA segment
Frontopolar artery
Orbitofrontal artery
Ophthalmic artery (ICA branch)
Pericallosal pial plexus
Pericallosal artery
Vertical (A2) ACA segment
Posterior cerebral artery (origin from ICA)
Pericallosal pial plexus
Choroid of globe

(Top) Digital subtraction internal carotid angiogram, lateral view, mid-arterial phase, shows the ACA and its major cortical branches. **(Bottom)** Late arterial phase, lateral view, shows the vascular plexi that delineate both the ocular choroid (supplied by branches of the ophthalmic artery) and the superior surface of the corpus callosum (the so-called pericallosal pial "blush").

AP DSA

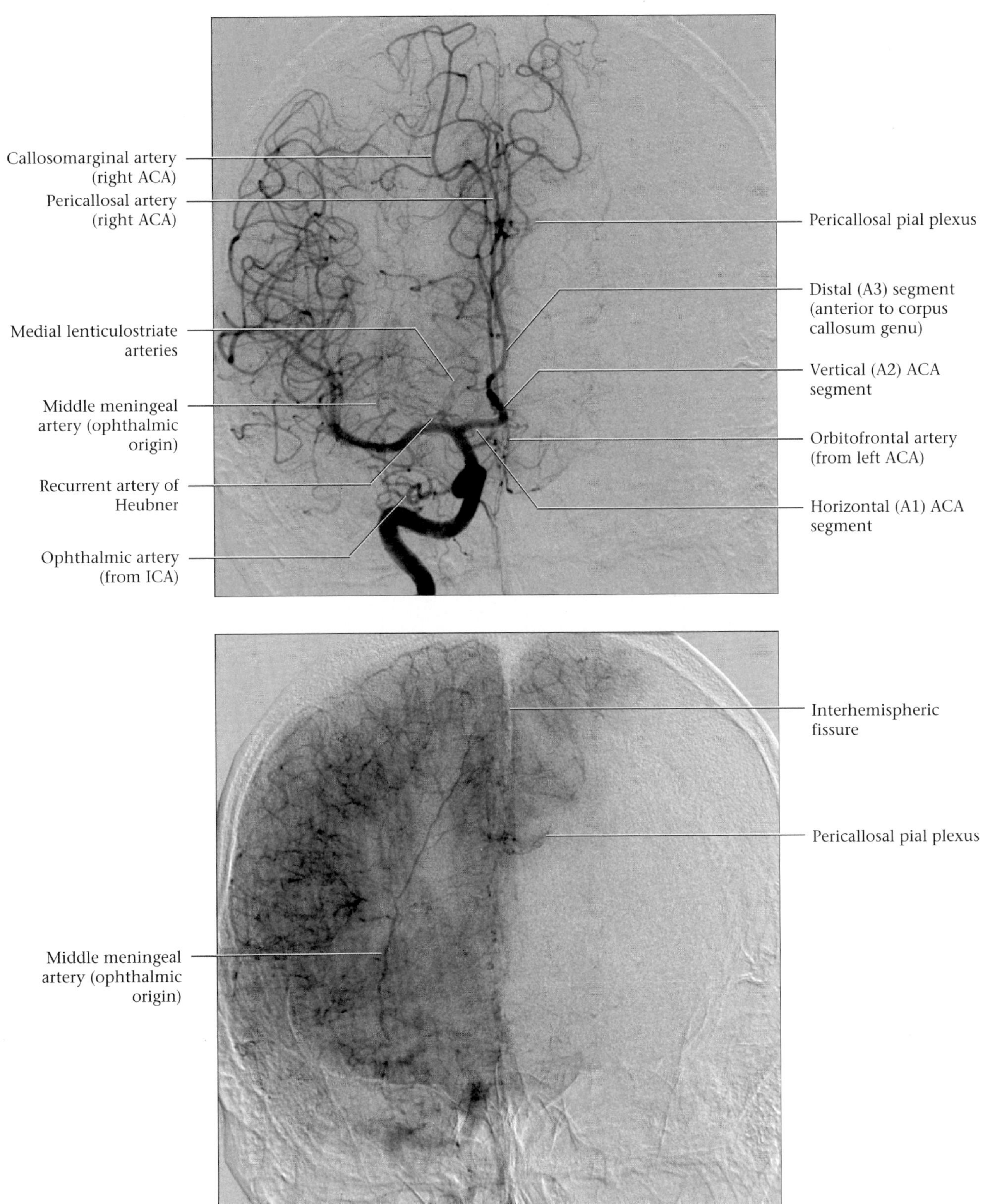

Callosomarginal artery (right ACA)
Pericallosal artery (right ACA)
Medial lenticulostriate arteries
Middle meningeal artery (ophthalmic origin)
Recurrent artery of Heubner
Ophthalmic artery (from ICA)
Pericallosal pial plexus
Distal (A3) segment (anterior to corpus callosum genu)
Vertical (A2) ACA segment
Orbitofrontal artery (from left ACA)
Horizontal (A1) ACA segment
Interhemispheric fissure
Pericallosal pial plexus
Middle meningeal artery (ophthalmic origin)

(Top) Digital subtraction right internal carotid angiogram, AP view, mid-arterial phase shows the ACA and its branches. Both distal ACAs fill from this injection because contrast has refluxed across the anterior communicating artery (which is not well seen on this projection). Note the ACAs are generally positioned in the midline, although they "wander" across the midline somewhat. This angiographic appearance is normal. **(Bottom)** Late arterial phase, AP view from the same series, shows the typical vascular "blush" formed by small branches of the pericallosal arteries as they course over the superior surface of the corpus callosum. Note that in this case, distal branches of both ACAs were filled when the right internal carotid artery was injected. The right middle meningeal artery is opacified because it originated from the ophthalmic artery, a normal variant seen in approximately 0.5% of cases.

ANTERIOR CEREBRAL ARTERY

MRA

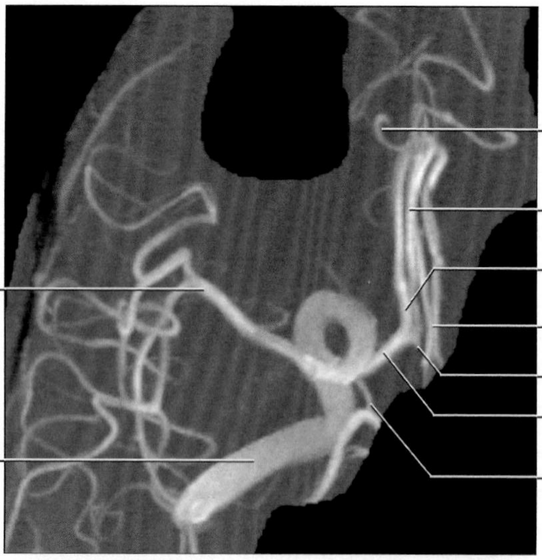

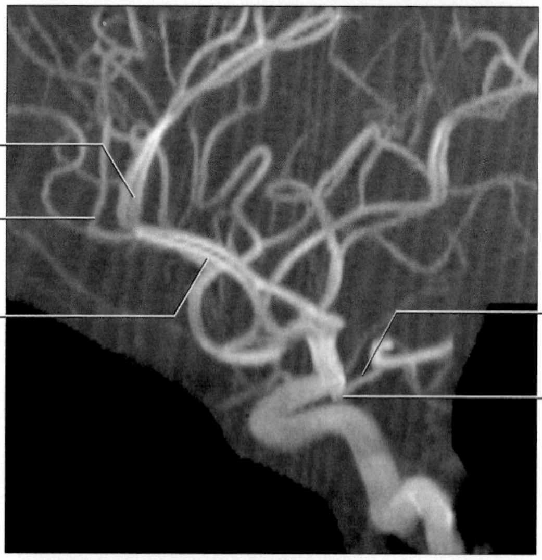

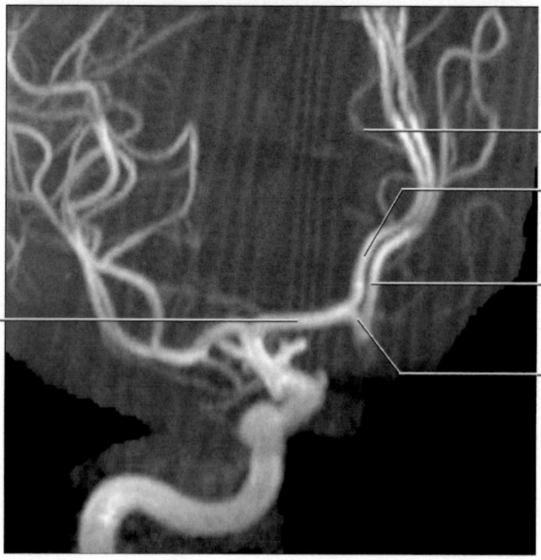

Callosomarginal artery
Pericallosal branch of right ACA
A2 segment, right ACA
A2 segment, left ACA
Anterior communicating artery
Right anterior cerebral artery, A1 segment
Posterior communicating artery
Right middle cerebral artery
Right internal carotid artery

Pericallosal branch of ACA
Callosomarginal branch of ACA
Anterior cerebral artery, A2 segment
Posterior communicating artery
Infundibulum of posterior communicating artery

Callosomarginal branch of ACA
A2 segment, right anterior cerebral artery
A2 segment, left anterior cerebral artery
A1 segment, anterior cerebral artery
Anterior communicating artery

(Top) Submentovertex view from 3D TOF MRA shows the right internal carotid artery and its branches. The major branches of the ACA are well seen although smaller branches (such as the medial lenticulostriate arteries and recurrent artery of Heubner) are not well delineated. **(Middle)** Lateral view of MRA demonstrates both anterior cerebral arteries and their major branches. **(Bottom)** Slightly oblique AP view of the right internal carotid artery circulation shows the ACA and ACoA, which is especially well seen. Short perforating branches are not visualized.

ANTERIOR CEREBRAL ARTERY

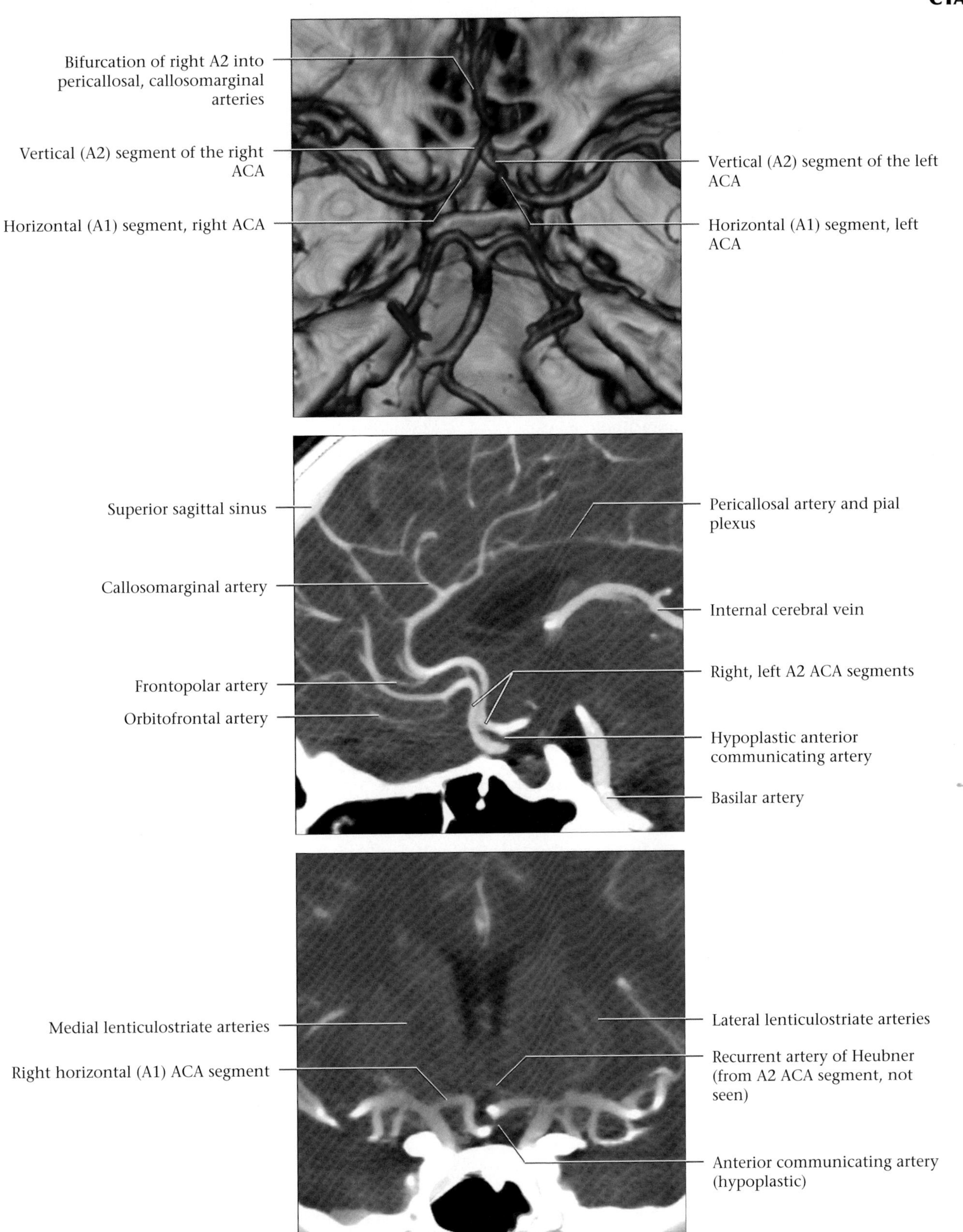

Bifurcation of right A2 into pericallosal, callosomarginal arteries
Vertical (A2) segment of the right ACA
Horizontal (A1) segment, right ACA
Vertical (A2) segment of the left ACA
Horizontal (A1) segment, left ACA
Superior sagittal sinus
Callosomarginal artery
Frontopolar artery
Orbitofrontal artery
Pericallosal artery and pial plexus
Internal cerebral vein
Right, left A2 ACA segments
Hypoplastic anterior communicating artery
Basilar artery
Medial lenticulostriate arteries
Right horizontal (A1) ACA segment
Lateral lenticulostriate arteries
Recurrent artery of Heubner (from A2 ACA segment, not seen)
Anterior communicating artery (hypoplastic)

(Top) Axial 3D color volume rendering of circle of Willis obtained using 64 detector row CT angiography. Both horizontal (A1) anterior cerebral artery (ACA) segments are symmetric. The anterior communicating artery is hypoplastic and not well seen on this view. The A2 (vertical) segment of both arteries within the interhemispheric fissure are seen in the midline. **(Middle)** Sagittal midline MIP image from same series clearly delineates both A2 segments as they course superiorly within the interhemispheric fissure in the cistern of the lamina terminalis. The corpus callosum genu can be faintly seen in this section, as well as CSF within the lateral ventricle. **(Bottom)** AP MIP section shows both horizontal (A1) ACA segments. Note hypoplastic anterior communicating artery, oriented in near-vertical plane. The ACoA course and configuration vary widely from patient to patient.

MIDDLE CEREBRAL ARTERY

Terminology

Abbreviations

- Middle cerebral artery (MCA)
- Internal carotid artery (ICA)

Synonyms

- Sylvian (lateral cerebral) fissure
- Insula (island of Reil)

Definitions

- Operculae = parts of the frontal, parietal, and temporal lobes that "overhang" and "enclose" the sylvian fissure

Gross Anatomy

Overview

- Larger, lateral terminal branch of supraclinoid ICA
- Four segments
  - Horizontal (M1) segment
  - Insular (M2) segments
  - Opercular (M3) segments
  - Cortical branches (M4) segments

Imaging Anatomy

Overview

- M2, M3 branches delineate insula, sylvian fissure

Anatomy Relationships

- **Horizontal (M1) segment**
  - Extends from terminal ICA bifurcation to sylvian fissure
  - Lies lateral to optic chiasm, behind olfactory trigone
  - Courses laterally under anterior perforated substance
  - Usually bi- or trifurcates just before sylvian fissure
  - Postbifurcation trunks enter sylvian fissure then turn upwards in a gentle curve (MCA "genu")
- **Insular (M2) segments**
  - Six to eight "stem" arteries arise from postbifurcation trunks, course superiorly within sylvian fissure, ramify over surface of insula
  - M2 segments end at top of sylvian fissure
- **Opercular (M3) segments**
  - M3 segments begin at top of sylvian fissure, course inferolaterally through sylvian fissure
  - Exit sylvian fissure at surface of brain
- **Cortical (M4) segments**
  - Exit sylvian fissure and ramify over lateral surface of hemisphere

Branches

- **Perforating branches** (lenticulostriate arteries), anterior temporal artery arise from M1
- **Cortical branches** (M4 segments)
  - Orbitofrontal (lateral frontobasal) artery
  - Prefrontal arteries
  - Precentral (prerolandic) artery
    - Runs between precentral and central sulci
  - Central sulcus (rolandic) artery
    - Runs within central (rolandic) sulcus
  - Postcentral sulcus (anterior parietal) artery
    - Runs in postcentral, then intraparietal sulcus
  - Posterior parietal artery
    - Exits posterior end of sylvian fissure
    - Runs posterosuperiorly along supramarginal gyrus
  - Angular artery
    - Most posterior branch exiting sylvian fissure
    - Runs posterosuperiorly over transverse temporal gyrus
  - Temporooccipital artery
    - Runs posteroinferiorly in superior temporal sulcus
  - Posterior temporal, medial temporal arteries
    - Extend inferiorly from sylvian fissure
    - Cross superior, middle temporal gyri

Vascular Territory

- Cortical branches
  - Considerable variation in territory of individual branches
  - Most common pattern
    - Supply most of lateral surface of cerebral hemispheres except for convexity and inferior temporal gyrus
    - Anterior tip of temporal lobe (variable)
- Penetrating branches
  - Medial lenticulostriate arteries (a few arise from proximal MCA)
    - Medial basal ganglia, caudate nucleus
    - Internal capsule
  - Lateral lenticulostriate arteries
    - Lateral putamen, caudate nucleus
    - External capsule

Normal Variants, Anomalies

- High variability in branching patterns
  - "Early" MCA bi- or trifurcation (within 1 cm of origin)
- True anomalies (hypoplasia, aplasia) rare
  - MCA duplication seen in 1-3% of cases
    - Large branch arises from distal ICA just prior to terminal bifurcation
    - Parallels main M1
  - Accessory MCA (rare)
    - Arises from anterior cerebral artery
    - High association with saccular aneurysm
  - Fenestrated MCA (rare)

Embryology

Embryologic Events

- Definitive appearance of MCA intimately related to formation of sylvian fissure, insula
- Fetal brain initially smooth, unsulcated; MCA branches lie over surface
- Shallow depressions on both sides of developing hemispheres appear at 8-12 weeks' gestation
- Depressions deepen, become overlapped by edges (operculae) of developing frontal, parietal, temporal lobes
  - MCA branches follow depressions, infolding brain
- Sylvian fissure forms, insula within its depths
- MCA branches curve up/over insula, then turn laterally, exit sylvian fissure, ramify over brain surface

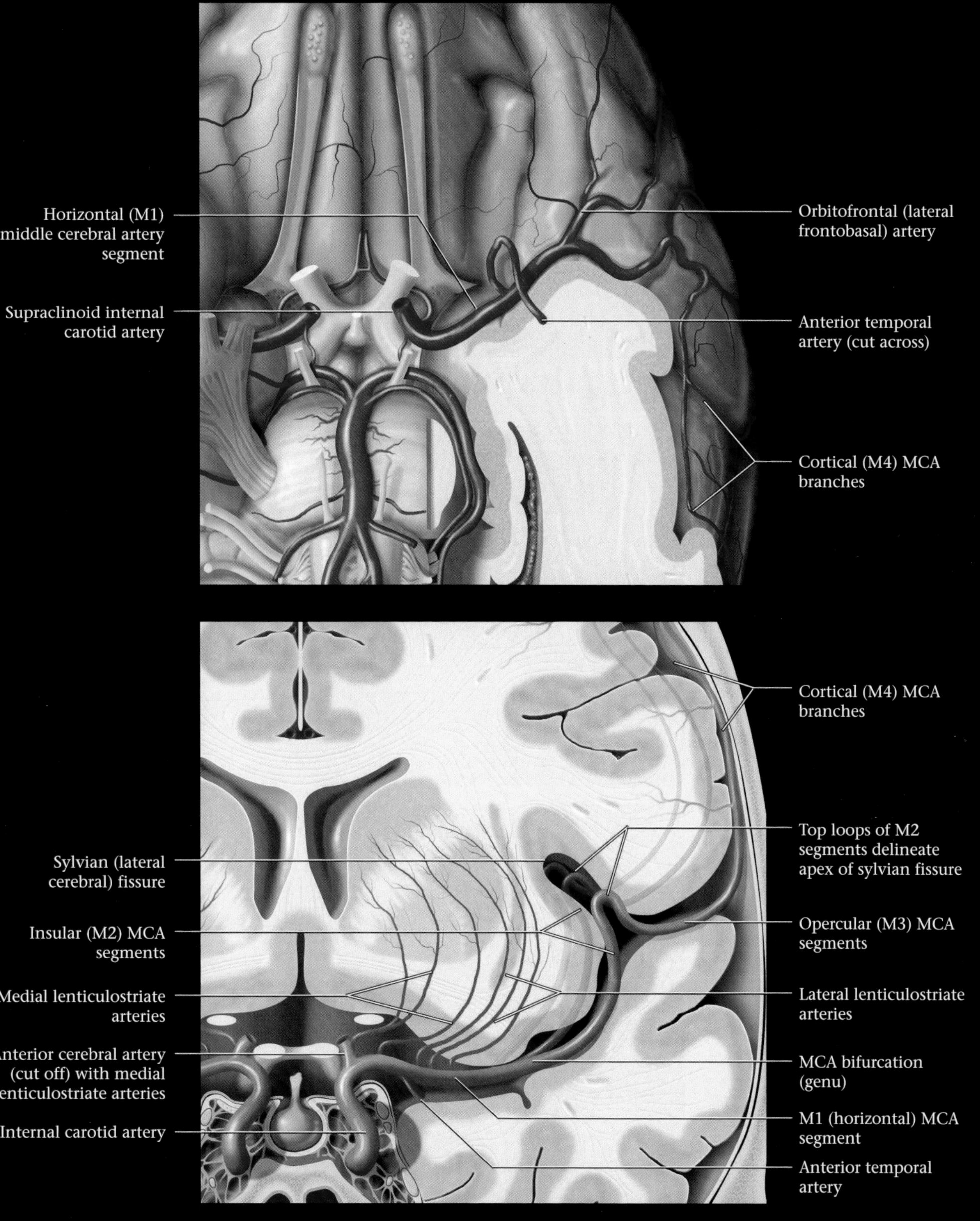

Horizontal (M1) middle cerebral artery segment
Supraclinoid internal carotid artery
Orbitofrontal (lateral frontobasal) artery
Anterior temporal artery (cut across)
Cortical (M4) MCA branches
Cortical (M4) MCA branches
Top loops of M2 segments delineate apex of sylvian fissure
Sylvian (lateral cerebral) fissure
Insular (M2) MCA segments
Opercular (M3) MCA segments
Medial lenticulostriate arteries
Lateral lenticulostriate arteries
Anterior cerebral artery (cut off) with medial lenticulostriate arteries
MCA bifurcation (genu)
Internal carotid artery
M1 (horizontal) MCA segment
Anterior temporal artery

(Top) The middle cerebral artery (MCA) and its relationship to adjacent structures is depicted on these graphics. Submentovertex view with the left temporal lobe sectioned through the temporal horn of the lateral ventricle is illustrated. The MCA supplies much of the lateral surface of the brain and is the larger of the two terminal branches of the internal carotid artery. **(Bottom)** AP view shows the MCA and its relationship to the adjacent brain. The MCA course through the Sylvian fissure and the M1-M4 segments are well-delineated. A few medial and numerous lateral lenticulostriate arteries arise from the top of the horizontal (M1) MCA segment, course superiorly through the anterior perforated substance, and supply the lateral basal ganglia + external capsule.

MIDDLE CEREBRAL ARTERY

LAT DSA

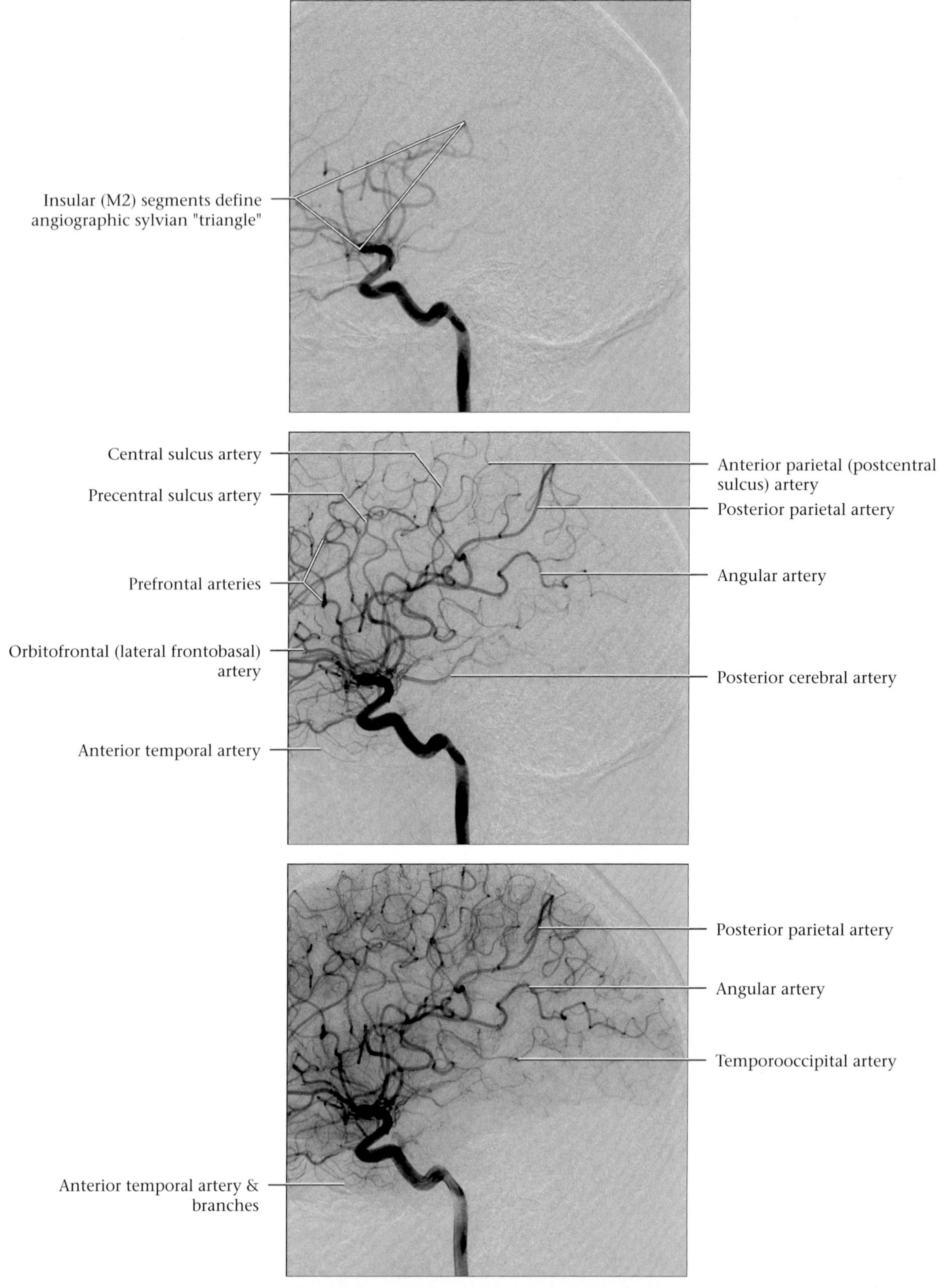
Insular (M2) segments define angiographic sylvian "triangle"
Central sulcus artery
Precentral sulcus artery
Prefrontal arteries
Orbitofrontal (lateral frontobasal) artery
Anterior temporal artery
Anterior parietal (postcentral sulcus) artery
Posterior parietal artery
Angular artery
Posterior cerebral artery
Posterior parietal artery
Angular artery
Temporooccipital artery
Anterior temporal artery & branches

(Top) Three lateral views of a left internal carotid angiogram show the middle cerebral artery (MCA), beginning with early arterial phase. Filling of the insular (M2) segments delineates the insula (sylvian "triangle"). **(Middle)** Mid-arterial phase shows filling of the opercular (M3) and cortical (M4) MCA segments. Transient filling of the ipsilateral posterior cerebral artery via the circle of Willis has occurred. **(Bottom)** Late arterial phase shows filling of the distal MCA branches with "brain stain" (diffuse vascular "blush") of the cortex. Note that only the most anterior aspect of the temporal lobe is opacified. Most of the temporal lobe is supplied by the posterior cerebral artery.

MIDDLE CEREBRAL ARTERY

AP DSA

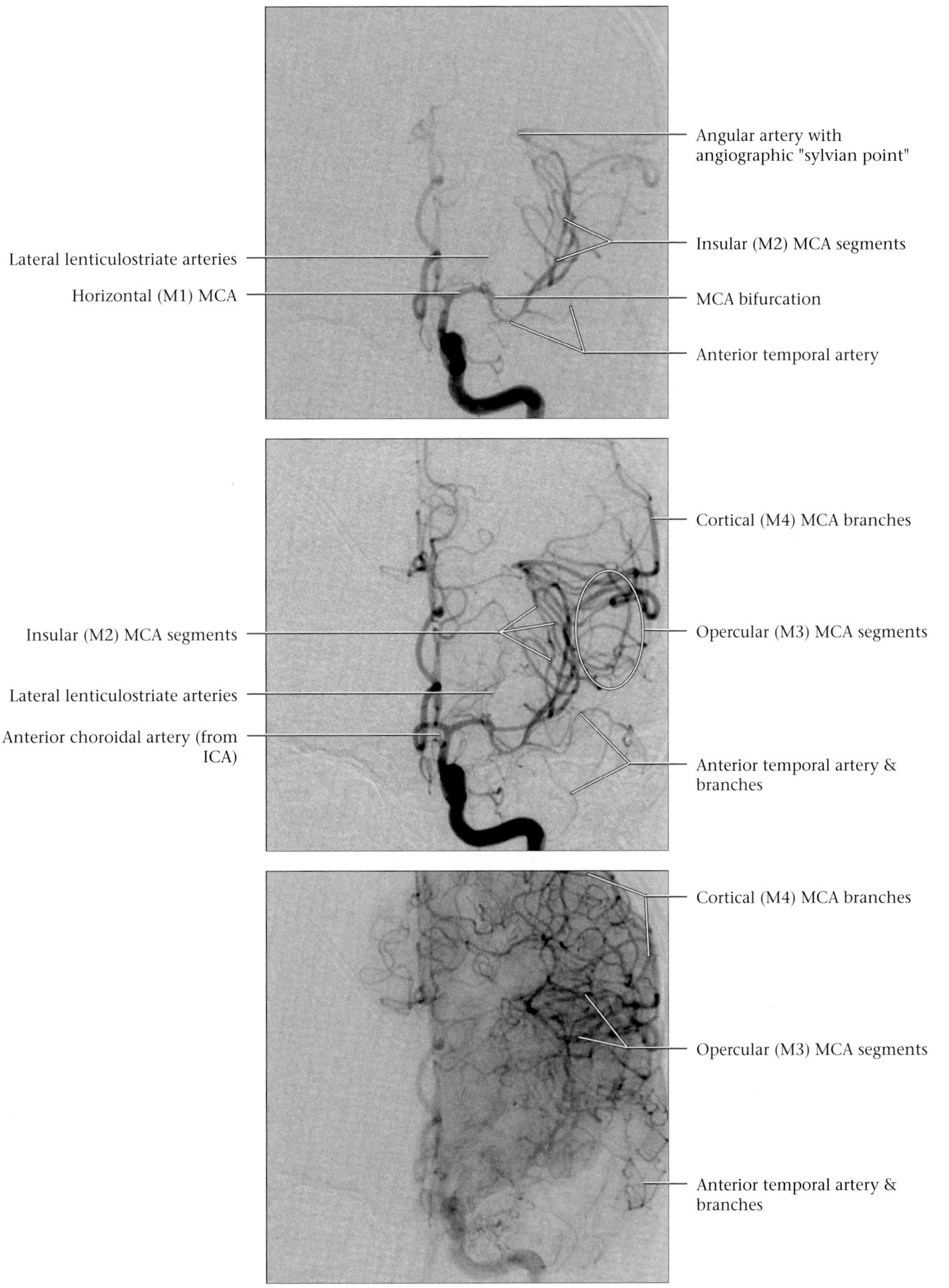
Angular artery with angiographic "sylvian point"
Insular (M2) MCA segments
Lateral lenticulostriate arteries
Horizontal (M1) MCA
MCA bifurcation
Anterior temporal artery
Cortical (M4) MCA branches
Insular (M2) MCA segments
Opercular (M3) MCA segments
Lateral lenticulostriate arteries
Anterior choroidal artery (from ICA)
Anterior temporal artery & branches
Cortical (M4) MCA branches
Opercular (M3) MCA segments
Anterior temporal artery & branches

(Top) Three AP views of left internal carotid angiogram illustrate normal middle cerebral artery (MCA) angiographic anatomy. Only the horizontal (M1) and insular (M2) segments are filled out on this early arterial phase image. The MCA bifurcates within 1 cm of its origin, a so-called "early bifurcating" MCA. The angiographic "sylvian point" is the highest, most medial insular loop of the MCA. **(Middle)** Mid-arterial phase demonstrates the insular (M2) and opercular (M3) MCA segments as well as early filling of some cortical (M4) MCA branches. **(Bottom)** Late arterial phase shows contrast has been washed out of the more proximal (M1, M2) MCA segments. The distal cortical (M4) MCA branches are now completely opacified. Note the "brain stain" caused by opacification of small branches within the basal ganglia as well as the cortex.

MIDDLE CEREBRAL ARTERY

MRA

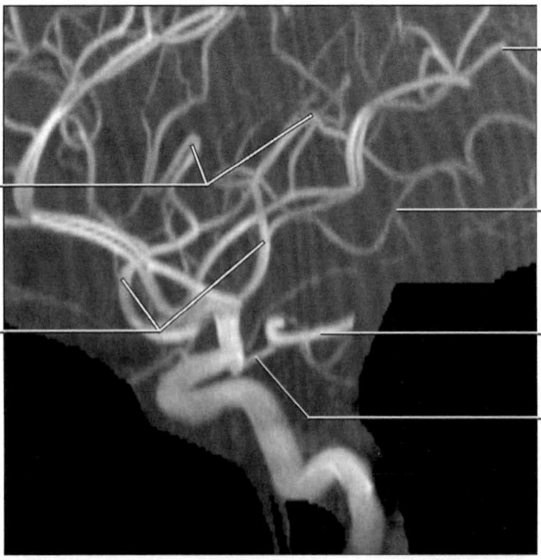

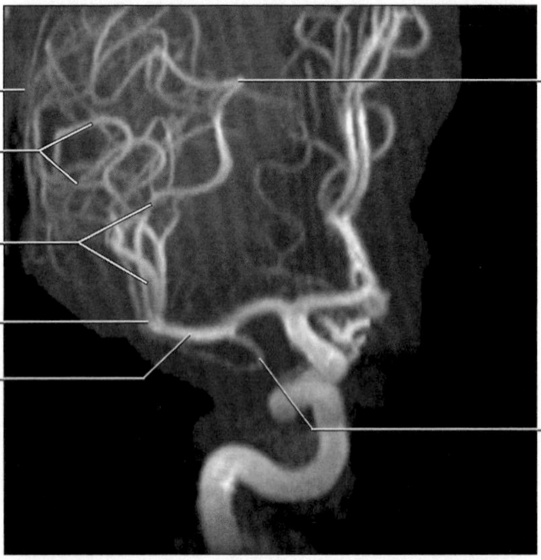

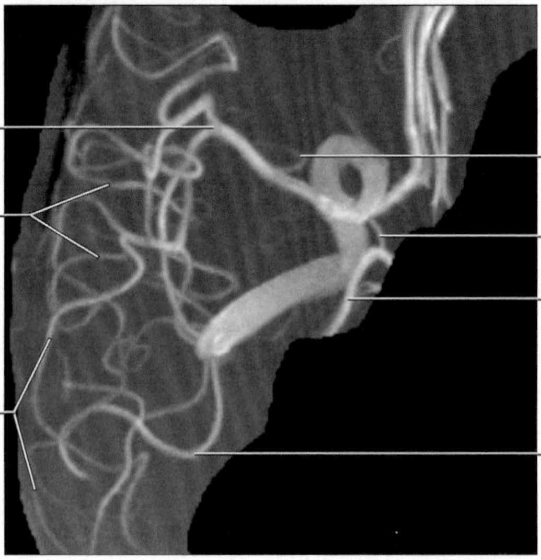

Apex of M2 loops define top of insula
Insular (M2) MCA segments
Angular artery
Temporooccipital artery
Posterior cerebral artery
Posterior communicating artery

Cortical (M4) MCA segments
Opercular (M3) MCA segments
Insular (M2) MCA segments
MCA trifurcation (genu)
Horizontal (M1) MCA segment
Angular artery with "sylvian point"
Anterior temporal artery

MCA bifurcation
Opercular (M3) MCA segments
Cortical (M4) MCA branches
Anterior temporal artery
Posterior communicating artery
Posterior cerebral artery
Angular artery with "sylvian point"

(Top) Three views of 3T MR angiogram are shown from top to bottom. Lateral view is shown on top. **(Middle)** AP view of the MR angiogram shows the MCA and its branches. The lateral lenticulostriate arteries are barely seen. **(Bottom)** Submentovertex view is optimal for visualizing the MCA bi- or trifurcation (genu) & the opercular (M3) segments. MCA aneurysms are often best delineated in this projection.

MIDDLE CEREBRAL ARTERY

3D-VRT CTA

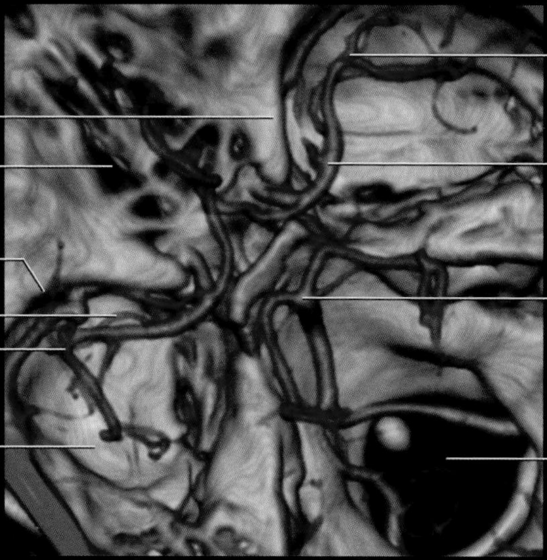

Lesser wing of left sphenoid bone
Cribriform plate
Greater wing of right sphenoid bone
Anterior temporal artery
MCA bifurcation
Middle cranial fossa
Left MCA bifurcation
Left horizontal (M1) MCA segment
Basilar artery bifurcation
Foramen magnum

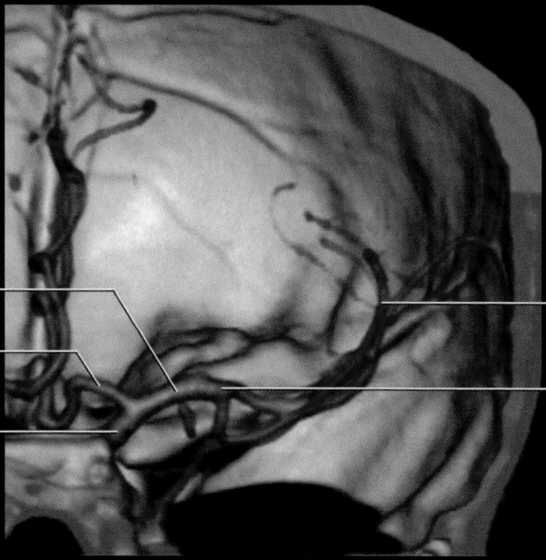

Horizontal (M1) segment of left MCA
Horizontal (A1) segment of left anterior cerebral artery
Supraclinoid internal carotid artery (ICA)
Insular (M2) MCA segments
MCA genu (bifurcation)

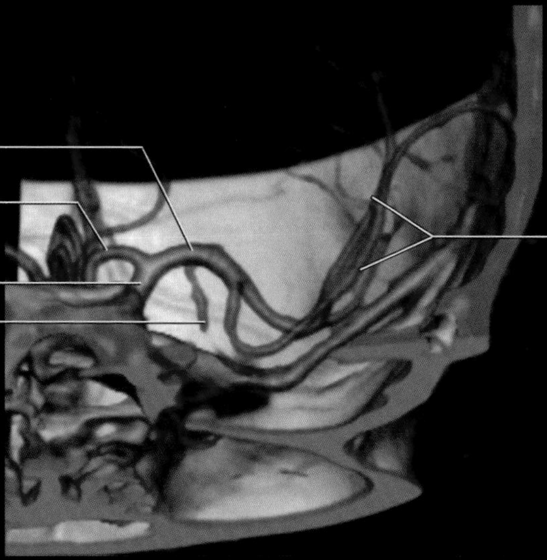

Horizontal (M1) MCA segment
Horizontal (A1) anterior cerebral artery segment
Supraclinoid ICA
Anterior temporal artery
Insular (M2) MCA segments

(Top) Three volume-rendered views of a CT angiogram show the circle of Willis & proximal intracranial arteries. CT angiogram with brain removed shows the relationship of both horizontal MCAs to the greater sphenoid wing. The vessels are viewed from the top down. **(Middle)** PA view shows the left internal carotid artery and its branches, viewed from behind. **(Bottom)** Viewed from behind at a slightly different angle, the anterior temporal artery and horizontal (M1) and insular (M2) segments are especially well seen. Note that it is difficult to see the more distal MCA branches on this examination. The proximal anterior and middle cerebral arteries, common sites for intracranial aneurysm formation, are exquisitely well visualized.

MIDDLE CEREBRAL ARTERY

CTA

MCA bifurcation
Insular (M2) MCA segments
Horizontal (M1) MCA segment
Left anterior cerebral artery

A2 ACA segments
Insular (M2) MCA segments

Anterior cerebral arteries (distal A2 segment, genu)
Opercular (M3) MCA segments
Pillars of fornix
Internal cerebral veins
Straight sinus

(Top) Three axial MIP views from a high-resolution CTA delineate the MCA & its branches. The lowest image, seen here, locates the MCA bifurcation precisely & shows the M1 segment especially well. **(Middle)** Section slightly above the top image shows the insular (M2) MCA segments, especially well seen on the left. **(Bottom)** Section through the foramen of Monro shows the opercular (M3) MCA segments bilaterally.

CTA

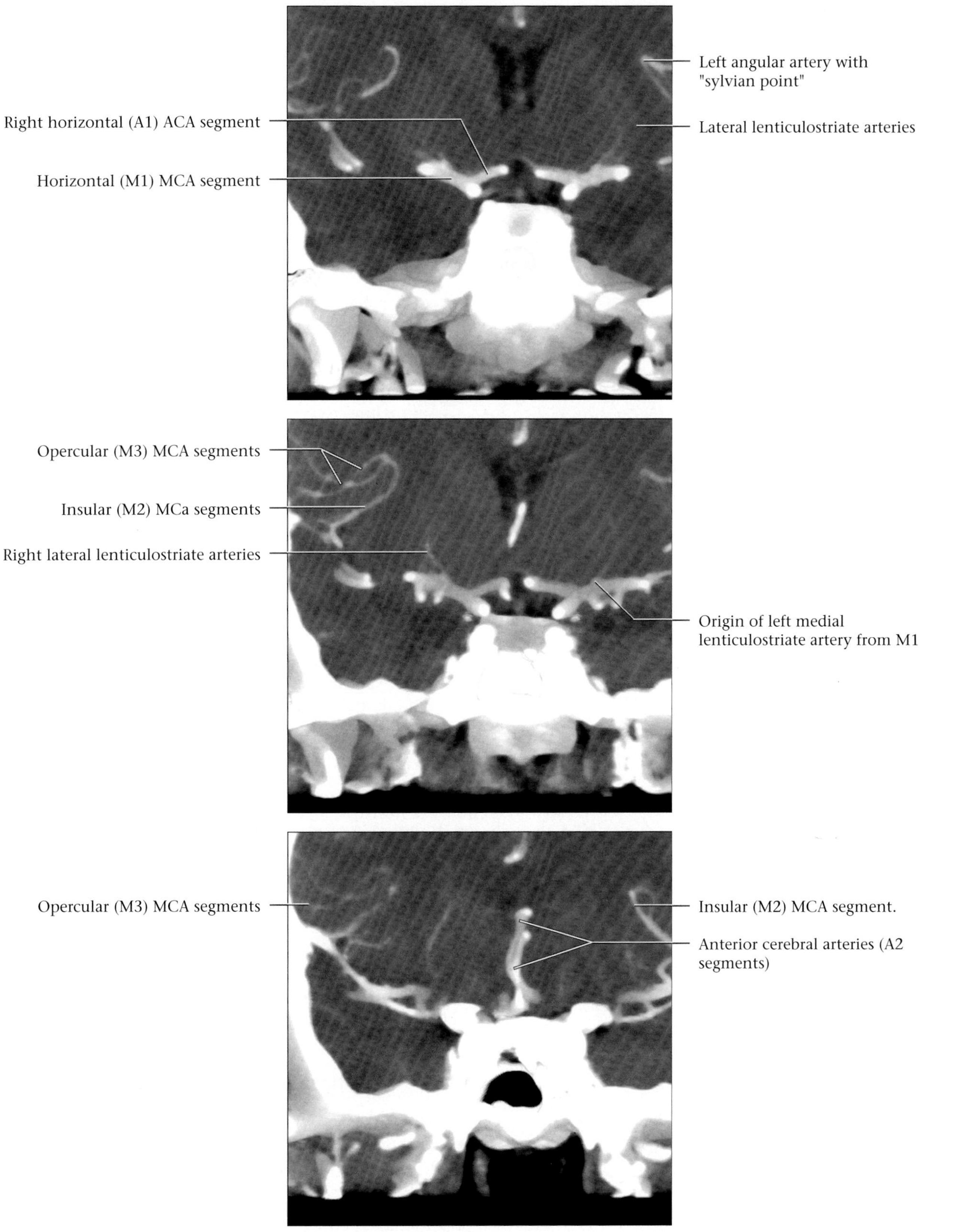
Left angular artery with "sylvian point"
Right horizontal (A1) ACA segment
Lateral lenticulostriate arteries
Horizontal (M1) MCA segment
Opercular (M3) MCA segments
Insular (M2) MCa segments
Right lateral lenticulostriate arteries
Origin of left medial lenticulostriate artery from M1
Opercular (M3) MCA segments
Insular (M2) MCA segment.
Anterior cerebral arteries (A2 segments)

(Top) Three coronal (AP) MIP images from CT angiogram demonstrate the lenticulostriate arteries especially well. CT angiogram through the bifurcation of the internal carotid arteries. **(Middle)** Slightly more anterior view shows origins of two prominent lenticulostriate arteries. The MCA gives rise to a few medial lenticulostriate arteries (most arise from the horizontal or A1 ACA segment). The more numerous group of perforating arteries, the lateral lenticulostriate arteries, arises from the mid- and distal M1 segments, and passes cephalad through the anterior perforated substance into the lateral basal ganglia and external capsule. **(Bottom)** Most anterior view shows the A2 segments of both anterior cerebral arteries as well as opercular (M3) MCA branches on the right and an insular (M2) segment on the left. Apex of insular loops marks the top of the insula.

POSTERIOR CEREBRAL ARTERY

Terminology

Abbreviations

- Posterior cerebral artery (PCA)
- Posterior communicating artery (PCoA)
- Basilar artery (BA)
- Internal carotid artery (ICA)

Gross Anatomy

Overview

- Main BA terminal branches = two PCAs
- Four segments
  - Precommunicating (P1 or mesencephalic) segment
  - Ambient (P2) segment
  - Quadrigeminal (P3) segment
  - Calcarine (P4) segment
- PCoAs connect PCA to ICA at P1/P2 junction

Imaging Anatomy

Overview

- PCAs sweep posterolaterally around midbrain

Anatomy Relationships

- **P1 (precommunicating) segment**
  - Extends laterally from BA bifurcation to junction with PCoA
  - Courses above cisternal segment of oculomotor nerve (CN3)
- **P2 (ambient) segment**
  - Extends from P1/PCoA junction
  - Curves around cerebral peduncle within ambient (perimesencephalic) cistern
  - Lies above tentorium, cisternal segment of trochlear nerve (CN4)
  - Parallels optic tract, basal vein of Rosenthal
- **P3 (quadrigeminal segment)**
  - Short segment within quadrigeminal cistern
  - Extends behind midbrain (quadrigeminal plate level) to calcarine fissure (occipital lobe)
- **P4 (calcarine) segment**
  - PCA terminates above tentorium, in calcarine fissure

Branches

- **Perforating (central) branches**
  - Posterior thalamoperforating arteries
    - Arise from P1, pass posterosuperiorly in interpeduncular fossa
    - Enter undersurface of midbrain
  - Thalamogeniculate arteries
    - Arise from P2, pass posteromedially into midbrain
  - Peduncular perforating arteries arise from P2, pass directly into cerebral peduncles
- **Ventricular/choroidal branches** (arise from P2)
  - Medial posterior choroidal artery
    - Curves around brainstem, enters tela choroidea and runs anteriorly along roof of third ventricle
  - Lateral posterior choroidal arteries
    - In lateral ventricle choroid plexus, curves anteriorly around thalamus
- **Cortical branches**
  - Anterior temporal artery arises from P2, courses anterolaterally under parahippocampal gyrus of inferior temporal lobe
  - Posterior temporal artery arises from P2, courses posteriorly
  - Distal PCA divides into two terminal trunks
    - Medial branches: Medial occipital artery, parietooccipital artery, calcarine artery, posterior splenial arteries
    - Lateral branches: Lateral occipital artery, temporal arteries

Vascular Territory

- Penetrating branches: Midbrain, thalami, posterior limb of internal capsule, optic tract
- Ventricular/choroidal branches: Choroid plexus of third/lateral ventricles, parts of thalami, posterior commissure, cerebral peduncles
- Splenial branches: Posterior body and splenium of corpus callosum
- Cortical branches: Posterior 1/3 of medial hemisphere surface; most of inferior temporal lobe, most of occipital lobe (including visual cortex)

Normal Variants, Anomalies

- "Fetal" origin of PCA
  - Large PCoA gives direct origin to PCA
  - P1 (precommunicating) PCA segment hypoplastic or absent
- Persistent carotid-basilar anastomoses
  - PCAs supplied by persistent trigeminal artery or proatlantal intersegmental artery

Anatomy-Based Imaging Issues

Imaging Pitfalls

- Absent PCA on vertebral angiogram usually due to "fetal" origin, not occlusion
  - Injection of ipsilateral carotid artery confirms presence of "fetal" PCA

Clinical Implications

Clinical Importance

- PCA occlusion causes homonymous hemianopsia

Embryology

Embryologic Events

- Definitive PCAs develop later than anterior, middle cerebral arteries
- Circulation to fetal cerebral hemispheres initially supplied entirely by embryonic ICA
- Proximal PCAs sprout from caudal division of embryonic ICA
- Vertebral, basilar arteries form from fusion of dorsal longitudinal neural arteries
- Anastomose with sprouting PCA stems
- Distal PCAs sprout from proximal stems

GRAPHICS

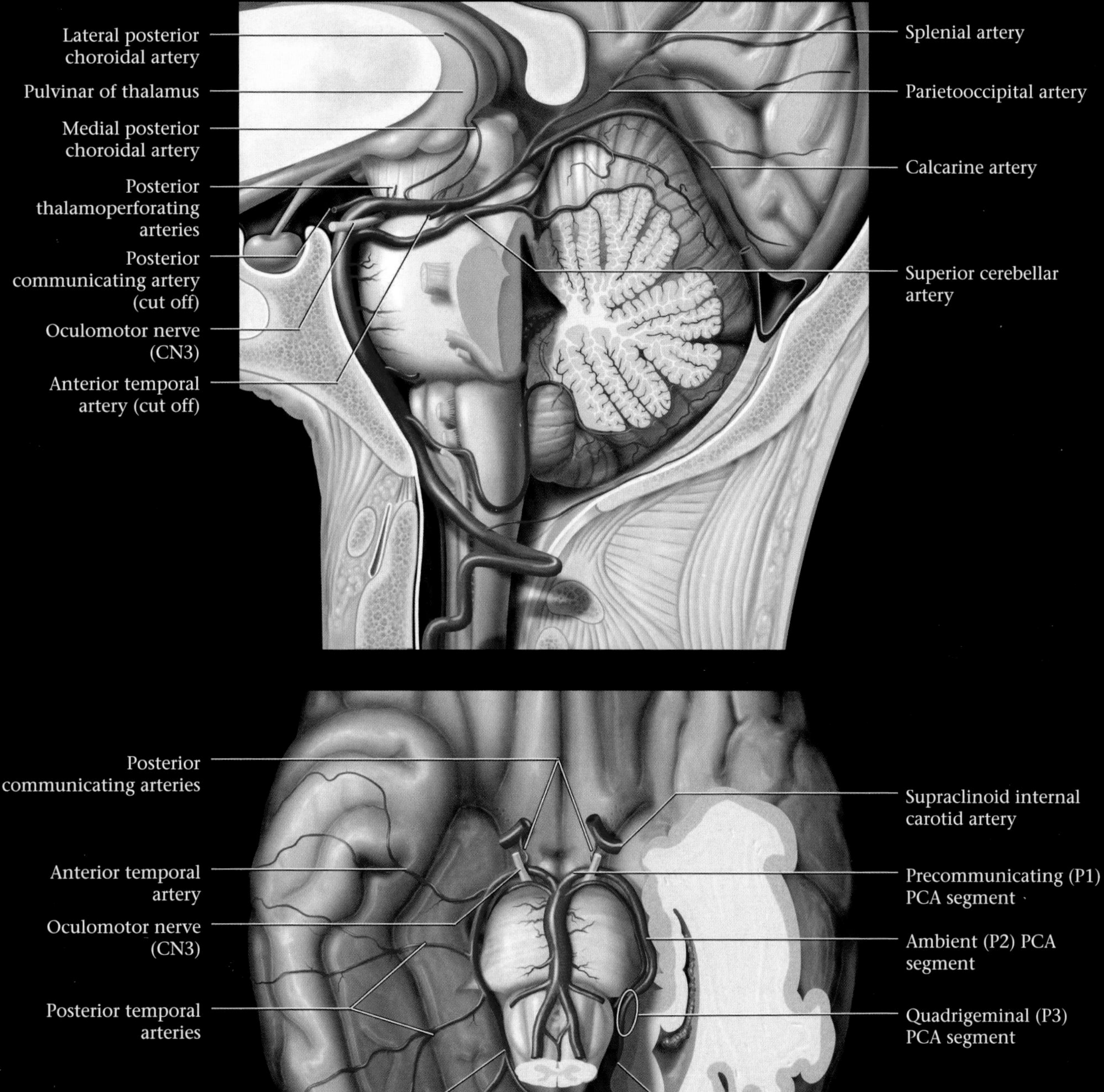
Lateral posterior choroidal artery
Pulvinar of thalamus
Medial posterior choroidal artery
Posterior thalamoperforating arteries
Posterior communicating artery (cut off)
Oculomotor nerve (CN3)
Anterior temporal artery (cut off)
Splenial artery
Parietooccipital artery
Calcarine artery
Superior cerebellar artery
Posterior communicating arteries
Anterior temporal artery
Oculomotor nerve (CN3)
Posterior temporal arteries
Calcarine (P4) PCA segment
Calcarine artery & branches
Supraclinoid internal carotid artery
Precommunicating (P1) PCA segment
Ambient (P2) PCA segment
Quadrigeminal (P3) PCA segment
Parietooccipital artery

(Top) Lateral graphic depicts the posterior cerebral artery and its branches. The tentorium and CN3 lie between the PCA above and the superior cerebellar artery below. The PCA has central (perforating), choroidal, and cortical branches as well as a small branch to the corpus callosum splenium. **(Bottom)** Submentovertex graphic shows the PCA and the relationship of its segments to the midbrain. The PCA supplies the occipital lobe and almost all of the inferior surface of the temporal lobe (except for its tip). The precommunicating (P1) PCA segment extends from the basilar bifurcation to the PCoA junction. The ambient (P2) segment swings posterolaterally around the midbrain. The quadrigeminal segment (P3) lies behind the midbrain. The PCA terminal segment is the calcarine (P4) segment.

POSTERIOR CEREBRAL ARTERY

LATERAL VA DSA

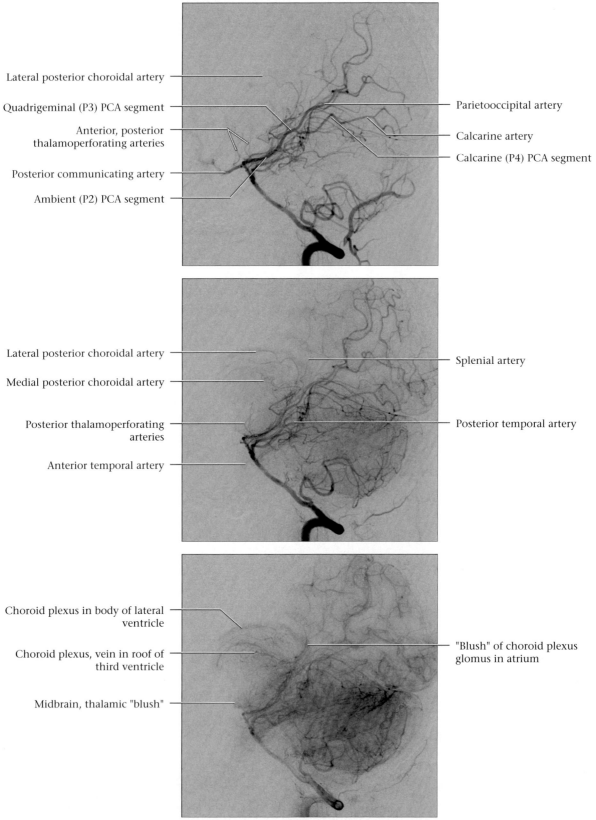

Lateral posterior choroidal artery
Quadrigeminal (P3) PCA segment
Anterior, posterior thalamoperforating arteries
Posterior communicating artery
Ambient (P2) PCA segment
Parietooccipital artery
Calcarine artery
Calcarine (P4) PCA segment

Lateral posterior choroidal artery
Medial posterior choroidal artery
Posterior thalamoperforating arteries
Anterior temporal artery
Splenial artery
Posterior temporal artery

Choroid plexus in body of lateral ventricle
Choroid plexus, vein in roof of third ventricle
Midbrain, thalamic "blush"
"Blush" of choroid plexus glomus in atrium

(Top) A series of three lateral views from a vertebrobasilar angiogram shows the PCA and its branches. Early arterial phase shows contrast reflux into the ipsilateral PCoA. Both anterior and posterior thalamoperforating arteries are opacified. The lateral posterior choroidal artery has a prominent "3" shape that allows it to be identified easily on this projection. The precommunicating (P1) PCA segment is not well seen but the P2 segment is shown as it curves around and behind the midbrain. **(Middle)** Mid-arterial phase shows the posterior thalamoperforating and choroidal arteries especially well. Note that PCA cortical branches are supplying the posterior third of the medial hemisphere surface. **(Bottom)** "Capillary" early venous phase shows a prominent vascular blush in lateral ventricle. Note "brain stain" depicting parietooccipital, midbrain PCA supply.

POSTERIOR CEREBRAL ARTERY

AP VA DSA

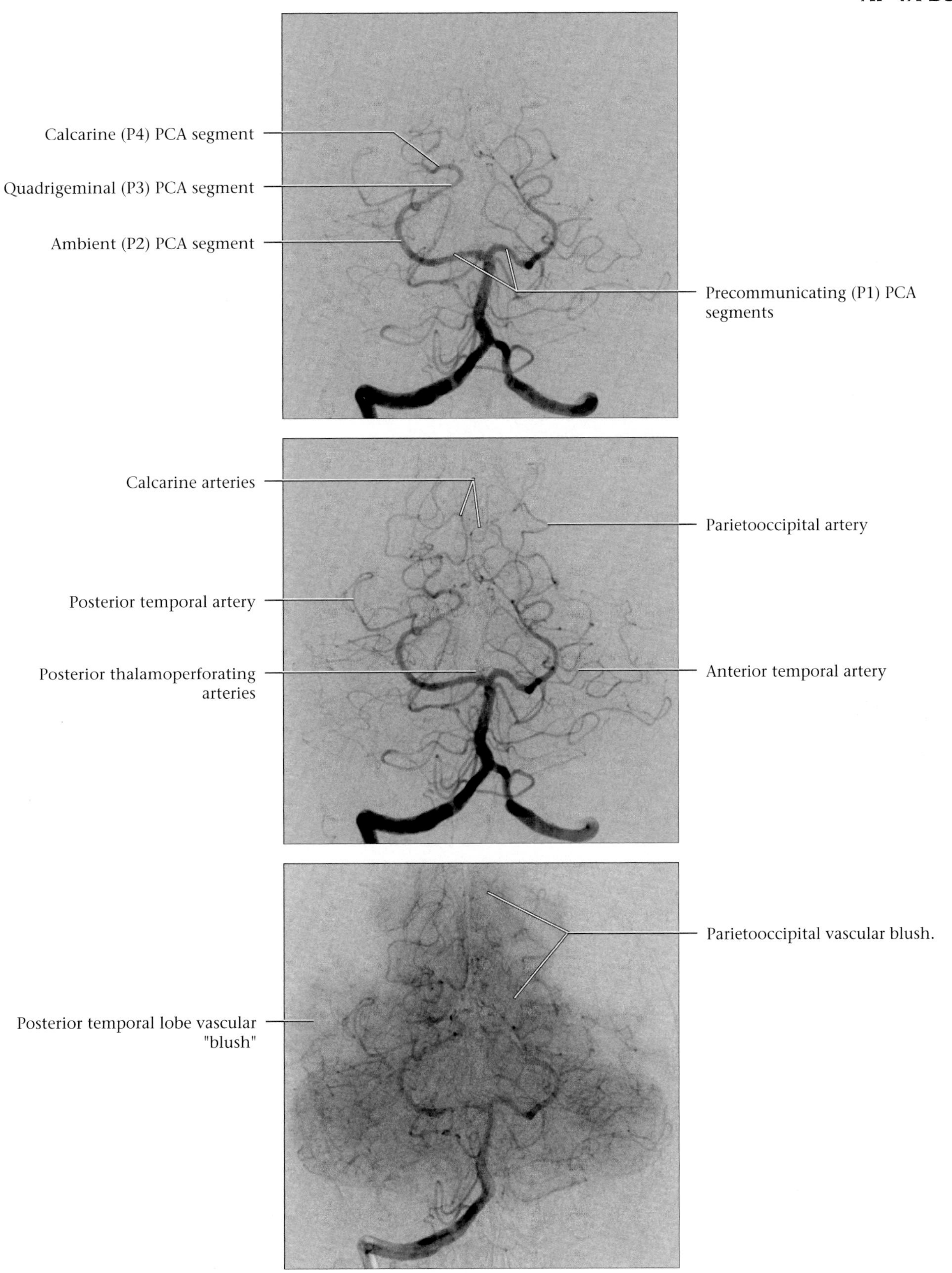
Calcarine (P4) PCA segment
Quadrigeminal (P3) PCA segment
Ambient (P2) PCA segment
Precommunicating (P1) PCA segments
Calcarine arteries
Parietooccipital artery
Posterior temporal artery
Posterior thalamoperforating arteries
Anterior temporal artery
Parietooccipital vascular blush.
Posterior temporal lobe vascular "blush"

(Top) A series of three AP views of a vertebrobasilar angiogram depict the PCA segments and their branches. The precommunicating (P1) segment is best seen in this projection. The PCAs sweep laterally and then posterosuperiorly around the midbrain. **(Middle)** Mid-arterial phase shows several of the cortical PCA branches especially well. In this view, anterior and posterior temporal arteries often overlap somewhat. In this projection the posterior thalamoperforating arteries are seen as a faint vascular blush lying just above the terminal basilar artery bifurcation. **(Bottom)** Late arterial phase shows the vascular blush of the PCA supply to the medial parietal and occipital lobes as well as the temporal lobes. The unopacified vertical "filling defect" is the dura of the falx cerebri that separates the two cerebral hemispheres.

POSTERIOR CEREBRAL ARTERY

LAT, AP ICA DSA

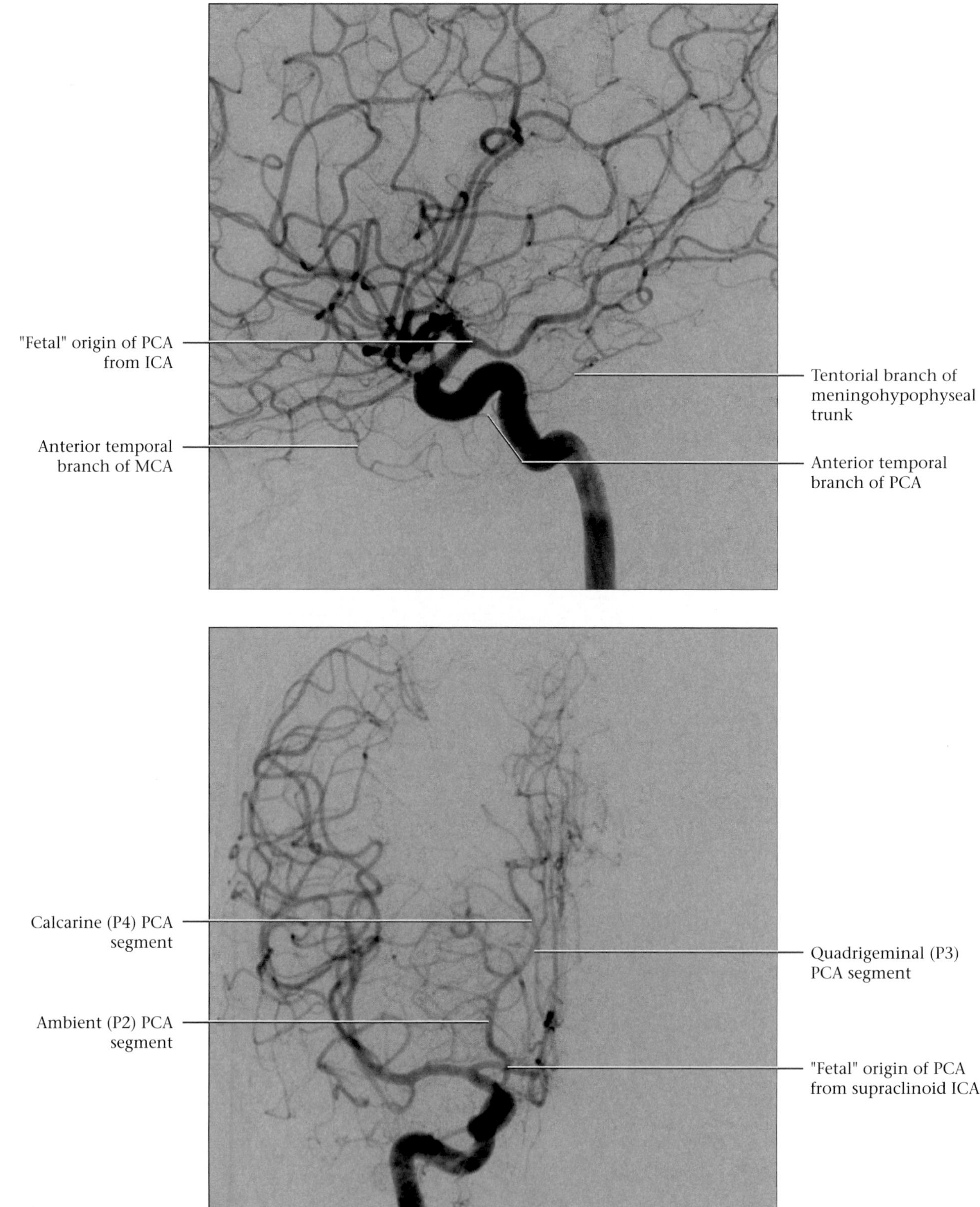
"Fetal" origin of PCA from ICA
Anterior temporal branch of MCA
Tentorial branch of meningohypophyseal trunk
Anterior temporal branch of PCA
Calcarine (P4) PCA segment
Ambient (P2) PCA segment
Quadrigeminal (P3) PCA segment
"Fetal" origin of PCA from supraclinoid ICA

(Top) A common normal variant is origin of the PCA from the supraclinoid internal carotid artery, sometimes termed a "fetal" origin of the PCA. In this instance the ipsilateral P2 segment is hypoplastic or absent and the potential for collateral flow through the circle of Willis is anatomically limited. The meningohypophyseal trunk, a branch of the cavernous ICA, is unusually prominent because it supplied a small dural arteriovenous fistula (not shown) at the transverse sinus/sigmoid sinus junction. **(Bottom)** AP view shows the PCA is opacified from the internal carotid injection. The vertebrobasilar angiogram in this patient (not illustrated) showed "absent" filling of the right PCA. The most common cause of this finding, as occurred in this case, is "fetal" origin of the PCA from the ICA instead of the vertebrobasilar system.

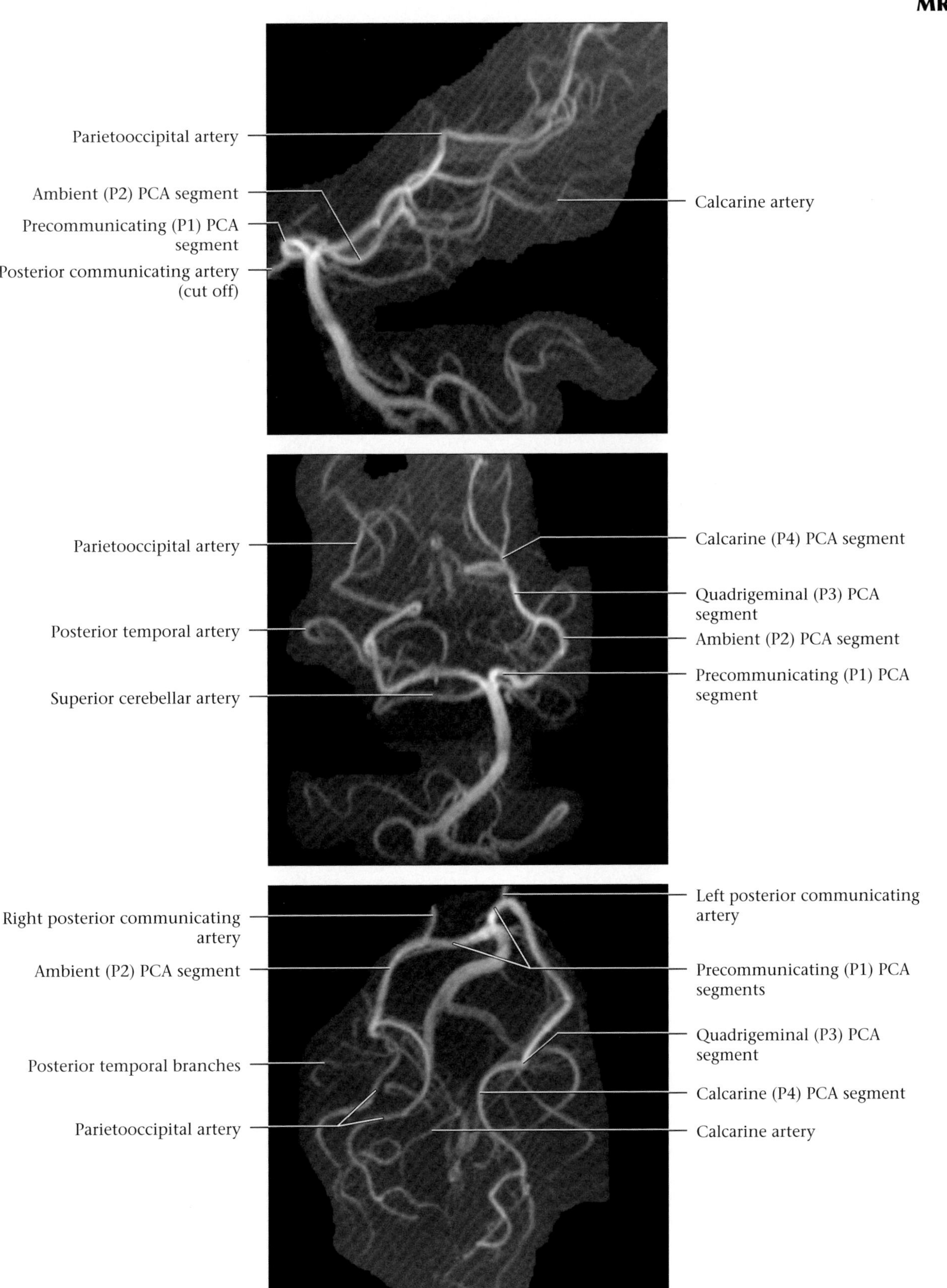

Parietooccipital artery
Ambient (P2) PCA segment
Precommunicating (P1) PCA segment
Posterior communicating artery (cut off)
Calcarine artery
Parietooccipital artery
Posterior temporal artery
Superior cerebellar artery
Calcarine (P4) PCA segment
Quadrigeminal (P3) PCA segment
Ambient (P2) PCA segment
Precommunicating (P1) PCA segment
Right posterior communicating artery
Ambient (P2) PCA segment
Posterior temporal branches
Parietooccipital artery
Left posterior communicating artery
Precommunicating (P1) PCA segments
Quadrigeminal (P3) PCA segment
Calcarine (P4) PCA segment
Calcarine artery

(Top) First of three views of an MRA obtained at 3T show the PCA and its major cortical branches. This slightly oblique lateral view shows the basilar bifurcation and the P1 segment. **(Middle)** AP view shows both PCAs as they sweep laterally and then posteriorly around the midbrain. Perforating arteries are not well seen on MRAs, even at 3T. **(Bottom)** Submentovertex view shows the PCA segments and distal cortical PCA branches especially well. The configuration of the PCA as it courses around the midbrain is highly variable. The P1 (precommunicating) segments vary significantly in both size, length, and tortuosity.

POSTERIOR CEREBRAL ARTERY

AP CTA

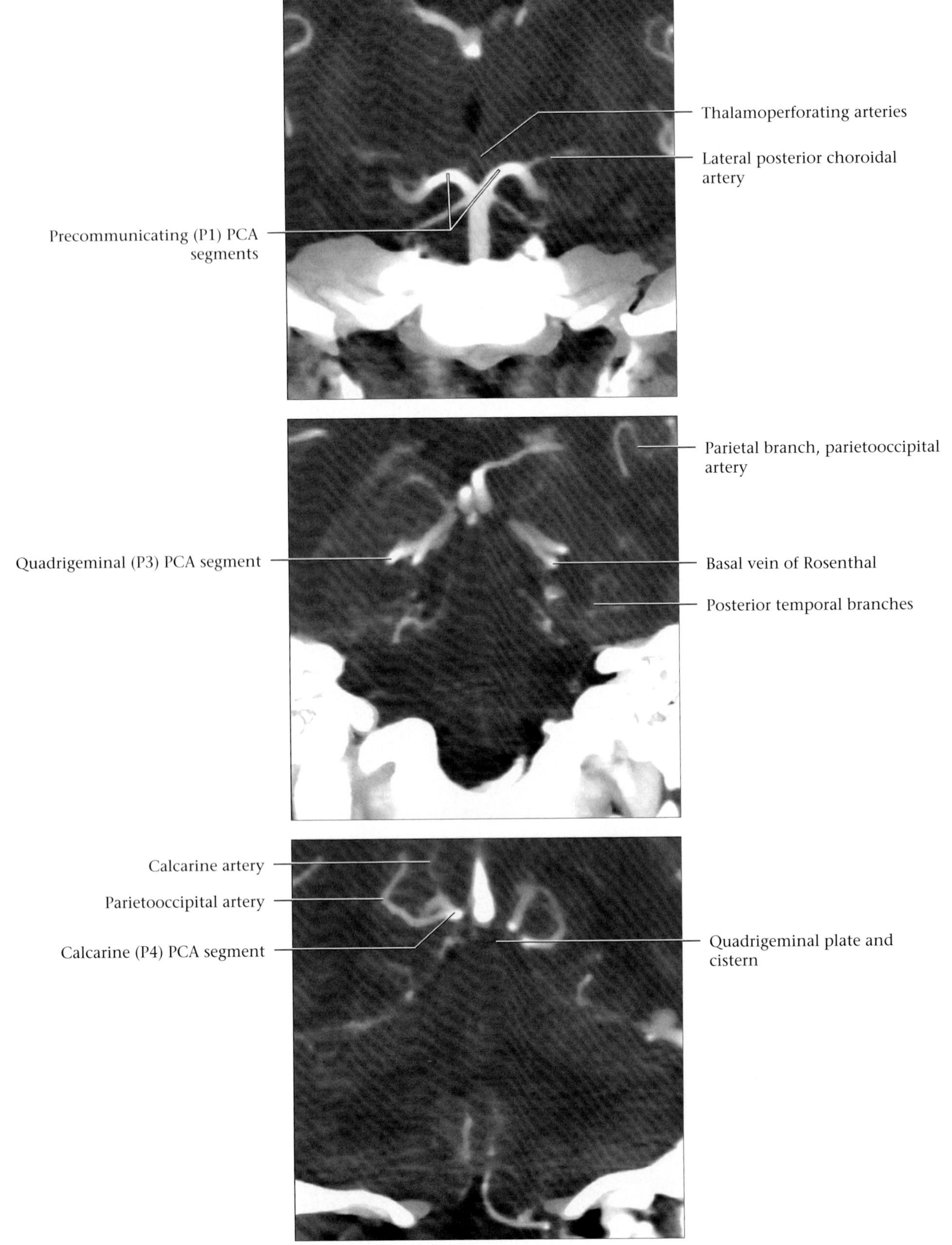
Thalamoperforating arteries
Lateral posterior choroidal artery
Precommunicating (P1) PCA segments
Parietal branch, parietooccipital artery
Quadrigeminal (P3) PCA segment
Basal vein of Rosenthal
Posterior temporal branches
Calcarine artery
Parietooccipital artery
Calcarine (P4) PCA segment
Quadrigeminal plate and cistern

(Top) Three coronal MIP reprojected views of a CTA depict the segments of the posterior cerebral artery and some of their branches. **(Middle)** The ambient (P2) PCA segments sweep posterosuperiorly around the midbrain just above the tentorium cerebelli. The quadrigeminal (P3) segment is relatively short and begins at the level of the dorsal midbrain near the quadrigeminal plate. The basal vein of Rosenthal is opacified on this CTA and should not be mistaken for the more laterally-located PCA. **(Bottom)** This section, shown at the anterior end of the calcarine fissure, depicts the terminal (P4) division of the right PCA into its lateral (parietooccipital) and more medial (calcarine) branches particularly well.

POSTERIOR CEREBRAL ARTERY

LATERAL CTA

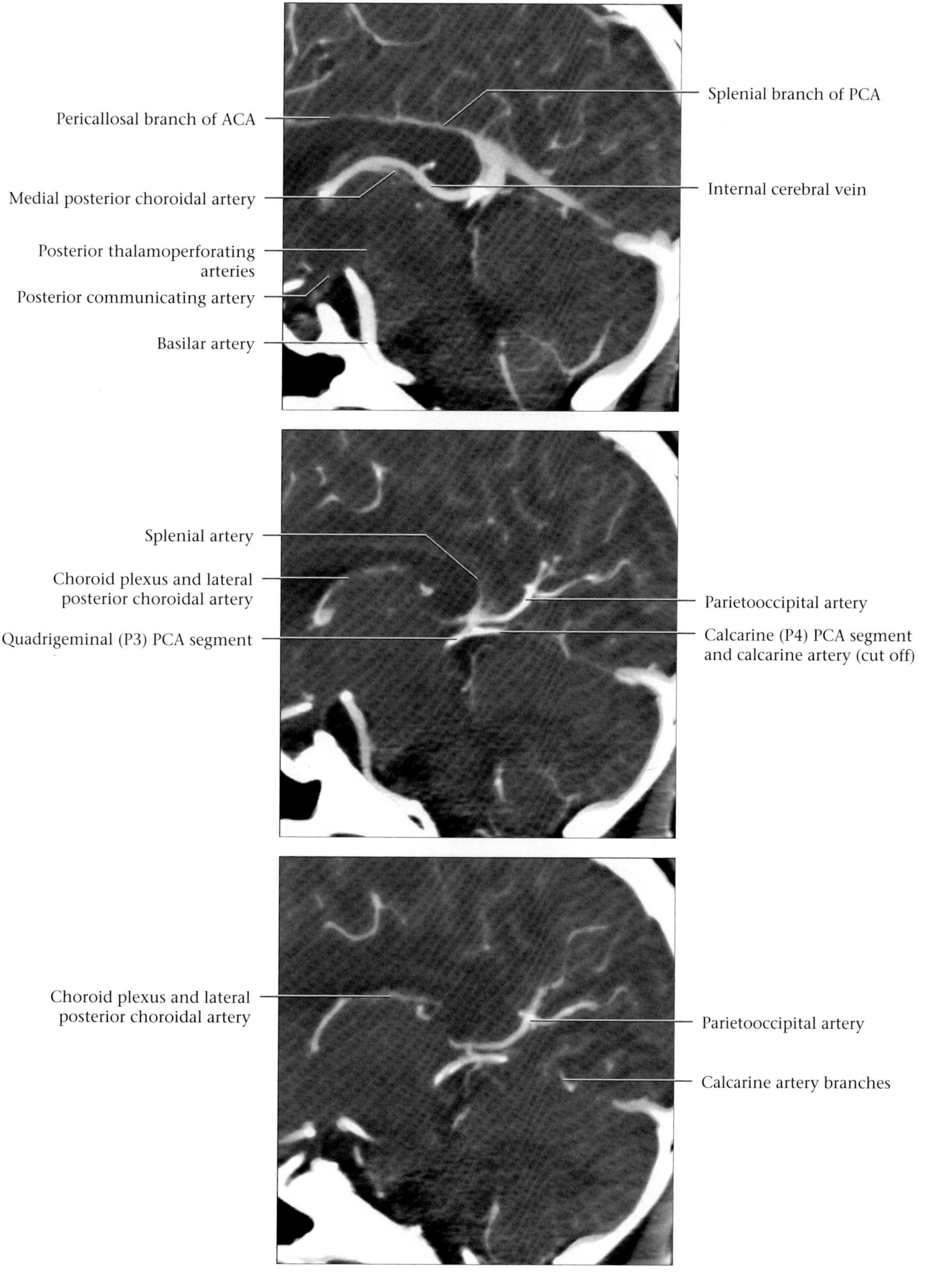
Pericallosal branch of ACA
Medial posterior choroidal artery
Posterior thalamoperforating arteries
Posterior communicating artery
Basilar artery
Splenial branch of PCA
Internal cerebral vein
Splenial artery
Choroid plexus and lateral posterior choroidal artery
Quadrigeminal (P3) PCA segment
Parietooccipital artery
Calcarine (P4) PCA segment and calcarine artery (cut off)
Choroid plexus and lateral posterior choroidal artery
Parietooccipital artery
Calcarine artery branches

(Top) First of six lateral views from a CTA depicts the PCA and its branches. The medial posterior choroidal artery is the small midline vessel lying just below the internal cerebral vein. Note the splenial branch of the PCA anastomoses above the corpus callosum with pericallosal branches from the ACA. When either vessel is occluded, this may provide an important source of potential collateral blood flow in addition to pial (watershed) collaterals. **(Middle)** Vascular blush of the choroid plexus in the lateral ventricle is seen here. It is supplied by the lateral posterior choroidal artery. **(Bottom)** The choroid plexus of the lateral ventricle, with its accompanying arteries and veins, "dives" inferiorly through the foramen of Monro.

POSTERIOR CEREBRAL ARTERY

LATERAL CTA

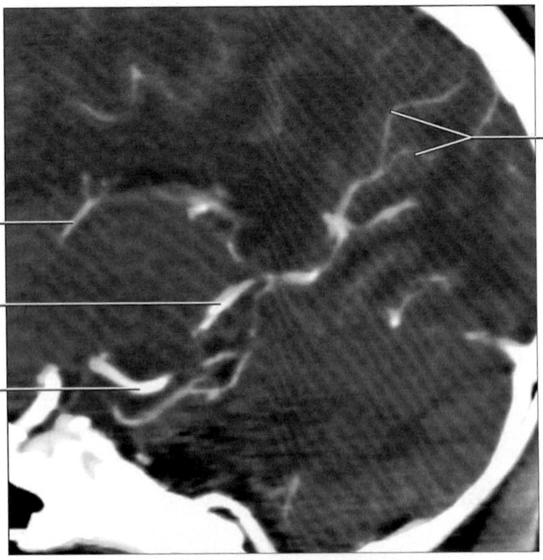

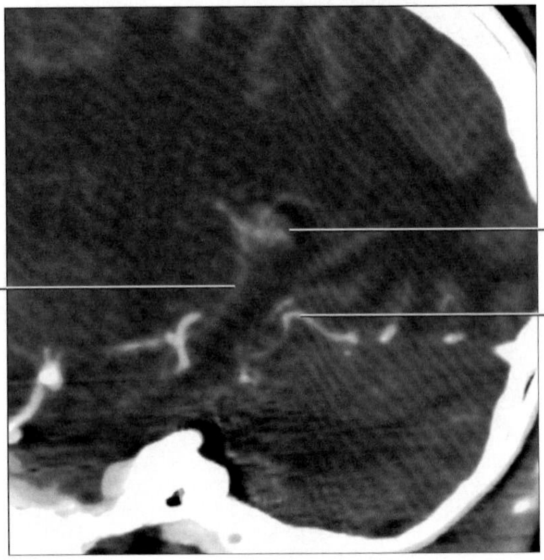

Parietal branches

Thalamostriate vein

Quadrigeminal (P3) PCA segment

Ambient (P2) PCA segment

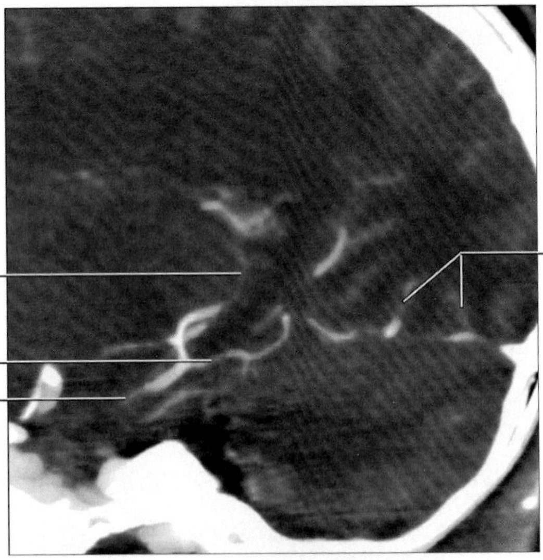

Calcarine branches

Lateral posterior choroidal artery

Posterior temporal artery

Anterior temporal artery

Choroid plexus glomus

Lateral posterior choroidal artery

Posterior temporal branches

(Top) More lateral section shows the parietal and occipital PCA branches very well. The posterior temporal artery is also seen here. **(Middle)** The lateral posterior choroidal artery originates from the P2 PCA segment and sweeps posterosuperiorly around the pulvinar of the thalamus to supply it as well as the choroid plexus. **(Bottom)** This section through the posterolateral thalamus and atrium of the lateral ventricle shows the lateral posterior choroidal artery and its supply to the glomus of the choroid plexus.

AXIAL CTA

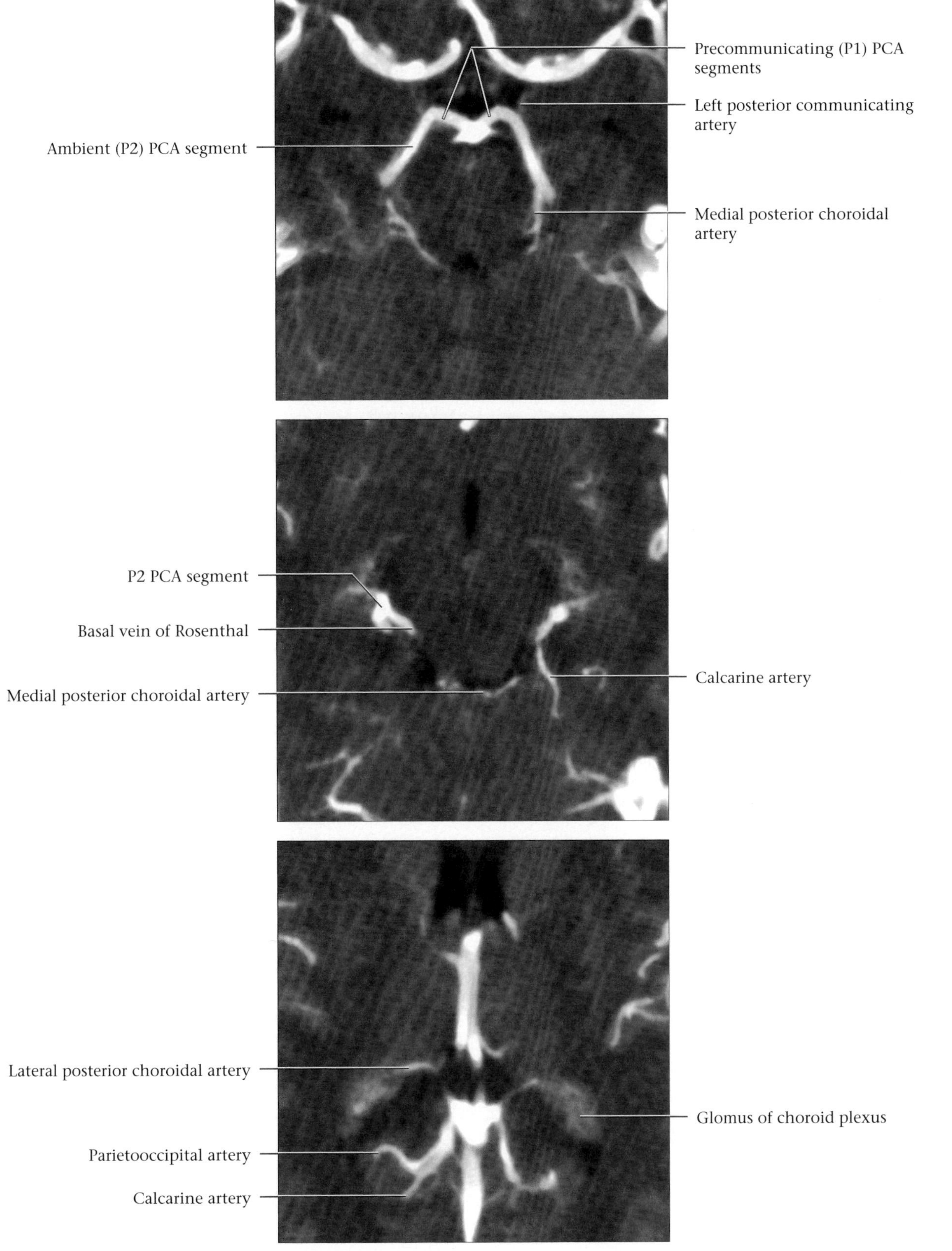
Precommunicating (P1) PCA segments
Left posterior communicating artery
Ambient (P2) PCA segment
Medial posterior choroidal artery
P2 PCA segment
Basal vein of Rosenthal
Calcarine artery
Medial posterior choroidal artery
Lateral posterior choroidal artery
Glomus of choroid plexus
Parietooccipital artery
Calcarine artery

(Top) First of three axial MIP reconstructions from CTA depicts the PCA segments especially well. Here, in the section through the circle of Willis, two small posterior communicating arteries are visualized. Both precommunicating (P1) PCA segments are quite prominent. **(Middle)** Section through the ambient and quadrigeminal cisterns shows their vascular contents, which include the P2 and P3 PCA segments as well as the more medially-positioned basal veins of Rosenthal. **(Bottom)** In this section near the tentorial apex, the lateral posterior choroidal arteries are seen as they supply the glomi of the choroid plexus. The terminal division of the PCA into its parietooccipital and calcarine branches occurs either in the distal quadrigeminal cistern or near the anterior aspect of the calcarine fissure.

VERTEBROBASILAR SYSTEM

Terminology

Abbreviations

- Vertebrobasilar (VB); vertebral artery (VA); basilar artery (BA)
- Superior cerebellar arteries (SCAs); posterior inferior cerebellar artery (PICA); anterior inferior cerebellar artery (AICA)
- Internal carotid artery (ICA)
- Anterior, posterior spinal arteries (ASA, PSA)

Gross Anatomy

Overview

- Four VA segments
  - Extraosseous (V1) segment (arch → C6)
  - Foraminal (V2) segment (C6 → C1)
  - Extraspinal (V3) segment (C1 → foramen magnum)
  - Intradural (V4) segment (intracranial)

Imaging Anatomy

Overview

- Ectasia, tortuosity, off-midline course, variations in configuration/branching patterns common

Anatomy Relationships

- **VA**
  - **V1**: Arises from subclavian artery, courses posterosuperiorly to enter C6 transverse foramen
  - **V2**
    - Ascends through C6-C3 transverse foramina
    - Turns superolaterally through the inverted "L-shaped" transverse foramen of axis (C2)
    - Courses short distance superiorly through C1 transverse foramen
  - **V3**
    - Exits top of atlas (C1) transverse foramen
    - Lies on top of C1 ring, curving posteromedially around atlantooccipital joint
    - As it passes around back of atlanto-occipital joint, turns sharply anterosuperiorly to pierce dura at foramen magnum
  - **V4**
    - After VA enters skull through foramen magnum, courses superomedially behind clivus
    - Unites with contralateral VA at/near pontomedullary junction to form BA
- **BA**
  - Courses superiorly in prepontine cistern (in front of pons, behind clivus)
  - Bifurcates into its terminal branches, PCAs, in interpeduncular or suprasellar cistern at/slightly above dorsum sellae

Branches

- **VA**
  - V1: Segmental cervical muscular, spinal branches
  - V2: Anterior meningeal artery, unnamed muscular/spinal branches
  - V3: Posterior meningeal artery
  - V4
    - Anterior, posterior spinal arteries
    - Perforating branches to medulla
    - **PICA**: Arises from distal VA, curves around/over tonsil, gives off perforating medullary, choroid, tonsillar, cerebellar branches
- **BA**
  - Pontine, midbrain perforating branches (numerous)
  - **AICA**
    - Lies ventromedial to CN7 and 8
    - Often loops into internal auditory meatus
  - **SCAs**
    - Arise from distal BA, course posterolaterally around midbrain below CN3, tentorium
    - Lie above CN5, often contact it
  - **PCAs** (terminal BA branches)

Vascular Territory

- VA
  - ASA: Upper cervical spinal cord, inferior medulla
  - PSA: Dorsal spinal cord to conus medullaris
  - Penetrating branches: Olives, inferior cerebellar peduncle, part of medulla
  - PICA: Lateral medulla, choroid plexus of fourth ventricle, tonsil, inferior vermis/cerebellum
- BA
  - Pontine perforating branches: Central medulla, pons, midbrain
  - AICA: IAC, CN7 and 8, anterolateral cerebellum
  - SCA: Superior vermis, superior cerebellar peduncle, dentate nucleus, brachium pontis, superomedial surface of cerebellum, upper vermis

Normal Variants, Anomalies

- Normal variants
  - VA: R/L variation in size, dominance common; aortic arch origin 5%
  - BA: Variation in course, branching patterns common (e.g., AICA/PICA may share common trunk)
- Anomalies
  - VA/BA may be fenestrated, duplicated (may have increased prevalence of aneurysms)
  - Embryonic carotid-basilar anastomoses (e.g., persistent trigeminal artery)

Embryology

Embryologic Events

- Plexiform longitudinal anastomoses between cervical intersegmental arteries → VA precursors
- Paired plexiform dorsal longitudinal neural arteries (LNAs) develop, form precursors of BA
- Transient anastomoses between dorsal longitudinal neural arteries, developing ICAs appear (primitive trigeminal/hypoglossal arteries, etc.)
- Definitive VAs arise from 7th cervical intersegmental arteries, anastomose with LNAs
- LNAs fuse as temporary connections with ICAs regress → definitive BA, VB circulation formed

GRAPHIC, 3D-VRT CTA

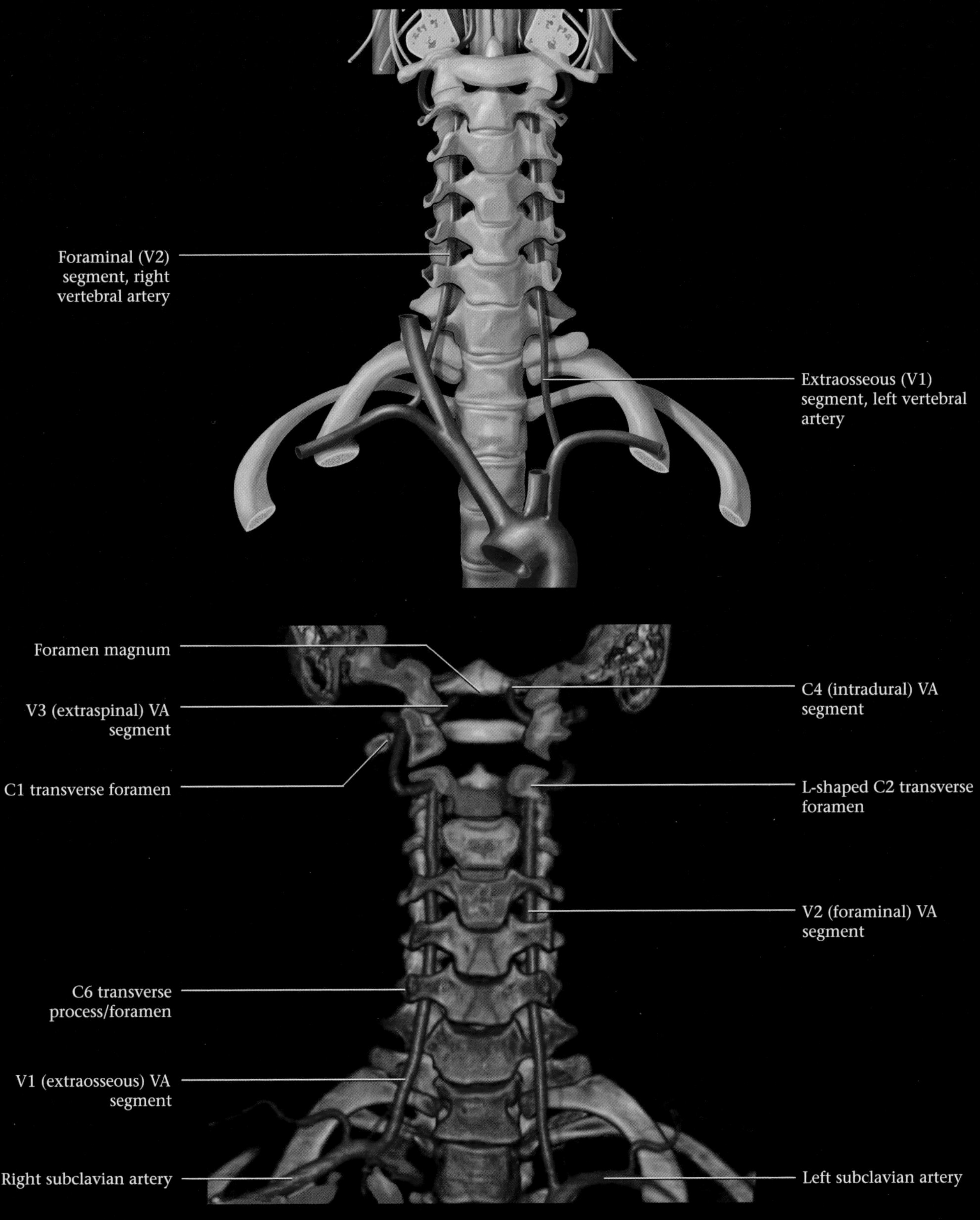

Foraminal (V2) segment, right vertebral artery
Extraosseous (V1) segment, left vertebral artery
Foramen magnum
V3 (extraspinal) VA segment
C1 transverse foramen
C4 (intradural) VA segment
L-shaped C2 transverse foramen
V2 (foraminal) VA segment
C6 transverse process/foramen
V1 (extraosseous) VA segment
Right subclavian artery
Left subclavian artery

(Top) Two of the three extracranial segments of the VAs and their relationship to the cervical spine are shown here in an AP graphic. The extraosseous (V1) VA segments extend from the superior aspect of the subclavian arteries to the C6 transverse foramina. The V2 (foraminal) segment extends from C6 to the VA exit from the C1 transverse foramina. **(Bottom)** For comparison with the graphic above, a 3D-VRT CTA shows the extracranial VAs. They originate from the superior aspect of the subclavian arteries. The VAs typically enter the transverse foramina of C6 and ascend almost vertically to C2, where they make a 90 degree turn laterally in the L-shaped C2 transverse foramen before ascending vertically again to C1.

GRAPHICS

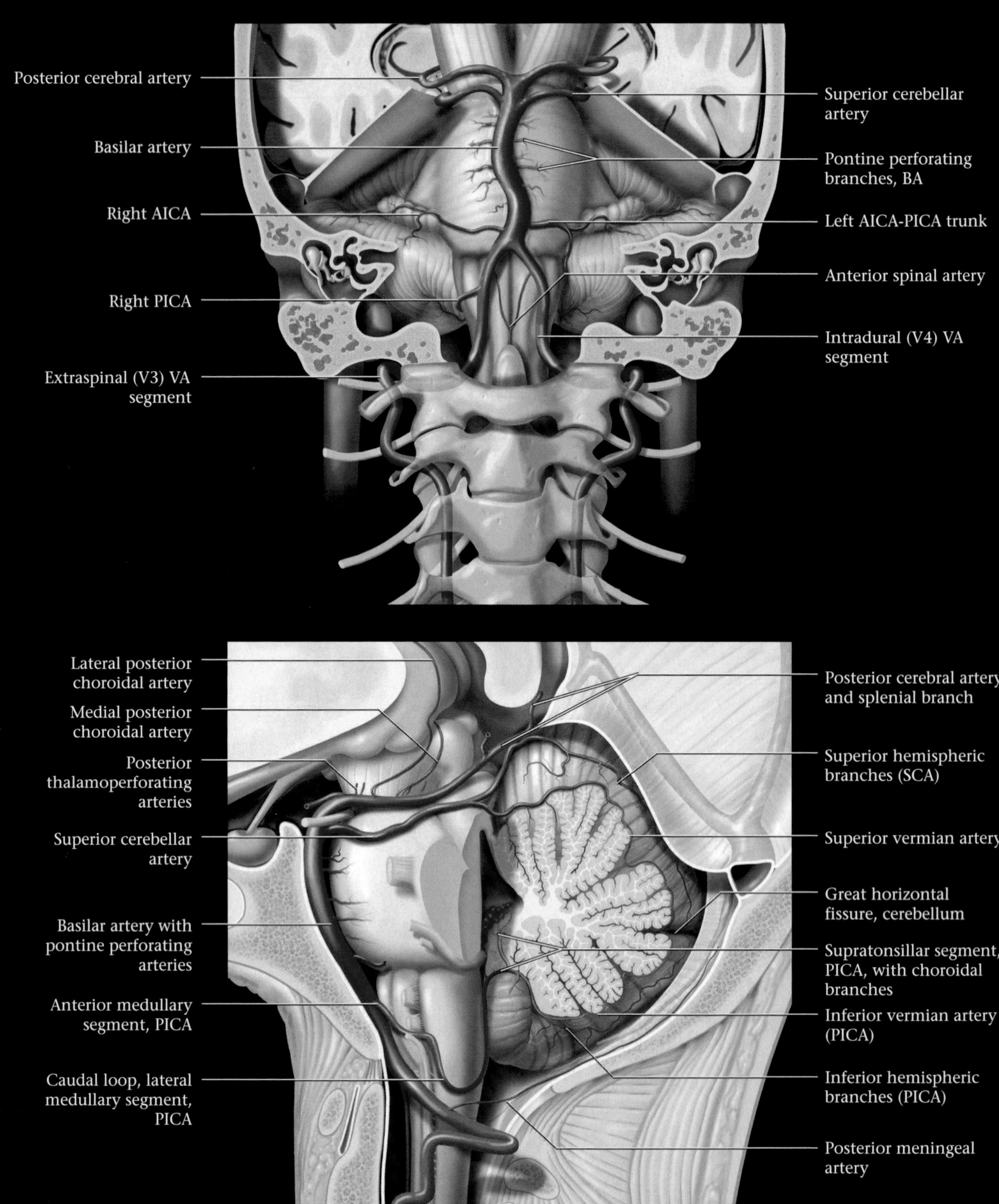

Posterior cerebral artery
Basilar artery
Right AICA
Right PICA
Extraspinal (V3) VA segment
Superior cerebellar artery
Pontine perforating branches, BA
Left AICA-PICA trunk
Anterior spinal artery
Intradural (V4) VA segment
Lateral posterior choroidal artery
Medial posterior choroidal artery
Posterior thalamoperforating arteries
Superior cerebellar artery
Basilar artery with pontine perforating arteries
Anterior medullary segment, PICA
Caudal loop, lateral medullary segment, PICA
Posterior cerebral artery and splenial branch
Superior hemispheric branches (SCA)
Superior vermian artery
Great horizontal fissure, cerebellum
Supratonsillar segment, PICA, with choroidal branches
Inferior vermian artery (PICA)
Inferior hemispheric branches (PICA)
Posterior meningeal artery

(Top) AP graphic depicts the distal cervical and intracranial VB system. V3 is the short extraspinal VA segment that extends from the top of C1 to the foramen magnum. V4 is the intradural (intracranial) segment. A right PICA originates from the VA. A combined AICA-PICA trunk is a common normal variant and is shown on the left. **(Bottom)** Lateral graphic depicts the VB system. Note relationship of PICA loops to medulla, cerebellar tonsil. Watershed between SCA, PICA is often near the great horizontal fissure of the cerebellum.

3D-VRT CTA

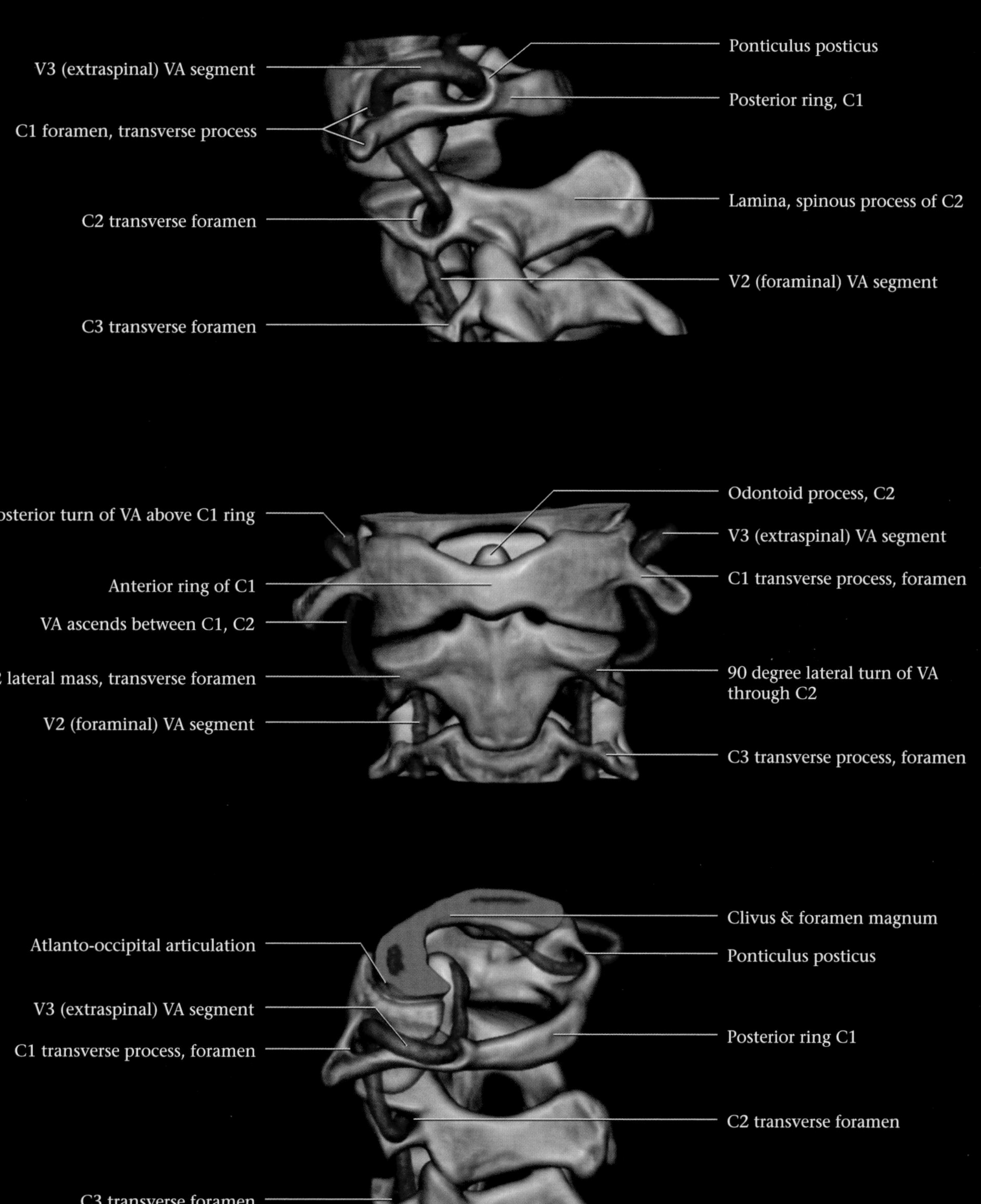
V3 (extraspinal) VA segment
C1 foramen, transverse process
C2 transverse foramen
C3 transverse foramen
Ponticulus posticus
Posterior ring, C1
Lamina, spinous process of C2
V2 (foraminal) VA segment
Posterior turn of VA above C1 ring
Anterior ring of C1
VA ascends between C1, C2
C2 lateral mass, transverse foramen
V2 (foraminal) VA segment
Odontoid process, C2
V3 (extraspinal) VA segment
C1 transverse process, foramen
90 degree lateral turn of VA through C2
C3 transverse process, foramen
Atlanto-occipital articulation
V3 (extraspinal) VA segment
C1 transverse process, foramen
C3 transverse foramen
Clivus & foramen magnum
Ponticulus posticus
Posterior ring C1
C2 transverse foramen

(Top) A series of three close-up views from the 3D-VRT CTA elegantly illustrate the relationship of the VA to the C1 and C2 vertebral bodies. Lateral projection shows the VA makes a 90 degree, "L-shaped" turn laterally through C2, then ascends between C2 and C1. After it exits the C1 transverse foramen it courses posteriorly above and along the C1 ring. A posterior bony ring (ponticulus posticus) is present in this case, a normal variant. **(Middle)** 3D-VRT CTA with close-up view shows the distal VA as it follows its complex course through the C2 and C1 transverse foramina. Here the VAs are shown from the AP (frontal) projection. **(Bottom)** The VA as it courses posterolaterally around the C1 lateral mass and above the C1 ring is clearly seen on this view. VA then turns anteromedially to enter foramen magnum. Note bony ring over right VA, a normal variant.

DSA

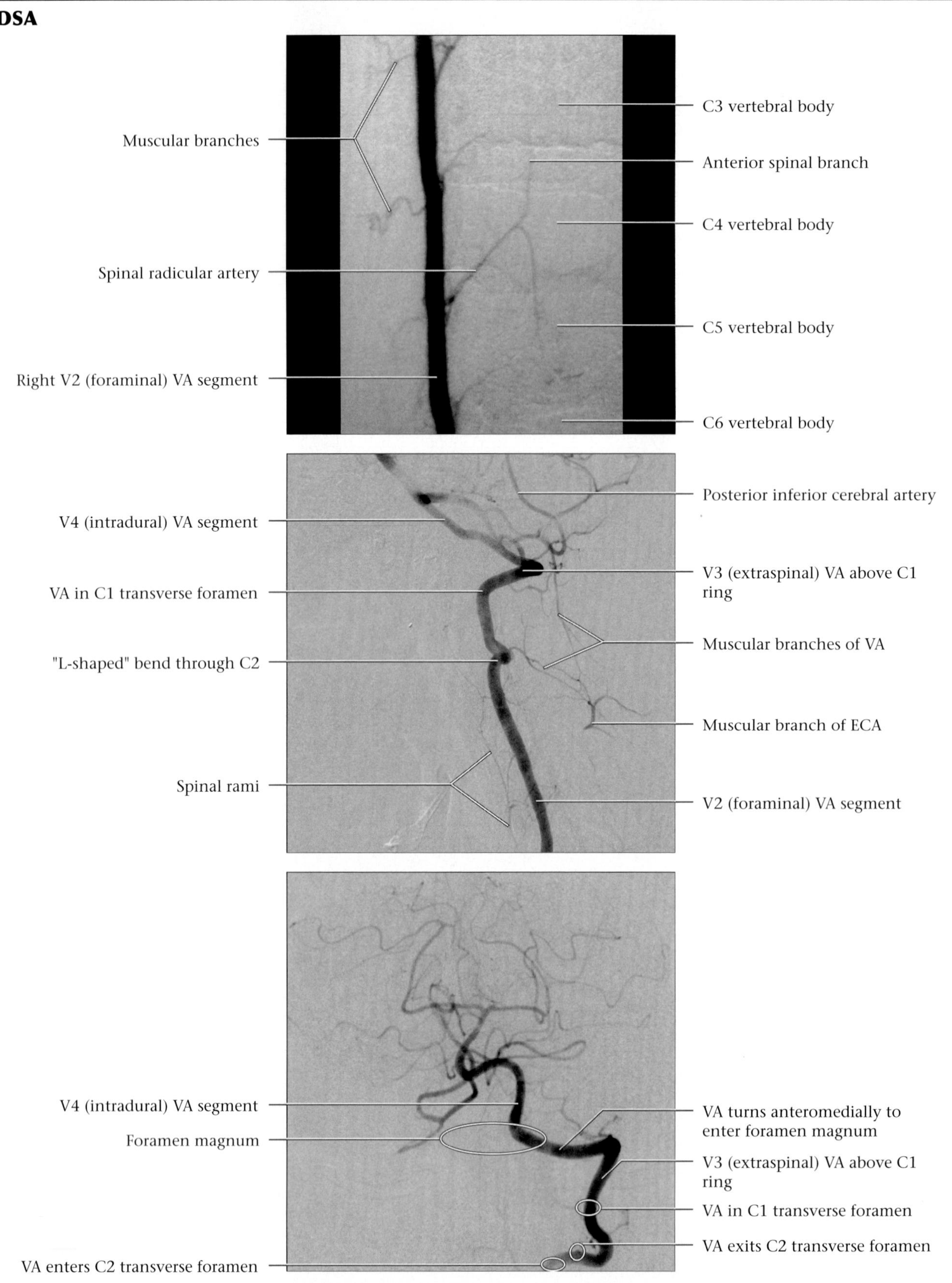

Muscular branches
Spinal radicular artery
Right V2 (foraminal) VA segment
C3 vertebral body
Anterior spinal branch
C4 vertebral body
C5 vertebral body
C6 vertebral body
V4 (intradural) VA segment
VA in C1 transverse foramen
"L-shaped" bend through C2
Spinal rami
Posterior inferior cerebral artery
V3 (extraspinal) VA above C1 ring
Muscular branches of VA
Muscular branch of ECA
V2 (foraminal) VA segment
V4 (intradural) VA segment
Foramen magnum
VA enters C2 transverse foramen
VA turns anteromedially to enter foramen magnum
V3 (extraspinal) VA above C1 ring
VA in C1 transverse foramen
VA exits C2 transverse foramen

(Top) Close-up AP view of right vertebral DSA shows the extracranial VA as it courses cephalad in the transverse foramina of C6 to C3. Segmental spinal rami and muscular branches arise from the V2 (foraminal) VA segment. Here, a prominent spinal ramus is large enough to reach the anterior median sulcus of the spinal cord where it divides into ascending and descending branches. These anastomose with the anterior spinal artery, which arises from the intradural VA. **(Middle)** Lateral DSA of vertebral angiogram shows the upper V2 (foraminal), V3 (extraspinal), and V4 (intradural) VA segments. Note prominent spinal arteries and anastomosis with muscular branches of the ECA. **(Bottom)** AP view shows VA course through the C2-C1 transverse foramina and above the C1 ring together with its anterior turn into the foramen magnum forming a "half square."

3D-VRT CTA

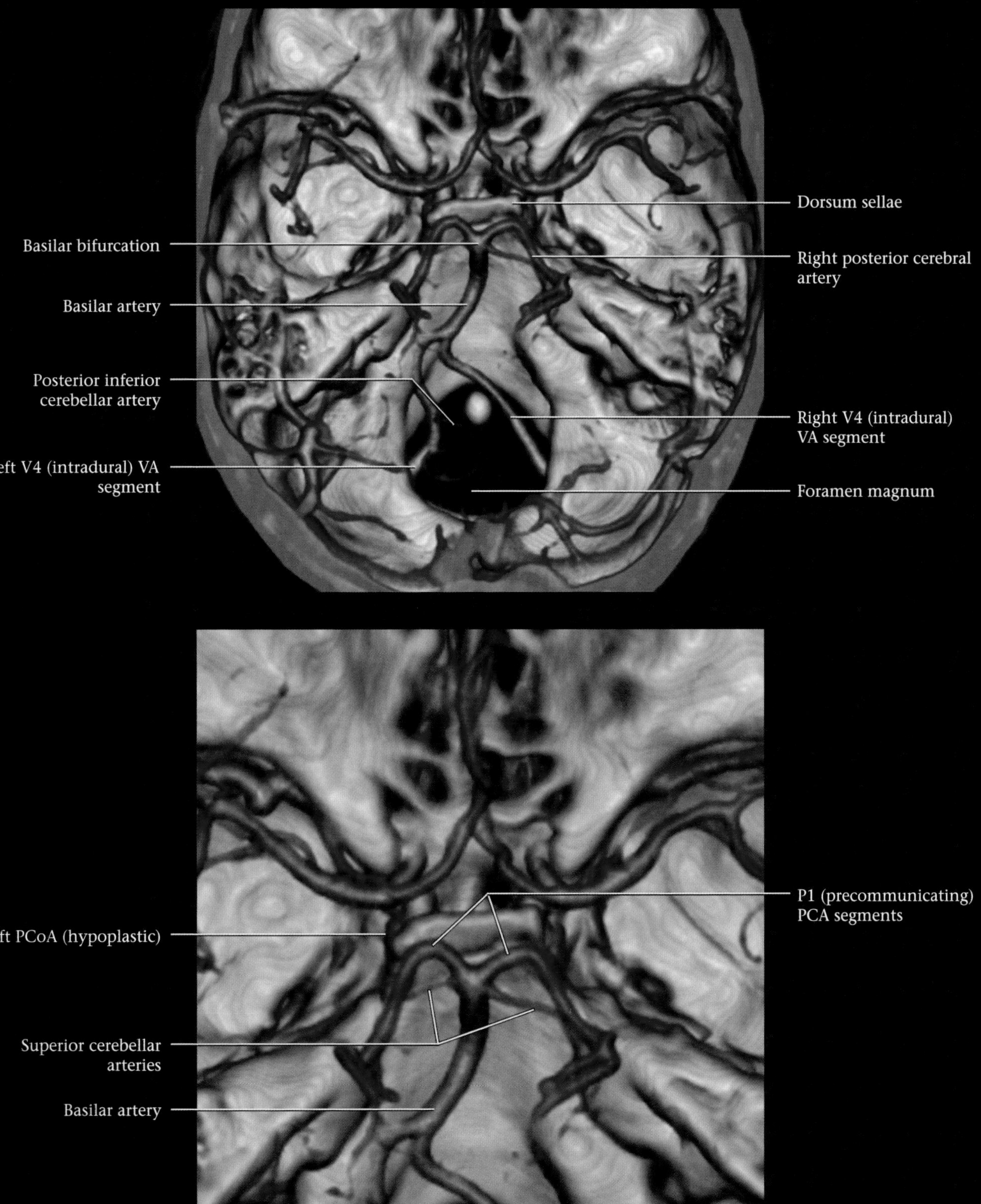

Dorsum sellae
Basilar bifurcation
Right posterior cerebral artery
Basilar artery
Posterior inferior cerebellar artery
Right V4 (intradural) VA segment
Left V4 (intradural) VA segment
Foramen magnum
P1 (precommunicating) PCA segments
Left PCoA (hypoplastic)
Superior cerebellar arteries
Basilar artery

(Top) 3D-VRT CTA of the intracranial circulation as seen from above. The skull and brain have been digitally removed to show the intracranial vertebrobasilar system and circle of Willis. The vertebral arteries pierce the dura at the foramen magnum and course anterosuperiorly to form the BA. The BA bifurcates about the level of the dorsum sellae into its two terminal branches, the posterior cerebral arteries. **(Bottom)** Close-up view shows the distal BA bifurcation. The superior cerebellar arteries arise just proximal to the bifurcation and are well seen here. The horizontal (P1) PCA segments are normal in size as both posterior communicating arteries (PCoAs) are small.

VERTEBROBASILAR SYSTEM

LATERAL DSA

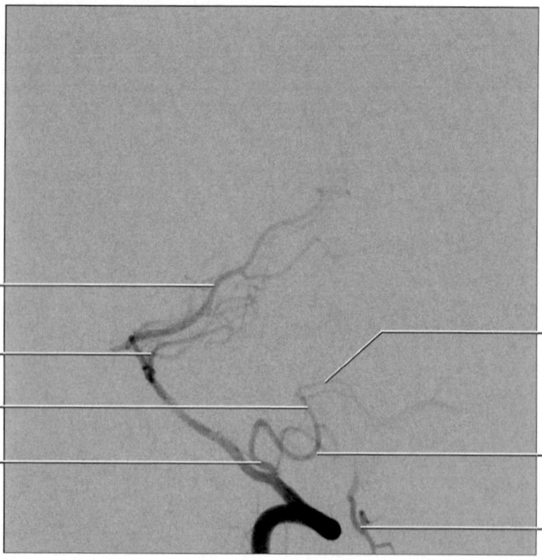

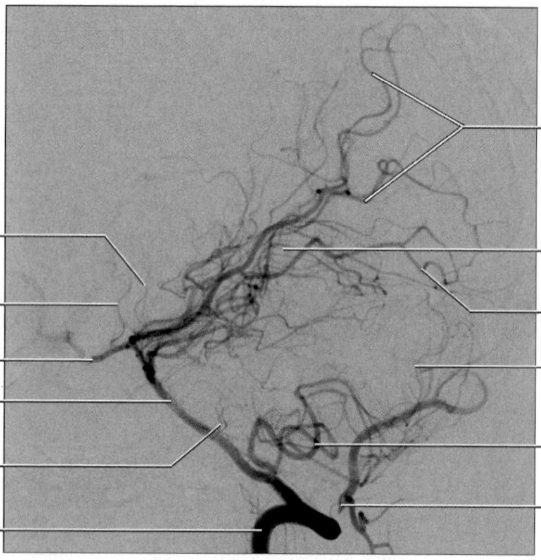

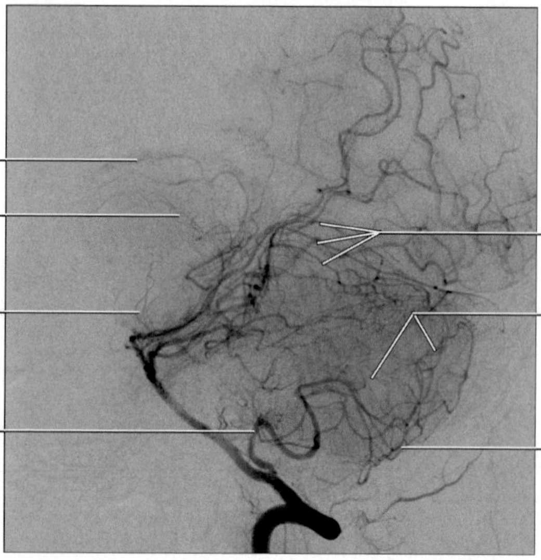

Posterior cerebral artery
Superior cerebellar artery (SCA)
PICA, posterior medullary segment
PICA, anterior medullary segment
PICA, supratonsillar segment
PICA, lateral medullary segment
Muscular branch of cervical VA ramus
Parietooccipital artery
Posterior thalamoperforating artery
Anterior thalamoperforating artery
Posterior communicating artery
Basilar artery
Basilar perforating arteries
V3 (extraspinal) VA segment
Superior vermian, cerebellar arteries
Calcarine artery (PCA branch)
Inferior vermian artery
Posterior inferior cerebellarl artery
Occipital artery (ECA branch)
Lateral posterior choroidal artery
Medial posterior choroidal artery
Thalamoperforating arteries
Posterior inferior cerebral artery
Superior hemispheric branches of SCA
PICA branches in great horizontal fissure of cerebellum
PICA hemispheric branches

(Top) Lateral view of a left vertebral DSA, early arterial phase, shows the intracranial vertebrobasilar system. PICA and its proximal loops are especially well seen. PICA has four segments and two distinct loops. The caudal or inferior loop is along the inferior medulla and may be as low as C2. The second (cranial) loop occurs as PICA courses above or across the cerebellar tonsil. **(Middle)** Mid-arterial phase shows distal branches of the VA and basilar artery. Note important vascular anastomosis between muscular branches of the VA and the occipital artery (an external carotid branch). The PCoA and its thalamoperforating branches are opacified. **(Bottom)** Late arterial phase shows normal vascular "blush" in territory supplied by the vertebrobasilar system. This includes the brainstem, vermis, cerebellum, occipital lobe, posterior thalami and some choroid plexus.

AP DSA

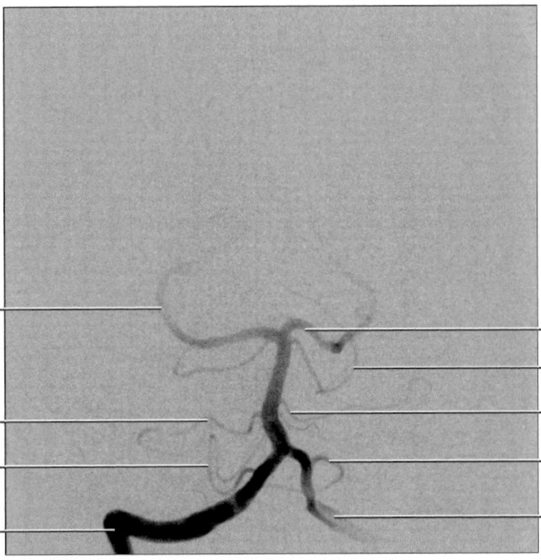

Right posterior cerebral artery
Left posterior cerebral artery
Superior cerebellar artery
Right AICA
Left AICA
Right PICA (posterior medullary segment)
Left PICA
Right vertebral artery
Unopacified blood in left VA

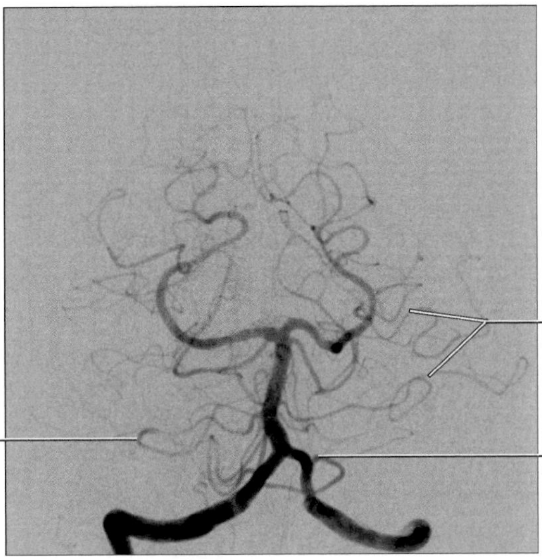

Cerebellar hemispheric branches
AICA looping into IAC
Anterior medullary segment of left PICA

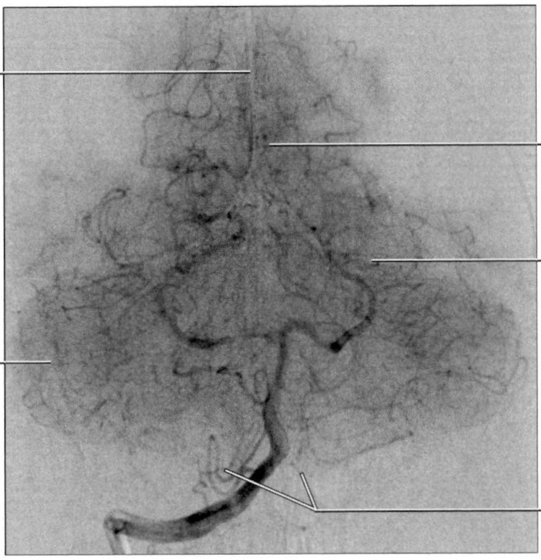

Falx cerebri
Calcarine cortex
Tentorium cerebelli
Cerebellar hemisphere
Cerebellar tonsils

(Top) AP view of right vertebral DSA, early arterial phase, shows origins of the major vertebral (VA) and basilar (BA) branches. Contrast has refluxed into the left VA, which is partially filled with unopacified blood. In this case, both the (PICAs) and (AICAs) arise separately, from the vertebral and basilar arteries respectively. **(Middle)** Mid-arterial phase shows the hemispheric branches of both PICAs, AICAs and superior cerebellar arteries. The right AICA is seen as it loops into the internal auditory canal (IAC). **(Bottom)** Later phase shows a dense vascular "blush" of the entire cerebellum and occipital lobes, and nicely demonstrates the vertebrobasilar vascular territory. The tentorium and falx are seen as thin, unopacified areas between the cerebellar hemispheres and occipital lobes.

VERTEBROBASILAR SYSTEM

MRA

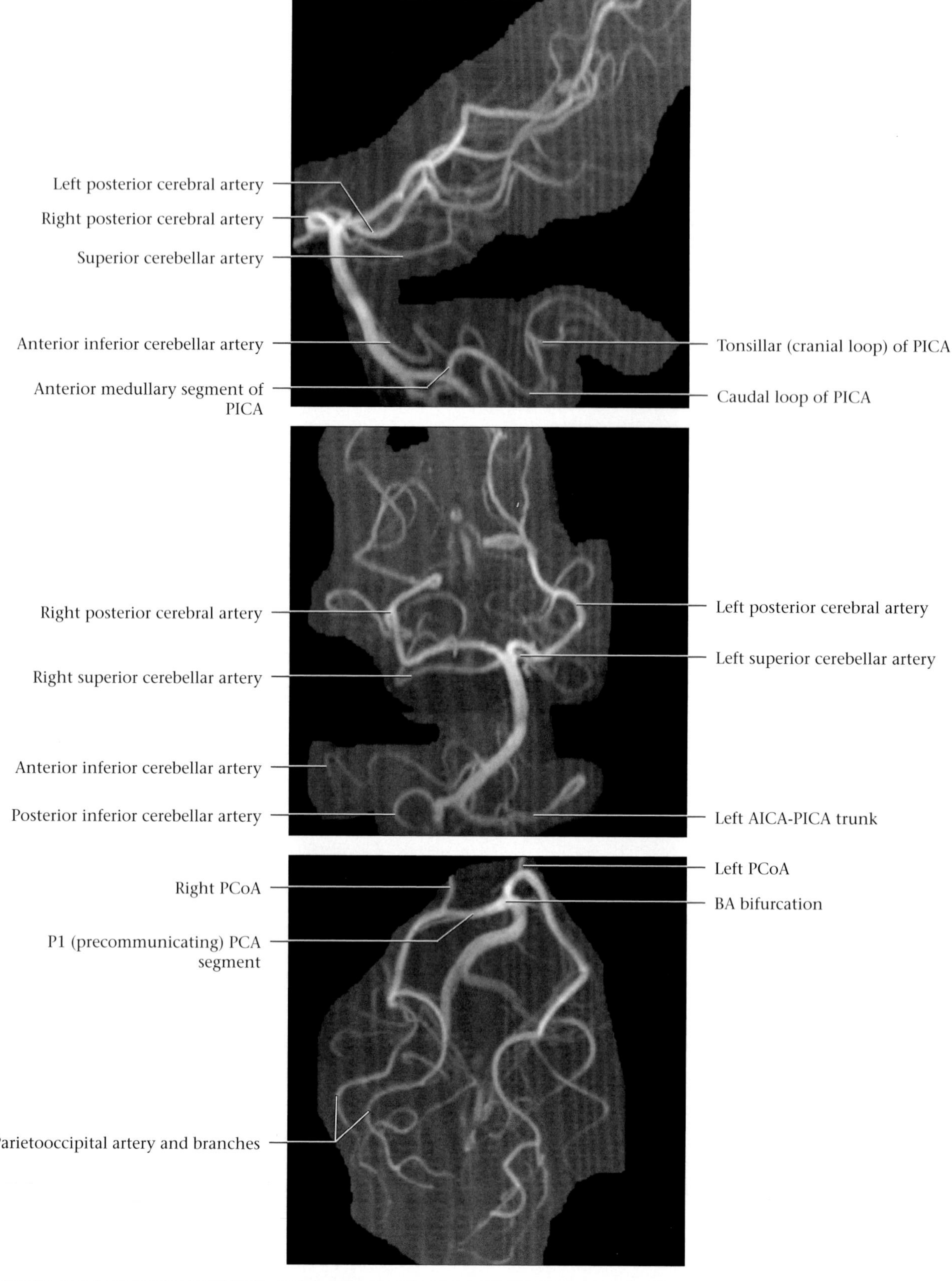

Left posterior cerebral artery
Right posterior cerebral artery
Superior cerebellar artery
Anterior inferior cerebellar artery
Anterior medullary segment of PICA
Tonsillar (cranial loop) of PICA
Caudal loop of PICA
Right posterior cerebral artery
Right superior cerebellar artery
Anterior inferior cerebellar artery
Posterior inferior cerebellar artery
Left posterior cerebral artery
Left superior cerebellar artery
Left AICA-PICA trunk
Right PCoA
P1 (precommunicating) PCA segment
Parietooccipital artery and branches
Left PCoA
BA bifurcation

(Top) Slightly oblique lateral view of an MRA shows the intracranial vertebrobasilar circulation. Here the posterior inferior and anterior inferior cerebellar arteries are especially well seen. **(Middle)** AP view shows the distal basilar bifurcation and more proximal branches. Two prominent superior cerebellar arteries are well seen here. On the left, a prominent VA branch is an AICA-PICA trunk. Common origin of these two branches from the VA is a frequent normal variant. **(Bottom)** Submentovertex view shows the basilar artery bifurcation especially well. The posterior cerebral and superior cerebellar branches are superimposed and loop laterally around the midbrain.

GRAPHICS

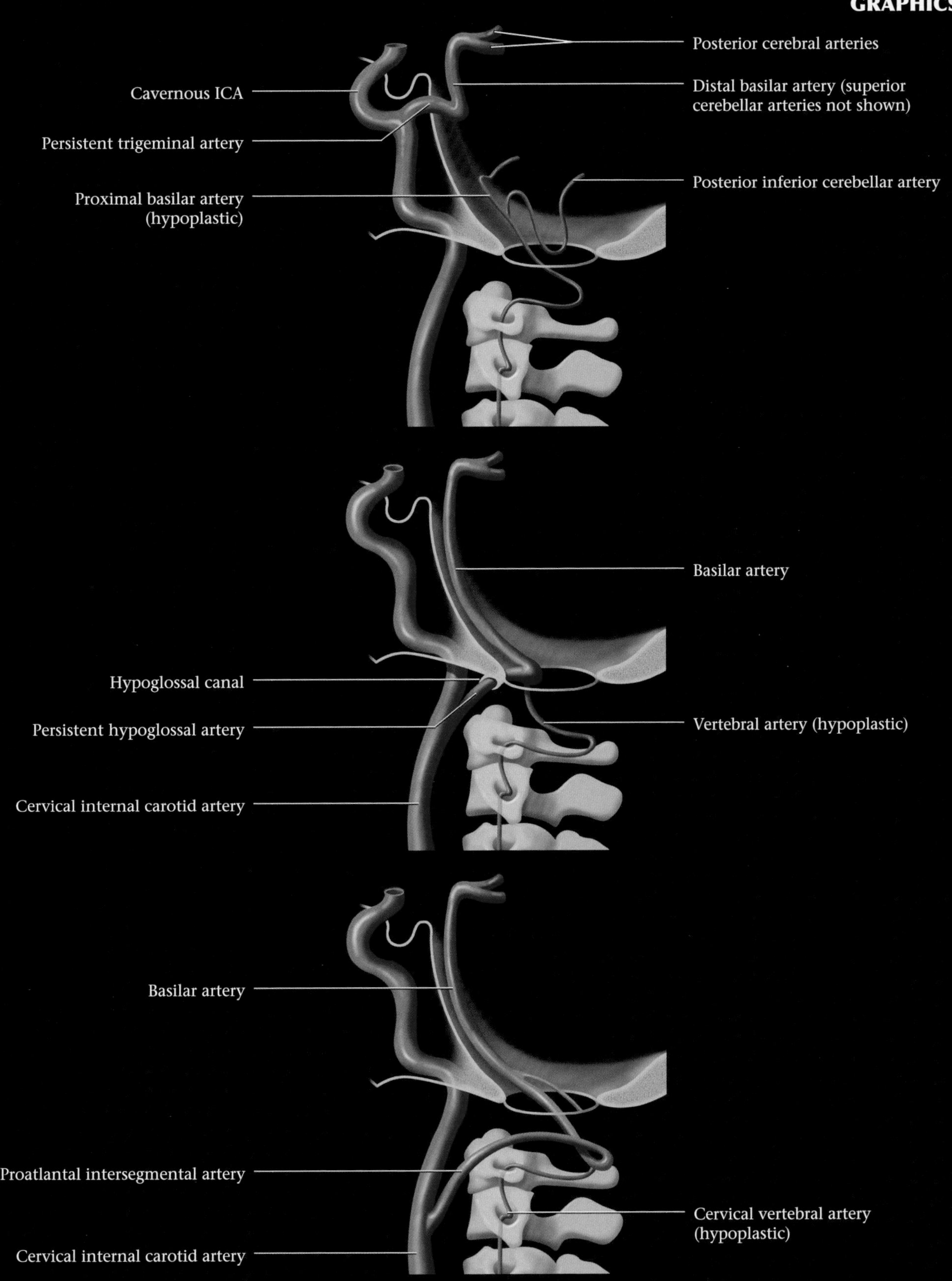
Posterior cerebral arteries
Cavernous ICA
Distal basilar artery (superior cerebellar arteries not shown)
Persistent trigeminal artery
Posterior inferior cerebellar artery
Proximal basilar artery (hypoplastic)
Basilar artery
Hypoglossal canal
Persistent hypoglossal artery
Vertebral artery (hypoplastic)
Cervical internal carotid artery
Basilar artery
Proatlantal intersegmental artery
Cervical vertebral artery (hypoplastic)
Cervical internal carotid artery

(Top) Persistent carotid-basilar anastomoses are depicted. This lateral graphic depicts a persistent trigeminal artery (PTA). Note typical "Neptune trident" appearance formed by ICA, PTA. A hypoplastic vertebral artery ends in PICA and AICA. The basilar artery between AICA and the PTA is absent. The posterior communicating artery is also absent. This is a Saltzman type I PTA. **(Middle)** Persistent (primitive) hypoglossal artery (PHA) is shown, originating from the ICA at C1-2 level and passing posterosuperiorly through an enlarged hypoglossal canal. The PHA does not traverse the foramen magnum and supplies the distal basilar artery. The ipsilateral VA is hypoplastic. **(Bottom)** Proatlantal intersegmental artery arises from the ICA at C2-3, courses posterosuperiorly between C1 and the occiput to join the VA.

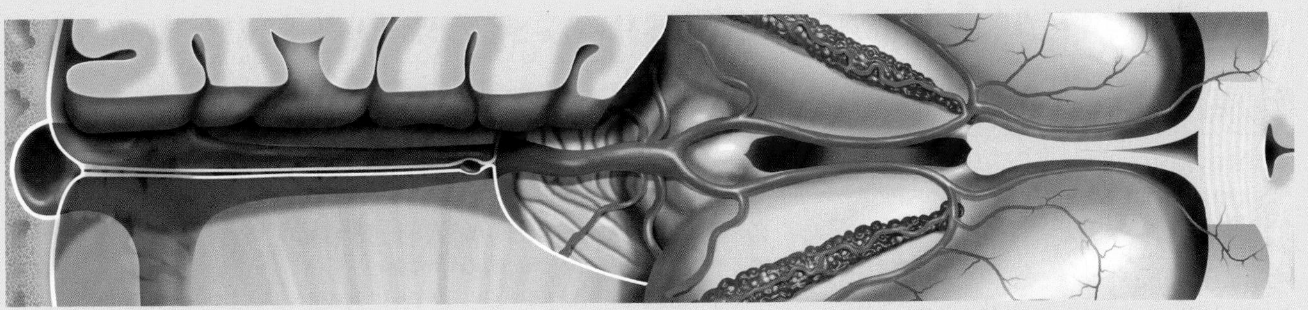

SECTION 8: Veins and Venous Sinuses

INTRACRANIAL VENOUS SYSTEM OVERVIEW

Terminology

Abbreviations

- Superior sagittal sinus (SSS)
- Inferior sagittal sinus (ISS)
- Internal cerebral vein (ICV)
- Straight sinus (SS)
- Great cerebral vein (vein of Galen, VofG)
- Transverse sinus (TS)
- Superior/inferior petrosal sinuses (SPS/IPS)
- Cavernous sinus (CS)
- Internal jugular vein (IJV)
- Basal vein of Rosenthal (BVR)
- Superficial, deep middle cerebral veins (SMCV; DMCV)

Definitions

- **Dural sinuses** are large, endothelial-lined trabeculated venous channels encased within folds/reflections of dura that define, form their walls
- **Cerebral veins** are thin-walled, valveless structures that cross SAS, pierce arachnoid/inner dura to enter dural venous sinus

Gross Anatomy

Overview

- **Dural venous sinuses** (divided into two groups)
  - **Anteroinferior group** (CS, SPS/IPS, clival, sphenoparietal)
  - **Posterosuperior group** (SSS, ISS, SS, TS, sigmoid, occipital)
- **Cerebral veins** (divided into 3 groups)
  - **Superficial ("external") veins** (3 subgroups)
    - Superior: 8-12 smaller cortical veins over hemispheres, vein of Trolard
    - Middle: SMCV, vein of Labbé
    - Inferior: DMCV, BVR
  - **Deep ("internal") veins**
    - Subependymal veins
    - ICVs (formed by thalamostriate, septal veins)
    - Great cerebral vein (VofG)
  - **Brainstem/posterior fossa veins** (3 subgroups)
    - Superior (galenic) group
    - Anterior (petrosal) group
    - Posterior (tentorial) group
- **Venous vascular territories**
  - More variable, less well-known than arterial territories
  - General concepts
    - Venous drainage generally radial, centrifugal (exception = deep cerebral structures)
    - Much of middle/superior brain surfaces (cortex, subcortical white matter) drained by cortical veins to SSS
    - Posterior/inferior temporal lobe, adjacent parietal lobe drained by vein of Labbé to TS
    - Insular cortex, parenchyma around sylvian (middle cerebral) fissure drained by sphenoparietal sinus to CS
    - Deep cerebral structures (central/deep white matter, basal ganglia) drained by medullary/subependymal veins to ICVs, VofG, SS; medial temporal lobe via DMCV/BVR to VofG

Anatomy Relationships

- **Dural venous sinuses**
  - Communicate with extracranial veins directly (via diploic veins in calvarium, emissary veins through basilar foramina)
  - Receive venous blood from superficial (cortical) veins, deep (subependymal) veins
- **Cerebral veins**
  - Superficial (cortical) veins lie in SAS, mainly follow sulci
  - Subependymal veins outline ventricles

Imaging Anatomy

Overview

- **Dural venous sinuses**
  - Visualization at DSA varies widely
    - Almost always: SSS, SS, TS, sigmoid sinus, internal jugular veins (IJVs)
    - Sometimes: ISS, SPS/IPS
    - Rare/inconstant: CS, sphenoparietal sinus, occipital sinus, clival (basal) venous plexus
- **Cerebral veins**
  - Superficial cortical veins almost always seen (number, configuration vary)
  - Deep veins almost always seen on late venous phase of DSA, only largest (e.g., thalamostriate veins) seen on MR/MRV
  - ICVs, VofG almost always seen on DSA, CTV, MRV

Anatomy-Based Imaging Issues

Imaging Recommendations

- Obtain source images for MR venogram perpendicular to main axis of dural sinus (e.g., coronal for SSS)
- MRV, CTV excellent for general overview of dural sinuses, cerebral veins but DSA best for detailed delineation

Imaging Pitfalls

- TSs often asymmetric, hypoplastic/atretic segment common (do not misdiagnose as occlusion)
- Saturation bands on MR disguise flow
- Jugular bulb flow often very asymmetric, turbulent (pseudolesion)
- Unopacified venous blood streaming into dural sinus on DSA should not be mistaken for filling defect (thrombus)
- "Giant" arachnoid granulations appear as round/ovoid CSF-equivalent filling defects in dural sinuses (especially TS), are a normal variant, should not be mistaken for thrombus
- Acute dural sinus, cortical vein thrombi isointense with brain on T1WI so T2* (GRE) or T1 C+ imaging very helpful
- Subacute clot is hyperintense on T1WI (do not mistake for enhancement)

INTRACRANIAL VENOUS SYSTEM OVERVIEW

GRAPHICS

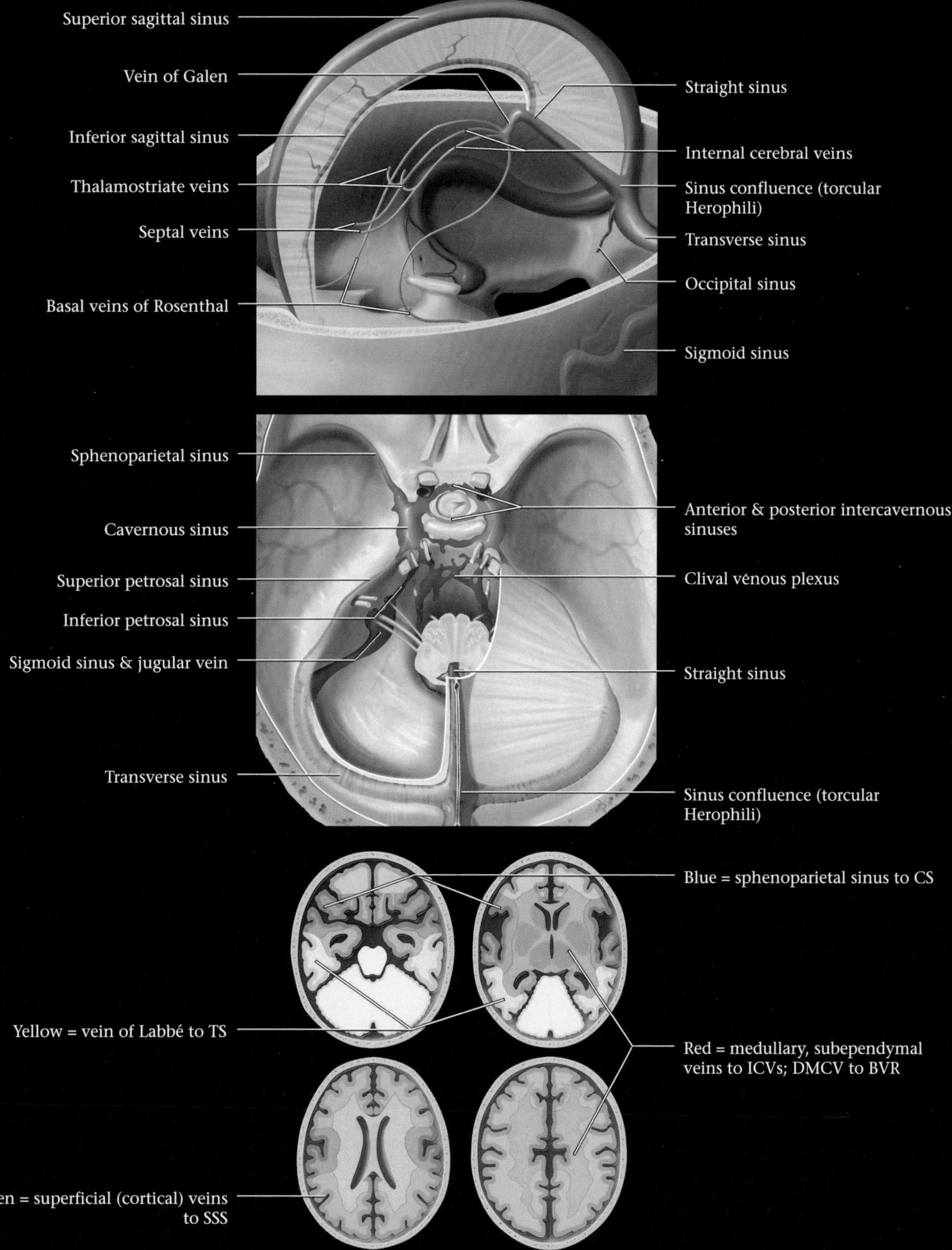

Superior sagittal sinus
Vein of Galen
Inferior sagittal sinus
Thalamostriate veins
Septal veins
Basal veins of Rosenthal
Straight sinus
Internal cerebral veins
Sinus confluence (torcular Herophili)
Transverse sinus
Occipital sinus
Sigmoid sinus
Sphenoparietal sinus
Cavernous sinus
Superior petrosal sinus
Inferior petrosal sinus
Sigmoid sinus & jugular vein
Transverse sinus
Anterior & posterior intercavernous sinuses
Clival venous plexus
Straight sinus
Sinus confluence (torcular Herophili)
Blue = sphenoparietal sinus to CS
Yellow = vein of Labbé to TS
Red = medullary, subependymal veins to ICVs; DMCV to BVR
Green = superficial (cortical) veins to SSS

(Top) A series of three graphics provides an overview of the intracranial veins and their drainage territories. The first of these, a 3D rendering of falx cerebri with major dural sinuses and deep veins, shows the interconnections between these two venous systems. **(Middle)** Intracranial view depicts the major dural venous sinuses as seen from top down. The cerebral hemispheres, midbrain and pons as well as the left half of the tentorium cerebelli have been removed. Note the numerous interconnections between both halves of the cavernous sinus, the clival venous plexus, and the petrosal sinuses. **(Bottom)** A series of four axial sections depicts typical venous drainage patterns of the cerebral hemispheres. In general, the deep white matter and basal ganglia are drained by the ICV and its tributaries (such as medullary veins).

INTRACRANIAL VENOUS SYSTEM OVERVIEW

AXIAL CECT

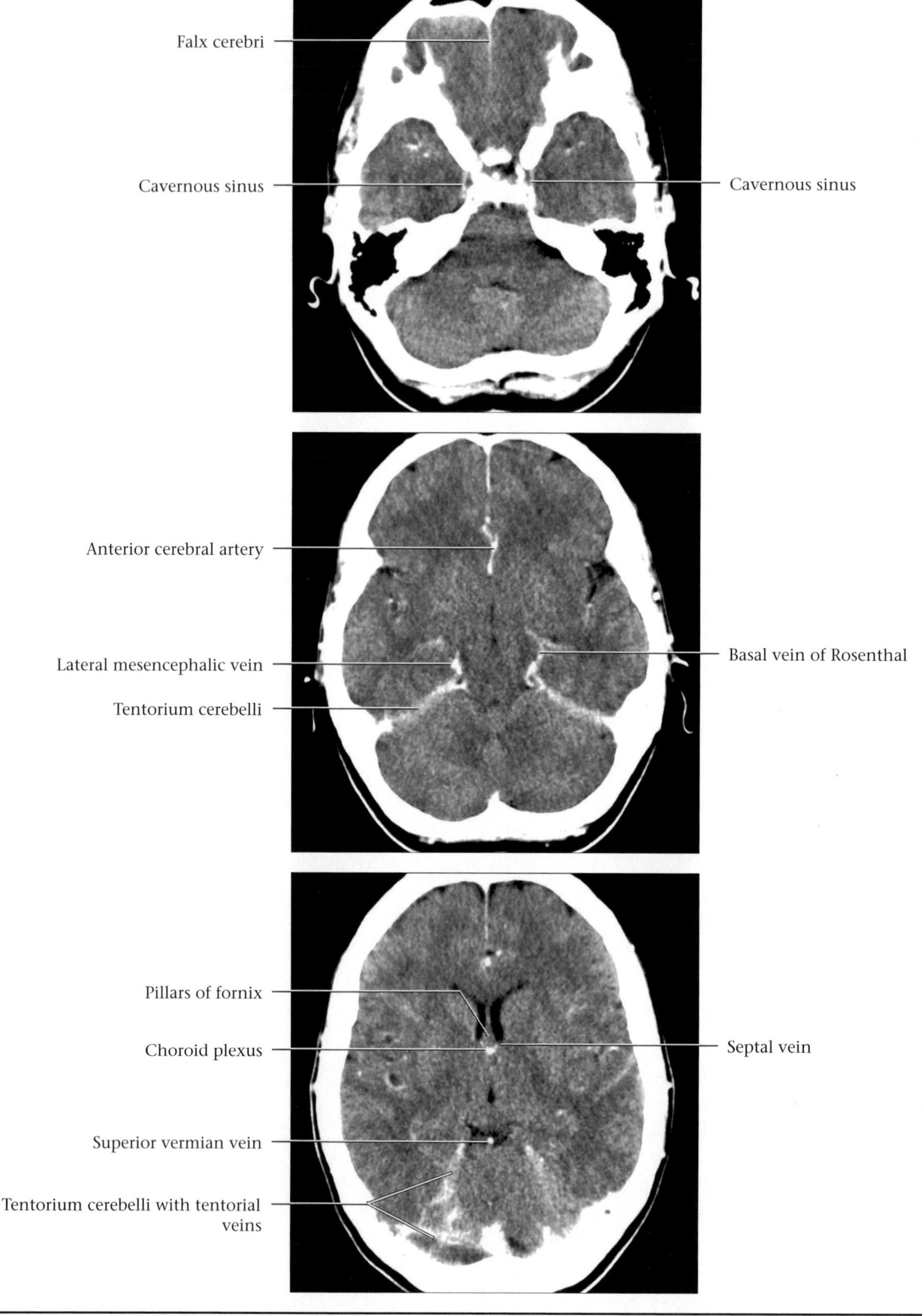
Falx cerebri
Cavernous sinus
Cavernous sinus
Anterior cerebral artery
Lateral mesencephalic vein
Basal vein of Rosenthal
Tentorium cerebelli
Pillars of fornix
Choroid plexus
Septal vein
Superior vermian vein
Tentorium cerebelli with tentorial veins

(Top) Series of six selected axial CECT images through the brain from inferior to superior are shown. Contrast in the lateral dural wall of the cavernous sinus is seen on this section. **(Middle)** Section through the midbrain shows dura of the tentorium cerebelli with adjacent basal veins of Rosenthal and lateral mesencephalic veins. **(Bottom)** Section through the foramen of Monro shows septal veins as they curve around the pillars of the fornix behind the frontal horns of both lateral ventricles. The larger, midline enhancing area represents choroid plexus as it is passing inferiorly from the lateral ventricles and forming the posterior border of the foramen of Monro. The anterior border is formed by the pillars of the fornix.

AXIAL CECT

Septal vein

Vein of Galen

Straight sinus

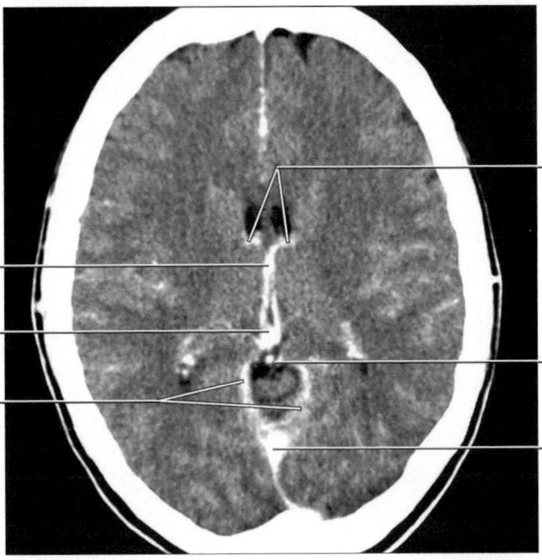

Thalamostriate veins

Internal cerebral veins (paired)

Vein of Galen

Precentral cerebellar vein

Apex of tentorium

Straight sinus

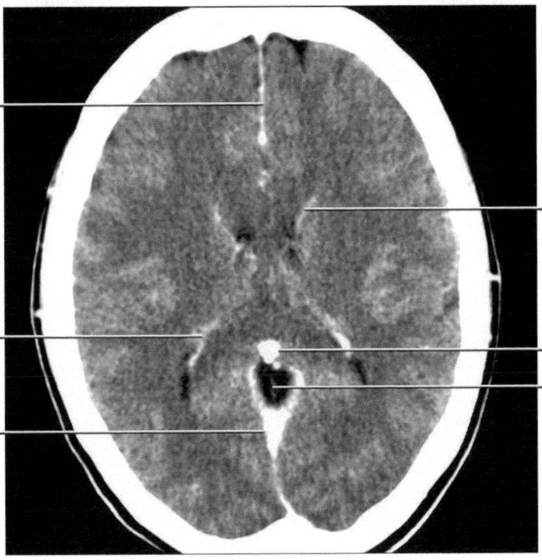

Falx cerebri

Anterior caudate vein

Choroid plexus, veins

Pineal gland (calcified)

Superior vermian cistern

Straight sinus

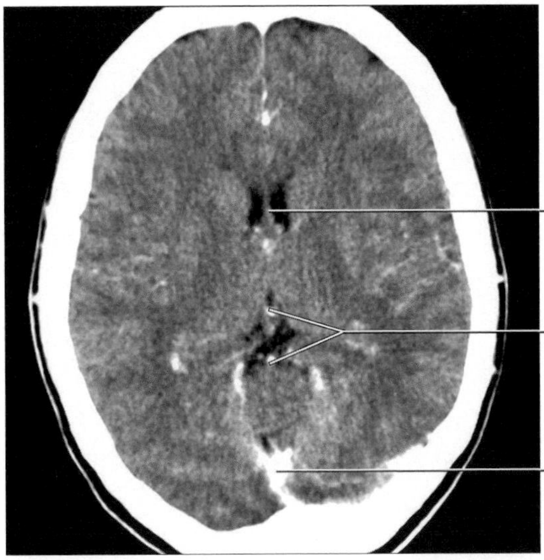

(Top) Scan at the level of the upper foramen of Monro. The vein of Galen, a "U-shaped" structure, is seen here with its anterior and posterior segments seen as two contrast-filled "dots" that curve above the pineal gland and under the corpus callosum splenium. **(Middle)** Section through the internal cerebral veins, paired paramedian structures, shows their extent from the thalamostriate tributaries anteriorly to the vein of Galen posteriorly. **(Bottom)** Scan through the upper ventricles and tentorial apex is depicted. Anterior caudate veins are subependymal tributaries of the thalamostriate veins. The septal and thalamostriate veins join to form the internal cerebral veins.

INTRACRANIAL VENOUS SYSTEM OVERVIEW

AXIAL T1 C+ MR

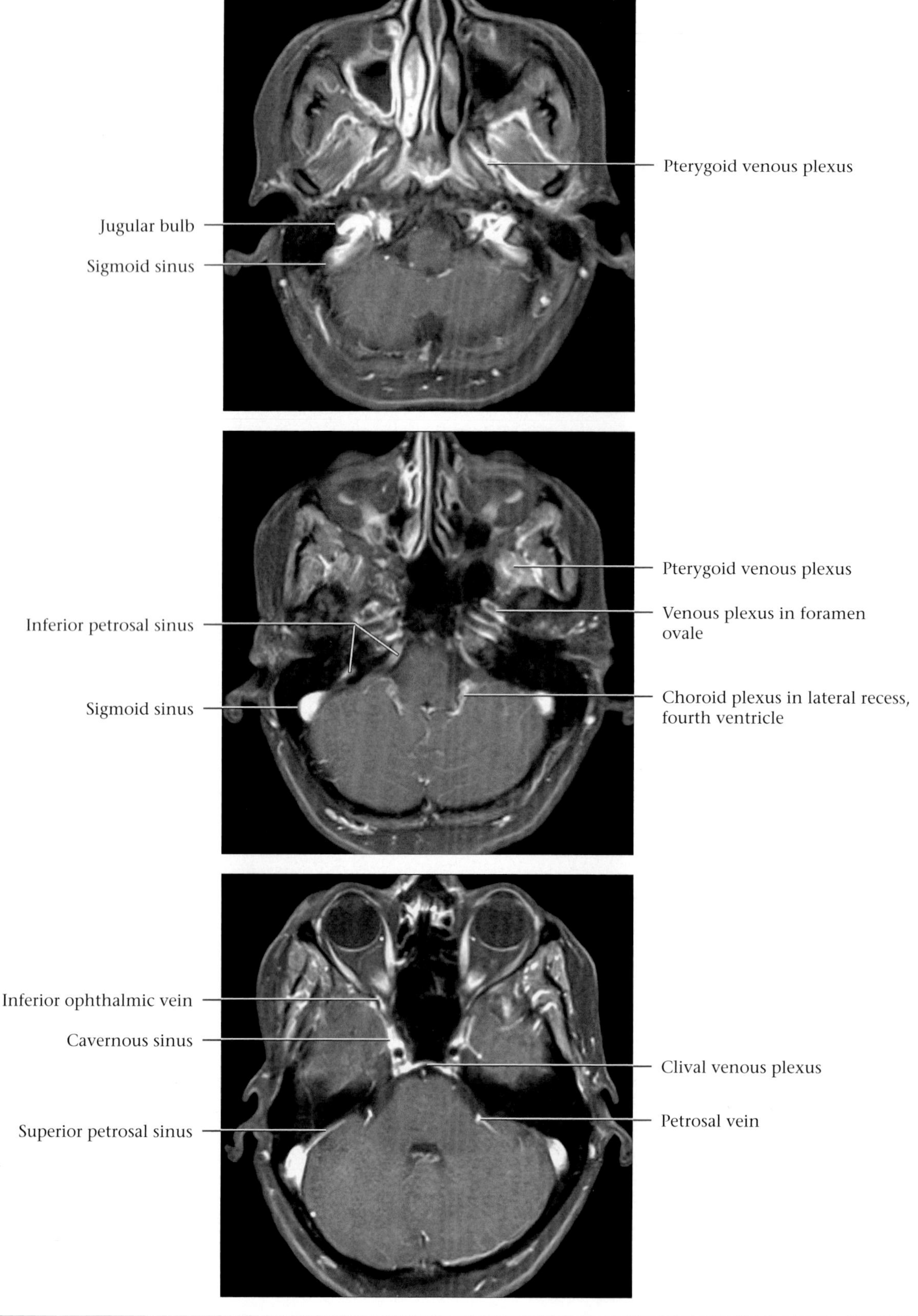

Pterygoid venous plexus
Jugular bulb
Sigmoid sinus
Pterygoid venous plexus
Venous plexus in foramen ovale
Inferior petrosal sinus
Choroid plexus in lateral recess, fourth ventricle
Sigmoid sinus
Inferior ophthalmic vein
Cavernous sinus
Clival venous plexus
Petrosal vein
Superior petrosal sinus

(Top) Series of nine axial T1 C+ MR scans from inferior to superior are depicted. Note inhomogeneous flow in the jugular bulb. This is normal and should not be mistaken for a mass or thrombus (jugular "pseudolesion"). **(Middle)** Section through the lateral recesses of the fourth ventricle shows the inferior petrosal sinuses, tributaries of the jugular bulb. The pterygoid venous plexus and the venous plexus in the foramen ovale are connected through the skull base to the cavernous sinus. These intra- to extracranial connections may provide an important source of collateral venous drainage if the CS becomes occluded. **(Bottom)** Section through the cavernous sinus shows connections with the clival plexus and the orbit (inferior ophthalmic vein). Petrosal veins in the cerebellopontine angle cistern are prominent but normal in this case.

INTRACRANIAL VENOUS SYSTEM OVERVIEW

AXIAL T1 C+ MR

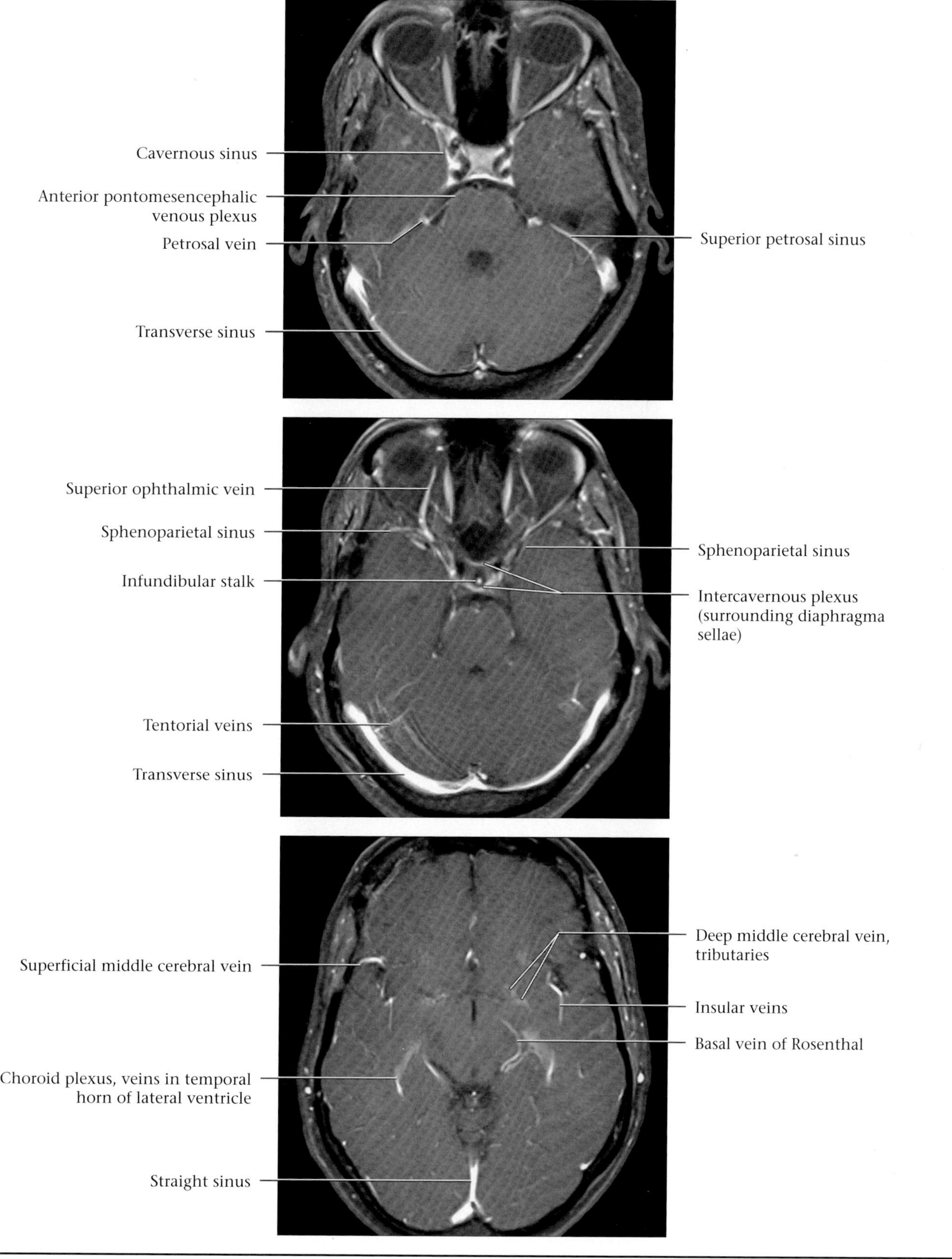
Cavernous sinus
Anterior pontomesencephalic venous plexus
Petrosal vein
Transverse sinus
Superior petrosal sinus
Superior ophthalmic vein
Sphenoparietal sinus
Infundibular stalk
Tentorial veins
Transverse sinus
Sphenoparietal sinus
Intercavernous plexus (surrounding diaphragma sellae)
Superficial middle cerebral vein
Choroid plexus, veins in temporal horn of lateral ventricle
Straight sinus
Deep middle cerebral vein, tributaries
Insular veins
Basal vein of Rosenthal

(Top) The cavernous sinus is especially well seen on this scan. Again note prominent petrosal veins in the upper cerebellopontine angle cisterns. The faint enhancement seen along the anterior belly of the pons is the anterior pontomesencephalic venous plexus and is normal, should not be mistaken for meningitis or leptomeningeal carcinomatosis. **(Middle)** Section through the upper cavernous sinus shows the intercavernous plexus surrounding the opening of the diaphragma sellae, which contains the infundibular stalk. Superior ophthalmic vein drains posteriorly into the cavernous sinus. **(Bottom)** Section through upper vermis shows the left BVR curving around midbrain, coursing posteriorly towards its confluence with the ICVs at the vein of Galen. The SMCV drains into the sphenoparietal sinus (shown on the lower section, above). DMCV drains into BVR and VofG.

INTRACRANIAL VENOUS SYSTEM OVERVIEW

AXIAL T1 C+ MR

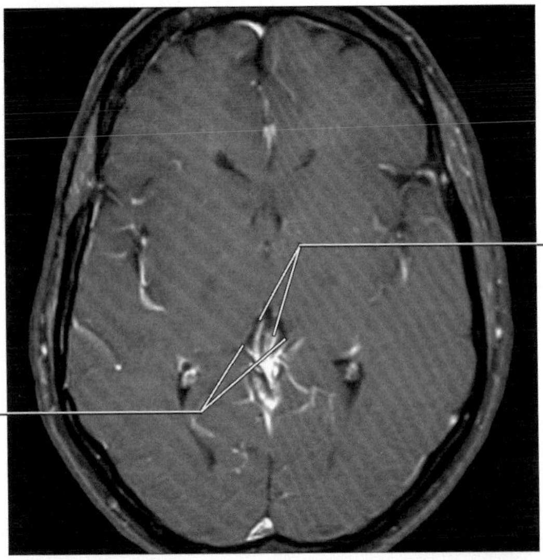

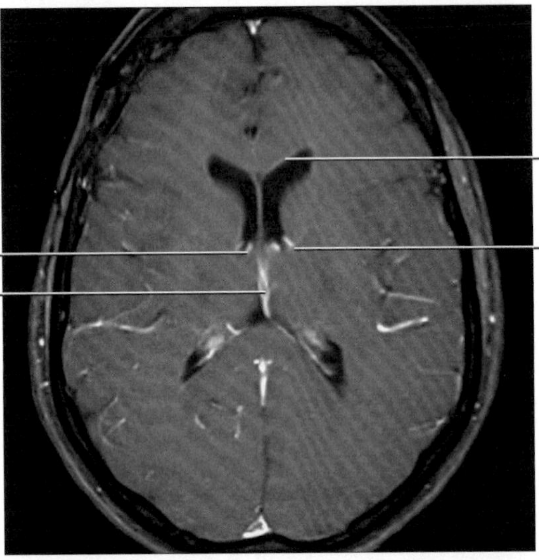

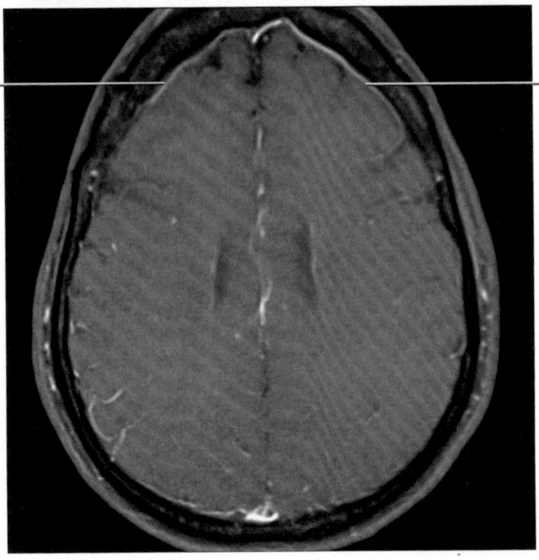

Internal cerebral veins

Basal veins of Rosenthal

Septal vein

Thalamostriate vein

Anterior caudate vein

Internal cerebral veins

Cortical vein

Cortical vein

(Top) The paired internal cerebral veins as they terminate in the vein of Galen are shown. Note the basal veins of Rosenthal terminating with the ICVs to form the great cerebral vein (of Galen). **(Middle)** Section through the foramen of Monro shows the septal, anterior caudate vein and thalamostriate tributaries of the internal cerebral veins. **(Bottom)** Most cephalad section shows prominent frontal superficial cortical veins, tributaries of the superior sagittal sinus.

INTRACRANIAL VENOUS SYSTEM OVERVIEW

LAT, OBL & AP MRV

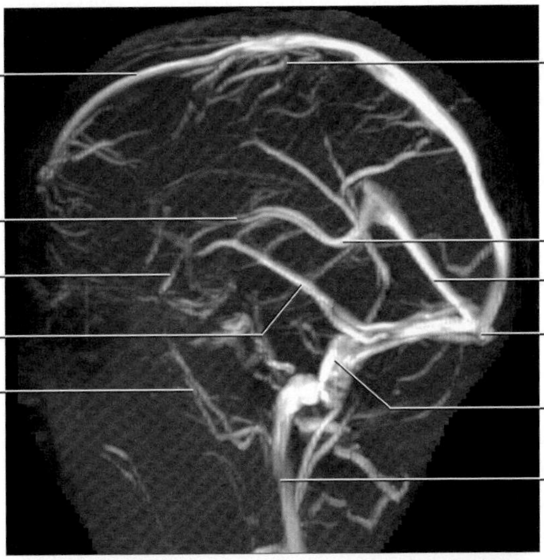

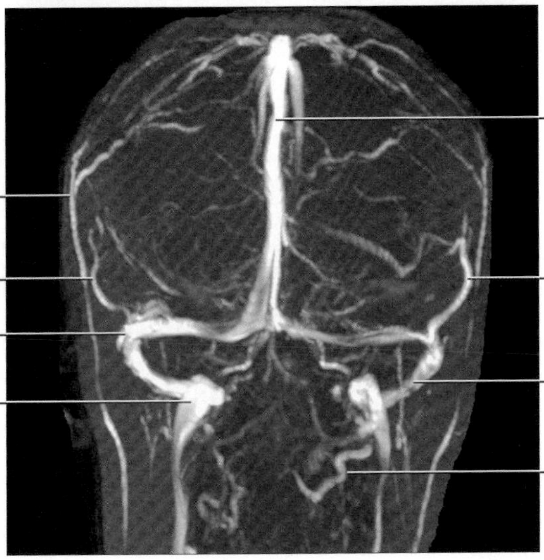

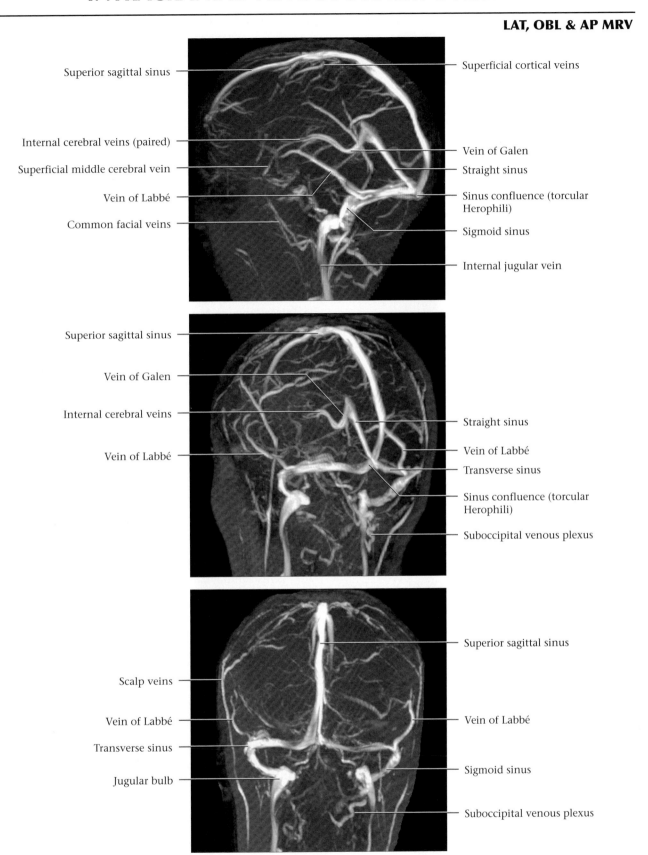

Superior sagittal sinus
Internal cerebral veins (paired)
Superficial middle cerebral vein
Vein of Labbé
Common facial veins
Superficial cortical veins
Vein of Galen
Straight sinus
Sinus confluence (torcular Herophili)
Sigmoid sinus
Internal jugular vein

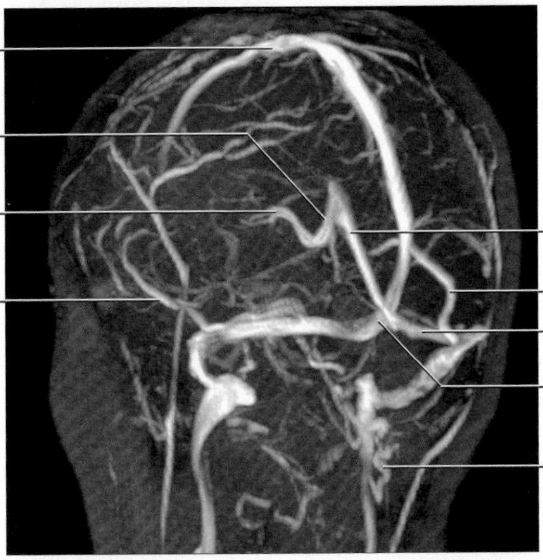

Superior sagittal sinus
Vein of Galen
Internal cerebral veins
Vein of Labbé
Straight sinus
Vein of Labbé
Transverse sinus
Sinus confluence (torcular Herophili)
Suboccipital venous plexus

Scalp veins
Vein of Labbé
Transverse sinus
Jugular bulb
Superior sagittal sinus
Vein of Labbé
Sigmoid sinus
Suboccipital venous plexus

(Top) Lateral view from an MRV demonstrates cerebral venous drainage. Dural venous sinuses and superficial cortical veins are well depicted on this lateral view. **(Middle)** Oblique view of the MRV shows dural sinuses draining posteroinferiorly to torcular Herophili, which splits into two nearly symmetric transverse sinuses. **(Bottom)** AP view shows superimposed superior sagittal and straight sinuses, which demonstrates slight but normal asymmetry of transverse sinuses. Larger (left) and smaller (right) veins of Labbé are seen here as they drain into the TS. The vein of Labbé can be quite large and drain a significant territory over the inferolateral cerebral hemisphere. If the TS becomes occluded, the vein of Labbé may also thrombose and cause a large venous infarct.

DURAL SINUSES

Terminology

Abbreviations

- Internal cerebral vein (ICV)
- Superior/inferior petrosal sinuses (SPS/IPS)

Gross Anatomy

Anatomy Relationships

- Endothelial-lined, contained within outer (periosteal), inner (meningeal) dural layers
- Often fenestrated, septated, multi-channeled
- Contain arachnoid granulations, villi
  - Extension of subarachnoid space (SAS) + arachnoid through dural wall into lumen of venous sinus
  - Returns cerebrospinal fluid (CSF) to venous circulation

Imaging Anatomy

Overview

- **Superior sagittal sinus (SSS)**
  - Appears as curvilinear structure that hugs inner calvarial vault
    - Originates from ascending frontal veins anteriorly
    - Runs posteriorly in midline at junction of falx cerebri with calvarium
  - Collects superficial cortical veins, increases in diameter as it courses posteriorly
  - Terminates at venous sinus confluence (often runs off midline posteriorly)
  - Important hemispheric tributary: Vein of Trolard
- **Inferior sagittal sinus (ISS)**
  - Smaller, inconstant channel in inferior (free) margin of falx cerebri
  - Lies above corpus callosum, from which it receives tributaries
  - Terminates at falcotentorial apex, joining with vein of Galen (VofG) to form straight sinus
- **Straight sinus (SS)**
  - Runs from falcotentorial apex posteroinferiorly to sinus confluence
  - Receives tributaries from falx, tentorium, cerebral hemispheres
- **Torcular Herophili (venous sinus confluence)**
  - Formed from union of SSS, SS, transverse sinuses
  - Often asymmetric, interconnections between TS highly variable
- **Transverse (lateral) sinuses (TSs)**
  - Contained between attachment of tentorial leaves to calvarium
  - Extends laterally from torcular to posterior border of petrous temporal bone
  - Often asymmetric (right side usually larger than left)
  - Hypoplastic/atretic segment common
  - Tributaries from tentorium, cerebellum, inferior temporal/occipital lobes
  - Important tributary: Vein of Labbé
- **Sigmoid sinuses**
  - Anteroinferior continuation of TSs
  - Gentle S-shaped inferior curve
  - Terminate by becoming internal jugular veins
- **Cavernous sinuses (CS)**
  - Irregularly-shaped, trabeculated venous compartment along sides of sella turcica
  - Contained within a prominent lateral, thin (often inapparent) medial dural wall
  - Extends from superior orbital fissure anteriorly to clivus and petrous apex posteriorly
  - Contains cavernous ICA, CN6 (inside CS itself) and 3, 4, V1 and V2 (within lateral dural wall)
  - Tributaries include superior/inferior ophthalmic veins, sphenoparietal sinus
  - Communicate inferiorly with pterygoid venous plexus, medially with contralateral CS, posteriorly with superior/inferior petrosal sinus, clival venous plexus
  - Inconstantly visualized at digital subtraction angiography
- **Miscellaneous dural venous sinuses**
  - Superior petrosal sinus (runs along petrous ridge from CS to sigmoid sinus)
  - Inferior petrosal sinus (runs along petrooccipital fissure from clival venous plexus to jugular bulb)
  - Sphenoparietal sinus (runs along lesser sphenoid wing from sylvian fissure to CS or IPS)
  - Occipital sinus (from foramen magnum to torcular)
  - Clival venous plexus (network of veins along clivus from dorsum sellae to foramen magnum)

Normal Variants, Anomalies

- Common variants
  - Absent anterior SSS (may begin posteriorly near coronal suture)
  - "Off-midline" SSS terminating directly in TS
  - Absence or hypoplasia of part/all of TS
  - Jugular bulbs can vary greatly in size, configuration (can be "high-riding", have jugular diverticulum, dehiscent jugular bulb)
  - "Giant" arachnoid granulations (round/ovoid CSF-equivalent filling defects in dural sinuses)
- Anomalies
  - Persistent embryonic falcine sinus (usually with VofG malformation)
  - Lambdoid-torcular inversion with high sinus confluence (with Dandy-Walker spectrum)

Anatomy-Based Imaging Issues

Imaging Recommendations

- Examine source images (not just reprojected views) of MRV/CTV
- DSA rarely required to diagnose dural sinus occlusion
- Acute dural sinus thrombus is isointense with brain on T1WI, profoundly hypointense on T2WI (may mimic "flow void") so T2* or T1 C+ imaging very helpful
- Subacute clot hyperintense on T1WI so pre-contrast scan needed to compare to T1 C+ images

Imaging Pitfalls

- TSs often asymmetric, hypoplastic/atretic segment common (do not misdiagnose as occlusion)
- Jugular bulbs often very asymmetric, turbulent flow (pseudoocclusion)

DURAL SINUSES

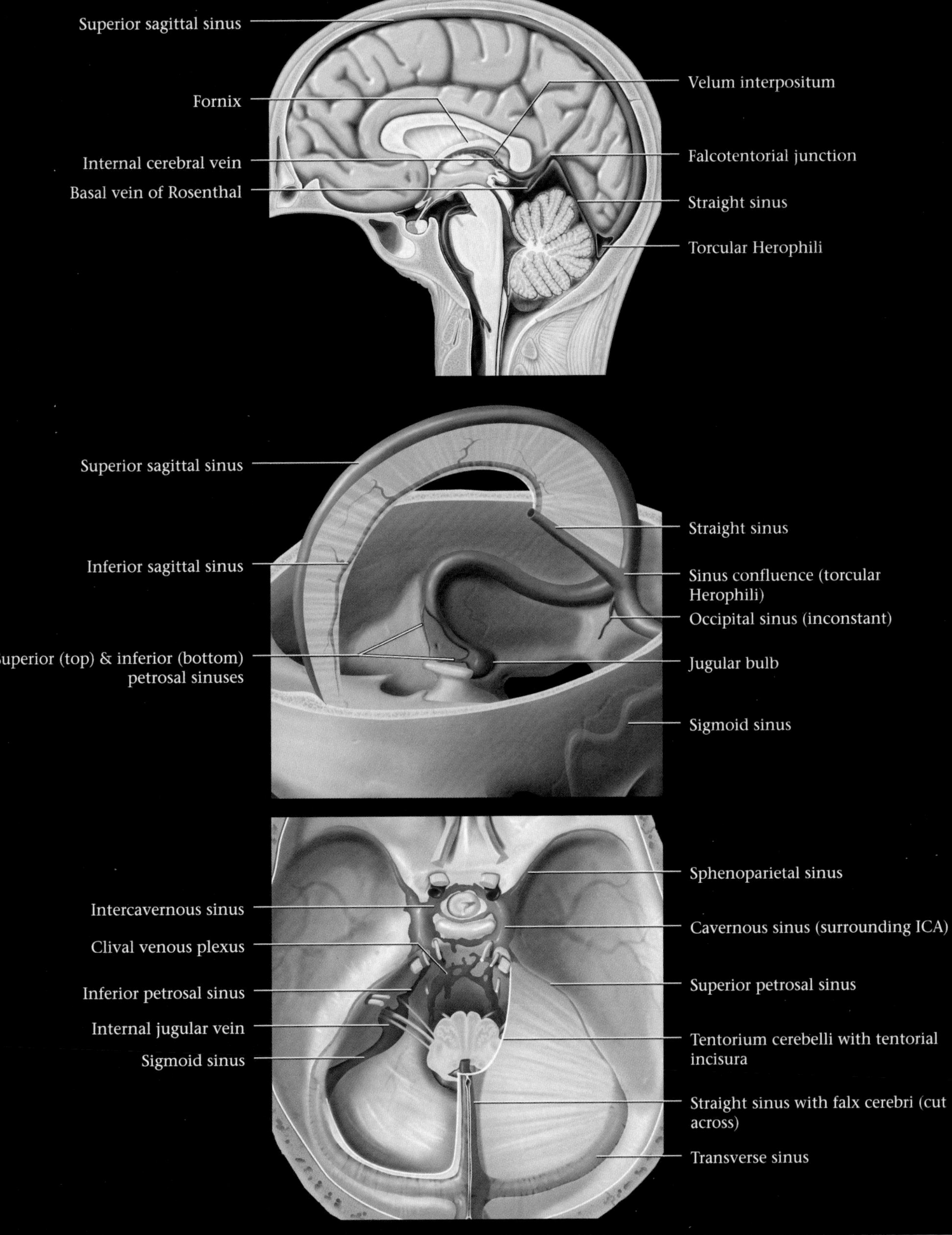
Superior sagittal sinus
Fornix
Internal cerebral vein
Basal vein of Rosenthal
Velum interpositum
Falcotentorial junction
Straight sinus
Torcular Herophili
Superior sagittal sinus
Inferior sagittal sinus
Superior (top) & inferior (bottom) petrosal sinuses
Straight sinus
Sinus confluence (torcular Herophili)
Occipital sinus (inconstant)
Jugular bulb
Sigmoid sinus
Intercavernous sinus
Clival venous plexus
Inferior petrosal sinus
Internal jugular vein
Sigmoid sinus
Sphenoparietal sinus
Cavernous sinus (surrounding ICA)
Superior petrosal sinus
Tentorium cerebelli with tentorial incisura
Straight sinus with falx cerebri (cut across)
Transverse sinus

(Top) A series of color graphics depict the major intracranial dural venous sinuses and their tributaries. This sagittal midline graphic shows an overview of the relationship of the midline venous sinuses to adjacent structures. The vein of Galen curves under the corpus callosum splenium, above the pineal gland, and joins the straight sinus at the falcotentorial junction. **(Middle)** The falx cerebri extends posteriorly from its origin at the crista galli to the falcotentorial junction. The superior sagittal sinus is enclosed in its superior borders and may begin as far anteriorly as the crista galli or as far posteriorly as the coronal suture. **(Bottom)** This image, with the brain removed and the sinuses at the skull base seen from above, shows the numerous interconnections between the cavernous sinus, clival venous plexus, sphenoparietal and petrosal sinuses.

GRAPHICS

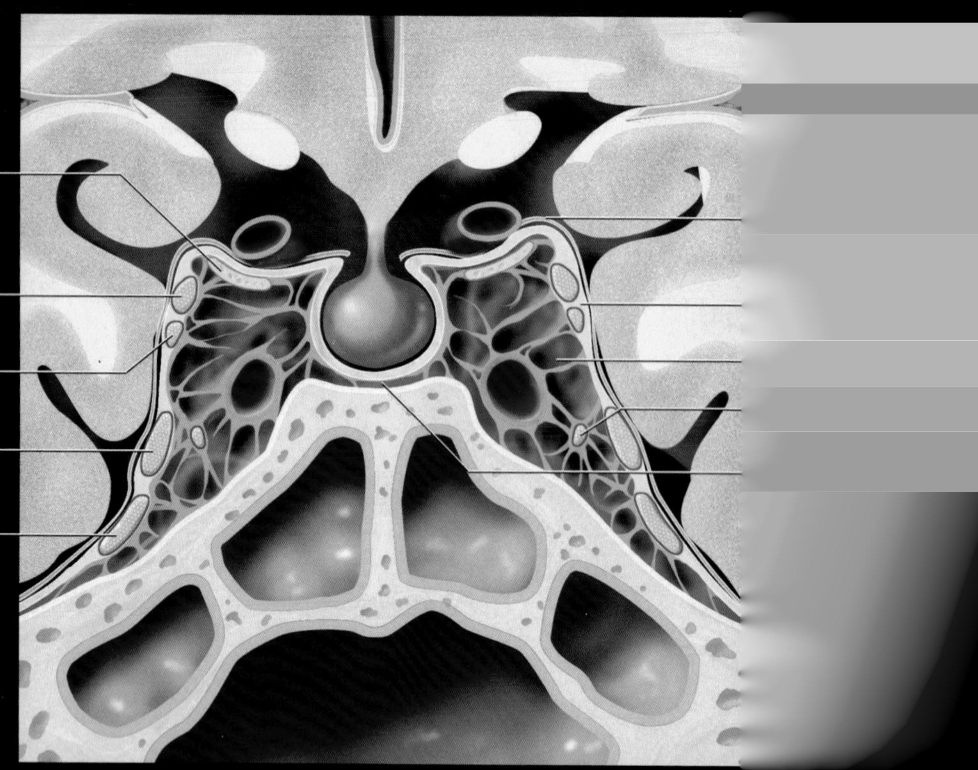

Anterior clinoid process (lesser sphenoid wing)
Oculomotor nerve
Trochlear nerve
First (ophthalmic) division, trigeminal nerve
Second (maxillary) division, trigeminal nerve

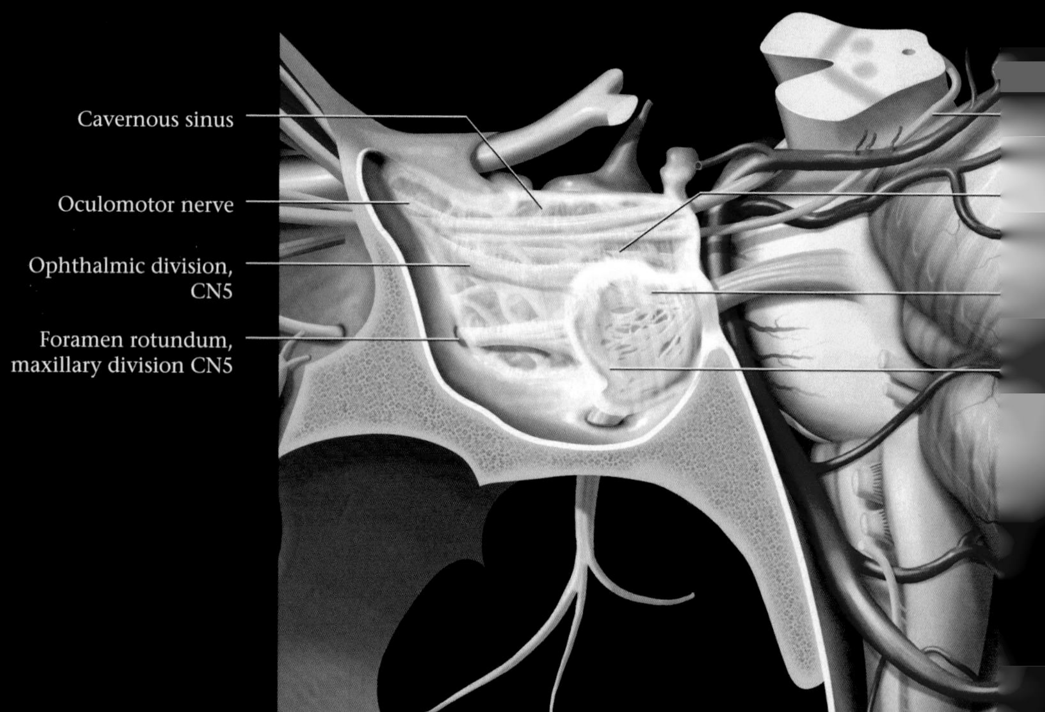

Cavernous sinus
Oculomotor nerve
Ophthalmic division, CN5
Foramen rotundum, maxillary division CN5

(Top) The cavernous sinus and its contents are shown in coronal section. The CS is fenestrat multi-channeled. The cavernous internal carotid artery and the abducens (CN6) nerve are th actually lie WITHIN the CS itself. Most of the cranial nerves are contained in the lateral dura medial dural wall is generally not apparent. **(Bottom)** Lateral view shows the dural-covered nerves (the internal carotid artery is not depicted). Meckel cave is a dura and arachnoid-line prepontine CSF cistern into the cavernous sinus. It contains the fascicles of the trigeminal n third (mandibular) division of CN5 exits the skull through the foramen ovale without passi

LAT ICA DSA

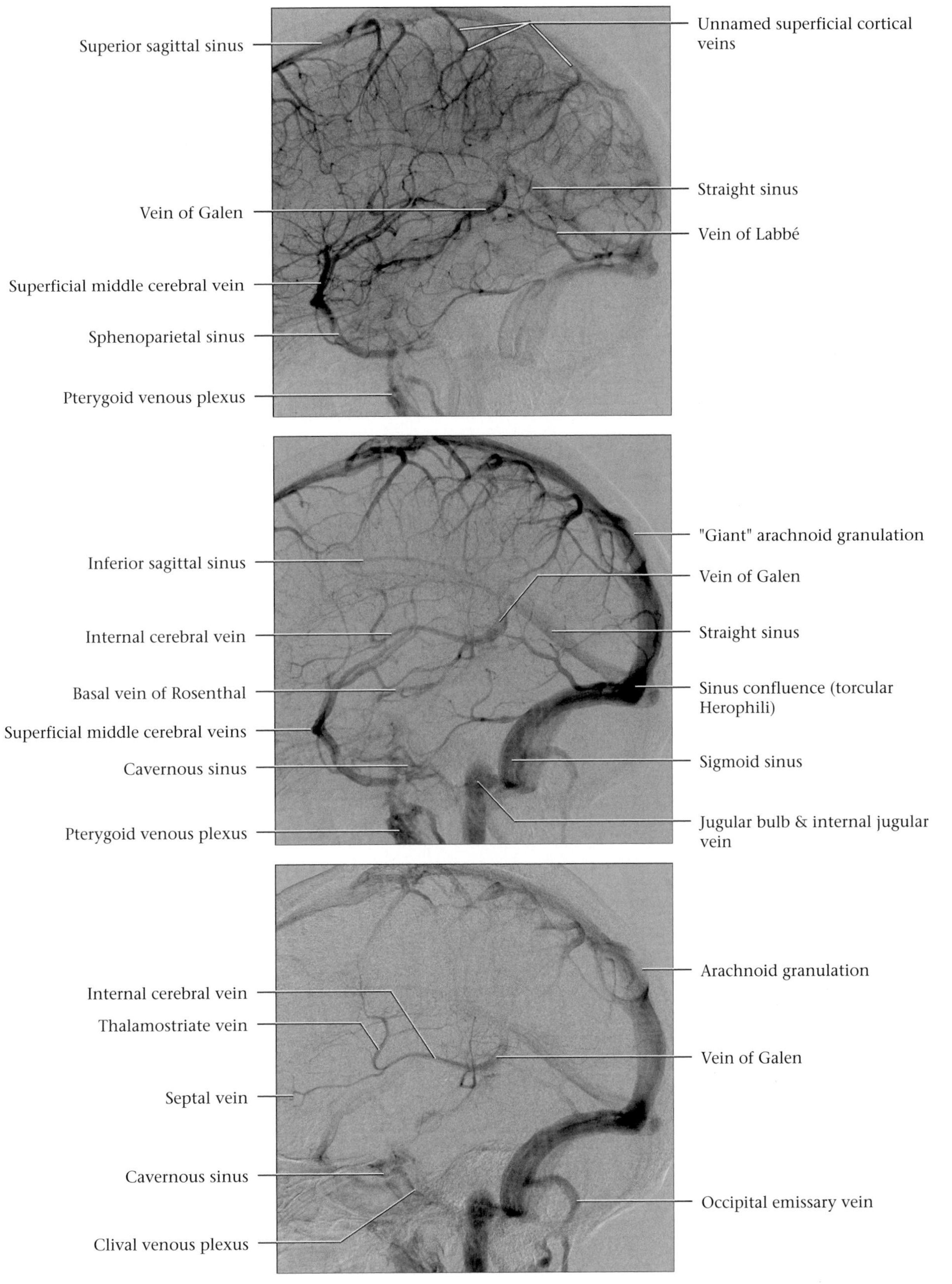
Superior sagittal sinus
Unnamed superficial cortical veins
Straight sinus
Vein of Galen
Vein of Labbé
Superficial middle cerebral vein
Sphenoparietal sinus
Pterygoid venous plexus
"Giant" arachnoid granulation
Inferior sagittal sinus
Vein of Galen
Internal cerebral vein
Straight sinus
Basal vein of Rosenthal
Sinus confluence (torcular Herophili)
Superficial middle cerebral veins
Sigmoid sinus
Cavernous sinus
Jugular bulb & internal jugular vein
Pterygoid venous plexus
Arachnoid granulation
Internal cerebral vein
Thalamostriate vein
Vein of Galen
Septal vein
Cavernous sinus
Occipital emissary vein
Clival venous plexus

(Top) Series of three lateral views of an internal carotid DSA are illustrated. Early venous phase shows the superficial cortical and anastomotic veins are most prominent and the venous sinuses are only faintly opacified. **(Middle)** Mid-venous phase shows prominent opacification of the dural venous sinuses. The cavernous sinus is well seen, along with its interconnections with the pterygoid venous plexus. **(Bottom)** Late venous phase shows contrast has been washed out of most of the cortical veins. The subependymal veins are quite prominent at this stage and are well seen with the disappearance of contrast from overlying cortical veins. A very prominent filling defect in the descending segment of the superior sagittal sinus, caused by a large arachnoid granulation, is now well seen. The transverse and sigmoid sinuses are a more common location for arachnoid granulations.

DURAL SINUSES

AP ICA DSA

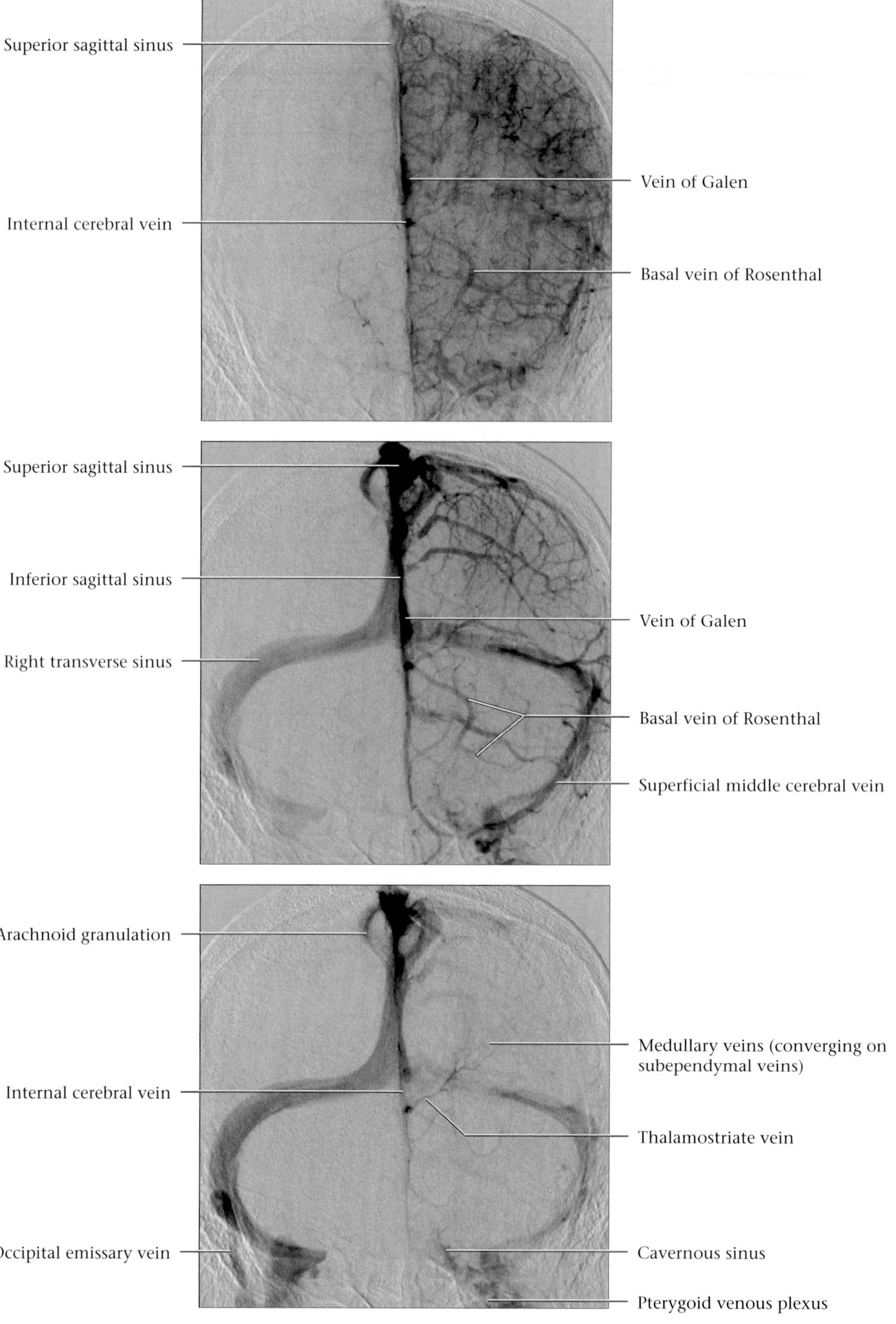
Superior sagittal sinus
Internal cerebral vein
Vein of Galen
Basal vein of Rosenthal
Superior sagittal sinus
Inferior sagittal sinus
Right transverse sinus
Vein of Galen
Basal vein of Rosenthal
Superficial middle cerebral vein
Arachnoid granulation
Internal cerebral vein
Medullary veins (converging on subependymal veins)
Thalamostriate vein
Occipital emissary vein
Cavernous sinus
Pterygoid venous plexus

(Top) Series of three AP venous phase angiograms are illustrated. Early venous phase shows prominent filling of numerous superficial cortical veins. The anterior aspect of the superior sagittal sinus is faintly opacified. If the AP view is perfectly straight, as it is in this case, the SSS, ISS, ICV, and VofG overlap in the midline. **(Middle)** Mid-venous phase shows major dural venous sinuses. The right transverse sinus is dominant and fills prominently even though contrast was injected into the left internal carotid artery. **(Bottom)** Late phase shows subependymal veins especially well. A less well-visualized segment of the left TS is seen, a normal variant that should not be mistaken for venous occlusion. Filling defect in the SSS is caused by a very large arachnoid granulation. The ICV arcs posteriorly to the VofG from its origin at the anterior thalamostriate vein.

DURAL SINUSES

OBL ICA DSA

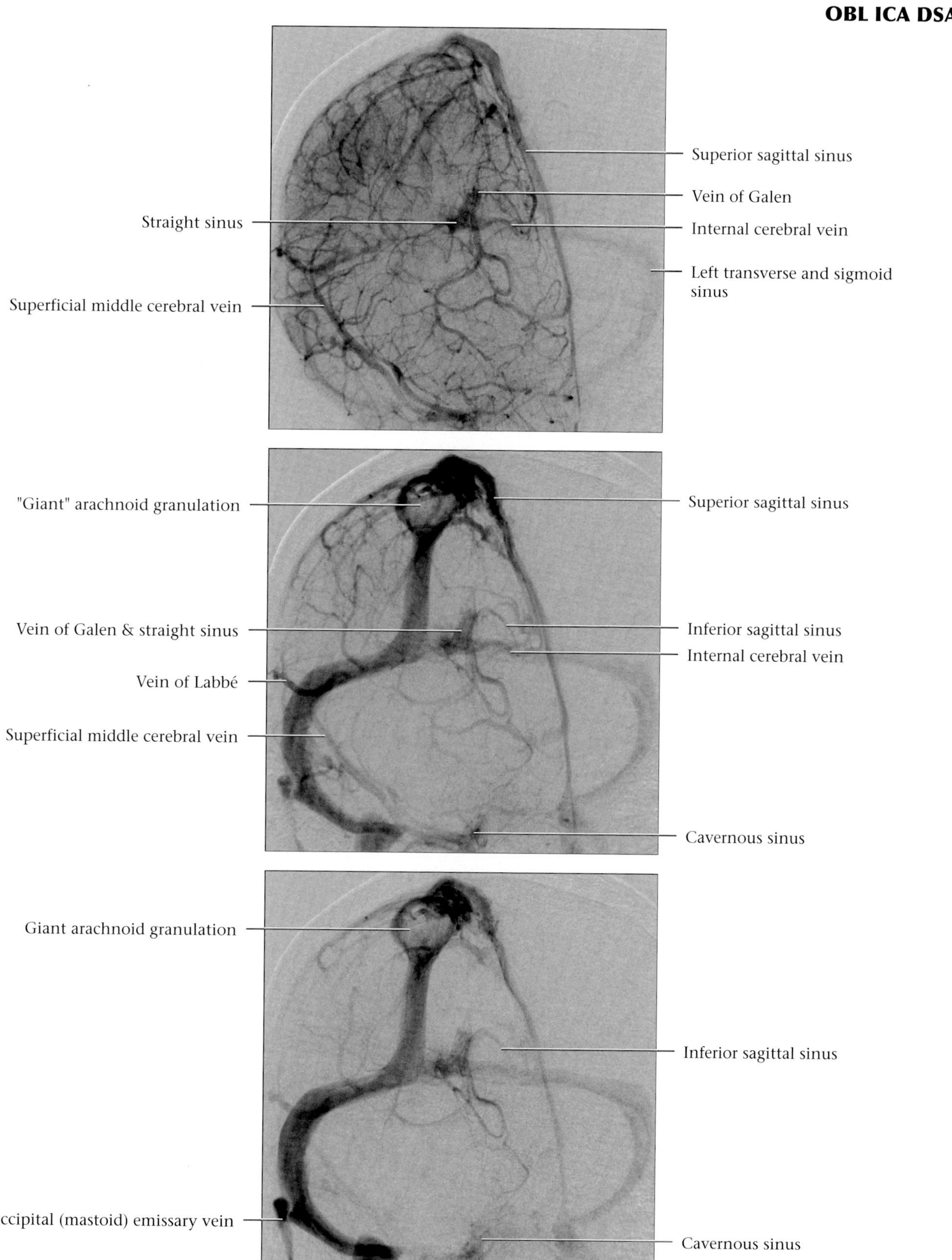
Superior sagittal sinus
Vein of Galen
Straight sinus
Internal cerebral vein
Left transverse and sigmoid sinus
Superficial middle cerebral vein
"Giant" arachnoid granulation
Superior sagittal sinus
Vein of Galen & straight sinus
Inferior sagittal sinus
Internal cerebral vein
Vein of Labbé
Superficial middle cerebral vein
Cavernous sinus
Giant arachnoid granulation
Inferior sagittal sinus
Occipital (mastoid) emissary vein
Cavernous sinus

(Top) A series of three oblique AP views of a right internal carotid DSA are illustrated. The early venous phase shows prominent superficial cortical veins. The superior sagittal and transverse sinuses are faintly opacified. This view is ideal for visualizing sinus occlusion. **(Middle)** In this mid-venous phase, both superficial and deep veins are visualized well, as are the major dural venous sinuses. In this case, the superior sagittal sinus arcs posteriorly all the way from the crista galli anteriorly to the sinus confluence posteriorly. **(Bottom)** Late venous phase shows a prominent filling defect in the superior sagittal sinus caused by a giant arachnoid granulation, a normal variant.

AXIAL T1 C+ MR

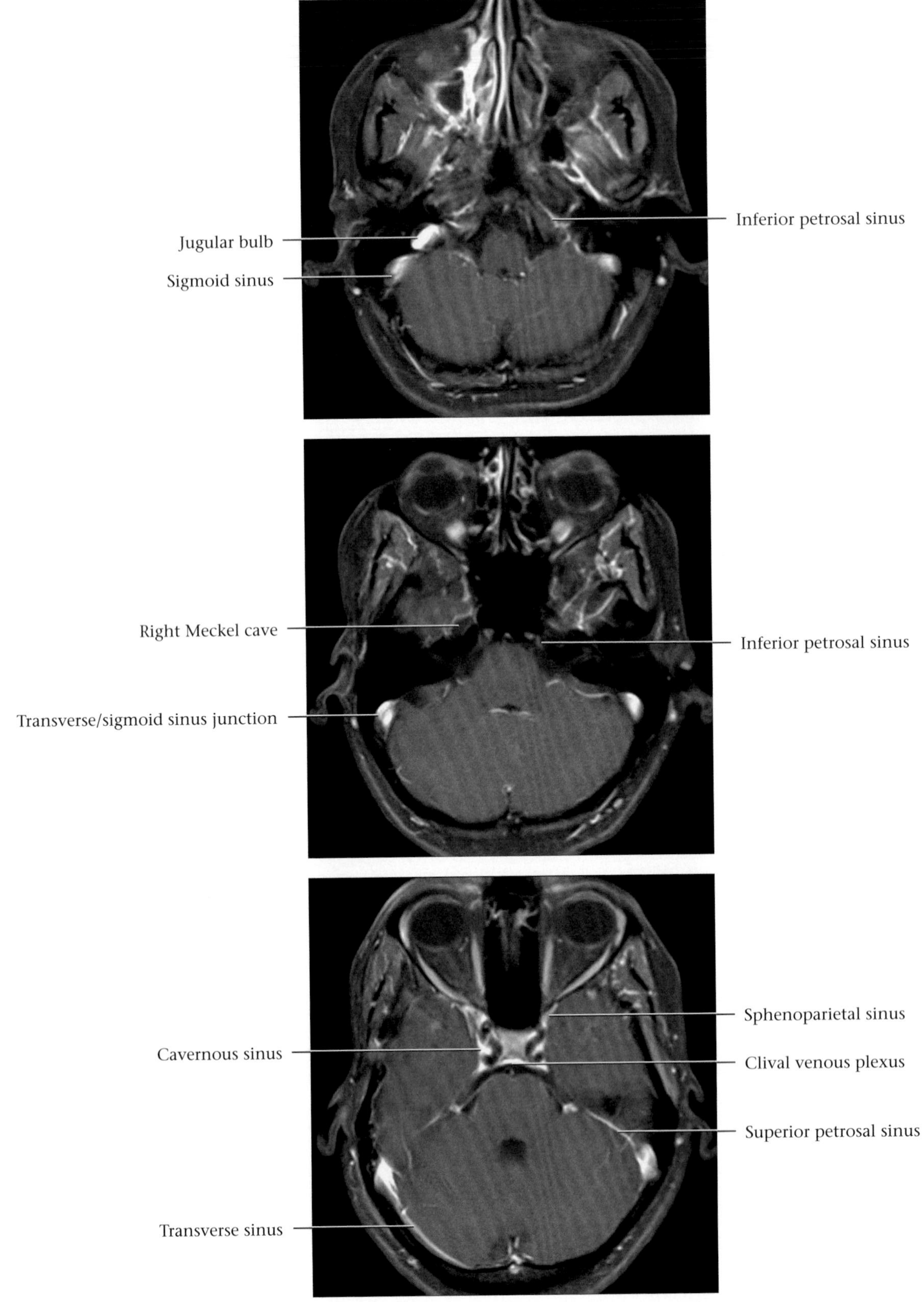
Jugular bulb
Sigmoid sinus
Inferior petrosal sinus
Right Meckel cave
Transverse/sigmoid sinus junction
Inferior petrosal sinus
Sphenoparietal sinus
Cavernous sinus
Clival venous plexus
Superior petrosal sinus
Transverse sinus

(Top) Series of nine axial T1 C+ MR scans from inferior to superior are illustrated. Section through the lower medulla and jugular foramen shows the sigmoid sinuses and right jugular bulb. Asymmetry of the jugular bulbs, seen here, is very common as is inhomogeneous flow and enhancement pattern. **(Middle)** Scan through the mid-pons includes the junction of the transverse with the sigmoid sinuses. **(Bottom)** Scan through the cavernous sinus shows its interconnections with the sphenoparietal sinuses anteriorly and the clival venous plexus posteriorly. The left superior petrosal sinus is shown draining into the transverse sinus.

DURAL SINUSES

AXIAL T1 C+ MR

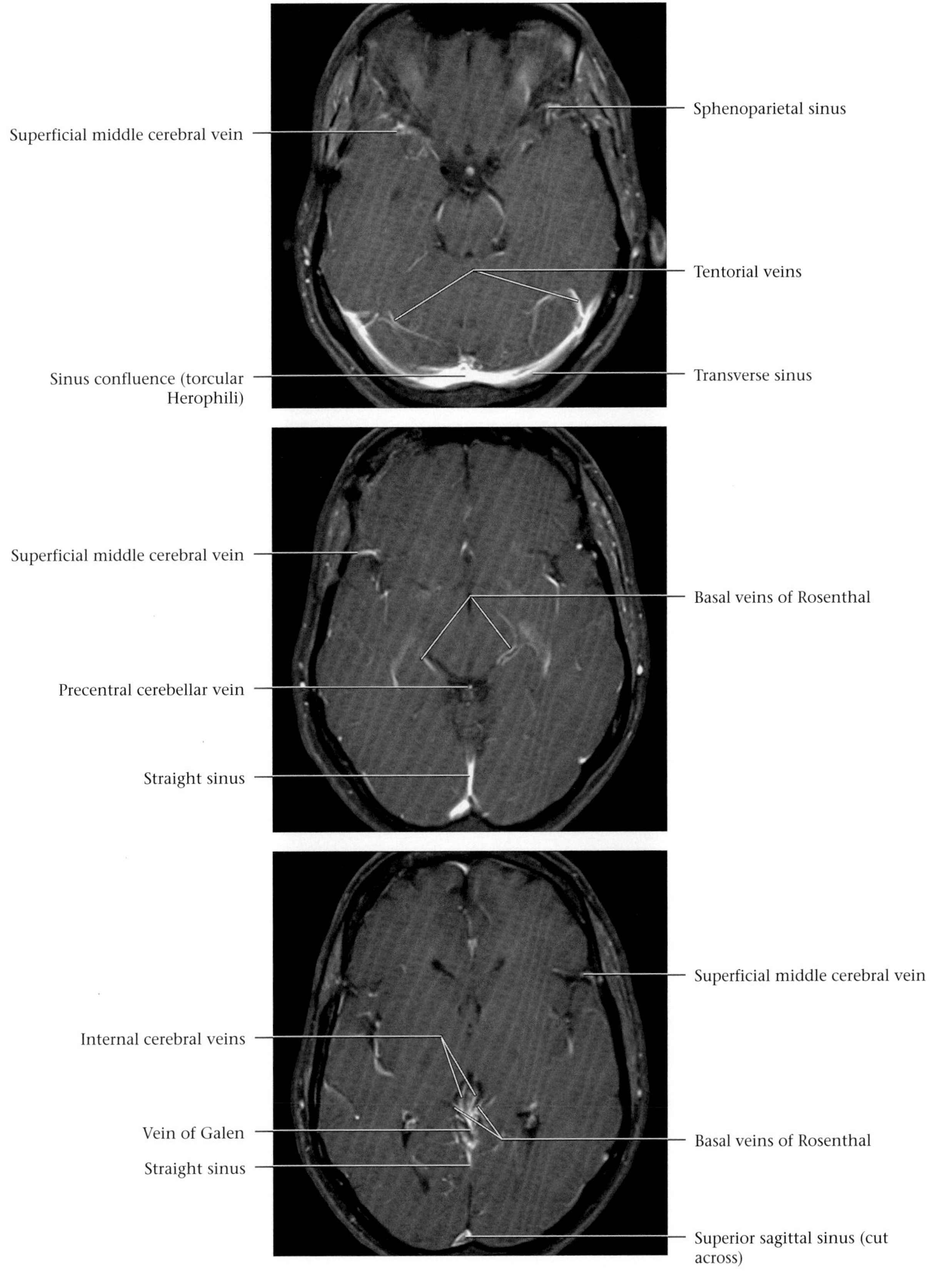
Superficial middle cerebral vein
Sphenoparietal sinus
Tentorial veins
Sinus confluence (torcular Herophili)
Transverse sinus
Superficial middle cerebral vein
Basal veins of Rosenthal
Precentral cerebellar vein
Straight sinus
Superficial middle cerebral vein
Internal cerebral veins
Vein of Galen
Basal veins of Rosenthal
Straight sinus
Superior sagittal sinus (cut across)

(Top) The superficial middle cerebral veins are shown on the right and the sphenoparietal sinus on the left. Note prominent tentorial veins draining into both transverse sinuses. **(Middle)** Section through the upper lateral cerebral (sylvian) fissure shows the superficial middle cerebral vein on the right. Both basal veins of Rosenthal are well seen. The junction between the straight sinus and torcular Herophili is included. **(Bottom)** Scan through the tentorial apex shows the internal cerebral veins and basal veins of Rosenthal forming the vein of Galen.

DURAL SINUSES

AXIAL T1 C+ MR

Superior sagittal sinus (anterior aspect)
Septal vein
Thalamostriate vein
Anterior caudate vein
Internal cerebral veins
Upper end of vein of Galen
Straight sinus
Superior sagittal sinus (posterior aspect)
Frontal cortical vein
Frontal cortical vein
Superior sagittal sinus
Superior sagittal sinus (anterior end)
Inferior sagittal sinus
Superior sagittal sinus (posterior end)

(Top) Scan through the foramen of Monro shows the thalamostriate and anterior caudate veins (cut across). The left septal vein is faintly seen in front of the frontal horn of the lateral ventricle. Both the small anterior and larger posterior aspects of the superior sagittal sinus are seen. **(Middle)** Section through the upper bodies of the lateral ventricles shows prominent unnamed frontal cortical veins draining into the anterior aspect of the superior sagittal sinus. Note "flow void" in the posterior aspect of the superior sagittal sinus, a normal finding caused by fast venous flow. **(Bottom)** The anterior and posterior aspects of the SSS are depicted on this upper section. A small portion of the inferior sagittal sinus can be identified in the interhemispheric fissure. The SSS increases in size as it passes posteriorly and collects cortical hemispheric veins

DURAL SINUSES

AP, LAT & OBL MRV

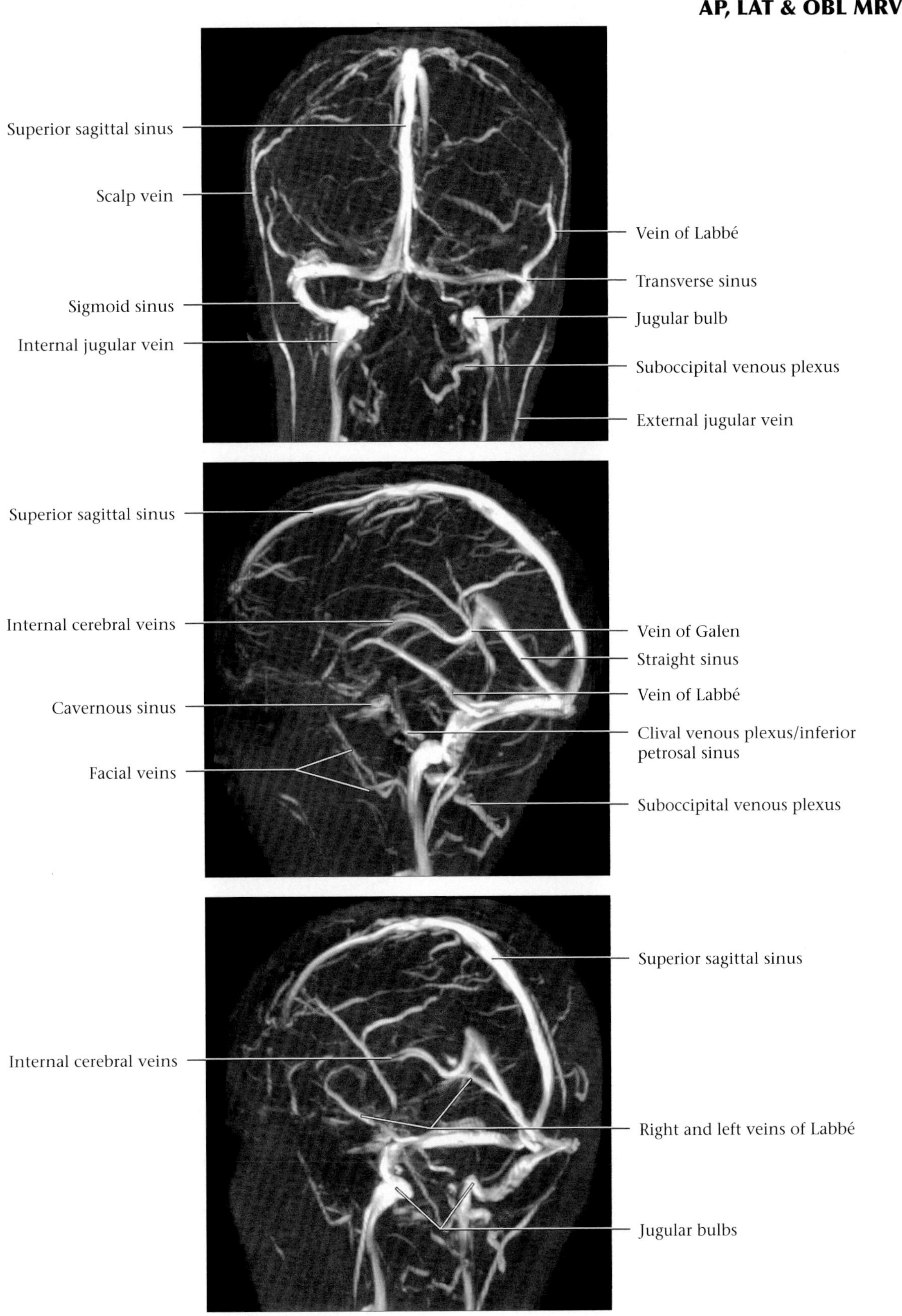

Superior sagittal sinus
Scalp vein
Sigmoid sinus
Internal jugular vein
Vein of Labbé
Transverse sinus
Jugular bulb
Suboccipital venous plexus
External jugular vein
Superior sagittal sinus
Internal cerebral veins
Cavernous sinus
Facial veins
Vein of Galen
Straight sinus
Vein of Labbé
Clival venous plexus/inferior petrosal sinus
Suboccipital venous plexus
Superior sagittal sinus
Internal cerebral veins
Right and left veins of Labbé
Jugular bulbs

(Top) AP view of an MR venogram depicts the major dural venous sinuses well. If large, anastomotic veins such as the vein of Labbé can be visualized on MRV. **(Middle)** Lateral view of the MRV shows the intracranial dural sinuses, anastomotic vein of Labbé, and some of the major extracranial veins. **(Bottom)** Oblique view of the MRV shows the transverse sinuses sweep anterolaterally from occipital protuberance to the posterior petrous bone where they join with superior petrosal sinus to form the sigmoid sinus. The superior sagittal sinus has a variable origin and may extend all the way from the crista galli to the sinus confluence. Some SSSs are formed near the coronal suture. In this case, the SSS is formed in the mid-frontal region by confluence of some prominent cortical veins. Note asymmetry of the jugular bulbs, a common normal variant.

SUPERFICIAL CEREBRAL VEINS

Terminology

Abbreviations

- Superficial middle cerebral vein (SMCV)
- Deep middle cerebral vein (DMCV)
- Vein of Trolard (VofT)
- Vein of Labbé (VofL)
- Basal vein of Rosenthal (BVR)
- Superior, inferior sagittal sinus (SSS; ISS)
- Cavernous sinus (CS)
- Sphenoparietal sinus (SPS)
- Great cerebral vein (of Galen, VofG)

Synonyms

- Cortical veins: Superficial or external veins

Gross Anatomy

Overview

- Highly variable in number and configuration
- Located within subarachnoid space (SAS), cisterns
- Organized anatomically into three groups (superior, middle, inferior)
- **Superior group**
  - 8-12 superficial cortical veins
  - Follow sulci, ascend to convexity
  - Cross subarachnoid space
  - Pierce arachnoid, inner dura, join SSS at right angles
- **Middle group**
  - **Superficial middle cerebral vein**
    - Inconstant, variable size/dominance
    - Begins over surface of lateral (sylvian) fissure
    - Collects numerous superficial veins from frontal, temporal, parietal operculae
    - Curves anteromedially around temporal lobe
    - Terminates in CS or SPS
- **Inferior group**
  - Orbital surface of frontal lobe drains superiorly to SSS
  - Temporal lobe, anterior cerebral veins anastomose with deep middle cerebral and basal veins
  - **Basal vein (of Rosenthal)**
    - Begins near anterior perforated substance
    - Receives anterior cerebral, DMCV tributaries (from insula, basal ganglia, parahippocampal gyrus)
    - Curves posteriorly around cerebral peduncles
    - Drains into great cerebral vein (of Galen)
- Three major named large **anastomotic cortical veins**
  - **Vein of Trolard**: Major superior anastomotic vein
  - **Vein of Labbé**: Major inferior anastomotic vein
  - **Superficial middle cerebral vein**: Major middle anastomotic vein

Anatomy Relationships

- Anastomotic veins
  - Have reciprocal relationship (if one is large, others typically smaller or absent)
  - Abundant anastomoses with each other as well as deep (internal) cerebral veins, orbit, extracranial venous plexi

Vascular Territories

- Superior group (cortical veins + SSS, ISS)
  - Superolateral hemispheric surfaces
  - Most of medial hemispheric surfaces between ISS, SSS
  - Most of frontal lobes except for perisylvian area
- Middle group (SMCV plus cavernous sinus)
  - Perisylvian area, anterior temporal lobes
- Inferior group
  - BVR: Inferior insula, basal ganglia, medial temporal lobes
  - VofL (plus TS): Posterior temporal, lower parietal lobes

Imaging Anatomy

Overview

- Highly variable in appearance with asymmetry between hemispheres common
- Superior group
  - Lateral DSA
    - Arranged in spoke-like pattern
    - Converge with SSS at right angles
    - Prominent VofT from sylvian fissure to SSS usually seen coursing over parietal lobe
  - AP DSA: "Stepladder" appearance from front to back
- Middle group
  - Lateral DSA: SMCV has single or multiple trunks that follow sylvian fissure, curve over temporal tip
  - AP DSA: SMCV drains into CS, SPS, or through foramen ovale into pterygoid venous plexus
- Inferior group
  - Lateral DSA: BVR curves somewhat inferiorly as it passes around midbrain
  - AP DSA: BVR curves laterally around midbrain to VofG

Anatomy-Based Imaging Issues

Imaging Recommendations

- MRV: Obtain source images perpendicular to veins of interest

Imaging Pitfalls

- VofT variable in size, position; may appear quite posterior on axial MR/CT scans

Embryology

Embryologic Events

- 8 weeks: Primitive, thin-walled plexus of undifferentiated vascular channels covers brain surface
  - Persistence of primitive leptomeningeal vascular plexus, paucity of normal cortical veins → Sturge-Weber syndrome
- 10-12 weeks: Progressive anastomosis, retrogressive differentiation causes plexi to coalesce into definitive cortical venous channels
  - Failure to coalesce → persistence of primitive, plexiform veins (common with malformations of cortical development)

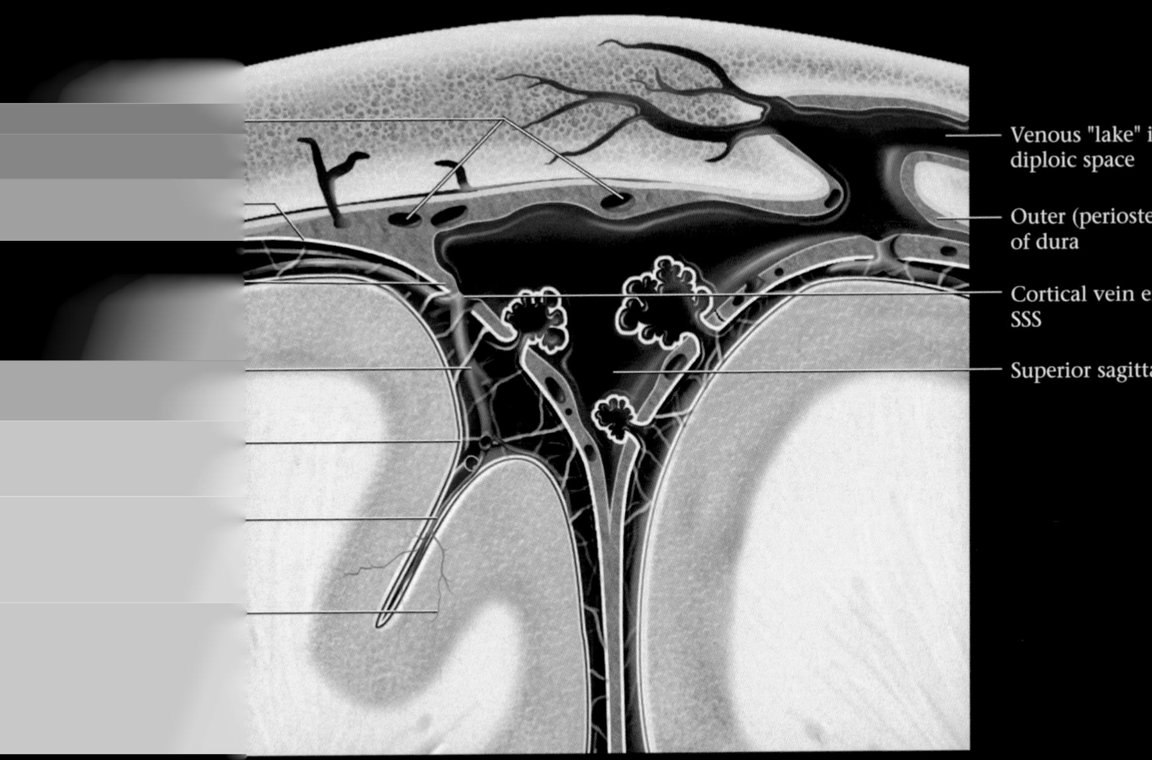
Venous "lake" in diploic space
Outer (periosteal) layer of dura
Cortical vein entering SSS
Superior sagittal sinus

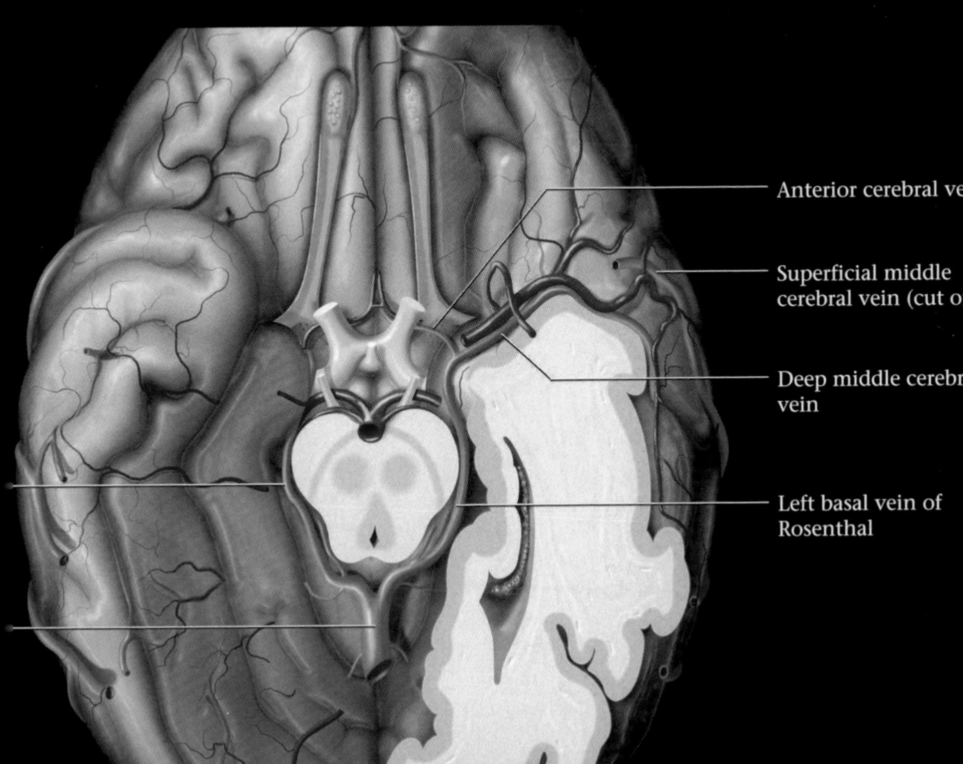
Anterior cerebral vein
Superficial middle cerebral vein (cut off)
Deep middle cerebral vein
Left basal vein of Rosenthal

rough the superior sagittal sinus depicts venous drainage of the superior hemispheres, etrating cortical veins collect venular tributaries, then exit the cortex and enter the ral sulcus). Cortical veins within the sulci collect numerous tiny draining veins and then wards the arachnoid. They pass through the arachnoid and inner (meningeal) dural layer thin the SAS, the veins are covered with a thin layer of cells that is continuous with the pia rachnoid. **(Bottom)** Inferior view shows major veins of the inferior brain, sylvian fissure. ebral vein (cut off) drains into the cavernous sinus (not shown). The anterior cerebral and

SUPERFICIAL CEREBRAL VEINS

GRAPHICS

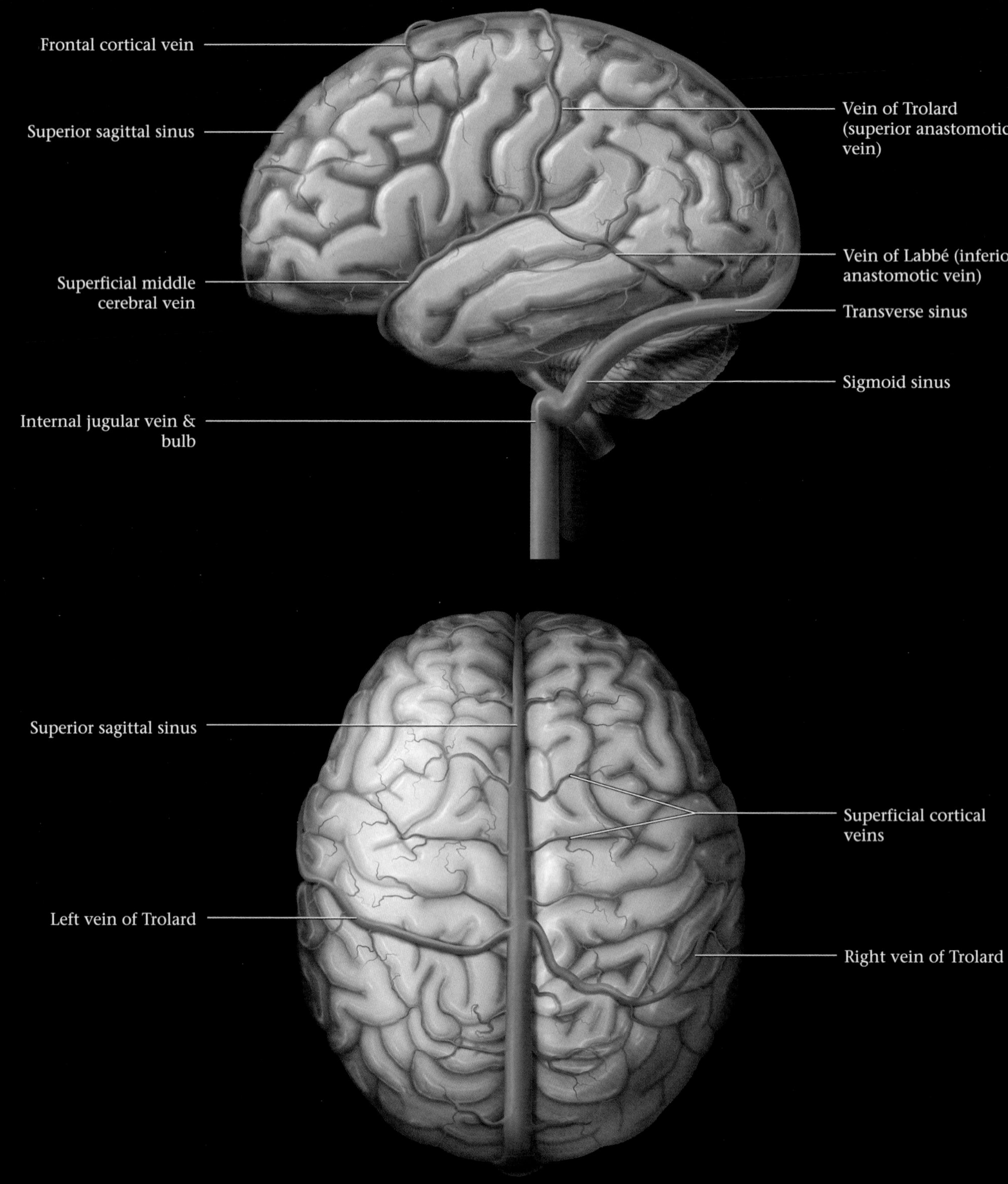
Frontal cortical vein
Superior sagittal sinus
Vein of Trolard (superior anastomotic vein)
Vein of Labbé (inferior anastomotic vein)
Superficial middle cerebral vein
Transverse sinus
Sigmoid sinus
Internal jugular vein & bulb
Superior sagittal sinus
Superficial cortical veins
Left vein of Trolard
Right vein of Trolard

(Top) Lateral graphic depicts the superficial cortical veins and their relationship to the dural venous sinuses. The three named anastomotic veins (superficial middle cerebral vein, vein of Trolard, vein of Labbé) are depicted here as all relatively similar in size. It is common to have one or two dominant anastomotic veins with hypoplasia of the other(s) present. **(Bottom)** Cortical venous tributaries of the SSS, seen from above. Two configurations of the vein of Trolard are depicted. On the left, the VofT courses directly superiorly from the sylvian fissure. On the right, the VofT sweeps more posteriorly.

SUPERFICIAL CEREBRAL VEINS

LAT ICA DSA

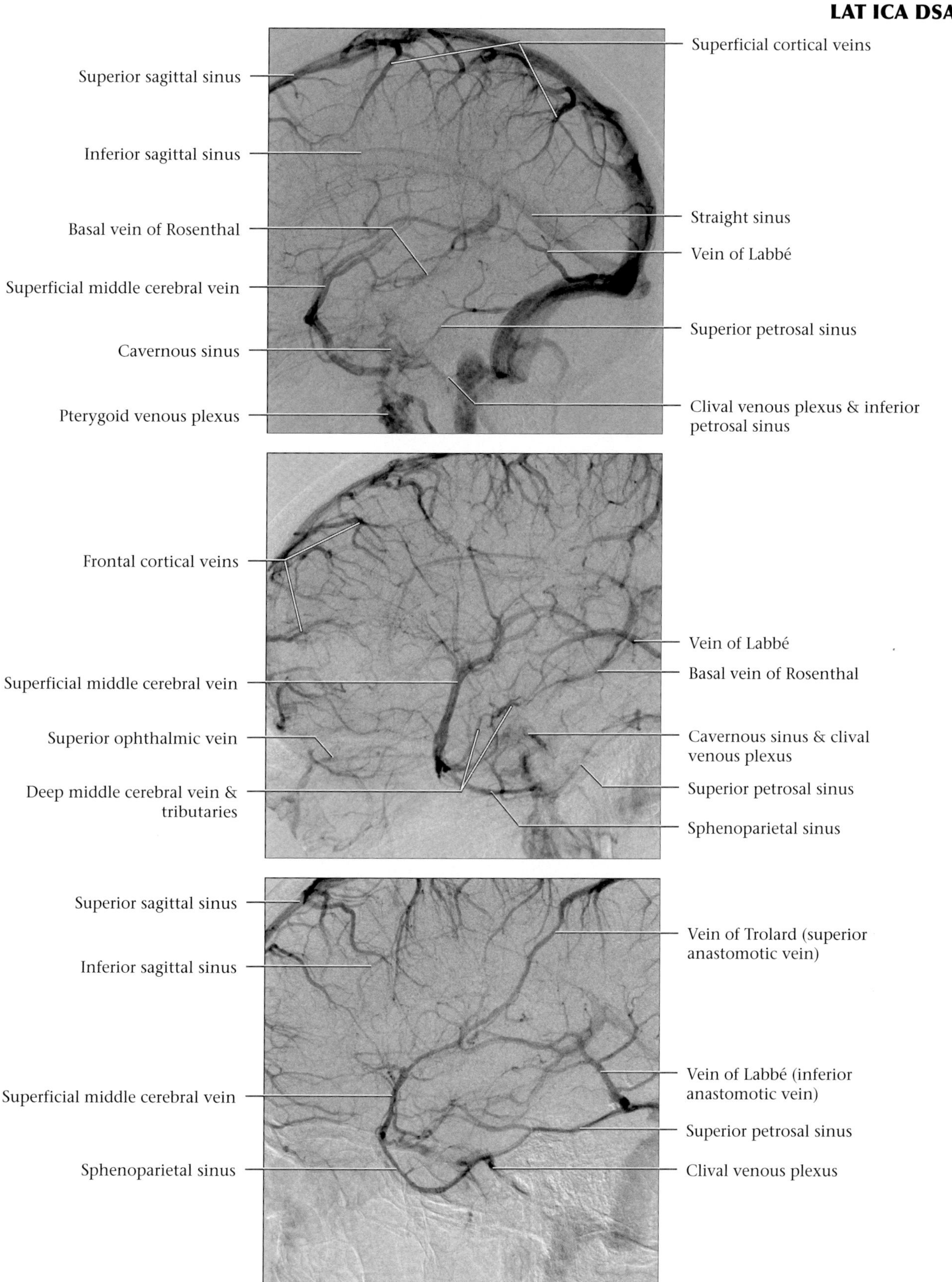
Superficial cortical veins
Superior sagittal sinus
Inferior sagittal sinus
Straight sinus
Basal vein of Rosenthal
Vein of Labbé
Superficial middle cerebral vein
Superior petrosal sinus
Cavernous sinus
Pterygoid venous plexus
Clival venous plexus & inferior petrosal sinus
Frontal cortical veins
Vein of Labbé
Basal vein of Rosenthal
Superficial middle cerebral vein
Superior ophthalmic vein
Cavernous sinus & clival venous plexus
Deep middle cerebral vein & tributaries
Superior petrosal sinus
Sphenoparietal sinus
Superior sagittal sinus
Vein of Trolard (superior anastomotic vein)
Inferior sagittal sinus
Vein of Labbé (inferior anastomotic vein)
Superficial middle cerebral vein
Superior petrosal sinus
Sphenoparietal sinus
Clival venous plexus

(Top) A series of three venous phase lateral ICA DSAs from different cases are shown to illustrate the superficial cerebral veins. Several superior cortical veins are present without a dominant, identifiable vein of Trolard. Here the superficial middle cerebral vein is large and a smaller vein of Labbé is present. The major drainage of the SMCV is into the pterygoid plexus, with a smaller pathway through a hypoplastic superior petrosal sinus into the sigmoid sinus. **(Middle)** In this case, a prominent superficial middle cerebral vein is present. Note filling of the superior ophthalmic vein, which communicates with the cavernous sinus (not well seen) and facial veins. **(Bottom)** In this case, all three anastomotic veins are visualized. All are approximately equal in size, with no dominant anastomotic pattern. This is a relatively unusual finding.

SUPERFICIAL CEREBRAL VEINS

AP DSA

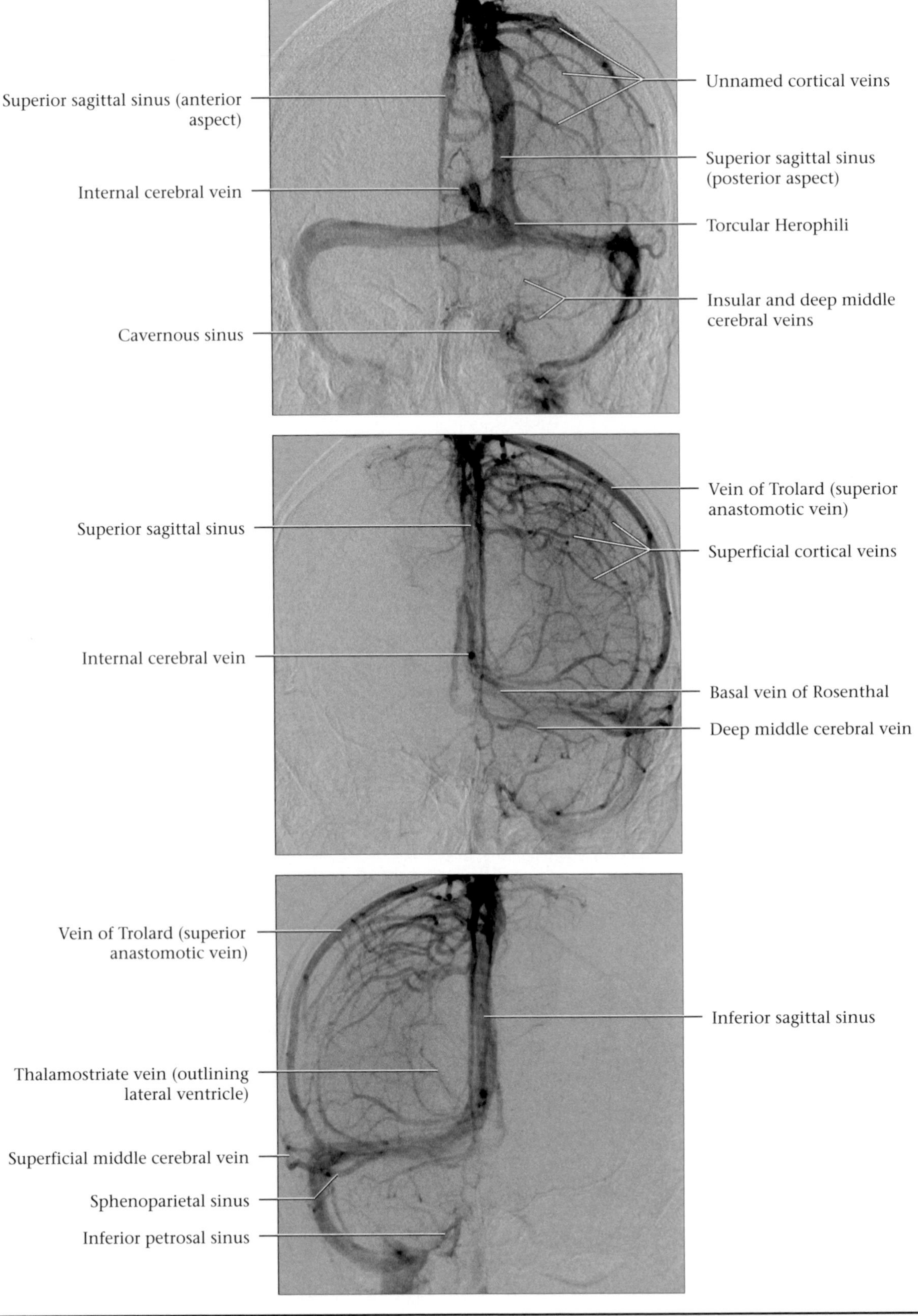
Superior sagittal sinus (anterior aspect)
Internal cerebral vein
Cavernous sinus
Unnamed cortical veins
Superior sagittal sinus (posterior aspect)
Torcular Herophili
Insular and deep middle cerebral veins
Superior sagittal sinus
Internal cerebral vein
Vein of Trolard (superior anastomotic vein)
Superficial cortical veins
Basal vein of Rosenthal
Deep middle cerebral vein
Vein of Trolard (superior anastomotic vein)
Thalamostriate vein (outlining lateral ventricle)
Superficial middle cerebral vein
Sphenoparietal sinus
Inferior petrosal sinus
Inferior sagittal sinus

(Top) A series of three AP venous phase angiograms are shown. Here, a slightly oblique view shows several unnamed cortical veins. On AP views, the cortical veins form a "stepladder" appearance as they drain from the hemispheric surface up to the superior sagittal sinus. The SSS increases in size as it passes from front to back. **(Middle)** A different case shows a very prominent vein of Trolard (superior anastomotic vein). Other unnamed smaller cortical veins have the classic "stepladder" appearance on this projection. **(Bottom)** This case has a prominent vein of Trolard (superior anastomotic vein) that originates at the sylvian fissure and passes superiorly over the hemisphere. A smaller superficial middle cerebral vein is seen draining into the sphenoparietal sinus. No vein of Labbé (inferior anastomotic vein) is seen. A small ISS is present, seen overlying the SSS.

SUPERFICIAL CEREBRAL VEINS

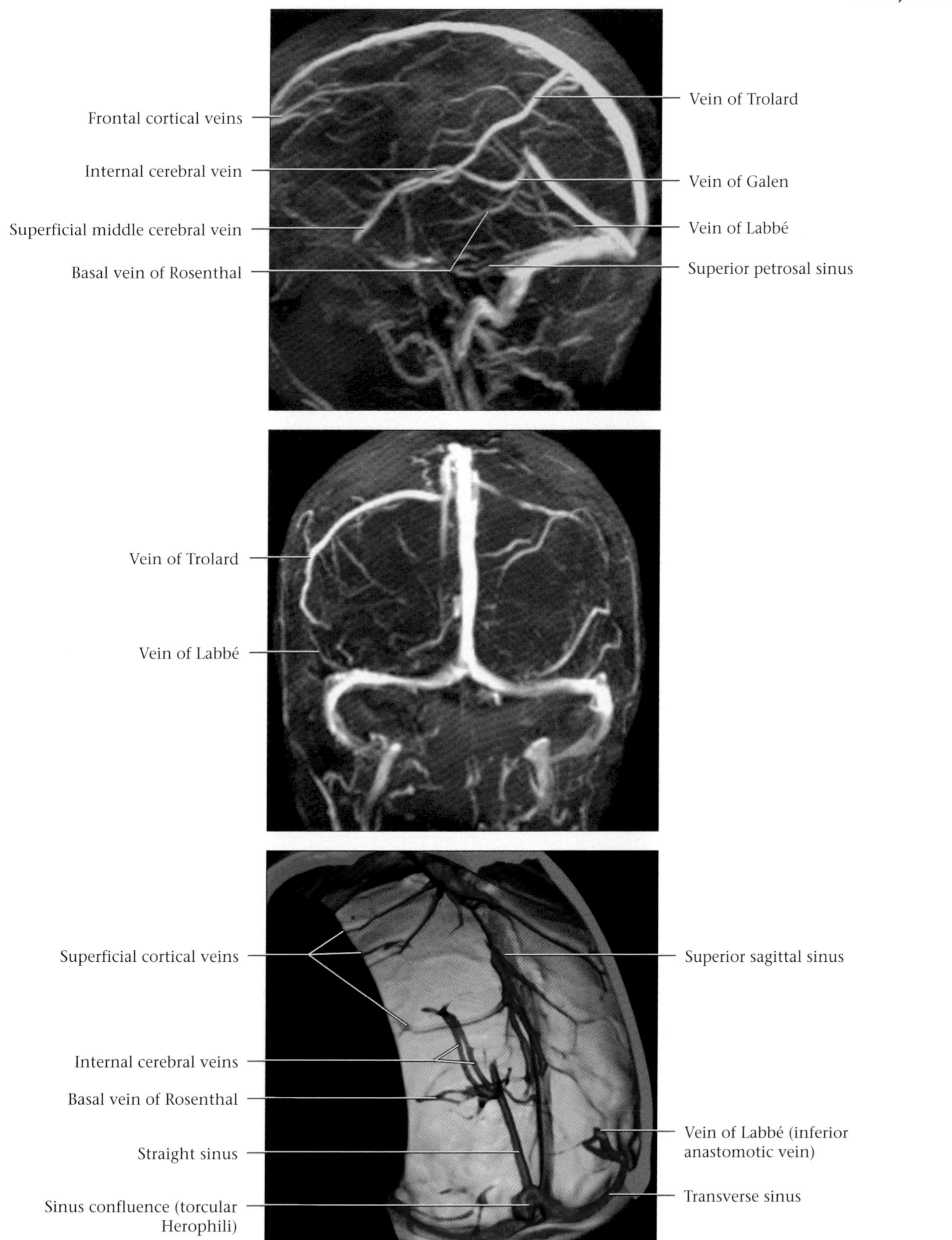
Frontal cortical veins
Internal cerebral vein
Superficial middle cerebral vein
Basal vein of Rosenthal
Vein of Trolard
Vein of Galen
Vein of Labbé
Superior petrosal sinus
Vein of Trolard
Vein of Labbé
Superficial cortical veins
Internal cerebral veins
Basal vein of Rosenthal
Straight sinus
Sinus confluence (torcular Herophili)
Superior sagittal sinus
Vein of Labbé (inferior anastomotic vein)
Transverse sinus

(Top) Lateral view MRV demonstrates prominent vein of Trolard and superficial middle cerebral vein. The vein of Labbé (inferior anastomotic vein), is relatively small. Prominent frontal veins contribute to the origin of the superior sagittal sinus. **(Middle)** AP view, MRV, shows a prominent right vein of Trolard. A small vein of Labbé is seen. In this case, the transverse sinuses are equal size. **(Bottom)** This cutaway view of a CT venogram shows the orientation of the superficial cortical veins to the superior sagittal sinus. The veins drain superiorly in an almost radial or "spoke wheel" pattern. When seen on a straight AP view, the cortical veins resemble a stepladder. In this case, there is no dominant superior anastomotic vein (of Trolard) and all the cortical veins are of relatively equal size. The BVR and ICVs are shown forming the vein of Galen.

DEEP CEREBRAL VEINS

Terminology

Abbreviations

- Septal, thalamostriate, internal cerebral veins (SV, TSV, ICV)
- Vein of Galen (VofG); basal vein of Rosenthal (BVR)
- Inferior sagittal sinus (ISS); straight sinus (SS)

Definitions

- Cavum veli interpositi: Space within double-layered tela choroidea of third ventricle, communicates posteriorly with quadrigeminal cistern

Gross Anatomy

Overview

- **Medullary veins**
  - Small, linear veins originate 1-2 cm below cortex
  - Course towards ventricles, terminate in subependymal veins
- **Subependymal veins**
  - **Septal veins**
    - Course posteriorly along septum pellucidum
    - Join with TSVs to form ICVs at interventricular foramen
  - **TSVs**
    - Receive caudate/terminal veins that course anteriorly between caudate nucleus, thalamus
    - Curve over caudate nuclei
    - Terminate at interventricular foramen (of Monro) by uniting with septal veins to form ICVs
- **Deep paramedian veins**
  - **ICVs**
    - Paired, paramedian
    - Course posteriorly in cavum veli interpositi
    - Terminate in rostral quadrigeminal cistern by uniting with each other, BVRs to form VofG
  - **VofG (great cerebral vein)**
    - Short, U-shaped midline vein formed from union of ICVs, BVRs
    - Curves posteriorly and superiorly under corpus callosum splenium in quadrigeminal cistern
    - Unites with ISS at falcotentorial apex to form SS

Anatomy Relationships

- Deep veins course under ventricular ependyma, define ventricular margins
- ICVs above third ventricle, pineal gland; under fornices, corpus callosum splenium

Vascular Territory

- ICVs, VofG and tributaries drain ovoid area surrounding lateral/third ventricles
- Caudate nuclei, putamen/globus pallidus, thalamus, internal capsule, deep cerebral (medullary) white matter, medial temporal lobes

Imaging Anatomy

Overview

- Medullary veins
  - On DSA appear as tiny, relatively uniform contrast-filled linear structures that terminate at right angles to the ventricular subependymal veins
- Subependymal veins
  - DSA, lateral view
    - "Dots" of contrast at subependymal/medullary vein junction define roof of lateral ventricle
  - DSA, AP view
    - TSV defines size, configuration of lateral ventricle; characteristic "double curve" appearance
    - BVR, tributary of VofG, begins at medial temporal lobe, curves around midbrain, looks like "frog leg"
  - T1 C+ MR usually shows TSV, caudate and septal veins; smaller subependymal veins usually inapparent
- Deep paramedian veins
  - DSA, lateral view
    - ICV follows gently undulating posterior course from foramen of Monro to VofG
    - VofG forms prominent arc, curving back/up around corpus callosum splenium
  - DSA, AP view
    - ICVs 1-2 mm off midline, seen as ovoid/elliptical collection of contrast
  - T1 C+ MR, axial view: ICVs seen as contrast-filled linear paramedian structures just above third ventricle
  - CTV/MRV: ICVs, VofG well seen

Normal Variants, Anomalies

- Variations common; true anomalies rare
- Vein of Galen malformation
  - Primitive median prosencephalic vein (MPV) persists as outlet for diencephalic, choroidal venous drainage
  - Persisting falcine sinus +/- absent/hypoplastic SS

Anatomy-Based Imaging Issues

Imaging Recommendations

- MRV/CTV delineate dural sinuses, large deep veins (e.g., ICV, BVR)
- DSA best for detailed delineation of deep veins/tributaries

Embryology

Embryologic Events

- 5th fetal week: Arterial supply to choroid plexus forms from meninx primitiva
- 7th-8th fetal week
  - Choroid plexus drains via single temporary midline vein (MPV)
  - MPV courses posteriorly toward developing interhemispheric dural plexus (falcine sinus)
- 10th week
  - ICVs annex drainage of choroid plexus
  - MPV regresses, caudal remnant unites with developing ICVs → definitive VofG formed

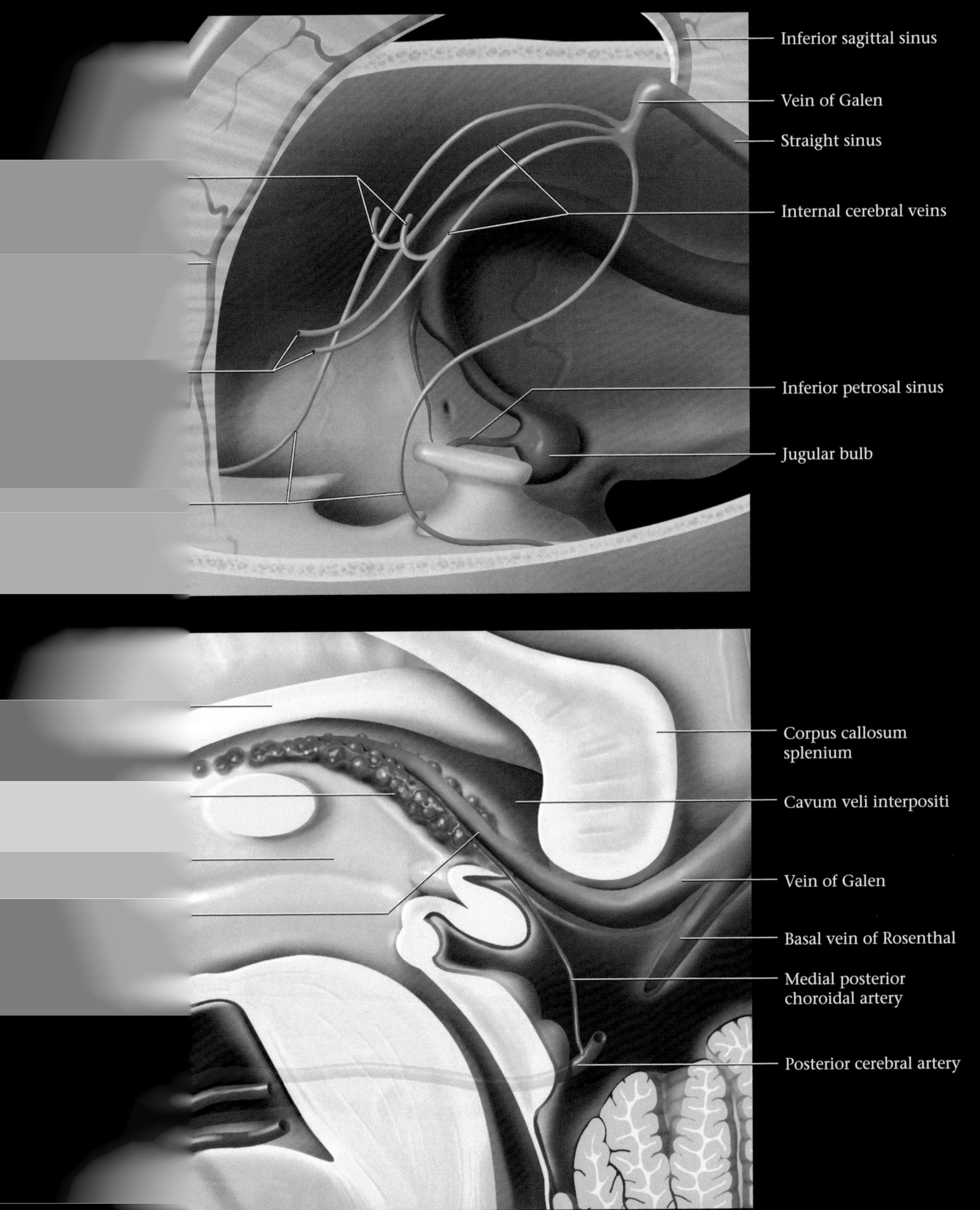
Inferior sagittal sinus
Vein of Galen
Straight sinus
Internal cerebral veins
Inferior petrosal sinus
Jugular bulb
Corpus callosum splenium
Cavum veli interpositi
Vein of Galen
Basal vein of Rosenthal
Medial posterior choroidal artery
Posterior cerebral artery

e major deep cerebral veins is illustrated. The septal and thalamostriate veins come together
ral veins. The ICVs and basal veins of Rosenthal are the major tributaries of the vein of
l sinus joins the vein of Galen near the apex of the falcotentorial junction. **(Bottom)**
epicts relationship of the internal cerebral vein to adjacent structures (there are two ICVs;
The ICV runs posteriorly in the cavum veli interpositi, which is within the double-layered
l ventricle (technically not above it). The ICVs lie above the pineal gland and body of the
fornix and corpus callosum splenium. The BVRs and ICVs unite to form the straight sinus

GRAPHICS

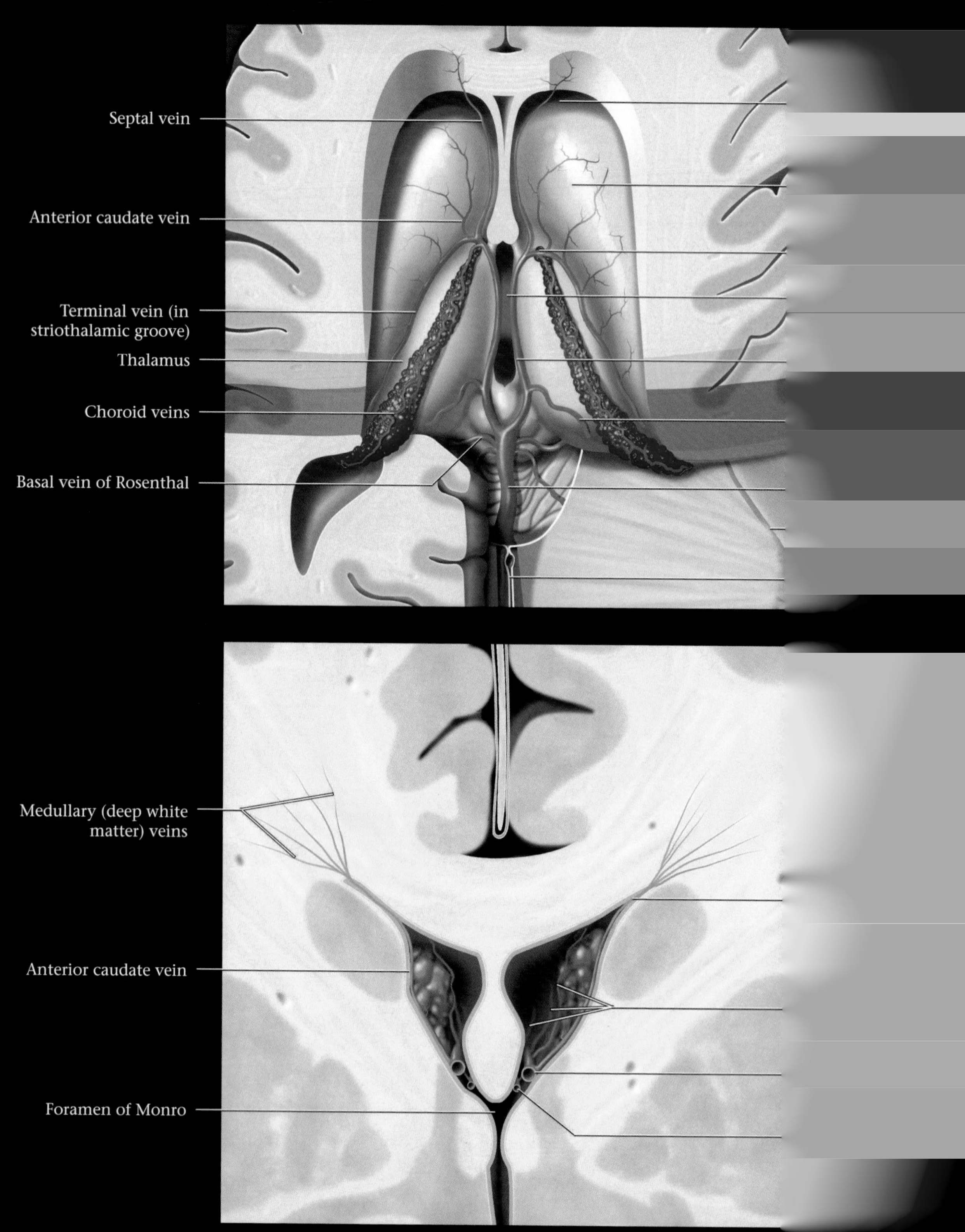

Septal vein
Anterior caudate vein
Terminal vein (in striothalamic groove)
Thalamus
Choroid veins
Basal vein of Rosenthal
Medullary (deep white matter) veins
Anterior caudate vein
Foramen of Monro

(Top) The deep (subependymal) veins are illustrated here as seen from the top down. The cc
fornices have been removed to show the lateral ventricles. The ICVs course posteriorly in th
just above the top of the third ventricle. **(Bottom)** Close-up coronal view of the lateral vent
between the medullary (deep white matter) and subependymal veins. Medullary veins conv
margins, drain into subependymal veins, and from there into the Galenic system. The inter
most prominent deep tributaries of the vein of Galen, which is formed by the junction of th

DEEP CEREBRAL VEINS

LAT & AP ICA DSA

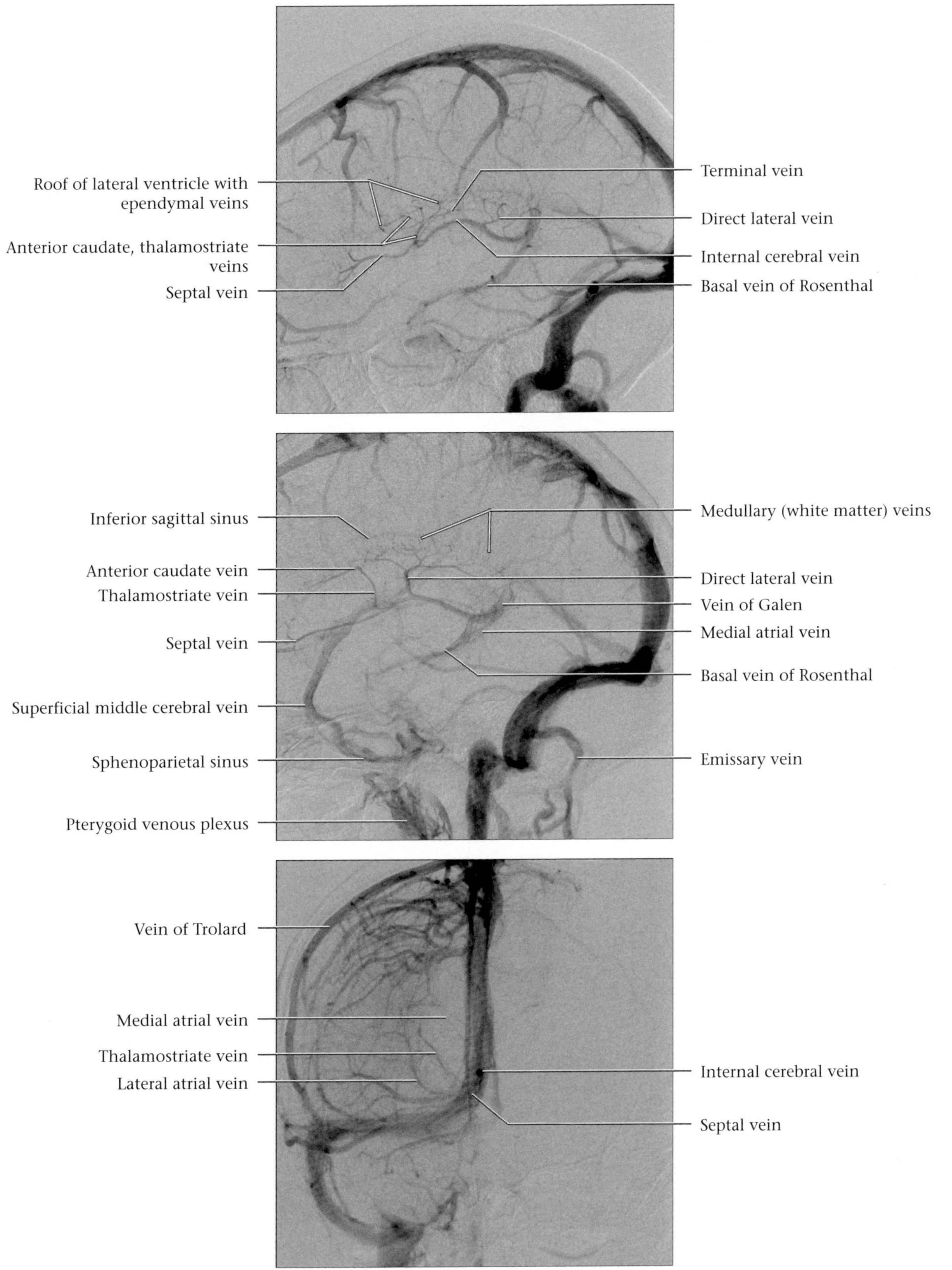
Roof of lateral ventricle with ependymal veins
Anterior caudate, thalamostriate veins
Septal vein
Terminal vein
Direct lateral vein
Internal cerebral vein
Basal vein of Rosenthal
Inferior sagittal sinus
Anterior caudate vein
Thalamostriate vein
Septal vein
Superficial middle cerebral vein
Sphenoparietal sinus
Pterygoid venous plexus
Medullary (white matter) veins
Direct lateral vein
Vein of Galen
Medial atrial vein
Basal vein of Rosenthal
Emissary vein
Vein of Trolard
Medial atrial vein
Thalamostriate vein
Lateral atrial vein
Internal cerebral vein
Septal vein

(Top) Two lateral DSA views from different patients, mid-venous phase, are shown. The deep white matter (medullary) veins converge on the ependymal veins, outlining the roof of the lateral ventricle (seen here as "dots" of contrast). **(Middle)** On the lateral view, venous phase, of this DSA, a long septal vein joins the thalamostriate and direct lateral veins well behind the foramen of Monro, a normal variant. The "brush-like" linear contrast collections seen near the roof of the lateral ventricle are the medullary (white matter) veins. **(Bottom)** AP view, mid-venous phase, of a DSA shows the thalamostriate vein as it outlines the lateral margin of the ventricle.

DEEP CEREBRAL VEINS

AXIAL T1 C+ MR

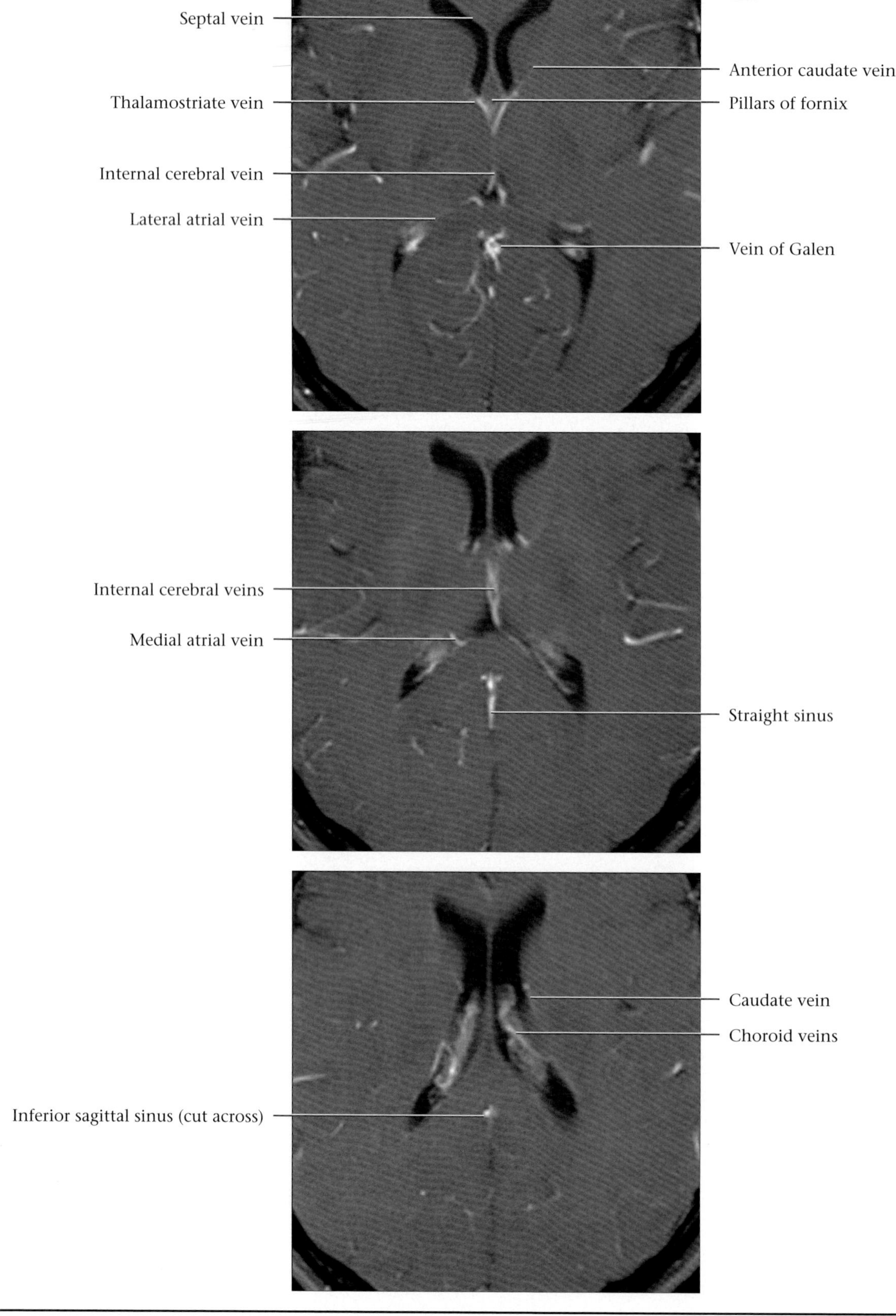
Septal vein
Anterior caudate vein
Thalamostriate vein
Pillars of fornix
Internal cerebral vein
Lateral atrial vein
Vein of Galen
Internal cerebral veins
Medial atrial vein
Straight sinus
Caudate vein
Choroid veins
Inferior sagittal sinus (cut across)

(Top) Series of three axial T1 C+ MR scans from inferior to superior is shown. Section through the foramen of Monro shows the septal veins as they curve posteriorly from the frontal horns around the pillars of the fornix. They join together with the thalamostriate veins to form the internal cerebral veins. **(Middle)** The paired internal cerebral veins are seen here as the course posteriorly in the velum interpositum, above the third ventricle. **(Bottom)** Scan through the bodies of the lateral ventricles shows the enhancing choroid plexus coursing anteriorly along the striothalamic groove. Choroid veins are the prominent tortuous vessels running over the choroid plexus.

DEEP CEREBRAL VEINS

CORONAL T1 C+ MR

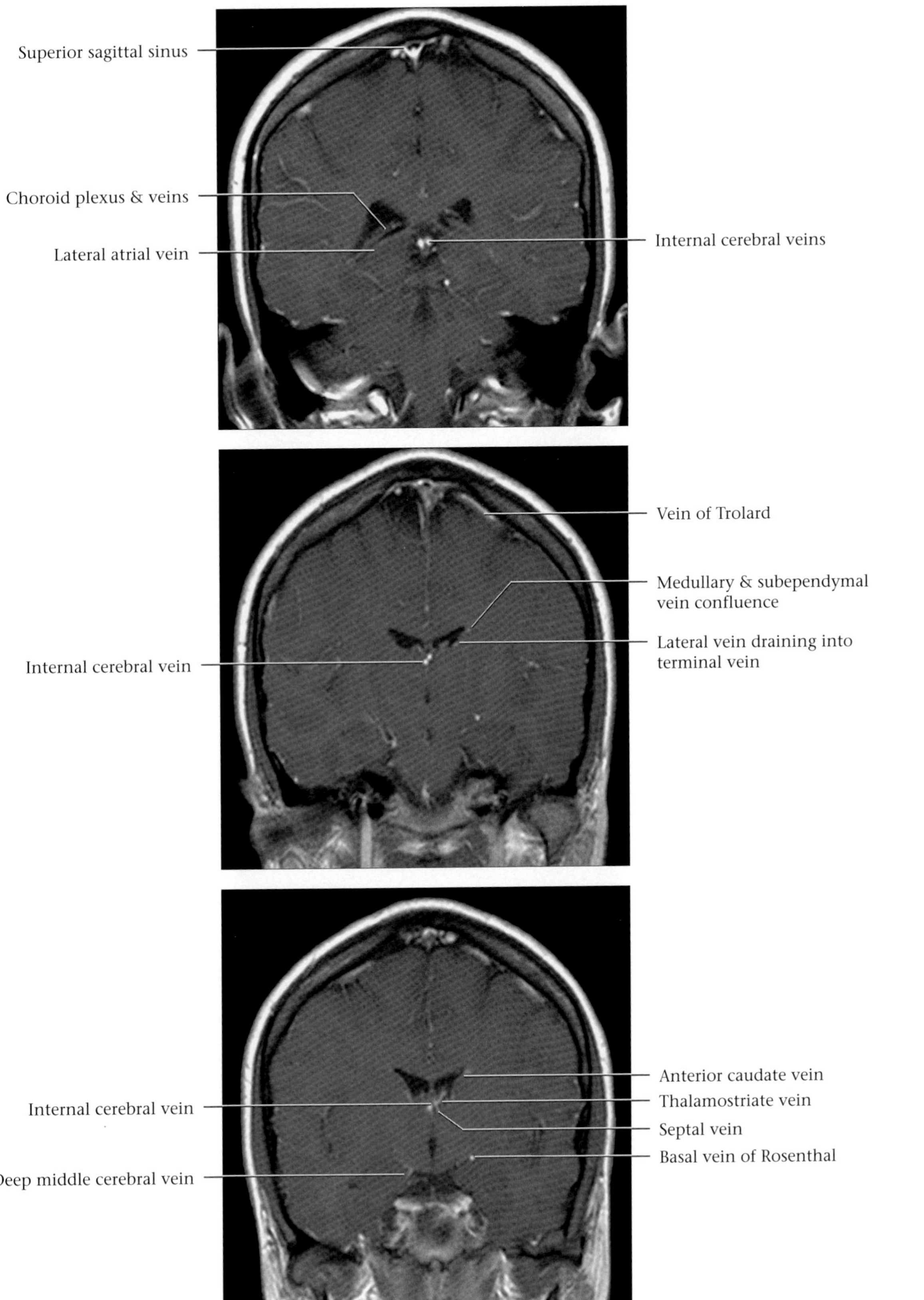
Superior sagittal sinus
Choroid plexus & veins
Lateral atrial vein
Internal cerebral veins
Vein of Trolard
Medullary & subependymal vein confluence
Lateral vein draining into terminal vein
Internal cerebral vein
Anterior caudate vein
Thalamostriate vein
Septal vein
Basal vein of Rosenthal
Internal cerebral vein
Deep middle cerebral vein

(Top) Series of three coronal T1 C+ scans from posterior to anterior are shown. Section through the atria of the lateral ventricles shows the choroid plexus and its veins as well as the internal cerebral veins coursing posteriorly within the velum interpositum. **(Middle)** Section through the bodies of the lateral ventricles shows faint enhancement along the superolateral margin of the ventricle representing confluence of the deep medullary (white matter) veins draining into a subependymal vein. **(Bottom)** Section just behind the foramen of Monro shows the septal and thalamostriate veins forming the internal cerebral vein.

DEEP CEREBRAL VEINS

CORONAL T2 MR

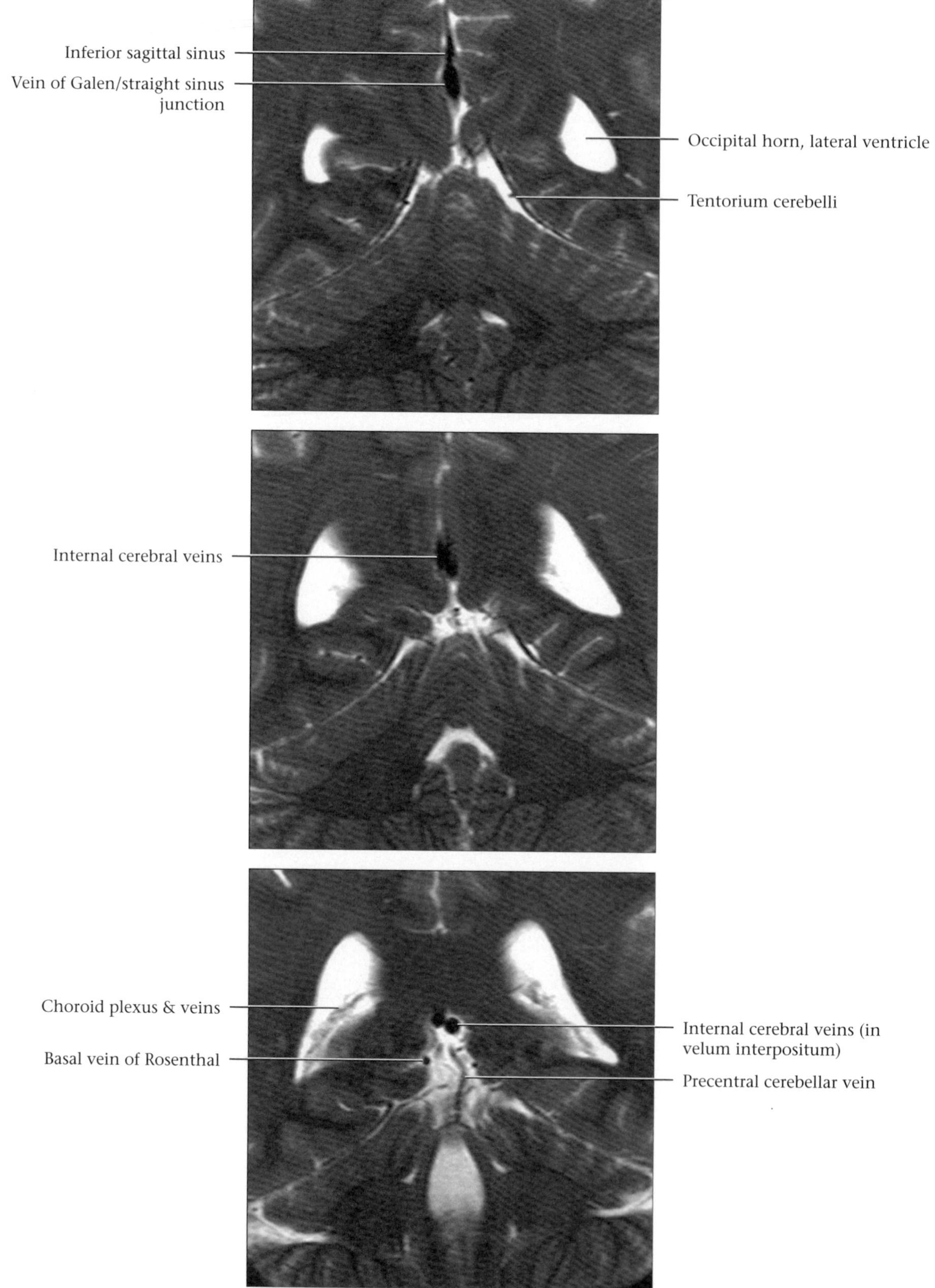
Inferior sagittal sinus
Vein of Galen/straight sinus junction
Occipital horn, lateral ventricle
Tentorium cerebelli
Internal cerebral veins
Choroid plexus & veins
Basal vein of Rosenthal
Internal cerebral veins (in velum interpositum)
Precentral cerebellar vein

(Top) Series of six coronal T2 MR images from posterior to anterior is shown. Section through the occipital horn of the lateral ventricle demonstrates confluence of the vein of Galen with the inferior sagittal sinus at the apex of the falcotentorial junction. **(Middle)** Internal cerebral veins are shown just prior to joining vein of Galen. **(Bottom)** Basal vein of Rosenthal and internal cerebral veins course posteriorly before anastomosing with vein of Galen. The precentral cerebellar vein courses superiorly in front of the central lobule of the vermis to join the vein of Galen. Even though it drains posterior fossa structures, this vein is generally considered part of the so-called "Galenic group" of veins.

DEEP CEREBRAL VEINS

CORONAL T2 MR

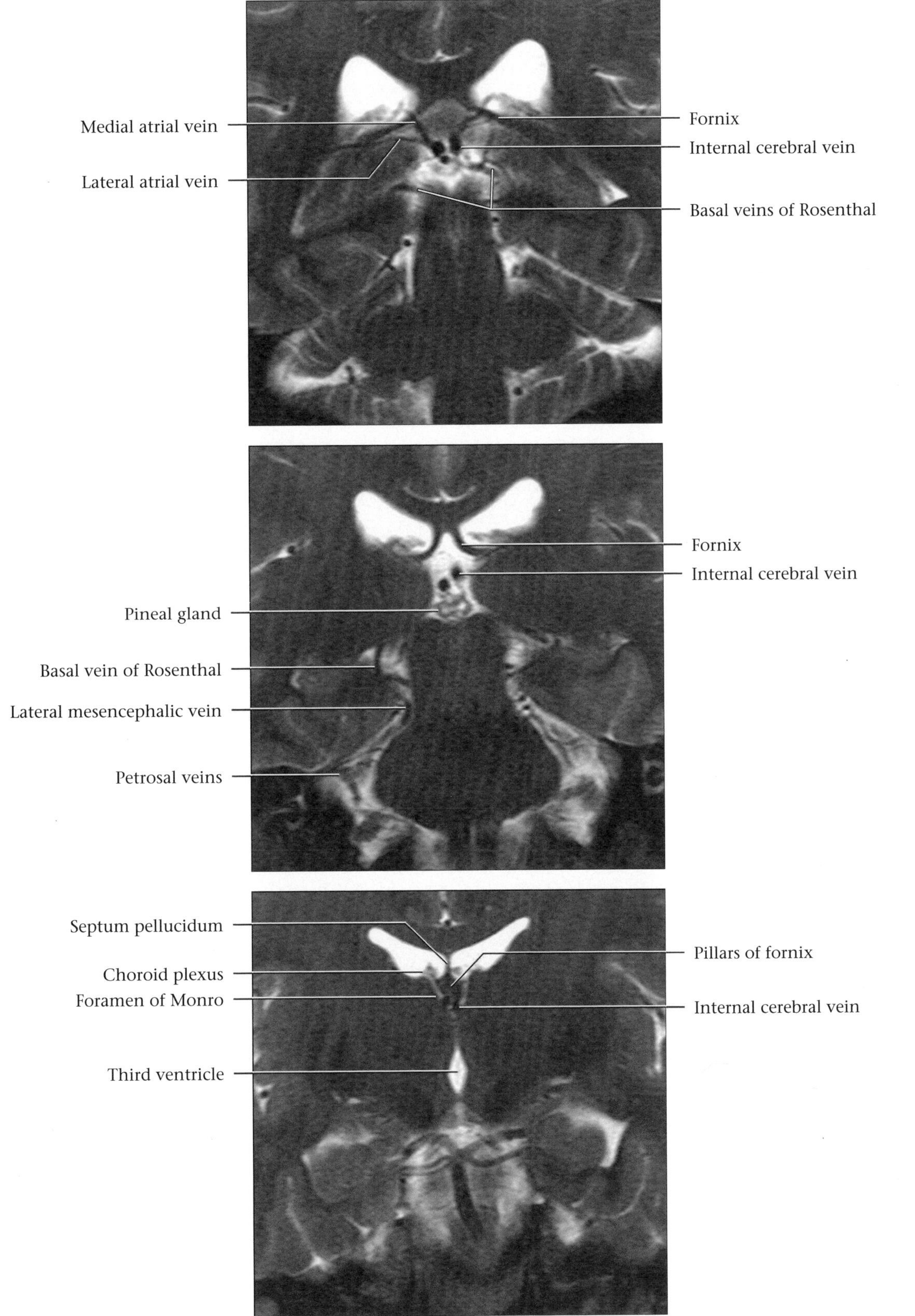
Medial atrial vein
Lateral atrial vein
Fornix
Internal cerebral vein
Basal veins of Rosenthal
Fornix
Internal cerebral vein
Pineal gland
Basal vein of Rosenthal
Lateral mesencephalic vein
Petrosal veins
Septum pellucidum
Choroid plexus
Foramen of Monro
Third ventricle
Pillars of fornix
Internal cerebral vein

(Top) Medial and lateral atrial veins drain into the internal cerebral veins. The basal veins of Rosenthal are seen here as they course superomedially around cerebral peduncles within the ambient and quadrigeminal cisterns. They will join the ICVs to form the vein of Galen. The BVRs are actually superficial cerebral veins, although their drainage pattern is into the deep venous system. **(Middle)** The internal cerebral veins are seen here as they course posteriorly within the velum interpositum, above a cystic pineal gland. The velum interpositum is a CSF-containing subarachnoid cistern and is anatomically an anterior extension of the quadrigeminal cistern. It lies beneath the fornices and above the third ventricle. Some posterior fossa veins are also seen in this section. **(Bottom)** Scan through the foramen of Monro shows origin of the internal cerebral veins.

DEEP CEREBRAL VEINS

AXIAL CTV

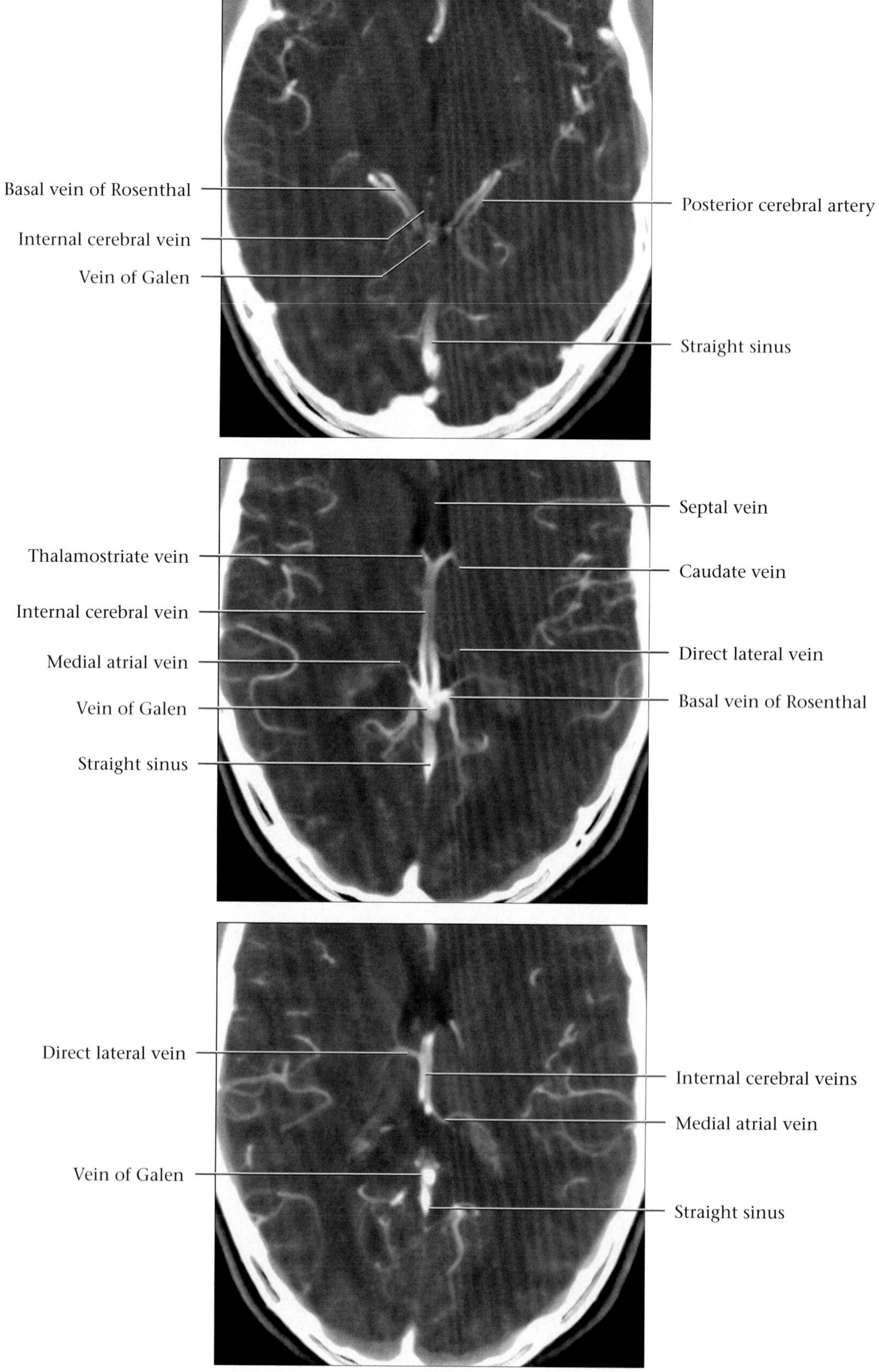
Basal vein of Rosenthal
Internal cerebral vein
Vein of Galen
Posterior cerebral artery
Straight sinus
Septal vein
Thalamostriate vein
Caudate vein
Internal cerebral vein
Medial atrial vein
Direct lateral vein
Vein of Galen
Basal vein of Rosenthal
Straight sinus
Direct lateral vein
Internal cerebral veins
Medial atrial vein
Vein of Galen
Straight sinus

(Top) First of three axial CT source images from a CT venogram are shown from inferior to superior. This section shows the basal veins of Rosenthal, posterior aspect of the internal cerebral veins, and vein of Galen. The BVRs, P2 posterior cerebral artery segments, and the trochlear nerve all course through the ambient cisterns and are in close proximity to one another. **(Middle)** This view shows the ICVs as they are formed from the thalamostriate and septal veins. Numerous ventricular tributaries are present. **(Bottom)** This view shows the internal cerebral veins, vein of Galen, and straight sinus. So-called "direct lateral" veins collect tributaries from the caudate body as they course along the stria terminalis, which demarcates the border between the caudate and thalamus. Sometimes these veins are quite prominent, as seen in this case.

DEEP CEREBRAL VEINS

AP CTV

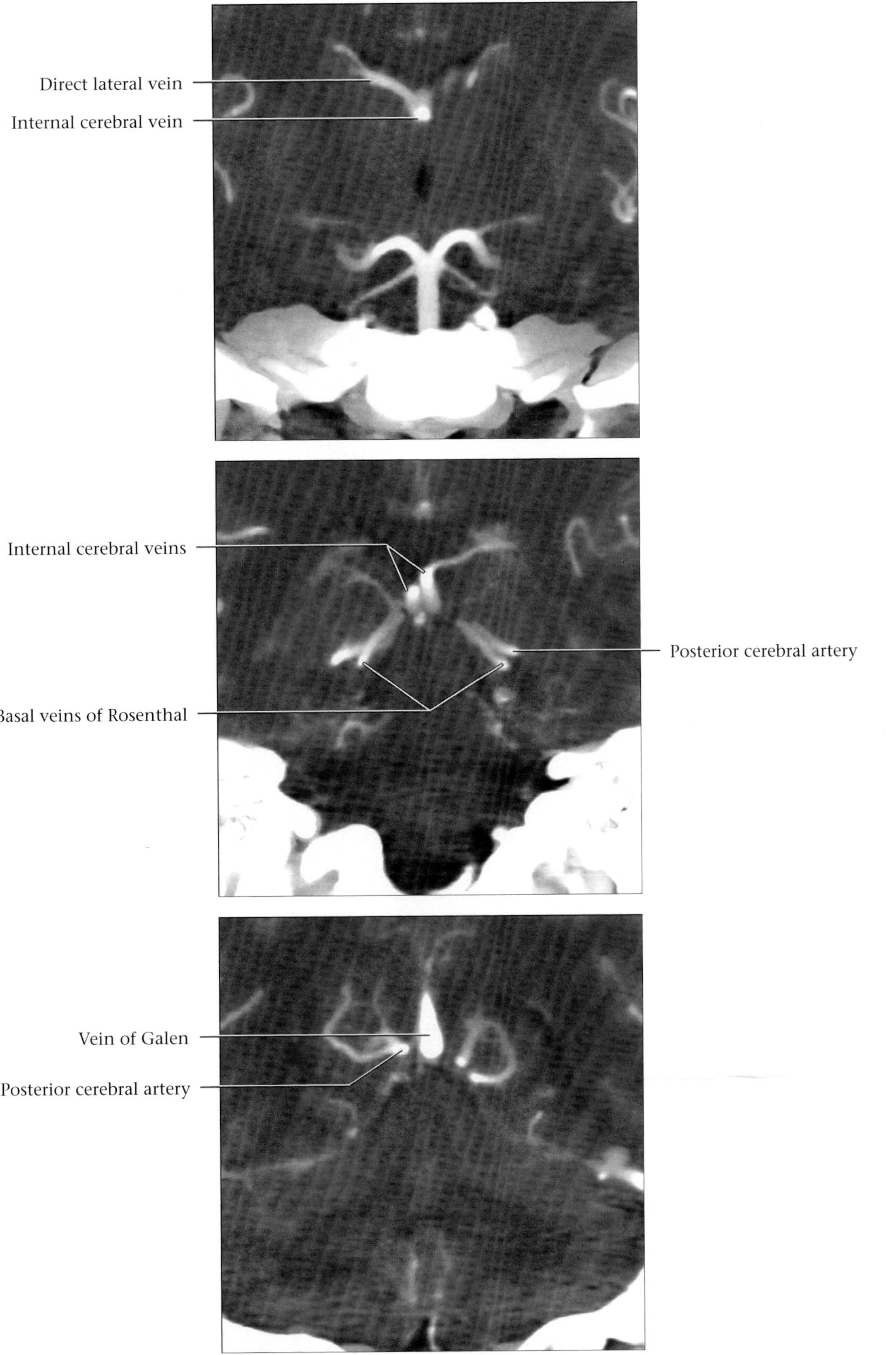
Direct lateral vein
Internal cerebral vein
Internal cerebral veins
Posterior cerebral artery
Basal veins of Rosenthal
Vein of Galen
Posterior cerebral artery

(Top) First of three AP views of CT venogram with section through the basilar bifurcation shows a large direct lateral vein draining into the internal cerebral vein. Its upper aspect runs along the caudate nucleus; its lower aspect curves over the thalamus. The stria terminalis is at the junction of these two segments. **(Middle)** The internal cerebral veins and both basal veins of Rosenthal are seen here just before they converge to form the vein of Galen. The posterior cerebral artery lies lateral to the BVRs. Both curve posteriorly around the midbrain, running in the ambient cistern. **(Bottom)** Image at the tentorial apex shows the vein of Galen. The posterior cerebral artery is seen here, dividing into its parietooccipital and calcarine arteries.

DEEP CEREBRAL VEINS

SAGITTAL CTV

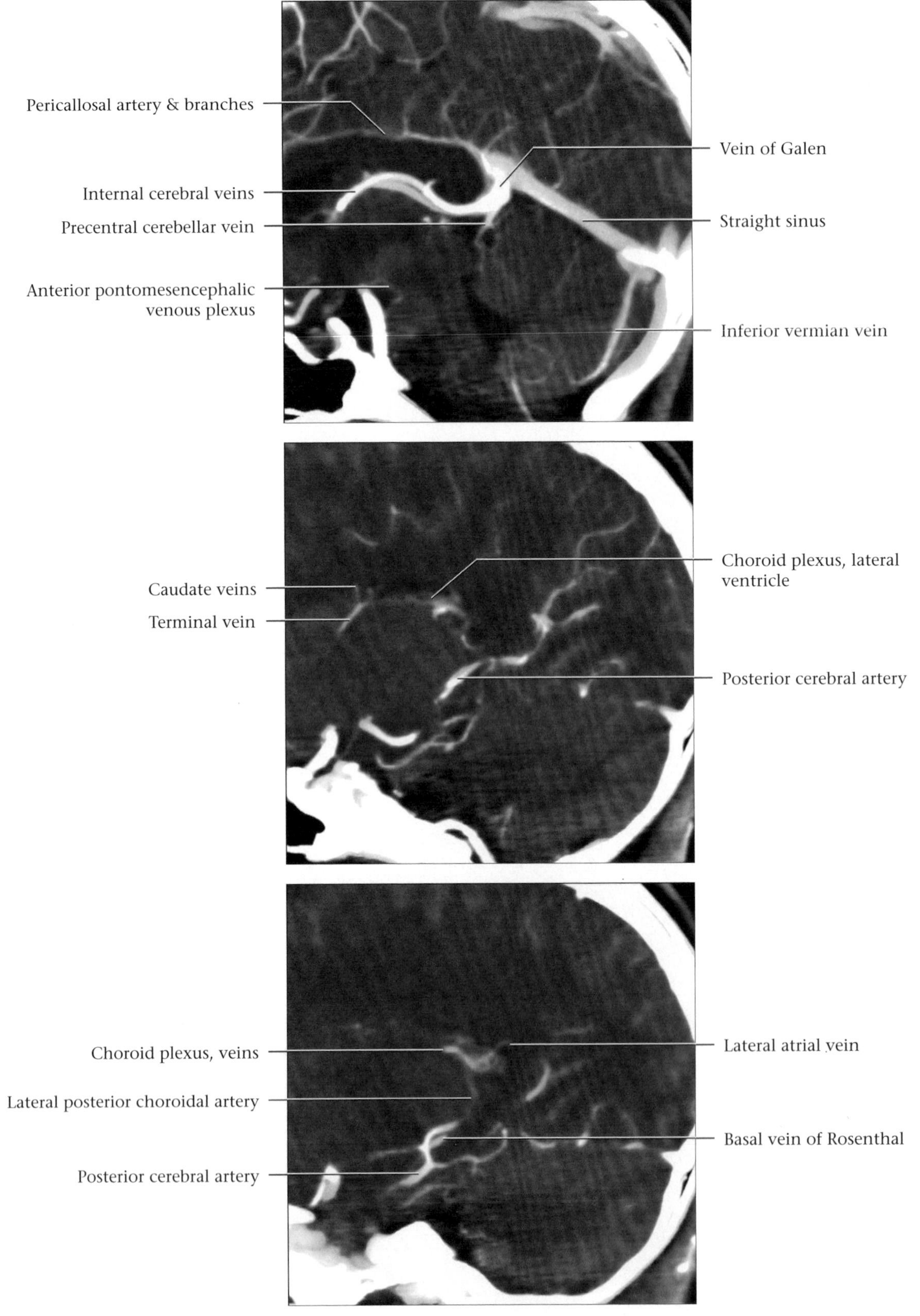
Pericallosal artery & branches
Internal cerebral veins
Precentral cerebellar vein
Anterior pontomesencephalic venous plexus
Vein of Galen
Straight sinus
Inferior vermian vein
Caudate veins
Terminal vein
Choroid plexus, lateral ventricle
Posterior cerebral artery
Choroid plexus, veins
Lateral posterior choroidal artery
Posterior cerebral artery
Lateral atrial vein
Basal vein of Rosenthal

(Top) Series of three sagittal views of a CT venogram are shown from medial to lateral. Midline view shows the internal cerebral veins as they follow a sinusoidal course, running posteriorly in the velum interpositum above the roof of the third ventricle. The vein of Galen and one of its tributaries, the precentral cerebellar vein, are well seen here. **(Middle)** Slightly more lateral view shows the choroid plexus of the lateral ventricle as it courses anteriorly along the striothalamic groove between the caudate nucleus and thalamus. This represents the stria terminalis. A so-called "terminal vein," seen here, may course along this groove and join the caudate and septal veins to form the thalamostriate vein. **(Bottom)** Both the basal vein of Rosenthal and posterior cerebral artery curve around the midbrain within the ambient cistern and are seen on this section.

DEEP CEREBRAL VEINS

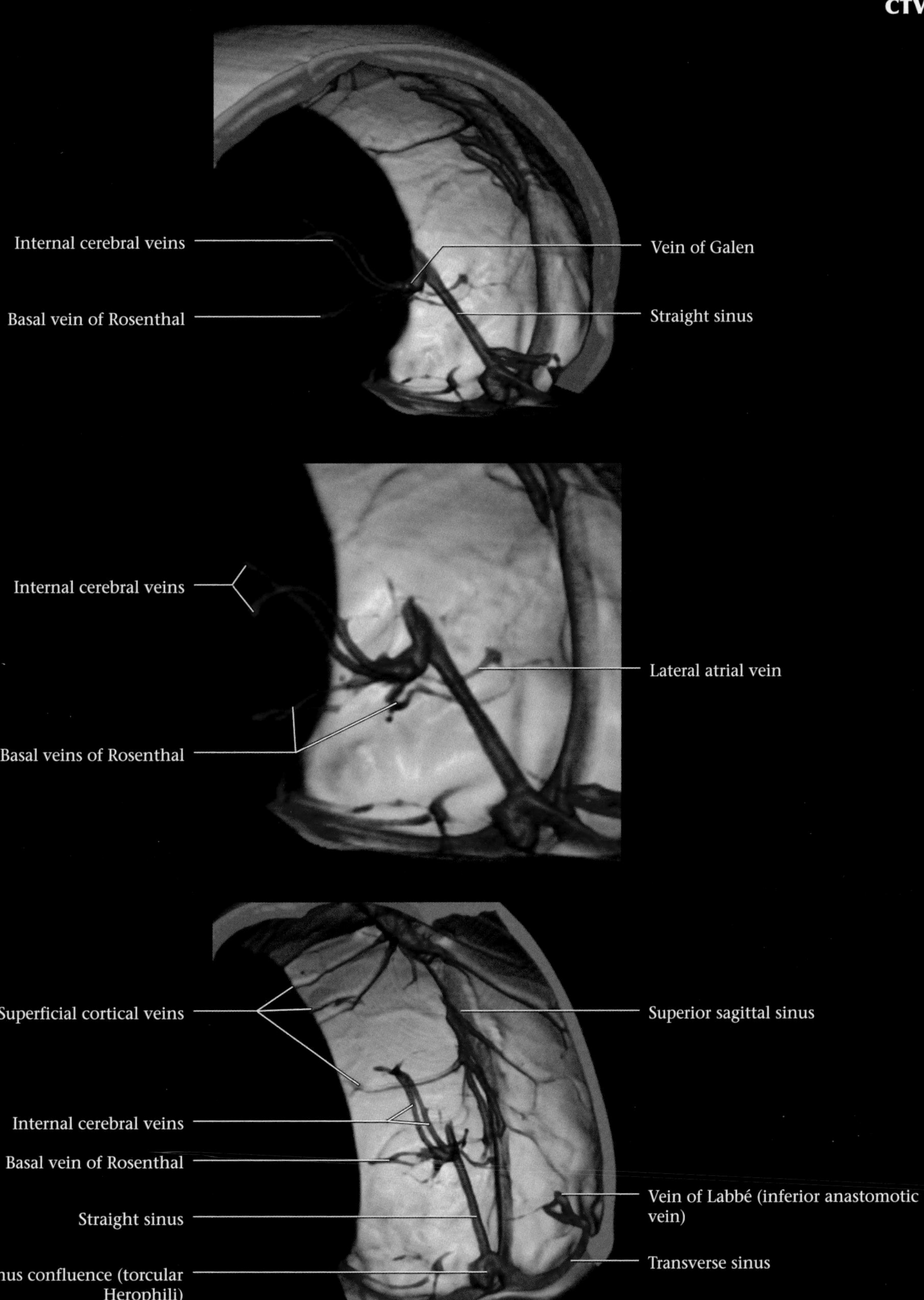
Internal cerebral veins
Vein of Galen
Basal vein of Rosenthal
Straight sinus
Internal cerebral veins
Lateral atrial vein
Basal veins of Rosenthal
Superficial cortical veins
Superior sagittal sinus
Internal cerebral veins
Basal vein of Rosenthal
Vein of Labbé (inferior anastomotic vein)
Straight sinus
Transverse sinus
Sinus confluence (torcular Herophili)

(Top) Three views of a CT venogram are shown. Overview image shows the internal cerebral veins and their relationship to the vein of Galen and straight sinus. **(Middle)** Close-up oblique view shows the internal cerebral veins and basal veins of Rosenthal as they join together at the vein of Galen. **(Bottom)** Cutaway view shows the relationship of the internal cerebral veins, vein of Galen, and straight sinus to the other major dural sinuses. Occlusion of the internal cerebral veins causes a venous infarct in the basal ganglia, internal capsule, and thalamus. An occluded vein of Galen and/or straight sinus may also cause this pattern. Because the deep white matter drains centrally into the subependymal veins, they may become congested and enlarged, with edema extending into the centrum semiovale.

DEEP CEREBRAL VEINS

MRV

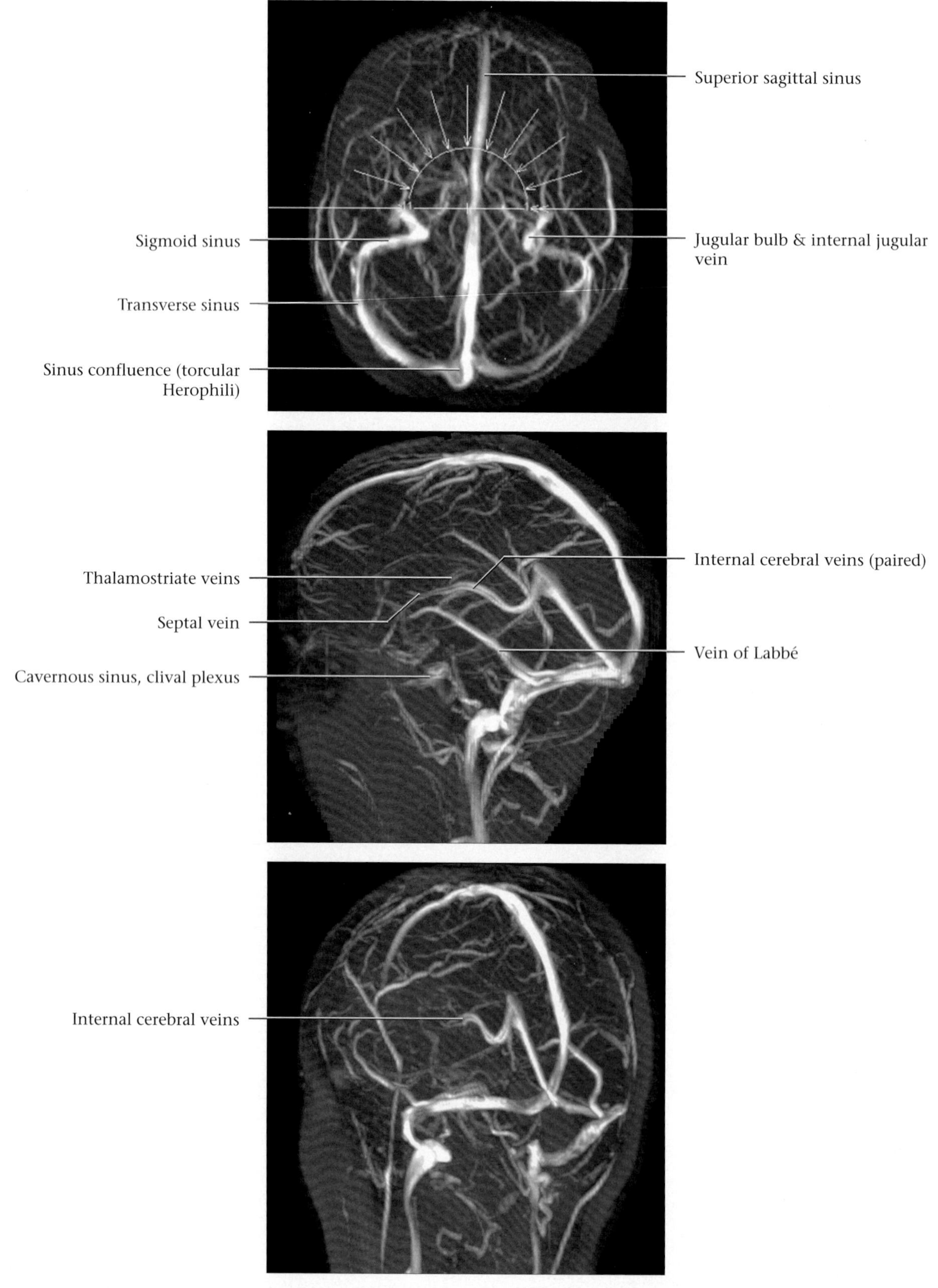
Superior sagittal sinus
Sigmoid sinus
Jugular bulb & internal jugular vein
Transverse sinus
Sinus confluence (torcular Herophili)
Internal cerebral veins (paired)
Thalamostriate veins
Septal vein
Vein of Labbé
Cavernous sinus, clival plexus
Internal cerebral veins

(Top) A series of three different projections from a 3T MR venogram is illustrated. The submentovertex view is especially good for evaluating patency of the major dural venous sinuses but overlap of many vessels largely obscures the deep cerebral veins. **(Middle)** Lateral view of the MRV demonstrates the major deep cerebral veins. Blood flow from deep venous system drains into internal cerebral vein before emptying into vein of Galen. This view is ideal for evaluating patency of the internal cerebral veins, vein of Galen and straight sinus. The subependymal and medullary veins are not generally visualized on standard MR venograms. **(Bottom)** Oblique AP view shows the major dural venous sinuses as well as the Galenic system. The normal sinusoidal course of the internal cerebral veins as well as their relationship to the vein of Galen are especially well seen.

DEEP CEREBRAL VEINS

MRV

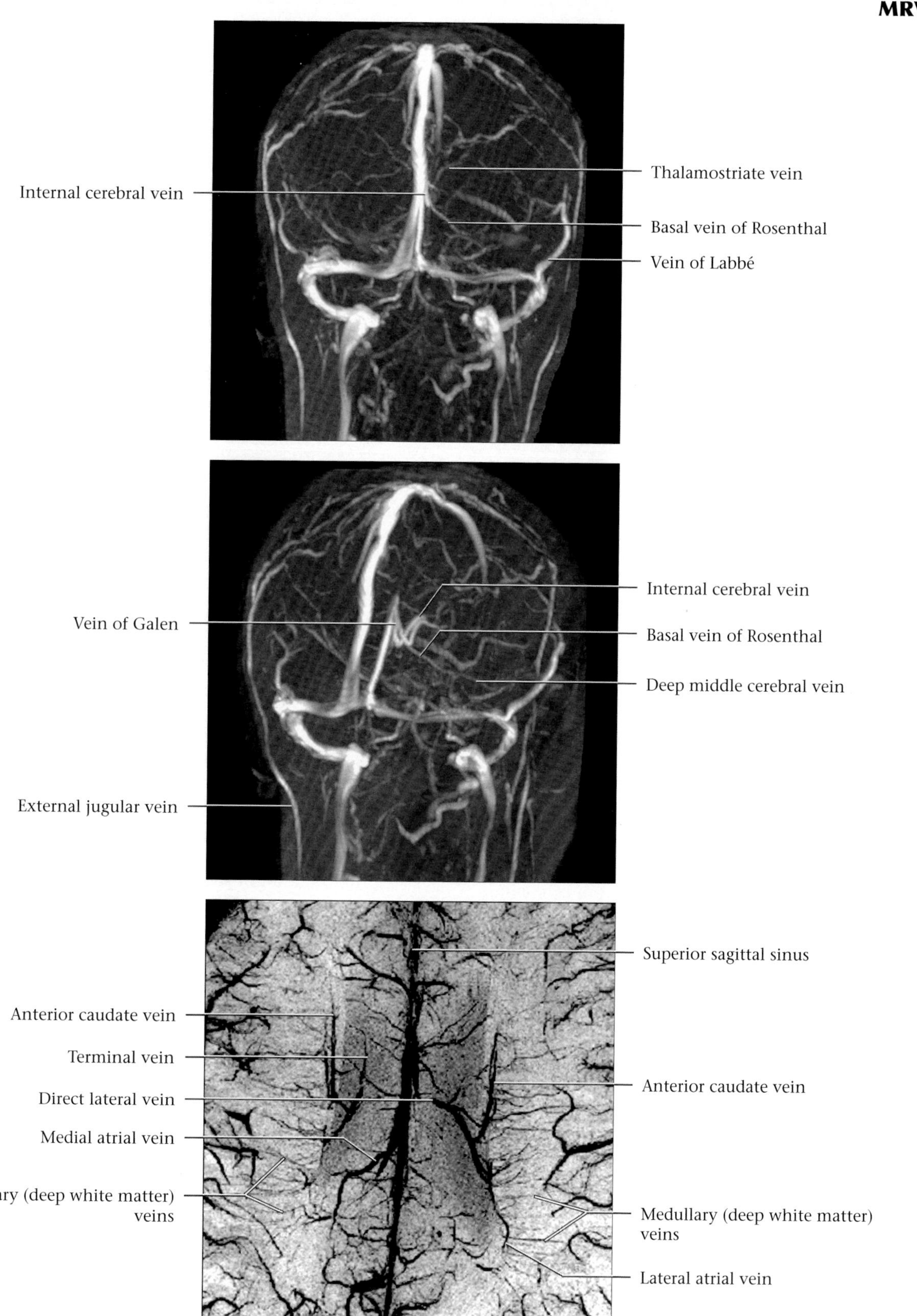
Internal cerebral vein
Thalamostriate vein
Basal vein of Rosenthal
Vein of Labbé
Vein of Galen
Internal cerebral vein
Basal vein of Rosenthal
Deep middle cerebral vein
External jugular vein
Superior sagittal sinus
Anterior caudate vein
Terminal vein
Direct lateral vein
Medial atrial vein
Medullary (deep white matter) veins
Anterior caudate vein
Medullary (deep white matter) veins
Lateral atrial vein

(Top) Straight AP view shows the internal cerebral vein is superimposed on the superior sagittal sinus. The thalamostriate vein, well seen here, defines the outer margin of the lateral ventricle. A prominent vein of Labbé is present on the left. **(Middle)** Oblique AP view demonstrates drainage of basal vein of Rosenthal into internal cerebral vein. One of its small but important tributaries, the deep middle cerebral vein, is well seen. **(Bottom)** Here a close-up view of axial contrast-enhanced susceptibility-weighted 3T MR venogram shows details of the deep venous drainage system and its tributaries. In this high-resolution study, the white matter (medullary) veins are seen converging on the subependymal veins at the margins of the lateral ventricles. The medullary (deep white matter veins) are not well seen on routine MRVs, even on 3T studies. (Courtesy J. Tsuruda, MD).

POSTERIOR FOSSA VEINS

Terminology

Abbreviations

- Vein of Galen (VofG)
- Precentral cerebellar vein (PCV)
- Anterior pontomesencephalic vein/venous plexus (APMV)
- Superior vermian vein (SVV)
- Inferior vermian vein (IVV)
- Cerebellopontine angle (CPA)
- Internal auditory canal (IAC)
- Superior petrosal sinus (SPS)
- Subarachnoid space (SAS)

Definitions

- Venous drainage for midbrain, pons, medulla, cerebellum, vermis

Gross Anatomy

Overview

- Three major posterior fossa/midbrain drainage systems
  - **Superior (galenic) group** drains up into vein of Galen, has three major named veins
    - **Precentral cerebellar vein**: Single, midline; lies between lingula/central lobule of vermis; terminates behind inferior colliculi by draining into VofG
    - **Superior vermian vein**: Originates near declive of vermis, courses up/over top of vermis (culmen), joins PCV and enters VofG
    - **Anterior pontomesencephalic vein**: Superficial venous plexus covers cerebral peduncles, anterior surface of pons
  - **Anterior (petrosal) group**
    - Petrosal vein: Prominent trunk in CPA that collects numerous tributaries from cerebellum, pons, medulla
  - **Posterior (tentorial) group**
    - **Inferior vermian veins**: Paired paramedian structures; curve posterosuperiorly under pyramis, uvula of vermis

Anatomy Relationships

- **PCV**
  - Courses over roof of fourth ventricle, anterior (superior) medullary velum in midline
  - Lies between lingula, central lobule of vermis
  - Upper end (at VofG level) lies below, behind quadrigeminal plate and pineal gland
- **SVV**
  - Courses over vermian apex
  - Lies under tentorium
- **APMV**
  - Lies under vertebrobasilar artery
  - Closely adherent to pial surface of pons
- **Petrosal vein**
  - Courses anterolaterally below CN5 (trigeminal nerve)
  - Enters SPS just above IAC

Vascular Territory

- Superior (galenic) group
  - Midbrain, pons, superior surface of cerebellar hemispheres, upper vermis
- Anterior (petrosal) group
  - Anterior (petrosal) surface of cerebellar hemispheres, lateral pons, brachium pontis, medulla, flocculus, nodulus
- Posterior (tentorial) group
  - Inferior/posterior surfaces of cerebellar hemispheres, inferior vermis, tonsils

Imaging Anatomy

Overview

- Superior ("galenic") group
  - Veins of this group generally course over superior surfaces of cerebellum, vermis as well as anterior surface of midbrain, pons and medulla
  - Superior cerebellar veins course over hemispheres
  - Galenic veins typically drain into VofG or directly into straight sinus (SS)
  - Cerebellar hemispheric veins also may drain laterally into transverse sinus (TS), SPS, or directly into small dural sinuses within tentorium
- Anterior (petrosal) group
  - Demarcates middle of cerebellopontine angle cistern
  - Petrosal vein courses superiorly to drain into SPS
- Posterior (tentorial) group
  - Demarcates inferior vermis

Normal Imaging

- DSA, lateral view
  - PCV: Anteriorly convex curve, lies halfway between tuberculum sellae and torcular Herophili
  - APMV: Outlines pons, midbrain; lies approximately 1 cm behind clivus at closest point
  - SVV: Outlines superior vermis; normally is 2-3 mm below straight sinus
  - IVV: Outlines inferior vermis; normally is at least 1 cm from inner table of skull
- DSA, AP view
  - Petrosal vein: May form prominent venous "star" in CPA cistern
  - SVVs/IVVs should lie in or near midline
- T1 C+ MR
  - APMV seen as faint plexiform enhancement along pial surface of pons, medulla
    - Seen on both sagittal, axial scans
- CECT
  - Axial: Scans cut obliquely through tentorium so superior cerebellar veins, SVVs appear as linear/serpentine areas of enhancement
  - Coronal: May show bridging veins crossing SAS between cerebellum/vermis, tentorium

Anatomy-Based Imaging Issues

Imaging Pitfalls

- APMV enhancement along pontine/medullary surface is normal; should not be mistaken for meningitis!

POSTERIOR FOSSA VEINS

GRAPHICS

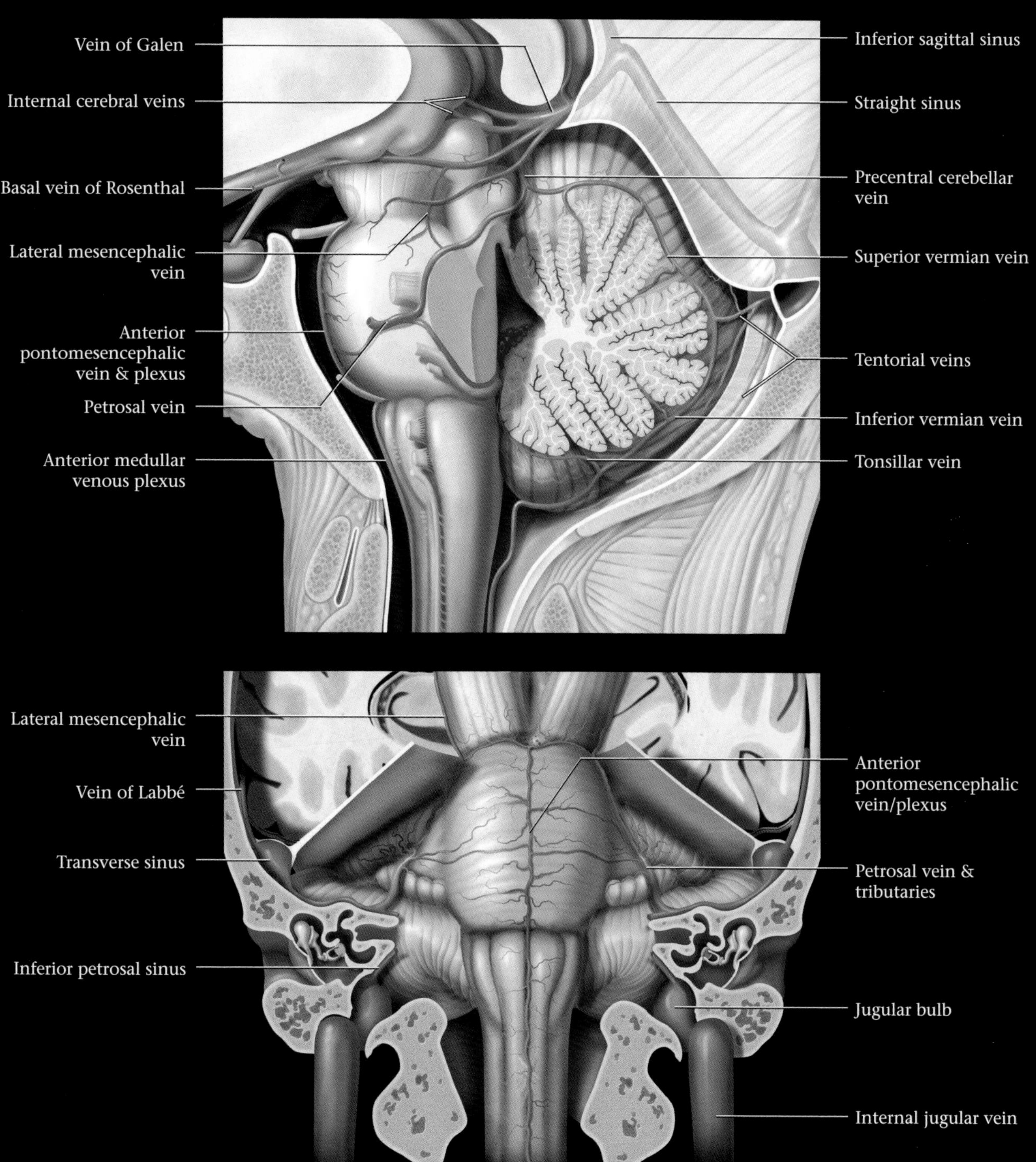

Vein of Galen
Internal cerebral veins
Basal vein of Rosenthal
Lateral mesencephalic vein
Anterior pontomesencephalic vein & plexus
Petrosal vein
Anterior medullar venous plexus
Inferior sagittal sinus
Straight sinus
Precentral cerebellar vein
Superior vermian vein
Tentorial veins
Inferior vermian vein
Tonsillar vein
Lateral mesencephalic vein
Vein of Labbé
Transverse sinus
Inferior petrosal sinus
Anterior pontomesencephalic vein/plexus
Petrosal vein & tributaries
Jugular bulb
Internal jugular vein

(Top) Sagittal graphic with cut through the vermis depicts normal posterior fossa venous drainage. The superior (galenic) group drains the upper cerebellum, vermis, and pons. The anterior (petrosal) group drains the lateral pons, cerebellum, medulla, and structures in the cerebellopontine angle cistern. The posterior (tentorial group) drains the inferior vermis and tentorium. **(Bottom)** AP graphic depicts major venous drainage of the pons, medulla, and anterolateral cerebellum. The anterior pontomesencephalic vein is actually a plexus of small veins covering the surface of the pons and medulla. The petrosal vein and its tributaries provide significant drainage for structures in the cerebellopontine angle cistern and anastomose with the lateral mesencephalic vein and superior petrosal sinus.

POSTERIOR FOSSA VEINS

LAT DSA

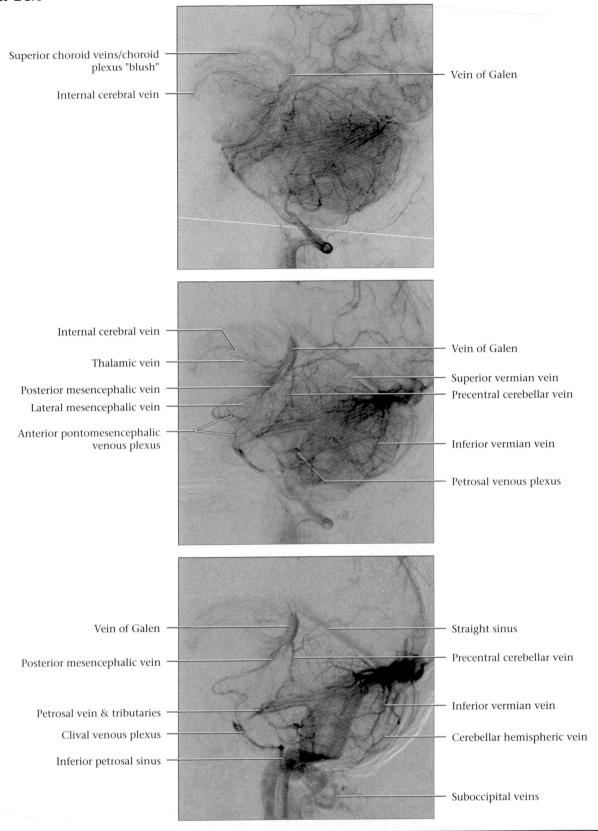

Superior choroid veins/choroid plexus "blush"
Internal cerebral vein
Vein of Galen

Internal cerebral vein
Thalamic vein
Posterior mesencephalic vein
Lateral mesencephalic vein
Anterior pontomesencephalic venous plexus
Vein of Galen
Superior vermian vein
Precentral cerebellar vein
Inferior vermian vein
Petrosal venous plexus

Vein of Galen
Posterior mesencephalic vein
Petrosal vein & tributaries
Clival venous plexus
Inferior petrosal sinus
Straight sinus
Precentral cerebellar vein
Inferior vermian vein
Cerebellar hemispheric vein
Suboccipital veins

(Top) Series of three lateral views of a vertebrobasilar DSA are shown. Late arterial/very early venous phase of a lateral DSA shows a prominent choroid plexus "blush" and early opacification of the internal cerebral vein, a normal finding on posterior fossa angiograms. **(Middle)** Mid-venous phase shows the anterior pontomesencephalic venous plexus outlining the belly of the pons and undersurface of the cerebral peduncles. Note numerous tiny pontine tributaries. **(Bottom)** Late venous phase shows prominent suboccipital veins, a normal finding. The clival venous plexus is opacified and is shown draining into the jugular vein via the inferior petrosal sinus. There is faint opacification of the superior sagittal sinus because the posterior cerebral arteries were opacified on the arterial phase of this study (not shown).

POSTERIOR FOSSA VEINS

AP VA DSA

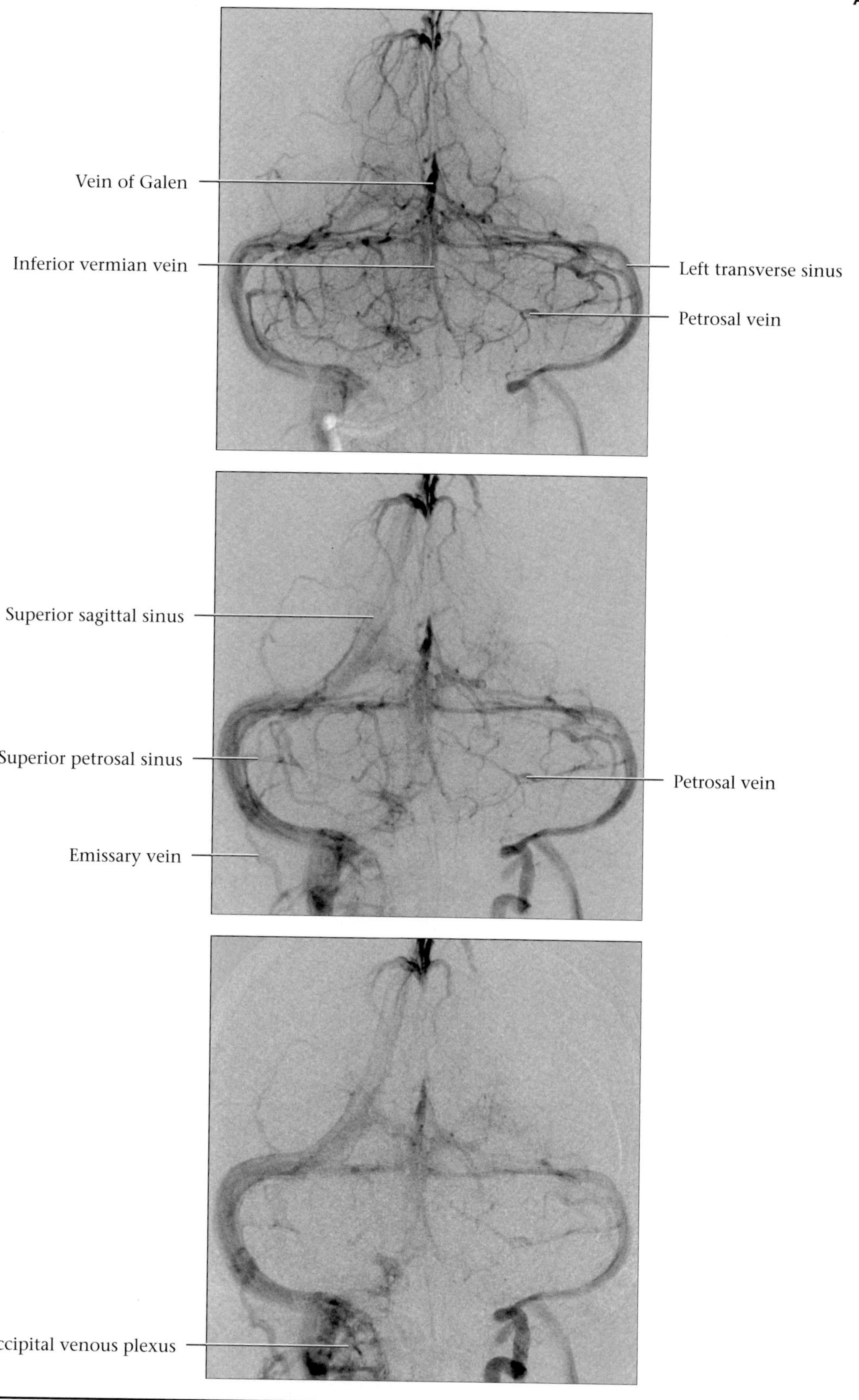
Vein of Galen
Inferior vermian vein
Left transverse sinus
Petrosal vein
Superior sagittal sinus
Superior petrosal sinus
Petrosal vein
Emissary vein
Suboccipital venous plexus

(Top) Series of three AP views of a vertebrobasilar DSA are shown. Early venous phase shows numerous cerebellar hemispheric and vermian veins as well as cortical veins of the occipital lobe (the posterior cerebral arteries were opacified on earlier arterial phase, not shown here). Note significant asymmetry between the sigmoid sinuses and jugular bulbs, a normal variant. **(Middle)** Mid-venous phase shows the petrosal veins draining into the superior petrosal sinuses, which in turn drain into the transverse sinuses. Note that the superior sagittal sinus deviates from the midline as it descends towards the right transverse sinus, a normal variant. **(Bottom)** Late venous phase shows opacification of very prominent suboccipital veins on the right, a normal finding.

POSTERIOR FOSSA VEINS

AXIAL T1 C+ MR

Internal jugular vein
Clival venous plexus
Marginal venous plexus of foramen magnum
Suboccipital venous plexus
Hypoglossal venous plexus
Jugular bulb
Sigmoid sinus
Emissary vein
Clival venous plexus
Inferior petrosal sinus
Choroid plexus of fourth ventricle in lateral recess
Inferior vermian veins (cut across)
Tonsillar vein

(Top) Series of six axial T1C+ fat-saturated MR scans through the posterior fossa are shown. Section through the foramen magnum shows the clival venous plexus and a striking marginal venous plexus around the rim of the foramen magnum. An inconstant dural sinus, the occipital sinus, may connect the marginal plexus with the torcular Herophili. Inhomogeneous signal within the IJV, as seen on this scan, is a normal finding. **(Middle)** Section through the jugular bulbs demonstrates the typical, normal side-to-side asymmetry and inhomogeneous enhancement. The enhancing structures medial to the bulbs are venous plexi that accompany CN12 as it passes through the hypoglossal canal. **(Bottom)** Scan through the lateral recesses of the fourth ventricle shows the inferior petrosal sinuses especially well. The IPS connects the clival venous plexus with the jugular bulb.

POSTERIOR FOSSA VEINS

AXIAL T1 C+ MR

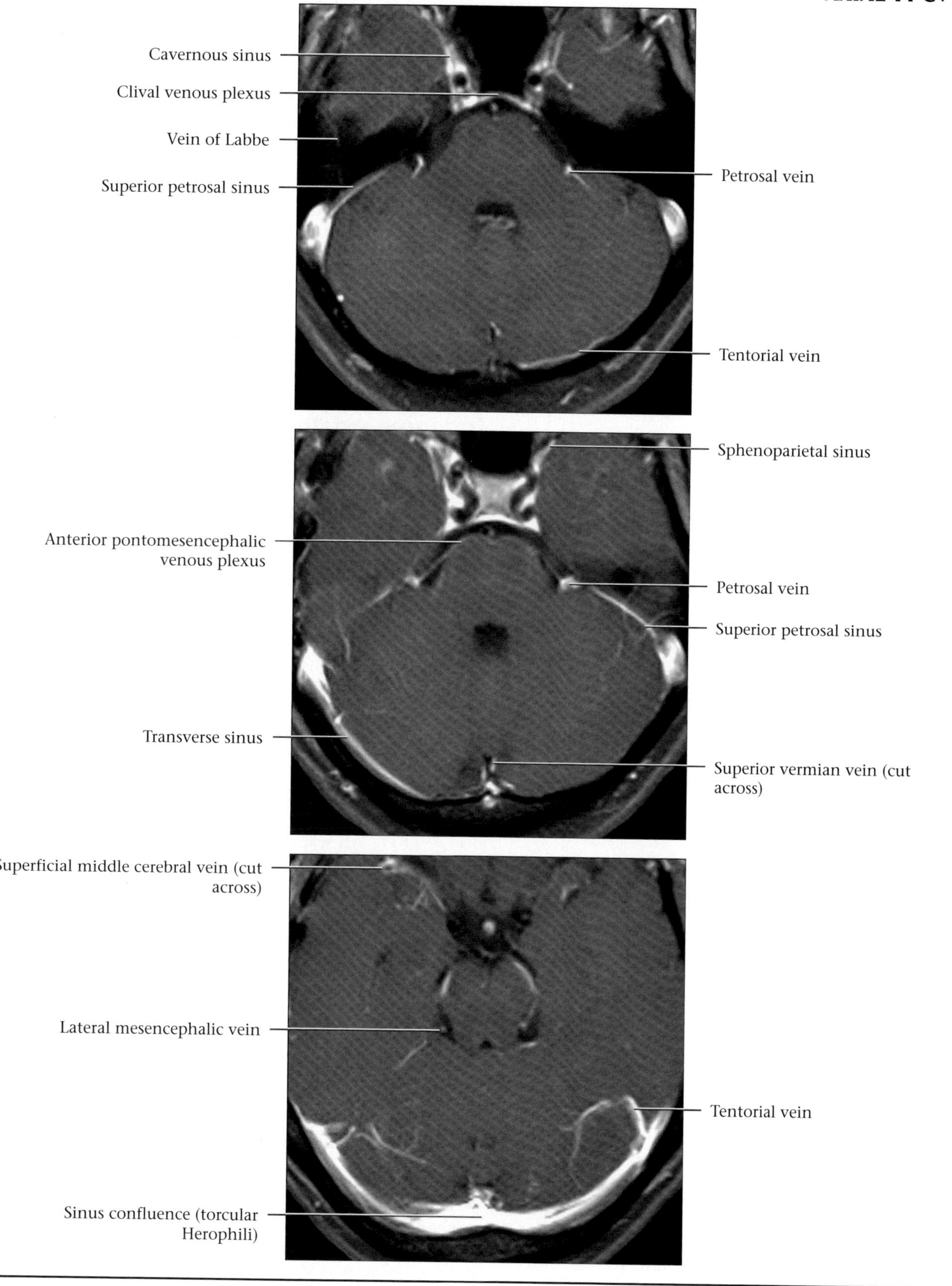
Cavernous sinus
Clival venous plexus
Vein of Labbe
Superior petrosal sinus
Petrosal vein
Tentorial vein
Sphenoparietal sinus
Anterior pontomesencephalic venous plexus
Petrosal vein
Superior petrosal sinus
Transverse sinus
Superior vermian vein (cut across)
Superficial middle cerebral vein (cut across)
Lateral mesencephalic vein
Tentorial vein
Sinus confluence (torcular Herophili)

(Top) Section through the upper petrous ridges shows the right superior petrosal sinus. A hypoplastic vein of Labbé is present. The prominent venous structures in the cerebellopontine angle cistern are petrosal veins. **(Middle)** Scan through the upper pons shows prominent petrosal veins bilaterally with numerous tributaries within the cerebellopontine angle cistern. The faint enhancement covering the pial surface of the pons is the anterior pontomesencephalic venous plexus and is a normal finding that should not be mistaken for meningitis. **(Bottom)** Scan through the upper cerebellum and midbrain shows very prominent tentorial veins that drain into the transverse sinuses.

EXTRACRANIAL VEINS

Terminology

Abbreviations

- Internal jugular vein (IJV)
- Internal carotid artery (ICA)
- Common carotid artery (CCA)
- Inferior, superior ophthalmic veins (IOV, SOV)
- Cavernous sinus (CS)

Definitions

- Extracranial veins include scalp, skull (diploic), face, neck veins

Gross Anatomy

Overview

- **Scalp veins** connect via emissary veins to cranial dural sinuses
  - Superficial temporal vein collects numerous scalp, auricular tributaries
    - Descends into parotid space
    - Together with maxillary vein forms retromandibular vein
- **Diploic veins**
  - Large, irregular endothelial-lined channels in diploic spaces of calvarium
  - May form large venous "lakes"
  - Connect freely with dural sinuses, meningeal veins
- **Emissary veins** connect intra- and extracranial veins
  - Traverse cranial apertures, foramina
  - Connect venous sinuses, extracranial veins
  - Highly variable
- **Orbital veins** (two major)
  - SOV connects face/orbit with CS
  - IOV is smaller, less conspicuous
- **Facial veins**
  - **Facial vein**
    - Begins at angle between eye, nose
    - Descends across masseter, curves around mandible
    - Joins IJV at hyoid level
    - Tributaries from orbit (supraorbital, superior ophthalmic veins), lips, jaw, facial muscles
  - **Deep facial vein**
    - Receives tributaries from deep face, connects facial vein with pterygoid plexus
  - **Pterygoid plexus**
    - Network of vascular channels in masticator space between temporalis/lateral pterygoid muscles
    - Connects cavernous sinuses, clival venous plexus with face/orbit tributaries
    - Drains into maxillary vein
  - **Retromandibular vein**
    - Formed from union of maxillary, superficial temporal veins
    - Lies within parotid space
    - Passes between external carotid artery (ECA) and CN7 to empty into IJV
- **Neck veins**
  - **External jugular vein**
    - From retromandibular, posterior auricular veins
    - Receives tributaries from scalp, ear, face
    - Size, extent highly variable
  - **Internal jugular vein**
    - Caudal continuation of sigmoid sinus
    - Jugular bulb = dilatation at origin
    - Courses inferiorly in carotid space posterolateral to ICA, CCA
    - Unites with subclavian vein to form brachiocephalic vein
    - Size highly variable; significant side-to-side asymmetry common
  - **Vertebral venous plexus**
    - Suboccipital venous plexus
    - Tributaries from basilar (clival) plexus, cervical musculature
    - Interconnects with sigmoid sinuses, cervical epidural venous plexus
    - Terminates in brachiocephalic vein

Imaging Anatomy

Overview

- Extracranial veins highly variable, inconstantly visualized on DSA/CTA/MRA
  - Scalp, emissary veins
    - Rarely opacified on normal DSA but often seen on fat-saturated T1 C+ MRs
    - May become prominent if dAVF, dural sinus occlusion, sinus pericranii present
  - Orbital veins
    - Flow in SOV is normally from EXTRA- to INTRACRANIAL
    - Rarely prominent at DSA unless vascular malformation (e.g., C-C fistula) or CS occlusion present (flow reverses)
  - Face, neck veins
    - Inconstantly visualized
    - Pterygoid plexus often prominent on both DSA, T1 C+ MR scans

Variations, Anomalies

- Extracranial venous drainage highly variable
- Sinus pericranii
  - Abnormal communication between dural venous sinus, extracranial veins
  - Seen as vascular scalp mass that communicates with dural sinus via transcalvarial vein (through well-defined bone defect)
  - Association with intracranial developmental venous anomaly common (+/- venous varix)

Anatomy-Based Imaging Issues

Imaging Pitfalls

- Diploic veins, venous "lakes" ("lacunae") may form sharply marginated, well-corticated skull lucencies (do not mistake for metastases or myeloma)
- Prominent, persistent SOV opacification on DSA is nearly always abnormal but normal on CECT, enhanced MR
- Asymmetric IJVs are common; one IJV may be many times the size of the contralateral IJV
- Extracranial venous plexuses (pterygoid, suboccipital) can normally be very prominent

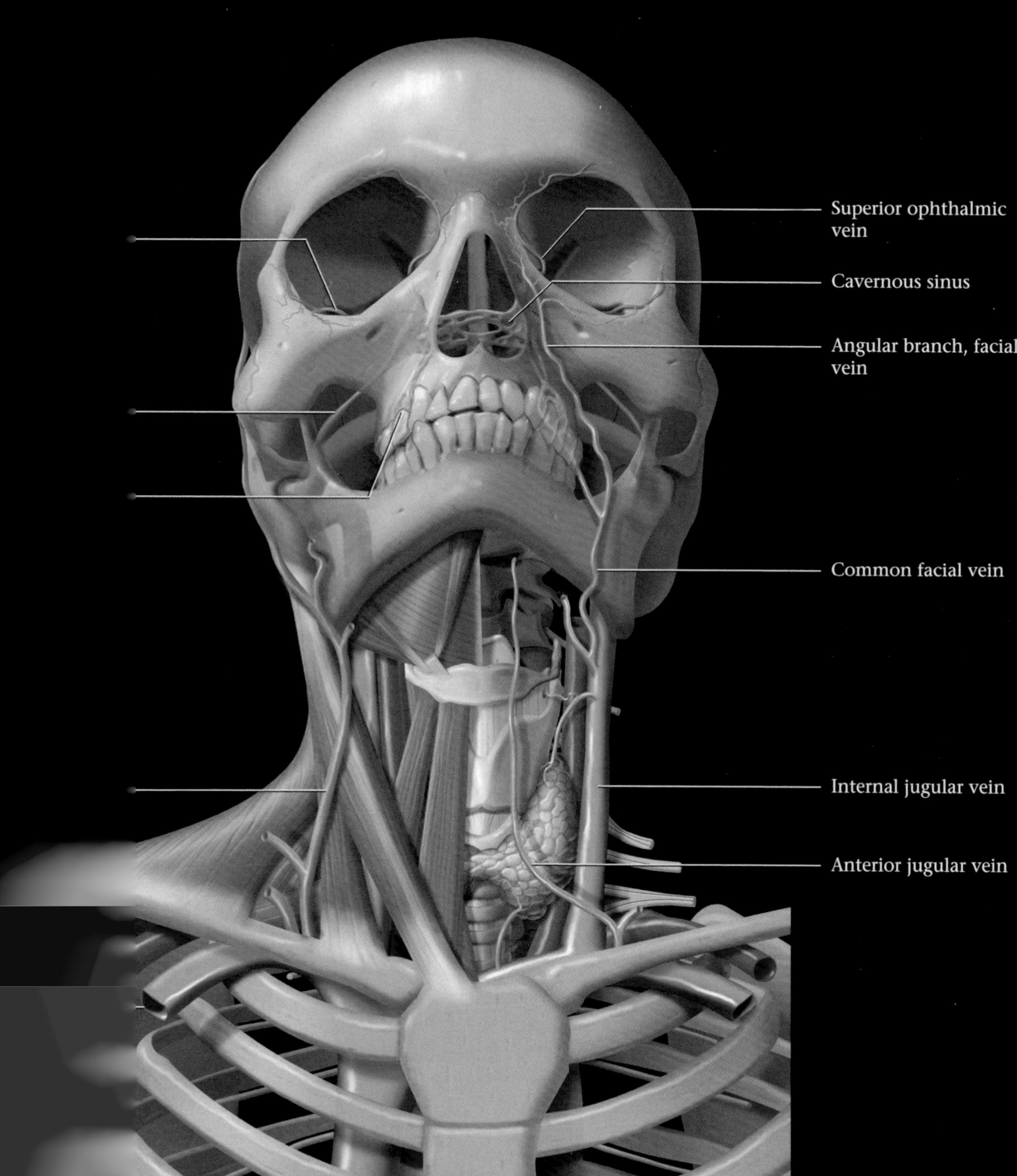

Superior ophthalmic vein
Cavernous sinus
Angular branch, facial vein
Common facial vein
Internal jugular vein
Anterior jugular vein

he extracranial venous system depicts the major neck veins, their drainage into the
ıumerous interconnections with the intracranial venous system. The pterygoid venous
s from the cavernous sinus and provides an important potential source of collateral venous

EXTRACRANIAL VEINS

GRAPHIC

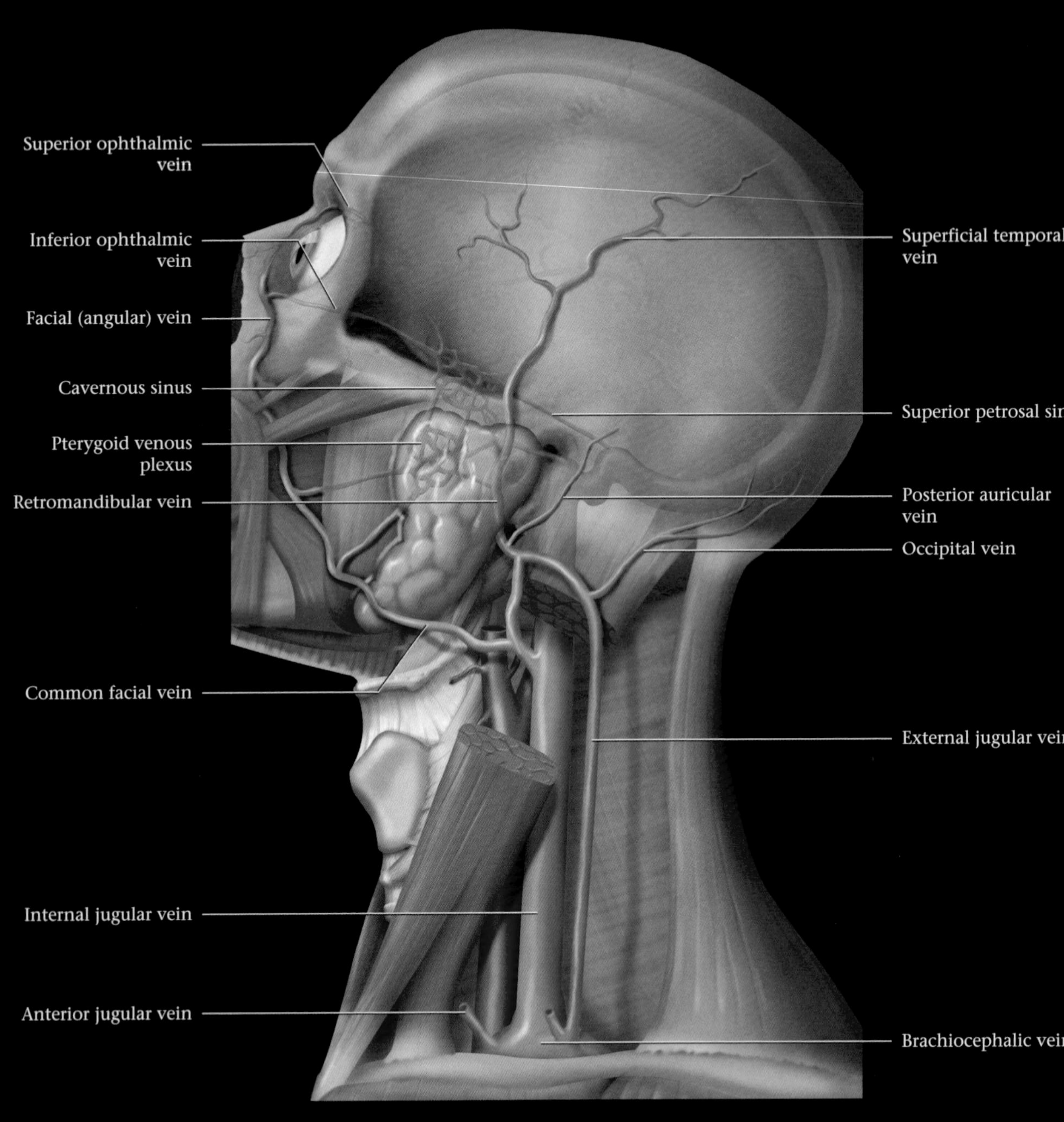
Superior ophthalmic vein
Inferior ophthalmic vein
Facial (angular) vein
Cavernous sinus
Pterygoid venous plexus
Retromandibular vein
Common facial vein
Internal jugular vein
Anterior jugular vein
Superficial temporal vein
Superior petrosal sin
Posterior auricular vein
Occipital vein
External jugular vei
Brachiocephalic vei

Sagittal graphic depicts the major extracranial veins of the scalp, face and neck. Significant tributaries are also show Numerous anastomoses between the intra- and extracranial veins provide a potential collateral pathway for venous drainage if a major dural sinus becomes thrombosed. Note collateral drainage from the cavernous sinus anteriorly (through the superior and inferior ophthalmic veins to the facial vein) as well as inferiorly (through basilar foramir to the pterygoid venous plexus) and posteriorly (through the superior and inferior petrosal sinuses). The internal ar external jugular veins also have significant interconnections. The deep vertebral venous plexus with its intra- and extraspinal anastomoses is not shown in this graphic.

SAGITTAL CECT

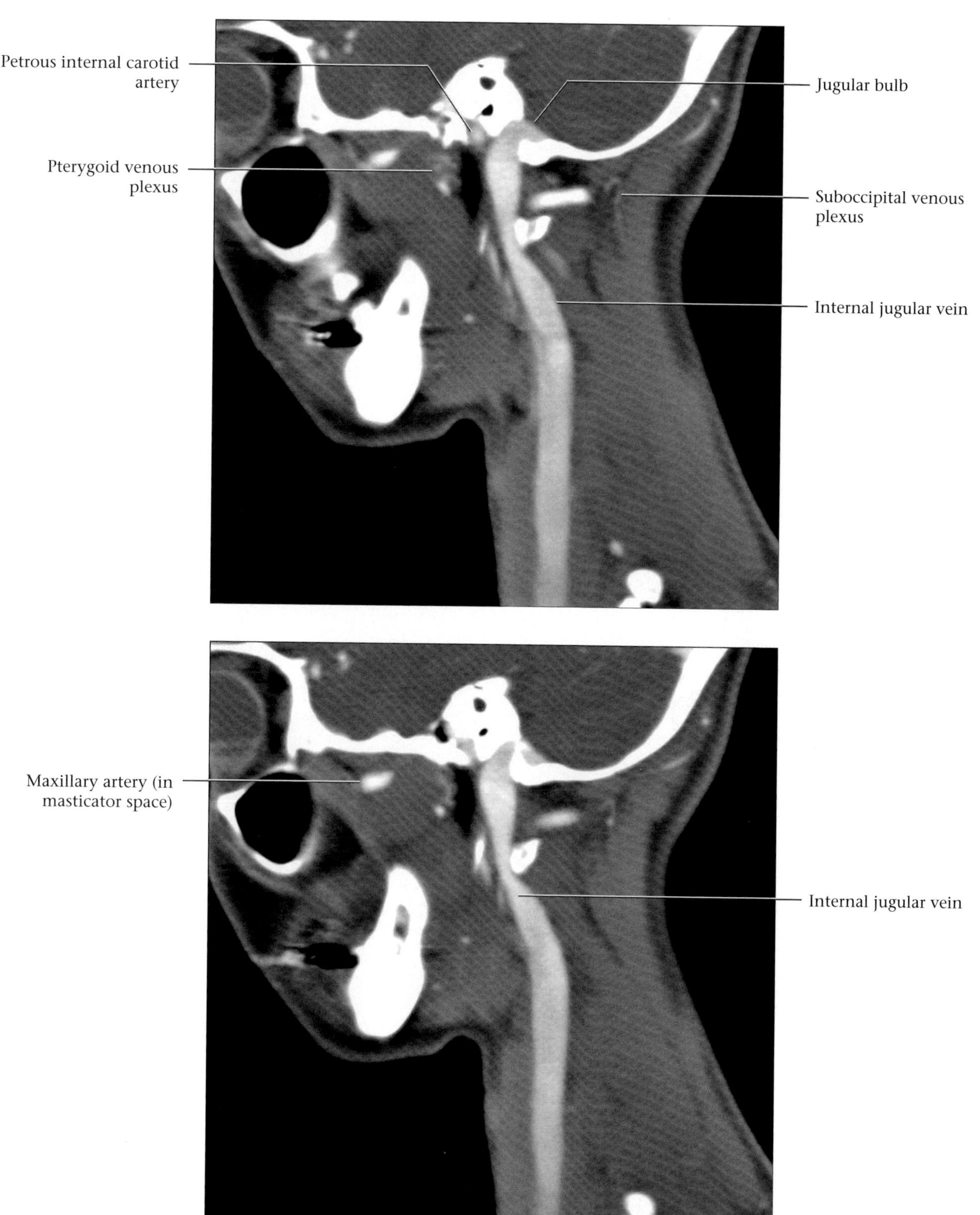
Petrous internal carotid artery
Jugular bulb
Pterygoid venous plexus
Suboccipital venous plexus
Internal jugular vein
Maxillary artery (in masticator space)
Internal jugular vein

(Top) Series of two reconstructed sagittal views from thin-section axial CECT scan shows the internal jugular vein and its relationship to the skull base. Note proximity of the IJV and jugular bulb to the petrous temporal bone and internal carotid artery. The IJV descends inferiorly within the carotid space. **(Bottom)** Internal jugular veins vary significantly in size. Significant side-to-side asymmetry is common. This IJV is average in size and configuration.

EXTRACRANIAL VEINS

CORONAL CECT

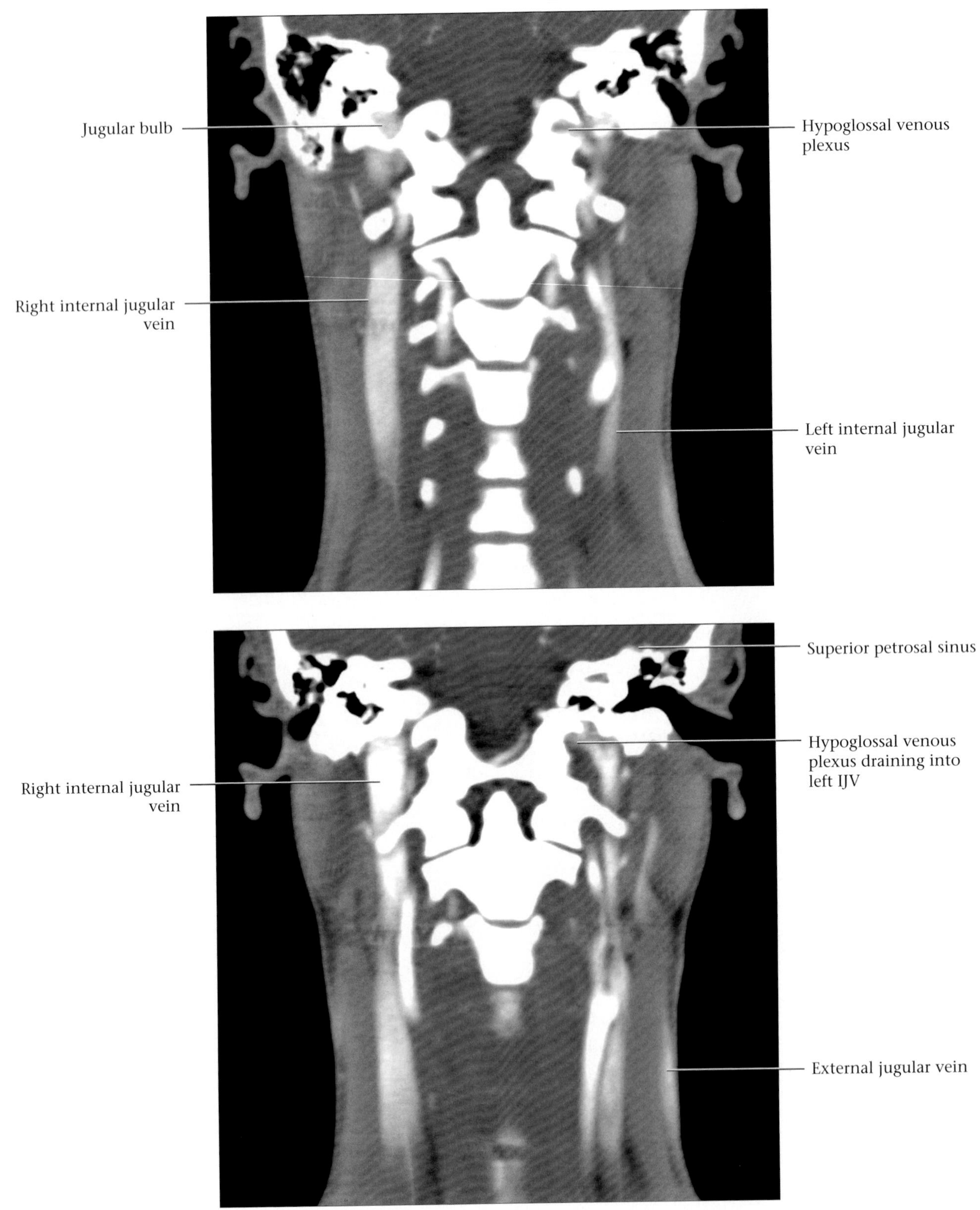
Jugular bulb
Hypoglossal venous plexus
Right internal jugular vein
Left internal jugular vein
Superior petrosal sinus
Hypoglossal venous plexus draining into left IJV
Right internal jugular vein
External jugular vein

(Top) A series of two coronal views from a thin-section CECT scan of the neck show the internal jugular veins and some tributaries that arise near the skull base. This view shows significant side-to-side asymmetry of the two IJVs, a common normal variant. **(Bottom)** Extensive interconnections between the intra- and extracranial venous systems are normally present. The hypoglossal venous plexus, petrosal sinuses, clival venous plexus, cavernous sinus and pterygoid plexus are extensively interconnected.

AXIAL T1 C+ MR

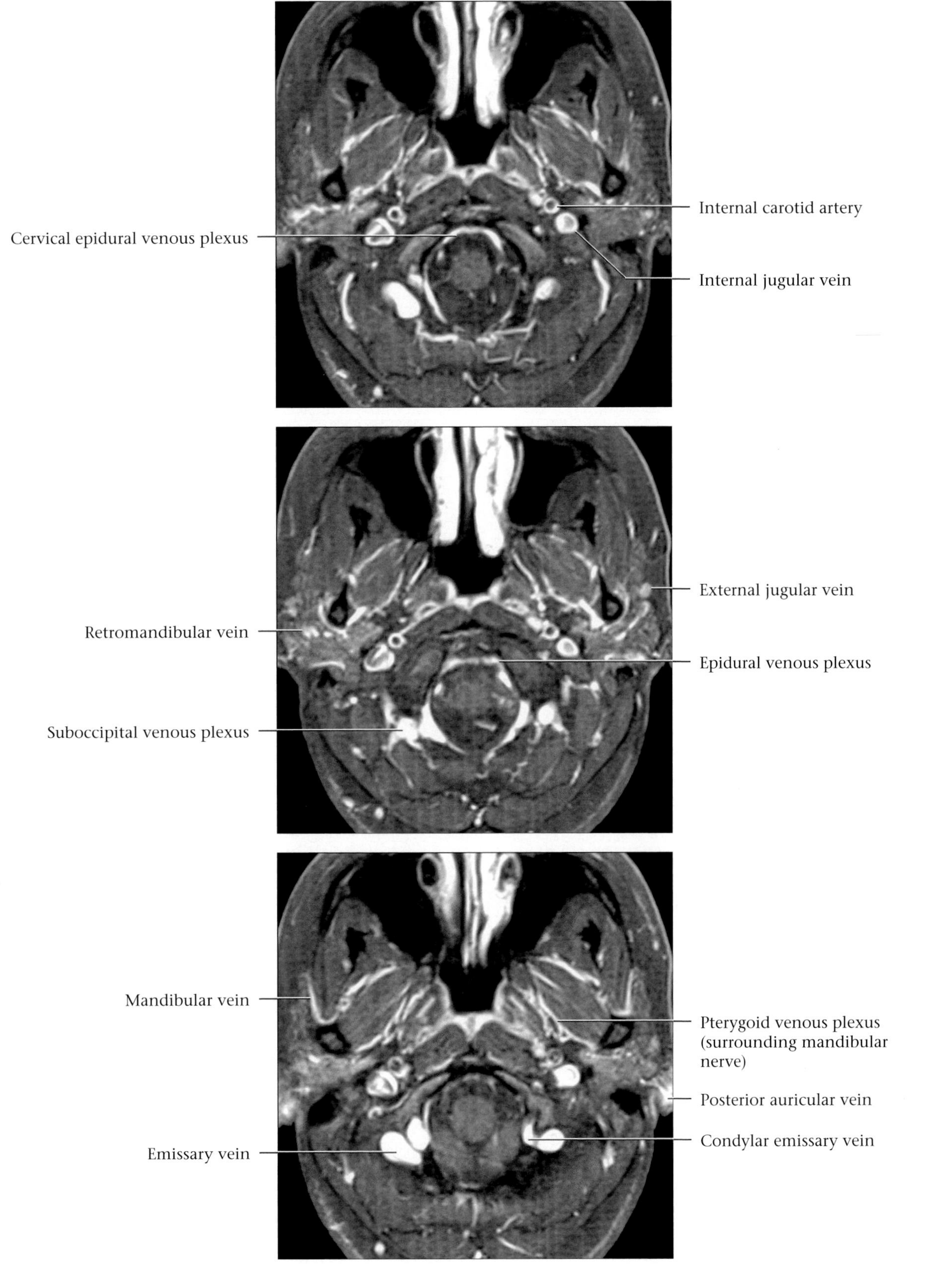
Internal carotid artery
Cervical epidural venous plexus
Internal jugular vein
External jugular vein
Retromandibular vein
Epidural venous plexus
Suboccipital venous plexus
Mandibular vein
Pterygoid venous plexus (surrounding mandibular nerve)
Posterior auricular vein
Condylar emissary vein
Emissary vein

(Top) A series of six axial T1 C+ MR scans are shown from inferior to superior. The upper cervical epidural venous plexus is seen on this section. Vessels within the carotid space are well-delineated. The cervical internal carotid artery lies anteromedial to the internal jugular vein in this space. **(Middle)** Section through the foramen magnum shows the interconnections between the lower clival, upper cervical epidural, and suboccipital venous plexi. Condylar emissary veins also connect the intra- and extracranial veins around the foramen magnum and upper cervical spinal canal. **(Bottom)** A more inferior section through the upper part of the extracranial internal jugular veins shows the inhomogeneous signal caused by spin dephasing. Unusually large condylar emissary veins are present, connecting with the suboccipital veins.

EXTRACRANIAL VEINS

AXIAL T1 C+ MR

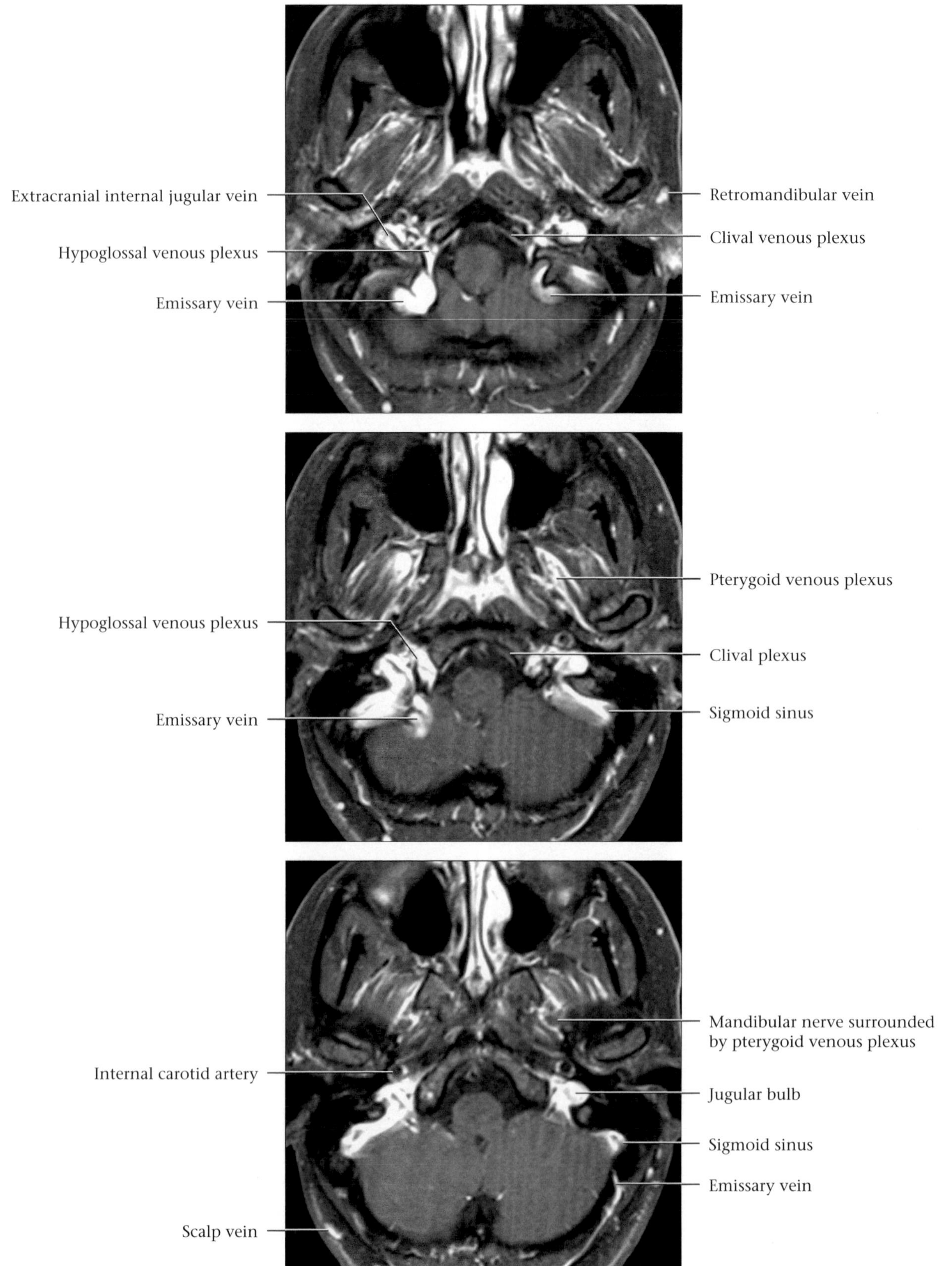
Extracranial internal jugular vein
Hypoglossal venous plexus
Emissary vein
Retromandibular vein
Clival venous plexus
Emissary vein
Pterygoid venous plexus
Hypoglossal venous plexus
Clival plexus
Emissary vein
Sigmoid sinus
Mandibular nerve surrounded by pterygoid venous plexus
Internal carotid artery
Jugular bulb
Sigmoid sinus
Emissary vein
Scalp vein

(Top) Scans continue superiorly. Section through the medulla, just above the foramen magnum, shows the hypoglossal venous plexus and its interconnections with the clival venous plexus and large condylar emissary veins. Note asymmetry of the jugular bulbs at this level, a common normal variant. **(Middle)** Section through the inferior clivus at the level of the hypoglossal canals shows prominent venous plexi traversing the hypoglossal canals. Note interconnections between the clival venous plexus and extracranial internal jugular vein via the hypoglossal venous plexi. **(Bottom)** This scan shows the jugular bulbs nicely.

CORONAL T1 C+ MR

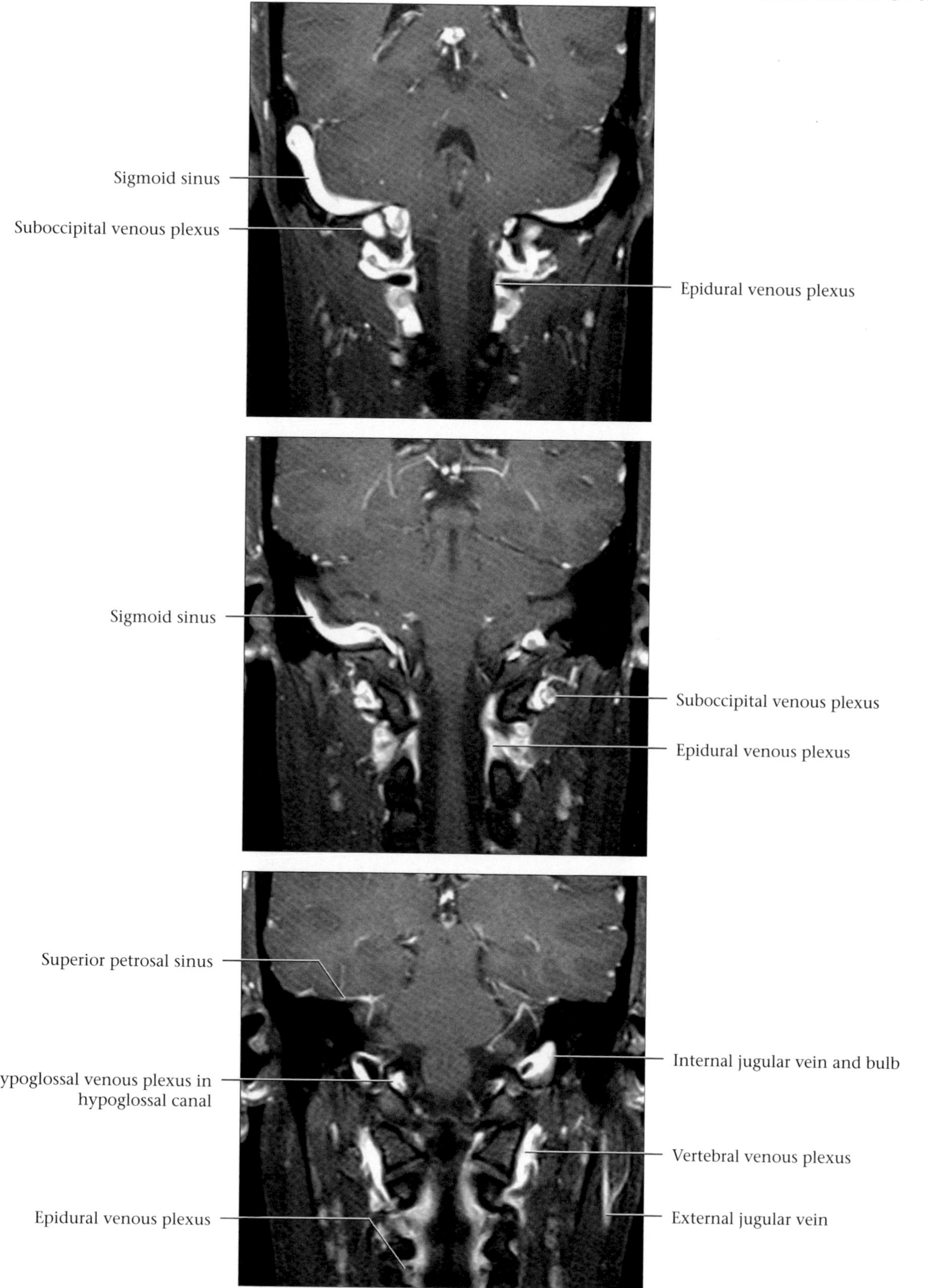
Sigmoid sinus
Suboccipital venous plexus
Epidural venous plexus
Sigmoid sinus
Suboccipital venous plexus
Epidural venous plexus
Superior petrosal sinus
Hypoglossal venous plexus in hypoglossal canal
Internal jugular vein and bulb
Vertebral venous plexus
Epidural venous plexus
External jugular vein

(Top) A series of six coronal fat-saturated T1 C+ MR scans from posterior to anterior demonstrate the numerous anastomoses between the posterior fossa dural venous sinuses and the extensive venous plexi that surround the upper cervical spine. These interconnections may provide a source for collateral venous drainage if the jugular vein becomes occluded. **(Middle)** Section through the cervicomedullary junction demonstrates prominent veins in and around the spine and posterior skull base. **(Bottom)** Section through the middle of the upper cervical spine and foramen magnum nicely demonstrates the numerous interconnections between prominent suboccipital veins, vertebral venous plexus and epidural venous plexus.

CORONAL T1 C+ MR

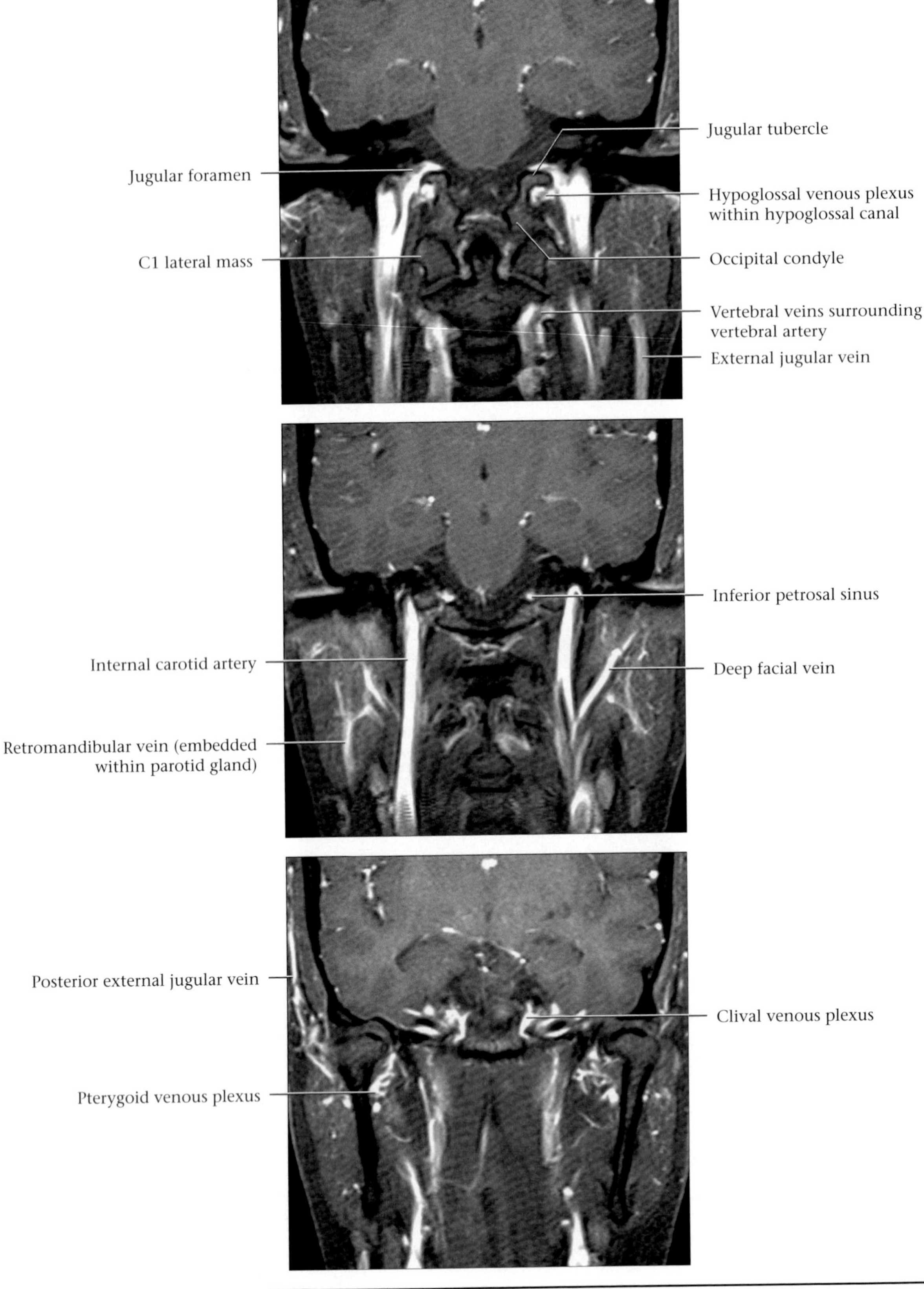
Jugular tubercle
Jugular foramen
Hypoglossal venous plexus within hypoglossal canal
C1 lateral mass
Occipital condyle
Vertebral veins surrounding vertebral artery
External jugular vein
Inferior petrosal sinus
Internal carotid artery
Deep facial vein
Retromandibular vein (embedded within parotid gland)
Posterior external jugular vein
Clival venous plexus
Pterygoid venous plexus

(Top) More anteriorly this section is directly through the jugular foramen. Note intensely enhancing internal jugular vein seen superolateral to the occipital condyles. The jugular tubercles and occipital condyles together resemble the outline of two eagles. The head of the eagle (jugular tubercle) separates the internal jugular bulb and vein from the hypoglossal canal and its venous plexus, nicely seen here. **(Middle)** Scan just anterior to the internal jugular veins shows the internal carotid artery running cephalad within the carotid space. The ICA lies anteromedial to the IJV. **(Bottom)** Scan through the mandibular condyles and lower clivus shows prominent enhancing veins under the skull base within the pterygoid muscles. These constitute the pterygoid venous plexus which is usually opacified on T1 C+ MR scans of the neck.

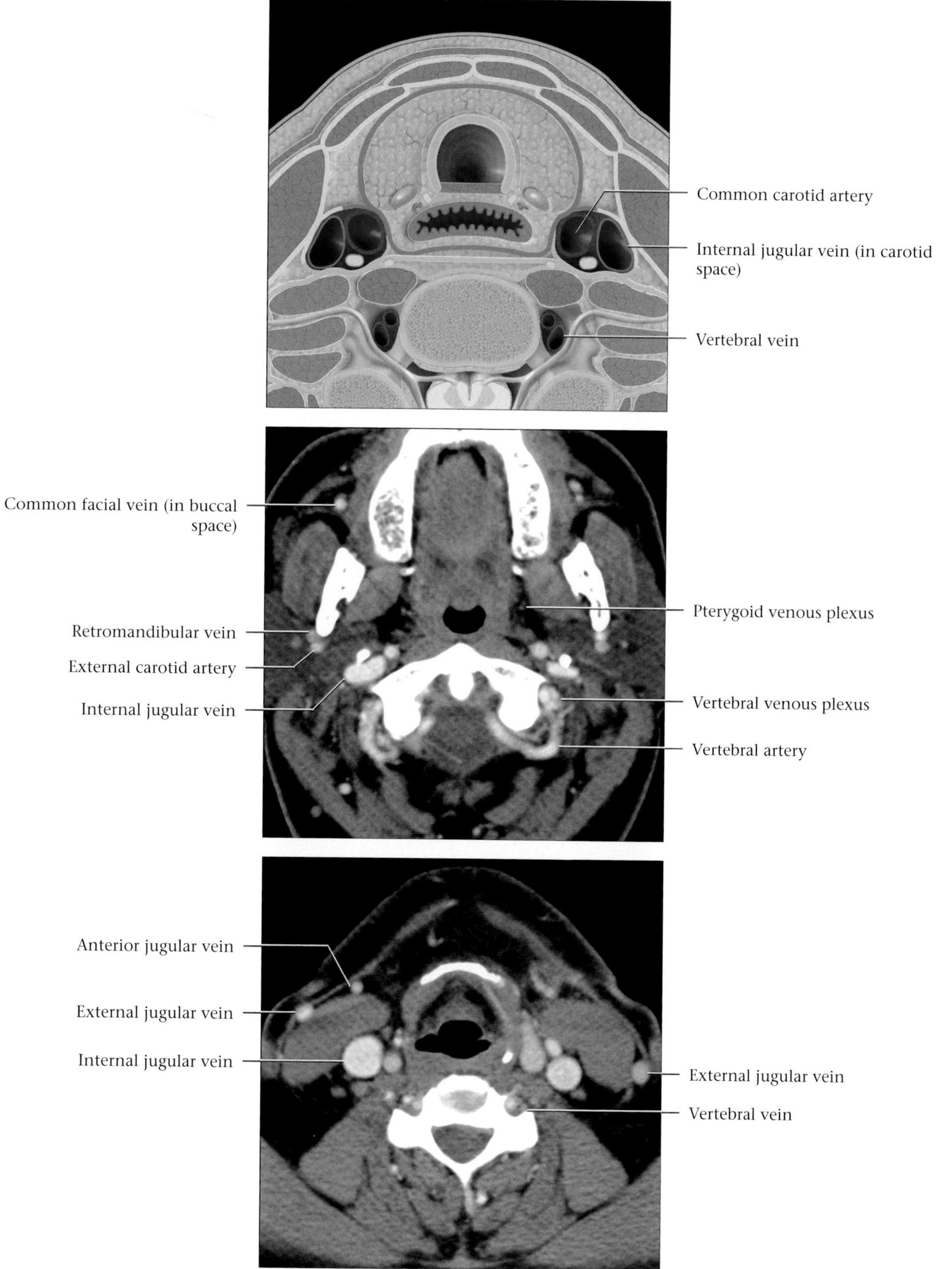
Common carotid artery
Internal jugular vein (in carotid space)
Vertebral vein
Common facial vein (in buccal space)
Retromandibular vein
External carotid artery
Internal jugular vein
Pterygoid venous plexus
Vertebral venous plexus
Vertebral artery
Anterior jugular vein
External jugular vein
Internal jugular vein
External jugular vein
Vertebral vein

(Top) Graphic and accompanying axial CECT scans depict the venous structures within the mid-neck. The internal jugular vein lies posterolateral to the carotid artery within the carotid space. **(Middle)** Axial CECT depicts the neck vessels at the C1 level. **(Bottom)** This image depicts the neck vessels at the level of the hyoid bone.

PART II

Head & Neck

Temporal Bone and Skull Base

Orbit, Nose and Sinuses

Suprahyoid and Infrahyoid Neck

Oral Cavity

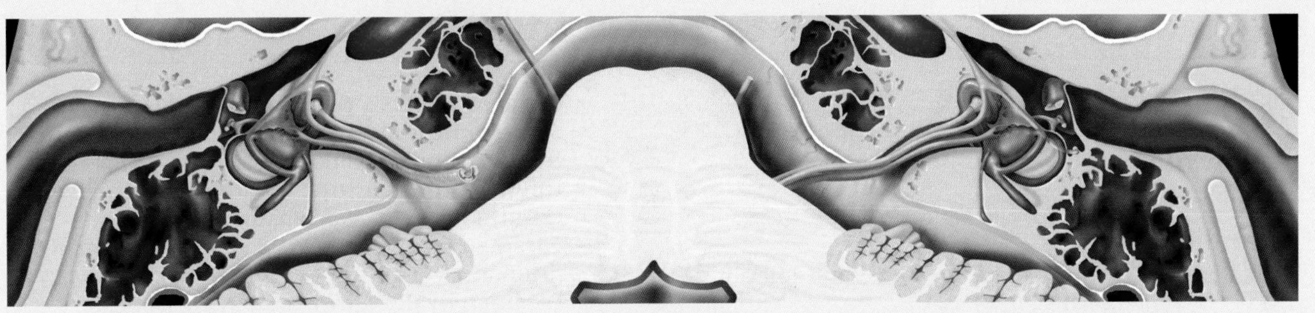

SECTION 1: Temporal Bone and Skull Base

SKULL BASE OVERVIEW

Terminology

Abbreviations

- Skull base (SB)

Definitions

- SB: Bony undulating surface which delimits inferior boundary of cranial vault

Imaging Anatomy

Overview

- **5 bones** make up base of skull
  - **Paired bones**: Frontal & temporal bones
  - **Unpaired bones**: Ethmoid, sphenoid & occipital bones
- **Two surfaces**
  - **Endocranial surface**: Faces brain, cisterns, cranial nerves (CN) & intracranial vessels
  - **Exocranial surface**: Faces extracranial head & neck
    - Anterior portion: Nasal cavity, frontal & ethmoid sinuses, orbits
    - Central portion: Anterior pharyngeal mucosal space, masticator, parotid & parapharyngeal spaces
    - Posterior portion: Posterior pharyngeal mucosal space, carotid, retropharyngeal, perivertebral spaces
- **Three regions**
  - Anterior, central & posterior skull base
  - **Anterior skull base (ASB)**
    - Anterolateral boundary: Frontal bones
    - Inferior relationships: Nasal vault, ethmoid & frontal sinuses; orbit and orbital canals
    - Superior relationships: Frontal lobes, CN1
    - ASB-CSB boundary: Lesser wing of sphenoid (sphenoid ridge) & planum sphenoidale
  - **Central skull base (CSB)**
    - Inferior relationships: Anterior roof of pharyngeal mucosal space, masticator, parotid & parapharyngeal spaces
    - Superior relationships: Temporal lobes, pituitary, cavernous sinus, Meckel cave, CN1-4, CN6, CNV1-3
    - CSB-PSB boundary: Dorsum sella & posterior clinoid processes medially, petrous ridges laterally
  - **Posterior skull base (PSB)**
    - Inferior relationships: Posterior pharyngeal mucosal space, carotid, retropharyngeal, perivertebral spaces
    - Superior relationships: Brainstem, cerebellum, CN7-8, CN9-12, transverse-sigmoid sinuses
    - Posterior boundary: Occipital bone

Internal Structures-Critical Contents

- **ASB**
  - Contents: Frontal, ethmoid bones
  - Foramina & structures transmitted
    - **Cribriform plate**: CN1, ethmoid arteries
- **CSB**
  - Contents: Sphenoid bone & anterior T-bones
  - Foramina & structures transmitted
    - **Optic canal**: CN2, ophthalmic artery (a)
    - **Superior orbital fissure**: CN3, CN4, CNV1 & CN6 & superior ophthalmic vein (v)
    - **Inferior orbital fissure**: Infraorbital a, v, nerve
    - **Carotid canal**: ICA, sympathetic plexus
    - **Foramen rotundum**: CNV2, artery of foramen rotundum & emissary veins
    - **Foramen ovale**: CNV3, lesser petrosal nerve, accessory meningeal branch maxillary artery & emissary vein
    - **Foramen spinosum**: Middle meningeal artery & vein, meningeal branch of mandibular nerve
    - **Foramen lacerum**: Not true foramen; cartilaginous floor of anteromedial horizontal petrous ICA canal
    - **Vidian canal**: Vidian artery & nerve
- **PSB**
  - Contents: Occipital & posterior T-bones
  - Foramina & structures transmitted
    - **Internal acoustic meatus**: CN7, CN8, labyrinthine a
    - **Hypoglossal canal**: CN12
    - **Foramen magnum**: Spinal portion CN11, vertebral arteries & medulla oblongata
    - **Jugular foramen**: **Pars nervosa:** CN9, Jacobson nerve & inferior petrosal sinus
    - **Jugular foramen**: **Pars vascularis:** CN10, Arnold nerve, CN11, jugular bulb & posterior meningeal a

Anatomy-Based Imaging Issues

Key Concepts or Questions

- Imaging of SB best done as combination of focused MR & bone CT
  - MR requires T1, T2 & T1 C+ with fat-saturation for full SB evaluation
  - Bone CT defines bone changes
- Suprahyoid neck spaces/structures abut SB allowing extracranial tumor to access intracranial area via perineural tumor
  - Masticator space: CNV3
  - Parotid space: CN7
  - Orbit: CNV1, CN3, 4, and 6
  - Sinus and nose, pterygopalatine fossa: CNV2

Imaging Recommendations

- **Bone CT**
  - Axial thin-slices with coronal reformations
  - Edge enhancing algorithm & wide window settings (> 2000 HU) necessary to evaluate bony anatomy
  - Narrow windows (200-400 HU) & smoothing algorithm to inspect regional soft tissues
  - If MR available, contrast unnecessary
- **MR**: Thin-slices (≤ 4 mm), axial & coronal, T1, T2 & T1 C+ fat-saturated
  - Pre-contrast T1 images use native fatty marrow for "contrast"
  - Use MRA & MRV for arteries and veins

Imaging Pitfalls

- Prominent foramen cecum, accessory foramina can be normal variants
- MR flow in jugular foramen may mimic a mass

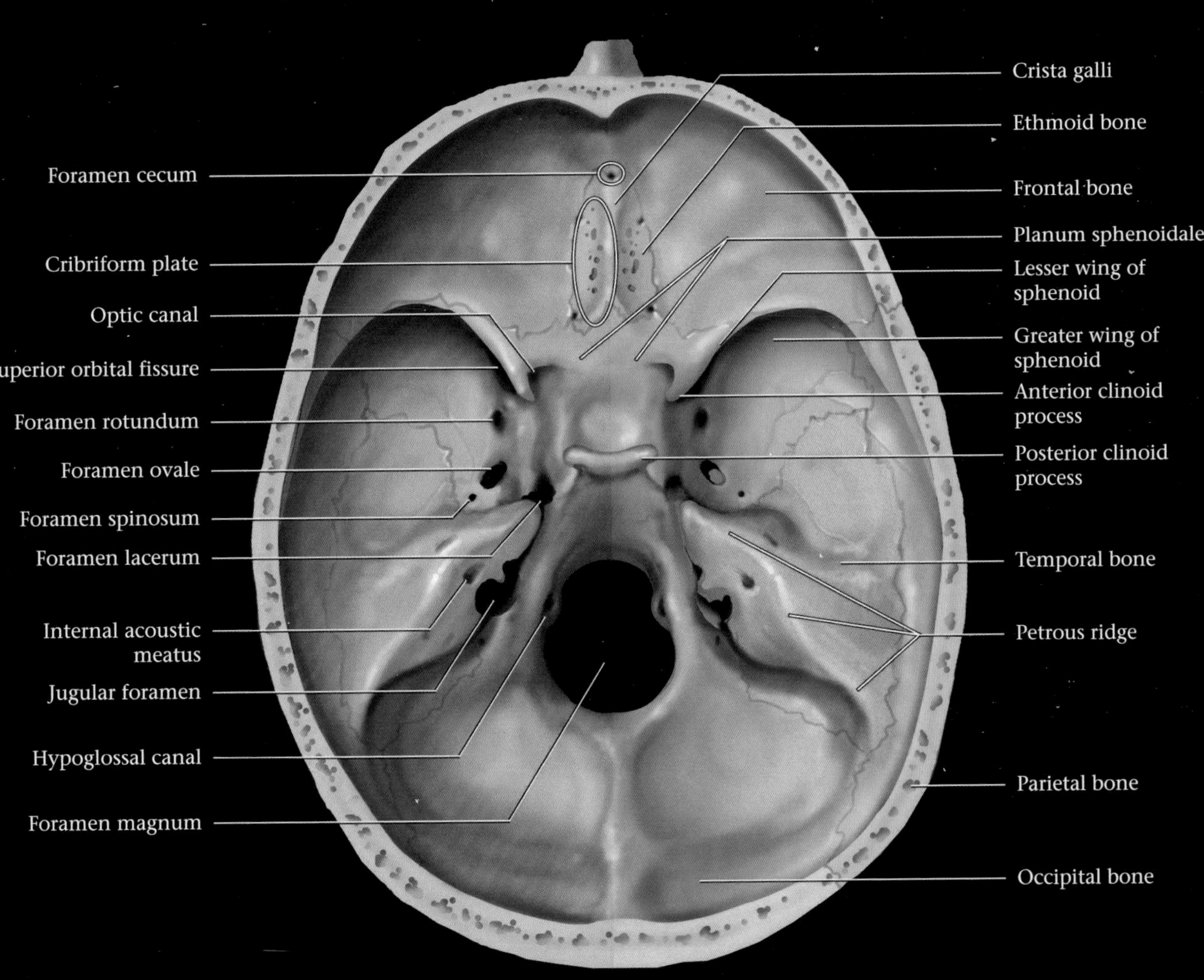
Foramen cecum
Cribriform plate
Optic canal
Superior orbital fissure
Foramen rotundum
Foramen ovale
Foramen spinosum
Foramen lacerum
Internal acoustic meatus
Jugular foramen
Hypoglossal canal
Foramen magnum
Crista galli
Ethmoid bone
Frontal bone
Planum sphenoidale
Lesser wing of sphenoid
Greater wing of sphenoid
Anterior clinoid process
Posterior clinoid process
Temporal bone
Petrous ridge
Parietal bone
Occipital bone

Graphic of endocranial skull base viewed from above with highlighted osseous landmarks labeled on the right. Important foramina are labeled on the left. The skull base is formed by the frontal, ethmoid, sphenoid, temporal, and occipital bones. The frontal, parietal, and occipital bones form the lateral vault of the cranium. The skull base is an undulating surface with grooves formed by the brain above and rough bony structures providing dural attachments. The lesser wing of the sphenoid and planum sphenoidale form the anterior skull base-central skull base border, while the petrous ridge and dorsum sella form the central skull base-posterior skull base boundary. The majority of important foramina are in the central skull base (sphenoid bone).

SKULL BASE OVERVIEW

GRAPHICS

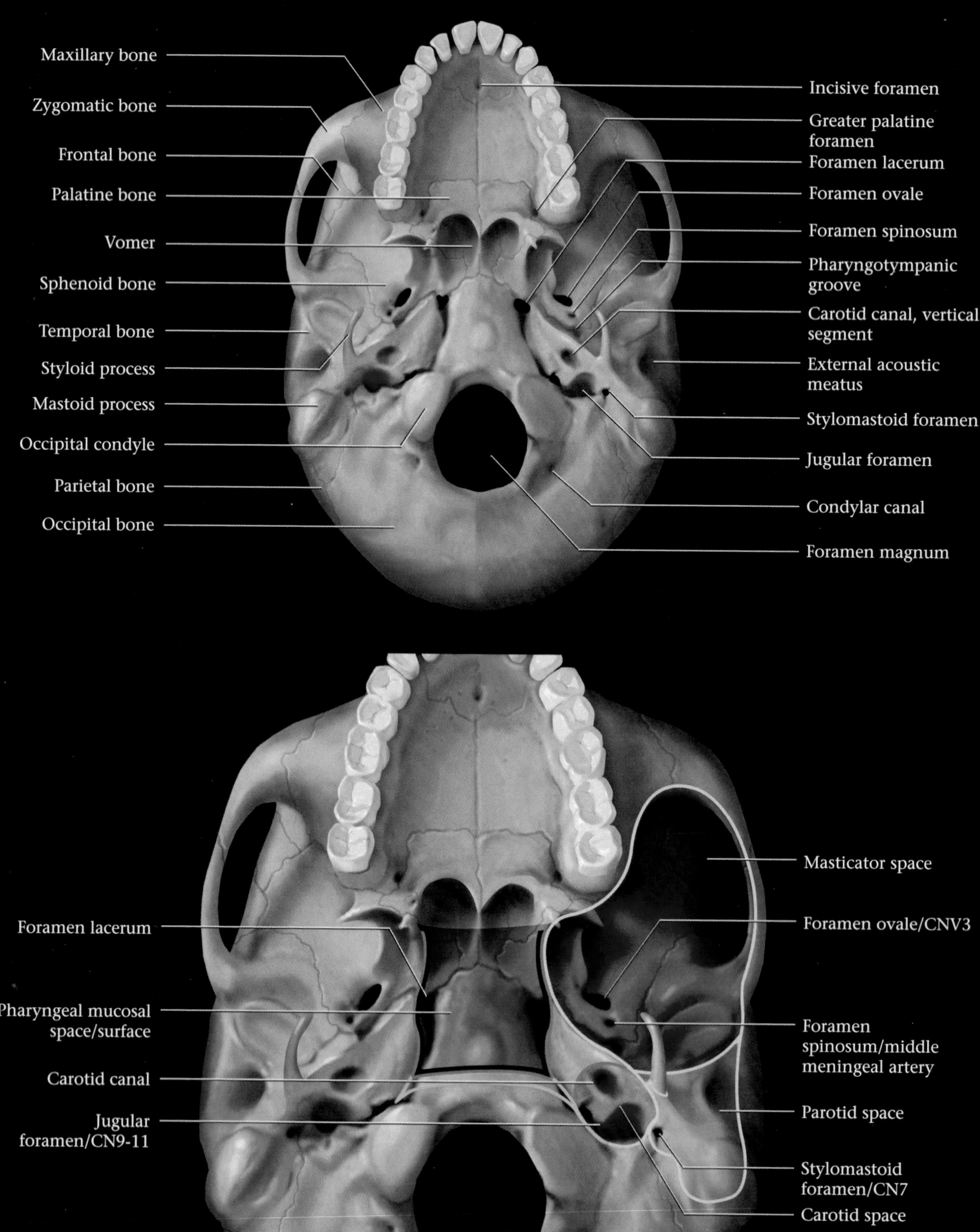
Maxillary bone
Zygomatic bone
Frontal bone
Palatine bone
Vomer
Sphenoid bone
Temporal bone
Styloid process
Mastoid process
Occipital condyle
Parietal bone
Occipital bone
Incisive foramen
Greater palatine foramen
Foramen lacerum
Foramen ovale
Foramen spinosum
Pharyngotympanic groove
Carotid canal, vertical segment
External acoustic meatus
Stylomastoid foramen
Jugular foramen
Condylar canal
Foramen magnum
Foramen lacerum
Pharyngeal mucosal space/surface
Carotid canal
Jugular foramen/CN9-11
Masticator space
Foramen ovale/CNV3
Foramen spinosum/middle meningeal artery
Parotid space
Stylomastoid foramen/CN7
Carotid space

(Top) Graphic of skull base viewed from below shows the complexity of exocranial skull base with bony landmarks labeled on the left and foramina labeled on the right. Note that in addition to the frontal, sphenoid, temporal, and occipital bones, the undersurface of the skull base is formed by maxilla, vomer, palatine and zygomatic bones. The ethmoid bone is not part of the exocranial skull base. **(Bottom)** Graphic of skull base viewed from below shows spaces of suprahyoid neck relationships to skull base. Four spaces have key interactions with skull base: Masticator, parotid, carotid and pharyngeal mucosal spaces. Parotid space (green) malignancy can follow CN7 into stylomastoid foramen. Masticator space (purple) receives CNV3 while CN9-12 enter the carotid space (red). The pharyngeal mucosal space abuts the foramen lacerum, which is covered by fibrocartilage in life.

AXIAL BONE CT

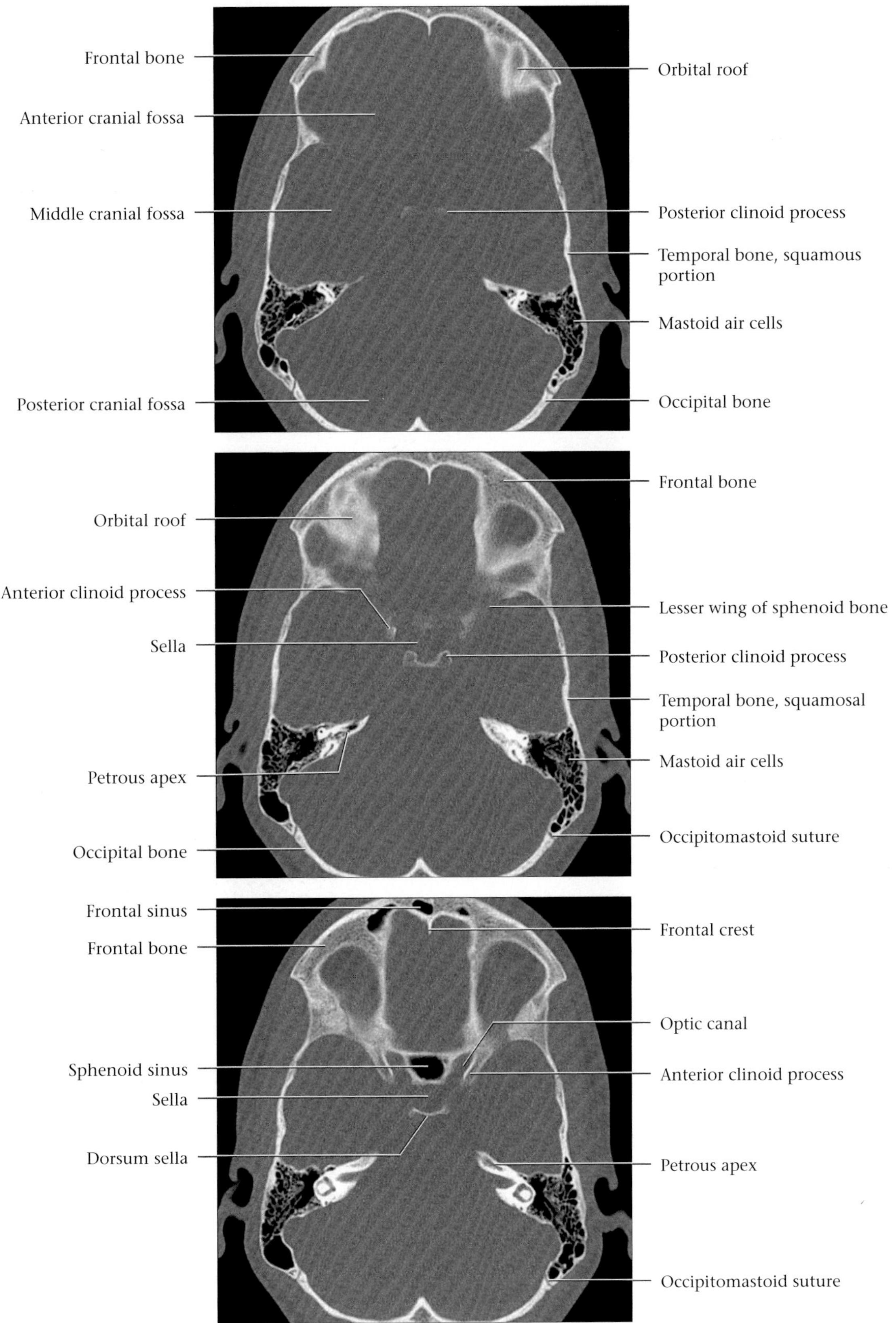
Frontal bone
Anterior cranial fossa
Middle cranial fossa
Posterior cranial fossa
Orbital roof
Posterior clinoid process
Temporal bone, squamous portion
Mastoid air cells
Occipital bone
Orbital roof
Anterior clinoid process
Sella
Petrous apex
Occipital bone
Frontal bone
Lesser wing of sphenoid bone
Posterior clinoid process
Temporal bone, squamosal portion
Mastoid air cells
Occipitomastoid suture
Frontal sinus
Frontal bone
Sphenoid sinus
Sella
Dorsum sella
Frontal crest
Optic canal
Anterior clinoid process
Petrous apex
Occipitomastoid suture

(Top) First of twelve axial bone CT images of skull base presented from superior to inferior. At level of orbital roof, brain within anterior, middle and posterior fossae is cradled above respective regions of skull base. Anterior skull base, central skull base, posterior skull base. **(Middle)** At level of the upper sella, the lesser wings of sphenoid and the planum sphenoidale, which demarcate the ASB-CSB border, are barely visible. More posterior, the petrous apices divide CSB from PSB. PSB houses the cerebellum, covered superiorly by tentorium cerebelli, which attaches to posterior clinoid processes. **(Bottom)** At the level of the anterior clinoid, the optic canals pass through the sphenoid bone, bounded by the anterior clinoid process laterally and the sphenoid sinus medially. The dorsum sella marks the anteromedial border of the PSB.

SKULL BASE OVERVIEW

AXIAL BONE CT

Frontal sinus
Superior orbital fissure
Optic canal (CN2)
Middle cranial fossa
Internal auditory canal (CN7 & 8)
Posterior cranial fossa
Frontal bone
Crista galli
Greater wing of sphenoid bone
Sphenoid sinus
Dorsum sella
Petrous apex
Temporal bone
Occipital bone

Superior orbital fissure
Petrooccipital fissure
Jugular bulb roof
Sigmoid sinus
Occipitomastoid suture
Frontal bone
Crista galli
Greater wing of sphenoid bone
Superior orbital fissure
Basisphenoid
Petrous apex
Cochlea
Mastoid air cells

Lamina papyracea
Anterior ethmoid artery canal
Superior orbital fissure
Petrooccipital fissure
Jugular bulb
Sigmoid sinus
Occipitomastoid suture
Foramen cecum remnant
Crista galli
Ethmoid air cells
Sphenoid sinus
Basisphenoid portion of clivus
Horizontal petrous ICA
Pars vascularis, jugular foramen
Pars nervosa, jugular foramen

(Top) In this image the crista galli superior tip is just visible. The optic canal transmits CN2 & ophthalmic artery to the orbit while the superior orbital fissure contains CN3, CN4, CNV1, CN6 & superior ophthalmic vein. Notice the close approximation of the optic canal and superior orbital fissure (SOF). The internal auditory canal is on the medial wall of the T-bone. **(Middle)** The crista galli provides attachment for falx cerebri and divides anterior aspect of ASB into 2 symmetric halves. Note that ethmoid air cells extend superior to cribriform plate. Sphenoid sinus is immediately below the sella and medial to superior orbital fissure. The apex of petrooccipital fissure is visible at medial tip of petrous apex. **(Bottom)** At the anterior base of crista galli is foramen cecum remnant. The petrooccipital fissure is the most common location for skull base chondrosarcoma.

AXIAL BONE CT

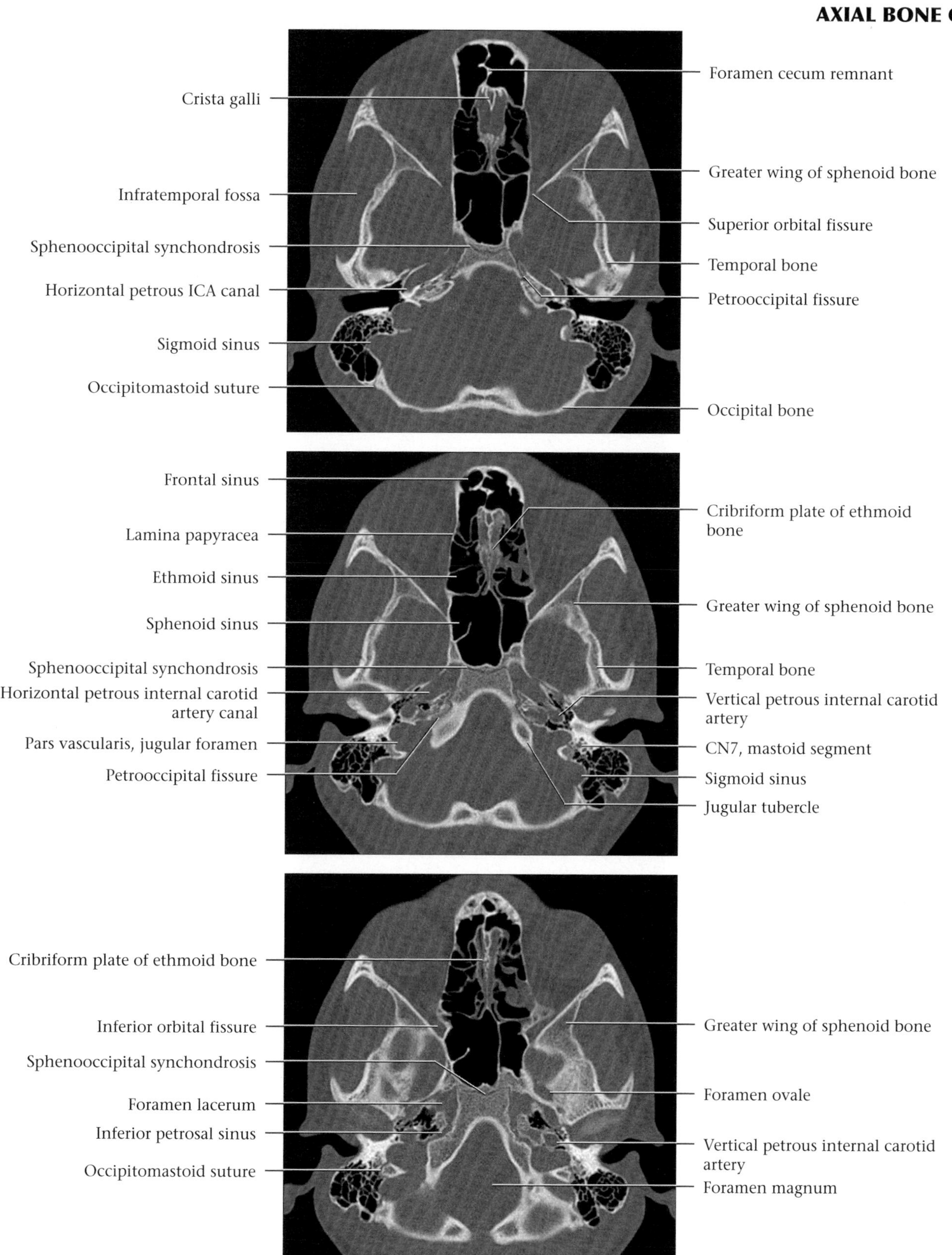
Crista galli
Foramen cecum remnant
Infratemporal fossa
Greater wing of sphenoid bone
Superior orbital fissure
Sphenooccipital synchondrosis
Temporal bone
Horizontal petrous ICA canal
Petrooccipital fissure
Sigmoid sinus
Occipitomastoid suture
Occipital bone
Frontal sinus
Cribriform plate of ethmoid bone
Lamina papyracea
Ethmoid sinus
Greater wing of sphenoid bone
Sphenoid sinus
Sphenooccipital synchondrosis
Temporal bone
Horizontal petrous internal carotid artery canal
Vertical petrous internal carotid artery
Pars vascularis, jugular foramen
CN7, mastoid segment
Petrooccipital fissure
Sigmoid sinus
Jugular tubercle
Cribriform plate of ethmoid bone
Inferior orbital fissure
Greater wing of sphenoid bone
Sphenooccipital synchondrosis
Foramen ovale
Foramen lacerum
Inferior petrosal sinus
Vertical petrous internal carotid artery
Occipitomastoid suture
Foramen magnum

(Top) At the level of the upper clivus the sphenooccipital synchondrosis is visible delineating the more anterior basisphenoid from the more posterior basiocciput. Posterolaterally the petrooccipital fissure is seen separating the more medial occipital bone from the more lateral temporal bone. **(Middle)** At the level of the cribriform plate of the ethmoid bone the frontal, ethmoid and sphenoid sinuses are all visible. Also note the vertical and horizontal segments of the petrous internal carotid arteries. **(Bottom)** Notice the inferior orbital fissure is bounded by the sphenoid sinus posteromedially and the greater wing of the sphenoid bone laterally. It contains the infraorbital artery, vein and nerve. The petrooccipital fissure has given way to the inferior petrosal sinus.

AXIAL BONE CT

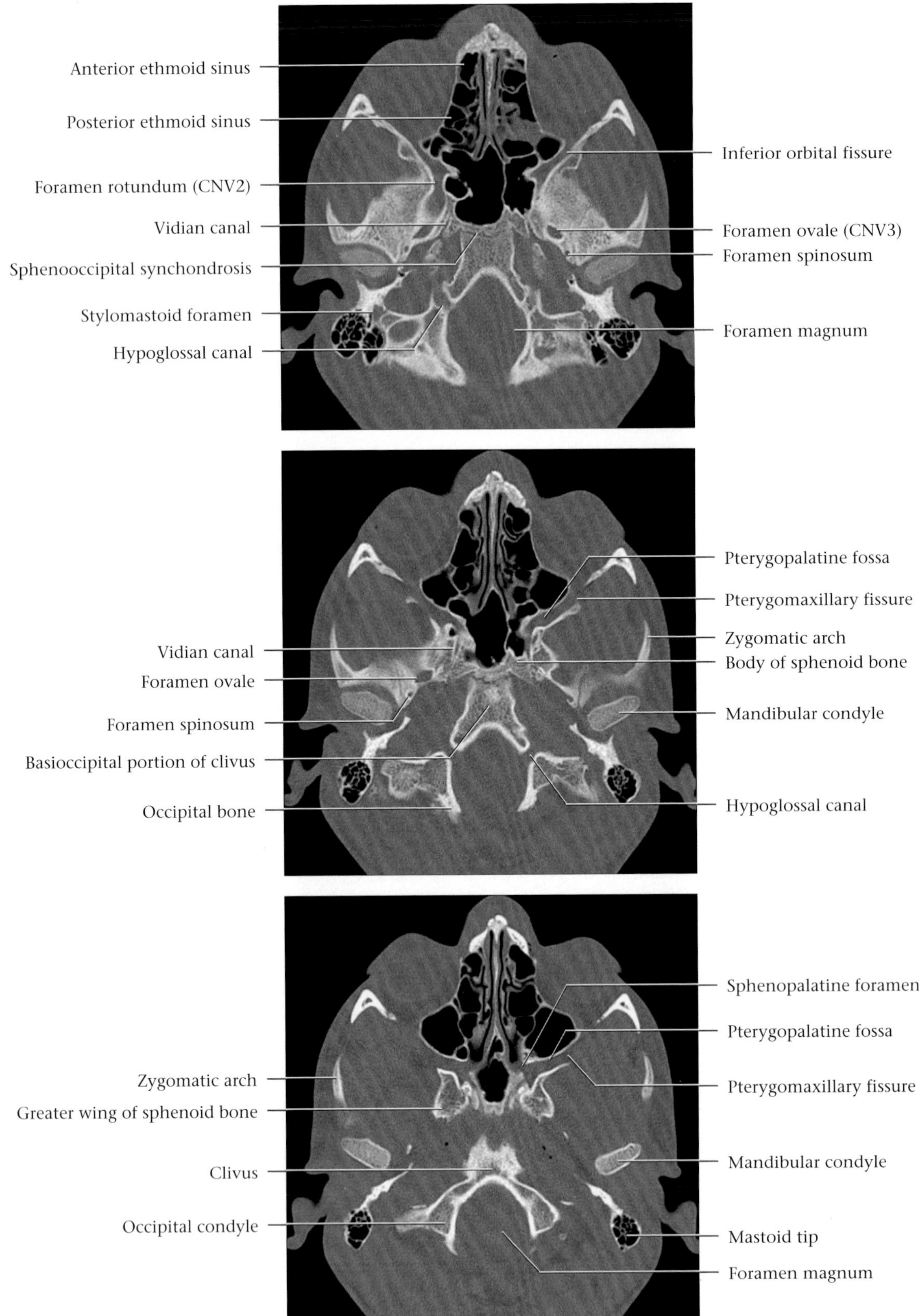
Anterior ethmoid sinus
Posterior ethmoid sinus
Foramen rotundum (CNV2)
Vidian canal
Sphenooccipital synchondrosis
Stylomastoid foramen
Hypoglossal canal
Inferior orbital fissure
Foramen ovale (CNV3)
Foramen spinosum
Foramen magnum
Vidian canal
Foramen ovale
Foramen spinosum
Basioccipital portion of clivus
Occipital bone
Pterygopalatine fossa
Pterygomaxillary fissure
Zygomatic arch
Body of sphenoid bone
Mandibular condyle
Hypoglossal canal
Zygomatic arch
Greater wing of sphenoid bone
Clivus
Occipital condyle
Sphenopalatine foramen
Pterygopalatine fossa
Pterygomaxillary fissure
Mandibular condyle
Mastoid tip
Foramen magnum

(Top) At the level of inferior orbital fissure and foramen rotundum the vidian canal is also seen. Foramen rotundum provides a conduit for CNV2 to access the cephalad margin of pterygopalatine fossa. CN3 traverses sphenoid bone via foramen ovale. The hypoglossal canal is seen in the inferior occipital bone. **(Middle)** This image is at the level of the hypoglossal canal in the low occipital bone. Anteriorly the pterygomaxillary fissure is the lateral opening of the pterygopalatine fossa. **(Bottom)** At the inferior margin of the foramen magnum the mastoid tips are still visible. The pterygopalatine fossa is well seen connecting medially with nasal cavity via sphenopalatine foramen and laterally with the masticator space through the pterygomaxillary fissure. The foramen rotundum and vidian canals also lead into the pterygopalatine fossa.

3D-VRT BONE CT

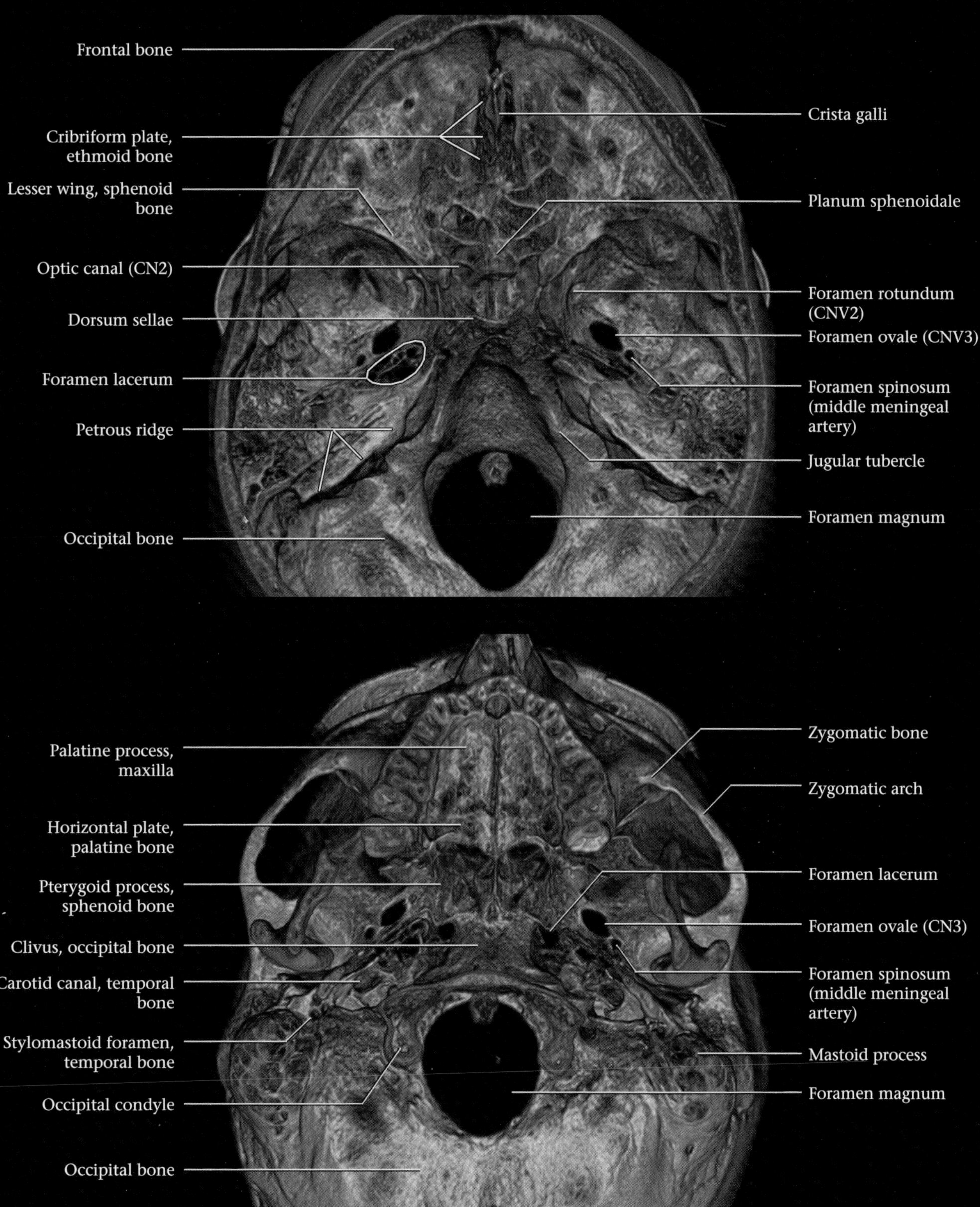
Frontal bone
Cribriform plate, ethmoid bone
Lesser wing, sphenoid bone
Optic canal (CN2)
Dorsum sellae
Foramen lacerum
Petrous ridge
Occipital bone
Crista galli
Planum sphenoidale
Foramen rotundum (CNV2)
Foramen ovale (CNV3)
Foramen spinosum (middle meningeal artery)
Jugular tubercle
Foramen magnum
Palatine process, maxilla
Horizontal plate, palatine bone
Pterygoid process, sphenoid bone
Clivus, occipital bone
Carotid canal, temporal bone
Stylomastoid foramen, temporal bone
Occipital condyle
Occipital bone
Zygomatic bone
Zygomatic arch
Foramen lacerum
Foramen ovale (CN3)
Foramen spinosum (middle meningeal artery)
Mastoid process
Foramen magnum

(Top) 3D-VRT image of osseous skull base from above. Anterior skull base is bounded by frontal bones anteriorly & lesser wing of sphenoid and planum sphenoidale posteriorly. Central skull base with its multitude of fissures & foramina, is made up of sphenoid bone & anterior temporal bone. It is bounded anteriorly by lesser wing of sphenoid & posterior planum sphenoidale & posteriorly by dorsum sellae & the petrous ridge. The posterior skull base extends from the dorsum sellae medially & the petrous ridges laterally to the occiput posteriorly. **(Bottom)** 3D-VRT image of osseous skull base from below highlights sphenoid bone with foramen ovale and spinosum and occipital bone with its occipital condyle. Notice frontal bone is not seen but instead maxillary, palatine and zygomatic bones are present anteriorly.

SAGITTAL BONE CT & T1 MR

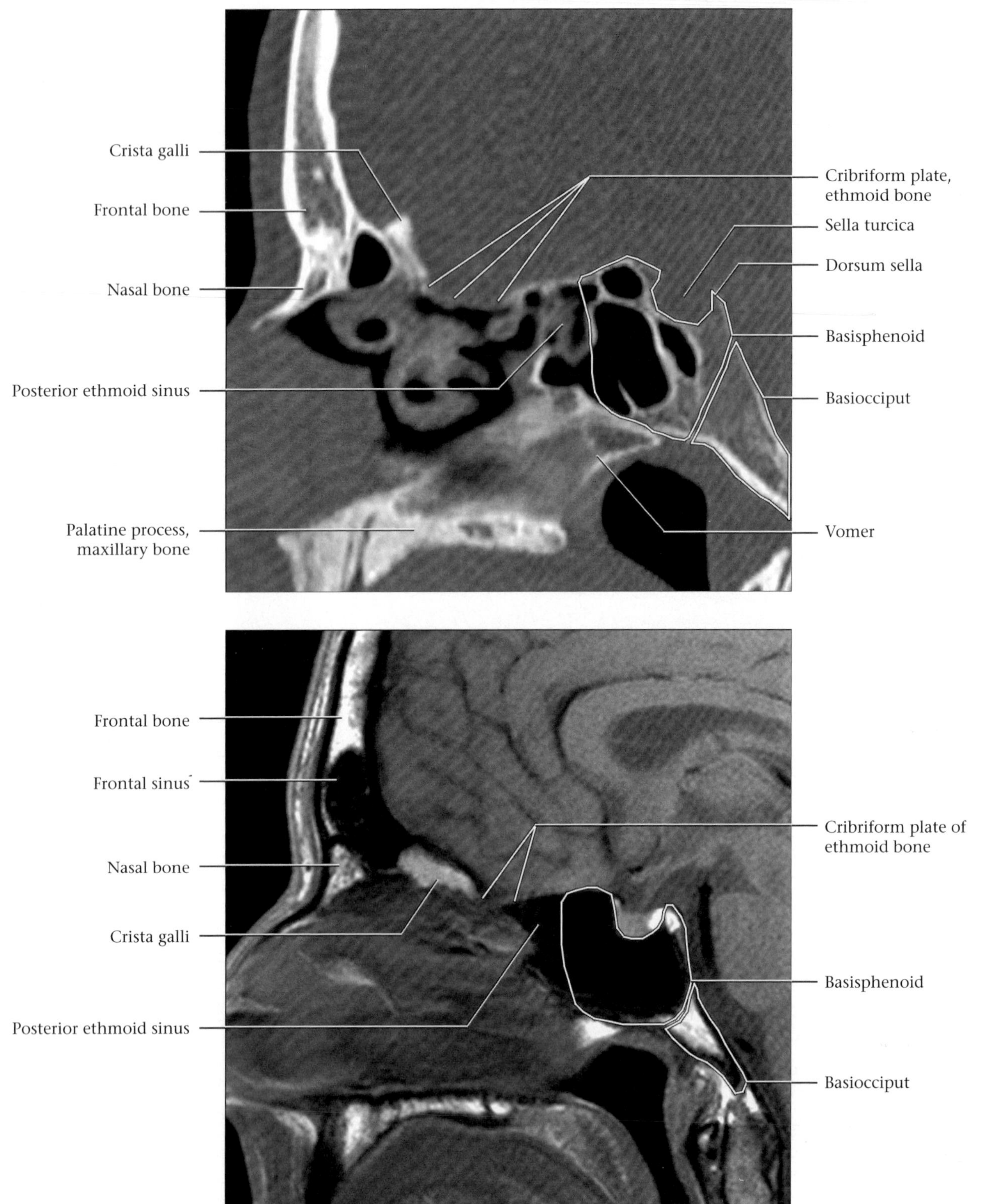
Crista galli
Frontal bone
Nasal bone
Posterior ethmoid sinus
Palatine process, maxillary bone
Cribriform plate, ethmoid bone
Sella turcica
Dorsum sella
Basisphenoid
Basiocciput
Vomer
Frontal bone
Frontal sinus
Nasal bone
Crista galli
Posterior ethmoid sinus
Cribriform plate of ethmoid bone
Basisphenoid
Basiocciput

(Top) Paramedian sagittal bone CT through anterior skull base shows the intimate relationship of the skull base to the paranasal sinuses. From anterior to posterior note the frontal and nasal bones, crista galli, cribriform plate basisphenoid and basiocciput. Notice that the sella is entirely embedded in the sphenoid bone. **(Bottom)** Paramedial sagittal T1 MR through the skull base shows the anterior, central and posterior skull base. The anterior skull base in this image is made up of frontal bone, crista galli and cribriform plate of ethmoid bone. The crista galli is high signal secondary to fatty marrow. The central skull base in the midline is often called the basisphenoid. It is made up of the sphenoid bone-sinus and cradles the pituitary gland. The sphenooccipital synchondrosis separates the basisphenoid from the basiocciput of the posterior skull base.

AXIAL T1 MR

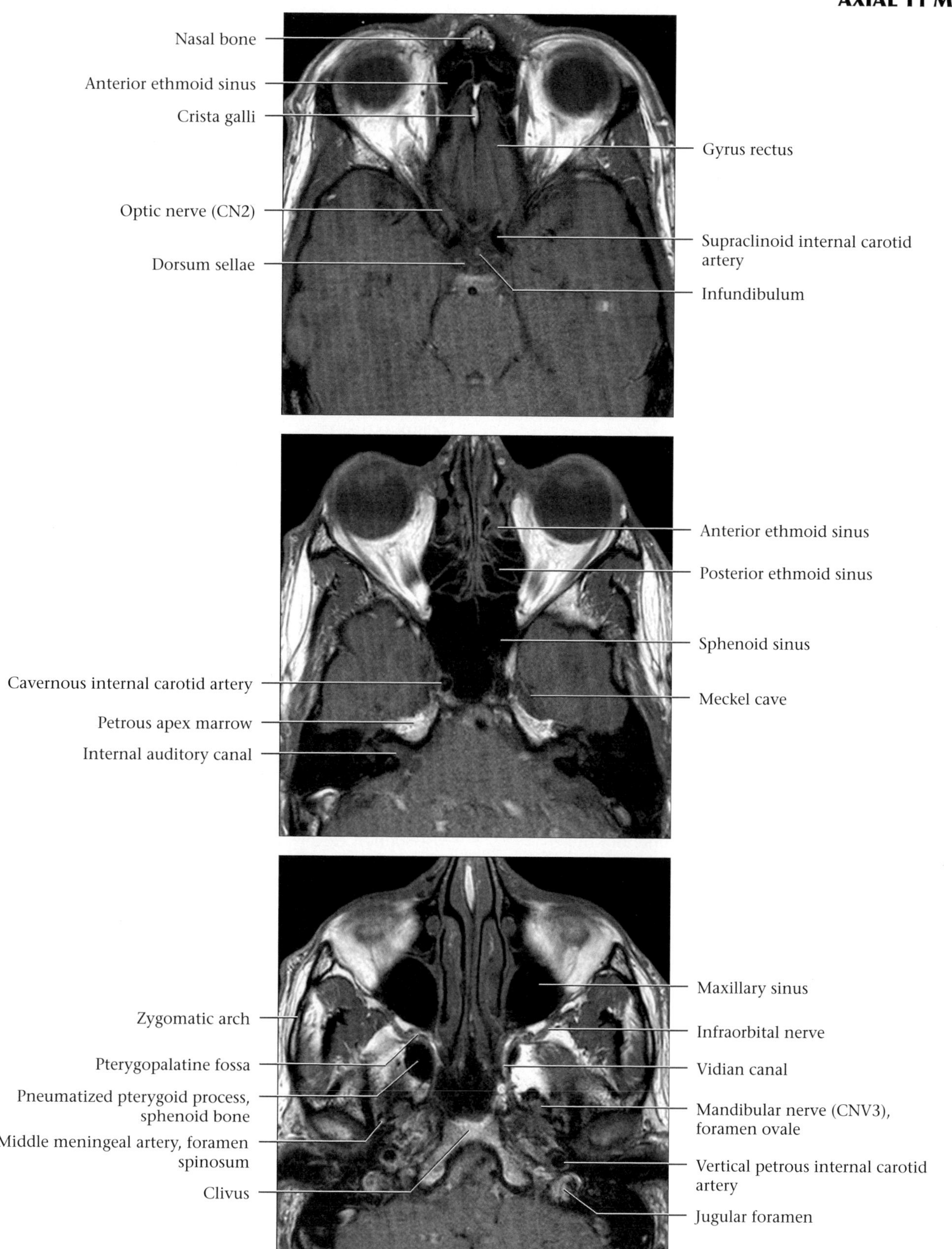

Nasal bone
Anterior ethmoid sinus
Crista galli
Gyrus rectus
Optic nerve (CN2)
Supraclinoid internal carotid artery
Dorsum sellae
Infundibulum
Anterior ethmoid sinus
Posterior ethmoid sinus
Sphenoid sinus
Cavernous internal carotid artery
Meckel cave
Petrous apex marrow
Internal auditory canal
Maxillary sinus
Zygomatic arch
Infraorbital nerve
Pterygopalatine fossa
Vidian canal
Pneumatized pterygoid process, sphenoid bone
Mandibular nerve (CNV3), foramen ovale
Middle meningeal artery, foramen spinosum
Vertical petrous internal carotid artery
Clivus
Jugular foramen

(Top) First of three axial T1 MR images through the skull base from superior to inferior shows the high signal fatty marrow in the crista galli. Adjacent to this are gyri recti of the frontal lobes. **(Middle)** Image through the cavernous sinus reveals ethmoid sinuses in the ethmoid bones of the anterior skull base and the sphenoid sinus in the sphenoid bone of the central skull base. The petrous apex fatty marrow is high signal with Meckel cave seen on its anterior margin. **(Bottom)** At the level of the pterygopalatine fossa the infraorbital nerve can be seen exiting anterolaterally. The vidian canal, another sphenoid bone structure, is visible connecting to the medial pterygopalatine fossa. Middle meningeal artery and CNV3 are noted passing through the foramen spinosum and ovale respectively. More posterolaterally the carotid canal and jugular foramen can be seen.

ANTERIOR SKULL BASE

Terminology

Abbreviations

- Anterior, central skull base (ASB, CSB)
- Greater wing (GWS) & lesser wing (LWS) of sphenoid

Definitions

- ASB: Skull base (SB) anterior to LWS & planum sphenoidale

Imaging Anatomy

Overview

- ASB is floor of anterior cranial fossa and roof of nose, ethmoid sinuses & orbits
- Bones forming ASB
  - Cribriform plate & ethmoid sinus roof of ethmoid bone centrally
  - Orbital plate of frontal bone laterally
  - Planum sphenoidale & lesser wing of sphenoid posteriorly
- Boundaries of ASB
  - Anterolaterally: Frontal bone
  - Posteriorly: LWS & planum sphenoidale
- Relationships of ASB
  - Superior: Frontal lobes, CN1
  - Inferior: Nasal vault & ethmoid sinus medially, orbit laterally

Bony Landmarks of Anterior Skull Base

- **Frontal crest:** Anterior midline ridge between frontal bones; falx cerebri attaches here
- **Crista galli:** Midline upward triangular process of ethmoid; anteroinferior falx cerebri attaches here
- **Anterior clinoid processes:** Medial aspect of LWS; free edge of tentorium cerebelli attaches here
- **Lesser wing of sphenoid:** Forms sphenoid ridge; separates anterior from central skull base
- **Planum sphenoidale:** Sphenoid bone superomedial plate anterior to tuberculum sellae

Foramina and Fissures of Anterior Skull Base

- **Foramen cecum**
  - Transmits: Variably transmits small emissary vein from nasal mucosa to superior sagittal sinus
  - Location: In margin between posterior aspect of frontal bone & anterior aspect of ethmoid
  - Relationships: Small midline pit found immediately anterior to crista galli
- **Anterior ethmoidal foramen**
  - Transmits: Anterior ethmoidal artery, vein, nerve
  - Location: Slit between ethmoid and frontal bones
  - Relationships: Just anterior to cribriform foramina
- **Posterior ethmoidal foramen**
  - Transmits: Posterior ethmoidal artery, vein, nerve
  - Location: Found at seam between sphenoid and ethmoid bones
  - Relationships: Just posterior to cribriform foramina
- **Foramina of cribriform plate**
  - Transmits: Afferent fibers from nasal mucosa to olfactory bulbs (CN1)
  - Location: ~ 20 perforations within cephalad ethmoid bone plate
  - Relationships: Medial aspect of ethmoid, supports olfactory bulbs

Development of Anterior Skull Base

- **Overview**
  - SB originates largely from cartilaginous precursors
    - Minimal contribution from membranous bone
  - > 100 ossification centers in SB development
  - Ossifies posterior to anterior & lateral to medial
  - Ossification is orderly & constant in 1st 2 years
    - Does not correspond to exact age however
- **Birth**: ASB develops primarily from cartilage with limited ossification at birth
  - Early ethmoid air cells may be seen but unossified crista galli is faint
- **1 month**: Ossification begins from ethmoidal labyrinth & turbinates; proceeds medially
- **3 months**: Roof of nasal cavity & tip of crista galli begin to ossify
  - Ethmoid air cells still inferior to cribriform plate
- **6 months**: Nasal roof is well-ossified; > 90% of patients have partial ossification nasal roof on every coronal CT image
  - Perpendicular plate of ethmoid begins to ossify
  - Ethmoid sinus extends above cribriform plate plane
- **12 months**: Crista galli is well-ossified; more than 70% of patients have ossified posterior cribriform plate
- **18 months**: Ethmoid air cells now extend above plane of cribriform plate and orbital plates of frontal bones help form early fovea ethmoidalis
- **24 months**: Fovea ethmoidalis achieves more mature appearance; perpendicular plate of ethmoid begins to fuse with ossified vomer, most patients still have a gap between nasal & ethmoid bones
- **> 24 months**
  - ASB nearly completely ossified; small gaps persist in nasal roof until early 3rd year
  - Foramen cecum ossifies as late as 5 years
  - Majority of cribriform plate & at least some of crista galli should be ossified

Anatomy-Based Imaging Issues

Key Concepts or Questions

- ASB ossification constant but variable in first 5 years
- Understanding of normal development will avoid confusion or misdiagnoses
- Anterior neuropore closes in 4th gestational week

Imaging Recommendations

- MR to search for anterior neuropore anomalies

Imaging Approaches

- Bone CT viewed at wide windows (> 2000 HU)
- Reformat at least two orthogonal planes

Imaging Pitfalls

- Apparent small gaps in ASB under age 3 are normal
- Do not confuse non-ossified foramen cecum for anterior neuropore anomaly
- Beware fatty marrow in crista galli or ossified falx cerebri is not pathology!

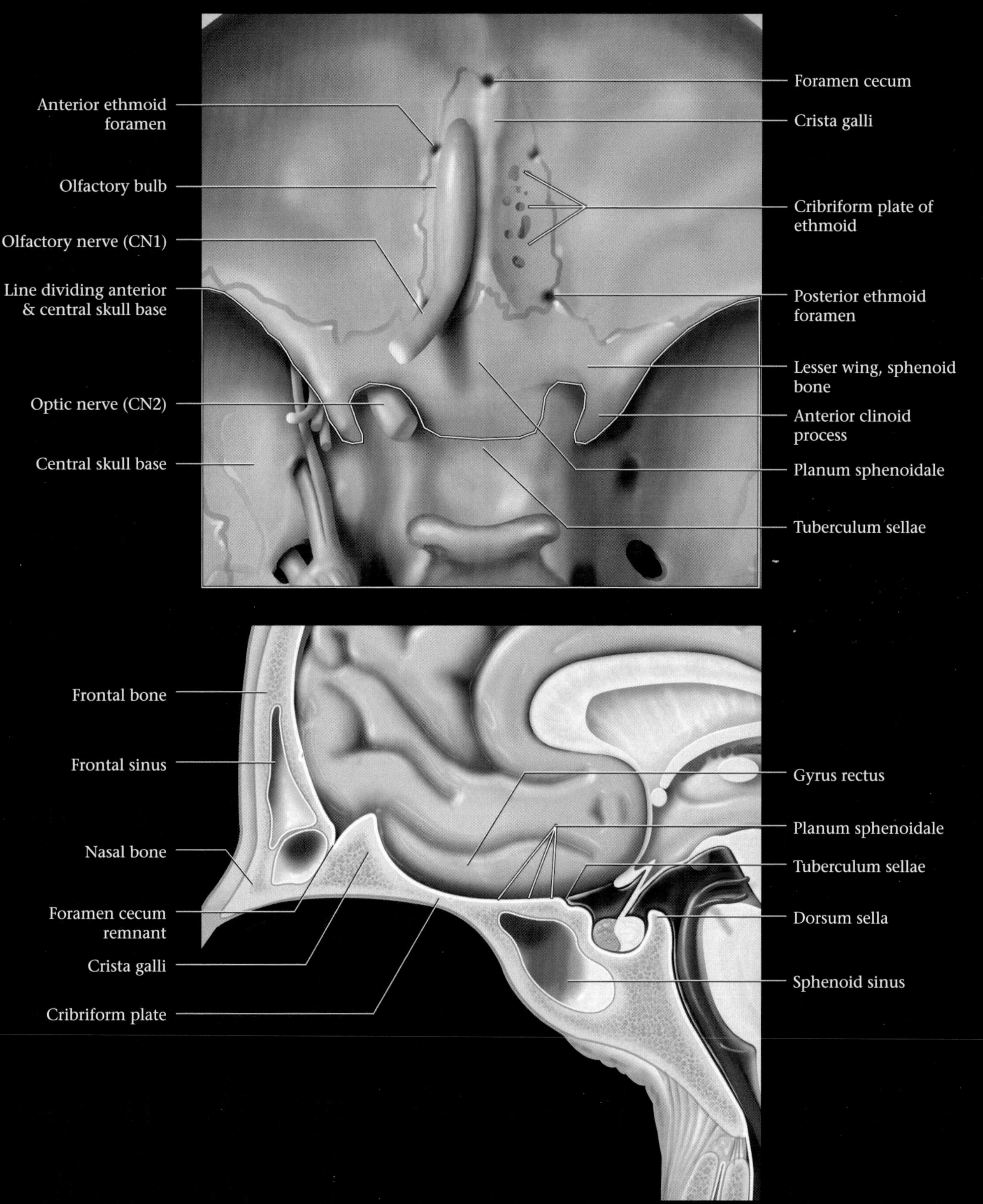

Anterior ethmoid foramen
Olfactory bulb
Olfactory nerve (CN1)
Line dividing anterior & central skull base
Optic nerve (CN2)
Central skull base
Foramen cecum
Crista galli
Cribriform plate of ethmoid
Posterior ethmoid foramen
Lesser wing, sphenoid bone
Anterior clinoid process
Planum sphenoidale
Tuberculum sellae
Frontal bone
Frontal sinus
Nasal bone
Foramen cecum remnant
Crista galli
Cribriform plate
Gyrus rectus
Planum sphenoidale
Tuberculum sellae
Dorsum sella
Sphenoid sinus

(Top) Graphic of anterior skull base seen from above shows olfactory bulb of CN1 laying on cribriform plate. Neural structures have been removed on right, allowing visualization of numerous perforations in the cribriform plate, through which afferent fibers from olfactory mucosa pass to form the olfactory bulb. Note the foramen cecum, a small pit anterior to the crista galli, bounded anteriorly by frontal bone, posteriorly by ethmoid bone. The posterior margin of the anterior skull base is formed by the lesser wing of sphenoid & planum sphenoidale. **(Bottom)** Sagittal graphic of anterior skull base shows midline vertical crista galli. Anterior to crista galli is foramen cecum remnant. Posterolateral to crista galli is horizontal cribriform plate. The planum sphenoidale is the posteromedial anterior skull base.

ANTERIOR SKULL BASE

GRAPHICS

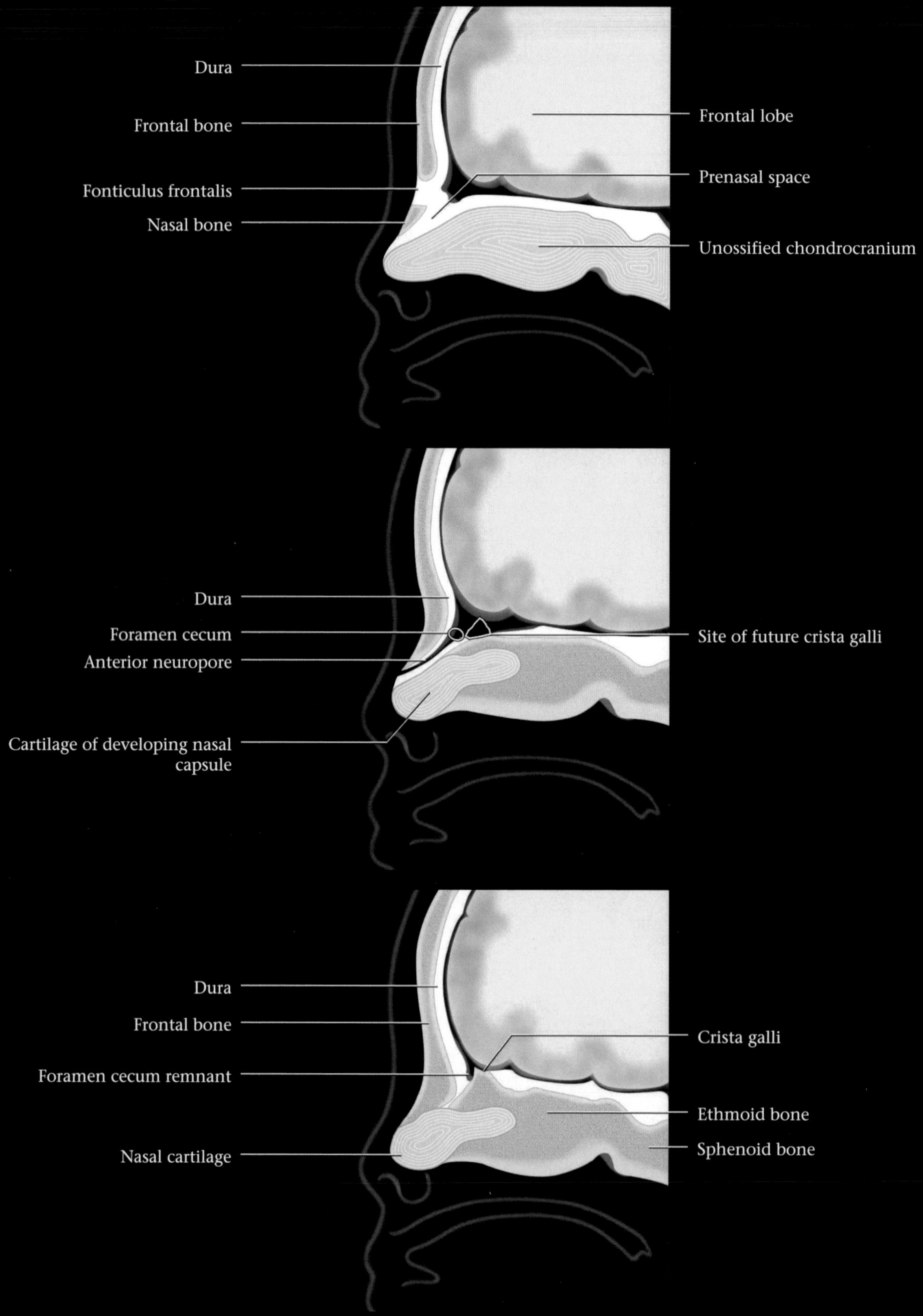

Dura
Frontal bone
Fonticulus frontalis
Nasal bone
Frontal lobe
Prenasal space
Unossified chondrocranium

Dura
Foramen cecum
Anterior neuropore
Cartilage of developing nasal capsule
Site of future crista galli

Dura
Frontal bone
Foramen cecum remnant
Nasal cartilage
Crista galli
Ethmoid bone
Sphenoid bone

(Top) Sagittal graphic of normal anterior skull base development. Fonticulus frontalis, a small ASB fontanelle, is normal cartilaginous gap between developing partially-ossified frontal & nasal bones. Prenasal space is also present at this time as a dura-filled space between developing nasal bones & cartilage of developing nasal capsule. Both sites can become location of a cephalocele. **(Middle)** Sagittal graphic of ASB slightly later in development. The fonticulus frontalis has closed & ossification of chondrocranium has proceeded from posterior to anterior. Prenasal space is now encased in bone & becomes foramen cecum. A normal stalk of dura extends through foramen cecum to skin (anterior neuropore). **(Bottom)** Sagittal graphic of ASB even later in development. Anterior neuropore has regressed. Foramen cecum will completely fuse by age 5.

ANTERIOR SKULL BASE

AXIAL BONE CT

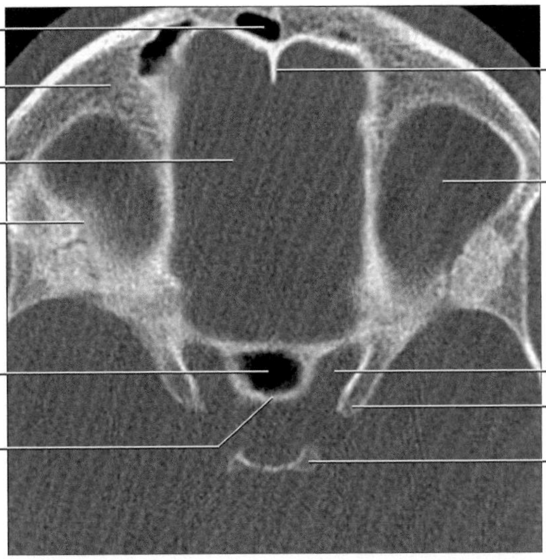

Frontal sinus
Frontal bone
Frontal lobe
Orbital roof
Sphenoid sinus
Tuberculum sellae
Frontal crest
Orbit
Optic canal
Anterior clinoid process
Dorsum sellae

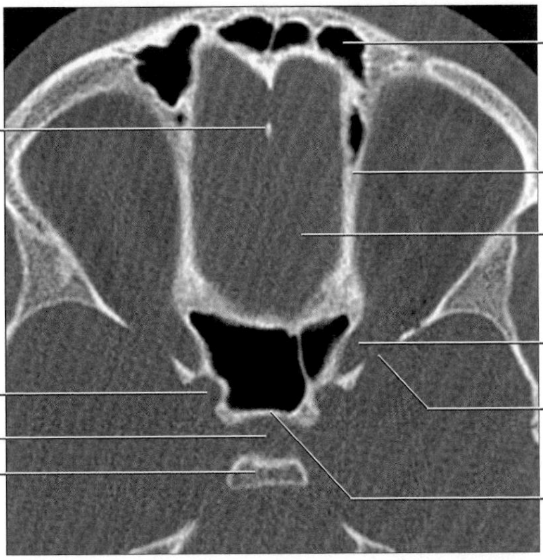

Crista galli
Cavernous internal carotid artery
Sella
Dorsum sella
Frontal sinus
Fovea ethmoidalis
Gyrus rectus
Optic canal
Superior orbital fissure
Tuberculum sellae

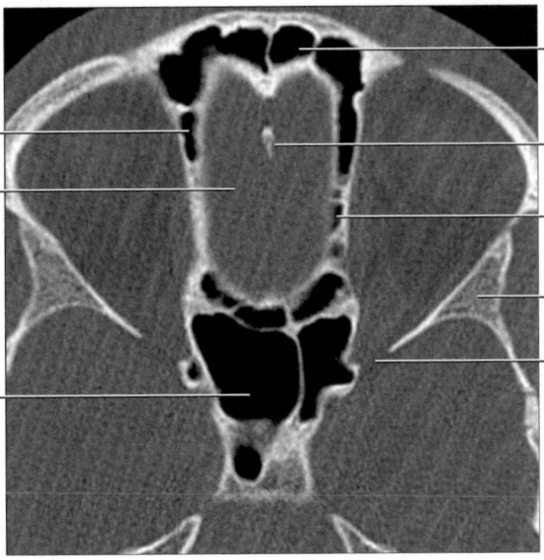

Anterior ethmoid air cells
Gyrus rectus
Sphenoid sinus
Frontal sinus
Crista galli
Posterior ethmoid air cells
Greater wing of sphenoid
Superior orbital fissure

(Top) First of nine axial bone CT images of anterior skull base from superior to inferior. This image is at the level of the orbital roof. Notice that the medial aspect of the frontal lobes extend more inferior than the lateral aspect. On this image, optic canal is seen passing medial to anterior clinoid process, lateral to the sphenoid sinus. The optic canal is thin and can be obscured by volume-averaging. **(Middle)** More inferiorly, cephalad tip of crista galli is seen in the midline where it and frontal crest give attachment to falx cerebri. Superior orbital fissure and optic canal are both visible. **(Bottom)** In this image the frontal, anterior and posterior ethmoid and sphenoid sinuses are all seen. Each sinus is named based on the bone in the skull base where it forms.

ANTERIOR SKULL BASE

AXIAL BONE CT

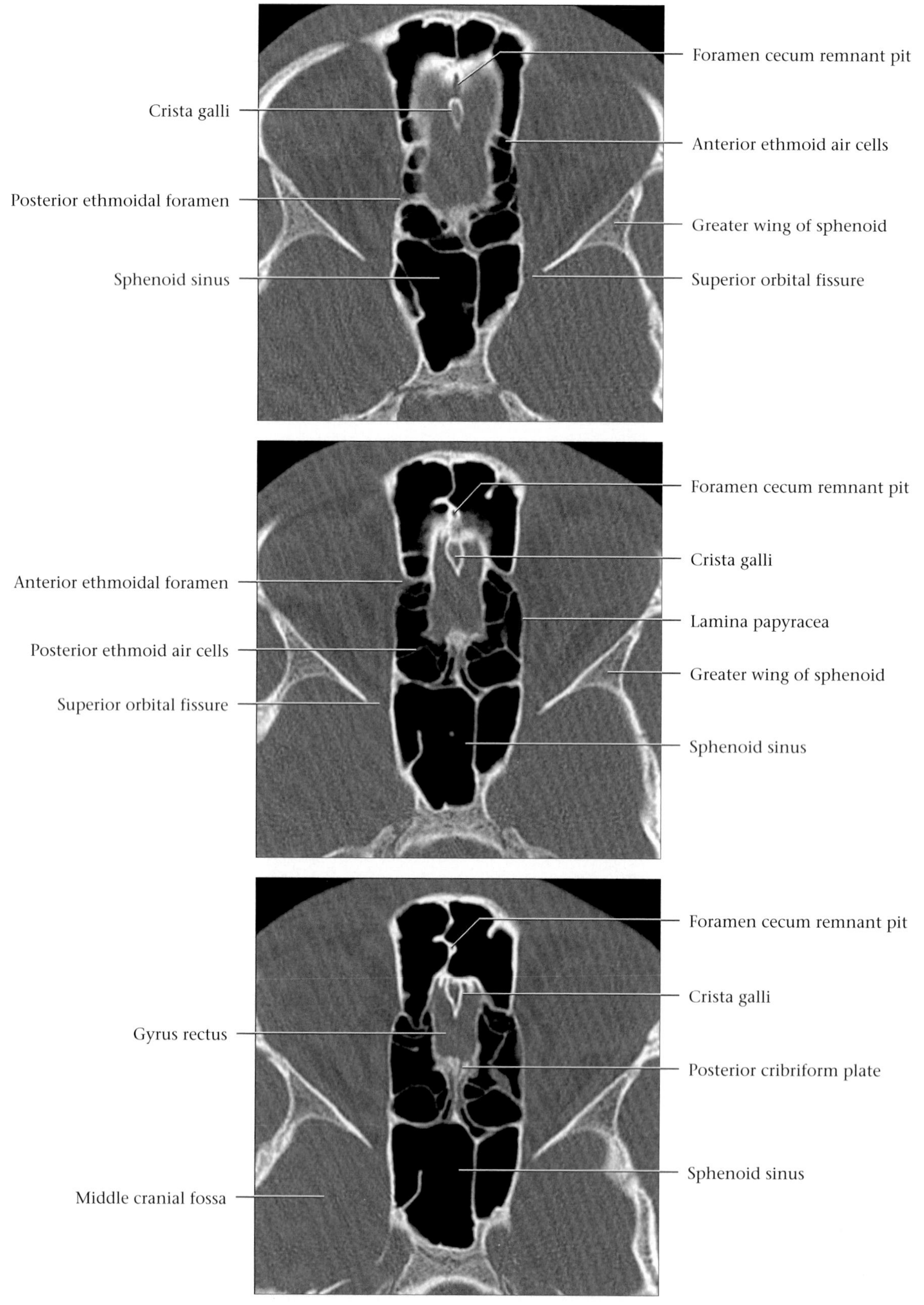
Foramen cecum remnant pit
Crista galli
Anterior ethmoid air cells
Posterior ethmoidal foramen
Greater wing of sphenoid
Sphenoid sinus
Superior orbital fissure
Foramen cecum remnant pit
Crista galli
Anterior ethmoidal foramen
Lamina papyracea
Posterior ethmoid air cells
Greater wing of sphenoid
Superior orbital fissure
Sphenoid sinus
Foramen cecum remnant pit
Crista galli
Gyrus rectus
Posterior cribriform plate
Sphenoid sinus
Middle cranial fossa

(Top) At this level the cephalad margin of the foramen cecum remnant pit is visible just anterior to the crista galli. The posterior ethmoidal foramen can be identified at the posterior margin of the cribriform plate (not seen on this image). Although not seen, the olfactory bulb is nestled between the ethmoid sinuses and the crista galli. **(Middle)** In this image the ethmoid air cells are laterally bounded by the lamina papyracea, the paper-thin medial wall of the orbit. The anterior ethmoidal foramen can also be seen bilaterally along the lateral wall of the ethmoid sinuses. This foramen contains the anterior ethmoidal artery, vein and nerve. **(Bottom)** In this image the posterior cribriform plate has come into view. Notice the cribriform plate is inferomedial to the ethmoid sinuses themselves.

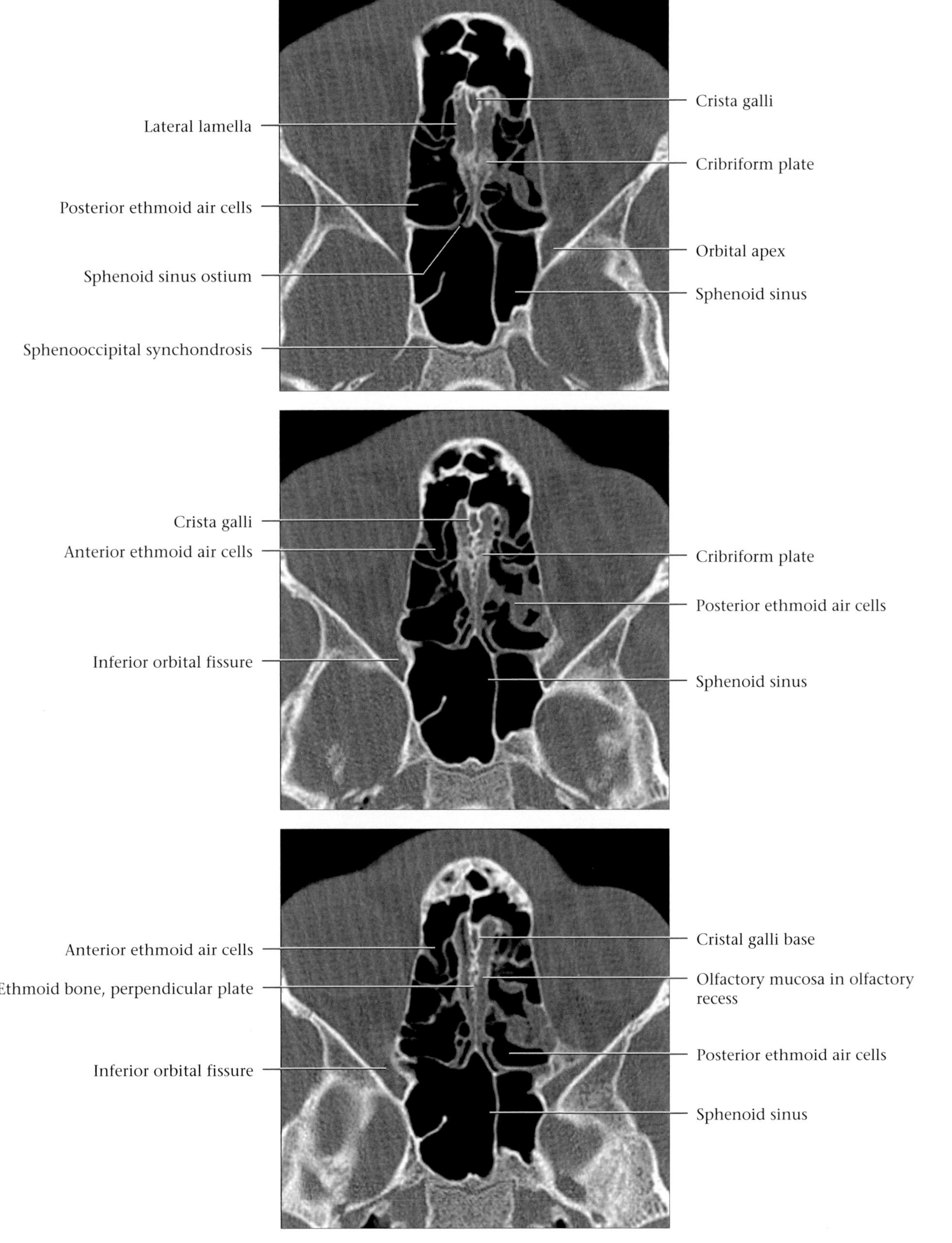

Lateral lamella
Posterior ethmoid air cells
Sphenoid sinus ostium
Sphenooccipital synchondrosis
Crista galli
Cribriform plate
Orbital apex
Sphenoid sinus
Crista galli
Anterior ethmoid air cells
Inferior orbital fissure
Cribriform plate
Posterior ethmoid air cells
Sphenoid sinus
Anterior ethmoid air cells
Ethmoid bone, perpendicular plate
Inferior orbital fissure
Cristal galli base
Olfactory mucosa in olfactory recess
Posterior ethmoid air cells
Sphenoid sinus

(Top) In this image through the cribriform plate the perforated bone is visible. Notice the lateral lamella represents the vertical bony wall of the ethmoid sinus that projects inferiorly from the fovea ethmoidalis (ethmoid sinus roof) down to the cribriform plate. This is far better seen on coronal sinus CT. **(Middle)** The cribriform plate has a variable relationship to the roof of the ethmoid sinuses (fovea ethmoidalis). The more inferior to fovea ethmoidalis the cribriform plate is found, the larger the dimension of the lateral lamella and the more easily a sinus surgery complication may occur. **(Bottom)** This image is found just below the cribriform plate. The perpendicular plate of the ethmoid bone if visible as is the olfactory mucosa in the olfactory recess of the nasal cavity. The olfactory mucosa is the site of origin of esthesioneuroblastoma.

CORONAL BONE CT

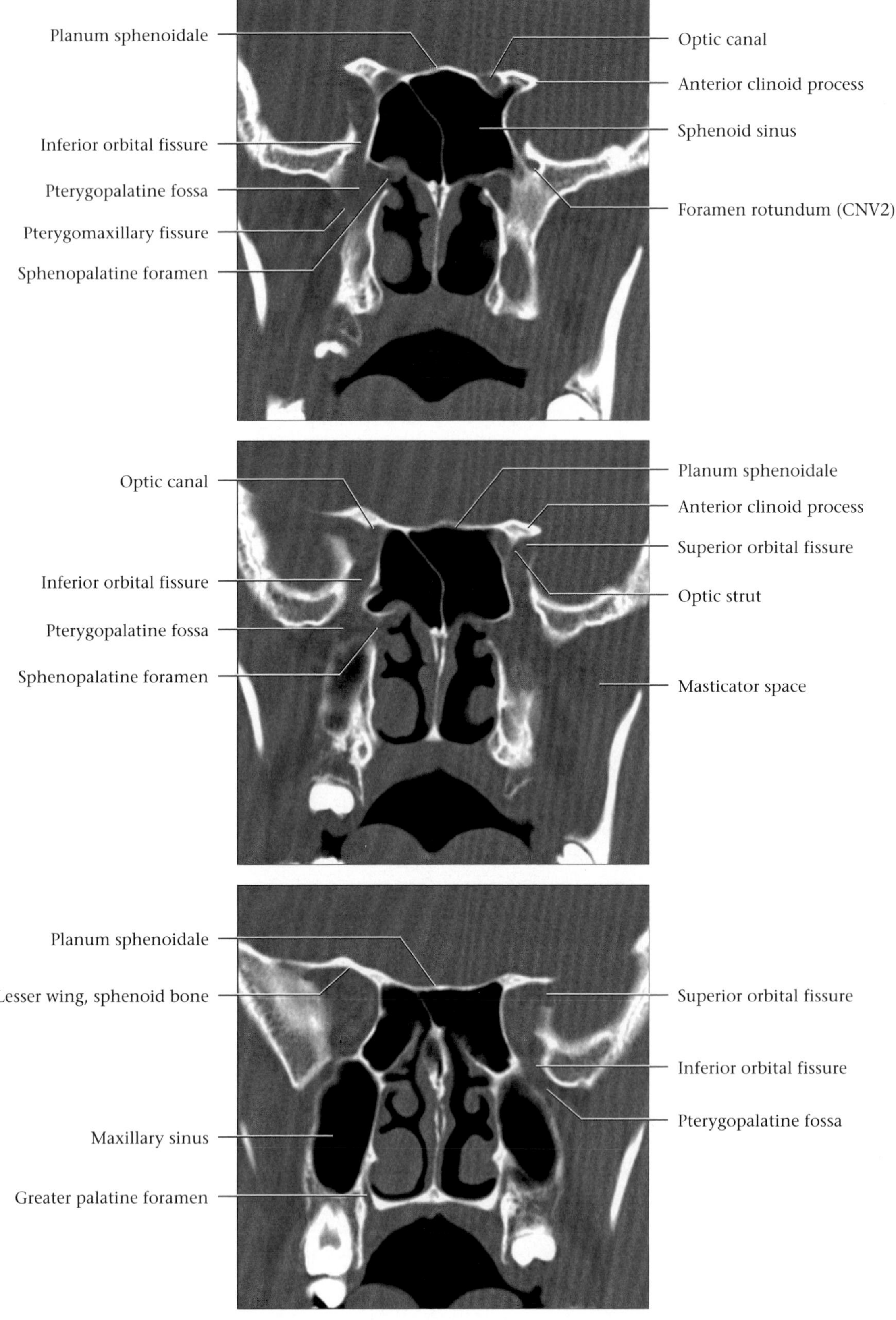
Planum sphenoidale
Optic canal
Anterior clinoid process
Sphenoid sinus
Inferior orbital fissure
Pterygopalatine fossa
Foramen rotundum (CNV2)
Pterygomaxillary fissure
Sphenopalatine foramen
Optic canal
Planum sphenoidale
Anterior clinoid process
Superior orbital fissure
Inferior orbital fissure
Optic strut
Pterygopalatine fossa
Sphenopalatine foramen
Masticator space
Planum sphenoidale
Lesser wing, sphenoid bone
Superior orbital fissure
Inferior orbital fissure
Pterygopalatine fossa
Maxillary sinus
Greater palatine foramen

(Top) First of six coronal sinus bone CT images presented from posterior to anterior shows the transition from central to anterior skull base. Notice the optic canal medial to the anterior clinoid processes. The inferior orbital fissure is seen inferolateral to the optic canal. The planum sphenoidale is the posterior sphenoid sinus roof. **(Middle)** Inferior to planum sphenoidale and lateral to the sphenoid sinus is the complex anatomy of the orbital apex. The most superomedial structure of the orbital apex is the optic canal, divided from superior orbital fissure by a small bony spur called the optic strut. The inferior orbital fissure communicates inferiorly with the pterygopalatine fossa. **(Bottom)** At level of orbital apex the lesser wing of the sphenoid bone is visible as the posterior orbital roof. The planum sphenoidale is the anterior roof of the sphenoid bone.

CORONAL BONE CT

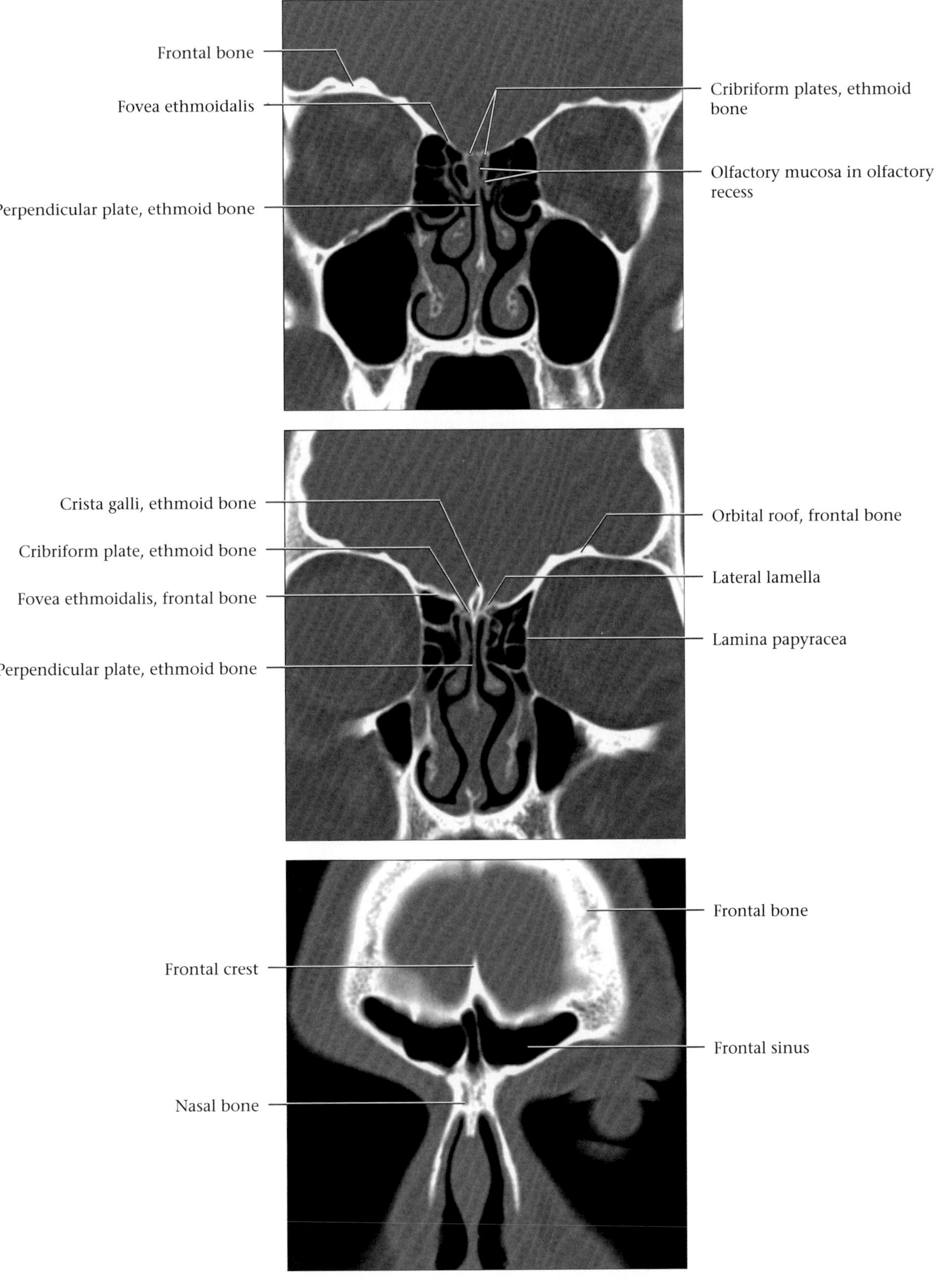
Frontal bone
Fovea ethmoidalis
Perpendicular plate, ethmoid bone
Cribriform plates, ethmoid bone
Olfactory mucosa in olfactory recess
Crista galli, ethmoid bone
Cribriform plate, ethmoid bone
Fovea ethmoidalis, frontal bone
Perpendicular plate, ethmoid bone
Orbital roof, frontal bone
Lateral lamella
Lamina papyracea
Frontal crest
Nasal bone
Frontal bone
Frontal sinus

(Top) At the level of the posterior cribriform plate the fovea ethmoidalis is seen sloping gradually toward the midline. In the midline the cribriform plates themselves are visible. **(Middle)** At the level of the crista galli it is possible to see the multiple pieces of the ethmoid bone. The crista galli is the most cephalad portion of the ethmoid bone, extending directly inferiorly into the perpendicular plate of the ethmoid bone. Just lateral to the base of the crista galli are the cribriform plates, lateral lamellae & fovea ethmoidalis portions of the frontal bone. **(Bottom)** In this image through the frontal bone & sinus note the anteroinferior nasal bone. Do not confuse the more anterosuperior frontal crest (part of frontal bones) with crista galli (part of ethmoid), not seen on this image.

AXIAL BONE CT DEVELOPMENT

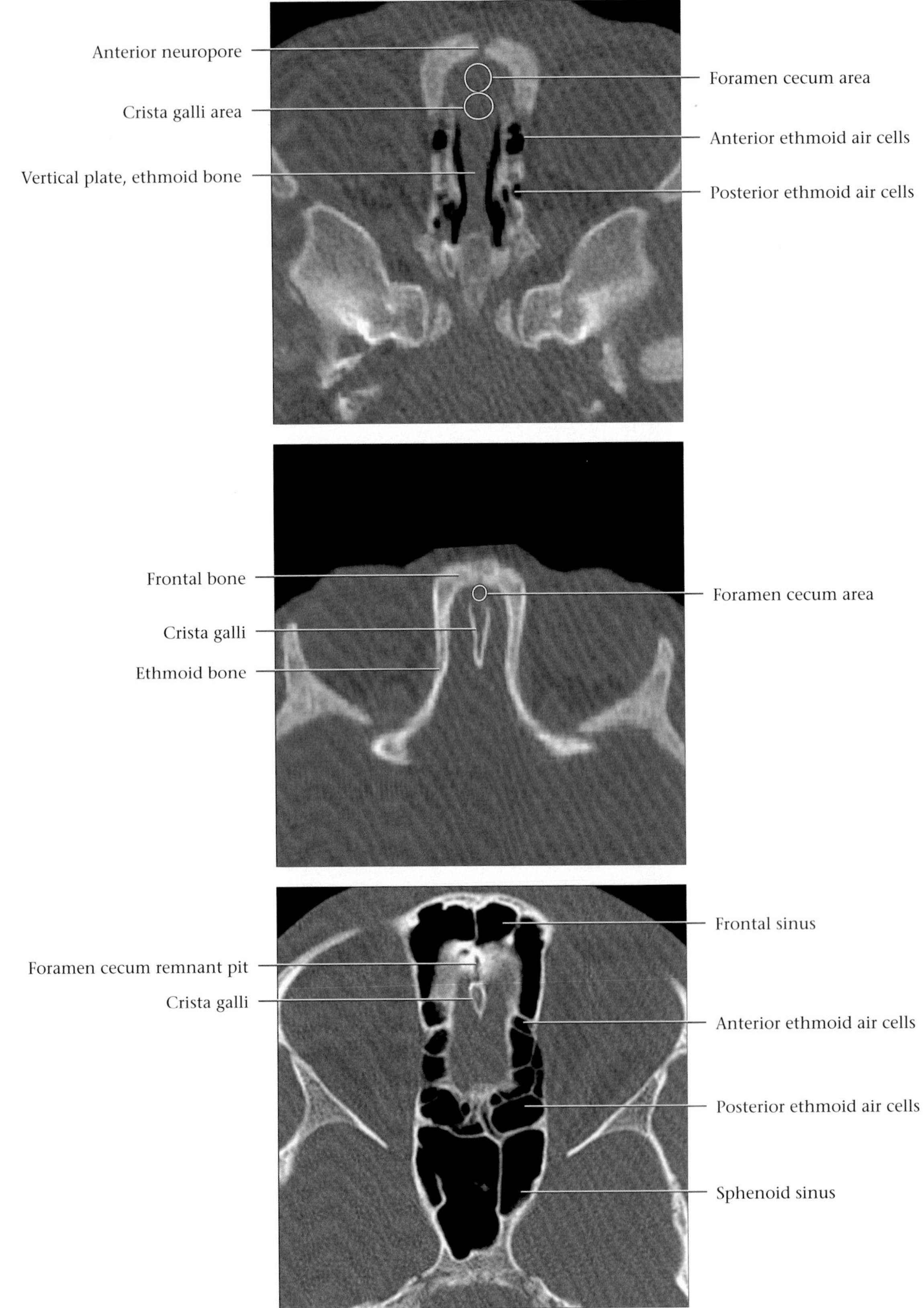
Anterior neuropore
Crista galli area
Vertical plate, ethmoid bone
Foramen cecum area
Anterior ethmoid air cells
Posterior ethmoid air cells
Frontal bone
Crista galli
Ethmoid bone
Foramen cecum area
Foramen cecum remnant pit
Crista galli
Frontal sinus
Anterior ethmoid air cells
Posterior ethmoid air cells
Sphenoid sinus

(Top) Axial bone CT through the anterior skull base in a newborn. The unossified gap between the nasal and frontal bones normally contains dura at this age and represents the regressing anterior neuropore. The area of the foramen cecum, crista galli, cribriform plate and perpendicular plate of the ethmoid bone are all normally unossified in the newborn. **(Middle)** Axial bone CT through the anterior skull base at 12 months. Crista galli is now well-ossified. The foramen cecum area is still not ossified. The foramen cecum is still open but the margins cannot be defined. **(Bottom)** Axial bone CT through the anterior skull base in an adult. The ethmoid air cells now extend far above the horizontal plane of the cribriform plate. Crista galli is thickened and heavily ossified. Although closed, the foramen cecum still demonstrates a small remnant pit.

CORONAL BONE CT DEVELOPMENT

Crista galli site
Cribriform plate site
Perpendicular plate, ethmoid bone

Cribriform plate
Crista galli
Fovea ethmoidalis
Anterior ethmoid air cells
Lateral lamella

Orbital roof, frontal bone
Crista galli
Fovea ethmoidalis, frontal bone
Cribriform plate, ethmoid bone
Lateral lamella
Olfactory recess with olfactory mucosa
Perpendicular plate, ethmoid bone

(Top) Coronal bone CT through the anterior skull base in a newborn. Anterior skull base is largely unossified, including crista galli, cribriform plate and perpendicular plate of ethmoid bone. There is a large gap between the orbital plates of frontal bones. Ethmoid air cells are not yet developed **(Middle)** Coronal bone CT through anterior skull base at 12 months. Ethmoid bone is now mostly ossified, particularly crista galli & posterior cribriform plate. Until age 2-3, unossified gaps in anterior cribriform plate & foramen cecum (not shown) can be normal. Note developing lateral lamella & fovea ethmoidalis are small. **(Bottom)** Coronal bone CT through anterior skull base in an adult. Anterior skull base is completely ossified. Ethmoid air cells extend superolateral to plane of the cribriform plate. Fovea ethmoidalis connected to cribriform plate by lateral lamella.

ANTERIOR SKULL BASE

CORONAL T2 MR DEVELOPMENT

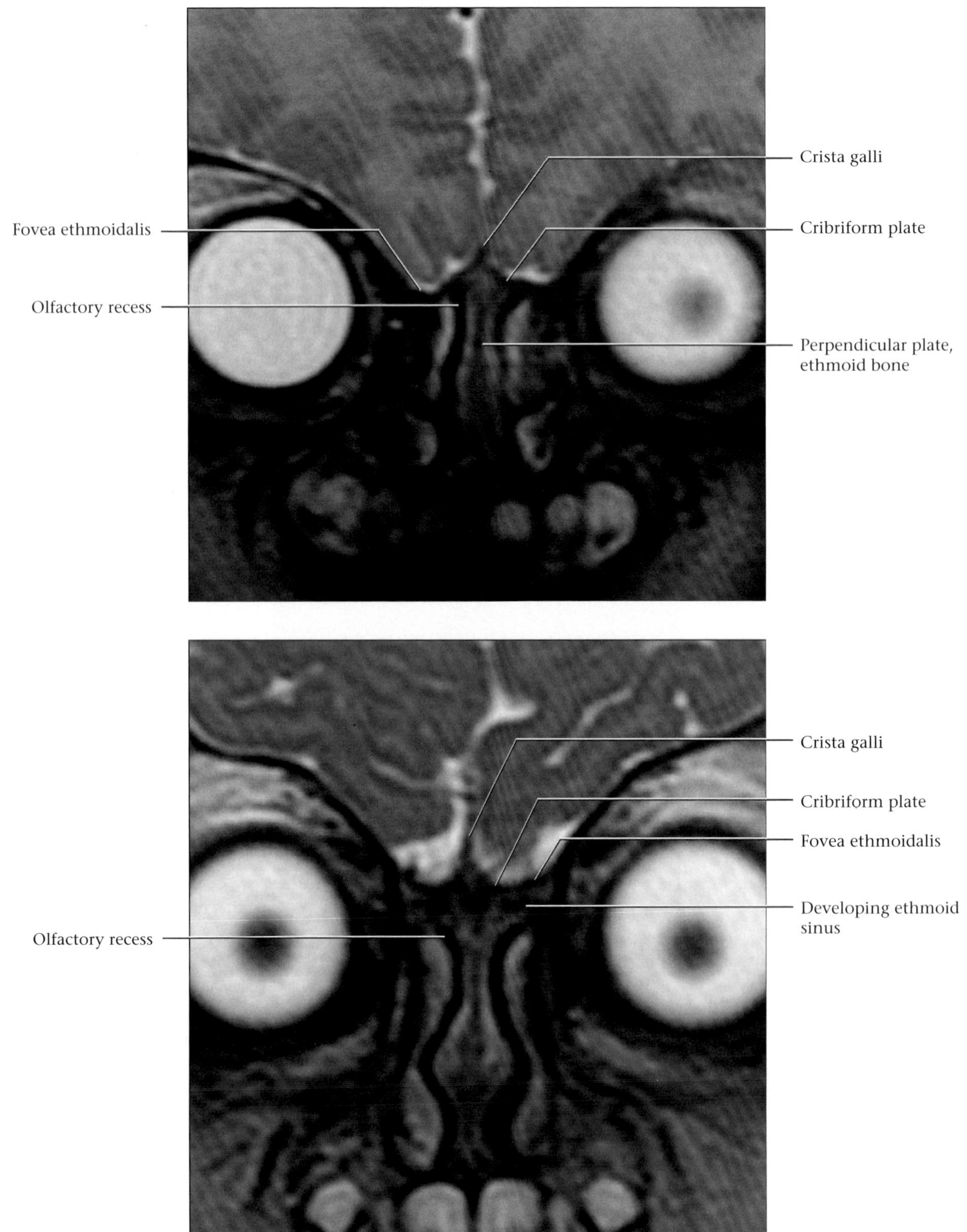
Crista galli
Fovea ethmoidalis
Cribriform plate
Olfactory recess
Perpendicular plate, ethmoid bone
Crista galli
Cribriform plate
Fovea ethmoidalis
Developing ethmoid sinus
Olfactory recess

(Top) Coronal T2 MR through the anterior skull base in a newborn. The anterior skull base is poorly ossified at birth. The cartilaginous crista galli and cribriform plate have an intermediate signal intensity. **(Bottom)** Coronal T2 MR through the anterior skull base at 6 months. Notice the distance between the cribriform plate-fovea ethmoidalis and the olfactory recess of the nose is enlarging with the development of ethmoid sinuses.

CORONAL T2 MR DEVELOPMENT

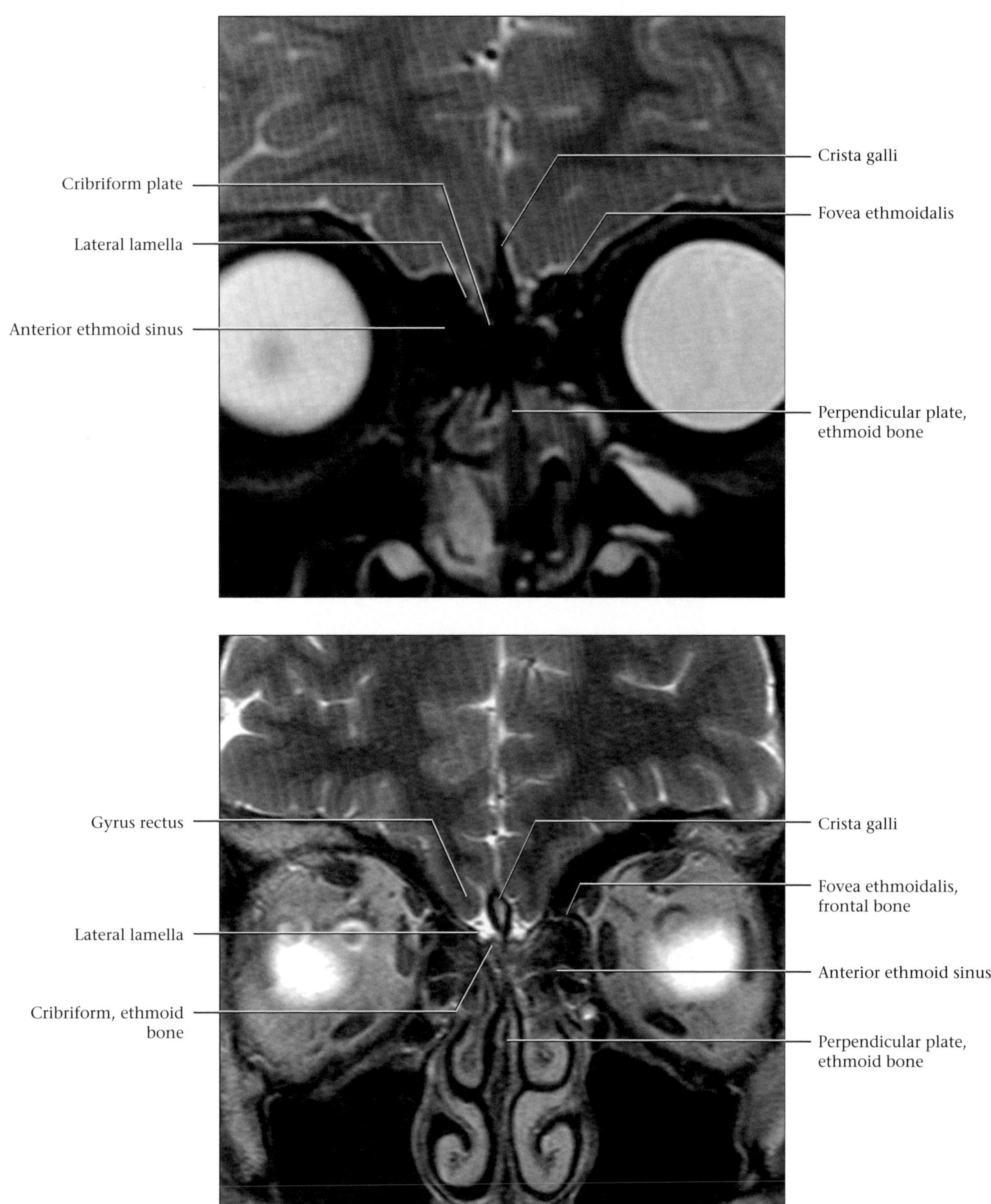

Cribriform plate
Lateral lamella
Anterior ethmoid sinus
Crista galli
Fovea ethmoidalis
Perpendicular plate, ethmoid bone
Gyrus rectus
Lateral lamella
Cribriform, ethmoid bone
Crista galli
Fovea ethmoidalis, frontal bone
Anterior ethmoid sinus
Perpendicular plate, ethmoid bone

(Top) Coronal T2 MR through the anterior skull base at 12 months. The crista galli, cribriform plate, lateral lamella and fovea ethmoidalis are largely ossified at this age. As a result the anterior skull base appears as low signal intensity form cortical bone. Notice the ethmoid sinus aeration now projects cephalad to the level of the crista galli base. The lateral lamella connects the fovea ethmoidalis to the lateral cribriform plate. **(Bottom)** Coronal T2 MR image through the anterior skull base in an adult. By adulthood, there is a significant amount of high signal fat in the well-ossified crista galli. Gyri recti appear to extend far more inferiorly than in childhood because the ethmoid air cell have enlarged superiorly.

SAGITTAL T1 MR DEVELOPMENT

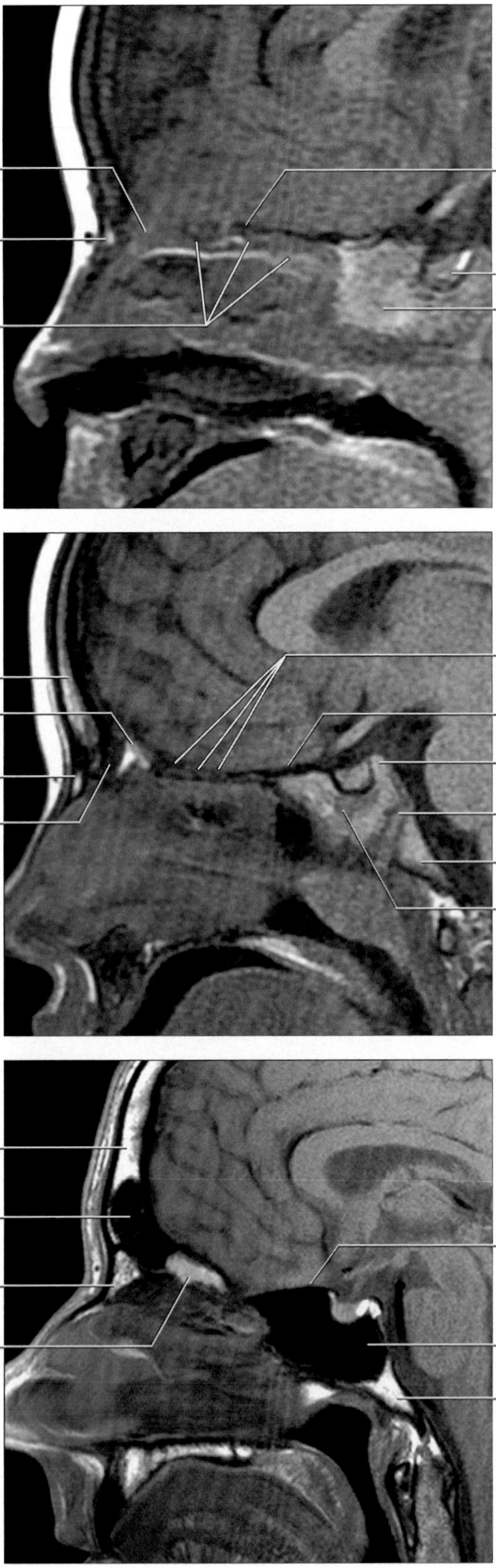

Foramen cecum
Fonticulus frontalis
Chondrocranium, anterior skull base
Cribriform plate/fovea ethmoidalis
Pituitary gland
Body, sphenoid bone

Frontal bone
Crista galli
Nasal bone
Foramen cecum
Cribriform plate
Planum sphenoidale
Dorsum sella
Sphenooccipital synchondrosis
Basiocciput (clivus)
Body of sphenoid bone

Frontal bone
Frontal sinus
Nasal bone
Crista galli
Planum sphenoidale
Sphenoid sinus
Basiocciput (clivus)

(Top) Sagittal T1 MR of anterior skull base in a 6 month old infant. The area of cribriform plate/fovea ethmoidalis has begun to ossify, hence the low signal line. Foramen cecum margins are difficult to discern as a result of absent ossification in the area. **(Middle)** Sagittal T1 MR of anterior skull base in 18 month old. There is rapid ossification of this area in 1st year of life. Note high signal fatty marrow in crista galli. Foramen cecum is visible anterior to crista galli, normally containing thin dural stalk that will obliterate by 5 years of age. **(Bottom)** Sagittal T1 MR of anterior skull base in an adult. Crista galli is readily visible because its fatty marrow. Foramen cecum is not seen because it is now fused. The frontal bone is distinguishable from the nasal bone anteriorly.

SAGITTAL T2 MR DEVELOPMENT

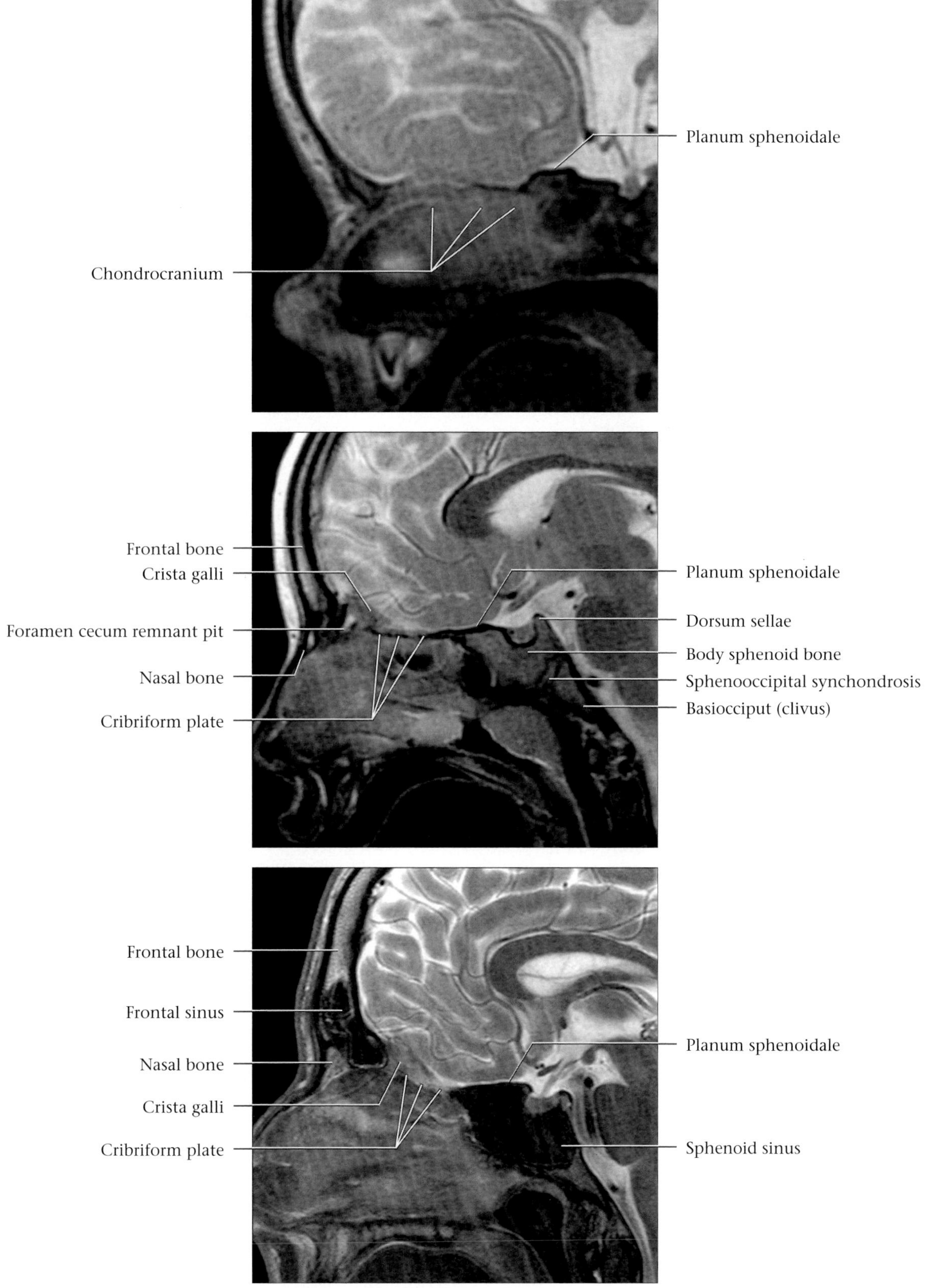
Planum sphenoidale
Chondrocranium
Frontal bone
Crista galli
Foramen cecum remnant pit
Nasal bone
Cribriform plate
Planum sphenoidale
Dorsum sellae
Body sphenoid bone
Sphenooccipital synchondrosis
Basiocciput (clivus)
Frontal bone
Frontal sinus
Nasal bone
Crista galli
Cribriform plate
Planum sphenoidale
Sphenoid sinus

(Top) Sagittal T2 MR of anterior skull base in a newborn. The chondrocranium is mostly intermediate signal intensity. Large "gaps" of the anterior skull base are seen because there is little ossification, particularly anteriorly. **(Middle)** Sagittal T2 MR of anterior skull base at 18 months. As anterior skull base progressively ossifies, crista galli becomes more conspicuous. The frontal and sphenoid bones are higher signal due to fatty marrow. Both the sphenoid and frontal sinuses continue to pneumatize well into the teenage years. Cribriform plate ossification is signaled by dark line anterior to planum sphenoidale. **(Bottom)** Sagittal T2 MR of anterior skull base in an adult. Crista galli is fully ossified and filled with high signal fatty marrow. Foramen cecum is fused & therefore not visible. The sphenoid sinus is fully pneumatized.

CENTRAL SKULL BASE

Terminology

Abbreviations

- Anterior, central, posterior skull base (ASB, CSB, PSB)
- Greater, lesser wings of sphenoid (GWS), (LWS)

Definitions

- CSB: Skull base posterior to LWS/planum sphenoidale & anterior to petrous ridge/dorsum sella

Imaging Anatomy

Overview

- CSB is floor of middle cranial fossa & roof of sphenoid sinus and GWS
- Bones forming CSB
  - Sphenoid bone, basisphenoid & GWS
  - Temporal bone anterior to petrous ridge
- Boundaries of CSB
  - Anteriorly boundary: Planum sphenoidale posterior margin (tuberculum sellae) medially & LWS laterally
  - Posterior boundary: Dorsum sella medially & petrous ridges laterally
- Relationships of CSB
  - Superior: Temporal lobes, pituitary, cavernous sinus, Meckel cave, CN1-4, CN6, CNV1-3
  - Inferior: Anterior roof of pharyngeal mucosal space, masticator, parotid & parapharyngeal spaces

Bony Landmarks of Central Skull Base

- **Sella turcica:** Contains pituitary gland
- **Anterior clinoid processes:** Extend posteromedially off lesser wing of sphenoid
- **Posterior clinoid processes:** Extend posterolaterally off dorsum sellae; attachment for tentorium cerebelli
- **Chiasmatic sulcus:** Just posteroinferior from posterior margin of planum sphenoidale; optic chiasm here
- **Tuberculum sellae:** Anterosuperior margin of sella turcica

Foramina and Fissures of Central Skull Base

- **Optic canal**
  - Transmits: CN2 with dura, arachnoid & pia, CSF & ophthalmic artery
  - Formed by LWS, superomedial to superior orbital fissure
- **Superior orbital fissure (SOF)**
  - Transmits: CN3, CN4, CNV1 & CN6 and superior ophthalmic vein
  - Formed by cleft between LWS & GWS
- **Inferior orbital fissure (IOF)**
  - Transmits: Infraorbital artery, vein & nerve
  - Formed by cleft between body of maxilla & GWS
- **Carotid canal**
  - Transmits: Internal carotid artery & sympathetic plexus
  - Formed by GWS & temporal bone
- **Foramen rotundum**
  - Transmits: CNV2, artery of foramen rotundum & emissary veins
  - Completely within sphenoid bone; superolateral to vidian canal
  - Provides direct connection to pterygopalatine fossa
- **Foramen ovale**
  - Transmits: CNV3, lesser petrosal nerve, accessory meningeal branch of maxillary artery & emissary vein
  - Completely within GWS
  - Provides direct connection to masticator space
- **Foramen spinosum**
  - Transmits: Middle meningeal artery & vein, meningeal branch of CNV3
  - Within GWS, posterolateral to foramen ovale
- **Foramen lacerum**
  - Not true foramen
  - Between temporal & sphenoid bones
  - Cartilaginous floor of medial part of horizontal petrous internal carotid artery canal
- **Vidian canal**
  - Transmits: Vidian artery and nerve
  - Formed by sphenoid bone, inferomedial to foramen rotundum

Development of Central Skull Base

- CSB formed by > 25 ossification centers
- Ossification occurs from posterior to anterior
- **Important ossification centers**: Orbitosphenoids, alisphenoids, pre- and postsphenoid, basiocciput
  - **Orbitosphenoids** ⇒ LWS, **alisphenoids** ⇒ GWS
  - **Presphenoid** and **postsphenoid** fuse at ~ 3 months
  - **Postsphenoid** and **basiocciput** fuse ⇒ clivus
- **Sphenooccipital synchondrosis**
  - Between postsphenoid and basiocciput
  - Responsible for most of postnatal SB growth
  - One of last sutures of SB to fuse
  - Open until 14 years, fuses by ~ 16 years in girls & ~ 18 years in boys

Variant Anatomy

- **Persistent craniopharyngeal canal**
  - Remnant of Rathke pouch
  - Vertical cleft in sphenoid body at site of fusion of pre- & postsphenoid; just posterior to tuberculum sellae area in adult
  - Extends from sella turcica to nasopharynx
- **Extensive pneumatization of sphenoid sinus**
  - Can cause endosinal vidian canals & foramen rotundum
  - Pneumatized clinoid processes
- **Canaliculus innominatus**
  - Variant canal for lesser superficial petrosal nerve, medial to foramen spinosum
- **Foramen of Vesalius**
  - Transmits emissary vein from cavernous sinus to pterygoid plexus
  - Anterior to foramen ovale

Anatomy-Based Imaging Issues

Imaging Pitfalls

- Beware sphenoid MR signal changes!
  - Sphenoid sinus: Low signal cartilage until 2 years → high signal fat until 6 years → low signal air (adult)
  - Clivus low signal until 25 years, then high signal fat
- Do not confuse pneumatized clinoid processes with vascular flow voids on MR

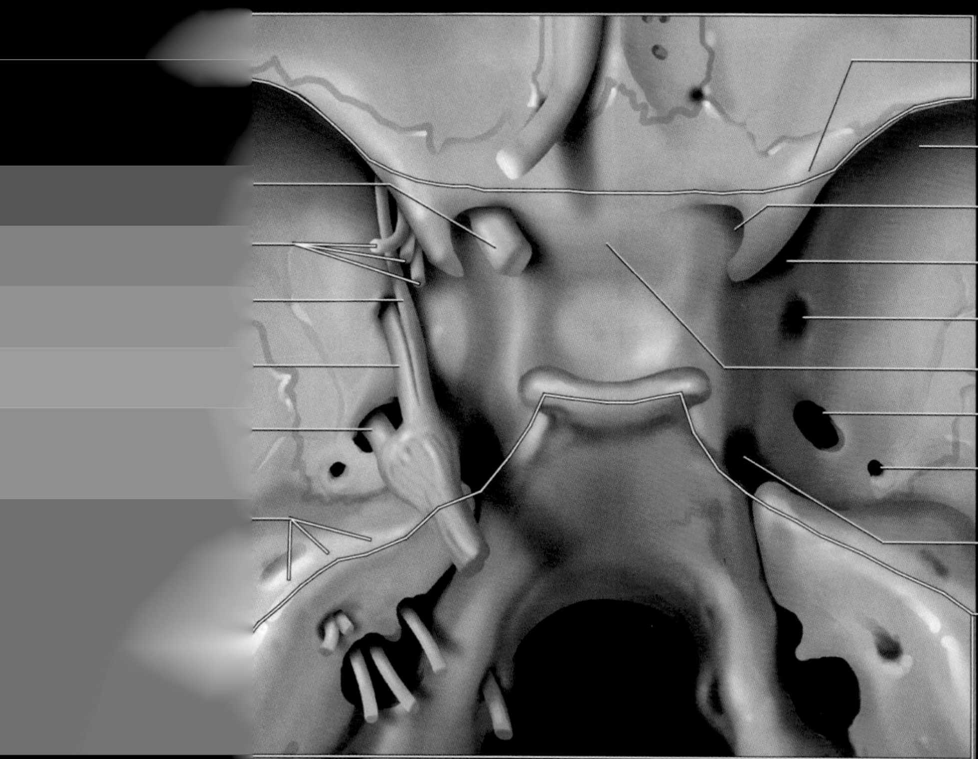
Lesser wing, sphenoid bone
Greater wing, sphenoid bone
Optical canal
Superior orbital fissure
Foramen rotundum
Tuberculum sellae
Foramen ovale
Foramen spinosum
Foramen lacerum
Posterior skull base

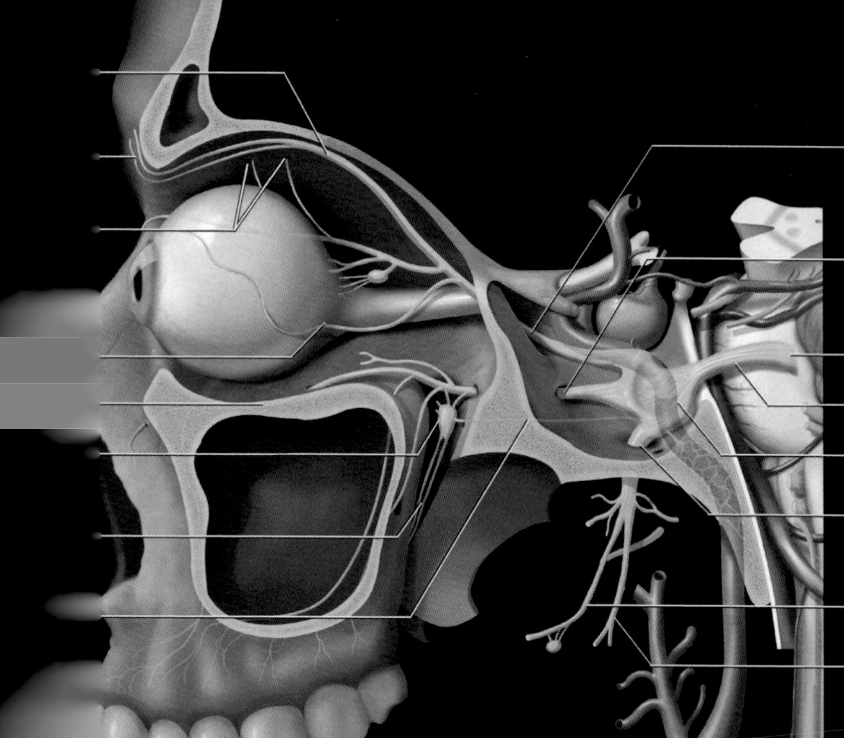
Ophthalmic division CN5 (CNV1) exiting superior orbital fissure
Maxillary division CN5 (CNV2) exiting foramen rotundum
Root entry zone
Preganglionic segment
Trigeminal ganglion
Mandibular division CN5 (CNV3) exiting foramen ovale
Lingual nerve
Inferior alveolar nerve

kull base from above shows important nerves on left. The numerous fissures & foramina of vn on right. Greater wing of sphenoid forms anterior wall of middle cranial fossa. The kull base is dorsum sella medially & petrous ridge laterally. **(Bottom)** Sagittal graphic r skull base depicts trigeminal nerve branches & exiting foramina. Ophthalmic division of iperior orbital fissure. Maxillary division of CN5 exits via foramen rotundum to become as drop the greater & lesser palatine nerves inferiorly to provide sensation for the hard & ivision of CN5 exits through foramen ovale, then divides into 2 main trunks, lingual &

GRAPHICS

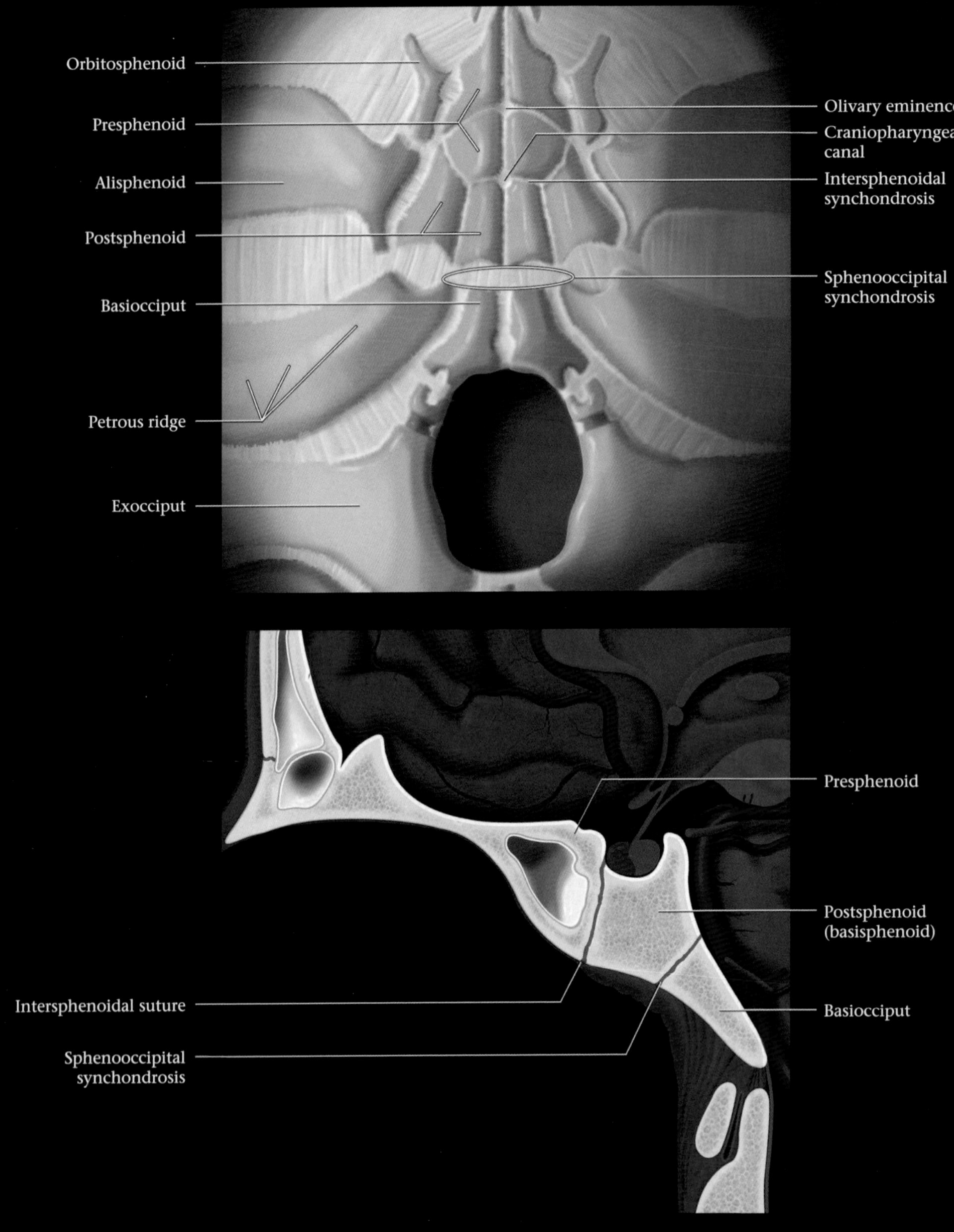

Orbitosphenoid
Presphenoid
Alisphenoid
Postsphenoid
Basiocciput
Petrous ridge
Exocciput
Olivary eminence
Craniopharyngeal canal
Intersphenoidal synchondrosis
Sphenooccipital synchondrosis
Presphenoid
Postsphenoid (basisphenoid)
Basiocciput
Intersphenoidal suture
Sphenooccipital synchondrosis

(Top) Schematic graphic of CSB from above shows its many ossification centers. Between ossification centers of presphenoid is cartilaginous gap called olivary eminence, obliterated shortly after birth. A persistent cleft, called craniopharyngeal canal can also be variably seen in intersphenoid synchondrosis. Do not confuse these variants with pathology. **(Bottom)** Lateral graphic of central skull base shows major ossification centers & location of sutures. Intersphenoidal suture closes at around 3 months age. At about age 2 years, presphenoid begins to demineralize & become pneumatized. Pneumatization progresses posteriorly into postsphenoid until about age 5-7. Sphenooccipital synchondrosis is one of last sutures to fuse at about age 16. It is the suture most responsible for growth of skull base.

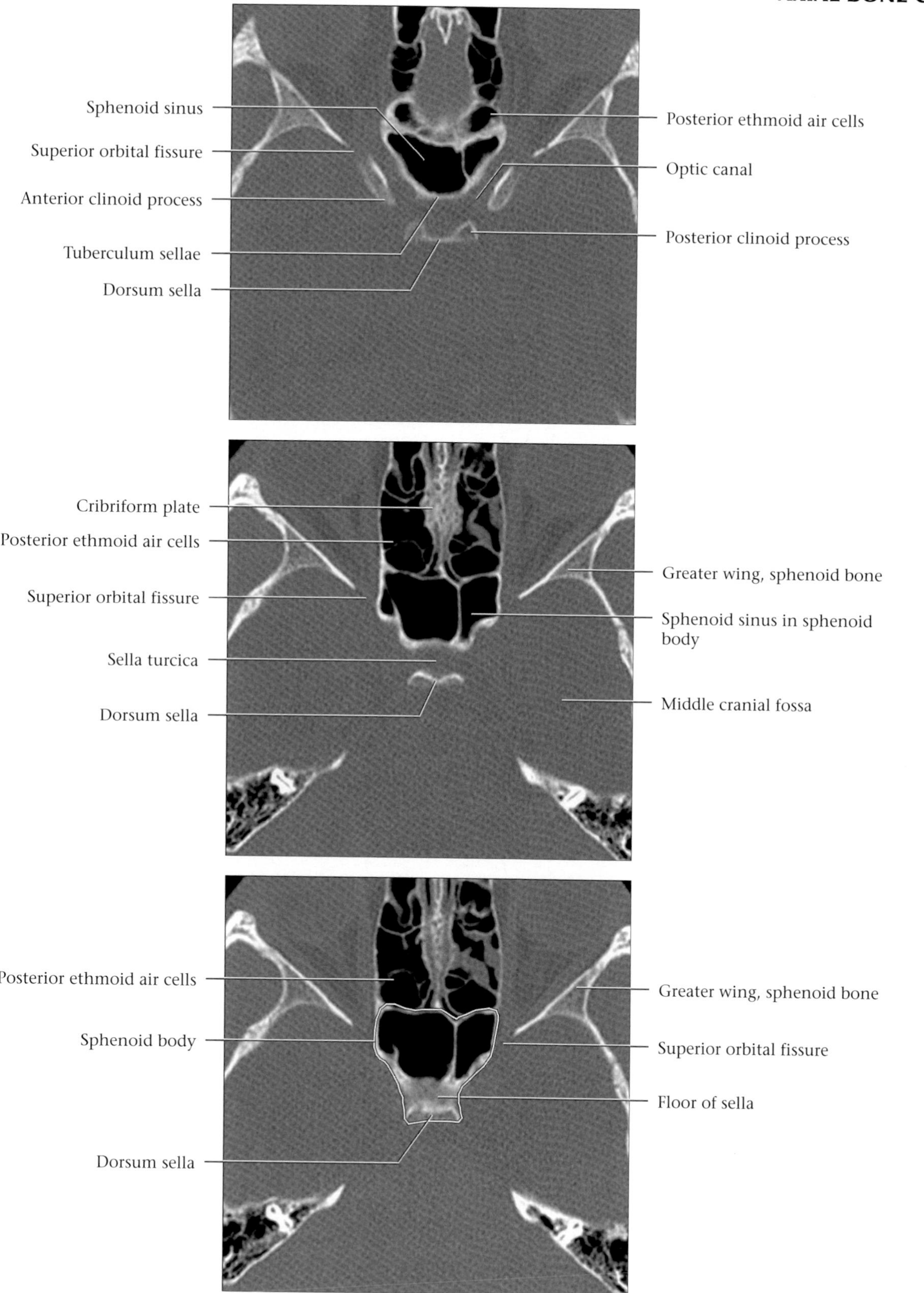

Sphenoid sinus
Superior orbital fissure
Anterior clinoid process
Tuberculum sellae
Dorsum sella
Posterior ethmoid air cells
Optic canal
Posterior clinoid process
Cribriform plate
Posterior ethmoid air cells
Superior orbital fissure
Sella turcica
Dorsum sella
Greater wing, sphenoid bone
Sphenoid sinus in sphenoid body
Middle cranial fossa
Posterior ethmoid air cells
Sphenoid body
Dorsum sella
Greater wing, sphenoid bone
Superior orbital fissure
Floor of sella

(Top) First of nine axial bone CT images of the central skull base presented from superior to inferior. Note that the posterior clinoids merge with the dorsum sella. The optic canal is bound by sphenoid sinus medially and anterior clinoid process laterally. Inferolateral to optic canal is superior orbital fissure. **(Middle)** At the level of sella turcica, the superior orbital fissure is seen as the medial opening of the orbit into the middle cranial fossa. It lies below optic canal, between the greater wing of the sphenoid and the sphenoid sinus. The sella turcica is bound by the dorsum sella posteriorly. **(Bottom)** In this image the body of the sphenoid bone is seen to be made up of the sphenoid sinus, sella turcica and the dorsum sella. Anterior to the sphenoid bone is the ethmoid bone.

AXIAL BONE CT

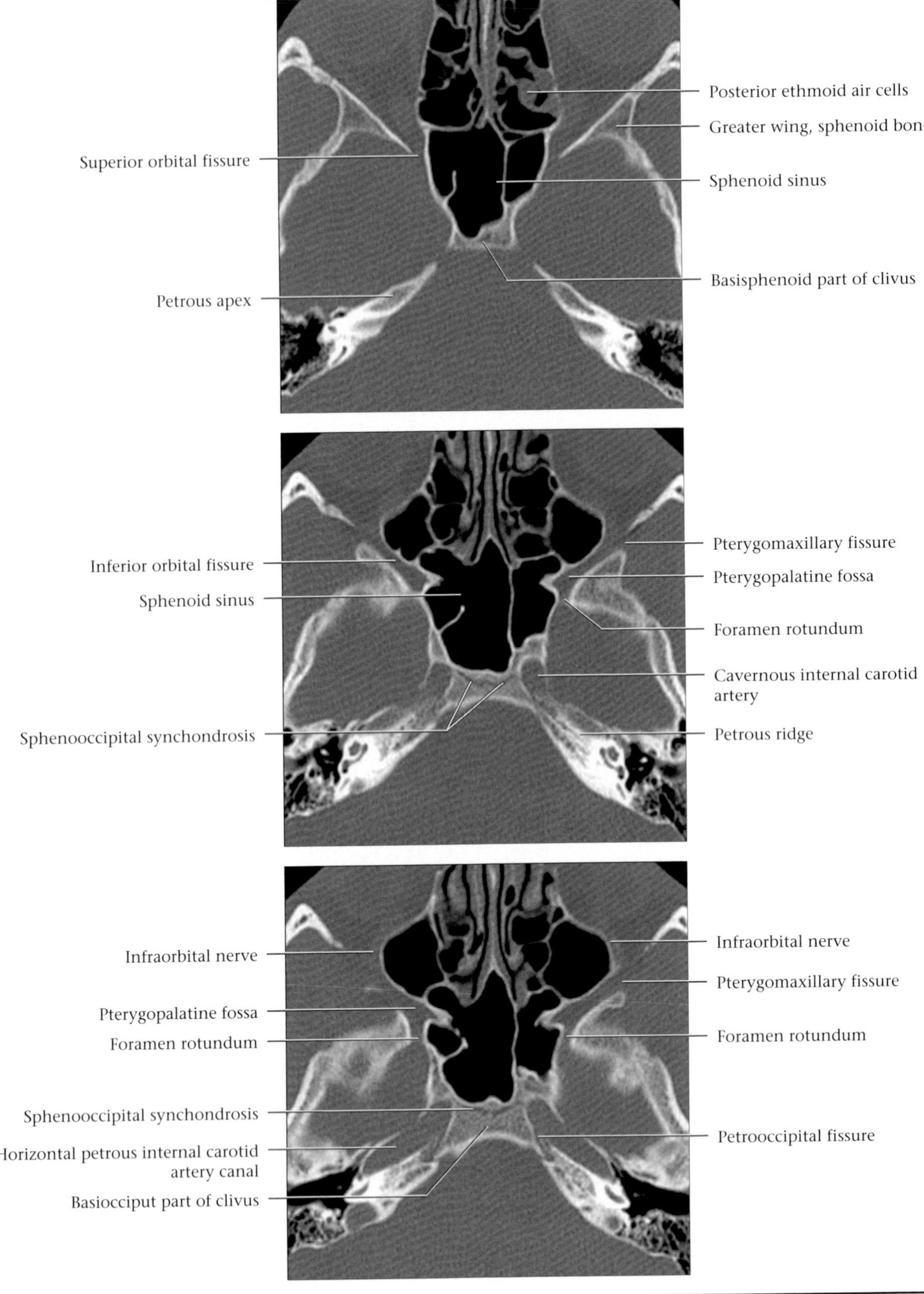
Posterior ethmoid air cells
Greater wing, sphenoid bone
Superior orbital fissure
Sphenoid sinus
Basisphenoid part of clivus
Petrous apex
Pterygomaxillary fissure
Inferior orbital fissure
Pterygopalatine fossa
Sphenoid sinus
Foramen rotundum
Cavernous internal carotid artery
Sphenooccipital synchondrosis
Petrous ridge
Infraorbital nerve
Infraorbital nerve
Pterygomaxillary fissure
Pterygopalatine fossa
Foramen rotundum
Foramen rotundum
Sphenooccipital synchondrosis
Petrooccipital fissure
Horizontal petrous internal carotid artery canal
Basiocciput part of clivus

(Top) In this image the clivus can be seen forming the medial posterior boundary of central skull base while the petrous ridge defines its lateral margin. **(Middle)** This image shows that pneumatization of sphenoid extending up to the sphenooccipital synchondrosis, which is partly unfused in this young adult. Note the foramen rotundum empties anteriorly into the pterygopalatine fossa which connects laterally with the masticator space through the pterygomaxillary fissure. **(Bottom)** At the level of foramen rotundum both pterygopalatine fossae are clearly visible. The maxillary division of trigeminal nerve (CNV2) exits the skull base through the foramen rotundum & continues as infraorbital nerve into orbit via inferior orbital fissure. Malignant tumors of the skin of the cheek, orbit & sinonasal area may all use CNV2 as a perineural route to gain intracranial access.

AXIAL BONE CT

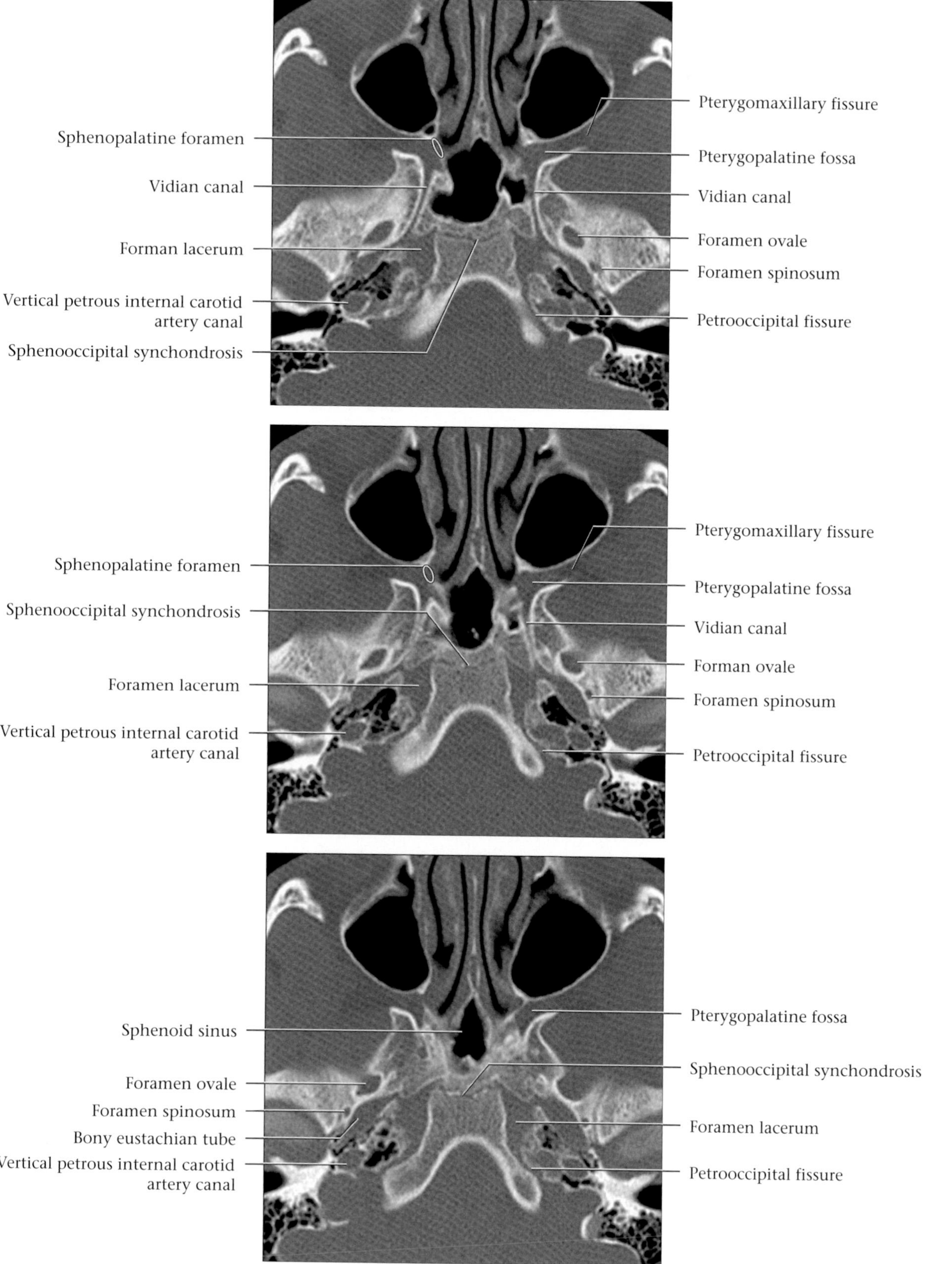
Sphenopalatine foramen
Vidian canal
Forman lacerum
Vertical petrous internal carotid artery canal
Sphenooccipital synchondrosis
Pterygomaxillary fissure
Pterygopalatine fossa
Vidian canal
Foramen ovale
Foramen spinosum
Petrooccipital fissure
Sphenopalatine foramen
Sphenooccipital synchondrosis
Foramen lacerum
Vertical petrous internal carotid artery canal
Pterygomaxillary fissure
Pterygopalatine fossa
Vidian canal
Forman ovale
Foramen spinosum
Petrooccipital fissure
Sphenoid sinus
Foramen ovale
Foramen spinosum
Bony eustachian tube
Vertical petrous internal carotid artery canal
Pterygopalatine fossa
Sphenooccipital synchondrosis
Foramen lacerum
Petrooccipital fissure

(Top) In this image the vidian canal is visible connecting pterygopalatine fossa anteriorly to carotid canal floor (foramen lacerum) posteriorly. A malignant tumor that has accessed the pterygopalatine fossa may reach the carotid canal of the skull base via perineural spread on the vidian nerve in the vidian canal. There is a medial connection between the pterygopalatine fossa & nose, the sphenopalatine foramen. Juvenile angiofibroma begins along the nasal margin of this foramen. **(Middle)** In this image note the foramen ovale is located in the greater wing of the sphenoid bone. Extracranial perineural malignancy on CNV3 enters the intracranial area via foramen ovale. **(Bottom)** In this image note the foramen spinosum is posterolateral to the foramen ovale in the greater wing of the sphenoid bone. The middle meningeal artery passes intracranially via the foramen spinosum.

CORONAL BONE CT

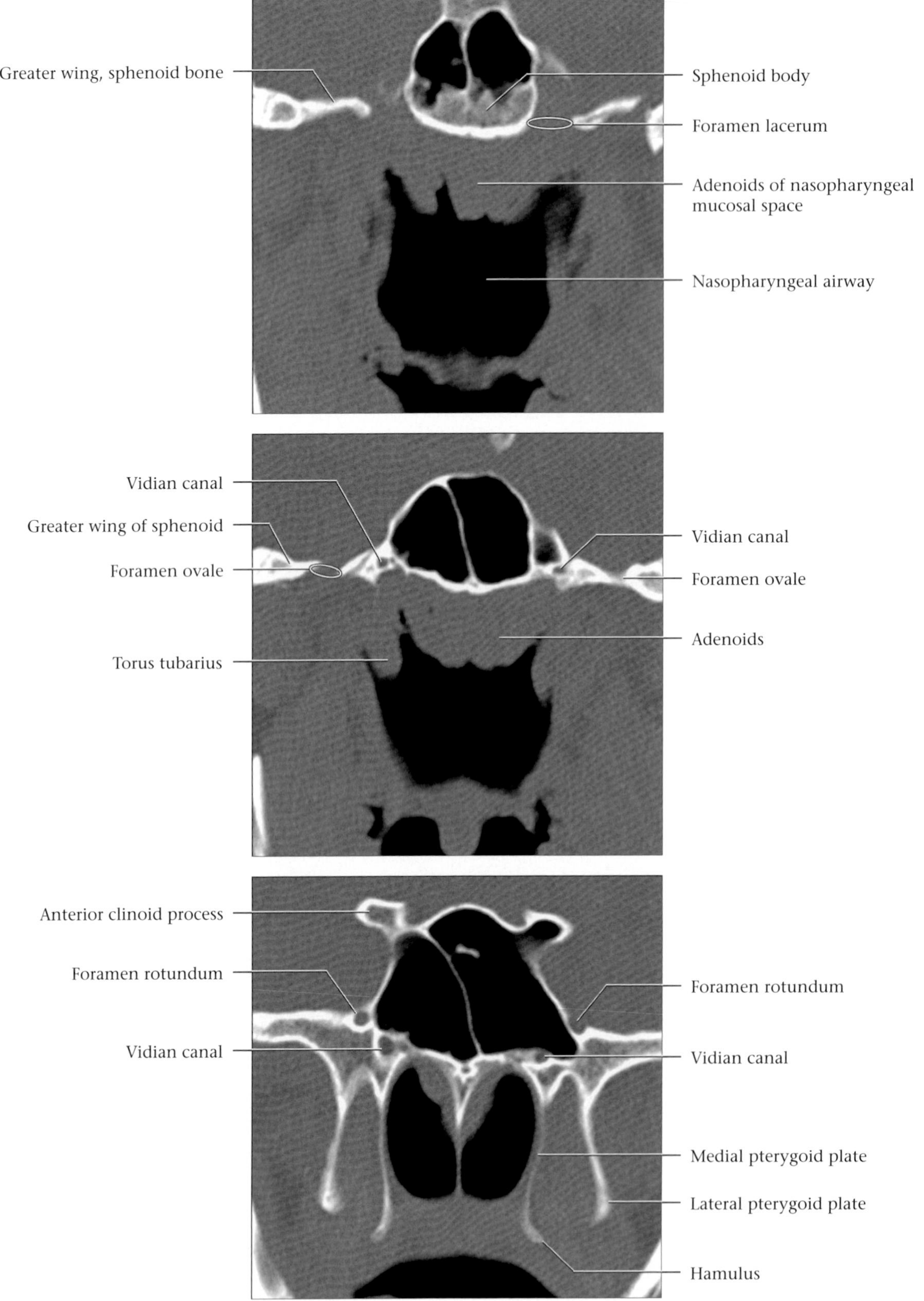
Greater wing, sphenoid bone
Sphenoid body
Foramen lacerum
Adenoids of nasopharyngeal mucosal space
Nasopharyngeal airway
Vidian canal
Greater wing of sphenoid
Foramen ovale
Vidian canal
Foramen ovale
Adenoids
Torus tubarius
Anterior clinoid process
Foramen rotundum
Vidian canal
Foramen rotundum
Vidian canal
Medial pterygoid plate
Lateral pterygoid plate
Hamulus

(Top) First of three coronal bone CT images of the central skull base presented from posterior to anterior. The foramen lacerum is seen as a large defect between the greater wing of the sphenoid bone and the sphenoid body. Foramen lacerum is not a true foramen. It represents the cartilaginous floor of the anteromedial horizontal segment of the petrous internal carotid artery canal. **(Middle)** In this image the foramen ovale is evident lateral to the vidian canal and anterolateral to foramen lacerum. It transmits CNV3 from the middle cranial fossa to the masticator space. **(Bottom)** More anteriorly, foramen rotundum and vidian canal are both seen running in the transverse plane. Both foramen rotundum and vidian canal open into the pterygopalatine fossa. Also note the pterygoid plates inferiorly.

AXIAL T1 C+ MR

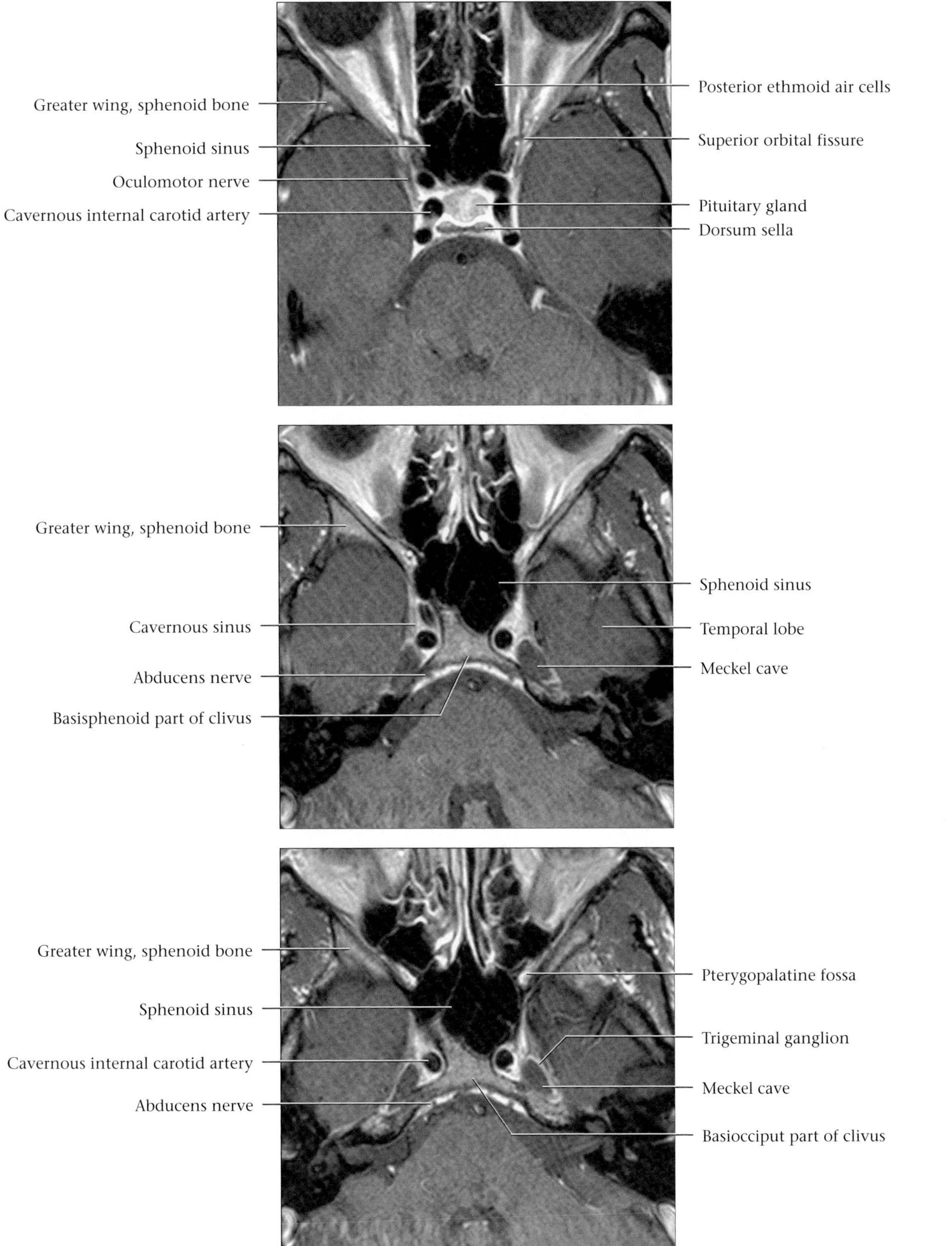

Greater wing, sphenoid bone
Sphenoid sinus
Oculomotor nerve
Cavernous internal carotid artery
Posterior ethmoid air cells
Superior orbital fissure
Pituitary gland
Dorsum sella
Greater wing, sphenoid bone
Cavernous sinus
Abducens nerve
Basisphenoid part of clivus
Sphenoid sinus
Temporal lobe
Meckel cave
Greater wing, sphenoid bone
Sphenoid sinus
Cavernous internal carotid artery
Abducens nerve
Pterygopalatine fossa
Trigeminal ganglion
Meckel cave
Basiocciput part of clivus

(Top) First of six axial T1 C+ MR images of the central skull base presented from superior to inferior. The enhancing venous plexus of the cavernous sinus is seen surrounding the cavernous internal carotid artery. Medially, the enhancing pituitary gland in the sella turcica is bound by the dorsum sella posteriorly and the sphenoid sinus anteriorly. **(Middle)** In this image the upper basisphenoid part of the clivus is seen. Cerebrospinal fluid-filled Meckel cave is seen along the posterior border of the cavernous sinus. **(Bottom)** In this image the basiocciput part of the clivus is visible. The upper clivus above the fused sphenooccipital synchondrosis is part of the sphenoid bone while the lower clivus is part of the occipital bone. Notice the marrow space of the clivus enhances.

CENTRAL SKULL BASE

AXIAL T1 C+ MR

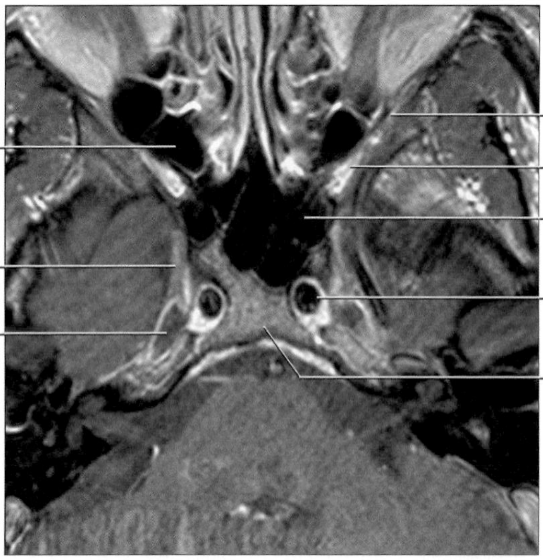

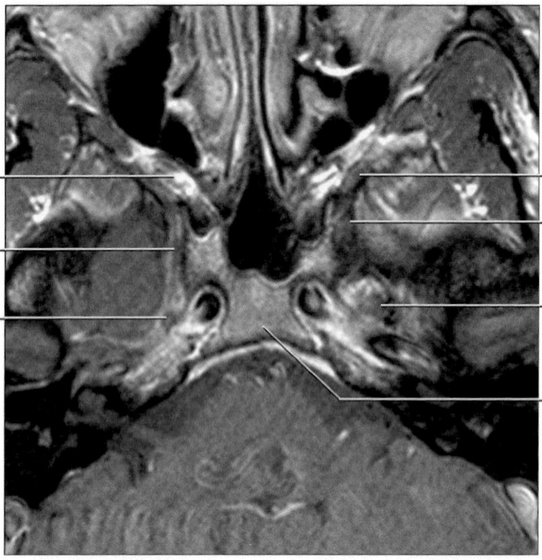

Maxillary sinus
Foramen rotundum
Meckel cave
Inferior orbital fissure
Pterygopalatine fossa
Sphenoid sinus
Anterior genu of horizontal petrous ICA
Clival occipital bone

Pterygopalatine fossa
Maxillary nerve (CN2)
Mandibular nerve (CNV3)
Maxillary nerve (CNV2)
Foramen rotundum
Mandibular nerve (CNV3)
Clival occipital bone

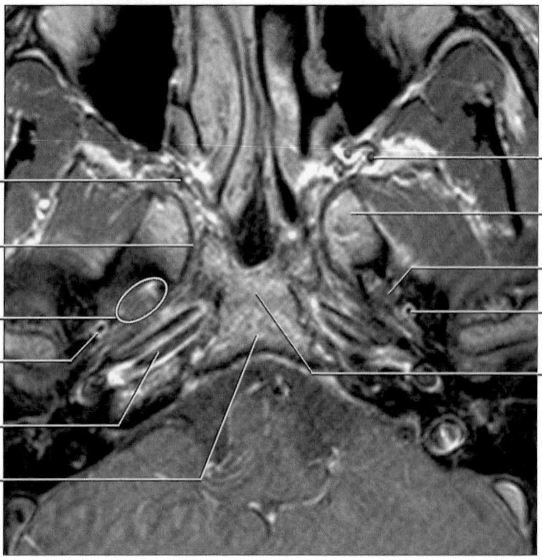

Pterygopalatine fossa
Vidian canal
CNV3 in foramen ovale
Middle meningeal artery in foramen spinosum
Horizontal petrous ICA
Clival occipital bone
Internal maxillary artery
Pterygoid process of sphenoid bone
CNV3 in foramen ovale
Middle meningeal artery in foramen spinosum
Body, sphenoid bone

(Top) Image through superior pterygopalatine fossa with its anterolateral connection to the inferior orbital fissure visible. The anteriorly projecting foramen rotundum can also be seen. The sphenoid bone is partially pneumatized (sphenoid sinus). **(Middle)** In this image the maxillary nerve (CNV2) is seen as a linear low intensity structure in the foramen rotundum on the right. On the left this same nerve can be seen exiting the foramen rotundum into the pterygopalatine fossa. **(Bottom)** At the level of the foramen ovale the mandibular nerve (CNV3) is seen bilaterally. Also note the middle meningeal artery passing through the foramen spinosum. The vidian canal is clearly visible medial to the foramen ovale. The clival occipital bone should be distinguished from the body of the sphenoid bone even though the sphenooccipital fissure cannot be discerned.

SAGITTAL T1 & T2 MR DEVELOPMENT

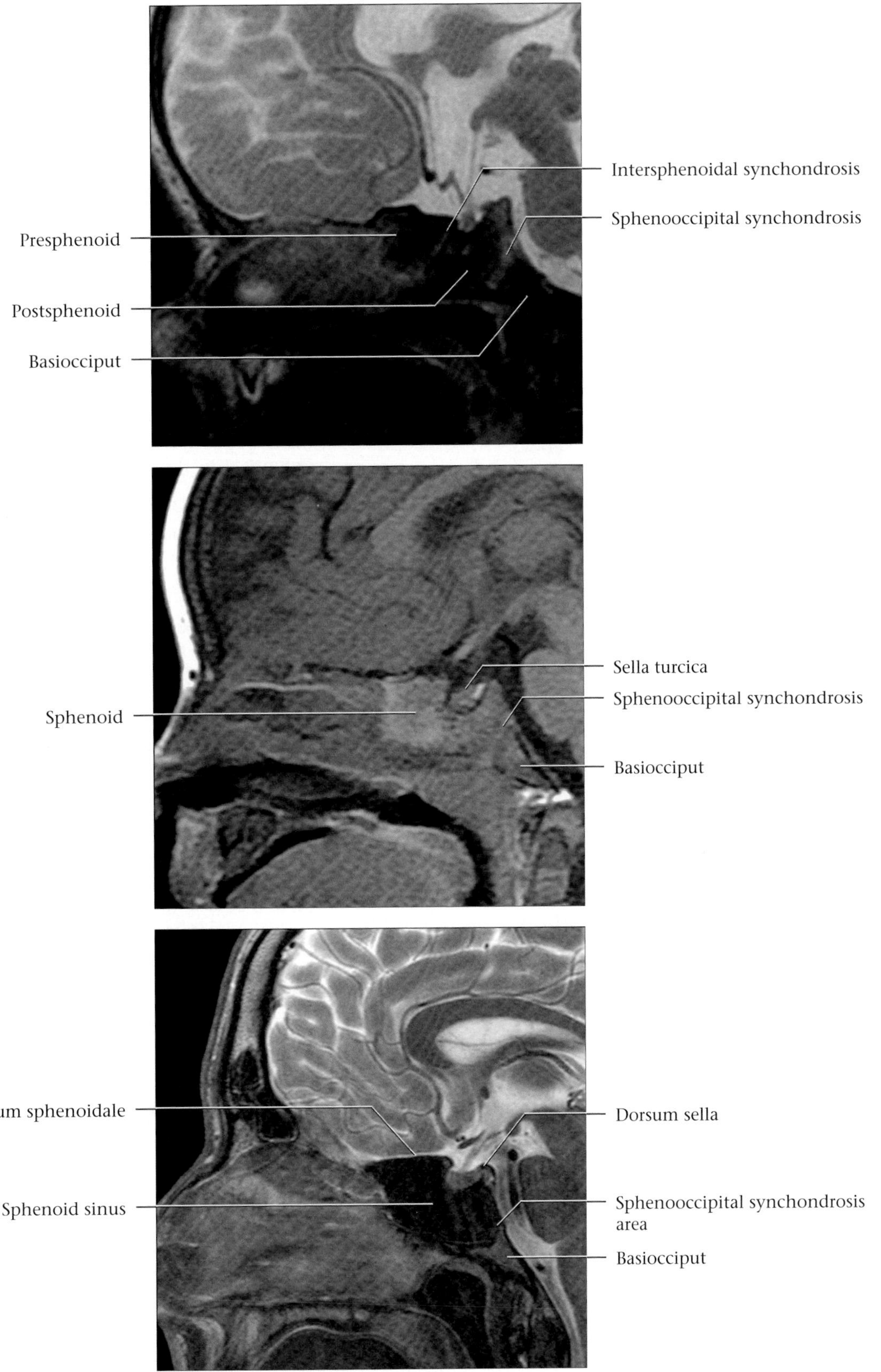
Intersphenoidal synchondrosis
Sphenooccipital synchondrosis
Presphenoid
Postsphenoid
Basiocciput
Sella turcica
Sphenooccipital synchondrosis
Sphenoid
Basiocciput
Planum sphenoidale
Dorsum sella
Sphenoid sinus
Sphenooccipital synchondrosis area
Basiocciput

(Top) Sagittal T2 MR of the CSB in a newborn shows the important synchondroses of this area. The intersphenoidal suture separates presphenoid from postsphenoid while the sphenooccipital synchondrosis separates postsphenoid from basiocciput. **(Middle)** Sagittal T1 MR of central skull base at 6 months. The intersphenoidal suture closes at about 3 months age resulting in formation of the sphenoid body from the presphenoid and postsphenoid. There is normal high signal fat within what used to be presphenoid. The sphenooccipital synchondrosis will remain open until adolescence. **(Bottom)** Sagittal T2 MR of central skull base in an adult. Typically, pneumatization extends throughout the entire sphenoid body up to the fused sphenooccipital synchondrosis. The sphenooccipital synchondrosis is one of last sutures of skull base to close. It fuses completely by about 16-18 years.

POSTERIOR SKULL BASE

Terminology

Abbreviations

- Posterior & central skull base (PSB, CSB)
- Temporal bone (TB)
- Jugular foramen (JF)

Definitions

- PSB: Skull base (SB) posterior to dorsum sella & petrous ridges

Imaging Anatomy

Overview

- PSB is made up of posterior temporal bones & occipital bone and transmits CN7-12, medulla oblongata & jugular vein
- Bones of PSB
  - Temporal bones posterior to petrous ridges
  - **Occipital bone** (3 parts)
    - **Basilar part** (basiocciput): Quadrilateral part anterior to foramen magnum
    - **Condylar part** (exoccipital): Occipital condyles here; lateral to foramen magnum
    - **Squamous part**: Large bony plate posterosuperior to foramen magnum
- Boundaries of PSB
  - Anterior boundary: Dorsum sella medially and petrous ridges laterally
  - Posterior boundary: Occipital bone
- Relationships of PSB
  - Inferior relationships: Posterior roof of pharyngeal mucosal space, carotid, parotid, retropharyngeal, perivertebral spaces & cervical spine
  - Superior relationships: Brainstem, cerebellum, CN7-8, CN9-12, transverse-sigmoid sinuses

Bony Landmarks of Posterior Skull Base

- **Petrous ridge of temporal bone**
  - Divides CSB from PSB
  - Attachment for fixed edge of tentorium cerebelli
- **Jugular tubercle**
  - Roof of hypoglossal canal seen well on coronal imaging
  - "Eagle's head" on coronal images is jugular tubercle

Foramina and Fissures of Posterior Skull Base

- **Internal acoustic meatus**
  - Transmits: CN7-8, labyrinthine artery
  - Opening in posterior wall TB superior to jugular foramen
  - Porus acusticus: Internal opening of internal acoustic meatus
- **Jugular foramen**
  - Two parts: Pars nervosa & pars vascularis partially divided by jugular spine
  - Between temporal & occipital bones
  - Carotid space extends directly up to JF
  - **Pars nervosa**
    - Transmits CN9, Jacobson nerve & inferior petrosal sinus
    - Anteromedial but contiguous with pars vascularis
  - **Pars vascularis**
    - Transmits CN10, Arnold nerve, CN11, jugular bulb & posterior meningeal artery
    - Larger than pars nervosa
- **Groove for sigmoid sinus**
  - Groove in medial mastoid temporal bone; cradles sigmoid sinus
- **Hypoglossal canal**
  - Transmits: CN12
  - Formed in condylar occipital bone
  - Inferomedial to jugular foramen
- **Foramen magnum**
  - Transmits: CN11 (cephalad component), vertebral arteries & medulla oblongata
  - Formed completely by occipital bone
- **Stylomastoid foramen**
  - Transmits: CN7
  - Found in exocranial skull base surface between mastoid tip & styloid process
  - Extends directly into parotid space

Development of Posterior Skull Base

- Occipital bone has 4 major ossification centers around foramen magnum
  - **Supraoccipital**, **basioccipital** & paired **exoccipital**
- PSB is nearly completely ossified by birth
- **Sutures of PSB** remain unfused until 2nd decade
  - Intraoccipital sutures fuses between 8 & 16 years
  - Petrooccipital & occipitomastoid sutures are among last to close (15-17 years)
- **Kerckring ossicle**
  - Small ovoid ossicle at posterior margin of FM
  - Unfused & separate in 50% of term newborns
  - Kerckring-supraoccipital suture fuses by 1 year

Variant Anatomy of Posterior Skull Base

- **Posterior condylar canal**
  - Inconstant canal for emissary vein & meningeal branch of ascending pharyngeal artery
  - One of largest emissary foramina of SB
- **Asymmetric petrous apices**
  - Can contain high signal fat or low signal air
- **Mastoid foramen**
  - Variably transmits emissary vein from sigmoid sinus
- **Persistent Kerckring ossicle**

Anatomy-Based Imaging Issues

Key Concepts or Questions

- PSB is largely ossified at birth but PSB sutures are last in SB to fuse
- PSB is intimately related to carotid & parotid spaces

Imaging Recommendations

- Bone CT with edge enhancement algorithm & wide windows (> 2000 HU)
- Use coronal imaging to examine normal "double eagles" of hypoglossal canal & jugular foramen area

Imaging Pitfalls

- Watch for asymmetric petrous apex air and/or fat
- Beware of jugular foramen pseudolesion from MR flow phenomenon
- Beware open synchondroses/suture as pseudofracture

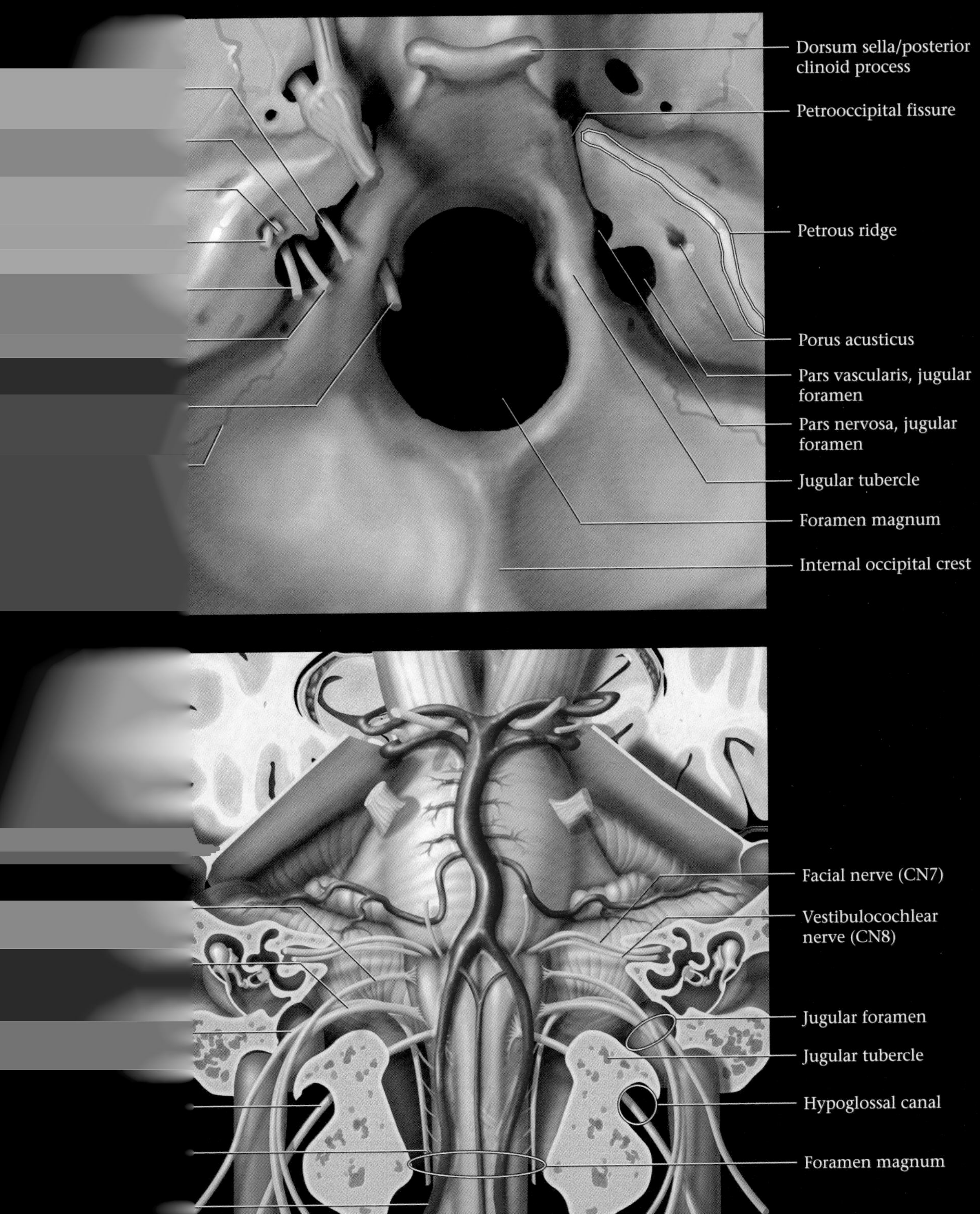
Dorsum sella/posterior clinoid process
Petrooccipital fissure
Petrous ridge
Porus acusticus
Pars vascularis, jugular foramen
Pars nervosa, jugular foramen
Jugular tubercle
Foramen magnum
Internal occipital crest
Facial nerve (CN7)
Vestibulocochlear nerve (CN8)
Jugular foramen
Jugular tubercle
Hypoglossal canal
Foramen magnum

r skull base as seen from above. Neural structures are shown on the left, bony landmarks on ary of posterior skull base is clivus medially and petrous ridge laterally. The major foramina , porus acusticus, jugular foramen and hypoglossal canal. Notice that the jugular foramen the petrooccipital fissure. **(Bottom)** Coronal graphic of posterior skull base viewed from the ouble eagle" appearance in the area of the hypoglossal canal. The jugular tubercle (eagle's e inferomedial hypoglossal canal from the jugular foramen. The hypoglossal nerve is found while CN9-11 traverse the skull base in the jugular foramen.

GRAPHIC & MR OF DURAL SINUSES

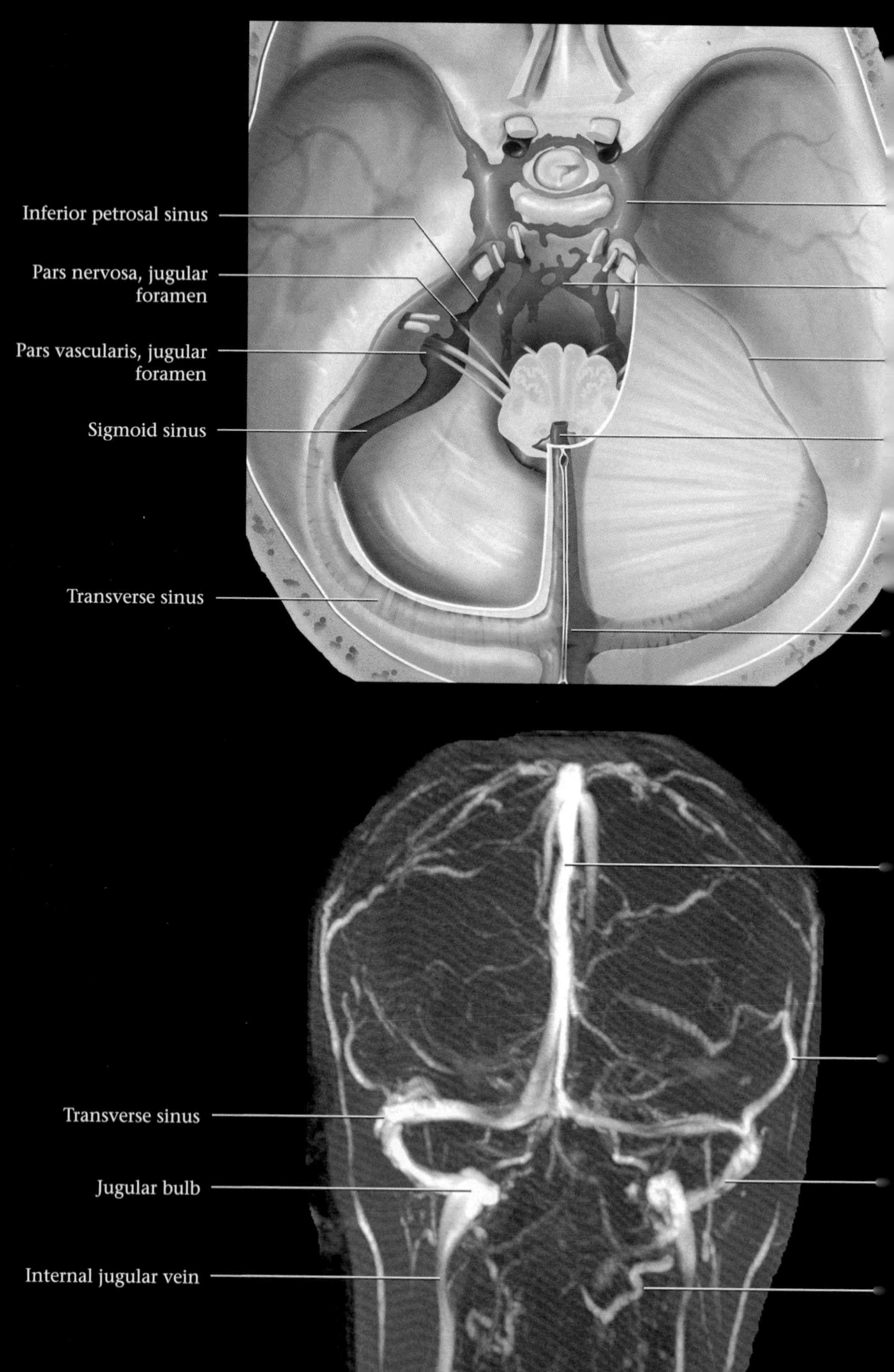

Inferior petrosal sinus
Pars nervosa, jugular foramen
Pars vascularis, jugular foramen
Sigmoid sinus
Transverse sinus
Transverse sinus
Jugular bulb
Internal jugular vein

(Top) Graphic of major dural venous sinuses and jugular foramen as seen from top down. T well as the left half of the tentorium cerebelli have been removed. Notice the transverse sin occipital bone while the sigmoid sinus is in the medial wall of the temporal bone. The two foramen are also visible. The anterior pars nervosa receives the glossopharyngeal nerve (CN has the vagus (CN10) & accessory (CN11) nerves passing through it. **(Bottom)** Coronal view venogram shows the transverse sinuses feeding through the sigmoid sinuses into the jugula bulb connects inferiorly with the internal jugular vein of the carotid space. The slight asym

AXIAL BONE CT

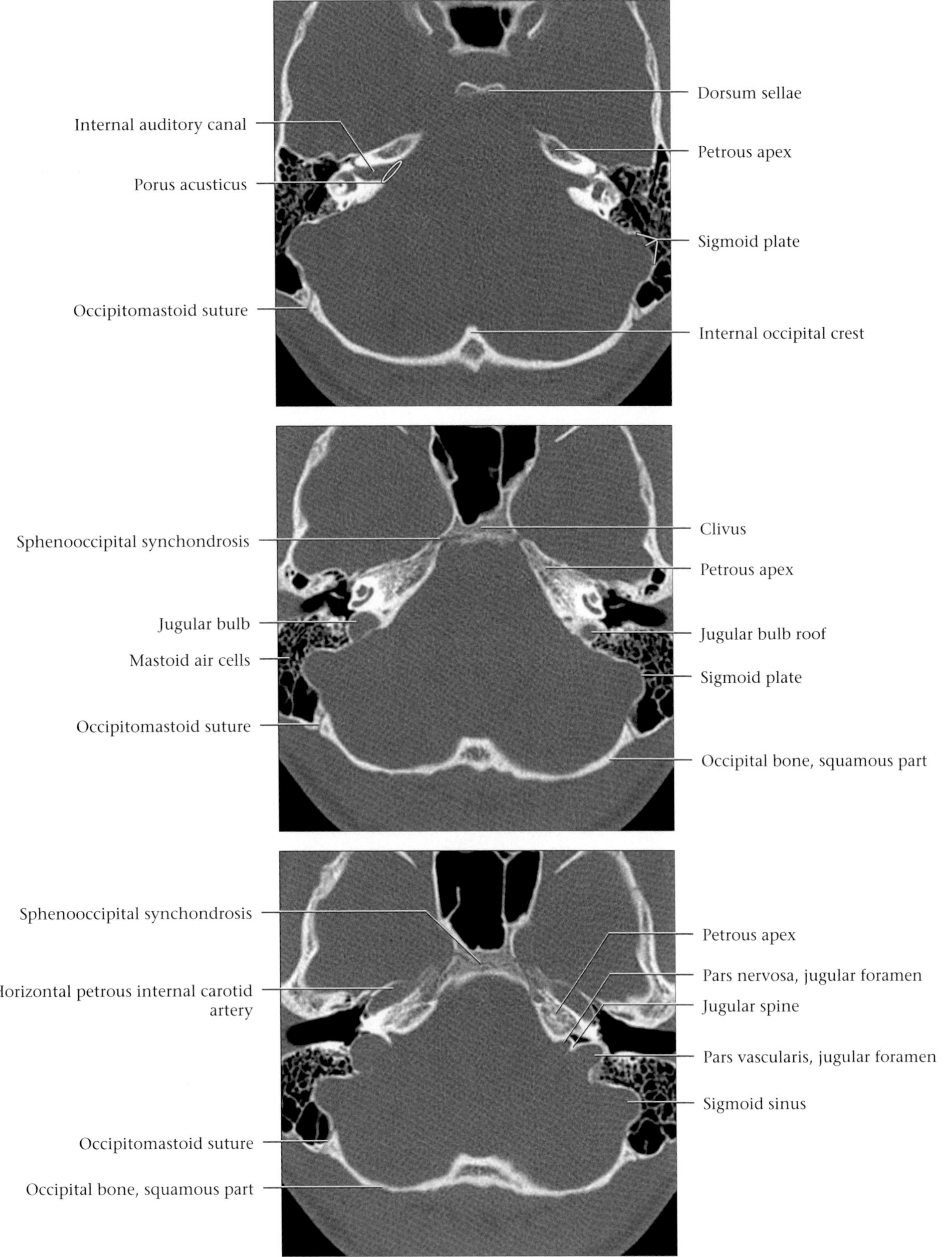
Dorsum sellae
Internal auditory canal
Petrous apex
Porus acusticus
Sigmoid plate
Occipitomastoid suture
Internal occipital crest
Clivus
Sphenooccipital synchondrosis
Petrous apex
Jugular bulb
Jugular bulb roof
Mastoid air cells
Sigmoid plate
Occipitomastoid suture
Occipital bone, squamous part
Sphenooccipital synchondrosis
Petrous apex
Pars nervosa, jugular foramen
Horizontal petrous internal carotid artery
Jugular spine
Pars vascularis, jugular foramen
Sigmoid sinus
Occipitomastoid suture
Occipital bone, squamous part

(Top) First of a nine axial bone CT images presented from superior to inferior shows the dorsum sella and the petrous temporal bone as the anterior margin of the posterior skull base. Posteriorly the midline is demarcated by the bony internal occipital crest which provides attachment for the falx cerebelli. Porus acusticus is the most superior foramen of posterior skull base and transmits CN7 and 8. **(Middle)** At the level of mid-cochlea the posterior cranial fossa is completely divided from middle cranial fossa by the clivus and petrous temporal bone. Laterally, the sigmoid plate separates the mastoid air cells from the sigmoid sinus. The jugular bulbs are visible bilaterally. **(Bottom)** At level of mid-jugular foramen note smaller anteromedial pars nervosa (CN9, Jacobsen nerve, inferior petrosal sinus) & larger pars vascularis (jugular bulb, Arnold nerve, CN10 and 11).

AXIAL BONE CT

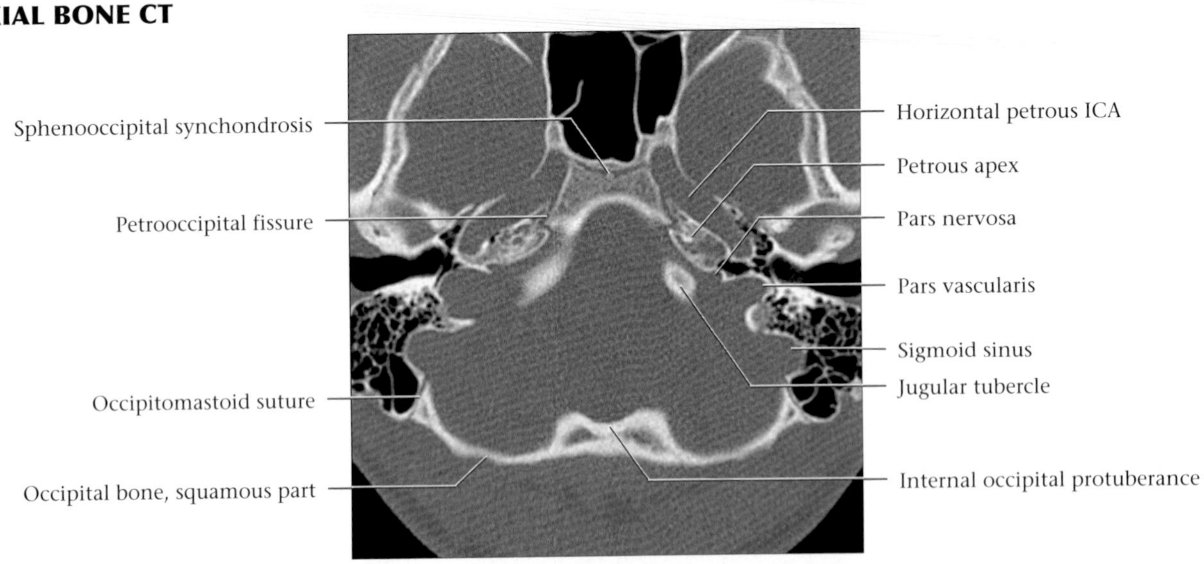

Sphenooccipital synchondrosis

Petrooccipital fissure

Occipitomastoid suture

Occipital bone, squamous part

Horizontal petrous ICA

Petrous apex

Pars nervosa

Pars vascularis

Sigmoid sinus

Jugular tubercle

Internal occipital protuberance

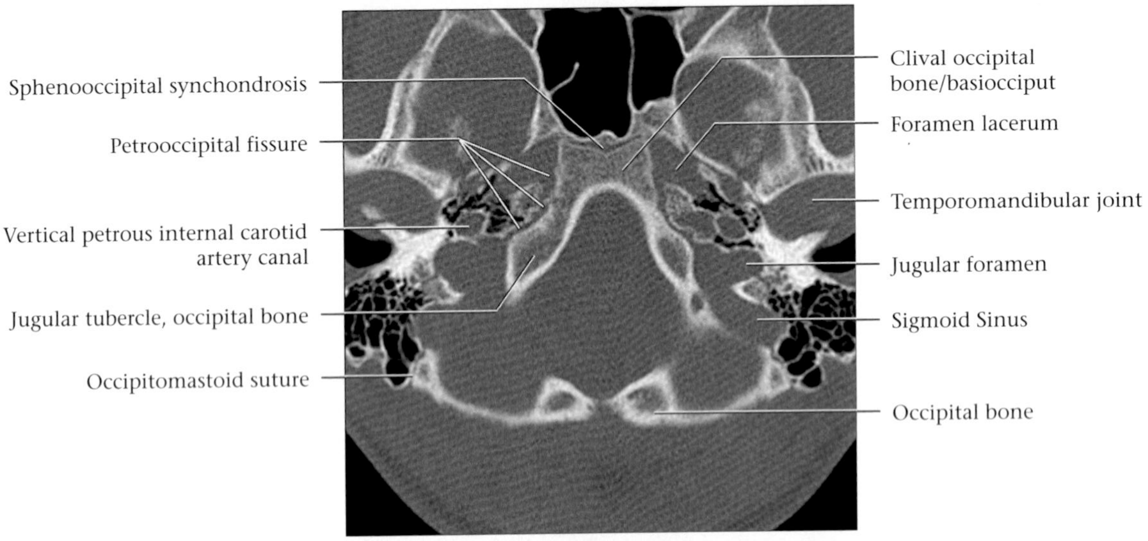

Sphenooccipital synchondrosis

Petrooccipital fissure

Vertical petrous internal carotid artery canal

Jugular tubercle, occipital bone

Occipitomastoid suture

Clival occipital bone/basiocciput

Foramen lacerum

Temporomandibular joint

Jugular foramen

Sigmoid Sinus

Occipital bone

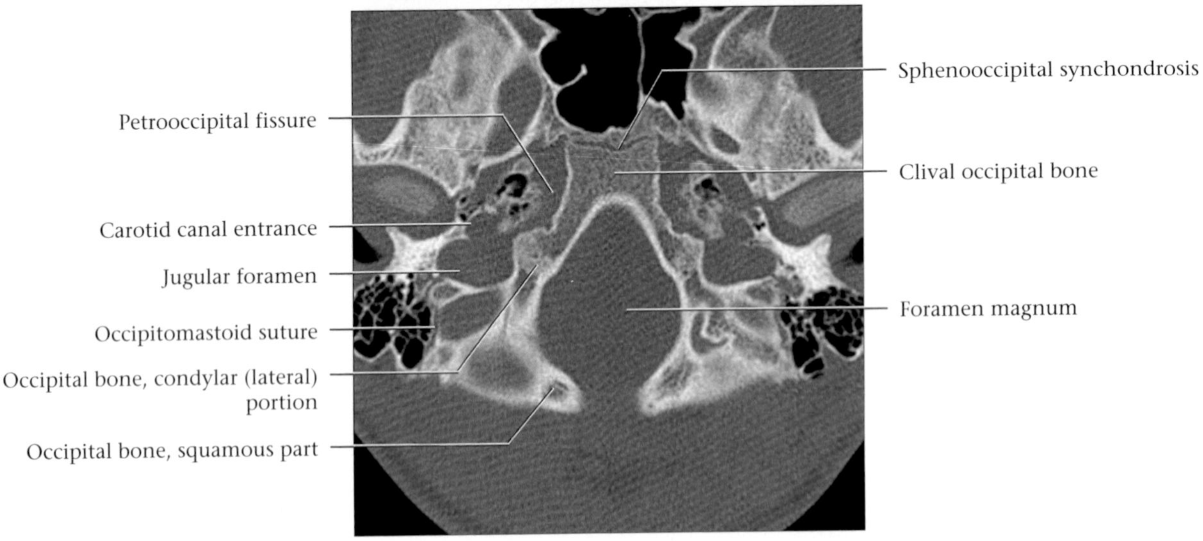

Petrooccipital fissure

Carotid canal entrance

Jugular foramen

Occipitomastoid suture

Occipital bone, condylar (lateral) portion

Occipital bone, squamous part

Sphenooccipital synchondrosis

Clival occipital bone

Foramen magnum

(Top) Image of posterior skull base shows the sphenooccipital synchondrosis, the petrooccipital fissure and the occipitomastoid suture all in the same plane. The sphenooccipital synchondrosis has not yet fused in this young adolescent. **(Middle)** Image through the jugular tubercle the clivus is made up almost completely of anterior occipital bone. The upper third of the clivus is above the sphenooccipital synchondrosis and is therefore part of the sphenoid bone. **(Bottom)** In this image the lower clivus (below the sphenooccipital synchondrosis) is clearly made up of occipital bone. The petrooccipital fissure separates the temporal bone from the occipital bone. The occipitomastoid suture separates the mastoid sinus from the squamosal portion of the occipital bone.

AXIAL BONE CT

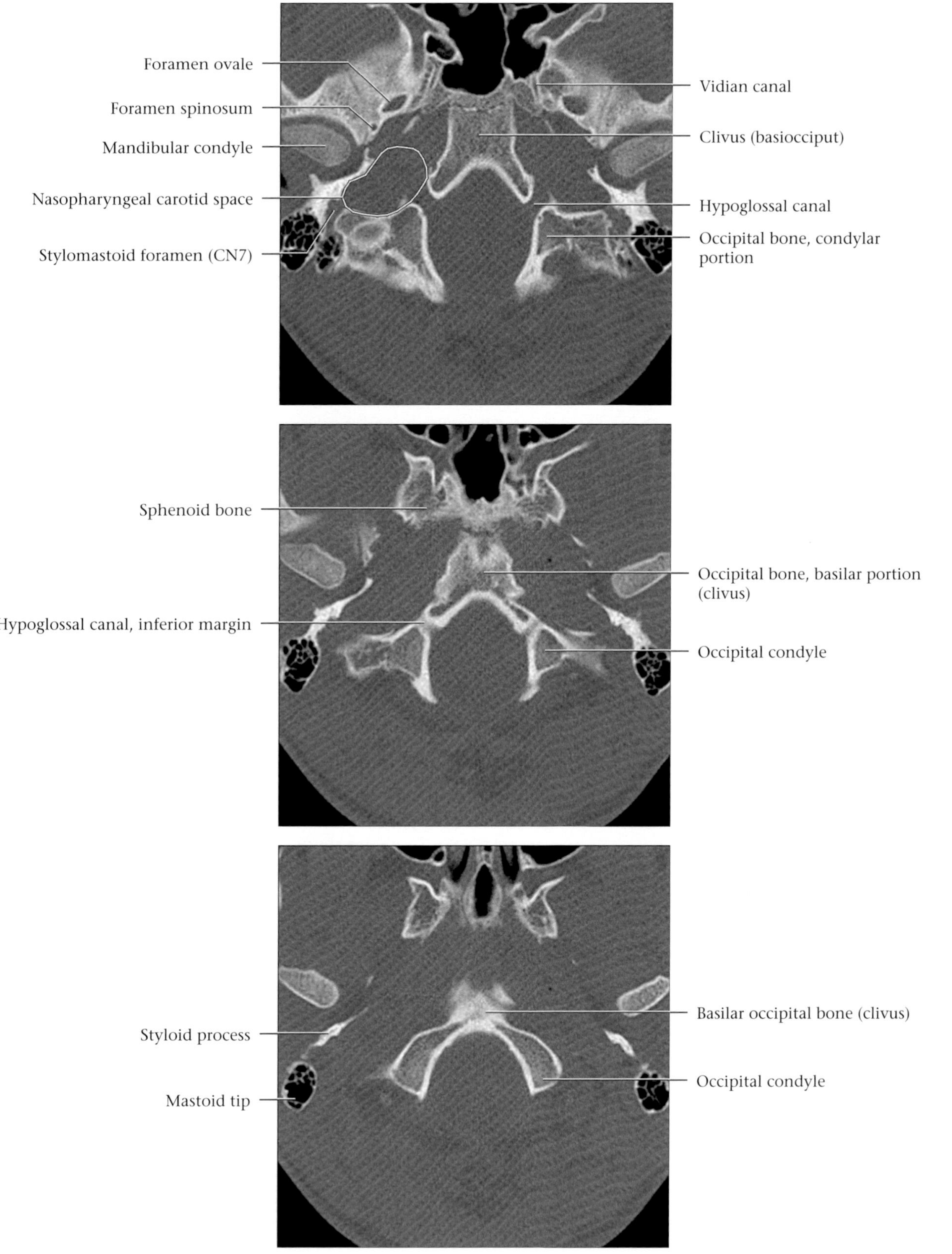
Foramen ovale
Foramen spinosum
Mandibular condyle
Nasopharyngeal carotid space
Stylomastoid foramen (CN7)
Vidian canal
Clivus (basiocciput)
Hypoglossal canal
Occipital bone, condylar portion
Sphenoid bone
Hypoglossal canal, inferior margin
Occipital bone, basilar portion (clivus)
Occipital condyle
Styloid process
Mastoid tip
Basilar occipital bone (clivus)
Occipital condyle

(Top) This image passes directly through the hypoglossal canal and stylomastoid foramen. This canal transmits only the hypoglossal nerve. Notice that as soon as the nerve exits the hypoglossal canal it immediately enters the nasopharyngeal carotid space to join the glossopharyngeal (CN9), vagus (CN10) and accessory (CN11) cranial nerves. **(Middle)** In this image the inferior margin of the hypoglossal canal runs within occipital bone, between the basilar (clival) and condylar portions. The inferior surface of the condylar occipital bone are the occipital condyles. **(Bottom)** In this image through the occipital condyle the inferior-most junction of the basilar (clival) occipital bone & the condylar occipital bone is visible. The occipital condyles rest the cranium upon the lateral masses of atlas (C1 vertebral body).

POSTERIOR SKULL BASE

CORONAL BONE CT

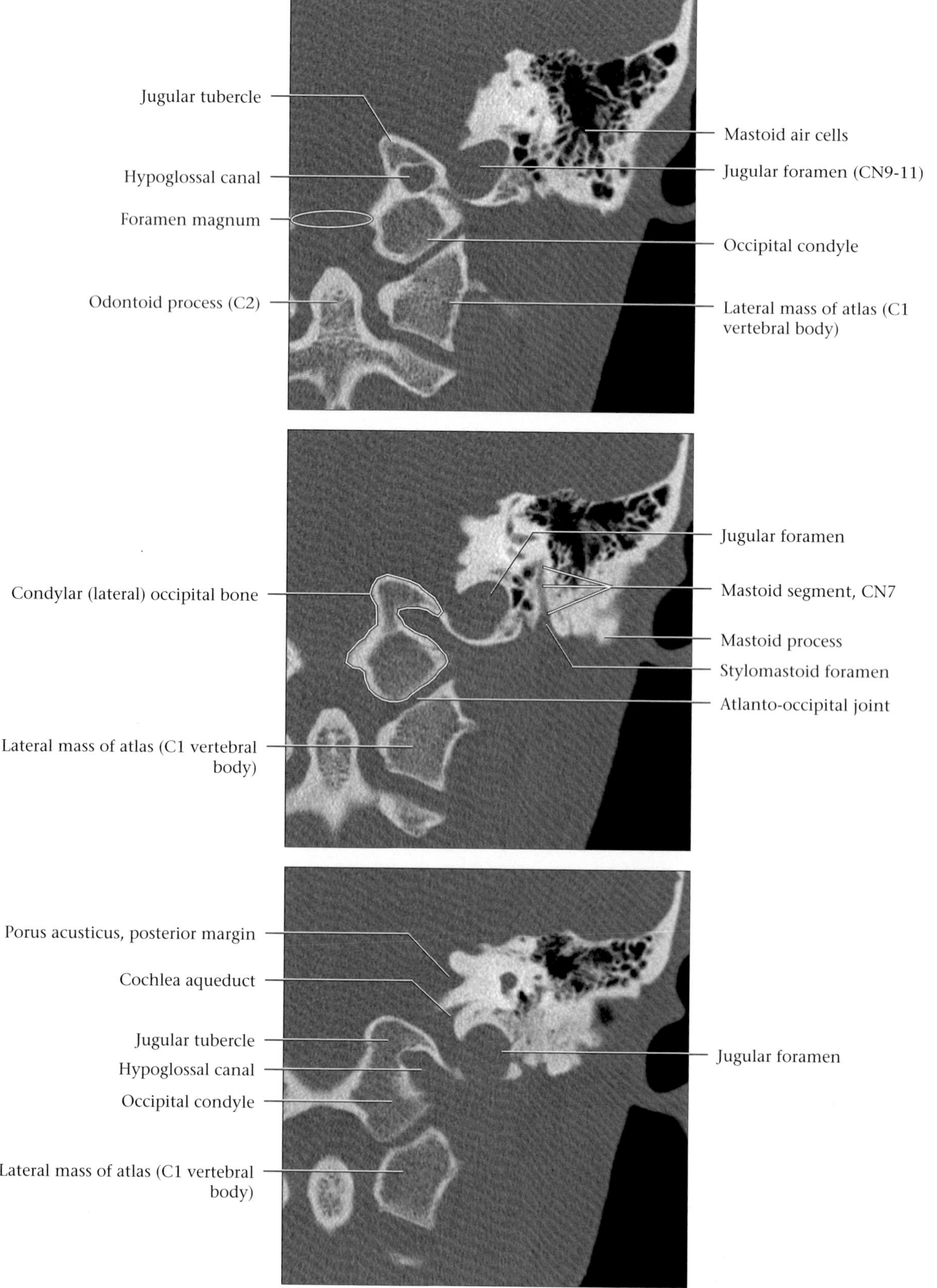
Jugular tubercle
Hypoglossal canal
Foramen magnum
Odontoid process (C2)
Mastoid air cells
Jugular foramen (CN9-11)
Occipital condyle
Lateral mass of atlas (C1 vertebral body)
Condylar (lateral) occipital bone
Lateral mass of atlas (C1 vertebral body)
Jugular foramen
Mastoid segment, CN7
Mastoid process
Stylomastoid foramen
Atlanto-occipital joint
Porus acusticus, posterior margin
Cochlea aqueduct
Jugular tubercle
Hypoglossal canal
Occipital condyle
Lateral mass of atlas (C1 vertebral body)
Jugular foramen

(Top) First of six coronal bone CT images of left posterior skull base presented from posterior to anterior. The hypoglossal canal passes through the condylar (lateral) portion of the occipital bone. In the coronal plane with both sides visible this area has been referred to as the "double eagle". Notice that the eagle's head & beak are the jugular tubercle. **(Middle)** In this image through the mastoid (descending) portion of intratemporal facial nerve canal the condylar part of the occipital bone is outlined. **(Bottom)** This image shows the classic "eagle" of posterior skull base with the "beak" of jugular tubercle separating the jugular foramen from the hypoglossal canal. Lesions of the hypoglossal canal affect the undersurface of the beak while lesions of the jugular foramen affect the external surface of the beak.

CORONAL BONE CT

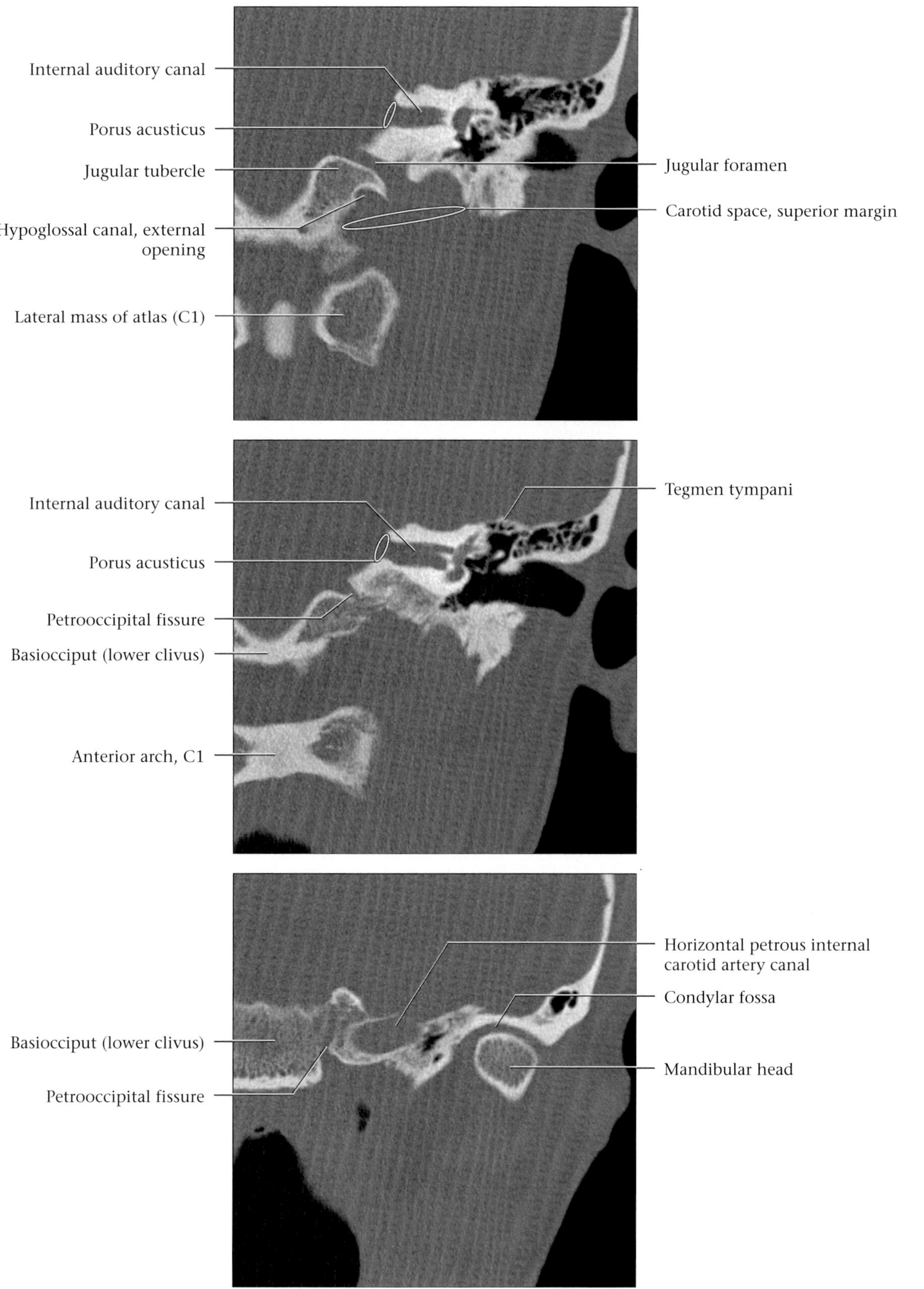
Internal auditory canal
Porus acusticus
Jugular tubercle
Hypoglossal canal, external opening
Lateral mass of atlas (C1)
Jugular foramen
Carotid space, superior margin
Internal auditory canal
Porus acusticus
Petrooccipital fissure
Basiocciput (lower clivus)
Anterior arch, C1
Tegmen tympani
Horizontal petrous internal carotid artery canal
Condylar fossa
Mandibular head
Basiocciput (lower clivus)
Petrooccipital fissure

(Top) In this image of left skull base and temporal bone notice both the hypoglossal canal and the jugular foramen "empty" into the cephalad carotid space. The upper carotid space therefore contains CN9-12 as well as the internal jugular vein. **(Middle)** In this image through the mid-internal auditory canal the petrooccipital fissure is visible separating the basioccipital portion of the occipital bone from the temporal bone. **(Bottom)** In this image through the condylar fossa of the temporomandibular joint the petrooccipital fissure is seen between the basiocciput and the temporal bone. The basiocciput is a large quadrilateral portion of the occipital bone that extends anterosuperiorly from the anterior margin of the foramen magnum to reach the sphenoid bone approximately 2/3 of the way up the clivus.

AXIAL T1 C+ MR

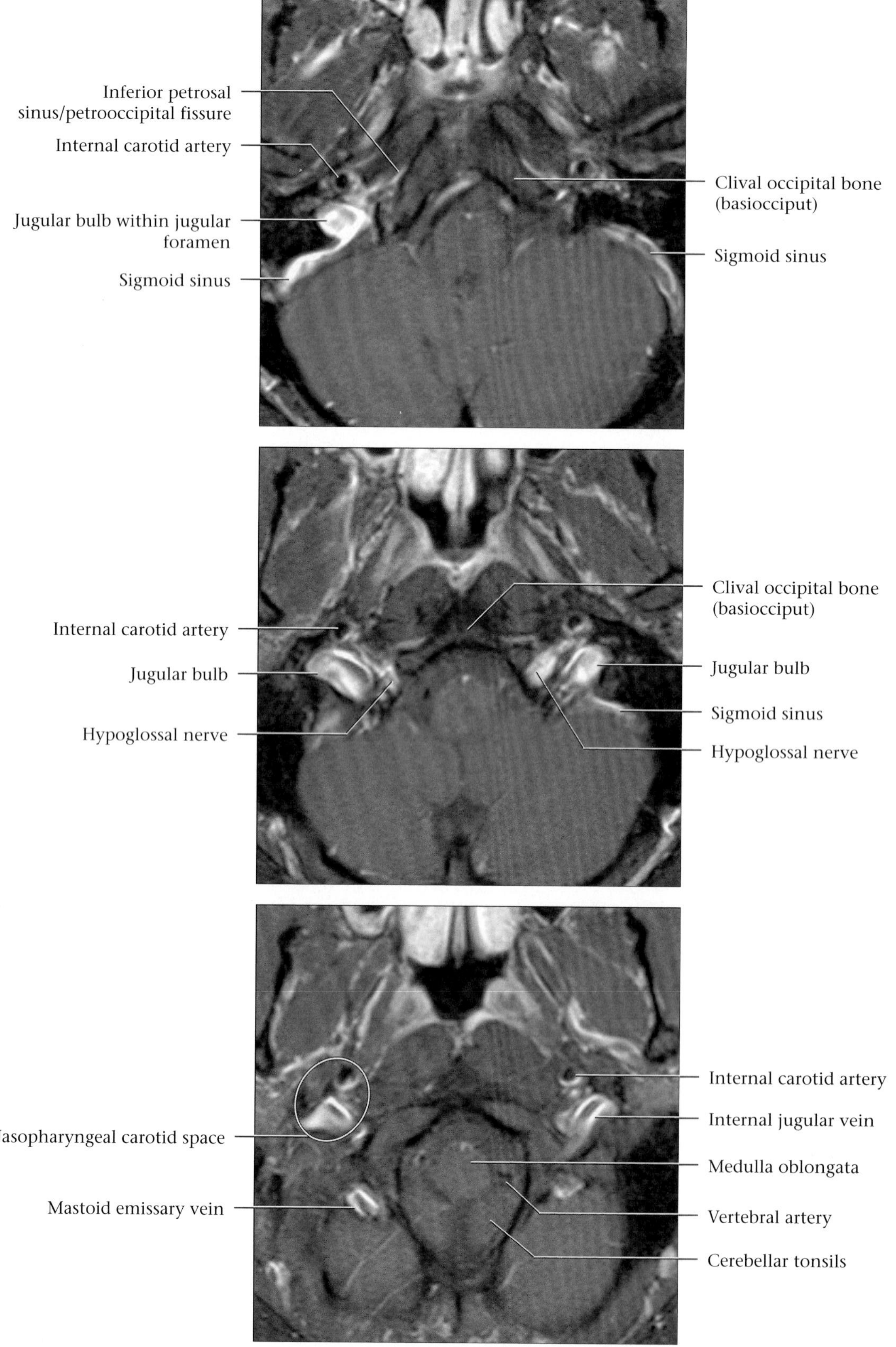

Inferior petrosal sinus/petrooccipital fissure
Internal carotid artery
Jugular bulb within jugular foramen
Sigmoid sinus
Clival occipital bone (basiocciput)
Sigmoid sinus
Clival occipital bone (basiocciput)
Internal carotid artery
Jugular bulb
Hypoglossal nerve
Jugular bulb
Sigmoid sinus
Hypoglossal nerve
Internal carotid artery
Internal jugular vein
Nasopharyngeal carotid space
Medulla oblongata
Mastoid emissary vein
Vertebral artery
Cerebellar tonsils

(Top) First of three axial fat-saturated T1 C+ MR images of the posterior skull base presented from superior to inferior. On the patient's right the high signal enhancing sigmoid sinus can be seen connecting anteromedially with the jugular bulb. **(Middle)** At the level of the hypoglossal canals the hypoglossal nerves can be seen as linear low intensity structures surrounded by the enhancing high signal basiocciput venous plexus. The complex signal seen in both jugular bulbs should not be mistaken for a lesion. **(Bottom)** At the level of the foramen magnum the internal jugular vein and internal carotid artery of the carotid space are visible. The vertebral arteries, medulla oblongata and inferior cerebellar tonsils are normally seen at this level.

CORONAL T1 C+ MR

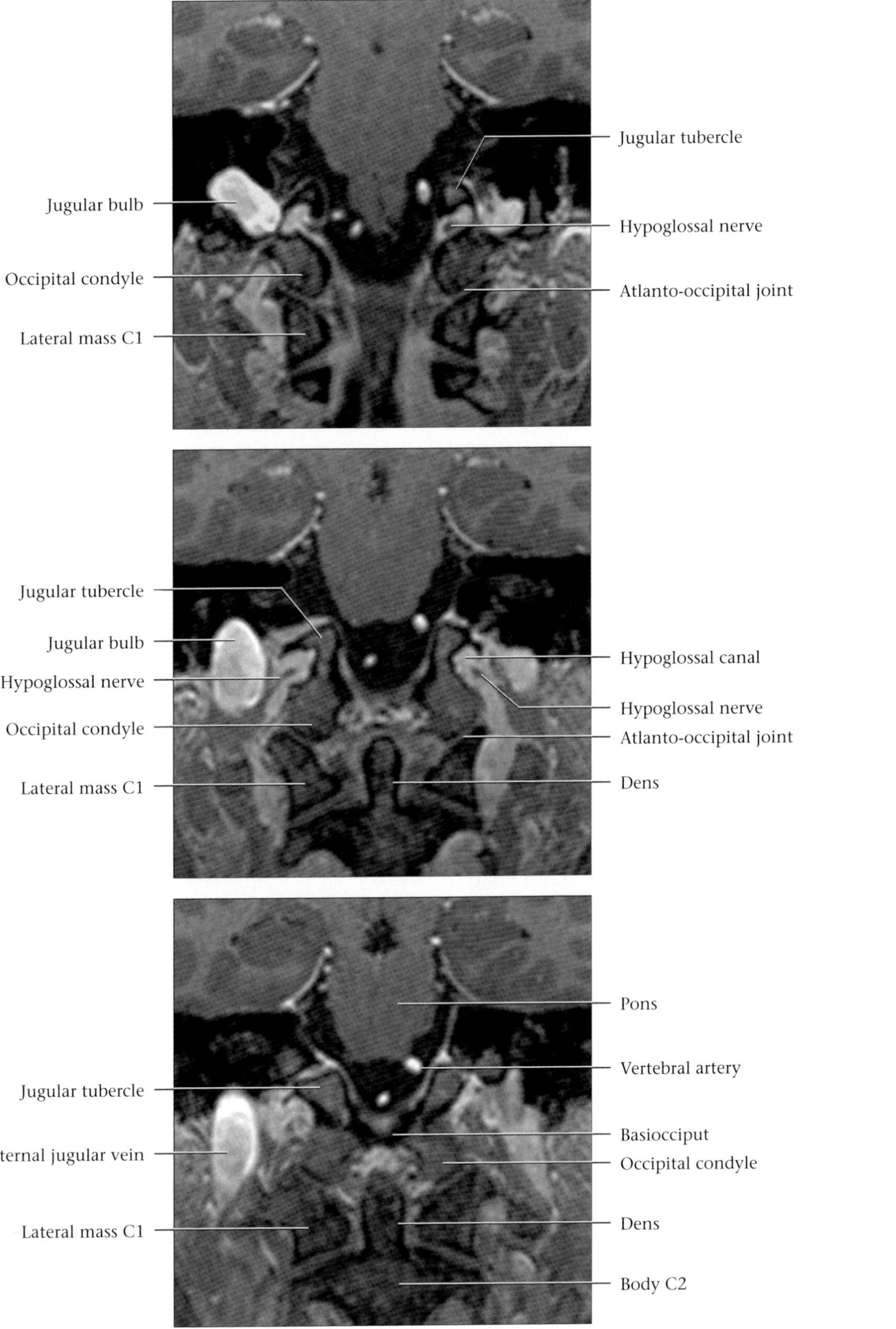
Jugular tubercle
Jugular bulb
Hypoglossal nerve
Occipital condyle
Atlanto-occipital joint
Lateral mass C1
Jugular tubercle
Jugular bulb
Hypoglossal canal
Hypoglossal nerve
Hypoglossal nerve
Occipital condyle
Atlanto-occipital joint
Lateral mass C1
Dens
Pons
Vertebral artery
Jugular tubercle
Basiocciput
Internal jugular vein
Occipital condyle
Dens
Lateral mass C1
Body C2

(Top) First of three coronal T1 C+ MR images of the posterior skull base presented from posterior to anterior shows the jugular bulb within the jugular foramen. The low signal hypoglossal nerve is seen just below the "eagle's head" in the hypoglossal canal. The high signal perineural basiocciput venous plexus is visible surrounding the hypoglossal nerve. **(Middle)** In this image the classic "double eagle heads" are visible (jugular tubercles) with the hypoglossal nerve seen exiting the inferior hypoglossal canal. **(Bottom)** In this image the anterior jugular tubercle can be seen meeting the inferior basiocciput. The jugular bulb has connected inferiorly with the internal jugular vein. The internal jugular vein is within the nasopharyngeal carotid space.

TEMPORAL BONE

Terminology

Abbreviations

- Temporal bone (T-bone)

Definitions

- T-bone: Paired bones located in posterolateral floor of middle & posterior cranial fossae made up of petrous pyramid & mastoid complex

Imaging Anatomy

Overview

- 5 bony parts to T-bone
  - Squamous: Forms lateral wall of middle cranial fossa
  - Mastoid: Aerated posterolateral T-bone
  - Petrous: Pyramidal shape medial T-bone containing inner ear, internal auditory canal & petrous apex
  - Tympanic: U-shaped bone forming bony EAC
  - Styloid: Forms styloid process after birth
- Major components of temporal bone
  - External auditory canal (EAC)
  - Middle ear-mastoid (ME-M)
  - Inner ear (IE)
  - Petrous apex (PA)
  - Internal auditory canal (IAC)
  - Facial nerve (CN7)
  - Petrous internal carotid artery (ICA)

Internal Structures-Critical Contents

- EAC: Tympanic bone medially, fibrocartilage laterally
  - Medial border is tympanic membrane
  - Nodal drainage to parotid chain
- Middle ear-mastoid
  - **Epitympanum** (attic): Middle ear above line from scutal tip to tympanic CN7
    - **Tegmen tympani**: Roof of middle ear cavity
    - **Prussak space** = lateral epitympanic recess
  - **Mesotympanum**: Middle ear proper
    - Posterior wall: 3 key structures = facial nerve recess, pyramidal eminence, sinus tympani
    - Medial wall: Lateral semicircular canal, tympanic segment CN7, oval & round window
  - **Hypotympanum**: Shallow trough in floor of ME
  - Mastoid sinus: 3 key structures
    - **Aditus ad antrum**: Connects epitympanum to mastoid antrum
    - **Mastoid antrum**: Large, central mastoid air cell
    - **Koerner septum**: Part of petrosquamosal suture running posterolaterally through mastoid air cells
- Inner ear components
  - **Bony labyrinth**: Bone confining cochlear, vestibule & semicircular canals
  - **Perilymphatic spaces**
    - Perilymphatic spaces include area in vestibule surrounding utricle & saccule, semicircular canals around semicircular ducts, within scala tympani & vestibuli of cochlea
    - **Perilymph** = fluid within bony labyrinth that "bathes" endolymph-containing membranous labyrinth structures
  - **Membranous labyrinth**
    - Includes vestibule (utricle & saccule), semicircular ducts, scala media of cochlea, endolymphatic duct & sac
    - Endolymph = fluid within structures of membranous labyrinth
  - **Cochlea**: ~ 2 1/2 turns; modiolus; 3 spiral chambers (scala tympani, scala vestibuli & scala media)
  - **Semicircular canals** (SCC), superior (S), lateral (L) & posterior (P)
    - SSCC: Projects cephalad; bony ridge over SSCC in roof of petrous pyramid called **arcuate eminence**
    - LSCC: Projects into middle ear with tympanic CN7 on under side
    - PSCC: Projects posteriorly parallel to petrous ridge
- Petrous apex: Anteromedial to inner ear
  - CN6 passes over superior margin of medial PA
- Intratemporal facial nerve
  - CN7 segments: IAC, labyrinthine, tympanic, mastoid segments
  - **Geniculate ganglion** = anterior genu
  - Posterior genu: Tympanic segment bends inferiorly to become mastoid segment
  - **Stylomastoid foramen**: CN7 exits skull base here
- Petrous internal carotid artery (ICA): C2 segment
  - ICA: Vertical & horizontal T-bone segments
  - Vertical segment: Rises to genu beneath cochlea
  - Horizontal segment: Projects anteromedially to turn cephalad as cavernous ICA
- Muscles of T-bone
  - **Tensor tympani muscle**
    - Dampens sound; hyperacusis if injured
    - Innervation: V3 branch
    - Location: Anteromedial wall, mesotympanum
    - Attachment: Tendon inserts on malleus
  - **Stapedius muscle**
    - Dampens sound; hyperacusis if injured
    - Innervation: CN7
    - Location: Muscle belly in pyramidal eminence
    - Attachment: Tendon attaches on head of stapes

Anatomy-Based Imaging Issues

Key Concepts or Questions

- Assign lesion to one of following T-bone areas: EAC, ME-M, IE, PA or intratemporal CN7
  - Construct location-specific differential diagnosis
  - Match imaging findings to differential diagnosis list

Embryology

Embryologic Events

- EAC forms from 1st branchial groove
- Tympanic cavity forms from 1st branchial pouch
- Ossicles form from 1st & 2nd branchial arch
- Endolymphatic system forms from otocyst
- Perilymphatic space & otic capsule forms from surrounding mesenchyme

Practical Implications

- In EAC atresia, IE spared as it forms from otocyst migration independent of EAC-ME formation

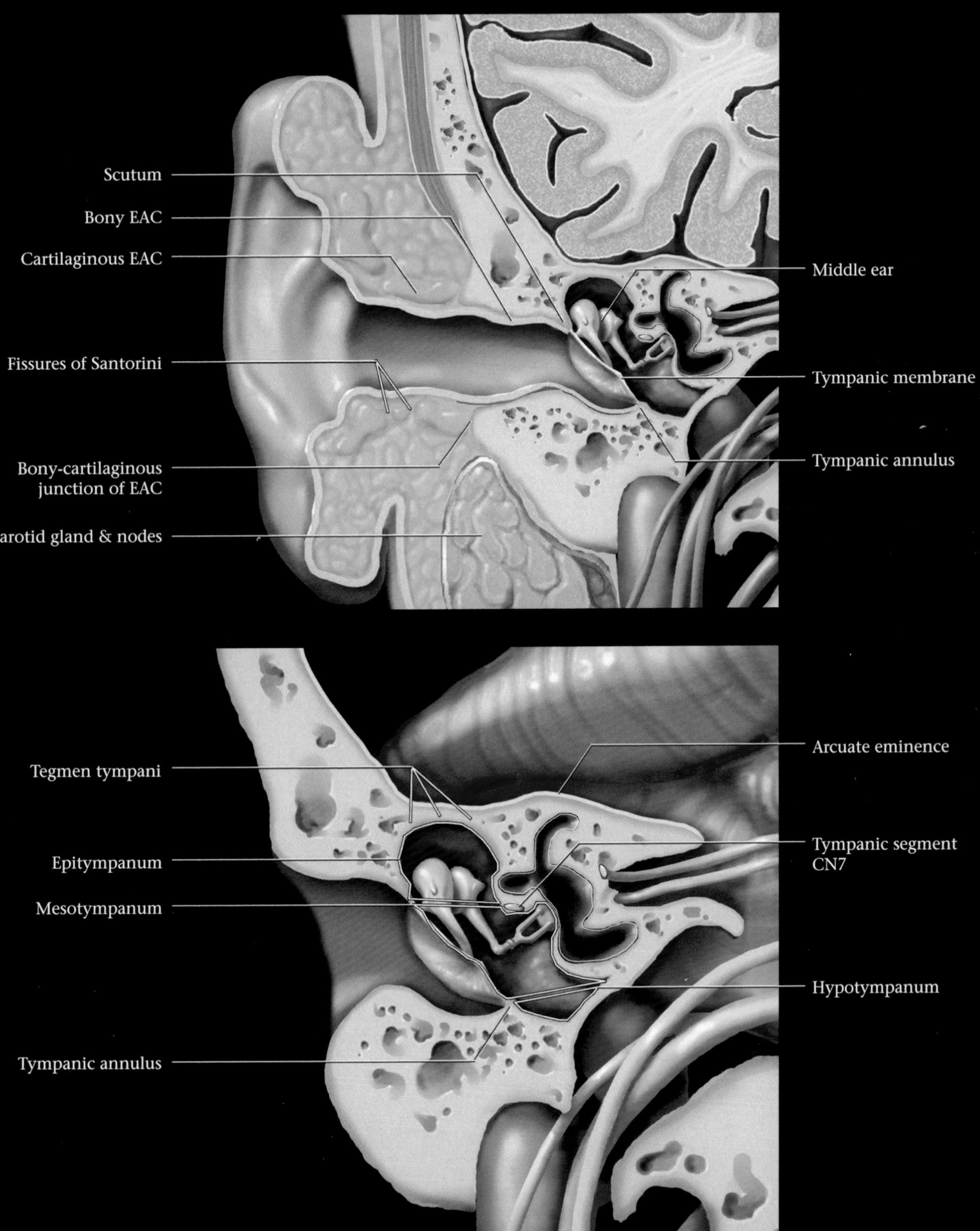
Scutum
Bony EAC
Cartilaginous EAC
Fissures of Santorini
Bony-cartilaginous junction of EAC
Parotid gland & nodes
Middle ear
Tympanic membrane
Tympanic annulus
Tegmen tympani
Epitympanum
Mesotympanum
Tympanic annulus
Arcuate eminence
Tympanic segment CN7
Hypotympanum

(Top) Coronal graphic of external & middle ear. The external auditory canal is made up of lateral cartilaginous and medial bony components. Infection of the EAC can penetrate inferomedially to the skull base and associated spaces via the fissures of Santorini (gaps in the EAC cartilage). External ear including EAC lymphatic drainage is to the parotid nodal chain. The medial margin of the EAC is the tympanic membrane which attaches to the scutum & tympanic annulus. **(Bottom)** Coronal magnified graphic of the middle ear. The middle ear is divided into 3 pieces, epitympanum, mesotympanum & hypotympanum. The epitympanum is defined as the middle ear cavity above a line drawn from the scutal tip & tympanic segment of CN7. Its roof is called the tegmen tympani. Mesotympanum extends from this line inferiorly to a line connecting tympanic annulus to base of cochlear promontory.

TEMPORAL BONE

GRAPHICS

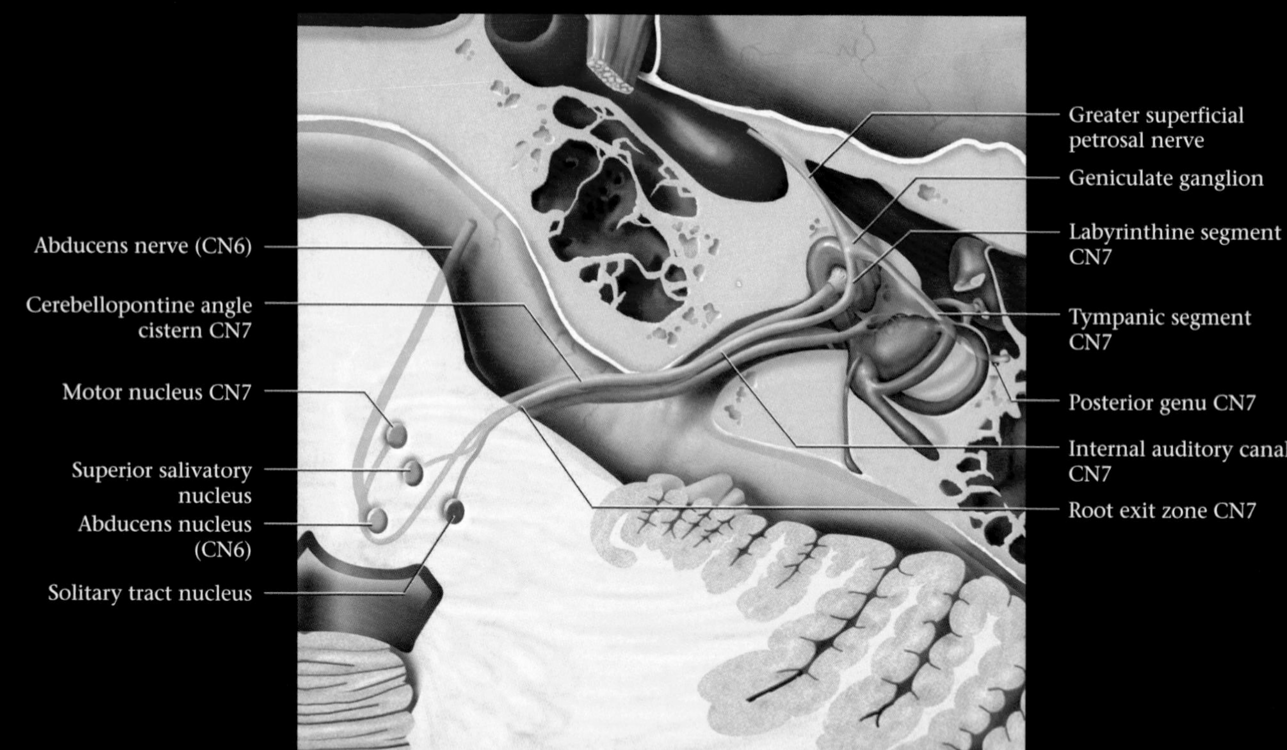
Abducens nerve (CN6)
Cerebellopontine angle cistern CN7
Motor nucleus CN7
Superior salivatory nucleus
Abducens nucleus (CN6)
Solitary tract nucleus
Greater superficial petrosal nerve
Geniculate ganglion
Labyrinthine segment CN7
Tympanic segment CN7
Posterior genu CN7
Internal auditory canal CN7
Root exit zone CN7

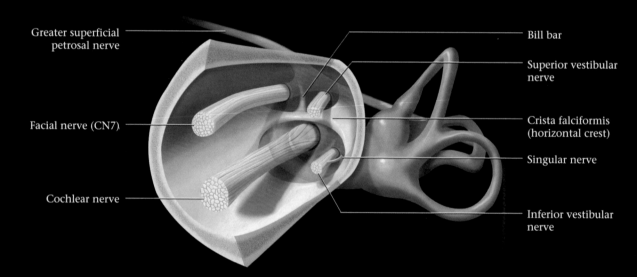

Greater superficial petrosal nerve
Facial nerve (CN7)
Cochlear nerve
Bill bar
Superior vestibular nerve
Crista falciformis (horizontal crest)
Singular nerve
Inferior vestibular nerve

(Top) Axial graphic of facial nerve from brainstem nuclei to posterior genu of temporal bone. The motor nucleus sends out its fibers to circle CN6 nucleus before reaching the root exit zone at pontomedullary junction. Superior salivatory nucleus sends parasympathetic secretomotor fibers to lacrimal, submandibular & sublingual glands. Solitary tract nucleus receives anterior 2/3 tongue taste information. **(Bottom)** Graphic depicting cranial nerve relationships in fundus of internal auditory canal. Notice the crista falciformis separates cochlear nerve & inferior vestibular nerve below from CN7 & superior vestibular nerve above. Also note Bill bar separating CN7 from the superior vestibular nerve. Bill bar is not visible on CT or MR imaging.

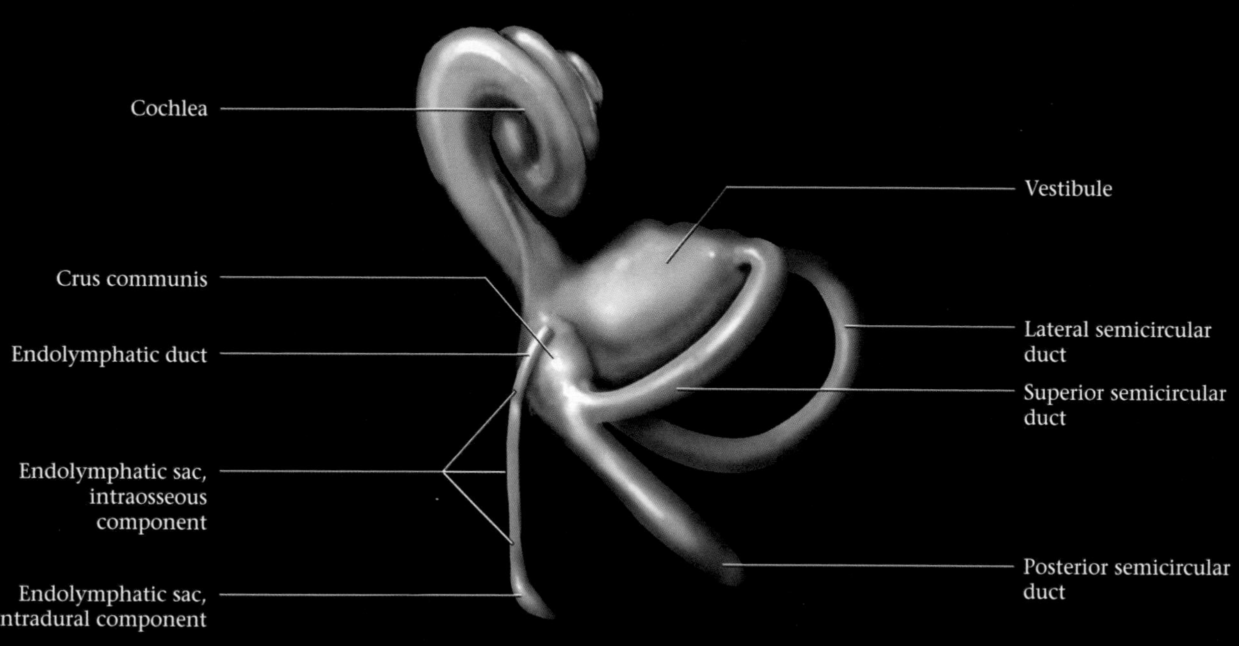
Cochlea
Crus communis
Endolymphatic duct
Endolymphatic sac, intraosseous component
Endolymphatic sac, intradural component
Vestibule
Lateral semicircular duct
Superior semicircular duct
Posterior semicircular duct

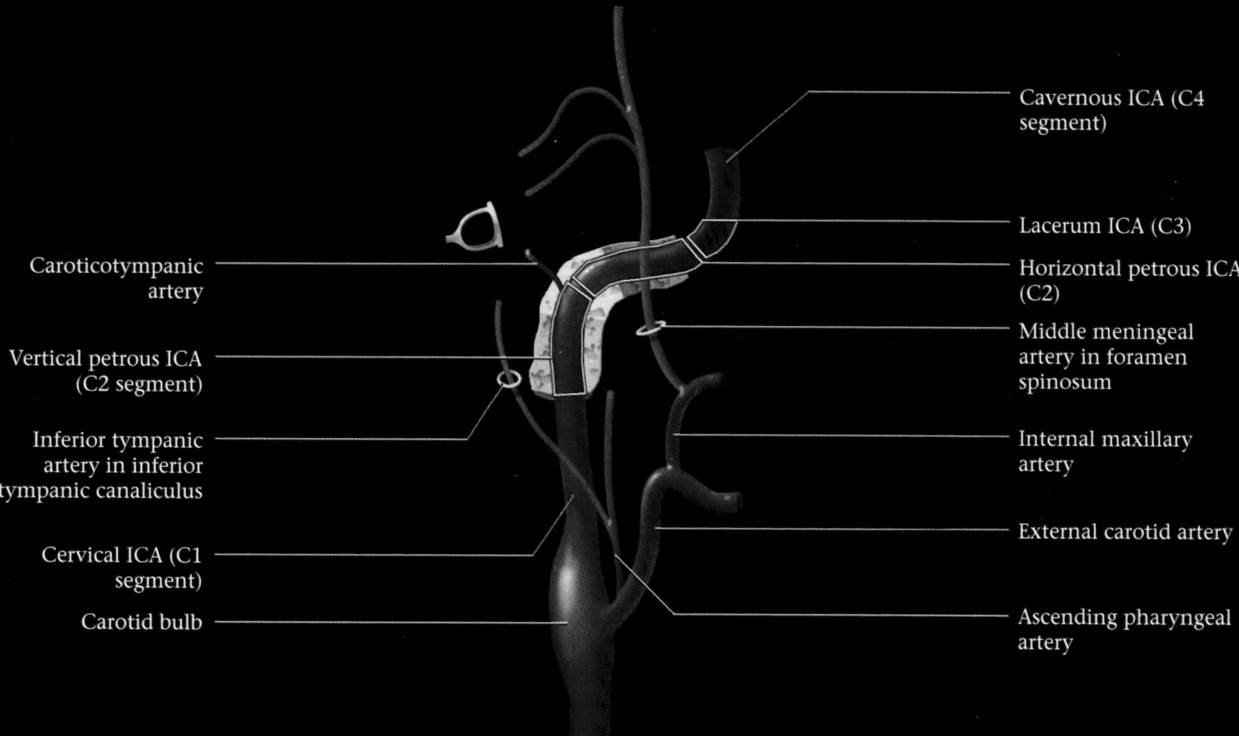
Caroticotympanic artery
Vertical petrous ICA (C2 segment)
Inferior tympanic artery in inferior tympanic canaliculus
Cervical ICA (C1 segment)
Carotid bulb
Cavernous ICA (C4 segment)
Lacerum ICA (C3)
Horizontal petrous ICA (C2)
Middle meningeal artery in foramen spinosum
Internal maxillary artery
External carotid artery
Ascending pharyngeal artery

(Top) Graphic of membranous labyrinth seen from above. Key elements of membranous labyrinth to consider include ~ 2 1/2 turns of the cochlea, the meeting point of the superior & posterior semicircular ducts (crus communis) & endolymphatic duct & sac. Note the endolymphatic duct has an intraosseous & intradural components. **(Bottom)** Sagittal graphic of petrous internal carotid artery. The cervical ICA enters the carotid canal of skull base to become the vertical petrous ICA (C2 subsegment ICA). It then turns anteromedially to become the horizontal petrous ICA (C2 subsegment ICA). The segment of the intracranial ICA just above the foramen lacerum is called the lacerum segment (C3 ICA segment). Note the inferior tympanic artery rise through the inferior tympanic canaliculus & middle meningeal artery arises off the internal maxillary artery passing through foramen spinosum.

AXIAL BONE CT

Squamous T-bone
Superior semicircular canal
Petrous apex
Mastoid air cells
Sigmoid sinus

Petrous apex
Internal auditory canal
Crus communis
Bony vestibular aqueduct
Mastoid antrum
Epitympanum
Aditus ad antrum
Koerner septum
Sigmoid plate

Labyrinthine segment CN7
Petrous apex
Porus acusticus of IAC
Vestibule
Fovea of bony vestibular aqueduct
Malleus head in epitympanum
Prussak space
Lateral semicircular canal
Koerner septum
Mastoid antrum
Posterior semicircular canal

(Top) First of twelve axial bone CT images of the left temporal bone presented from superior to inferior. Superior semicircular canal projects cephalad from inner ear. Bony cover over top of this semicircular canal is called arcuate eminence. **(Middle)** At the level of upper internal auditory canal the aditus ad antrum (L. "entrance to the cave") is seen connecting the epitympanum to mastoid antrum (L. "cave"). Notice Koerner septum separating the mastoid antrum from squamous portion of the mastoid air cells. **(Bottom)** At the level of the lateral semicircular canal the opening to the internal auditory canal, the porus acusticus is particularly well seen. The fovea of the bony vestibular aqueduct along the posterior wall of the T-bone houses the intradural endolymphatic sac. Prussak space is visible as the portion of the epitympanum lateral to the ossicles.

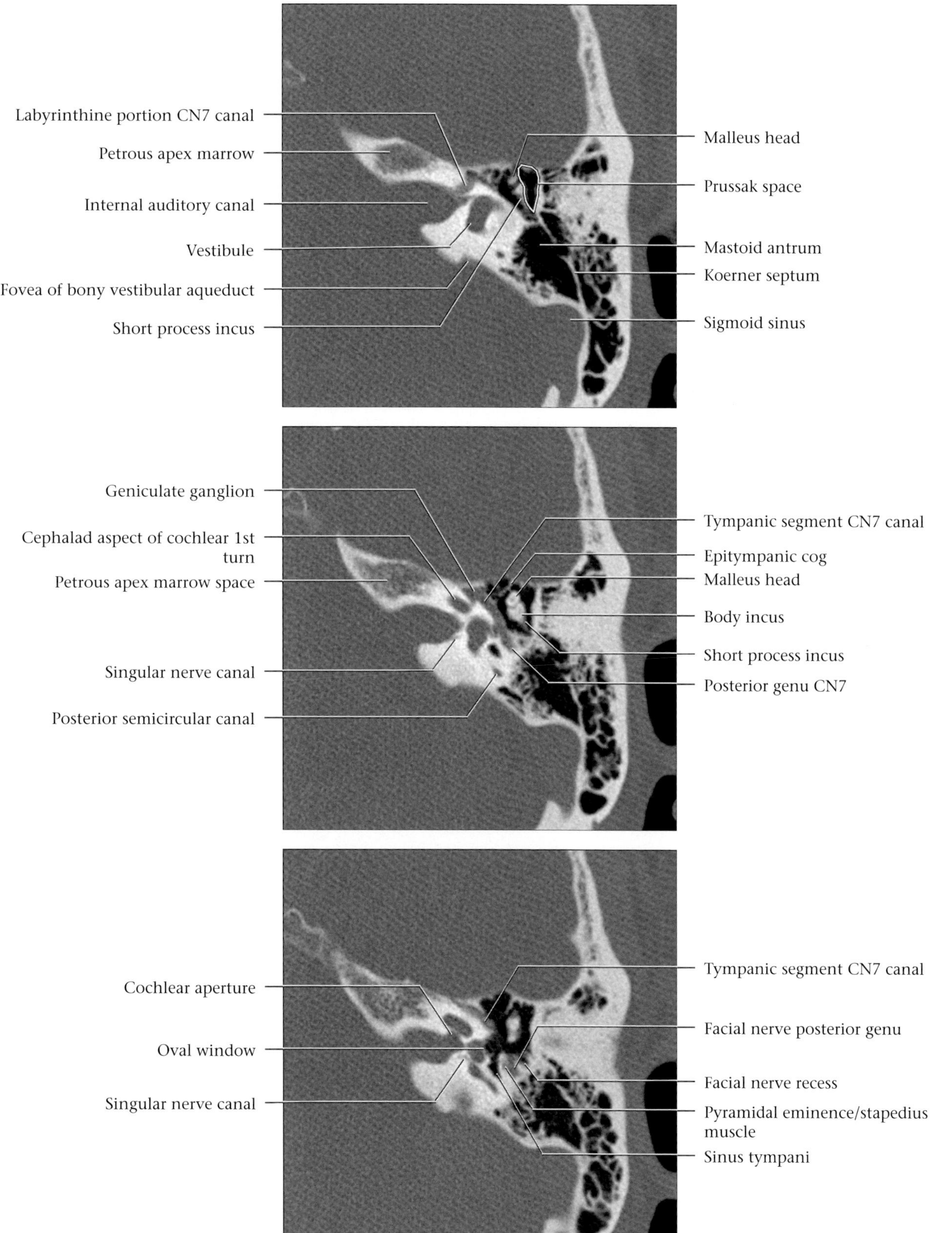
Labyrinthine portion CN7 canal
Petrous apex marrow
Internal auditory canal
Vestibule
Fovea of bony vestibular aqueduct
Short process incus
Malleus head
Prussak space
Mastoid antrum
Koerner septum
Sigmoid sinus
Geniculate ganglion
Cephalad aspect of cochlear 1st turn
Petrous apex marrow space
Singular nerve canal
Posterior semicircular canal
Tympanic segment CN7 canal
Epitympanic cog
Malleus head
Body incus
Short process incus
Posterior genu CN7
Cochlear aperture
Oval window
Singular nerve canal
Tympanic segment CN7 canal
Facial nerve posterior genu
Facial nerve recess
Pyramidal eminence/stapedius muscle
Sinus tympani

(Top) Image through the labyrinthine segment of the facial nerve shows this structure just cephalad to the cochlea. Prussak space is now visible as the lateral epitympanic recess. This is the first area the typical pars flaccida cholesteatoma involves in the middle ear. **(Middle)** In this image the tympanic segment of the facial nerve is seen from the anteromedial geniculate ganglion to the posterior genu where it changes to become the mastoid segment. The cog is seen crossing the anterior epitympanum. **(Bottom)** In this image three key structures on posterior wall of middle ear cavity are well seen. From medial to lateral they are the sinus tympani, pyramidal eminence and the facial nerve recess. Also note the oval window along the medial wall of the mesotympanum just anterior to the sinus tympani.

TEMPORAL BONE

AXIAL BONE CT

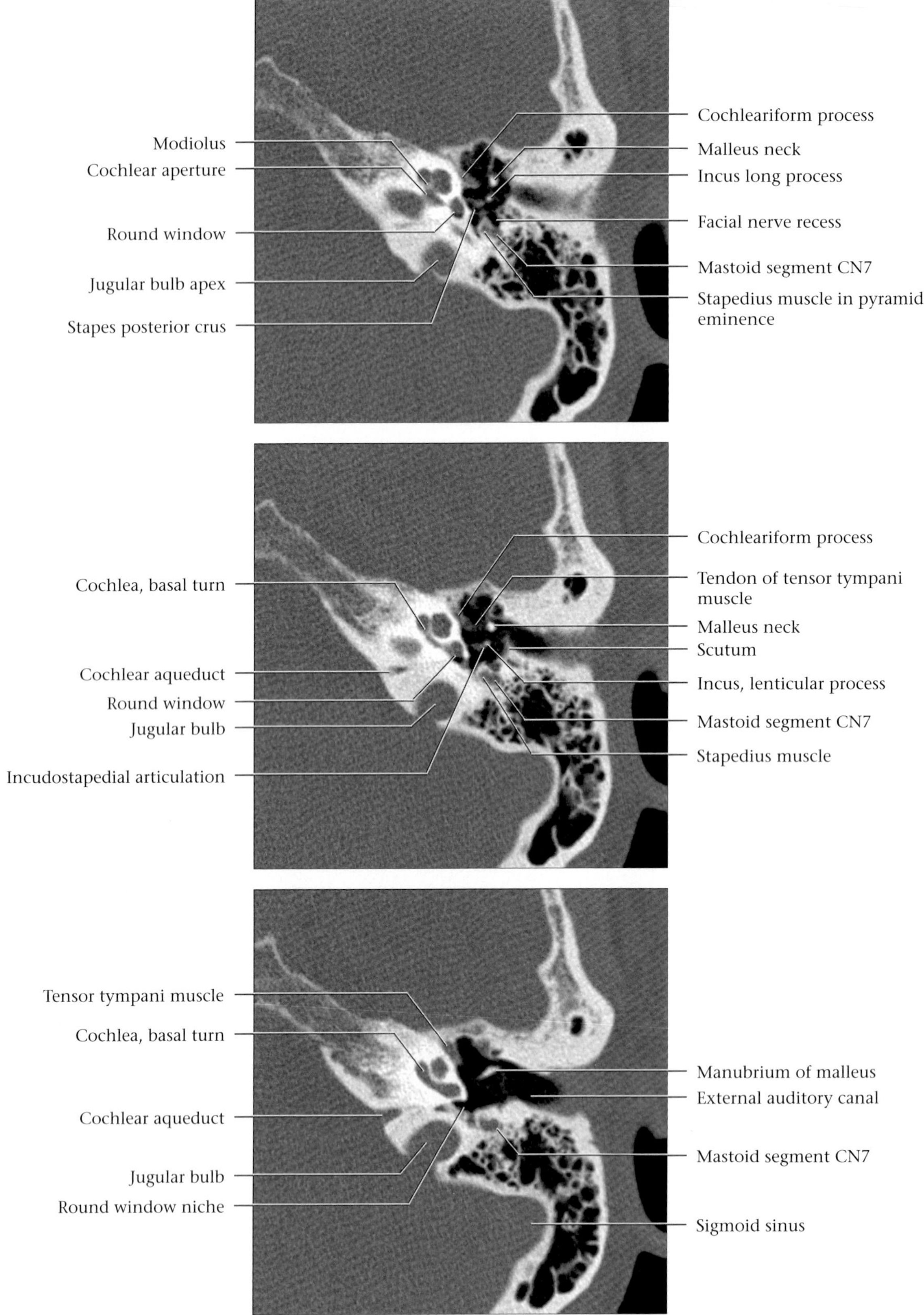
Modiolus
Cochlear aperture
Round window
Jugular bulb apex
Stapes posterior crus
Cochleariform process
Malleus neck
Incus long process
Facial nerve recess
Mastoid segment CN7
Stapedius muscle in pyramidal eminence
Cochlea, basal turn
Cochlear aqueduct
Round window
Jugular bulb
Incudostapedial articulation
Cochleariform process
Tendon of tensor tympani muscle
Malleus neck
Scutum
Incus, lenticular process
Mastoid segment CN7
Stapedius muscle
Tensor tympani muscle
Cochlea, basal turn
Cochlear aqueduct
Jugular bulb
Round window niche
Manubrium of malleus
External auditory canal
Mastoid segment CN7
Sigmoid sinus

(Top) Image at the level of the cochlear aperture the cochleariform process can be seen high on the cochlear promontory. The cochleariform process is the annulus through which the tendon of the tensor tympani muscle turns toward the more lateral malleus. Stapes crura visible. Stapedius muscle in pyramidal eminence is now distinguishable from mastoid segment of facial nerve. **(Middle)** Mid-cochlear image shows both the cochleariform process and the tendon of the tensor tympani muscle extending over to the malleus. The incudostapedial articulation is visible between the lenticular process of the incus & the stapes head. Also note the round window at the base of the basal turn of the cochlea. **(Bottom)** At the level of the low mesotympanum note the cochlear aqueduct on the medial wall inferior to the internal auditory canal. The manubrium of the malleus is also visible.

AXIAL BONE CT

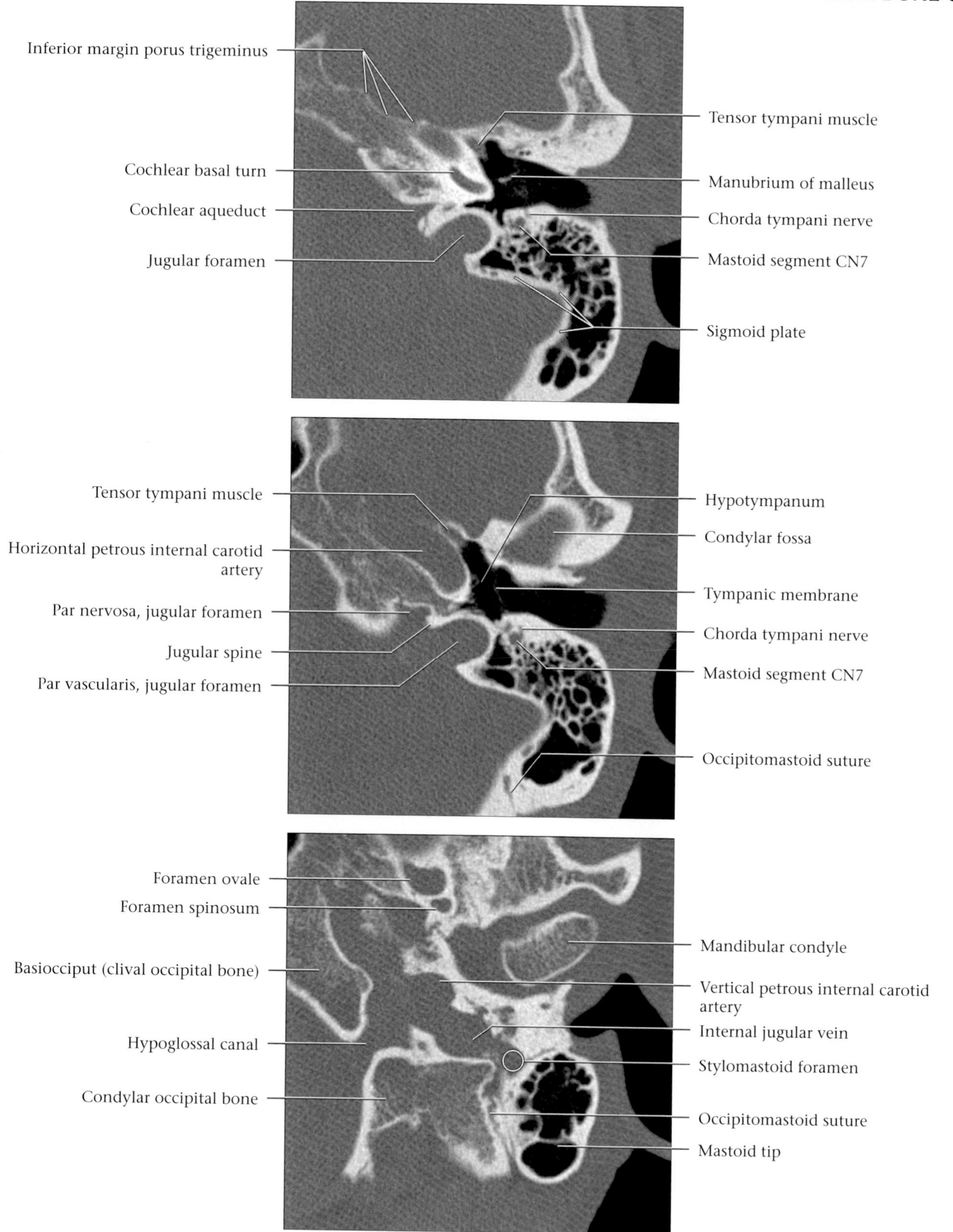
Inferior margin porus trigeminus
Cochlear basal turn
Cochlear aqueduct
Jugular foramen
Tensor tympani muscle
Manubrium of malleus
Chorda tympani nerve
Mastoid segment CN7
Sigmoid plate
Tensor tympani muscle
Horizontal petrous internal carotid artery
Par nervosa, jugular foramen
Jugular spine
Par vascularis, jugular foramen
Hypotympanum
Condylar fossa
Tympanic membrane
Chorda tympani nerve
Mastoid segment CN7
Occipitomastoid suture
Foramen ovale
Foramen spinosum
Basiocciput (clival occipital bone)
Hypoglossal canal
Condylar occipital bone
Mandibular condyle
Vertical petrous internal carotid artery
Internal jugular vein
Stylomastoid foramen
Occipitomastoid suture
Mastoid tip

(Top) In this image the normal cortex of the sigmoid plate is well seen. The sigmoid plate separates the mastoid air cells from the sigmoid sinus. Notice the cochlear aqueduct on the medial T-bone wall. **(Middle)** At the level of the hypotympanum normal gossamer tympanic membrane is just barely visible. The horizontal petrous internal carotid artery canal is seen running anteromedial toward the cavernous sinus. Notice the pars nervosa & par vascularis of the jugular foramen partially separated by the jugular spine. **(Bottom)** The mastoid tip is seen in this inferior image. Just anteromedial to the mastoid tip is the stylomastoid foramen where the facial nerve exists the skull base. Notice the entrance to the vertical segment of the petrous internal carotid artery canal just medial to the condylar fossa. The occipitomastoid suture should not be mistaken for a fracture line.

CORONAL BONE CT

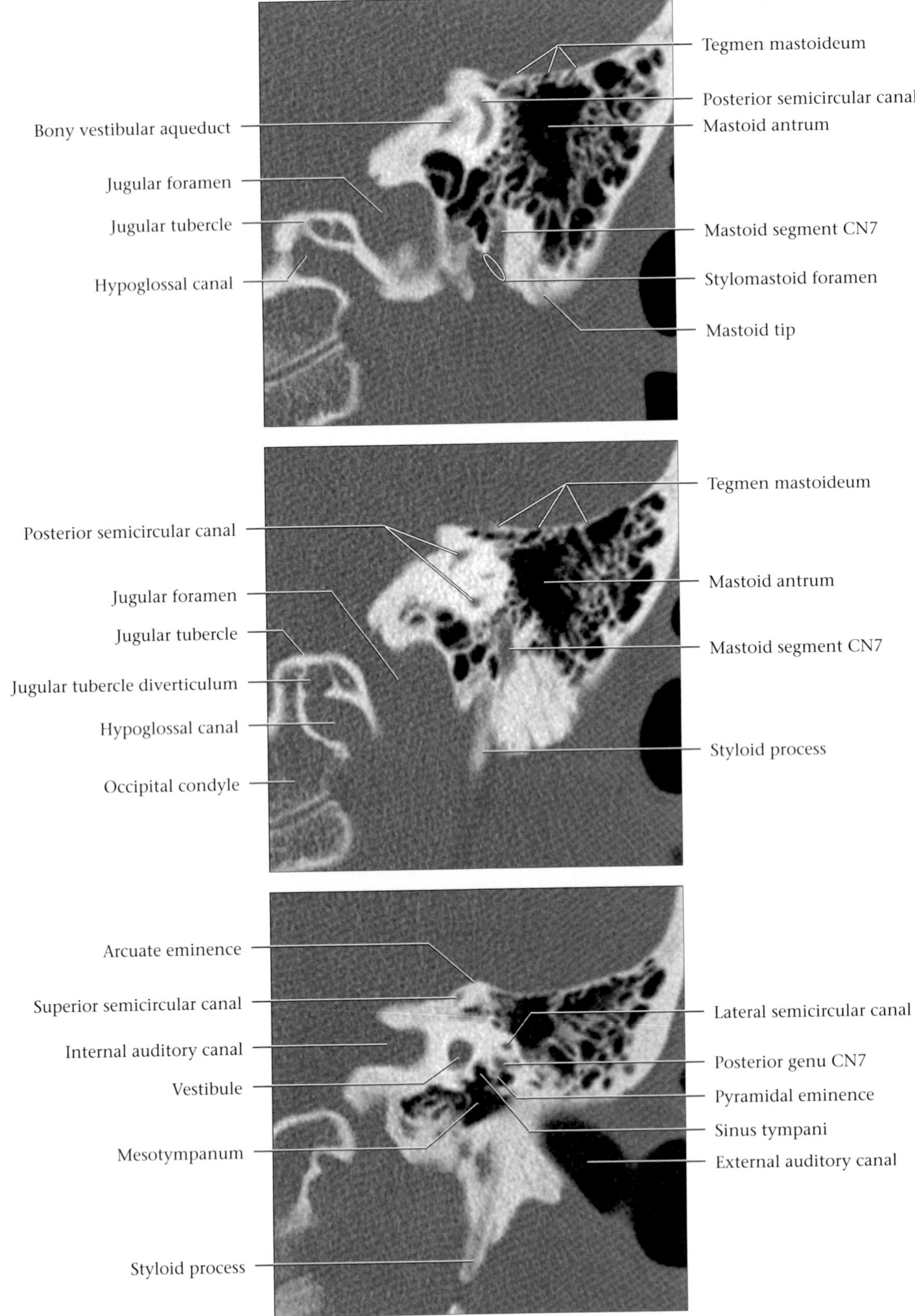
Tegmen mastoideum
Posterior semicircular canal
Mastoid antrum
Bony vestibular aqueduct
Jugular foramen
Jugular tubercle
Hypoglossal canal
Mastoid segment CN7
Stylomastoid foramen
Mastoid tip
Tegmen mastoideum
Posterior semicircular canal
Mastoid antrum
Jugular foramen
Jugular tubercle
Jugular tubercle diverticulum
Hypoglossal canal
Occipital condyle
Mastoid segment CN7
Styloid process
Arcuate eminence
Superior semicircular canal
Internal auditory canal
Vestibule
Mesotympanum
Styloid process
Lateral semicircular canal
Posterior genu CN7
Pyramidal eminence
Sinus tympani
External auditory canal

(Top) First of twelve coronal bone CT images presented from posterior to anterior. In this most posterior image the stylomastoid foramen and distal mastoid segment of the facial nerve can be seen to be protected by the mastoid tip. The mastoid sinus grows into this protective position in the first decade of life. **(Middle)** In this image the mid-mastoid segment of the facial nerve is seen. The jugular foramen and the hypoglossal canal are separated by the "eagle's beak", a portion of the jugular tubercle. **(Bottom)** In this image of posterior mesotympanum the 3 critical posterior wall structures are seen. From medial to lateral these structures are sinus tympani, pyramidal eminence & facial nerve recess with the posterior genu of CN7 in its depth. Note that it is possible to see the stapedius muscle as a small, round soft tissue density within pyramidal eminence.

CORONAL BONE CT

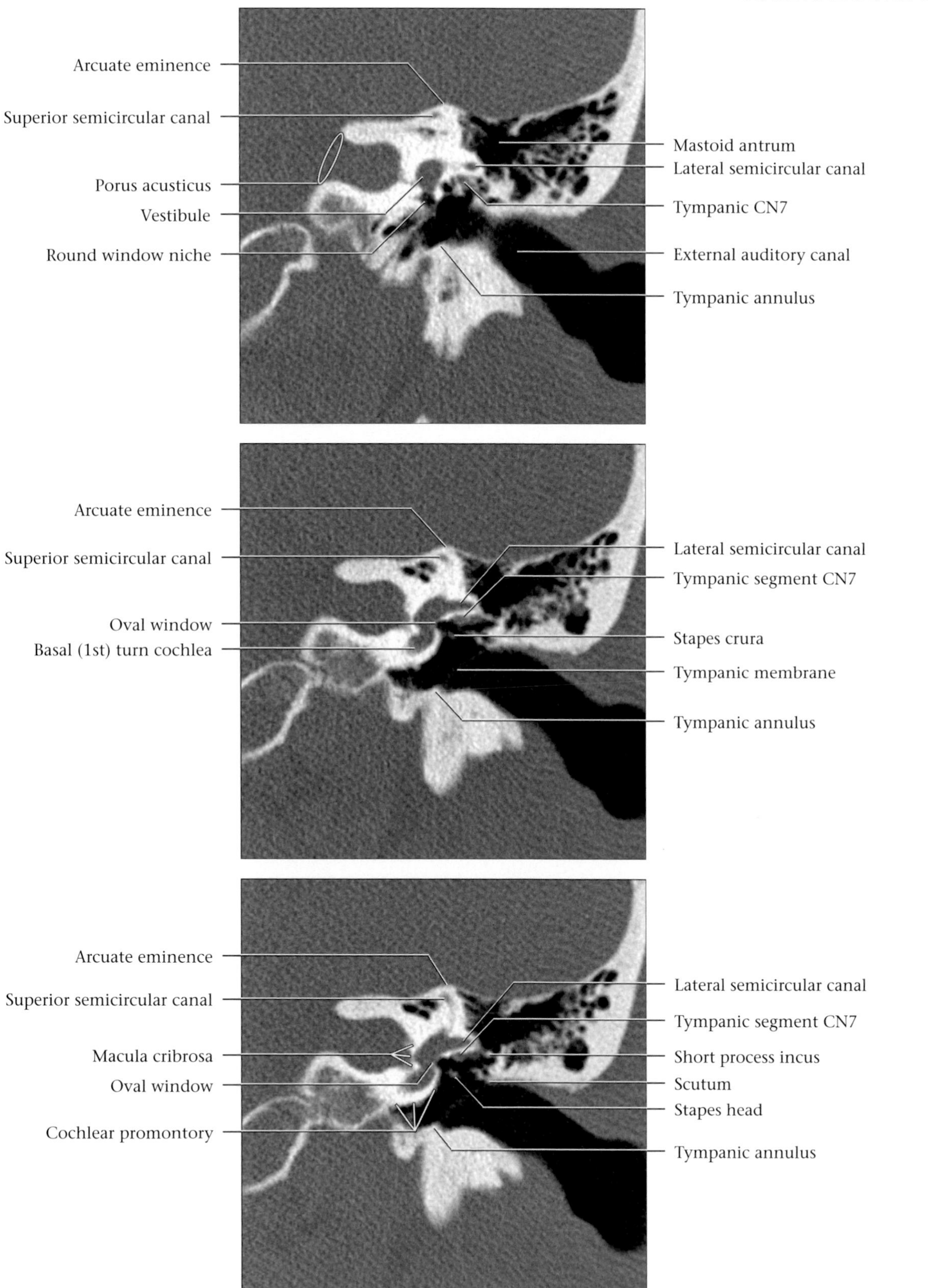
Arcuate eminence
Superior semicircular canal
Porus acusticus
Vestibule
Round window niche
Mastoid antrum
Lateral semicircular canal
Tympanic CN7
External auditory canal
Tympanic annulus
Arcuate eminence
Superior semicircular canal
Oval window
Basal (1st) turn cochlea
Lateral semicircular canal
Tympanic segment CN7
Stapes crura
Tympanic membrane
Tympanic annulus
Arcuate eminence
Superior semicircular canal
Macula cribrosa
Oval window
Cochlear promontory
Lateral semicircular canal
Tympanic segment CN7
Short process incus
Scutum
Stapes head
Tympanic annulus

(Top) In this image the posterior tympanic segment of the facial nerve is visible under the lateral semicircular canal. The round window niche is a small air-filled area off the medial mesotympanum that leads to the round window membrane. **(Middle)** At the level of the oval window niche the basal turn of the cochlea becomes visible. Notice the tympanic membrane is barely seen when it is normal. Its inferior attachment, the tympanic annulus is a useful landmark separating the middle ear from the medial external ear. **(Bottom)** In this image the short process of the incus is seen projecting posteriorly into the aditus ad antrum. Both the tympanic membrane attachments can be seen, the superior scutum and the inferior tympanic annulus. Notice the cochlear promontory projects out into the mesotympanum. Glomus tympanicum paragangliomas occur here.

CORONAL BONE CT

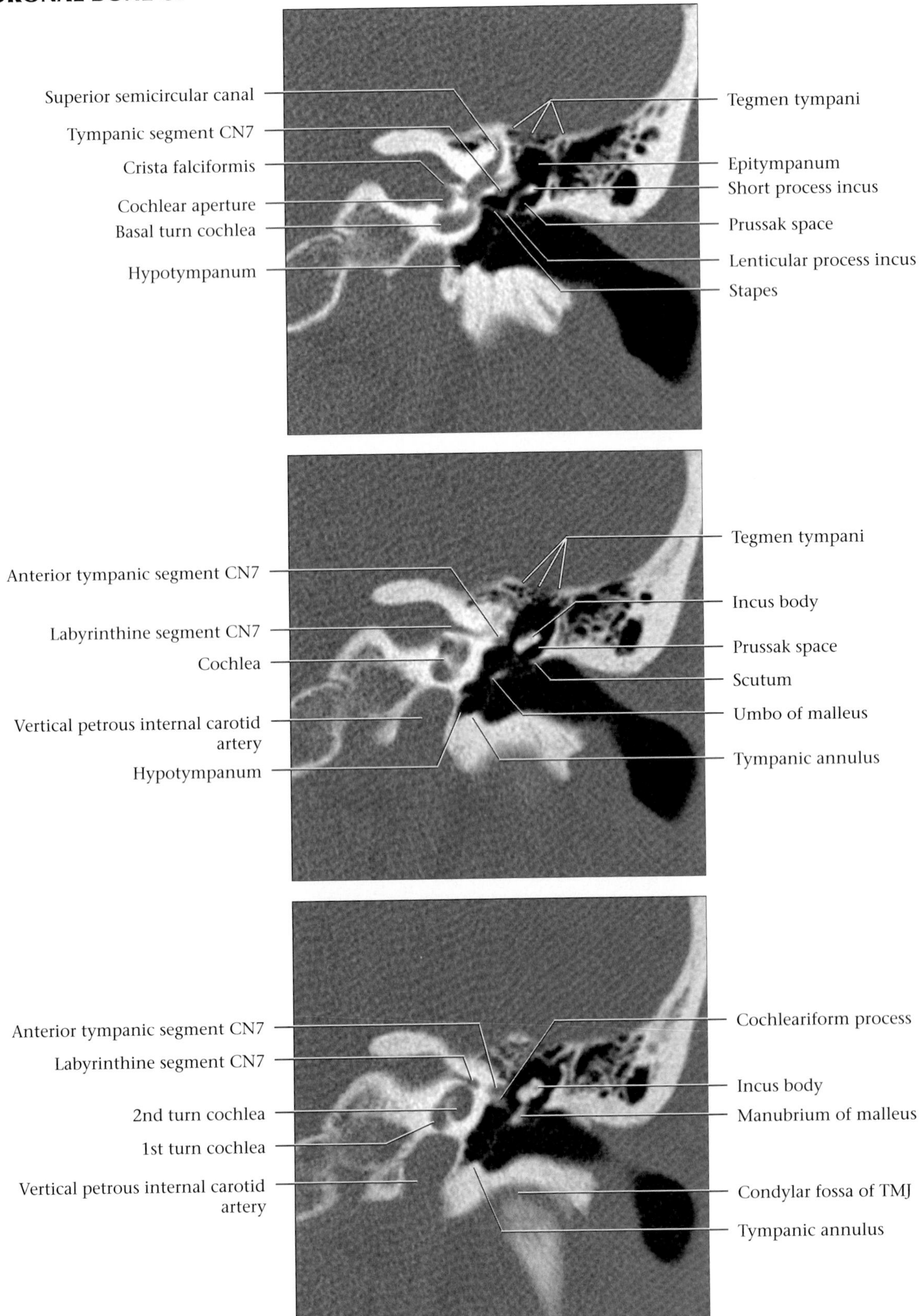

Superior semicircular canal
Tympanic segment CN7
Crista falciformis
Cochlear aperture
Basal turn cochlea
Hypotympanum
Tegmen tympani
Epitympanum
Short process incus
Prussak space
Lenticular process incus
Stapes
Anterior tympanic segment CN7
Labyrinthine segment CN7
Cochlea
Vertical petrous internal carotid artery
Hypotympanum
Tegmen tympani
Incus body
Prussak space
Scutum
Umbo of malleus
Tympanic annulus
Anterior tympanic segment CN7
Labyrinthine segment CN7
2nd turn cochlea
1st turn cochlea
Vertical petrous internal carotid artery
Cochleariform process
Incus body
Manubrium of malleus
Condylar fossa of TMJ
Tympanic annulus

(Top) Image through the mid-mesotympanum shows the more superior epitympanum with the long and short processes of the incus forming the medial margin and the lateral epitympanic wall the lateral margin of Prussak space. Pars flaccida cholesteatoma involve the middle ear cavity first in Prussak space. **(Middle)** In this image the tegmen tympani (L. "roof of the cave") can be seen as the superior wall of the epitympanum. Note its normal variable thickness. Just above the cochlea the facial nerve canal is seen emerging from the fundus of the internal auditory canal to become the labyrinthine segment CN7. **(Bottom)** Three key structures are seen together in this image, the labyrinthine segment CN7, anterior tympanic CN7 and the cochleariform process. Note the tendon of the tensor tympani muscles projecting from the cochleariform process to attach to the malleus.

CORONAL BONE CT

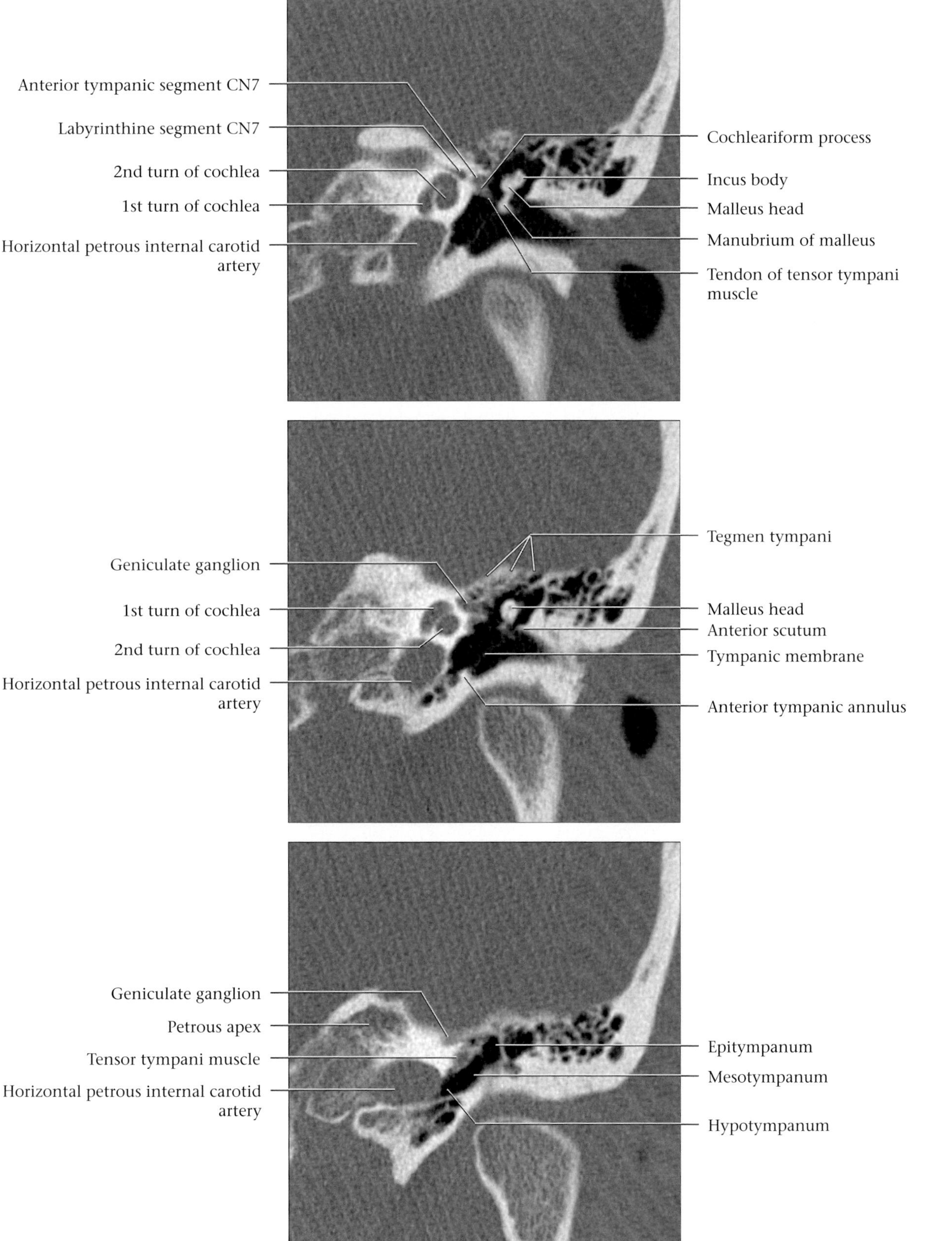

Anterior tympanic segment CN7
Labyrinthine segment CN7
2nd turn of cochlea
1st turn of cochlea
Horizontal petrous internal carotid artery
Cochleariform process
Incus body
Malleus head
Manubrium of malleus
Tendon of tensor tympani muscle
Geniculate ganglion
1st turn of cochlea
2nd turn of cochlea
Horizontal petrous internal carotid artery
Tegmen tympani
Malleus head
Anterior scutum
Tympanic membrane
Anterior tympanic annulus
Geniculate ganglion
Petrous apex
Tensor tympani muscle
Horizontal petrous internal carotid artery
Epitympanum
Mesotympanum
Hypotympanum

(Top) The labyrinthine segment of CN7 is seen here merging together with the anterior tympanic CN7 above the cochlea. The cochleariform process and tendon of the tensor tympani muscle are both visible. The petrous internal carotid horizontal segment can be seen below the cochlea. **(Middle)** In this image the tegmen tympani is thick and well-defined. The geniculate ganglion in the geniculate fossa is seen on the superolateral cochlea with the horizontal petrous internal carotid artery below the cochlea. Both the scutum and tympanic annulus are visible between the gossamer tympanic membrane. **(Bottom)** In the most anterior middle ear cavity the ossicles are not seen. The geniculate ganglion in the geniculate fossa along with the tensor tympanic muscle are visible. The horizontal petrous internal carotid artery is now projecting anteromedially.

SAGITTAL T2 MR

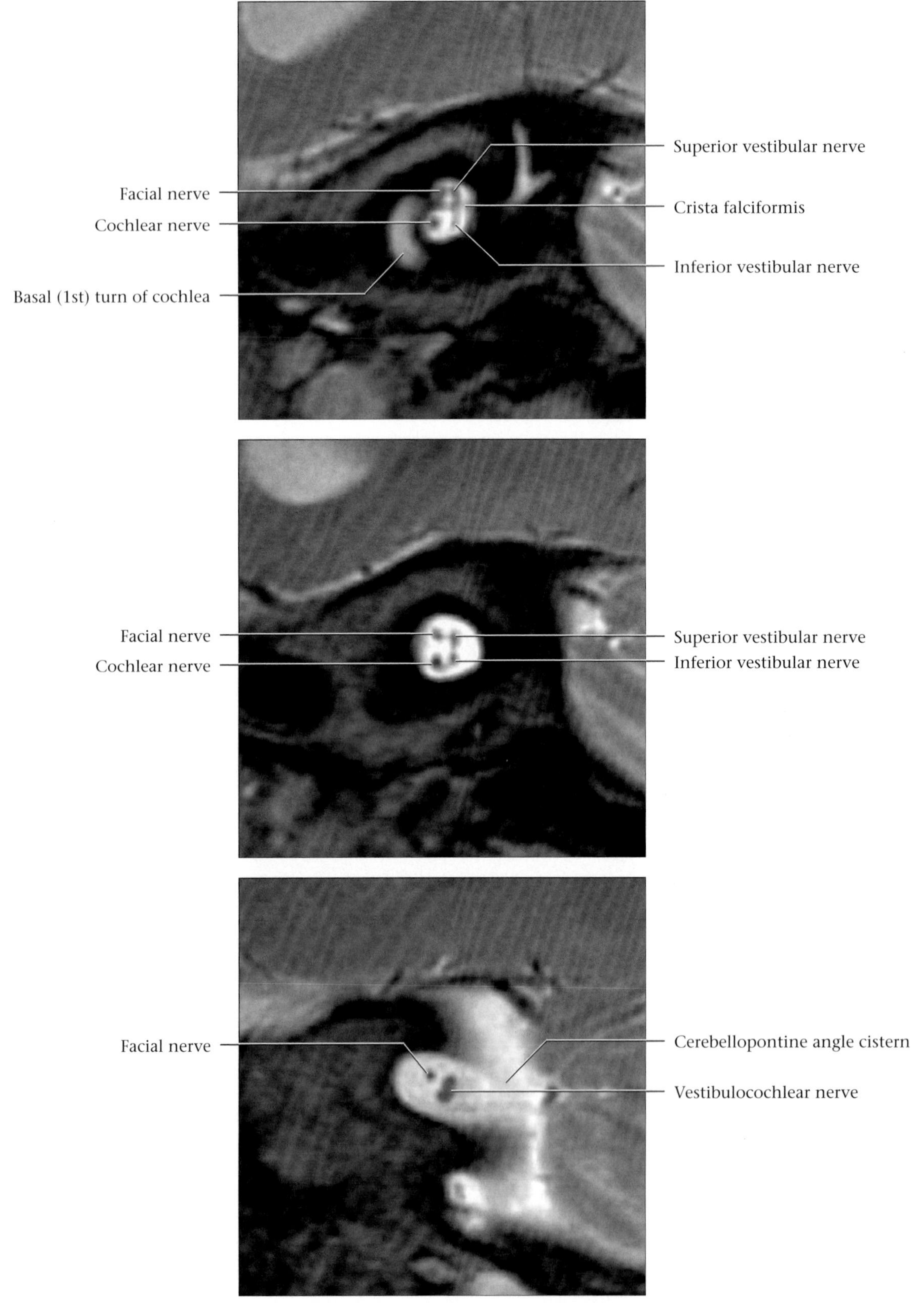
Facial nerve
Cochlear nerve
Basal (1st) turn of cochlea
Superior vestibular nerve
Crista falciformis
Inferior vestibular nerve
Facial nerve
Cochlear nerve
Superior vestibular nerve
Inferior vestibular nerve
Facial nerve
Cerebellopontine angle cistern
Vestibulocochlear nerve

(Top) First of three high-resolution oblique sagittal T2 MR images presented from lateral to medial of internal auditory canal shows facial nerve to be anterosuperior & cochlear nerve to be anteroinferior. This fundal view reveals crista falciformis seen as a vague low signal line dividing CN7 & the superior vestibular nerve from the cochlear and inferior vestibular nerves. **(Middle)** In the mid-internal auditory canal four discrete nerves are visible. Notice the anterosuperior facial nerve is normally slightly smaller than the anteroinferior cochlear nerve. The superior and inferior vestibular nerves are often joined by connecting fibers as in this example. **(Bottom)** At the level of the porus acusticus the vestibulocochlear nerve has the appearance of a "catcher's mitt" with the facial nerve looking like the "ball in the mitt".

AXIAL T2 MR

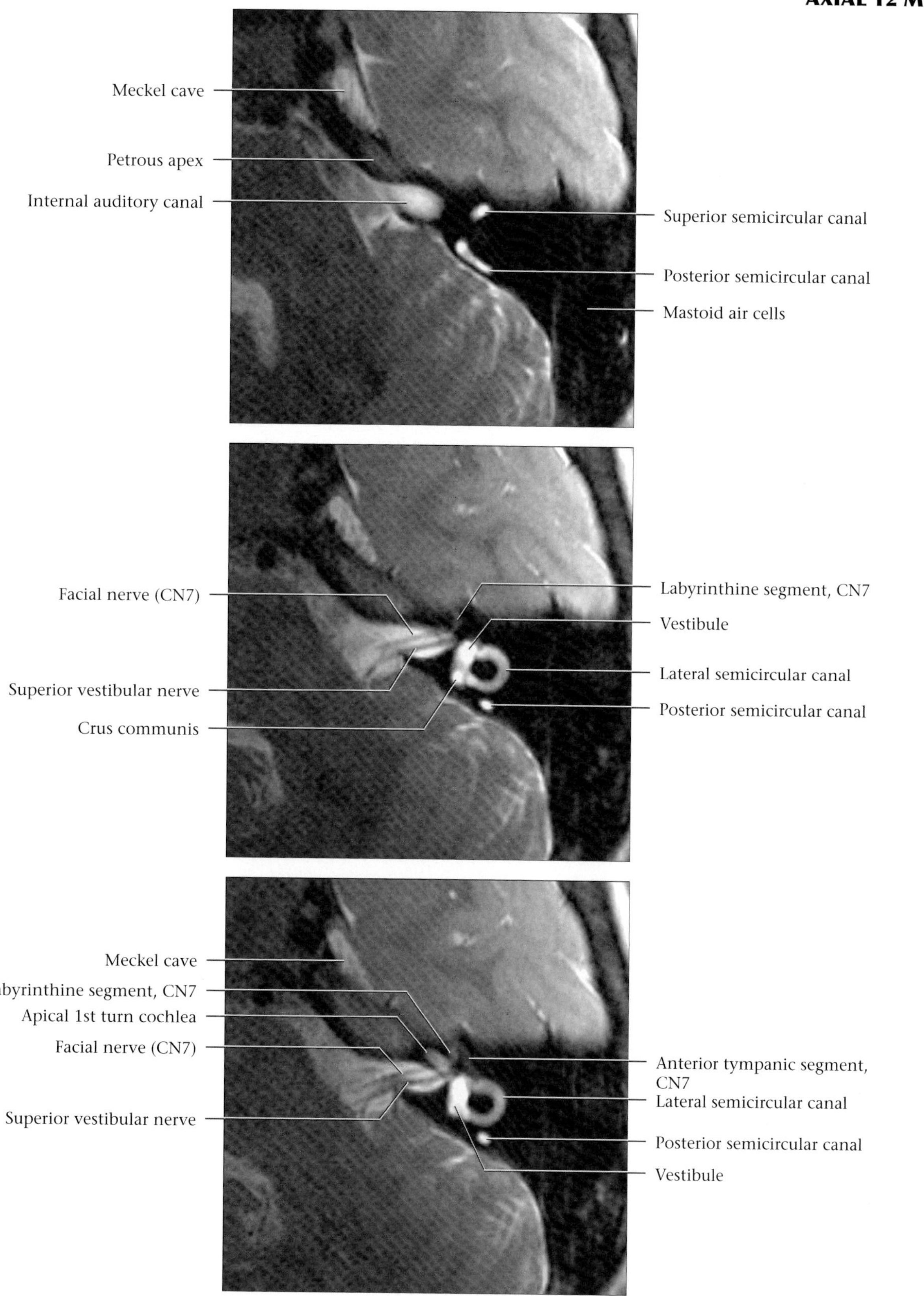
Meckel cave
Petrous apex
Internal auditory canal
Superior semicircular canal
Posterior semicircular canal
Mastoid air cells
Facial nerve (CN7)
Superior vestibular nerve
Crus communis
Labyrinthine segment, CN7
Vestibule
Lateral semicircular canal
Posterior semicircular canal
Meckel cave
Labyrinthine segment, CN7
Apical 1st turn cochlea
Facial nerve (CN7)
Superior vestibular nerve
Anterior tympanic segment, CN7
Lateral semicircular canal
Posterior semicircular canal
Vestibule

(Top) First of six axial high-resolution thin-section T2 MR images presented from superior to inferior through the left temporal bone shows the superior internal auditory canal and semicircular canals. **(Middle)** In this image the facial nerve is visible anterior to the superior vestibular nerve in the superior aspect of the internal auditory canal. The fluid spaces of the membranous labyrinth are high signal within the dark signal of the bony labyrinth. **(Bottom)** In this image the labyrinthine and anterior tympanic segments of the facial nerve are visible. As they are not surrounded by cerebrospinal fluid as is CN7 in the internal auditory canal they are more difficult to see.

AXIAL T2 MR

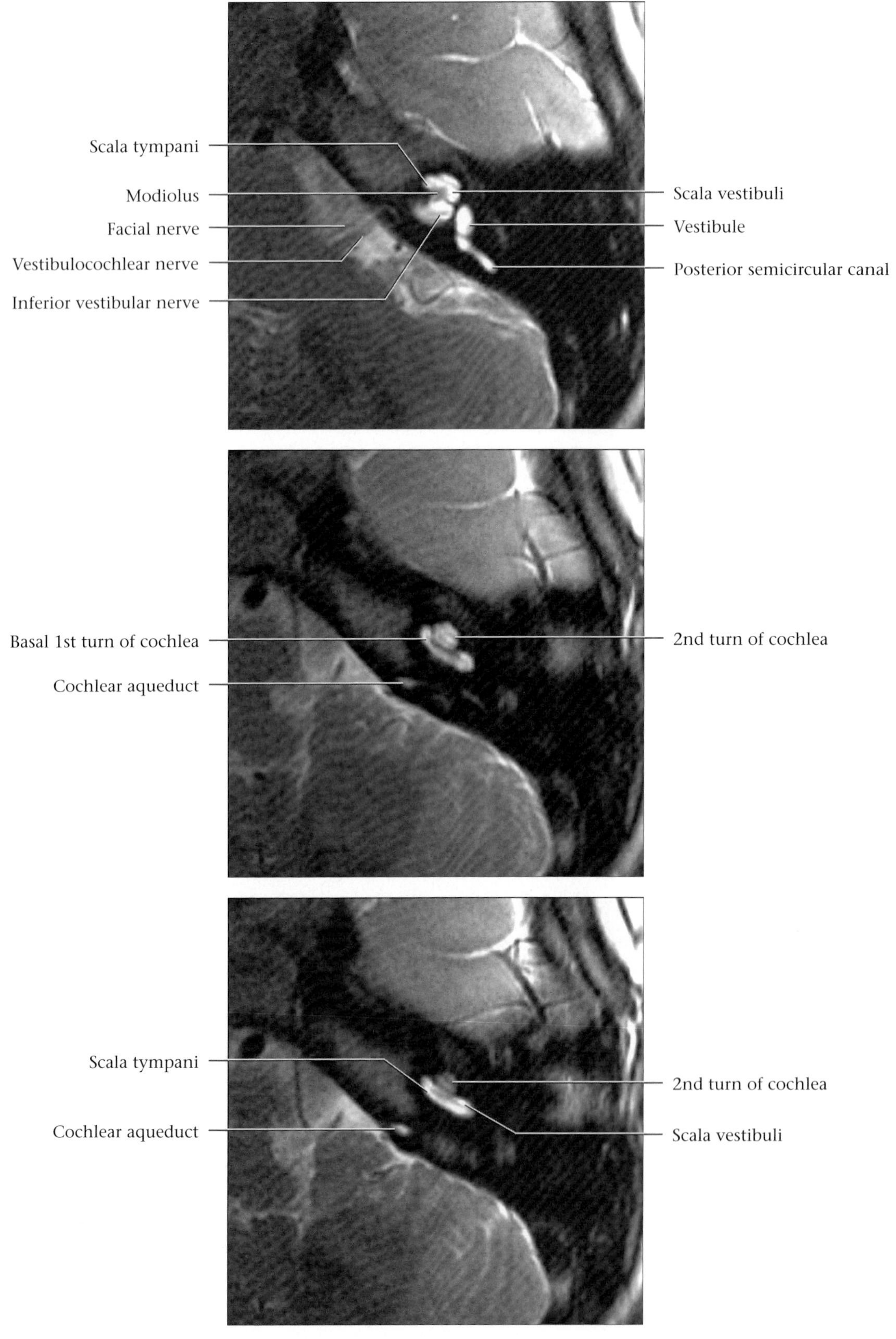

Scala tympani
Modiolus
Facial nerve
Vestibulocochlear nerve
Inferior vestibular nerve
Scala vestibuli
Vestibule
Posterior semicircular canal
Basal 1st turn of cochlea
Cochlear aqueduct
2nd turn of cochlea
Scala tympani
Cochlear aqueduct
2nd turn of cochlea
Scala vestibuli

(Top) In this image through the cochlear aperture the modiolus of the cochlea is seen as an intermediate signal structure at the hub of the cochlea. The two larger cochlear chambers of the are visible. The anterior chamber is the scala vestibuli while the posterior chamber is the scala tympani. The scala media is not routinely resolvable. **(Middle)** In this image both the first and second turns of the cochlea are visible. The osseous spiral lamina within the cochlea is seen as a fine low signal line within the fluid of the cochlear membranous labyrinth. **(Bottom)** The cochlear aqueduct is a tubular-shaped structure on the medial wall of the temporal bone inferior to the internal auditory canal. No definite function can be assigned to this structure.

CORONAL T2 MR

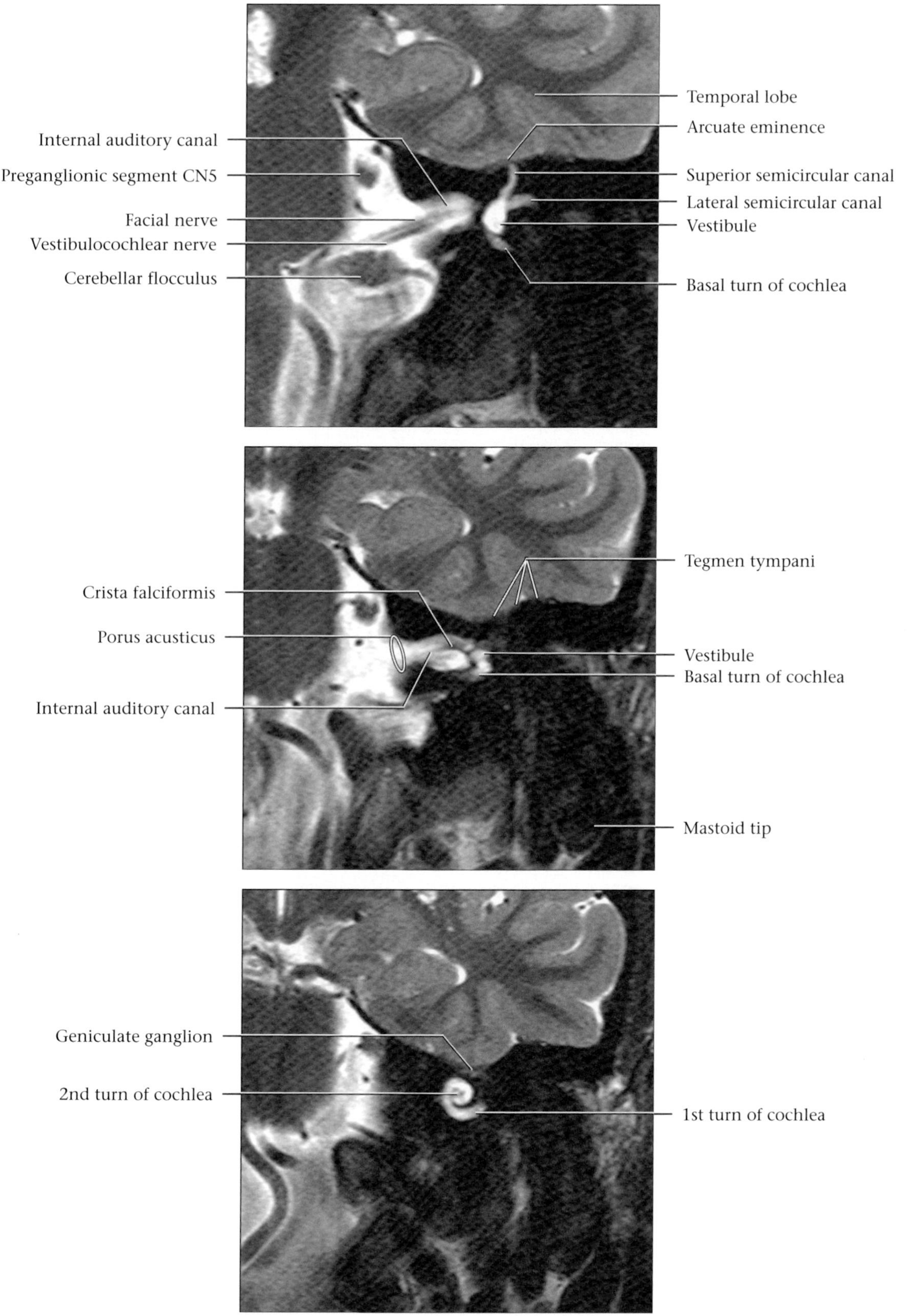
Temporal lobe
Arcuate eminence
Internal auditory canal
Preganglionic segment CN5
Superior semicircular canal
Lateral semicircular canal
Facial nerve
Vestibule
Vestibulocochlear nerve
Cerebellar flocculus
Basal turn of cochlea
Tegmen tympani
Crista falciformis
Porus acusticus
Vestibule
Basal turn of cochlea
Internal auditory canal
Mastoid tip
Geniculate ganglion
2nd turn of cochlea
1st turn of cochlea

(Top) First of three coronal T2 MR images of the left ear presented from posterior to anterior. The membranous labyrinth of the inner ear is visible as high signal fluid. Notice the superior and lateral semicircular canals adjacent to the vestibule. **(Middle)** In this image through the internal auditory canal an unusually long crista falciformis is seen in the fundus. The area of the tegmen tympani is marked but no landmarks in the middle ear are visible because both air and bone are low signal on MR imaging. **(Bottom)** At the level of the cochlea the snail shape is particularly obvious displaying both the first and second turns. The geniculate ganglion is barely visible above and lateral to the cochlea. Again note the lack of middle ear definable structures.

COCHLEA

Terminology

Abbreviations

- Temporal bone (T-bone)

Definitions

- Cochlea: (L. "snail shell") coiled, tapered tube inside the inner ear, responsible for transmitting sound to organ of Corti (sensory organ of hearing)

Imaging Anatomy

Overview

- Inner ear organization: 3 components
  - **Bony labyrinth**: Bone confining cochlea, vestibule & semicircular canals
  - **Perilymphatic spaces**: Area in vestibule surrounding utricle & saccule, semicircular canals around semicircular ducts & within scala tympani & vestibuli of cochlea
    - **Perilymph** "bathes" membranous labyrinth structures
  - **Membranous labyrinth**
    - Vestibular utricle & saccule, semicircular ducts, scala media of cochlea, endolymphatic duct & sac all contain endolymph
    - **Endolymph** is functional fluid within structures of membranous labyrinth; bathes & nourishes its sensory epithelium

Internal Structures-Critical Contents

- Cochlea contains ~ 2 ½ turns
- **Cochlear aperture**: Opening to cochlea from IAC fundus
- **Modiolus**: Central bony axis of cochlea
  - Houses spiral ganglion (cell bodies of cochlear nerve)
- **Osseous spiral lamina**: Thin bony plate projecting to basilar membrane from modiolus
  - Provides supportive function & allows organized transmission of cochlear nerve fibers to each segment of cochlea
- 3 spiral chambers of cochlea
  - **Scala tympani**
    - Posterior chamber of cochlea
    - Descending spiral containing perilymph
  - **Scala vestibuli**
    - Anterior chamber of cochlea
    - Ascending spiral containing perilymph
    - Perilymph connects to subarachnoid space via cochlear aqueduct
  - **Scala media** (cochlear duct)
    - Separated from anterior scala vestibuli by vestibular (Reissner) membrane
    - Separated from posterior scala tympani by basilar membrane
    - Contains organ of Corti (hearing apparatus); sits on basilar membrane
- Cochlear nerve cell bodies = spiral ganglion
  - **Spiral ganglion** bipolar cells
  - Send antegrade axon to organ of Corti
  - Send retrograde axon to form cochlear nerve

Anatomy-Based Imaging Issues

Key Concepts or Questions

- Creation of hearing
  - Movement of stapes results in transmission of fluid waves via oval window through vestibule to cochlear recess
  - Cochlear recess fluid wave transmitted to scala vestibuli (ascending spiral) of cochlea
  - Fluid waves (sound waves) enter perilymph of scala vestibuli and are then transmitted via vestibular membrane into endolymph of cochlear duct
  - This transmission causes displacement of basilar membrane, which stimulates hair cell receptors in organ of Corti
  - Hair cell movement generates electronic potentials converted to action potentials in cochlear nerve
    - High frequency sounds converted at cochlear base
    - Low frequency sound converted at cochlear apex

Imaging Recommendations

- T-bone CT: Evaluates bony aspects of cochlear diseases
  - Otosclerosis, labyrinthine ossificans, bony details of complex inner ear dysplasias
- T-bone MR: Evaluates membranous labyrinth diseases
  - T1 C+ MR: Labyrinthitis, intralabyrinthine schwannoma
  - T2 high-resolution MR: Cochlear nerve size in cochlear implant candidates

Clinical Implications

Clinical Importance

- Cochlea responsible for hearing as it transforms fluid motion into electrical energy
  - Any disease that affects cochlear nuclei, cochlear nerve, cochlea can cause sensorineural hearing loss

Embryology

Embryologic Events

- Cochlea development occurs between 3rd & 8th fetal weeks
- **Otic placode** (3rd week) invaginates to becomes otic pit (4th week)
- **Otic pit** becomes otocyst (otic vesicle) at week 5
- **Otocyst** migrates to inner ear location during week 5
- Cochlear duct (scala media) forms (6th week)
- 2 1/2 turn cochlea forms (by end of 8th week)
- Fetus "hears" by 24th week with maturation of organ of Corti

Practical Implications

- Inner ear forms as separate event from external & middle ear
  - EAC atresia usually presents with normal inner ear
- Injury to organ of Corti may occur long after cochlear infrastructure forms
  - Normal cochlea on imaging often seen in setting of profound sensorineural hearing loss

GRAPHICS

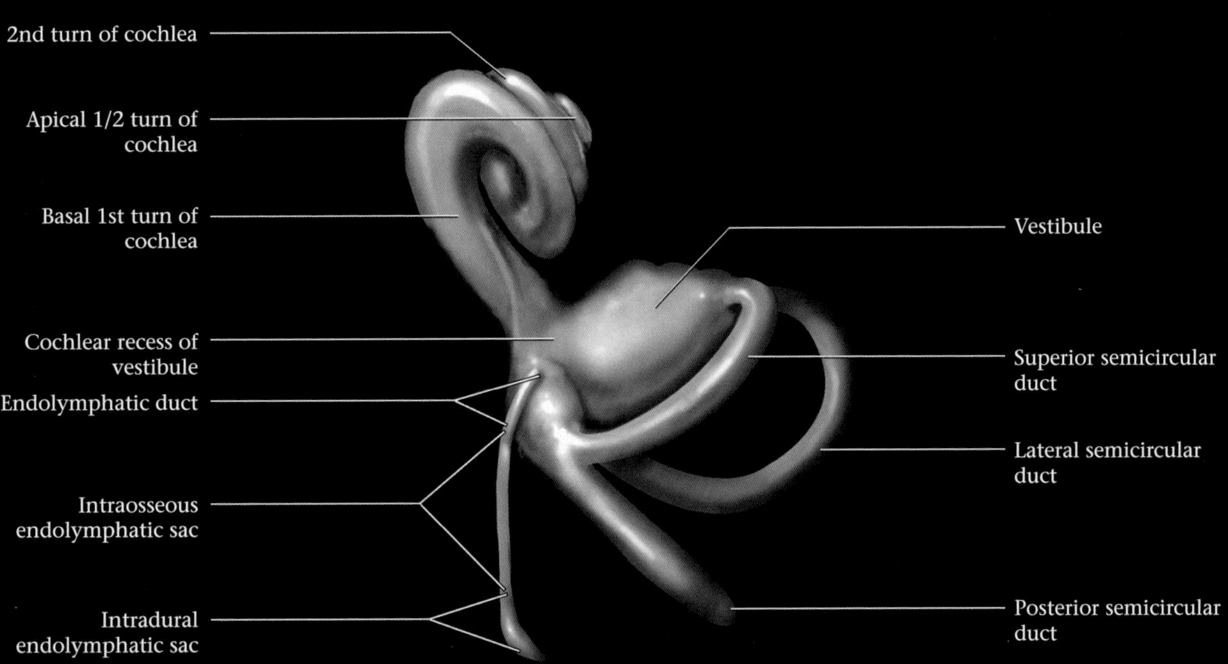

2nd turn of cochlea
Apical 1/2 turn of cochlea
Basal 1st turn of cochlea
Cochlear recess of vestibule
Endolymphatic duct
Intraosseous endolymphatic sac
Intradural endolymphatic sac
Vestibule
Superior semicircular duct
Lateral semicircular duct
Posterior semicircular duct

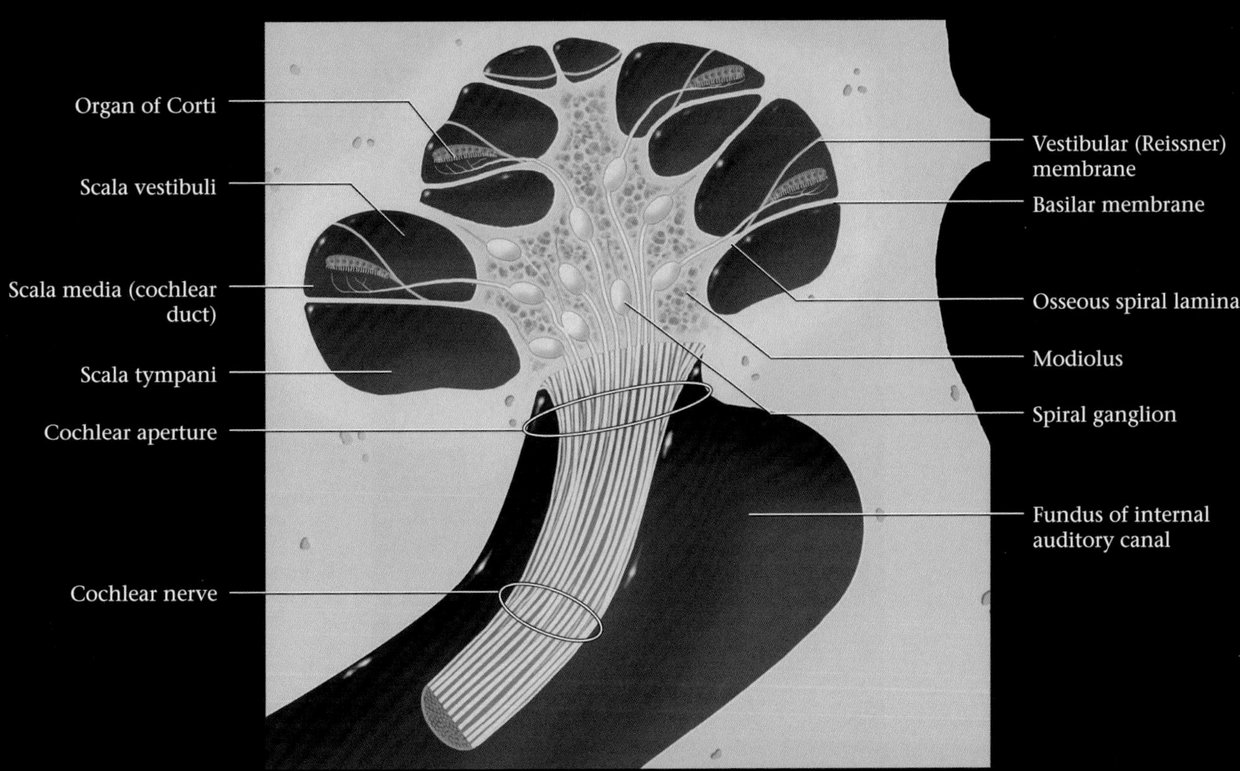

Organ of Corti
Scala vestibuli
Scala media (cochlear duct)
Scala tympani
Cochlear aperture
Cochlear nerve
Vestibular (Reissner) membrane
Basilar membrane
Osseous spiral lamina
Modiolus
Spiral ganglion
Fundus of internal auditory canal

(Top) Graphic of fluid spaces of inner ear viewed from above. The endolymph-filled structures include the vestibular utricle & saccule, semicircular ducts, scala media of cochlea, endolymphatic duct & sac. The perilymph-filled areas include the vestibule surrounding the utricle & saccule, between semicircular ducts & walls of the semicircular canals, within the vestibular aqueduct surrounding the endolymphatic duct and the scala tympani and vestibuli. **(Bottom)** Graphic of axial view of cochlea shows the 3 scalar chambers, scala media, scala vestibuli & scala tympani. Notice the bipolar cell bodies of the spiral ganglia within the modiolus send distal fibers to the organ of Corti and proximal fibers into the cochlear nerve. The cochlear nerve passes through the cochlear aperture into the fundus of the internal auditory canal.

COCHLEA

AXIAL BONE CT

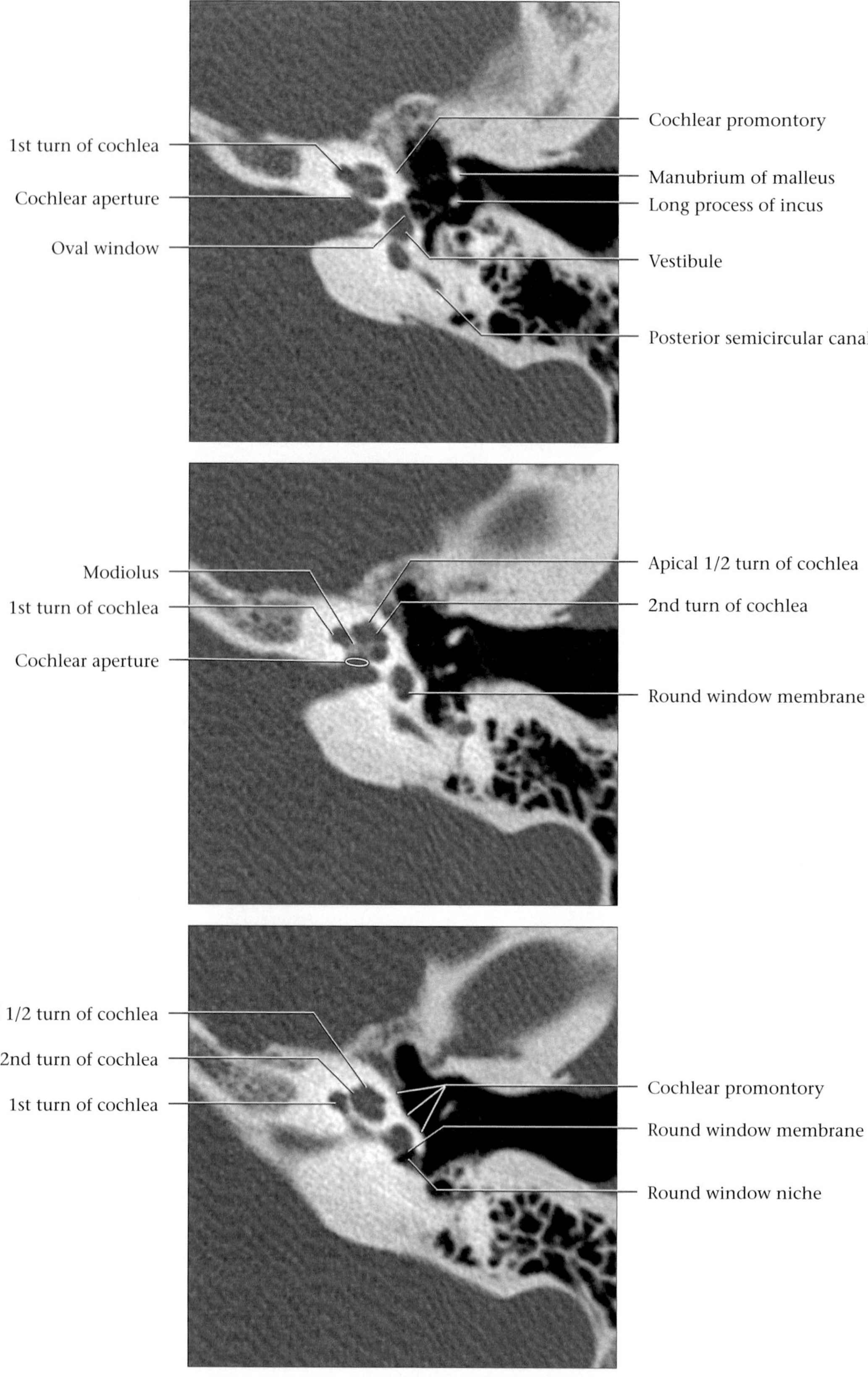
1st turn of cochlea
Cochlear aperture
Oval window
Cochlear promontory
Manubrium of malleus
Long process of incus
Vestibule
Posterior semicircular canal
Modiolus
1st turn of cochlea
Cochlear aperture
Apical 1/2 turn of cochlea
2nd turn of cochlea
Round window membrane
Apical 1/2 turn of cochlea
2nd turn of cochlea
1st turn of cochlea
Cochlear promontory
Round window membrane
Round window niche

(Top) First of three axial bone CT images presented from superior to inferior shows the membranous labyrinth fluid space of the cochlea as low density compared to the high density bony labyrinth. **(Middle)** In this image through the mid-cochlea the full cochlear aperture is visible at the base of the cochlea. Just inside the cochlear base the modiolus is seen. The modiolus looks like a higher density crown-shaped structure. Notice that the cochlear turns are well seen in this image. **(Bottom)** In this image through the basal 1st turn of the cochlea it is possible to see the posterolateral origin of the basal turn at the round window membrane. The middle ear wall of the cochlea is referred to as the cochlear promontory.

COCHLEA

AXIAL T2 MR

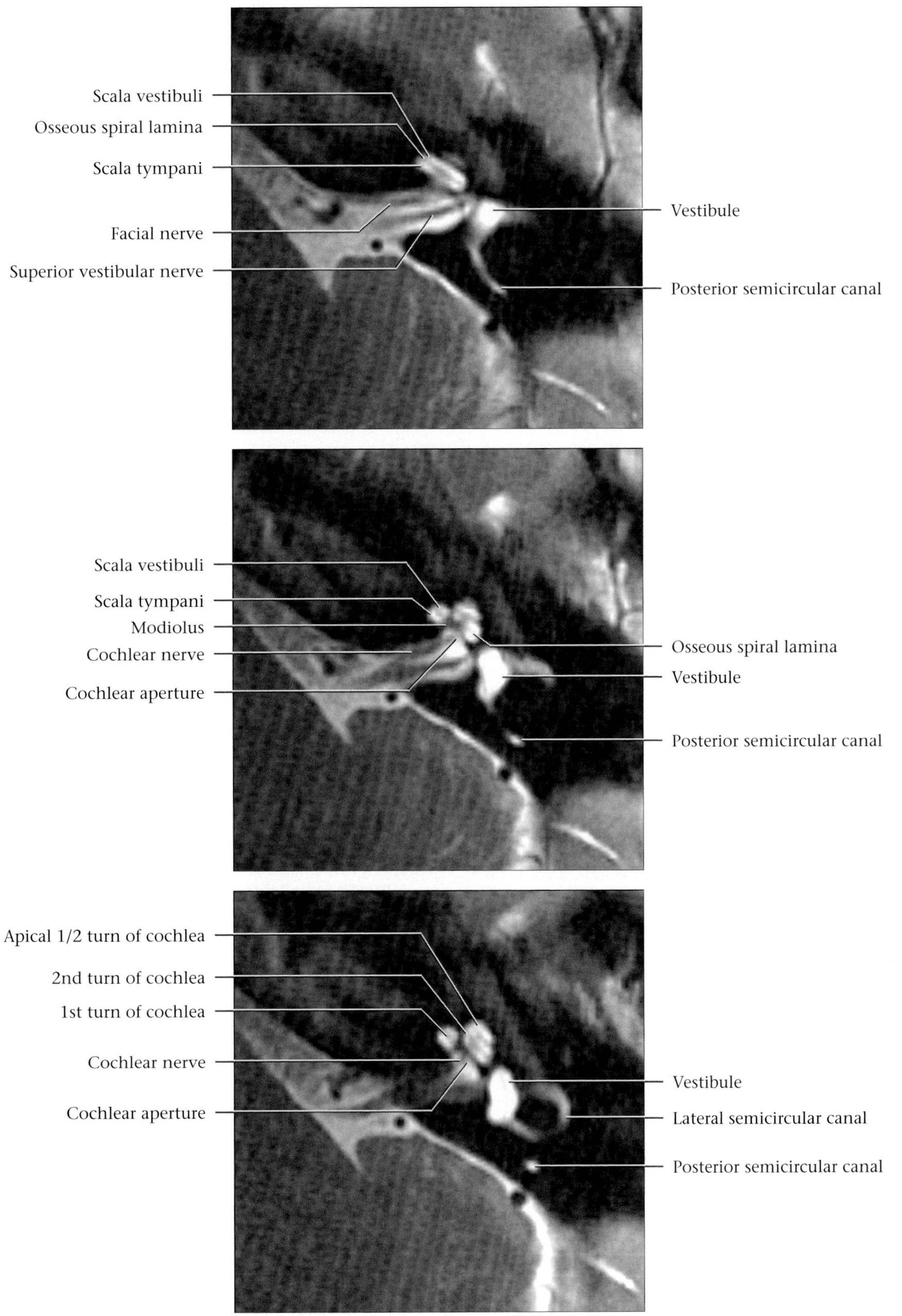
Scala vestibuli
Osseous spiral lamina
Scala tympani
Facial nerve
Superior vestibular nerve
Vestibule
Posterior semicircular canal
Scala vestibuli
Scala tympani
Modiolus
Cochlear nerve
Cochlear aperture
Osseous spiral lamina
Vestibule
Posterior semicircular canal
Apical 1/2 turn of cochlea
2nd turn of cochlea
1st turn of cochlea
Cochlear nerve
Cochlear aperture
Vestibule
Lateral semicircular canal
Posterior semicircular canal

(Top) First of 3 axial T2 MR images of inner ear presented from superior to inferior reveals high signal membranous labyrinth within the low signal bony labyrinth. The cochlea is divided by osseous spiral lamina into an anterior scala vestibuli & a posterior scala tympani. Note that the scala vestibuli & tympani have equal transverse dimensions. **(Middle)** In this image through the mid-cochlea the cochlear nerve is visible in the anteroinferior IAC. The cochlear nerve exits the fundus of the internal auditory canal to enter the cochlea through the cerebrospinal fluid filled cochlear aperture. The modiolus is visible as a intermediate intensity structure at the cochlear base. **(Bottom)** The 1st and 2nd turns and the apical 1/2 turn of the cochlea are all visible on this image. Also notice the cochlear nerve in the cochlear aperture on its way to the modiolus.

INTRATEMPORAL FACIAL NERVE

Terminology

Abbreviations

- Facial nerve: CN7

Definitions

- Intratemporal facial nerve: CN7 as it passes through temporal bone from its entrance into internal auditory canal (IAC) to its exit at stylomastoid foramen

Imaging Anatomy

Overview

- CN7 enters temporal bone as a mixed cranial nerve with motor, parasympathetic & taste functions
- Intratemporal segment is one of four
  - Intra-axial, cisternal & extracranial are other three
- Intratemporal CN7 extends from porus acusticus of IAC to stylomastoid foramen

Internal Structures-Critical Contents

- CN7 intratemporal segment divided into four subsegments: IAC, labyrinthine, tympanic & mastoid
- **IAC segment intracranial CN7**
  - Extent: Porus acusticus to IAC fundus
  - Relationship: Anterosuperior position above crista falciformis
  - Branches: None
- **Labyrinthine segment intratemporal CN7**
  - Extent: Connects fundal CN7 to geniculate ganglion
  - Relationship: Passes through bony labyrinth just superior to cochlea
  - Branches: None
- **Geniculate ganglion** (anterior genu)
  - Extent: Single site anterosuperior to cochlea
  - Branches: Greater superficial petrosal nerve
- **Tympanic segment intratemporal CN7** (horizontal segment)
  - Extent: Connects anterior to posterior genu
  - Relationship: Passes immediately under lateral semicircular canal
  - Branches: None
- **Posterior genu**
  - Extent: Elbow of CN7 turning tympanic segment into mastoid segment
- **Mastoid segment intratemporal CN7**
  - Extent: Connects posterior genu to stylomastoid foramen
  - Relationship: Passes inferiorly in bone just posterior to facial nerve recess
  - Branches: Stapedius nerve & chorda tympani nerve
- **Facial nerve branches**
  - **Greater superficial petrosal nerve**
    - Arises from geniculate ganglion, passing anteromedially to exit T-bone via facial hiatus
    - Carries parasympathetic fibers on way to lacrimal gland
  - **Stapedius nerve**
    - Arise from high mastoid segment CN7
    - Provides motor innervation to stapedius muscle
  - **Chorda tympani nerve**
    - Arises from lower mastoid segment of CN7
    - Arches anterosuperiorly to enter middle ear cavity
    - Courses across middle ear cavity passing between malleus & incus
    - Exits anterior wall of middle ear cavity
    - Carries taste fibers from anterior 2/3 tongue retrograde & parasympathetic fibers antegrade to sublingual & submandibular glands
  - **Terminal motor branches**
    - Beyond chorda tympani branch of CN7 mastoid segment has only motor fibers
    - Pure motor CN7 exits stylomastoid foramen to become extracranial CN7
- Facial nerve arteries
  - Superficial petrosal branch (petrosal artery) of middle meningeal artery supplies greater superficial petrosal nerve & geniculate ganglion
  - Stylomastoid branch of posterior auricular artery supplies mastoid & tympanic segments of CN7

Anatomy-Based Imaging Issues

Key Concepts or Questions

- In all temporal bone imaging studies (CT or MR), radiologist **must** inspect entire course of facial nerve!

Imaging Recommendations

- Enhanced, thin-section fat-saturated MR best for peripheral facial nerve paralysis
  - If lesion found along intratemporal segments of CN7, T-bone CT vital to further assess anatomy & characterize lesion
- In peripheral facial nerve paralysis, be sure scan includes brainstem, CPA, IAC, T-bone & **parotid**

Imaging Pitfalls

- Imaging routine Bell palsy unnecessary
- Mild enhancement of labyrinthine segment, geniculate ganglion & anterior tympanic segment of CN7 is normal on enhanced T1 MR
  - Results from circumneural arteriovenous plexus
  - This enhancement may be amplified by fundal acoustic schwannoma

Clinical Implications

Clinical Importance

- Peripheral facial nerve paralysis results from injury to "peripheral facial nerve"
  - "Peripheral facial nerve" defined as CN7 from its brainstem nucleus, through CPA, IAC, temporal bone to extracranial component
  - Injury to specific locations along peripheral facial nerve results in CN7 paralysis with addition location-specific symptoms
    - If lesion occurs proximal to geniculate ganglion, lacrimation, sound dampening & taste affected
    - If CN6 also injured, lesion should be in pons
    - If CN8 also injured, lesion should be in CPA-IAC
    - If lacrimation, sound dampening & taste variably affected, intratemporal lesion most likely
    - If CN7 special functions spared but peripheral CN7 paralysis present, parotid space implicated

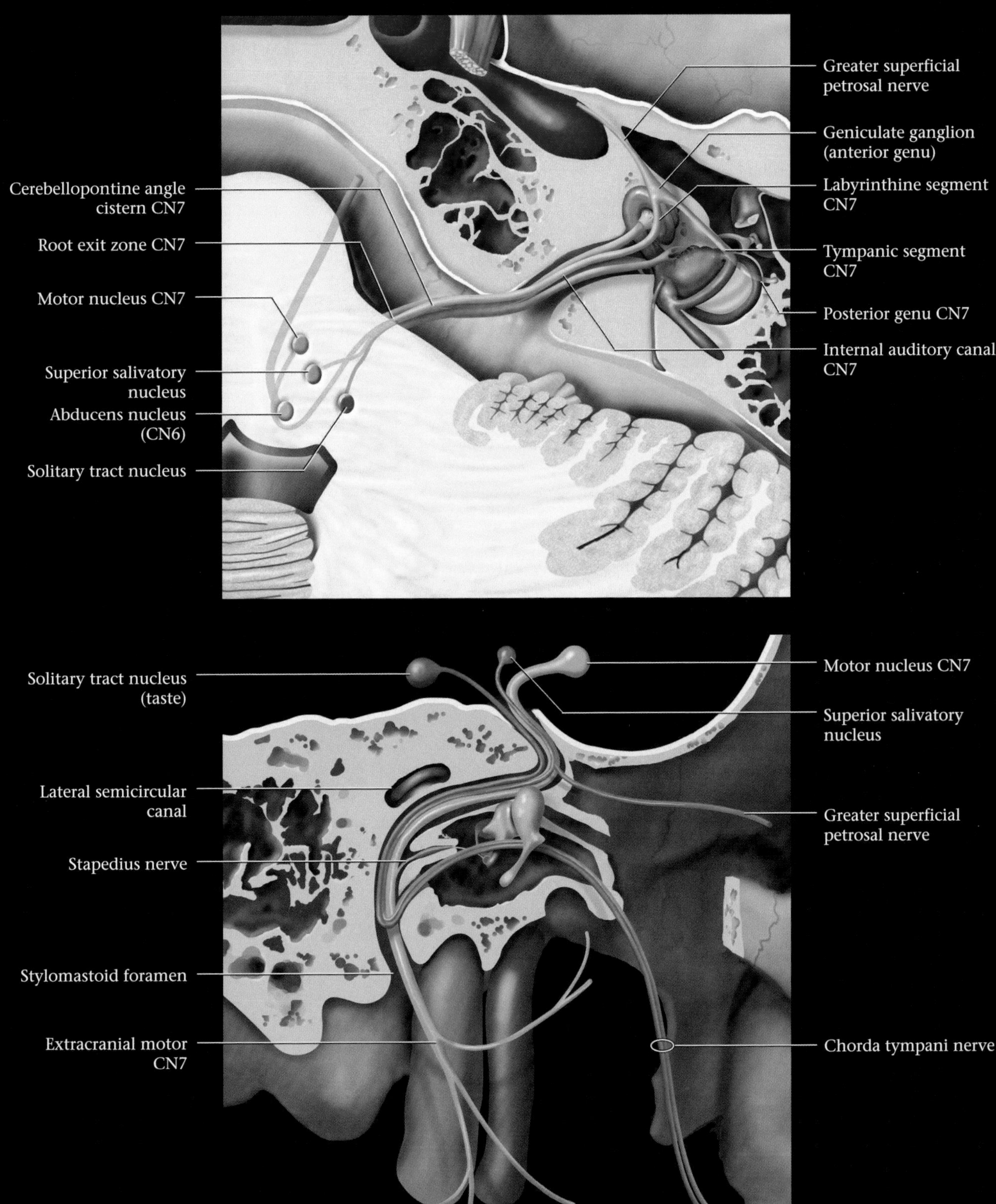
Cerebellopontine angle cistern CN7
Root exit zone CN7
Motor nucleus CN7
Superior salivatory nucleus
Abducens nucleus (CN6)
Solitary tract nucleus
Greater superficial petrosal nerve
Geniculate ganglion (anterior genu)
Labyrinthine segment CN7
Tympanic segment CN7
Posterior genu CN7
Internal auditory canal CN7
Solitary tract nucleus (taste)
Lateral semicircular canal
Stapedius nerve
Stylomastoid foramen
Extracranial motor CN7
Motor nucleus CN7
Superior salivatory nucleus
Greater superficial petrosal nerve
Chorda tympani nerve

(Top) Axial graphic of CN7 from brainstem nuclei to upper mastoid segment. Motor nucleus sends out fibers to circle CN6 nucleus before reaching root exit zone at pontomedullary junction. Superior salivatory nucleus sends parasympathetic secretomotor fibers to lacrimal, submandibular & sublingual glands. Solitary tract nucleus receives anterior 2/3 tongue taste information. **(Bottom)** Sagittal graphic depicts intratemporal CN7. Motor fibers pass through T-bone, "giving rise to" stapedius nerve to stapedius muscle, then exits via stylomastoid foramen. Parasympathetic fibers from superior salivatory nucleus reach lacrimal gland via greater superficial petrosal nerve and submandibular & sublingual glands via chorda tympanic nerve. Anterior 2/3 tongue taste fibers come via chorda tympani nerve. Note chorda tympani nerve branches from mastoid segment above stylomastoid foramen.

INTRATEMPORAL FACIAL NERVE

AXIAL BONE CT

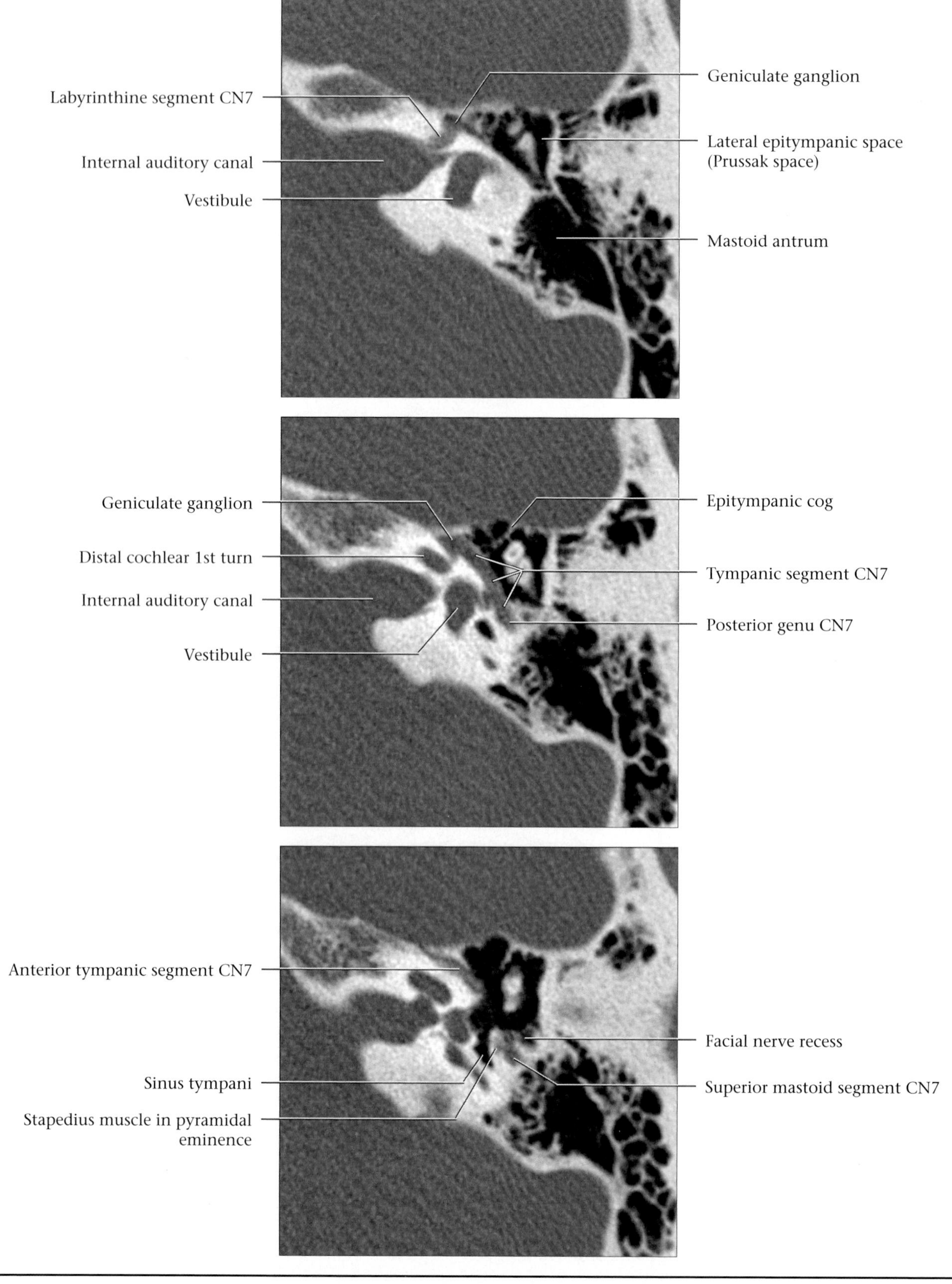
Labyrinthine segment CN7
Internal auditory canal
Vestibule
Geniculate ganglion
Lateral epitympanic space (Prussak space)
Mastoid antrum
Geniculate ganglion
Distal cochlear 1st turn
Internal auditory canal
Vestibule
Epitympanic cog
Tympanic segment CN7
Posterior genu CN7
Anterior tympanic segment CN7
Sinus tympani
Stapedius muscle in pyramidal eminence
Facial nerve recess
Superior mastoid segment CN7

(Top) First of six axial bone CT images of left ear presented from superior to inferior. In this image the labyrinthine segment of the facial nerve can be seen as a semilunar canal that exits the anterosuperior fundus of the internal auditory canal and terminates in the geniculate ganglion. This curved canal is in the bony labyrinth just above the cochlea. **(Middle)** In this image the entire course of the tympanic segment of the facial nerve is seen from its origin in the geniculate ganglion to its junction with the posterior genu. The tympanic segment of CN7 passes under the lateral semicircular canal. **(Bottom)** The superior mastoid segment of the facial nerve is seen in this image posterior to the facial nerve recess in the posterior wall of the middle ear cavity. Do not mistake the stapedius muscle for the mastoid segment of CN7.

AXIAL BONE CT

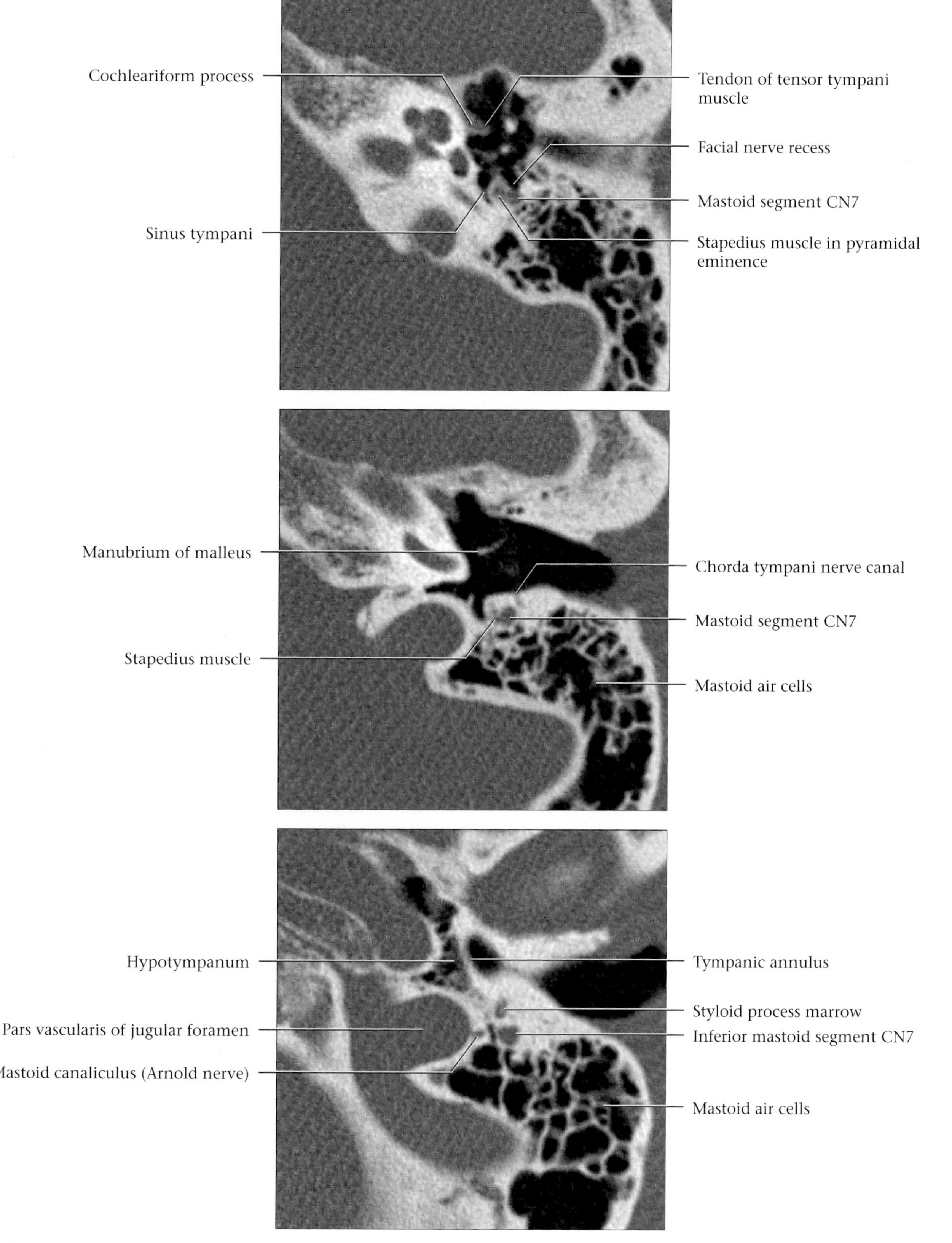

Cochleariform process
Tendon of tensor tympani muscle
Facial nerve recess
Mastoid segment CN7
Sinus tympani
Stapedius muscle in pyramidal eminence
Manubrium of malleus
Chorda tympani nerve canal
Mastoid segment CN7
Stapedius muscle
Mastoid air cells
Hypotympanum
Tympanic annulus
Styloid process marrow
Pars vascularis of jugular foramen
Inferior mastoid segment CN7
Mastoid canaliculus (Arnold nerve)
Mastoid air cells

(Top) The posterior wall of the middle ear cavity has 3 important contours. From medial to lateral they are the sinus tympani, pyramidal eminence and facial nerve recess. The mastoid segment of CN7 is found just posterior to the facial nerve recess while the belly of the stapedius muscle is seen just medial to this at the base of the pyramidal eminence. **(Middle)** At the level of the low mesotympanum the mastoid segment of CN7 is visible in the posterior wall of the middle ear. The inferior aspect of the belly of the stapedius muscle is seen just medial to the mastoid segment of CN7. Also notice the chorda tympani nerve exiting into the middle ear cavity. **(Bottom)** At the level of low mastoid segment of the facial nerve the styloid process marrow is seen anteriorly. Also note the mastoid canaliculus (canal of Arnold nerve) emerging from the lateral jugular foramen.

CORONAL BONE CT

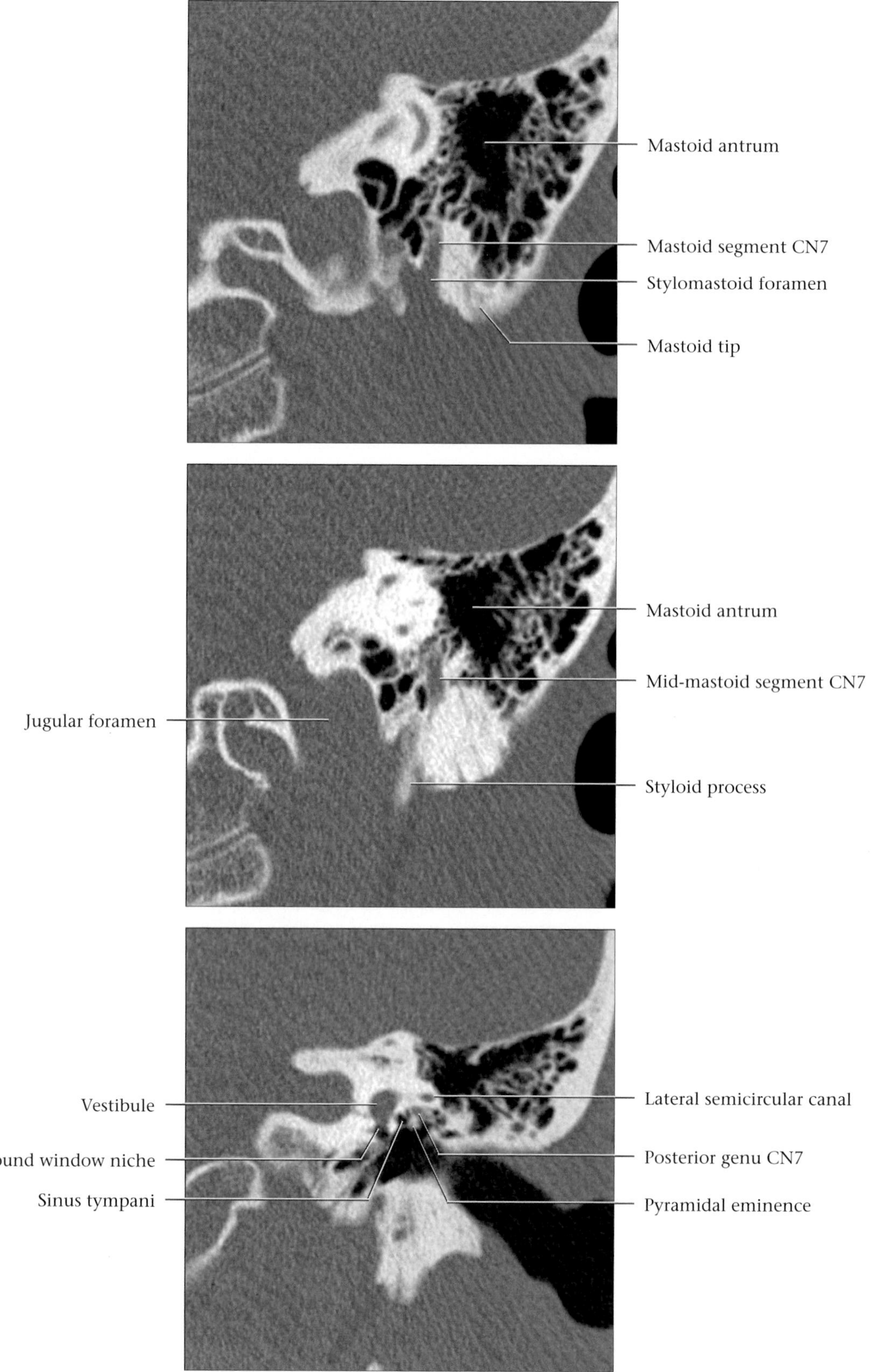
Mastoid antrum
Mastoid segment CN7
Stylomastoid foramen
Mastoid tip
Mastoid antrum
Mid-mastoid segment CN7
Jugular foramen
Styloid process
Vestibule
Round window niche
Sinus tympani
Lateral semicircular canal
Posterior genu CN7
Pyramidal eminence

(Top) First of six coronal bone CT images of the left ear presented from posterior to anterior. In this image the low mastoid segment of the facial nerve is visible. The stylomastoid foramen marks the transition from mastoid to extracranial segments of the facial nerve. The chorda tympani nerve exits from this area. **(Middle)** In this image the mid-mastoid segment of the facial nerve is seen just posterior to the facial nerve recess. The stapedius nerve exits in this area. **(Bottom)** The posterior genu can be seen just lateral to the pyramidal eminence. The posterior margin of the lateral semicircular canal is also visible on this image as are the sinus tympani and pyramidal eminence.

CORONAL BONE CT

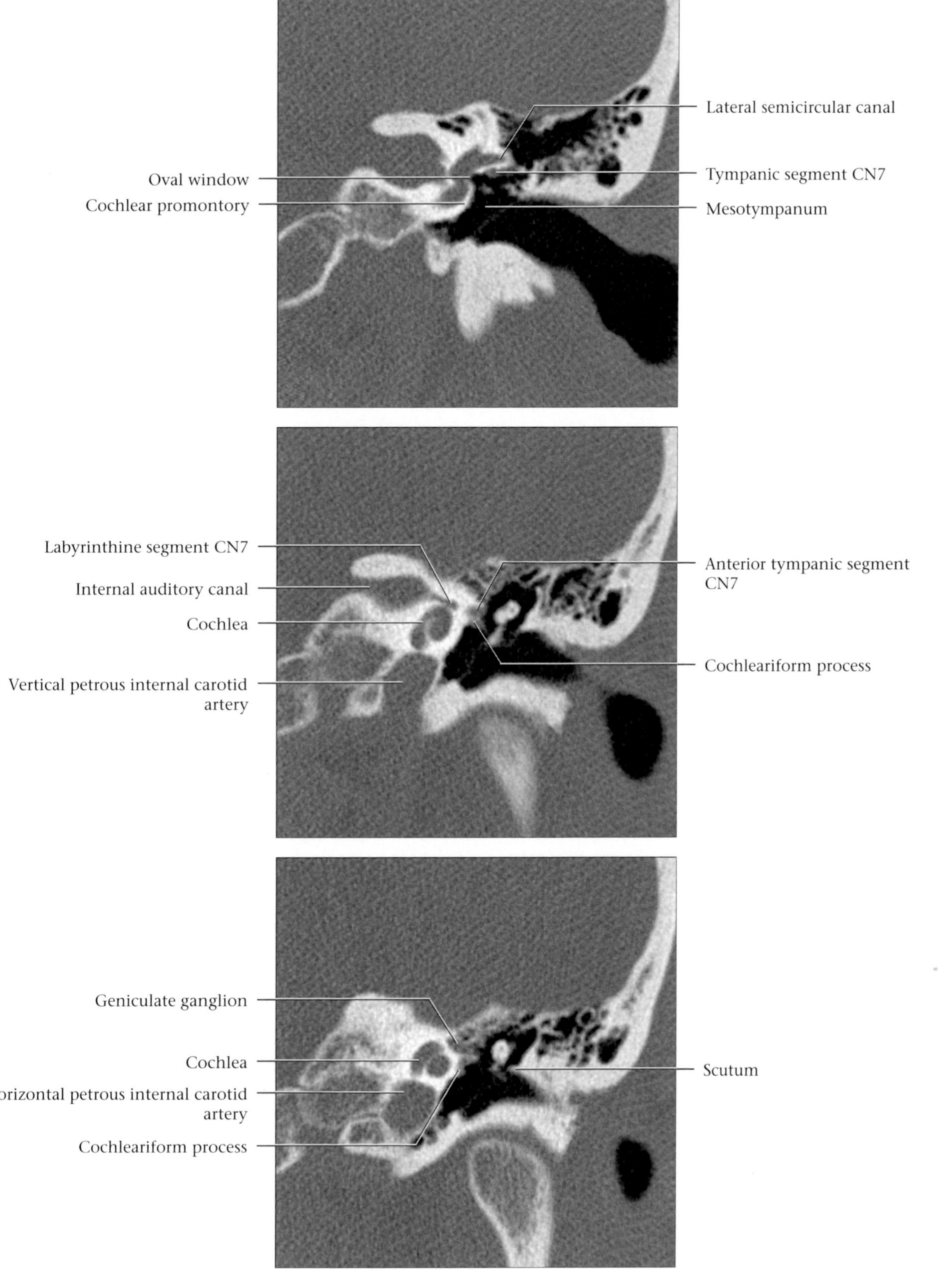
Lateral semicircular canal
Oval window
Tympanic segment CN7
Cochlear promontory
Mesotympanum
Labyrinthine segment CN7
Anterior tympanic segment CN7
Internal auditory canal
Cochlea
Cochleariform process
Vertical petrous internal carotid artery
Geniculate ganglion
Cochlea
Scutum
Horizontal petrous internal carotid artery
Cochleariform process

(Top) The mid-tympanic segment of CN7 is seen along the inferior surface of the lateral semicircular canal. A thin bony covering for CN7 is visible. Notice the position of the nerve relative to the inferomedial oval window. When oval window atresia is present, the tympanic segment is seen closer to or within the oval window niche as a associated finding. **(Middle)** In this image the labyrinthine segment of CN7 can be seen to exit the anterosuperior internal auditory canal. Also note the anterior tympanic segment of CN7 canal high on the medial wall of the middle ear cavity. Just inferiorly on the medial wall is the cochleariform process which through which the tendon of the tensor tympani tendon passes. **(Bottom)** Superolateral to the cochlea the geniculate ganglion is visible.

INTRATEMPORAL FACIAL NERVE

AXIAL BONE CT CHORDA TYMPANI NERVE

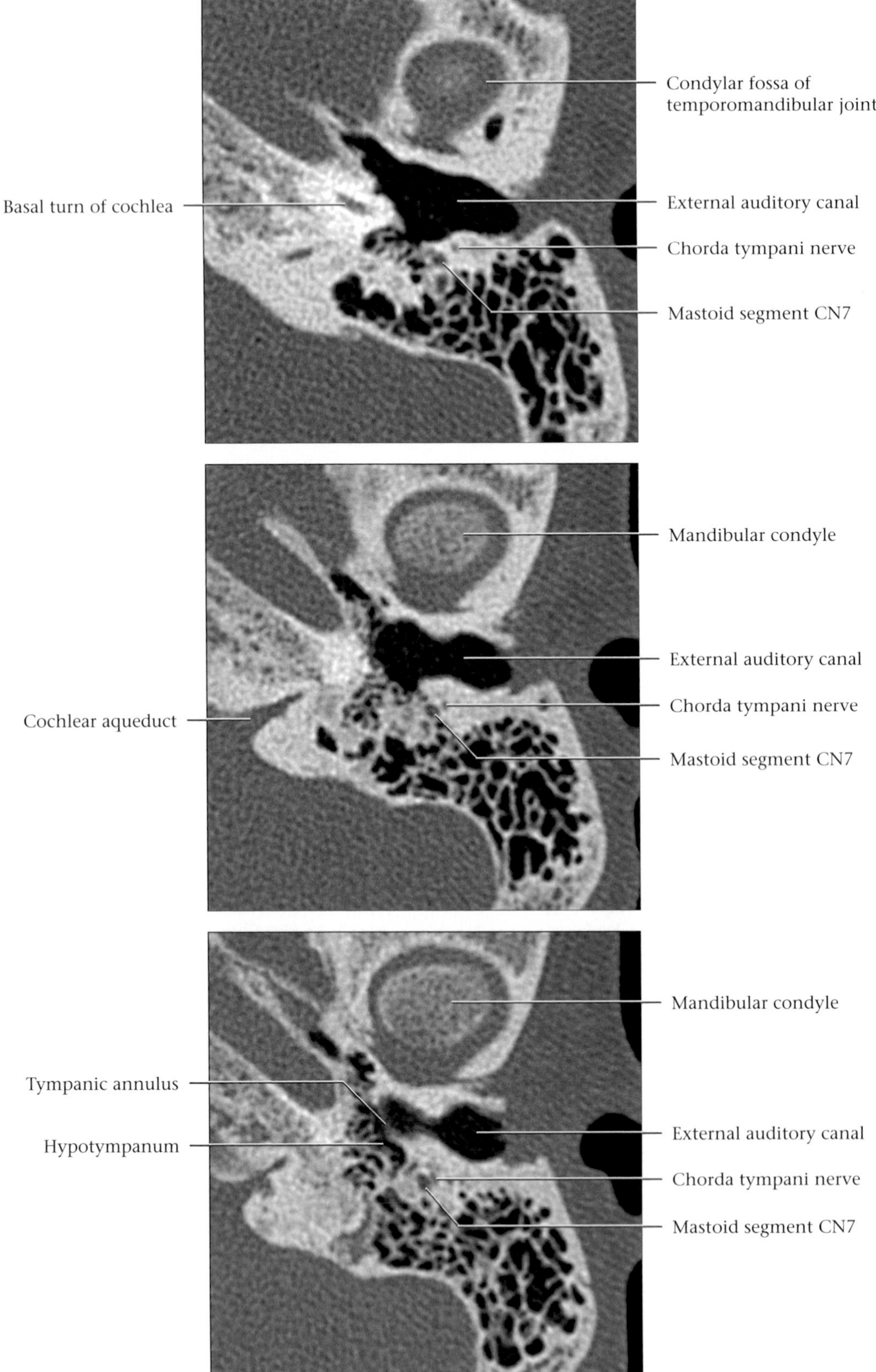
Condylar fossa of temporomandibular joint
Basal turn of cochlea
External auditory canal
Chorda tympani nerve
Mastoid segment CN7
Mandibular condyle
External auditory canal
Cochlear aqueduct
Chorda tympani nerve
Mastoid segment CN7
Mandibular condyle
Tympanic annulus
Hypotympanum
External auditory canal
Chorda tympani nerve
Mastoid segment CN7

(Top) First of three magnified axial bone CT images of the left ear presented from superior to inferior demonstrating the canal of the chorda tympani nerve. In this image the chorda tympani nerve is seen just before exiting into the middle ear cavity. Remember the chorda tympani nerve contains efferent parasympathetic fibers to submandibular and sublingual glands as well as afferent anterior 2/3 tongue taste fibers. **(Middle)** In this image the chorda tympani nerve can be seen approaching its origin from the low mastoid segment of the facial nerve. **(Bottom)** The chorda tympani nerve is visible in this image budding from the lateral margin of the low mastoid segment of the facial nerve. Notice that this image is taken through the upper margin of the tympanic annulus and is therefore at the level of the hypotympanum.

CORONAL BONE CT CHORDA TYMPANI NERVE

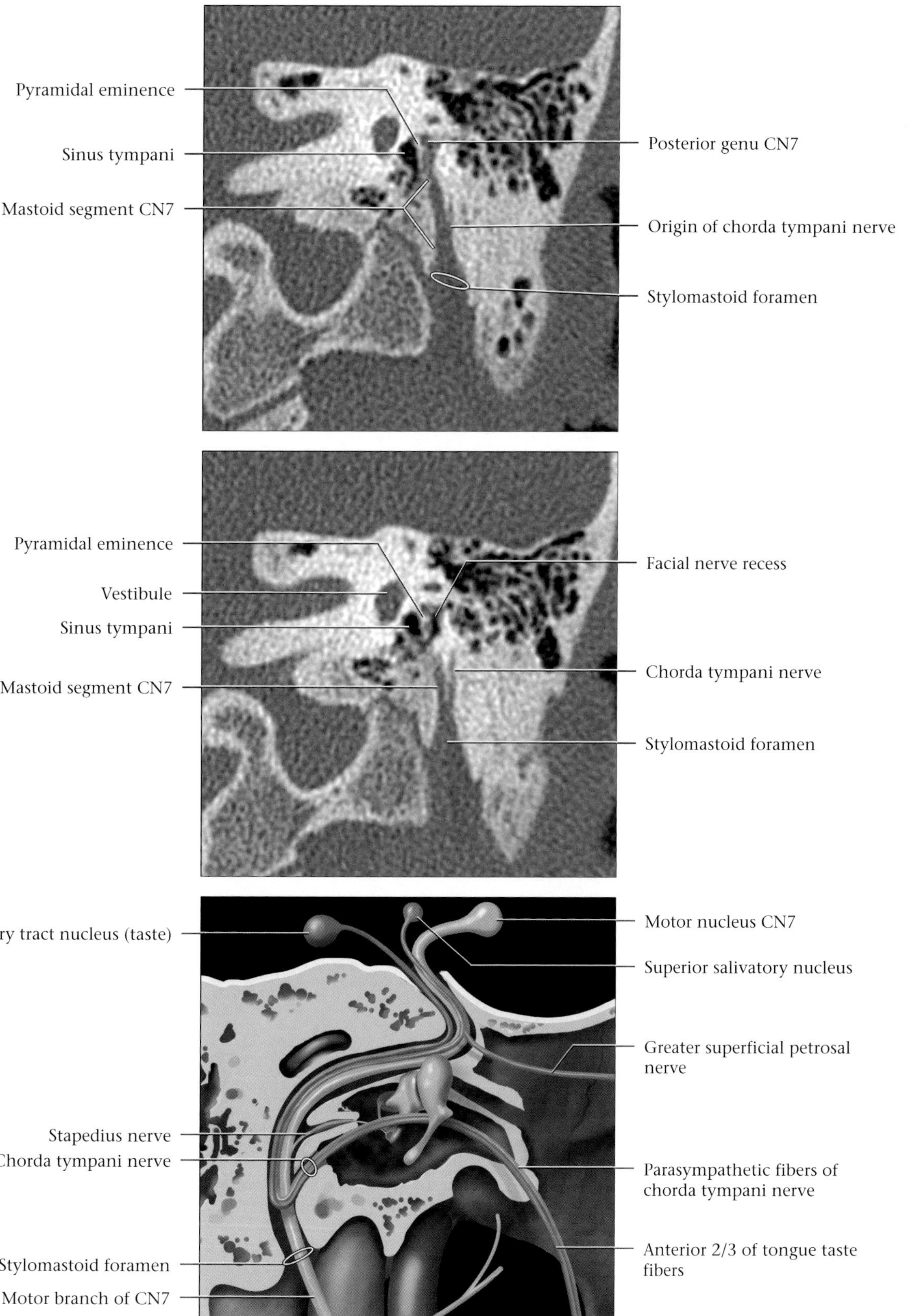

Pyramidal eminence
Sinus tympani
Mastoid segment CN7
Posterior genu CN7
Origin of chorda tympani nerve
Stylomastoid foramen
Pyramidal eminence
Vestibule
Sinus tympani
Mastoid segment CN7
Facial nerve recess
Chorda tympani nerve
Stylomastoid foramen
Solitary tract nucleus (taste)
Stapedius nerve
Chorda tympani nerve
Stylomastoid foramen
Motor branch of CN7
Motor nucleus CN7
Superior salivatory nucleus
Greater superficial petrosal nerve
Parasympathetic fibers of chorda tympani nerve
Anterior 2/3 of tongue taste fibers

(Top) First of two coronal bone CT images of the left ear presented from posterior to anterior shows the mastoid segment of the facial nerve from its origin at the posterior genu and its skull base exit at the stylomastoid foramen. The site of origin of the chorda tympani nerve from the mastoid segment can be seen along its lateral margin. **(Middle)** This image reveals the distal mastoid segment of the facial nerve. The canal of the chorda tympani nerve is visible as a cephalad projecting channel branching from the lateral mastoid segment. **(Bottom)** Magnified sagittal graphic of intratemporal CN7 & its branches. Chorda tympani branch of CN7 is seen approximately 2/3 of way down mastoid segment of facial nerve. Note the chorda tympani nerve has efferent parasympathetic fibers to submandibular & sublingual gland and efferent taste fibers from anterior 2/3 of tongue.

INTRATEMPORAL FACIAL NERVE

AXIAL T2 MR

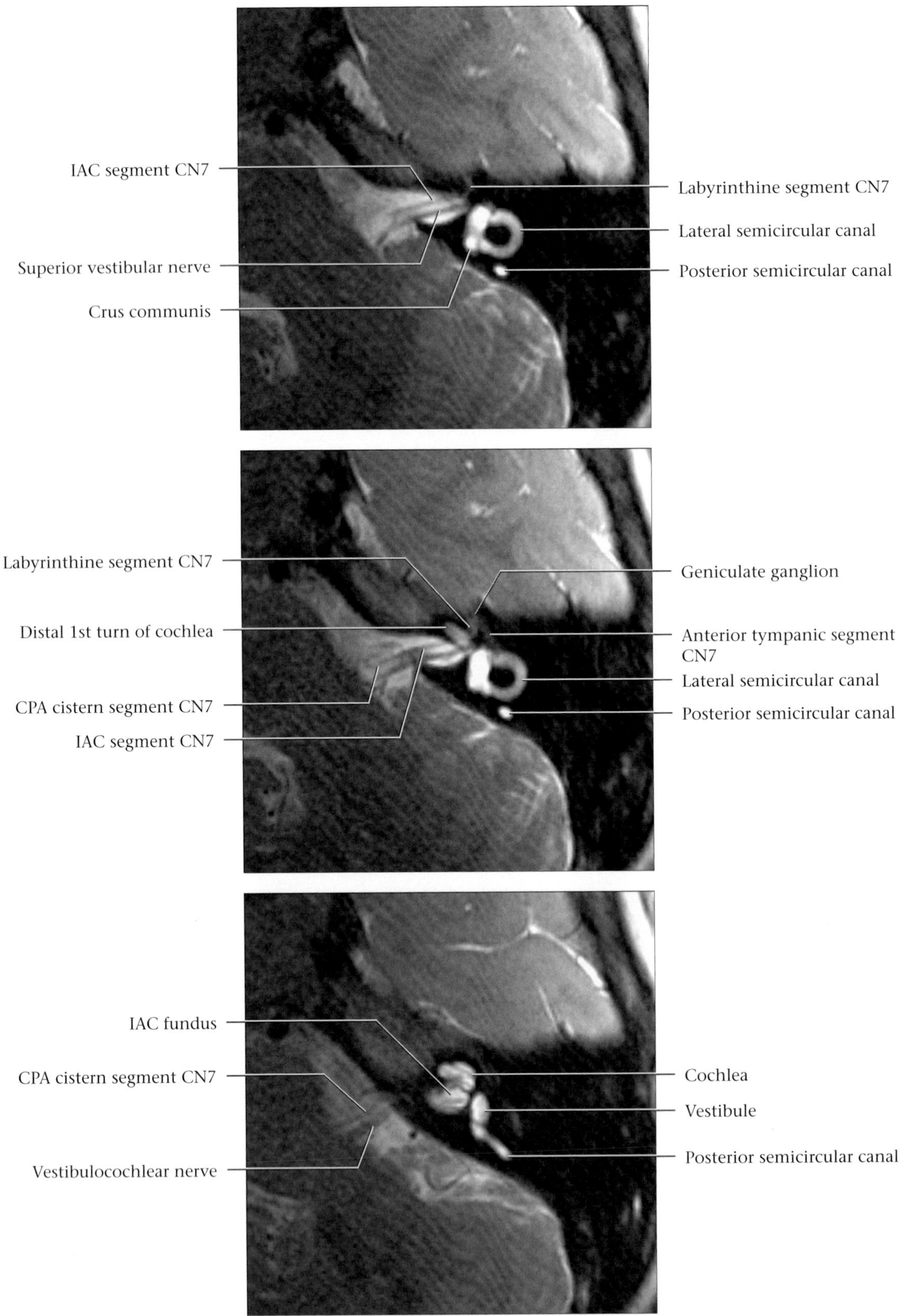
IAC segment CN7
Superior vestibular nerve
Crus communis
Labyrinthine segment CN7
Lateral semicircular canal
Posterior semicircular canal
Labyrinthine segment CN7
Distal 1st turn of cochlea
CPA cistern segment CN7
IAC segment CN7
Geniculate ganglion
Anterior tympanic segment CN7
Lateral semicircular canal
Posterior semicircular canal
IAC fundus
CPA cistern segment CN7
Vestibulocochlear nerve
Cochlea
Vestibule
Posterior semicircular canal

(Top) First of three axial high-resolution thin-section T2 MR images of left ear presented from superior to inferior. In this image the internal auditory canal segment of the facial nerve is visible in the anterosuperior quadrant. At the fundus of the IAC the anterior curving soft tissue structure is the labyrinthine segment of the facial nerve. **(Middle)** In this image the labyrinthine segment can be seen passing just superior to the cochlea in the bony labyrinth. It terminates in the geniculate ganglion (anterior genu), then turns and becomes the tympanic segment of the facial nerve which projects posterolaterally to run underneath the lateral semicircular canal. **(Bottom)** The CPA cistern segment of the facial nerve is visible in this image just anterior to the vestibulocochlear nerve. This more anterior position persists across the cerebellopontine angle cistern.

AXIAL T1 C+ MR

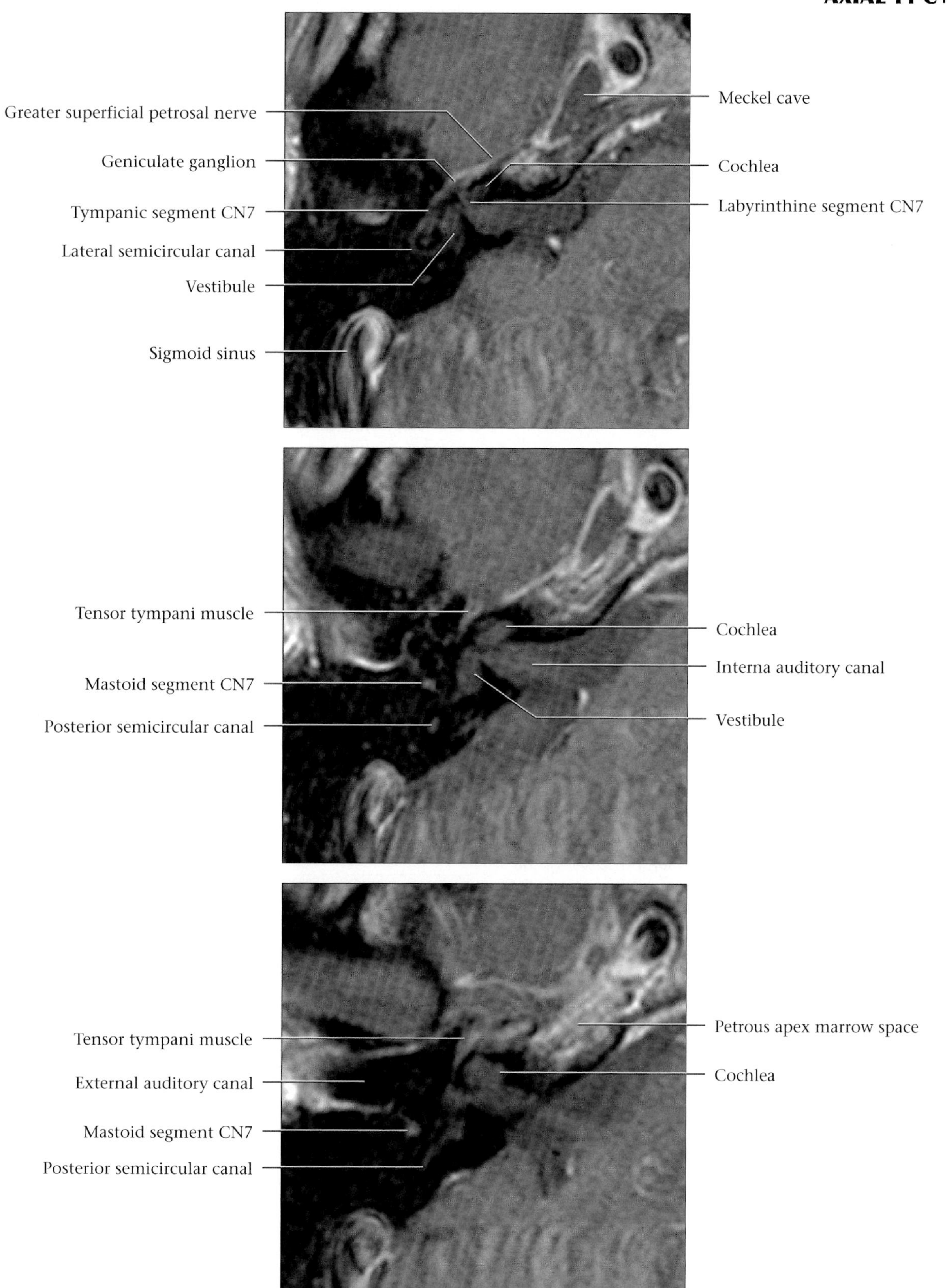
Greater superficial petrosal nerve
Geniculate ganglion
Tympanic segment CN7
Lateral semicircular canal
Vestibule
Sigmoid sinus
Meckel cave
Cochlea
Labyrinthine segment CN7
Tensor tympani muscle
Mastoid segment CN7
Posterior semicircular canal
Cochlea
Interna auditory canal
Vestibule
Tensor tympani muscle
External auditory canal
Mastoid segment CN7
Posterior semicircular canal
Petrous apex marrow space
Cochlea

(Top) First of three axial T1 C+ MR images without fat-saturation of the right temporal bone presented from superior to inferior. These magnified 3T MR images amplify areas of enhancement. Notice the circumneural arteriovenous plexus enhancing the greater superficial petrosal nerve, geniculate ganglion and anterior tympanic segment of the facial nerve. The labyrinthine segment does not normally enhance. **(Middle)** In this image the tensor tympani muscle is enhancing just below the anterior tympanic segment of the facial nerve (not seen on this image). Do not mistake one for the other. The superior mastoid segment of the facial nerve and the area of the posterior genu may also enhance normally. **(Bottom)** The superior mastoid segment of CN7 is seen normally enhancing in this image. The circumneural arteriovenous plexus is thought to be responsible for this appearance.

MIDDLE EAR AND OSSICLES

Terminology

Abbreviations

- Temporal bone (T-bone)
- Middle ear (ME)

Definitions

- Ossicles: 3 smallest bones in human body (malleus, incus & stapes) in the middle ear that amplify sound vibrations, conveying them from tympanic membrane to oval window
- Middle ear: Six-sided cavity between external ear & inner ear, containing 3 ossicles, 2 muscles & opening to eustachian tube

Imaging Anatomy

Anatomy Relationships

- ME sits in T-bone between external & inner ears

Internal Structures-Critical Contents

- **Middle ear subdivisions**
  - **Epitympanum** (attic): Tegmen tympani is roof with floor defined by line between scutum & tympanic segment of facial nerve
    - **Prussak space**: Lateral epitympanic recess
    - **Anterior epitympanic recess**: Epitympanic recess anteromedial to epitympanic "cog"; medial wall is anterior tympanic segment CN7
    - **Tegmen tympani** (L. for "roof of cavity"): Thin bony roof between epitympanum & middle cranial fossa dura
    - **Aditus ad antrum** (L. for "entrance to cave"): Connects epitympanum of middle ear to mastoid antrum
  - **Mesotympanum**: Middle ear cavity between line connecting scutum & tympanic segment CN7 above & line connecting tympanic annulus & base of cochlear promontory below
    - Posterior wall (posterior tympanum) has 3 important structures: Facial nerve recess, pyramidal eminence & sinus tympani
    - Medial wall: Lateral semicircular canal, tympanic segment CN7, oval & round window found here
  - **Hypotympanum**: Shallow trough in floor of middle ear cavity
- **Middle ear muscles**
  - **Tensor tympani muscle**
    - Muscle found anteroinferior to anterior tympanic segment CN7
    - Tendon passes through cochleariform process, then attaches to neck of malleus
    - Innervated by CNV3
  - **Stapedius muscle**
    - Muscle found just medial to upper mastoid segment CN7
    - Tendon emerges from apex of pyramidal eminence, then attaches to head or posterior crura of stapes
    - Innervated by CN7 motor branch of mastoid segment
- **Ossicles of middle ear**
  - **Malleus** (hammer)
    - Location: Anterior epitympanum & mesotympanum
    - Components: Head, neck, lateral process, anterior process & manubrium
    - Ligaments: Superior, anterior, lateral mallear ligaments & tendon of tensor tympani muscle
  - **Incus** (anvil)
    - Location: Posterior epitympanum & mesotympanum
    - Components: Body, short, long & **lenticular processes**
    - Ligament: Posterior incudal ligament
  - **Stapes** (stirrup)
    - Location: Medial mesotympanum
    - Components: Head, anterior & posterior crura & footplate
    - Ligament: Ligament of stapedius muscle attaches to stapes
    - **Stapes superstructure**: Stapes portion derived from 2nd branchial arch = head, crura, tympanic portion of footplate
    - Vestibular portion of footplate of stapes & annular ligament derived from otic capsule
- **Tympanic membrane** (TM)
  - Separates external from middle ear
  - Upper 1/3 = **pars flaccida**; lower 2/3 = **pars tensa**
  - Malleus umbo & lateral process embedded in TM
  - Three layers of TM
    - External layer continuous with skin of EAC = ectoderm
    - Inner layer continuous with middle ear mucosa = endoderm
    - Intermediate fibrous layer = mesoderm
  - Superior attachment: **Scutum** (L. for "shield")
  - Inferior attachment: **Tympanic annulus**

Clinical Implications

Clinical Importance

- EAC-tympanic membrane-ossicles-oval window
  - Conductive chain disruption results in conductive hearing loss

Embryology

Embryologic Events

- EAC forms from 1st branchial groove
- Middle ear forms from 1st branchial pouch
- Ossicles form from 1st & 2nd branchial arches
  - 1st branchial arch: Head & neck of malleus, body & short process of incus
  - 2nd branchial arch: Manubrium of malleus, long & lenticular processes of incus, stapes superstructure

Practical Implications

- EAC atresia is 1st & 2nd branchial apparatus lesion
- Ossicular rotation & deformity part of imaging appearance
- Oval window atresia may or may not be associated with EAC atresia

MIDDLE EAR AND OSSICLES

GRAPHICS

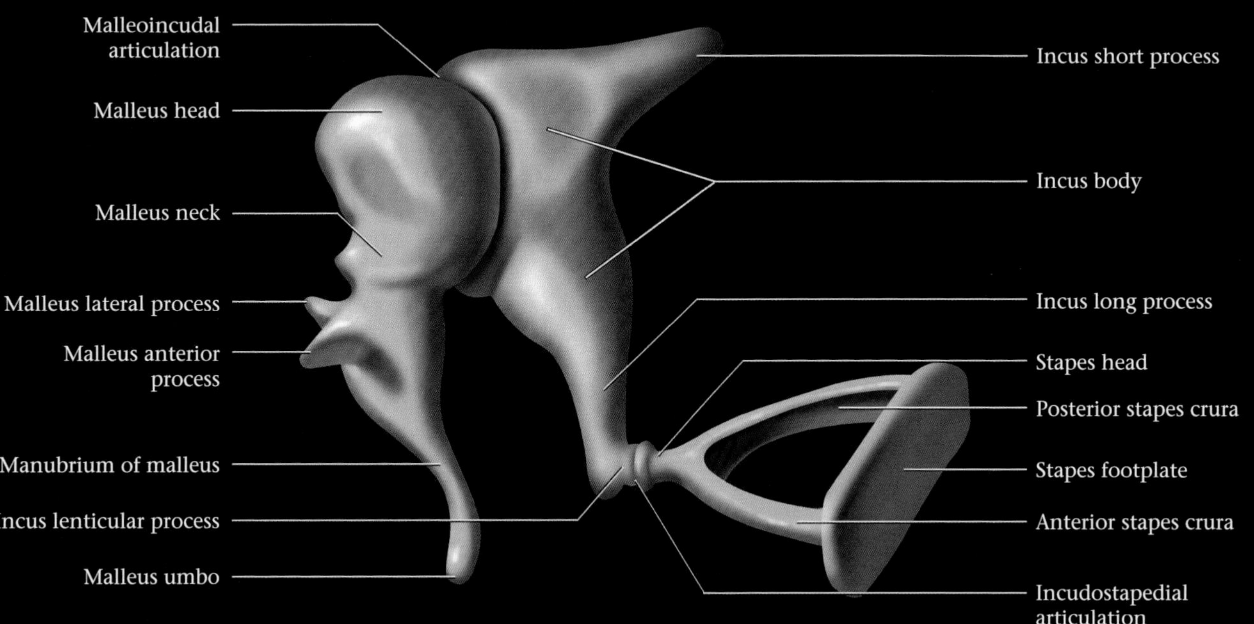

Malleoincudal articulation
Malleus head
Malleus neck
Malleus lateral process
Malleus anterior process
Manubrium of malleus
Incus lenticular process
Malleus umbo
Incus short process
Incus body
Incus long process
Stapes head
Posterior stapes crura
Stapes footplate
Anterior stapes crura
Incudostapedial articulation

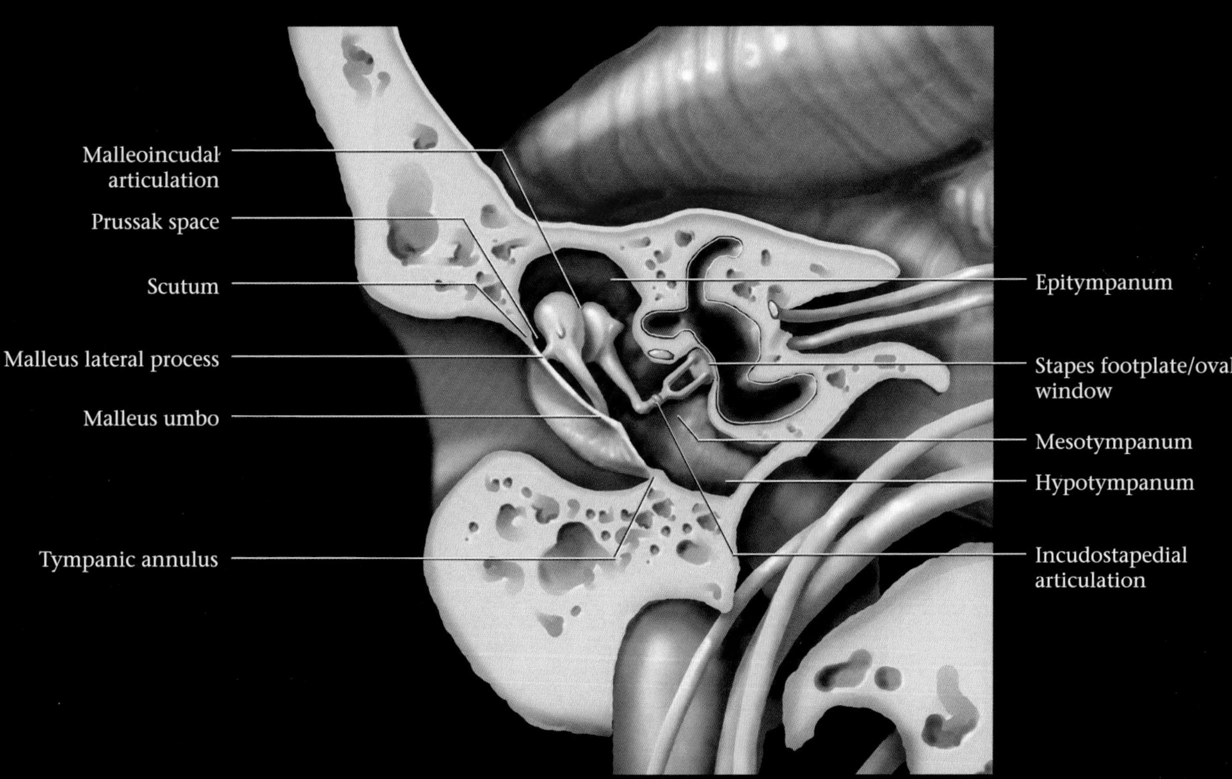

Malleoincudal articulation
Prussak space
Scutum
Malleus lateral process
Malleus umbo
Tympanic annulus
Epitympanum
Stapes footplate/oval window
Mesotympanum
Hypotympanum
Incudostapedial articulation

(Top) Graphic of right middle ear ossicles viewed from front. The anterolateral malleus has a head, neck, manubrium with lateral & anterior processes. The incus is the largest ossicle with a large body, a short & a long process and a lenticular process. The lenticular process & stapes hub meet at 90 degree angle. The stapes has a head, crura & a footplate. The space between stapes crura is called the obturator foramen. **(Bottom)** Coronal graphic of right temporal bone shows the conductive chain from the tympanic membrane to the oval window. Notice the lateral process and umbo of the malleus are embedded in the tympanic membrane. The TM is attached superiorly to the scutum & the tympanic annulus inferiorly. The two joints between the ossicles are the malleoincudal and the incudostapedial articulations.

MIDDLE EAR AND OSSICLES

AXIAL BONE CT

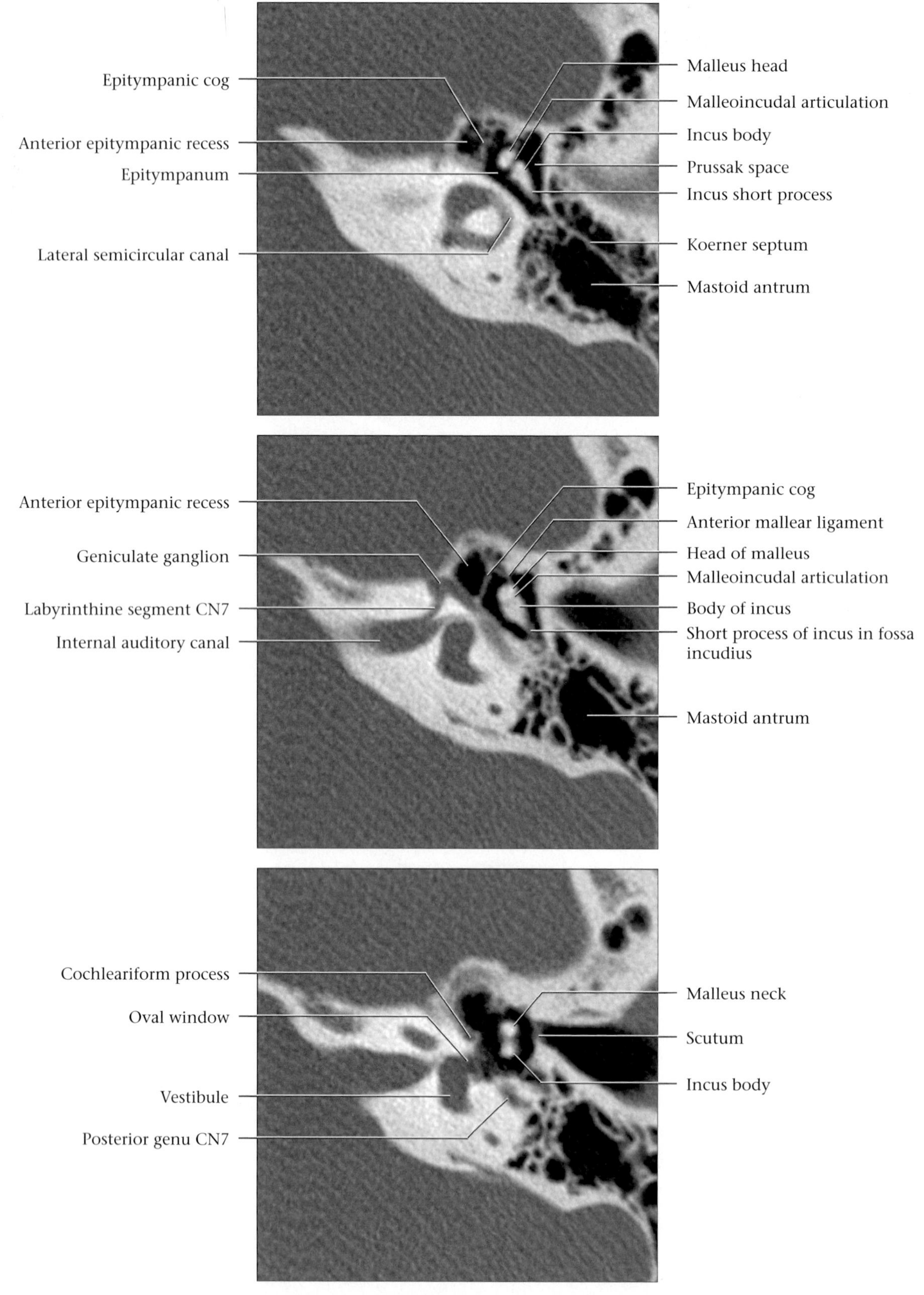

Epitympanic cog
Anterior epitympanic recess
Epitympanum
Lateral semicircular canal
Malleus head
Malleoincudal articulation
Incus body
Prussak space
Incus short process
Koerner septum
Mastoid antrum
Anterior epitympanic recess
Geniculate ganglion
Labyrinthine segment CN7
Internal auditory canal
Epitympanic cog
Anterior mallear ligament
Head of malleus
Malleoincudal articulation
Body of incus
Short process of incus in fossa incudius
Mastoid antrum
Cochleariform process
Oval window
Vestibule
Posterior genu CN7
Malleus neck
Scutum
Incus body

(Top) First of six magnified axial bone CT images of the left ear from superior to inferior shows malleus head articulating with the body of the incus at the malleoincudal articulation. Prussak space (lateral epitympanic recess) is seen lateral to the ossicles. The short process of the incus is "pointing" into the aditus ad antrum. **(Middle)** In this image through the level of the geniculate ganglion it is possible to see the anterior epitympanic recess defined by the epitympanic cog laterally and the anterior tympanic segment of the facial nerve. Diseases affecting this area may cause facial nerve paralysis. **(Bottom)** At the level of the oval window the malleus neck and incus body are seen in the upper mesotympanum. The facial nerve is transitioning from its tympanic segment to its mastoid segment as the posterior genu.

AXIAL BONE CT

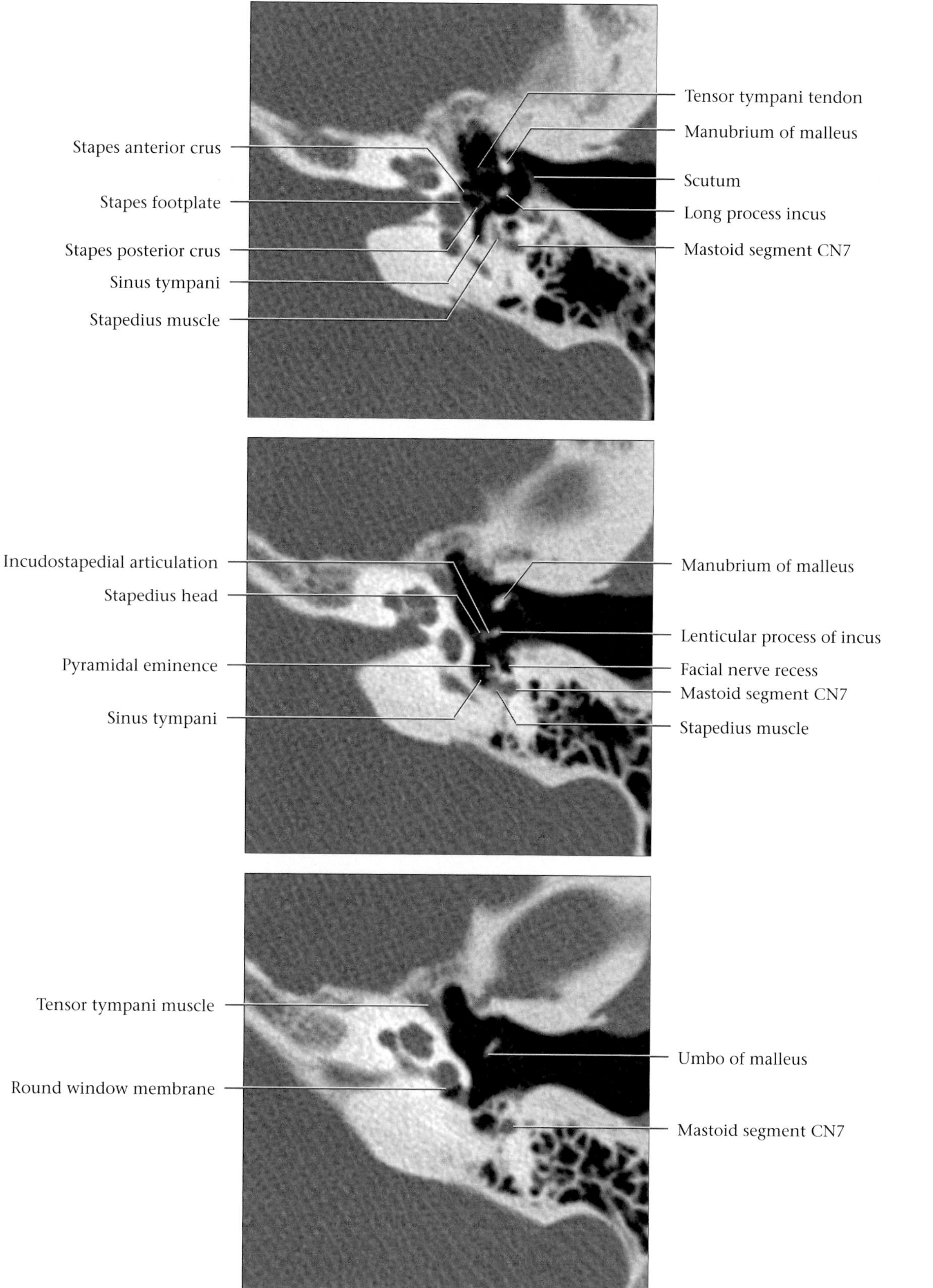
Tensor tympani tendon
Manubrium of malleus
Scutum
Long process incus
Mastoid segment CN7
Stapes anterior crus
Stapes footplate
Stapes posterior crus
Sinus tympani
Stapedius muscle
Incudostapedial articulation
Stapedius head
Pyramidal eminence
Sinus tympani
Manubrium of malleus
Lenticular process of incus
Facial nerve recess
Mastoid segment CN7
Stapedius muscle
Tensor tympani muscle
Round window membrane
Umbo of malleus
Mastoid segment CN7

(Top) In this image the anterior & posterior crura of the stapes are visible with the stapes footplate/oval window in between. The tensor tympani tendon can be seen reaching from the cochleariform process to the manubrium of the malleus. Both the stapedius muscle & the mastoid segment of the facial nerve are seen in the posterior tympanum wall. **(Middle)** In this image the ridges & recesses of the posterior tympanum are well seen. From medial to lateral they are the sinus tympani, pyramidal eminence & facial nerve recess. Behind these structures observe the stapedius muscle & the mastoid segment of CN7. Note the incudostapedial articulation connecting the lenticular process of the incus to the head of the stapes. **(Bottom)** The inferior tip of the manubrium is the umbo. At the round window membrane level the mastoid segment of CN7 is now seen without the stapedius muscle.

MIDDLE EAR AND OSSICLES

CORONAL BONE CT

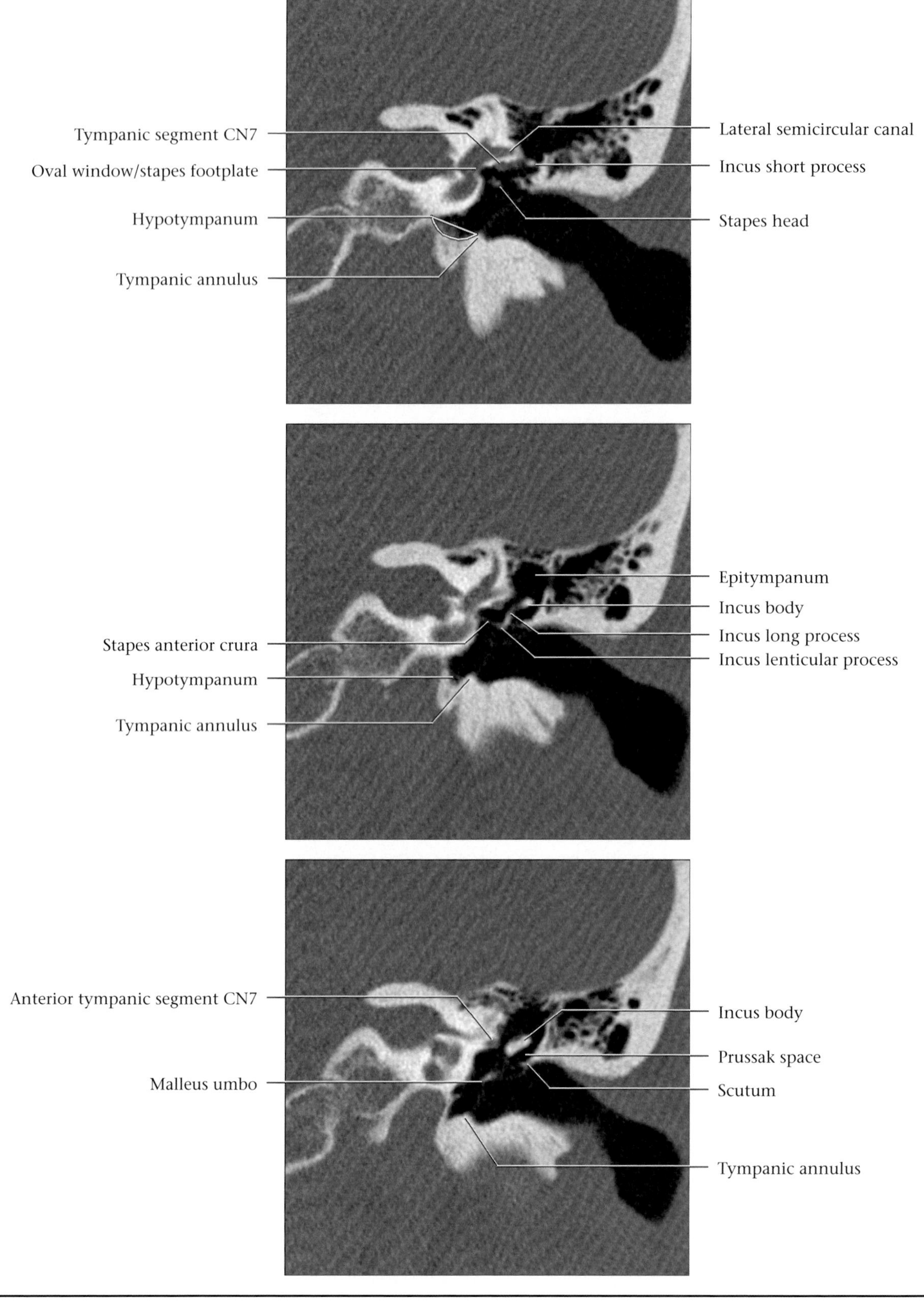
Tympanic segment CN7
Oval window/stapes footplate
Hypotympanum
Tympanic annulus
Lateral semicircular canal
Incus short process
Stapes head
Epitympanum
Incus body
Incus long process
Incus lenticular process
Stapes anterior crura
Hypotympanum
Tympanic annulus
Anterior tympanic segment CN7
Malleus umbo
Incus body
Prussak space
Scutum
Tympanic annulus

(Top) First of six coronal bone CT images of the left ear presented from posterior to anterior. In this image through the oval window notice how thin the normal stapes footplate is. **(Middle)** At the level of the anterior oval window margin the body, long process and lenticular process of the incus can be seen. **(Bottom)** In this image the body of the incus is seen at same level as umbo of malleus. The tympanic membrane is barely visible strung between the superior scutum and inferior tympanic annulus. The epitympanum is defined as the area of the middle ear cavity above a line drawn between the tip of the scutum and the tympanic segment of the facial nerve.

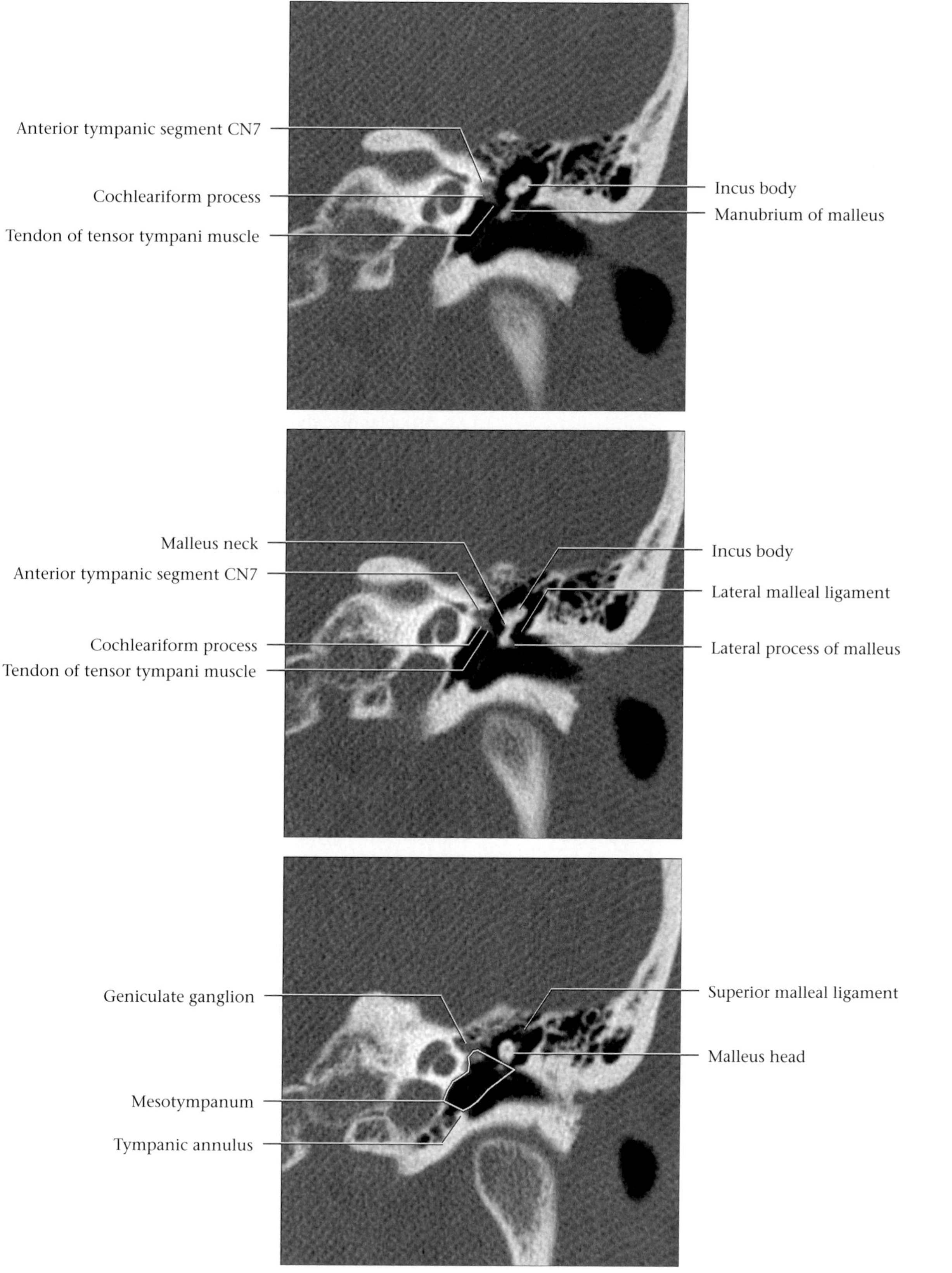
Anterior tympanic segment CN7
Cochleariform process
Tendon of tensor tympani muscle
Incus body
Manubrium of malleus
Malleus neck
Anterior tympanic segment CN7
Cochleariform process
Tendon of tensor tympani muscle
Incus body
Lateral malleal ligament
Lateral process of malleus
Geniculate ganglion
Mesotympanum
Tympanic annulus
Superior malleal ligament
Malleus head

(Top) In this image through the anterior tympanic cavity the tendon of the tensor tympani muscle is seen turning 90 degrees in the cochleariform process, then projecting over to the manubrium of the malleus. **(Middle)** The lateral process of the malleus and the umbo are both embedded in the medial surface of the tympanic membrane. The tendon of the tensor tympani muscle inserts on the medial surface of the manubrium of the malleus. **(Bottom)** In this image the head of the malleus can be seen in the anterior epitympanum. The mesotympanum can be defined as the middle ear cavity below the line connecting the tympanic segment of the facial nerve and the inferior tip of the scutum and above the line connecting the superior tip of the tympanic annulus and the inferior margin of the cochlear promontory.

TEMPOROMANDIBULAR JOINT

Terminology

Abbreviations

- Temporomandibular joint (TMJ)

Definitions

- **TMJ**: Articulation between mandible & temporal bone

Imaging Anatomy

Overview

- Complex diarthrodial joint with 2 functional movements
  - Rotatory movement in inferior compartment between mandibular condyle & articular disc
  - Sliding (translational) component in superior compartment between disc & mandibular fossa

Internal Structures-Critical Contents

- **Articular surfaces of TMJ**
  - Undersurface of squamosal portion of T-bone contains mandibular fossa & articular eminence
    - **Mandibular fossa** (articular fossa) located anterior to external auditory meatus
    - **Articular eminence** (articular tubercle) located anterior to mandibular fossa
  - **Mandibular condyle**
    - Condylar head & neck: Posterior protrusion from ramus of mandible
- **Articular disc**
  - Oval "dumbbell-shaped" plate
    - Disc superior surface: Concavoconvex to fit articular eminence & mandibular fossa
    - Disc inferior surface: Concave to conform to condylar head
  - **Intermediate zone** of disc found between anterior & posterior bands
  - **Anterior band**
    - Anteriorly attaches to joint capsule
    - Portion is integrated into superior aspect of lateral pterygoid muscle
  - **Posterior band**: Posterior disc margin is bilaminar = **bilaminar zone**
    - **Superior portion** composed of **loose** fibroelastic tissue; attached to posterior mandibular fossa
    - **Inferior portion** composed of **taut** fibrous material; attached to posterior margin of mandibular condyle
  - Medially & laterally disc attaches to joint capsule as well as medial & lateral mandibular condyle
- **TMJ compartments**
  - Disc creates superior & inferior compartments
  - **Superior joint compartment**
    - Between disc & mandibular fossa of T-bone
  - **Inferior joint compartment**
    - Between disc & condyle; two distinct recesses
    - **Anterior recess**: Anterior to condylar head
    - **Posterior recess**: Posterior to condylar head, deep to posterior insertion of articular disc onto posterior condylar neck
- **TMJ capsule & ligaments**
  - **Joint capsule**
    - Funnel-shaped
    - Extends inferiorly from temporal bone to attach to condylar neck
  - **TMJ ligaments**
    - Temporomandibular ligament: Lateral ligament attached to tubercle on zygoma root above & lateral surface of mandibular neck below
    - Sphenomandibular ligament: Medial ligament that attaches above on spine of sphenoid & below to lingula of mandibular foramen

MR Appearances of TMJ

- **Articular disc**
  - Articular disc: Low signal on both T1 & T2
- **Articular disc movement**
  - Initially upon mouth opening, inferior joint rotates
  - When mouth fully opens, mandibular condyle slides forwards & downwards onto articular eminence
  - Articular disc slides in same direction until its posterior fibroelastic attachments are stretched to their limits
- **Closed mouth sagittal MR**
  - Disc is "sigmoid shaped" in anterior half of joint space on sagittal closed mouth MR
  - Junction between low signal posterior band of disc & intermediate signal bilaminar zone is at "12 o'clock" position relative to mandibular condyle
  - Anterior band is located immediately inferior to articular eminence
- **Open mouth sagittal MR**
  - Disc is "bow tie shaped" anteroinferiorly beneath condylar eminence & above mandibular condyle

Anatomy-Based Imaging Issues

Imaging Recommendations

- Most TMJ imaging is requested for internal derangement (abnormal disc position) or TMJ degenerative disorders
- MR is best imaging modality to evaluate TMJ soft tissues, especially articular disc
- Sagittal MR is mainstay of TMJ imaging evaluation
  - Coronal closed mouth T1, sagittal T1 & T2 with closed & open mouth acquisitions needed
  - Fat-saturated T2 best for evaluation of joint effusion
- Bone CT may be needed to assess osseous structures
  - Multislice bone CT scan with 1 mm axial images
  - Sagittal & coronal reformations helpful

Imaging Pitfalls

- In cases with apparent limited motion between open and closed mouth series, look closely for articular disc abnormalities

Clinical Implications

Clinical Importance

- "TMJ disorder" is general term including both abnormalities of TMJ itself & muscles of mastication
- Estimated to cost $30 billion a year in lost productivity in USA

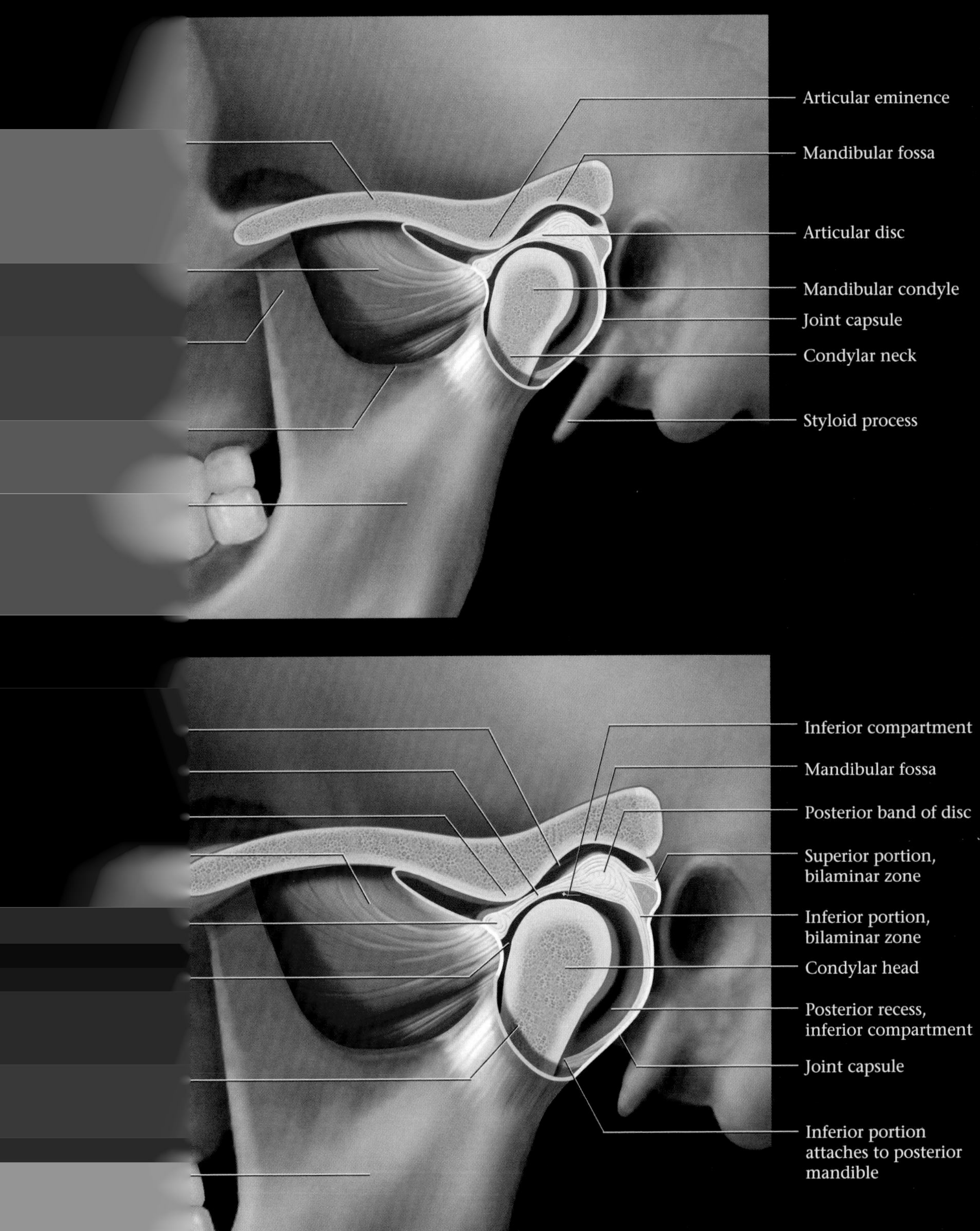
Articular eminence
Mandibular fossa
Articular disc
Mandibular condyle
Joint capsule
Condylar neck
Styloid process
Inferior compartment
Mandibular fossa
Posterior band of disc
Superior portion, bilaminar zone
Inferior portion, bilaminar zone
Condylar head
Posterior recess, inferior compartment
Joint capsule
Inferior portion attaches to posterior mandible

ws the relationship of the condylar head to base of skull at TMJ. Key global features of the lar condyle, articular disc, mandibular fossa and the articular eminence. **(Bottom)** of the TMJ shows the articular disc with its anterior and posterior bands. The thinner part ese bands is called the intermediate zone. The disc separates the joint into a superior and an ote the anterior band connecting to the lateral pterygoid muscle. The posterior margin of red to as the bilaminar zone, with the superior strut attaching to the posterior mandibular

3D-VRT BONE CT

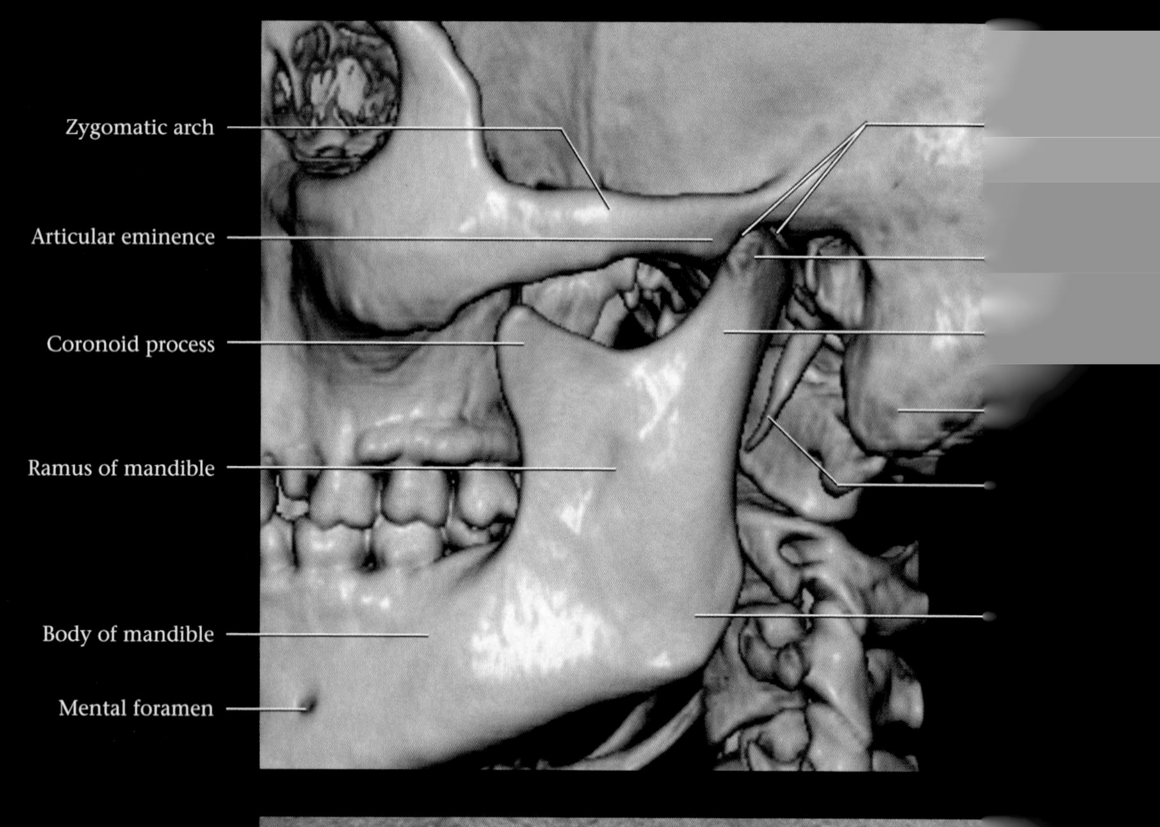
Zygomatic arch
Articular eminence
Coronoid process
Ramus of mandible
Body of mandible
Mental foramen

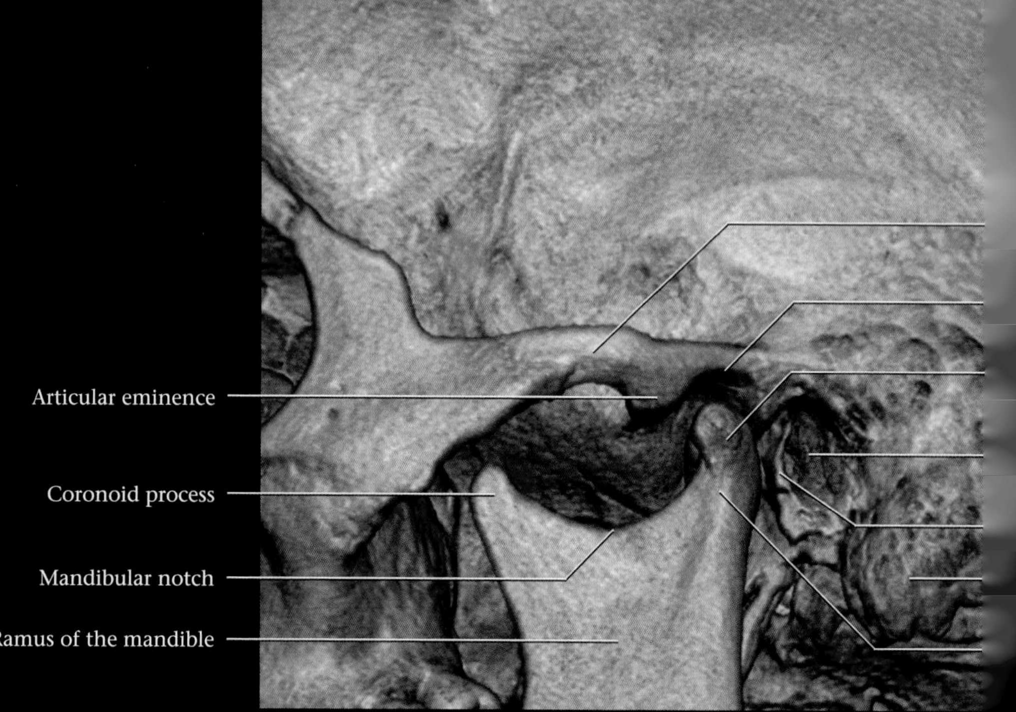
Articular eminence
Coronoid process
Mandibular notch
Ramus of the mandible

(Top) Sagittal 3D-VRT image shows the osseous anatomy of TMJ. The condylar head is situa fossa deep to the posterior zygomatic arch. The zygomatic arch provides some protection lat setting of trauma. The TMJ must be fully evaluated on all mandibular trauma cases to ensur mandibular condyle has occurred. **(Bottom)** Sagittal 3D-VRT magnified image shows the os area. In this closed or occlusal position, the condylar head is within the mandibular fossa. Ir position (not shown), the condylar head slides anteroinferiorly onto the articular eminence. relationship between the condylar head and tympanic bone of the external auditory canal.

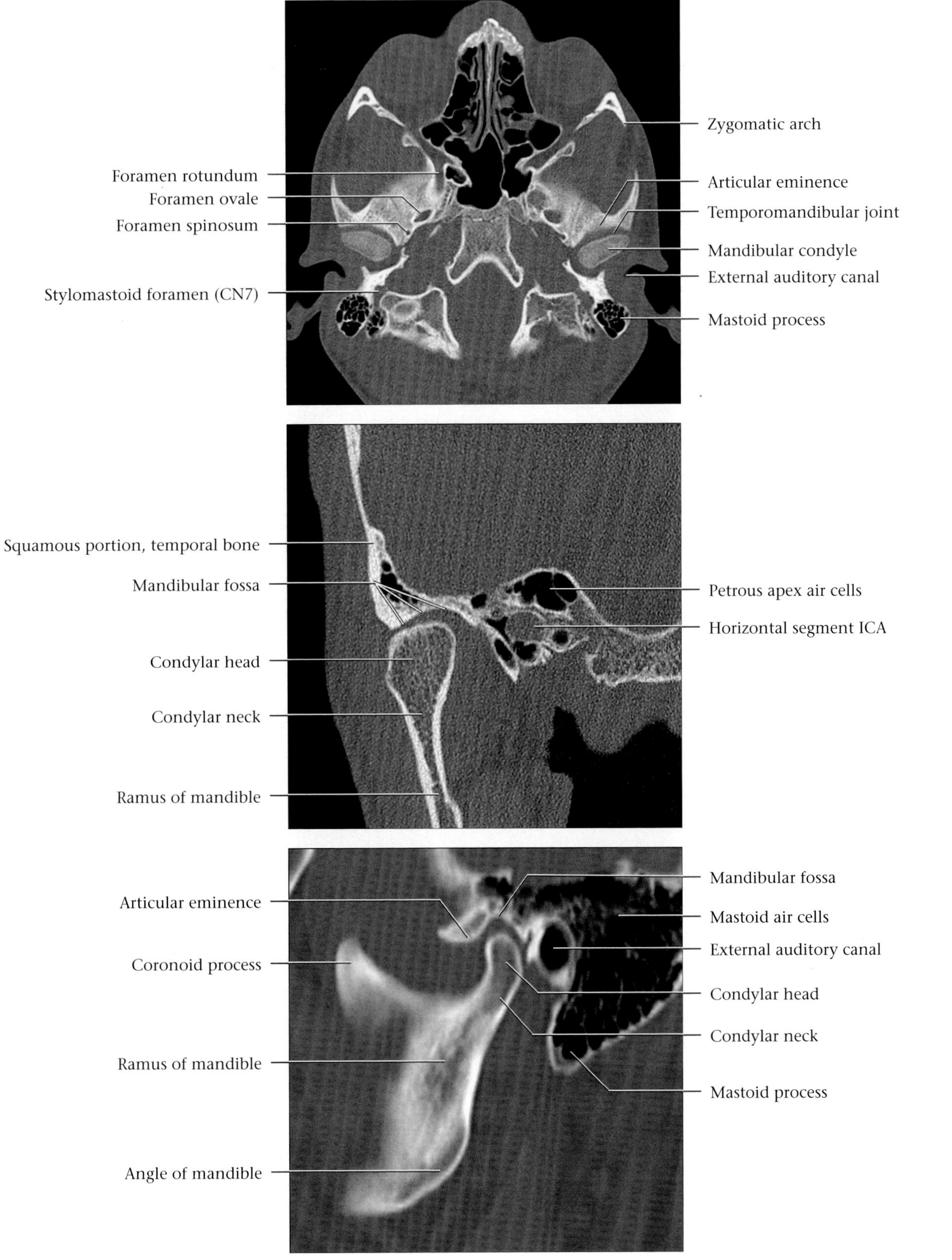

Zygomatic arch
Foramen rotundum
Foramen ovale
Foramen spinosum
Articular eminence
Temporomandibular joint
Mandibular condyle
External auditory canal
Stylomastoid foramen (CN7)
Mastoid process
Squamous portion, temporal bone
Mandibular fossa
Petrous apex air cells
Horizontal segment ICA
Condylar head
Condylar neck
Ramus of mandible
Mandibular fossa
Articular eminence
Mastoid air cells
External auditory canal
Coronoid process
Condylar head
Condylar neck
Ramus of mandible
Mastoid process
Angle of mandible

(Top) Axial bone CT image shows the relationship of the mandibular condyles to the articular eminences of the TMJ. Foramen spinosum, transmitting the middle meningeal artery is immediately anteromedial to the TMJ. In this plane, the articular eminence is seen as posterior attachment of zygomatic arch. **(Middle)** Coronal bone CT image of the right TMJ shows the coronal relationship of right mandibular condyle and fossa of the TMJ. The coronal plane in closed mouth position shows horizontal segment of carotid canal medial to TMJ and variable aeration of temporal bone air cells superior to the TMJ. **(Bottom)** Sagittal bone CT reformatted image shows the sagittal relationship of osseous TMJ, with the mandibular condyle normally seated within mandibular fossa in closed mouth position.

SAGITTAL T1 MR

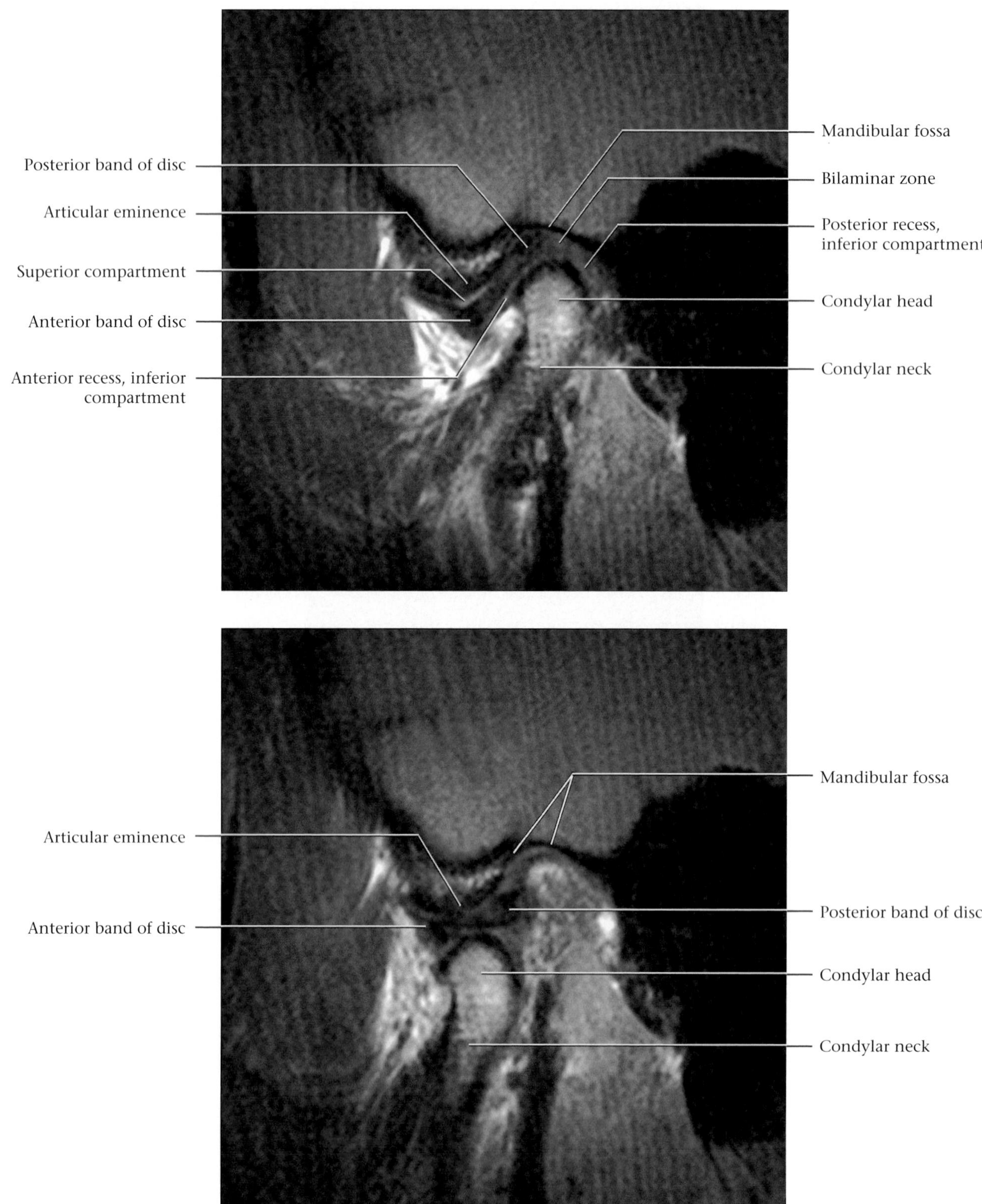

Posterior band of disc
Articular eminence
Superior compartment
Anterior band of disc
Anterior recess, inferior compartment
Mandibular fossa
Bilaminar zone
Posterior recess, inferior compartment
Condylar head
Condylar neck
Articular eminence
Anterior band of disc
Mandibular fossa
Posterior band of disc
Condylar head
Condylar neck

(Top) Closed mouth sagittal T1 MR image shows the condylar head seated in the mandibular fossa. The low signal articular disc has a "sigmoid shape" & is seen in the anterior half of the joint space. The junction between the low signal posterior band of the disc & intermediate signal of the bilaminar zone is normally found at "12 o'clock" relative to the condylar head in the closed mouth position. **(Bottom)** Open mouth sagittal T1 MR image. The condylar head has translated anteroinferiorly onto the articular eminence. The articular disc has moved to a position between the articular eminence & mandibular condyle, taking on a "bow tie" appearance. Both disc & mandibular condyle must complete this anterior movement for the TMJ to function normally. When the disc fails to complete this movement, internal derangement of the TMJ results. (Images courtesy Juan Fuentes, MD).

TEMPOROMANDIBULAR JOINT

SAGITTAL T2 MR

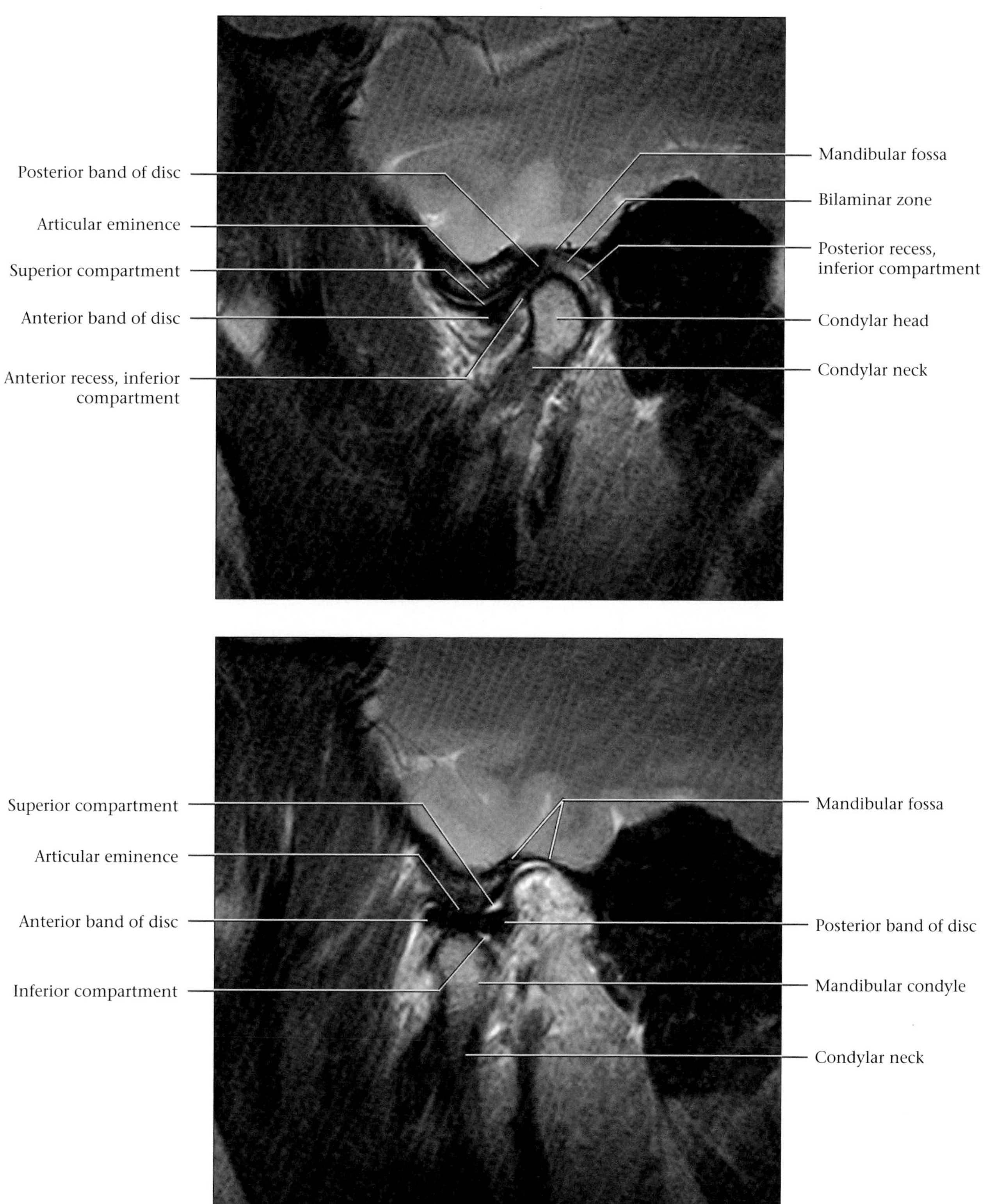
Posterior band of disc
Articular eminence
Superior compartment
Anterior band of disc
Anterior recess, inferior compartment
Mandibular fossa
Bilaminar zone
Posterior recess, inferior compartment
Condylar head
Condylar neck
Superior compartment
Articular eminence
Anterior band of disc
Inferior compartment
Mandibular fossa
Posterior band of disc
Mandibular condyle
Condylar neck

(Top) Closed mouth sagittal T2 MR image shows the condylar head seated in mandibular fossa. The low signal articular disc is has a "sigmoid shape" & is seen in the anterior half of the joint space. Notice that the the junction between the low signal posterior band of the disc & the intermediate signal of the bilaminar zone is normally found at "12 o'clock" relative to the condylar head in the closed mouth position. **(Bottom)** Open mouth T2 MR sagittal image reveals the condylar head has translated anteroinferiorly onto the articular eminence. The disc has also moved to a position between the articular eminence & mandibular condyle, taking on a "bow tie" appearance in the process. Both disc & mandibular condyle must complete this anteroinferior movement for the TMJ to function normally. (Images courtesy Juan Fuentes, MD).

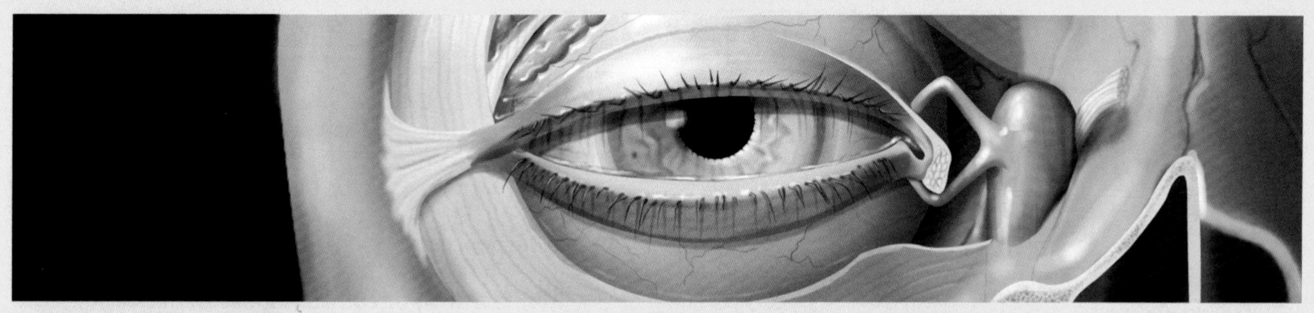

SECTION 2: Orbit, Nose and Sinuses

ORBIT OVERVIEW

Terminology

Abbreviations

- Cranial nerves
  - Optic nerve (CN2)
  - Oculomotor nerve (CN3)
  - Trochlear nerve (CN4)
  - Trigeminal nerve (CN5)
    - Branches (V1, V2 and V3)
  - Abducens nerve (CN6)
- Orbital structures
  - Superior/inferior ophthalmic veins (SOV/IOV)
  - Superior/inferior orbital fissures (SOF/IOF)
  - Extra-ocular muscles (EOM)

Imaging Anatomy

Internal Structures-Critical Contents

- **Intraorbital nerves**
  - CN2: Discussed separately
  - CN3: Motor to medial, superior, and inferior recti, and levator palpebrae; parasympathetic motor to iris
  - CN4: Motor to superior oblique
  - CN6: Motor to lateral rectus
  - CN5: Sensory from orbit and eyelids (V1)
- **Ophthalmic artery**
  - Major arterial supply of the orbit
  - First intradural branch of internal carotid artery (ICA); passes through optic canal, pierces dural sheath laterally at apex
  - Major branches: Central retinal, posterior ciliary, muscular, lacrimal, supraorbital, ethmoidal, and nasofrontal
- **Ophthalmic veins**
  - SOV: Located between CN2 and superior rectus; drains through superior fissure into cavernous sinus
  - IOV: Located adjacent to inferior rectus; drains through inferior fissure into pterygoid plexus
- **Extraocular muscles**
  - **Recti**
    - Superior, inferior, lateral, medial
    - Origins at annulus of Zinn
    - Insertions at corneoscleral surface
  - **Superior oblique**
    - Origin at medial margin of annulus of Zinn
    - Passes through trochlea at superomedial rim
    - Inserts posterolaterally on sclera superiorly
  - **Inferior oblique**
    - Origin at anteroinferior orbital rim
    - Insertion posterolaterally on sclera inferiorly
  - **Levator palpebrae superioris**
    - Origin at annulus of Zinn
    - Courses above superior rectus, divides in two
    - Superior aponeurosis insertion at upper eyelid
    - Inferior Müller insertion at tarsal plate
- **Nasolacrimal apparatus**
  - **Lacrimal gland**
    - Orbital lobe: Larger, lies in bony fossa at anterior aspect of superotemporal orbit
    - Palpebral lobe: Smaller, lies inferiorly, separated by levator aponeurosis
  - Drainage via puncta at medial lower lids → canaliculi → lacrimal sac → nasolacrimal duct
- **Anterior periorbita**
  - **Tarsal plates**
    - Dense connective tissue plates within eyelids
  - **Orbital septum**
    - Fascia arising from orbital periosteum
    - Inserts into aponeurosis and fascia of lids at margins of superior and inferior tarsi

Anatomy-Based Imaging Issues

Key Concepts or Questions

- Approach to orbital lesions
  - Localize to region and involved structures
    - Globe: Intraocular vs. transscleral
    - Optic nerve vs. nerve-sheath complex
    - Intraconal vs. conal vs. extraconal orbit
    - Lacrimal gland: Unilateral vs. bilateral (systemic)
    - Isolated vs. multifocal vs. trans-spatial process
    - Intracranial: Direct extension vs. secondary
  - Assess CT, MR, and/or ultrasound characteristics
    - Solid or cystic; heterogeneity
    - Fluid, fat, blood, or soft tissue
    - Bony remodeling vs. destruction
    - Well-defined vs. infiltrative
    - Degree and homogeneity of enhancement

Imaging Recommendations

- General comments
  - CT & MR are complementary techniques; both indicated for evaluation of complex lesions
- CT
  - Excellent evaluation of orbit aided by natural contrast between fat, bone, air & soft tissues
  - Easily detects calcifications
  - Noncontrast CT alone for thyroid orbitopathy
- MR
  - Optimal soft tissue contrast for globe, optic nerve, orbital structures, and intracranial findings
  - Stronger gradients, faster sequences, surface coils, routine use of fat suppression ± gadolinium improve image quality
- Ultrasound
  - First line modality for intraocular lesions
  - Noninvasive, readily available

Imaging Approaches

- Imaging protocols
  - CT
    - Axial + coronal planes; thin-sections (≤ 2 mm)
    - Multislice isovoxel acquisition with MPR
    - Soft tissue algorithm; bone in at least one plane
    - Contrast for masses or inflammatory disease
    - Noncontrast only when in conjunction with MR
  - MR
    - Axial: Above orbital roof to orbital floor
    - Coronal: Back of pons through globe
    - Thin-section (3-4 mm); small FOV (12-16 cm)
    - T1 pre-contrast (axial + coronal)
    - STIR or T2 FSE fat-saturation (axial + coronal)
    - T1 C+ with fat-saturation (axial + coronal)
    - Whole brain axial FLAIR and T1 C+

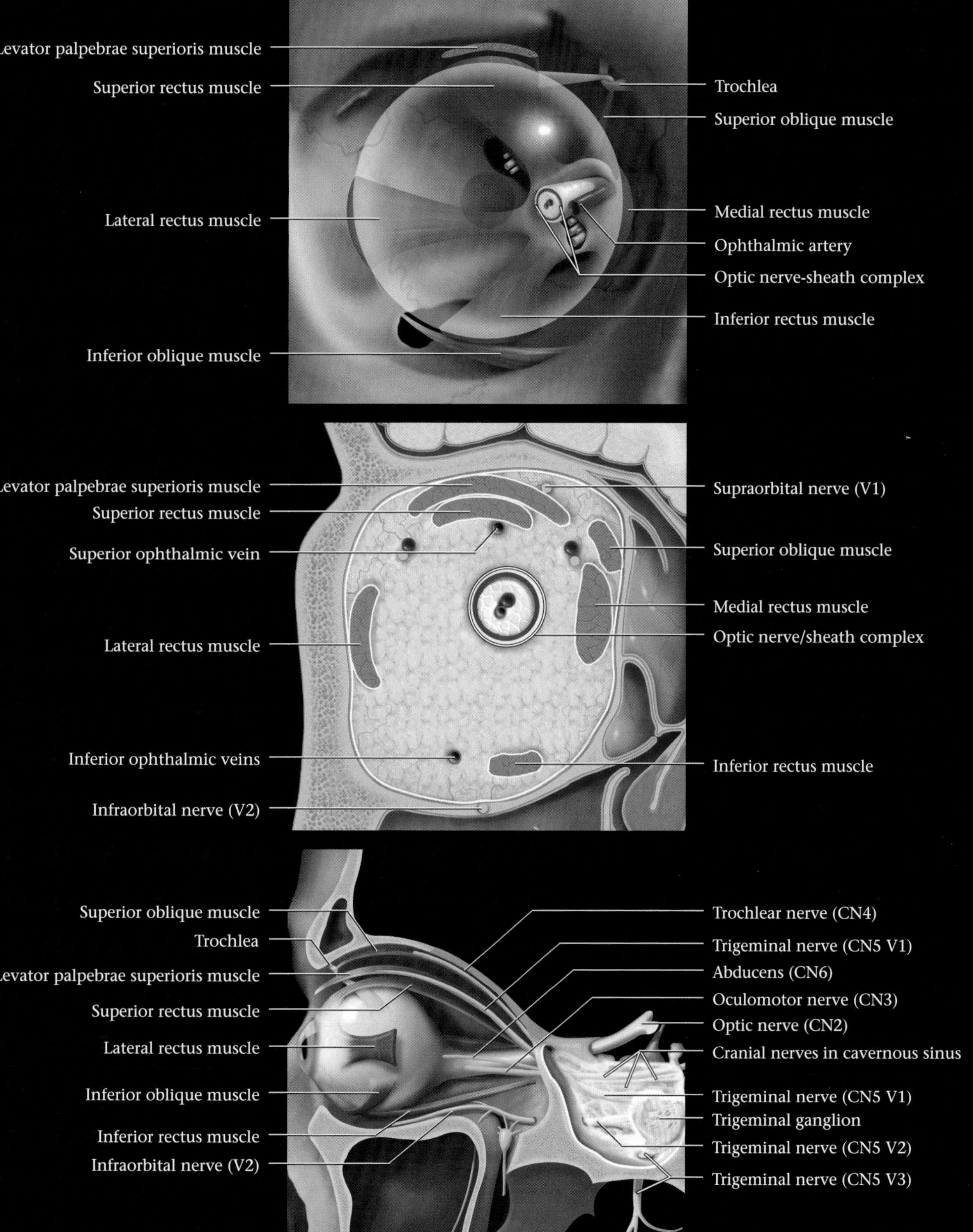

Levator palpebrae superioris muscle
Superior rectus muscle
Trochlea
Superior oblique muscle
Lateral rectus muscle
Medial rectus muscle
Ophthalmic artery
Optic nerve-sheath complex
Inferior rectus muscle
Inferior oblique muscle
Levator palpebrae superioris muscle
Superior rectus muscle
Superior ophthalmic vein
Supraorbital nerve (V1)
Superior oblique muscle
Medial rectus muscle
Lateral rectus muscle
Optic nerve/sheath complex
Inferior ophthalmic veins
Inferior rectus muscle
Infraorbital nerve (V2)
Superior oblique muscle
Trochlea
Levator palpebrae superioris muscle
Superior rectus muscle
Lateral rectus muscle
Inferior oblique muscle
Inferior rectus muscle
Infraorbital nerve (V2)
Trochlear nerve (CN4)
Trigeminal nerve (CN5 V1)
Abducens (CN6)
Oculomotor nerve (CN3)
Optic nerve (CN2)
Cranial nerves in cavernous sinus
Trigeminal nerve (CN5 V1)
Trigeminal ganglion
Trigeminal nerve (CN5 V2)
Trigeminal nerve (CN5 V3)

(Top) Frontal graphic of the right orbit. The rectus muscles originate at the annulus of Zinn at the orbital apex and insert at the corneoscleral junction of the eye, forming a muscle cone. The superior oblique muscle courses through the trochlea, providing for the angled pulley motion of this muscle. The inferior oblique inserts at the inferolateral aspect of the eye. **(Middle)** Coronal graphic of the right orbit. The optic nerve-sheath complex courses in the intraconal space behind the eye. Branches of CN3-6, branches of the ophthalmic artery, and ophthalmic veins are located in the intraconal and extraconal spaces. **(Bottom)** Lateral graphic of the left orbit. Intricate mechanics and innervation of the EOMs provide for complementary and complex control of eye motion. CN2-6 enter the orbit via complex foramina.

ORBIT OVERVIEW

CORONAL T1 MR

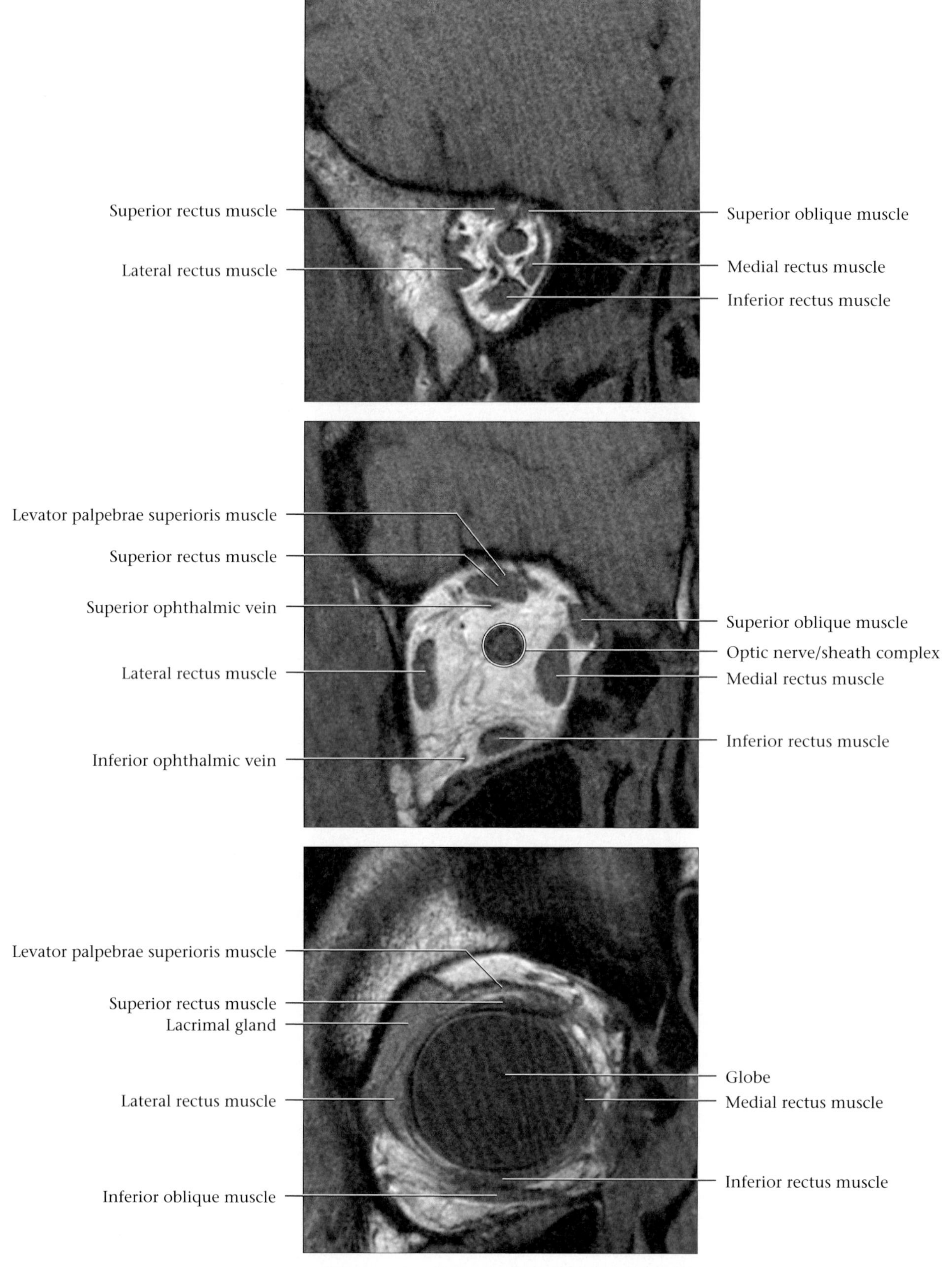

Superior rectus muscle
Lateral rectus muscle
Superior oblique muscle
Medial rectus muscle
Inferior rectus muscle
Levator palpebrae superioris muscle
Superior rectus muscle
Superior ophthalmic vein
Lateral rectus muscle
Inferior ophthalmic vein
Superior oblique muscle
Optic nerve/sheath complex
Medial rectus muscle
Inferior rectus muscle
Levator palpebrae superioris muscle
Superior rectus muscle
Lacrimal gland
Lateral rectus muscle
Inferior oblique muscle
Globe
Medial rectus muscle
Inferior rectus muscle

(Top) First of three coronal T1 MR images presented from posterior to anterior at the level of the orbital apex shows close proximity of extraocular muscles, nerve-sheath complex and ophthalmic vessels. **(Middle)** Image in the mid-orbit shows the muscle cone formed by the EOMs, with the nerve-sheath complex centrally in the intraconal space. Complex and variable branches of the ophthalmic artery are seen as small flow voids within the intraconal and extraconal fat. **(Bottom)** Image at the level of the globe shows the flattened and thinned tendinous contours of the EOMs near their insertions. The inferior oblique muscle is evident at this level. The lacrimal gland is isointense and located in the anterior aspect of the superotemporal extraconal space.

ORBIT OVERVIEW

OBLIQUE SAGITTAL T1 MR

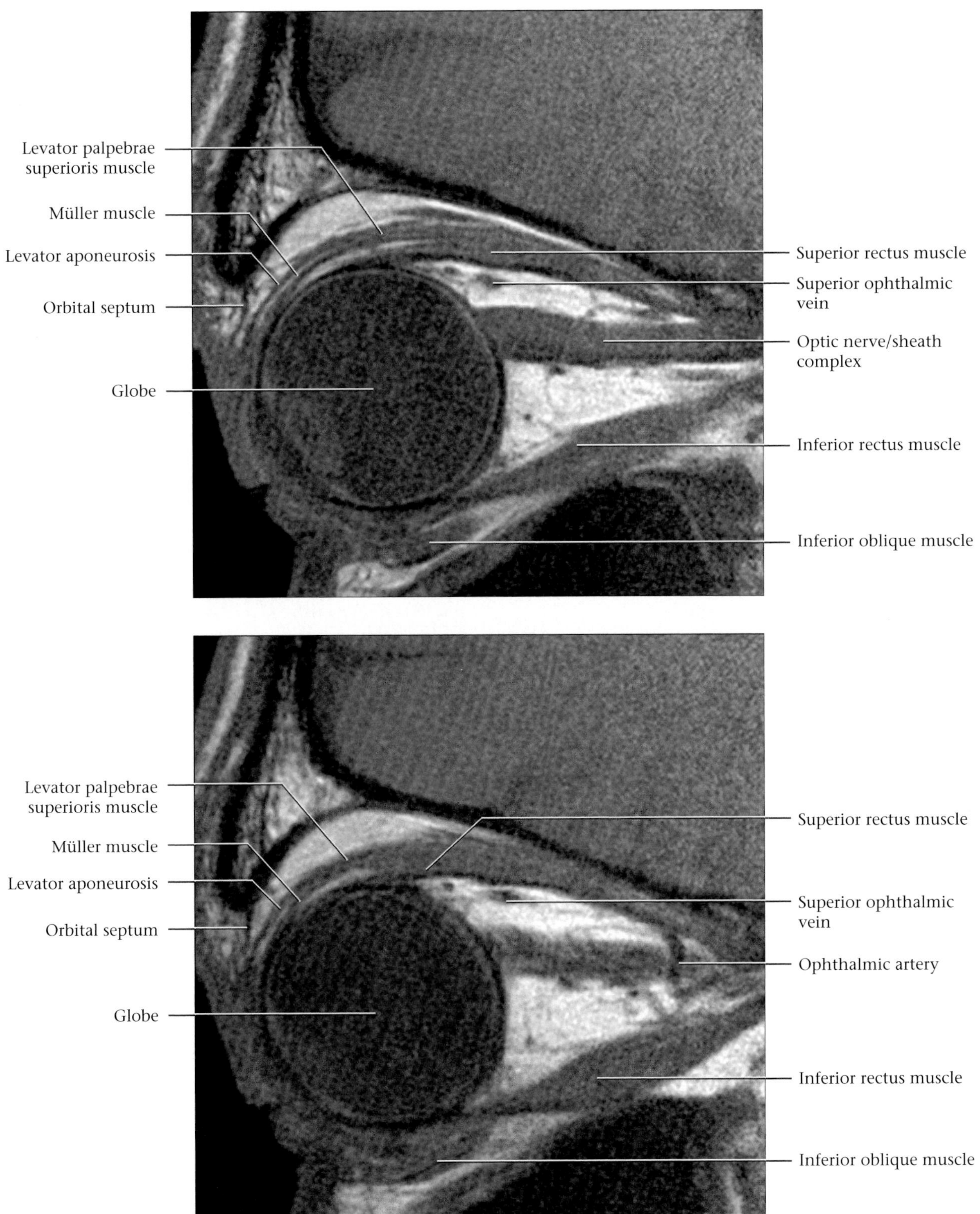

Levator palpebrae superioris muscle
Müller muscle
Levator aponeurosis
Orbital septum
Globe
Superior rectus muscle
Superior ophthalmic vein
Optic nerve/sheath complex
Inferior rectus muscle
Inferior oblique muscle
Levator palpebrae superioris muscle
Müller muscle
Levator aponeurosis
Orbital septum
Globe
Superior rectus muscle
Superior ophthalmic vein
Ophthalmic artery
Inferior rectus muscle
Inferior oblique muscle

(Top) First of two oblique sagittal T1 MR images at the mid-orbit, from medial to lateral. The intimate relationship between the superior oblique and levator palpebrae superioris muscles is evident in this plane. The distinct division of the Müller muscle and levator aponeurosis anteriorly is evident. Inferiorly, the inferior oblique muscle is seen in oblique cross-section, distinct from the inferior oblique muscle. **(Bottom)** Image at the lateral aspect of the orbital apex shows the ophthalmic artery as it exits the dural sheath laterally and courses over the nerve-sheath complex. The orbital septum is visible as a discrete low signal fibrous band that separates the preseptal periorbita from the remainder of the orbit. The SOV is visible in its expected location.

BONY ORBIT AND FORAMINA

Terminology

Abbreviations

- **Bones, foramina, and fissures**
  - Greater wing of sphenoid (GWS)
  - Lesser wing of sphenoid (LWS)
  - Optic canal (OpC)
  - Superior orbital fissure (SOF)
  - Inferior orbital fissure (IOF)
  - Foramen rotundum (FR)
  - Foramen ovale (FO)
  - Vidian canal (VC)
  - Pterygopalatine fossa (PPF)
- **Cranial nerves**
  - Optic nerve (CN2)
  - Oculomotor nerve (CN3)
  - Trochlear nerve (CN4)
  - Trigeminal nerve (CN5)
    - Ophthalmic branch (V1)
    - Maxillary branch (V2)
    - Mandibular branch (V3)
  - Abducens nerve (CN6)
- **Vessels**
  - Ophthalmic artery (OA)
  - Superior ophthalmic vein (SOV)
  - Inferior ophthalmic vein (IOV)

Definitions

- MPR: 2D multiplanar reformations

Gross Anatomy

Bones of the Orbit

- **Frontal bone**
  - Forms superior rim and anterior portion of roof (orbital process)
- **Zygomatic bone**
  - Forms inferolateral rim, anterior portion of lateral wall (orbital process), and anterior portion of lateral floor (maxillary process)
- **Maxillary bone**
  - Forms inferomedial rim (frontal process) & anterior portion of inferomedial wall (orbital surface)
- **Nasal bone**
  - Forms bridge of nose
  - Anteromedial to frontal process of maxillary bone
- **Ethmoid bone**
  - Forms mid portion of medial wall
  - Very thin bone (lamina papyracea)
- **Lacrimal bone**
  - Forms anterior portion of medial wall, just posterior to frontal process of maxillary bone
  - Fossa for lacrimal sac
- **Sphenoid bone**
  - Forms posterior portion of lateral wall (GWS) and posterior portion of medial roof (LWS)
  - Complex contours between GWS and LWS create elaborate apical fissures
- **Palatine bone**
  - Forms small portion of inferomedial wall posteriorly
  - Located between orbital portions of ethmoid & maxillary bones

Imaging Anatomy

Anatomy Relationships

- **Major foramina**
  - **Optic canal**
    - Formed completely by LWS
    - Separated from SOF by optic strut
  - **Superior orbital fissure**
    - Formed by LWS medially, GWS laterally
    - Primary connection orbit ↔ intracranial
  - **Inferior orbital fissure**
    - Formed by GWS and zygomatic bone laterally, maxillary and ethmoid bones medially
    - Mostly contiguous with SOF, separated only at posterior aspect by short bony roof of FR
    - Anterior continuation of FR

Internal Structures-Critical Contents

- **Contents of foramina**
  - **Optic canal**: CN2 and OA
  - **Superior orbital fissure**: CN3, 4, 5 (V1), & 6, SOV
  - **Inferior orbital fissure**: CN5 (V2), IOV
  - **Foramen rotundum**: CN5 (V2)-proximal segment
  - **Foramen ovale**: CN5 (V3)
  - **Supraorbital foramen**: Supraorbital nerve (V1)
  - **Infraorbital foramen**: Infraorbital nerve (V2)

Anatomy-Based Imaging Issues

Key Concepts or Questions

- **Pathways of orbit-sinus disease spread**
  - Orbit → intracranial
    - SOF and IOF: Common pathway; extends into cavernous sinus and Meckel cave, involves CN3-6
    - OpC: Involves optic nerve, dura
  - Orbit → deep face
    - SOF and IOF: Communicate with PPF
  - Sinus → orbit
    - Ethmoid: Common pathway via lamina papyracea
    - Frontal: Especially post-obstructive process

Imaging Recommendations

- CT
  - Preferred for assessing bony structures and foramina
- MR
  - Preferred for evaluation of tumor and inflammation
  - Foramina not as easily seen as CT, but can be discerned by superimposing image of CT

Imaging Pitfalls

- Assessing foramina
  - Optic canal oriented obliquely
    - Complete ring not visible in coronal plane
    - MPR orthogonal to long axis may be required to demonstrate intact canal
  - FR and VC often mistaken
    - FR appears superolateral in coronal plane
    - FR appears short compared to longer/curvilinear VC
- Artifacts
  - Dental artifact troublesome on direct coronal images
    - Axial multislice source with coronal MPR preferred if dental amalgam present

BONY ORBIT AND FORAMINA

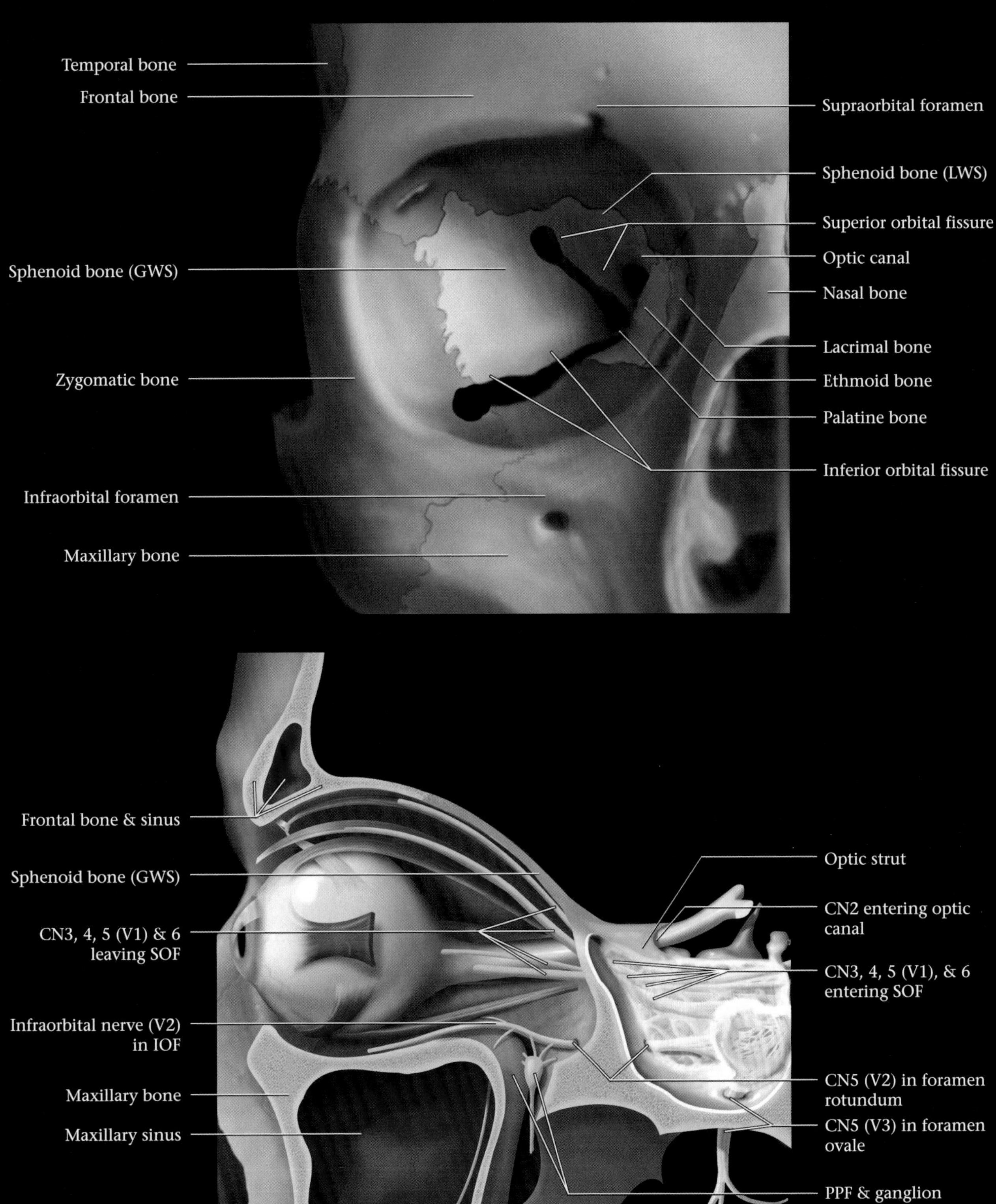

Temporal bone
Frontal bone
Supraorbital foramen
Sphenoid bone (LWS)
Superior orbital fissure
Optic canal
Sphenoid bone (GWS)
Nasal bone
Lacrimal bone
Zygomatic bone
Ethmoid bone
Palatine bone
Inferior orbital fissure
Infraorbital foramen
Maxillary bone
Frontal bone & sinus
Optic strut
Sphenoid bone (GWS)
CN2 entering optic canal
CN3, 4, 5 (V1) & 6 leaving SOF
CN3, 4, 5 (V1), & 6 entering SOF
Infraorbital nerve (V2) in IOF
CN5 (V2) in foramen rotundum
Maxillary bone
CN5 (V3) in foramen ovale
Maxillary sinus
PPF & ganglion

(Top) Frontal graphic of the bones of the right orbit. A total of seven embryologically distinct bones contribute to the bony orbit. The complex orbital fissures and optic canal at the apex are formed largely by the wings of the sphenoid bone and associated relationships. **(Bottom)** Lateral graphic of the left orbit. The optic nerve (CN2) is relatively isolated in the optic canal, whereas the superior orbital fissure transmits CN3, 4, 5 (V1), and 6 as they course forward from the cavernous sinus and Meckel cave. The other branches of CN5 also contribute to the complexity of the central skull base as they pass through their respective foramina.

BONY ORBIT AND FORAMINA

AXIAL BONE CT

Nasal bone
Maxillary bone (frontal process)
Nasolacrimal duct
Lacrimal bone
Maxillary bone and sinus
Zygomatic bone
Inferior orbital fissure
Pterygopalatine fossa
Foramen rotundum
Foramen rotundum

Nasomaxillary suture
Lacrimal bone
Ethmoid bone (lamina papyracea)
Sphenozygomatic suture
Greater wing of sphenoid
Sphenotemporal suture
Superior orbital fissure
Central sphenoid bone and sinus

Frontal bone
Frontal recess
Zygomatic bone
Ethmoid sinus
Greater wing of sphenoid
Superior orbital fissure
Optic canal
LWS (optic strut)
Sella turcica

(Top) First of three axial bone CT images presented from inferior to superior. The short, horizontally oriented foramen rotundum is seen at the posterior margin of the PPF, with the IOF extending anterolaterally in roughly the same plane. Anteriorly, relationships between the medial bony orbit and nasolacrimal structures are evident. **(Middle)** Image at the level of the mid-orbit. The SOF is seen as a gap at the orbital apex. The thin ethmoid bone forms the bulk of the medial orbital wall. **(Bottom)** Image at the level of the upper orbit. The optic canals show characteristic angles as the nerves approach the chiasm, which is located above the sella. The SOF is inferior and lateral to the optic canal, from which it is separated by the bony optic strut of the LWS. Sinus air space within the paramedian portions of the frontal bones is seen anteriorly.

BONY ORBIT AND FORAMINA

CORONAL BONE CT

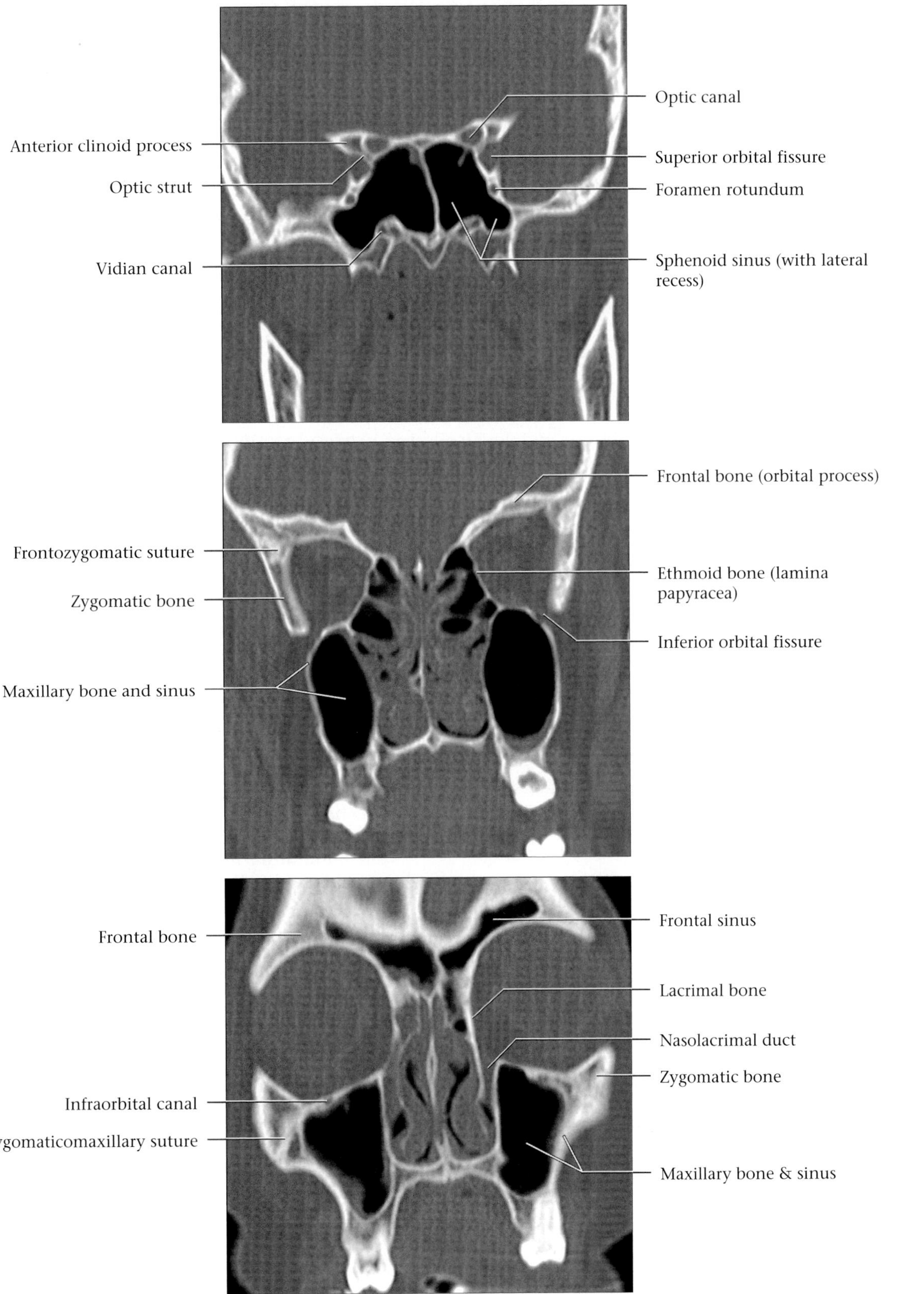

Optic canal
Anterior clinoid process
Superior orbital fissure
Optic strut
Foramen rotundum
Vidian canal
Sphenoid sinus (with lateral recess)
Frontal bone (orbital process)
Frontozygomatic suture
Ethmoid bone (lamina papyracea)
Zygomatic bone
Inferior orbital fissure
Maxillary bone and sinus
Frontal sinus
Frontal bone
Lacrimal bone
Nasolacrimal duct
Zygomatic bone
Infraorbital canal
Zygomaticomaxillary suture
Maxillary bone & sinus

(Top) First of three coronal bone CT images presented from posterior to anterior. The obliquely oriented optic canals show characteristic ovoid shape. The SOF is located inferolaterally relative to the optic canal, with the optic strut and attached clinoid process of the LWS separating the two. Further inferolaterally is the foramen rotundum. The vidian canal is inferior and medial to rotundum, noting a prominent lateral recess of the sphenoid sinus separating the two foramina. **(Middle)** Image at the level of the mid-orbit. Contours of the bony orbit, including integrity of the thin lamina papyracea of the medial wall, are best seen in this plane. **(Bottom)** Image at the level of the anterior orbit. Contours of the bony orbital rim are best evaluated in the coronal plane. The nasolacrimal structures, as well as anterior sinonasal spaces, are well demonstrated.

OPTIC NERVE/SHEATH COMPLEX

Terminology

Abbreviations

- Optic nerve-sheath complex (ONSC)
- Optic nerve (CN2)
- Ophthalmic artery (OA)
- Superior/inferior ophthalmic vein (SOV/IOV)

Definitions

- Optic nerve, chiasm & tract: Afferent visual CNS pathways that extend from retina to visual nuclei of midbrain
- Optic sheath: Dural encasement of intraorbital CN2

Gross Anatomy

Overview

- **Optic nerve and tract**
  - Anatomically a CNS tract
    - Composed of oligodendrocytes
  - Different from other cranial nerves
    - Composed of Schwann cells
- **Optic sheath**
  - Dural encasement of nerve
    - Contiguous with intracranial dura
    - All 3 membrane layers of meninges present including pia, arachnoid & dura mater
  - CSF-filled arachnoid space surrounds nerve
    - Contiguous with suprasellar cistern
    - Transmits intracranial pressure changes

Imaging Anatomy

Extent

- **Optic nerve**
  - From optic nerve head to chiasm
  - Optic nerve segments
    - **Intraocular**: Within nerve head (1 mm)
    - **Orbital**: Nerve head to optic canal (30 mm)
    - **Canalicular**: Within optic canal (10 mm)
    - **Cisternal**: Optic canal to optic chiasm (10 mm)
- **Optic chiasm**
  - Within suprasellar cistern
    - Just anterior to pituitary stalk
  - Decussation of half of axons
    - Represents nasal portion of retina
    - Each half of visual field from each eye is afferent to contralateral visual cortex
- **Optic tract**
  - From optic chiasm to visual nuclei of midbrain

Anatomy Relationships

- Optic canal
  - Transmits ONSC and OA
  - Separated from superior fissure by optic strut

Internal Structures-Critical Contents

- **Vascular supply**
  - **Ophthalmic artery**
    - First intradural branch of ICA
    - Major arterial supply to orbit
    - Passes through optic canal in dural sheath
    - Exits sheath laterally at orbital apex
  - **Central retinal artery**
    - Major branch of OA, supplies retina
    - Enters CN2 ≈ 1 cm posterior to nerve head
  - **Central retinal vein**
    - Accompanies central retinal artery
    - Drains directly into cavernous sinus

Anatomy-Based Imaging Issues

Key Concepts or Questions

- **Orientation of optic nerve**
  - **Intraorbital segment**
    - Posteromedial oblique sagittal long axis
    - Roughly horizontal plane
    - Position varies with eye movement
    - Nerve longer than distance from apex to globe, tends to form an "S-shaped" contour
  - **Canalicular segment**
    - Oblique axis results in non-orthogonal "ovoid" cross sectional appearance on coronal images
  - **Cisternal segment**
    - Angle changes relative to intraorbital segment as it courses posteriorly
    - Oblique sagittal long axis ≈ 30° medially and superiorly

Imaging Recommendations

- Routine orbital approach appropriate for most nerve/sheath lesions
- Special circumstances
  - **Sheath mass** (possible meningioma)
    - May benefit from noncontrast CT to detect calcification
    - Additional brain imaging may be necessary to define extent of intra-axial tumor
  - **Inflammatory nerve work-up** (optic neuritis)
    - Requires concomitant brain imaging
    - High incidence of demyelinating disease

Imaging Approaches

- Dedicated optic nerve MR imaging
  - Axial sequences
    - 3.0 mm, anterior fossa floor through floor of orbit
  - Coronal sequences
    - 3.5 mm, back of pons through globe
  - T1WI, STIR, and T1 C+ with fat suppression
    - Both axial and coronal
    - May substitute axial T2WI FSE + fat suppression for STIR

Imaging Pitfalls

- Motion artifacts on MR
  - Common due to irrepressible eye motion
- Surface coils
  - Generally not adequate to visualize entire ONSC

Clinical Implications

Nerve vs. sheath masses

- Important distinction, very different therapies
- Best with coronal STIR and T1 C+ with fat suppression

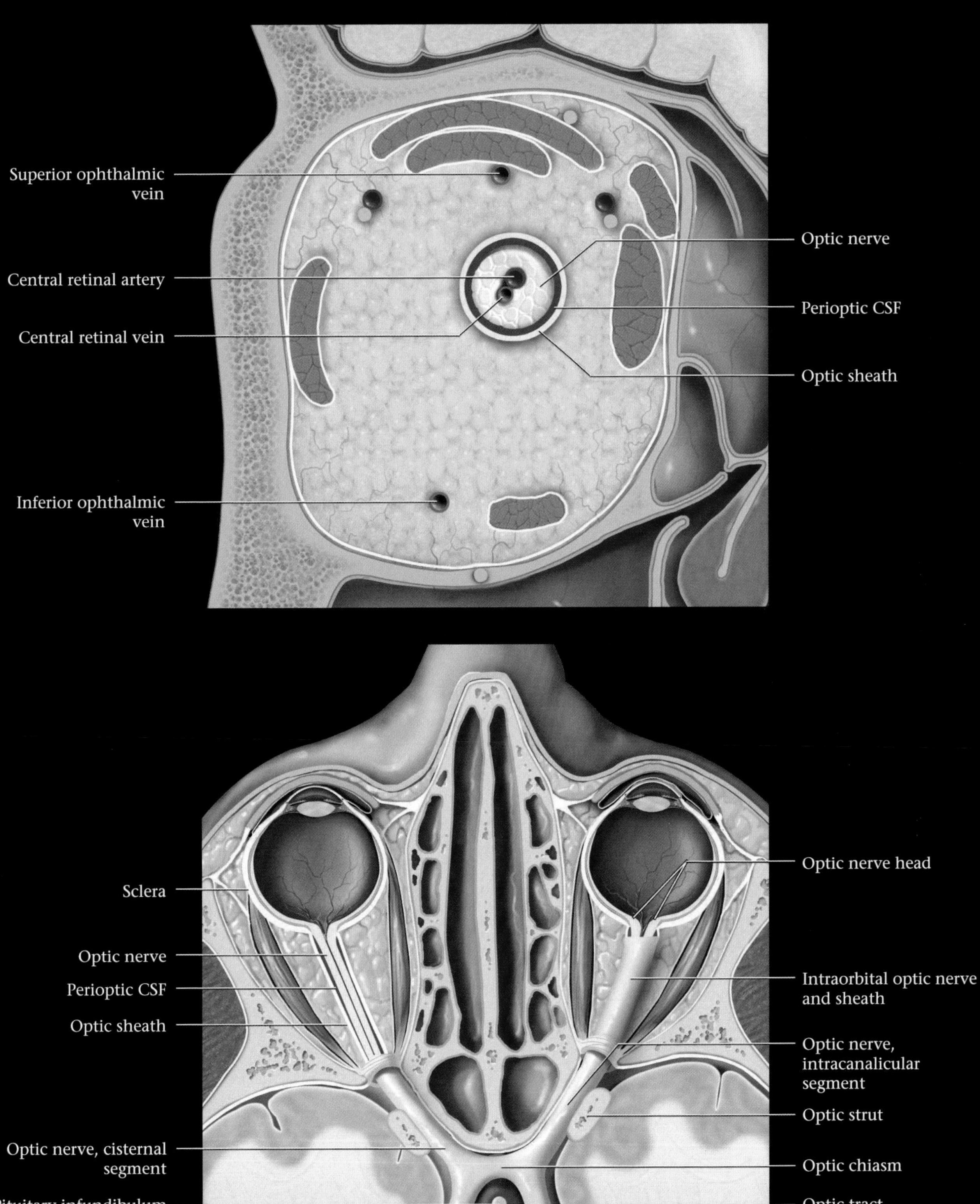
Superior ophthalmic vein
Central retinal artery
Central retinal vein
Inferior ophthalmic vein
Optic nerve
Perioptic CSF
Optic sheath
Sclera
Optic nerve
Perioptic CSF
Optic sheath
Optic nerve, cisternal segment
Pituitary infundibulum
Optic nerve head
Intraorbital optic nerve and sheath
Optic nerve, intracanalicular segment
Optic strut
Optic chiasm
Optic tract

(Top) Coronal graphic of the mid-orbit depicting the optic nerve-sheath complex. The nerve is bathed by a thin layer of CSF which is contained by the dural optic sheath. The central retinal vessels are external to the optic sheath posteriorly in the orbit, and pierce the dura in the mid-portion of the nerve to travel within the substance of the nerve anteriorly. **(Bottom)** Axial graphic of the intraorbital and intracranial segments of CN2. The extra-axial optic pathways can be segmented (posterior to anterior) into optic tract, optic chiasm, cisternal nerve, intracanalicular nerve, and intraorbital nerve. The optic sheath is a dural reflection that is contiguous with intracranial dura mater. Note the relationship of the pituitary infundibulum to the optic chiasm.

OPTIC NERVE/SHEATH COMPLEX

CORONAL & AXIAL T1 MR

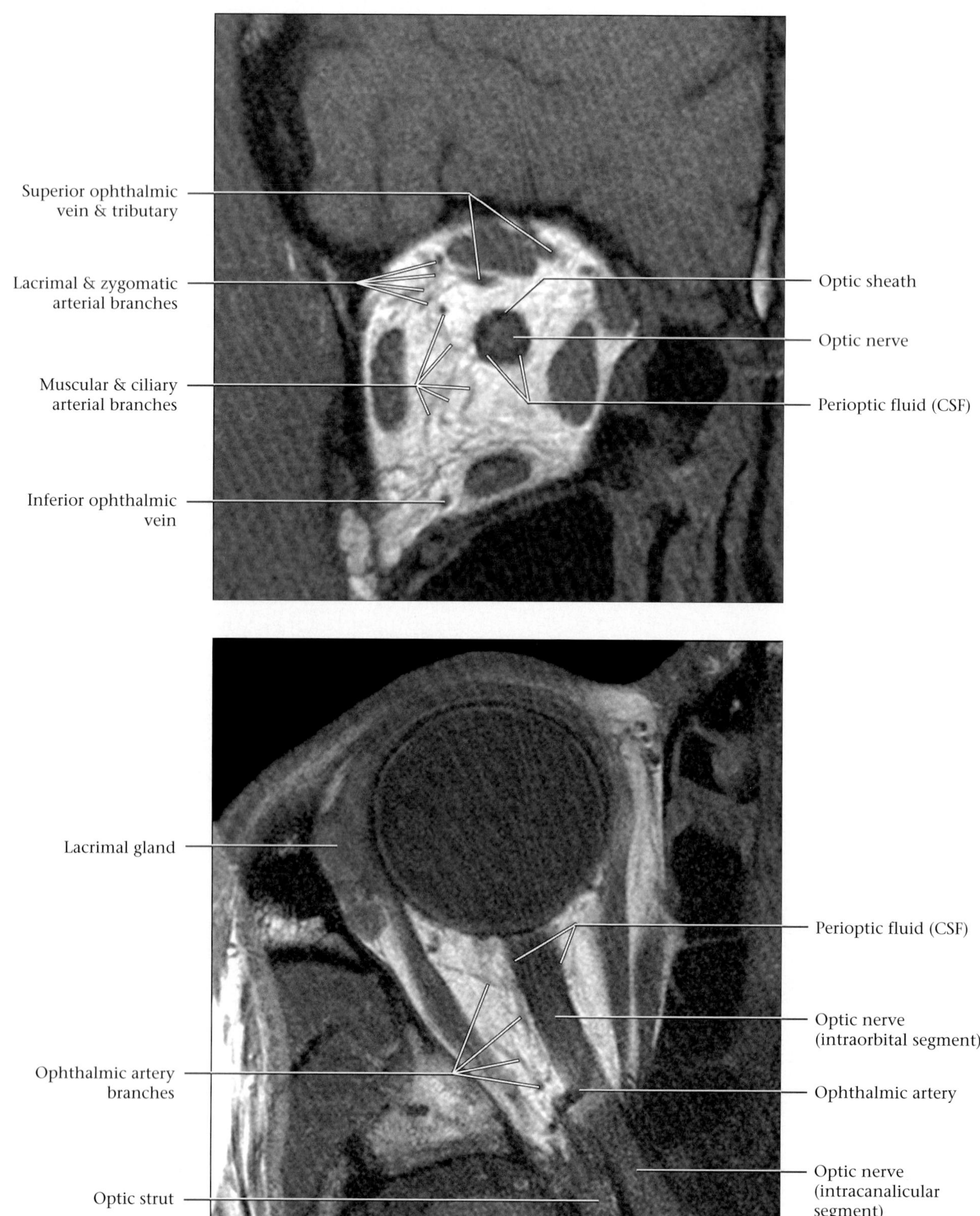
Superior ophthalmic vein & tributary
Lacrimal & zygomatic arterial branches
Muscular & ciliary arterial branches
Inferior ophthalmic vein
Optic sheath
Optic nerve
Perioptic fluid (CSF)
Lacrimal gland
Ophthalmic artery branches
Optic strut
Perioptic fluid (CSF)
Optic nerve (intraorbital segment)
Ophthalmic artery
Optic nerve (intracanalicular segment)

(Top) Coronal high-resolution T1 MR of the intraconal orbit. The optic nerve/sheath complex is centered within the EOM cone. Perioptic fluid is contiguous with intracranial CSF, and is seen as hypointense signal between the nerve centrally and the dural sheath peripherally. Intraconal branches of the ophthalmic artery are in proximity with the nerve/sheath complex; considerable variation exists in the order and anastomotic connections of these branches. **(Bottom)** Axial high-resolution T1 MR of the mid-orbit. The optic nerve/sheath complex angles medially within the muscle cone as it courses toward the optic canal. The ophthalmic artery is visible near the apex as it exits laterally from within the dural sheath just beyond the optic canal.

OPTIC NERVE/SHEATH COMPLEX

CORONAL & AXIAL STIR MR

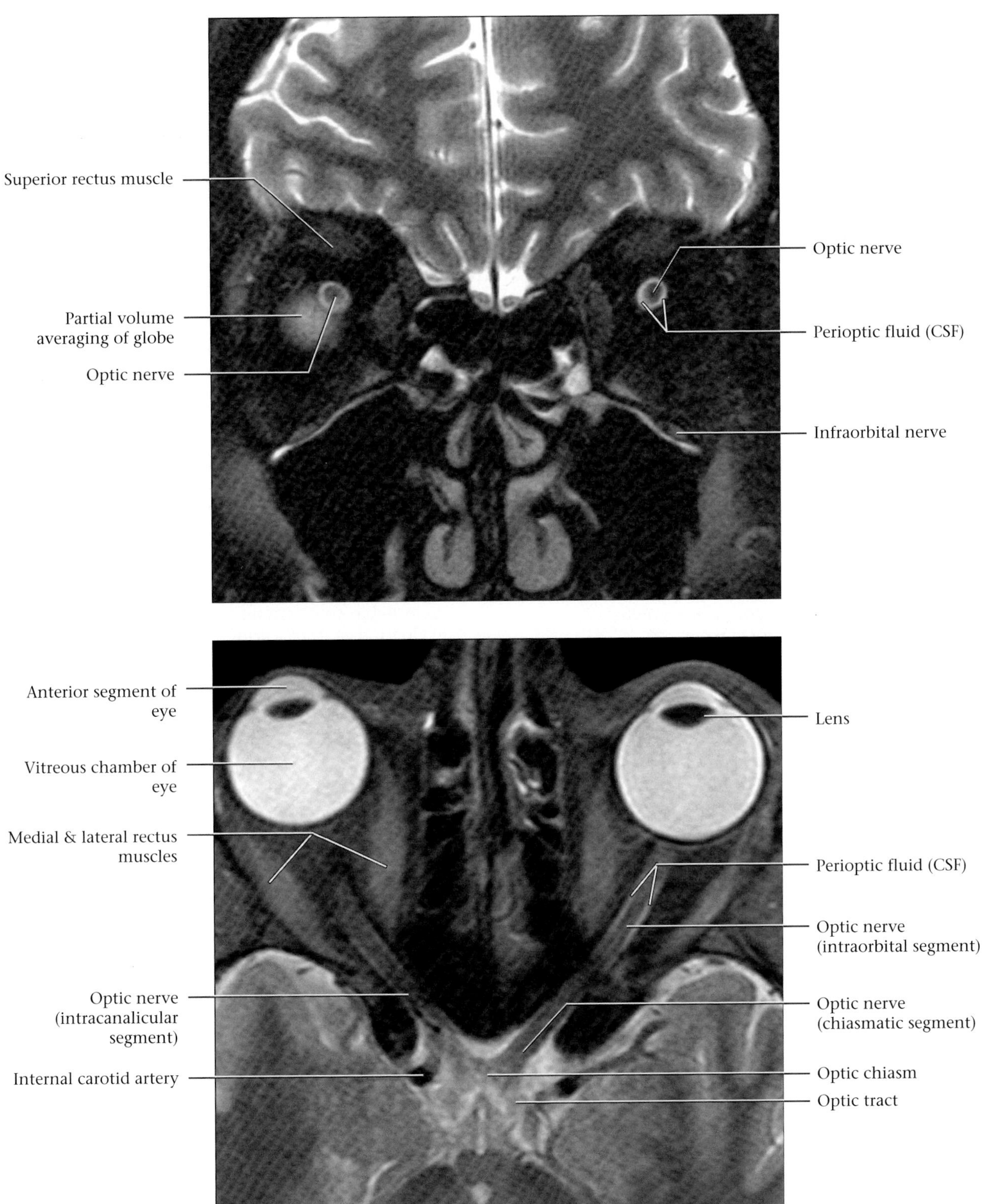
Superior rectus muscle
Partial volume averaging of globe
Optic nerve
Optic nerve
Perioptic fluid (CSF)
Infraorbital nerve
Anterior segment of eye
Vitreous chamber of eye
Medial & lateral rectus muscles
Optic nerve (intracanalicular segment)
Internal carotid artery
Lens
Perioptic fluid (CSF)
Optic nerve (intraorbital segment)
Optic nerve (chiasmatic segment)
Optic chiasm
Optic tract

(Top) Coronal T2 STIR image of the orbits. STIR technique provides reliable and effective suppression of intraorbital fat, making the fluid signal of the perioptic cerebrospinal fluid appear conspicuous. Extraocular muscles appear relatively hypointense on STIR. Remember the arachnoid space surrounding the optic nerve is contiguous with the suprasellar cistern. Its size will therefore vary with intracranial pressure. **(Bottom)** Axial T2 STIR image of the orbits. A slightly oblique plane allows for demonstration of both intraorbital and cisternal segments of CN2. Because of the normal angulation of the nerves proximally, the chiasm and tracts are usually demonstrated on images superior to those depicting the intraorbital nerves. The anterior segment of the eye includes both the anterior and posterior chambers in front of the lens.

GLOBE

Gross Anatomy

Segments

- **Anterior segment of globe**
  - Portion of eye in front of anterior margin of vitreous (hyaloid face)
    - Ciliary body, suspensory ligaments and lens
    - Anterior and posterior chambers
    - Iris
    - Cornea
- **Posterior segment of globe**
  - Vitreoretinal portion of the eye and its layers
    - Vitreous chamber
    - Retina
    - Choroid
    - Sclera

Chambers

- **Anterior chamber**
  - Major chamber of anterior segment
  - Between cornea and iris
  - Filled with aqueous humor which provides nutrition and structure
- **Posterior chamber**
  - Small potential space posterior to iris and anterior to lens/ligament complex
  - Contiguous with anterior chamber through pupil
- **Vitreous chamber**
  - Large chamber that fills posterior segment
  - Filled with viscoelastic transparent gel

Tunicae

- **Tunica interna (retina)**
  - Multilayered sensorineural organ
    - Photoreceptor cells (rods and cones) overlie pigment epithelium at outermost layer
    - Bipolar and ganglion cells form inner layer (next to vitreous), & assemble & convey sensory signals
  - Regions and extent
    - **Macula**: Central portion, daylight & color vision
    - **Fovea**: Macular center, highest spatial resolution
    - **Peripheral**: Outer portion, night vision & motion
    - **Ora serrata**: Anterior margin of retina
- **Tunica vasculosa (uvea)**
  - Pigmented, vascular loose connective tissue
  - **Choroid**
    - Layer between retina and sclera
    - Vascular supply to photoreceptor layer
  - **Ciliary body**
    - Uveal structure anterior to ora serrata
    - Attached to lens via zonule fibers
    - Contractile function provides for lens accommodation
    - Source of aqueous production
  - **Iris**
    - Thin elastic tissue overlying lens
    - Sphincter muscle provides pupillary response
- **Tunica fibrosa (sclera)**
  - Outer fibrous layer
  - Attachment site for extraocular muscles
  - Contiguous with dura of optic sheath as well as fibrous diaphragm (lamina cribrosa) at nerve head
  - Contiguous with cornea anteriorly

Imaging Anatomy

Overview

- Primary imaging approaches
  - Direct funduscopy is first line technique
  - Sonography readily available at most eye clinics
- Cross-sectional modalities (MR and CT)
  - Particularly useful in eyes with opaque media (i.e., obscured by vitreous or aqueous opacity)
  - Routine imaging as part of orbital evaluation
    - Extraocular extension of ocular disease
    - Ocular involvement of orbital process

Internal Structures-Critical Contents

- **Anterior segment**
  - Aqueous chambers exhibit fluid signal
  - Lens moderately hyperdense on CT, isodense on T1WI, hypodense relative to fluid on T2WI
  - Ciliary body and iris variably distinguishable but not diagnostic detail
- **Posterior segment**
  - Vitreous chamber exhibits fluid signal

Anatomy-Based Imaging Issues

Imaging Recommendations

- CT
  - Preferred in some circumstances
  - Evaluation of calcification (e.g., retinoblastoma)
  - Evaluation in a child without sedation
- MR
  - Preferred for evaluation of extraocular extent of disease
  - T2WI useful for evaluating vitreous and aqueous chambers; otherwise limited utility in eye
  - T1WI pre- and post-contrast better for assessing uveoretinal structures
  - Surface coils improve signal and resolution in globe but may be limited in assessment of posterior orbit

Imaging Pitfalls

- MR
  - Irrepressible globe movement results in ubiquitous motion artifact

Embryology

Embryologic Events

- **Optic fissure**
  - Extends along inferonasal aspect of optic disc & stalk
  - Fissure fusion (about 5th week) required for normal globe and nerve formation
  - Failure of fusion results in coloboma
- **Primary vitreous**
  - Embryonic fibrovascular hyaloid, with hyaloid artery in Cloquet canal
  - Normally regresses about 7 months gestation
    - Visible in premature infant
  - Failure of regression results in persistent hyperplastic primary vitreous

GRAPHIC & SAGITTAL T1 MR

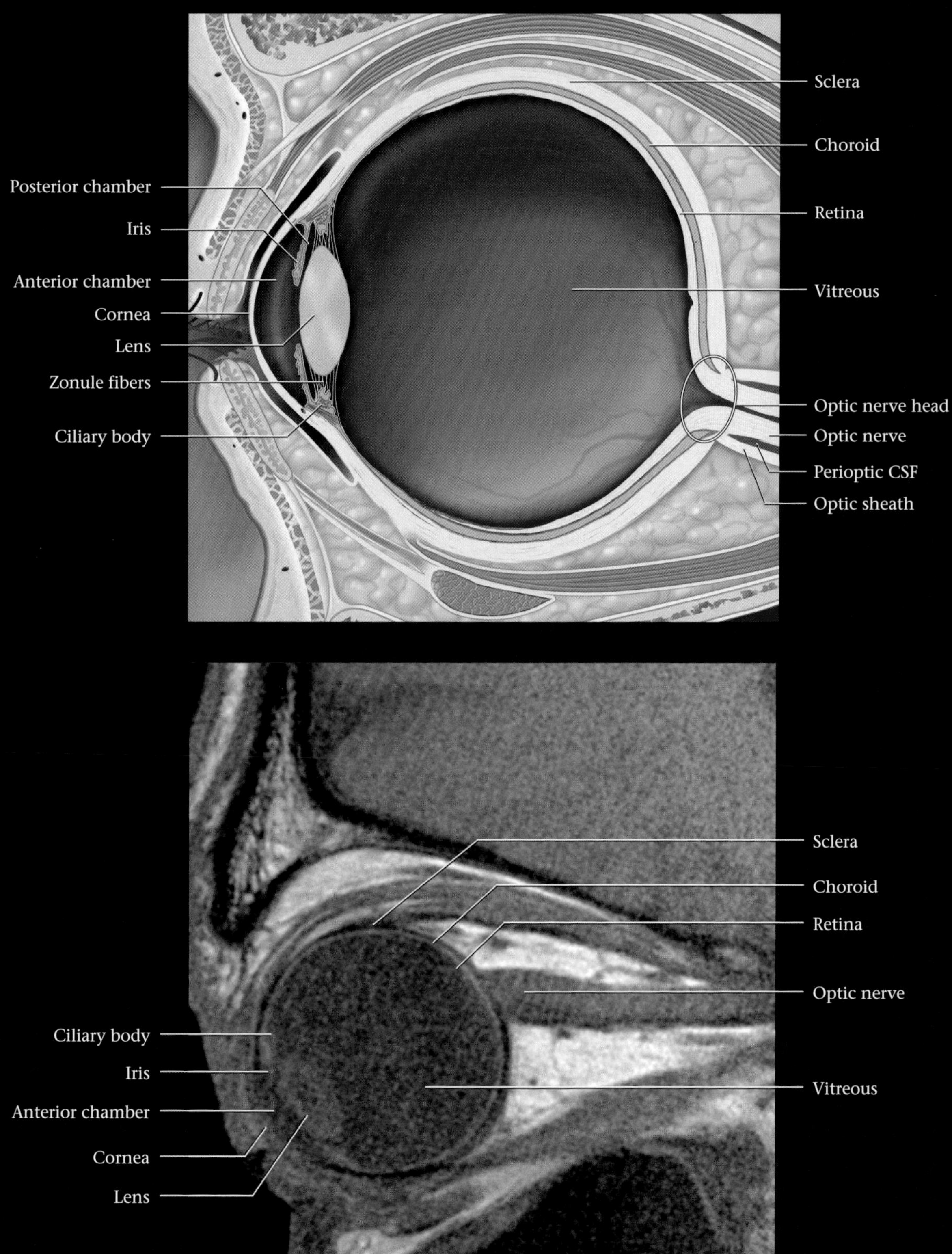
Sclera
Choroid
Retina
Vitreous
Optic nerve head
Optic nerve
Perioptic CSF
Optic sheath
Posterior chamber
Iris
Anterior chamber
Cornea
Lens
Zonule fibers
Ciliary body
Sclera
Choroid
Retina
Optic nerve
Vitreous
Ciliary body
Iris
Anterior chamber
Cornea
Lens

(Top) Sagittal graphic shows that the anterior and posterior chambers of the anterior segment are contiguous through the pupil. The choroid and iris are anterior extensions of the uveal tract. The posterior segment is filled by the vitreous chamber. The retina and sclera are contiguous with the optic nerve and sheath, respectively, at the nerve head. **(Bottom)** Sagittal T1 MR shows that the aqueous filled anterior chamber and vitreous filled posterior chamber exhibit essentially pure fluid signal. The lens is distinguishable; the iris and ciliary body are identifiable but not reliably diagnostic on routine MR imaging. The pigmented choroid may be seen as a thin hyperintense layer on high-resolution T1.

SINONASAL OVERVIEW

Terminology

Abbreviations

- Sinonasal (SN)

Definitions

- SN: Nasal cavity, paranasal sinuses (maxillary, frontal, ethmoid, and sphenoid), and surrounding structures

Imaging Anatomy

Overview

- Nasal cavity: Triangle divided in midline by septum
  - Roof: Cribriform plate
  - Floor: Hard and soft palate
  - Lateral: Lateral nasal wall with attached turbinates
  - Nasal septum
    - Bony septum: Perpendicular plate of ethmoid posterosuperiorly and vomer posteroinferiorly
    - Cartilage: Septal cartilage anteriorly
  - Turbinates
    - Bony superior, middle, and inferior turbinates project inferomedially into nasal cavity
    - Define region below as superior, middle, and inferior meati, respectively
    - Middle turbinate attaches superiorly to cribriform plate via vertical lamella and posteriorly and laterally to lamina papyracea via basal lamella
  - Meati
    - **Superior meatus**: Receives drainage from posterior ethmoid cells at sphenoethmoidal recess
    - **Middle meatus: Ethmoid bulla**: Large ethmoid air cell positioned at superior aspect of ostiomeatal complex (OMC), receives drainage from anterior ethmoid air cells
    - **Middle meatus: Hiatus semilunaris**: Semilunar region between uncinate process and ethmoid bulla, receives drainage from anterior ethmoid air cells and maxillary sinus via infundibulum
    - **Inferior meatus**: Receives drainage from nasolacrimal duct anteriorly

Extent

- Nasal cavity and paranasal sinuses aerate the maxillary, frontal, sphenoid, and ethmoid bones

Anatomy Relationships

- **Maxillary sinus**: Paired air cells within maxillary bone
  - Drain via maxillary ostium located along superior aspect of medial wall into infundibulum then into hiatus semilunaris at the middle meatus
- **Ethmoid sinus**: Paired groups of 3-18 air cells within ethmoid labyrinths
  - Separated into anterior and posterior groups separated by basal lamella (lateral attachment of middle turbinate to lamina papyracea)
  - Ethmoid bulla: Dominant anterior ethmoid air cell that protrudes inferomedially into infundibulum or hiatus semilunaris
  - Anterior drainage: Anterior recess of hiatus semilunaris and middle meatus via ethmoid bulla
  - Posterior drainage: Superior meatus and sphenoethmoidal recess
- **Frontal sinus**: Paired air cells within frontal bone
  - Drainage through frontal recess into middle meatus
- **Sphenoid sinus**: Paired air cells within sphenoid bone
  - Drainage into sphenoethmoidal recess
- Extramural paranasal air cells
  - **Infraorbital ethmoid cells (Haller)** = ethmoid cells that extend into inferomedial orbital floor
  - **Agger nasi cells** = most anterior air cells that involve lacrimal bone or maxilla
  - **Sphenoethmoidal cells (Onodi)** = posterior ethmoid air cells with prominent superolateral pneumatization; close relationship to optic nerve

Internal Structures-Critical Contents

- **Pterygopalatine fossa (PPF)**
  - Major crossroads between nasal cavity, masticator space, orbit, and middle cranial fossa
- **Sphenoethmoidal recess (SER)**
  - Receives drainage from sphenoid sinus and variable drainage from posterior ethmoid air cells
- **Olfactory tract and bulb**
  - Nasal mucosa and sensory nerves traverse cribriform plate and synapse with secondary neurons in olfactory bulb and olfactory tracts

Anatomy-Based Imaging Issues

Key Concepts or Questions

- Majority of SN imaging depicts complete absence or sporadic (nonobstructive) mild disease

Imaging Recommendations

- Common rhinosinusitis symptoms case best imaged with NECT, bone algorithm
  - Multislice CT can acquire 1 mm axial sections & reconstruct coronal & sagittal images
- Sinusitis complications can be imaged with CECT, but CEMR better evaluates surrounding structures

Imaging Approaches

- Coronal sinus CT used in presurgical work-up and follow-up of inflammatory sinonasal disease
- MR: If enhanced scan needed to define complex inflammatory or neoplastic disease, use enhanced MR
  - Fat-saturation should be utilized on at least one post-contrasted sequence

Imaging Pitfalls

- **Be aware of variations in sinus pneumatization**

Clinical Implications

Clinical Importance

- Rhinosinusitis accounts for over 2 million office visits and $2 billion in direct medical costs yearly

Embryology

Embryologic Events

- Paranasal sinuses develop as diverticula from the nasal vault with a contiguous mucosal surface

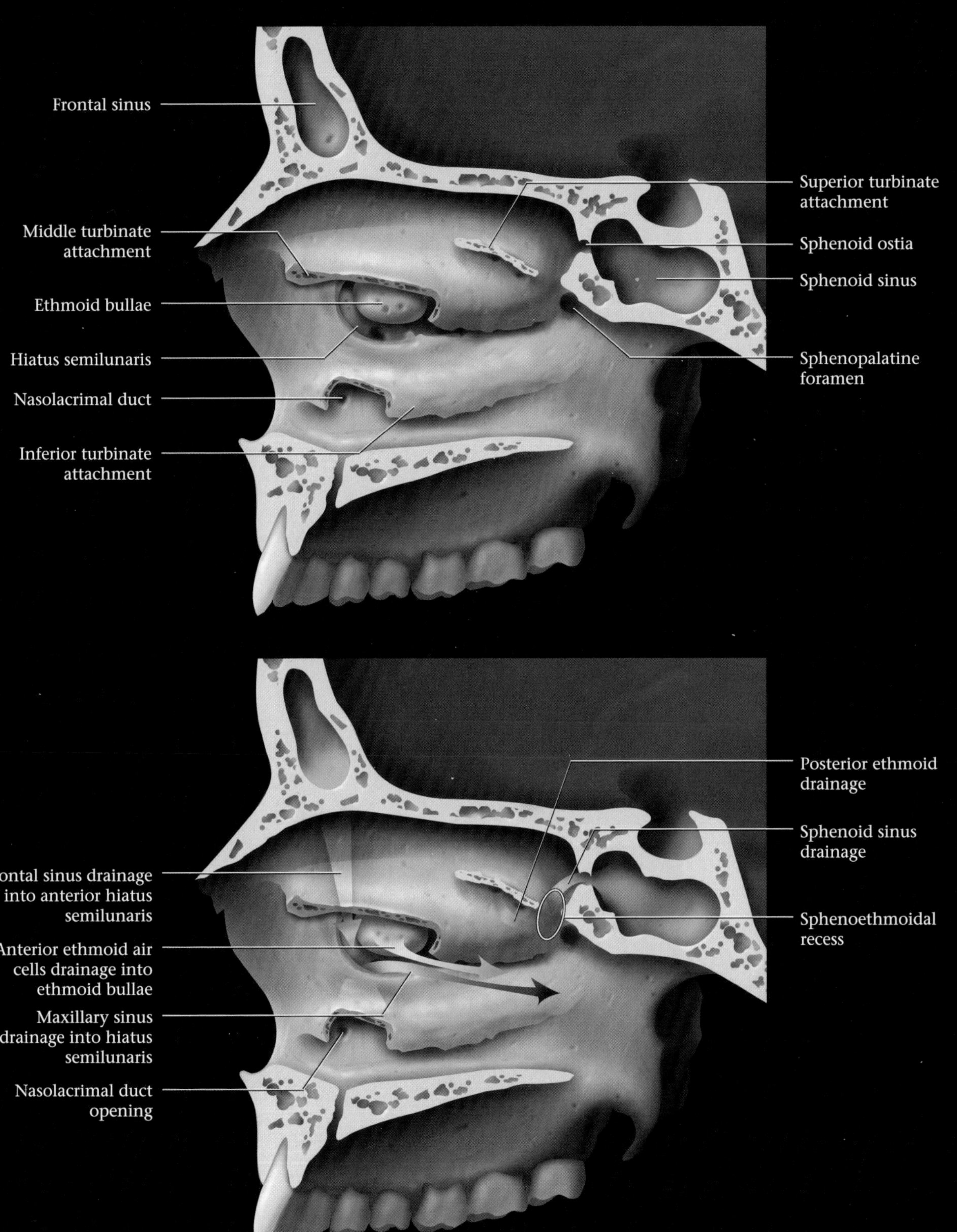

Frontal sinus
Middle turbinate attachment
Ethmoid bullae
Hiatus semilunaris
Nasolacrimal duct
Inferior turbinate attachment
Superior turbinate attachment
Sphenoid ostia
Sphenoid sinus
Sphenopalatine foramen
Frontal sinus drainage into anterior hiatus semilunaris
Anterior ethmoid air cells drainage into ethmoid bullae
Maxillary sinus drainage into hiatus semilunaris
Nasolacrimal duct opening
Posterior ethmoid drainage
Sphenoid sinus drainage
Sphenoethmoidal recess

(Top) Sagittal graphic demonstrates the osseous anatomy of the lateral wall of the nose. The superior and middle turbinate have been resected. The ethmoid bullae and hiatus semilunaris are seen below the middle turbinate attachment. The nasolacrimal duct empties into the anterior aspect of the inferior meatus. **(Bottom)** Sagittal graphic of the lateral wall of the nose shows the drainage pathways of the sinuses. The sphenoid and posterior ethmoid sinuses drain into the sphenoethmoidal recess in the posterior nasal cavity. The maxillary sinus drains via the maxillary infundibulum while the anterior ethmoids mostly drain through the concha bullosa into the ostiomeatal complex/middle meatus. The frontal sinus drains into the anterior middle meatus through the nasofrontal drainage system.

AXIAL BONE CT

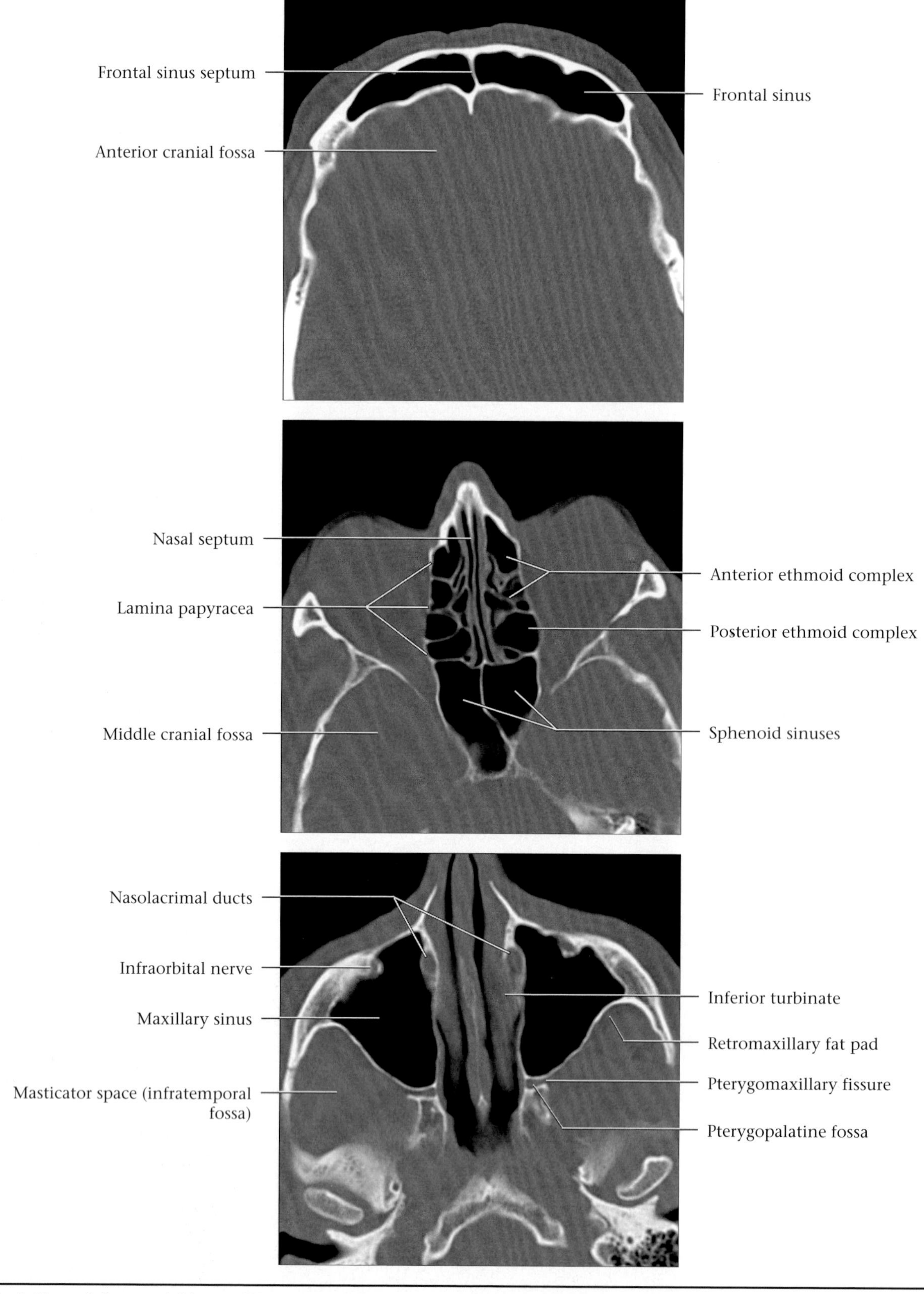
Frontal sinus septum
Frontal sinus
Anterior cranial fossa
Nasal septum
Anterior ethmoid complex
Lamina papyracea
Posterior ethmoid complex
Middle cranial fossa
Sphenoid sinuses
Nasolacrimal ducts
Infraorbital nerve
Inferior turbinate
Maxillary sinus
Retromaxillary fat pad
Pterygomaxillary fissure
Masticator space (infratemporal fossa)
Pterygopalatine fossa

(Top) First of three axial bone CT images of the sinuses presented from superior to inferior. This image shows the frontal sinuses, with their midline septum, and thin posterior wall, separating the sinuses from the anterior cranial fossa. Frontal sinus disease can extend posteriorly into the cranial vault. **(Middle)** This image shows the ethmoid air cells and sphenoid sinuses. The thin lamina papyracea is the lateral wall of the ethmoid sinuses. Ethmoid air cell disease can extend through the lamina papyracea to create a post-septal subperiosteal abscess. **(Bottom)** This image through the maxillary sinuses shows their intimate relationship to the nasolacrimal ducts, pterygopalatine fossa and retromaxillary fat pad. Notice the infraorbital nerve anteriorly just before it exits through the infraorbital foramen.

CORONAL BONE CT

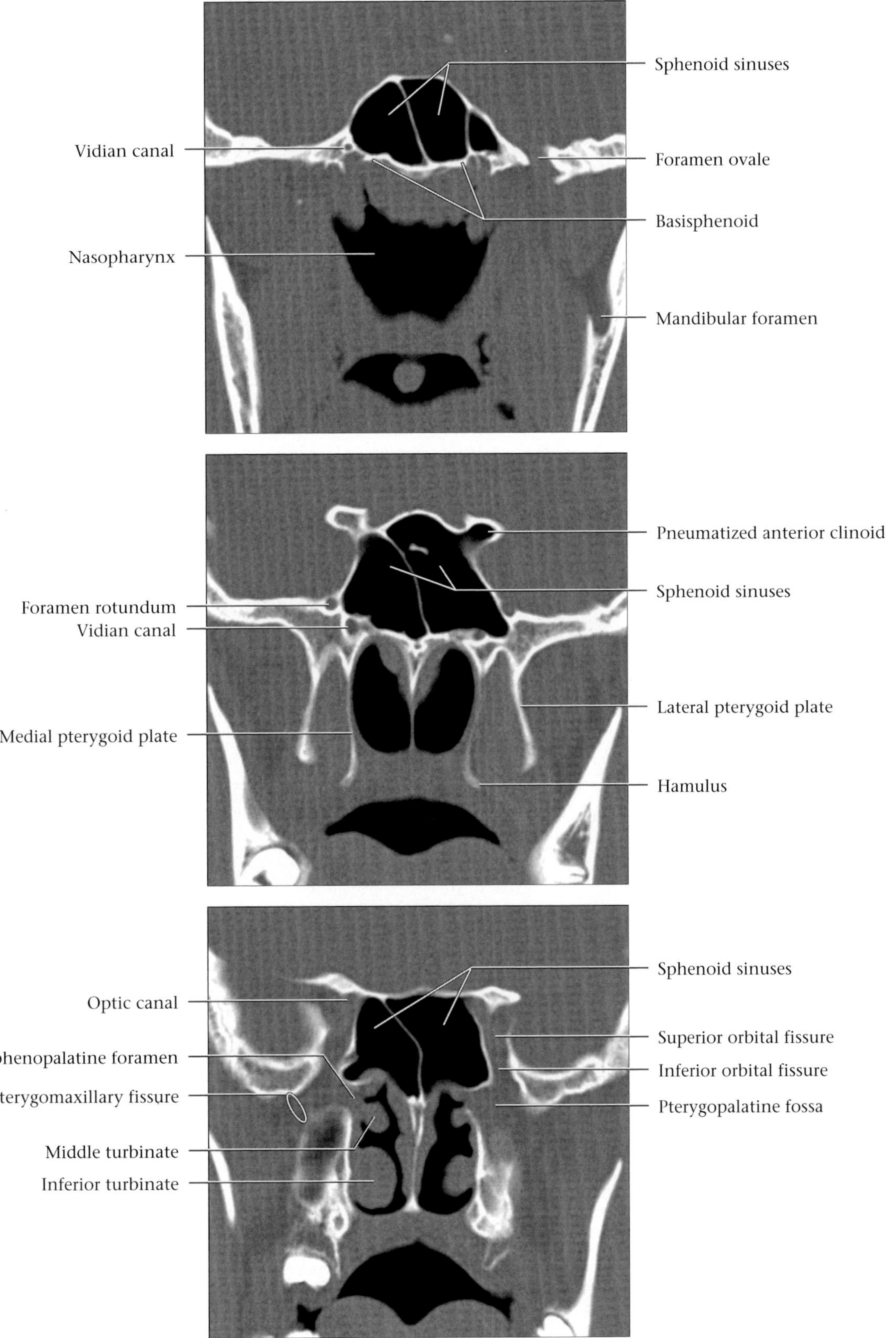
Sphenoid sinuses
Vidian canal
Foramen ovale
Basisphenoid
Nasopharynx
Mandibular foramen
Pneumatized anterior clinoid
Sphenoid sinuses
Foramen rotundum
Vidian canal
Lateral pterygoid plate
Medial pterygoid plate
Hamulus
Sphenoid sinuses
Optic canal
Superior orbital fissure
Sphenopalatine foramen
Inferior orbital fissure
Pterygomaxillary fissure
Pterygopalatine fossa
Middle turbinate
Inferior turbinate

(Top) First of nine coronal bone CT noncontrasted images through the paranasal sinuses are presented from posterior to anterior. This image shows the sphenoid sinuses, superior to the nasopharynx. **(Middle)** This image shows the pterygoid plates, posterior to the maxillary sinuses. Inferolateral to the sphenoid sinus note the foramen rotundum and the vidian canal. **(Bottom)** This image shows the complex anatomic landscape surrounding the PPF. The lateral exit of the PPF is the pterygomaxillary fissure through which it exits into the masticator space. Superiorly the PPF exits into the inferior orbital fissure. The medial exit from the PPF is through the foramen rotundum into the posterolateral nose.

CORONAL BONE CT

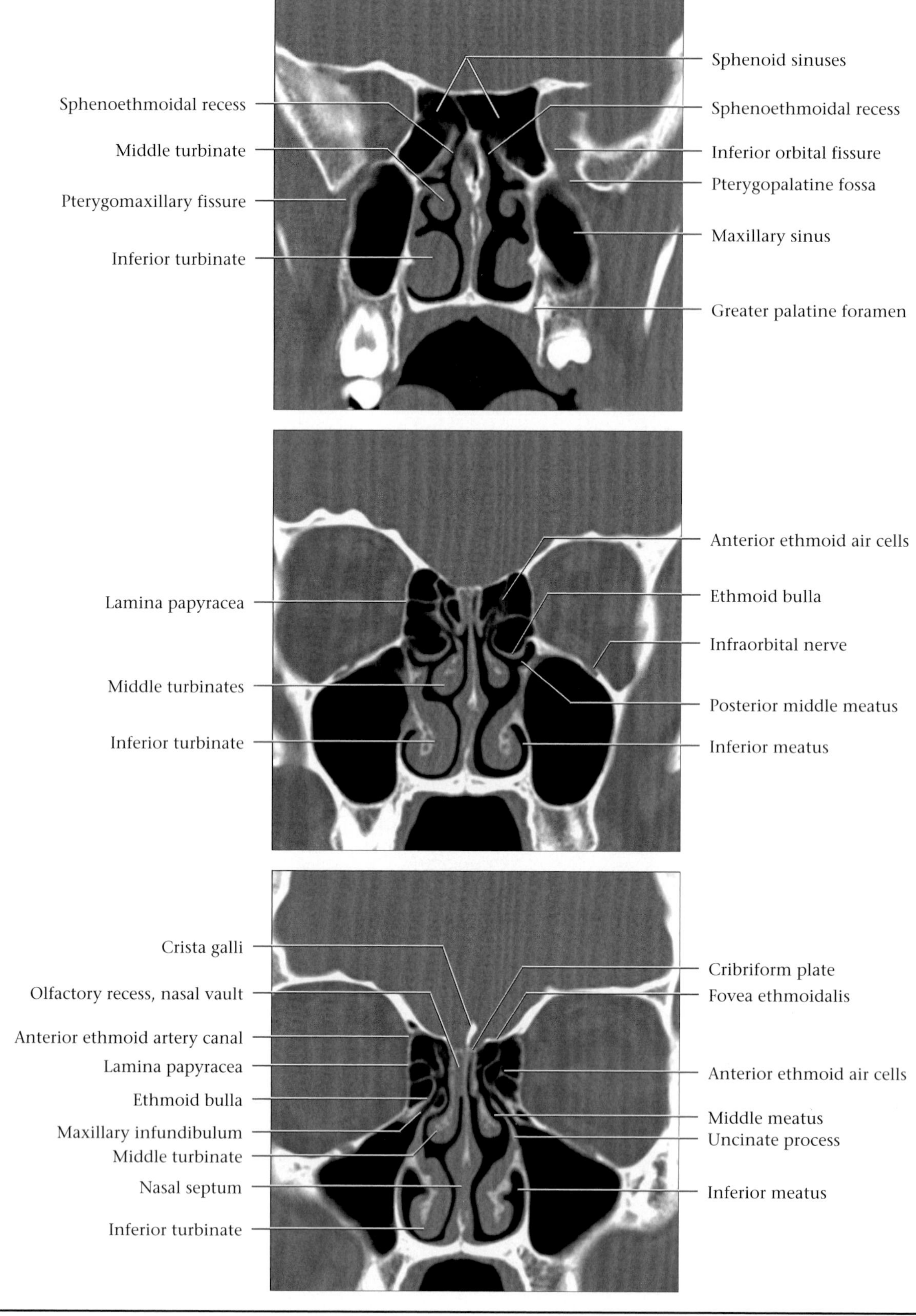
Sphenoid sinuses
Sphenoethmoidal recess
Sphenoethmoidal recess
Middle turbinate
Inferior orbital fissure
Pterygopalatine fossa
Pterygomaxillary fissure
Maxillary sinus
Inferior turbinate
Greater palatine foramen
Anterior ethmoid air cells
Ethmoid bulla
Lamina papyracea
Infraorbital nerve
Middle turbinates
Posterior middle meatus
Inferior turbinate
Inferior meatus
Crista galli
Cribriform plate
Olfactory recess, nasal vault
Fovea ethmoidalis
Anterior ethmoid artery canal
Lamina papyracea
Anterior ethmoid air cells
Ethmoid bulla
Middle meatus
Maxillary infundibulum
Uncinate process
Middle turbinate
Nasal septum
Inferior meatus
Inferior turbinate

(Top) In this image the sphenoethmoidal recess is visible as vertical air-filled slits in the posterosuperior nose into which both the posterior ethmoid sinus and the sphenoid sinus empty. Note the greater palatine canal exiting the lateral hard-soft palate junction. Perineural malignancy may travel from the palate to the pterygopalatine fossa via the greater palatine nerve. **(Middle)** In this image through the anterior ethmoid air cells the ethmoid bulla is seen projecting inferiorly into the middle meatus. The shared wall with between the anterior ethmoid air cells and the orbit is paper thin, hence the term lamina papyracea. **(Bottom)** Image through the ostiomeatal complex shows the maxillary infundibulum draining the maxillary sinuses into the middle meatus. The uncinate process, middle meatus, maxillary infundibulum and ethmoid bulla are the components of OMC.

CORONAL BONE CT

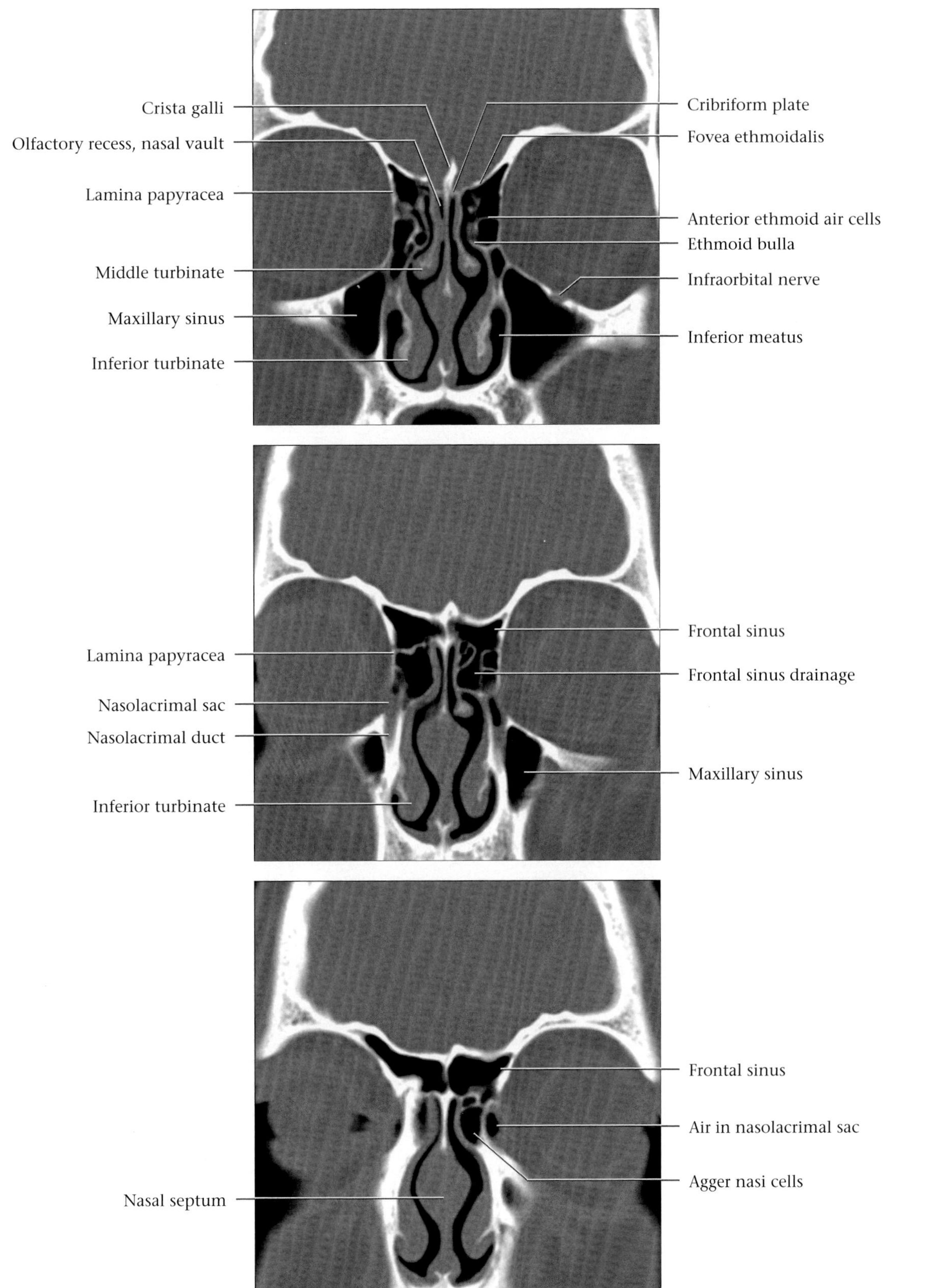
Crista galli
Olfactory recess, nasal vault
Lamina papyracea
Middle turbinate
Maxillary sinus
Inferior turbinate
Cribriform plate
Fovea ethmoidalis
Anterior ethmoid air cells
Ethmoid bulla
Infraorbital nerve
Inferior meatus
Lamina papyracea
Nasolacrimal sac
Nasolacrimal duct
Inferior turbinate
Frontal sinus
Frontal sinus drainage
Maxillary sinus
Nasal septum
Frontal sinus
Air in nasolacrimal sac
Agger nasi cells

(Top) In this image through the anterior aspect of the anterior ethmoid complex the fovea ethmoidalis (roof of ethmoid), cribriform plate and crista galli can all be seen along the roof of the sinuses and nose from lateral to medial. The olfactory recess of the nasal vault contains the nasal mucosa. From the nasal mucosa arises esthesioneuroblastoma. **(Middle)** This image shows the close relationship of the nasolacrimal ducts to the maxillary sinuses. Remember the nasolacrimal duct drains into the anterior recess of the inferior turbinate. **(Bottom)** In this image through the frontal sinuses the anteroinferior extramural ethmoid air cells also called the agger nasi air cells can be seen. Notice the normal air-filled left nasolacrimal sac just lateral to the agger nasi cells.

SAGITTAL BONE CT

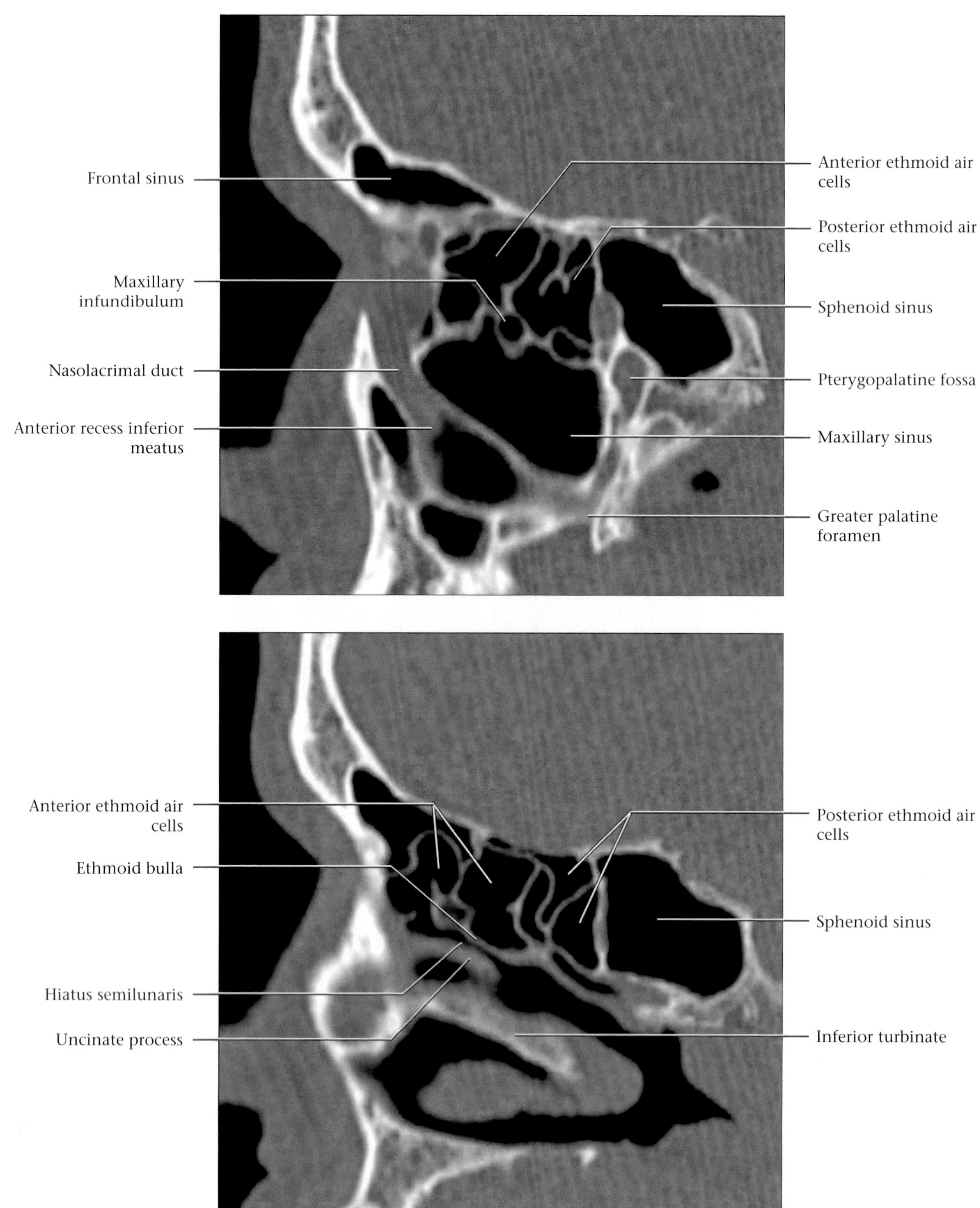
Frontal sinus
Maxillary infundibulum
Nasolacrimal duct
Anterior recess inferior meatus
Anterior ethmoid air cells
Posterior ethmoid air cells
Sphenoid sinus
Pterygopalatine fossa
Maxillary sinus
Greater palatine foramen
Anterior ethmoid air cells
Ethmoid bulla
Hiatus semilunaris
Uncinate process
Posterior ethmoid air cells
Sphenoid sinus
Inferior turbinate

(Top) First of four sagittal bone CT noncontrasted images through the paranasal sinuses presented from lateral to medial. This image shows the nasolacrimal duct, draining into the inferior meatus. Also note the pterygopalatine fossa posterior to the maxillary sinus. **(Bottom)** In this image the uncinate process can be seen just inferior to the ethmoid bulla. The gap between these two structures is the hiatus semilunaris.

SAGITTAL BONE CT

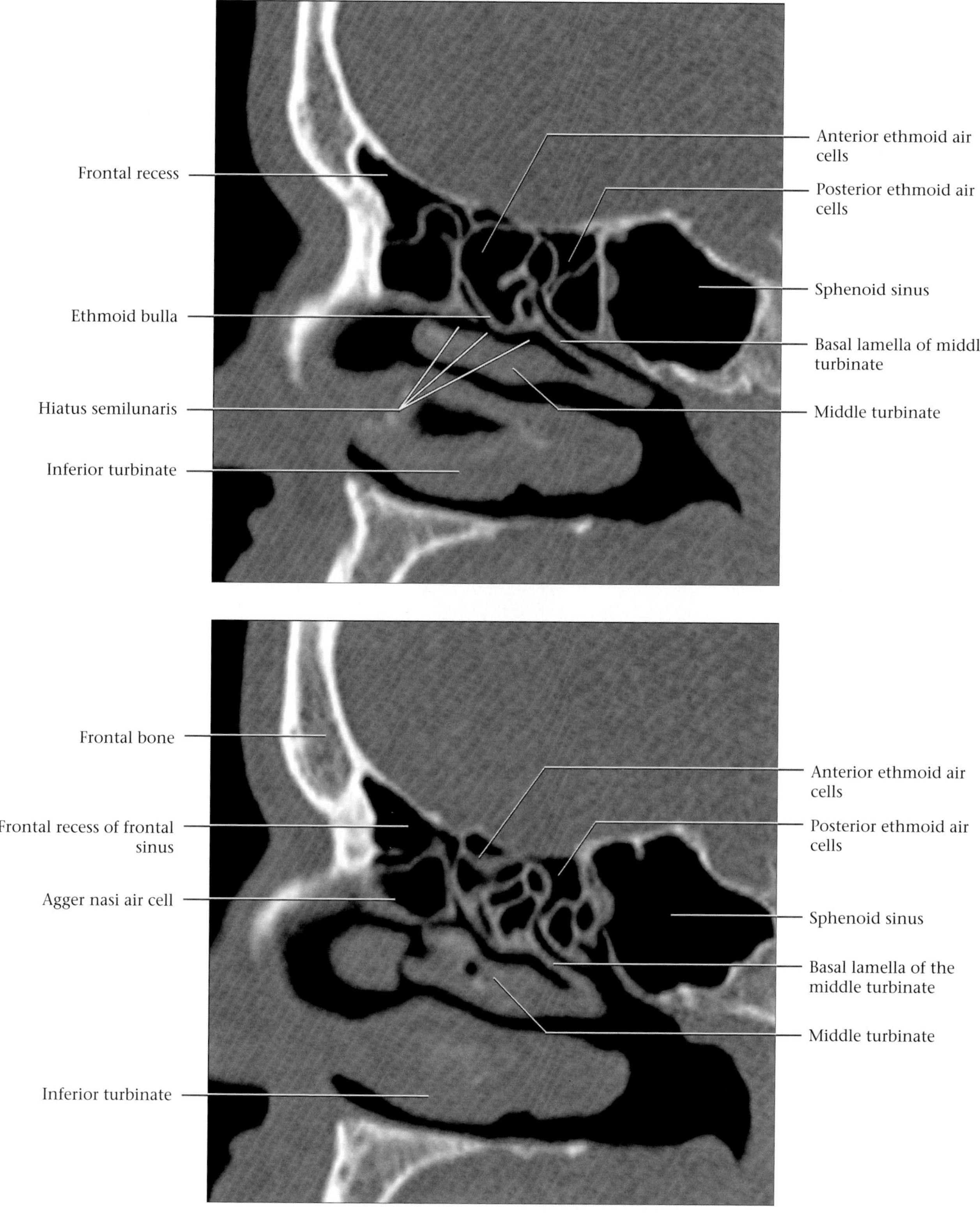
Frontal recess
Ethmoid bulla
Hiatus semilunaris
Inferior turbinate
Anterior ethmoid air cells
Posterior ethmoid air cells
Sphenoid sinus
Basal lamella of middle turbinate
Middle turbinate
Frontal bone
Frontal recess of frontal sinus
Agger nasi air cell
Inferior turbinate
Anterior ethmoid air cells
Posterior ethmoid air cells
Sphenoid sinus
Basal lamella of the middle turbinate
Middle turbinate

(Top) This image shows the middle and inferior turbinates, as well as the basal lamella of the middle turbinate. **(Bottom)** In this image the anteroinferior ethmoid air cell (agger nasi cells) are seen extending anteroinferiorly to the frontal recess of the frontal sinus. If this cell is infected, the frontal sinus recess and frontal sinus will also become infected secondarily.

AXIAL T1 MR

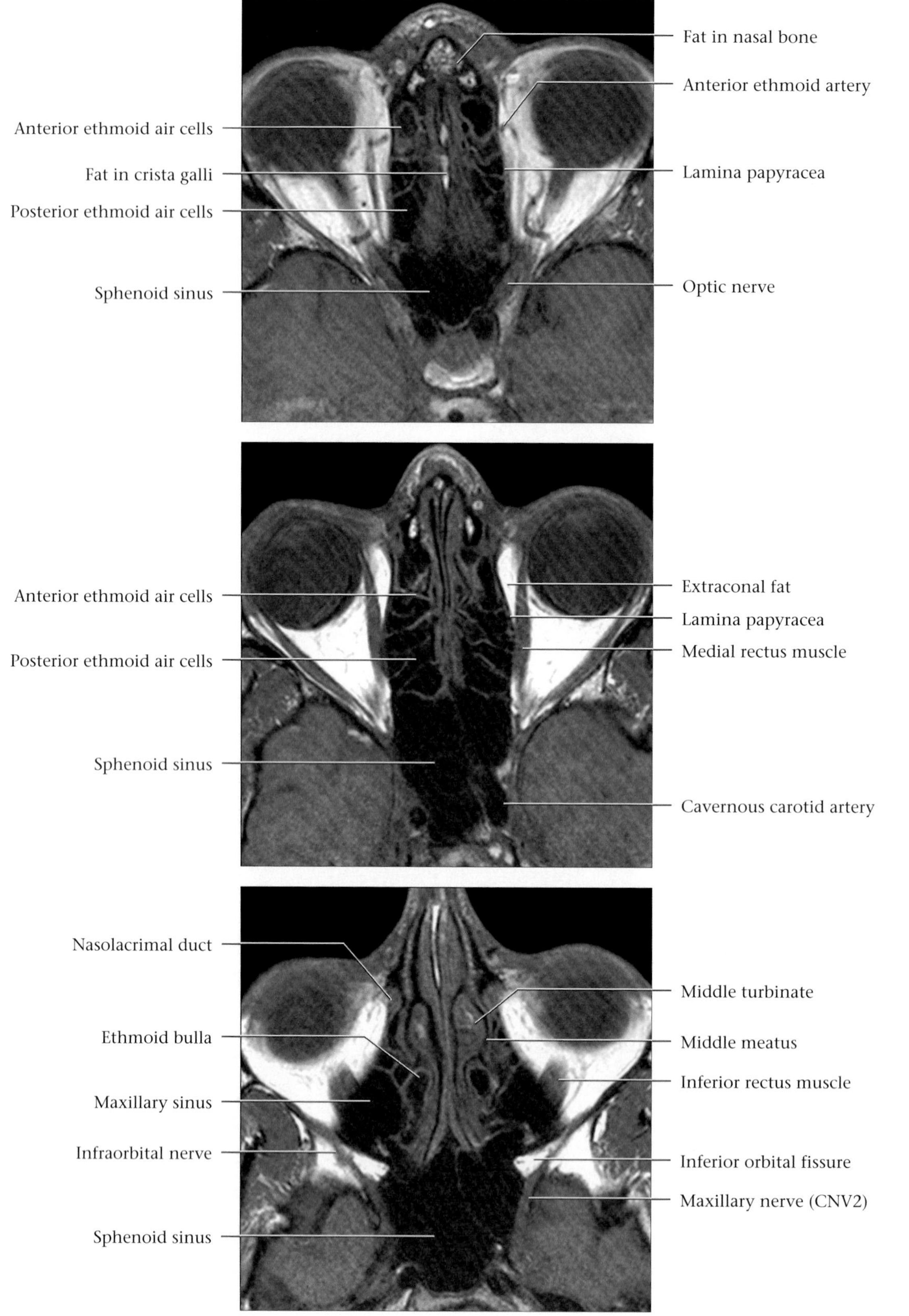

Fat in nasal bone
Anterior ethmoid artery
Anterior ethmoid air cells
Fat in crista galli
Lamina papyracea
Posterior ethmoid air cells
Sphenoid sinus
Optic nerve
Anterior ethmoid air cells
Extraconal fat
Lamina papyracea
Medial rectus muscle
Posterior ethmoid air cells
Sphenoid sinus
Cavernous carotid artery
Nasolacrimal duct
Middle turbinate
Ethmoid bulla
Middle meatus
Inferior rectus muscle
Maxillary sinus
Infraorbital nerve
Inferior orbital fissure
Maxillary nerve (CNV2)
Sphenoid sinus

(Top) First of six axial pre-contrasted T1 MR images presented from superior to inferior, through the paranasal sinuses and the nasal vault. In this image the anterior ethmoid artery is visible piercing the lamina papyracea into the anterior ethmoid air cells. **(Middle)** In this image through the mid-globes the close relationship of the ethmoid air cells to extraconal fat and medial rectus muscle is seen. The thin lateral wall of the ethmoid sinus (lamina papyracea) is is all that separates the orbit from the sinus. If the ethmoid sinuses become infected, inadequate treatment can lead to orbital infection. **(Bottom)** In this image through the superior portion of the maxillary sinus the ethmoid bulla, middle meatus and middle turbinate are seen in the axial plane. Notice the fluid-filled normal nasolacrimal duct in the anterior aspect of the lateral nasal wall.

AXIAL T1 MR

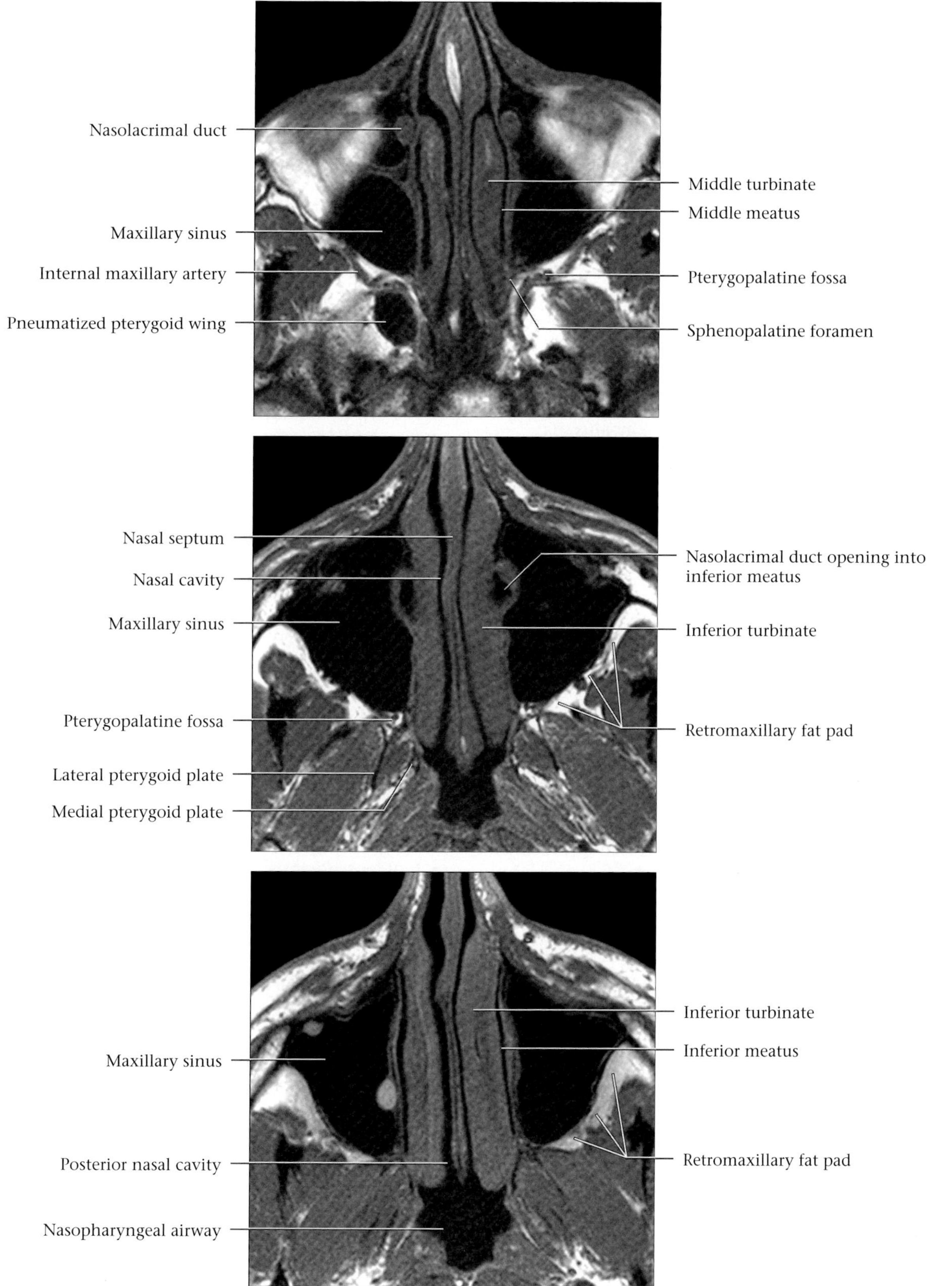
Nasolacrimal duct
Maxillary sinus
Internal maxillary artery
Pneumatized pterygoid wing
Middle turbinate
Middle meatus
Pterygopalatine fossa
Sphenopalatine foramen
Nasal septum
Nasal cavity
Maxillary sinus
Pterygopalatine fossa
Lateral pterygoid plate
Medial pterygoid plate
Nasolacrimal duct opening into inferior meatus
Inferior turbinate
Retromaxillary fat pad
Maxillary sinus
Posterior nasal cavity
Nasopharyngeal airway
Inferior turbinate
Inferior meatus
Retromaxillary fat pad

(Top) At the level of the pterygopalatine fossa the internal maxillary artery can be seen as its principal occupant. The medial exit from the pterygopalatine fossa is the sphenopalatine foramen. Juvenile angiofibroma originates along the nasal margin of the sphenopalatine foramen. Often the first route of spread for this tumor is through this foramen into the pterygopalatine fossa. **(Middle)** In this image the nasolacrimal duct is visible emptying inferiorly into the anterior recess of the inferior meatus. The inferior turbinate is the largest of the turbinates and can be mistaken for a mass when large and asymmetric. **(Bottom)** At the level of the mid-maxillary sinus the posterior nasal cavity can be seen in direct continuity with the nasopharyngeal airway. The retromaxillary fat pad sits behind the maxillary sinus. It is the superior extension of the buccal space.

OSTIOMEATAL UNIT (OMU)

Terminology

Abbreviations

- Ostiomeatal unit (OMU), ostiomeatal complex (OMC)

Definitions

- OMU: Complex anatomic region where drainage of frontal, anterior ethmoid and maxillary sinuses occurs

Imaging Anatomy

Overview

- OMU includes superomedial maxillary sinus, maxillary infundibulum, uncinate process, ethmoid bulla, hiatus semilunaris and middle meatus

Extent

- OMU is area superolateral to middle meatus that receives drainage of frontal, anterior ethmoid and maxillary sinuses

Anatomy Relationships

- **Middle meatus** is most complicated of meati, receiving drainage from multiple sinuses
  - **Anterior ethmoid air cells** drain mostly into **ethmoid bulla**
    - **Ethmoid bulla**: Large ethmoid air cell positioned at superior aspect of OMU, immediately superior to hiatus semilunaris
  - **Frontal sinus** drains into anterior aspect of middle meatus
    - If uncinate process inserts on middle turbinate or skull base, frontal sinus drains through **frontal recess** into ethmoid infundibulum then middle meatus
    - If uncinate process inserts on lamina papyracea, frontal recess drains into anterior middle meatus directly
    - **Frontal recess**: Drainage funnel for frontal sinus
  - **Maxillary sinus** drains through maxillary infundibulum into middle meatus via maxillary ostium
- **Hiatus semilunaris**: Semilunar trough between tip of uncinate process and ethmoid bulla seen best from endoscopic vantage point
  - Hiatus semilunaris difficult to see on coronal sinus CT

Internal Structures-Critical Contents

- **Middle meatus**: Space between middle turbinate and medial wall of maxillary sinus
- **Maxillary infundibulum**: Drainage channel of maxillary sinus
  - Defined laterally by orbit and medially by uncinate process
  - Drains into middle meatus via **maxillary ostium**
- **Uncinate process**: Upper medial maxillary sinus wall
  - Defines medial wall of maxillary infundibulum
- **Ethmoid bulla**: Dominant anterior ethmoid air cell that protrudes inferomedially into infundibulum and upper middle meatus
- Normal aeration variants in vicinity of OMU
  - **Concha bullosa**: Aeration of nasal turbinate, most commonly **middle turbinate**
    - When inflamed, concha bullosa may obstruct OMU at middle meatus
    - Complete obstructive OMU pattern with frontal, maxillary, and anterior ethmoid opacification
  - **Haller cell** (infraorbital ethmoid air cell): Air cell located inferolateral to orbit and lateral to maxillary infundibulum
    - When inflamed, may obstruct maxillary infundibulum creating isolated maxillary infundibular pattern of sinus disease
    - Infundibular pattern: Only maxillary sinus is diseased with sparing of ethmoid sinuses
  - **Agger nasi** air cell: Most anterior ethmoid air cells
    - Found lateral to lamina papyracea, adjacent to frontal recess
    - When inflamed, agger nasi air cell may obstruct frontal recess causing isolated opacification of frontal sinus without involving anterior ethmoid or maxillary sinuses

Anatomy-Based Imaging Issues

Key Concepts or Questions

- Sinus CT used in presurgical work-up and follow-up of inflammatory sinonasal disease

Imaging Recommendations

- Common rhinosinusitis symptom cases are best imaged with bone algorithm CT
  - Coronal plane CT optimally depicts OMU

Imaging Approaches

- Multislice scanners can acquire thin (1 mm) supine sections with reconstruction of coronal and sagittal images
- If older scanner is available only, prone hyperextended coronal acquisitions may be preferable to move potential fluid in maxillary sinus away from OMU

Clinical Implications

Clinical Importance

- Sinus disease is single most common chronic complaint in USA
  - OMU is most important anatomic region for potential surgical treatment
- Clinical presentation of OMU obstruction
  - Facial fullness, pressure, loss of sense of smell and postnasal drainage
- OMU can also be obstructed secondary to anatomic variations or local noninfectious inflammatory processes such as allergic rhinitis

Function-Dysfunction

- Normal mucociliary pattern within paranasal sinuses is movement of secretions towards natural ostia
- Recirculation disorders may result despite endoscopic creation of surgical ostia

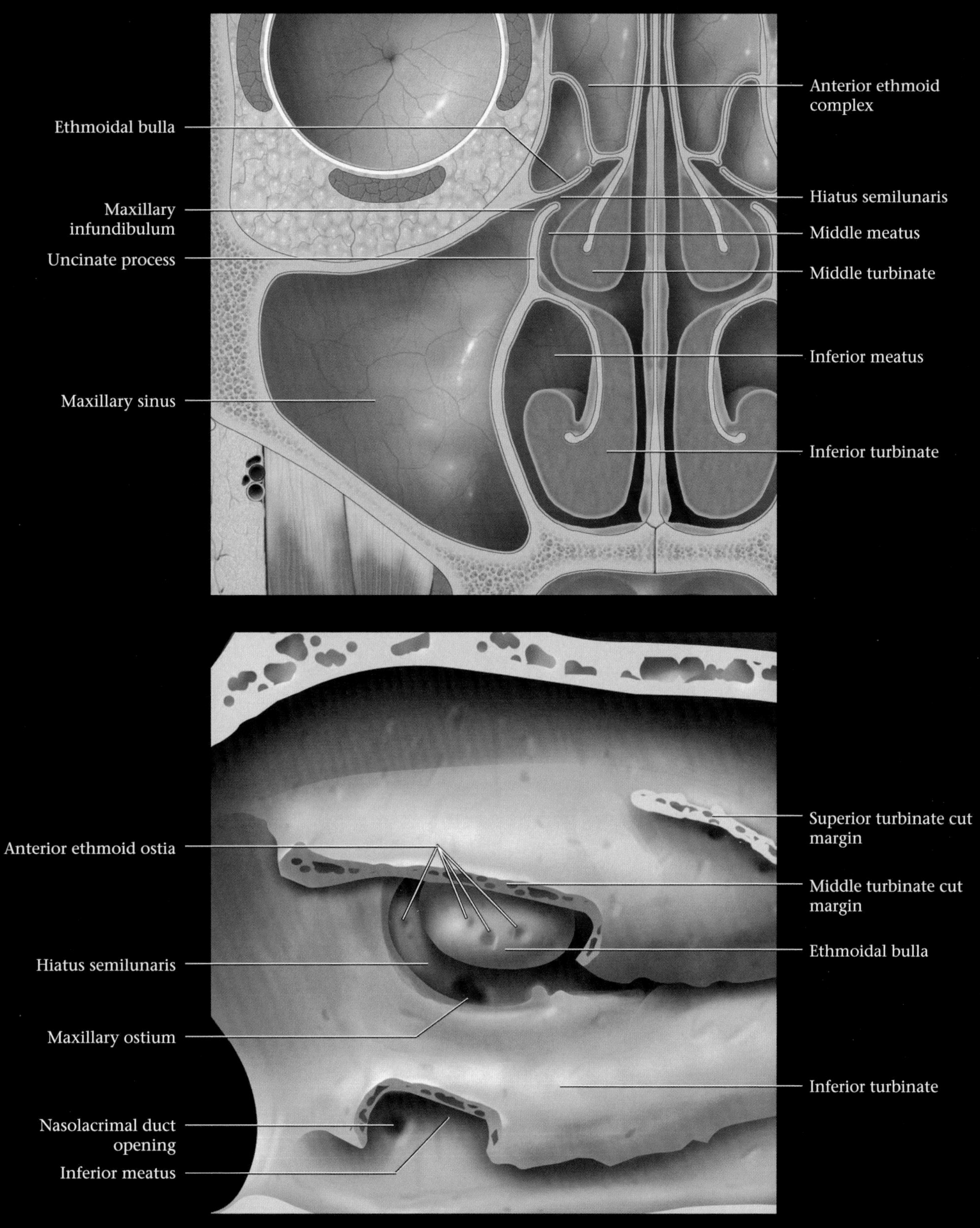
Ethmoidal bulla
Maxillary infundibulum
Uncinate process
Maxillary sinus
Anterior ethmoid complex
Hiatus semilunaris
Middle meatus
Middle turbinate
Inferior meatus
Inferior turbinate
Anterior ethmoid ostia
Hiatus semilunaris
Maxillary ostium
Nasolacrimal duct opening
Inferior meatus
Superior turbinate cut margin
Middle turbinate cut margin
Ethmoidal bulla
Inferior turbinate

(Top) Coronal graphic of magnified right sinonasal area illustrates the important structures of the ostiomeatal unit. Note the maxillary infundibulum provides drainage for the maxillary sinus while the ethmoid bulla (dominant ethmoid air cell of anterior ethmoid complex) protrudes inferomedially into the upper middle meatus. The middle meatus is the key area of drainage of normal secretions of the anterior ethmoid sinuses and the maxillary sinus. **(Bottom)** Graphic of lateral wall of nose focused on the region of the middle meatus with the superior turbinate removed as well as part of the middle turbinate. Note anterior ethmoid ostia drain into middle meatus as does the maxillary sinus via maxillary infundibulum. The nasolacrimal duct drains into the inferior meatus.

OSTIOMEATAL UNIT (OMU)

CORONAL BONE CT

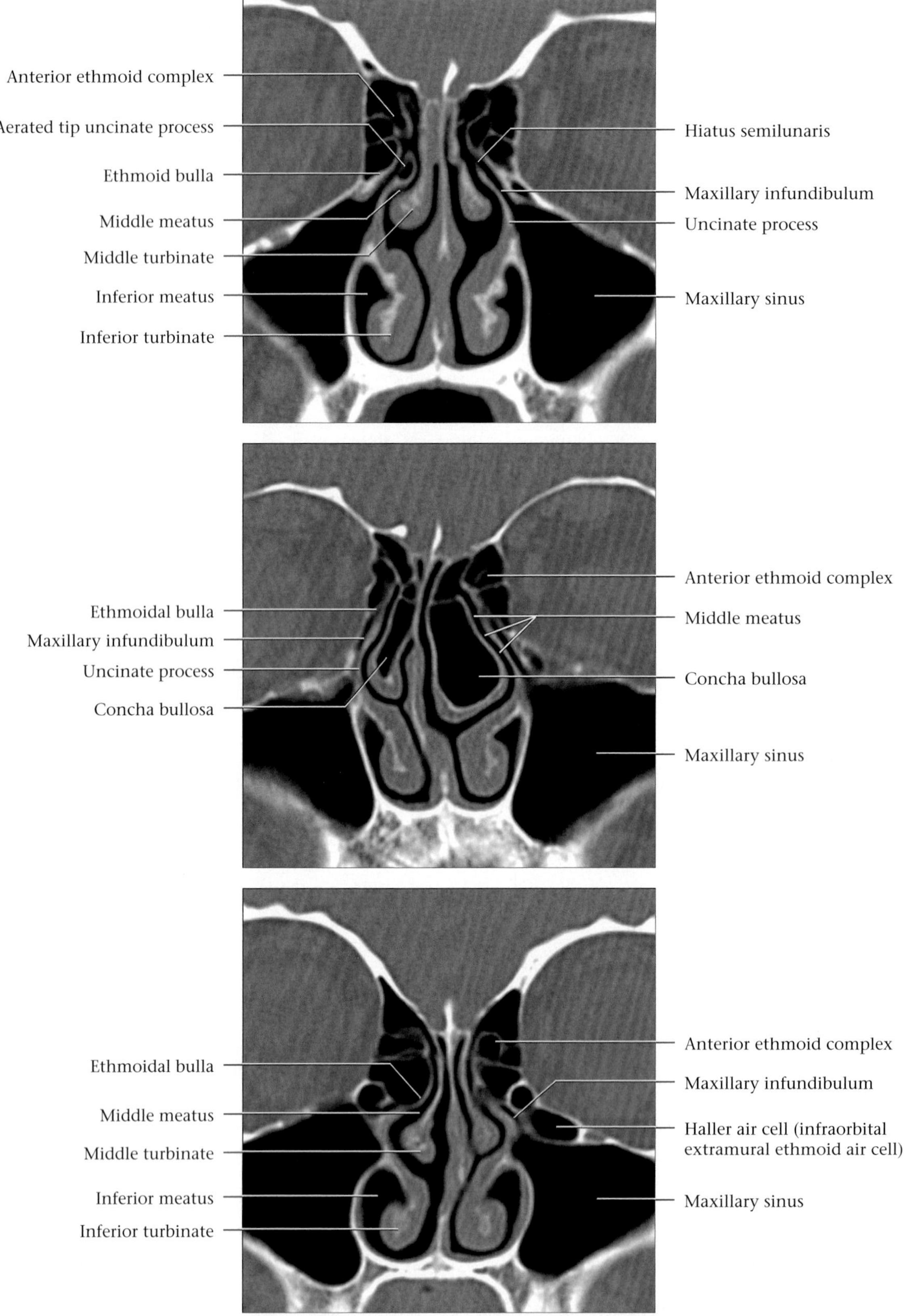
Anterior ethmoid complex
Aerated tip uncinate process
Ethmoid bulla
Middle meatus
Middle turbinate
Inferior meatus
Inferior turbinate
Hiatus semilunaris
Maxillary infundibulum
Uncinate process
Maxillary sinus
Ethmoidal bulla
Maxillary infundibulum
Uncinate process
Concha bullosa
Anterior ethmoid complex
Middle meatus
Concha bullosa
Maxillary sinus
Ethmoidal bulla
Middle meatus
Middle turbinate
Inferior meatus
Inferior turbinate
Anterior ethmoid complex
Maxillary infundibulum
Haller air cell (infraorbital extramural ethmoid air cell)
Maxillary sinus

(Top) First of three coronal bone CT images through the normal ostiomeatal complex. This image shows the typical appearance of the maxillary infundibulum and ethmoid bulla. Notice the right superior tip of the uncinate process is pneumatized. **(Middle)** In this image bilateral aerated uncomplicated concha bullosa are visible. Notice the the attenuated maxillary infundibulum. If the concha bullosa becomes infected (complicated), early obstruction of the middle meatus causes opacification of the ipsilateral maxillary, anterior ethmoid and frontal sinuses. **(Bottom)** Image through a normal ostiomeatal unit with Haller air cell (infraorbital air cell) seen protruding into maxillary infundibulum. If the Haller cell becomes infected it can cause an "infundibular pattern" of sinus disease where the maxillary sinus is opacified without ethmoid involvement.

SAGITTAL BONE CT

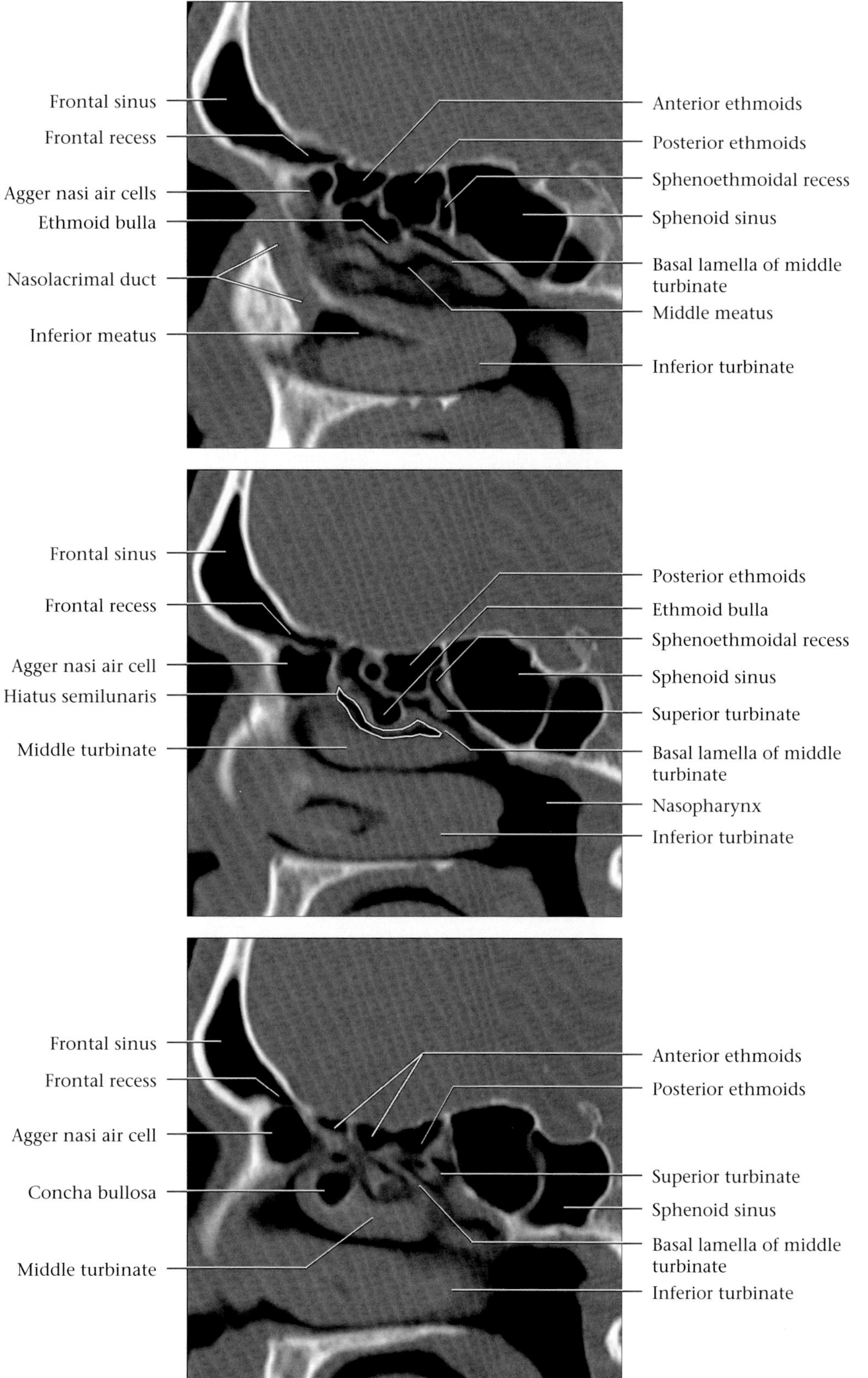
Frontal sinus
Frontal recess
Agger nasi air cells
Ethmoid bulla
Nasolacrimal duct
Inferior meatus
Anterior ethmoids
Posterior ethmoids
Sphenoethmoidal recess
Sphenoid sinus
Basal lamella of middle turbinate
Middle meatus
Inferior turbinate
Frontal sinus
Frontal recess
Agger nasi air cell
Hiatus semilunaris
Middle turbinate
Posterior ethmoids
Ethmoid bulla
Sphenoethmoidal recess
Sphenoid sinus
Superior turbinate
Basal lamella of middle turbinate
Nasopharynx
Inferior turbinate
Frontal sinus
Frontal recess
Agger nasi air cell
Concha bullosa
Middle turbinate
Anterior ethmoids
Posterior ethmoids
Superior turbinate
Sphenoid sinus
Basal lamella of middle turbinate
Inferior turbinate

(Top) First of three sagittal bone CT reformations of the sinonasal region presented from lateral to medial demonstrating the structures of the ostiomeatal unit and its vicinity. In this image the middle meatus can be seen just inferior to the ethmoid bulla. The nasolacrimal duct is visible emptying inferiorly into the anterior aspect of the inferior meatus. **(Middle)** In this image middle and inferior turbinates, as well as the basal lamella of the middle turbinate are seen. Also note the curvilinear hiatus semilunaris. The frontal recess is visible extending around the agger nasi air cell. The sphenoethmoidal recess receives the secretions of the posterior ethmoid and sphenoid sinuses. **(Bottom)** Notice the air cell in the anterior middle turbinate (concha bullosa) in this image. The basal lamella of the middle turbinate is also visible.

PTERYGOPALATINE FOSSA

Terminology

Abbreviations
- Pterygopalatine fossa (PPF)

Synonyms
- Sphenopalatine fossa

Definitions
- **PPF**: Major crossroads deep within deep face between the nasal cavity, oral cavity, masticator space, orbit, and the middle cranial fossa

Gross Anatomy

Overview
- Pterygopalatine fossa is a 3 dimensional box
  - Anterior wall: Posterior wall of maxillary sinus
  - Posterior wall: Pterygoid plates and inferior aspect of lesser wing of sphenoid bone
  - Roof: Inferior orbital fissure
  - Floor: Narrowing to palatine canals
  - Medial wall: Perpendicular plate of palatine bone with sphenopalatine foramen
  - Lateral wall: Narrowing to pterygomaxillary fissure

Imaging Anatomy

Overview
- PPF is important anatomic landmark for potential routes of spread of disease throughout deep face

Extent
- Small, but important deep face cavity with osseous borders

Anatomy Relationships
- Boundaries
  - Anterior: Posterior wall maxillary sinus
  - Posterior: Pterygoid process of sphenoid bone
  - Medial: Perpendicular plate of palatine bone

Internal Structures-Critical Contents
- Pterygopalatine ganglion
- Maxillary nerve (CNV2) enters via foramen rotundum
- Distal internal maxillary artery enters via pterygomaxillary fissure

Anatomy-Based Imaging Issues

Key Concepts or Questions
- Communications
  - **Pterygomaxillary fissure**: Lateral opening into nasopharyngeal masticator space, between the maxilla and lateral pterygoid plate
  - **Sphenopalatine foramen**: Medial opening into superior meatus; covered with mucosa
  - **Foramen rotundum**: Posterior opening to middle cranial fossa that transmits maxillary nerve (CNV2)
  - **Vidian canal**: Posterior opening below foramen rotundum that extends posteriorly to foramen lacerum (transmits vidian nerve)
  - **Inferior orbital fissure**: Anterior opening into orbit (transmits infraorbital nerve and artery)
  - **Pterygopalatine canal**: Inferior canal leading to greater & lesser palatine foramina to oral cavity (transmits descending palatine nerve and artery)

Imaging Recommendations
- Like many lesions near skull base, both bone CT (for bone evaluation) and enhance MR (for soft tissue evaluation) may be required for complete evaluation of PPF mass

Imaging Approaches
- Thin (1 mm or less), bone algorithm, noncontrasted axial sections best delimitate osseous structures surrounding PPF
- Contrasted MR of deep face best evaluates soft tissue abnormalities of PPF
  - Similar to many lesions of extra-cranial head and neck, often pre-contrasted T1 MR series best show lesions of PPF

Imaging "Sweet Spots"
- Axial T1 weighted pre-contrasted images often best demonstrate subtle lesions of the PPF
- Similar to most of head and neck imaging, clinical information is critical

Imaging Pitfalls
- Beware of fat-saturation artifact
  - Blooming at air-tissue interface may obscure PPF as result of maxillary sinus air directly anterior to PPF
- Dental amalgam artrifact may also obscure subtle lesions of PPF

Clinical Implications

Clinical Importance
- PPF serves as crossroads of deep face
  - **Perineural tumor** from hard-soft palate may follow **palatine nerves** superiorly into PPF
  - **Perineural tumor** from cheek skin, maxillary sinus or orbit may follow **infraorbital nerve** to PPF
  - PPF tumor may access intracranial compartment via foramen ovale or vidian canal

Function-Dysfunction
- Pterygopalatine ganglion contains post-synaptic parasympathetic nerve cell bodies and sympathetic fibers
  - Parasympathetic fibers from superior salivatory nucleus in brainstem enter via vidian nerve, greater superficial petrosal nerve, and nervus intermediate root of facial nerve
  - Sympathetic fibers from vidian nerve communicate autonomic impulses to greater and lesser palatine nerves and branches of CNV2
    - Supplying lacrimal gland, glands of nasal cavity, paranasal sinus, and roof of oral cavity

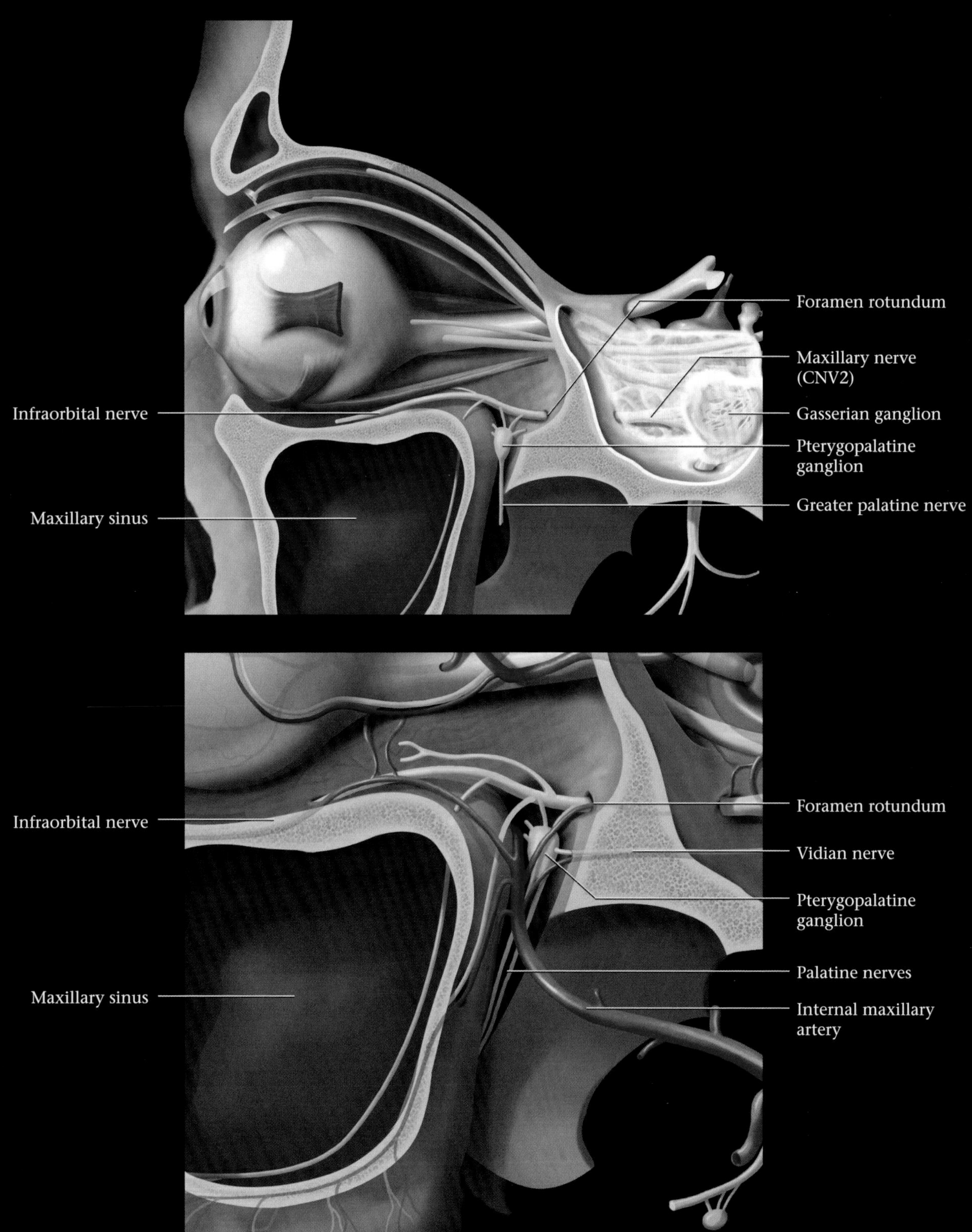

Foramen rotundum
Maxillary nerve (CNV2)
Infraorbital nerve
Gasserian ganglion
Pterygopalatine ganglion
Maxillary sinus
Greater palatine nerve
Foramen rotundum
Infraorbital nerve
Vidian nerve
Pterygopalatine ganglion
Palatine nerves
Maxillary sinus
Internal maxillary artery

(Top) Sagittal graphic demonstrates the anatomic landscape surrounding the pterygopalatine fossa. This image shows the close relationship of the pterygopalatine fossa to the inferior orbital foramen, and its important transiting structures superiorly, as well as the vital intracranial structures posteriorly, the cavernous sinus, and Meckel cave, with the Gasserian ganglion. **(Bottom)** Magnified sagittal graphic demonstrates the structures traversing the pterygopalatine fossa. This important crossroads of the deep face allows a potential pathway for disease between the orbit, sinonasal cavity, masticator space, and the intracranial cavity. The internal maxillary artery supplies the foramina surrounding the fossa and the nervous structures are shown along their pathway from the face to the intracranial cavity through this central deep face location.

PTERYGOPALATINE FOSSA

AXIAL BONE CT

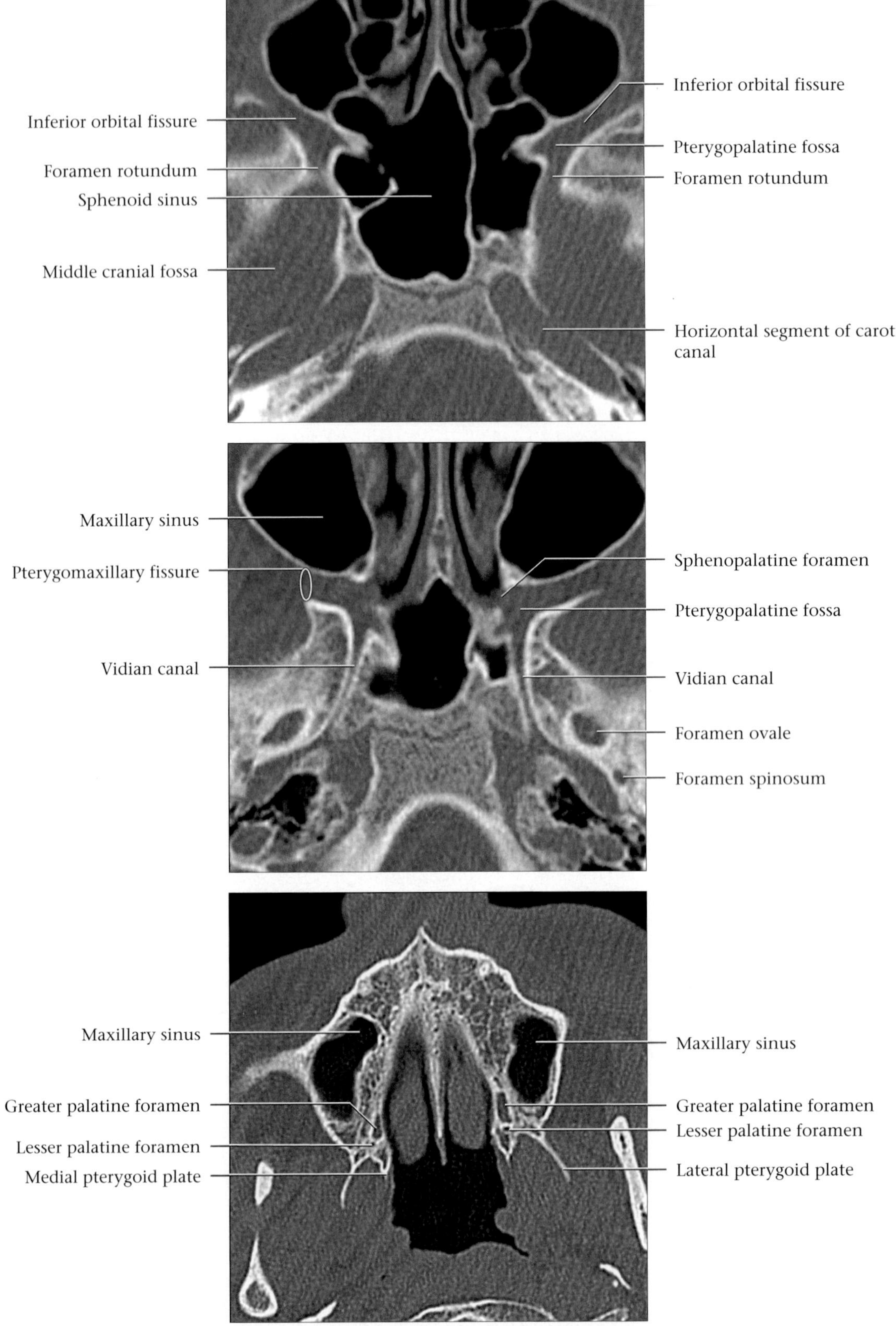

Inferior orbital fissure
Foramen rotundum
Sphenoid sinus
Middle cranial fossa
Inferior orbital fissure
Pterygopalatine fossa
Foramen rotundum
Horizontal segment of carotid canal
Maxillary sinus
Pterygomaxillary fissure
Vidian canal
Sphenopalatine foramen
Pterygopalatine fossa
Vidian canal
Foramen ovale
Foramen spinosum
Maxillary sinus
Greater palatine foramen
Lesser palatine foramen
Medial pterygoid plate
Maxillary sinus
Greater palatine foramen
Lesser palatine foramen
Lateral pterygoid plate

(Top) First of three axial bone CT images presented from superior to inferior through the pterygopalatine fossa and surrounding structures. This image shows the foramen rotundum through which the maxillary nerves traverse. Note the close relationship of the lateral walls of the sphenoid sinus to the superior aspect of the pterygopalatine fossa. **(Middle)** Image through the pterygopalatine fossa demonstrates this crossroads of the deep face. The vidian canals are visible connecting the pterygopalatine fossa to the petrous carotid canal. Don't mistake the vidian canal for the superolateral foramen rotundum. **(Bottom)** This inferior image demonstrates the greater and lesser palatine foramen, which transmit the greater and lesser palatine nerves respectively from the pterygopalatine fossa inferiorly to the palate.

PTERYGOPALATINE FOSSA

CORONAL BONE CT

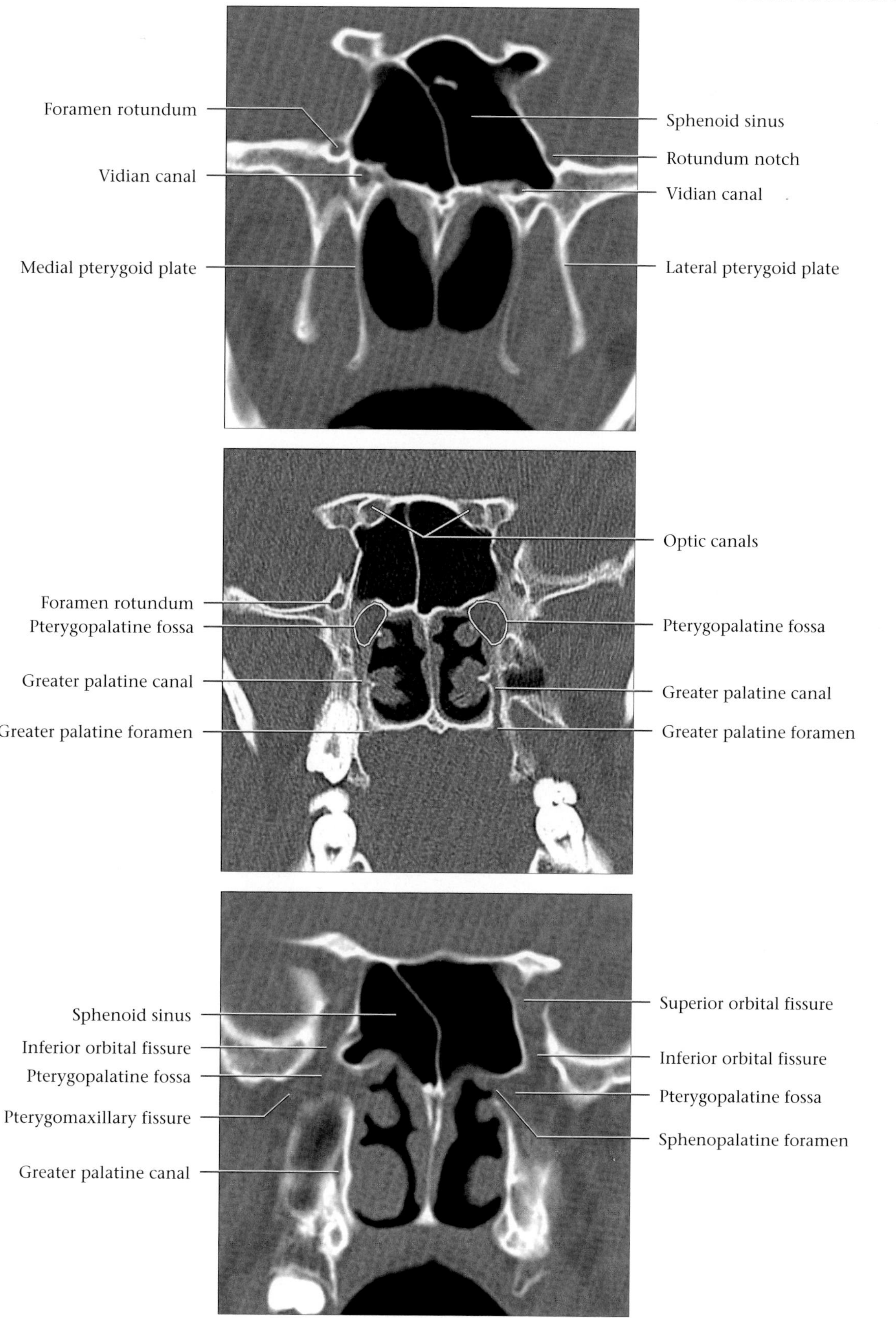
Foramen rotundum
Vidian canal
Medial pterygoid plate
Sphenoid sinus
Rotundum notch
Vidian canal
Lateral pterygoid plate
Optic canals
Foramen rotundum
Pterygopalatine fossa
Greater palatine canal
Greater palatine foramen
Pterygopalatine fossa
Greater palatine canal
Greater palatine foramen
Sphenoid sinus
Inferior orbital fissure
Pterygopalatine fossa
Pterygomaxillary fissure
Greater palatine canal
Superior orbital fissure
Inferior orbital fissure
Pterygopalatine fossa
Sphenopalatine foramen

(Top) First of three coronal bone CT images presented from posterior to anterior. This image shows the communication routes from the pterygopalatine fossa to the middle cranial fossa. Foramen rotundum is seen in the normal position, superior and lateral to the vidian canal. **(Middle)** Image through the posterior pterygopalatine fossa and through the vertical aspect of the greater palatine canal shows this canal connecting the pterygopalatine fossa above with the greater palatine foramen below. The greater palatine nerve which provides sensory innervation to the posterior 2/3 of the soft palate uses the greater palatine to canal to access the palate. **(Bottom)** Image through the anterior pterygoid fossa shows the communication routes to the nasal vault and infratemporal fossa. The sphenopalatine foramen is covered by mucosa, but is a potential route of spread of disease.

PTERYGOPALATINE FOSSA

SAGITTAL BONE CT

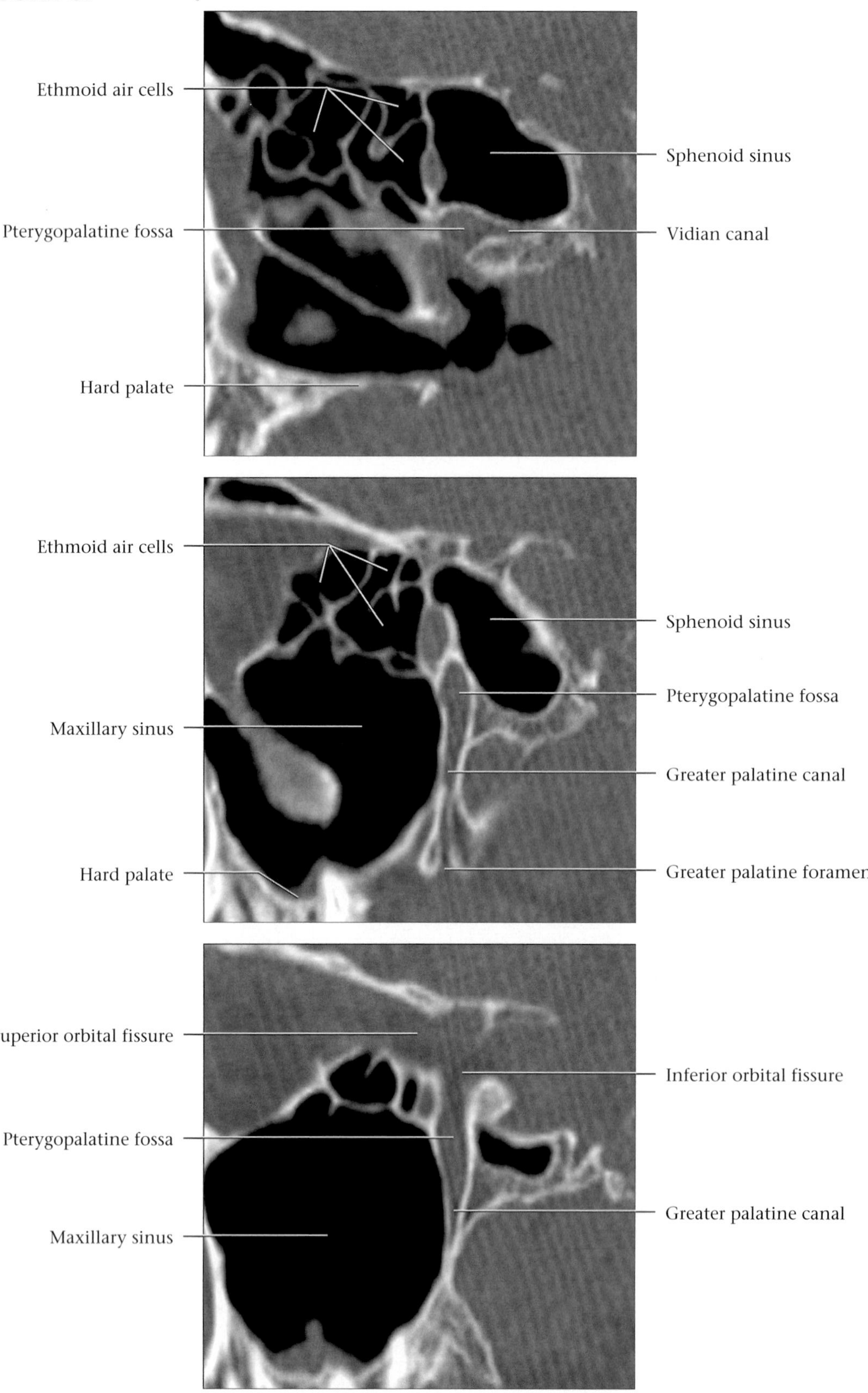
Ethmoid air cells
Sphenoid sinus
Pterygopalatine fossa
Vidian canal
Hard palate
Ethmoid air cells
Sphenoid sinus
Pterygopalatine fossa
Maxillary sinus
Greater palatine canal
Hard palate
Greater palatine foramen
Superior orbital fissure
Inferior orbital fissure
Pterygopalatine fossa
Greater palatine canal
Maxillary sinus

(Top) First of three sagittal bone CT images through the pterygopalatine fossa from medial to lateral. This image show the medial pterygopalatine fossa, and the anterior vidian canal extending posteriorly towards the foramen lacerum. Notice the well-aerated sphenoid sinus seen immediately superior to the pterygopalatine fossa. **(Middle)** This image nicely demonstrates the greater palatine canal, extending inferiorly from the pterygopalatine canal to the palate. This again demonstrates the importance of the PPF, with potential routes of spread of diease from the oral cavity, sinonasal region, orbit, infratemporal fossa, and intracranial cavity. **(Bottom)** This image demonstrates the greater palatine canal, extending inferiorly from the pterygopalatine canal to the palate. The superior orbital fissure, is an important connection between the pterygopalatine fossa and the orbit.

PTERYGOPALATINE FOSSA

AXIAL T1 MR

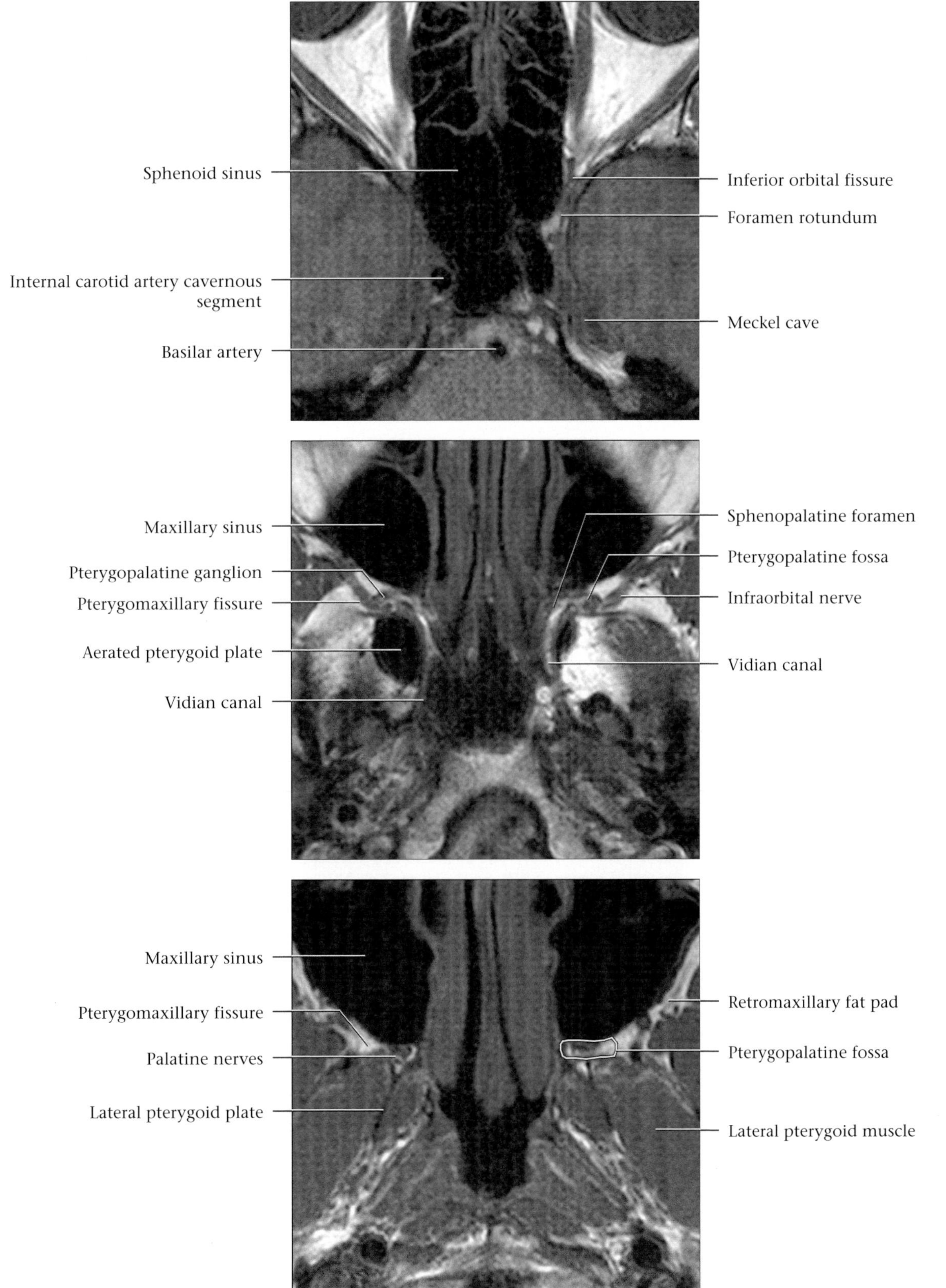

Sphenoid sinus
Inferior orbital fissure
Foramen rotundum
Internal carotid artery cavernous segment
Meckel cave
Basilar artery
Maxillary sinus
Sphenopalatine foramen
Pterygopalatine fossa
Pterygopalatine ganglion
Pterygomaxillary fissure
Infraorbital nerve
Aerated pterygoid plate
Vidian canal
Vidian canal
Maxillary sinus
Retromaxillary fat pad
Pterygomaxillary fissure
Palatine nerves
Pterygopalatine fossa
Lateral pterygoid plate
Lateral pterygoid muscle

(Top) First of three axial T1 MR images presented from superior to inferior. This image shows the foramen rotundum, transmitting cranial nerve V2 from the cavernous sinus to the pterygopalatine fossa. The borders of the cavernous sinus are shown to be concave in this normal case, anterior to Meckel cave, containing the cavernous segments of the internal carotid arteries. **(Middle)** This image shows the pterygopalatine fossa and its connections to the deep face. Medially it communicates with the nose through the sphenopalatine foramen. Laterally it communicates with the masticator space via the pterygomaxillary fissure. The vidian canal connects the petrous carotid canal to the pterygopalatine fossa. **(Bottom)** In this image the inferior pterygopalatine fossa is visible with the palatine nerves visible as low signal dots in the fat of the fossa.

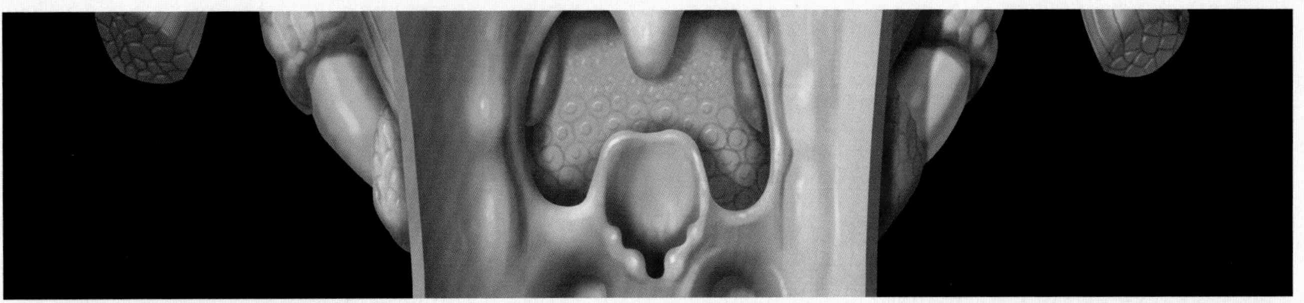

SECTION 3: Suprahyoid and Infrahyoid Neck

SUPRAHYOID AND INFRAHYOID NECK OVERVIEW

Terminology

Abbreviations

- Suprahyoid neck (SHN)
- Infrahyoid neck (IHN)

Definitions

- SHN: Spaces from skull base to hyoid bone (excluding orbit, sinuses & oral cavity) including parapharyngeal (PPS), pharyngeal mucosal (PMS), masticator (MS), parotid (PS), carotid (CS), buccal (BS), retropharyngeal (RPS) & perivertebral (PVS) spaces
- IHN: Spaces below hyoid bone with some continuing into mediastinum including visceral space (VS), posterior cervical space (PCS), anterior cervical space (ACS), CS, RPS & PVS

Imaging Anatomy

Overview

- **Key** to understanding SHN & IHN spaces is **fascia**
- 3 layers of deep cervical fascia cleave neck into spaces
  - **Superficial layer, deep cervical fascia (SL-DCF)**
    - SHN: Around MS & PS; part of carotid sheath
    - IHN: Invests neck by surrounding strap, sternocleidomastoid & trapezius muscles
  - **Middle layer, deep cervical fascia (ML-DCF)**
    - SHN: ML-DCF defines PMS deep margin; contributes to carotid sheath
    - IHN: Circumscribes VS; part of carotid sheath
  - **Deep layer, deep cervical fascia (DL-DCF)**
    - SHN & IHN: Surrounds perivertebral space
    - SHN & IHN: Contributes to carotid sheath
    - SHN & IHN: **Alar fascia** is slip of DL-DCF providing lateral wall to RPS & DS; also posterior wall to RPS separating RPS from DS

Spaces of Suprahyoid & Infrahyoid Neck

- **Parapharyngeal space**
  - Location: SHN from skull base to posterior submandibular space
  - Contents: Fat & pterygoid venous plexus
  - Importance: Pattern of displacement helps define SHN mass space of origin
- **Pharyngeal mucosal space**
  - Location: SHN space medial to PPS, anterior to RPS
  - Contents: Mucosa, minor salivary glands, PMS lymphatic ring, constrictor muscles
    - Nasopharyngeal, oropharyngeal & hypopharyngeal mucosal surfaces
    - PMS of nasopharynx: Torus tubarius, adenoids, superior constrictor & levator palatini muscles
    - PMS of oropharynx: Anterior & posterior tonsillar pillars, palatine & lingual tonsils, soft palate
  - Fascia: PMS on airway side of ML-DCF
  - Importance: Squamous cell carcinoma & NHL here
- **Masticator space**
  - Location: Anterolateral to PPS in SHN
  - Contents: Ramus & condyle of mandible, CNV3, masseter, medial & lateral pterygoid & temporalis muscles, pterygoid venous plexus
  - Fascia: MS surrounded by SL-DCF
  - Importance: Perineural tumor on CNV3; sarcoma
- **Parotid space**
  - Location: Lateral to PPS in SHN
  - Contents: Parotid gland, extracranial CN7, nodes, retromandibular vein, external carotid artery
  - Fascia: PS surrounded by SL-DCF
  - Importance: Intraparotid CN7; parotid nodes; perineural tumor on CN7
- **Carotid space**
  - Location: Posterior to PPS in SHN; lateral to VS & RPS in IHN
    - Begins at inferior jugular foramen & carotid canal of skull base; extends to aortic arch
  - Contents: CN9-12, internal jugular vein, carotid artery
  - Fascia: All 3 layers, deep cervical fascia
  - Importance: CN10 & carotid here; squamous cell carcinoma nodes along superficial margin
- **Retropharyngeal space**
  - Location: Posterior to PMS in SHN & VS in IHN
    - Begins at clivus; traverses SHN-IHN to T3 level
  - Contents: Nodes & fat in SHN; no nodes in IHN
  - Fascia: Anterior fascia is ML-DCF, lateral & posterior fascia is DL-DCF (alar fascia)
  - Importance: Inferior communication with DS allows infection access to mediastinum
- **Danger space**
  - Posterior to RPS in SHN & IHN; continues inferiorly into mediastinum
- **Perivertebral space**
  - Location: Behind RPS & around spine in SHN & IHN
    - Defined from skull base above to clavicle below
  - Contents: Prevertebral & paraspinal components
    - Prevertebral: Vertebral body, veins & arteries, prevertebral & scalene muscles, brachial plexus & phrenic nerve
    - Paraspinal: Posterior elements of vertebra, levator scapulae & paraspinal muscles
  - Fascia: Surrounded by DL-DCF
    - Divided by DL-DCF slip into prevertebral & paraspinal components
  - Importance: PVS malignancy may be epidural
- **Visceral space**
  - Location: IHN only; extends into mediastinum
  - Contents: Thyroid & parathyroids, paratracheal nodes, esophagus, trachea, recurrent laryngeal nerve
  - Fascia: VS surrounded by ML-DCF
  - Importance: Trachea & esophagus traverse VS
- **Posterior cervical space**
  - Location: SHN PCS begins at mastoid tip, extends to clavicle; most PCS volume in IHN
  - Contents: Fat, CN11, spinal accessory nodes
  - Fascia: Between SL- & DL-DCF
  - Importance: Spinal accessory nodal diseases

Key Spatial Relationships

- **SHN spaces surrounding PPS**
  - Medial is PMS: PMS mass displaces PPS laterally
  - Anterior is MS: MS mass displaces PPS posteriorly
  - Lateral is PS: PS mass displaces PPS medially
  - Posterior is CS: CS mass displaces PPS anteriorly
  - Posteromedial is lateral RPS: Lateral RPS nodal mass displaces PPS anterolaterally

SUPRAHYOID AND INFRAHYOID NECK OVERVIEW

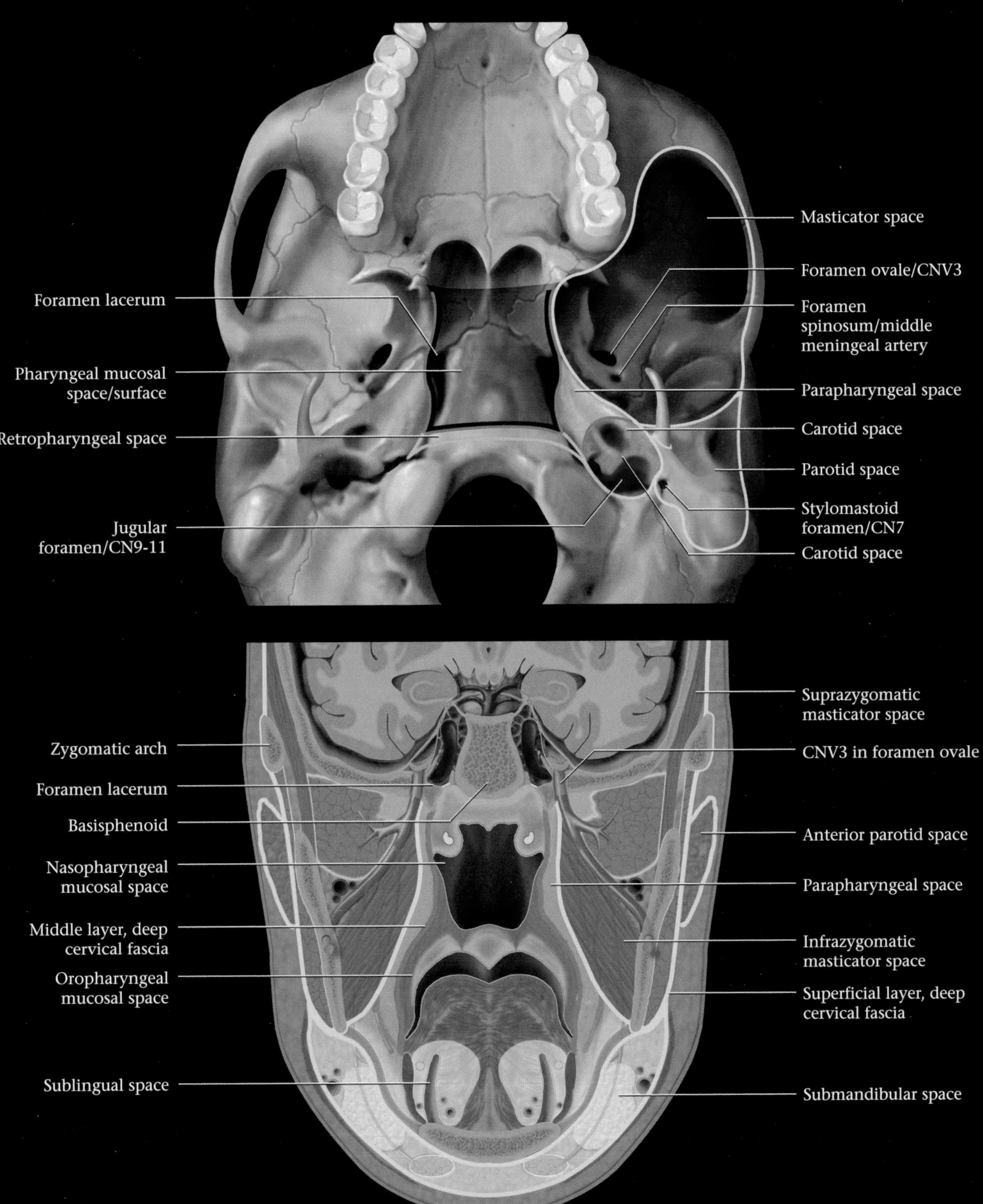
Masticator space
Foramen ovale/CNV3
Foramen spinosum/middle meningeal artery
Foramen lacerum
Pharyngeal mucosal space/surface
Parapharyngeal space
Retropharyngeal space
Carotid space
Parotid space
Stylomastoid foramen/CN7
Jugular foramen/CN9-11
Carotid space
Suprazygomatic masticator space
Zygomatic arch
CNV3 in foramen ovale
Foramen lacerum
Basisphenoid
Anterior parotid space
Nasopharyngeal mucosal space
Parapharyngeal space
Middle layer, deep cervical fascia
Infrazygomatic masticator space
Oropharyngeal mucosal space
Superficial layer, deep cervical fascia
Sublingual space
Submandibular space

(Top) Graphic of skull base from below shows spaces of suprahyoid neck relationships to skull base. Four spaces have key interactions with skull base, masticator, parotid, carotid and pharyngeal mucosal spaces. PS (green) malignancy can follow CN7 into stylomastoid foramen. MS (purple) receives CNV3 while CN9-12 enter the CS (red). The PMS abuts the foramen lacerum, which is covered by fibrocartilage in life. Also note that the superficial layer of deep cervical fascia (yellow line) surrounds the MS & PS and middle layer is on non-airway side of PMS (pink line). **(Bottom)** Coronal graphic of suprahyoid neck spaces as they interact with the skull base. The masticator space has the largest area of abutment with the skull base, including CNV3. The pharyngeal mucosal space abuts the basisphenoid and foramen lacerum.

SUPRAHYOID AND INFRAHYOID NECK OVERVIEW

GRAPHICS

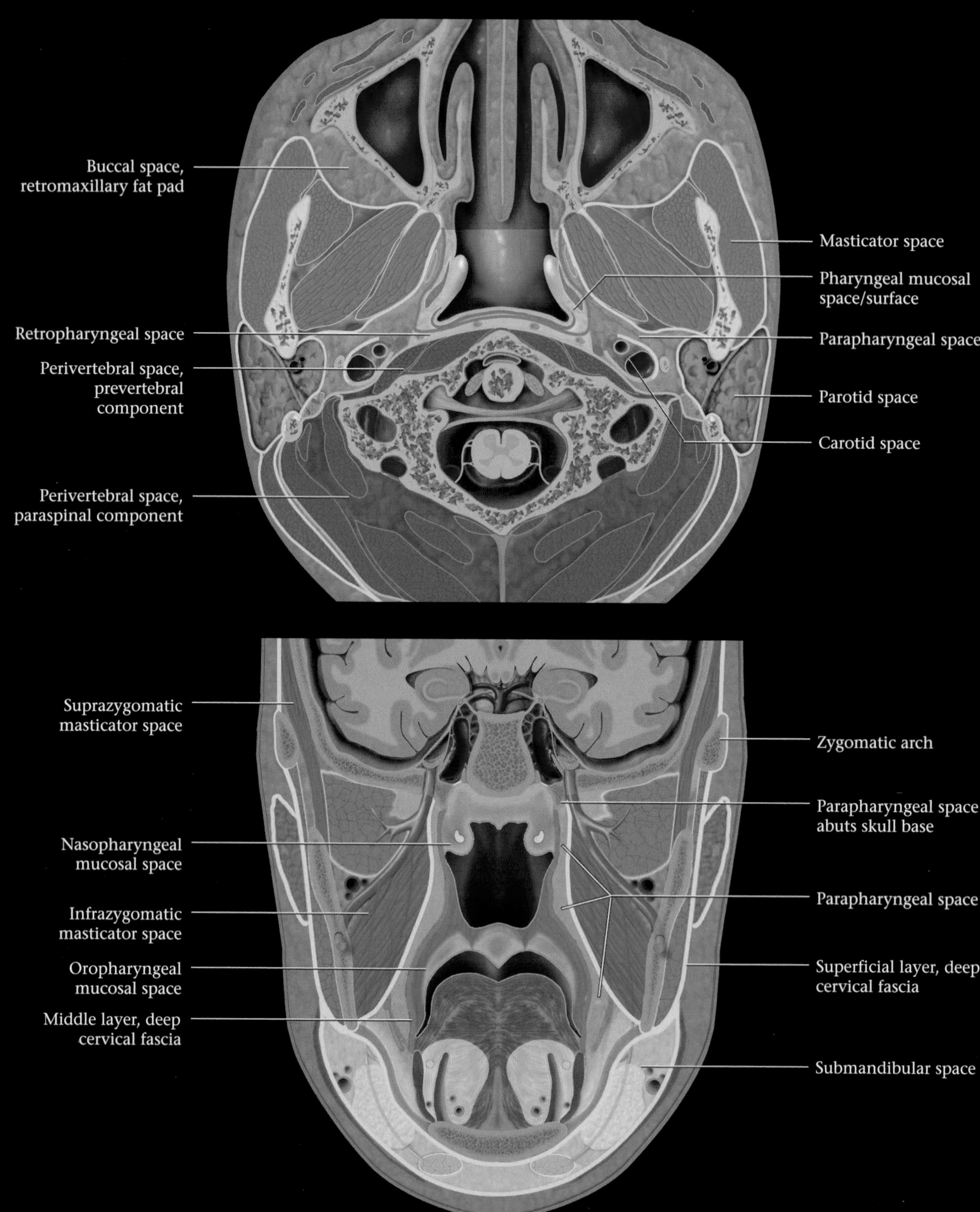

Buccal space, retromaxillary fat pad
Masticator space
Pharyngeal mucosal space/surface
Retropharyngeal space
Parapharyngeal space
Perivertebral space, prevertebral component
Parotid space
Carotid space
Perivertebral space, paraspinal component
Suprazygomatic masticator space
Zygomatic arch
Parapharyngeal space abuts skull base
Nasopharyngeal mucosal space
Parapharyngeal space
Infrazygomatic masticator space
Oropharyngeal mucosal space
Superficial layer, deep cervical fascia
Middle layer, deep cervical fascia
Submandibular space

(Top) Axial graphic depicting the spaces of the suprahyoid neck. Surrounding the paired fat-filled parapharyngeal spaces are the four critical paired spaces of this region, the pharyngeal mucosal, masticator, parotid and carotid spaces. The retropharyngeal and perivertebral spaces are the midline non-paired spaces. A PMS mass pushes the PPS laterally; MS mass pushes PPS posteriorly; PS mass pushes PPS medially; CS mass pushes PPS anteriorly. **(Bottom)** Coronal graphic of parapharyngeal space. The parapharyngeal spaces are paired fat-filled spaces in the more lateral aspect of the suprahyoid neck. This space abuts the skull base between the masticator and pharyngeal mucosal spaces. There are no important structures at the point of intersection between the PPS and the skull base. Inferiorly the PPS communicates inferiorly with the posterior submandibular space.

GRAPHICS

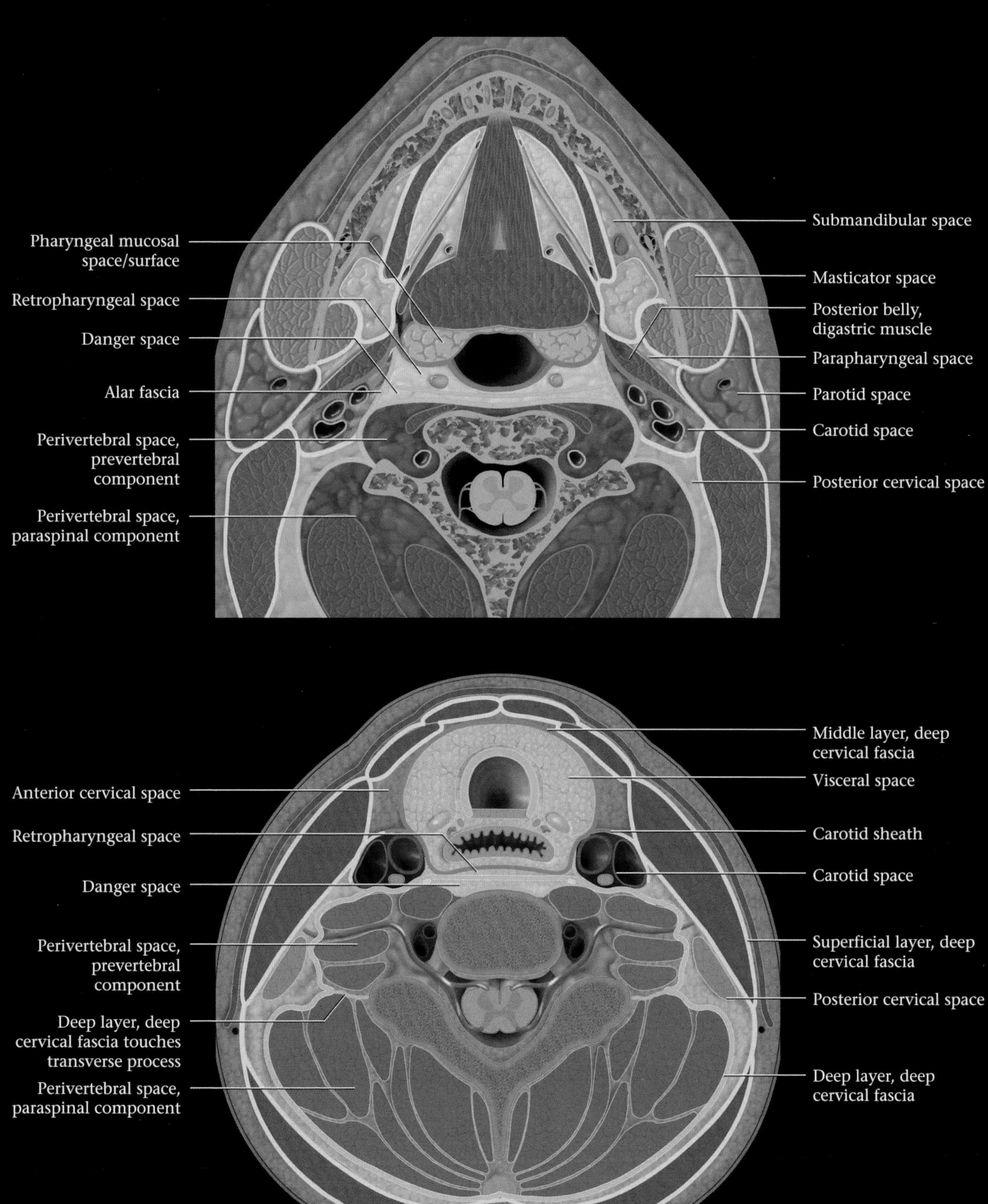
Pharyngeal mucosal space/surface
Retropharyngeal space
Danger space
Alar fascia
Perivertebral space, prevertebral component
Perivertebral space, paraspinal component
Submandibular space
Masticator space
Posterior belly, digastric muscle
Parapharyngeal space
Parotid space
Carotid space
Posterior cervical space
Anterior cervical space
Retropharyngeal space
Danger space
Perivertebral space, prevertebral component
Deep layer, deep cervical fascia touches transverse process
Perivertebral space, paraspinal component
Middle layer, deep cervical fascia
Visceral space
Carotid sheath
Carotid space
Superficial layer, deep cervical fascia
Posterior cervical space
Deep layer, deep cervical fascia

(Top) Axial graphic of the suprahyoid neck spaces at the level of the oropharynx. The superficial (yellow line), middle (pink line) and deep (turquoise line) layers of deep cervical fascia outline the suprahyoid neck spaces. Notice the lateral borders of the retropharyngeal & danger spaces are called the alar fascia and represents a slip of the deep layer of deep cervical fascia. **(Bottom)** Axial graphic depicting the fascia and spaces of the infrahyoid neck. The three layers of deep cervical fascia are present in the suprahyoid and infrahyoid neck. The carotid sheath is made up of all 3 layers of deep cervical fascia (tri-color line around carotid space). Notice the deep layer completely circles the perivertebral space, diving in laterally to divide it into prevertebral and a paraspinal components.

SUPRAHYOID AND INFRAHYOID NECK OVERVIEW

GRAPHICS

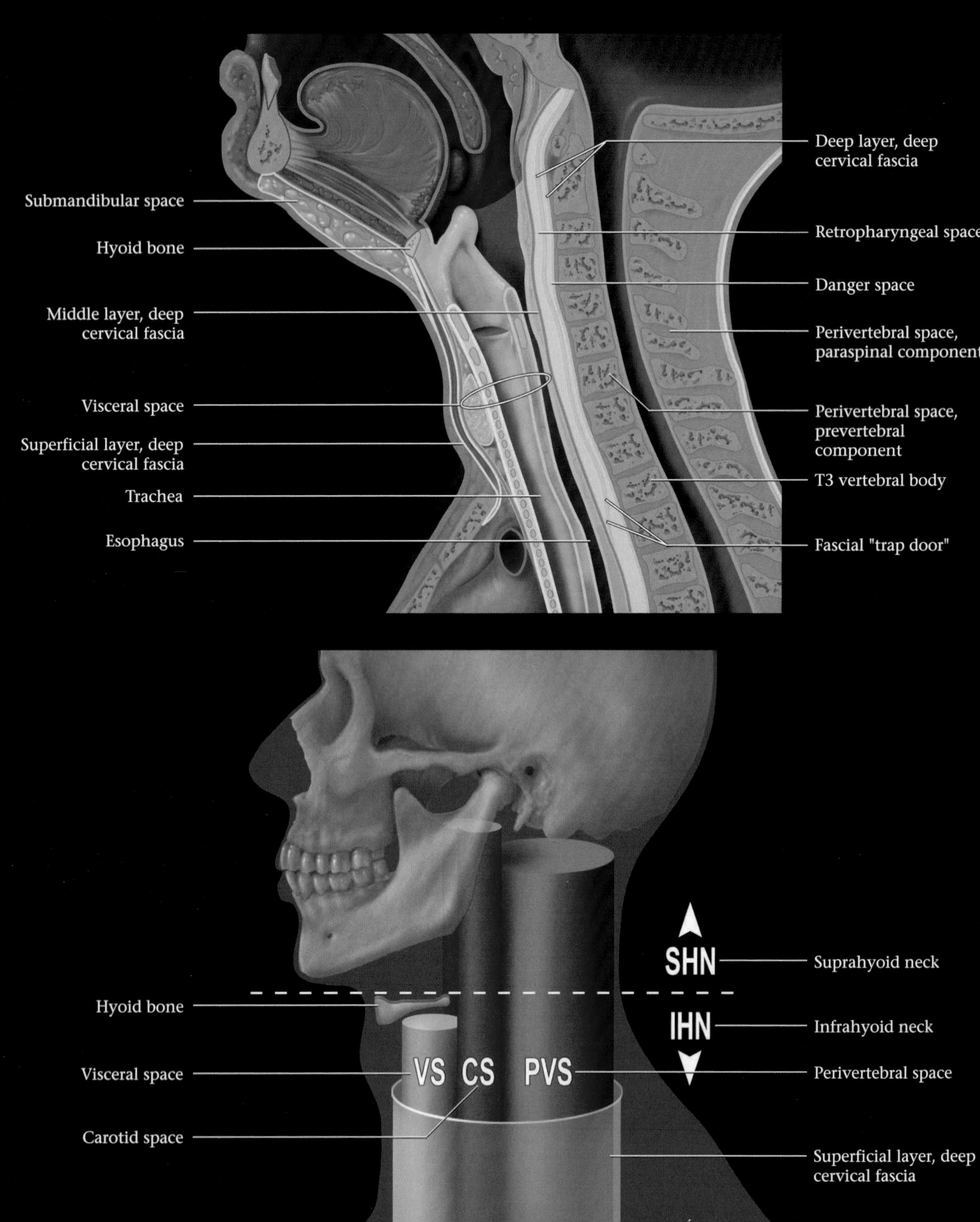

Deep layer, deep cervical fascia
Submandibular space
Retropharyngeal space
Hyoid bone
Danger space
Middle layer, deep cervical fascia
Perivertebral space, paraspinal component
Visceral space
Perivertebral space, prevertebral component
Superficial layer, deep cervical fascia
T3 vertebral body
Trachea
Esophagus
Fascial "trap door"
SHN
Suprahyoid neck
Hyoid bone
IHN
Infrahyoid neck
Visceral space
VS
CS
PVS
Perivertebral space
Carotid space
Superficial layer, deep cervical fascia

(Top) Sagittal graphic depicting longitudinal spatial relationships of the infrahyoid neck. Anteriorly the visceral space is seen surrounded by middle layer of deep cervical fascia. Just anterior to the vertebral column the retropharyngeal and danger spaces run inferiorly toward the mediastinum. Notice the fascial "trap door" found at the approximate level of T3 vertebral body that serves as a conduit from the retropharyngeal to the danger space. Retropharyngeal space infection or tumor may access the mediastinum via this route of spread. **(Bottom)** Lateral graphic of extracranial head and neck showing the spaces as "tubes" as they traverse the area. This is particularly true of the carotid spaces which reach from the skull base to the aortic arch. Both the visceral and perivertebral spaces continue inferiorly into the thorax.

AXIAL CECT SUPRAHYOID NECK

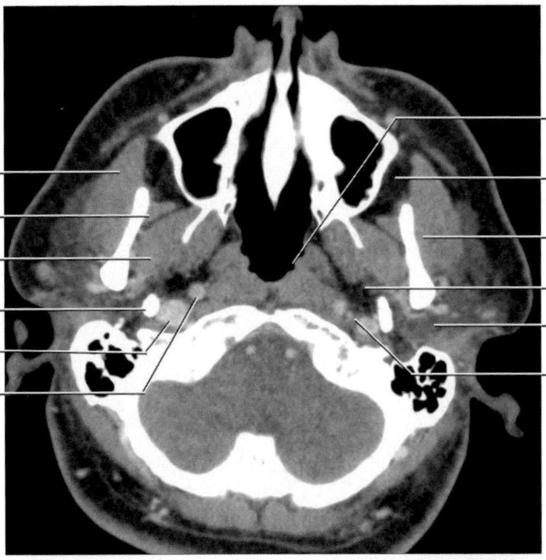

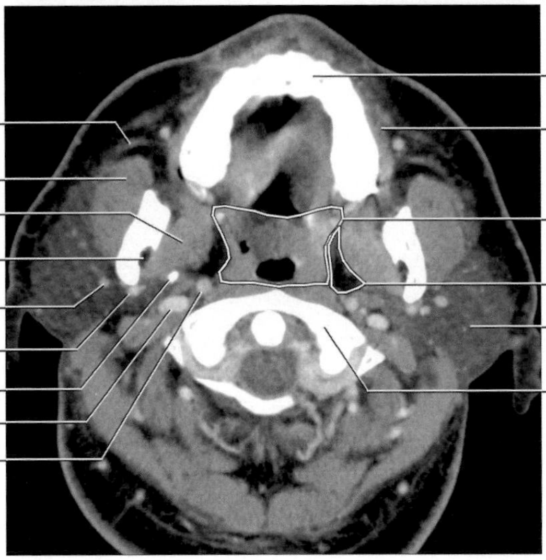

Masseter muscle
Temporalis muscle
Lateral pterygoid muscle
Styloid process
Internal jugular vein
Internal carotid artery
Pharyngeal mucosal space/surface
Retromaxillary fat pad (buccal space)
Masticator space
Parapharyngeal space
Parotid space
Carotid space

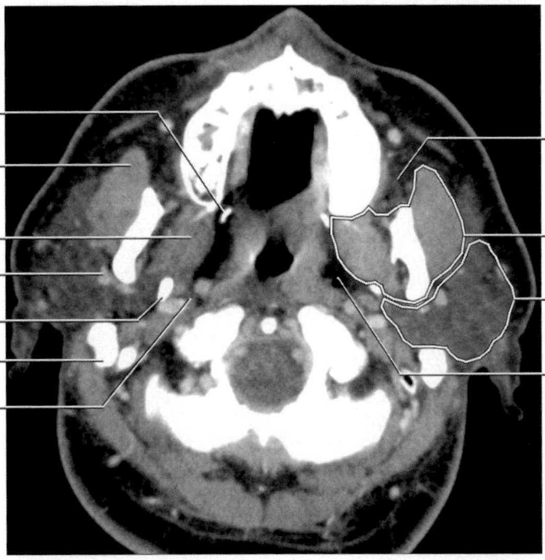

Hamulus, medial pterygoid plate
Masseter muscle
Medial pterygoid muscle
Retromandibular vein
Styloid process
Mastoid tip
Carotid space
Retromaxillary fat pad (buccal space)
Masticator space
Parotid space
Parapharyngeal space

Parotid duct
Masseter muscle
Medial pterygoid muscle
Mandibular foramen
Retromandibular vein
External carotid artery
Styloid process
Internal jugular vein
Internal carotid artery
Maxillary ridge
Buccinator muscle
Pharyngeal mucosal space
Parapharyngeal space
Parotid space
Anterior arch C1

(Top) First of 12 axial contrast-enhanced CT images of both the suprahyoid & infrahyoid aspect of the extracranial head & neck presented from superior to inferior. This image at the level of the nasopharynx shows the four key spaces surrounding the parapharyngeal space, the pharyngeal mucosal, masticator, parotid and carotid spaces. **(Middle)** In this image at level of inferior maxillary sinus the styloid process is seen anterolateral to the carotid space. The superficial layer of deep cervical fascia defines the masticator and parotid spaces. The more anterior buccal space has no fascial definition. **(Bottom)** At the level of the maxillary ridge the area of the pharyngeal mucosal space is outlined between the paired fat-filled parapharyngeal spaces. Posterior to the pharyngeal mucosal space are the tightly packed retropharyngeal and perivertebral spaces.

AXIAL CECT SUPRAHYOID NECK

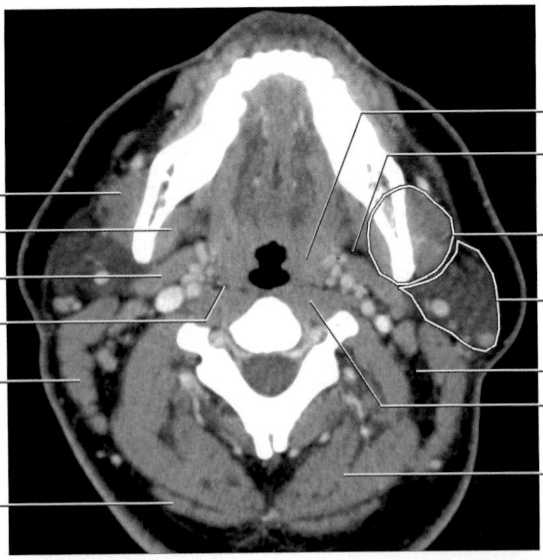

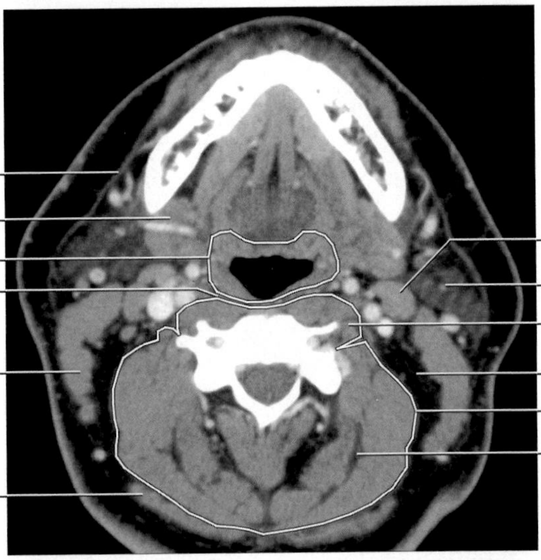

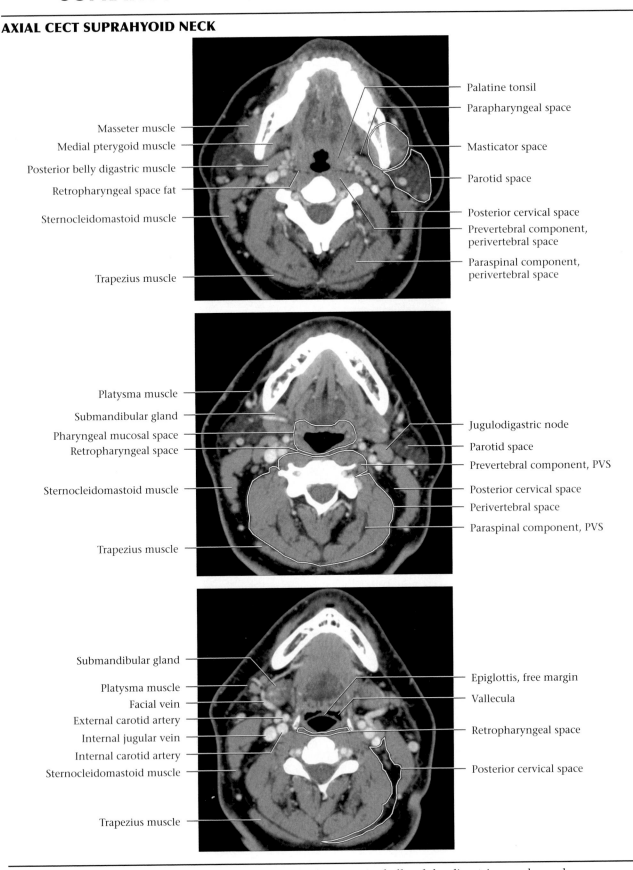

Masseter muscle
Medial pterygoid muscle
Posterior belly digastric muscle
Retropharyngeal space fat
Sternocleidomastoid muscle
Trapezius muscle
Palatine tonsil
Parapharyngeal space
Masticator space
Parotid space
Posterior cervical space
Prevertebral component, perivertebral space
Paraspinal component, perivertebral space

Platysma muscle
Submandibular gland
Pharyngeal mucosal space
Retropharyngeal space
Sternocleidomastoid muscle
Trapezius muscle
Jugulodigastric node
Parotid space
Prevertebral component, PVS
Posterior cervical space
Perivertebral space
Paraspinal component, PVS

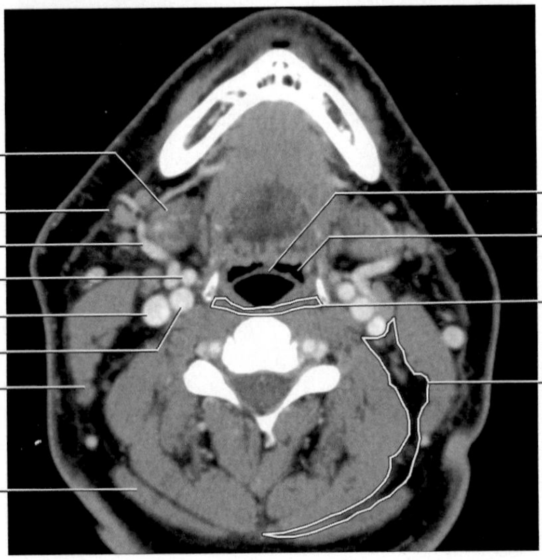

Submandibular gland
Platysma muscle
Facial vein
External carotid artery
Internal jugular vein
Internal carotid artery
Sternocleidomastoid muscle
Trapezius muscle
Epiglottis, free margin
Vallecula
Retropharyngeal space
Posterior cervical space

(Top) In this image at the level of the mandibular body the posterior belly of the digastric muscle can be seen dividing the parotid tail from the carotid space. The direction of displacement of this muscle can define whether a lesion is in the parotid space (posteromedial displacement) or in the carotid space (anterolateral displacement). **(Middle)** In this image through the low oropharynx the pharyngeal mucosal space has been outline anterior to the perivertebral space. The space between the two is the retropharyngeal space. The alar fascia that makes up the lateral borders of the retropharyngeal space are not shown. **(Bottom)** At the level of the free margin of epiglottis the retropharyngeal space is outline behind the pharyngeal mucosal space. The posterior cervical space contains fat, accessory cranial nerve (CN11) and the spinal accessory nodal chain (level 5 nodes).

AXIAL CECT INFRAHYOID NECK

Platysma muscle
Hyoid bone
Prevertebral muscles
Common carotid artery
Internal jugular vein
Sternocleidomastoid muscle
Levator scapulae muscle
Paraspinal muscles
Trapezius muscle
Submandibular space
Prevertebral component, perivertebral space
Carotid space
Vagus nerve location
Posterior cervical space
Paraspinal component, perivertebral space

Platysma muscle
Prevertebral strap muscles
Thyroid cartilage
External jugular vein
Sternocleidomastoid muscle
Prevertebral muscles
Levator scapulae muscle
Paraspinal muscles
Trapezius muscle
Submandibular space
Retropharyngeal space fat
Sympathetic chain location
Posterior cervical space
Paraspinal component, perivertebral space

Platysma muscle
Infrahyoid strap muscles
Sternocleidomastoid muscle
External jugular vein
Prevertebral muscles
Vertebral artery/vein
Levator scapulae muscle
Trapezius muscle
Anterior cervical space
Visceral space
Carotid space
Posterior cervical space
Prevertebral component, perivertebral space
Retropharyngeal space fat

(Top) Axial CT image at the level of the hyoid bone shows the carotid space now contains the common carotid artery, internal jugular vein and vagus nerve only. The large, fat-filled submandibular space is seen anteriorly. **(Middle)** In this image at the level of the supraglottis of the larynx the large sternocleidomastoid and trapezius muscles are seen in the lateral neck. Both muscles are innervated by the accessory cranial nerve. **(Bottom)** In this image at the level of the glottis of the larynx the visceral space contains the hypopharynx, larynx and infrahyoid strap muscles. Just behind the hypopharynx is the retropharyngeal space which contains only fat in the infrahyoid neck. Notice that the inferior extension of the submandibular space into the infrahyoid neck is the anterior cervical space.

AXIAL CECT INFRAHYOID NECK

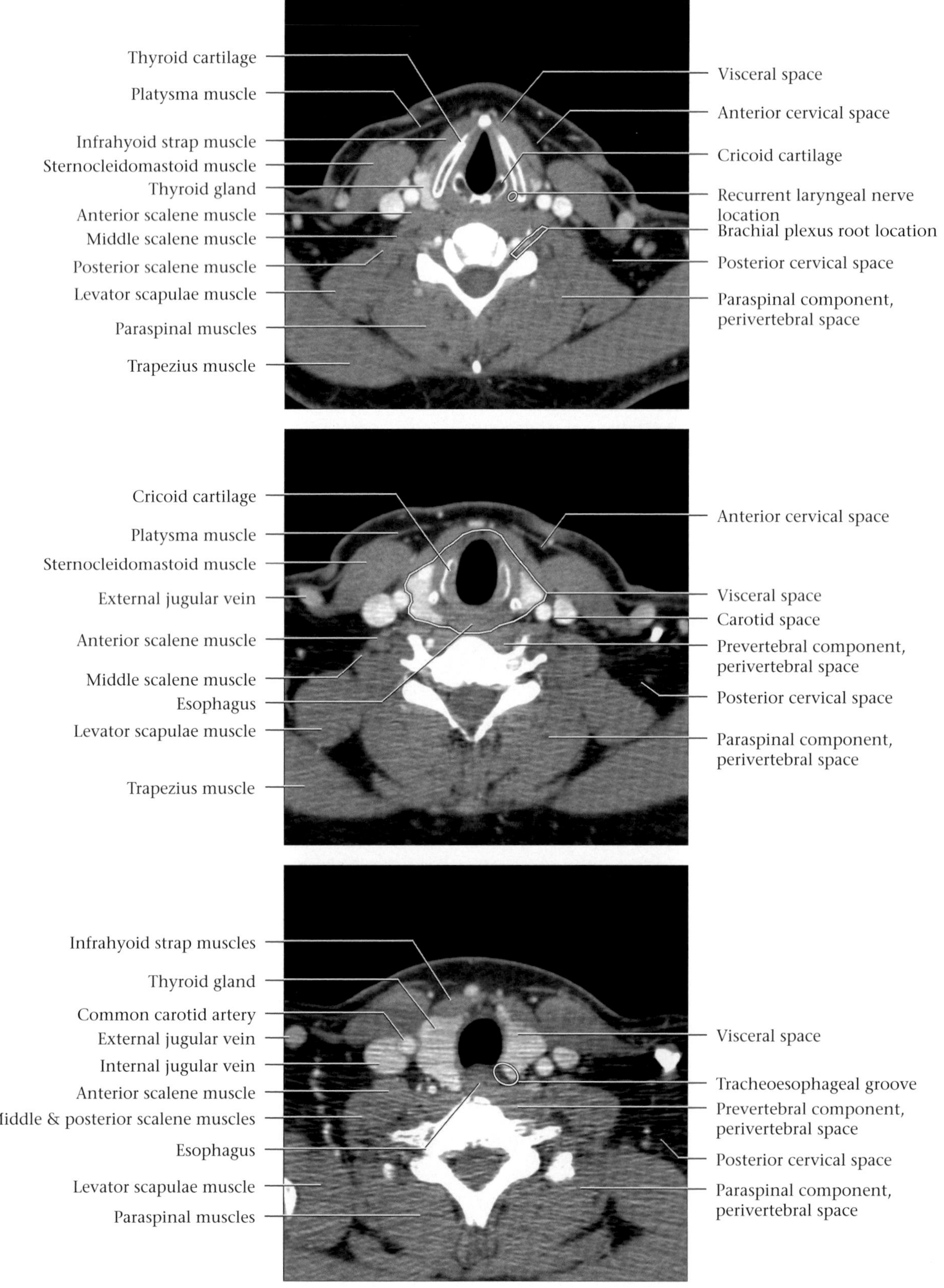

Thyroid cartilage
Platysma muscle
Infrahyoid strap muscle
Sternocleidomastoid muscle
Thyroid gland
Anterior scalene muscle
Middle scalene muscle
Posterior scalene muscle
Levator scapulae muscle
Paraspinal muscles
Trapezius muscle
Visceral space
Anterior cervical space
Cricoid cartilage
Recurrent laryngeal nerve location
Brachial plexus root location
Posterior cervical space
Paraspinal component, perivertebral space
Cricoid cartilage
Platysma muscle
Sternocleidomastoid muscle
External jugular vein
Anterior scalene muscle
Middle scalene muscle
Esophagus
Levator scapulae muscle
Trapezius muscle
Anterior cervical space
Visceral space
Carotid space
Prevertebral component, perivertebral space
Posterior cervical space
Paraspinal component, perivertebral space
Infrahyoid strap muscles
Thyroid gland
Common carotid artery
External jugular vein
Internal jugular vein
Anterior scalene muscle
Middle & posterior scalene muscles
Esophagus
Levator scapulae muscle
Paraspinal muscles
Visceral space
Tracheoesophageal groove
Prevertebral component, perivertebral space
Posterior cervical space
Paraspinal component, perivertebral space

(Top) At cricoid cartilage level the visceral space now contains the upper thyroid gland. The low density brachial plexus root projects anterolaterally from the neural foramen to pass between the anterior and middle scalene muscles in the prevertebral component of perivertebral space. **(Middle)** In this image the visceral space contains the high density thyroid gland, the upper cervical esophagus and the cricoid cartilage. The middle layer of the deep cervical fascia circumscribes the visceral space. **(Bottom)** At the level of upper cervical trachea the visceral space is filled with thyroid gland, parathyroid glands (not visible), trachea & cervical esophagus. The area of tracheoesophageal groove contains the recurrent laryngeal nerve & the paratracheal nodal chain. It is via the paratracheal nodal chain that differentiated thyroid carcinoma accesses the mediastinum.

AXIAL CECT CERVICOTHORACIC JUNCTION

Infrahyoid strap muscles
Thyroid gland
Prevertebral muscles
Anterior scalene muscle
Brachial plexus root
Middle scalene muscle
Posterior scalene muscle
Levator scapulae muscle
Paraspinal muscles
Trapezius muscle
Visceral space
Carotid space
Posterior cervical space
Prevertebral component, perivertebral space
Vertebral artery
Paraspinal component, perivertebral space

Prevertebral muscles
Anterior scalene muscle
Middle scalene muscle
Vertebral artery
Levator scapulae muscle
Paraspinal muscles
Trapezius muscle
Visceral space
Carotid space
Posterior cervical space
Brachial plexus root
First rib
Paraspinal component, perivertebral space

Infrahyoid strap muscle
Internal jugular vein
Anterior scalene muscle
Subclavian artery
Brachial plexus roots
Middle scalene muscle
Lung apex
Trapezius muscle
Visceral space
Vertebral vein
Vertebral artery
Second rib
Paraspinal component, perivertebral space

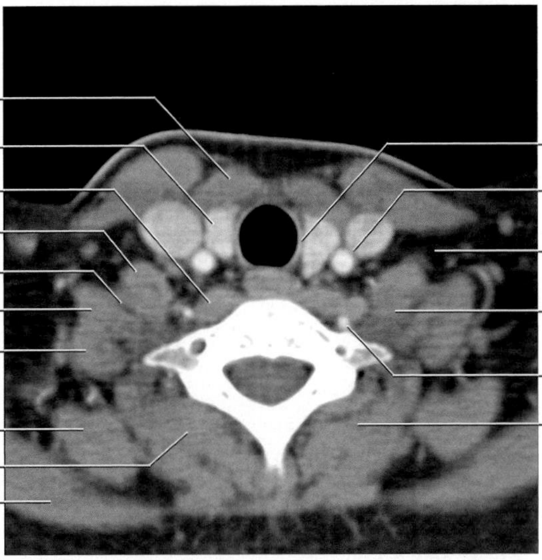

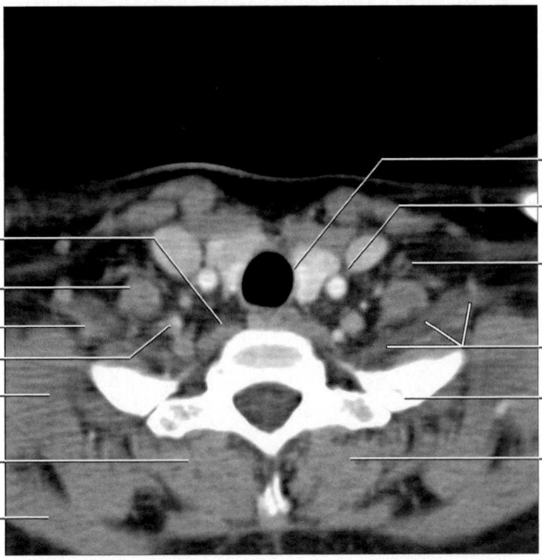

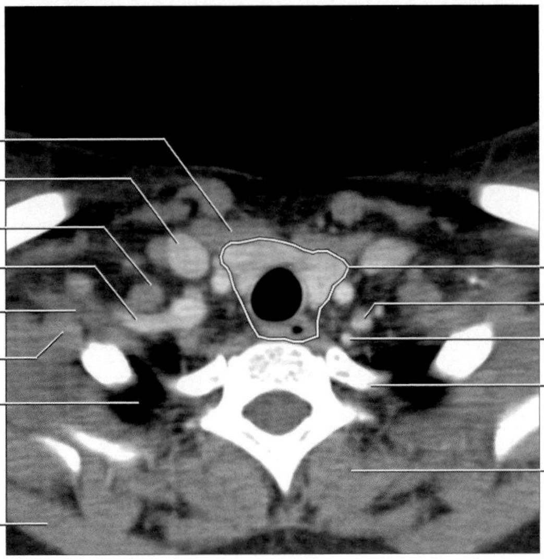

(Top) First of three axial CECT images through the lower cervical neck and cervicothoracic junction presented from superior to inferior shows the anterior, middle and posterior scalene muscles in the prevertebral component of the perivertebral space. Notice the brachial plexus roots between the anterior and middle scalene muscles. **(Middle)** At the level of the first thoracic vertebral body and first rib the anterior scalene is clearly visibile anterior to the roots of the brachial plexus. The visceral space contains the thyroid gland, parathyroid glands (not visible on CT), the cervical esophagus and trachea. **(Bottom)** In this image at the level of the lung apices the visceral space is outlined by the middle layer of deep cervical fascia. The right subclavian artery passes between the anterior and middle scalene muscles along with the brachial plexus roots.

SUPRAHYOID AND INFRAHYOID NECK OVERVIEW

AXIAL T1 MR

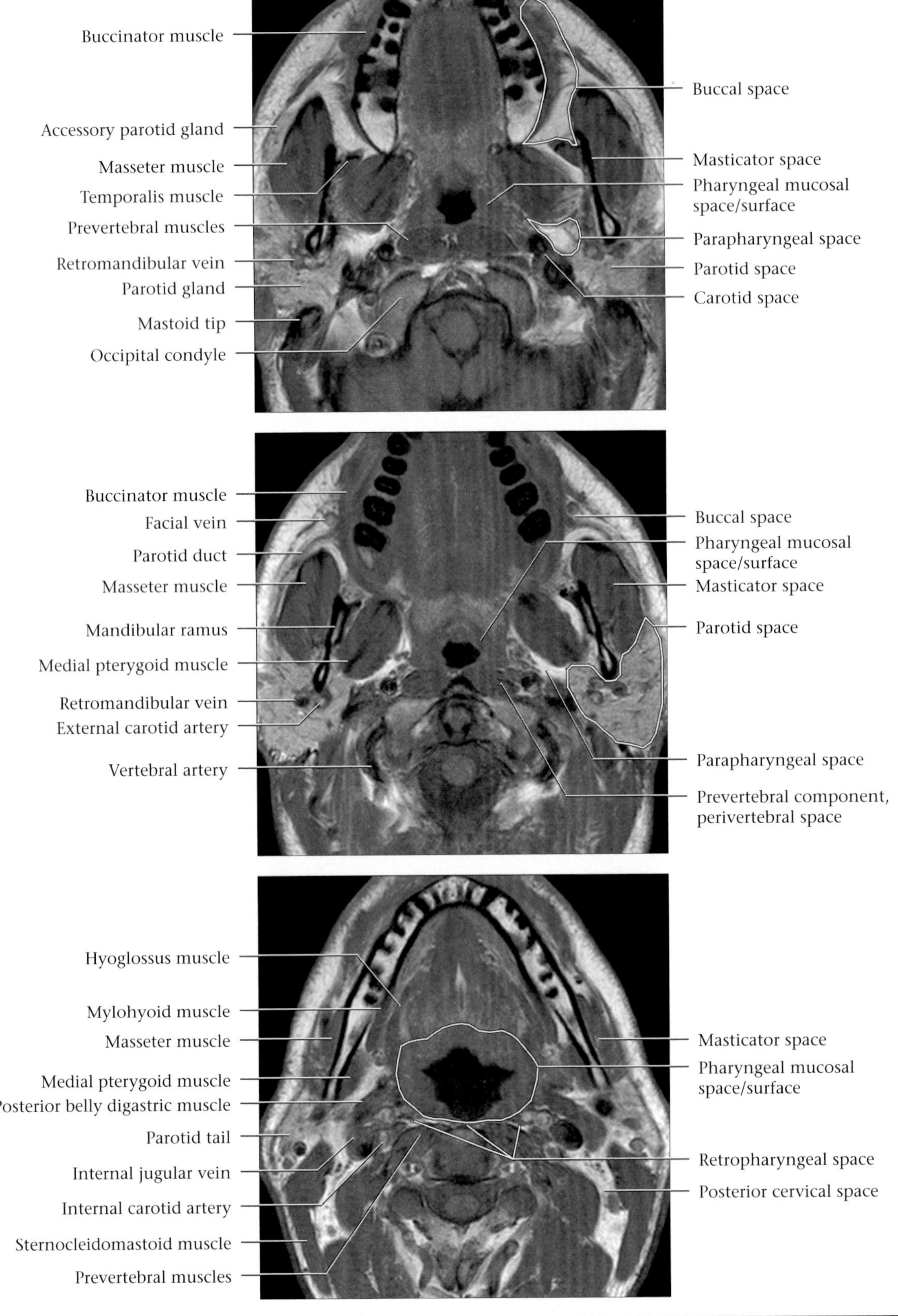
Buccinator muscle
Accessory parotid gland
Masseter muscle
Temporalis muscle
Prevertebral muscles
Retromandibular vein
Parotid gland
Mastoid tip
Occipital condyle
Buccal space
Masticator space
Pharyngeal mucosal space/surface
Parapharyngeal space
Parotid space
Carotid space
Buccinator muscle
Facial vein
Parotid duct
Masseter muscle
Mandibular ramus
Medial pterygoid muscle
Retromandibular vein
External carotid artery
Vertebral artery
Buccal space
Pharyngeal mucosal space/surface
Masticator space
Parotid space
Parapharyngeal space
Prevertebral component, perivertebral space
Hyoglossus muscle
Mylohyoid muscle
Masseter muscle
Medial pterygoid muscle
Posterior belly digastric muscle
Parotid tail
Internal jugular vein
Internal carotid artery
Sternocleidomastoid muscle
Prevertebral muscles
Masticator space
Pharyngeal mucosal space/surface
Retropharyngeal space
Posterior cervical space

(Top) First of 6 axial T1 MR images of the suprahyoid & infrahyoid neck presented from superior to inferior. In this image the buccal space is outlined on left. There is no fascial margin to the buccal space. The parapharyngeal space is seen as 2 fat-filled areas surrounded by the pharyngeal mucosal, masticator, parotid & carotid spaces. **(Middle)** In this image at mandibular teeth level the parotid space is seen posterior to the masticator space. Both are surrounded by the superficial layer of deep cervical fascia. **(Bottom)** In this image the pharyngeal mucosal space is made up of the anterior lingual & lateral palatine tonsils. Fat stripe behind the pharyngeal mucosal space is the retropharyngeal space. Behind the retropharyngeal space is the prevertebral component of the perivertebral space. The posterior belly of digastric muscle separates carotid from parotid space.

AXIAL T1 MR

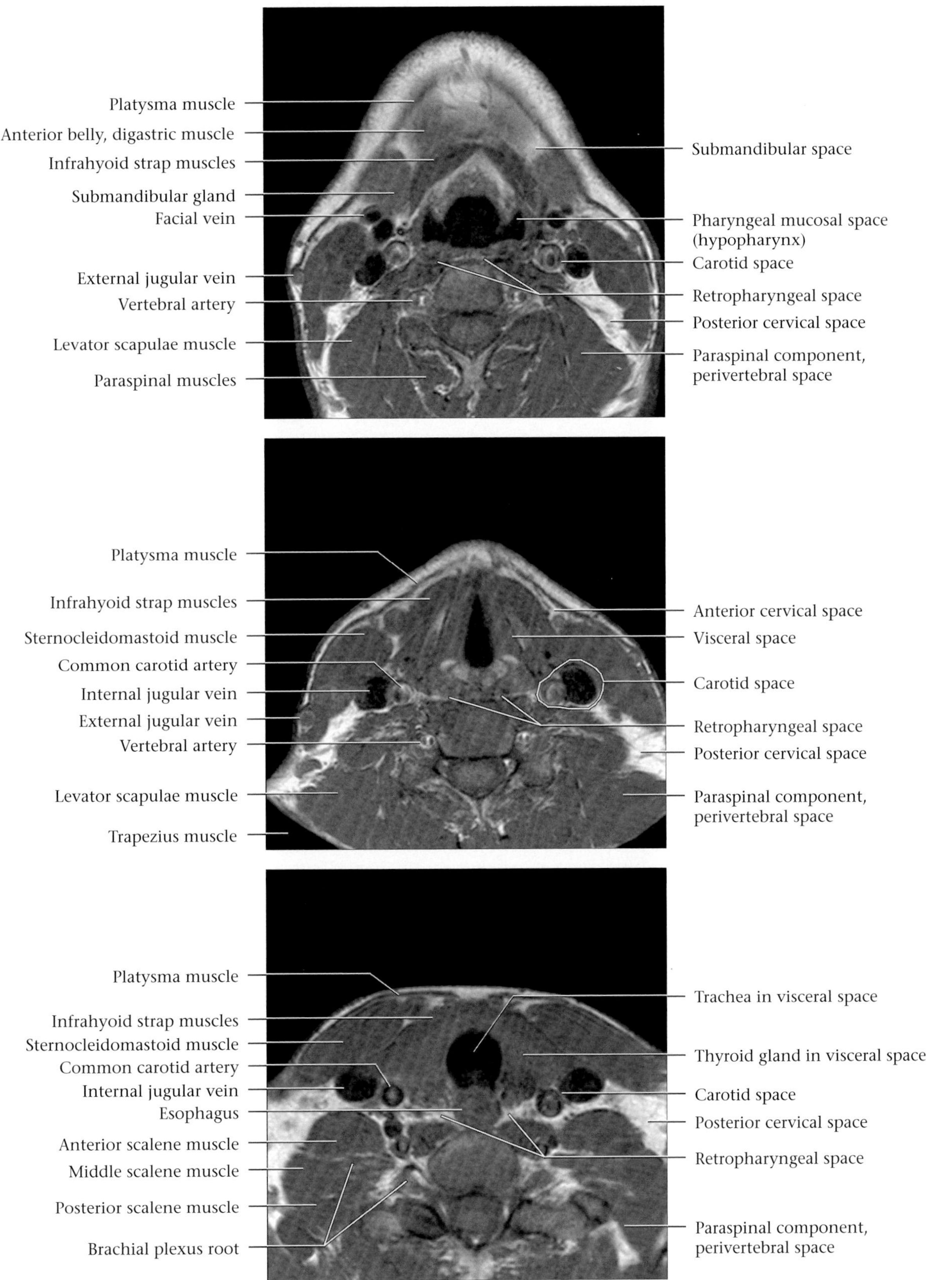
Platysma muscle
Anterior belly, digastric muscle
Infrahyoid strap muscles
Submandibular gland
Facial vein
External jugular vein
Vertebral artery
Levator scapulae muscle
Paraspinal muscles
Submandibular space
Pharyngeal mucosal space (hypopharynx)
Carotid space
Retropharyngeal space
Posterior cervical space
Paraspinal component, perivertebral space
Platysma muscle
Infrahyoid strap muscles
Sternocleidomastoid muscle
Common carotid artery
Internal jugular vein
External jugular vein
Vertebral artery
Levator scapulae muscle
Trapezius muscle
Anterior cervical space
Visceral space
Carotid space
Retropharyngeal space
Posterior cervical space
Paraspinal component, perivertebral space
Platysma muscle
Infrahyoid strap muscles
Sternocleidomastoid muscle
Common carotid artery
Internal jugular vein
Esophagus
Anterior scalene muscle
Middle scalene muscle
Posterior scalene muscle
Brachial plexus root
Trachea in visceral space
Thyroid gland in visceral space
Carotid space
Posterior cervical space
Retropharyngeal space
Paraspinal component, perivertebral space

(Top) In this image the visceral space of the infrahyoid neck is visible. The middle layer of deep cervical fascia circumscribes the visceral space. The visceral space at this level contains the infrahyoid strap muscles, pyriform sinuses & epiglottis. **(Middle)** At the level of true vocal cords both the anterior & posterior cervical spaces are seen. Note the anterior cervical space is a direct extension of the submandibular space into the infrahyoid neck. The carotid space is surrounded by the carotid sheath. The common carotid artery, internal jugular vein & vagus nerve are found in the infrahyoid carotid space. **(Bottom)** At the level of the upper trachea the thyroid gland is now the largest structure in the visceral space. The parathyroid glands, cervical trachea and esophagus, paratracheal nodes and recurrent laryngeal nerve are all in the visceral space.

AXIAL T2 MR

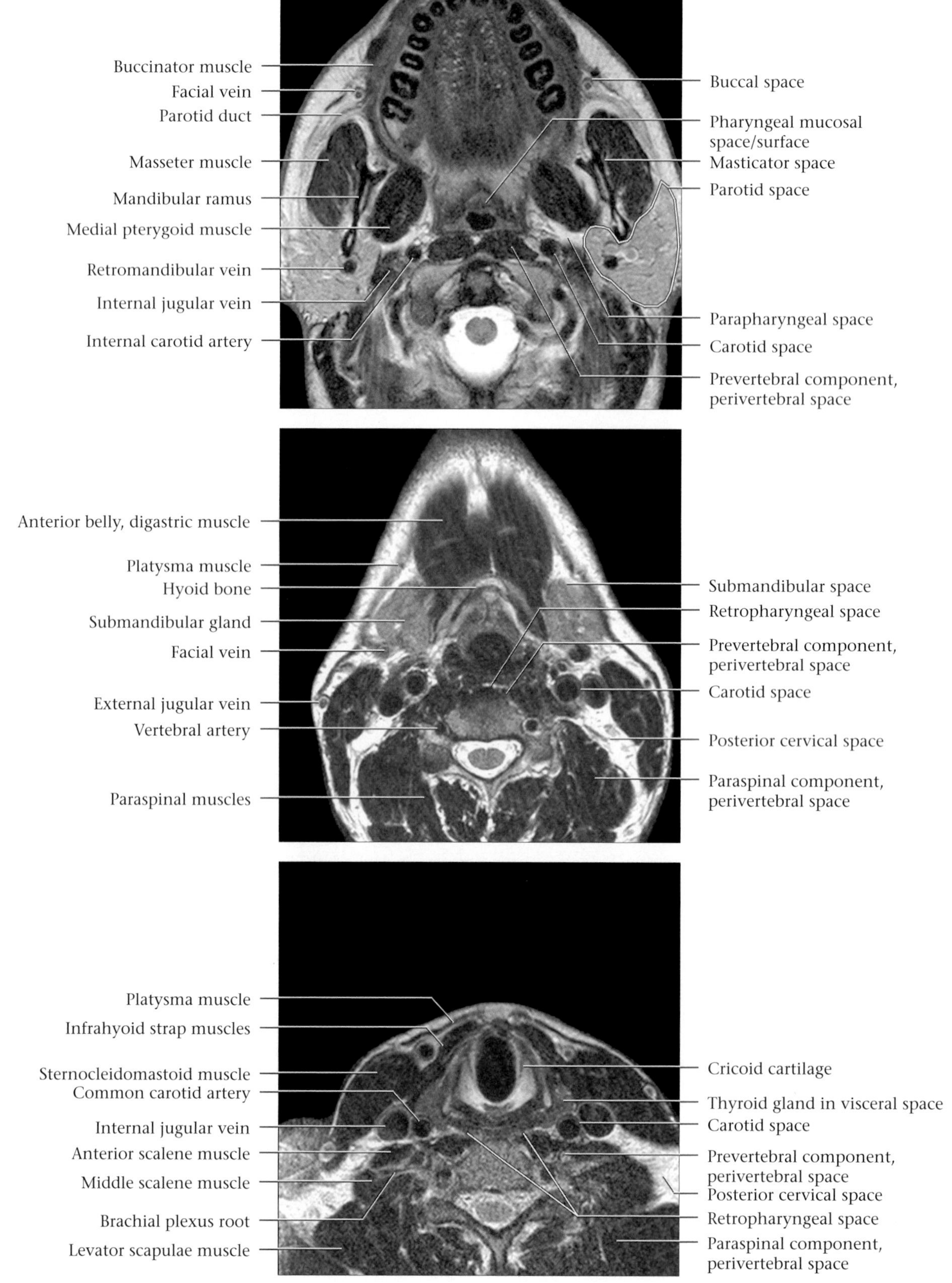

Buccinator muscle
Facial vein
Parotid duct
Masseter muscle
Mandibular ramus
Medial pterygoid muscle
Retromandibular vein
Internal jugular vein
Internal carotid artery
Buccal space
Pharyngeal mucosal space/surface
Masticator space
Parotid space
Parapharyngeal space
Carotid space
Prevertebral component, perivertebral space
Anterior belly, digastric muscle
Platysma muscle
Hyoid bone
Submandibular gland
Facial vein
External jugular vein
Vertebral artery
Paraspinal muscles
Submandibular space
Retropharyngeal space
Prevertebral component, perivertebral space
Carotid space
Posterior cervical space
Paraspinal component, perivertebral space
Platysma muscle
Infrahyoid strap muscles
Sternocleidomastoid muscle
Common carotid artery
Internal jugular vein
Anterior scalene muscle
Middle scalene muscle
Brachial plexus root
Levator scapulae muscle
Cricoid cartilage
Thyroid gland in visceral space
Carotid space
Prevertebral component, perivertebral space
Posterior cervical space
Retropharyngeal space
Paraspinal component, perivertebral space

(Top) First of three axial T2 MR images of the neck at the level of the maxillary alveolar ridge shows the 4 key spaces surrounding the fat-filled parapharyngeal space. These important four spaces are the pharyngeal mucosal, masticator, parotid & carotid spaces. The parotid & masticator spaces are circumscribed by superficial layer of deep cervical fascia. **(Middle)** In this image at the level of hyoid bone the large submandibular glands are visible in the submandibular space deep to the platysma muscle. **(Bottom)** At the level of the cricoid cartilage the prevertebral & paraspinal components of the perivertebral space can be seen. The brachial plexus roots exit the prevertebral component between the anterior & middle scalene muscles to enter the posterior cervical space fat on their way to the axilla.

SUPRAHYOID AND INFRAHYOID NECK OVERVIEW

CORONAL T1 MR

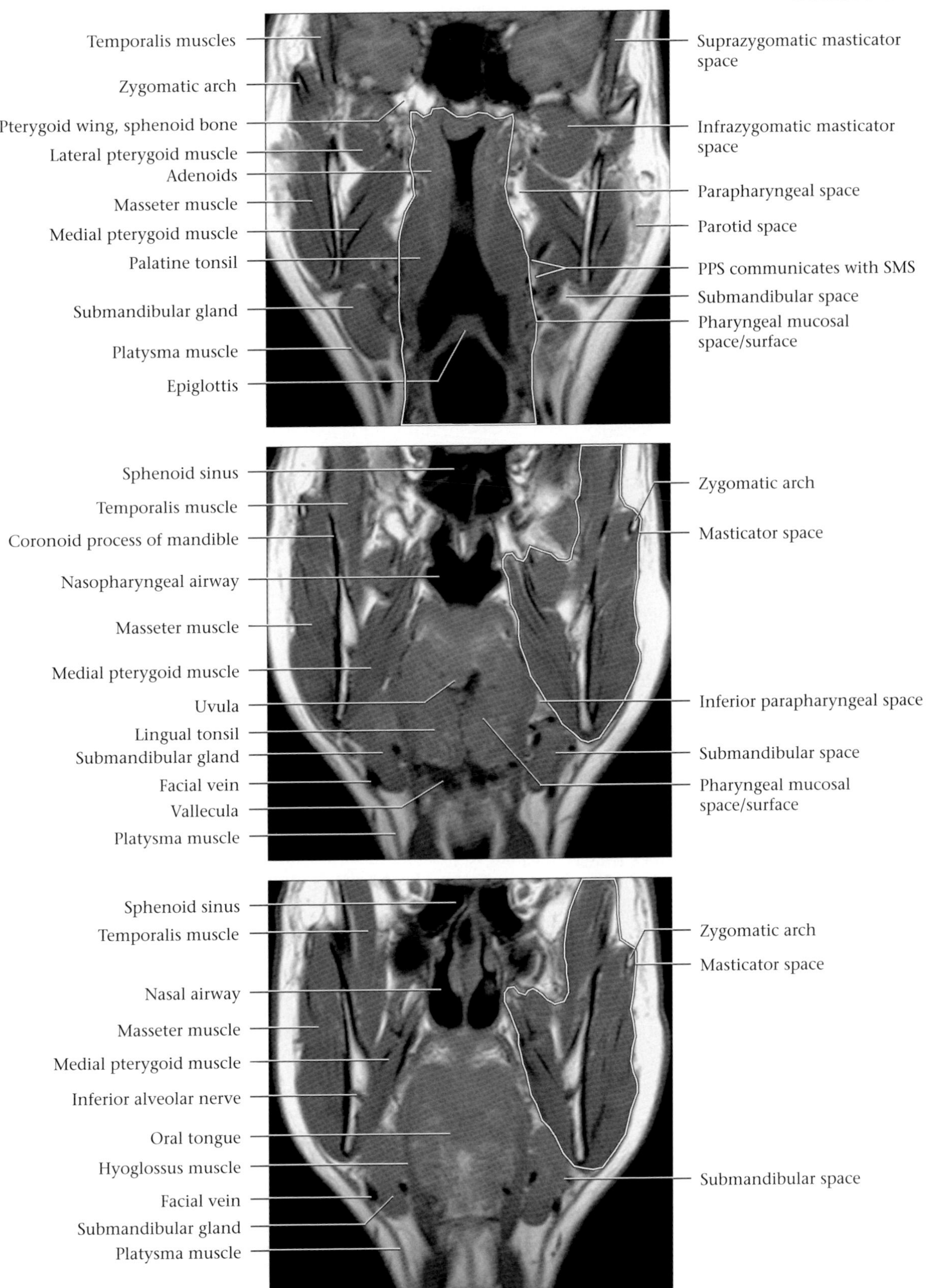

Temporalis muscles
Zygomatic arch
Pterygoid wing, sphenoid bone
Lateral pterygoid muscle
Adenoids
Masseter muscle
Medial pterygoid muscle
Palatine tonsil
Submandibular gland
Platysma muscle
Epiglottis
Suprazygomatic masticator space
Infrazygomatic masticator space
Parapharyngeal space
Parotid space
PPS communicates with SMS
Submandibular space
Pharyngeal mucosal space/surface
Sphenoid sinus
Temporalis muscle
Coronoid process of mandible
Nasopharyngeal airway
Masseter muscle
Medial pterygoid muscle
Uvula
Lingual tonsil
Submandibular gland
Facial vein
Vallecula
Platysma muscle
Zygomatic arch
Masticator space
Inferior parapharyngeal space
Submandibular space
Pharyngeal mucosal space/surface
Sphenoid sinus
Temporalis muscle
Nasal airway
Masseter muscle
Medial pterygoid muscle
Inferior alveolar nerve
Oral tongue
Hyoglossus muscle
Facial vein
Submandibular gland
Platysma muscle
Zygomatic arch
Masticator space
Submandibular space

(Top) First of three coronal T1 MR images presented from posterior to anterior shows the pharyngeal mucosal space extending from nasopharynx to hypopharynx. It is from the pharyngeal mucosal space that the most common malignancies of the head & neck arise, squamous cell carcinoma from the mucosa, non-Hodgkin lymphoma from the tonsils & minor salivary gland malignancy from the minor salivary glands. **(Middle)** In this image the masticator space has been outlined. Remember this space has a suprazygomatic & an infrazygomatic component. Since there is no "horizontal fascia" between the zygomatic arch, diseases may spread within the masticator space between the suprazygomatic & infrazygomatic components. **(Bottom)** In this image through the posterior nose 3 of the major muscles of mastication are visible, the masseter, medial pterygoid and temporalis muscles.

PARAPHARYNGEAL SPACE

Terminology

Abbreviations

- Parapharyngeal space (PPS)

Synonyms

- Parapharyngeal space has been called "prestyloid parapharyngeal space"
  - Carotid space called "post-styloid parapharyngeal space" in this alterative terminology
  - Carotid space preferred terminology

Definitions

- **Parapharyngeal space**: Central, fat-filled spaces in lateral suprahyoid neck (SHN) around which most of important spaces are located
  - These surrounding important spaces are pharyngeal mucosal space (PMS), masticator space (MS), parotid space (PS) and carotid space (CS)

Imaging Anatomy

Overview

- PPS contents are limited, therefore few lesions actually begin in this location
  - Diseases of PPS usually arise in adjacent spaces (PMS, MS, PS, CS), spreading secondarily into PPS
- Importance of PPS is its conspicuity on CT and MR as well as its direction of displacement by mass lesions of surrounding spaces
  - **PPS displacement pattern helps define actual space of origin**
    - PMS mass lesion pushes PPS laterally
    - MS mass lesion pushes PPS posteriorly
    - PS mass lesion pushes PPS medially
    - CS mass lesion pushes PPS anteriorly
    - Lateral retropharyngeal space mass (nodal) pushes PPS anterolaterally
  - Combining center of mass lesion with displacement direction of PPS yields strong impression of "space of origin" of SHN mass lesion

Extent

- Crescent-shaped fat-filled space in craniocaudal dimension extends from skull base above to superior cornu of hyoid bone inferiorly

Anatomy Relationships

- As fatty tube separating other SHN spaces from one another, PPS functions as "elevator shaft" through which infection and tumor from these adjacent spaces may travel from skull base to hyoid bone
- Inferiorly there is **no fascia** separating inferior PPS from submandibular space (SMS)
  - Open communication between inferior PPS and posterior SMS therefore exists
- Superiorly PPS interacts with skull base in bland triangular area on inferior surface of petrous apex
  - **No exiting skull base foramina** are found in this area of attachment
- Surrounding spaces include
  - PMS medially
  - MS anterolaterally
  - PS laterally
  - CS posteriorly
  - RPS posteromedially

Internal Structures-Critical Contents

- PPS has **no** mucosa, muscle, bone, nodes or major salivary gland tissue within its boundaries
  - Consequently few things primarily begin in PPS
- **Critical PPS contents**
  - **Fat**: Key constituent making PPS easily identifiable even with larger SHN mass lesions
  - Minor salivary glands (ectopic, rare)
  - Internal maxillary artery
  - Ascending pharyngeal artery
  - Pterygoid venous plexus (small portion, mostly MS)

Fascial of Parapharyngeal Space

- Fascial margins of PPS are complex; made up of different layers of deep cervical fascia
  - Medial fascial margin of PPS
    - Made up of middle layer, deep cervical fascia as it curves around lateral margin of PMS
  - Lateral fascial margin of PPS
    - Formed by medial slip of superficial layer of deep cervical fascia along deep border of MS & PS
  - Posterior fascial margin of PPS
    - Formed by deep layer of deep cervical fascia on anterolateral margin of retropharyngeal space and anterior part of carotid sheath (made up of components of all 3 layers of deep cervical fascia)

Anatomy-Based Imaging Issues

Key Concepts or Questions

- Because of limited normal anatomic contents of PPS, few lesions primarily arise in PPS
  - Rare lesions found in PPS include benign mixed tumor (from minor salivary gland rests in PPS), lipoma and atypical second branchial cleft cyst
  - To say lesion is primary to PPS, it must be completely surrounded by PPS fat
  - In most cases where lesion is thought to be primary to PPS, careful observation will find connection to one of surrounding spaces (usually PS)
- **PPS fat displacement** is **key imaging relationship** used in evaluation of SHN mass lesions

Imaging Recommendations

- MR better delineates skull base, meningeal & perineural lesions
  - Fat-saturated contrast-enhanced T1 MR may make PPS fat difficult to see

Imaging Pitfalls

- Remember most lesions of PPS arise from adjacent SHN spaces

Clinical Implications

Clinical Importance

- Since PPS empties inferiorly into SMS, PPS lesion may present as "angle of mandible" mass

GRAPHICS

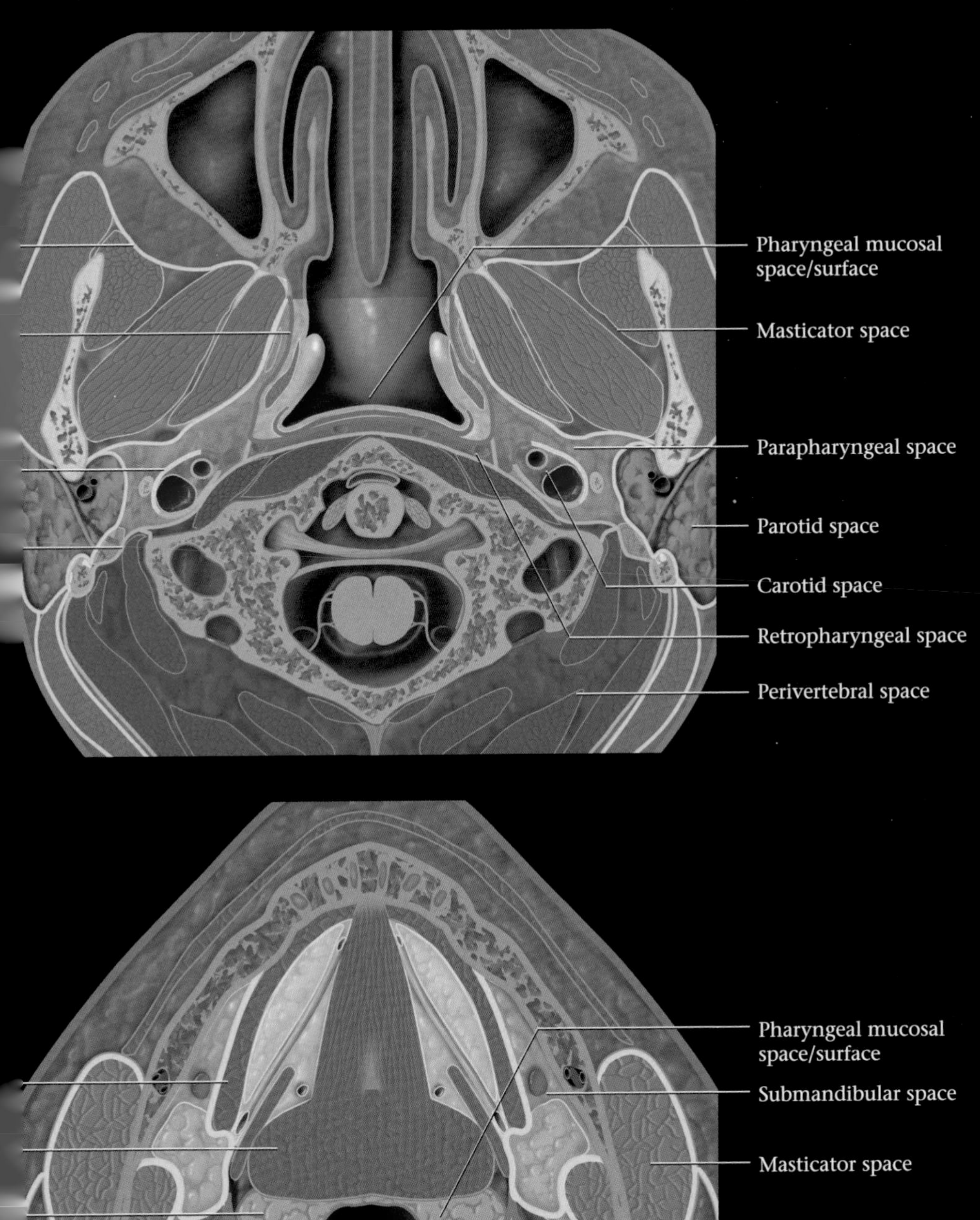
Pharyngeal mucosal space/surface
Masticator space
Parapharyngeal space
Parotid space
Carotid space
Retropharyngeal space
Perivertebral space
Pharyngeal mucosal space/surface
Submandibular space
Masticator space
Parapharyngeal space
Parotid space
Carotid space
Retropharyngeal space

normal parapharyngeal space at the level of the nasopharynx demonstrating the complex t only contents. The surrounding pharyngeal mucosal, masticator, parotid and carotid nass lesions push into the parapharyngeal space. The resulting displacement pattern of the y be helpful in defining the space of origin of a mass in the suprahyoid neck. **(Bottom)** of the low oropharynx shows the slip of parapharyngeal space fat is just anterolateral to the stric muscle. Inferior to this level the parapharyngeal space communicates anteriorly with Yellow lines in the drawing represent superficial layer, pink lines middle and aquamarine

GRAPHICS

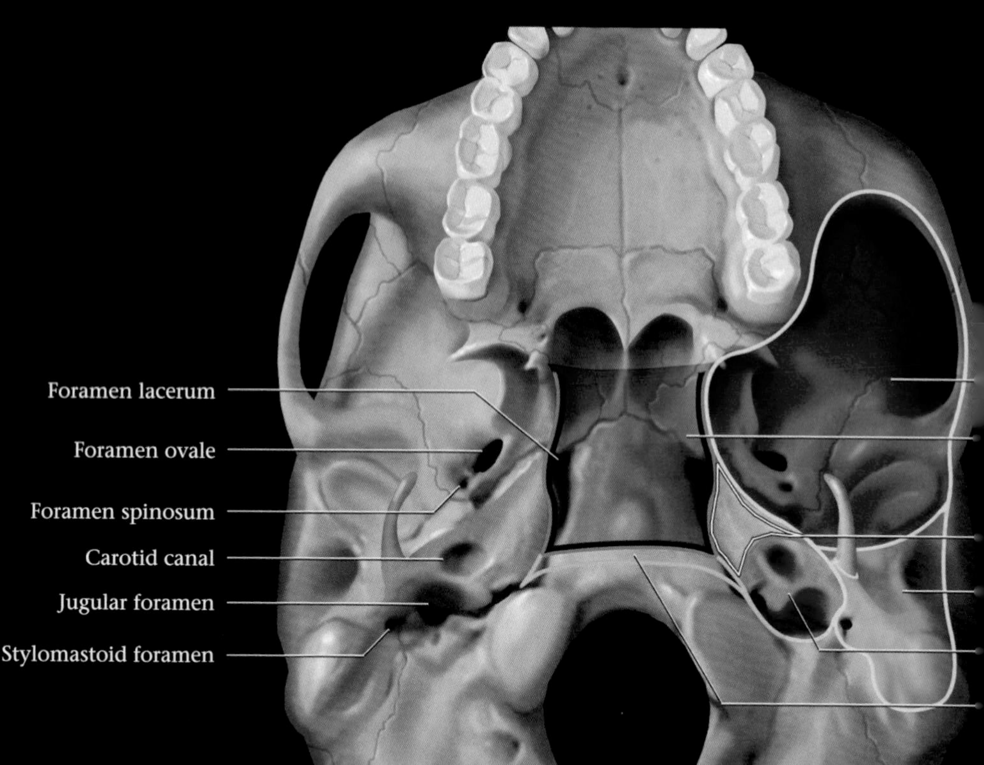

Foramen lacerum
Foramen ovale
Foramen spinosum
Carotid canal
Jugular foramen
Stylomastoid foramen

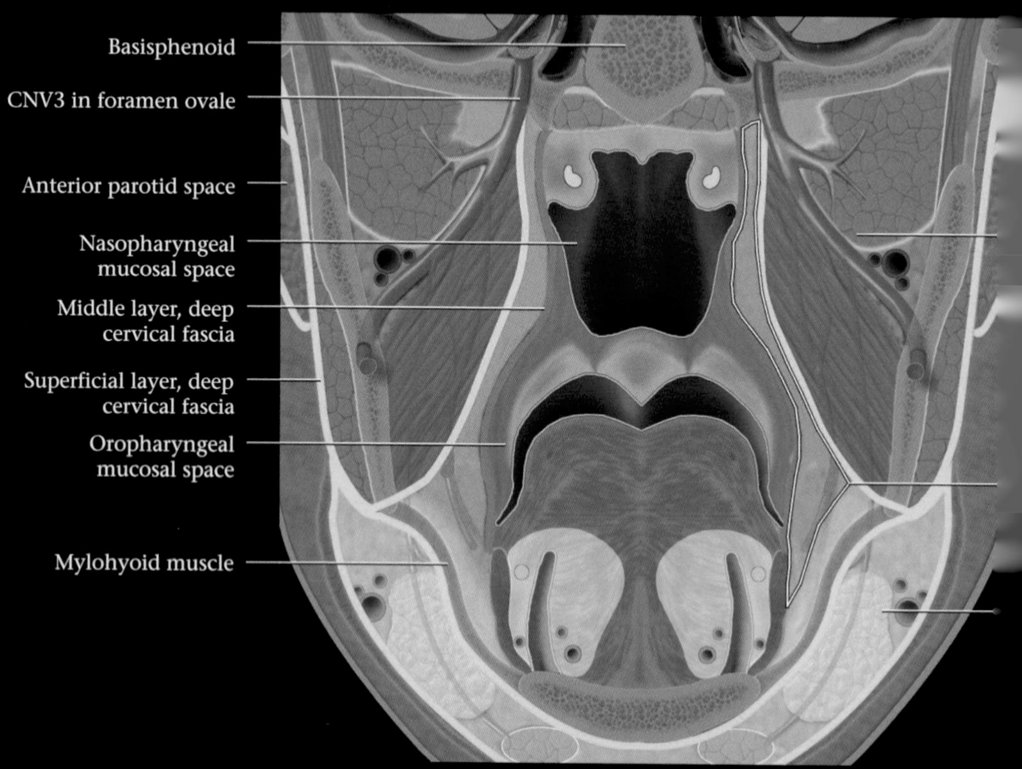

Basisphenoid
CNV3 in foramen ovale
Anterior parotid space
Nasopharyngeal mucosal space
Middle layer, deep cervical fascia
Superficial layer, deep cervical fascia
Oropharyngeal mucosal space
Mylohyoid muscle

(Top) Axial graphic of the suprahyoid neck spaces interaction with the skull base highlighti space. Notice that the parapharyngeal space abuts the inferior surface of the skull base in an structures. **(Bottom)** Coronal graphic of suprahyoid neck spaces as they interact with the sk submandibular space inferiorly. The parapharyngeal space interacts with no critical structure base. Inferiorly it "empties" into the posterior submandibular space along the posterior marg muscle. As a consequence of this anatomic arrangement it is possible for an infection or a m breaks into the parapharyngeal space to present inferiorly as an "angle of mandible" mass.

AXIAL CECT

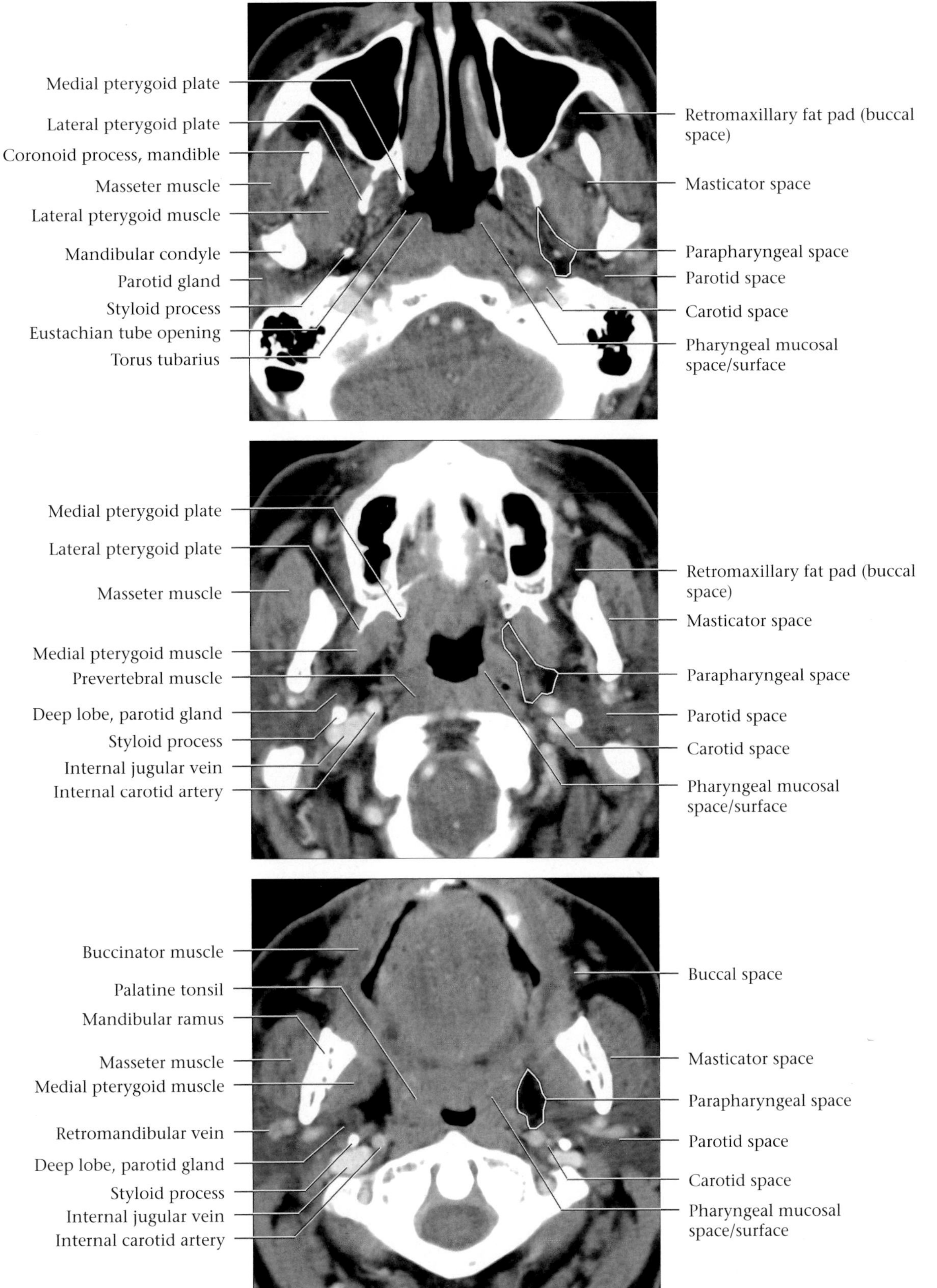
Medial pterygoid plate
Lateral pterygoid plate
Coronoid process, mandible
Masseter muscle
Lateral pterygoid muscle
Mandibular condyle
Parotid gland
Styloid process
Eustachian tube opening
Torus tubarius
Retromaxillary fat pad (buccal space)
Masticator space
Parapharyngeal space
Parotid space
Carotid space
Pharyngeal mucosal space/surface
Medial pterygoid plate
Lateral pterygoid plate
Masseter muscle
Medial pterygoid muscle
Prevertebral muscle
Deep lobe, parotid gland
Styloid process
Internal jugular vein
Internal carotid artery
Retromaxillary fat pad (buccal space)
Masticator space
Parapharyngeal space
Parotid space
Carotid space
Pharyngeal mucosal space/surface
Buccinator muscle
Palatine tonsil
Mandibular ramus
Masseter muscle
Medial pterygoid muscle
Retromandibular vein
Deep lobe, parotid gland
Styloid process
Internal jugular vein
Internal carotid artery
Buccal space
Masticator space
Parapharyngeal space
Parotid space
Carotid space
Pharyngeal mucosal space/surface

(Top) First of six contrast-enhanced axial CT images of the suprahyoid neck presented from superior to inferior shows the superior end of the parapharyngeal space just before it abuts the skull base. Notice the 4 major spaces surrounding the parapharyngeal space, the pharyngeal mucosal, masticator, parotid and carotid spaces. **(Middle)** In this image at the level of the inferior maxillary sinus the complex shape of the parapharyngeal space is visible. Notice the lateral margin of the parapharyngeal space is the deep lobe of the parotid gland. **(Bottom)** In this mid-oropharynx image the parapharyngeal space has the palatine tonsil on its entire medial border. It is easy to see that a squamous cell carcinoma of the palatine tonsil that is deeply invasive would immediately enter the parapharyngeal space fat, pushing it from medial to lateral.

PARAPHARYNGEAL SPACE

AXIAL CECT

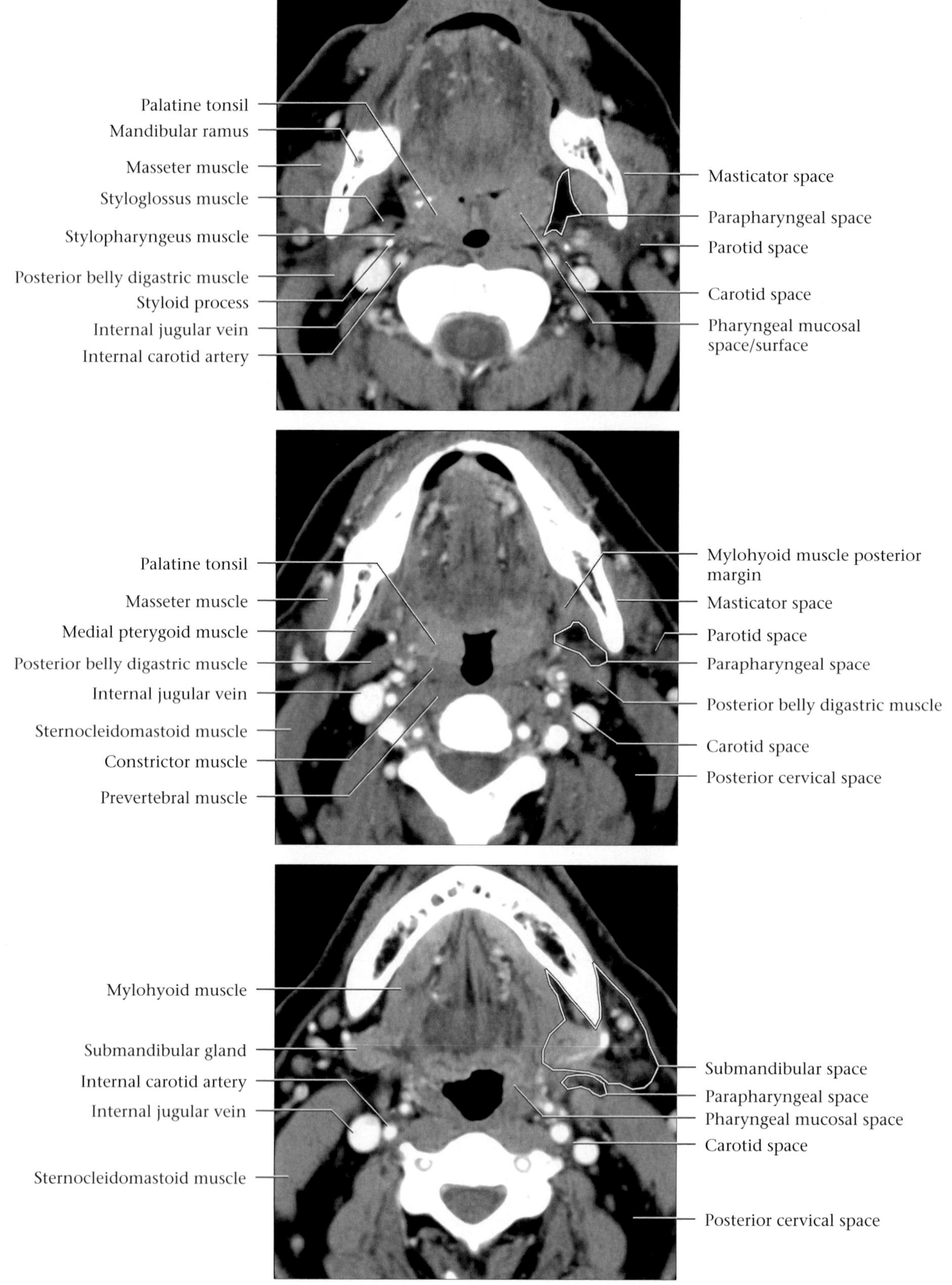

Palatine tonsil
Mandibular ramus
Masseter muscle
Styloglossus muscle
Stylopharyngeus muscle
Posterior belly digastric muscle
Styloid process
Internal jugular vein
Internal carotid artery
Masticator space
Parapharyngeal space
Parotid space
Carotid space
Pharyngeal mucosal space/surface
Palatine tonsil
Masseter muscle
Medial pterygoid muscle
Posterior belly digastric muscle
Internal jugular vein
Sternocleidomastoid muscle
Constrictor muscle
Prevertebral muscle
Mylohyoid muscle posterior margin
Masticator space
Parotid space
Parapharyngeal space
Posterior belly digastric muscle
Carotid space
Posterior cervical space
Mylohyoid muscle
Submandibular gland
Internal carotid artery
Internal jugular vein
Sternocleidomastoid muscle
Submandibular space
Parapharyngeal space
Pharyngeal mucosal space
Carotid space
Posterior cervical space

(Top) In this image the parapharyngeal space points anteriorly toward the submandibular space. On more inferior images it will communicate with the posterosuperior submandibular space in this area. Notice the stylopharyngeus and styloglossus muscle on the posterior margin of the parapharyngeal space. **(Middle)** At the level of the mandibular body the parapharyngeal space is seen entering the superior submandibular space just anterior to the posterior belly of the digastric muscles and just posterior to the mylohyoid muscle. **(Bottom)** In this image through the superior submandibular space it is possible to see the most inferior parapharyngeal space merging with the submandibular space. Remember there is no fascia separating the inferior parapharyngeal, posterior submandibular and sublingual spaces at the posterior margin of the mylohyoid muscle.

PARAPHARYNGEAL SPACE

AXIAL T1 MR

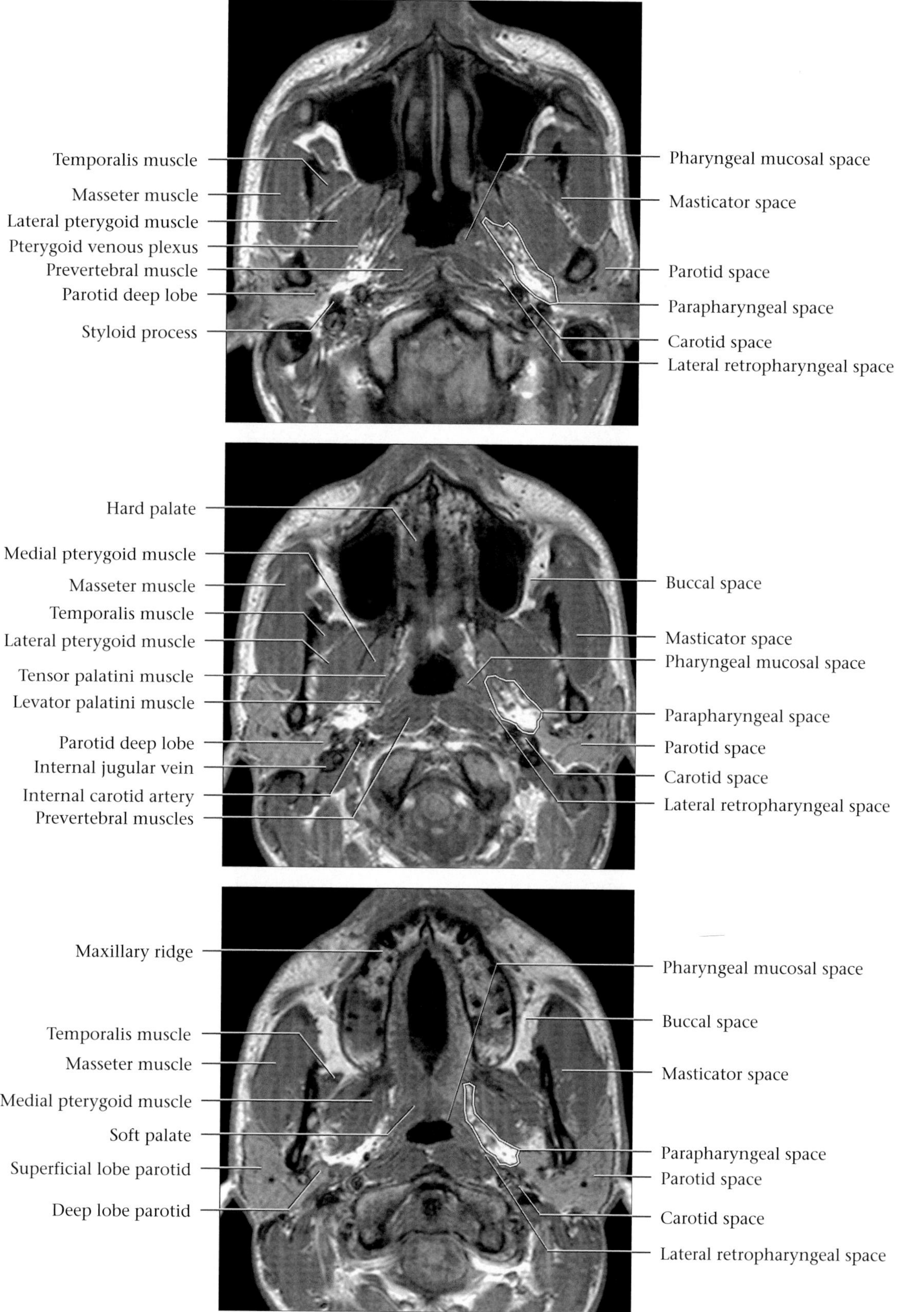

Temporalis muscle
Masseter muscle
Lateral pterygoid muscle
Pterygoid venous plexus
Prevertebral muscle
Parotid deep lobe
Styloid process
Pharyngeal mucosal space
Masticator space
Parotid space
Parapharyngeal space
Carotid space
Lateral retropharyngeal space
Hard palate
Medial pterygoid muscle
Masseter muscle
Temporalis muscle
Lateral pterygoid muscle
Tensor palatini muscle
Levator palatini muscle
Parotid deep lobe
Internal jugular vein
Internal carotid artery
Prevertebral muscles
Buccal space
Masticator space
Pharyngeal mucosal space
Parapharyngeal space
Parotid space
Carotid space
Lateral retropharyngeal space
Maxillary ridge
Temporalis muscle
Masseter muscle
Medial pterygoid muscle
Soft palate
Superficial lobe parotid
Deep lobe parotid
Pharyngeal mucosal space
Buccal space
Masticator space
Parapharyngeal space
Parotid space
Carotid space
Lateral retropharyngeal space

(Top) First of six axial T1 MR images of the suprahyoid neck presented from superior to inferior shows the parapharyngeal space at the level of the nasopharynx. Here the surrounding spaces include the pharyngeal mucosal, masticator, parotid and carotid spaces. Notice the lateral retropharyngeal space is on the posteromedial aspect of the parapharyngeal space. **(Middle)** In this image at the level of the hard palate the posterior margins of the tensor and levator palatini muscles are visible along the anteromedial margin of the parapharyngeal space on the right. **(Bottom)** At the level of the maxillary ridge the parapharyngeal space on the left is surrounded in clockwise order by the medial pterygoid muscle, deep lobe of parotid, internal carotid artery, lateral pharynx and the soft palate.

AXIAL T1 MR

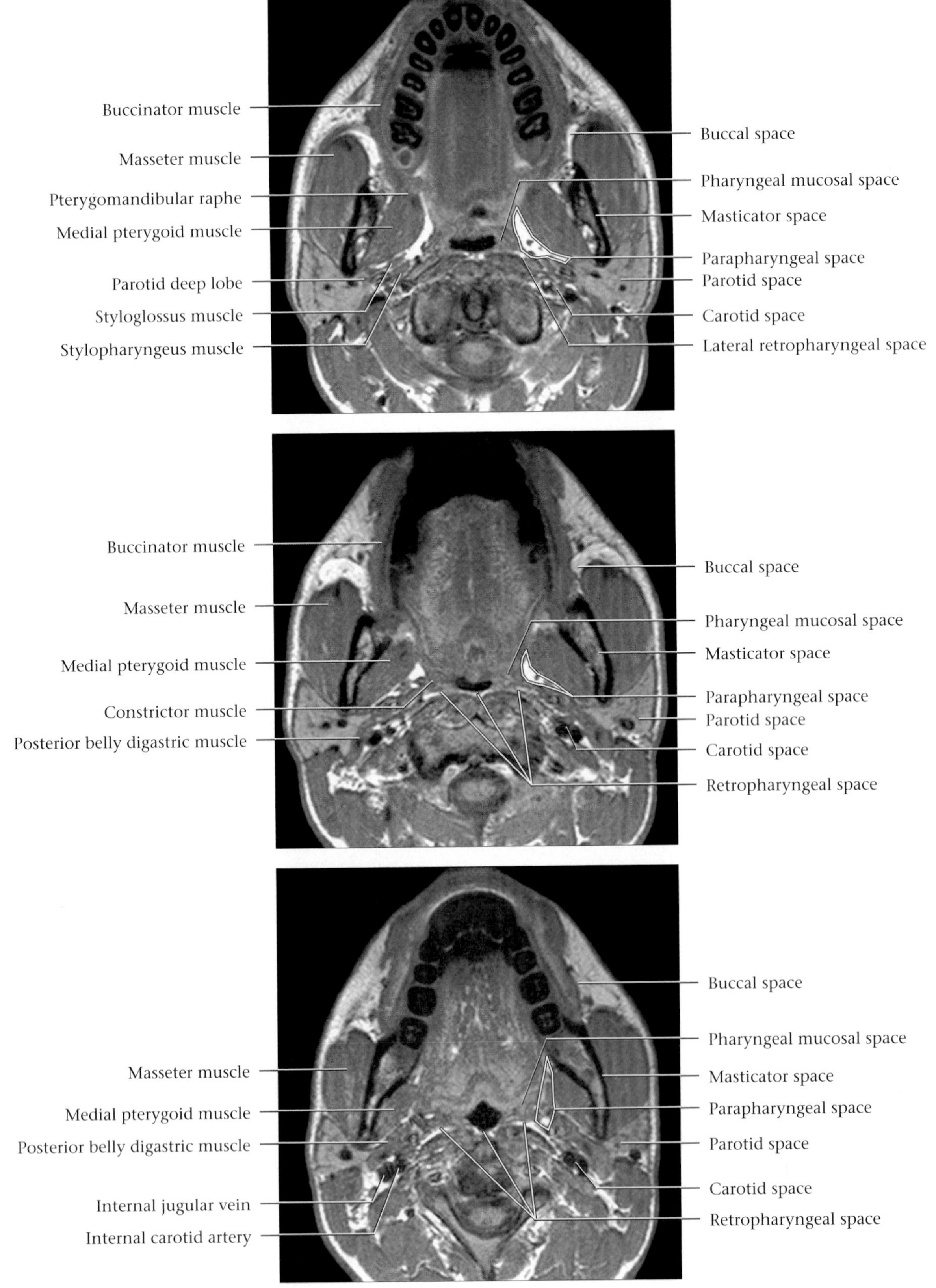

Buccinator muscle
Masseter muscle
Pterygomandibular raphe
Medial pterygoid muscle
Parotid deep lobe
Styloglossus muscle
Stylopharyngeus muscle
Buccal space
Pharyngeal mucosal space
Masticator space
Parapharyngeal space
Parotid space
Carotid space
Lateral retropharyngeal space
Buccinator muscle
Masseter muscle
Medial pterygoid muscle
Constrictor muscle
Posterior belly digastric muscle
Buccal space
Pharyngeal mucosal space
Masticator space
Parapharyngeal space
Parotid space
Carotid space
Retropharyngeal space
Masseter muscle
Medial pterygoid muscle
Posterior belly digastric muscle
Internal jugular vein
Internal carotid artery
Buccal space
Pharyngeal mucosal space
Masticator space
Parapharyngeal space
Parotid space
Carotid space
Retropharyngeal space

(Top) In this image at the level of the maxillary teeth the PPS takes on a crescentic shape as it bends around the medial pterygoid muscle of the masticator space. The pharyngeal mucosal space makes up the medial border of the PPS. Posteromedially the lateral retropharyngeal space is found while the carotid space makes up the PPS posterolateral border. The deep lobe of the parotid gland makes up the lateral margin of the PPS. **(Middle)** In this image at the level of the mid-oropharynx the parapharyngeal space becomes smaller along its inferior margin. **(Bottom)** In this image at the level of the mandibular teeth the parapharyngeal space is visible "pointing" anteriorly where it joins the posterosuperior margin of the submandibular space. Parapharyngeal abscess and tumor may access the submandibular space via this route.

CORONAL T1 MR

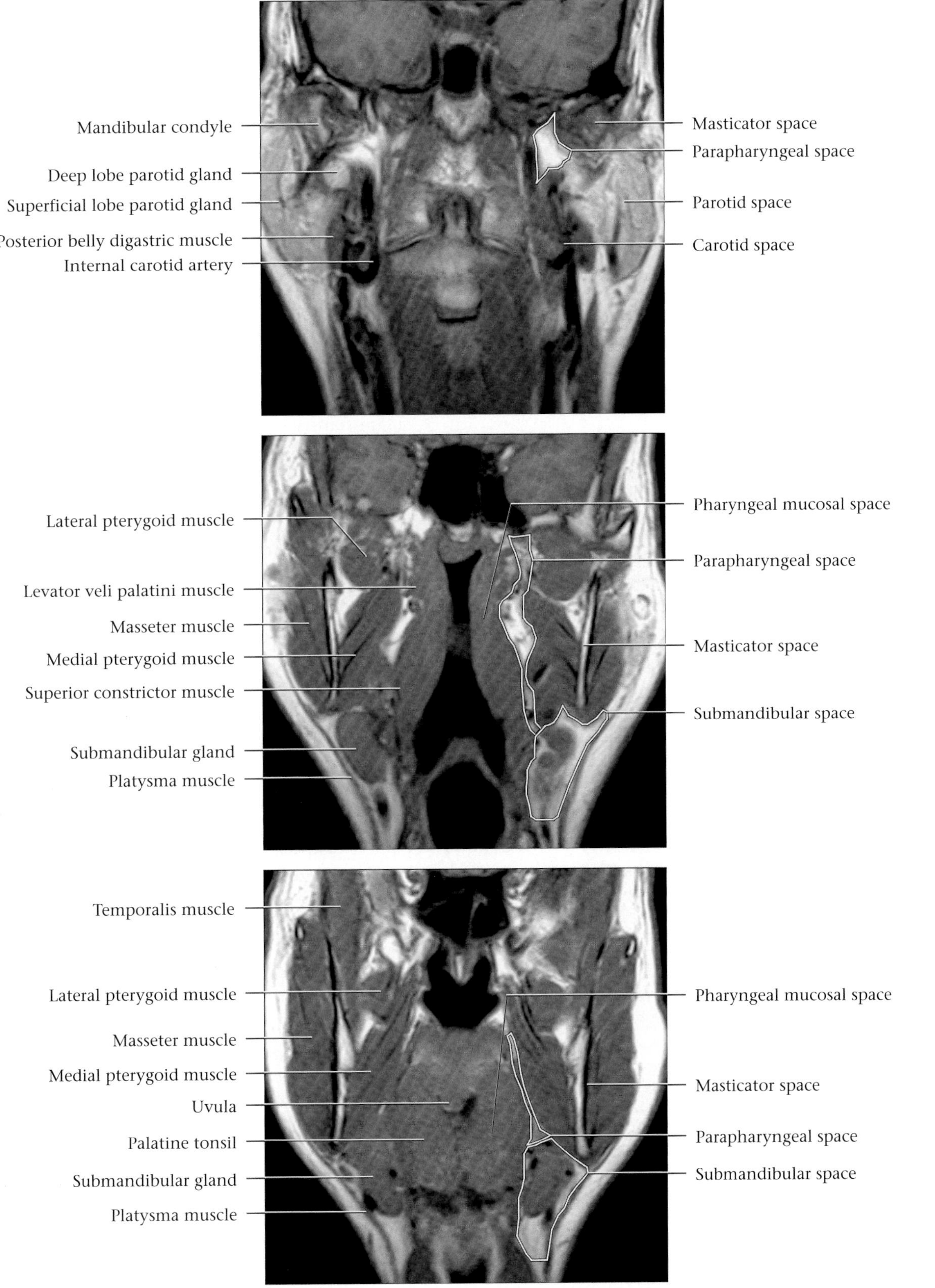

Mandibular condyle
Deep lobe parotid gland
Superficial lobe parotid gland
Posterior belly digastric muscle
Internal carotid artery
Masticator space
Parapharyngeal space
Parotid space
Carotid space
Lateral pterygoid muscle
Levator veli palatini muscle
Masseter muscle
Medial pterygoid muscle
Superior constrictor muscle
Submandibular gland
Platysma muscle
Pharyngeal mucosal space
Parapharyngeal space
Masticator space
Submandibular space
Temporalis muscle
Lateral pterygoid muscle
Masseter muscle
Medial pterygoid muscle
Uvula
Palatine tonsil
Submandibular gland
Platysma muscle
Pharyngeal mucosal space
Masticator space
Parapharyngeal space
Submandibular space

(Top) First of three coronal T1 MR images of the suprahyoid neck presented from posterior to anterior. In this image through the mandibular condyles the posterior parapharyngeal space is seen medial to the deep lobe of the parotid gland. **(Middle)** In this image the PPS is visible from its superior area of skull base abutment to its inferior merging with the submandibular space. Note the site of abutment with the skull base contains no vital structures. Remember there is no fascia present between the inferior PPS and the posterior submandibular space. **(Bottom)** In this image through the anterior parapharyngeal space the connection between the parapharyngeal space and submandibular space is seen. Submandibular space disease, especially abscess, may at times spread superiorly into the parapharyngeal space via this connection.

PHARYNGEAL MUCOSAL SPACE

Terminology

Abbreviations

- Pharyngeal mucosal space (PMS)

Definitions

- **PMS:** Nasopharyngeal, oropharyngeal & hypopharyngeal surface structures on airway side of middle layer of deep cervical fascia

Imaging Anatomy

Overview

- PMS is conceptual construct to complete map of spaces of suprahyoid neck
  - PMS alternative term: Pharyngeal mucosal surface
- There is **no fascia on surface of PMS**, so it is not a true fascia-enclosed space

Extent

- PMS is a continuous mucosal sheet defined from nasopharynx to hypopharynx (includes soft palate)
- Nasopharyngeal, oropharyngeal & hypopharyngeal mucosal space components
  - See larynx anatomy for hypopharynx anatomy

Anatomy Relationships

- Airway side of PMS has no fascial border
- Posterior to PMS is retropharyngeal space (RPS)
- Lateral to PMS is parapharyngeal space (PPS)
- Skull base relationship to PMS
  - Broad area of attachment to skull base present
  - Attachment area includes posterior basisphenoid (sphenoid sinus floor), anterior basiocciput (anterior clivus)
  - Also includes **foramen lacerum**
    - Foramen lacerum: Cartilaginous floor of anterior horizontal petrous internal carotid artery
    - Represents perivascular route for nasopharyngeal carcinoma to access intracranial structures

Internal Structures-Critical Contents

- **Mucosal surface of pharynx**
- **PMS lymphatic ring**: Lymphatic ring of tissue of PMS that declines in size with advancing age
  - Synonym: Waldeyer ring
  - Nasopharynx: **Adenoids**
  - Oropharynx, lateral wall: **Palatine (faucial) tonsil**
  - Oropharynx, base of tongue: **Lingual tonsil**
- **Minor salivary glands**
  - Soft palate mucosa has highest concentration
- **Pharyngobasilar fascia**
  - Tough aponeurosis that connects superior constrictor muscle to skull base
  - Posterosuperior margin notch = **sinus of Morgagni**
    - Levator palatini muscle & eustachian tube pass through this notch on way from skull base to PMS
- **Pharyngeal mucosal space muscles**
  - Superior, middle & inferior constrictor muscles
  - Salpingopharyngeus muscle
  - Levator palatini muscle, distal end
- **Torus tubarius**: Cartilaginous end of eustachian tube

Fascia of Pharyngeal Mucosal Space

- **Middle layer, deep cervical fascia** (ML-DCF) represents deep margin of PMS
  - In nasopharynx ML-DCF encircles lateral & posterior margins of pharyngobasilar fascia
  - In oropharynx ML-DCF on deep margin of superior & middle constrictor muscles
  - In hypopharynx ML-DCF on deep margin of inferior constrictor muscle

Anatomy-Based Imaging Issues

Key Concepts or Questions

- What imaging findings define a lesion as primary to pharyngeal mucosal space?
  - Lesion is designated primary to PMS under following circumstances
    - Lesion center is **medial to parapharyngeal space**
    - PMS mass **pushes PPS fat from medial to lateral**
    - PMS mass **disrupts normal PMS mucosal & submucosal architecture**

Imaging Recommendations

- CECT or MR can both successfully image PMS
- If skull base invasion or perineural tumor suspected, T1 C+ fat-saturated MR best
- Bone CT may then be added to delineate skull base bone changes & tumor matrix

Imaging Approaches

- If malignant tumor of PMS suspected, remember to stage primary tumor & nodes in cervical neck

Imaging Pitfalls

- Most common error in interpreting images of PMS is labeling normal asymmetry as tumor
- Lateral pharyngeal recess is notoriously asymmetric & may have fluid within it
- Variable amounts of lymphoid tissue can also create misimpression of tumor

Clinical Implications

Clinical Importance

- Referring MD can see PMS surface well
  - Use clinical impressions as part of imaging report
- Most common lesion of PMS is squamous cell carcinoma (SCCa)
  - Become familiar with routes of spread of SCCa by specific primary tumor site
  - Become familiar with staging criteria for each specific primary tumor site
- If not obviously SCCa, **differential diagnosis of PMS mass** relies heavily on normal PMS contents
  - From mucosa: Squamous cell carcinoma
  - From lymphoid tissue: Non-Hodgkin lymphoma
  - From minor salivary glands: Minor salivary gland malignancies (uncommon)
  - From constrictor or levator palatini muscles: Rhabdomyosarcoma (rare)

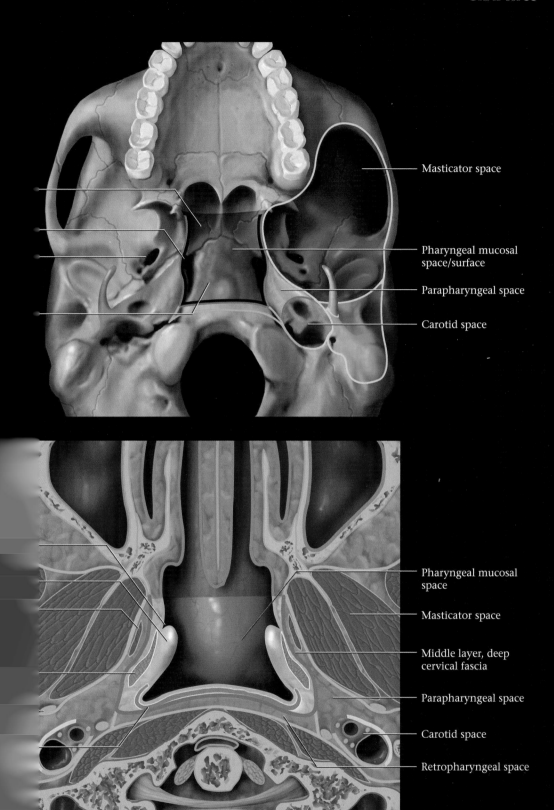

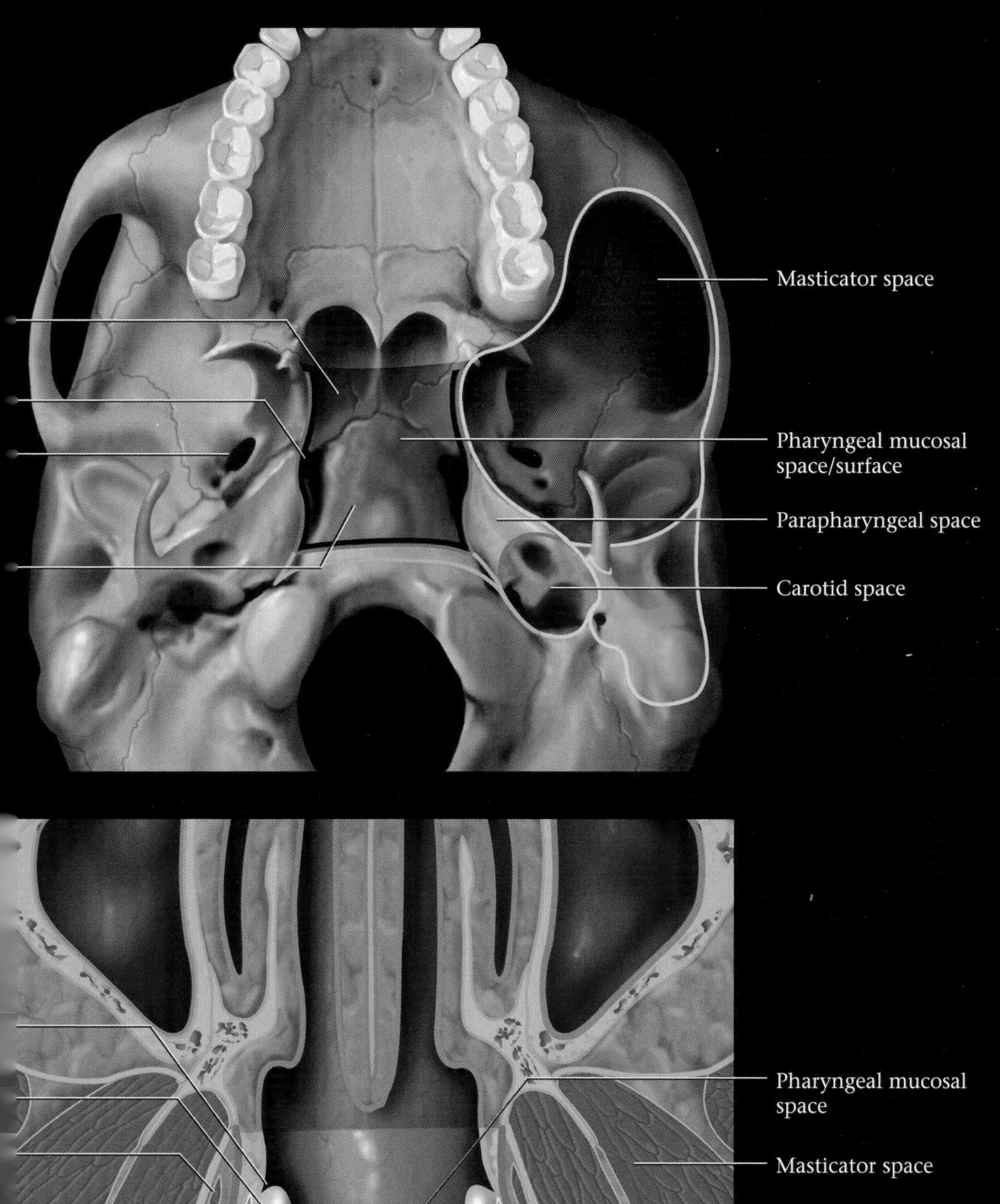

Masticator space
Pharyngeal mucosal space/surface
Parapharyngeal space
Carotid space
Pharyngeal mucosal space
Masticator space
Middle layer, deep cervical fascia
Parapharyngeal space
Carotid space
Retropharyngeal space

se from below shows spaces of suprahyoid neck relationships to skull base with emphasis on
pace. Notice the pharyngeal mucosal space butts a broad area of the sphenoid and occipital
um, the cartilaginous floor to the anteromedial horizontal petrous internal carotid artery
nent area. Malignant tumors of the nasopharyngeal mucosal space can access the
via the foramen lacerum. **(Bottom)** Axial graphic of the nasopharyngeal mucosal space (in
pharyngeal constrictor and levator veli palatini muscles are within the space. The middle
a provides a deep margin to the space. The retropharyngeal space is behind and the

GRAPHICS

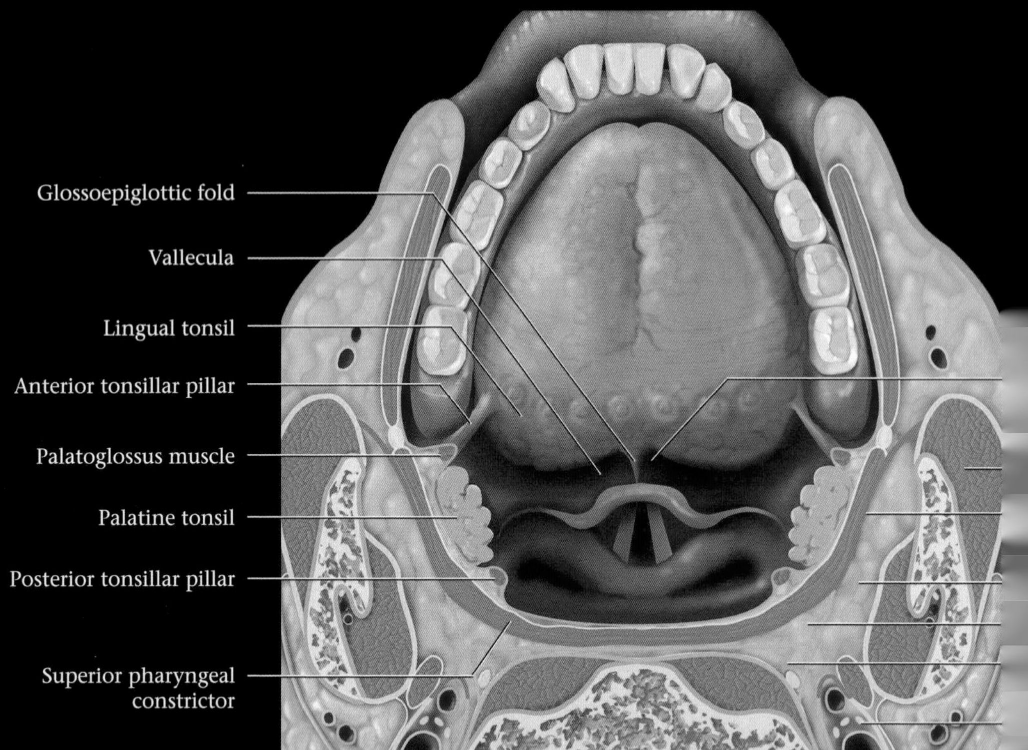
Glossoepiglottic fold
Vallecula
Lingual tonsil
Anterior tonsillar pillar
Palatoglossus muscle
Palatine tonsil
Posterior tonsillar pillar
Superior pharyngeal constrictor

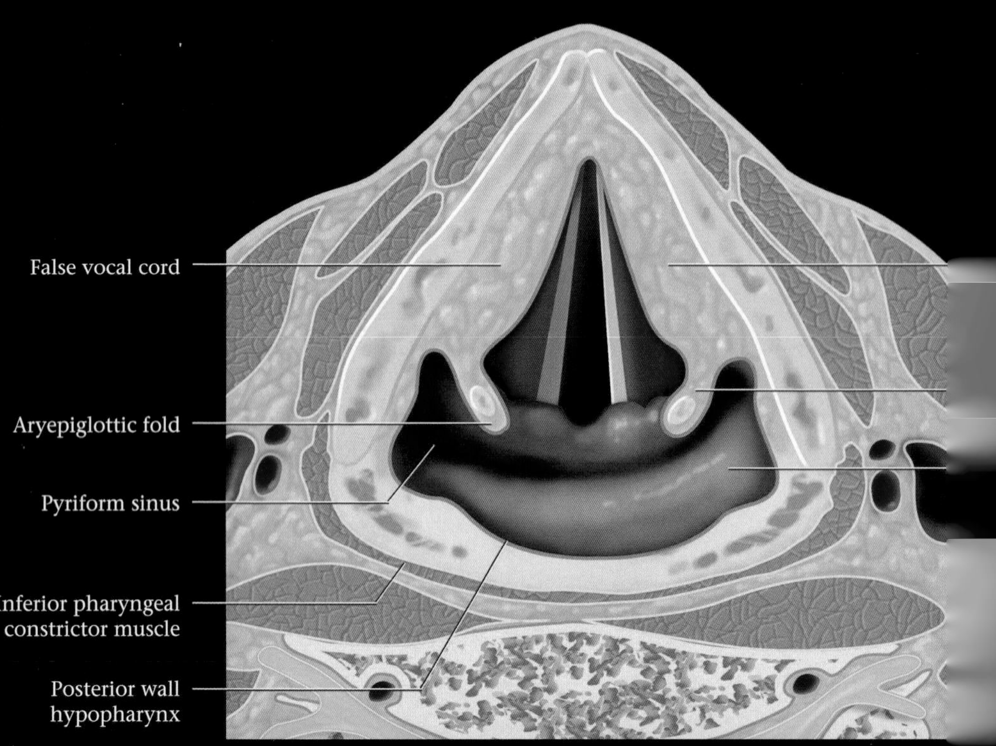
False vocal cord
Aryepiglottic fold
Pyriform sinus
Inferior pharyngeal constrictor muscle
Posterior wall hypopharynx

(Top) Axial graphic of the oropharyngeal mucosal space (in blue) viewed from above reveals constrictor, the tonsillar pillars along with the palatine and lingual tonsils are all occupants layer of deep cervical fascia provides a deep margin to the space. The retropharyngeal space parapharyngeal space is lateral to the pharyngeal mucosal space. **(Bottom)** Axial graphic of aspect of the pharyngeal mucosal space. At the level of the supraglottis the hypopharynx is sinus & posterior wall. Notice that the posterior wall of the aryepiglottic fold is in the hypop anterior wall is in the supraglottic larynx. For this reason this area is commonly referred to a

GRAPHICS

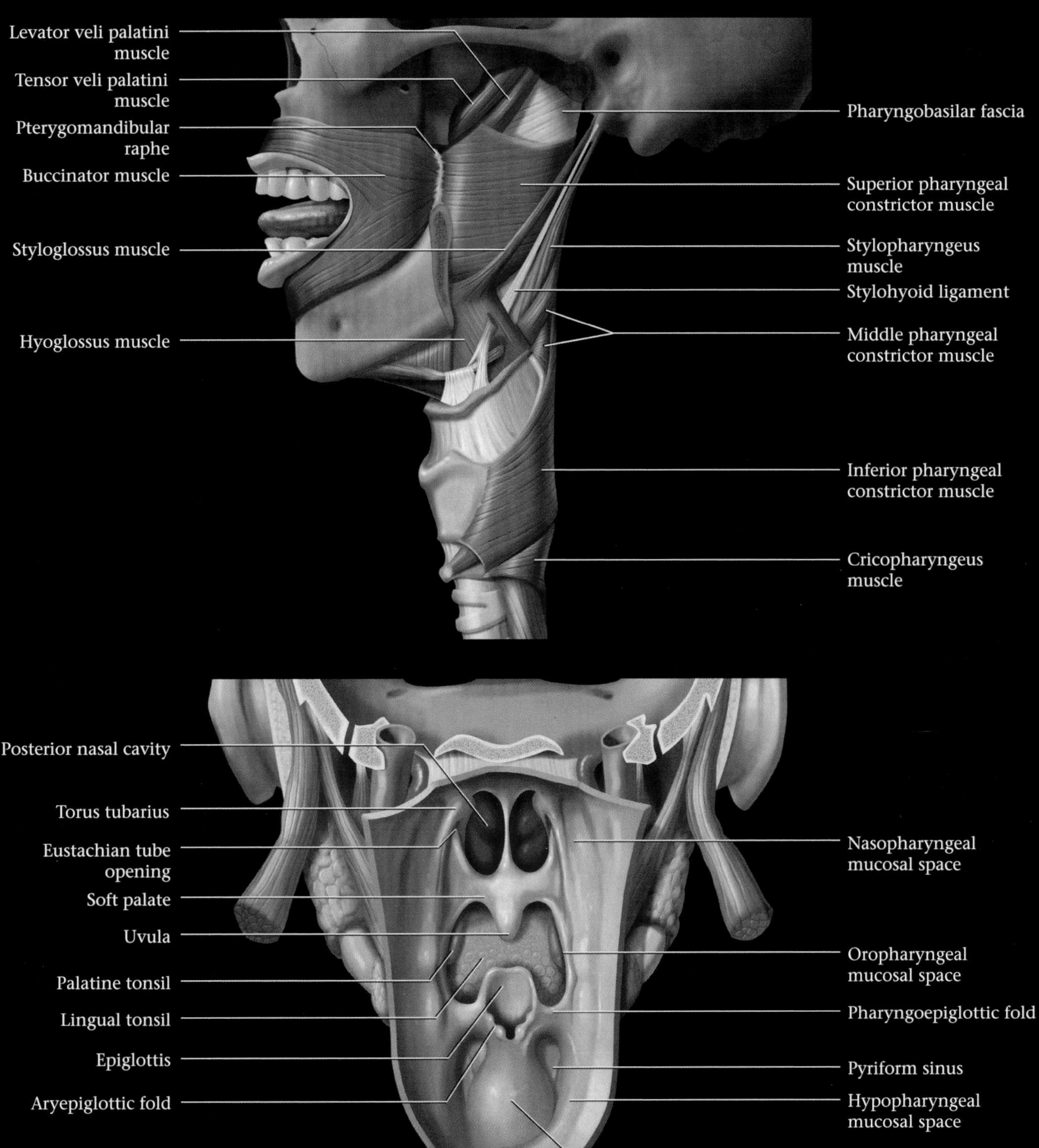
Levator veli palatini muscle
Tensor veli palatini muscle
Pterygomandibular raphe
Buccinator muscle
Styloglossus muscle
Hyoglossus muscle
Pharyngobasilar fascia
Superior pharyngeal constrictor muscle
Stylopharyngeus muscle
Stylohyoid ligament
Middle pharyngeal constrictor muscle
Inferior pharyngeal constrictor muscle
Cricopharyngeus muscle
Posterior nasal cavity
Torus tubarius
Eustachian tube opening
Soft palate
Uvula
Palatine tonsil
Lingual tonsil
Epiglottis
Aryepiglottic fold
Thyroid gland
Cervical esophagus
Nasopharyngeal mucosal space
Oropharyngeal mucosal space
Pharyngoepiglottic fold
Pyriform sinus
Hypopharyngeal mucosal space
Postcricoid hypopharynx

(Top) Lateral graphic showing the major muscles of the pharyngeal mucosal space. Notice the superior, middle and inferior pharyngeal constrictor muscles are in the posterior wall of the pharyngeal mucosal space from the nasopharynx through the oropharynx to the hypopharynx. The pharyngobasilar fascia attaches the superior pharyngeal constrictor to the skull base. The distal end of the levator veli palatini muscle is on the airway side of the middle layer of deep cervical fascia, making it a part of the pharyngeal mucosal space. **(Bottom)** Graphic of the pharyngeal mucosal space/surface seen from behind shows this space can be divided into nasopharyngeal, oropharyngeal and hypopharyngeal areas. The lymphatic ring of the pharyngeal mucosal space contains the nasopharyngeal adenoids and the oropharyngeal palatine and lingual tonsils.

GENERIC PMS MASS

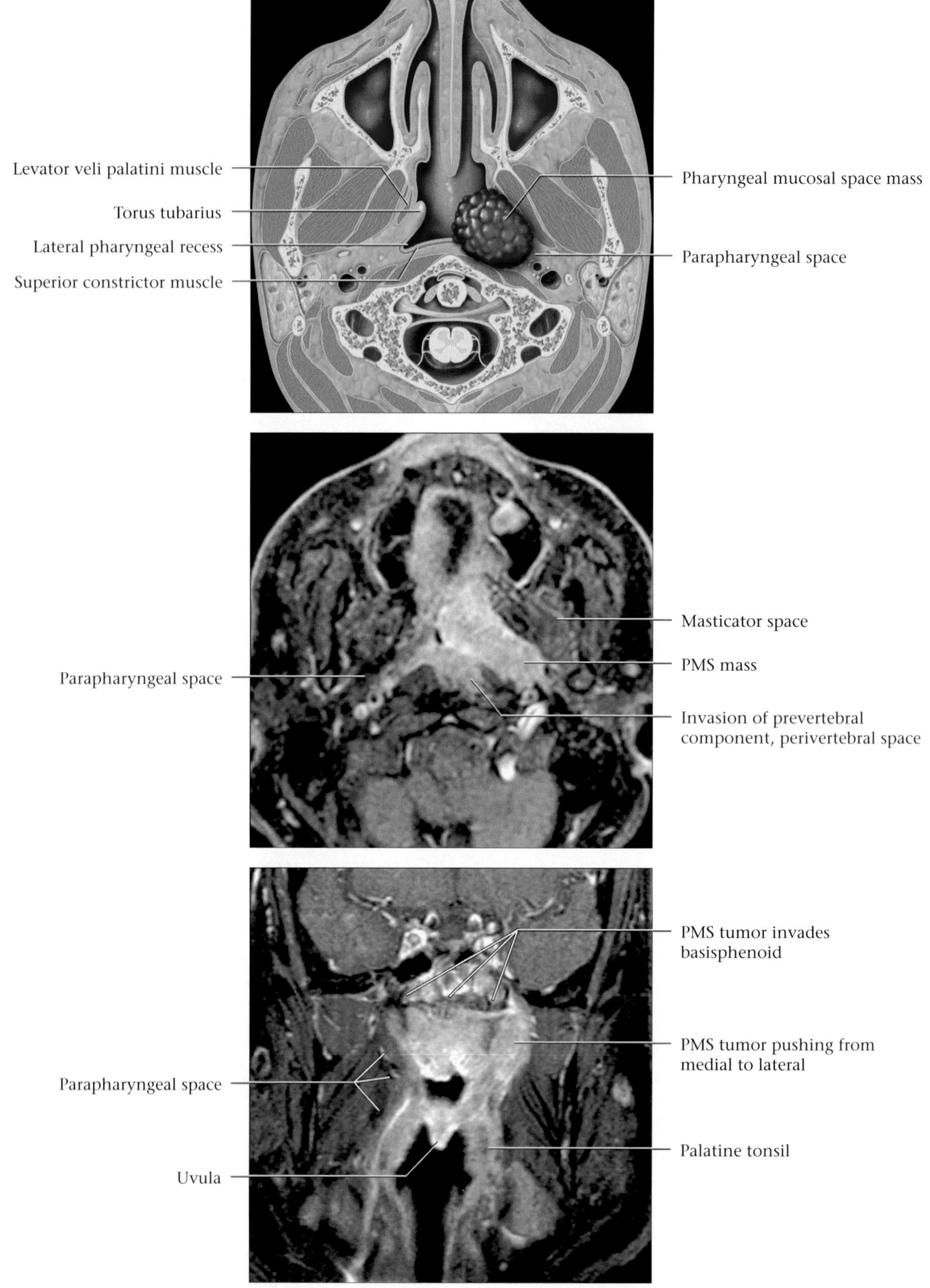

Levator veli palatini muscle
Torus tubarius
Lateral pharyngeal recess
Superior constrictor muscle
Pharyngeal mucosal space mass
Parapharyngeal space
Masticator space
PMS mass
Parapharyngeal space
Invasion of prevertebral component, perivertebral space
PMS tumor invades basisphenoid
PMS tumor pushing from medial to lateral
Parapharyngeal space
Palatine tonsil
Uvula

(Top) Axial graphic of a generic pharyngeal mucosal space mass demonstrates the disruption of the normal architecture of the surface of the pharynx with bulging of the mass into the pharyngeal airway. Also notice the deep margin of the mass is displacing the parapharyngeal space fat from medial to lateral. **(Middle)** In this illustrative case of squamous cell carcinoma of the nasopharyngeal aspect of the pharyngeal mucosal space the tumor can be seen disrupting the mucosal surface of the nasopharynx while pushing into the parapharyngeal space from medial to lateral. The parapharyngeal space is more difficult to see because this is a fat-saturated T1 enhanced MR image. **(Bottom)** In this coronal fat-saturated T1 enhanced MR image of nasopharyngeal carcinoma the area of abutment & invasion of the skull base by this PMS tumor are clearly visible.

BARIUM SWALLOW

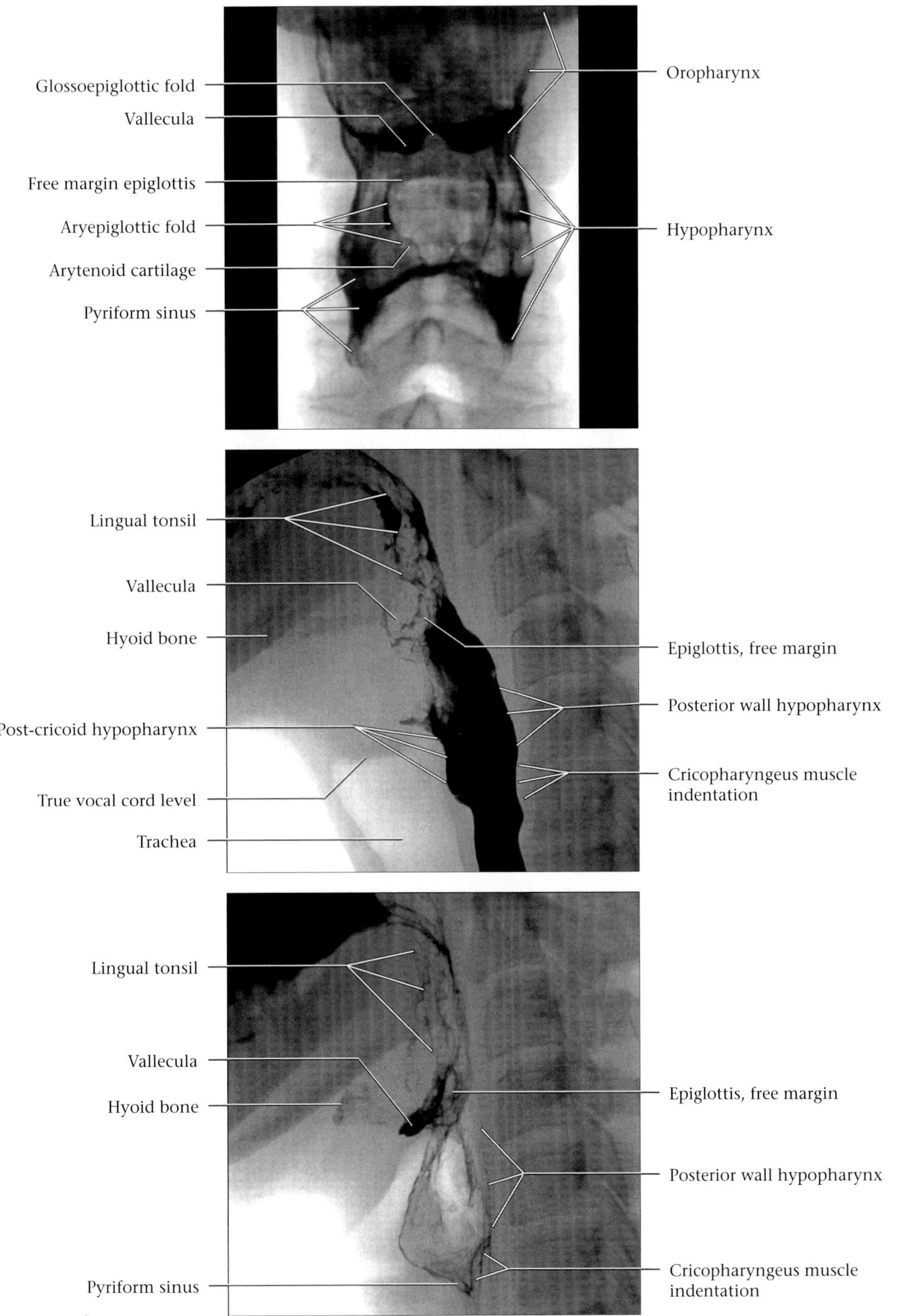
Glossoepiglottic fold
Vallecula
Free margin epiglottis
Aryepiglottic fold
Arytenoid cartilage
Pyriform sinus
Oropharynx
Hypopharynx
Lingual tonsil
Vallecula
Hyoid bone
Post-cricoid hypopharynx
True vocal cord level
Trachea
Epiglottis, free margin
Posterior wall hypopharynx
Cricopharyngeus muscle indentation
Lingual tonsil
Vallecula
Hyoid bone
Pyriform sinus
Epiglottis, free margin
Posterior wall hypopharynx
Cricopharyngeus muscle indentation

(Top) Anteroposterior barium swallow image focused on the low oropharyngeal and hypopharyngeal mucosal space surfaces. Notice the hypopharynx extends from the level of the vallecula and glossoepiglottic fold superiorly to the inferior margin of the pyriform sinus. **(Middle)** In this lateral view of a barium swallow the irregular surface of the lingual tonsil is recognized along the posterior margin of the tongue. The post-cricoid area and the posterior wall of the hypopharynx make up two of the three major subsites within the hypopharynx. The third subsite is the pyriform sinus. **(Bottom)** In this lateral barium swallow image the indentation of the cricopharyngeus muscle is particularly well seen. Remember the inferior margin of the vallecula marks the transition from oropharynx to hypopharynx.

PHARYNGEAL MUCOSAL SPACE

AXIAL T1 MR

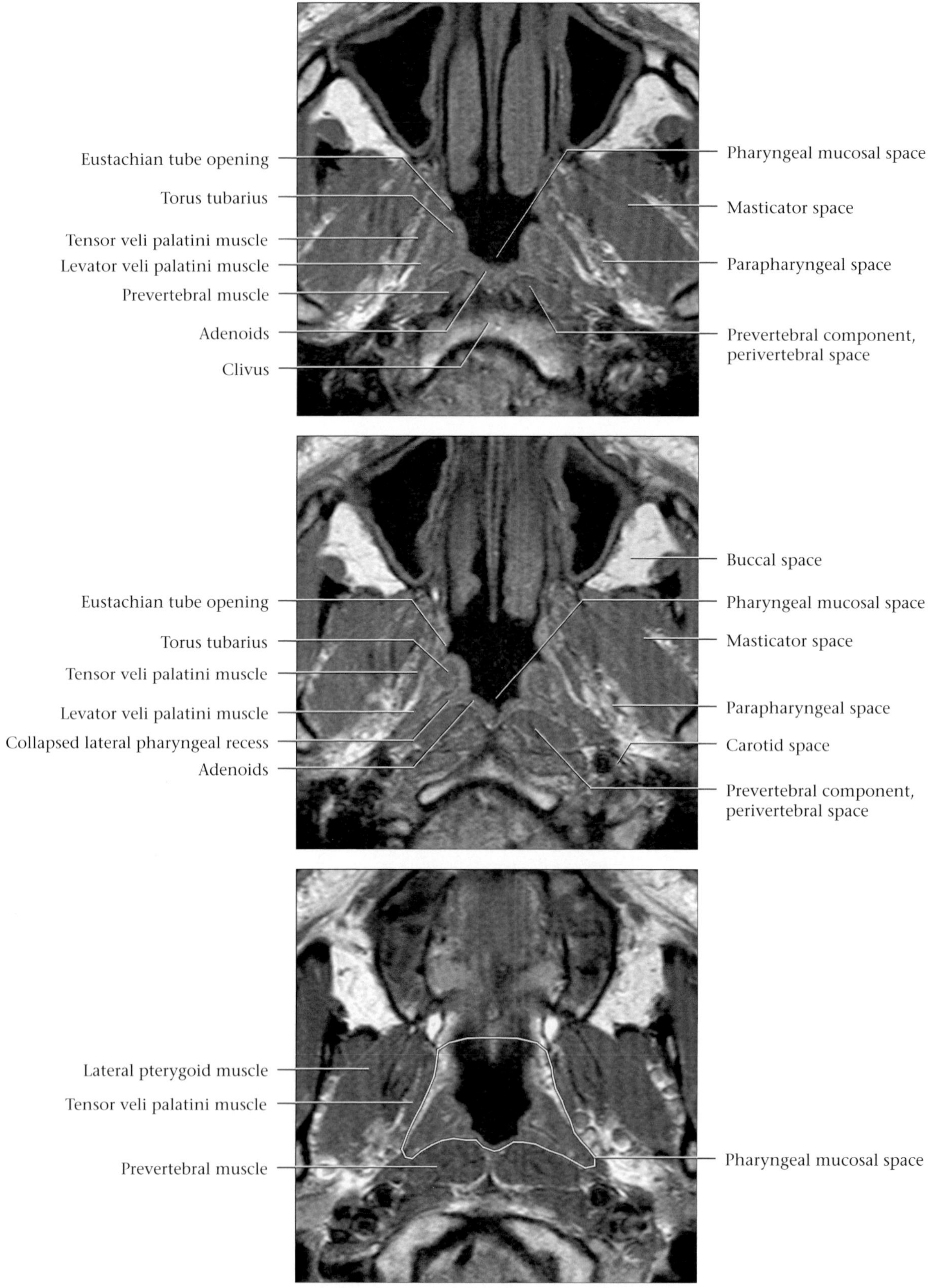
Eustachian tube opening
Torus tubarius
Tensor veli palatini muscle
Levator veli palatini muscle
Prevertebral muscle
Adenoids
Clivus
Pharyngeal mucosal space
Masticator space
Parapharyngeal space
Prevertebral component, perivertebral space
Eustachian tube opening
Torus tubarius
Tensor veli palatini muscle
Levator veli palatini muscle
Collapsed lateral pharyngeal recess
Adenoids
Buccal space
Pharyngeal mucosal space
Masticator space
Parapharyngeal space
Carotid space
Prevertebral component, perivertebral space
Lateral pterygoid muscle
Tensor veli palatini muscle
Prevertebral muscle
Pharyngeal mucosal space

(Top) First of six axial T1 unenhanced MR images presented from superior to inferior shows the pharyngeal mucosal space at the level of the nasopharynx. Notice the torus tubarius (distal cartilaginous eustachian tube) & the nasopharyngeal adenoids. The lateral pharyngeal recess is collapsed & therefore not visible on imaging. **(Middle)** In this image the levator veli palatini muscle is seen transitioning to the pharyngeal side of the middle layer of deep cervical fascia (not seen). It does so over the superior margin of the pharyngobasilar fascia in the sinus of Morgagni. The tensor veli palatini muscle does not enter the pharyngeal mucosal space. **(Bottom)** In this image through the inferior maxillary sinuses the area of the pharyngeal mucosal space is outlined. Remember the middle layer of deep cervical fascia forms the lateral & posterior deep margins of the PMS.

AXIAL T1 MR

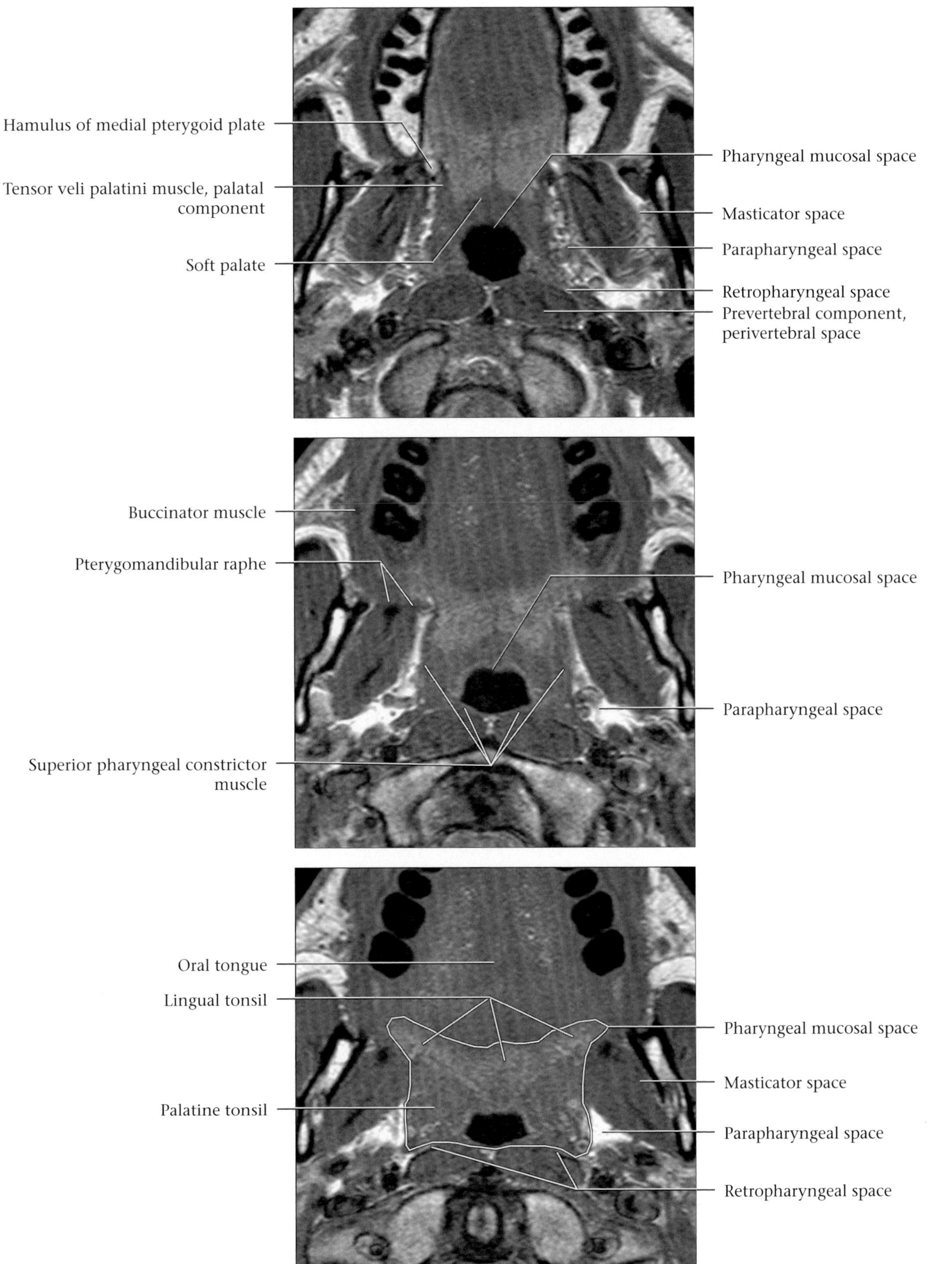
Hamulus of medial pterygoid plate
Tensor veli palatini muscle, palatal component
Soft palate
Pharyngeal mucosal space
Masticator space
Parapharyngeal space
Retropharyngeal space
Prevertebral component, perivertebral space
Buccinator muscle
Pterygomandibular raphe
Superior pharyngeal constrictor muscle
Pharyngeal mucosal space
Parapharyngeal space
Oral tongue
Lingual tonsil
Palatine tonsil
Pharyngeal mucosal space
Masticator space
Parapharyngeal space
Retropharyngeal space

(Top) At the level of the maxillary alveolar ridge the tensor veli palatini muscle is seen turning around the hamulus of the medial pterygoid plate to enter the anterolateral soft palate. Notice that posterior to the pharyngeal mucosal space the thin fat stripe of the retropharyngeal space is just visible in front of the prevertebral component of the perivertebral space. **(Middle)** At the level of the maxillary teeth the pharyngeal mucosal space of the superior oropharynx is seen. Note the superior margin of the palatine tonsil along with the soft palate itself. The superior pharyngeal constrictor muscle is present along the margins of the PMS just inside the middle layer of deep cervical fascia which cannot be seen with imaging. **(Bottom)** In the mid-oropharynx the lingual and palatine tonsils of the PMS lymphatic ring fill the pharyngeal mucosal space.

AXIAL T2 MR

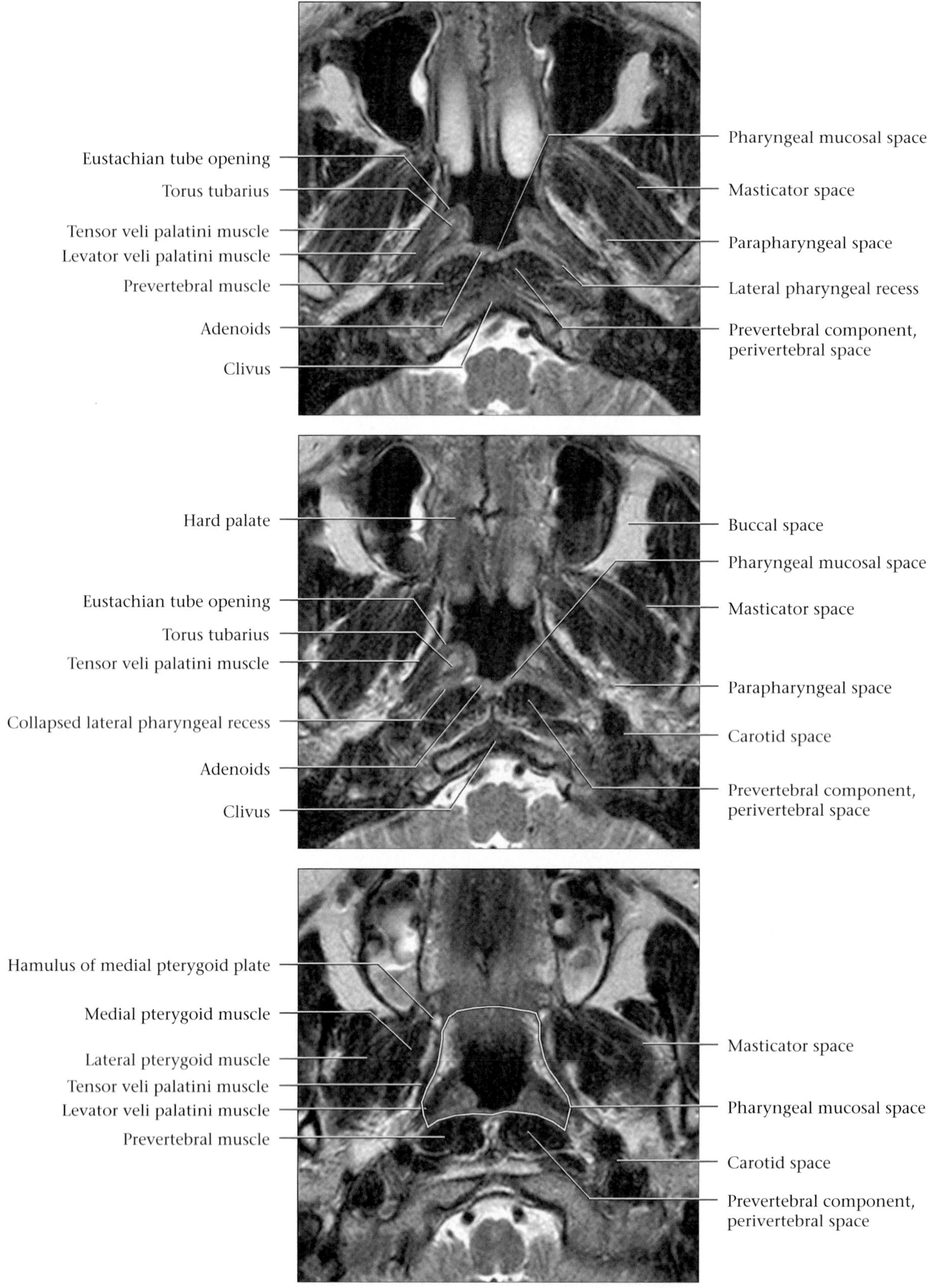

Eustachian tube opening
Torus tubarius
Tensor veli palatini muscle
Levator veli palatini muscle
Prevertebral muscle
Adenoids
Clivus
Pharyngeal mucosal space
Masticator space
Parapharyngeal space
Lateral pharyngeal recess
Prevertebral component, perivertebral space
Hard palate
Eustachian tube opening
Torus tubarius
Tensor veli palatini muscle
Collapsed lateral pharyngeal recess
Adenoids
Clivus
Buccal space
Pharyngeal mucosal space
Masticator space
Parapharyngeal space
Carotid space
Prevertebral component, perivertebral space
Hamulus of medial pterygoid plate
Medial pterygoid muscle
Lateral pterygoid muscle
Tensor veli palatini muscle
Levator veli palatini muscle
Prevertebral muscle
Masticator space
Pharyngeal mucosal space
Carotid space
Prevertebral component, perivertebral space

(Top) First of nine axial T2 unenhanced MR images presented from superior to inferior shows the pharyngeal mucosal space at the level of the nasopharynx. Notice the torus tubarius (distal cartilaginous eustachian tube) & the nasopharyngeal adenoids. The lateral pharyngeal recess is collapsed & therefore not visible on imaging. **(Middle)** In this image the levator veli palatini muscle is seen transitioning to the pharyngeal side of the middle layer of deep cervical fascia (not seen). It does so over the superior margin of the pharyngobasilar fascia in the sinus of Morgagni. The tensor veli palatini muscle does not enter the pharyngeal mucosal space. **(Bottom)** In this image through the inferior maxillary sinuses the area of the pharyngeal mucosal space is outlined.

AXIAL T2 MR

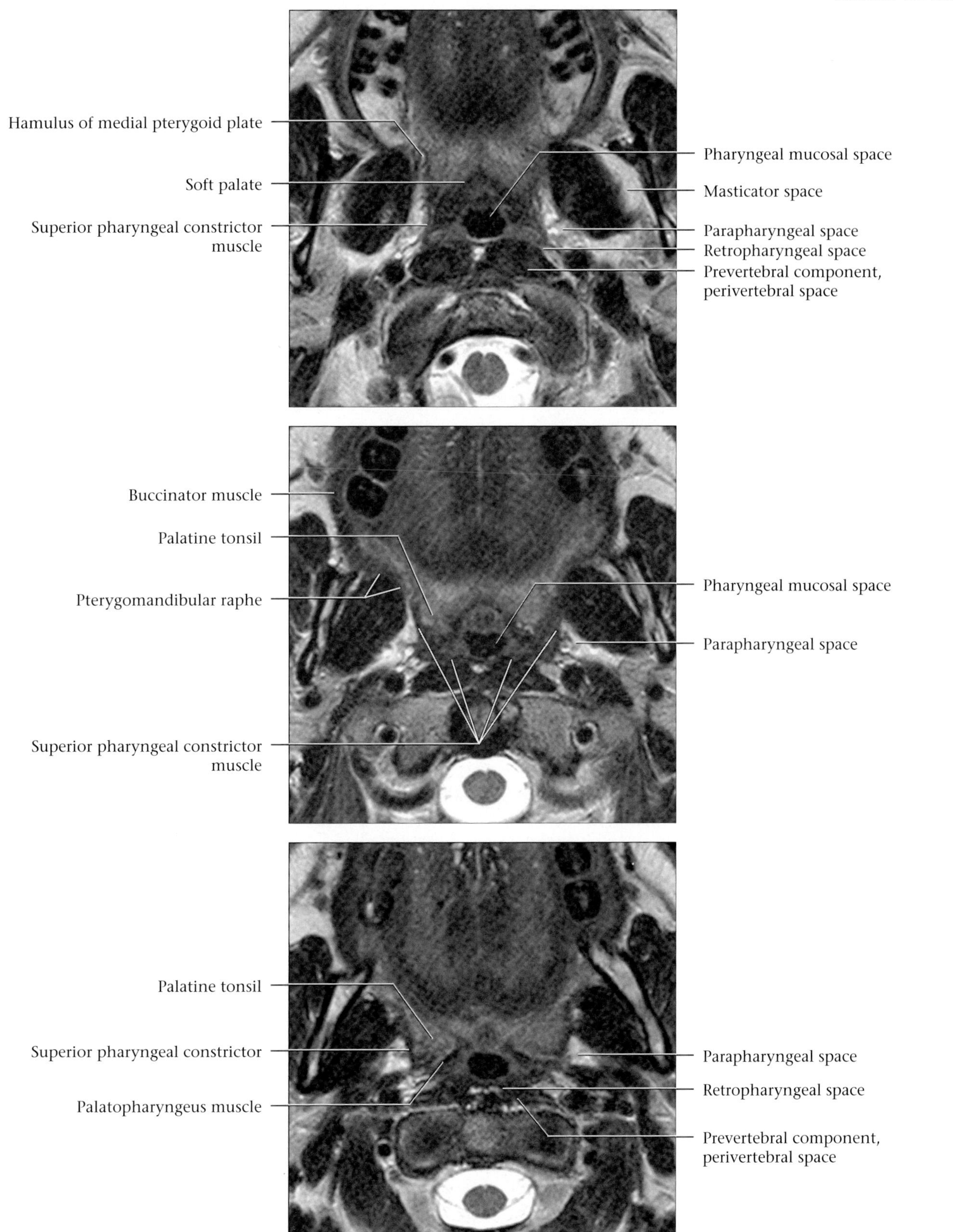
Hamulus of medial pterygoid plate
Soft palate
Superior pharyngeal constrictor muscle
Pharyngeal mucosal space
Masticator space
Parapharyngeal space
Retropharyngeal space
Prevertebral component, perivertebral space
Buccinator muscle
Palatine tonsil
Pterygomandibular raphe
Pharyngeal mucosal space
Parapharyngeal space
Superior pharyngeal constrictor muscle
Palatine tonsil
Superior pharyngeal constrictor
Palatopharyngeus muscle
Parapharyngeal space
Retropharyngeal space
Prevertebral component, perivertebral space

(Top) At the level of the soft palate the pharyngeal mucosal space is seen with the parapharyngeal space along its lateral borders. The retropharyngeal space is very thin at this level but it is present between the posterior pharyngeal mucosal space and the prevertebral component of the perivertebral space. **(Middle)** At the level of the maxillary teeth the pharyngeal mucosal space of the superior oropharynx is visible. Note the superior margin of the palatine tonsil. The superior pharyngeal constrictor muscle is present along the margins of the PMS just inside the middle layer of deep cervical fascia which cannot be seen with imaging. **(Bottom)** In this image through the mid-oropharynx the palatine tonsil is the main occupant of the pharyngeal mucosal space. The retropharyngeal space fat stripe is seen posteriorly while the parapharyngeal spaces are lateral.

AXIAL T2 MR

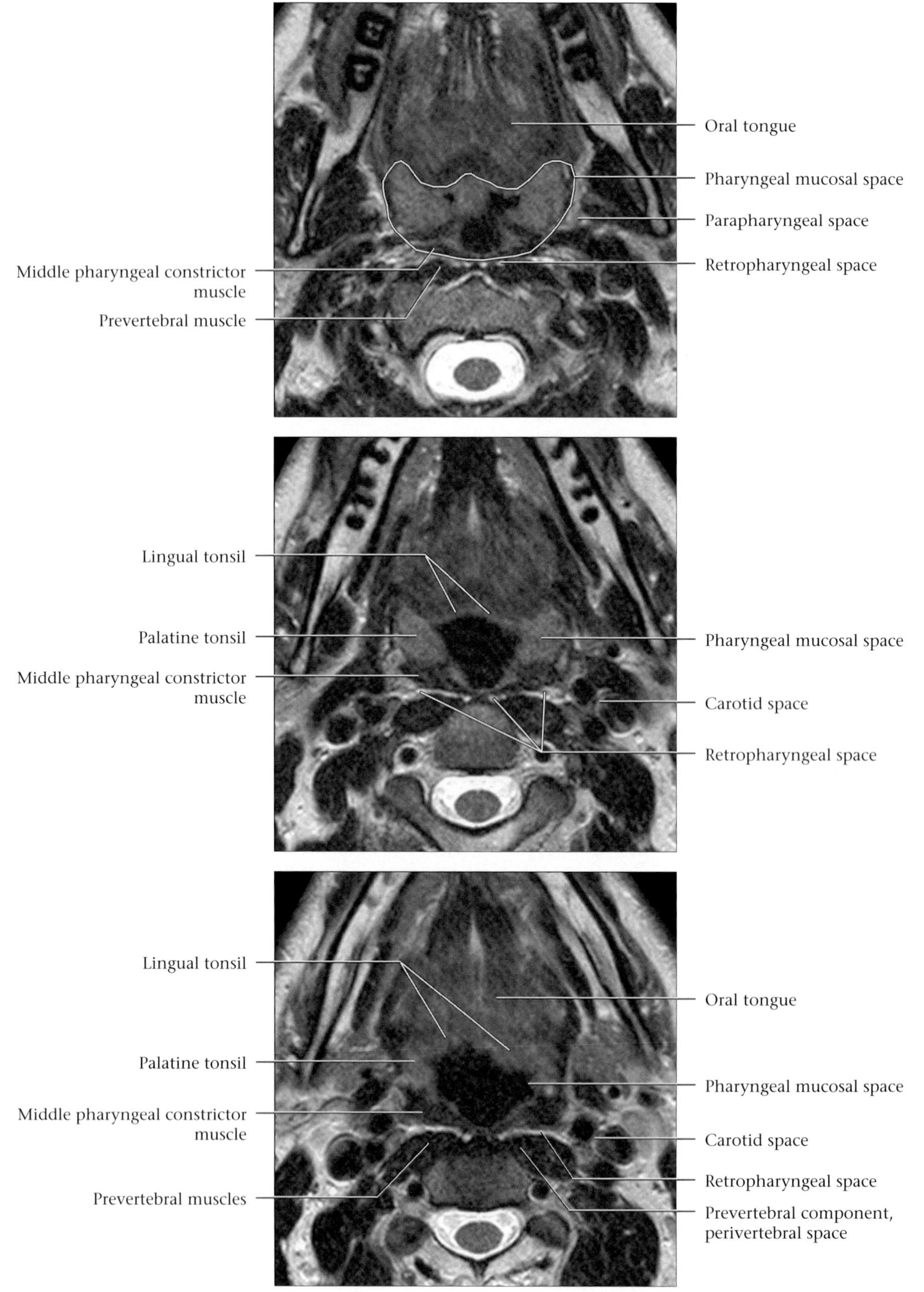

Oral tongue
Pharyngeal mucosal space
Parapharyngeal space
Retropharyngeal space
Middle pharyngeal constrictor muscle
Prevertebral muscle
Lingual tonsil
Palatine tonsil
Middle pharyngeal constrictor muscle
Pharyngeal mucosal space
Carotid space
Retropharyngeal space
Lingual tonsil
Oral tongue
Palatine tonsil
Pharyngeal mucosal space
Middle pharyngeal constrictor muscle
Carotid space
Retropharyngeal space
Prevertebral muscles
Prevertebral component, perivertebral space

(Top) At the level of the mandibular teeth the pharyngeal mucosal space contains the lingual and palatine tonsils. Anterior to the lingual tonsil is the oral tongue of the oral cavity. **(Middle)** In this image the retropharyngeal space fat stripe is clearly seen posterior to the pharyngeal mucosal space. Behind the retropharyngeal space is the prevertebral component of the perivertebral space. A posterior pharyngeal wall squamous cell carcinoma may directly invade the retropharyngeal space or spread via lymphatics to the retropharyngeal nodes. **(Bottom)** Low in the oropharynx thicker lingual tonsillar tissue can be seen along with an attenuated palatine tonsil. Remember the lingual tonsil is located in the oropharynx, not the oral cavity.

GRAPHIC & CORONAL T1 C+ MR

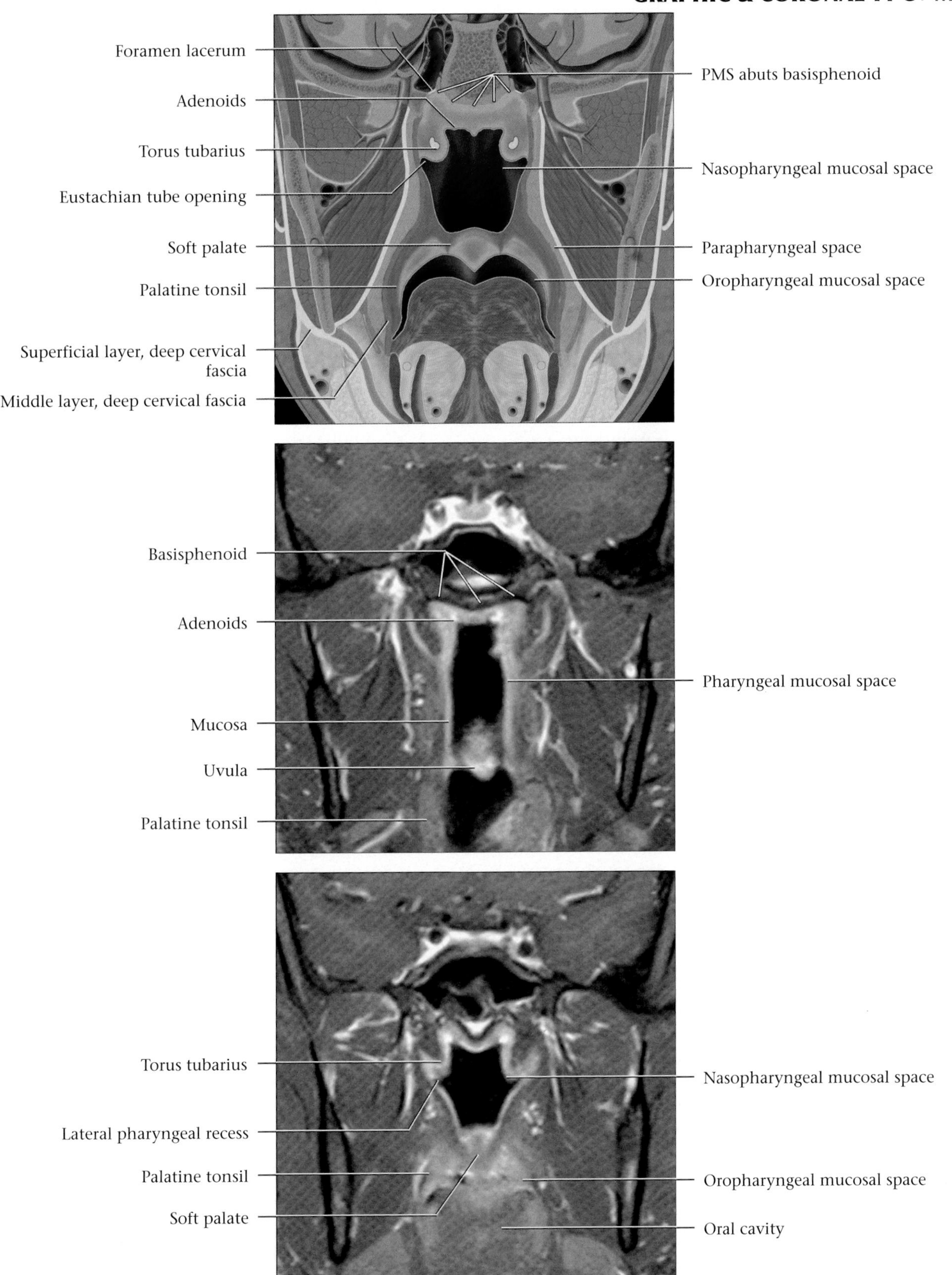
Foramen lacerum
Adenoids
Torus tubarius
Eustachian tube opening
Soft palate
Palatine tonsil
Superficial layer, deep cervical fascia
Middle layer, deep cervical fascia
PMS abuts basisphenoid
Nasopharyngeal mucosal space
Parapharyngeal space
Oropharyngeal mucosal space
Basisphenoid
Adenoids
Mucosa
Uvula
Palatine tonsil
Pharyngeal mucosal space
Torus tubarius
Lateral pharyngeal recess
Palatine tonsil
Soft palate
Nasopharyngeal mucosal space
Oropharyngeal mucosal space
Oral cavity

(Top) Coronal graphic of nasopharyngeal and oropharyngeal mucosal space. Notice the middle layer of deep cervical fascia defining the lateral margin of the pharyngeal mucosal space. The parapharyngeal spaces are paired fatty spaces lateral to the pharyngeal mucosal space. **(Middle)** Coronal enhanced fat-saturated T1 MR image shows the pharyngeal mucosal space surface enhances. Notice that the roof of the nasopharyngeal mucosal space abuts the basisphenoid. Remember that a nasopharyngeal carcinoma that begins in the roof of the nasopharynx will often have invaded the sphenoid sinus at the time of presentation. **(Bottom)** Coronal enhanced fat-saturated T1 MR image reveals the enhancing sheet of mucosa with the torus tubarius (cartilaginous eustachian tube) and lateral pharyngeal recess.

MASTICATOR SPACE

Terminology

Abbreviations

- Masticator space (MS)

Definitions

- Large, paired anterolateral spaces of suprahyoid neck (SHN) containing muscles of mastication, posterior body & ramus of mandible & of CNV3
- Surgical terms
  - Infratemporal fossa: MS area deep to zygomatic arch, superficial to pterygomaxillary fissure
  - Temporal fossa: Suprazygomatic MS

Imaging Anatomy

Overview

- MS is large SHN space spanning area from high parietal calvarium (suprazygomatic MS) above to mandibular angle below
- **Suprazygomatic MS**: Contains only belly of temporalis muscle
- **Infrazygomatic MS**: MS "proper"; containing masseter, medial & lateral pterygoids, CNV3 & ramus/posterior body of mandible

Extent

- Craniocaudal extent of MS is more extensive than commonly recognized
- On its cephalad margin MS reaches high on parietal calvarium at top of suprazygomatic MS

Anatomy Relationships

- Abuts skull base with **foramen ovale** & **foramen spinosum** included

Internal Structures-Critical Contents

- **Muscles of mastication**
  - **Masseter**: Originates from zygomatic arch; inserts lateral surface of ramus/angle of mandible
  - **Temporalis**: Originates from suprazygomatic MS; inserts on medial surface of coronoid process & anterior surface of mandibular ramus
  - **Medial pterygoid**: Originates from medial surface lateral pterygoid plate & palatine bone pyramidal process; inserts medial surface mandibular ramus
  - **Lateral pterygoid**: Originates from greater wing of sphenoid (superior head) & lateral surface of lateral pterygoid plate (inferior head); inserts capsule & articular disk of TMJ (superior head) & neck of mandible (inferior head)
- **Mandibular division, trigeminal nerve (V3)**
  - **Masticator nerve branch** (proximal V3 motor to muscles of mastication)
  - **Mylohyoid nerve branch** (motor to anterior belly of digastric and mylohyoid muscles)
  - **Inferior alveolar nerve branch** (V3 sensory to mandible & chin)
  - **Lingual nerve** (V3 sensory to anterior 2/3 tongue, floor of mouth)
  - **Auriculotemporal nerve** (V3 sensory to EAC/TMJ)
- **Ramus and posterior body of mandible**
  - Coronoid process: Temporalis muscle inserts here
  - Condylar process: Mandibular condyle neck & head
  - Temporomandibular joint is within MS but considered separately
- **Pterygoid venous plexus** along posterior border of lateral pterygoid muscle & parapharyngeal space

Fascia of Masticator Space

- **Superficial layer, deep cervical fascia** (SL-DCF) splits along inferior mandible, creating "sling" enclosing MS
  - **Medial fascial slip** runs along deep surface of pterygoid muscles
    - This slip of SL-DCF inserts on undersurface of skull base just medial to foramen ovale
  - **Lateral slip SL-DCF** covers surface of masseter muscle, attaching to zygomatic arch
    - Slip continues cephalad over surface of temporalis muscle to top of suprazygomatic MS
  - **No horizontal fascia** exists deep to zygomatic arch
    - MS lesions pass freely in cranial-caudal directions under zygomatic arch

Anatomy-Based Imaging Issues

Key Concepts or Questions

- What imaging features define a lesion as primary to the masticator space?
  - Center of MS lesion must be in muscles of mastication-mandibular ramus
  - MS lesions displace parapharyngeal space from anterior to posterior

Imaging Recommendations

- CECT or MR can both easily image MS
- Enhanced multiplanar MR better for **perineural V3 spread** and intracranial disease manifestations
- If lesion affects skull base or mandible, add bone CT to delineate bony involvement and tumor matrix

Imaging Approaches

- When MS tumor is identified, imaging must include entire course of **CNV3** in search of perineural tumor
- Image distal to mental foramen of mandible and proximal to lateral pons, including mandibular foramen, foramen ovale and Meckel cave

Imaging Pitfalls

- MS pseudolesions
  - Pterygoid venous plexus asymmetry may appear as infiltrating, enhancing "lesion"
  - V3 motor atrophy of muscles of mastication makes normal contralateral MS look like "lesion"
  - Asymmetric accessory parotid gland may appear as unilateral "mass" over surface of masseter muscle

Clinical Implications

Clinical Importance

- **Trismus** (jaw spasm from masticator muscle spasm) is primary symptom of MS tumor or infection
- Primary MS tumor is **sarcoma**
- Remember to look for perineural V3 tumor whenever MS mass is identified!

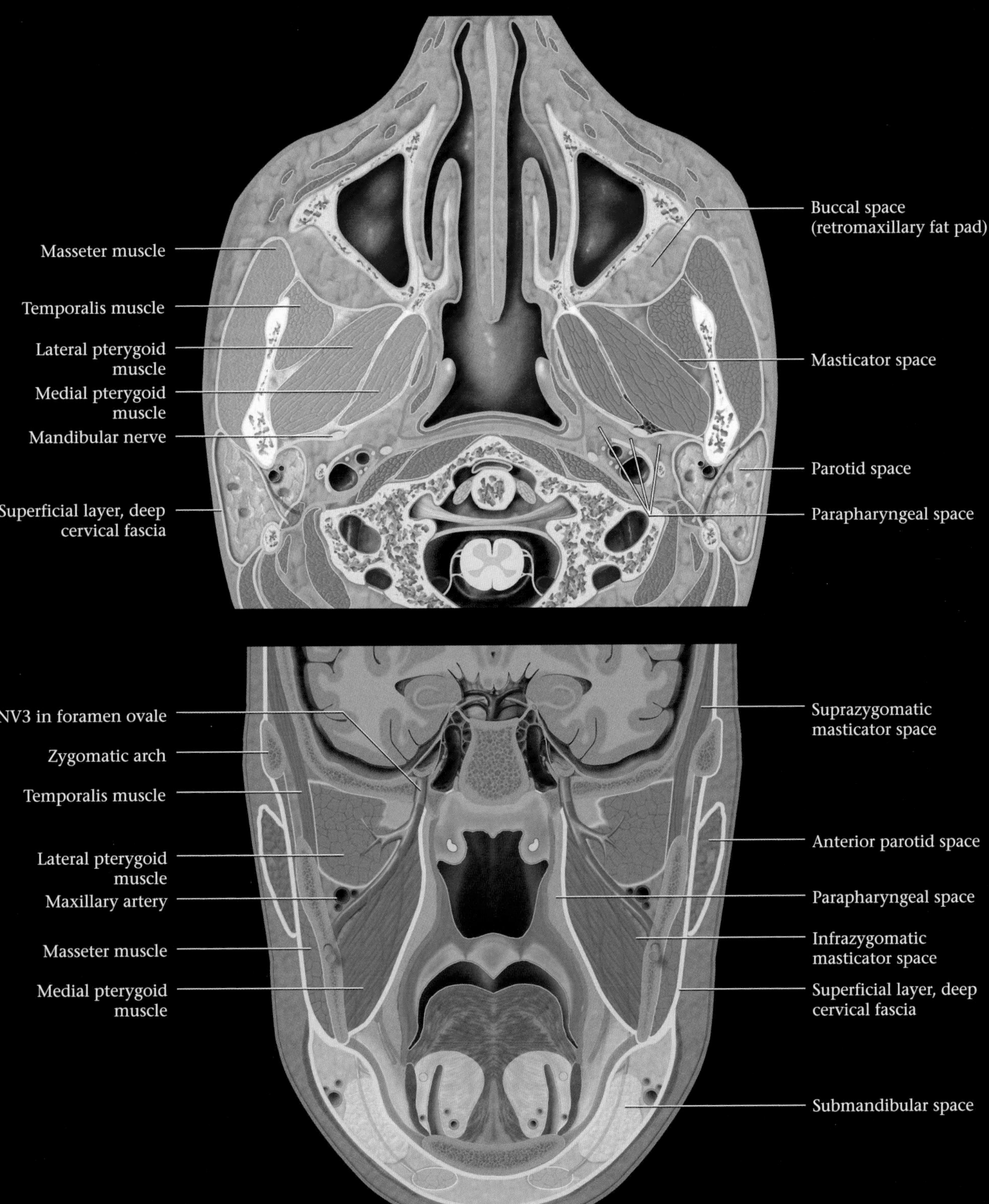
Masseter muscle
Temporalis muscle
Lateral pterygoid muscle
Medial pterygoid muscle
Mandibular nerve
Superficial layer, deep cervical fascia
Buccal space (retromaxillary fat pad)
Masticator space
Parotid space
Parapharyngeal space
CNV3 in foramen ovale
Zygomatic arch
Temporalis muscle
Lateral pterygoid muscle
Maxillary artery
Masseter muscle
Medial pterygoid muscle
Suprazygomatic masticator space
Anterior parotid space
Parapharyngeal space
Infrazygomatic masticator space
Superficial layer, deep cervical fascia
Submandibular space

(Top) Axial graphic shows the masticator space enclosed by superficial layer, deep cervical fascia (yellow line). The muscles of mastication from medial to lateral are the medial & lateral pterygoid, temporalis & masseter muscles. Note the mandibular nerve (CNV3 main trunk) lies just posterior to medial pterygoid muscle inside the superficial layer of deep cervical fascia. The buccal space is anterior while the parapharyngeal and parotid space are posterior to the masticator space. **(Bottom)** Coronal graphic of MS reveals a suprazygomatic & infrazygomatic component. Notice the superficial layer of deep cervical fascia attaches to the skull base just medial to the foramen ovale. There is no "horizontal fascia" beneath the zygomatic arch preventing spread of masticator space disease superiorly into the suprazygomatic masticator space.

MASTICATOR SPACE

GRAPHICS

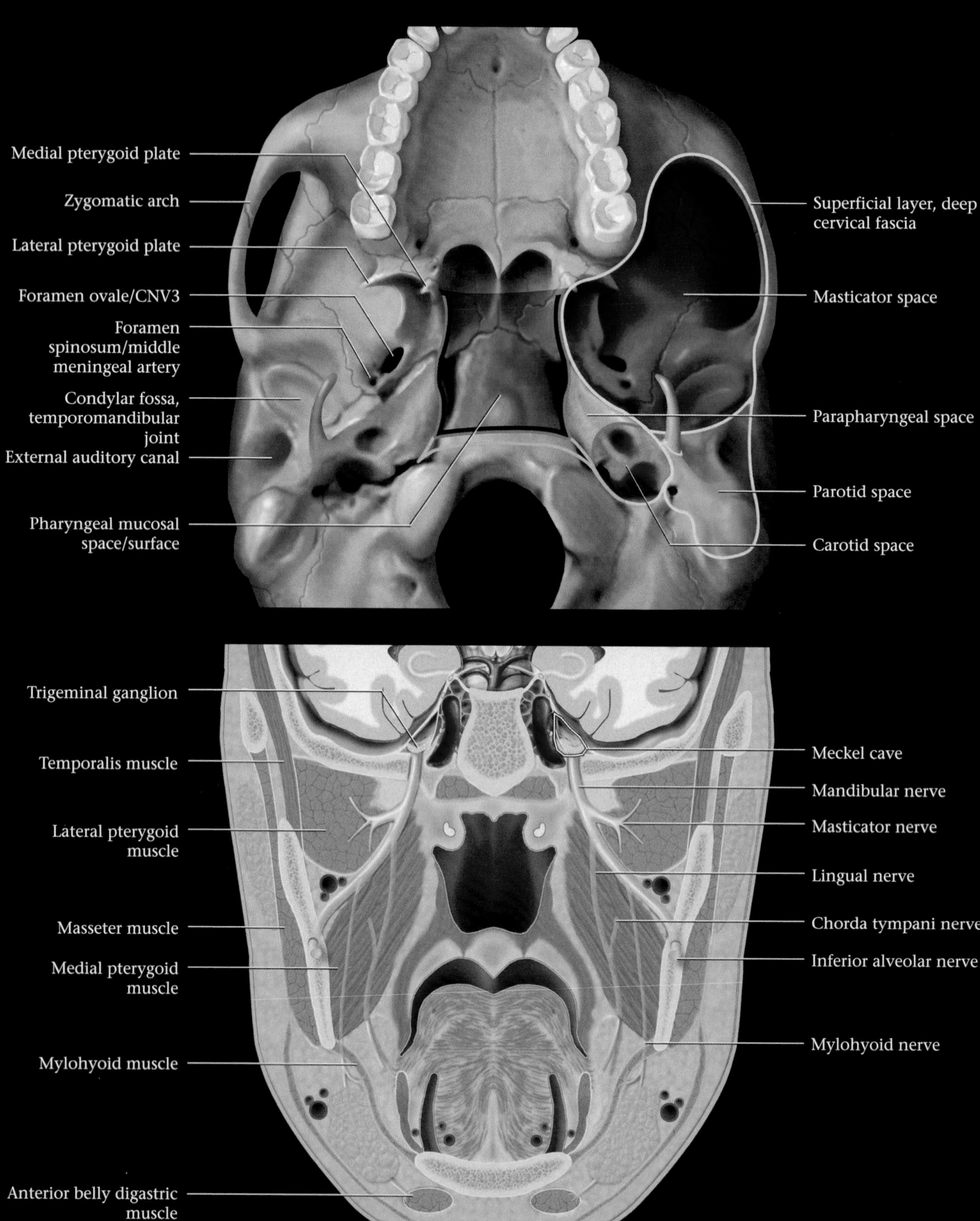
Medial pterygoid plate
Zygomatic arch
Lateral pterygoid plate
Foramen ovale/CNV3
Foramen spinosum/middle meningeal artery
Condylar fossa, temporomandibular joint
External auditory canal
Pharyngeal mucosal space/surface
Superficial layer, deep cervical fascia
Masticator space
Parapharyngeal space
Parotid space
Carotid space
Trigeminal ganglion
Temporalis muscle
Lateral pterygoid muscle
Masseter muscle
Medial pterygoid muscle
Mylohyoid muscle
Anterior belly digastric muscle
Meckel cave
Mandibular nerve
Masticator nerve
Lingual nerve
Chorda tympani nerve
Inferior alveolar nerve
Mylohyoid nerve

(Top) Graphic of skull base viewed from below shows the masticator space abutting the sphenoid and temporal bones. The masticator space (purple) has a broad abutment with the skull base. CNV3 enters the masticator space through foramen ovale while the foramen spinosum conveys the middle meningeal artery into the intracranial compartment. Notice that the temporomandibular joint is within the confines of the masticator space. **(Bottom)** Coronal graphic of the mandibular division of the trigeminal nerve. Note CNV3 exits skull base through foramen ovale without entering the cavernous sinus. The 2 motor branches from CNV3 are the masticator nerve (to muscles of mastication) and the mylohyoid nerve (to mylohyoid and anterior belly of digastric muscle). The main sensory branches are the lingual and inferior alveolar nerves.

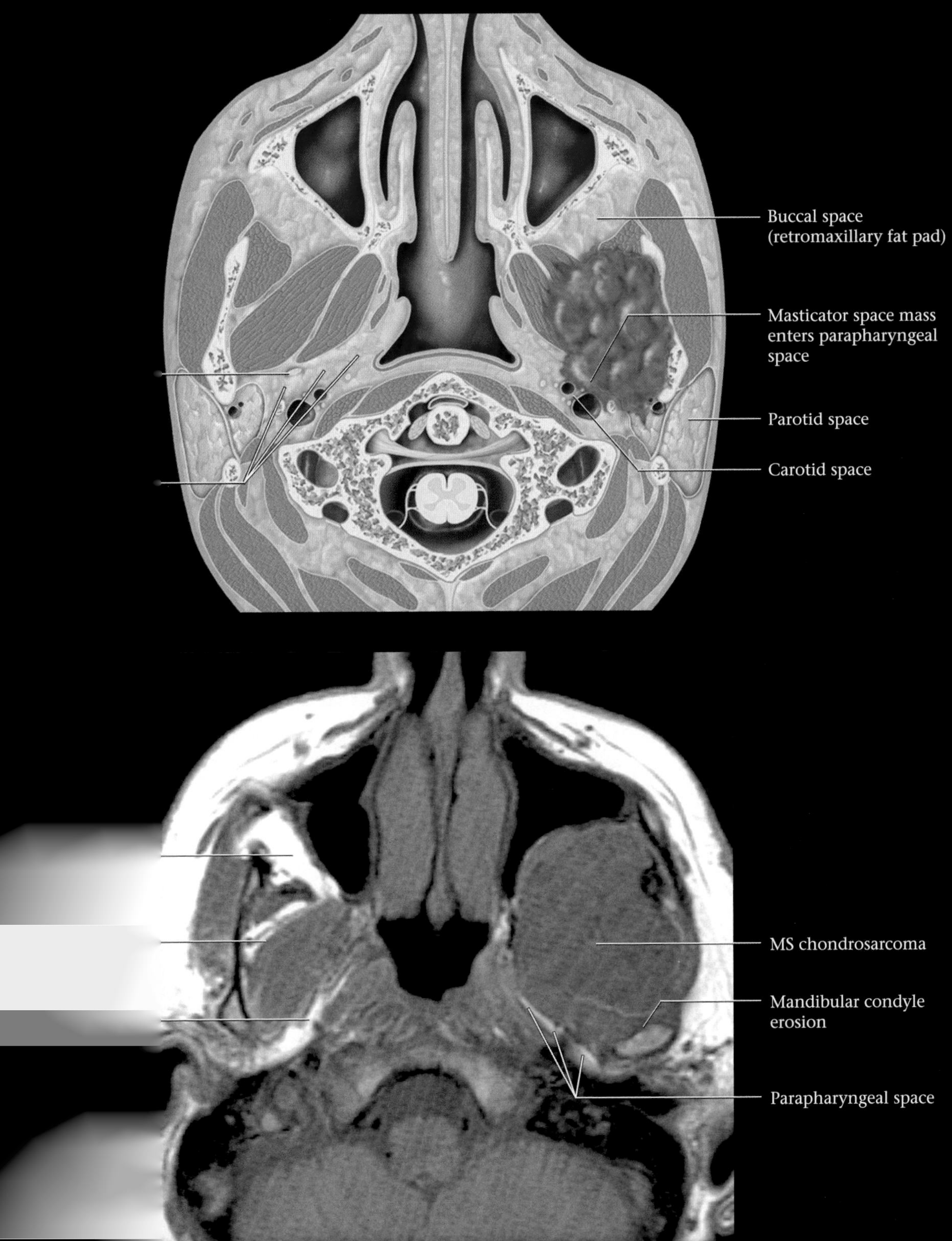
Buccal space
(retromaxillary fat pad)
Masticator space mass
enters parapharyngeal
space
Parotid space
Carotid space
MS chondrosarcoma
Mandibular condyle
erosion
Parapharyngeal space

level of the low nasopharynx demonstrates a generic masticator space mass invading the
n anterior to posterior. Notice the mandibular nerve is engulfed by the tumor. Masticator
nasticator muscles and erode the posterior body, ramus or condylar process of the
T1 unenhanced MR image through the nasopharynx shows a large mass of the masticator
arapharyngeal space from anterior to posterior, invades the muscles of mastication and
ndyle. The differential diagnosis of primary tumors of the masticator space includes
n lymphoma. In this case, the tumor was a chondrosarcoma.

PERINEURAL CNV3 MALIGNANCY

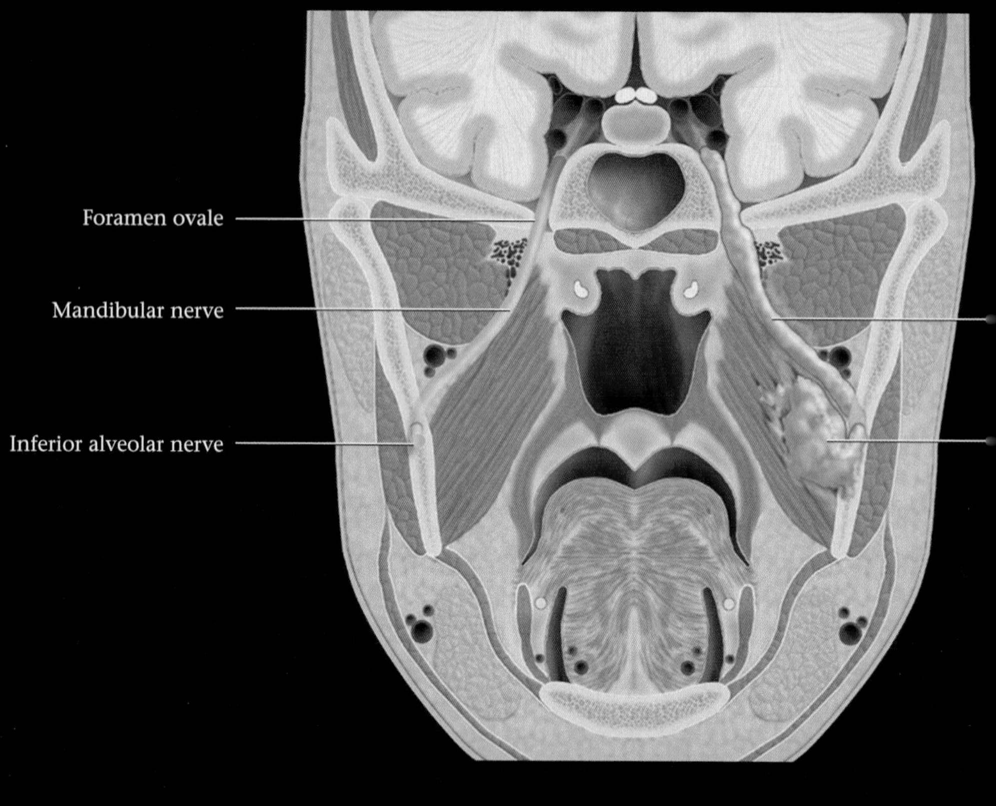

Foramen ovale
Mandibular nerve
Inferior alveolar nerve

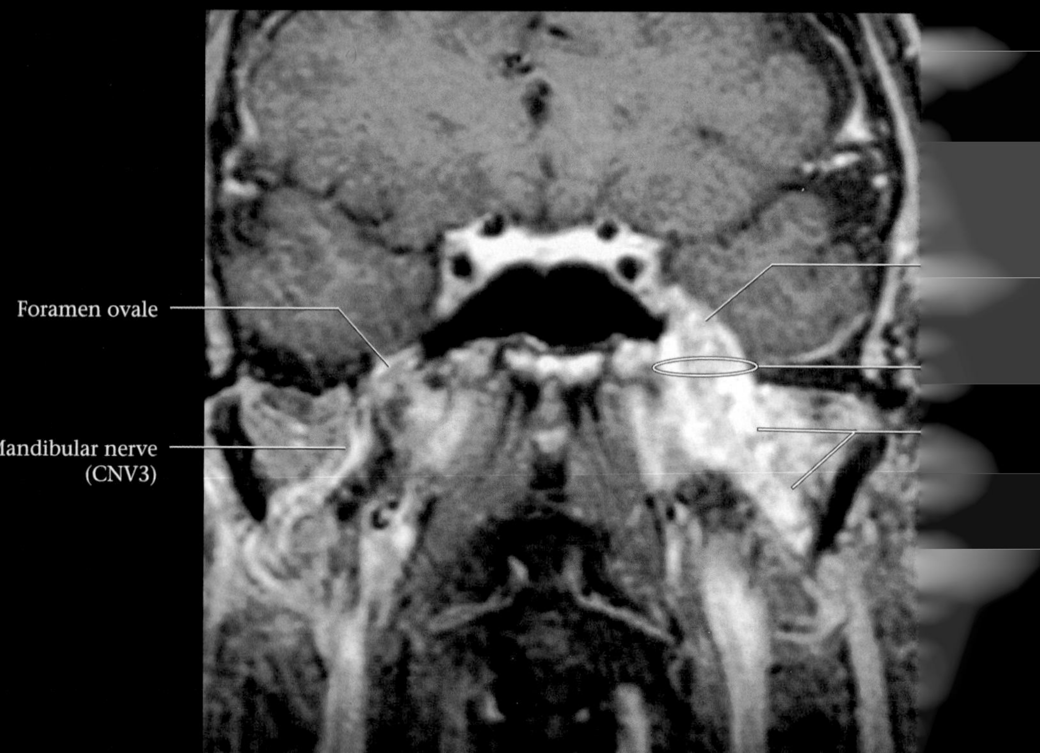

Foramen ovale
Mandibular nerve
(CNV3)

(Top) Coronal graphic of the suprahyoid neck focused on the masticator space and the mar drawing a generic masticator space malignancy if visible invading the lower masticator spac mandible and spreading via a perineural route up the mandibular nerve through the forame intracranial compartment. Both primary masticator space malignancy and squamous cell ca cavity can access the intracranial compartment in this manner. **(Bottom)** Coronal T1 enhar image through the foramen ovale shows enhancing perineural malignant tumor spreading masticator space along the mandibular nerve. Notice the enlarged left foramen ovale and th

AXIAL CECT

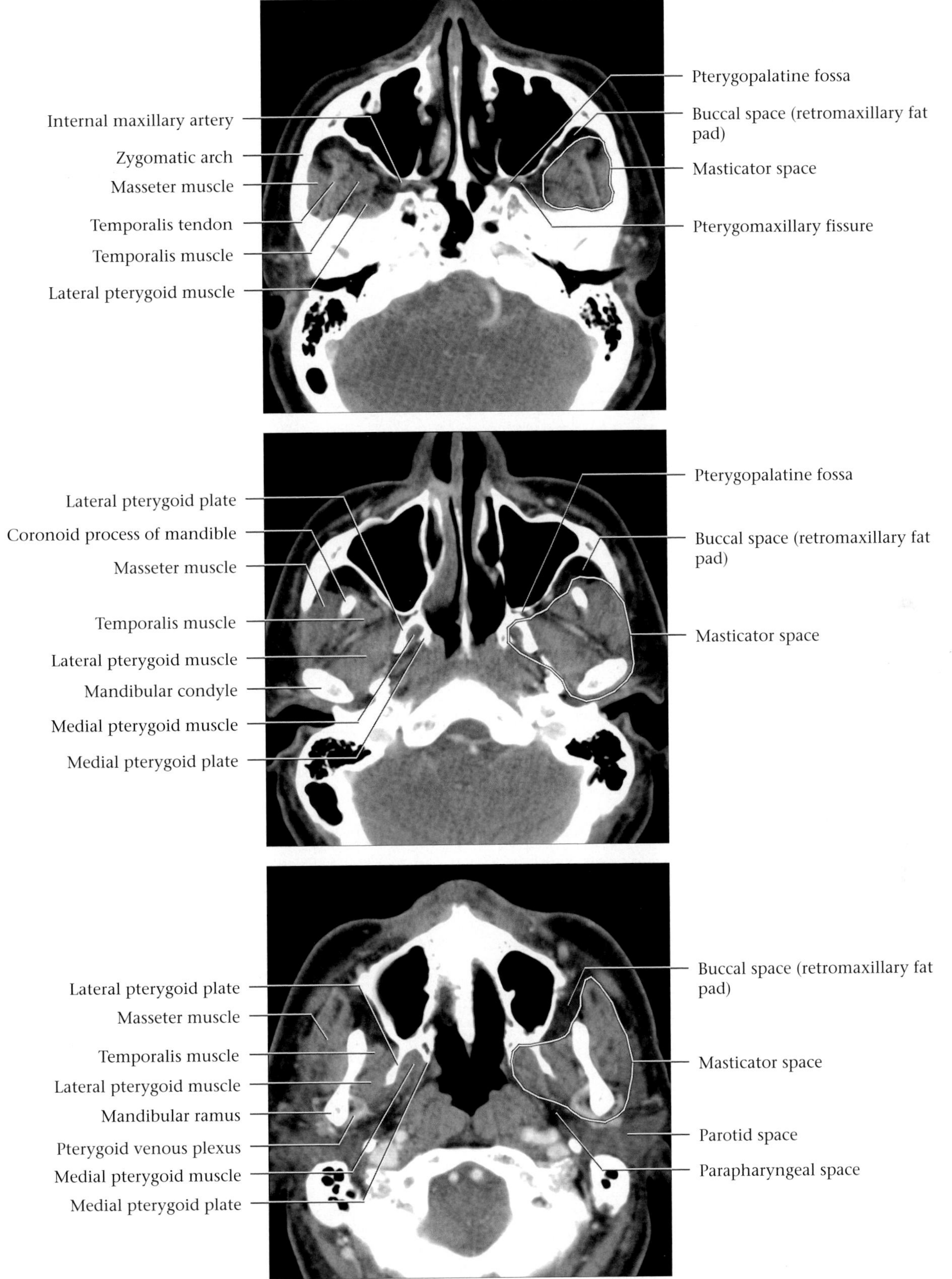
Internal maxillary artery
Zygomatic arch
Masseter muscle
Temporalis tendon
Temporalis muscle
Lateral pterygoid muscle
Pterygopalatine fossa
Buccal space (retromaxillary fat pad)
Masticator space
Pterygomaxillary fissure
Lateral pterygoid plate
Coronoid process of mandible
Masseter muscle
Temporalis muscle
Lateral pterygoid muscle
Mandibular condyle
Medial pterygoid muscle
Medial pterygoid plate
Pterygopalatine fossa
Buccal space (retromaxillary fat pad)
Masticator space
Lateral pterygoid plate
Masseter muscle
Temporalis muscle
Lateral pterygoid muscle
Mandibular ramus
Pterygoid venous plexus
Medial pterygoid muscle
Medial pterygoid plate
Buccal space (retromaxillary fat pad)
Masticator space
Parotid space
Parapharyngeal space

(Top) First of six axial CECT images presented from superior to inferior shows the masticator space medial to the zygomatic arch. Notice the masseter muscle arising from the inferior margin of the zygomatic arch. Also note the superior head of the lateral pterygoid muscle. **(Middle)** At the level of the mandibular condyles the MS contains the muscles of mastication & temporomandibular joint. Note the inferior head of the lateral pterygoid muscle arising from the lateral surface of the lateral pterygoid plate. The medial pterygoid muscle arises from the pterygoid fossa. **(Bottom)** In this image through the low maxillary sinuses the masticator space is seen between the more anterior buccal space and the more posterior parapharyngeal and parotid spaces. Notice the pterygoid venous plexus as the enhancing area along the posterolateral margin of the MS.

MASTICATOR SPACE

AXIAL CECT

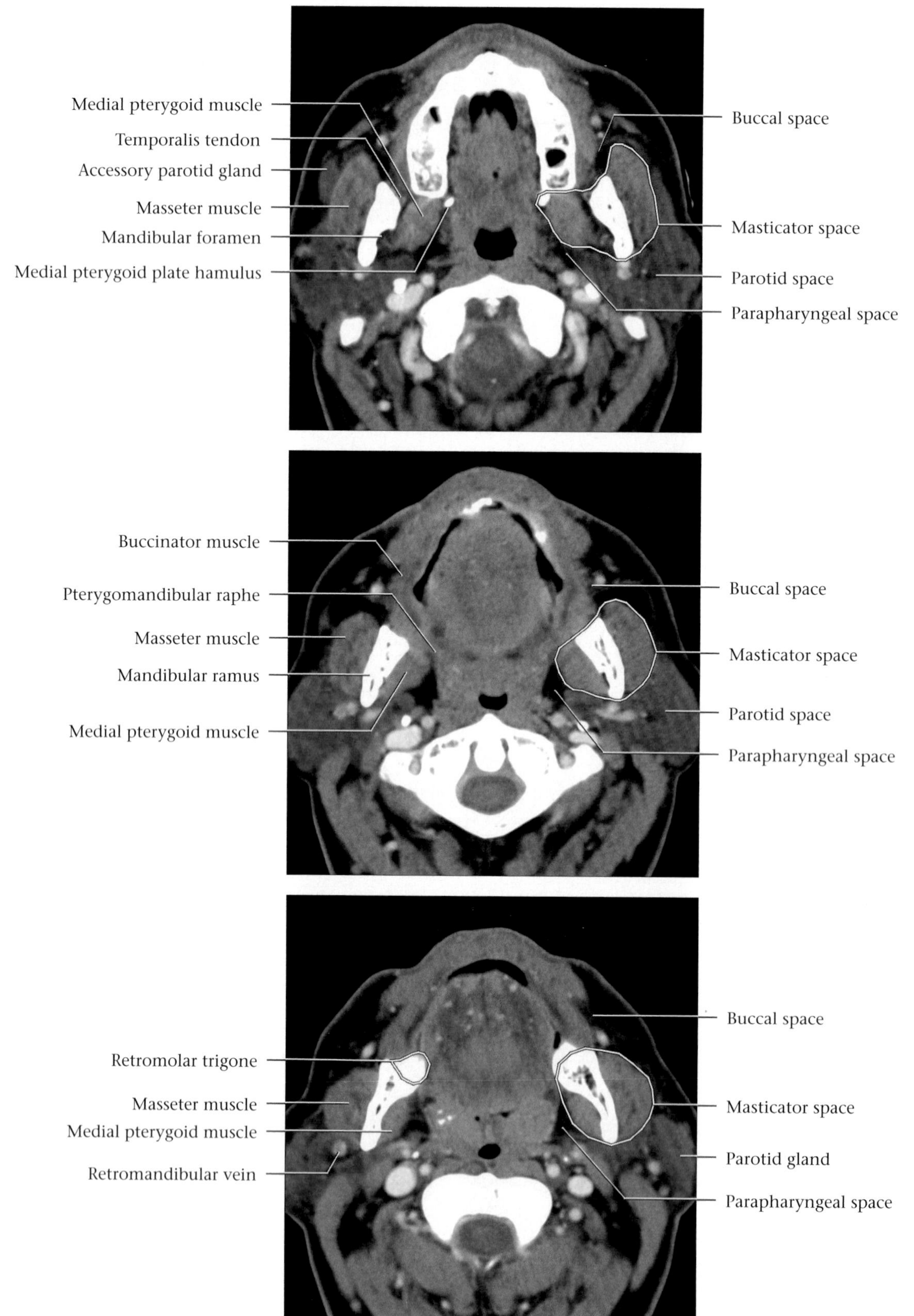
Medial pterygoid muscle
Temporalis tendon
Accessory parotid gland
Masseter muscle
Mandibular foramen
Medial pterygoid plate hamulus
Buccal space
Masticator space
Parotid space
Parapharyngeal space
Buccinator muscle
Pterygomandibular raphe
Masseter muscle
Mandibular ramus
Medial pterygoid muscle
Buccal space
Masticator space
Parotid space
Parapharyngeal space
Retromolar trigone
Masseter muscle
Medial pterygoid muscle
Retromandibular vein
Buccal space
Masticator space
Parotid gland
Parapharyngeal space

(Top) In this image through the maxillary ridge the mandibular foramen is seen. The inferior alveolar nerve enters the mandible in this location. Note the hamulus of the medial pterygoid plate which acts as a pulley for the tendon of the tensor veli palatini muscle & is site of superior attachment of pterygomandibular raphe. **(Middle)** In this image the attachment of the medial pterygoid is visible along the medial ramus. Remember the pterygomandibular raphe is the tendinous point of junction between the buccinator muscle and the superior constrictor muscle. **(Bottom)** In this image the retromolar triangle is seen. Notice the retromolar trigone sits on the anterior surface of the masticator space. If a squamous cell carcinoma arises in the retromolar trigone the masticator space may be directly invaded. From there, perineural tumor spread on CNV3 may occur.

AXIAL T1 MR

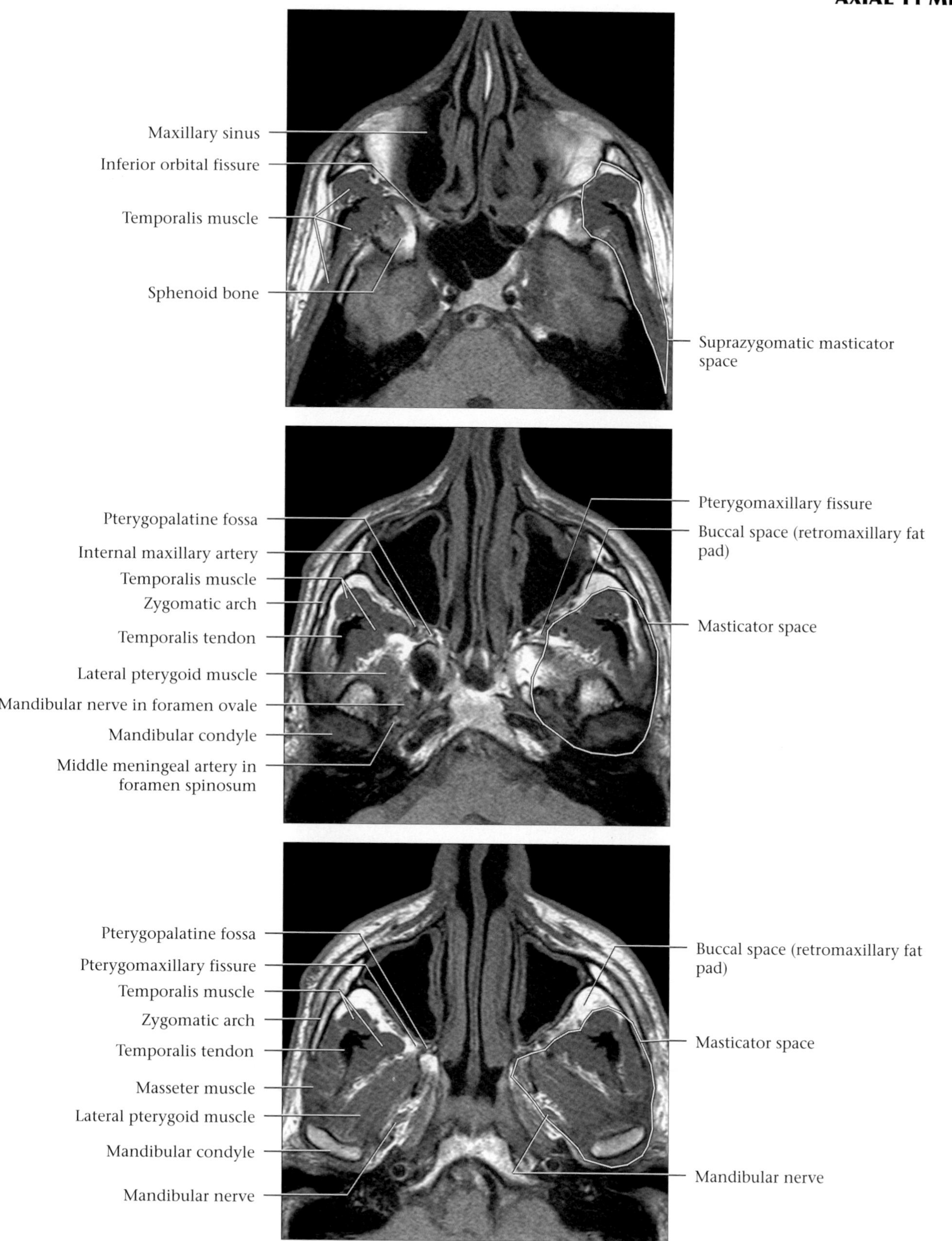
Maxillary sinus
Inferior orbital fissure
Temporalis muscle
Sphenoid bone
Suprazygomatic masticator space
Pterygopalatine fossa
Internal maxillary artery
Temporalis muscle
Zygomatic arch
Temporalis tendon
Lateral pterygoid muscle
Mandibular nerve in foramen ovale
Mandibular condyle
Middle meningeal artery in foramen spinosum
Pterygomaxillary fissure
Buccal space (retromaxillary fat pad)
Masticator space
Pterygopalatine fossa
Pterygomaxillary fissure
Temporalis muscle
Zygomatic arch
Temporalis tendon
Masseter muscle
Lateral pterygoid muscle
Mandibular condyle
Mandibular nerve
Buccal space (retromaxillary fat pad)
Masticator space
Mandibular nerve

(Top) First of six axial T1 MR images presented from superior to inferior. In this image above the zygomatic arch the suprazygomatic masticator space is seen. Notice that the temporalis muscle & fat are the only occupants of this portion of the masticator space. **(Middle)** In this image the mandibular nerve (CNV3) can be visualized within the foramen ovale. The middle meningeal artery can be seen posterolateral to foramen ovale within the foramen spinosum. The pterygopalatine fossa opens laterally through the pterygomaxillary fissure into the MS. **(Bottom)** In this image the mandibular nerve is visible along the posteromedial border of the lateral pterygoid muscle. The temporalis muscle & its hypointense tendon fill the anterolateral masticator space. The lateral pterygoid muscle inferior head originates from the lateral surface of lateral pterygoid plate.

AXIAL T1 MR

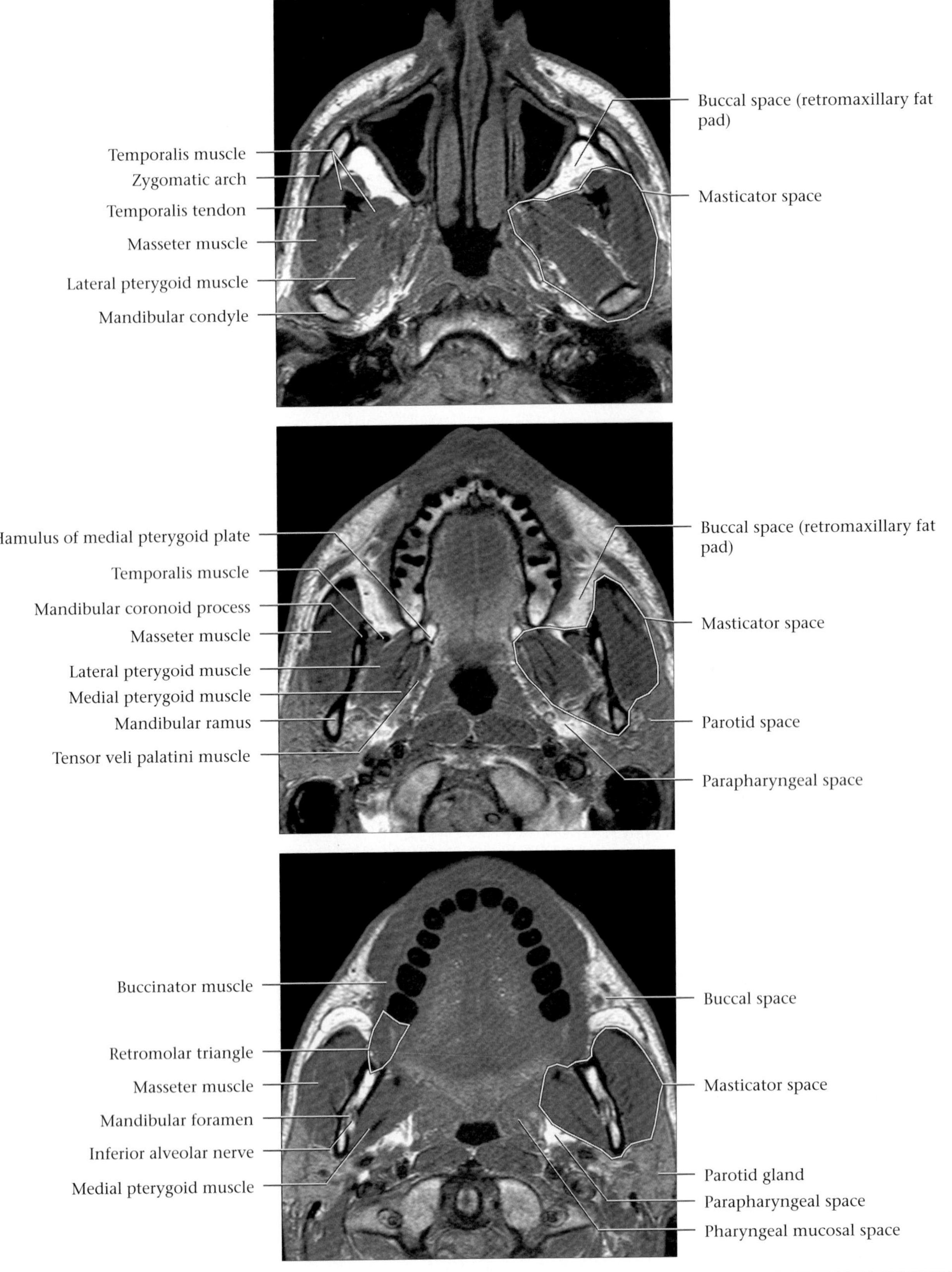
Temporalis muscle
Zygomatic arch
Temporalis tendon
Masseter muscle
Lateral pterygoid muscle
Mandibular condyle
Buccal space (retromaxillary fat pad)
Masticator space
Hamulus of medial pterygoid plate
Temporalis muscle
Mandibular coronoid process
Masseter muscle
Lateral pterygoid muscle
Medial pterygoid muscle
Mandibular ramus
Tensor veli palatini muscle
Buccal space (retromaxillary fat pad)
Masticator space
Parotid space
Parapharyngeal space
Buccinator muscle
Retromolar triangle
Masseter muscle
Mandibular foramen
Inferior alveolar nerve
Medial pterygoid muscle
Buccal space
Masticator space
Parotid gland
Parapharyngeal space
Pharyngeal mucosal space

(Top) In this image the masseter muscle is seen arising from the inferior surface of the zygomatic arch. The retromaxillary fat pad (superior buccal space) is visible anterior to the masticator space. **(Middle)** Image at the level of the maxillary ridge the temporalis muscle is seen inserting on the medial surface of the coronoid process of the mandible. The tensor veli palatini muscle approaches the hamulus of the medial pterygoid plate where it will turn medially to the soft palate. **(Bottom)** Image at the level of the mandibular teeth, the inferior alveolar nerve can be seen entering the mandibular foramen. The retromolar triangle represents the mucosal surface behind the 3rd mandibular molar and in front of the anterior mandibular ramus. Squamous cell carcinoma of the retromolar triangle when invasive readily involves the masticator space.

CORONAL T1 MR

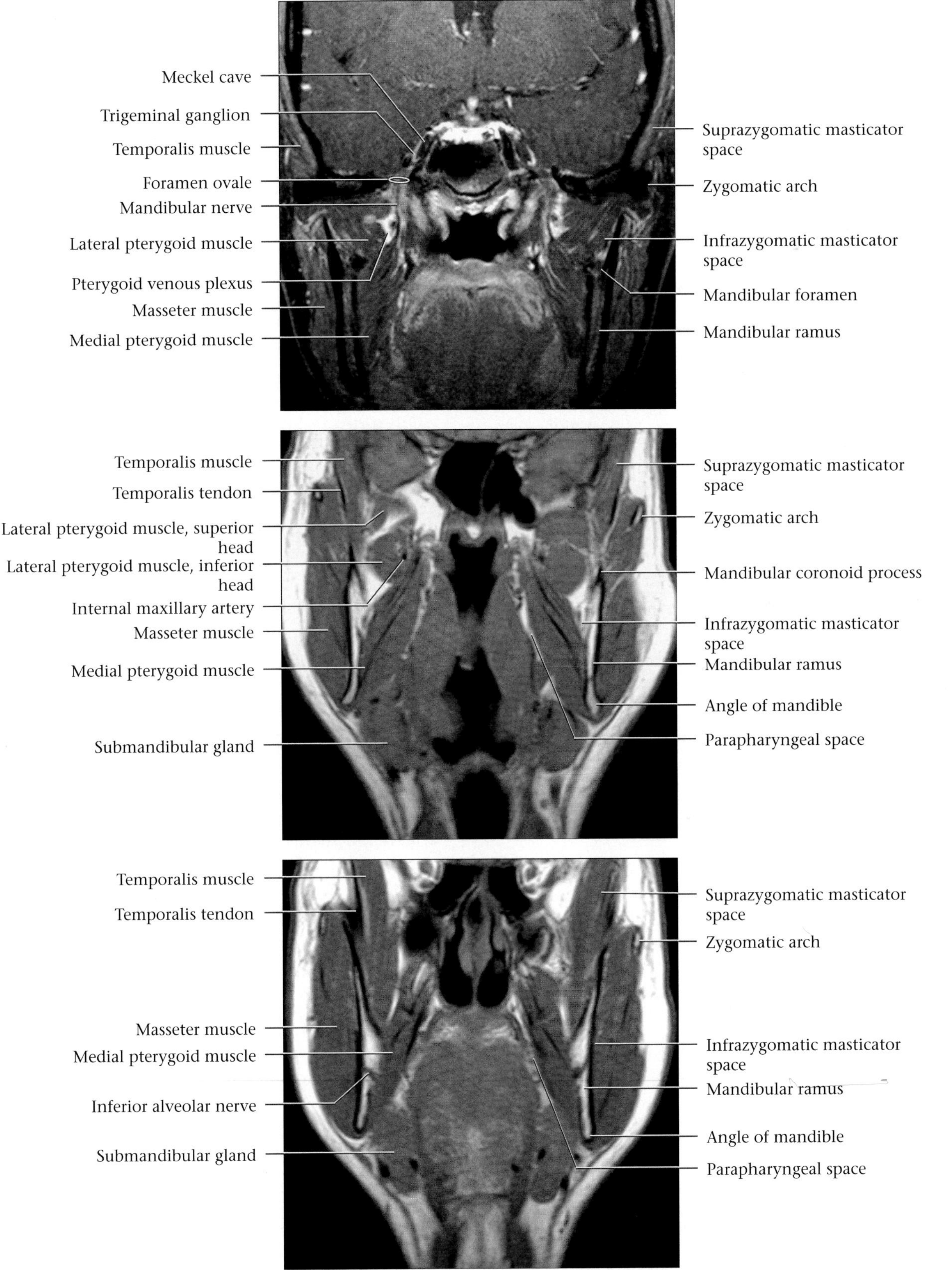
Meckel cave
Trigeminal ganglion
Temporalis muscle
Foramen ovale
Mandibular nerve
Lateral pterygoid muscle
Pterygoid venous plexus
Masseter muscle
Medial pterygoid muscle
Suprazygomatic masticator space
Zygomatic arch
Infrazygomatic masticator space
Mandibular foramen
Mandibular ramus
Temporalis muscle
Temporalis tendon
Lateral pterygoid muscle, superior head
Lateral pterygoid muscle, inferior head
Internal maxillary artery
Masseter muscle
Medial pterygoid muscle
Submandibular gland
Suprazygomatic masticator space
Zygomatic arch
Mandibular coronoid process
Infrazygomatic masticator space
Mandibular ramus
Angle of mandible
Parapharyngeal space
Temporalis muscle
Temporalis tendon
Masseter muscle
Medial pterygoid muscle
Inferior alveolar nerve
Submandibular gland
Suprazygomatic masticator space
Zygomatic arch
Infrazygomatic masticator space
Mandibular ramus
Angle of mandible
Parapharyngeal space

(Top) Coronal T1 enhanced fat-saturated MR image shows the mandibular nerve (main trunk CNV3) descending through foramen ovale. Although not visible, the masticator nerve (motor to muscles of mastication) branches off the mandibular nerve shortly after it exits the foramen ovale. **(Middle)** Coronal T1 unenhanced MR image reveals the superior and inferior heads of the lateral pterygoid muscles. Also note the medial pterygoid muscle arises from the pterygoid fossa above and inserts on the medial ramus and angle of the mandible. **(Bottom)** Coronal T1 unenhanced MR image through the posterior nose shows masseter muscle arising from the inferior surface of the zygomatic arch and inserting on the lateral ramus and angle of the mandible. Notice the inferior alveolar nerve as a focal low signal focus within the high signal fatty marrow of the mandible.

PAROTID SPACE

Terminology

Abbreviations

- Parotid space (PS)

Definitions

- **PS**: Paired lateral suprahyoid neck spaces enclosed by superficial layer deep cervical fascia containing parotid glands, nodes & extracranial facial nerve branches

Imaging Anatomy

Extent

- PS extends from external auditory canal (EAC) & mastoid tip superiorly to below angle of mandible (parotid tail)
  - Parotid tail inserts inferiorly between platysma & sternocleidomastoid muscle in area of posterior submandibular space

Anatomy Relationships

- Parapharyngeal space (PPS) is directly medial to PS
- Masticator space (MS) is anterior to PS
- Carotid space (CS) is separated from upper PS by posterior belly digastric muscle

Internal Structures-Critical Contents

- **Parotid gland**
  - Superficial lobe represents ~ 2/3 of parotid space
  - Deep lobe projects into lateral PPS
- **Extracranial facial nerve (CN7)**
  - Exits stylomastoid foramen as single trunk; ramifies within PS lateral to retromandibular vein
  - Ramifying intraparotid facial nerve creates surgical plane between superficial & deep lobes
  - Intraparotid facial nerve **not visible** with CT or MR except proximally with high-resolution 3T MR
- **External carotid artery**
  - Medial, smaller vessel of 2 seen just behind mandibular ramus in PS
- **Retromandibular vein**
  - Lateral, larger of 2 vessels seen just behind mandibular ramus in parotid
  - Intraparotid facial nerve branches course just lateral to retromandibular vein
- **Intraparotid lymph nodes**
  - ~ 20 lymph nodes found in each parotid gland
  - Parotid nodes are 1st order drainage for EAC, pinna & surrounding scalp
- **Parotid duct**
  - Emerges from anterior PS, runs along surface of masseter muscle
  - Duct then arches through buccal space to pierce buccinator muscle at level of upper 2nd molar
- **Accessory parotid glands**
  - Project over surface of masseter muscles
  - Present in ~ 20% of normal anatomic dissections

Fascia of Parotid Space

- Superficial layer of deep cervical fascia (SL-DCF) surrounds parotid space

Anatomy-Based Imaging Issues

Key Concepts or Questions

- What imaging features define a **primary parotid space lesion**?
  - Center of lesion is within parotid gland
  - If larger mass lesion of deep lobe, mass displaces PPS from lateral to medial with widening of stylomandibular gap

Imaging Recommendations

- CECT or MR can both readily image PS
- T1 C+ fat-saturated axial & coronal MR better for perineural CN7 spread

Imaging Approaches

- Small, superficial lobe PS lesions need no imaging
  - Needle aspiration to confirm benign mixed tumor with superficial parotidectomy sufficient
- If inflammation-infection of PS suspected, CECT best
  - Angle gantry to avoid dental amalgam & visualize parotid duct looking for cause of obstruction
  - 2-3 mm CT slice thickness recommended
- If tumor suspected, T1 C+ fat-saturated MR best
  - Look for perineural facial nerve tumor along intratemporal segments CN7
  - T-bone CT helps define associated bony changes

Imaging Pitfalls

- Parotid gland becomes progressively more fatty with advancing age
  - Parotid glands appear similar to soft tissue in children
- Parotid tail mass must be identified as intraparotid or excision may injure facial nerve
  - Parotid tail area defined by superficial platysma, deep sternocleidomastoid & carotid space
- Facial nerve plane in parotid can only be estimated

Clinical Implications

Clinical Importance

- Intraparotid facial nerve although invisible to imager is key PS structure
- Try to assess relationship of mass lesion to estimated facial nerve plane (lateral to retromandibular vein)
  - Superficial, deep or in plane of intraparotid CN7?
  - Evidence of perineural tumor affecting CN7?
- Parotid tumors: Benign mixed tumor (75%), Warthin tumor (5%), adenoid cystic carcinoma (5%), mucoepidermoid carcinoma (5%), other (10%)

Embryology

Embryologic Events

- Parotid space undergoes **late encapsulation** in embryogenesis

Practical Implications

- Late encapsulation results in intraparotid lymph nodes
- Parotid nodes are 1st-order drainage for malignancies of adjacent scalp, EAC & deep face

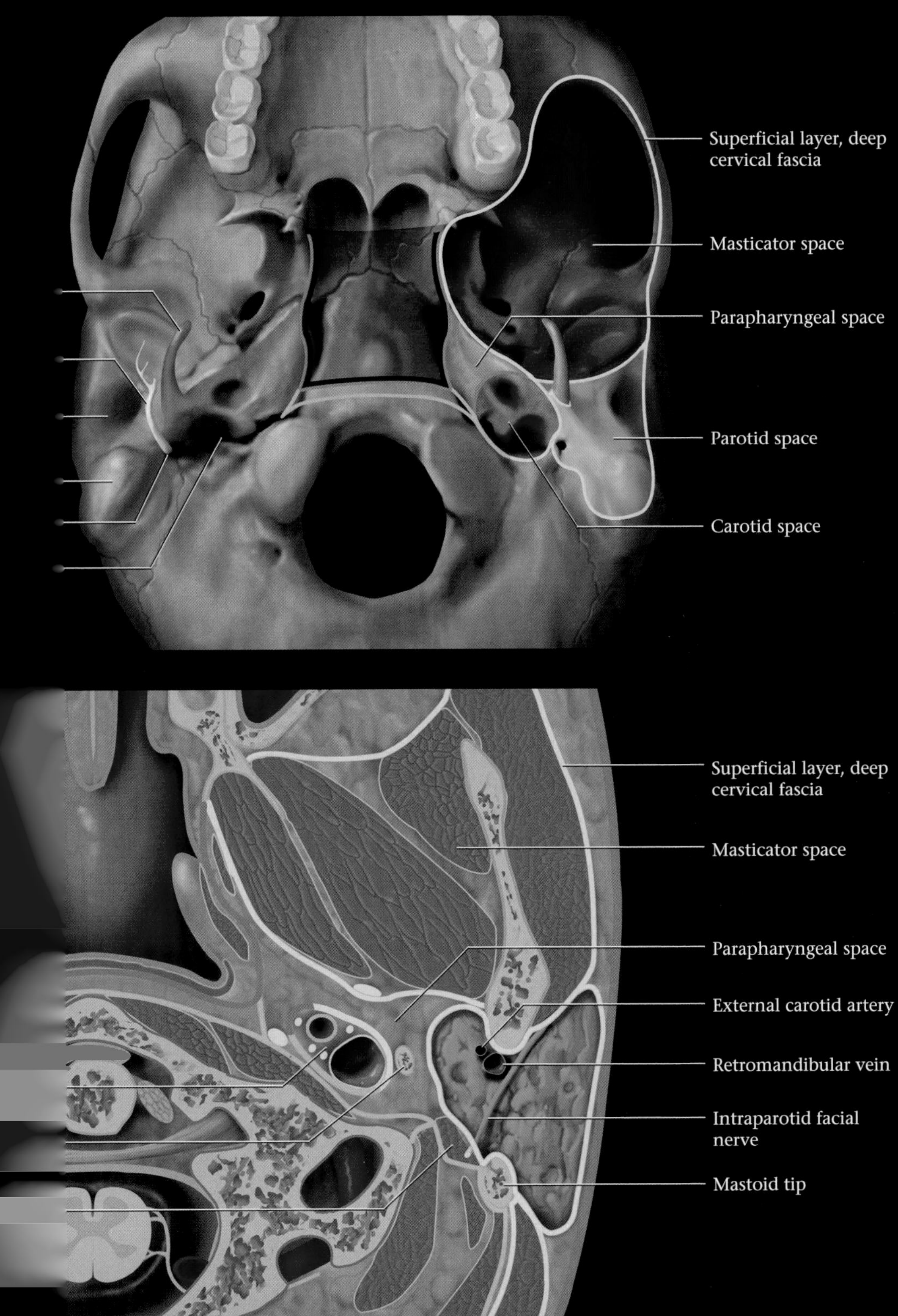

Superficial layer, deep cervical fascia
Masticator space
Parapharyngeal space
Parotid space
Carotid space
Superficial layer, deep cervical fascia
Masticator space
Parapharyngeal space
External carotid artery
Retromandibular vein
Intraparotid facial nerve
Mastoid tip

ll base viewed from below illustrating the interaction between the parotid space & the skull he stylomastoid foramen at the skull base, just posterior to the styloid process and lateral to PS is the most lateral space in the nasopharyngeal & oropharyngeal area, extending from l above to the level of the mandibular angle below. **(Bottom)** Axial graphic of the PS at the . The PS contains from medial to lateral the external carotid artery, retromandibular vein & otid CN7 creates a surgical plane that divides the gland into superficial & deep lobes. he deep lobe will displace the parapharyngeal space fat medially. PS is enclosed by the

GRAPHICS

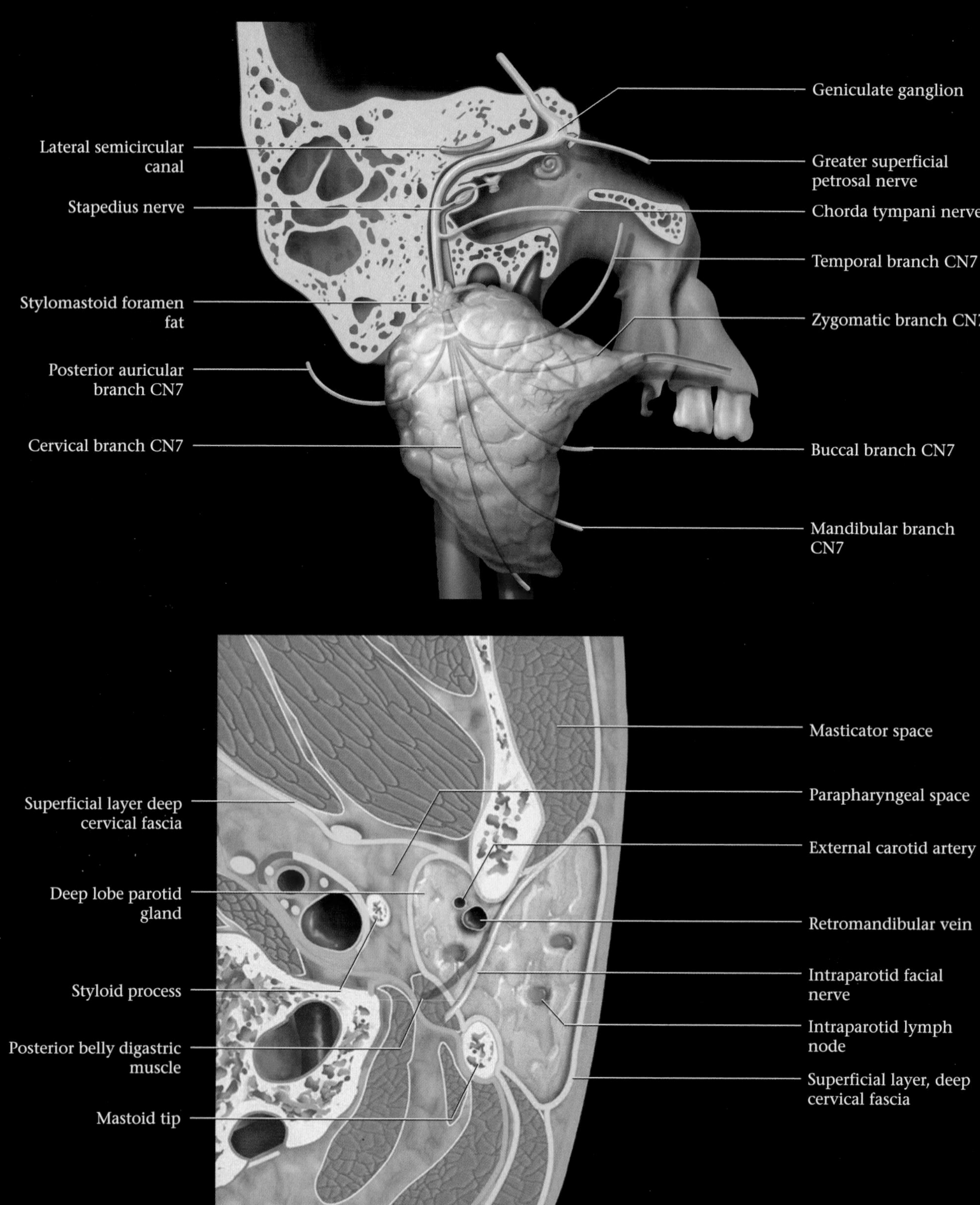

Lateral semicircular canal
Stapedius nerve
Stylomastoid foramen fat
Posterior auricular branch CN7
Cervical branch CN7
Geniculate ganglion
Greater superficial petrosal nerve
Chorda tympani nerve
Temporal branch CN7
Zygomatic branch CN7
Buccal branch CN7
Mandibular branch CN7
Masticator space
Superficial layer deep cervical fascia
Parapharyngeal space
External carotid artery
Deep lobe parotid gland
Retromandibular vein
Intraparotid facial nerve
Styloid process
Intraparotid lymph node
Posterior belly digastric muscle
Superficial layer, deep cervical fascia
Mastoid tip

(Top) Sagittal graphic of the parotid gland & facial nerve. The facial nerve exits the skull base at the stylomastoid foramen, then enters the parotid gland where it ramifies into six major branches. The plane of the facial nerve branches within the parotid gland is used by the surgeons to define a superficial and a deep lobe of the parotid. This is a surgically defined, not a radiologically defined, delineation. **(Bottom)** Axial graphic of the PS at the level of C1 vertebral body. The intraparotid course of the facial nerve extends from just medial to the mastoid tip to a position just lateral to the retromandibular vein. Late embryologic encapsulation of the parotid gland accounts for intraparotid lymph nodes, which serve as first-order drainage for malignancies of the deep face, scalp and external ear. The normal parotid gland contains ~ 20 nodes.

GENERIC PAROTID SPACE MASS

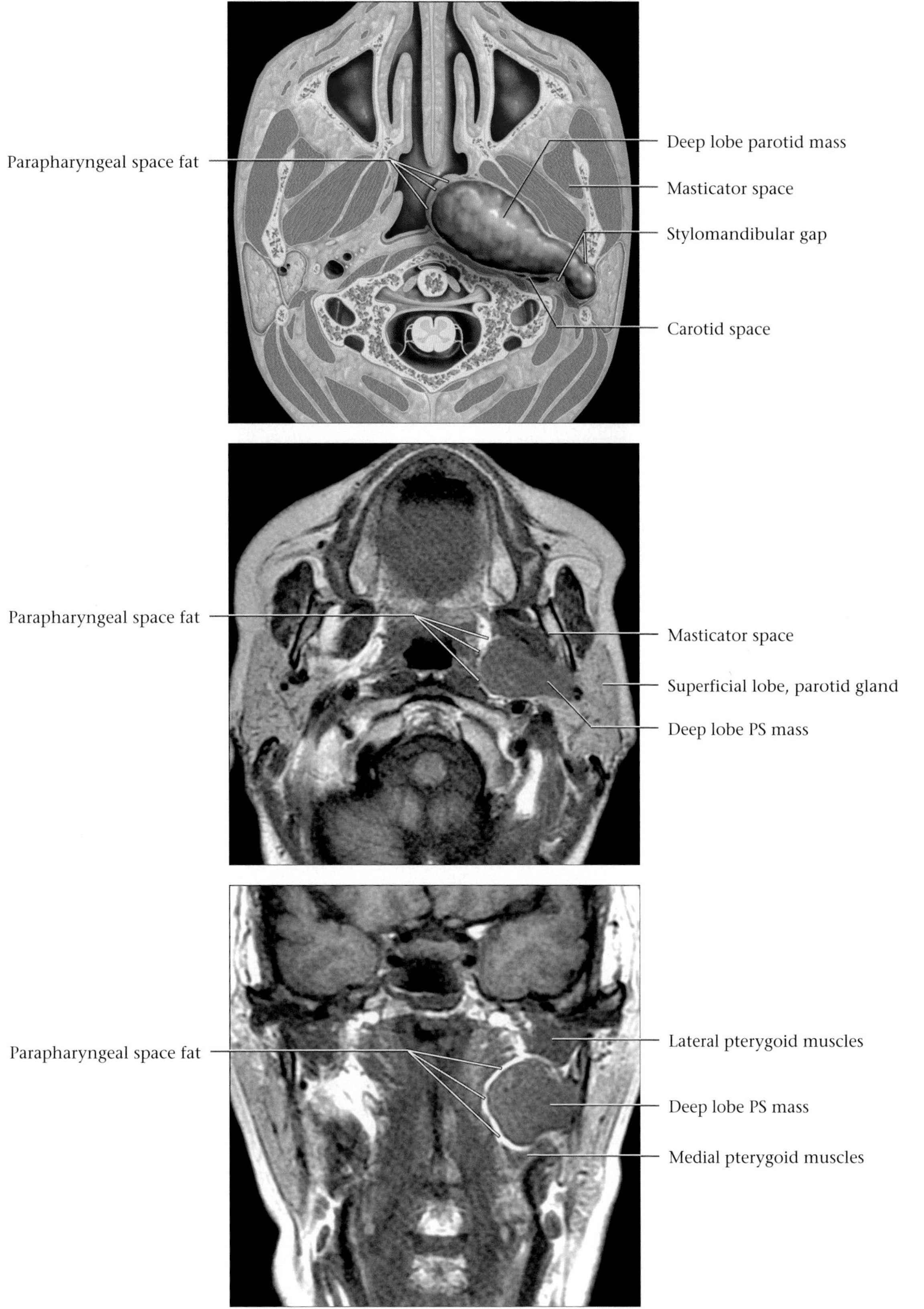
Parapharyngeal space fat
Deep lobe parotid mass
Masticator space
Stylomandibular gap
Carotid space
Parapharyngeal space fat
Masticator space
Superficial lobe, parotid gland
Deep lobe PS mass
Parapharyngeal space fat
Lateral pterygoid muscles
Deep lobe PS mass
Medial pterygoid muscles

(Top) Axial graphic of generic deep lobe of parotid gland mass demonstrates medial displacement of the parapharyngeal space fat. Notice also the slight enlargement of the stylomandibular gap. Smaller lesions of the superficial lobe of the parotid gland are easily identified as intraparotid. Larger deep lobe lesions may be more difficult to identify as PS in origin. **(Middle)** Axial T1 MR through the maxillary ridge reveals a pear-shaped mass arising from the deep lobe of the parotid gland. This benign mixed tumor enlarges medially, displacing the parapharyngeal space from lateral to medial. **(Bottom)** Coronal T1 MR of a large benign mixed tumor enlarging medially from its origin in the deep lobe of the parotid gland. Note the crescent of parapharyngeal space fat arching medially and still visible despite the large size of this deep lobe tumor.

PERINEURAL PAROTID SPACE MALIGNANCY

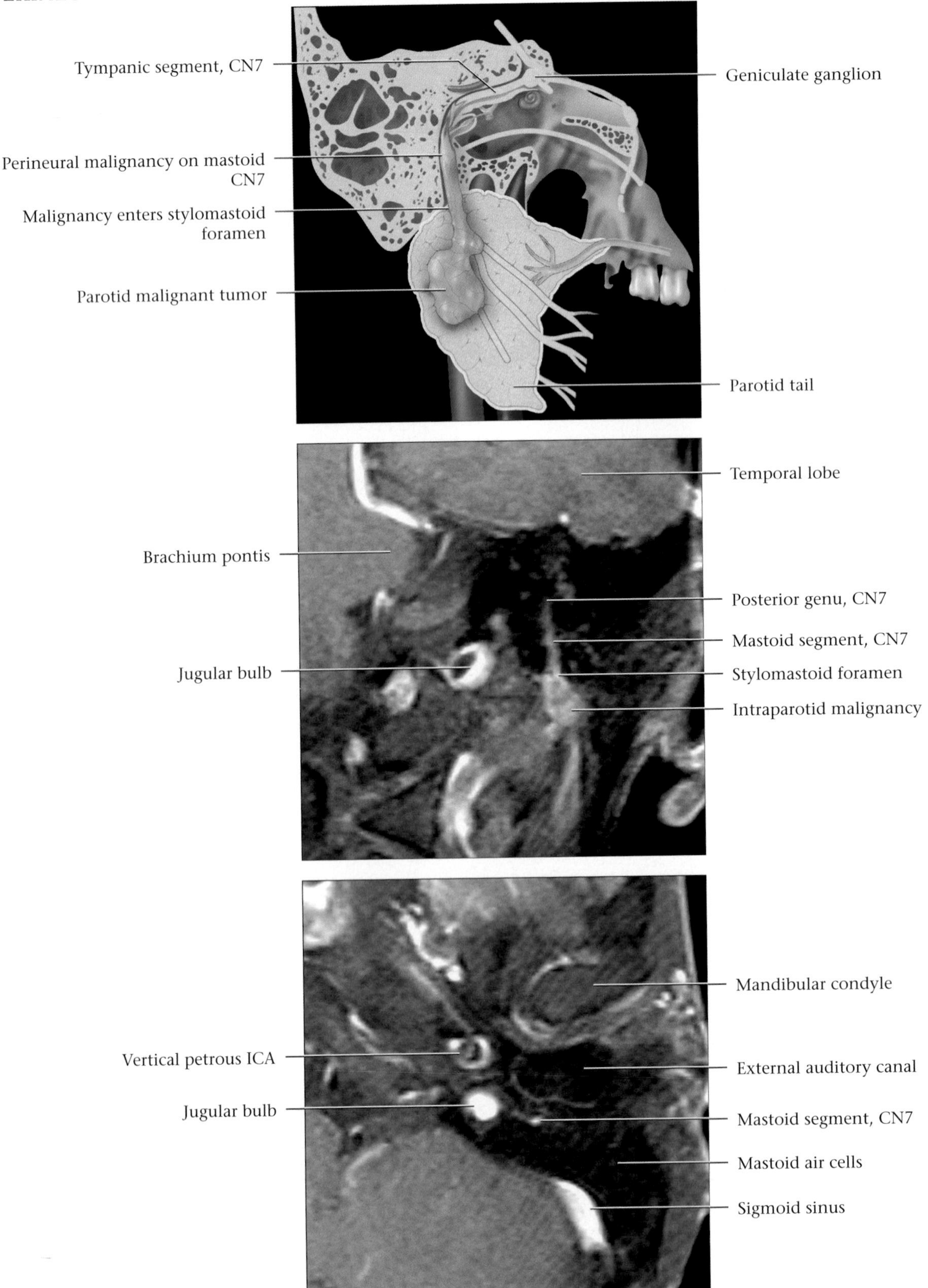
Tympanic segment, CN7
Geniculate ganglion
Perineural malignancy on mastoid CN7
Malignancy enters stylomastoid foramen
Parotid malignant tumor
Parotid tail
Temporal lobe
Brachium pontis
Posterior genu, CN7
Mastoid segment, CN7
Jugular bulb
Stylomastoid foramen
Intraparotid malignancy
Mandibular condyle
Vertical petrous ICA
External auditory canal
Jugular bulb
Mastoid segment, CN7
Mastoid air cells
Sigmoid sinus

(Top) Sagittal graphic of a generic parotid malignancy affecting intraparotid facial nerve. The tumor spreading along CN7 through the stylomastoid foramen to the proximal mastoid segment within the temporal bone. If left untreated, such perineural malignant tumor will eventually access the intracranial compartment via the internal auditory canal. **(Middle)** Coronal T1 enhanced fat-saturated MR of the left temporal bone shows an enhancing adenoid cystic carcinoma of the parotid gland spreading into the lower flared portion of the stylomastoid foramen. This malignant tumor then spreads in a perineural fashion up the mastoid segment of the facial nerve to the posterior genu. **(Bottom)** Axial enhanced T1 fat-saturated MR image reveals an enlarged enhancing mastoid segment of CN7 as a result of perineural spread of adenoid cystic carcinoma from the parotid space.

AXIAL CECT

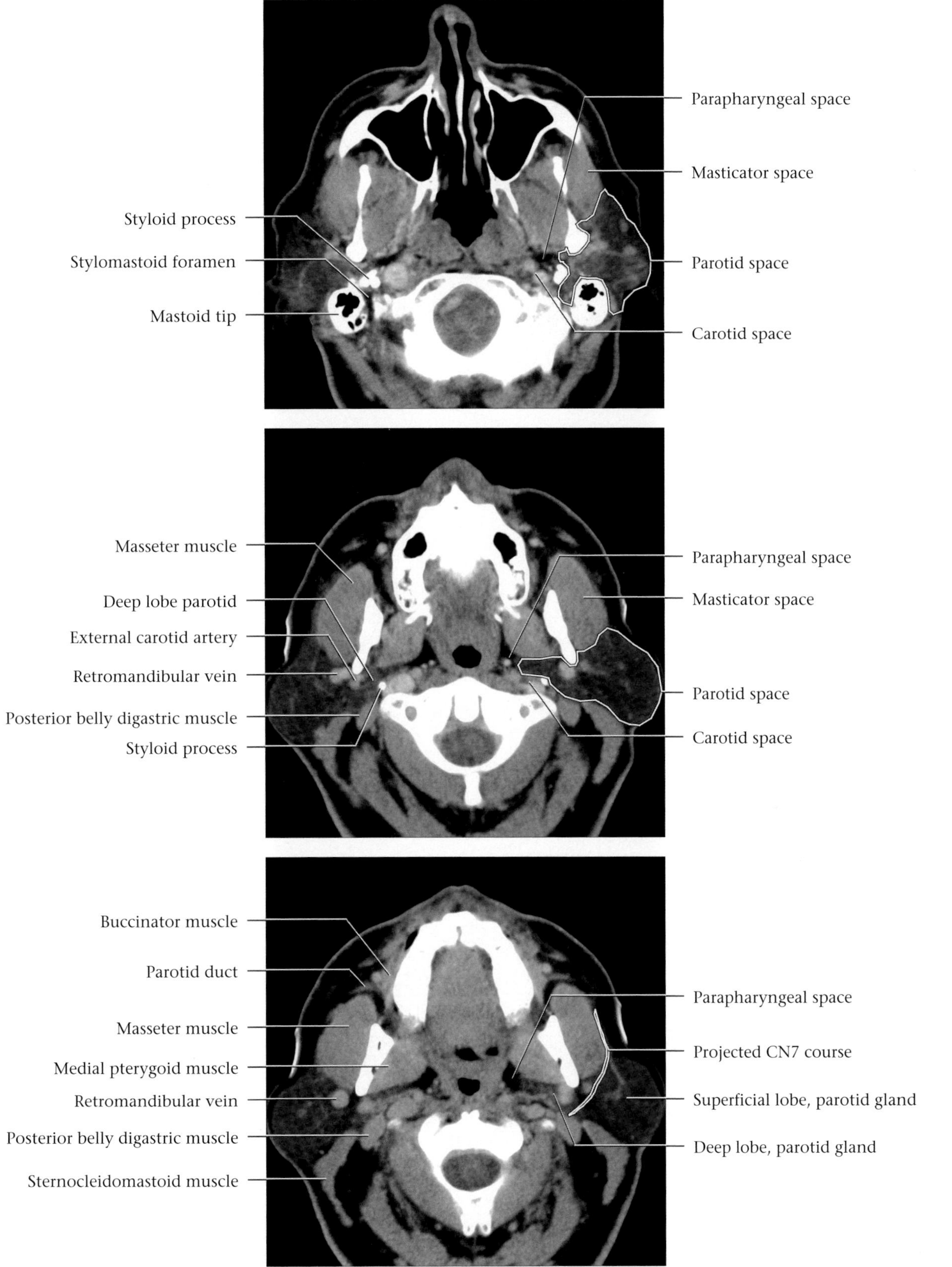
Parapharyngeal space
Masticator space
Styloid process
Stylomastoid foramen
Parotid space
Mastoid tip
Carotid space
Masseter muscle
Parapharyngeal space
Masticator space
Deep lobe parotid
External carotid artery
Retromandibular vein
Parotid space
Posterior belly digastric muscle
Carotid space
Styloid process
Buccinator muscle
Parotid duct
Parapharyngeal space
Masseter muscle
Projected CN7 course
Medial pterygoid muscle
Retromandibular vein
Superficial lobe, parotid gland
Posterior belly digastric muscle
Deep lobe, parotid gland
Sternocleidomastoid muscle

(Top) First of six axial CECT images presented superior to inferior. This image shows the right stylomastoid foramen with low attenuation fat contained within. The facial nerve is not visualized on CT images. If perineural tumor is present, stylomastoid foramen fat will be replaced by tumor. **(Middle)** In this image the deep lobe of the parotid gland can be seen projecting through the stylomandibular gap to abut the parapharyngeal space. Note the medial external carotid artery and more lateral retromandibular vein. **(Bottom)** In this image, the parotid duct is seen piecing the buccinator muscle just lateral to the 2nd maxillary molar. The projected course of the extracranial CN7 lateral to the retromandibular vein & over the surface of the masseter muscle is drawn. Note the large size of the superficial lobe compared to the deep lobe of the parotid.

PAROTID SPACE

AXIAL CECT

Masseter muscle
Medial pterygoid muscle
Retromandibular vein
External carotid artery
Sternocleidomastoid muscle
Posterior belly of digastric muscle
Parapharyngeal space
Masticator space
Parotid space
Carotid space

Platysma muscle
Deep lobe parotid
Posterior belly digastric muscle
Internal jugular vein
Internal carotid artery
Parapharyngeal space
Masticator space
Parotid space
Carotid space

Mylohyoid muscle
Platysma muscle
Submandibular gland
Parotid tail
Sternocleidomastoid muscle
Submandibular space
Parotid space
Posterior cervical space

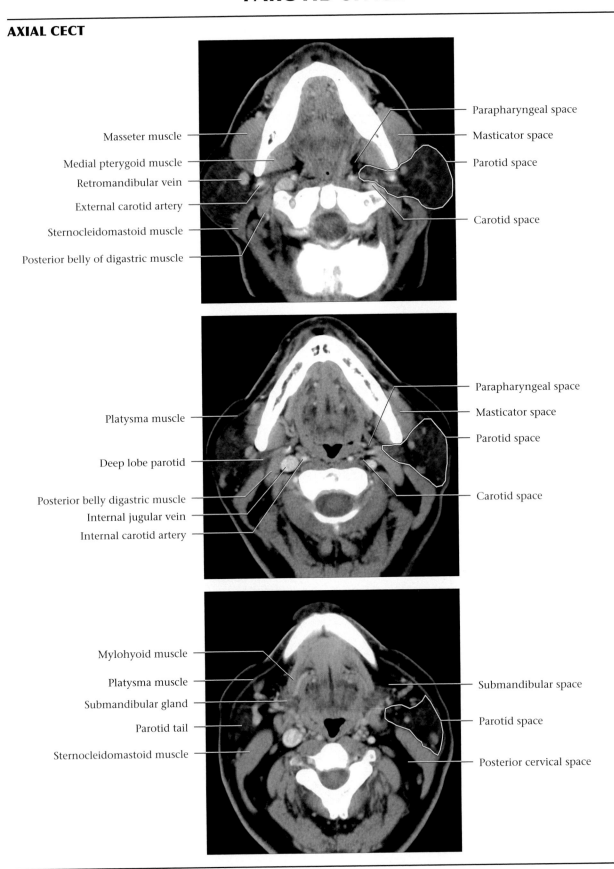

(Top) In this image at the level of the mid-oropharynx the larger laterally placed retromandibular vein can be distinguished from the more medial external carotid artery. Remember that the intraparotid facial nerve cannot be seen on CECT but its path can be projected along a line just lateral to the retromandibular vein and out over the surface of the masseter muscle. **(Middle)** At the level of the mandibular angle the parotid space is now separated from the carotid space by the posterior belly of the digastric muscle. Note the platysma muscle is now visible over the surface of the parotid gland. **(Bottom)** Just below the mandible the parotid tail is visible projecting into the posterior aspect of the submandibular space. Excisional biopsy of a low lying mass, unrecognized as being in the parotid tail, may result in facial nerve injury.

AXIAL T1 MR

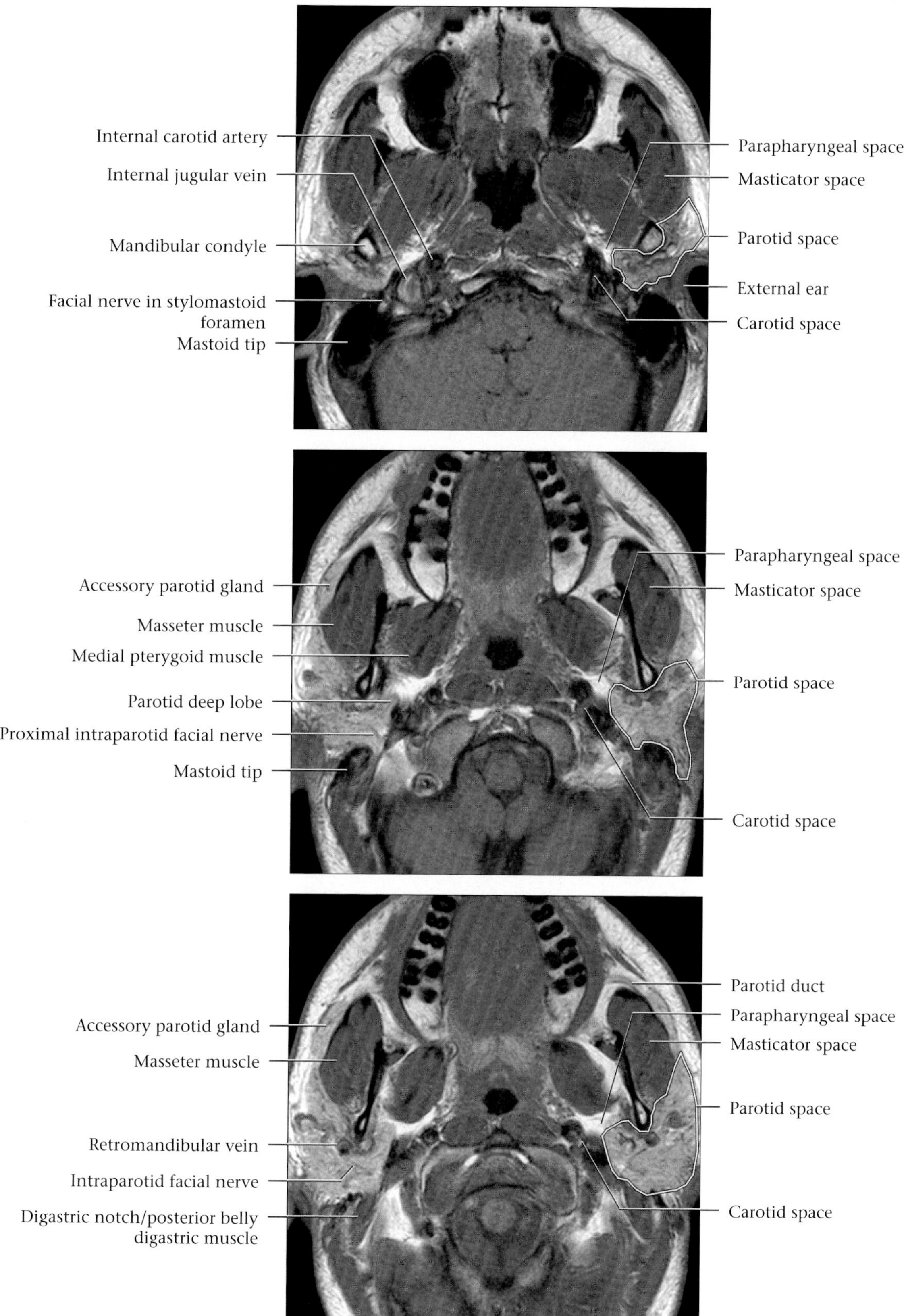

Internal carotid artery
Internal jugular vein
Mandibular condyle
Facial nerve in stylomastoid foramen
Mastoid tip
Parapharyngeal space
Masticator space
Parotid space
External ear
Carotid space
Accessory parotid gland
Masseter muscle
Medial pterygoid muscle
Parotid deep lobe
Proximal intraparotid facial nerve
Mastoid tip
Parapharyngeal space
Masticator space
Parotid space
Carotid space
Accessory parotid gland
Masseter muscle
Retromandibular vein
Intraparotid facial nerve
Digastric notch/posterior belly digastric muscle
Parotid duct
Parapharyngeal space
Masticator space
Parotid space
Carotid space

(Top) First of six axial T1 MR images presented superior to inferior shows the right facial nerve exiting the stylomandibular foramen. There is fat in the lower flared aspect of the stylomastoid foramen so the main trunk of the facial nerve is visible. **(Middle)** In this image the proximal intraparotid facial nerve is seen on the right. Note the accessory parotid gland overlying the right masseter muscle bilaterally. **(Bottom)** At the level of the maxillary ridge a branch of the intraparotid facial nerve is seen projecting anterolaterally around the lateral margin of the retromandibular vein. Usually not visible on routine imaging, the intraparotid facial nerve and its branches follow a predictable course anterolaterally around the lateral margin of the retromandibular vein, from there anteriorly along the lateral surface of the masseter muscle.

PAROTID SPACE

AXIAL T1 MR

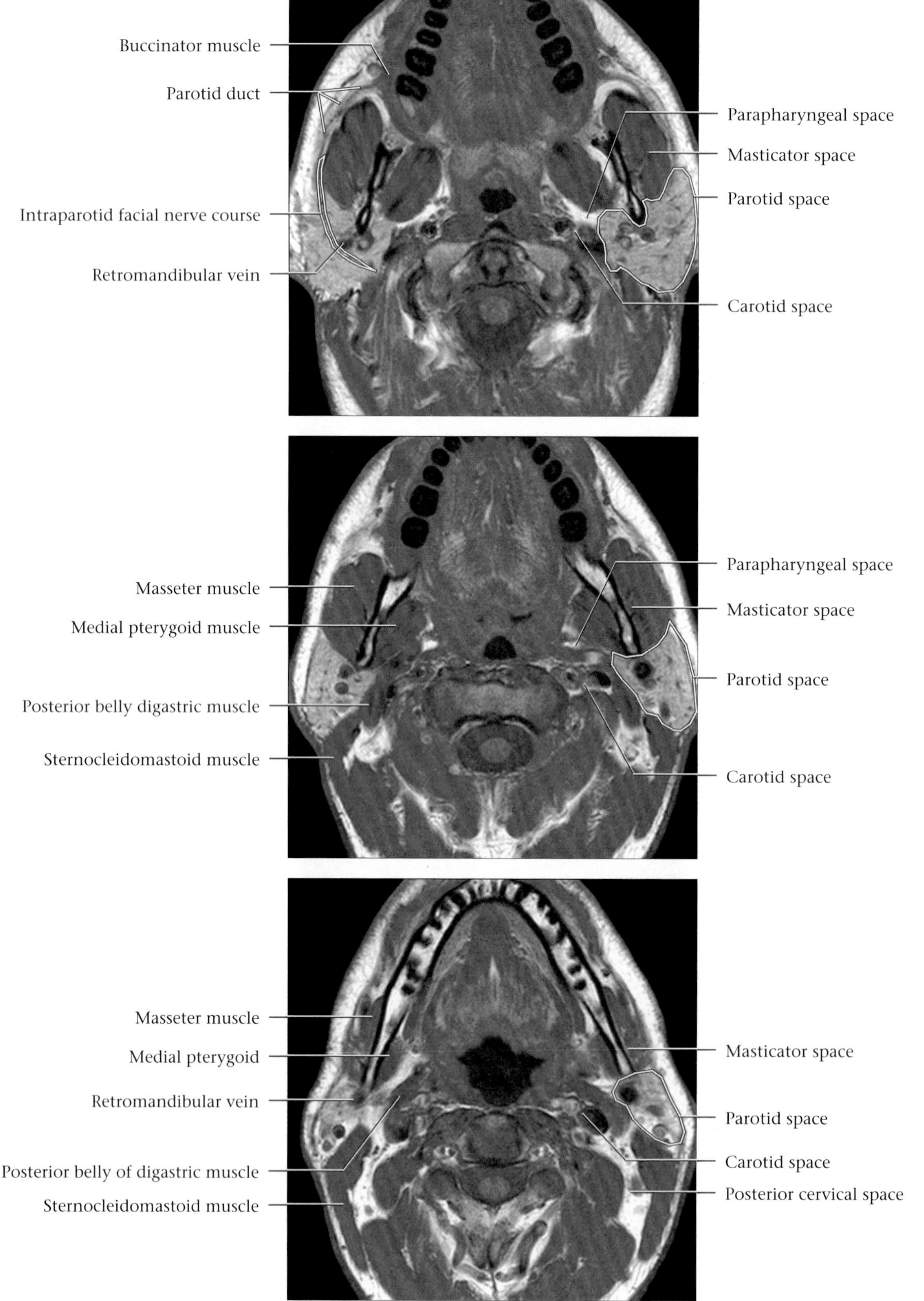
Buccinator muscle
Parotid duct
Intraparotid facial nerve course
Retromandibular vein
Parapharyngeal space
Masticator space
Parotid space
Carotid space
Masseter muscle
Medial pterygoid muscle
Posterior belly digastric muscle
Sternocleidomastoid muscle
Parapharyngeal space
Masticator space
Parotid space
Carotid space
Masseter muscle
Medial pterygoid
Retromandibular vein
Posterior belly of digastric muscle
Sternocleidomastoid muscle
Masticator space
Parotid space
Carotid space
Posterior cervical space

(Top) At the level of the maxillary teeth the parotid space is visible posterolateral to the masticator space. Remember that both the masticator & parotid spaces are circumscribed by superficial layer of deep cervical fascia. Note the projected intraparotid facial nerve course drawn on the right. **(Middle)** In this image the posterior belly of the digastric muscle is seen on the posteromedial boundary of the parotid space, separating the PS from the carotid space. The posterior belly of the digastric muscle is innervated by a branch of the facial nerve. **(Bottom)** In this image the parotid gland is seen at the mandibular angle. The posterior belly of the digastric muscle is seen between the parotid tail & the carotid space on the left. When a parotid space mass is present, the medial displacement of the posterior belly of the digastric muscle helps define its location.

AXIAL T2 FS MR

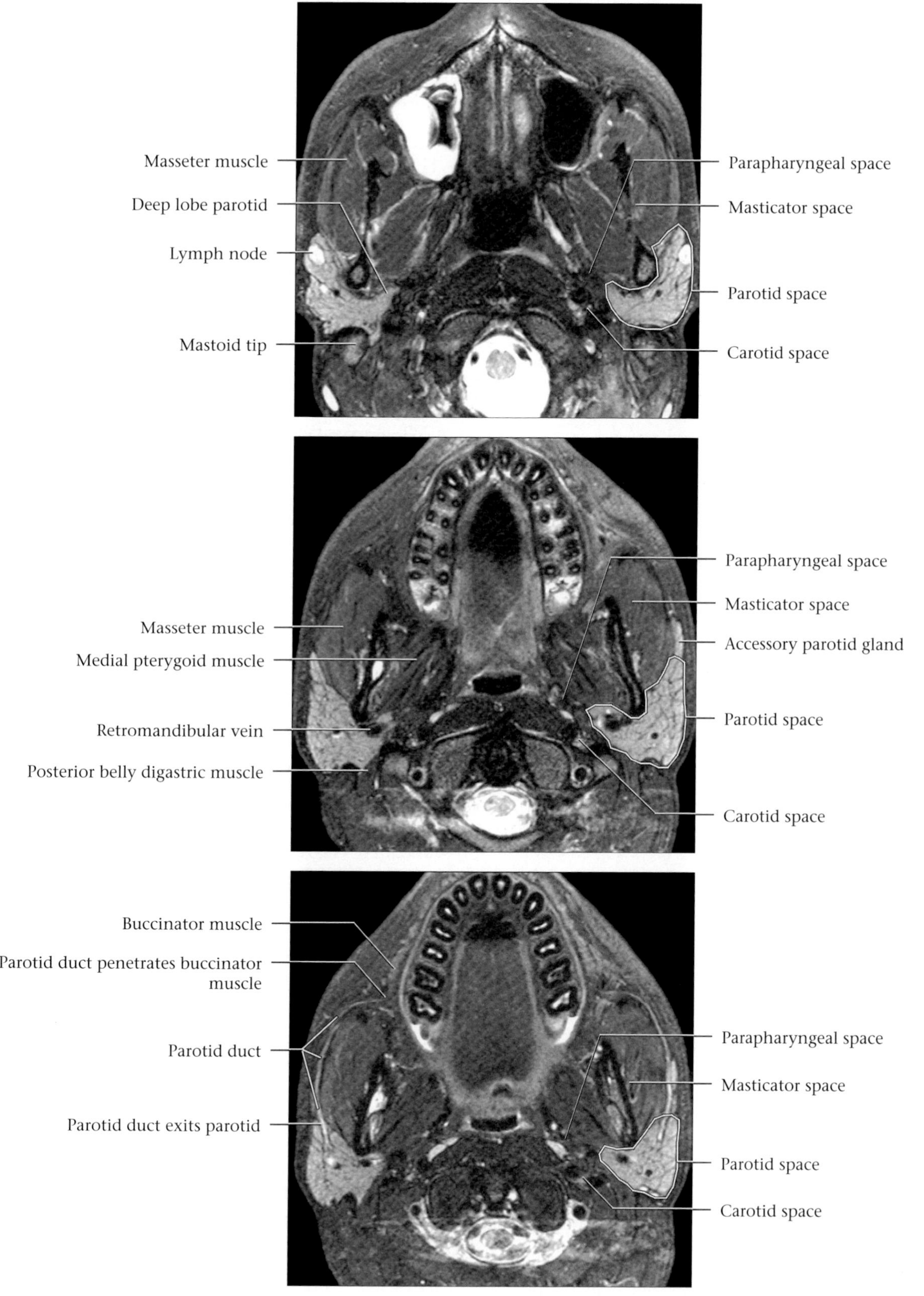
Masseter muscle
Deep lobe parotid
Lymph node
Mastoid tip
Parapharyngeal space
Masticator space
Parotid space
Carotid space
Parapharyngeal space
Masticator space
Accessory parotid gland
Parotid space
Carotid space
Masseter muscle
Medial pterygoid muscle
Retromandibular vein
Posterior belly digastric muscle
Buccinator muscle
Parotid duct penetrates buccinator muscle
Parotid duct
Parotid duct exits parotid
Parapharyngeal space
Masticator space
Parotid space
Carotid space

(Top) First of three axial T2 fat-saturated MR images presented superior to inferior shows the adult parotid gland is higher signal than the surrounding muscles of the suprahyoid neck. A few sporadic high signal intraparotid nodes are present at this level. The parapharyngeal space fat is low signal because of the fat-saturation MR sequence. **(Middle)** The parotid space often abuts the accessory parotid gland that may be seen over the surface of the masseter muscle. Both are within the superficial layer of deep cervical fascia. **(Bottom)** In this image at the level of the maxillary teeth the high signal linear parotid duct is easily visualized extending anteriorly from the parotid gland along the surface of the masseter muscle to penetrate the buccinator muscle.

CAROTID SPACE

Terminology

Abbreviations

- Carotid space (CS)
- Suprahyoid neck (SHN) and infrahyoid neck (IHN)

Definitions

- Paired, tubular spaces surrounded by carotid sheath that contain carotid arteries, internal jugular veins, **cranial nerves (CN) 9-12 (SHN) & CN10 (IHN)**

Imaging Anatomy

Overview

- Carotid space travels from inferior margins of jugular foramen-carotid canal above to aortic arch below
- SHN carotid space contains CN9-12, internal carotid artery and internal jugular vein
- IHN carotid space contains CN10 only, common carotid artery, internal jugular vein; internal jugular nodal chain is closely associated with its outer surface

Extent

- CS defined from skull base (carotid canal and jugular foramen) to aortic arch below
- CS can be divided into its major segments
  - Nasopharyngeal, oropharyngeal, cervical and mediastinal segments

Anatomy Relationships

- **SHN carotid space adjacent spaces**
  - Retropharyngeal space (RPS) medial
  - Perivertebral space posterior
  - Parotid space lateral
  - Parapharyngeal space (PPS) anterior
- **IHN carotid space adjacent spaces**
  - Visceral space and RPS medial
  - Perivertebral space posterior
  - Anterior cervical space anterior
  - Posterior cervical space lateral

Internal Structures-Critical Contents

- **SHN carotid space**
  - **Internal carotid artery (ICA)**
  - **Internal jugular vein (IJV)**
  - **Cranial nerves 9-12 in nasopharyngeal CS**
  - Only CN10 remains in CS from oropharyngeal CS inferiorly
  - CN10 located in posterior notch formed by ICA and IJV
  - **Sympathetic plexus** between medial CS and lateral RPS
- **IHN carotid space**
  - **Common carotid artery (CCA)**
  - **Internal jugular vein**
  - **Vagus nerve**
  - Internal jugular nodal chain closely associated but **not** in infrahyoid neck carotid space

Fascia of Carotid Space

- **Carotid sheath** made from components of **all 3 layers of deep cervical fascia**
  - Suprahyoid carotid space: Carotid sheath incomplete or less substantial
  - Infrahyoid carotid space: Carotid sheath well-defined, tenacious fascia

Anatomy-Based Imaging Issues

Key Concepts or Questions

- What imaging features define a lesion as primary to carotid space?
  - **Lesion in SHN carotid space**
    - Center of lesion is within area of ICA-IJV, posterior to PPS
    - Lesion displaces PPS fat anteriorly
    - Pushes posterior belly of digastric muscle laterally
    - If in nasopharyngeal CS, pushes styloid process anterolaterally
    - When mass begins in posterior SHN CS (vagal schwannoma, neurofibroma, paraganglioma), ICA is pushed anteriorly as mass enlarges
  - **Lesion in IHN carotid space**
    - May engulf CCA and IJV or push them apart
    - May splay external carotid artery (ECA) and ICA (carotid body paraganglioma)
- What are statistically common lesions found in the carotid space?
  - Paraganglioma, schwannoma, IJV thrombosis & carotid artery dissection-pseudoaneurysm

Imaging Recommendations

- CECT or MR both can easily identify normal CS anatomy and CS lesions
- If using MR, remember to acquire unenhanced T1 (to look for high velocity flow voids of paraganglioma)
- MRA and MRV may be helpful in defining the normal and diseased vessels of CS (ICA dissection; pseudoaneurysm; IJV thrombosis)

Imaging Approaches

- Remember that CS runs from jugular foramen-carotid canal of skull base above to aortic arch below
- If imaging CS because of **left** vagal neuropathy, must reach aortopulmonic window inferiorly

Imaging Pitfalls

- Normal vascular flow phenomenon of IJV may mimic schwannoma or thrombosis

Clinical Implications

Clinical Importance

- **CN9-12** and **carotid artery** are vital structures in carotid space

Function-Dysfunction

- **Injury to nasopharyngeal CS** may result in complex cranial neuropathy involving some combination of **CN9-12**
- **Vagus nerve injury**: Vocal cord paralysis
- Carotid artery proximity to internal jugular nodal chain makes injury from squamous cell carcinoma extranodal tumor likely

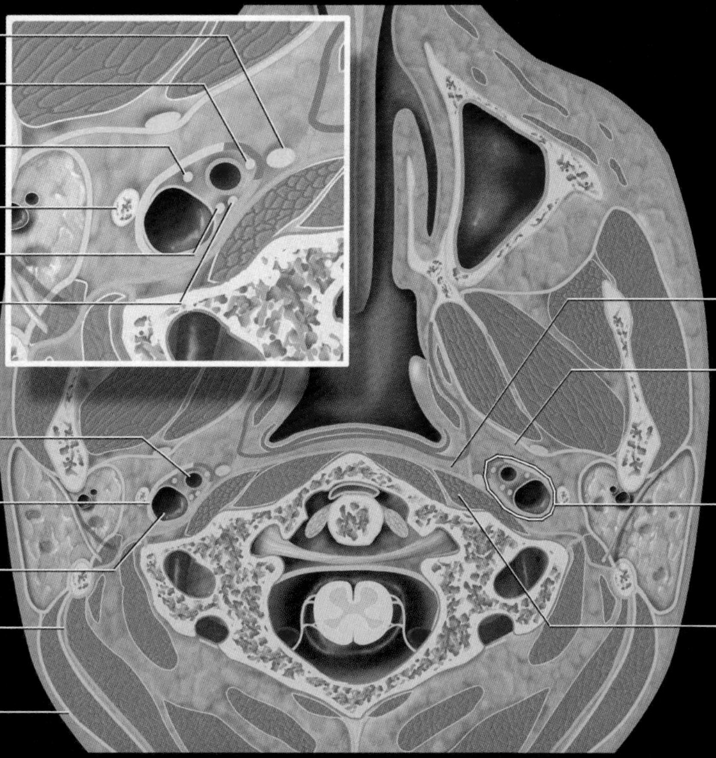

CAROTID SPACE

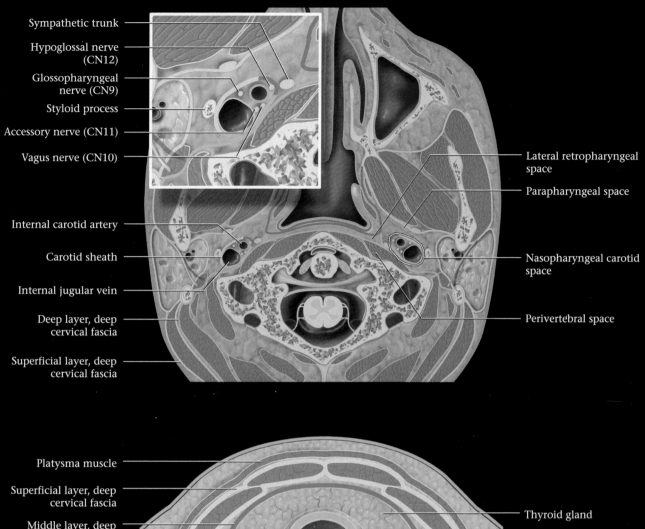

Sympathetic trunk
Hypoglossal nerve (CN12)
Glossopharyngeal nerve (CN9)
Styloid process
Accessory nerve (CN11)
Vagus nerve (CN10)
Internal carotid artery
Carotid sheath
Internal jugular vein
Deep layer, deep cervical fascia
Superficial layer, deep cervical fascia
Lateral retropharyngeal space
Parapharyngeal space
Nasopharyngeal carotid space
Perivertebral space

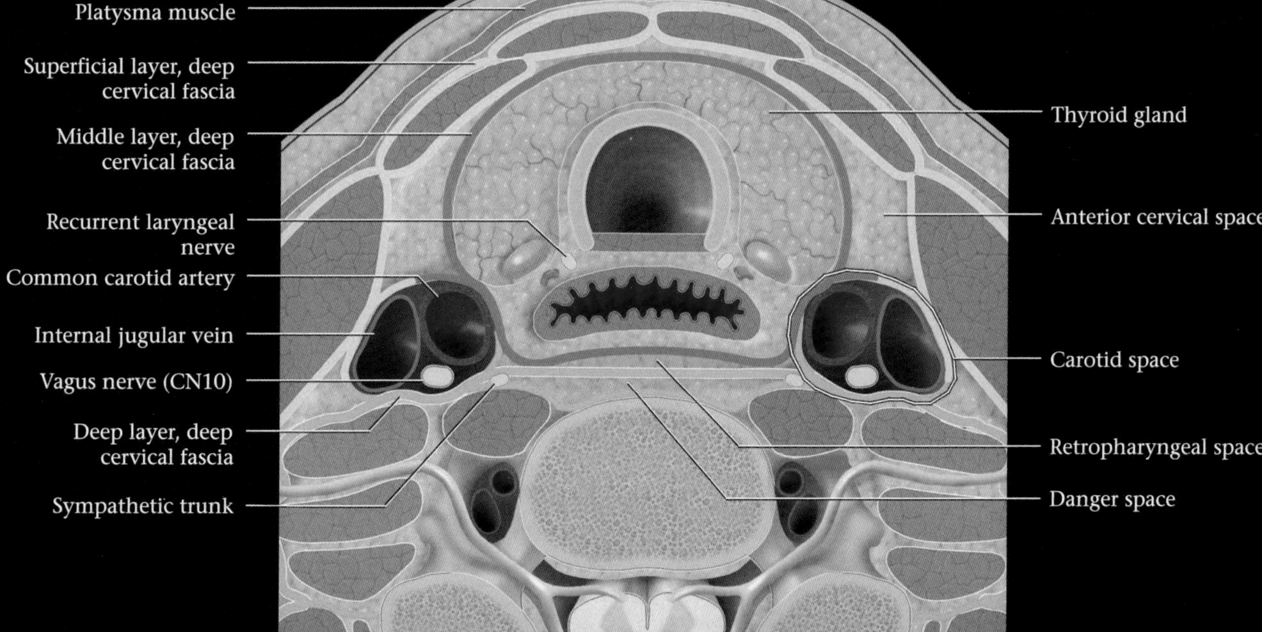
Platysma muscle
Superficial layer, deep cervical fascia
Middle layer, deep cervical fascia
Recurrent laryngeal nerve
Common carotid artery
Internal jugular vein
Vagus nerve (CN10)
Deep layer, deep cervical fascia
Sympathetic trunk
Thyroid gland
Anterior cervical space
Carotid space
Retropharyngeal space
Danger space

(Top) Axial graphic of the suprahyoid neck at the level of C1 vertebral body with insert showing magnified carotid space. The suprahyoid carotid space contains CN9-12, the internal carotid artery & the internal jugular vein. The carotid sheath is made up of components of all 3 layers of deep cervical fascia (tri-color line around carotid space). In the suprahyoid neck the carotid sheath is less substantial than in the infrahyoid neck. The sympathetic trunk runs just medial to the carotid space. **(Bottom)** Axial graphic of the carotid space in the infrahyoid neck. Note that the carotid sheath contains all 3 layers of the deep cervical fascia (tri-color line). In the infrahyoid neck the carotid sheath is tenacious throughout its length. The infrahyoid carotid space contains the common carotid artery, internal jugular vein and only the vagus cranial nerve.

CAROTID SPACE

GRAPHICS

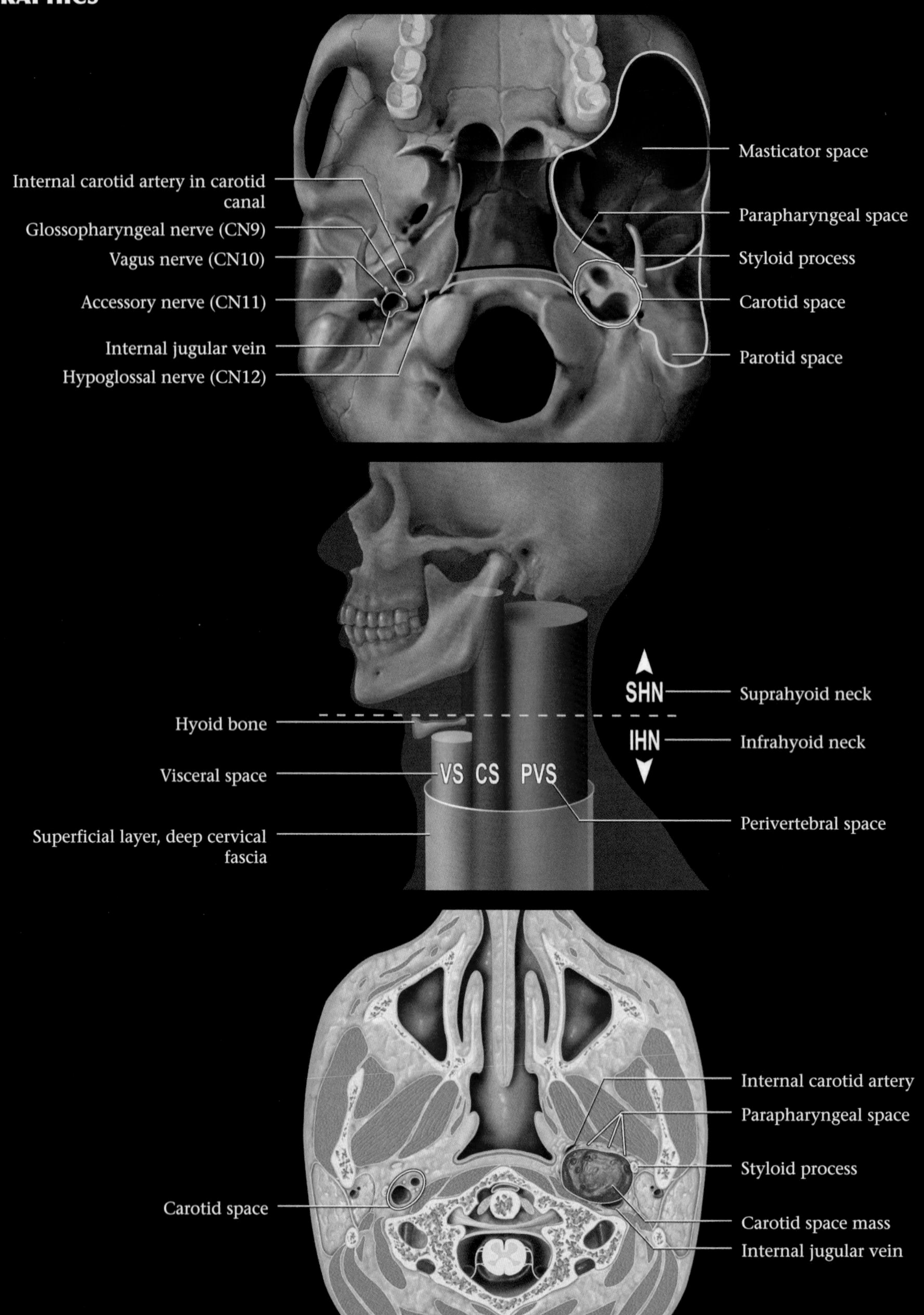
Internal carotid artery in carotid canal
Glossopharyngeal nerve (CN9)
Vagus nerve (CN10)
Accessory nerve (CN11)
Internal jugular vein
Hypoglossal nerve (CN12)
Masticator space
Parapharyngeal space
Styloid process
Carotid space
Parotid space
Hyoid bone
Visceral space
Superficial layer, deep cervical fascia
SHN
IHN
VS
CS
PVS
Suprahyoid neck
Infrahyoid neck
Perivertebral space
Carotid space
Internal carotid artery
Parapharyngeal space
Styloid process
Carotid space mass
Internal jugular vein

(Top) Axial graphic of skull base viewed from below illustrating the interaction between the carotid space & the skull base. The nasopharyngeal CS is inferior continuation of carotid canal, jugular foramen & hypoglossal canal. Internal carotid artery, internal jugular vein & CN9-12 are found within CS. The carotid sheath is depicted as a tri-color line because it is formed from all 3 layers of deep cervical fascia. **(Middle)** Lateral oblique graphic of the neck showing the CS as a tube running from skull base to the aortic arch. The CS is divided at hyoid bone level into a suprahyoid & infrahyoid portions. Suprahyoid CS has CN9-12 within it & the infrahyoid CS has only vagus nerve inside. **(Bottom)** Axial graphic shows a generic CS mass. A CS mass displaces the parapharyngeal space fat anteriorly as well as lifts the styloid process anterolaterally.

CECT & MRA OF CS VESSELS

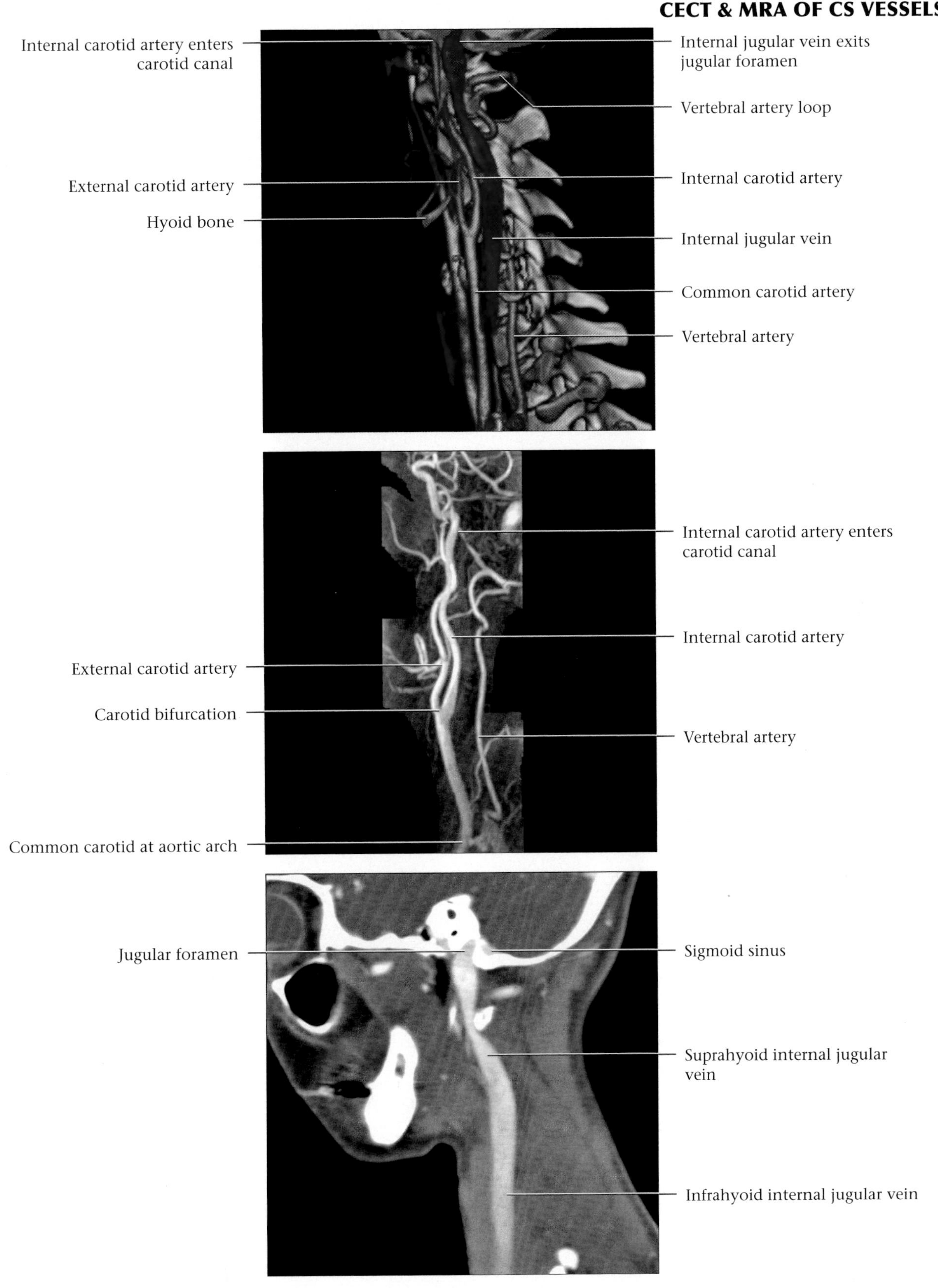
Internal carotid artery enters carotid canal
Internal jugular vein exits jugular foramen
Vertebral artery loop
External carotid artery
Internal carotid artery
Hyoid bone
Internal jugular vein
Common carotid artery
Vertebral artery
Internal carotid artery enters carotid canal
Internal carotid artery
External carotid artery
Carotid bifurcation
Vertebral artery
Common carotid at aortic arch
Jugular foramen
Sigmoid sinus
Suprahyoid internal jugular vein
Infrahyoid internal jugular vein

(Top) Lateral view 3D-VRT CECT reconstruction of major vessels of the neck. The hyoid bone is approximately at the level of the carotid bifurcation with the internal carotid artery found in the suprahyoid carotid space and the common carotid artery found within the infrahyoid carotid space. **(Middle)** Lateral view of extracranial MRA shows the carotid artery from the arch below to the supraclinoid area above. Remember that the carotid artery extends in the carotid space throughout this entire distance. **(Bottom)** Sagittal reformation of CECT of the extracranial head and neck shows the internal jugular vein from its emergence from the jugular foramen above to the clavicle level below. Thrombosis of this vessel can mimic infection (acute thrombophlebitis) or tumor (chronic thrombosis).

AXIAL CECT

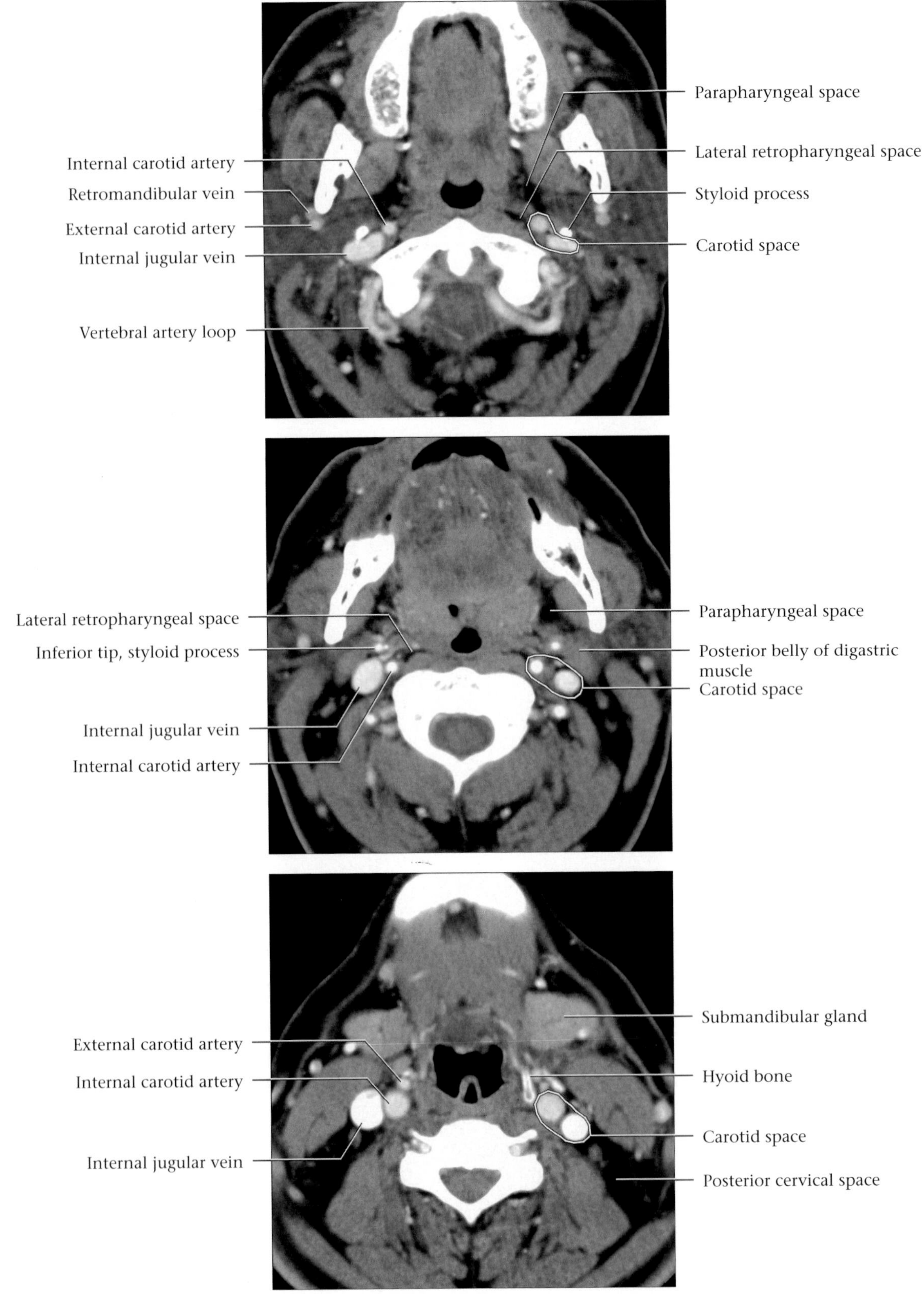

Internal carotid artery
Retromandibular vein
External carotid artery
Internal jugular vein
Vertebral artery loop
Parapharyngeal space
Lateral retropharyngeal space
Styloid process
Carotid space
Lateral retropharyngeal space
Inferior tip, styloid process
Internal jugular vein
Internal carotid artery
Parapharyngeal space
Posterior belly of digastric muscle
Carotid space
External carotid artery
Internal carotid artery
Internal jugular vein
Submandibular gland
Hyoid bone
Carotid space
Posterior cervical space

(Top) First of six axial CECT images presented from superior to inferior. In this image at the level of C1 vertebral body the nasopharyngeal carotid space contains the internal carotid artery, internal jugular vein and CN9-12. Notice that the CS is posterior to the styloid process. At the level of the nasopharynx a carotid space mass will push from posterior to anterior into the parapharyngeal space and displace the styloid process anterolaterally. **(Middle)** In this image at the level of the mid-oropharynx the posterior belly of the digastric muscle is visible anterolateral to the carotid space. A CS mass here would push this muscle anterolaterally and the parapharyngeal space anteriorly. **(Bottom)** At the level of the hyoid bone the carotid bifurcation can be seen. At this level only the vagus nerve is left within the CS.

CAROTID SPACE

AXIAL CECT

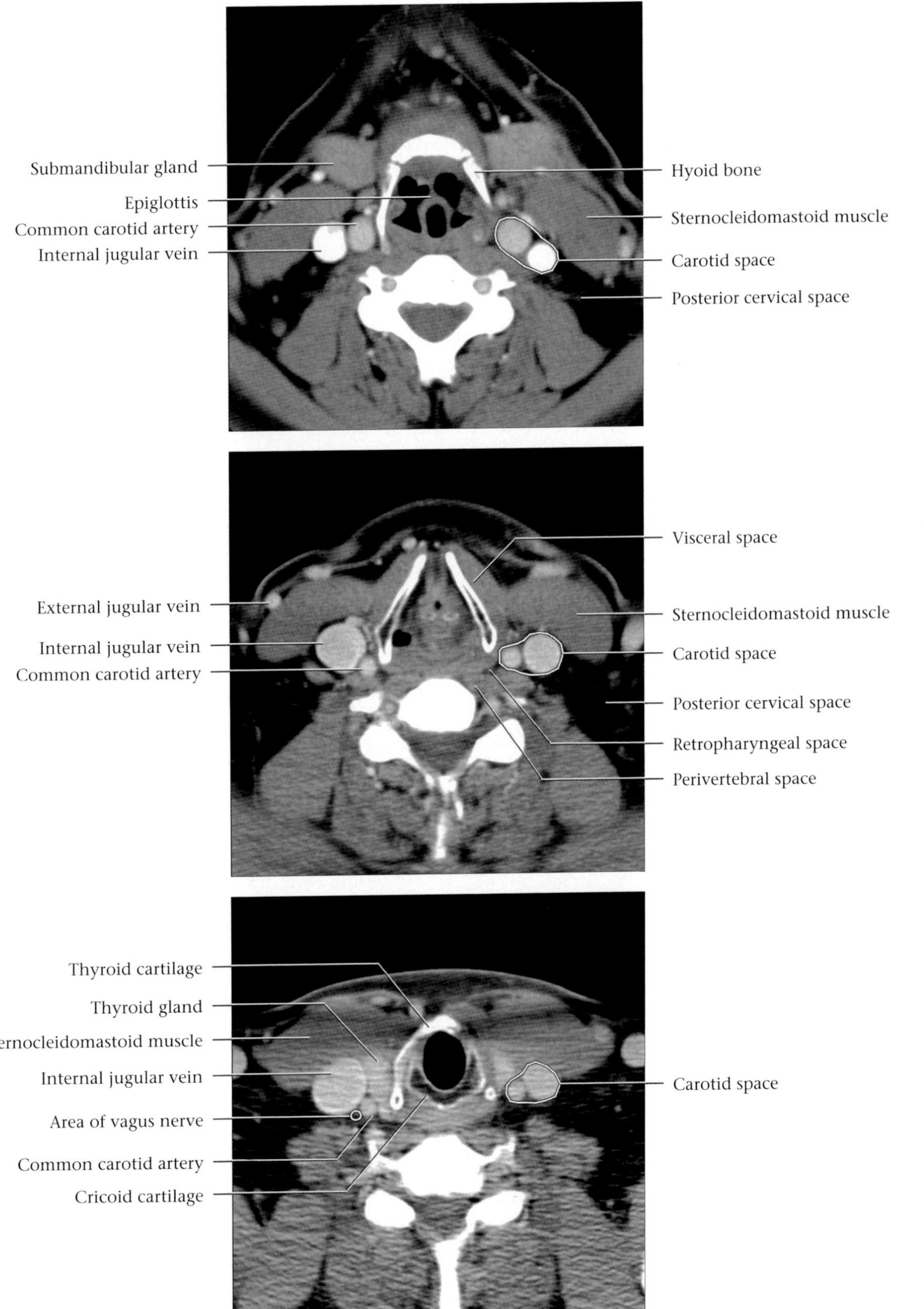
Submandibular gland
Epiglottis
Common carotid artery
Internal jugular vein
Hyoid bone
Sternocleidomastoid muscle
Carotid space
Posterior cervical space
External jugular vein
Internal jugular vein
Common carotid artery
Visceral space
Sternocleidomastoid muscle
Carotid space
Posterior cervical space
Retropharyngeal space
Perivertebral space
Thyroid cartilage
Thyroid gland
Sternocleidomastoid muscle
Internal jugular vein
Area of vagus nerve
Common carotid artery
Cricoid cartilage
Carotid space

(Top) At the level of the hyoid bone the carotid space has only the common carotid artery, internal jugular vein and vagus nerve within it. Notice that despite the high resolution nature of this CT image, it is not possible to see the vagus nerve or the carotid sheath. **(Middle)** In this image through the infrahyoid aspect of the carotid space the surrounding deep tissue anatomy can be seen. Posterolateral to the carotid space the large fat-filled posterior cervical space is visible. Posteromedial the perivertebral space is found. Medial to the CS is the visceral space and the retropharyngeal space. Anteriorly resides the sternocleidomastoid muscle. **(Bottom)** At the level of the cricoid cartilage the infrahyoid carotid space contains the common carotid artery, internal jugular vein and vagus nerve. Despite its large size the vagal trunk cannot be seen.

RETROPHARYNGEAL SPACE

Terminology

Abbreviations

- Retropharyngeal space (RPS)

Definitions

- RPS: Midline space just posterior to pharynx & cervical esophagus running from skull base to T3 vertebral level in mediastinum

Imaging Anatomy

Overview

- RPS is fat-filled space in posterior midline of neck that can be identified on imaging from skull base to upper mediastinum
- Upper-most RPS (nasopharyngeal portion) is "tight"
  - In RPS abscess path of least resistance is inferiorly
- **RPS nodes only found in suprahyoid neck RPS**

Extent

- Skull base to T3 vertebral body level in upper mediastinum

Anatomy Relationships

- **Suprahyoid neck (SHN) RPS**
  - Pharyngeal mucosal space (PMS) is anterior
  - Danger space (DS) is directly posterior to RPS
  - Carotid space is lateral to RPS
- **Infrahyoid neck (IHN) RPS**
  - Hypopharynx & cervical esophagus are anterior
  - Danger space is directly posterior to RPS
    - RPS empties via "fascial trap door" into DS inferiorly at ~ T3 level
  - Carotid space is lateral to RPS

Internal Structures-Critical Contents

- **Suprahyoid neck RPS** (skull base to hyoid bone)
  - Fat is primary occupant of SHN RPS
  - **RPS lymph nodes**
    - **Lateral group**: Also called nodes of Rouviere
    - **Medial group**: Less often visible on imaging
- **Infrahyoid neck RPS** (hyoid bone to T3 vertebral body in mediastinum)
  - **Fat only** in IHN RPS
  - No RPS nodes below hyoid bone!

Fascia of Retropharyngeal Space

- RPS has complex fascial margins
- Anterior wall fascia: Middle layer, deep cervical fascia
  - Fascia is just behind constrictor muscle of pharyngeal mucosal space
- Posterior wall fascia: Deep layer, deep cervical fascia
  - Fascia is just anterior to prevertebral muscles of perivertebral space
  - Two slips present with danger space between
- Lateral fascial wall: Slip of deep layer, deep cervical fascial called **alar fascia**
- **Median raphe** divides RPS into two halves
  - Relatively weak fascial slip that is present more consistently in superior RPS

Anatomy-Based Imaging Issues

Key Concepts or Questions

- What radiologic findings define a lesion as primary to retropharyngeal space?
  - **Unilateral-nodal SHN mass**
    - Centered posteromedial to parapharyngeal space (PPS) & directly medial to carotid space
    - Encroaches on PPS from posteromedial to anterolateral (mimics carotid space mass)
  - **"Extranodal" mass in SHN or IHN** (pus or tumor filling RPS)
    - Rectangular-shaped mass centered behind PMS
    - Mass anterior to prevertebral muscles
    - Mass flattens & remains anterior to prevertebral muscles as it enlarges
    - Contrast with perivertebral space mass which elevates prevertebral muscles as it enlarges
- **SHN RPS lesion imaging appearances**
  - Lesion begins most commonly in RPS nodes
  - Seen on CT or MR as unilateral RPS mass
  - If extranodal disease (edema, infection or tumor), will fill RPS from side to side
- **IHN RPS lesion imaging appearances**
  - Originates in SHN RPS, spreads inferiorly into IHN
  - Fills entire IHN RPS from side to side
  - Remember to look at SHN RPS if you find IHN RPS disease

Imaging Approaches

- **CECT best** imaging tool in evaluation of **RPS infection**
- **MR imaging** far more sensitive to presence of **RPS tumor adenopathy**

Imaging Pitfalls

- RPS & DS are indistinguishable on CT or MR imaging
  - Best to consider DS as conduit for RPS disease into mediastinum only
    - Otherwise, describe lesions in RPS only & ignore DS from imaging perspective
- Lateral RPS nodal mass may mimic carotid space mass
  - Look for mass medial to carotid space (CS)
  - Mass displacement of CS is posterolaterally
  - Both RPS & CS displace parapharyngeal space anteriorly
- Not all fluid in RPS is abscess
  - Internal jugular vein thrombosis & longus colli tendonitis can both cause RPS edema
  - Non-abscess fluid: No enhancement of wall; minimal mass effect

Clinical Implications

Clinical Importance

- RPS nodes are seeded by pharyngitis
  - Once seeded they react, suppurate & eventually rupture to create RPS abscess
- Squamous cell carcinoma of nasopharynx and posterior wall of oropharynx & hypopharynx drain into RPS nodal chain

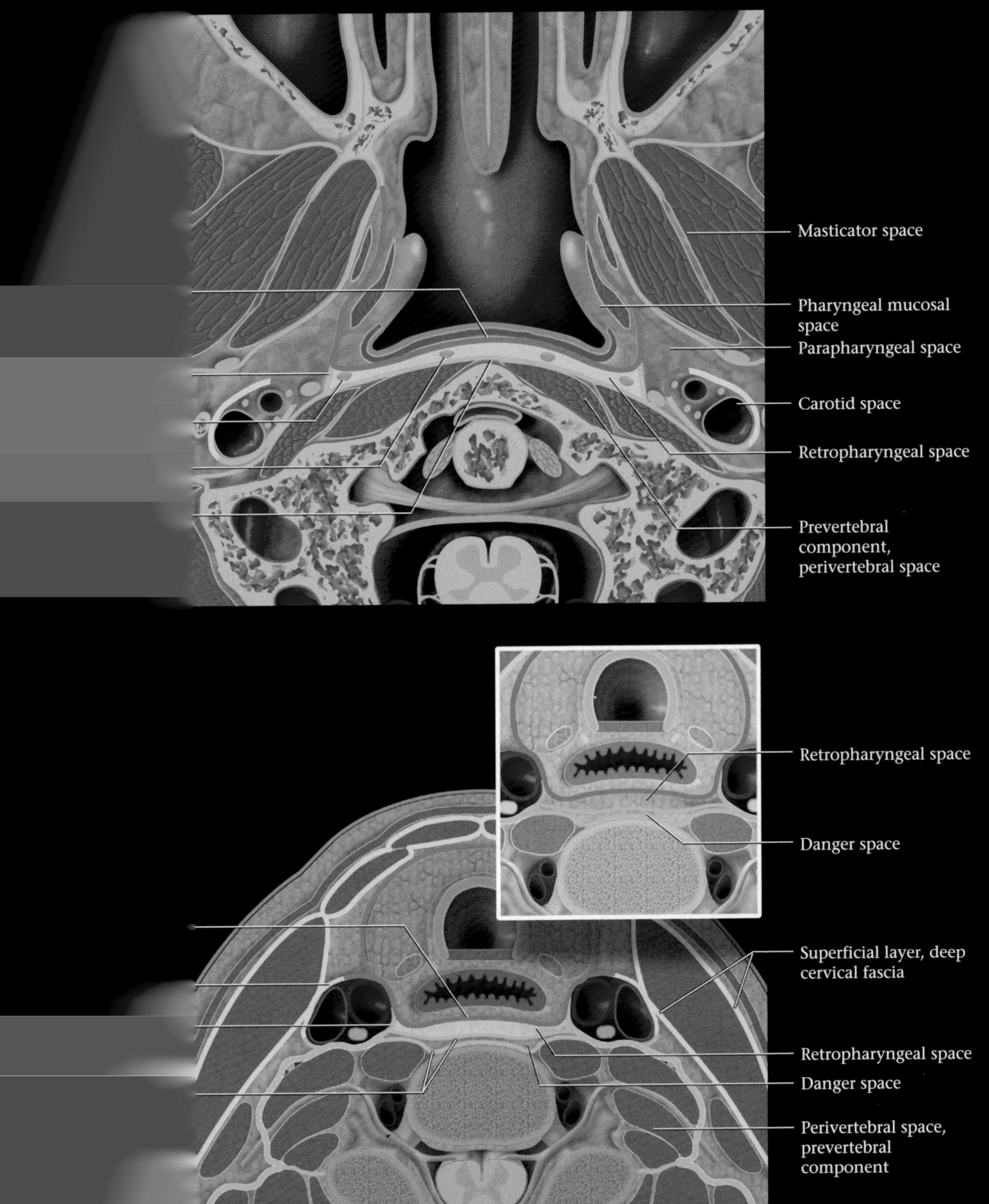
Masticator space
Pharyngeal mucosal space
Parapharyngeal space
Carotid space
Retropharyngeal space
Prevertebral component, perivertebral space
Retropharyngeal space
Danger space
Superficial layer, deep cervical fascia
Retropharyngeal space
Danger space
Perivertebral space, prevertebral component

retropharyngeal space in suprahyoid neck. In the suprahyoid neck the retropharyngeal
ral retropharyngeal nodes. Notice the middle layer of deep cervical fascia is the anterior
e deep layer of deep cervical fascia is the posterior border. The lateral wall is a slip of the
fascia. **(Bottom)** Axial graphic depicting the fascia that make up the borders of the
er spaces in the infrahyoid neck. The deep layer of deep cervical fascia is important as it
all of the retropharyngeal space, both the anterior and posterior wall of the danger space
h spaces (alar fascia). Notice that there is only fat in the infrahyoid RPS. Nodes are only

RETROPHARYNGEAL SPACE

GRAPHICS

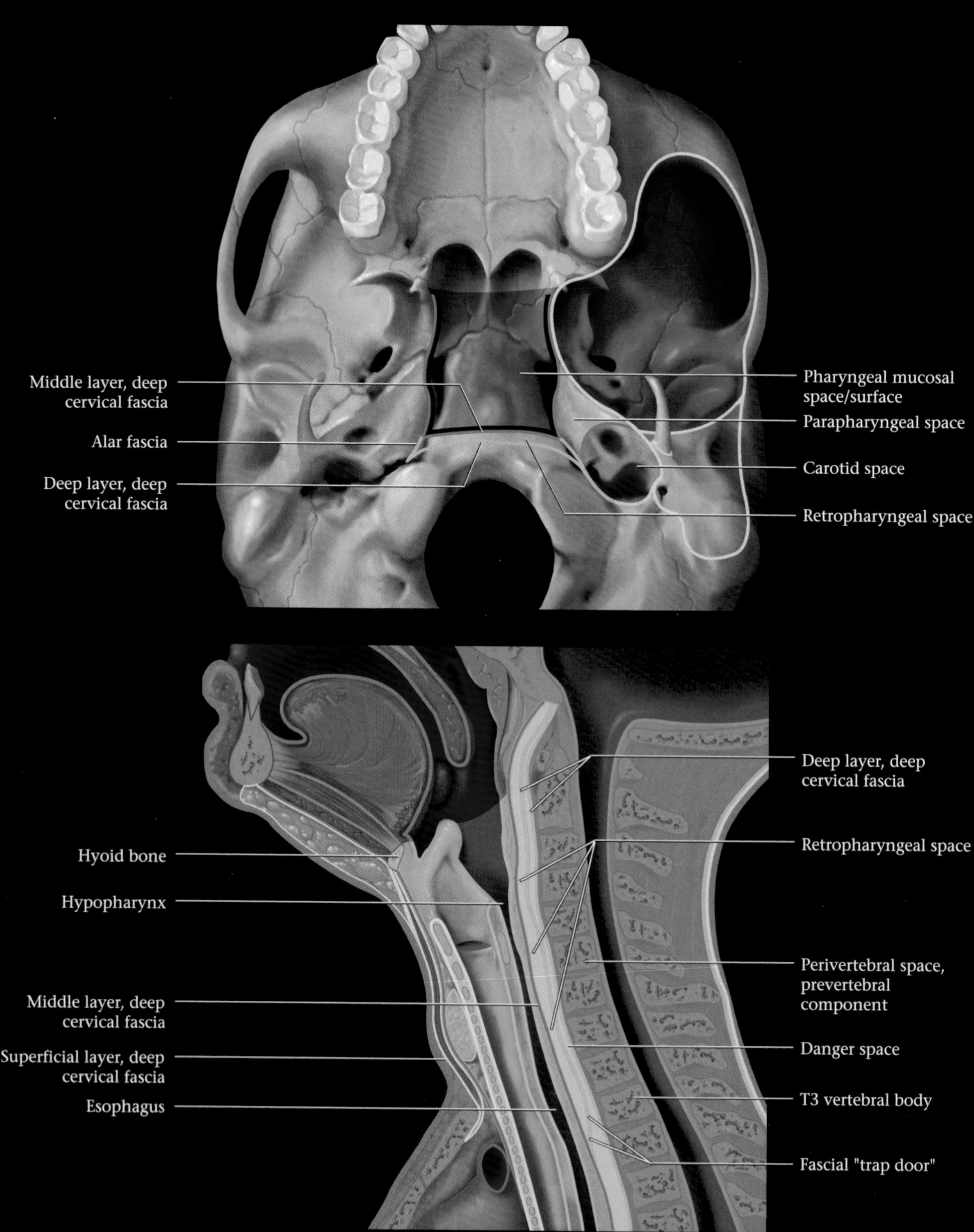
Middle layer, deep cervical fascia
Alar fascia
Deep layer, deep cervical fascia
Pharyngeal mucosal space/surface
Parapharyngeal space
Carotid space
Retropharyngeal space
Hyoid bone
Hypopharynx
Middle layer, deep cervical fascia
Superficial layer, deep cervical fascia
Esophagus
Deep layer, deep cervical fascia
Retropharyngeal space
Perivertebral space, prevertebral component
Danger space
T3 vertebral body
Fascial "trap door"

(Top) Axial graphic of skull base from below showing the abutment of the retropharyngeal space with the skull base. Notice that the retropharyngeal space abuts the external surface of the basiocciput in an area where there are no foramina. **(Bottom)** Sagittal graphic depicting longitudinal spatial relationships of the infrahyoid neck with emphasis on the retropharyngeal and danger spaces. Seen just anterior to the vertebral column the retropharyngeal and danger spaces run inferiorly from the skull base towards the mediastinum. Notice the fascial "trap door" found at the approximate level of T3 vertebral body that serves as a conduit from the retropharyngeal to the danger space. Retropharyngeal space infection or tumor may access the mediastinum via this route of spread.

AXIAL SHN RPS GENERIC MASS

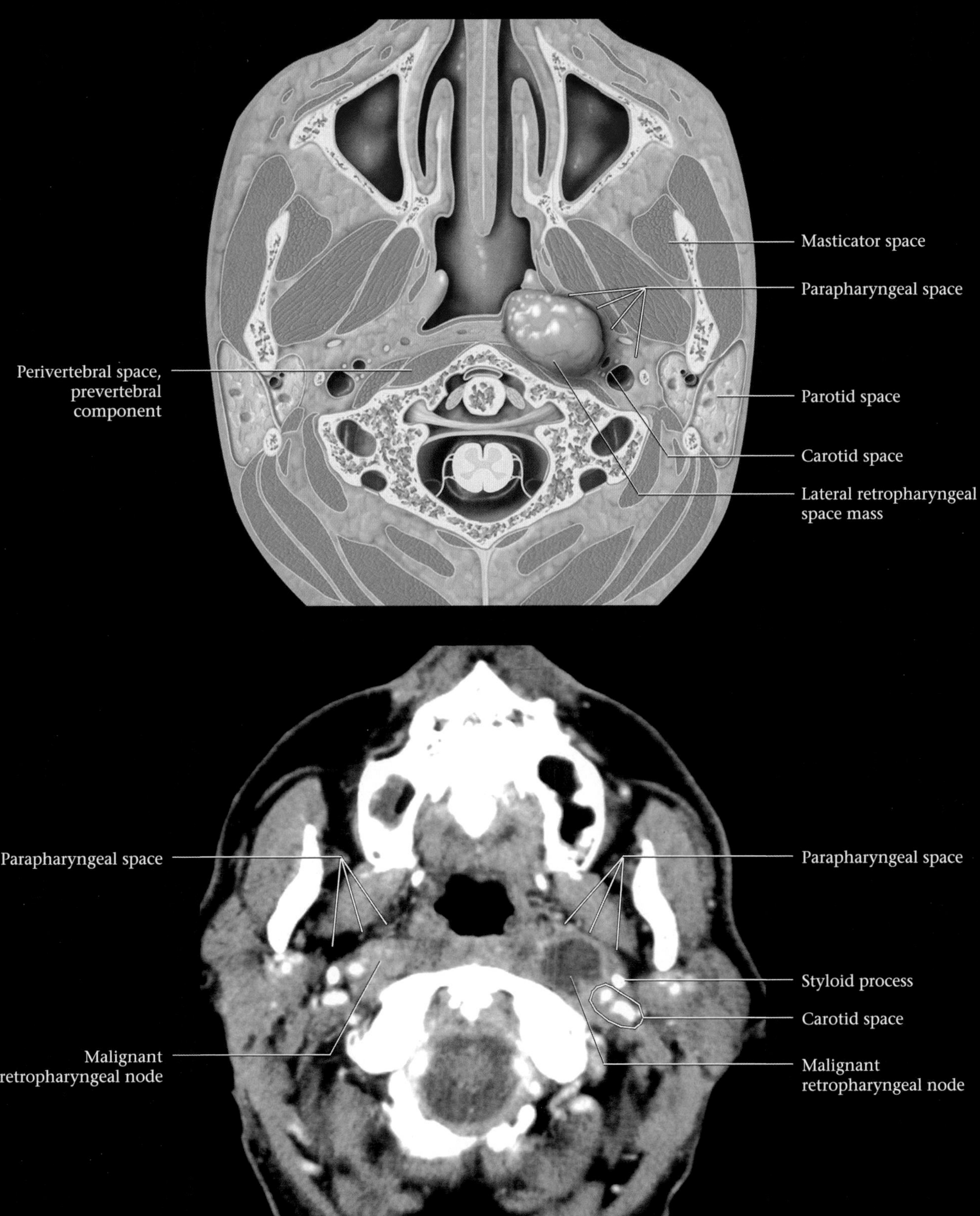
Masticator space
Parapharyngeal space
Perivertebral space, prevertebral component
Parotid space
Carotid space
Lateral retropharyngeal space mass
Parapharyngeal space
Parapharyngeal space
Styloid process
Carotid space
Malignant retropharyngeal node
Malignant retropharyngeal node

(Top) Axial graphic depicting a generic mass beginning in the lateral retropharyngeal nodal group of the retropharyngeal space. Notice that the lateral retropharyngeal space mass displaces the carotid space posterolaterally and the parapharyngeal space anteriorly. This mass lesion can be mistaken for a carotid space mass if the imager is not cognizant of its more medial location. **(Bottom)** Axial enhanced CT at the level of the low nasopharynx reveals bilateral malignant lateral retropharyngeal lymph nodes from a posterior oropharyngeal wall squamous cell carcinoma (not shown). The larger left-sided necrotic node displaces the parapharyngeal space anteriorly and the carotid space posterolaterally. The smaller right-sided node has not yet caused significant mass effect on either the parapharyngeal or carotid spaces.

AXIAL IHN RPS GENERIC MASS

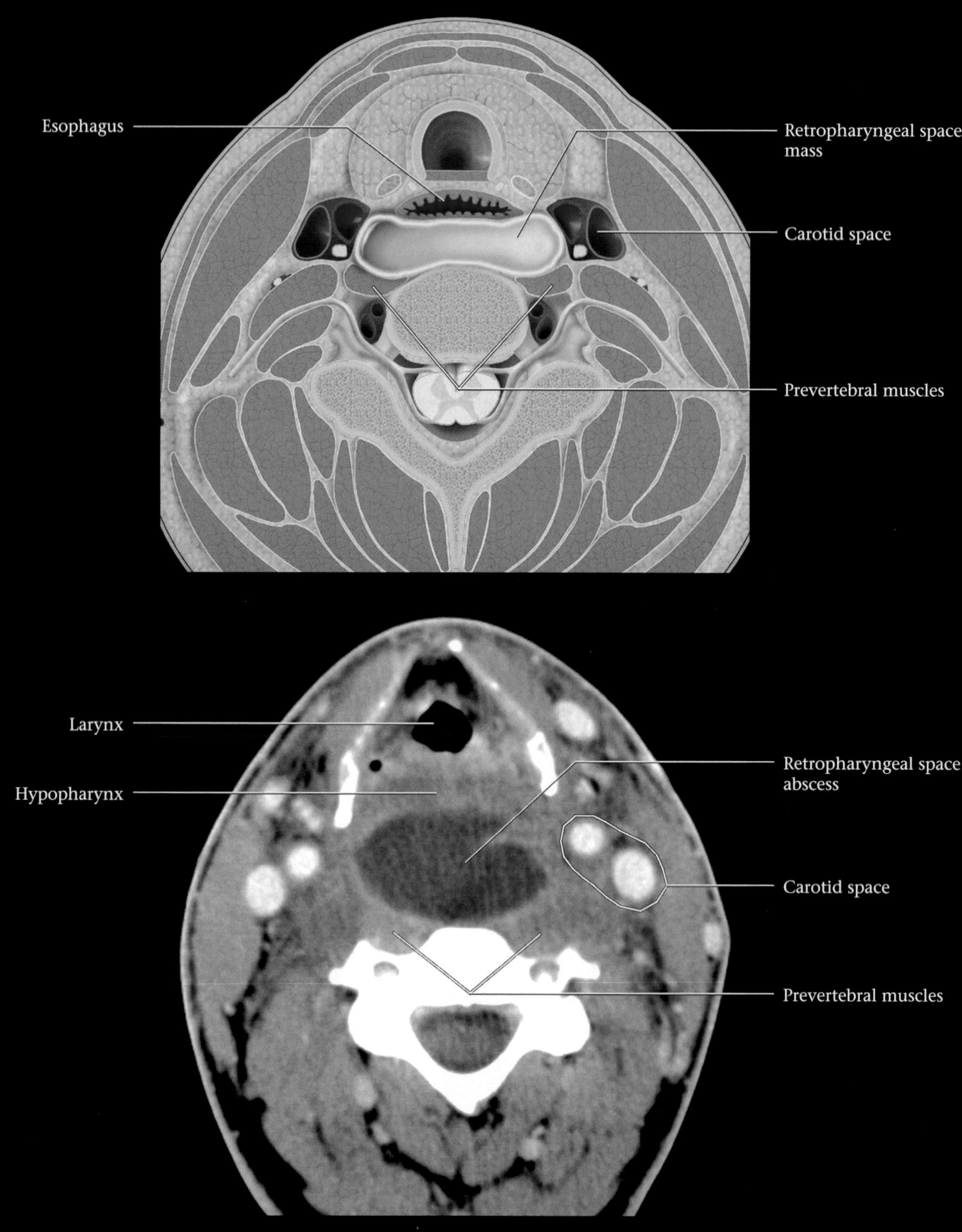

Esophagus
Retropharyngeal space mass
Carotid space
Prevertebral muscles
Larynx
Hypopharynx
Retropharyngeal space abscess
Carotid space
Prevertebral muscles

(Top) Axial graphic of generic retropharyngeal space mass lesion in the infrahyoid neck. Note the anterior displacement of the visceral space and the lateral displacement of the carotid spaces. The prevertebral muscles are flattened, not elevated. **(Bottom)** Axial enhanced CT at the level of the infrahyoid neck supraglottic larynx demonstrates an abscess filling the retropharyngeal space. This ovoid-shaped abscess displaces the visceral space (hypopharynx/larynx) anteriorly and the carotid spaces laterally. The prevertebral muscles are posterior to the abscess cavity.

AXIAL CECT

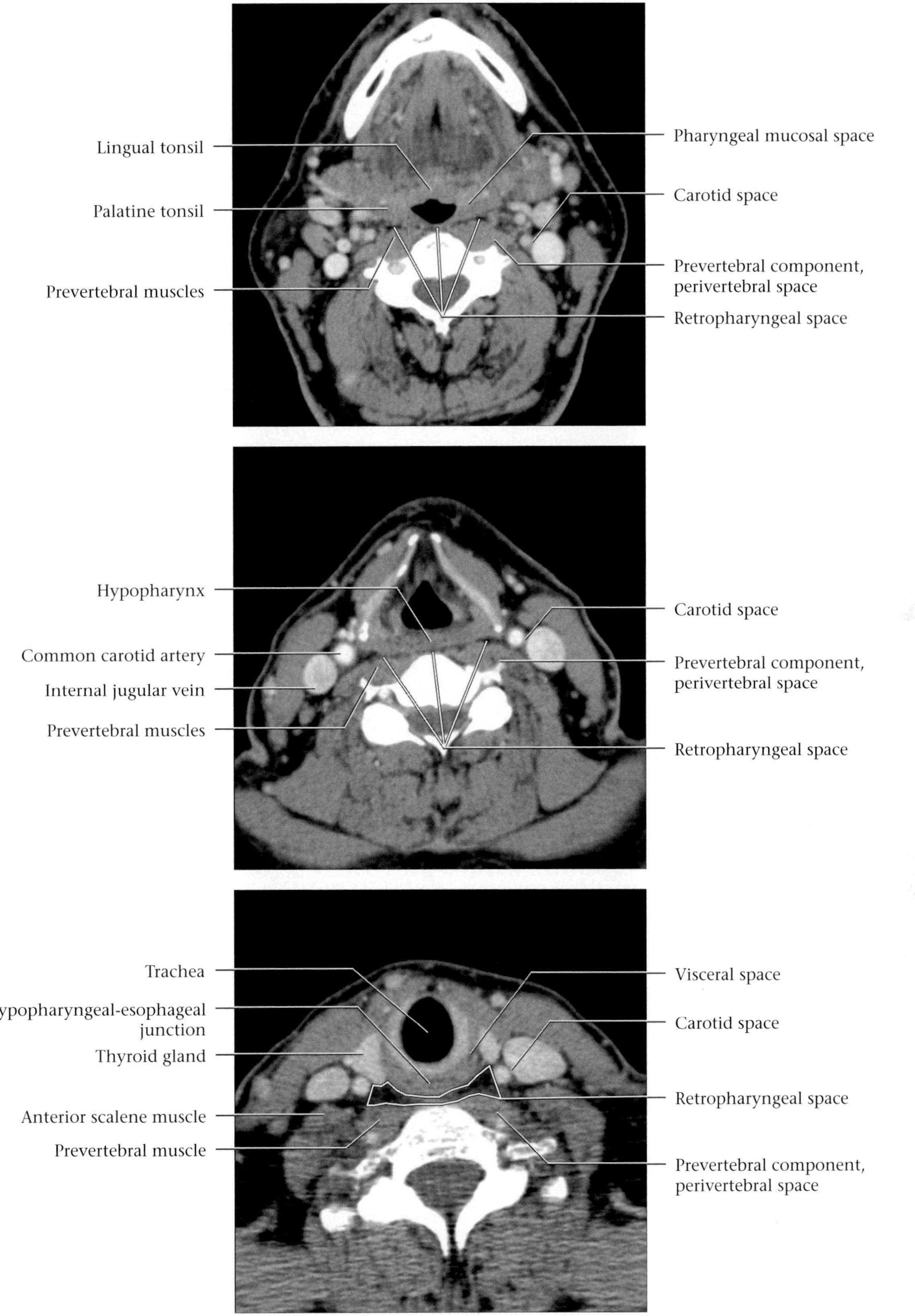

Lingual tonsil
Palatine tonsil
Prevertebral muscles
Pharyngeal mucosal space
Carotid space
Prevertebral component, perivertebral space
Retropharyngeal space
Hypopharynx
Common carotid artery
Internal jugular vein
Prevertebral muscles
Carotid space
Prevertebral component, perivertebral space
Retropharyngeal space
Trachea
Hypopharyngeal-esophageal junction
Thyroid gland
Anterior scalene muscle
Prevertebral muscle
Visceral space
Carotid space
Retropharyngeal space
Prevertebral component, perivertebral space

(Top) First of three axial CECT images of the neck. This image at the level of the low oropharynx shows the stripe of fat behind the pharyngeal mucosal space that represents the retropharyngeal space. Posterior to the retropharyngeal space is the prevertebral portion of the perivertebral space. Lateral to it are the carotid spaces. **(Middle)** In this image at the level of the supraglottis the stripe of fat behind the larynx & hypopharynx is the retropharyngeal space. The carotid spaces are at the lateral margin of the RPS bilaterally. **(Bottom)** At the level of the mid-infrahyoid neck the retropharyngeal space is larger and more obvious than in the suprahyoid neck. Anterior is the visceral space with the hypopharyngeal-esophageal junction abutting the RPS. The prevertebral component of the perivertebral space is posterior to the RPS.

AXIAL T1 MR

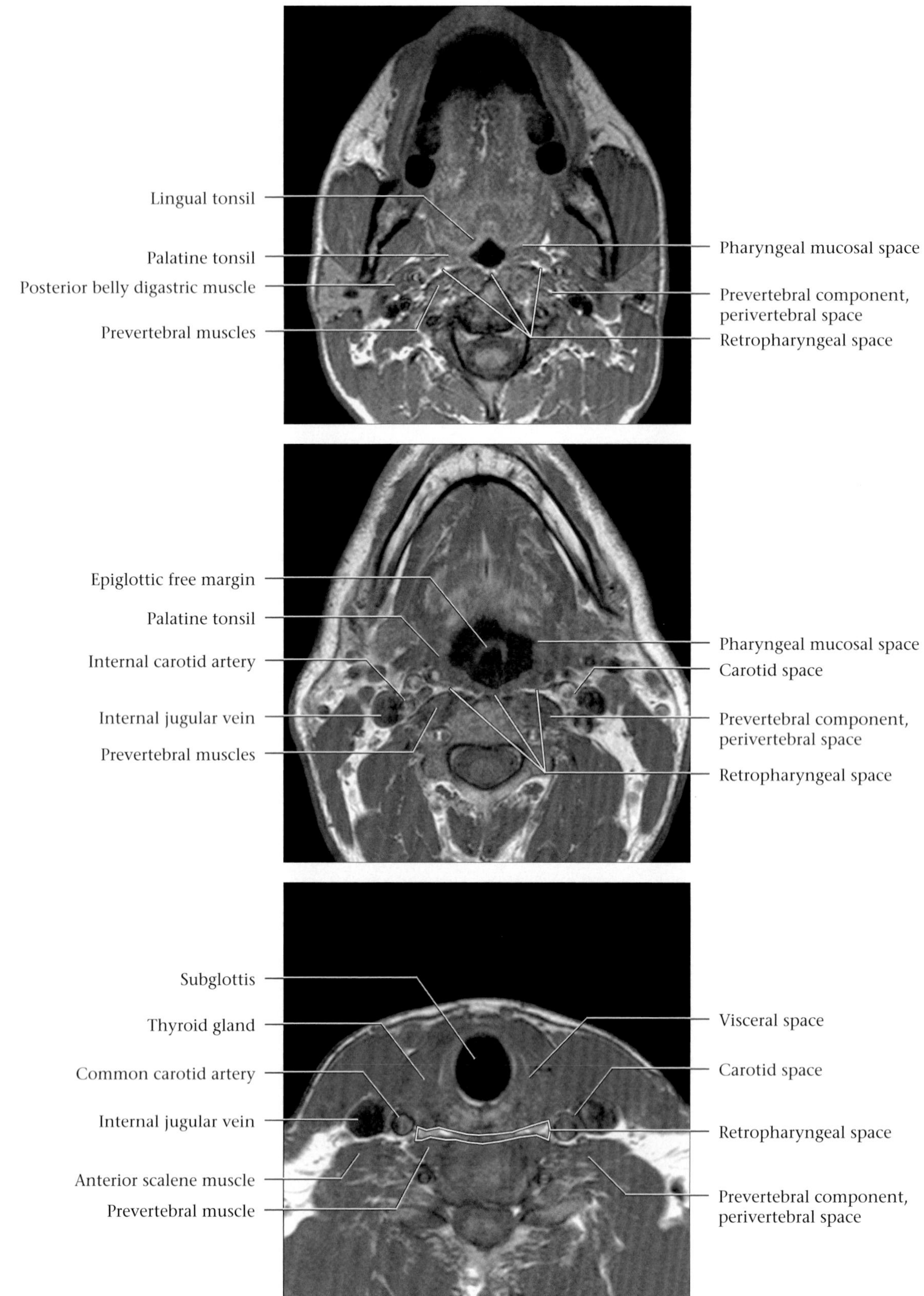

Lingual tonsil
Palatine tonsil
Posterior belly digastric muscle
Prevertebral muscles
Pharyngeal mucosal space
Prevertebral component, perivertebral space
Retropharyngeal space
Epiglottic free margin
Palatine tonsil
Internal carotid artery
Internal jugular vein
Prevertebral muscles
Pharyngeal mucosal space
Carotid space
Prevertebral component, perivertebral space
Retropharyngeal space
Subglottis
Thyroid gland
Common carotid artery
Internal jugular vein
Anterior scalene muscle
Prevertebral muscle
Visceral space
Carotid space
Retropharyngeal space
Prevertebral component, perivertebral space

(Top) First of three axial T1 MR images of the extracranial head and neck. This image at the level of the oropharynx shows a thin stripe of high signal fat behind the pharyngeal mucosal space that represents the retropharyngeal space. Posterior to the retropharyngeal space is the prevertebral portion of the perivertebral space. **(Middle)** In this image at the level of the low oropharynx, the high signal stripe of fat behind the oropharyngeal mucosal space is the retropharyngeal space. The carotid spaces are at the lateral margin of the RPS bilaterally. The prevertebral muscles in the perivertebral space are directly posterior to the RPS. **(Bottom)** In this image at the level of the mid-infrahyoid neck the RPS is easily seen between the carotid spaces. The visceral space is anterior and the prevertebral component of the perivertebral space posterior to the RPS.

AXIAL BONE CT & T2 MR

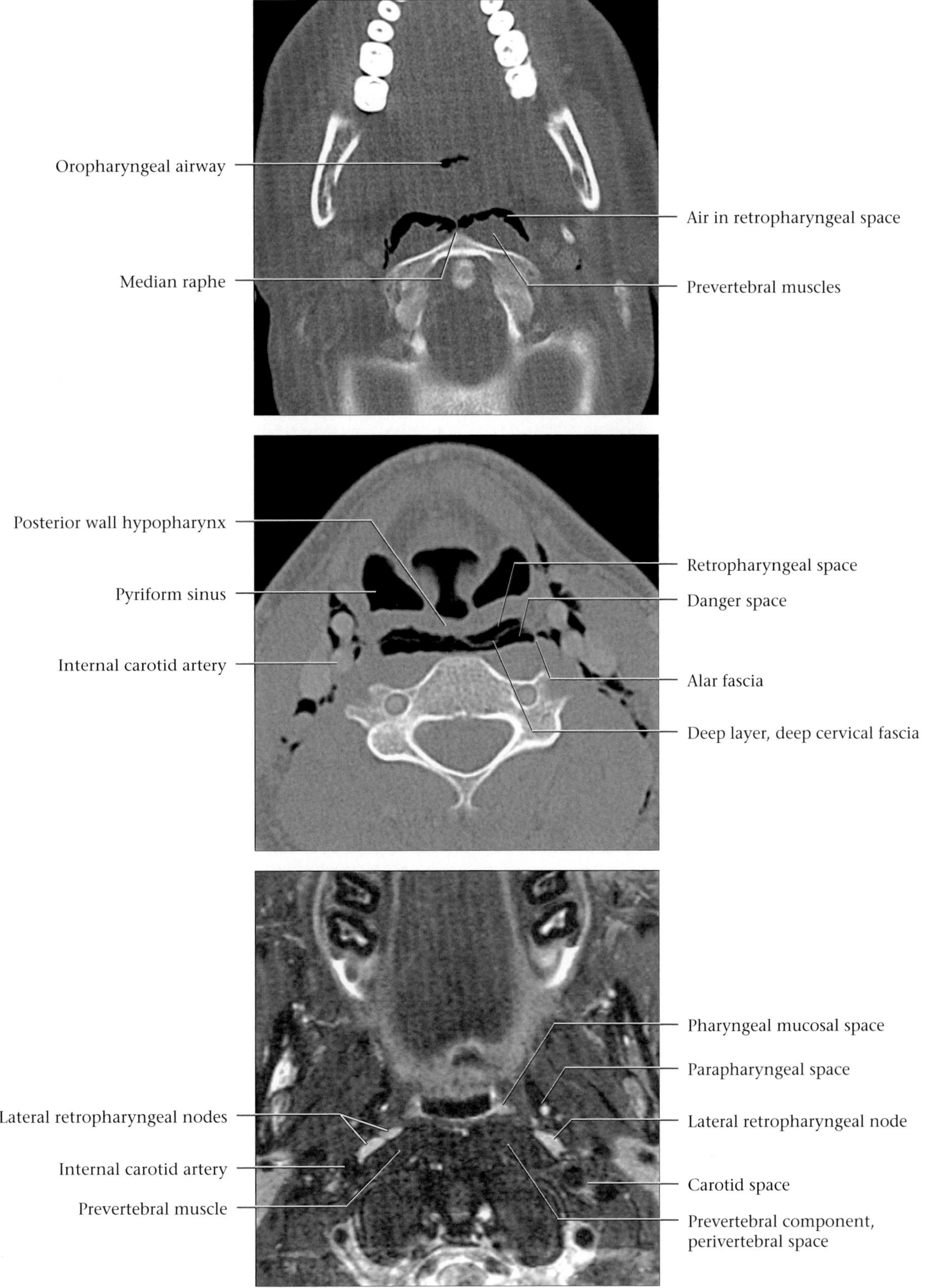
Oropharyngeal airway
Air in retropharyngeal space
Median raphe
Prevertebral muscles
Posterior wall hypopharynx
Retropharyngeal space
Pyriform sinus
Danger space
Internal carotid artery
Alar fascia
Deep layer, deep cervical fascia
Pharyngeal mucosal space
Parapharyngeal space
Lateral retropharyngeal nodes
Lateral retropharyngeal node
Internal carotid artery
Carotid space
Prevertebral muscle
Prevertebral component, perivertebral space

(Top) Axial bone CT through mid-oropharynx in a trauma patient shows air has collected in the retropharyngeal space, allowing the median raphe to be seen. The median raphe functions as an attachment of the constrictor muscles. In addition it provides an initial barrier to spread of disease from side to side in the retropharyngeal space. **(Middle)** Axial bone CT at level of the supraglottis in trauma patient shows air in the retropharyngeal and danger spaces. Air allows identification of the lateral alar fascia and the anterior slip of deep layer of deep cervical fascia that separates these 2 spaces. **(Bottom)** Axial fat-saturated T2 MR through the low nasopharynx in a young adolescent reveals normal lateral RPS nodes bilaterally. Notice these nodes are positioned just medial to the internal carotid artery and posteromedial to the fat-saturated parapharyngeal space.

PERIVERTEBRAL SPACE

Terminology

Abbreviations

- Perivertebral space (PVS)

Synonyms

- Perivertebral space: Prevertebral space
  - Historic prevertebral space term include soft tissues behind vertebral column
  - Perivertebral space term adopted to include all tissues under deep layer of deep cervical fascia (DL-DCF), both in front of & behind vertebral column

Definitions

- **PVS**: Cylindrical space surrounding vertebral column extending from skull base to upper mediastinum bounded by deep layer, deep cervical fascia subdivided into prevertebral & paraspinal components
- Perivertebral space: Peri (Gr. for around) the vertebra

Imaging Anatomy

Extent

- PVS extends from skull base above to T4 in posterior mediastinum
- Some anatomists describe PVS as discrete anatomic space to level of coccyx

Anatomy Relationships

- **PVS consists of 2 major components**
  - Prevertebral portion or space
  - Paraspinal portion or space
- **Prevertebral-PVS** sits directly behind retropharyngeal throughout extracranial H&N
  - Anterolateral to prevertebral-PVS is carotid space
  - Lateral to prevertebral-PVS is anterior aspect of posterior cervical space
- **Paraspinal-PVS** is deep to posterior cervical space & posterior to transverse processes of cervical spine

Internal Structures-Critical Contents

- **Prevertebral-PVS or prevertebral space**
  - Prevertebral muscles (longus colli & capitis)
  - Scalene muscles (anterior, middle & posterior)
  - Brachial plexus roots
  - Phrenic nerve (C3-C5)
  - Vertebral artery & vein
  - Vertebral body
- **Paraspinal-PVS or prevertebral space**
  - Paraspinal muscles
  - Posterior elements, vertebral column
- **Brachial plexus** (BP), proximal aspect
  - Brachial plexus has complex spatial anatomy
  - C5-T1 roots leave cervical neural foramina, pass between anterior & middle scalene of prevertebral-PVS
  - BP roots pass through opening in DL-DCF, pass into posterior cervical space on their way to axilla

Fascia of Perivertebral Space

- **DL-DCF completely circumscribes PVS**
  - Anterior portion arches from cervical spine transverse process across prevertebral muscles to opposite transverse process
    - Anterior DL-DCF called "**the carpet**" by surgeons
    - Pharynx slides up & down on this smooth, "carpet-like" surface
    - "Carpet" is tenacious, with infection or tumor of PVS redirected into **epidural space** by this fascia
    - Pharyngeal malignancy blocked from accessing PVS by this tough fascia
  - Posterior portion DL-DCF arches over surface of paraspinal muscles to attach to nuchal ligament of spinous process of vertebral body

Anatomy-Based Imaging Issues

Key Concepts or Questions

- What imaging findings define a mass lesion as primary to prevertebral-PVS?
  - Mass is centered within prevertebral muscles or corpus of vertebral body
  - Mass lifts prevertebral muscles anteriorly (RPS mass pushes them posteriorly)

Imaging Approaches

- Lateral plain film
  - Quick check on prevertebral soft tissue swelling & on integrity of cervical vertebral bodies
- CECT with soft tissue & bone algorithm & sagittal reformation
  - Best exam to look at cervical soft tissue & bones
- Cervical spine MR best to assess epidural disease

Imaging Pitfalls

- **Hypertrophic levator scapulae muscle** (LSM): Mistaken for enhancing mass or recurrent tumor
  - Secondary to CN11 injury (during neck dissection)
    - Sternocleidomastoid (SCM) & trapezius atrophy
    - LSM hypertrophies to help lift arm
  - Imaging findings
    - LSM enlarges, may enhance
    - SCM & trapezius small, fatty infiltrated

Clinical Implications

Clinical Importance

- Prevertebral-PVS contains important structures
  - Proximal brachial plexus, phrenic nerve, vertebral arteries
- Most PVS lesions originate in vertebral body (infection or metastatic tumor)
  - Vertebral body is usually diseased when PVS lesion is found
- Prevertebral-PVS disease may involve epidural space
  - If infection or malignancy breaks out of cervical vertebral body into prevertebra-PVS, 1st obstruction to spread is deep layer of deep cervical fascia
  - Path of least resistance of spreading pus or tumor is deep through neural foramen into epidural space
  - When prevertebral PVS disease is found on imaging, **always check for epidural space extension!**

PERIVERTEBRAL SPACE

GRAPHICS

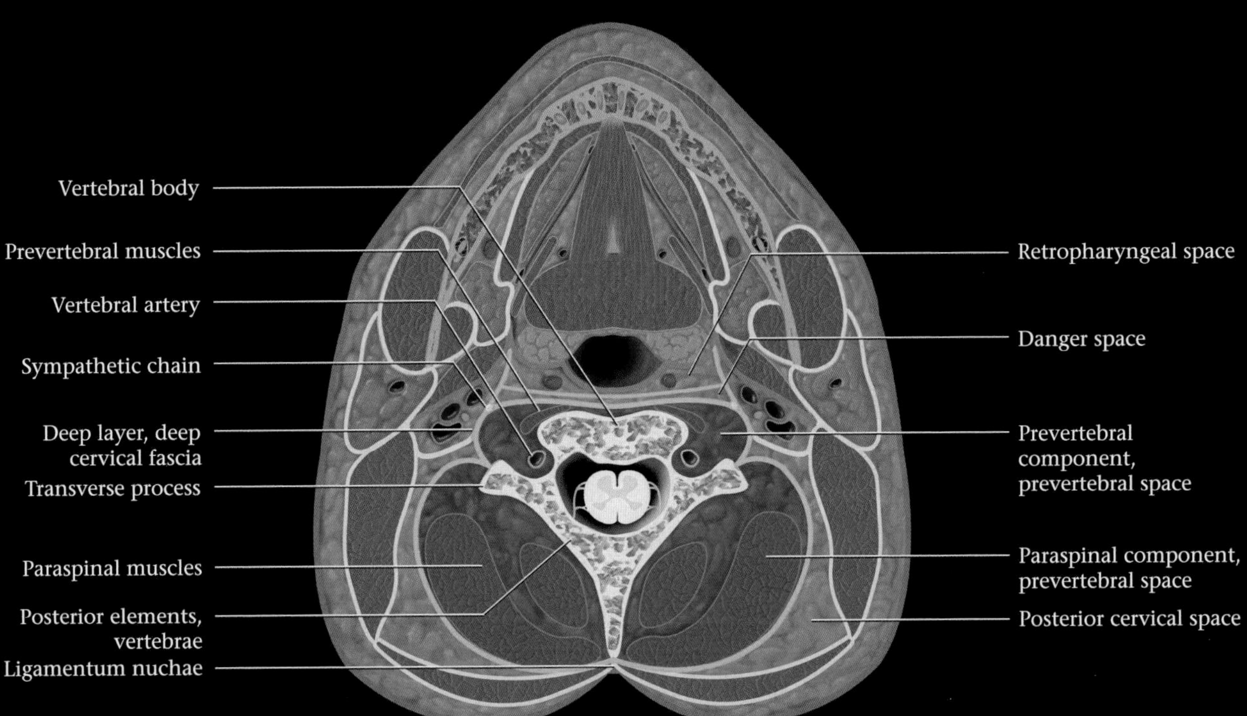
Vertebral body
Prevertebral muscles
Vertebral artery
Sympathetic chain
Deep layer, deep cervical fascia
Transverse process
Paraspinal muscles
Posterior elements, vertebrae
Ligamentum nuchae
Retropharyngeal space
Danger space
Prevertebral component, prevertebral space
Paraspinal component, prevertebral space
Posterior cervical space

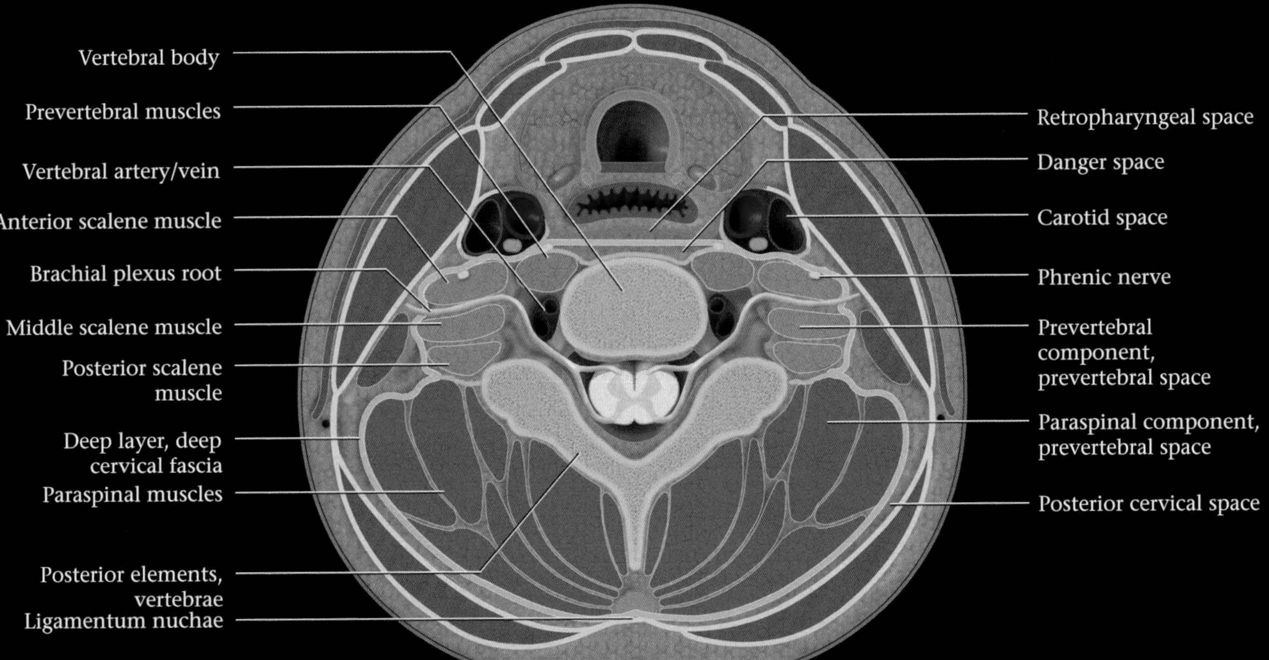
Vertebral body
Prevertebral muscles
Vertebral artery/vein
Anterior scalene muscle
Brachial plexus root
Middle scalene muscle
Posterior scalene muscle
Deep layer, deep cervical fascia
Paraspinal muscles
Posterior elements, vertebrae
Ligamentum nuchae
Retropharyngeal space
Danger space
Carotid space
Phrenic nerve
Prevertebral component, prevertebral space
Paraspinal component, prevertebral space
Posterior cervical space

(Top) Axial graphic through the level of the oropharynx shows prevertebral and paraspinal components of the perivertebral space beneath the deep layer of deep cervical fascia. Notice this fascia curves medially to touch the spinous processes of the vertebral, dividing the perivertebral space into a prevertebral and paraspinal components. The danger and retropharyngeal spaces are anterior to the perivertebral space while the posterior cervical space is lateral and posterior. **(Bottom)** Axial graphic through the thyroid bed shows prevertebral & paraspinal components of the perivertebral space beneath the deep layer of deep cervical fascia. Notice this fascia curves medially to touch the spinous processes of the vertebral, dividing the perivertebral space into a prevertebral and paraspinal components. The prevertebral component is key as it contains brachial plexus roots.

PERIVERTEBRAL SPACE

GRAPHICS

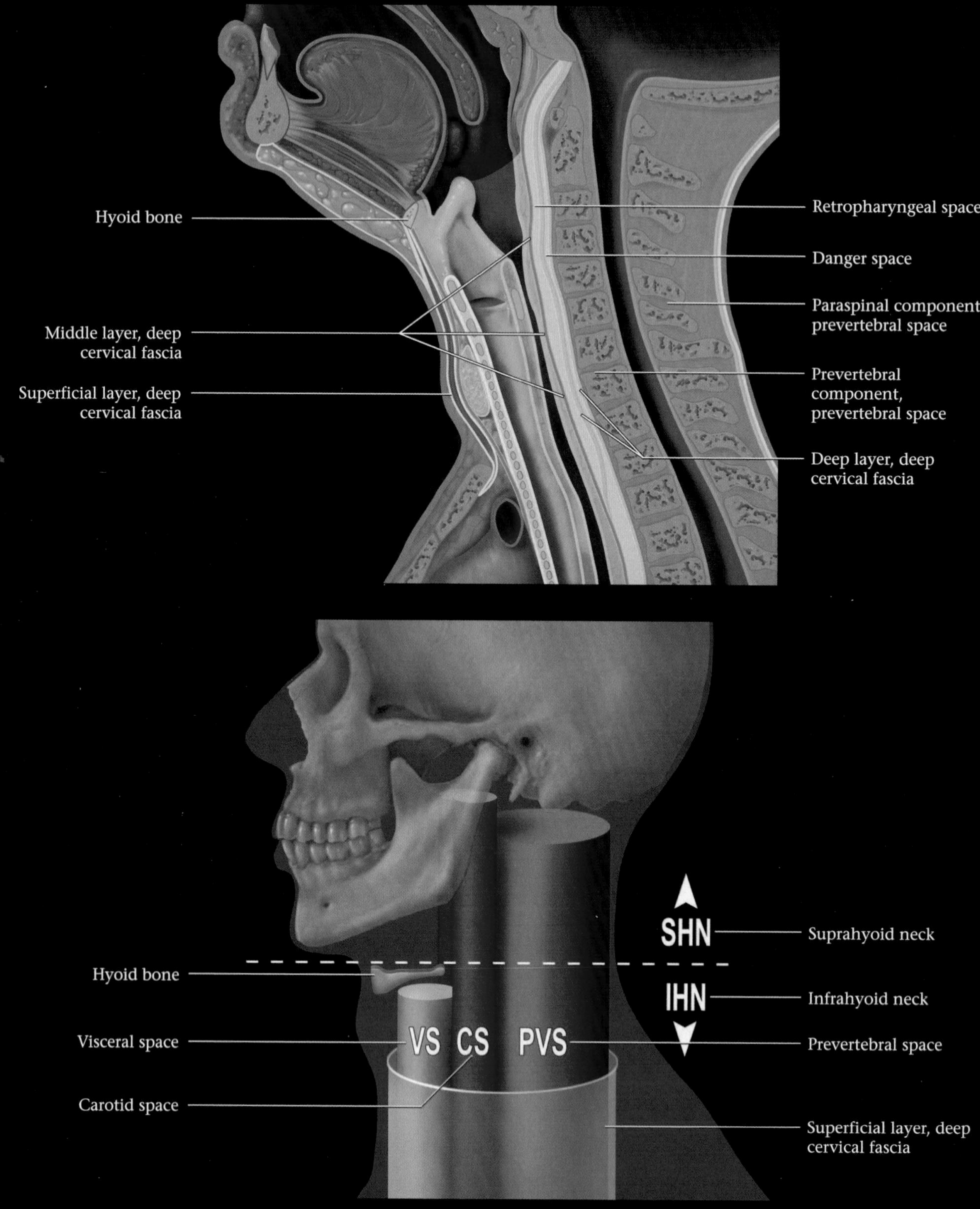
Hyoid bone
Middle layer, deep cervical fascia
Superficial layer, deep cervical fascia
Retropharyngeal space
Danger space
Paraspinal component, prevertebral space
Prevertebral component, prevertebral space
Deep layer, deep cervical fascia
SHN
IHN
Suprahyoid neck
Infrahyoid neck
Hyoid bone
Visceral space
Carotid space
VS
CS
PVS
Prevertebral space
Superficial layer, deep cervical fascia

(Top) Sagittal graphic depicting midline longitudinal spatial relationships of the infrahyoid neck. In the midline only the vertebral body is seen in the prevertebral component of the perivertebral space. Just anterior to the vertebral column the retropharyngeal and danger spaces run inferiorly toward the mediastinum. In the midline paraspinal component of the perivertebral space only the spinous processes are visible. **(Bottom)** Lateral graphic of extracranial head and neck showing the spaces as "tubes" as they traverse the area. The perivertebral space is shown as a tube of tissue that projects from the skull base inferiorly into the thorax. Notice the superficial layer of deep cervical fascia envelops all the spaces of the extracranial head and neck below the hyoid bone.

GENERIC PVS SUPRAHYOID MASS

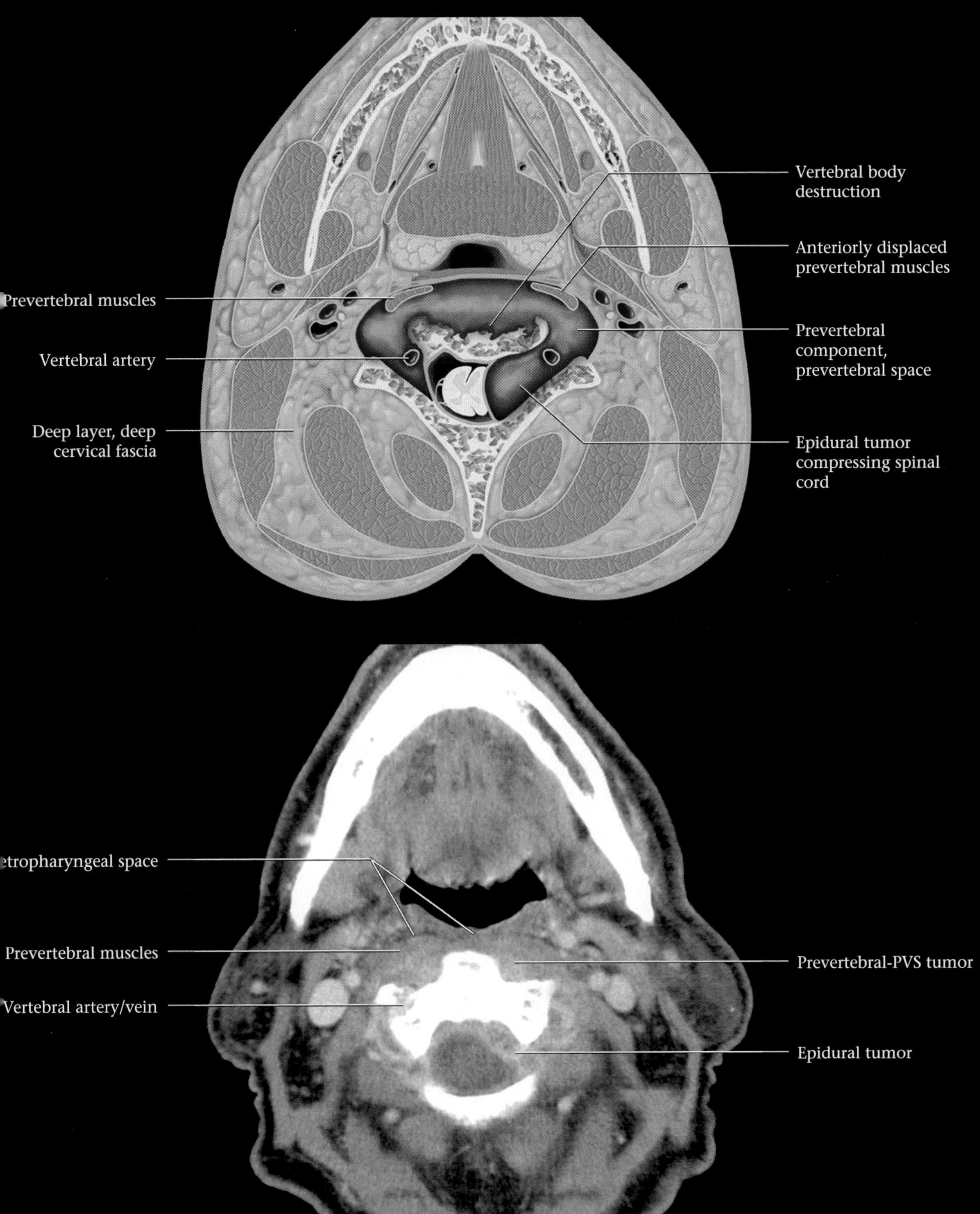
Vertebral body destruction
Anteriorly displaced prevertebral muscles
Prevertebral muscles
Prevertebral component, prevertebral space
Vertebral artery
Deep layer, deep cervical fascia
Epidural tumor compressing spinal cord
etropharyngeal space
Prevertebral muscles
Prevertebral-PVS tumor
Vertebral artery/vein
Epidural tumor

op) Axial graphic through the oropharynx reveals a generic suprahyoid neck perivertebral space mass involving the tebral body. Notice the vertebral body destruction and the elevation of the prevertebral muscles. The vertebral eries are engulfed by the tumor. In addition the tumor is confined by the deep layer of deep cervical fascia, forcing centrally into the epidural space where it is causing spinal cord compression. **(Bottom)** Axial contrast-enhanced CT nonstrates an enhancing malignant tumor involving prevertebral component of the perivertebral space. The nor remains confined to the perivertebral space by the deep layer of deep cervical fascia. Consequently the tumor ead centrally into the epidural space where it may cause cord compression.

PERIVERTEBRAL SPACE

GENERIC PVS INFRAHYOID MASS

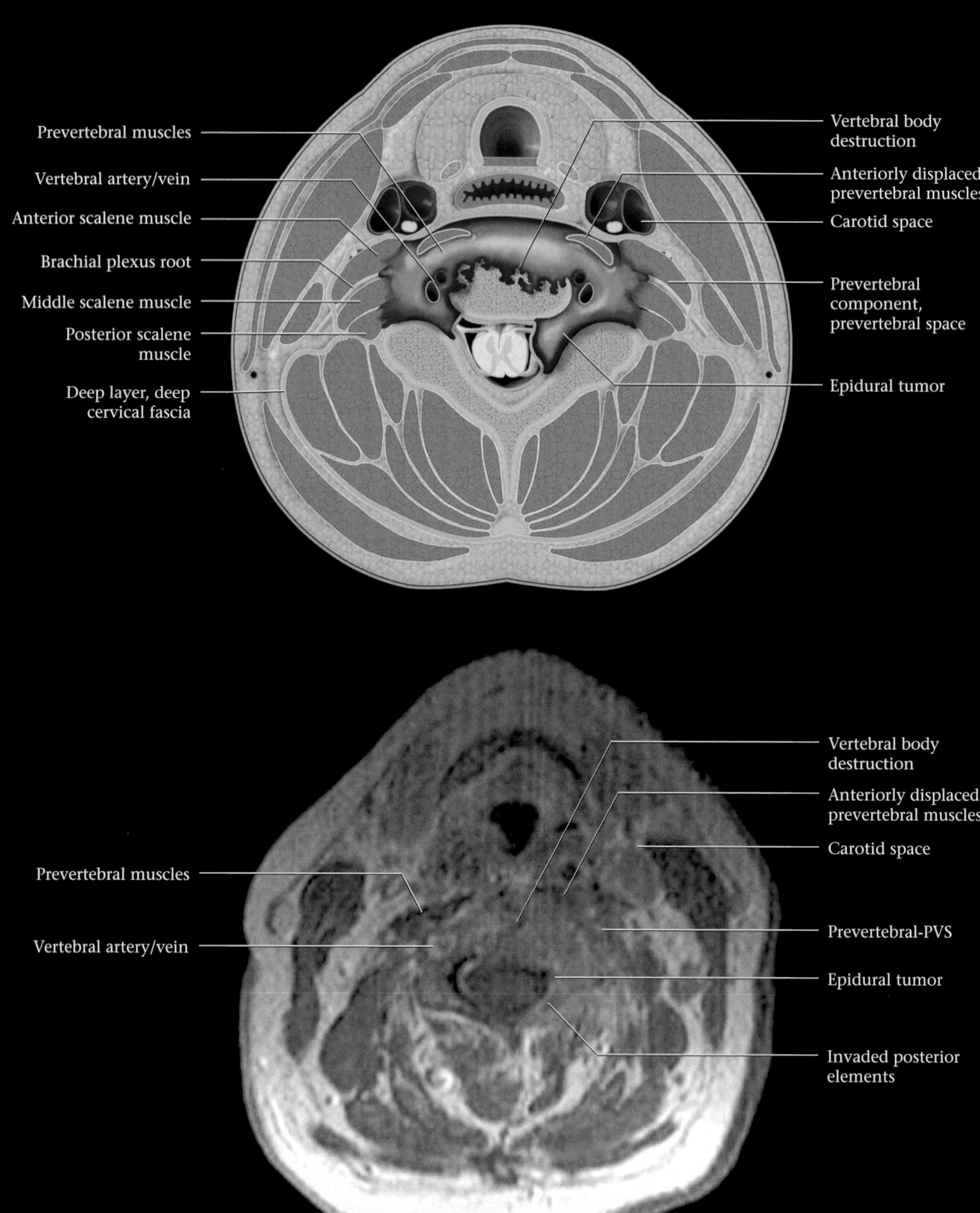
Prevertebral muscles
Vertebral artery/vein
Anterior scalene muscle
Brachial plexus root
Middle scalene muscle
Posterior scalene muscle
Deep layer, deep cervical fascia
Vertebral body destruction
Anteriorly displaced prevertebral muscles
Carotid space
Prevertebral component, prevertebral space
Epidural tumor
Prevertebral muscles
Vertebral artery/vein
Vertebral body destruction
Anteriorly displaced prevertebral muscles
Carotid space
Prevertebral-PVS
Epidural tumor
Invaded posterior elements

(Top) Axial graphic through the thyroid bed shows a generic infrahyoid neck perivertebral space mass arising out of the vertebral body. Notice the vertebral body destruction and the elevation of the prevertebral muscles. The vertebral artery and vein as well as the brachial plexus roots are engulfed by the tumor. In addition the tumor is confined by the deep layer of deep cervical fascia, forcing it centrally into the epidural space. **(Bottom)** Axial T1 enhanced MR image without fat saturation shows an enhancing metastatic tumor involving the vertebral body and its posterior elements on the left with extensive epidural tumor visible. The vertebral artery is engulfed by the tumor and the left prevertebral muscles are displaced anteriorly. Notice that the tumor remains confined to the perivertebral space by the deep layer of deep cervical fascia.

AXIAL CECT

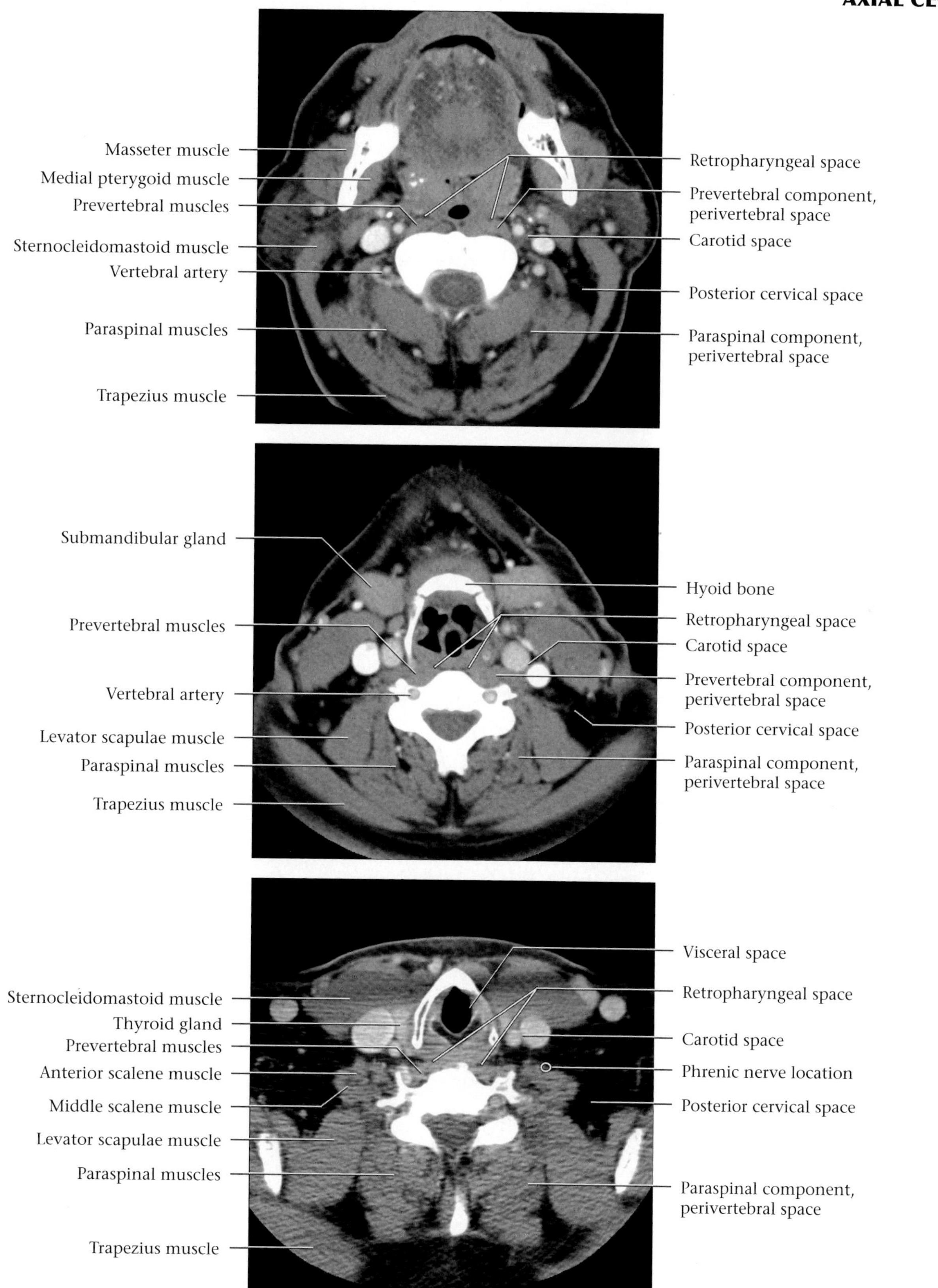
Masseter muscle
Medial pterygoid muscle
Prevertebral muscles
Sternocleidomastoid muscle
Vertebral artery
Paraspinal muscles
Trapezius muscle
Retropharyngeal space
Prevertebral component, perivertebral space
Carotid space
Posterior cervical space
Paraspinal component, perivertebral space
Submandibular gland
Prevertebral muscles
Vertebral artery
Levator scapulae muscle
Paraspinal muscles
Trapezius muscle
Hyoid bone
Retropharyngeal space
Carotid space
Prevertebral component, perivertebral space
Posterior cervical space
Paraspinal component, perivertebral space
Sternocleidomastoid muscle
Thyroid gland
Prevertebral muscles
Anterior scalene muscle
Middle scalene muscle
Levator scapulae muscle
Paraspinal muscles
Trapezius muscle
Visceral space
Retropharyngeal space
Carotid space
Phrenic nerve location
Posterior cervical space
Paraspinal component, perivertebral space

(Top) First of six axial CECT images through the extracranial head and neck chosen to highlight the normal features of the perivertebral space. This image at the level of the C2 vertebral body shows the prevertebral component of the perivertebral space contains the prevertebral muscles, vertebral body and vertebral artery only. The retropharyngeal space fat stripe is visible anteriorly. **(Middle)** In this image at the level of the hyoid bone the levator scapulae muscles and the paraspinal muscles along with the posterior elements of the vertebral body are the principal occupants of the paraspinal component of the perivertebral space. **(Bottom)** At the level of the cricoid cartilage the scalene muscles are visible. The phrenic nerve location is marked on the left to remind the imager of its presence even though it is not visible on imaging.

PERIVERTEBRAL SPACE

AXIAL CECT

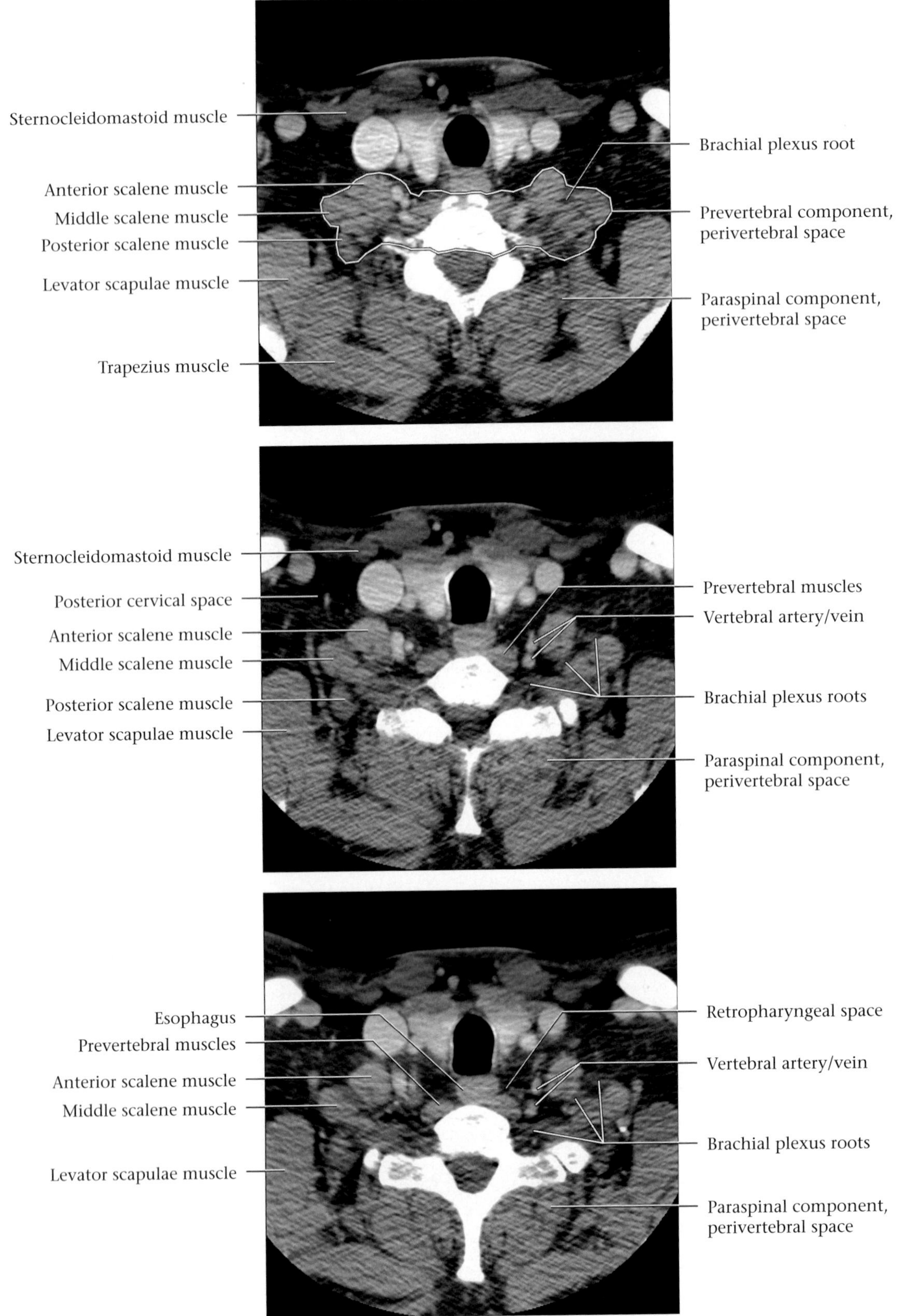
Sternocleidomastoid muscle
Anterior scalene muscle
Middle scalene muscle
Posterior scalene muscle
Levator scapulae muscle
Trapezius muscle
Brachial plexus root
Prevertebral component, perivertebral space
Paraspinal component, perivertebral space
Sternocleidomastoid muscle
Posterior cervical space
Anterior scalene muscle
Middle scalene muscle
Posterior scalene muscle
Levator scapulae muscle
Prevertebral muscles
Vertebral artery/vein
Brachial plexus roots
Paraspinal component, perivertebral space
Esophagus
Prevertebral muscles
Anterior scalene muscle
Middle scalene muscle
Levator scapulae muscle
Retropharyngeal space
Vertebral artery/vein
Brachial plexus roots
Paraspinal component, perivertebral space

(Top) At the level of the upper thyroid bed the scalene muscles are seen in the prevertebral component of the perivertebral space. The anterior band of deep layer of deep cervical fascia is referred to as the "carpet". **(Middle)** In this image at the level of the mid-thyroid bed the low density ovoid brachial plexus roots can be seen emerging from the cervical neural foramina to pass anterolaterally between the anterior and middle scalene muscles in the prevertebral component of the perivertebral space. **(Bottom)** At the level of the low-thyroid bed the low density brachial plexus roots are visible passing anterolaterally between the anterior and middle scalene muscles in the prevertebral component of the perivertebral space. These roots continue through openings in the deep layer of deep cervical fascia into the posterior cervical space on their way to the axillary apex.

AXIAL T2 FS & CORONAL STIR MR

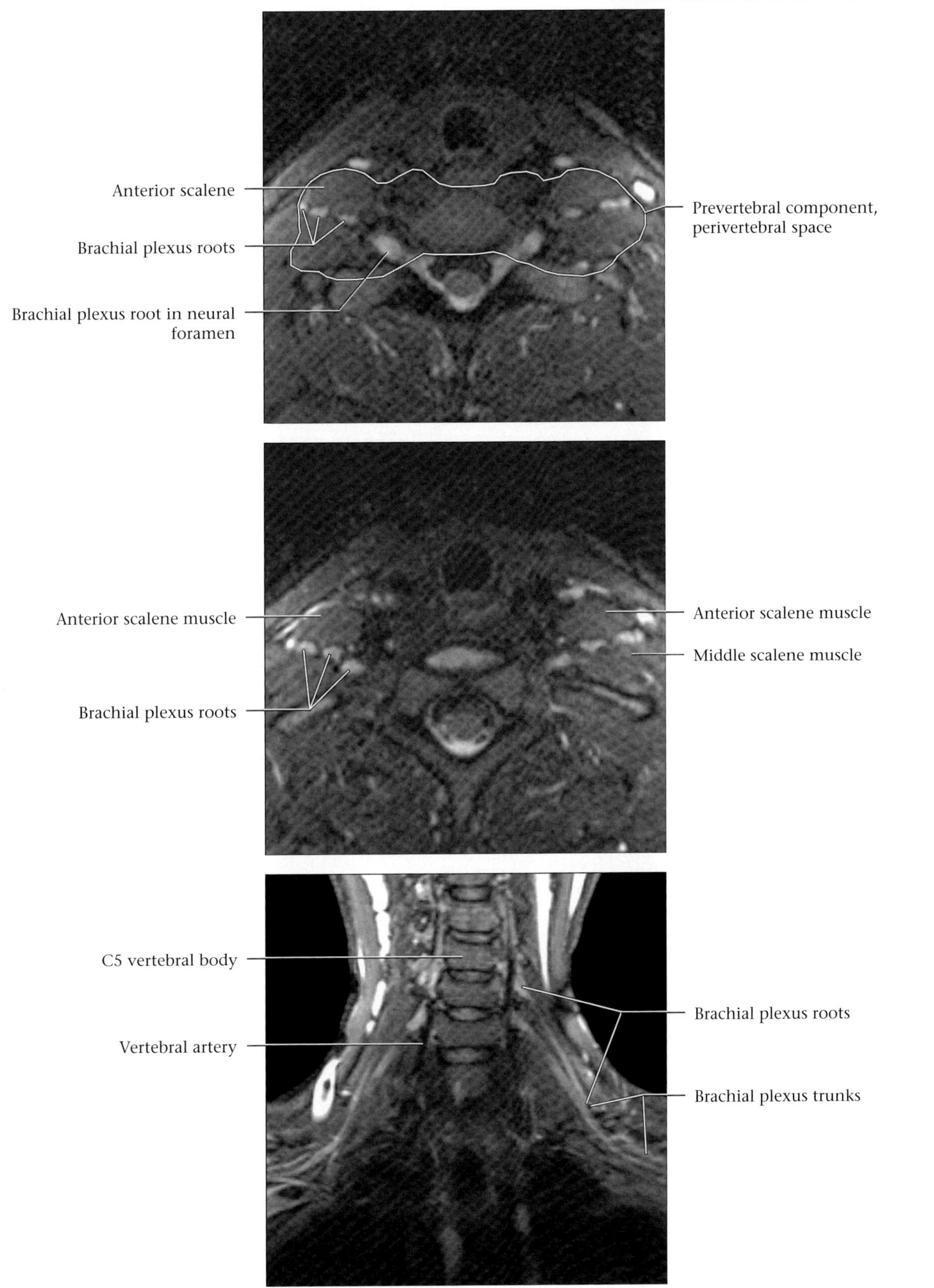
Anterior scalene
Brachial plexus roots
Brachial plexus root in neural foramen
Prevertebral component, perivertebral space
Anterior scalene muscle
Brachial plexus roots
Anterior scalene muscle
Middle scalene muscle
C5 vertebral body
Vertebral artery
Brachial plexus roots
Brachial plexus trunks

(Top) Axial T2 fat-saturated MR image at level of thyroid gland shows the normal high signal brachial plexus roots between anterior & middle scalene muscles. Notice a single root passes through the neural foramen bilaterally. Brachial plexus arises from ventral rami of C5 through T1. **(Middle)** In this axial T2 fat-saturated MR image the anterior & middle scalene muscles can be seen on the anterior & posterior sides of the high signal brachial plexus roots. Distally the 5 roots become 3 trunks (upper, middle & lower) as they emerge from their interscalene muscle location. **(Bottom)** Coronal STIR MR through the lower cervical vertebral bodies shows both the 5 brachial plexus roots & the 3 trunks in the same plane. The pneumonic "Robert Taylor Drinks Cold Beer" reminds us that the brachial plexus transitions from Roots to Trunks to Divisions to Cords to end in Branches.

POSTERIOR CERVICAL SPACE

Terminology

Abbreviations

- Posterior cervical space (PCS)

Definitions

- **PCS**: Posterolateral fat-containing space in neck with complex fascial boundaries that extends from posterior mastoid tip to clavicle

Imaging Anatomy

Overview

- Posterolateral fat-filled space just deep & posterior to sternomastoid muscle
- Lesions of PCS arise from spinal accessory nodal chain
    - Infection, inflammation & tumor involving these nodes constitute vast majority of lesions in PCS

Extent

- PCS extends from small superior component near mastoid tip to broader base at level of clavicle
- When viewed from side, appears as "tilting tent"

Anatomy Relationships

- Superficial space lies superficial to PCS
- Deep to PCS is perivertebral space
    - Anterior PCS is superficial to prevertebral component of perivertebral space
    - Posterior PCS is superficial to paraspinal component of perivertebral space
- Anteromedial to PCS is carotid space

Internal Structures-Critical Contents

- **Fat** is primary occupant of PCS
- **Accessory nerve** (CN11)
- **Spinal accessory lymph node chain**
    - In node level numbering system this is **level 5**
    - Level 5 spinal accessory nodes (SAN) further subdivided into A & B levels at hyoid bone
        - **Level 5A**: SAN above cricoid cartilage level
        - **Level 5B**: SAN below cricoid cartilage level
- **Pre-axillary brachial plexus**
    - Segment of brachial plexus emerging from anterior & middle scalene gap passes through PCS
    - Leaves PCS with axillary artery into axillary fat
- **Dorsal scapular nerve**
    - Arises from brachial plexus (spinal nerves C4 & C5)
    - Motor innervation to rhomboid & levator scapulae muscles

Fascia of Posterior Cervical Space

- Complex fascial boundaries surround PCS
    - Superficial: Superficial layer of deep cervical fascia
    - Deep: Deep layer of deep cervical fascia
    - Anteromedial: Carotid sheath (all 3 layers, deep cervical fascia)

Other Related Anatomic Information

- **Posterior triangle**
    - Definition: Region of cervical neck posterolateral to sternomastoid muscle & anteromedial to trapezius muscle
    - Subdivided by inferior belly of omohyoid muscle into occipital & subclavian triangles
- **Occipital triangle**
    - Boundaries: Anteromedial sternomastoid muscle; posterolateral trapezius muscle; inferior is inferior belly of omohyoid muscle
    - Contents: Fat, accessory nerve (CN11), dorsal scapular nerves & spinal accessory nodes
    - Occipital triangle is majority of PCS
- **Subclavian triangle**
    - Boundaries: Superior inferior belly of omohyoid muscle; anteromedial sternocleidomastoid muscle; posterolateral trapezium muscle
    - Contents: 3rd portion of subclavian artery, cervical brachial plexus
    - Subclavian triangle is lower, smaller portion of PCS

Anatomy-Based Imaging Issues

Key Concepts or Questions

- What are criteria for defining a cervical neck mass lesion as primary to PCS?
    - Lesion must be **centered within fat of PCS**
    - Lesion displaces carotid space anteromedially
    - Lesion elevates sternocleidomastoid muscle
    - Lesion flattens deeper perivertebral space structures
- How can you tell a internal jugular from SAN?
    - Within infrahyoid PCS
        - Spinal accessory nodes are in fat of PCS with slip of fat separating them from carotid space
        - Internal jugular nodes abut carotid space
    - Within suprahyoid PCS
        - Internal jugular & spinal accessory nodal chain converge cephalad toward jugulodigastric group
        - Differentiating internal jugular from spinal accessory adenopathy tougher in suprahyoid area
        - Nodes that abut anterior, lateral or posterior to carotid space, consider internal jugular nodes
        - If node has fat slip separating it from carotid space, consider spinal accessory nodes

Clinical Implications

Clinical Importance

- CN11 runs in floor of PCS
- Spinal accessory nodes are main normal occupants of posterior cervical space

Function-Dysfunction

- Accessory cranial neuropathy results when CN11 injured
    - Most commonly injured during neck dissection for malignant SCCa nodes
    - Less commonly injured by extranodal spread of squamous cell carcinoma
    - Dysfunction: Sternomastoid & trapezius muscle paresis
        - Acute denervation: Muscles may swell & enhance
        - Chronic denervation: Muscles atrophy & fatty infiltrate
        - Levator scapulae muscle hypertrophies
        - Patient has difficulty lifting arm

GRAPHICS

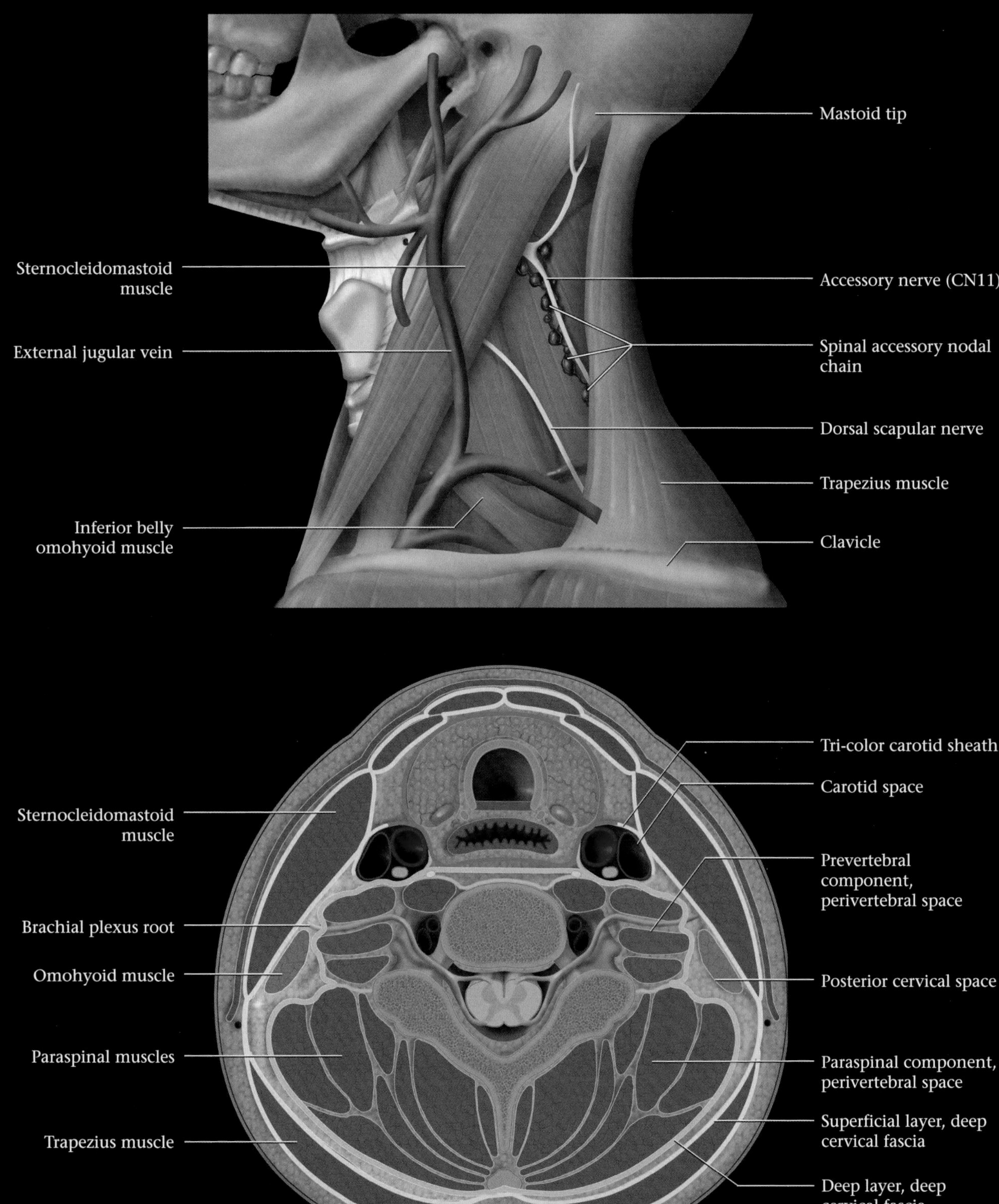
Mastoid tip
Sternocleidomastoid muscle
Accessory nerve (CN11)
External jugular vein
Spinal accessory nodal chain
Dorsal scapular nerve
Trapezius muscle
Inferior belly omohyoid muscle
Clavicle
Tri-color carotid sheath
Carotid space
Sternocleidomastoid muscle
Prevertebral component, perivertebral space
Brachial plexus root
Omohyoid muscle
Posterior cervical space
Paraspinal muscles
Paraspinal component, perivertebral space
Superficial layer, deep cervical fascia
Trapezius muscle
Deep layer, deep cervical fascia

(Top) Lateral graphic if extracranial head & neck shows the posterior cervical space as a "tilting tent" with its superior margin at the level of the mastoid tip and its inferior border at the clavicle. Notice it has two main nerves in its floor, the accessory nerve (CN11) and the dorsal scapular nerve. The spinal accessory nodal chain is its key occupant with regards to the kind of lesions found in the PCS. **(Bottom)** Axial graphic through the thyroid bed of the infrahyoid neck depicts the posterior cervical space with its complex fascial borders. The superficial layer of deep cervical fascia is its superficial border while the deep layer of deep cervical fascia is its deep border. Note the tri-color carotid sheath is its anteromedial border. The brachial plexus roots travel through the PCS on their way to the axillary apex.

PCS NODAL STATIONS/DISEASES

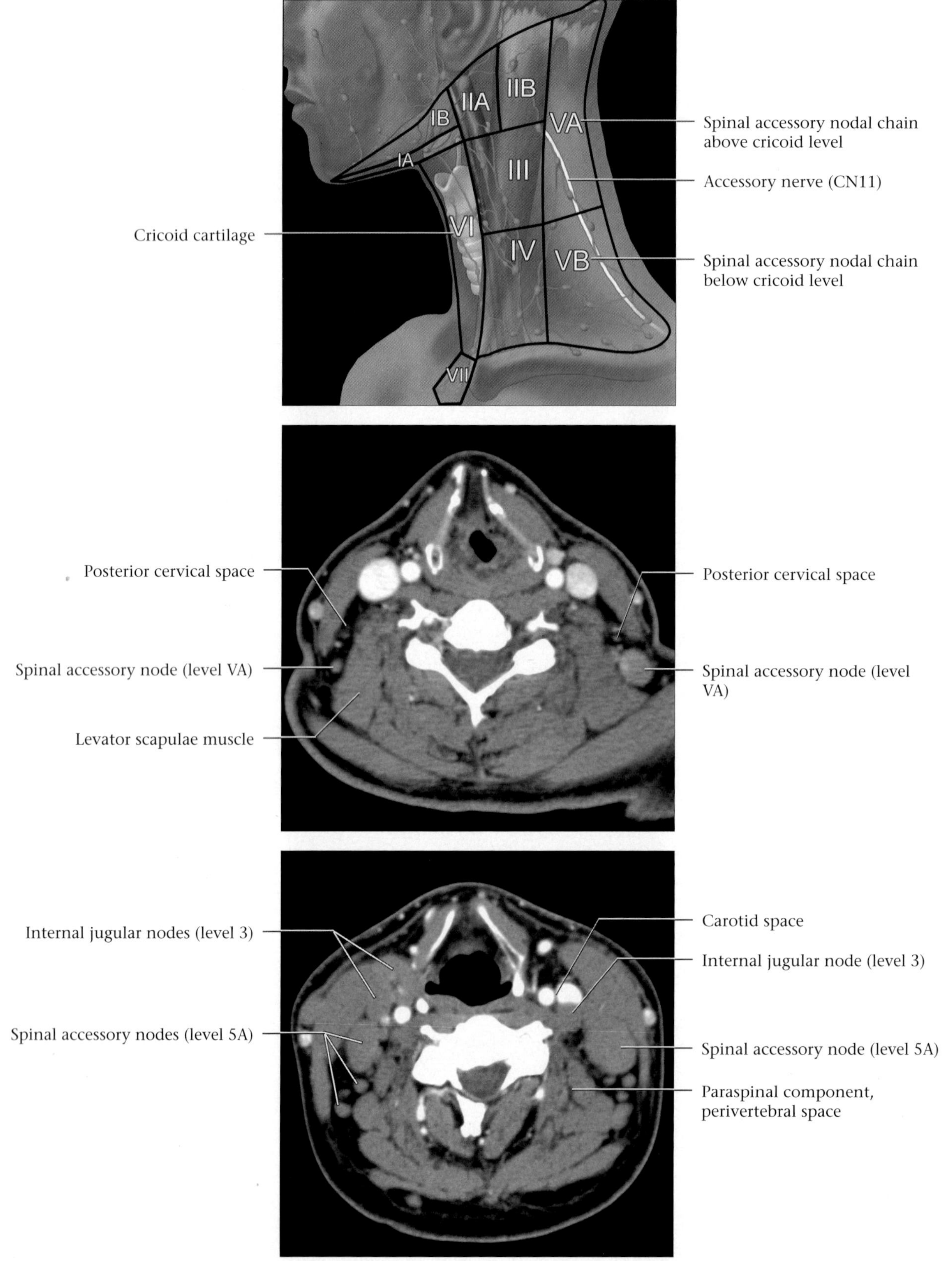
IB
IIA
IIB
VA
IA
III
VI
IV
VB
VII
Spinal accessory nodal chain above cricoid level
Accessory nerve (CN11)
Cricoid cartilage
Spinal accessory nodal chain below cricoid level
Posterior cervical space
Spinal accessory node (level VA)
Levator scapulae muscle
Posterior cervical space
Spinal accessory node (level VA)
Internal jugular nodes (level 3)
Spinal accessory nodes (level 5A)
Carotid space
Internal jugular node (level 3)
Spinal accessory node (level 5A)
Paraspinal component, perivertebral space

(Top) Oblique graphic of the extracranial head and neck depicting the principal nodal chains and their assigned levels. The spinal accessory chain (level 5) is divided at axial level of the cricoid cartilage into upper level 5B and lower level 5A groups. Level 2, 3 & 4 nodes are in the internal jugular chain. **(Middle)** Axial CECT image of the cervical neck at the level of the supraglottis shows bilateral level 5A nodes in the posterior cervical space of the neck. They are considered 5A because they are in the posterior cervical space above the cricoid cartilage. **(Bottom)** In this image in a patient with non-Hodgkin lymphoma nodes can be seen both in the internal jugular and spinal accessory nodal chains. Notice that there is fat and internal jugular nodes between the spinal accessory chain and the carotid space.

GENERIC MASS IN PCS

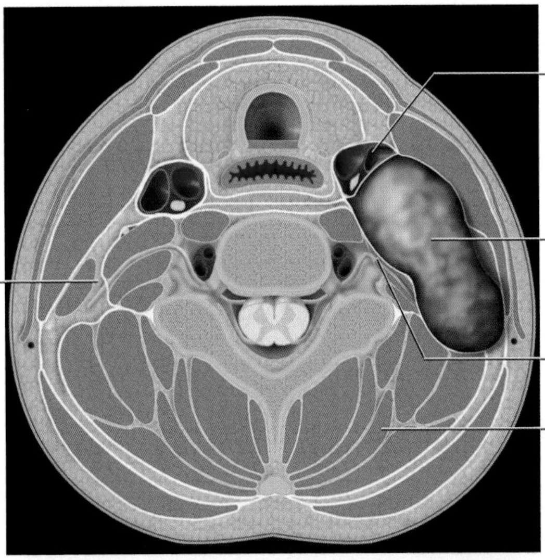

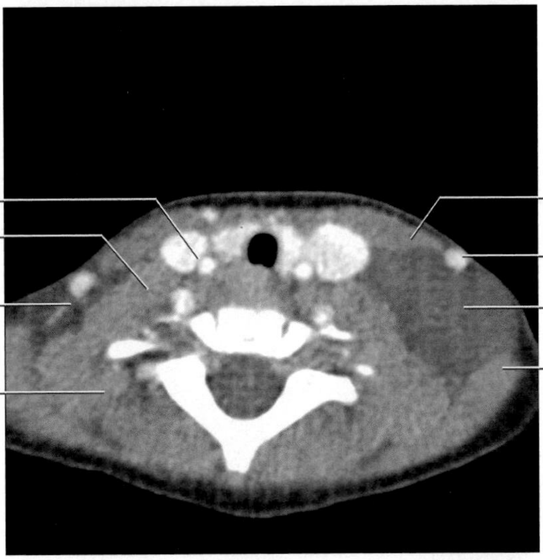

Carotid space

Posterior cervical space

Generic posterior cervical space mass

Prevertebral component, perivertebral space

Paraspinal component, perivertebral space

Carotid space

Prevertebral component, perivertebral space

Posterior cervical space

Paraspinal component, perivertebral space

Sternocleidomastoid muscle

External jugular vein

PCS lymphatic malformation

Trapezius muscle

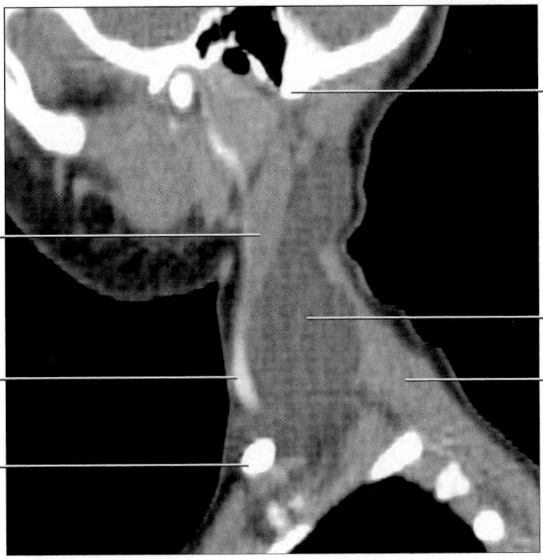

Mastoid tip

Sternocleidomastoid muscle

PCS lymphatic malformation

External jugular vein

Trapezius muscle

Clavicle

(Top) Axial graphic in the infrahyoid neck showing a generic mass in the posterior cervical space on the left. Notice the lesion is centered within fat of PCS. A PCS mass typically displaces the carotid space anteromedially, elevates the sternocleidomastoid muscle and flattens the deeper perivertebral space structures. **(Middle)** In this axial CECT image at the level of the thyroid bed a lymphatic malformation is seen filling the left posterior cervical space. **(Bottom)** CECT sagittal reformation reveals a posterior cervical space lymphatic malformation. The image is presented to show the "tilted tent" shape of the posterior cervical space from its superior margin at the mastoid tip to its inferior margin at the clavicle.

POSTERIOR CERVICAL SPACE

AXIAL CECT

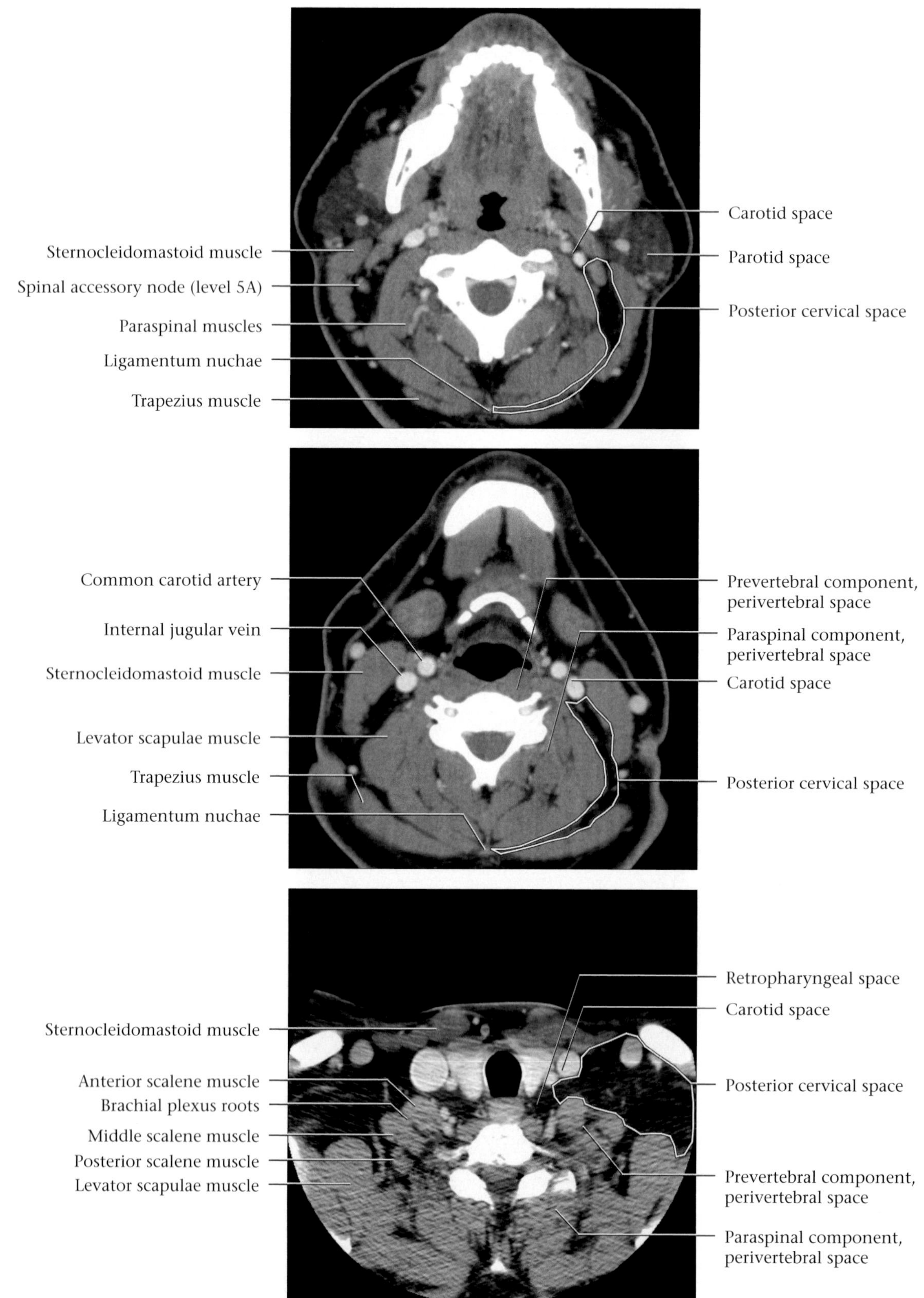

Sternocleidomastoid muscle
Spinal accessory node (level 5A)
Paraspinal muscles
Ligamentum nuchae
Trapezius muscle
Carotid space
Parotid space
Posterior cervical space
Common carotid artery
Internal jugular vein
Sternocleidomastoid muscle
Levator scapulae muscle
Trapezius muscle
Ligamentum nuchae
Prevertebral component, perivertebral space
Paraspinal component, perivertebral space
Carotid space
Posterior cervical space
Sternocleidomastoid muscle
Anterior scalene muscle
Brachial plexus roots
Middle scalene muscle
Posterior scalene muscle
Levator scapulae muscle
Retropharyngeal space
Carotid space
Posterior cervical space
Prevertebral component, perivertebral space
Paraspinal component, perivertebral space

(Top) First of three axial CECT at the level of the mid-oropharynx shows the fat-filled posterior cervical space. Notice the posteromedial extension of the posterior cervical space between the paraspinal muscles and the trapezius where it reaches as far as the ligamentum nuchae. **(Middle)** In this CECT image at the level of the hyoid bone the anteromedial border of the posterior cervical space abuts the carotid space. Deep to the posterior cervical space is the paraspinal component of the perivertebral space. The lateral-most muscle in the paraspinal muscle group is the levator scapulae muscle. **(Bottom)** At the level of the clavicle the posterior cervical space is visible enlarging in the inferolateral direction to meet the axillary apex. Notice the brachial plexus roots must traverse the PCS as they emerge from between the anterior and middle scalene muscles.

CORONAL T1 MR

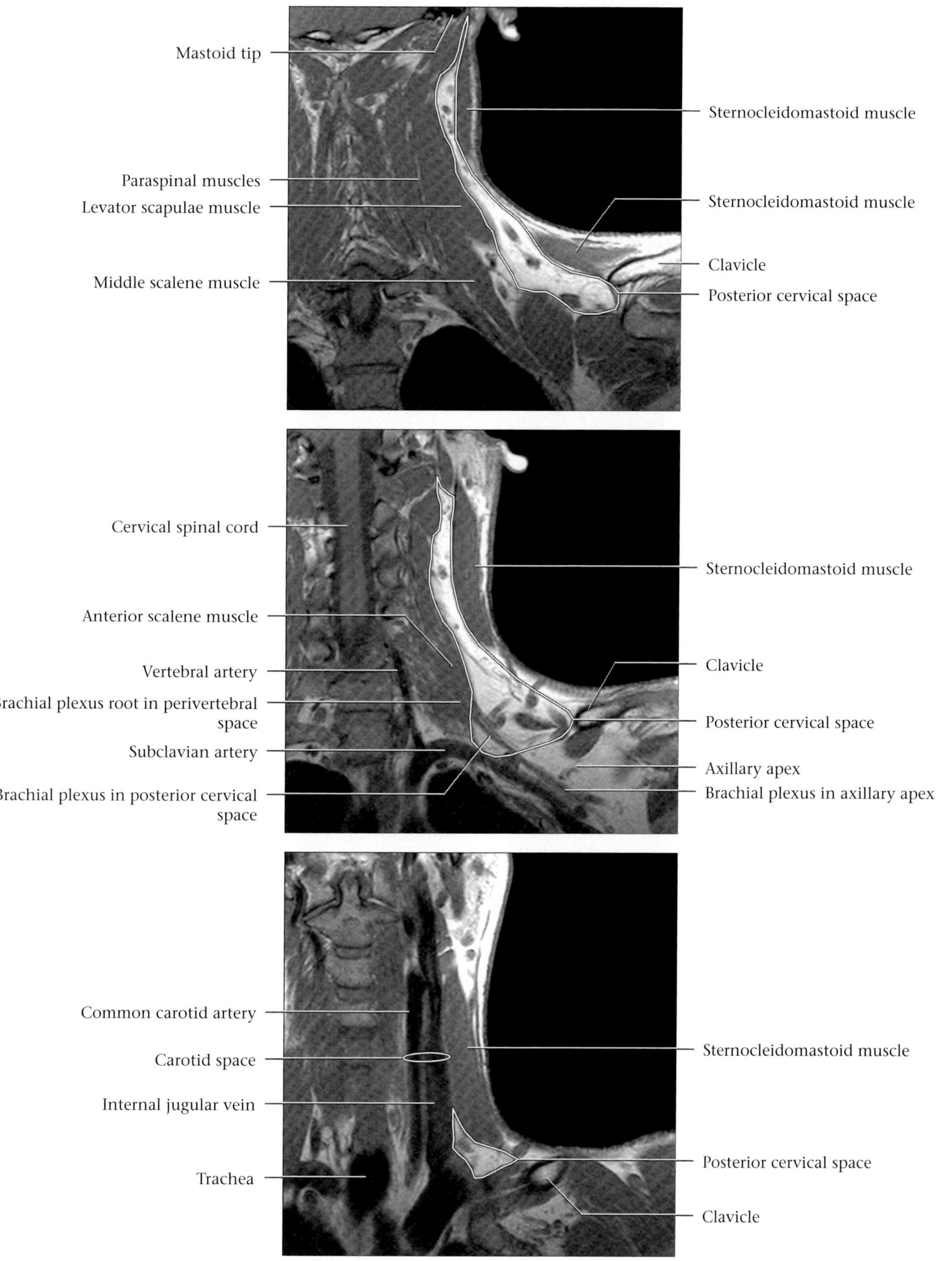
Mastoid tip
Sternocleidomastoid muscle
Paraspinal muscles
Levator scapulae muscle
Sternocleidomastoid muscle
Clavicle
Middle scalene muscle
Posterior cervical space
Cervical spinal cord
Sternocleidomastoid muscle
Anterior scalene muscle
Clavicle
Vertebral artery
Brachial plexus root in perivertebral space
Posterior cervical space
Subclavian artery
Axillary apex
Brachial plexus in posterior cervical space
Brachial plexus in axillary apex
Common carotid artery
Carotid space
Sternocleidomastoid muscle
Internal jugular vein
Posterior cervical space
Trachea
Clavicle

(Top) First of three coronal T1 MR images presented from posterior to anterior of the extracranial head and neck emphasizing the anatomy of the posterior cervical space. In this image the PCS is seen spanning the distance between the mastoid tip superiorly and the axillary apex inferolaterally. A few scattered level 5 spinal accessory lymph nodes are seen in the high signal fat of the PCS. **(Middle)** In this image through the cervical spinal cord the brachial plexus roots are visible exiting the perivertebral space into the PCS on their way to the axillary apex. Lymph node disease of the lower spinal accessory chain in the PCS can affect the brachial plexus. **(Bottom)** In this image through the carotid space the most anteroinferior aspect of the posterior cervical space is seen.

VISCERAL SPACE

Terminology

Abbreviations

- Visceral space (VS)

Definitions

- **VS**: Cylindrical space in midline infrahyoid neck (IHN) enclosed by middle layer, deep cervical fascia

Imaging Anatomy

Overview

- Cylindrical space in core of IHN extending from hyoid bone to upper mediastinum
- **Contains IHN viscera** (larynx, trachea, hypopharynx, esophagus, thyroid & parathyroid glands)

Extent

- VS stretches length of IHN from hyoid bone above to superior mediastinum below

Anatomy Relationships

- **VS is largest space of IHN**
- Lateral to VS are paired anterior cervical spaces
- Posterolateral to VS are paired carotid spaces (CS)
- Posterior to VS is retropharyngeal space (RPS)

Internal Structures-Critical Contents

- **Thyroid gland**
  - Two lobes connected by isthmus
- **Parathyroid glands**
  - 4 glands, 2 pairs behind upper & lower poles of thyroid gland
  - Superior 2 glands consistent in location
  - Inferior 2 glands less reliable in location
    - May be normally found in cervicothoracic junction or superior mediastinum
- **Cervical trachea & esophagus**
- **Recurrent laryngeal nerve**
  - Left: Recurs at level of arch where it passes through aortopulmonic window
  - Right: Recurs in most inferior IHN around right subclavian artery
  - In tracheoesophageal groove on way up to larynx
- **VS lymph nodes (level VI group)**
  - Paratracheal lymph node group
    - **First order drainage for thyroid malignancy**
    - Serves as primary conduit for nodal spread into superior mediastinum
  - Prelaryngeal lymph node group
  - Pretracheal lymph node group

Fascia

- **Middle layer, deep cervical fascia** (ML-DCF) completely encloses visceral space
- ML-DCF also referred to as "visceral fascia"

Anatomy-Based Imaging Issues

Key Concepts or Questions

- What imaging clues define a mass lesion as primary to visceral space?
- Lesion may originate in thyroid, parathyroid (tracheoesophageal groove), trachea or esophageus
  - **Thyroid mass lesion**
    - Mass surrounded at least in part by thyroid tissue
    - CS displaced laterally with trachea & esophagus displaced to opposite side of neck
  - **Parathyroid (tracheoesophageal groove) mass lesion**
    - Mass centered between thyroid lobe anteriorly & longus colli muscle posteriorly
    - Displaces thyroid lobe anteriorly & CS anterolaterally
    - Mass may originate from parathyroid gland, paratracheal node or recurrent laryngeal nerve
  - **Cervical tracheal mass lesion**
    - Mass centered in tracheal wall
    - Displaces thyroid laterally & esophagus posteriorly
  - **Cervical esophageal mass lesion**
    - Mass centered in midline, posterior VS immediately posterior to trachea
    - Displaces trachea & thyroid gland anteriorly

Imaging Approaches

- **Ultrasound** ± needle aspiration biopsy is **first best single approach** to lesions of VS
- If differentiated thyroid carcinoma, nuclear medicine (I-131) diagnostic study is then done
  - If suspected nodes from clinical examination or I-131 study, cross-sectional imaging usually done in presurgical period
  - MR is preferred imaging tool to stage superior mediastinum as it prevents iodine load delaying iodine-based nuclear medicine therapy
  - If suspect VS malignancy, image to carina to include level VI (paratracheal, prelaryngeal & pretracheal) nodes & superior mediastinal nodes (level VII)
- All other lesions of VS that require cross-sectional imaging, easier to cover neck to carina with CECT

Imaging Pitfalls

- Patulous esophagus may project from behind left tracheal margin, mimicking parathyroid adenoma
- Ending VS cross-sectional imaging at cervicothoracic junction is significant imaging mistake
  - **Multiple VS lesions require imaging to carina**
    - When staging VS tumor, especially differentiated thyroid carcinoma, must evaluate upper mediastinal nodes (level VII)
    - Distal vagal neuropathy requires continuing to carina if on **left**
    - Searching for "ectopic parathyroid adenoma" includes upper mediastinal search

Clinical Implications

Clinical Importance

- VS mass symptoms depend of structures involved
  - Recurrent laryngeal nerve: Distal vagal neuropathy with isolated vocal cord paralysis; hoarseness
  - Cervical esophagus: Dysphagia; solid food intolerance
  - Cervical trachea: Stridor, shortness of breath

VISCERAL SPACE

GRAPHICS

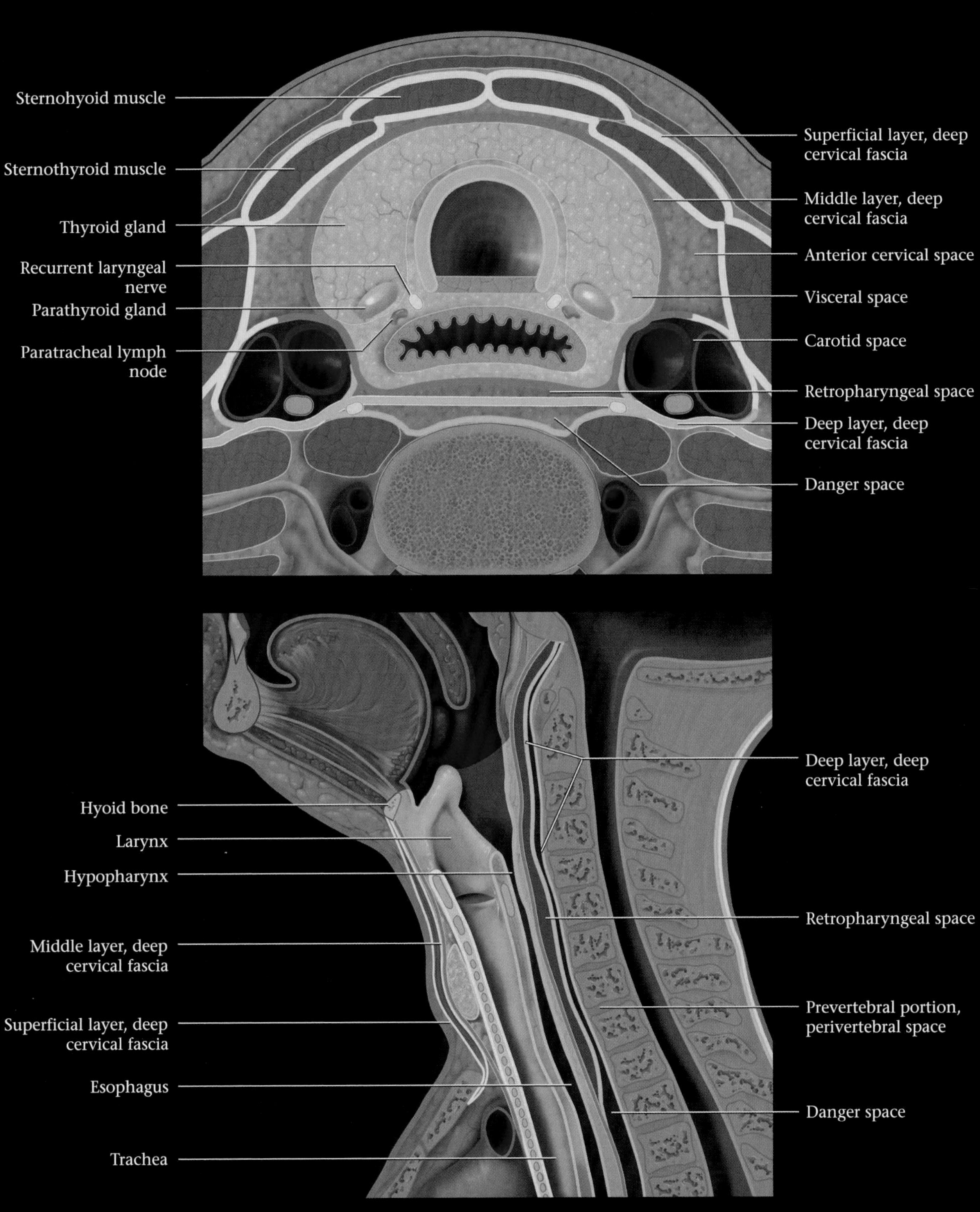
Sternohyoid muscle
Sternothyroid muscle
Thyroid gland
Recurrent laryngeal nerve
Parathyroid gland
Paratracheal lymph node
Superficial layer, deep cervical fascia
Middle layer, deep cervical fascia
Anterior cervical space
Visceral space
Carotid space
Retropharyngeal space
Deep layer, deep cervical fascia
Danger space
Hyoid bone
Larynx
Hypopharynx
Middle layer, deep cervical fascia
Superficial layer, deep cervical fascia
Esophagus
Trachea
Deep layer, deep cervical fascia
Retropharyngeal space
Prevertebral portion, perivertebral space
Danger space

(Top) Axial graphic shows visceral space defined by middle layer of deep cervical fascia (pink). Middle layer of deep cervical fascia, also called "visceral fascia," runs along deep surface of strap muscles, merges anteriorly with superficial layer of deep cervical fascia (yellow) & splits to encapsulate thyroid gland. Middle layer of deep cervical fascia also forms anterior margin of retropharyngeal space & contributes to carotid sheath. Recurrent laryngeal nerve lies in tracheoesophageal groove & injury results in vocal cord paralysis & hoarseness. **(Bottom)** Sagittal graphic shows longitudinal relationships of infrahyoid neck. Note visceral space (orange) is the only space unique to infrahyoid neck extending from hyoid bone to superior mediastinum. Visceral space is cylindrical space in anterior midline neck surrounded by middle layer of deep cervical fascia (pink).

AXIAL CECT

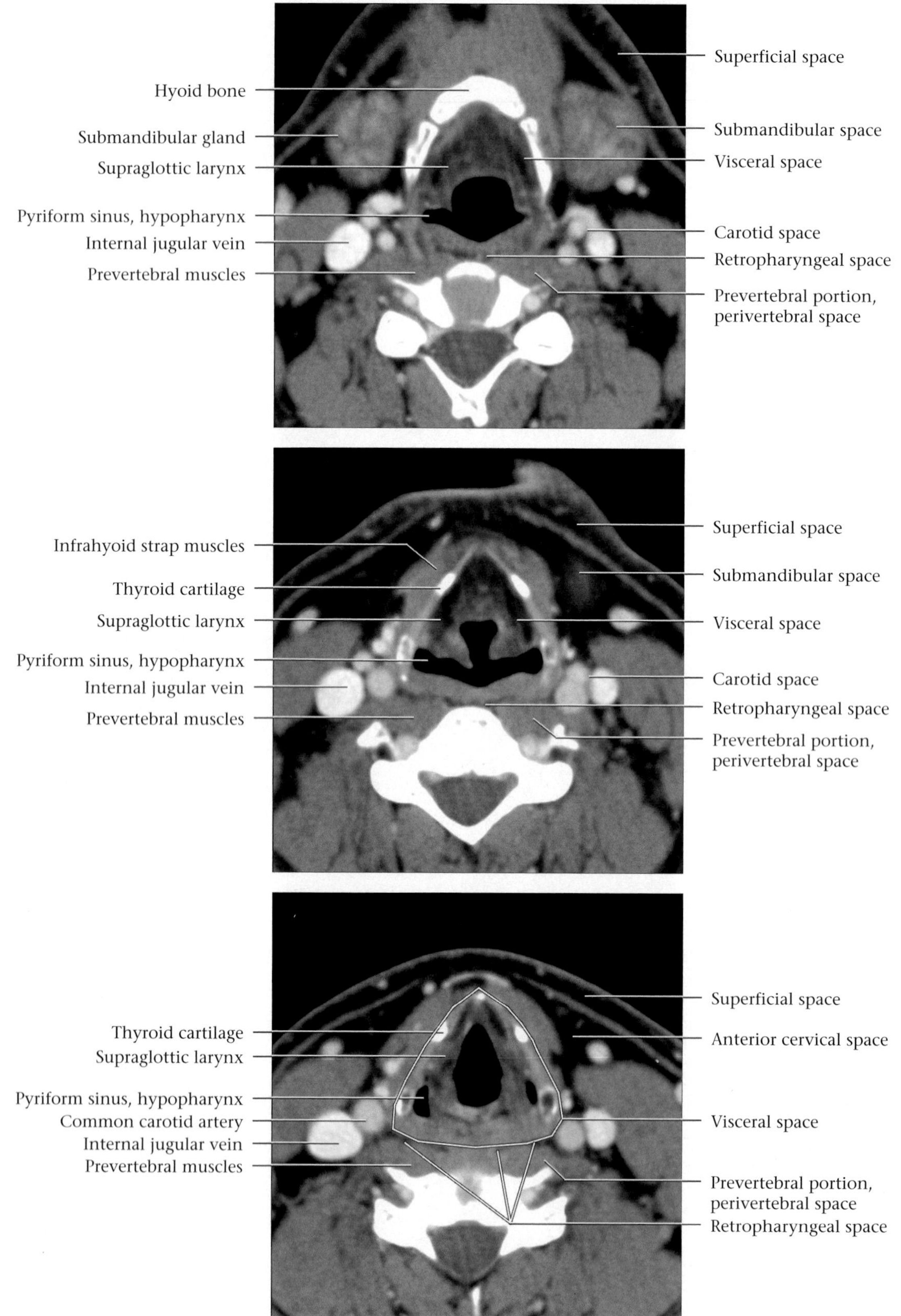

Hyoid bone
Submandibular gland
Supraglottic larynx
Pyriform sinus, hypopharynx
Internal jugular vein
Prevertebral muscles
Superficial space
Submandibular space
Visceral space
Carotid space
Retropharyngeal space
Prevertebral portion, perivertebral space
Infrahyoid strap muscles
Thyroid cartilage
Supraglottic larynx
Pyriform sinus, hypopharynx
Internal jugular vein
Prevertebral muscles
Superficial space
Submandibular space
Visceral space
Carotid space
Retropharyngeal space
Prevertebral portion, perivertebral space
Thyroid cartilage
Supraglottic larynx
Pyriform sinus, hypopharynx
Common carotid artery
Internal jugular vein
Prevertebral muscles
Superficial space
Anterior cervical space
Visceral space
Prevertebral portion, perivertebral space
Retropharyngeal space

(Top) First of six axial CECT images presented from superior to inferior of visceral space shows hyoid bone which represents superior extent of visceral space. This cylindrical space in midline infrahyoid neck is enclosed by middle layer of deep cervical fascia & extends to superior mediastinum. Submandibular space is continuous with anterior cervical space. **(Middle)** This image shows visceral space contains larynx & hypopharynx at this level. It is bordered posteriorly by retropharyngeal space & posterolaterally by carotid spaces. **(Bottom)** This image shows visceral space is completely enclosed by middle layer of deep cervical fascia, represented by line drawing. Paired anterior cervical spaces are lateral to visceral space & are continuous with submandibular spaces superiorly. Retropharyngeal space is seen as stripe of fat between posterior hypopharynx & prevertebral muscles.

VISCERAL SPACE

AXIAL CECT

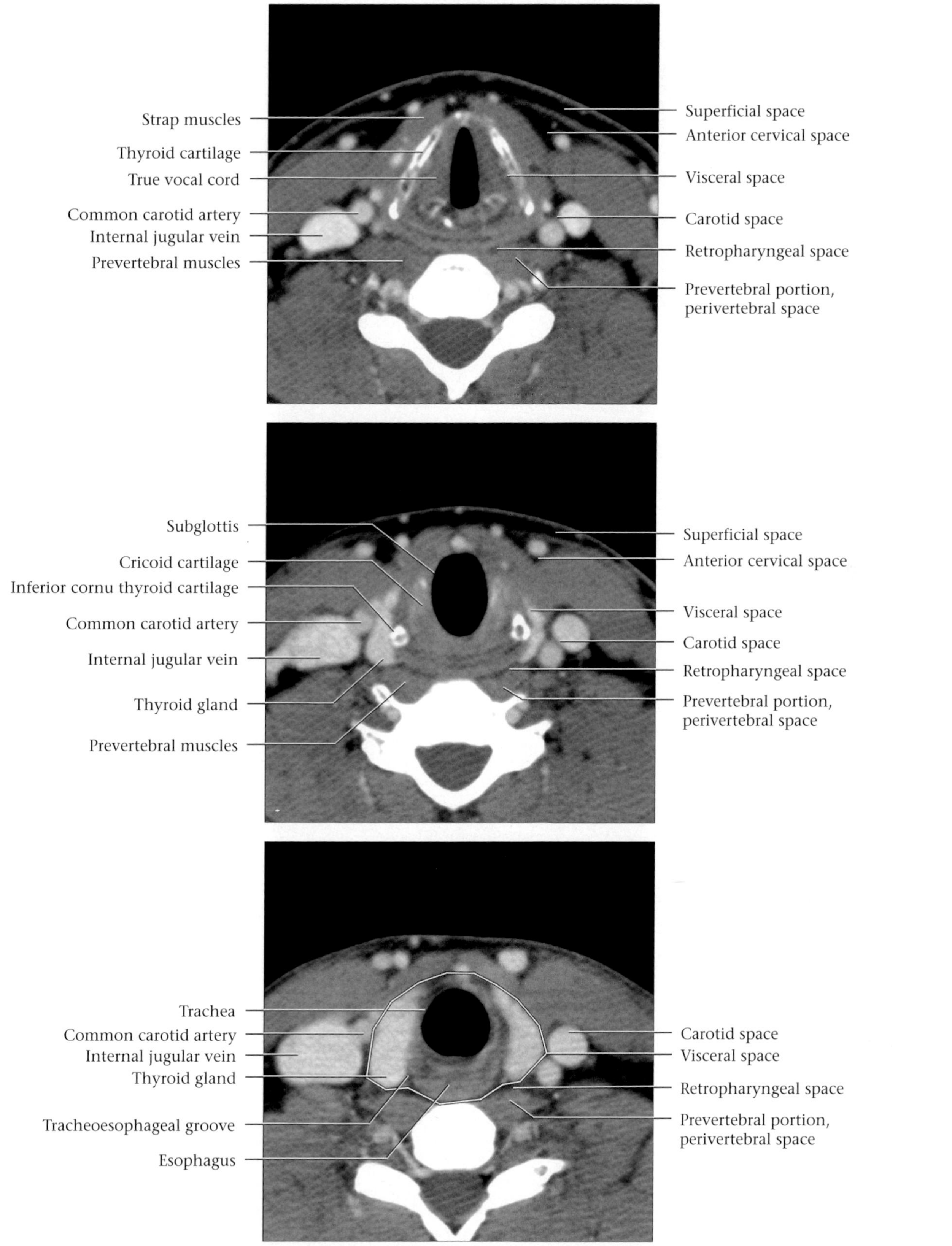
Strap muscles
Thyroid cartilage
True vocal cord
Common carotid artery
Internal jugular vein
Prevertebral muscles
Superficial space
Anterior cervical space
Visceral space
Carotid space
Retropharyngeal space
Prevertebral portion, perivertebral space
Subglottis
Cricoid cartilage
Inferior cornu thyroid cartilage
Common carotid artery
Internal jugular vein
Thyroid gland
Prevertebral muscles
Superficial space
Anterior cervical space
Visceral space
Carotid space
Retropharyngeal space
Prevertebral portion, perivertebral space
Trachea
Common carotid artery
Internal jugular vein
Thyroid gland
Tracheoesophageal groove
Esophagus
Carotid space
Visceral space
Retropharyngeal space
Prevertebral portion, perivertebral space

(Top) Image at level of glottis shows visceral space in anterior midline surrounded by anterior cervical space, carotid space & retropharyngeal space. Recurrent laryngeal nerve is located in tracheoesophageal groove but cannot be seen on conventional imaging. Injury of this nerve results in vocal cord paralysis & imaging should extend to carina in patients with left-sided injury. **(Middle)** Image at subglottic larynx level shows upper thyroid lobes. **(Bottom)** Image at thyroid gland level shows inferior visceral space which includes esophagus & trachea. Thyroid disease is one of most common lesions of visceral space & is often best evaluated by ultrasound. If differentiated thyroid disease is present, nuclear medicine I-131 study is next best study. CECT may delay therapy in patients planned for iodine-based nuclear medicine therapy.

VISCERAL SPACE

CORONAL CECT & THYROID MASS GRAPHIC

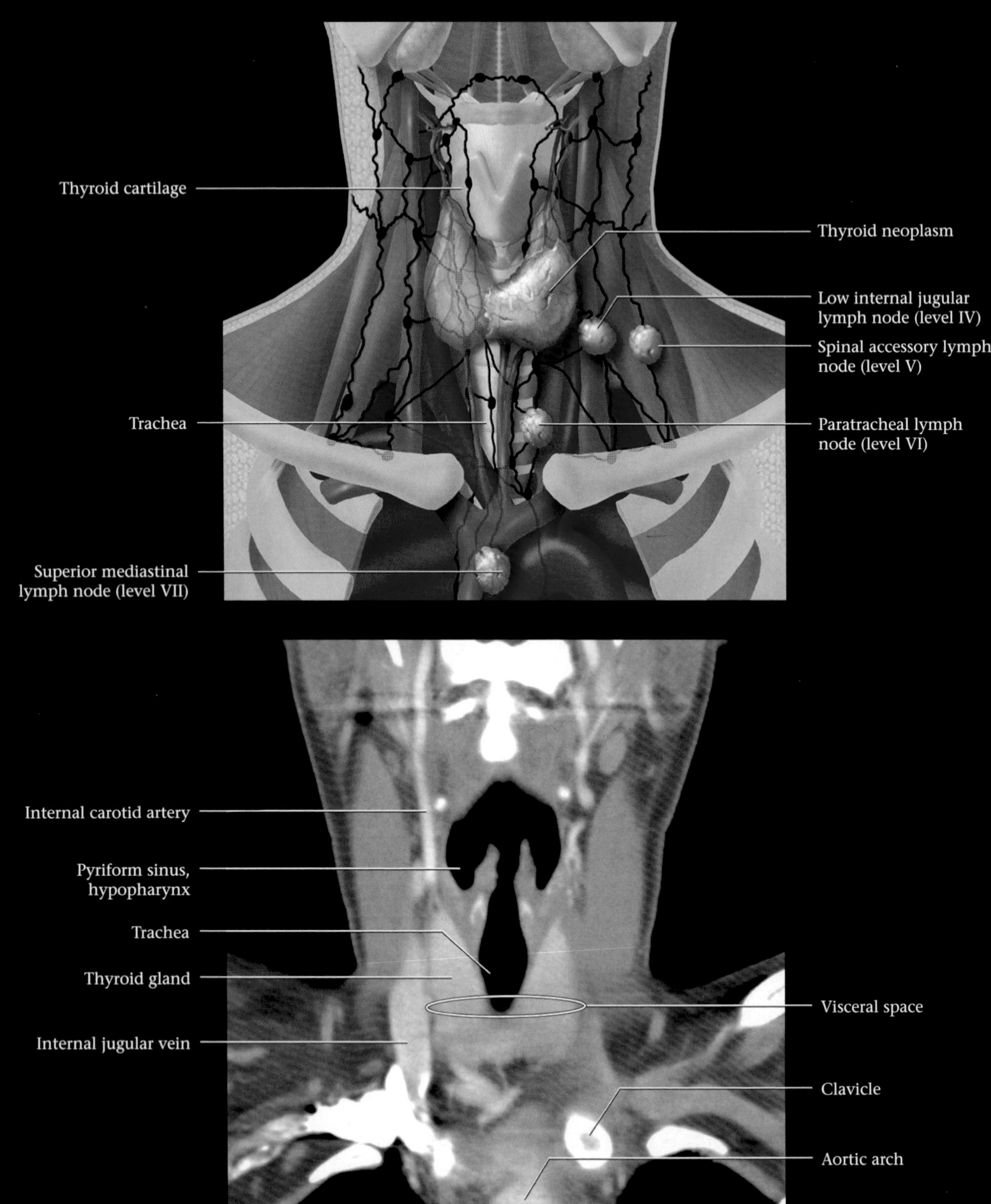
Thyroid cartilage
Thyroid neoplasm
Low internal jugular lymph node (level IV)
Spinal accessory lymph node (level V)
Trachea
Paratracheal lymph node (level VI)
Superior mediastinal lymph node (level VII)
Internal carotid artery
Pyriform sinus, hypopharynx
Trachea
Thyroid gland
Visceral space
Internal jugular vein
Clavicle
Aortic arch

(Top) Coronal graphic shows a typical VS mass, differentiated thyroid carcinoma, within left lobe of thyroid gland. Several metastatic lymph nodes are seen including paratracheal lymph nodes (within visceral space), superior mediastinal, low internal jugular & spinal accessory chain lymph nodes. Paratracheal lymph node group is first order drainage for thyroid malignancy & serves as main conduit for nodal spread into superior mediastinum. **(Bottom)** Coronal CECT image shows chevron shape of thyroid gland to best advantage. Visceral space contents includes larynx, hypopharynx, trachea, esophagus, thyroid & parathyroid glands. Recurrent laryngeal nerves & paratracheal (level VI) lymph nodes are other important visceral space structures. Ending imaging at cervicothoracic junction is an important imaging mistake. Many VS lesions require imaging to carina.

SAGITTAL ANATOMY & GENERIC VS MASS GRAPHIC

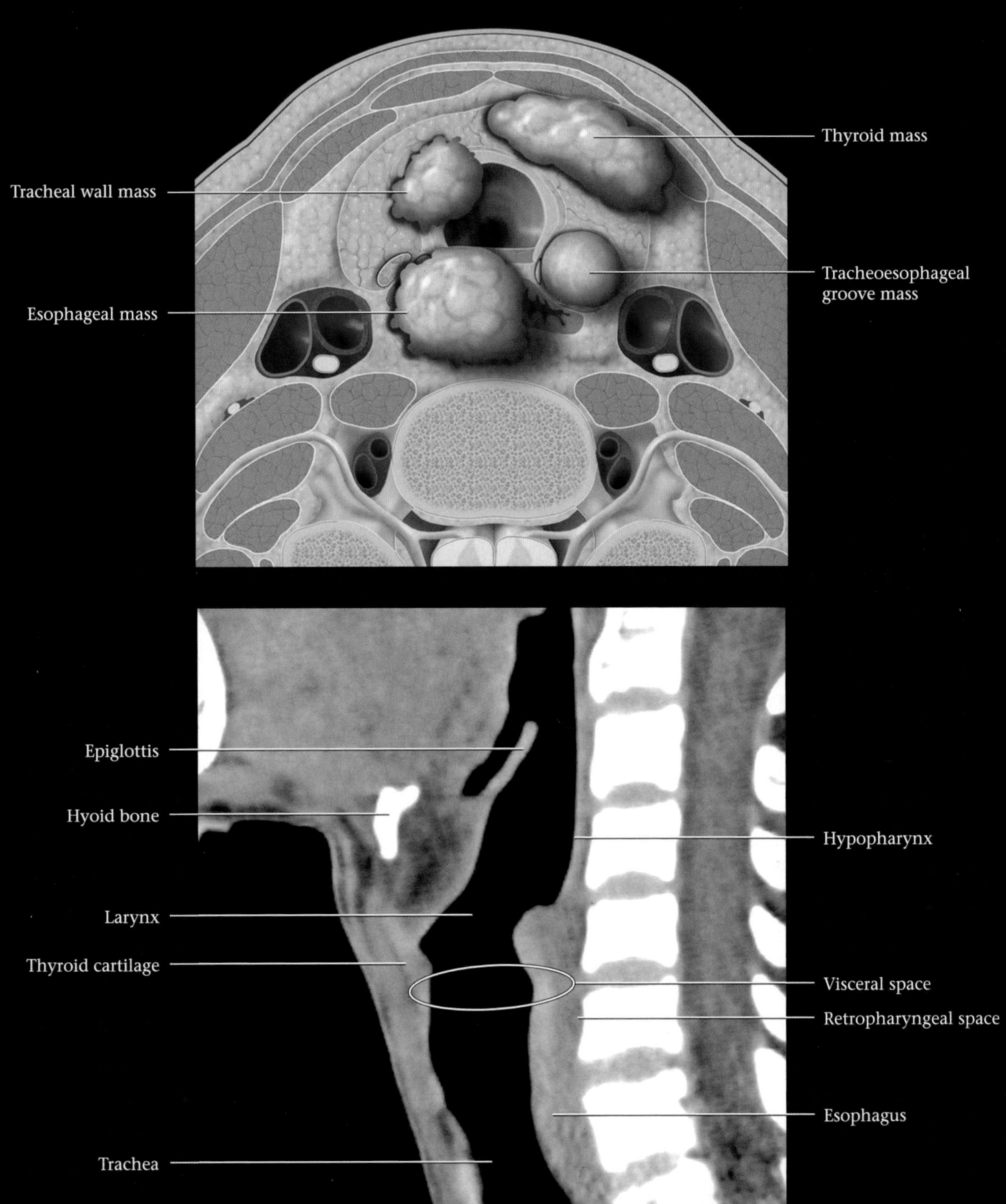

Thyroid mass
Tracheal wall mass
Tracheoesophageal groove mass
Esophageal mass
Epiglottis
Hyoid bone
Hypopharynx
Larynx
Thyroid cartilage
Visceral space
Retropharyngeal space
Esophagus
Trachea

(Top) Axial graphic shows four distinct generic visceral space mass locations. Thyroid mass is defined by mass at least partially surrounded by thyroid tissue. A mass involving tracheoesophageal groove typically results in recurrent laryngeal nerve injury. Differential considerations for tracheoesophageal groove lesion include a malignant paratracheal lymph node (often from differentiated thyroid carcinoma), parathyroid adenoma, traumatic dislocation of cricothyroid joint, recurrent laryngeal nerve schwannoma or patulous esophagus. Tracheal wall mass is centered in tracheal wall & displaces thyroid gland laterally & esophagus posteriorly. An esophageal mass is typically midline & displaces trachea & thyroid anteriorly. **(Bottom)** Sagittal NECT reformation shows visceral space in midline infrahyoid neck, anterior to retropharyngeal space.

HYPOPHARYNX-LARYNX

Terminology

Abbreviations
- Aryepiglottic fold (AE fold)
- True vocal cord (TVC); false vocal cord (FVC)

Synonyms
- Hypopharynx = laryngopharynx

Definitions
- Hypopharynx: Caudal continuation of pharyngeal mucosal space, between oropharynx & esophagus
- Larynx: Junction of upper & lower airway

Imaging Anatomy

Extent
- Hypopharynx: Extends from level of glossoepiglottic & pharyngoepiglottic folds superiorly to inferior cricoid cartilage (cricopharyngeus muscle)
  - Oropharynx above, cervical esophagus below
- Larynx: Cranial margin at level of glossoepiglottic & pharyngoepiglottic folds with caudal margin defined by lower edge of cricoid
  - Oropharynx above, trachea below

Internal Structures-Critical Contents
- **Hypopharynx** consists of 3 regions
  - **Pyriform sinus:** Anterolateral recess of HP
    - Between inner surface of thyrohyoid membrane (above), thyroid cartilage (below) & lateral AE fold
    - Pyriform sinus apex (inferior tip) at level of TVC
    - Anteromedial margin of pyriform sinus is posterolateral wall of AE fold ("marginal supraglottis")
  - **Posterior wall:** Inferior continuation of posterior oropharynx wall
  - **Post-cricoid region:** Anterior wall of lower hypopharynx
    - Interface between hypopharynx & larynx
    - Extends from cricoarytenoid joints to lower edge of cricoid cartilage
  - Pharyngeal plexus (CN9-10 branches) provides all motor & most sensory to hypopharynx
- **Laryngeal cartilages**
  - **Thyroid cartilage:** Largest laryngeal cartilage; "shields" larynx
    - Two anterior laminae meet anteriorly at acute angle
    - Superior thyroid notch at anterior superior aspect
    - Superior cornua are elongated & narrow, attach to thyrohyoid ligament
    - Inferior cornua are short & thick, articulating medially with sides of cricoid cartilage
  - **Cricoid cartilage:** Only complete ring in endolarynx, provides structural integrity
    - Two portions, posterior lamina & anterior arch
    - "Signet ring" band anterior & "signet" posterior
    - Lower border of cricoid cartilage is junction between larynx above & trachea below
  - **Arytenoid cartilage:** Paired pyramidal cartilages that sit atop posterior cricoid cartilage
    - Vocal & muscular processes are at level of TVC
    - Vocal processes: Anterior projections of arytenoids where posterior margins of TVC attach
  - Corniculate cartilage: Rests on top of superior process of arytenoid cartilage, within AE folds
- **Supraglottis of endolarynx**
  - Extends from tip of epiglottis above to laryngeal ventricle below
  - Contains vestibule, epiglottis, pre-epiglottic fat, AE folds, FVC, paraglottic space, arytenoid cartilages
  - **Epiglottis:** Leaf-shaped cartilage, larynx lid with free margin (suprahyoid), fixed portion (infrahyoid)
    - Petiole is "stem" of leaf which attaches epiglottis to thyroid lamina via thyroepiglottic ligament
    - Hyoepiglottic ligament attaches epiglottis to hyoid; glossoepiglottic fold is midline mucous membrane covering hyoepiglottic ligament
  - **Pre-epiglottic space:** Fat-filled space between hyoid bone anteriorly & epiglottis posteriorly
  - **AE folds:** Projects from cephalad tip of arytenoid cartilages to inferolateral margin of epiglottis
    - Represents superolateral margin of supraglottis, dividing it from pyriform sinus (hypopharynx)
  - **False vocal cords:** Mucosal surfaces of laryngeal vestibule of supraglottis
    - Beneath FVC are paired paraglottic spaces
  - **Paraglottic spaces:** Paired fatty regions beneath false & true vocal cords
    - Superiorly they merge into pre-epiglottic space
    - Terminates inferiorly at under surface of TVC
- **Glottis of endolarynx**
  - TVC & anterior & posterior commissures
    - **TVC:** Only soft tissue structures of glottic region
    - Comprised of thyroarytenoid muscle (medial fibers are "vocalis muscle")
    - Anterior commissure: Midline, anterior meeting point of TVC
- **Subglottis of endolarynx**
  - Subglottis extends from under surface of TVC to inferior surface of cricoid cartilage
  - Mucosal surface of subglottic area is closely applied to cricoid cartilage
  - **Conus elasticus:** Fibroelastic membrane extends from medial margin of TVC above to cricoid below
  - **Quadrangular membrane:** Fibrous membrane extends from upper arytenoid & corniculate cartilages (posteriorly) to lateral margin epiglottis (anteriorly); medial margin of paraglottic space

Embryology

Embryologic Events
- Larynx has two embryologically distinct portions separated at laryngeal ventricle
- Supraglottic larynx forms from primitive buccopharyngeal anlage & has rich lymphatics
- Glottic & subglottic larynx forms from tracheobronchial buds & has few lymphatics

Practical Implications
- Supraglottic SCCa have a much higher incidence of nodal metastases at presentation compared to glottic & subglottic SCCa

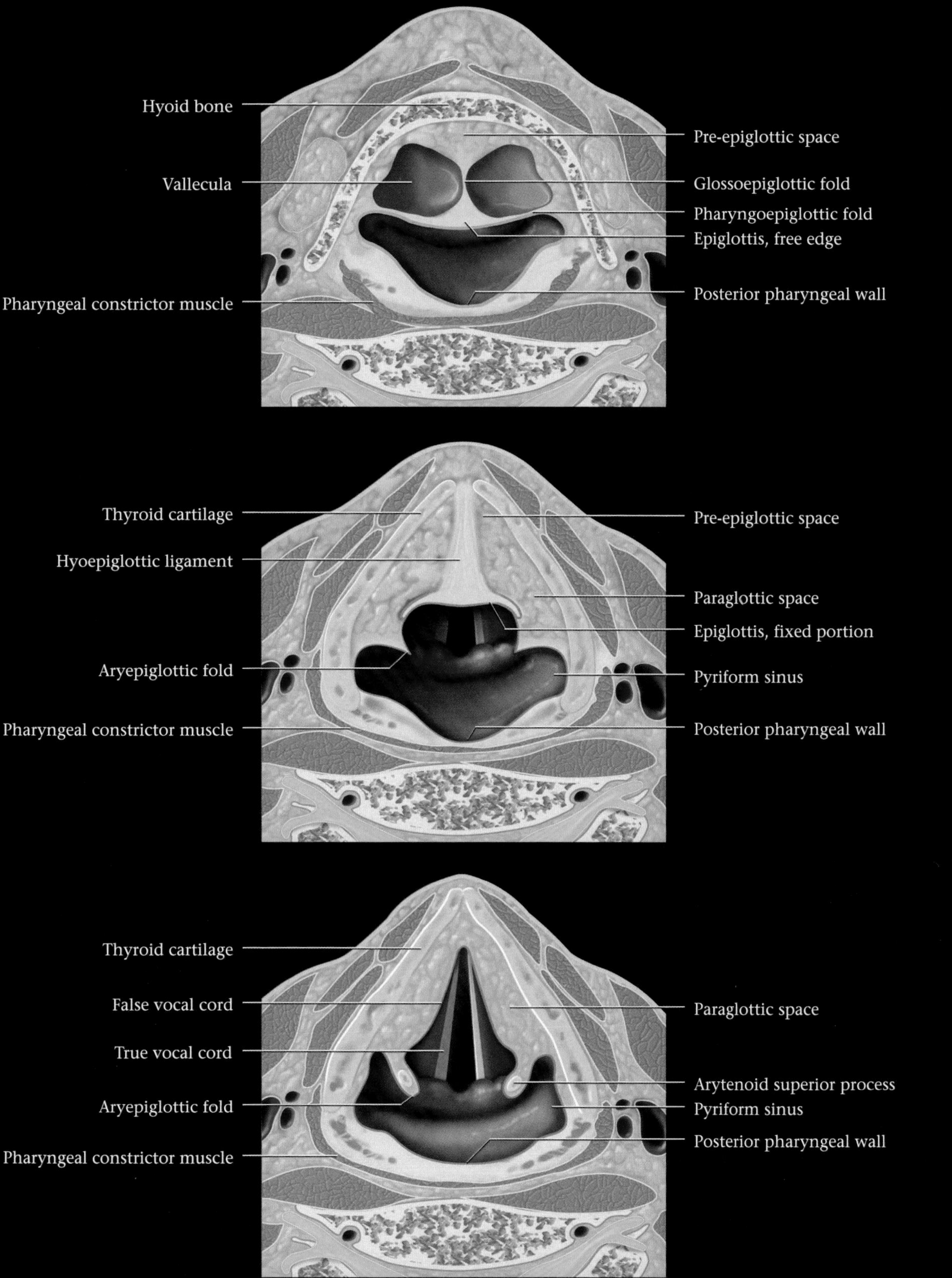
Hyoid bone
Vallecula
Pharyngeal constrictor muscle
Pre-epiglottic space
Glossoepiglottic fold
Pharyngoepiglottic fold
Epiglottis, free edge
Posterior pharyngeal wall
Thyroid cartilage
Hyoepiglottic ligament
Aryepiglottic fold
Pharyngeal constrictor muscle
Pre-epiglottic space
Paraglottic space
Epiglottis, fixed portion
Pyriform sinus
Posterior pharyngeal wall
Thyroid cartilage
False vocal cord
True vocal cord
Aryepiglottic fold
Pharyngeal constrictor muscle
Paraglottic space
Arytenoid superior process
Pyriform sinus
Posterior pharyngeal wall

(Top) First of six axial graphics of larynx & hypopharynx from superior to inferior shows roof of hypopharynx at hyoid bone level & high supraglottic structures. Free edge of epiglottis is attached to hyoid bone via hyoepiglottic ligament which is covered by glossoepiglottic fold, a ridge of mucous membrane. **(Middle)** Graphic at mid-supraglottic level shows hyoepiglottic ligament dividing lower pre-epiglottic space. No fascia separates pre-epiglottic space from paraglottic space. These two endolaryngeal spaces are submucosal locations where tumors hide from clinical detection. Aryepiglottic fold represents junction between larynx & hypopharynx. **(Bottom)** Graphic at low supraglottic level shows false vocal cords (FVC) formed by mucosal surfaces of laryngeal vestibule. Paraglottic space is beneath FVC, a common location for submucosal tumor spread.

HYPOPHARYNX-LARYNX

GRAPHICS

Thyroid cartilage
Vocalis muscle
Thyroarytenoid muscle
Pyriform sinus apex
Cricoid cartilage
Post-cricoid hypopharynx
Anterior commissure
Vocal ligament
Vocal process, arytenoid cartilage
Arytenoid cartilage
Thyroarytenoid gap
Posterior cricoarytenoid muscle

Thyroid cartilage
Cricoid cartilage
Pharyngeal constrictor muscle
Longus capitis muscle
Undersurface of true vocal cord
Cricothyroid space
Posterior cricoarytenoid muscle
Post-cricoid hypopharynx
Posterior wall, hypopharynx

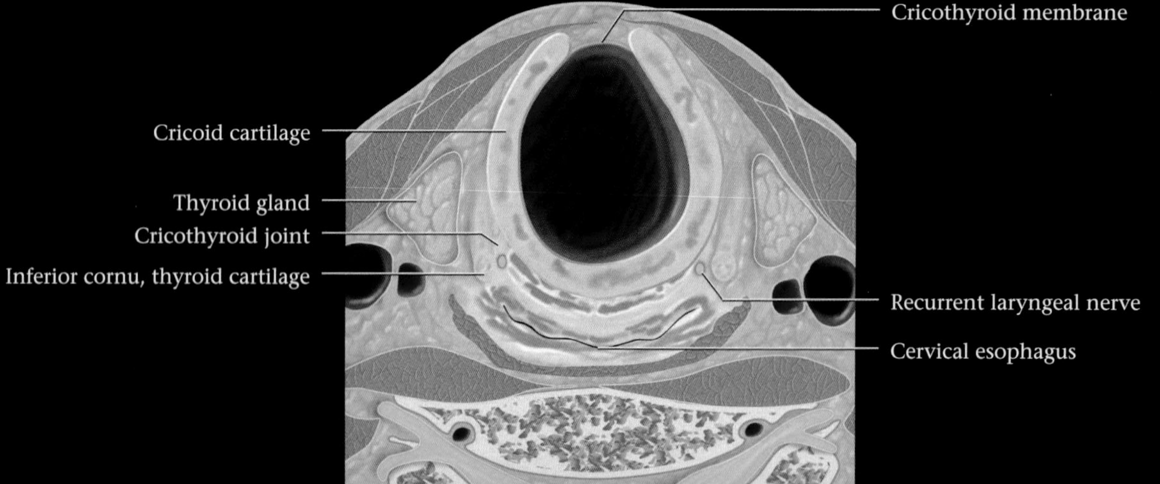
Cricothyroid membrane
Cricoid cartilage
Thyroid gland
Cricothyroid joint
Inferior cornu, thyroid cartilage
Recurrent laryngeal nerve
Cervical esophagus

(Top) Graphic at glottic, true vocal cord level shows thyroarytenoid muscle which makes up bulk of true vocal cord. Medial fibers of thyroarytenoid muscle are known as vocalis muscle. Pyriform sinus apex is seen at glottic level. Thyroarytenoid gap is location where tumors may spread between larynx & hypopharynx. **(Middle)** Graphic at level of undersurface of true vocal cord shows posterior lamina of cricoid cartilage. Post-cricoid hypopharynx represents anterior wall of lower hypopharynx & extends from cricoarytenoid joints to lower edge of cricoid cartilage at cricopharyngeus muscle. Posterior wall of hypopharynx represents inferior continuation of posterior oropharyngeal wall & extends to cervical esophagus. **(Bottom)** Graphic at subglottic level shows cricothyroid joint immediately adjacent to recurrent laryngeal nerve, located in tracheoesophageal groove.

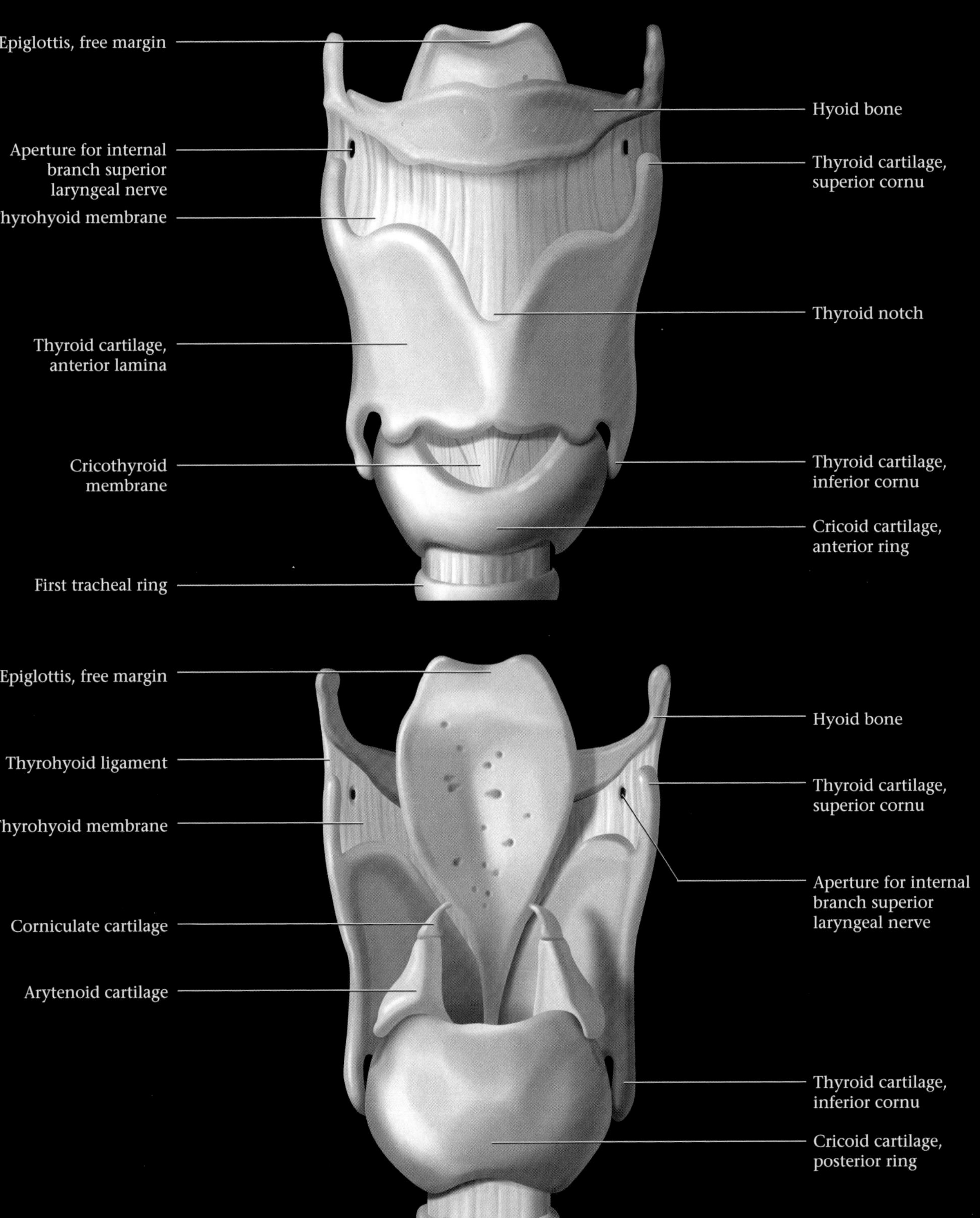
Epiglottis, free margin
Hyoid bone
Aperture for internal branch superior laryngeal nerve
Thyroid cartilage, superior cornu
Thyrohyoid membrane
Thyroid notch
Thyroid cartilage, anterior lamina
Cricothyroid membrane
Thyroid cartilage, inferior cornu
Cricoid cartilage, anterior ring
First tracheal ring
Epiglottis, free margin
Hyoid bone
Thyrohyoid ligament
Thyroid cartilage, superior cornu
Thyrohyoid membrane
Aperture for internal branch superior laryngeal nerve
Corniculate cartilage
Arytenoid cartilage
Thyroid cartilage, inferior cornu
Cricoid cartilage, posterior ring

(Top) Anterior view of laryngeal cartilage which provides structural framework for soft tissues of larynx to drape over. Note two large anterior laminae of thyroid cartilage "shield" the larynx. Thyrohyoid membrane contains an aperture through which internal branch of superior laryngeal nerve & associated vessels course. Mixed (external) laryngoceles herniate through thyrohyoid membrane to extend into submandibular space. **(Bottom)** Posterior view shows arytenoid cartilage sitting on top of posterior cricoid cartilage. True vocal cord attaches to vocal process of arytenoid cartilage & forms glottis. Epiglottis is a leaf-shaped cartilage which forms lid of larynx & contains fixed & free margins. Cricoid cartilage is only complete ring in endolarynx & provides structural integrity. Lower border of cricoid represents junction between larynx above & trachea below.

HYPOPHARYNX-LARYNX

GRAPHICS

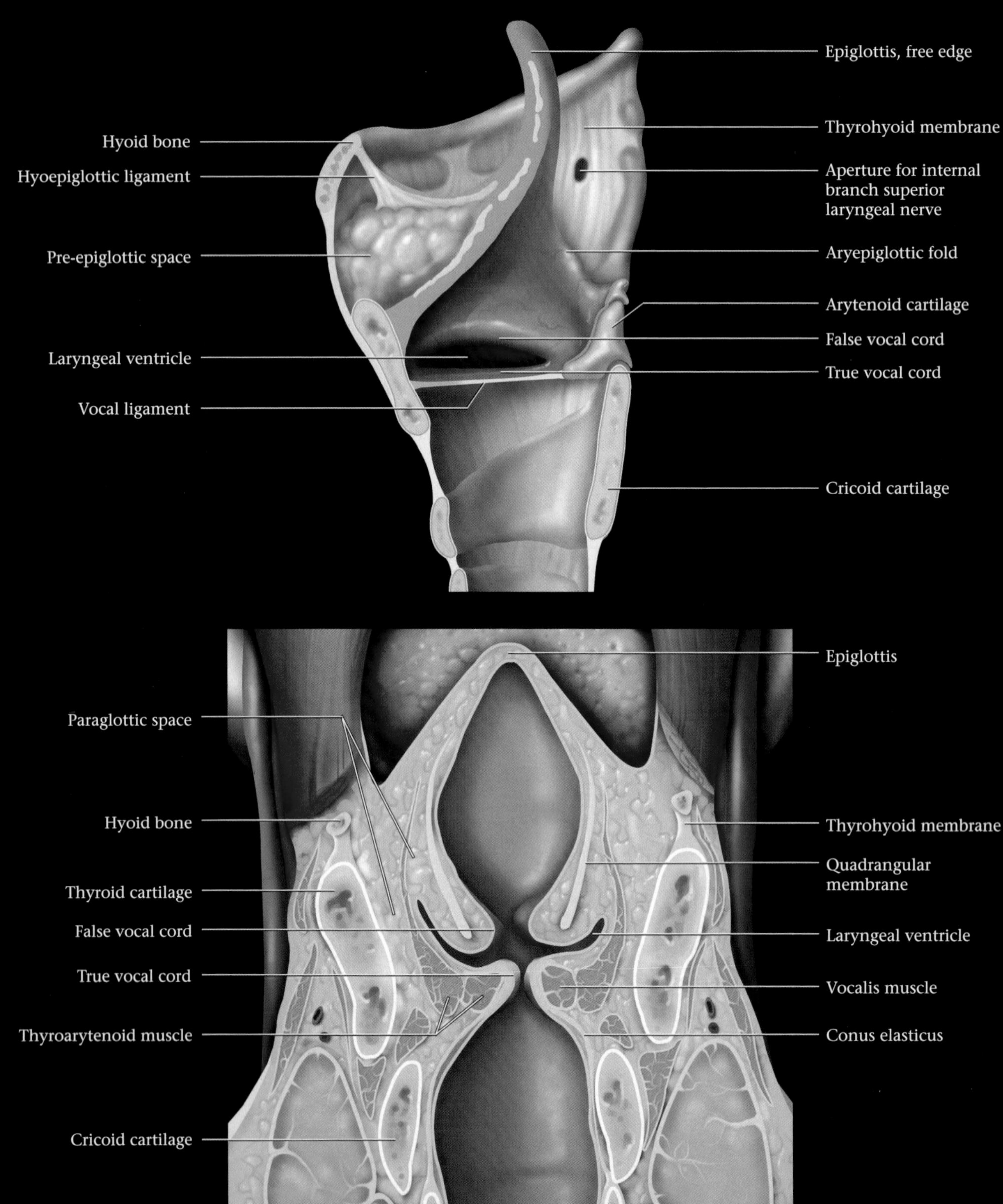
Epiglottis, free edge
Thyrohyoid membrane
Hyoid bone
Hyoepiglottic ligament
Aperture for internal branch superior laryngeal nerve
Pre-epiglottic space
Aryepiglottic fold
Arytenoid cartilage
False vocal cord
Laryngeal ventricle
True vocal cord
Vocal ligament
Cricoid cartilage
Epiglottis
Paraglottic space
Hyoid bone
Thyrohyoid membrane
Quadrangular membrane
Thyroid cartilage
False vocal cord
Laryngeal ventricle
True vocal cord
Vocalis muscle
Thyroarytenoid muscle
Conus elasticus
Cricoid cartilage

(Top) Sagittal graphic of midline larynx shows laryngeal ventricle, air-space which separates false vocal cords above with true vocal cords below. Aryepiglottic folds project from tip of arytenoid cartilage to inferolateral margin of epiglottis. Aryepiglottic folds represent junction between supraglottis & hypopharynx. Medial wall of aryepiglottic fold is endolaryngeal while posterolateral wall is anteromedial margin of pyriform sinus. **(Bottom)** Coronal graphic posterior view shows false & true vocal cords separated by laryngeal ventricle. Quadrangular membrane is a fibrous membrane which extends from upper arytenoid & corniculate cartilages to lateral epiglottis. Conus elasticus is a fibroelastic membrane which extends from vocal ligament of true vocal cord to cricoid. There membranes represent a relative barrier to tumor spread but are not seen on conventional imaging.

REFORMATTED CT & GRAPHIC

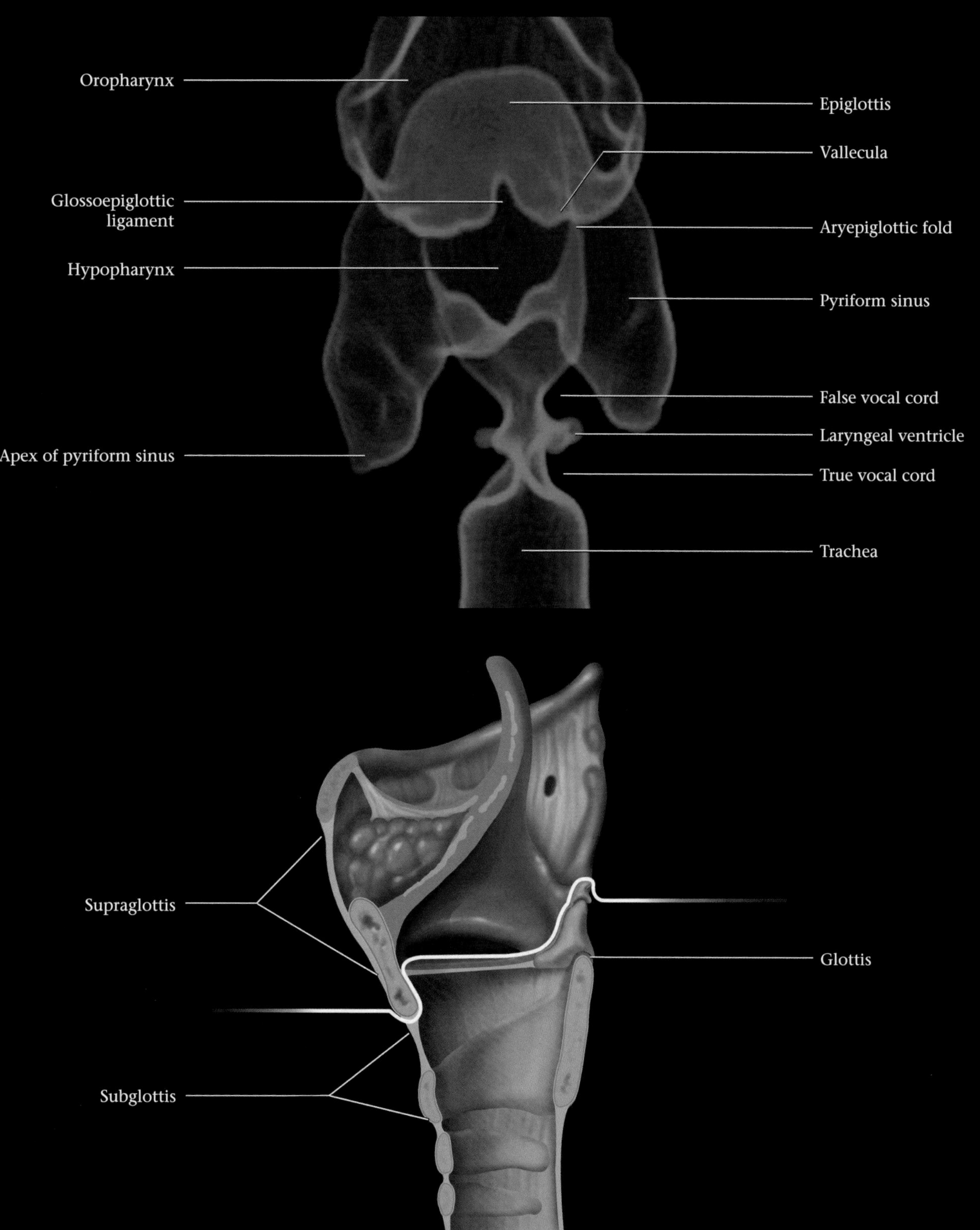

Oropharynx
Epiglottis
Vallecula
Glossoepiglottic ligament
Aryepiglottic fold
Hypopharynx
Pyriform sinus
False vocal cord
Laryngeal ventricle
Apex of pyriform sinus
True vocal cord
Trachea
Supraglottis
Glottis
Subglottis

(Top) Coronal 3D reformatted CT image shows mucosal surfaces of larynx & hypopharynx. Pyriform sinus represents anterolateral recess of hypopharynx & is most common location for hypopharyngeal tumors. Pyriform sinus apex (inferior tip) lies at level of true vocal cord which allows pyriform sinus tumors access to true vocal cords. (Courtesy of Christine Glastonbury, MBBS). **(Bottom)** Sagittal graphic of larynx shows two separate embryologically defined regions, separated at laryngeal ventricle. Supraglottis (purple) forms from primitive buccopharyngeal anlage & has rich lymphatics that drain to upper internal jugular nodes. Glottis & subglottis (green) form from tracheobronchial buds & have sparse lymphatics, drain to internal jugular & paratracheal nodes. Supraglottic tumors have much higher incidence of nodal metastases at presentation than glottic & subglottic tumors.

AXIAL CECT CORDS ABDUCTED (APART)

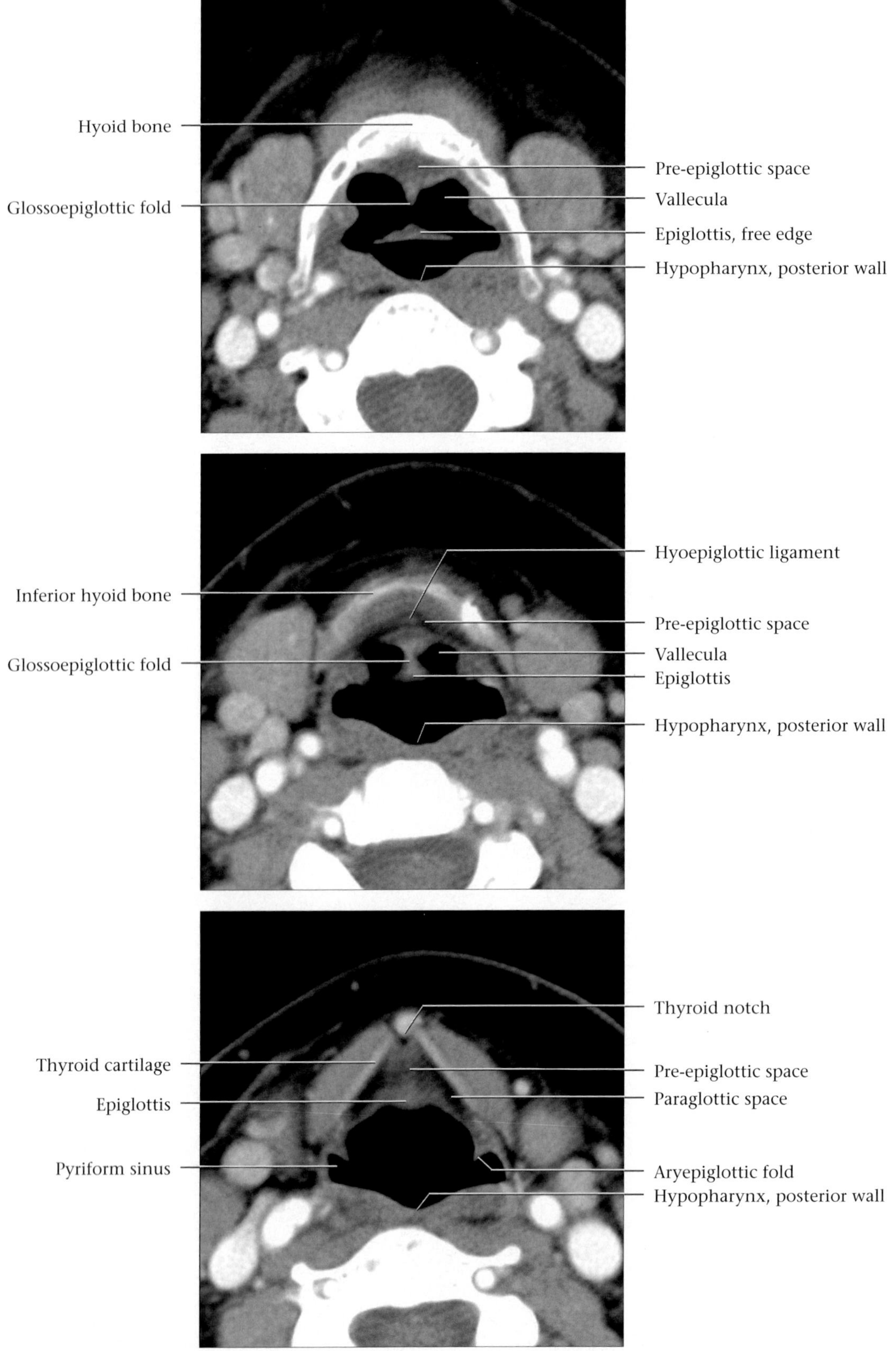
Hyoid bone
Glossoepiglottic fold
Pre-epiglottic space
Vallecula
Epiglottis, free edge
Hypopharynx, posterior wall
Hyoepiglottic ligament
Inferior hyoid bone
Glossoepiglottic fold
Pre-epiglottic space
Vallecula
Epiglottis
Hypopharynx, posterior wall
Thyroid notch
Thyroid cartilage
Epiglottis
Pyriform sinus
Pre-epiglottic space
Paraglottic space
Aryepiglottic fold
Hypopharynx, posterior wall

(Top) First of nine axial CECT images presented from superior to inferior of larynx & hypopharynx with patient in quiet respiration. Hyoid bone represents the level of the roof of larynx & hypopharynx. Glossoepiglottic & pharyngoepiglottic folds represent transition from oropharynx above to larynx & hypopharynx below. **(Middle)** Image of high supraglottic level of larynx shows C-shaped pre-epiglottic space, a common location for tumors to hide. If supraglottic tumor extends to pre-epiglottic space, it becomes a T3 tumor. **(Bottom)** Image of high supraglottic level shows pre-epiglottic & paraglottic spaces are continuous, with no intervening fascia. This allows tumors to spread submucosally in these locations. Aryepiglottic fold, part of larynx, represents transition between larynx & hypopharynx. Posterolateral wall of aryepiglottic fold is anteromedial margin of pyriform sinus.

AXIAL CECT CORDS ABDUCTED (APART)

Thyroid cartilage
Pyriform sinus
Thyroid notch
Thyroepiglottic ligament
Paraglottic space
Aryepiglottic fold
Hypopharynx, posterior wall

Thyroid cartilage
Strap muscles
Paraglottic space
False vocal cord
Hypopharynx, posterior wall

Anterior commissure
Thyroid cartilage
Posterior commissure
Thyroarytenoid gap
Hypopharynx
True vocal cord
Vocal process, arytenoid
Arytenoid cartilage
Cricoid cartilage

(Top) Image of mid-supraglottic level shows thyroepiglottic ligament dividing the pre-epiglottic space. Aryepiglottic folds are at margin of pyriform sinus & larynx & a tumor primary to aryepiglottic fold is considered a "marginal supraglottic" tumor. **(Middle)** Image of low supraglottic level shows false vocal cord level. Paraglottic space represents deep fatty space beneath false vocal cords. Tumors that cross laryngeal ventricle & involve false & true vocal cords are considered transglottic. **(Bottom)** Image at glottic level shows true vocal cords in abduction in quiet respiration. True vocal cord level is identified on CT when arytenoid & cricoid cartilages are seen & muscle fills inferior paraglottic space. Anterior & posterior commissures of true vocal cords should be less than 1 mm in normal patients. Post-cricoid hypopharynx is typically collapsed.

AXIAL CECT CORDS ABDUCTED (APART)

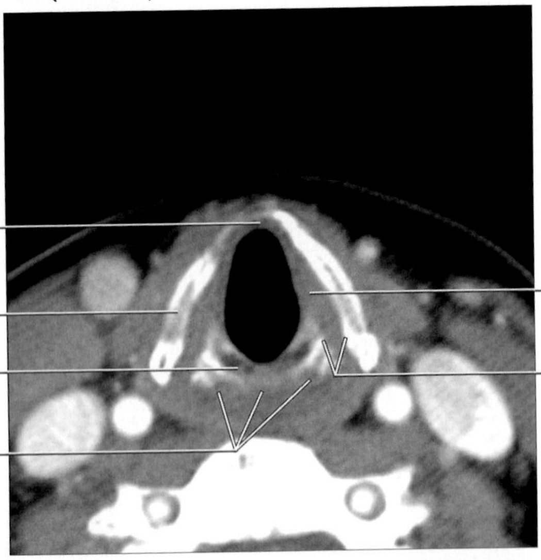

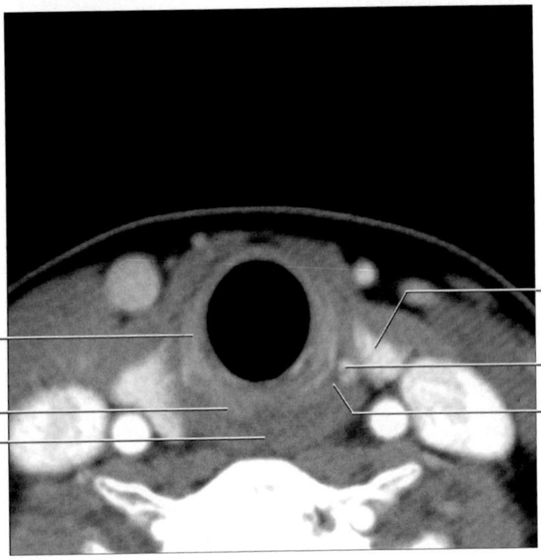

Anterior commissure
Thyroid cartilage
Cricoid cartilage
Post-cricoid hypopharyngeal wall
Undersurface of true cord
Cricothyroid space

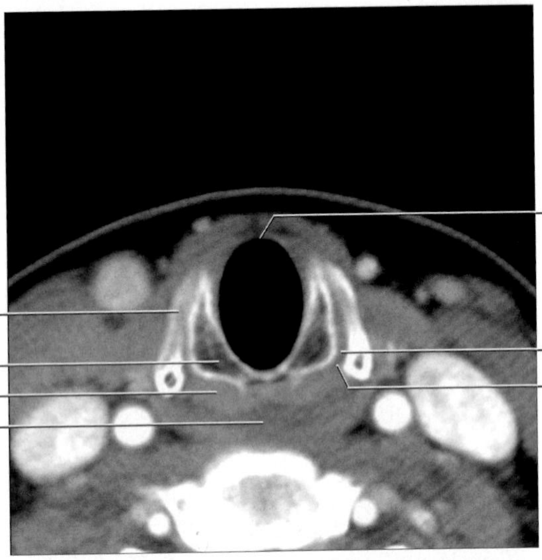

Cricothyroid membrane
Thyroid cartilage
Cricoid cartilage
Posterior cricoarytenoid muscle
Hypopharynx
Cricothyroid joint
Location of recurrent laryngeal nerve

Thyroid gland
Cricoid cartilage
Inferior cornu, thyroid cartilage
Posterior cricoarytenoid muscle
Hypopharynx/esophagus junction
Location of recurrent laryngeal nerve

(Top) In this image through the undersurface of true cord level the cricothyroid space is seen. Lack of arytenoid cartilage identifies undersurface of true cord level. **(Middle)** Image more inferior shows subglottic level with cricoid ring nearly complete. Cricoid is only complete cartilage ring in larynx & provides structural integrity. Dislocations of cricothyroid joint may result in vocal cord paralysis secondary to recurrent laryngeal nerve injury. There may be associated atrophy of posterior cricoarytenoid muscle on involved side of vocal cord paralysis. **(Bottom)** At the level of the inferior cricoid cartilage the inferior margin of larynx & hypopharynx are transitioning to the trachea & cervical esophagus. Mucosa along subglottis should be no more than 1mm in normal patients. If thickened mucosa, raises concern for tumor.

AXIAL CECT CORDS ADDUCTED (TOGETHER)

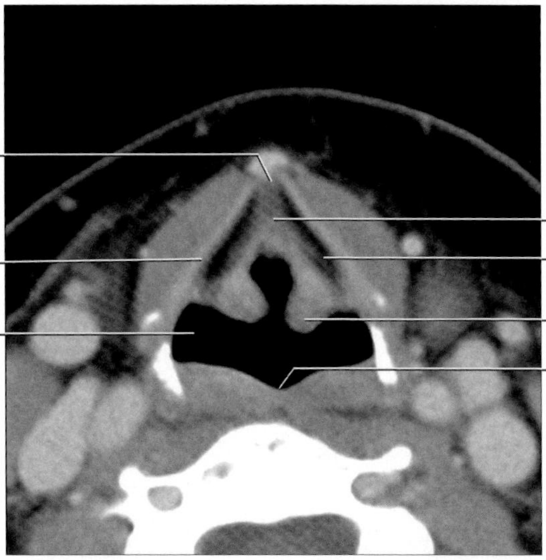

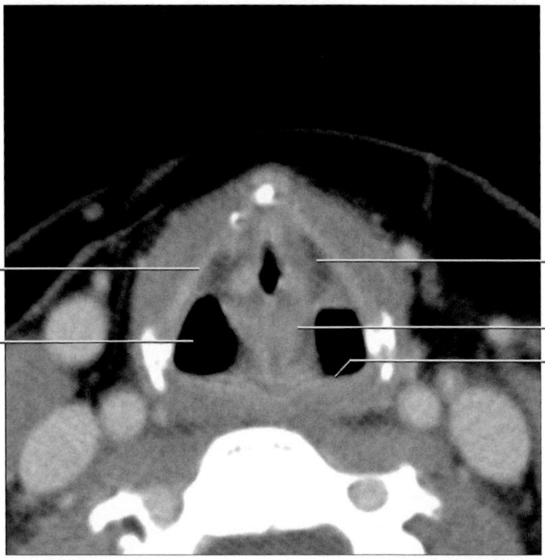

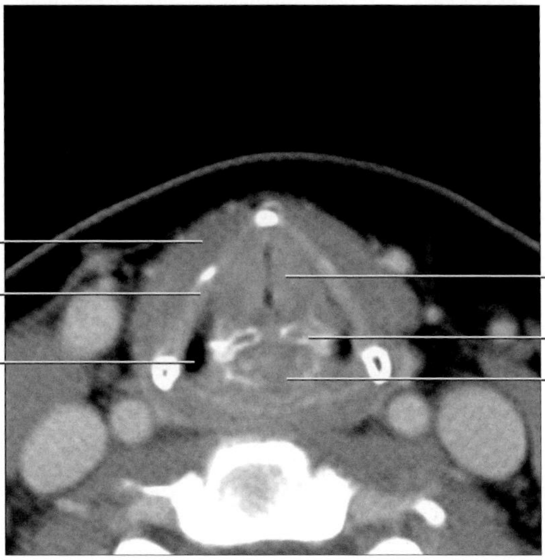

Thyroid notch
Thyroid cartilage
Pyriform sinus
Thyroepiglottic ligament
Paraglottic space
Aryepiglottic fold
Posterior wall, hypopharynx

Thyroid cartilage
Pyriform sinus
Paraglottic space
Aryepiglottic fold
Posterior wall, hypopharynx

Strap muscles
Thyroid cartilage
Pyriform sinus
True vocal cord
Arytenoid cartilage
Cricoid cartilage

(Top) First of three axial CECT images from superior to inferior in patient with breath holding shows adduction of false & true vocal cords as well as aryepiglottic folds. **(Middle)** Image at low supraglottic level shows level of false vocal cords in adduction. Note mucosa of aryepiglottic folds contacts posterior hypopharyngeal wall. **(Bottom)** Image at glottic level shows adduction of true vocal cords. With breath holding, true vocal cords oppose in midline. A cord that remains paramedian is either paralyzed or mechanically fixed. Vocal cord paralysis typically results in a paramedian true vocal cords with associated abnormal location of arytenoid cartilage which is fixed in an anterior-medial position. With breath holding, paralyzed cord remains fixed while opposite normal cord crosses midline in attempt to close glottis. There may be an associated patulous pyriform sinus.

CORONAL NECT

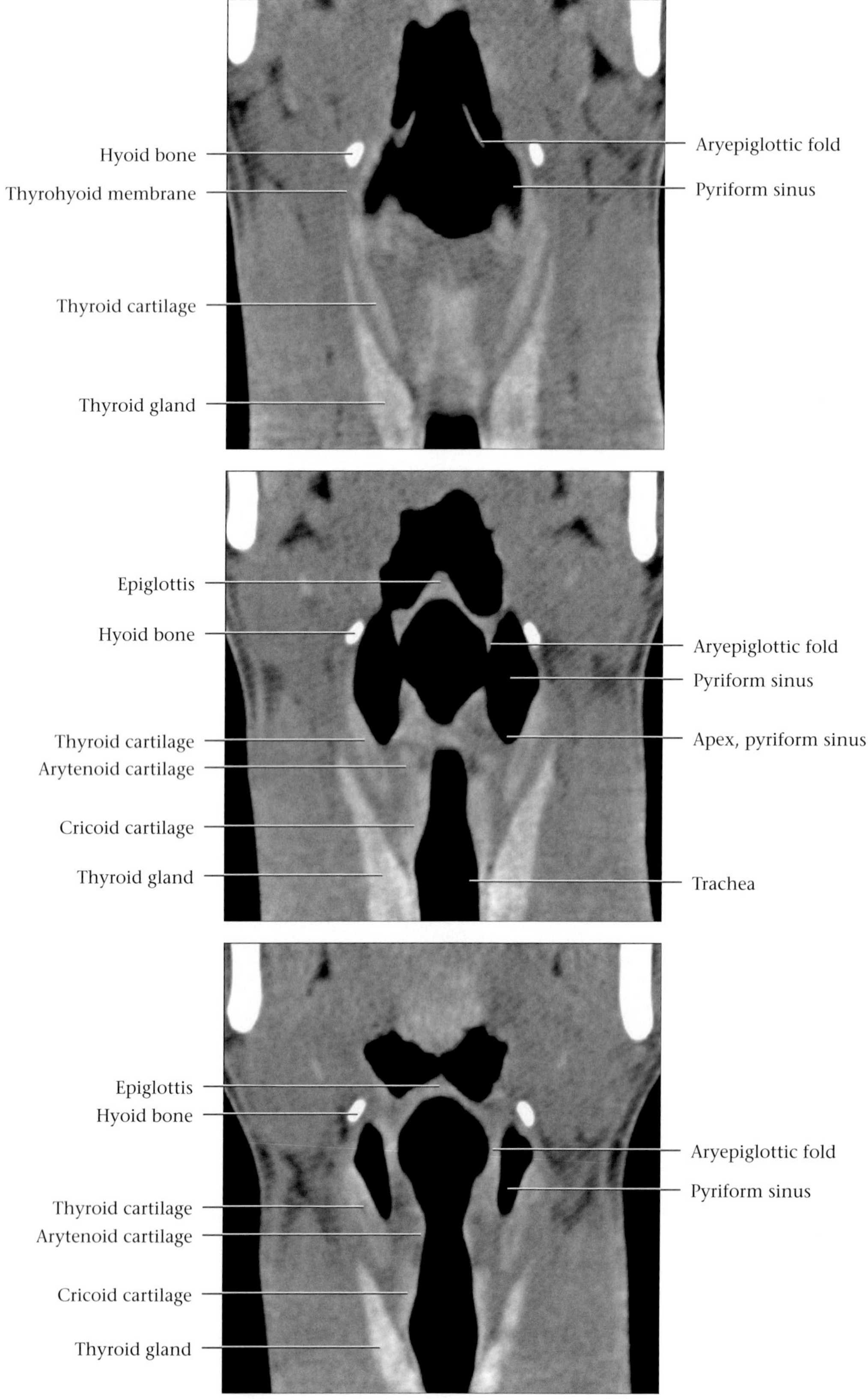
Hyoid bone
Thyrohyoid membrane
Thyroid cartilage
Thyroid gland
Aryepiglottic fold
Pyriform sinus
Epiglottis
Hyoid bone
Thyroid cartilage
Arytenoid cartilage
Cricoid cartilage
Thyroid gland
Aryepiglottic fold
Pyriform sinus
Apex, pyriform sinus
Trachea
Epiglottis
Hyoid bone
Thyroid cartilage
Arytenoid cartilage
Cricoid cartilage
Thyroid gland
Aryepiglottic fold
Pyriform sinus

(Top) First of six NECT coronal reformation images of larynx & hypopharynx presented from posterior to anterior shows hyoid bone which represents the level of the roof of larynx & hypopharynx. CT is particularly good for evaluation of patients with diseases of larynx & hypopharynx as these patients often have difficulty with secretions, coughing & swallowing making a short exam time vital. **(Middle)** Image more anterior shows laryngeal cartilages. These cartilages are variably ossified in adults which makes pathologic conditions such as cartilage invasion difficult to diagnose with certainty. Apex of pyriform sinus extends inferiorly to level of true vocal cord. **(Bottom)** In this Image aryepiglottic folds are well seen as they extend from lateral epiglottis to arytenoid cartilage. Pyriform sinus is most common location for tumors of hypopharynx.

CORONAL NECT

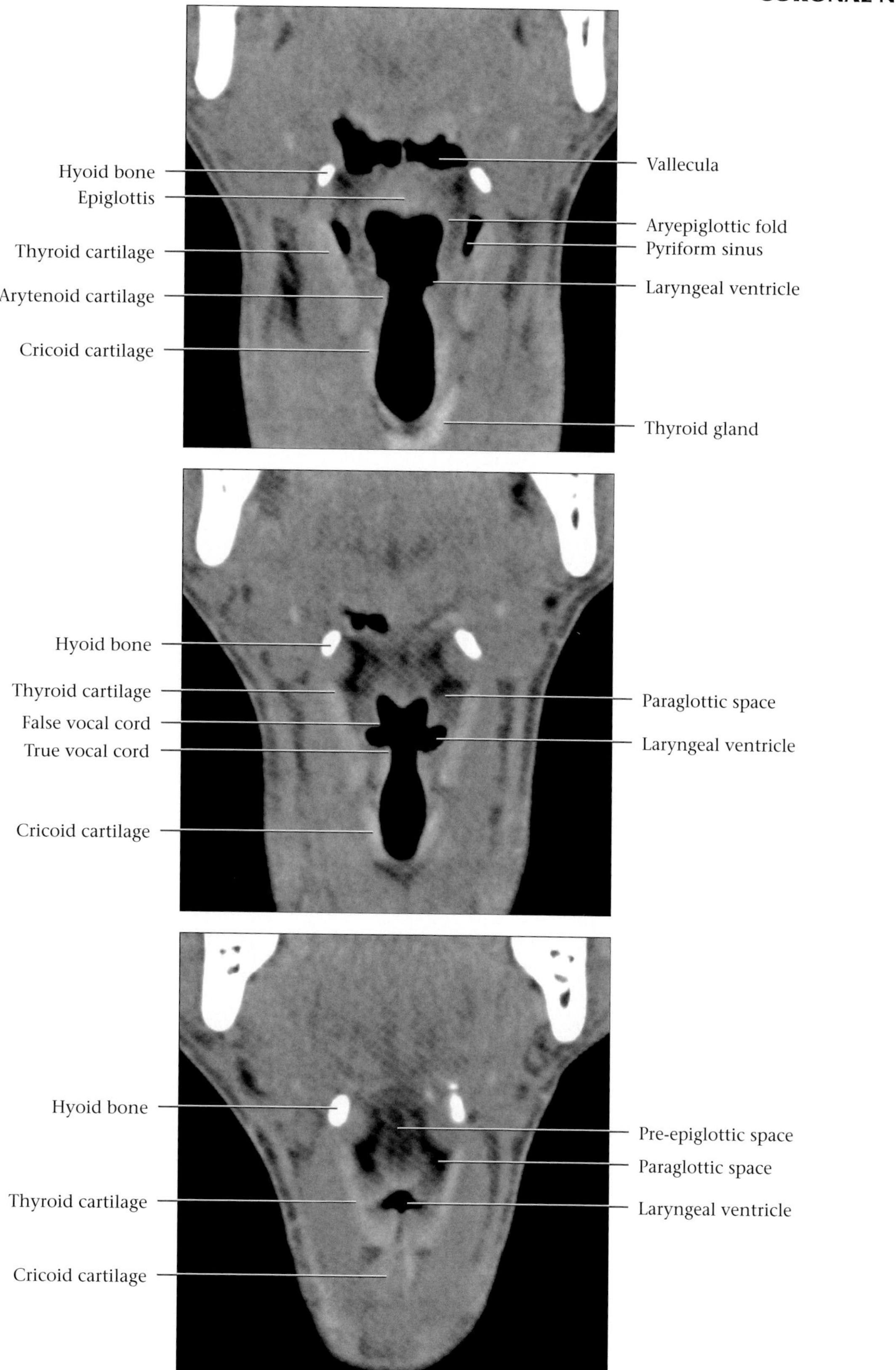

Hyoid bone
Epiglottis
Thyroid cartilage
Arytenoid cartilage
Cricoid cartilage
Vallecula
Aryepiglottic fold
Pyriform sinus
Laryngeal ventricle
Thyroid gland
Hyoid bone
Thyroid cartilage
False vocal cord
True vocal cord
Cricoid cartilage
Paraglottic space
Laryngeal ventricle
Hyoid bone
Thyroid cartilage
Cricoid cartilage
Pre-epiglottic space
Paraglottic space
Laryngeal ventricle

(Top) This image shows the fixed portion of epiglottis in midline. Aryepiglottic fold which represents junction between larynx anteriorly & hypopharynx posteriorly is noted. **(Middle)** In this image the laryngeal ventricle is visible as an air space between false vocal cords above & true vocal cords below. When a tumor crosses laryngeal ventricle to involve true & false cords it is transglottic, which has important treatment implications. Coronal imaging is particularly useful for evaluation of transglottic disease. **(Bottom)** This image reveals pre-epiglottic fat to be continuous with paraglottic fat. These are the most important spaces of endolarynx as they allow submucosal spread of tumors which is undetectable by clinical exam.

SAGITTAL NECT

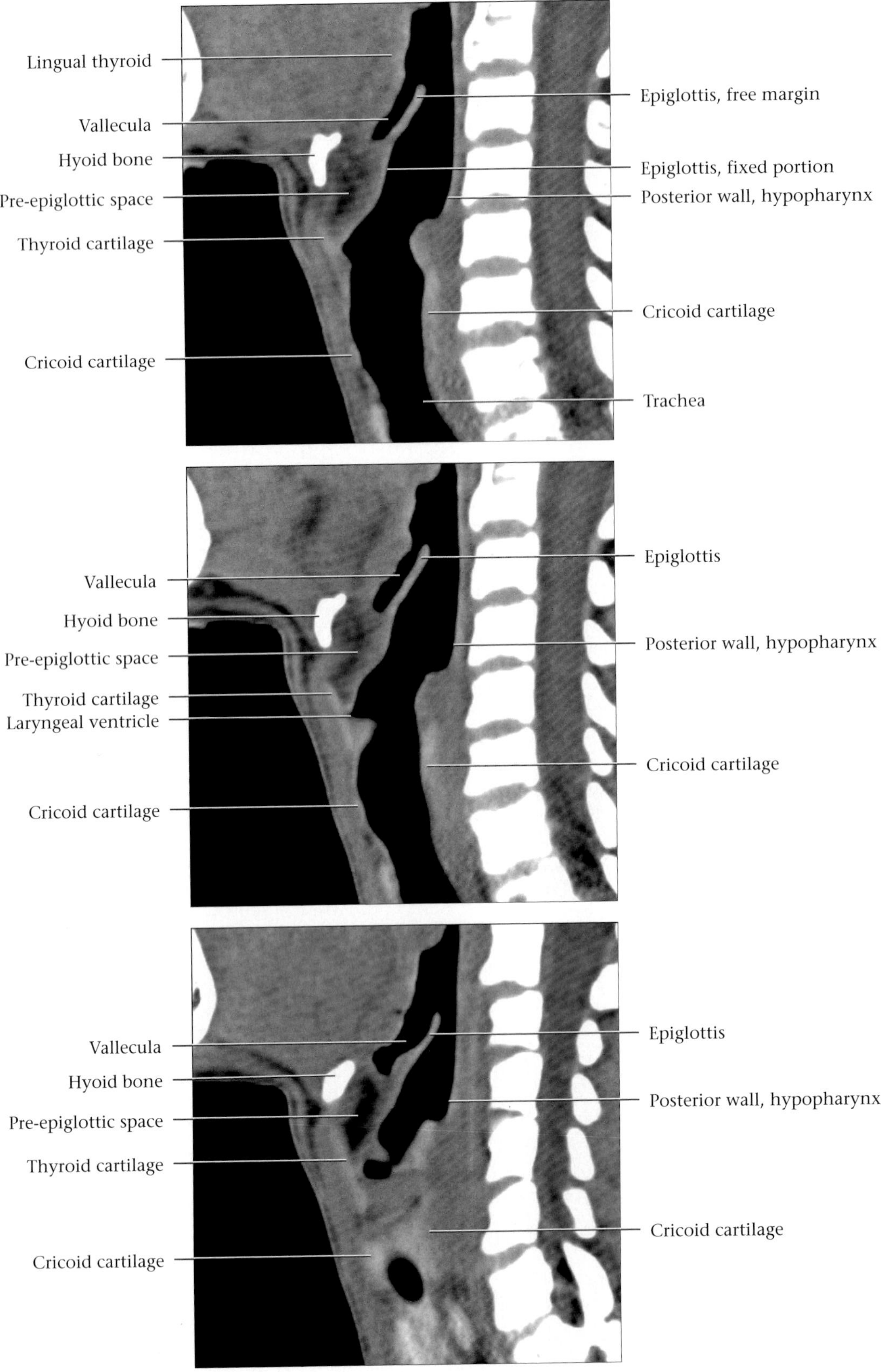
Lingual thyroid
Vallecula
Hyoid bone
Pre-epiglottic space
Thyroid cartilage
Cricoid cartilage
Epiglottis, free margin
Epiglottis, fixed portion
Posterior wall, hypopharynx
Cricoid cartilage
Trachea
Vallecula
Hyoid bone
Pre-epiglottic space
Thyroid cartilage
Laryngeal ventricle
Cricoid cartilage
Epiglottis
Posterior wall, hypopharynx
Cricoid cartilage
Vallecula
Hyoid bone
Pre-epiglottic space
Thyroid cartilage
Cricoid cartilage
Epiglottis
Posterior wall, hypopharynx
Cricoid cartilage

(Top) First of three sagittal NECT images from medial to lateral shows midline larynx & hypopharynx. Pre-epiglottic fat is seen at midline posterior & inferior to hyoid bone. Diseases of posterior hypopharyngeal wall are well seen on sagittal imaging. Sagittal imaging also helps define cranial to caudal extent of lesions. **(Middle)** Image more lateral shows laryngeal ventricle, the air space that separates false vocal cords above from true vocal cords below. **(Bottom)** Image more lateral shows laryngeal cartilages. Laryngeal cartilage is variably ossified in adults which makes disease of the cartilage difficult to evaluate, particularly cartilage invasion from tumors & traumatic injury. Cricoid cartilage is only complete ring in larynx & provides structural integrity. It has a signet ring shape with the larger signet portion projecting posteriorly.

AXIAL T1 MR

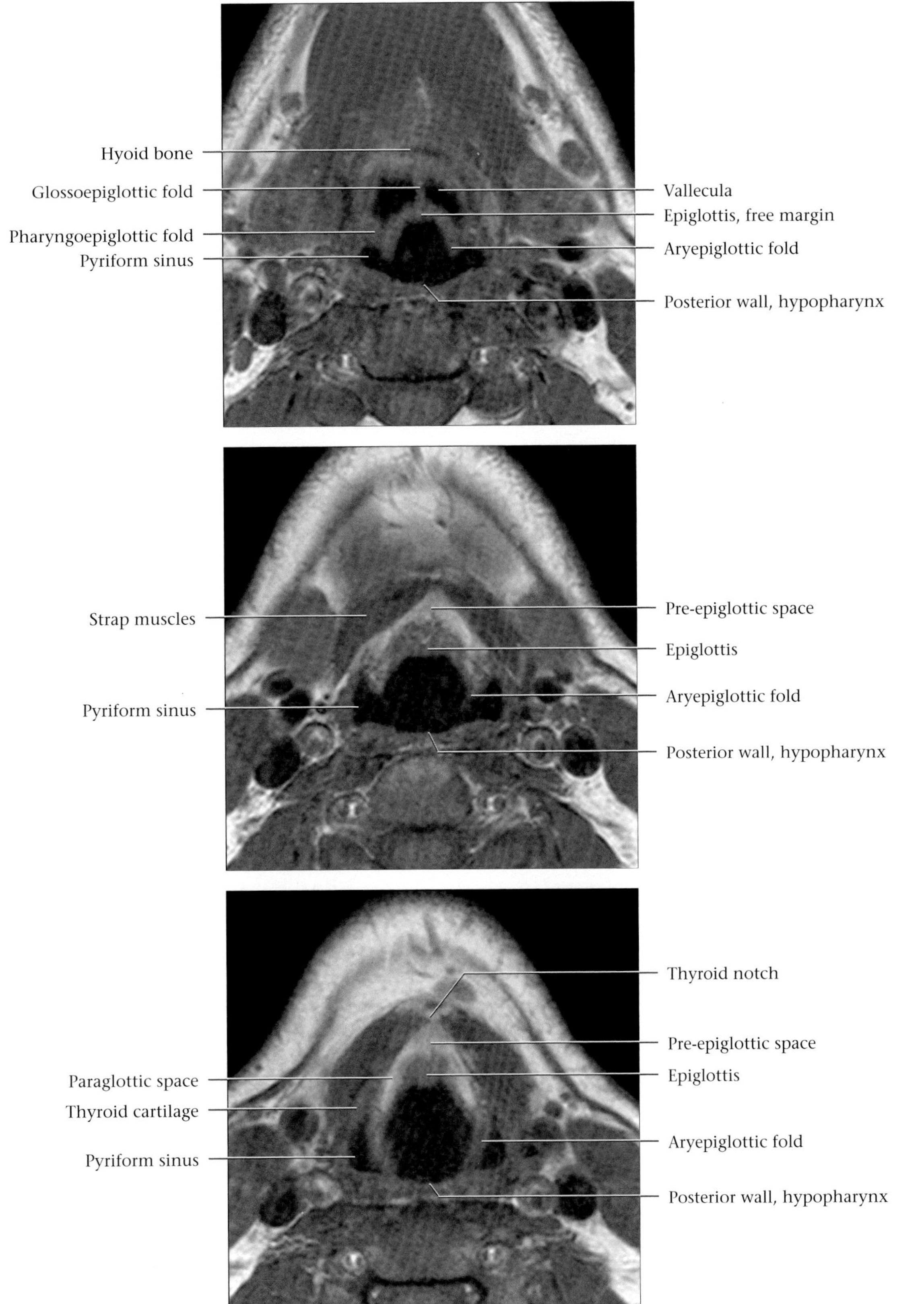
Hyoid bone
Glossoepiglottic fold
Pharyngoepiglottic fold
Pyriform sinus
Vallecula
Epiglottis, free margin
Aryepiglottic fold
Posterior wall, hypopharynx
Strap muscles
Pyriform sinus
Pre-epiglottic space
Epiglottis
Aryepiglottic fold
Posterior wall, hypopharynx
Thyroid notch
Pre-epiglottic space
Epiglottis
Paraglottic space
Thyroid cartilage
Pyriform sinus
Aryepiglottic fold
Posterior wall, hypopharynx

(Top) First of six axial T1 MR images from superior to inferior of larynx & hypopharynx with patient in quiet respiration shows roof of larynx which is defined by epiglottis, glossoepiglottic & pharyngoepiglottic folds. MR is typically reserved for answering specific questions such as cartilage invasion rather than as a first imaging study of a patient with larynx or hypopharynx disease. **(Middle)** Image at level of high supraglottis shows C-shaped fat filled pre-epiglottic space & fixed portion of epiglottis. Cartilage is variably ossified which make it somewhat difficult to visualize on T1 MR images. **(Bottom)** Image at mid-supraglottic level shows fat of pre-epiglottic space continuous with fat of paraglottic space. Lack of fascia between these two submucosal spaces allows tumor to travel from one to the other & hide from clinical detection.

AXIAL T1 MR

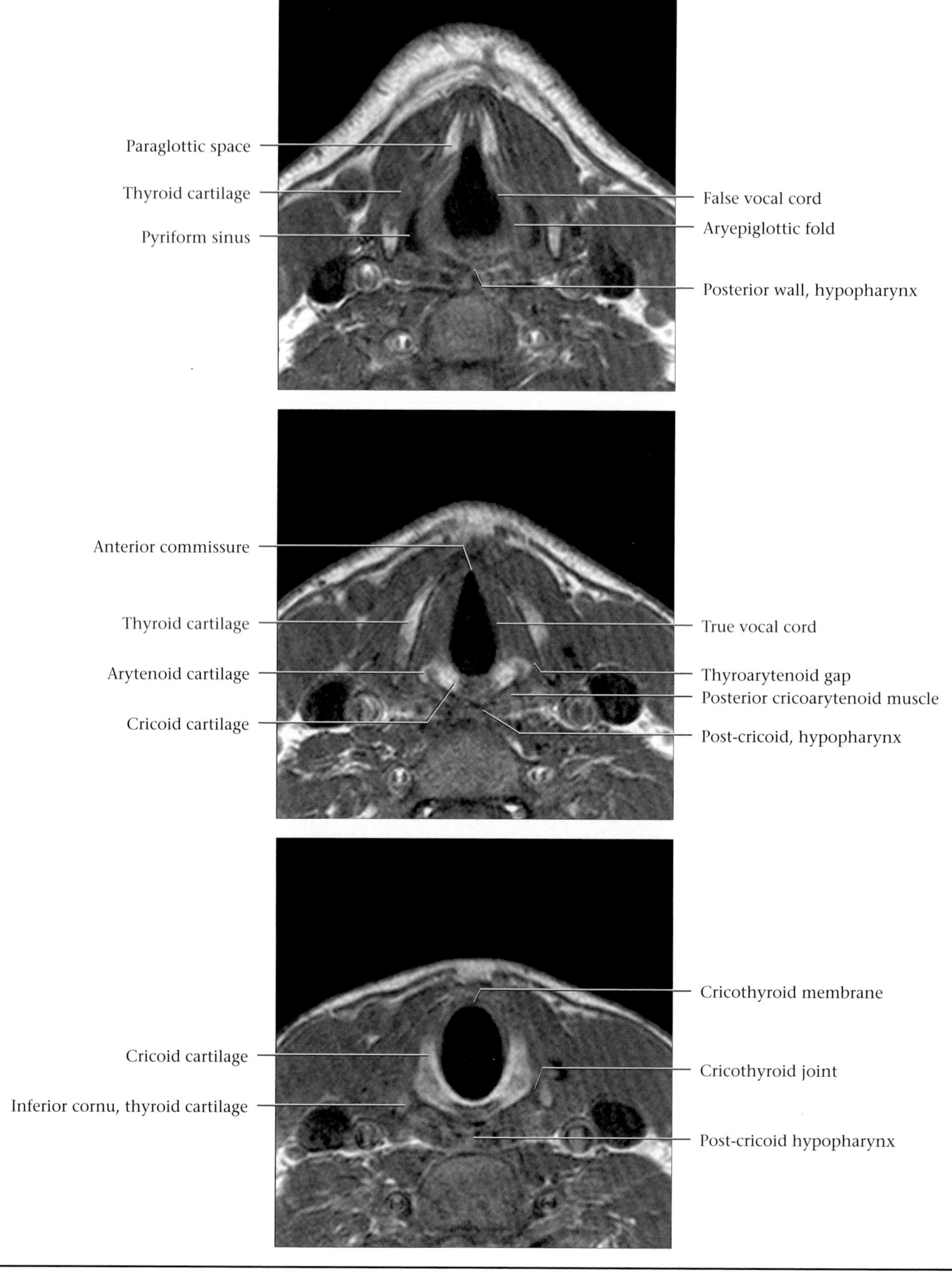

Paraglottic space
Thyroid cartilage
Pyriform sinus
False vocal cord
Aryepiglottic fold
Posterior wall, hypopharynx
Anterior commissure
Thyroid cartilage
Arytenoid cartilage
Cricoid cartilage
True vocal cord
Thyroarytenoid gap
Posterior cricoarytenoid muscle
Post-cricoid, hypopharynx
Cricothyroid membrane
Cricoid cartilage
Inferior cornu, thyroid cartilage
Cricothyroid joint
Post-cricoid hypopharynx

(Top) Image at level of low supraglottis demonstrates false vocal cords & aryepiglottic folds. Paraglottic space beneath false vocal cords is primarily fat filled. Aryepiglottic folds often contact posterior wall of hypopharynx in normal patients. **(Middle)** Image at glottic level shows muscle in paraglottic space beneath true vocal cords. Both cricoid & arytenoid cartilage are seen at true vocal cords level. Thyroarytenoid muscle makes up bulk of true vocal cords. Posterior cricoarytenoid muscle is often atrophied in patients with vocal cord paralysis. **(Bottom)** Image at subglottic level shows large, broad posterior cricoid cartilage. Cricothyroid joint is where recurrent laryngeal nerve is located. Dislocation of this joint is associated with recurrent laryngeal nerve injury. Post-cricoid hypopharynx extends from cricoarytenoid joints to lower cricoid cartilage.

SAGITTAL T1 MR

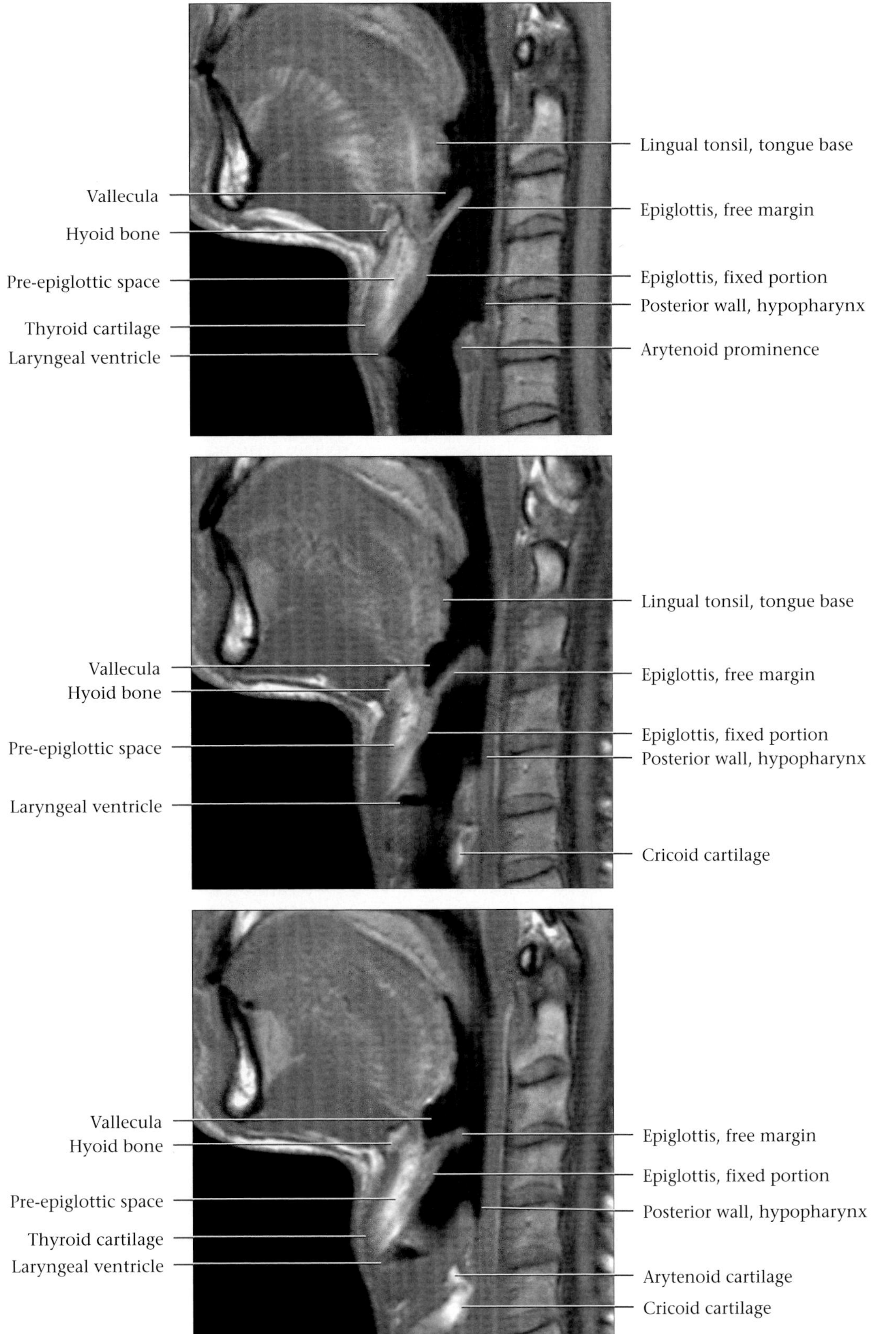

Lingual tonsil, tongue base
Vallecula
Epiglottis, free margin
Hyoid bone
Pre-epiglottic space
Epiglottis, fixed portion
Posterior wall, hypopharynx
Thyroid cartilage
Arytenoid prominence
Laryngeal ventricle
Lingual tonsil, tongue base
Vallecula
Epiglottis, free margin
Hyoid bone
Epiglottis, fixed portion
Pre-epiglottic space
Posterior wall, hypopharynx
Laryngeal ventricle
Cricoid cartilage
Vallecula
Epiglottis, free margin
Hyoid bone
Epiglottis, fixed portion
Pre-epiglottic space
Posterior wall, hypopharynx
Thyroid cartilage
Laryngeal ventricle
Arytenoid cartilage
Cricoid cartilage

(Top) First of three sagittal T1 MR images from medial to lateral of larynx & hypopharynx shows midline structures. Pre-epiglottic space is T1 hyperintense as it is primarily fat-filled. Free margin (suprahyoid) & fixed portion (infrahyoid) of epiglottis is well visualized making sagittal imaging useful for evaluation of epiglottic lesions. **(Middle)** Image just lateral to midline shows laryngeal ventricle which is important as it is the air-space that separates false vocal cords above from true vocal cords below. Knowing if a tumor crosses the laryngeal ventricle is vital for surgical planning. **(Bottom)** Paramedial image through the cricoarytenoid joint shows arytenoid cartilage sitting on top of posterior cricoid cartilage. Traumatic dislocation of arytenoid cartilage may mimic vocal cord paralysis clinically & on imaging.

THYROID GLAND

Imaging Anatomy

Overview

- "H" or "U" shaped gland in anterior cervical neck formed from 2 elongated lateral lobes with superior & inferior poles connected by median isthmus
- 40% of people have **pyramidal lobe** ascending from isthmus area toward hyoid bone

Extent

- Extends from level of 5th cervical vertebra to 1st thoracic vertebra

Anatomy Relationships

- Thyroid gland lies anterior & lateral to trachea in **visceral space** of infrahyoid neck
- Posteromedially is **tracheoesophageal groove** (paratracheal nodes, recurrent laryngeal nerve, parathyroid glands)
- Posterolaterally are carotid spaces
- Anteriorly are infrahyoid strap muscles
- Anterolaterally are sternocleidomastoid muscles
- Parathyroid glands lie close to deep surface of thyroid gland; may be intracapsular

Internal Structures-Critical Contents

- **Thyroid gland**
  - Two **lateral lobes** each ≈ 4 cm in height
    - Each lobe has upper & lower pole
    - Lateral lobes are commonly asymmetric
  - Lateral lobes joined by midline **isthmus**
- **Arterial supply to thyroid gland**
  - **Superior thyroid arteries**
    - Superior thyroid artery is 1st anterior branch of external carotid artery
    - Runs superficially on anterior border of lateral lobe, sending a branch deep into gland before curving toward isthmus where it anastomoses with contralateral artery
    - Proximal course closely associated with superior laryngeal nerve
  - **Inferior thyroid arteries**
    - Arises from thyrocervical trunk, a branch of subclavian artery
    - Ascends vertically, then curves medially to enter tracheoesophageal groove in plane posterior to carotid space
    - Most of its branches penetrate posterior aspect of lateral thyroid lobe
    - Closely associated with recurrent laryngeal nerve
  - **Thyroidea ima** occasionally present (3%)
    - Single vessel originating from aortic arch or innominate artery
    - Enters thyroid gland at inferior border of isthmus
- **Venous drainage of thyroid gland**
  - 3 pairs of veins arise from venous plexus on surface of thyroid gland
  - Superior & middle thyroid veins drain into internal jugular vein
  - Inferior thyroid veins end in left brachiocephalic vein
- **Lymphatic drainage from thyroid gland**
  - Lymphatic drainage is extensive & multidirectional
  - Image-based nodal classification: **Level 6**
  - Initial lymphatic drainage courses to periglandular nodes
    - Prelaryngeal, pretracheal & paratracheal nodes along recurrent laryngeal nerve
    - Paratracheal nodes drain along recurrent laryngeal nerve into mediastinum
    - Regional drainage occurs laterally into internal jugular chain (level 2-4) & spinal accessory chain (level 5), higher in the neck along internal jugular vein

Fascia

- **Middle layer of deep cervical fascia** surrounds visceral space & ensheathes thyroid gland
- Thyroid gland has inner **true capsule**
  - True capsule is thin & adheres closely to gland
  - Extension of capsule into gland forms numerous septae, dividing gland into lobes & lobules

Embryology

Embryologic Events

- Thyroid is first endocrine gland in body to develop (~ 24th gestational day)
- Thyroid gland originates from 1st & 2nd pharyngeal pouches (medial anlage)
- Originates as proliferation of endodermal epithelial cells on median surface of developing pharyngeal floor termed **foramen cecum**
- Bilobed thyroid gland descends anterior to pharyngeal gut along **thyroglossal duct**
  - Tubular duct later solidifies then obliterates entirely (gestational weeks 7-10)
- Inferior descent of thyroid gland carries it anterior to hyoid bone & laryngeal cartilages
- As it descends it takes on its mature shape, with a median isthmus connecting 2 lateral lobes
- Lateral thyroid lobes may form from 4th & 6th branchial pouches (lateral anlagen)

Practical Implications

- **Thyroglossal duct cyst** results from failure of involution of portion of thyroglossal duct
  - Occurs anywhere along course of thyroglossal duct from foramen cecum at tongue base to just anterior to thyroid lobes
  - Most occur in midline in vicinity of hyoid bone
  - When infrahyoid, most commonly paramedian, just dorsal to lateral thyroid lobe
  - Often have thyroid tissue in wall
- **Thyroid tissue remnants** from sequestration of thyroid tissue along thyroglossal duct
  - Seen anywhere along course of thyroglossal duct from foramen cecum to superior mediastinum
  - Pyramidal lobe of thyroid is midline normal variant remnant of this process
  - **Ectopic thyroid gland** from incomplete descent of thyroid into low neck
    - Seen anywhere along course from foramen cecum in tongue base to superior mediastinum
    - Most common location in neck is just deep to foramen cecum in tongue base = **lingual thyroid**

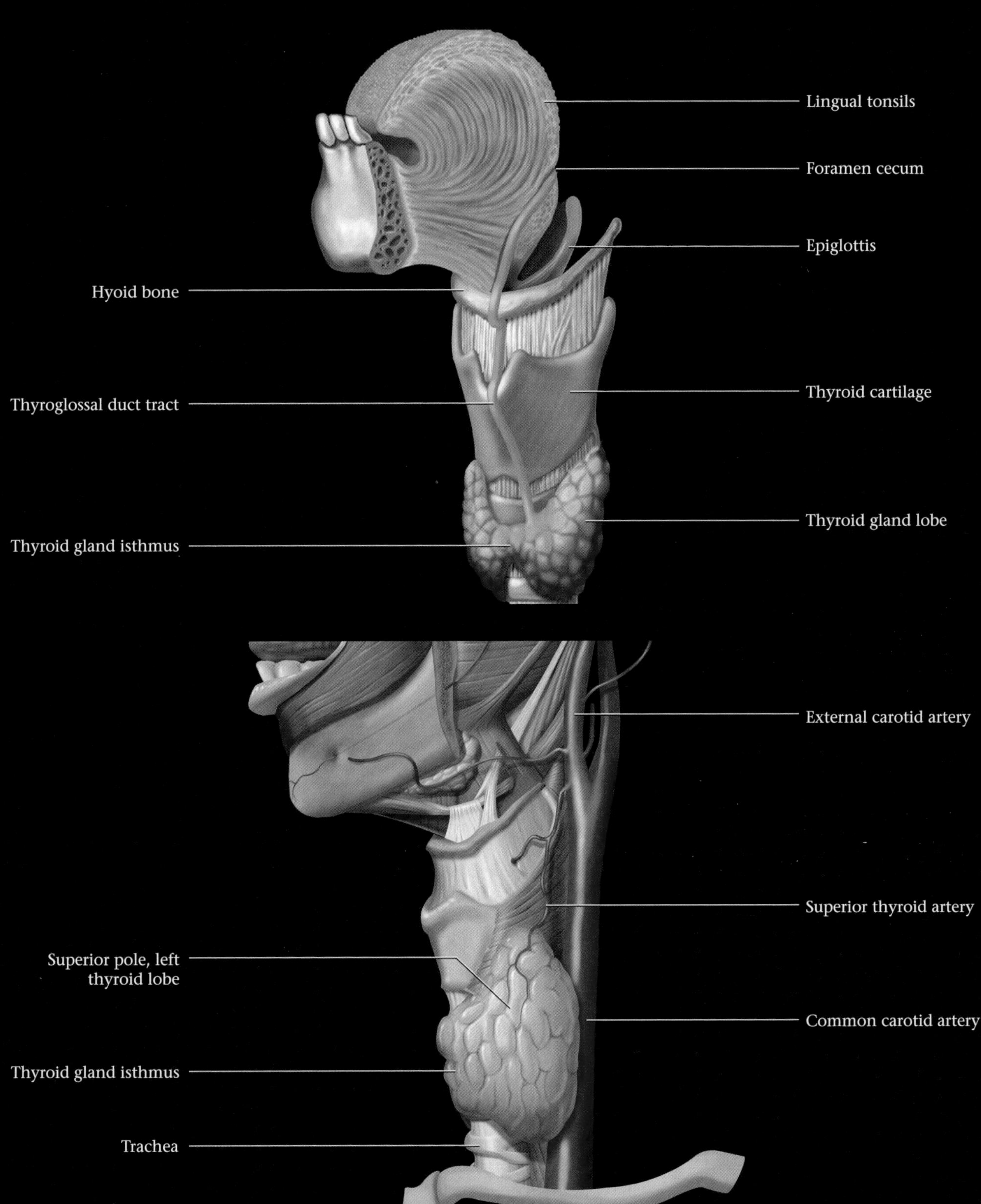
Lingual tonsils
Foramen cecum
Epiglottis
Hyoid bone
Thyroglossal duct tract
Thyroid cartilage
Thyroid gland lobe
Thyroid gland isthmus
External carotid artery
Superior thyroid artery
Superior pole, left thyroid lobe
Common carotid artery
Thyroid gland isthmus
Trachea

(Top) Sagittal oblique graphic displays thyroglossal duct tract as it traverses the cervical neck from its origin at the foramen cecum to its termination in the anterior & lateral visceral space of the infrahyoid neck. The medial thyroid anlage arises from the paramedian aspect of the 1st & 2nd branchial pouches (foramen cecum area), then descends inferiorly through the tongue base, floor of mouth, around and in front of the hyoid bone, through the area of the infrahyoid strap muscles to a final position in the thyroid bed of the visceral space. Thyroglossal duct cyst (failure of involution of duct) or thyroid tissue remnants may be found anywhere along this tract. **(Bottom)** Oblique graphic of the infrahyoid neck shows the superior thyroid artery as the first branch of the external carotid artery. Its proximal course closely associated with superior laryngeal nerve.

THYROID GLAND

GRAPHICS

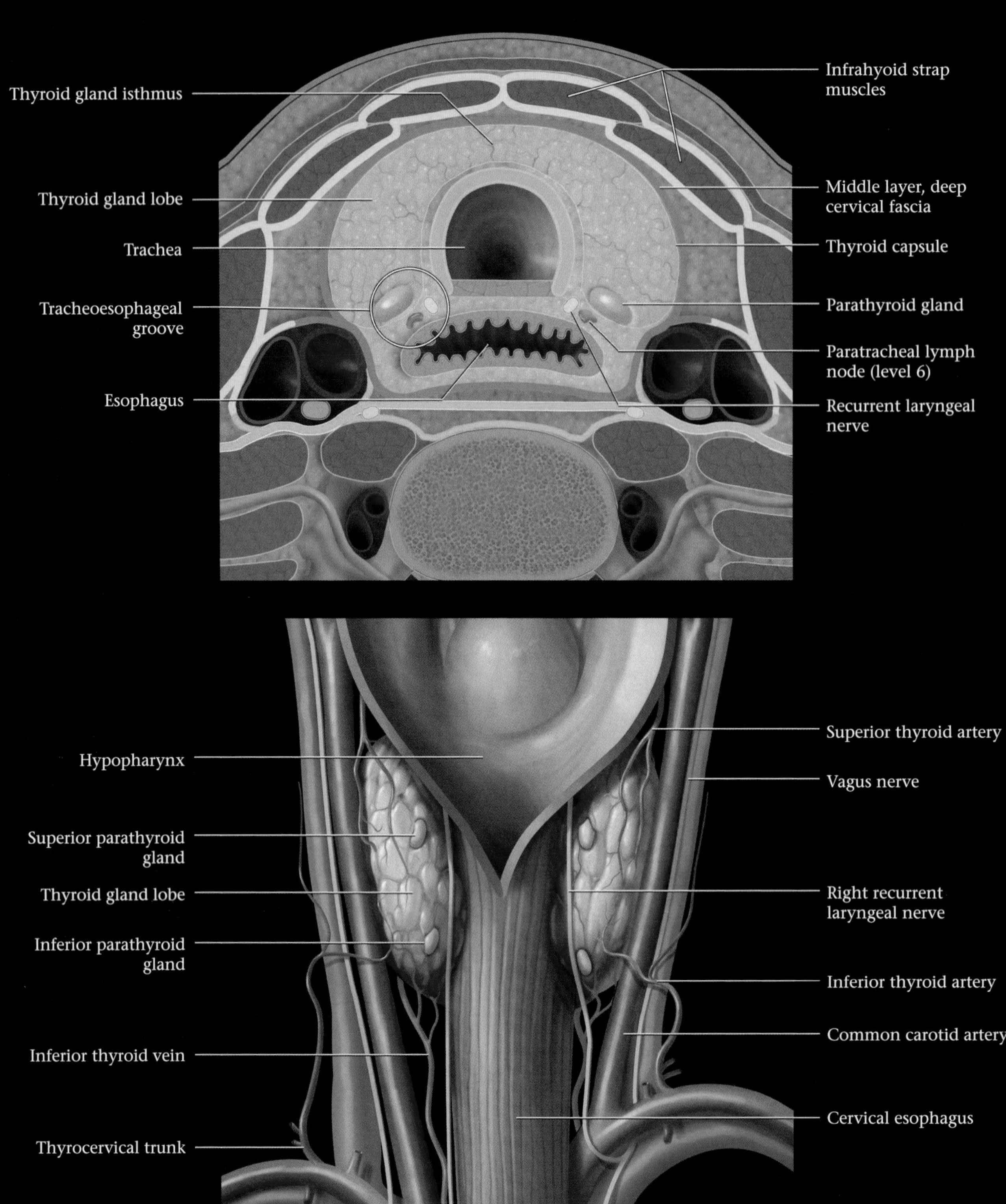
Thyroid gland isthmus
Thyroid gland lobe
Trachea
Tracheoesophageal groove
Esophagus
Infrahyoid strap muscles
Middle layer, deep cervical fascia
Thyroid capsule
Parathyroid gland
Paratracheal lymph node (level 6)
Recurrent laryngeal nerve
Hypopharynx
Superior parathyroid gland
Thyroid gland lobe
Inferior parathyroid gland
Inferior thyroid vein
Thyrocervical trunk
Superior thyroid artery
Vagus nerve
Right recurrent laryngeal nerve
Inferior thyroid artery
Common carotid artery
Cervical esophagus

(Top) Axial graphic at thyroid level, depicts the thyroid lobes & isthmus in the anterior visceral space wrapping around the trachea. Notice that there are three key structures found in the area of the tracheoesophageal groove, the recurrent laryngeal nerve, the paratracheal lymph node chain and the parathyroid gland. The parathyroid glands may be inside or outside of the thyroid capsule. **(Bottom)** Coronal graphic views the thyroid and parathyroid glands from behind. The drawing depicts the typical anatomic relationships of the paired superior and inferior parathyroid glands closely applied to the posterior lobes of the thyroid gland. Note the arterial supply to superior and inferior thyroid lobes, the superior and inferior thyroid arteries respectively.

AXIAL CECT

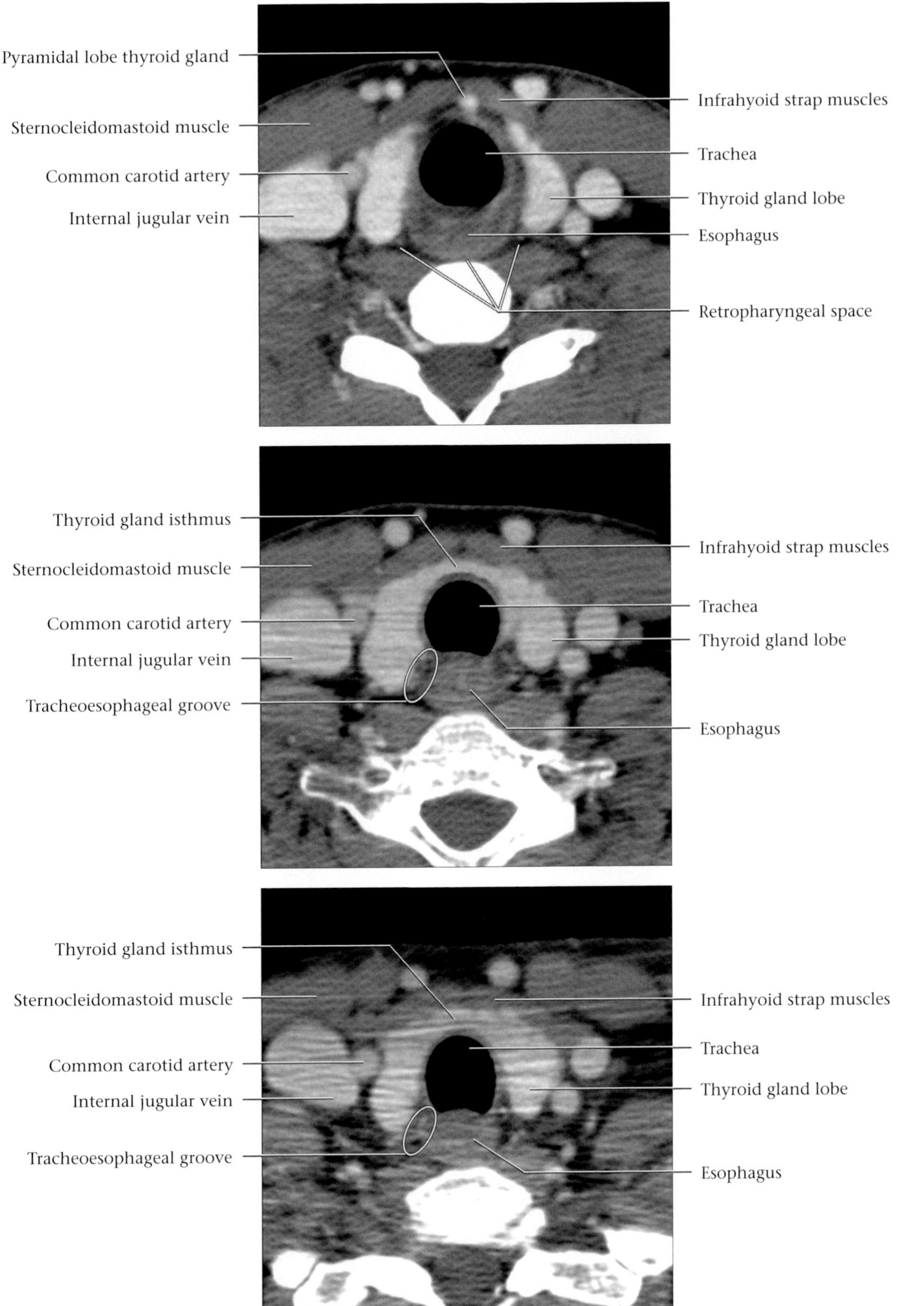
Pyramidal lobe thyroid gland
Sternocleidomastoid muscle
Common carotid artery
Internal jugular vein
Infrahyoid strap muscles
Trachea
Thyroid gland lobe
Esophagus
Retropharyngeal space
Thyroid gland isthmus
Sternocleidomastoid muscle
Common carotid artery
Internal jugular vein
Tracheoesophageal groove
Infrahyoid strap muscles
Trachea
Thyroid gland lobe
Esophagus
Thyroid gland isthmus
Sternocleidomastoid muscle
Common carotid artery
Internal jugular vein
Tracheoesophageal groove
Infrahyoid strap muscles
Trachea
Thyroid gland lobe
Esophagus

(Top) First of three axial CECT images presented from superior to inferior shows a small superiorly projecting pyramidal lobe in the anterior midline just beneath the infrahyoid strap muscles. Notice the retropharyngeal space fat stripe extends posterior to the thyroid lobes and esophagus. **(Middle)** In this image the thyroid gland isthmus is visible arching from thyroid lobe to thyroid lobe across the anterior surface of the trachea beneath the infrahyoid strap muscles. The thyroid lobes are found along the lateral margin of the trachea. **(Bottom)** The thyroid gland isthmus is prominent on this image. The tracheoesophageal groove has been circled. Remember that the recurrent laryngeal nerve, paratracheal nodes and parathyroid glands can all be normally found in this location. None of these structures are normally visible on routine enhanced CT images.

THYROID GLAND

CORONAL CECT

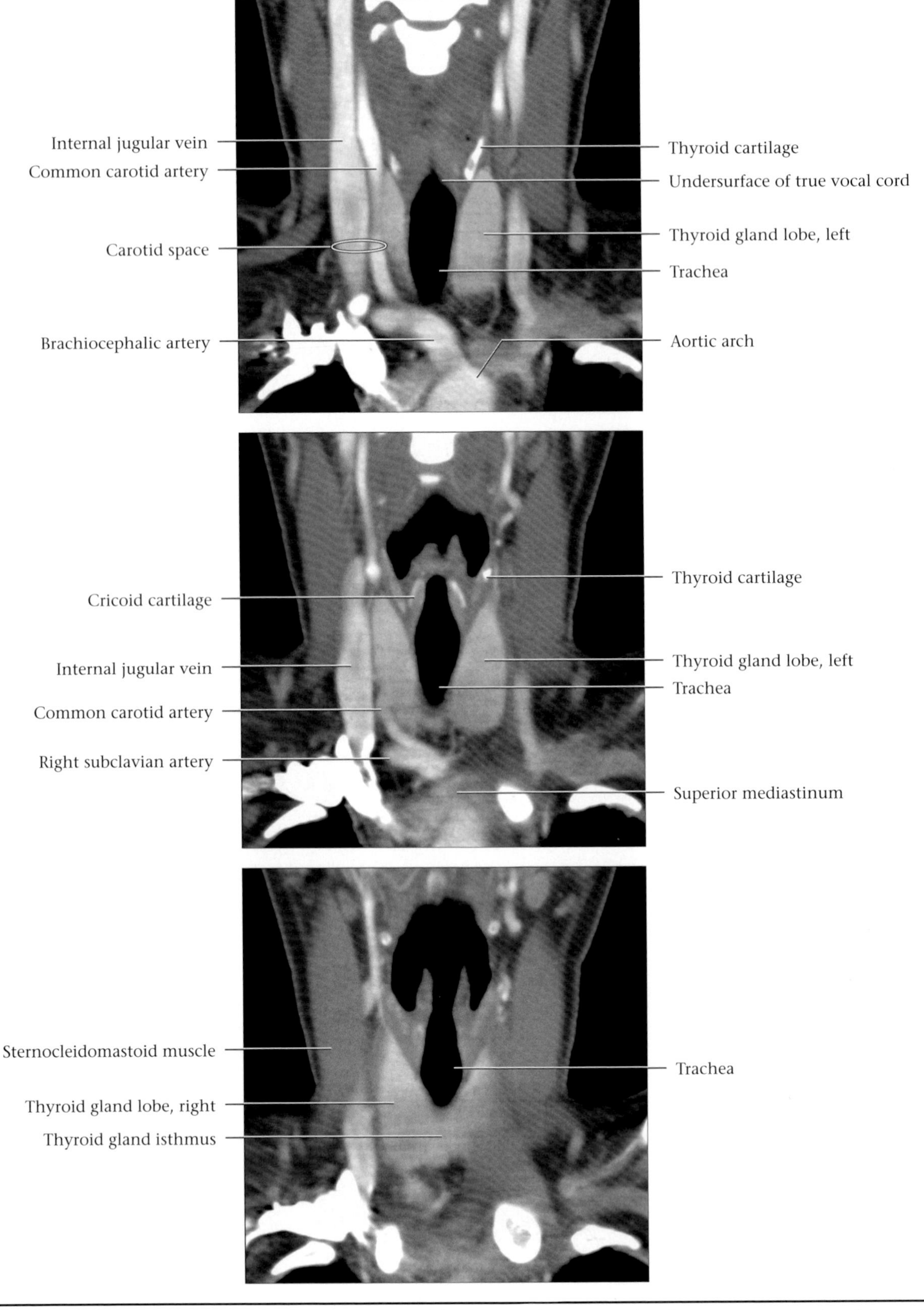

Internal jugular vein
Common carotid artery
Carotid space
Brachiocephalic artery
Thyroid cartilage
Undersurface of true vocal cord
Thyroid gland lobe, left
Trachea
Aortic arch
Cricoid cartilage
Internal jugular vein
Common carotid artery
Right subclavian artery
Thyroid cartilage
Thyroid gland lobe, left
Trachea
Superior mediastinum
Sternocleidomastoid muscle
Thyroid gland lobe, right
Thyroid gland isthmus
Trachea

(Top) First of three coronal CECT reformations presented from posterior to anterior demonstrates the two lobes of the thyroid gland with the trachea on their medial borders. Lateral to each of the thyroid lobes are the carotid spaces containing the vagus nerve, common carotid artery and internal jugular vein. **(Middle)** In this image the chevron-shaped lobes of the thyroid gland are particularly well seen. Notice the intimate relationship between the superomedial thyroid gland and the larynx. Remember that thyroid gland malignancy first order nodes are the paratracheal nodes. The paratracheal nodes drain inferiorly into the superior mediastinum. Consequently it is important for the radiologist to image to the aortic arch in cases of thyroid gland malignancy. **(Bottom)** The isthmus of the thyroid gland is visible just anterior to the trachea in this image.

ULTRASOUND

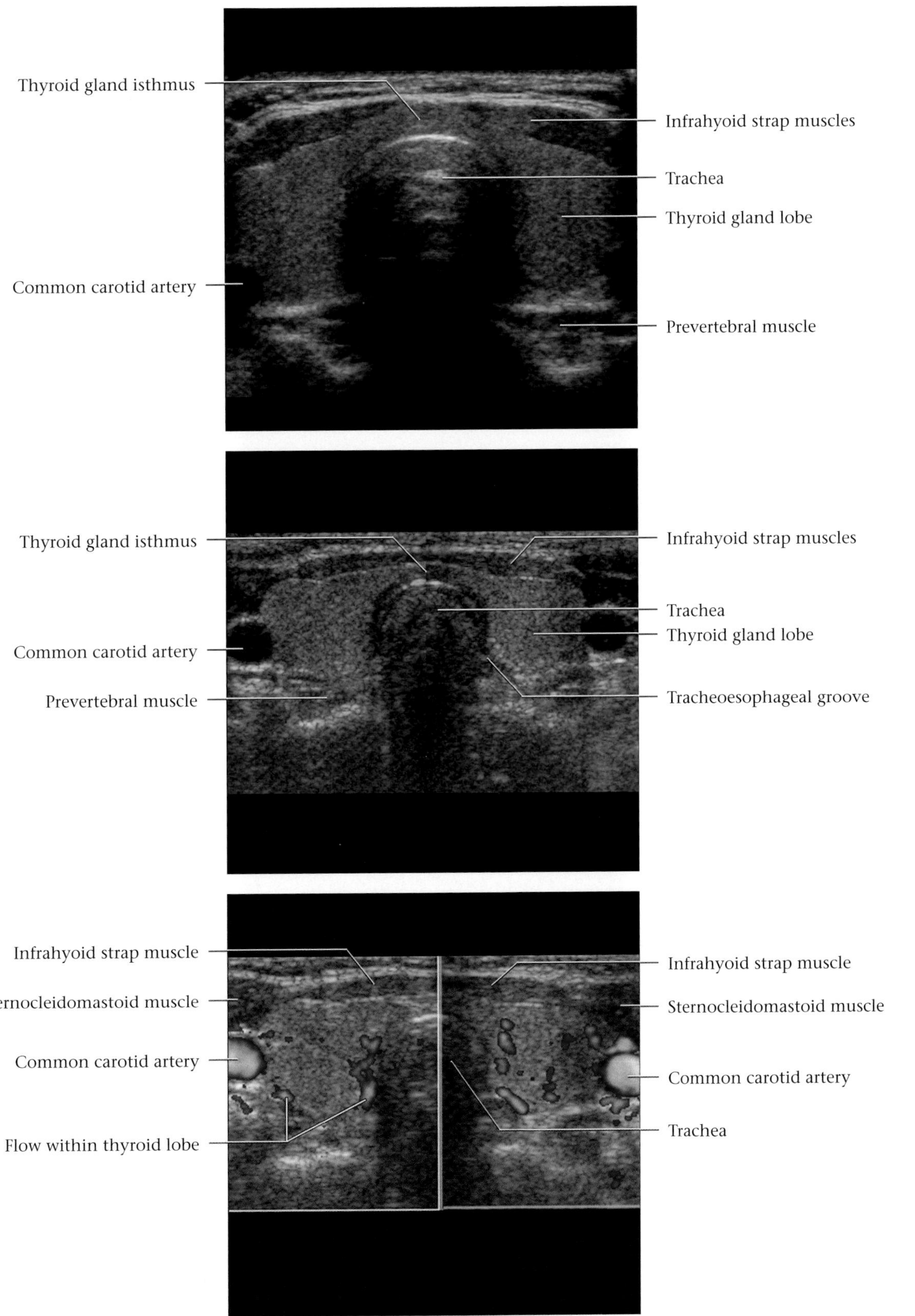
Thyroid gland isthmus
Infrahyoid strap muscles
Trachea
Thyroid gland lobe
Common carotid artery
Prevertebral muscle
Thyroid gland isthmus
Infrahyoid strap muscles
Trachea
Thyroid gland lobe
Common carotid artery
Prevertebral muscle
Tracheoesophageal groove
Infrahyoid strap muscle
Sternocleidomastoid muscle
Common carotid artery
Flow within thyroid lobe
Infrahyoid strap muscle
Sternocleidomastoid muscle
Common carotid artery
Trachea

(Top) In this transverse grayscale ultrasound image the thyroid gland isthmus is visible arching from thyroid lobe to thyroid lobe across the anterior surface of the trachea beneath the infrahyoid strap muscles. Notice that the tracheoesophageal grooves & cervical esophagus are not seen due to shadowing from air in the trachea. **(Middle)** Higher resolution transverse grayscale ultrasound image constructed from individual scans of both sides of the neck shows the tracheoesophageal grooves as a result of angling of the transducer at the time of scan acquisition. **(Bottom)** Power Doppler images of both sides of the neck at the level of the thyroid lobes shows flow in both common carotid arteries. The normal power Doppler image of the thyroid demonstrates sporadic flow within the thyroid lobes secondary to branches of intrathyroid vessels.

ULTRASOUND

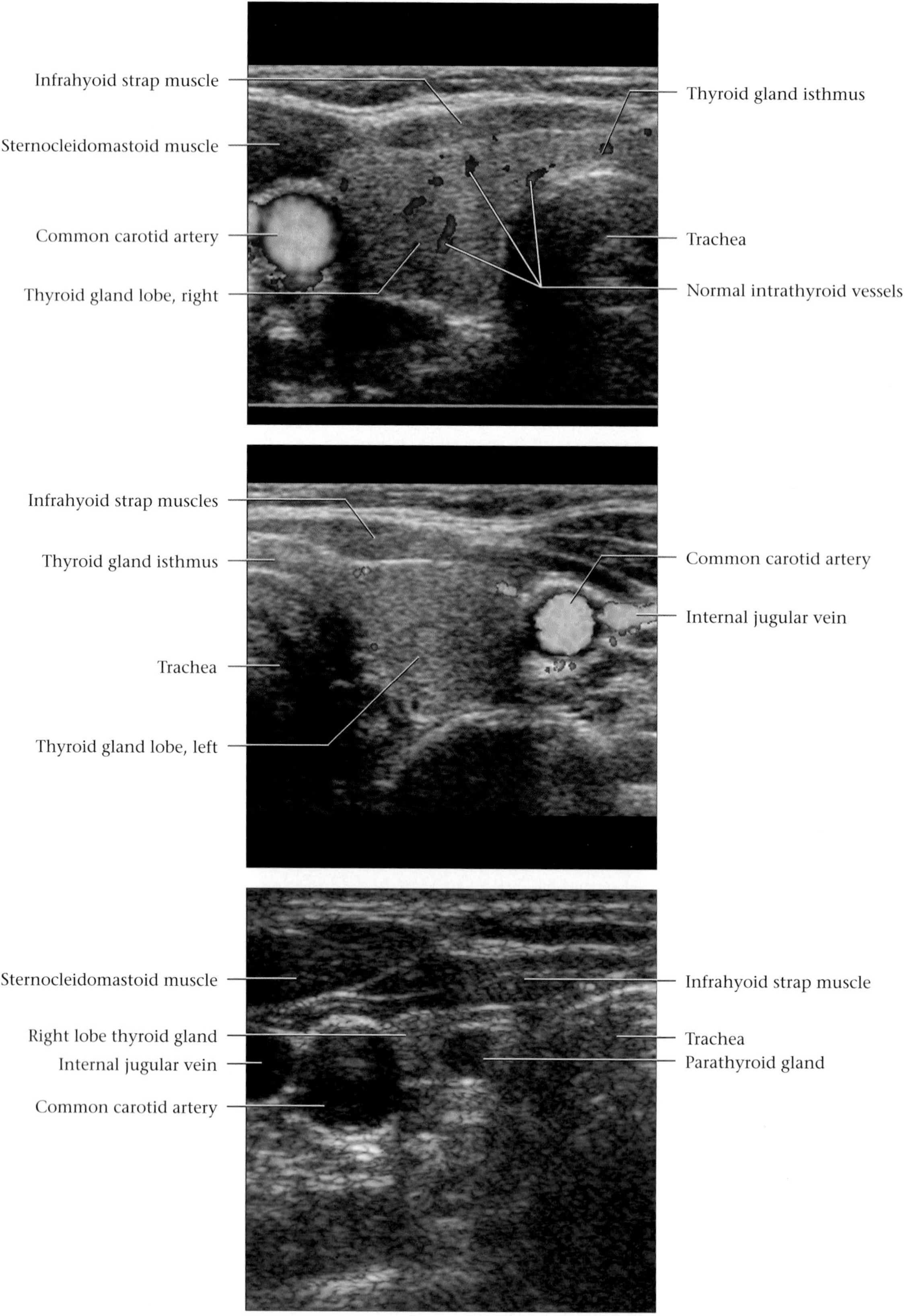

Infrahyoid strap muscle
Sternocleidomastoid muscle
Common carotid artery
Thyroid gland lobe, right
Thyroid gland isthmus
Trachea
Normal intrathyroid vessels
Infrahyoid strap muscles
Thyroid gland isthmus
Trachea
Thyroid gland lobe, left
Common carotid artery
Internal jugular vein
Sternocleidomastoid muscle
Right lobe thyroid gland
Internal jugular vein
Common carotid artery
Infrahyoid strap muscle
Trachea
Parathyroid gland

(Top) In this transverse power Doppler ultrasound image through the right thyroid lobe the, high flow within the common carotid is visible along the lateral margin of the right thyroid lobe. The focal sporadic areas of high flow within the thyroid lobe and isthmus represent normal intrathyroidal vessels. **(Middle)** Transverse color Doppler ultrasound image of the left thyroid lobe shows high flow in the common carotid artery and internal jugular vein. Color Doppler provides directional and flow information. The colored areas within the thyroid lobe represent intrathyroidal vessels. **(Bottom)** In this transverse grayscale sonographic image of the right neck shows a well-circumscribed hypoechoic right superior parathyroid gland medial to common carotid artery and posterior to superior right thyroid lobe.

GRAPHICS OF THYROID LESIONS

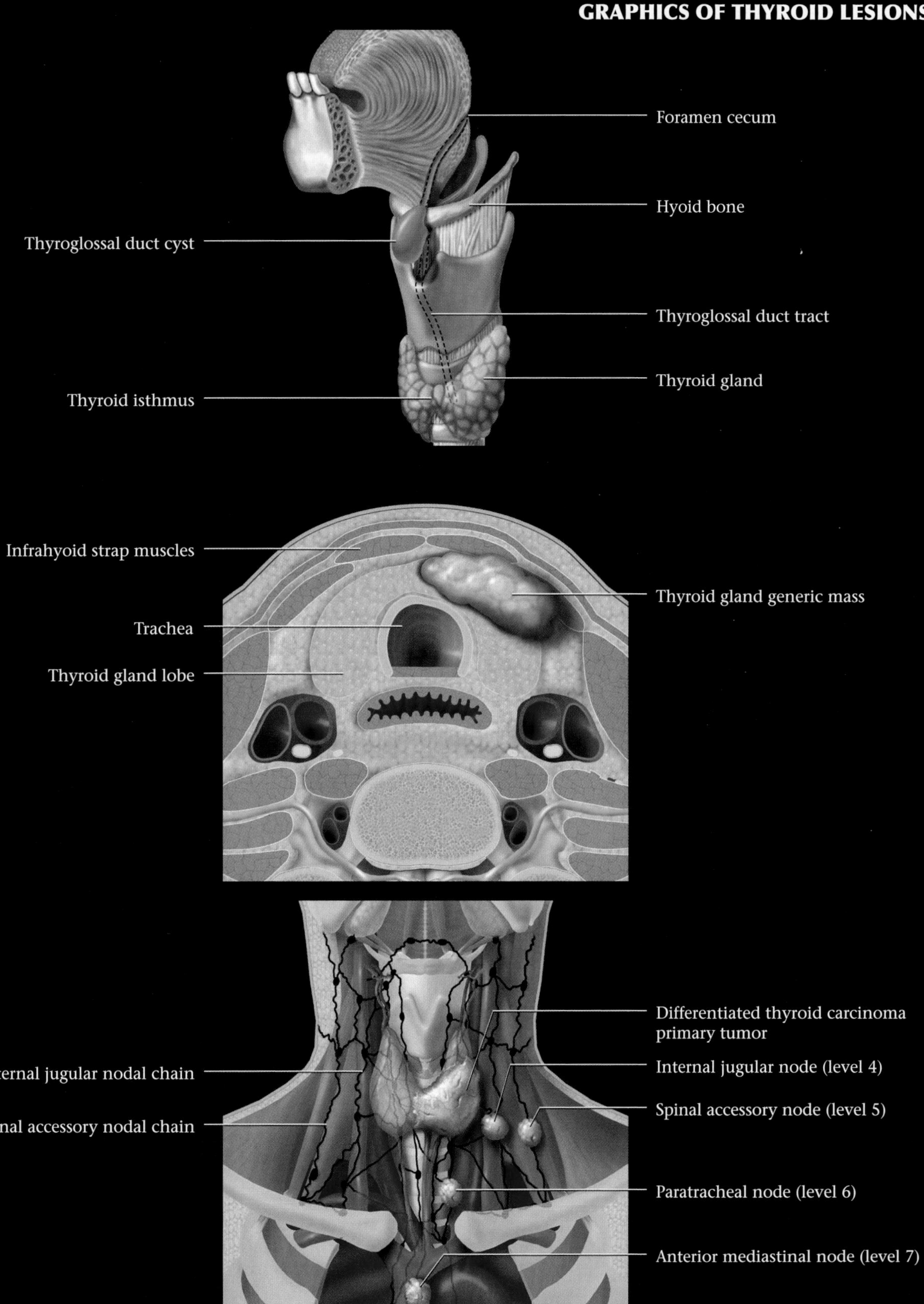
Foramen cecum
Hyoid bone
Thyroglossal duct cyst
Thyroglossal duct tract
Thyroid gland
Thyroid isthmus
Infrahyoid strap muscles
Thyroid gland generic mass
Trachea
Thyroid gland lobe
Differentiated thyroid carcinoma primary tumor
Internal jugular node (level 4)
Internal jugular nodal chain
Spinal accessory node (level 5)
Spinal accessory nodal chain
Paratracheal node (level 6)
Anterior mediastinal node (level 7)

(Top) Oblique sagittal graphic of a thyroglossal duct cyst that occurs at the level of the hyoid bone along the thyroglossal duct tract. Thyroglossal duct cysts and thyroid remnants can be found anywhere along the tract of the thyroglossal duct from the level of the foramen cecum to the superior mediastinum. **(Middle)** Axial graphic through the thyroid bed shows a generic intrathyroid mass. The lesion appears to arise out of the left thyroid lobe, lifting the infrahyoid strap muscles. **(Bottom)** Coronal graphic of the infrahyoid neck and superior mediastinum shows a left thyroid lobe and isthmus differentiated thyroid carcinoma primary. Notice that in addition to nodal metastases in the internal jugular and spinal accessory chains there are also nodal metastases in the paratracheal and superior mediastinal nodal groups.

PARATHYROID GLANDS

Terminology

Abbreviations

- Parathyroid gland (PTG)

Definitions

- **PTG**: Posterior visceral space (VS) endocrine glands that control calcium metabolism by producing parathormone

Imaging Anatomy

Anatomy Relationships

- PTG closely applied to posterior surface of thyroid lobes within visceral space
- PTG extracapsular (outside thyroid capsule) in most cases
- PTG in vicinity of tracheoesophageal groove

Internal Structures-Critical Contents

- **Parathyroid glands**
  - Small lentiform glands posterior to thyroid glands in visceral space
  - Normal measurements
    - Approximately 6 mm length, 3-4 mm transverse & 1-2 mm in anteroposterior diameter
  - **Normal number = 4**, two superior & two inferior
    - May be as many as 12 total PTGs
  - **Superior PTG normal locations**
    - Lie on posterior border of middle 1/3 of thyroid 75% of time
    - 25% found behind upper or lower 1/3 of thyroid
    - 7% found below inferior thyroidal artery
    - Rarely found behind pharynx or esophagus
  - **Inferior PTG normal locations**
    - Inferior glands lie lateral to lower pole of thyroid gland (50%)
    - 15% lie within 1 cm of inferior thyroid poles
    - 35% position is variable residing anywhere from angle of mandible to lower anterior mediastinum
    - Intrathyroidal PTG are rare
  - **PTG arterial supply**
    - Superior PTG supplied by **superior thyroid artery**
    - Inferior PTG supplied by **inferior thyroid artery**

Fascia

- Visceral space & its contents including PTGs are surrounded by **middle layer of deep cervical fascia**

Parathyroid Gland Microscopic Anatomy

- PTG are composed of chief cells & oxyphil cells
- Cells are embedded within fibrous capsule & mixed with adipose tissue
- Oxyphil cell function unknown
- **Chief cells** manufacture **parathormone** (PTH)
  - PTH regulates concentration of calcium in interstitial fluids
  - Serum calcium levels regulate secretion of PTH

Anatomy-Based Imaging Issues

Imaging Approaches

- Imaging for pre-operative localization of parathyroid adenoma (PTA)
  - Ultrasonography
    - Best 1st examination for localizing most PTA
    - Use high-resolution linear array transducer (7.5-10 MHz)
    - Identifies 95% of PTA weighing > 1 gram
  - Cross-sectional imaging (CT or MR)
    - Used for anatomic localization of ectopic PTA discovered with radionuclide exam
  - Nuclear scintigraphy
    - Tc-99m sestamibi concentrates in PTA
    - Very useful study when **ectopic PTA** is suspected from negative surgical exploration

Clinical Implications

Clinical Importance

- Primary hyperparathyroidism with hypercalcemia is most commonly secondary to PTA
  - Less common cause is parathyroid hyperplasia
- Imaging of PTG is primarily to find PTA
- Imaging & surgical challenges arise when PTG affected is ectopic

Embryology

Embryologic Events

- **Superior PTG** develop from **4th branchial pouch** along with primordium of **thyroid gland**
  - Less than 2% of superior PTG are **ectopic**
- **Inferior PTG** develop from **3rd branchial pouch** along with anlage of **thymus**
  - Descend variable distance with thymic anlage in thymopharyngeal duct tract
  - May descend into anterior mediastinum as far as pericardium

Practical Implications

- Abnormal PTG descent may cause inferior PTG to occupy "ectopic" sites
  - May be of critical importance when searching for parathyroid adenoma
    - In cases where surgical exploration for PTA is done without imaging, no PTA may be found if PTG is ectopic
  - **Most frequent ectopic site** is just **below inferior thyroid pole**
  - Less commonly PT may migrate into superior mediastinum with thymus creating ectopic mediastinal PTA
  - Rarely PTG does not descend significantly which creates ectopic in upper cervical neck PTA
  - Rarest reported locations include retropharyngeal, retro-esophageal & posterior mediastinal PTA

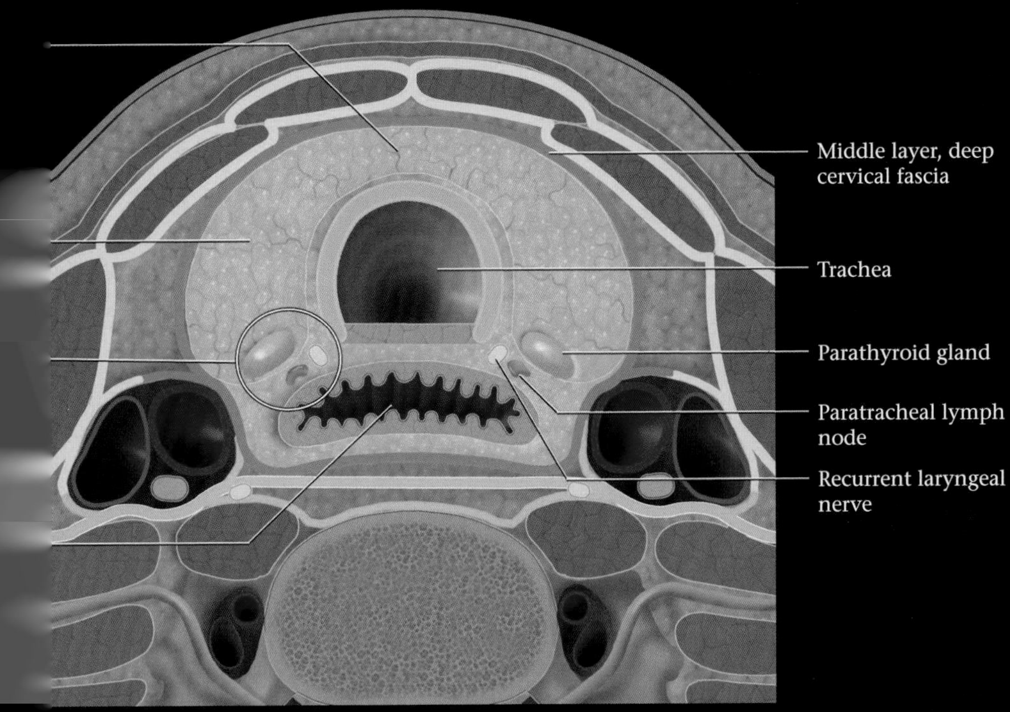
Middle layer, deep cervical fascia
Trachea
Parathyroid gland
Paratracheal lymph node
Recurrent laryngeal nerve

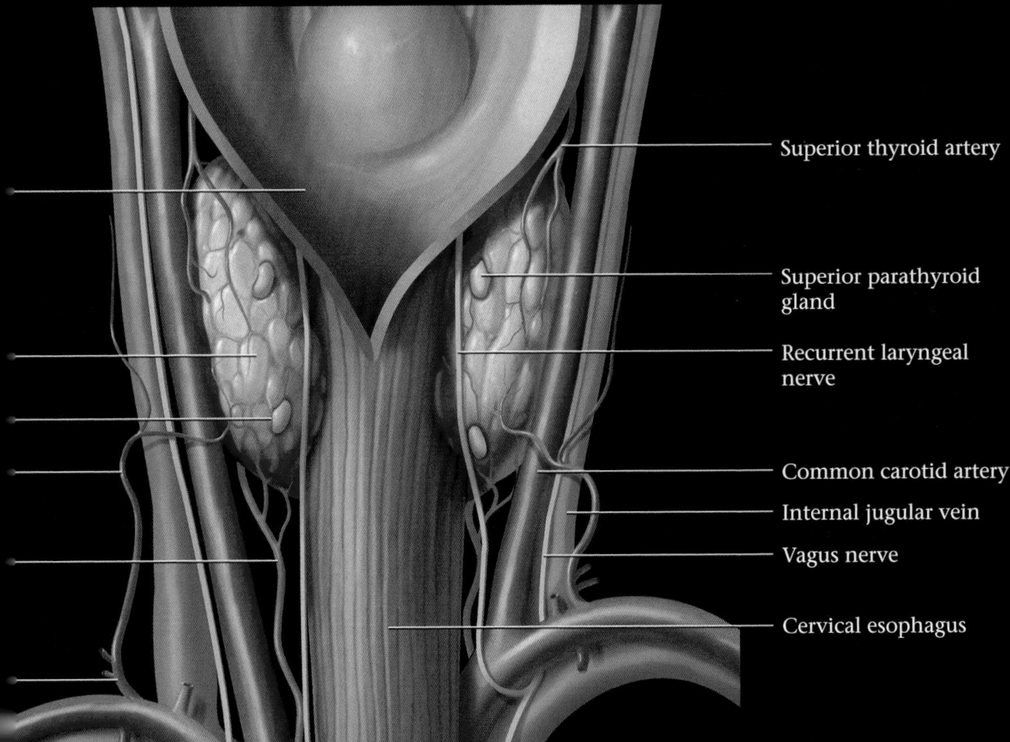
Superior thyroid artery
Superior parathyroid gland
Recurrent laryngeal nerve
Common carotid artery
Internal jugular vein
Vagus nerve
Cervical esophagus

roid level, depicts the superior parathyroid glands in the visceral space just posterior to the t there are three key structures found in the area of the tracheoesophageal groove, the the paratracheal lymph node chain and the parathyroid gland. **(Bottom)** Coronal graphic thyroid glands and thyroid gland from behind. The drawing depicts the typical anatomic d superior and inferior parathyroid glands in the visceral space. Note the arterial supply to thyroid glands, the superior and inferior thyroid arteries respectively. It is easy to see why a l esophagus, thyroid or parathyroid gland could present with vocal cord paralysis.

GRAPHICS OF PARATHYROID GLAND EMBRYOLOGY

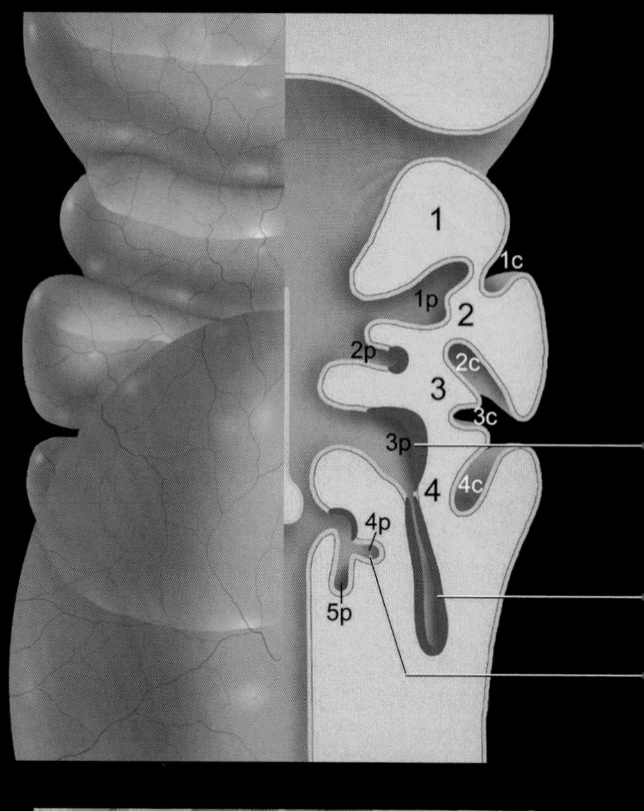
1
1c
1p
2
2p
2c
3
3c
3p
4
4c
4p
5p

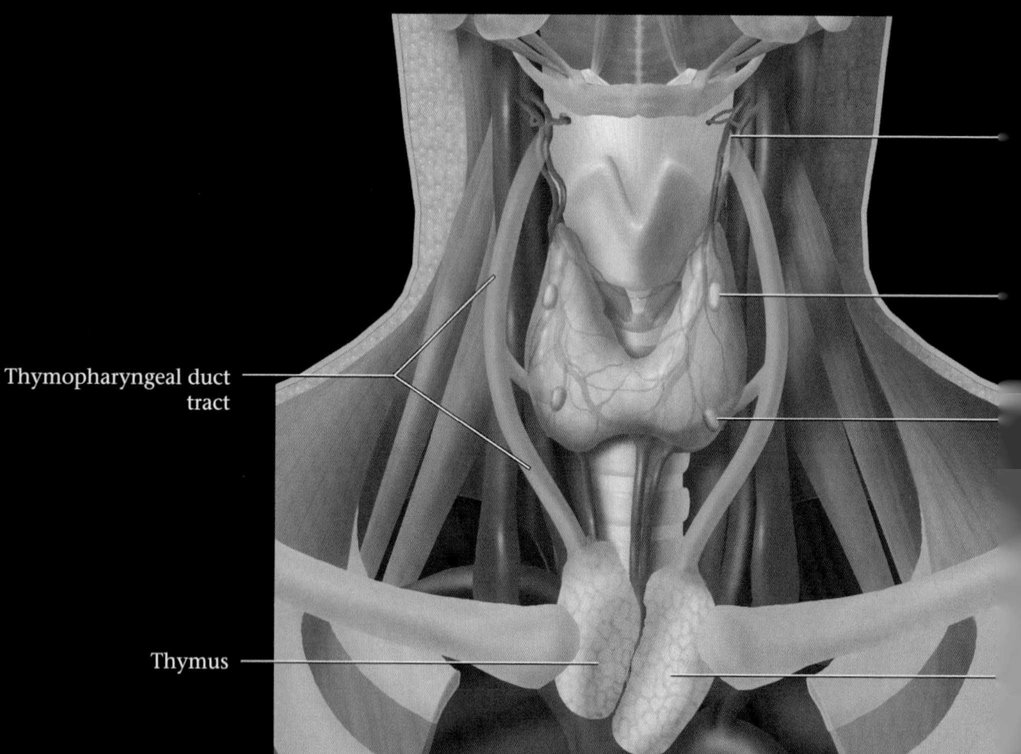
Thymopharyngeal duct tract
Thymus

(Top) Anteroposterior graphic of 6 week old fetus shows embryologic anatomy of branchial
The superior parathyroid glands develop from the 4th branchial pouches, along with primo
superior glands & the thyroid gland migrate caudally along the thyroglossal duct. The inferi
develop from 3rd branchial pouches along with anlage of thymus. The inferior glands & pri
caudally along the thymopharyngeal duct. **(Bottom)** Anteroposterior graphic of the cervical
the inferomedial migration of thymic primordia & inferior parathyroid glands along paired
tracts. Note the tracts extend from lateral hypopharyngeal area to anterior mediastinum. Va
parathyroid glands may result in ectopic locations along the thymopharyngeal duct tracts.

ULTRASOUND

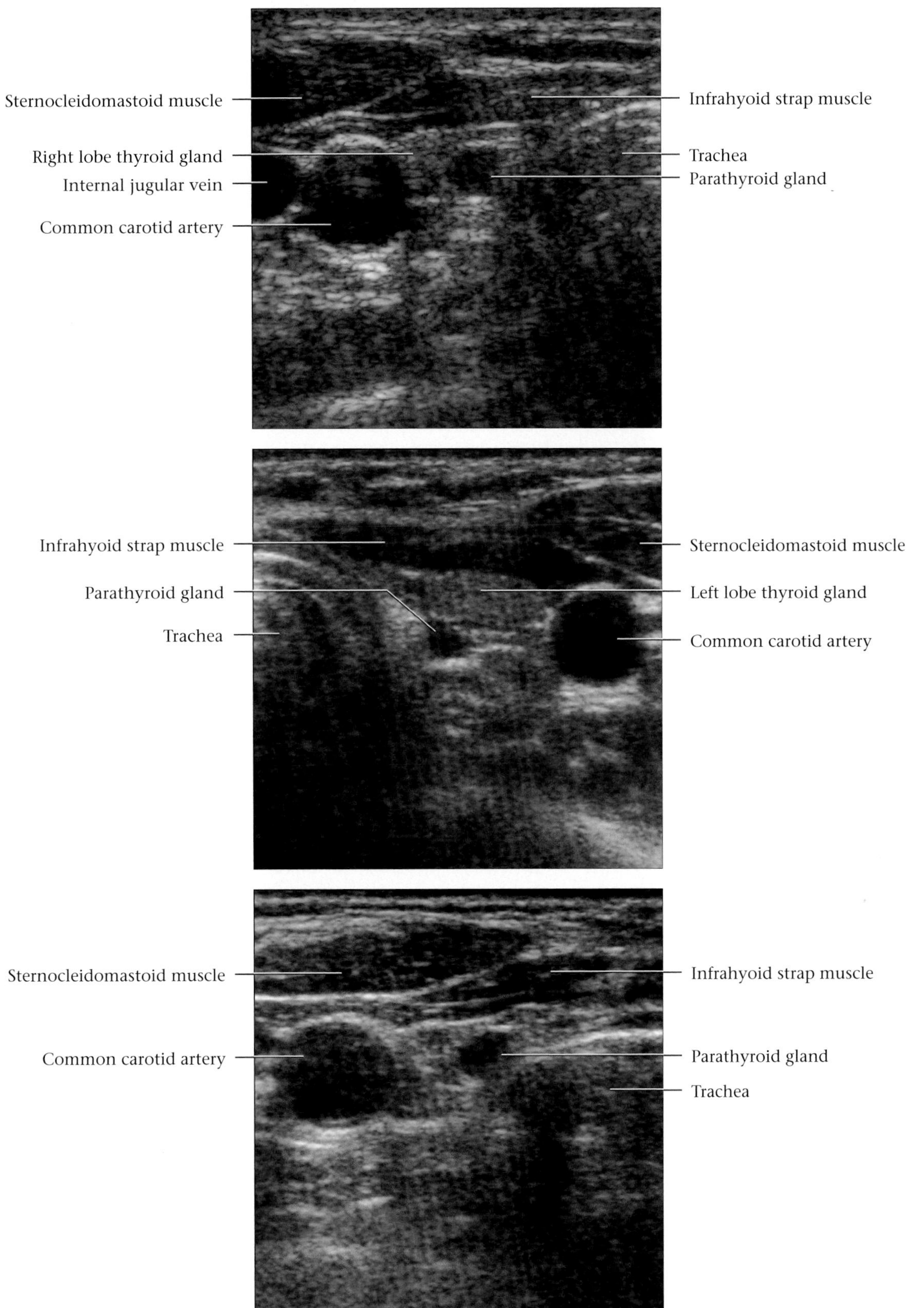
Sternocleidomastoid muscle
Right lobe thyroid gland
Internal jugular vein
Common carotid artery
Infrahyoid strap muscle
Trachea
Parathyroid gland
Infrahyoid strap muscle
Parathyroid gland
Trachea
Sternocleidomastoid muscle
Left lobe thyroid gland
Common carotid artery
Sternocleidomastoid muscle
Common carotid artery
Infrahyoid strap muscle
Parathyroid gland
Trachea

(Top) First of three transverse, grayscale sonographic image of right neck shows a well-circumscribed hypoechoic right superior parathyroid gland medial to common carotid artery and posterior to superior right thyroid lobe. **(Middle)** Image of left neck at the level of the thyroid gland shows the left inferior parathyroid gland as a hypoechoic ovoid lesion closely applied to posterior right thyroid lobe. The esophagus is not seen due to shadowing from the trachea, however the parathyroid gland is positioned within the tracheoesophageal groove. **(Bottom)** Image of right neck, demonstrates a right inferior parathyroid gland medial to common carotid artery, lateral to cervical trachea and inferior to right thyroid lobe.

GENERIC TRACHEOESOPHAGEAL GROOVE MASS

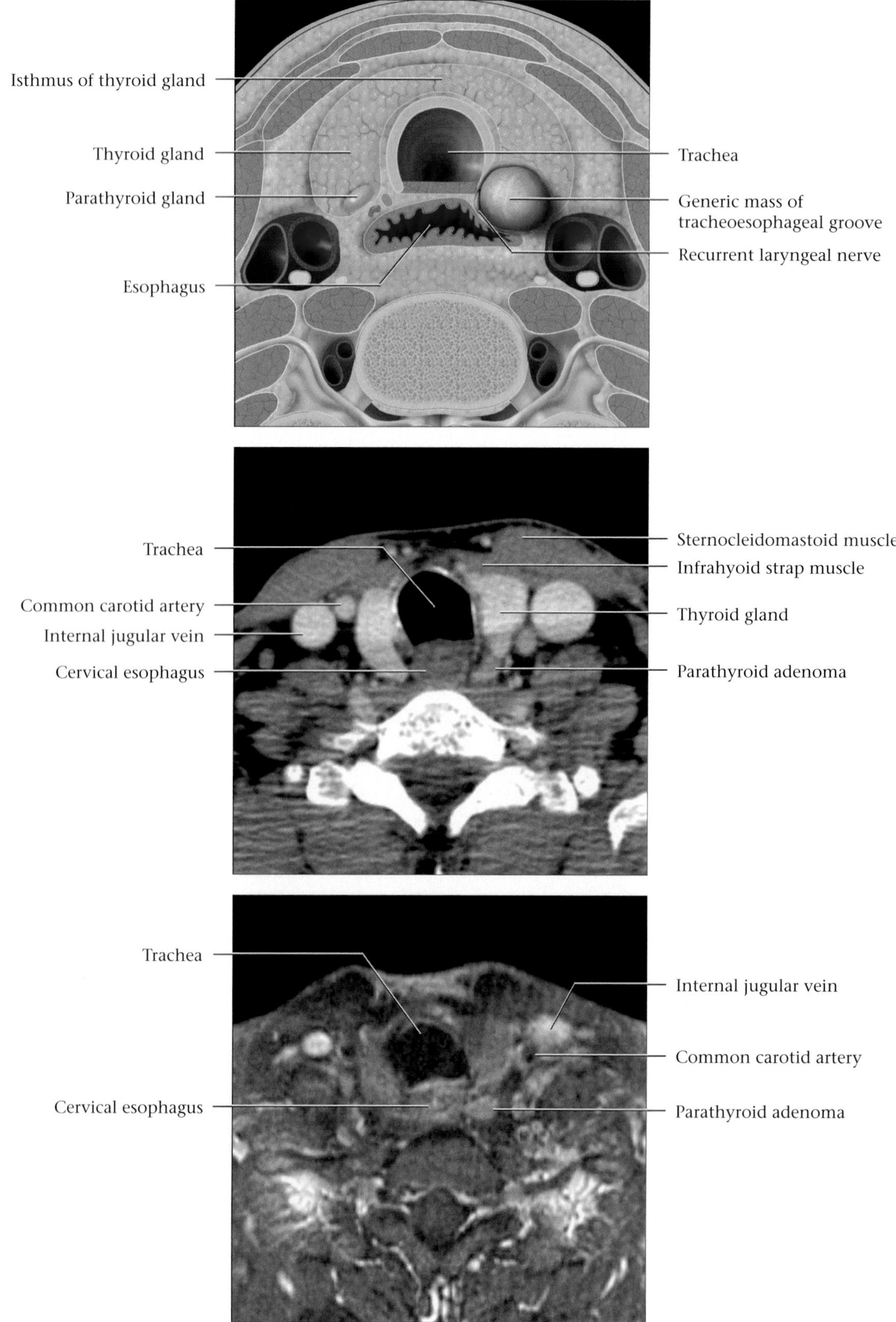
Isthmus of thyroid gland
Thyroid gland
Parathyroid gland
Esophagus
Trachea
Generic mass of tracheoesophageal groove
Recurrent laryngeal nerve
Trachea
Common carotid artery
Internal jugular vein
Cervical esophagus
Sternocleidomastoid muscle
Infrahyoid strap muscle
Thyroid gland
Parathyroid adenoma
Trachea
Cervical esophagus
Internal jugular vein
Common carotid artery
Parathyroid adenoma

(Top) Axial graphic shows a well-circumscribed generic mass in the left tracheoesophageal groove, causing mass effect on recurrent laryngeal nerve, esophagus, trachea and left thyroid lobe. Parathyroid adenoma, recurrent laryngeal nerve schwannoma and nodal disease in the paratracheal nodal chain all could cause such an appearance. **(Middle)** Axial CECT image at the level of thyroid gland shows an enhancing parathyroid adenoma in the left tracheoesophageal groove, posterior to left thyroid lobe. In a patient with hypercalcemia and elevated parathormone, this location and appearance is diagnostic. **(Bottom)** Axial T1 contrast-enhanced fat-saturated MR image at the level of the thyroid bed demonstrates an enhancing parathyroid adenoma posterior to the left lobe of the thyroid in the left tracheoesophageal groove.

ECTOPIC PARATHYROID ADENOMA

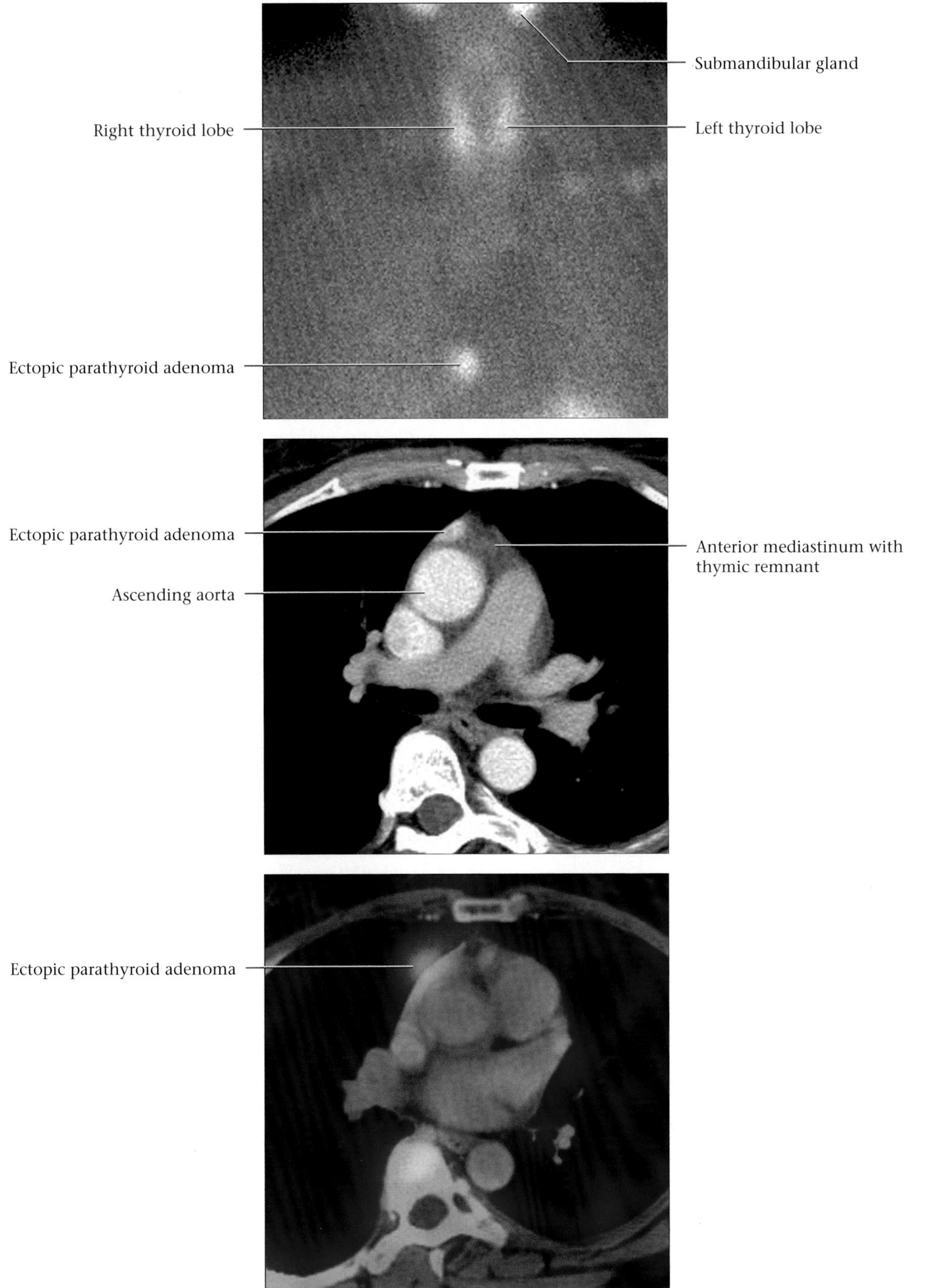
Submandibular gland
Right thyroid lobe
Left thyroid lobe
Ectopic parathyroid adenoma
Ectopic parathyroid adenoma
Anterior mediastinum with thymic remnant
Ascending aorta
Ectopic parathyroid adenoma

(Top) Hypercalcemic patient with elevated parathormone underwent Tc-99m Sestamibi nuclear medicine scan. In this 120 minute delayed scan an area of persistent concentration of isotope is visible in the mediastinum. In this clinical setting an ectopic parathyroid adenoma can be diagnosed. Persistent activity is also visualized in thyroid and submandibular salivary glands. CECT is ordered for presurgical localization. **(Middle)** Axial CECT image at the level of main pulmonary artery demonstrates an enhancing parathyroid adenoma in the anterior mediastinum, anterior to ascending aorta. **(Bottom)** Axial fusion image of CECT and Tc-99m Sestamibi nuclear medicine scan at the level of left atrium, shows ectopic radiotracer activity in an anterior mediastinal parathyroid adenoma.

CERVICAL TRACHEA AND ESOPHAGUS

Terminology

Definitions

- Cervical trachea: Air-conveying flexible tube made of cartilage & fibromuscular membrane connecting larynx to lungs
- Cervical esophagus: Muscular food & fluid-conveying tube connecting pharynx to stomach

Imaging Anatomy

Overview

- Trachea
  - 10-13 cm tube extending in midline from inferior larynx at ≈ 6th cervical vertebral body to carina at upper margin of 5th thoracic vertebral body (carina)
- Esophagus
  - 25 cm tube extending in midline from inferior hypopharynx at ≈ 6th cervical vertebral body to 11th thoracic vertebral body
  - Descends behind trachea & thyroid, lying in front of lower cervical vertebrae
    - Inclines slightly to left in lower cervical neck & upper mediastinum, returning to midline at T5 vertebral body level

Anatomy Relationships

- **Cervical trachea**
  - Anterior structures: Infrahyoid strap muscles; isthmus of thyroid gland (2nd-4th tracheal cartilages)
  - Lateral structures: Lobes of thyroid gland
    - Tracheoesophageal groove structures: Recurrent laryngeal nerve, paratracheal nodes, parathyroid glands
  - Posterior structure: Cervical esophagus
- **Cervical esophagus**
  - Anterior structure: Cervical trachea
  - Anterolateral structures: Tracheoesophageal groove structures
  - Lateral structures: Carotid spaces
  - Posterior structures: Retropharyngeal/danger spaces

Internal Structures-Critical Contents

- **Cervical trachea**
  - **Cartilage anatomy**
    - Each cartilage is "imperfect ring" of cartilage surrounding anterior two-thirds of trachea
    - Flat deficient posterior portion is completed with fibromuscular membrane
    - Cross-sectional shape of trachea is that of letter D, with flat side posterior
    - Smooth muscle fibers in posterior membrane (trachealis muscle) attach to free ends of tracheal cartilages & provide alteration in tracheal cross-sectional area
    - Hyaline cartilage calcifies with age
  - **First tracheal cartilage**
    - Broadest of all tracheal cartilages
    - Often bifurcates at one end & is connected by cricotracheal ligament to inferior cricoid cartilage
  - **Cervical tracheal mucosa**
    - Continuous sheet from larynx above
    - Layer of pseudostratified ciliated columnar epithelium interspersed with goblet cells with both lying on basal lamina
    - Cilia propel mucus towards laryngeal inlet (1,000 beats per minute)
    - Minor salivary glands sporadically distributed in tracheal mucosa
  - **Blood supply**: Inferior thyroid arteries & veins
  - **Lymphatic drainage**: Level VI pretracheal & paratracheal nodes
- **Cervical esophagus**
  - Begins at lower border of cricoid cartilage as continuation of hypopharynx
    - Upper limit is defined by cricopharyngeus muscle, which encircles it from front to back
  - **Cervical esophageal mucosa**
    - Non-keratinized stratified squamous epithelium
  - **Blood supply**: Inferior thyroid arteries & veins
  - **Lymphatic drainage**: Level VI paratracheal nodes

Fascia

- Middle layer, deep cervical fascia surrounds visceral space with trachea & esophagus inside

Anatomy-Based Imaging Issues

Imaging Approaches

- **Cervical trachea**
  - **Multislice CT** with sagittal & coronal reformations exam of choice for trachea
- **Cervical esophagus**
  - **Air-contrast barium swallow** is **primary diagnostic tool** in esophageal evaluation
  - Multislice CECT for esophageal tumor staging

Clinical Implications

Clinical Importance

- Cervical tracheal lesions present with shortness of breath & stridor
  - May be treated for asthma prior to diagnosis
- Cervical esophageal lesions present with dysphagia
  - Aspiration pneumonia may occur prior to diagnosis

Embryology

Embryologic Events

- During 4th gestational week respiratory primordium begins with formation of laryngotracheal groove that extends lengthwise in floor of gut just caudal to pharyngeal pouches
- Groove then deepens into laryngotracheal diverticulum whose ventral ectoderm become larynx & trachea
- Lateral furrows develop on either side of laryngotracheal diverticulum, then deepen to form laryngotracheal tube
- Tracheoesophageal septum then develops caudally to cranially, separating respiratory system from esophagus

CERVICAL TRACHEA AND ESOPHAGUS

BARIUM SWALLOW

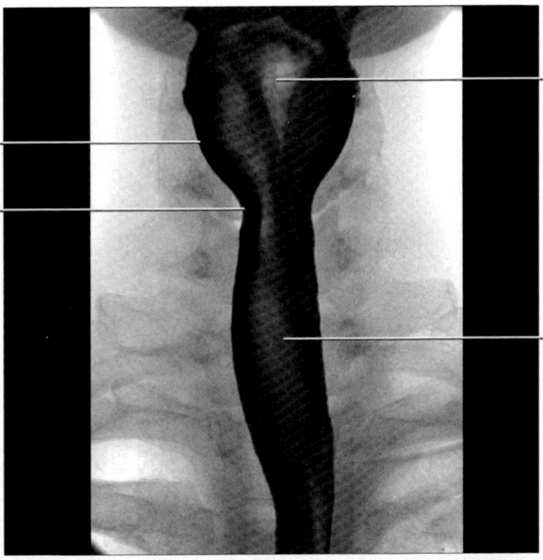

Larynx
Hypopharynx
Junction of hypopharynx & esophagus
Cervical esophagus

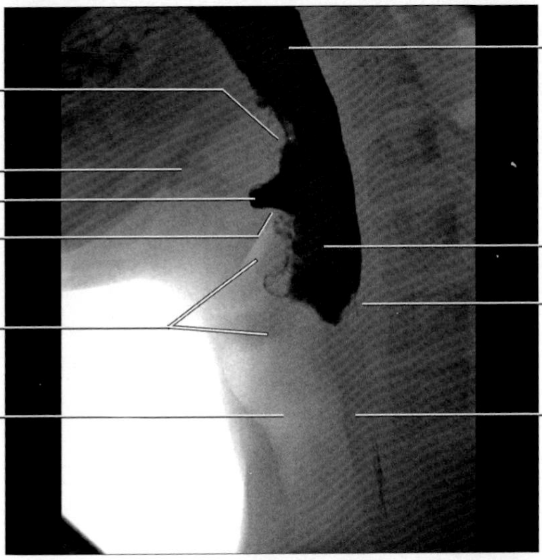

Oropharynx
Lingual tonsil
Hyoid bone
Vallecula
Epiglottis
Hypopharynx
Cricopharyngeus muscle indentation
Larynx
Trachea
Esophagus

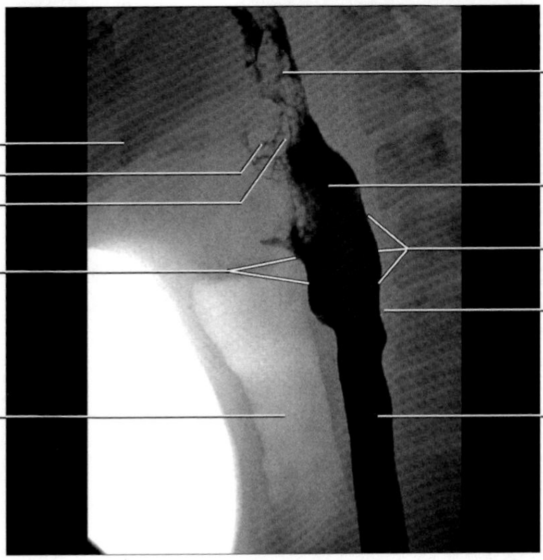

Oropharynx
Hyoid bone
Vallecula
Epiglottis
Hypopharynx
Posterior wall hypopharynx
Post-cricoid hypopharynx
Cricopharyngeus muscle indentation
Trachea
Esophagus

(Top) Frontal view of a normal barium swallow shows barium deflected around the larynx which appears as a filling defect. Inferior cricoid cartilage delineates inferior larynx & hypopharynx on CT studies as well as junction of hypopharynx with cervical esophagus. **(Middle)** Lateral view of barium swallow of upper pharynx shows junction of oropharynx & hypopharynx at hyoid bone. Lingual tonsil (base of tongue) causes a lobulated impression upon anterior oropharynx. Epiglottis closes during swallowing to protect larynx from aspiration. Valleculae are recesses between tongue & epiglottis. **(Bottom)** Lateral view of barium swallow shows hypopharynx & cervical esophagus posterior to larynx & trachea. Hypopharynx extends from hyoid bone to cricopharyngeus muscle. Cricopharyngeus muscle demarcates hypopharynx from cervical esophagus on barium studies & is typically located at C5/6 level.

CERVICAL TRACHEA AND ESOPHAGUS

GRAPHICS

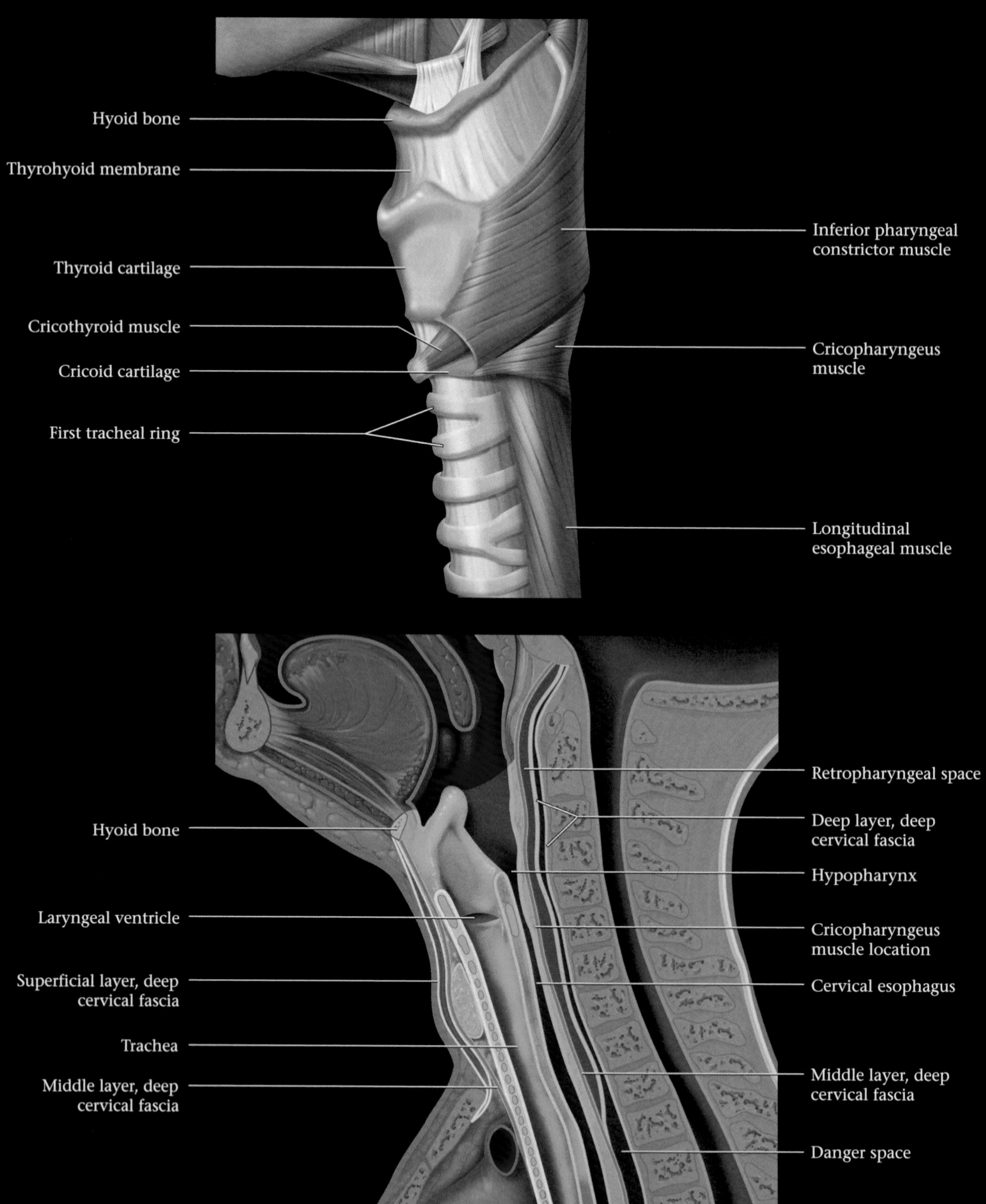

Hyoid bone
Thyrohyoid membrane
Thyroid cartilage
Cricothyroid muscle
Cricoid cartilage
First tracheal ring
Inferior pharyngeal constrictor muscle
Cricopharyngeus muscle
Longitudinal esophageal muscle
Hyoid bone
Laryngeal ventricle
Superficial layer, deep cervical fascia
Trachea
Middle layer, deep cervical fascia
Retropharyngeal space
Deep layer, deep cervical fascia
Hypopharynx
Cricopharyngeus muscle location
Cervical esophagus
Middle layer, deep cervical fascia
Danger space

(Top) Lateral graphic shows junction of larynx & hypopharynx with trachea & esophagus. Cricopharyngeus muscle, which separates hypopharynx from cervical esophagus is part of the inferior constrictor muscle. Esophagus is composed of outer longitudinal muscles & an inner circular muscle layer (not shown). First tracheal ring is broadest of all tracheal cartilages & is often merged to cricoid cartilage or second tracheal ring. Mucosal portions of posterior trachea are separated from esophagus by a thin layer of connective tissue, often called the "party wall" as it separates trachea anteriorly from esophagus posteriorly. **(Bottom)** Sagittal graphic shows longitudinal relationships of infrahyoid neck. Note middle layer of deep cervical fascia (pink) encircles trachea & esophagus as part of visceral space. Trachea & esophagus are inferior continuation of airway & pharynx.

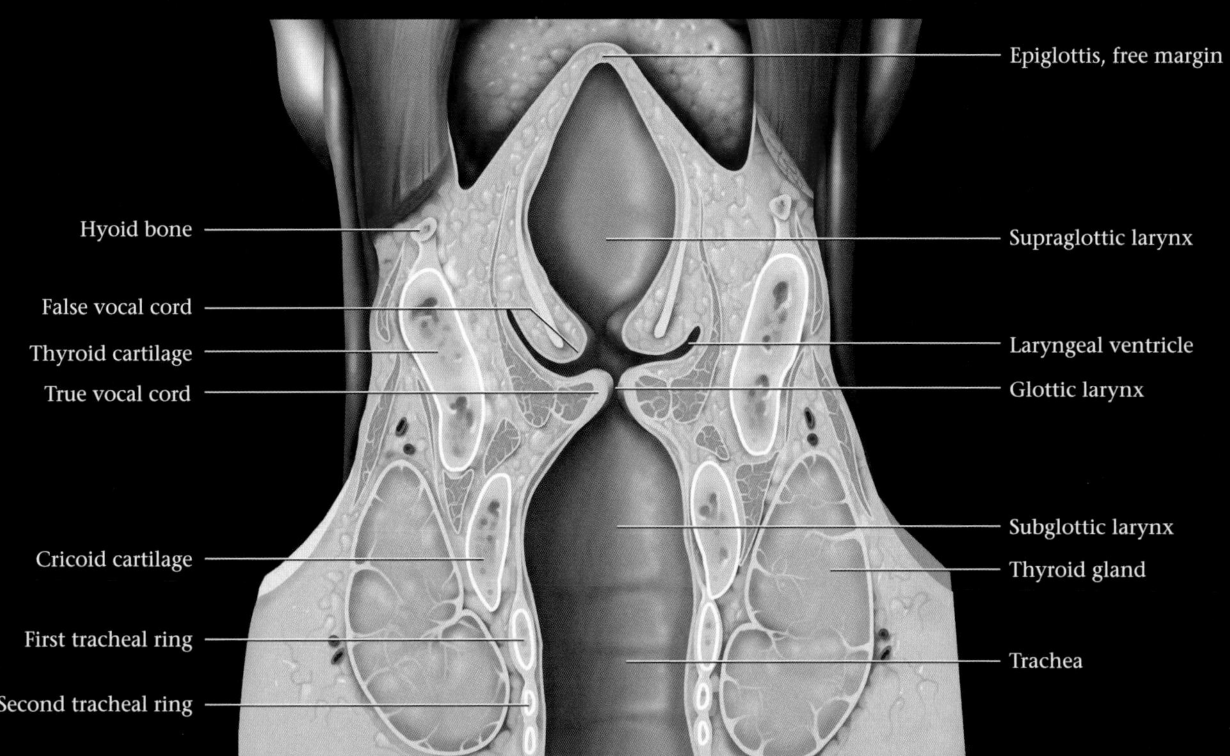
Epiglottis, free margin
Hyoid bone
Supraglottic larynx
False vocal cord
Thyroid cartilage
True vocal cord
Laryngeal ventricle
Glottic larynx
Subglottic larynx
Cricoid cartilage
Thyroid gland
First tracheal ring
Trachea
Second tracheal ring

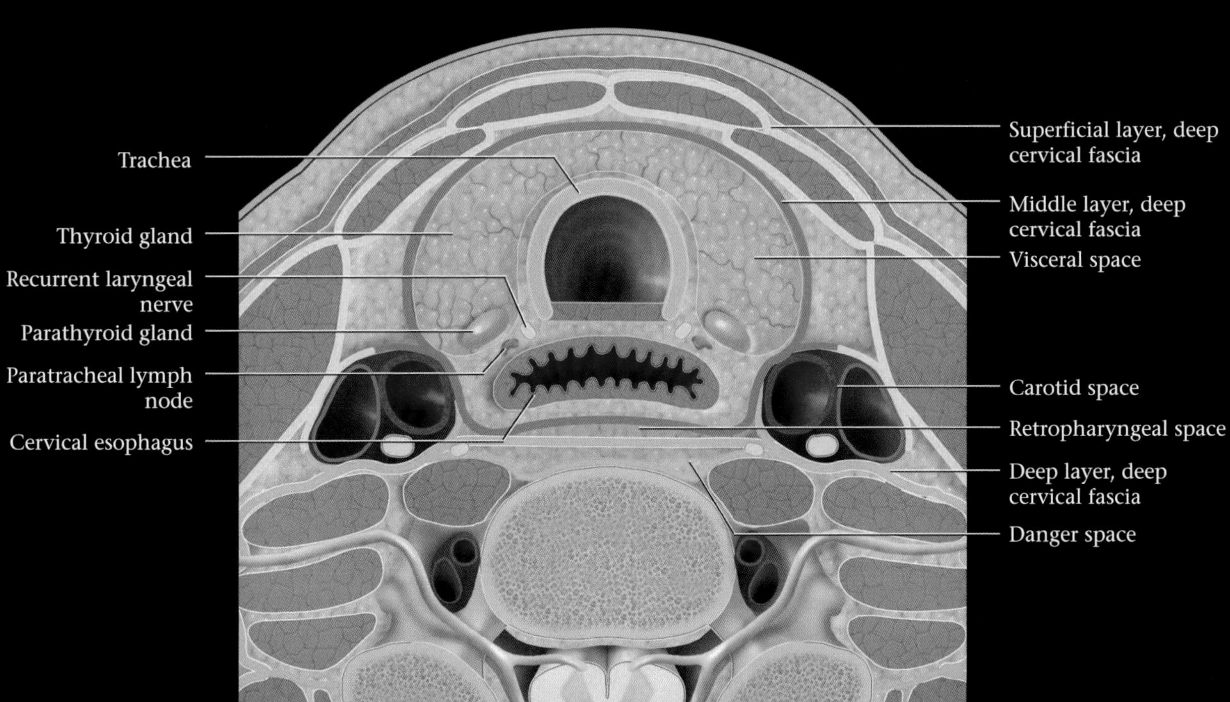
Superficial layer, deep cervical fascia
Trachea
Middle layer, deep cervical fascia
Thyroid gland
Visceral space
Recurrent laryngeal nerve
Parathyroid gland
Paratracheal lymph node
Carotid space
Cervical esophagus
Retropharyngeal space
Deep layer, deep cervical fascia
Danger space

(Top) Coronal graphic shows larynx & trachea. Supraglottic larynx includes epiglottis, aryepiglottic folds, false vocal cords & pre-epiglottic & paraglottic spaces. Glottic larynx includes true vocal cords. Subglottic larynx is separated from trachea at inferior cricoid cartilage. First tracheal ring is located 1.5-2 cm below true vocal cords & is broadest of all cartilage rings. Second, third & fourth tracheal rings are surrounded by thyroid gland, anteriorly & laterally. Coronal & sagittal reformatted images are particularly helpful in evaluation of tracheal stenosis & other disorders. **(Bottom)** Axial graphic shows layers of deep cervical fascia in infrahyoid neck. Note middle layer of deep cervical fascia as it surrounds visceral space. Important components of tracheoesophageal groove include recurrent laryngeal nerve, paratracheal nodes & parathyroid glands.

CERVICAL TRACHEA AND ESOPHAGUS

AXIAL CECT

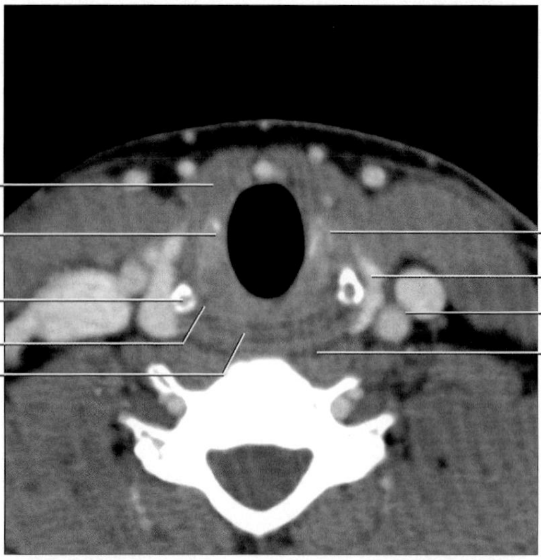

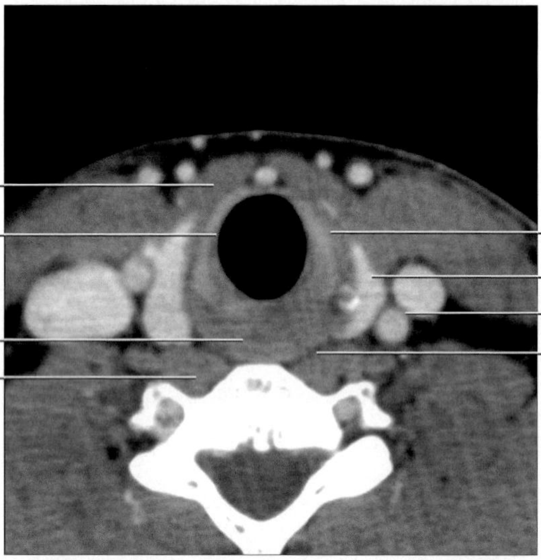

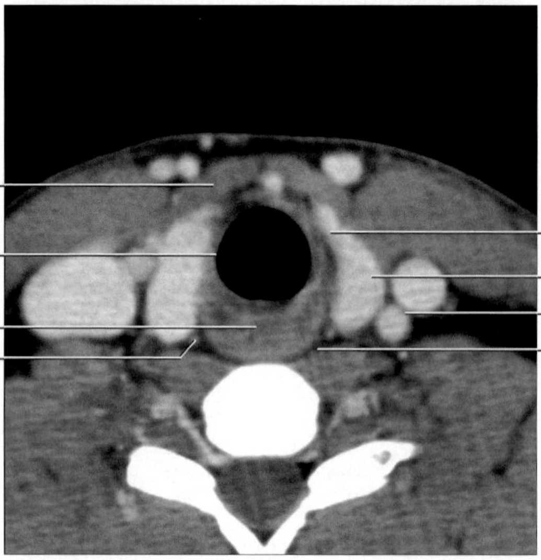

Strap muscles
Inferior cricoid cartilage
Thyroid cartilage, inferior cornu
Cricothyroid joint
Hypopharynx
Visceral space
Superior thyroid gland
Carotid space
Retropharyngeal space

Strap muscles
Inferior cricoid cartilage
Hypopharynx/esophagus junction
Prevertebral muscles
Visceral space
Superior thyroid gland
Carotid space
Retropharyngeal space

Strap muscles
Trachea
Esophagus
Tracheoesophageal groove
Visceral space
Thyroid gland
Carotid space
Retropharyngeal space

(Top) First of six axial CECT images from superior to inferior shows inferior larynx & hypopharynx & transition to cervical trachea & esophagus. Inferior larynx & hypopharynx are defined by inferior cricoid cartilage on cross-sectional imaging. This image shows subglottic larynx, area from undersurface of true vocal cords to inferior surface of cricoid cartilage. Cricothyroid joint lies adjacent to recurrent laryngeal nerve & dislocation of this joint may result in vocal cord paralysis. **(Middle)** This image shows junction of hypopharynx & larynx which is defined by cricopharyngeus muscle on barium swallow studies. This muscle is an inferior portion of inferior pharyngeal constrictor muscle & is typically present at C5/6. **(Bottom)** Image more inferior shows cervical trachea & esophagus. The upper second through fourth tracheal rings are surrounded by thyroid gland.

AXIAL CECT

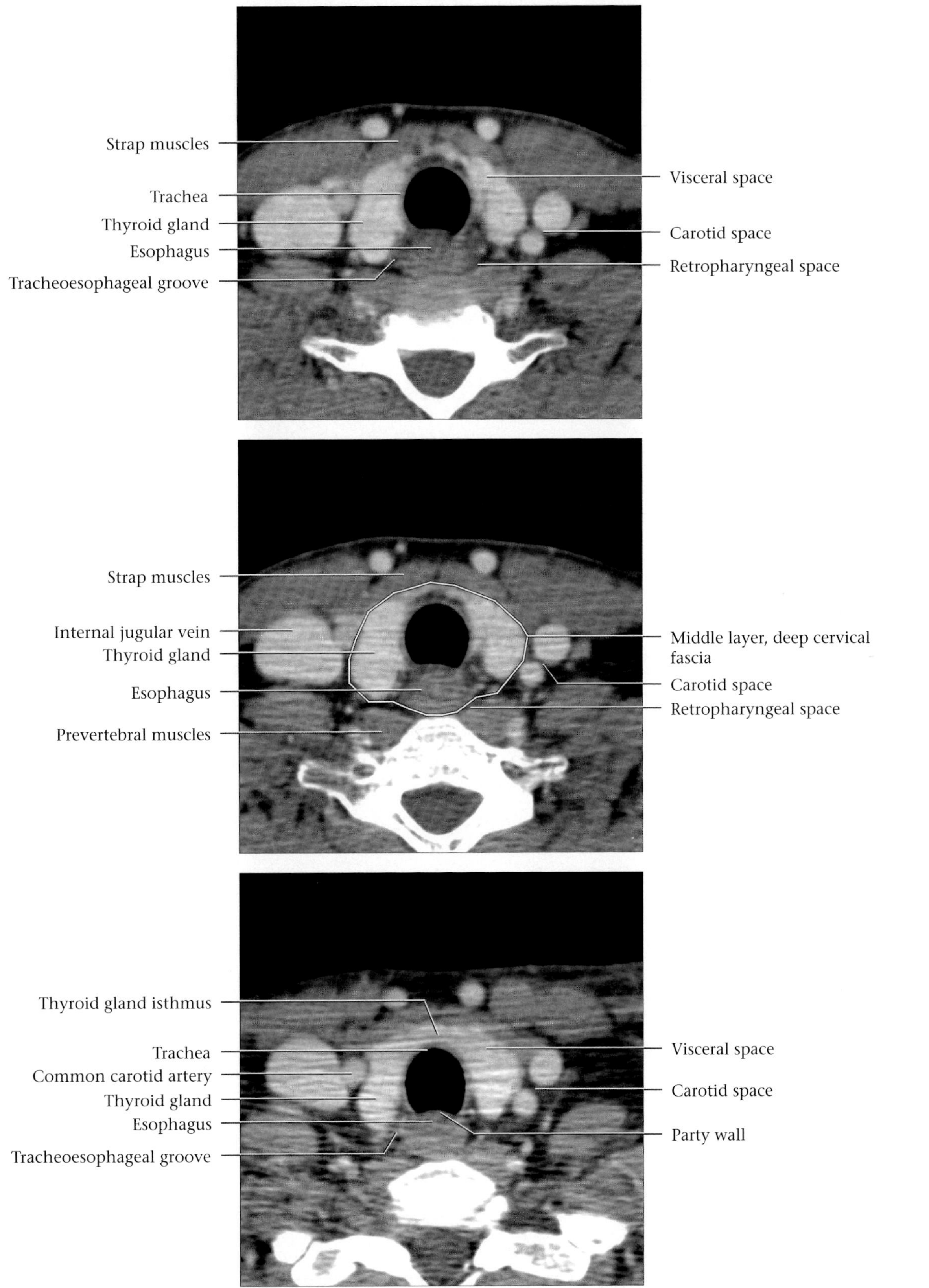
Strap muscles
Trachea
Thyroid gland
Esophagus
Tracheoesophageal groove
Visceral space
Carotid space
Retropharyngeal space
Strap muscles
Internal jugular vein
Thyroid gland
Esophagus
Prevertebral muscles
Middle layer, deep cervical fascia
Carotid space
Retropharyngeal space
Thyroid gland isthmus
Trachea
Common carotid artery
Thyroid gland
Esophagus
Tracheoesophageal groove
Visceral space
Carotid space
Party wall

(Top) Image more inferior shows cervical trachea & esophagus within inferior visceral space. Cervical trachea is bordered anteriorly by infrahyoid strap muscles, anteriorly & laterally by thyroid gland & tracheoesophageal groove structures & posteriorly by esophagus. Esophagus is bordered anteriorly by cervical trachea, anterolaterally by tracheoesophageal groove structures, laterally by carotid spaces & posteriorly by retropharyngeal space. **(Middle)** This image shows middle layer of deep cervical fascia encircling the visceral space. **(Bottom)** This image shows the "party wall", the thin layer of connective tissue that separates mucosal portions of posterior trachea from anterior esophagus. Tracheoesophageal groove structures include recurrent laryngeal nerve, paratracheal lymph nodes & parathyroid glands.

GENERIC TRACHEAL MASS GRAPHIC & CECT

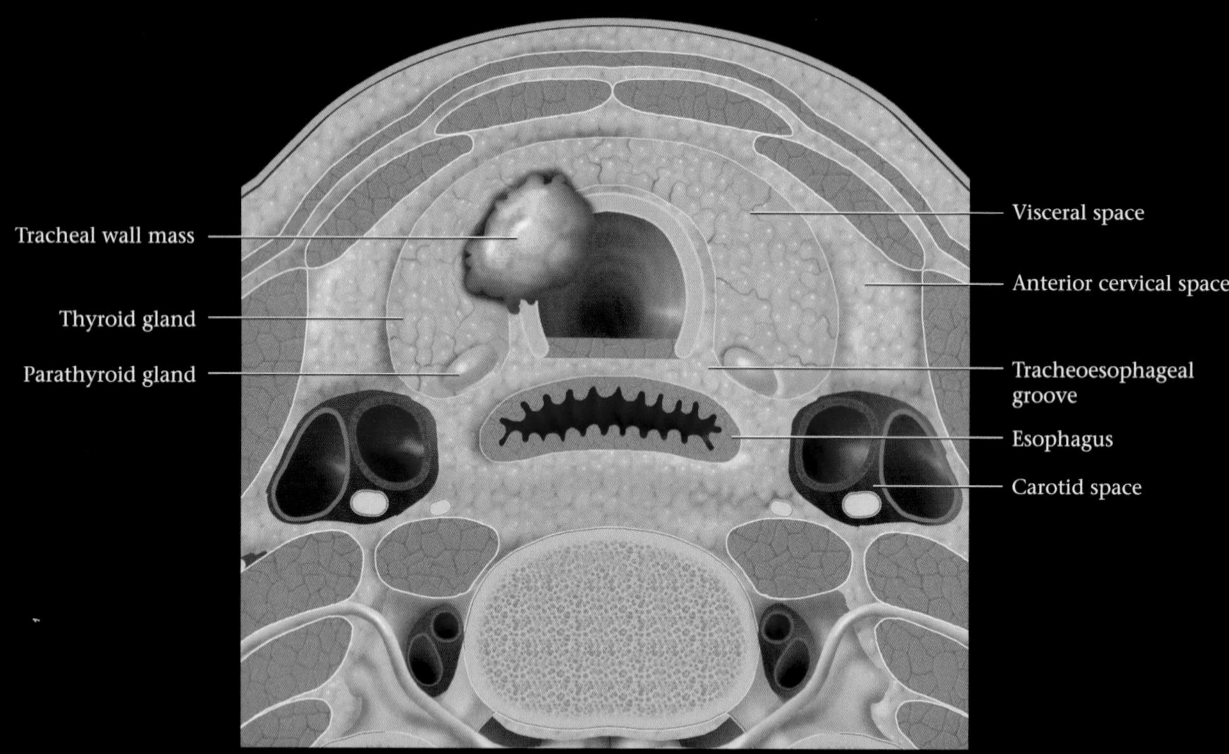
Tracheal wall mass
Thyroid gland
Parathyroid gland
Visceral space
Anterior cervical space
Tracheoesophageal groove
Esophagus
Carotid space

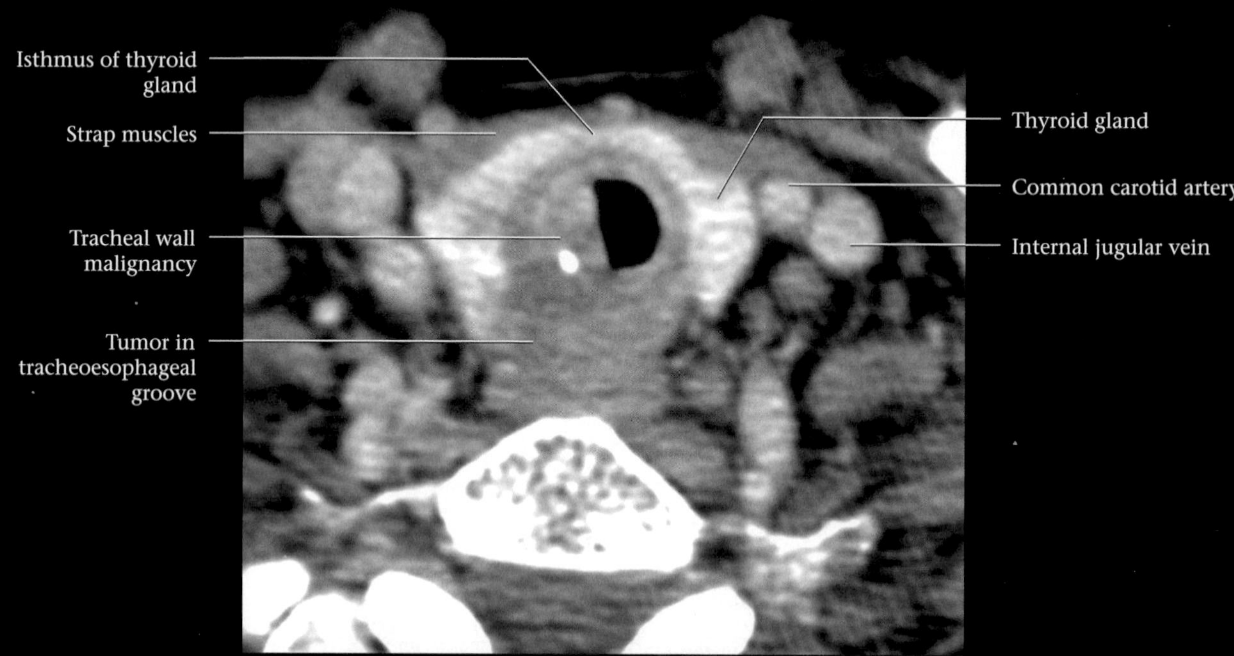
Isthmus of thyroid gland
Strap muscles
Tracheal wall malignancy
Tumor in tracheoesophageal groove
Thyroid gland
Common carotid artery
Internal jugular vein

(Top) Axial graphic shows a generic tracheal wall mass. A mass within the tracheal wall typically displaces thyroid gland laterally & esophagus posteriorly. Primary tumors of the trachea are rare, representing 2% of upper airway tumors. Most common primary malignant tumors include squamous cell carcinomas (SCCa) & adenoid cystic carcinomas. SCCa usually arise in lower trachea & carina. Adenoid cystic carcinomas are usually located on posterolateral tracheal wall. **(Bottom)** Axial CECT image demonstrates a right tracheal wall adenoid cystic carcinoma that has spread posteriorly to involve the right tracheoesophageal groove and anterior wall of the cervical esophagus. Such lesions can be relatively asymptomatic until stridor supervenes.

GENERIC ESOPHAGEAL MASS GRAPHIC & CECT

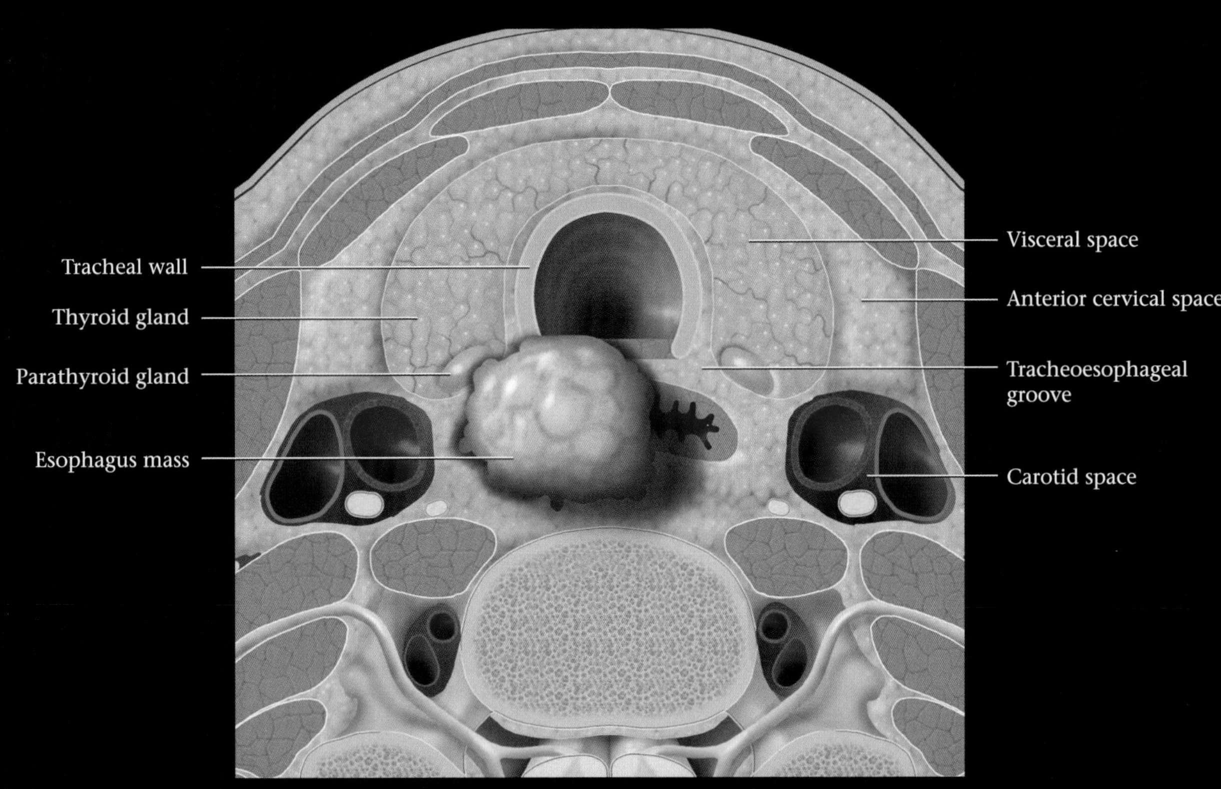
Tracheal wall
Thyroid gland
Parathyroid gland
Esophagus mass
Visceral space
Anterior cervical space
Tracheoesophageal groove
Carotid space

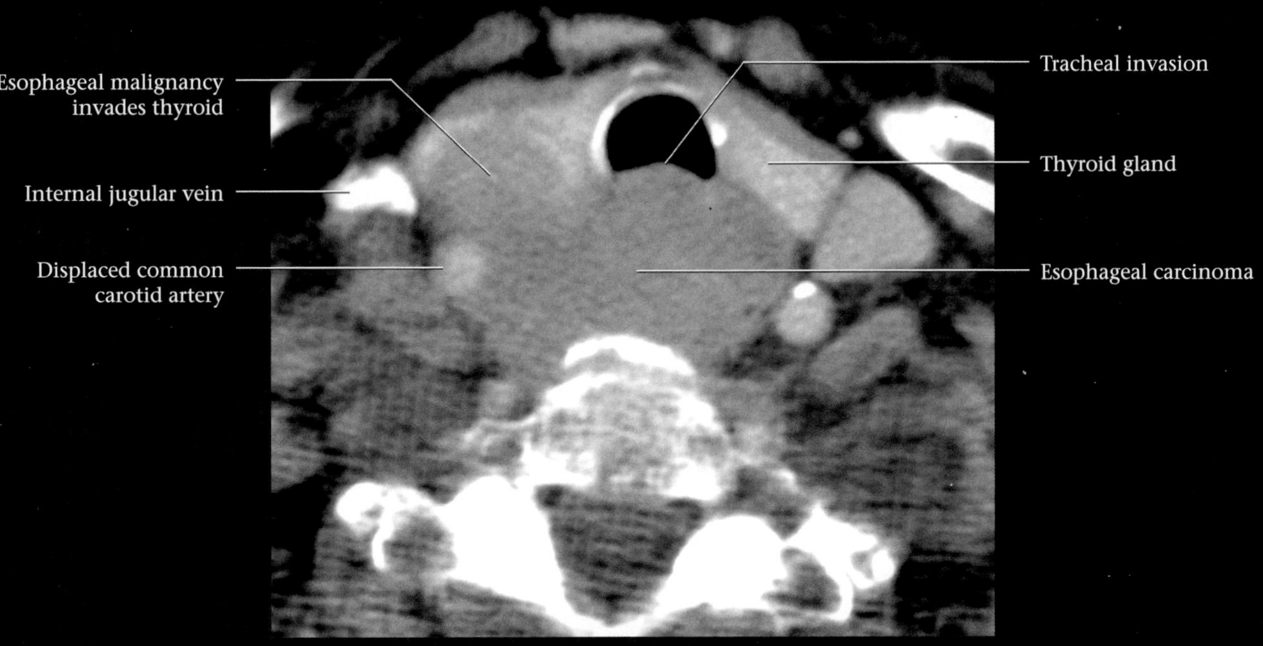
Esophageal malignancy invades thyroid
Internal jugular vein
Displaced common carotid artery
Tracheal invasion
Thyroid gland
Esophageal carcinoma

(Top) Axial graphic of a generic esophageal mass which is typically midline & displaces trachea & thyroid gland anteriorly. 90% of esophageal carcinomas are squamous cell carcinoma while the remainder are adenocarcinoma related to Barrett esophagus. CT is particularly useful to define extent of disease & associated metastases, typically to peri-esophageal, paratracheal, supraclavicular & mediastinal lymph nodes & the liver. Leiomyoma is most common benign tumor of the esophagus & is usually incidentally discovered. **(Bottom)** Axial CECT through the lower thyroid bed in the cervical neck reveals a large retrotracheal invasive mass (esophageal carcinoma) that has lifted the trachea and left thyroid lobe anteriorly. The right common carotid artery is displaced laterally. The tumor has invaded the right thyroid lobe and the posterior trachea.

CERVICAL LYMPH NODES

Terminology

Abbreviations

- Internal jugular chain (IJC)

Synonyms

- Internal jugular chain: Deep cervical chain
- Spinal accessory chain (SAC): Posterior triangle chain

Definitions

- **Jugulodigastric node**: "Sentinel" (highest) node, found at apex of IJC at angle of mandible
- **"Signal" (Virchow) node**: Node found at bottom of IJC in supraclavicular fossa

Imaging Anatomy

Overview

- Differentiation between benign or "reactive" nodes vs pathological nodes
  - Morphology: Oval nodes with central fatty hila
  - Size criteria
    - < 1.5 cm for IJC nodes near the angle of the mandible
    - < .8 mm for retropharyngeal nodes
    - < 1 cm for all other nodal groups

Internal Structures-Critical Contents

- **Imaging-based nodal classification**
  - **Level I: Submental & submandibular nodes**
    - Level IA: Submental nodes: Found between anterior bellies of digastric muscles
    - Level IB: Submandibular nodes: Found around submandibular glands in submandibular space
  - **Level II: Upper IJC nodes** from posterior belly of digastric muscle to hyoid bone
    - Level IIA: Level II node anterior, medial, lateral or posterior to internal jugular vein (IJV); if posterior to IJV, node must be inseparable from IJV
    - Level IIA contains jugulodigastric nodal group
    - Level IIB: Level II node posterior to IJV with fat plane visible between node & IJV
  - **Level III: Mid-IJC nodes** from hyoid bone to inferior margin of cricoid cartilage
  - **Level IV: Low IJC nodes** from inferior cricoid margin to clavicle
  - **Level V: Nodes of posterior cervical space (SAC)**
    - SAC nodes lie posterior to back margin of sternocleidomastoid muscle
    - Level VA: Upper SAC nodes from skull base to bottom of cricoid cartilage
    - Level VB: Lower SAC nodes from cricoid to clavicle
  - **Level VI: Nodes of visceral space** found from hyoid bone above to top of manubrium below
    - Includes prelaryngeal, pretracheal and **paratracheal** subgroups
  - **Level VII: Superior mediastinal nodes** found between carotid arteries from top of manubrium above to innominate vein below
- Other nodal groups not included in standard imaging-based nodal classification
  - **Parotid nodal group**: Intraglandular or extraglandular
    - Both intraglandular & extraglandular nodes are within fascia circumscribing parotid space
    - Drains into upper IJC nodes (level II)
    - Most common tumors to involve this group are skin SCCa, melanoma & parotid malignancy
  - **Retropharyngeal (RPS) nodal group**: 2 subgroups
    - Medial RPS nodes: Found in paramedian RPS in suprahyoid neck (SHN)
    - Lateral RPS nodes: Found in lateral RPS in SHN, lateral to prevertebral muscles, medial to ICA
    - Drainage pattern: Receive drainage from posterior pharynx; drains into high IJC
  - **Facial nodal group**
    - Mandibular nodes: Found along external mandibular surface
    - Buccinator nodes: In buccal space
    - Infraorbital nodes: In nasolabial fold
    - Malar nodes: On malar eminence
    - Retrozygomatic nodes: Deep to zygomatic arch

Anatomy-Based Imaging Issues

Imaging Approaches

- SCCa nodal staging: CECT or T1 C+ MR
  - Scan extent: Skull base to clavicles
- PET-CT utility in H & N SCCa nodal work-up
  - Small active malignant node identification & treatment planning
- Differentiated thyroid carcinoma: MR preferred
  - Scan extent: Skull base to **carina**

Clinical Implications

Clinical Importance

- Presence of malignant SCCa nodes in staging associated with 50% ↓ in long term survival
  - If extranodal spread present, further 50% ↓
- IJC is final common pathway for all lymphatics of upper aerodigestive tract & neck
  - Since IJC empties into subclavian vein, IJV or thoracic duct, SCCa does not normally drain directly into mediastinum
  - Neck imaging to stage SCCa: Skull base to clavicles
- **Retropharyngeal space nodal group**
  - Reactive appearing RPS nodes commonly seen in younger patients on brain MR exam
  - Important when identified on imaging in SCCa setting, as often clinically silent
- When **"signal" node** (lowest IJC) found on imaging without upper neck nodes, primary is not in neck
- **Parotid nodal group**
  - Receives lymph drainage from external auditory canal, eustachian tube, skin of lateral forehead & temporal region, posterior cheek, gums & buccal mucous membrane (especially due to skin squamous cell carcinoma & melanoma)
  - Parotidectomy & nodal dissection of neck are necessary if malignancy of superficial ear area presents as cervical neck malignant adenopathy

CERVICAL LYMPH NODES

GRAPHICS

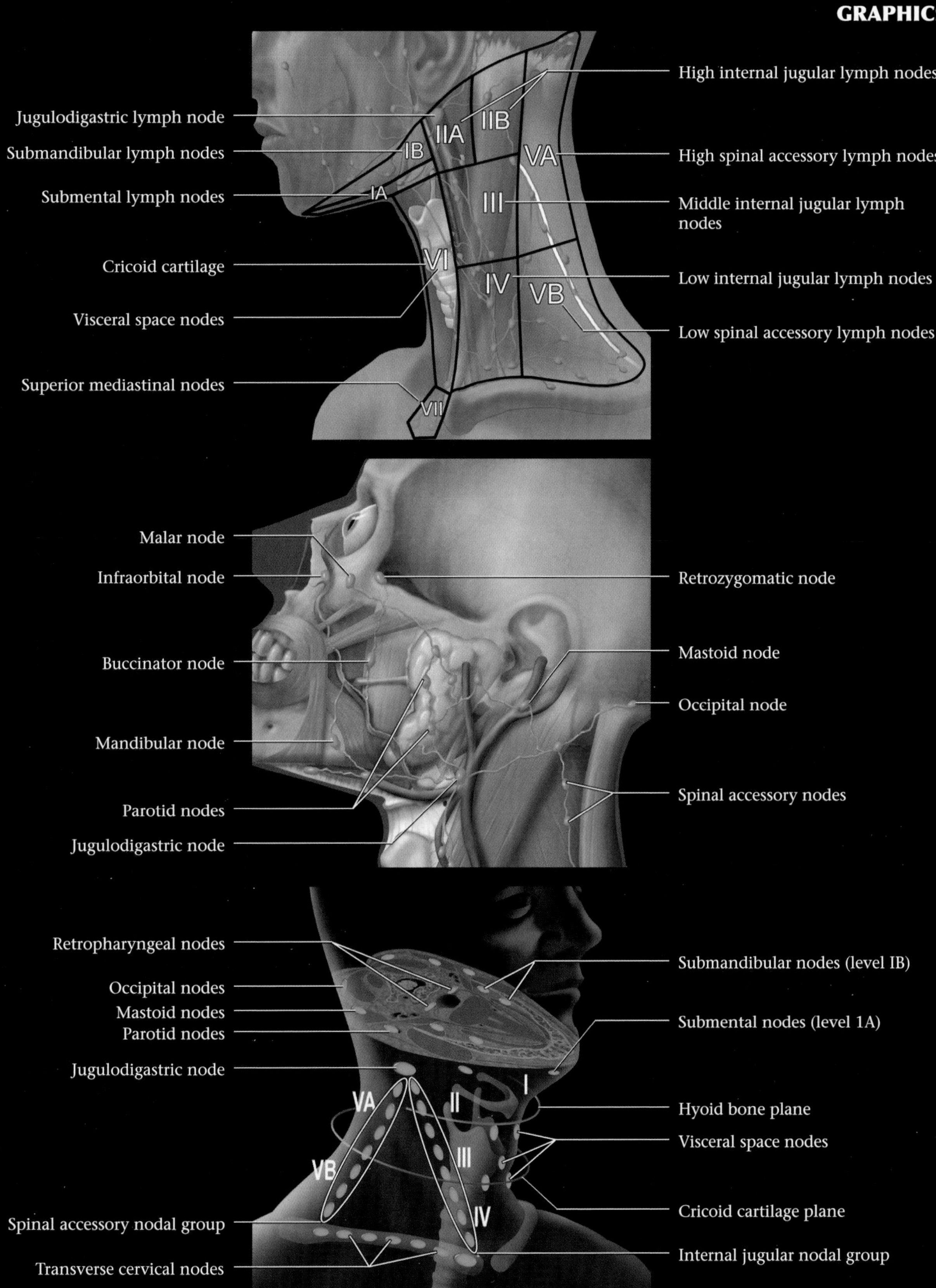

Jugulodigastric lymph node
Submandibular lymph nodes
Submental lymph nodes
Cricoid cartilage
Visceral space nodes
Superior mediastinal nodes
High internal jugular lymph nodes
High spinal accessory lymph nodes
Middle internal jugular lymph nodes
Low internal jugular lymph nodes
Low spinal accessory lymph nodes
IA
IB
IIA
IIB
VA
III
VI
IV
VB
VII
Malar node
Infraorbital node
Buccinator node
Mandibular node
Parotid nodes
Jugulodigastric node
Retrozygomatic node
Mastoid node
Occipital node
Spinal accessory nodes
Retropharyngeal nodes
Occipital nodes
Mastoid nodes
Parotid nodes
Jugulodigastric node
Spinal accessory nodal group
Transverse cervical nodes
Submandibular nodes (level IB)
Submental nodes (level 1A)
Hyoid bone plane
Visceral space nodes
Cricoid cartilage plane
Internal jugular nodal group
I
II
VA
III
VB
IV

(Top) Lateral oblique graphic of the neck shows the anatomic locations for the major nodal groups of the neck. Division of the internal jugular nodal chain into high, middle and low regions is defined by the level of the hyoid bone and cricoid cartilage. Similarly, the spinal accessory nodal chain is divided into high & low regions by the level of the cricoid cartilage. **(Middle)** Lateral view of facial nodes plus parotid nodes. None of these nodes bear level numbers but instead must be described by their anatomic location. **(Bottom)** Lateral oblique graphic of cervical neck depicts an axial slice through the suprahyoid neck. Note the retropharyngeal nodes behind the pharynx are often clinically occult. The hyoid bone (blue arc) & cricoid cartilage (orange circle) planes are highlighted as they serve to subdivide the internal jugular & spinal accessory nodal group levels.

CERVICAL LYMPH NODES

ULTRASOUND

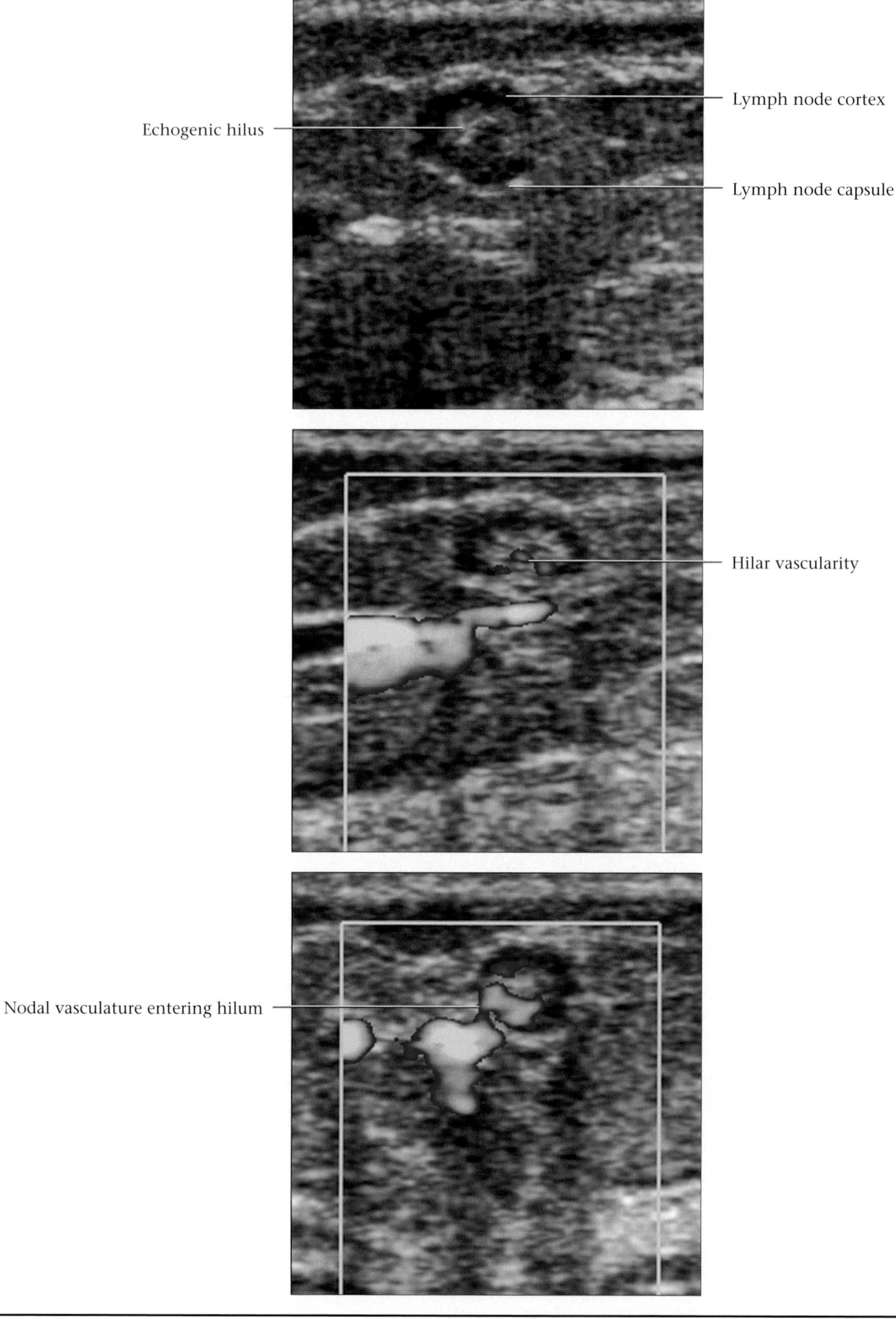
Lymph node cortex
Echogenic hilus
Lymph node capsule
Hilar vascularity
Nodal vasculature entering hilum

(Top) Grayscale ultrasound image shows the normal sonographic features of lymph nodes, which are typically oval in shape, with unsharp borders and a prominent echogenic hilus. Large round nodes with effacement of the echogenic hilus and sharpening of the borders, are findings typical of pathologic nodes. These findings however, should not be used individually as sole diagnostic criteria. Ancillary findings of soft tissue edema or matting of lymph nodes may also be seen with infection, malignancy or radiation changes. **(Middle)** Ultrasound image with power Doppler, demonstrates power Doppler signal at the lymph node hilum. Vascularity of the hilum is a normal sonographic finding. **(Bottom)** Ultrasound image with power Doppler, demonstrates linear power Doppler signal in the central hilum of the node, which represents the nodal artery and vein which enter at the hilum.

AXIAL CECT

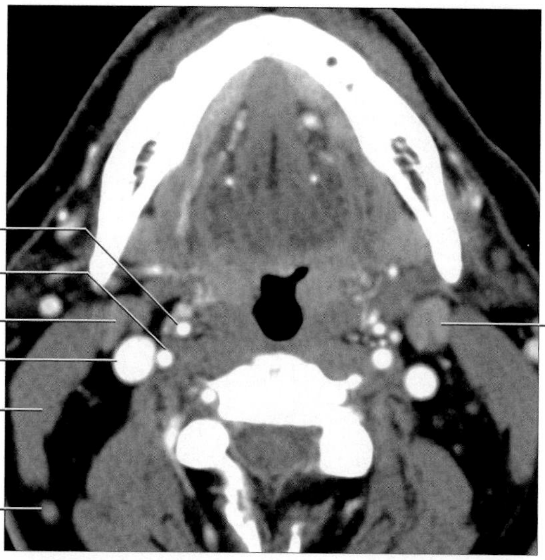

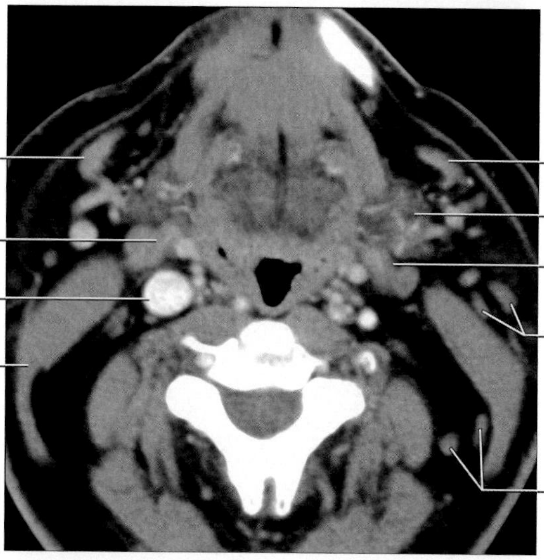

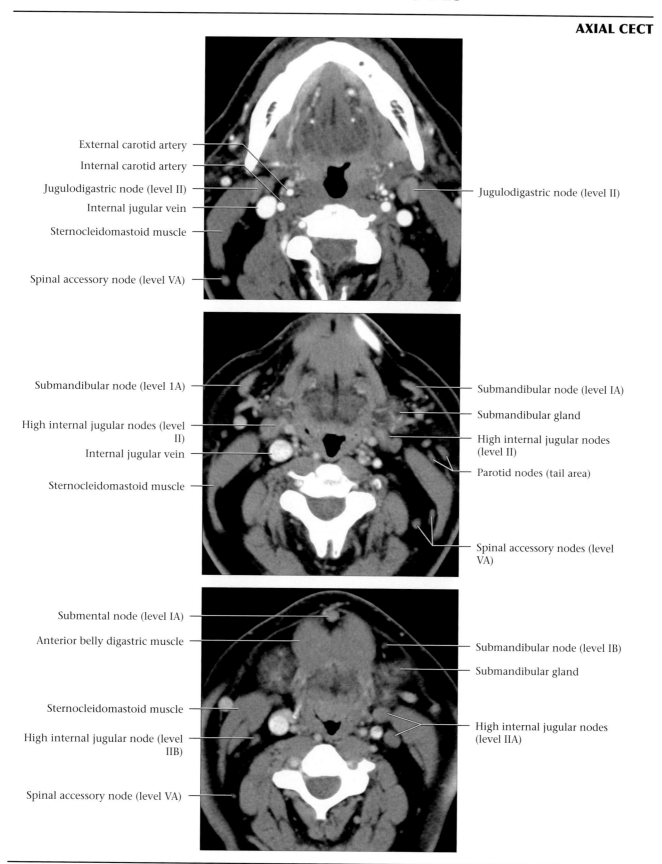

External carotid artery
Internal carotid artery
Jugulodigastric node (level II)
Internal jugular vein
Sternocleidomastoid muscle
Spinal accessory node (level VA)
Jugulodigastric node (level II)

Submandibular node (level 1A)
High internal jugular nodes (level II)
Internal jugular vein
Sternocleidomastoid muscle
Submandibular node (level IA)
Submandibular gland
High internal jugular nodes (level II)
Parotid nodes (tail area)
Spinal accessory nodes (level VA)

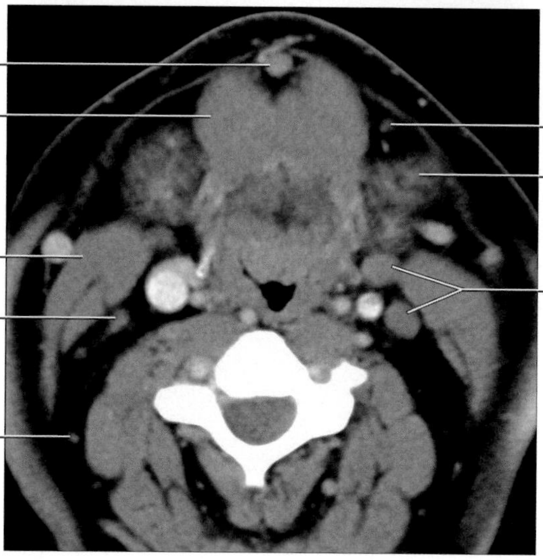

Submental node (level IA)
Anterior belly digastric muscle
Sternocleidomastoid muscle
High internal jugular node (level IIB)
Spinal accessory node (level VA)
Submandibular node (level IB)
Submandibular gland
High internal jugular nodes (level IIA)

(Top) First of three axial CECT images of the suprahyoid neck presented from superior to inferior demonstrates lymph nodes in the internal jugular (level II) and spinal accessory chains (level V). The jugulodigastric node is the highest or "sentinel" node of the internal jugular chain. **(Middle)** In this image the internal jugular & spinal accessory lymph nodes are seen along with submandibular nodes (level IA) anterolateral to the submandibular glands in submandibular space. Note the internal jugular nodes are closely applied to the carotid space while the spinal accessory nodes are in the posterior cervical space. **(Bottom)** In this image just above the hyoid bone a submental (level IA) node is seen between the anterior bellies of digastric muscles. Note also the submandibular (level IB), high internal jugular (level IIA & IIB) & spinal accessory (level VA) nodes.

AXIAL T1 & T2 MR

Submandibular node (level IB)
Submandibular gland
Lingual tonsil
High internal jugular node (level IIA)
High internal jugular node (level IIA)

Submandibular node (level IB)
Submandibular gland
Lingual tonsil
Internal jugular chain node
Internal jugular chain node
Oropharynx

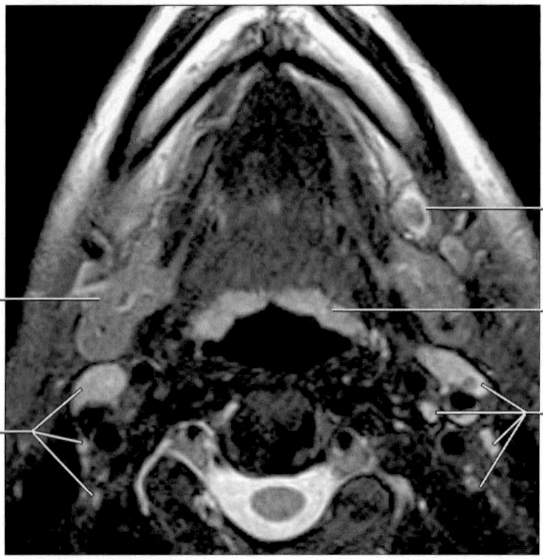

Submandibular node (level IB)
Submandibular gland
Lingual tonsil
High internal jugular nodes (level IIA)
High internal jugular nodes (level IIA)

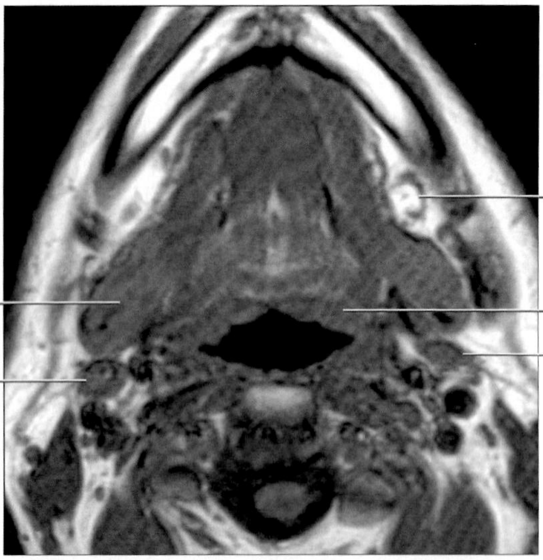

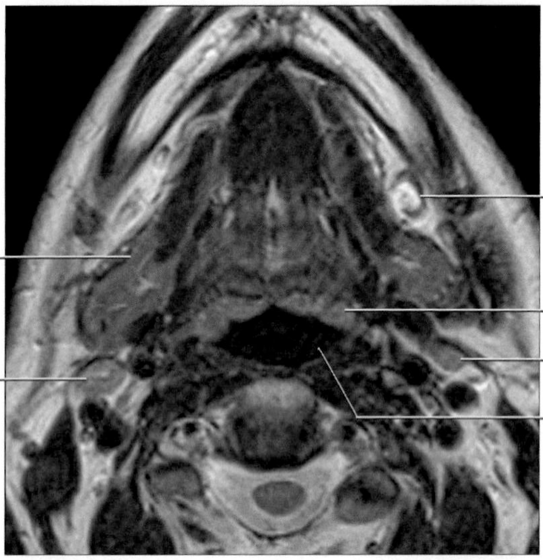

(Top) Axial T1 MR image through low oropharynx shows characteristic low T1 signal of lymph nodes. A prominent submandibular node with a fatty hilum is seen on the left. Level IIA internal jugular nodes are observed bilaterally. **(Middle)** Axial T2 MR image at level of low oropharynx bilateral high internal jugular nodes as intermediate signal intensity. **(Bottom)** Axial T2 MR image with fat saturation creates increased conspicuity of lymph nodes. The smaller high internal jugular nodes surrounding the carotid space are easily identified on this fat-saturated T2 image. STIR MR sequences create the same level of nodal conspicuity. Lingual tonsil tissue is also made more conspicuous with the fat-saturation T2 sequence.

RETROPHARYNGEAL NODES

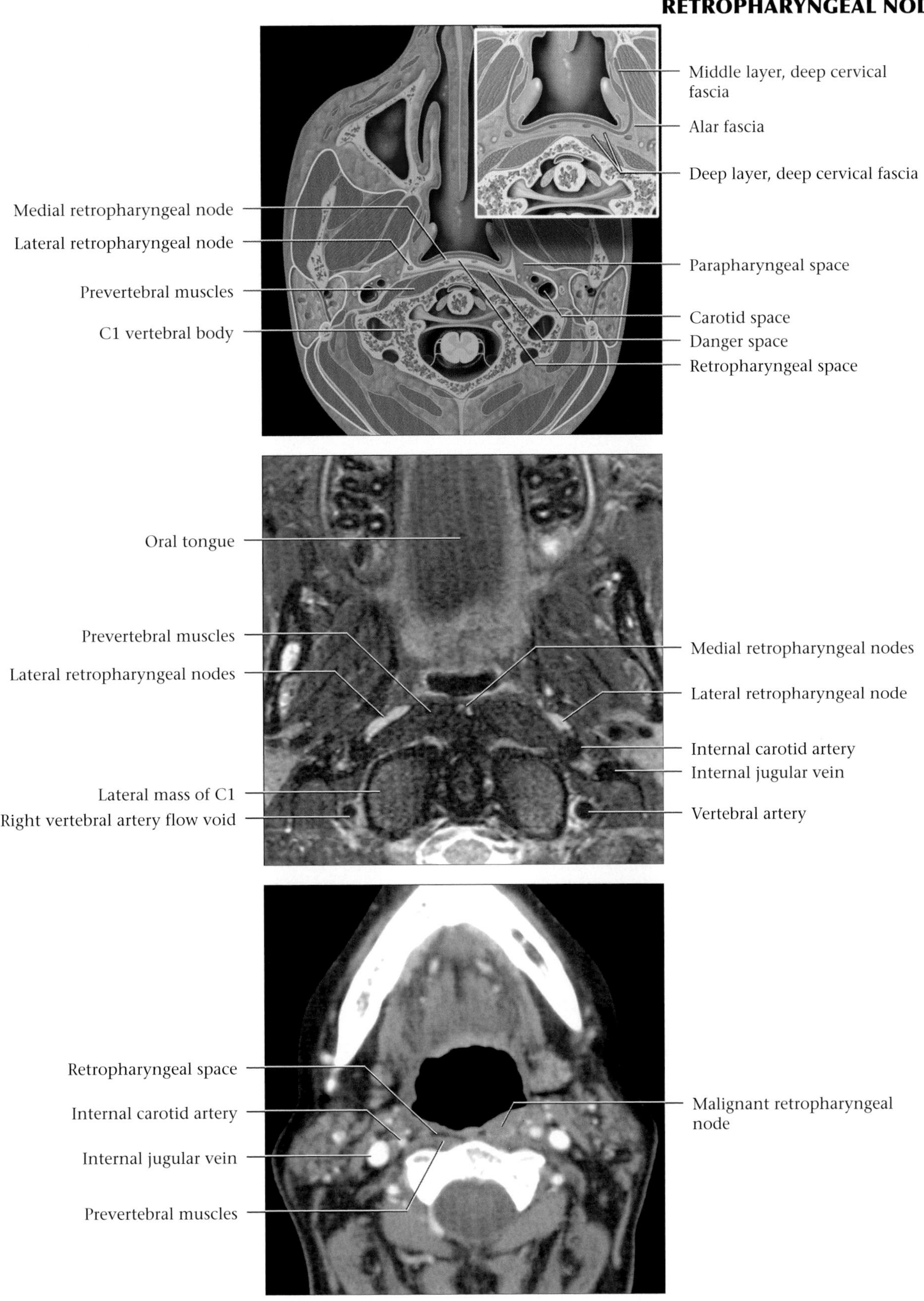
Middle layer, deep cervical fascia
Alar fascia
Deep layer, deep cervical fascia
Medial retropharyngeal node
Lateral retropharyngeal node
Prevertebral muscles
C1 vertebral body
Parapharyngeal space
Carotid space
Danger space
Retropharyngeal space
Oral tongue
Prevertebral muscles
Lateral retropharyngeal nodes
Lateral mass of C1
Right vertebral artery flow void
Medial retropharyngeal nodes
Lateral retropharyngeal node
Internal carotid artery
Internal jugular vein
Vertebral artery
Retropharyngeal space
Internal carotid artery
Internal jugular vein
Prevertebral muscles
Malignant retropharyngeal node

(Top) Axial graphic at the base of skull, demonstrates the typical location of medial and lateral retropharyngeal nodes. Medial retropharyngeal nodes are found in the paramedian retropharyngeal space of the suprahyoid neck. Lateral retropharyngeal nodes are lateral to the prevertebral muscles, and medial to the internal carotid artery. **(Middle)** Axial T2 MR image with fat-saturation shows the location of both medial & lateral retropharyngeal lymph nodes. Note the lateral group is located on the anterolateral surface of the prevertebral muscles, just medial to the carotid space. **(Bottom)** Axial CECT at the level of the low oropharynx reveals a small medial retropharyngeal node in a patient with a posterior wall hypopharynx squamous cell carcinoma (not shown). Central low density allows diagnosis of malignant node despite small size.

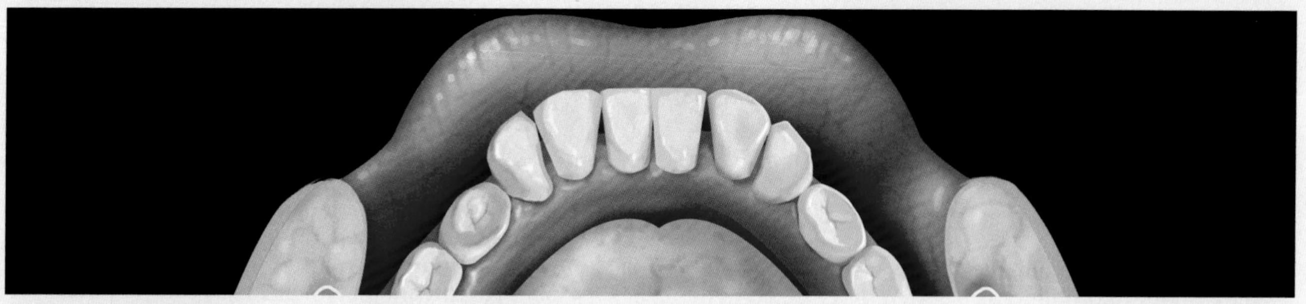

SECTION 4: Oral Cavity

ORAL CAVITY OVERVIEW

Terminology

Abbreviations

- Oral cavity (OC)

Definitions

- OC: Area of suprahyoid neck below sinonasal region and anterior to oropharynx

Imaging Anatomy

Overview

- OC is separated from oropharynx by soft palate, anterior tonsillar pillars and circumvallate papillae
- Suggested approach to OC imaging anatomy is to consider 4 distinct regions
  - **Oral mucosal space/surface (OMS)**
  - **Sublingual space (SLS)**: Non-fascial lined area superomedial to mylohyoid muscle
  - **Submandibular space (SMS)**: SMS is located inferolateral to mylohyoid muscle
  - **Root of tongue (ROT)**: Made up of genioglossus-geniohyoid complex & lingual septum

Anatomy Relationships

- Oral cavity regional relationships
  - Superior: Hard palate, maxillary alveolar ridge
  - Lateral: Cheek-buccal space
  - Inferior: Mylohyoid muscle (floor of mouth), mandibular alveolar ridge and teeth
  - Posterior: Soft palate, anterior tonsillar pillars & lingual tonsil (tongue base)
- Sublingual space relationships
  - SLS in oral tongue between mylohyoid muscle inferolaterally and genioglossus medially
  - Both SLS communicate anteriorly beneath frenulum
    - Form "**horizontal horseshoe**" in deep oral tongue
  - Posteriorly SLS empties into posterosuperior aspect of SMS and inferior parapharyngeal space (PPS)
  - No fascia separates posterior SLS from SMS and inferior PPS
    - Direct communication allows spread of disease among these 3 spaces
- Submandibular space relationships
  - SMS is a "**vertical horseshoe**" space between hyoid bone below and mylohyoid muscle sling above
  - SMS communicates posteriorly with inferior PPS and posterior SLS
  - SMS continues inferiorly as anterior cervical space
- Root of tongue relationships
  - Inferiorly ROT ends at mylohyoid sling
  - Anteriorly ends at mandibular symphysis

Internal Structures-Critical Contents

- **Oral tongue**
  - Oral tongue: Anterior 2/3 of tongue
    - Base of tongue: Posterior 1/3 of tongue (lingual tonsil of oropharynx)
  - Root of tongue: Deep muscles of oral tongue (genioglossus and geniohyoid) + lingual septum
  - **Extrinsic tongue muscles**
    - **Genioglossus**: Large, fan-shaped muscle arising anteriorly from superior mental spine on inner surface of symphysis menti of mandible; inserts along entire length of under surface of tongue
    - **Hyoglossus**: Thin & quadrilateral shaped arising from body & greater cornu of hyoid bone; passes vertically upward to insert into side of tongue
    - Styloglossus and palatoglossus
- **Mylohyoid muscle**
  - Forms **floor of mouth**
  - Separates lower OC into SMS and SLS except along posterior margin
  - Arises from **mylohyoid line** of mandible
  - **Mylohyoid cleft** at junction of anterior 1/3 and posterior 2/3 of mylohyoid muscle
    - May be prominent with fat ± vessels ± accessory salivary tissue
- **Oral mucosal space/surface**
  - Lines entire OC including buccal (cheeks), gingival (gums), palatal and lingual surfaces
  - Subepithelial collections of **minor salivary glands** found all over OC
    - Most common locations are inner surface of lip, buccal mucosa and palate
  - **Retromolar trigone**: Small triangular shaped region of mucosa behind last molar on mandibular ramus
    - Anatomical crossroads of OC, oropharynx, soft palate, buccal space, floor of mouth, masticator space and PPS
- **Sublingual space**
  - Lingual nerve: V3 sensory combined with CN7 chorda tympani nerve (anterior 2/3 of tongue taste)
  - Distal CN9 and CN12 (motor to tongue)
  - Lingual artery and vein
  - Sublingual glands and ducts
  - Hyoglossus muscle anterior margin projects into posterior SLS
  - Deep portion of submandibular gland and submandibular gland duct
- **Submandibular space**
  - Large superficial portion of submandibular gland
  - Submental (level IA) and submandibular (level IB) lymph node groups
  - Facial vein and artery
  - Inferior loop of CN12
  - Anterior belly of digastric muscles
- **Pterygomandibular raphe**
  - Fibrous band extending from posterior mandibular mylohyoid line to medial pterygoid plate hamulus
  - Buccinator and superior pharyngeal constrictor meet at pterygomandibular raphe
  - Lies beneath mucosa of retromolar trigone
  - Perifascial route of spread for SCCa

Fascia

- SLS is **not** lined by fascia
- SMS is lined by superficial layer of deep cervical fascia
  - Deeper slip of fascia runs along external surface of mylohyoid muscle and more shallow slip parallels deep margin of platysma
  - No fascia separates posterior SMS and SLS from inferior parapharyngeal space

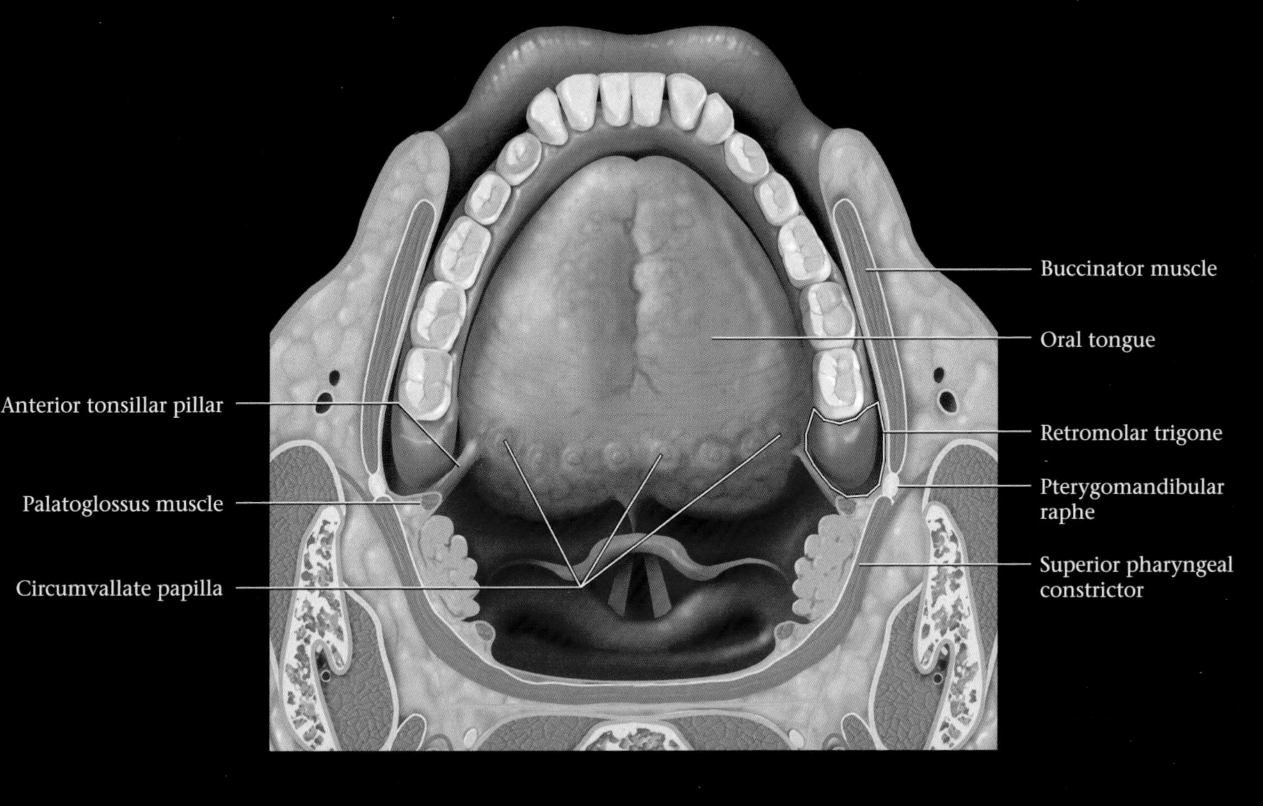
Buccinator muscle
Oral tongue
Anterior tonsillar pillar
Retromolar trigone
Palatoglossus muscle
Pterygomandibular raphe
Circumvallate papilla
Superior pharyngeal constrictor

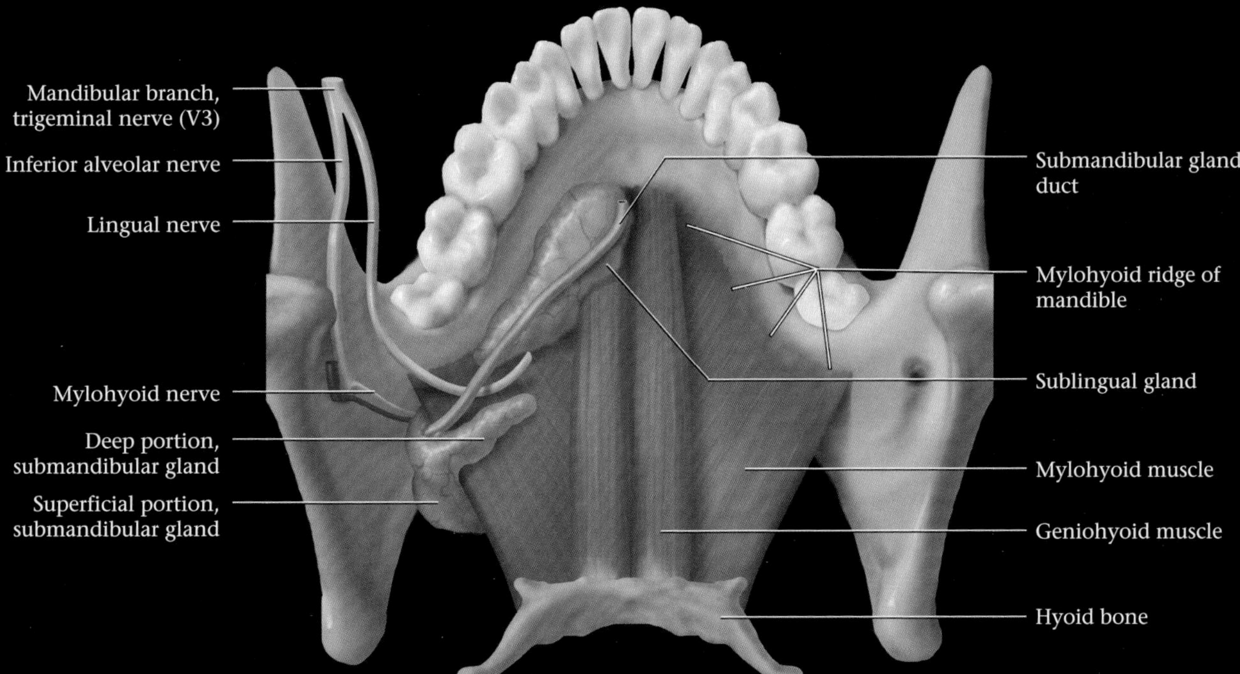
Mandibular branch, trigeminal nerve (V3)
Inferior alveolar nerve
Lingual nerve
Submandibular gland duct
Mylohyoid ridge of mandible
Sublingual gland
Mylohyoid nerve
Deep portion, submandibular gland
Superficial portion, submandibular gland
Mylohyoid muscle
Geniohyoid muscle
Hyoid bone

(Top) View from above of oral mucosal space/surface shaded in blue. Notice the circumvallate papilla, a superficial line of taste buds, divides anterior oral cavity from posterior oropharynx. The lingual tonsil is part of oropharynx, not the oral cavity. The pterygomandibular raphe connects the posterior margin of buccinator muscle to anterior margin of the superior pharyngeal constrictor muscle. It also represents a key route of perifascial spread of squamous cell carcinoma of the retromolar trigone. **(Bottom)** Drawing of floor of mouth from above. The mylohyoid muscle sling is the principal structure of the floor of the mouth. This muscle attaches to the hyoid bone inferiorly & the mylohyoid ridge of the medial mandibular cortex. Superomedial to the mylohyoid muscle is the sublingual space while the submandibular space is inferolateral to this muscle.

ORAL CAVITY OVERVIEW

GRAPHICS

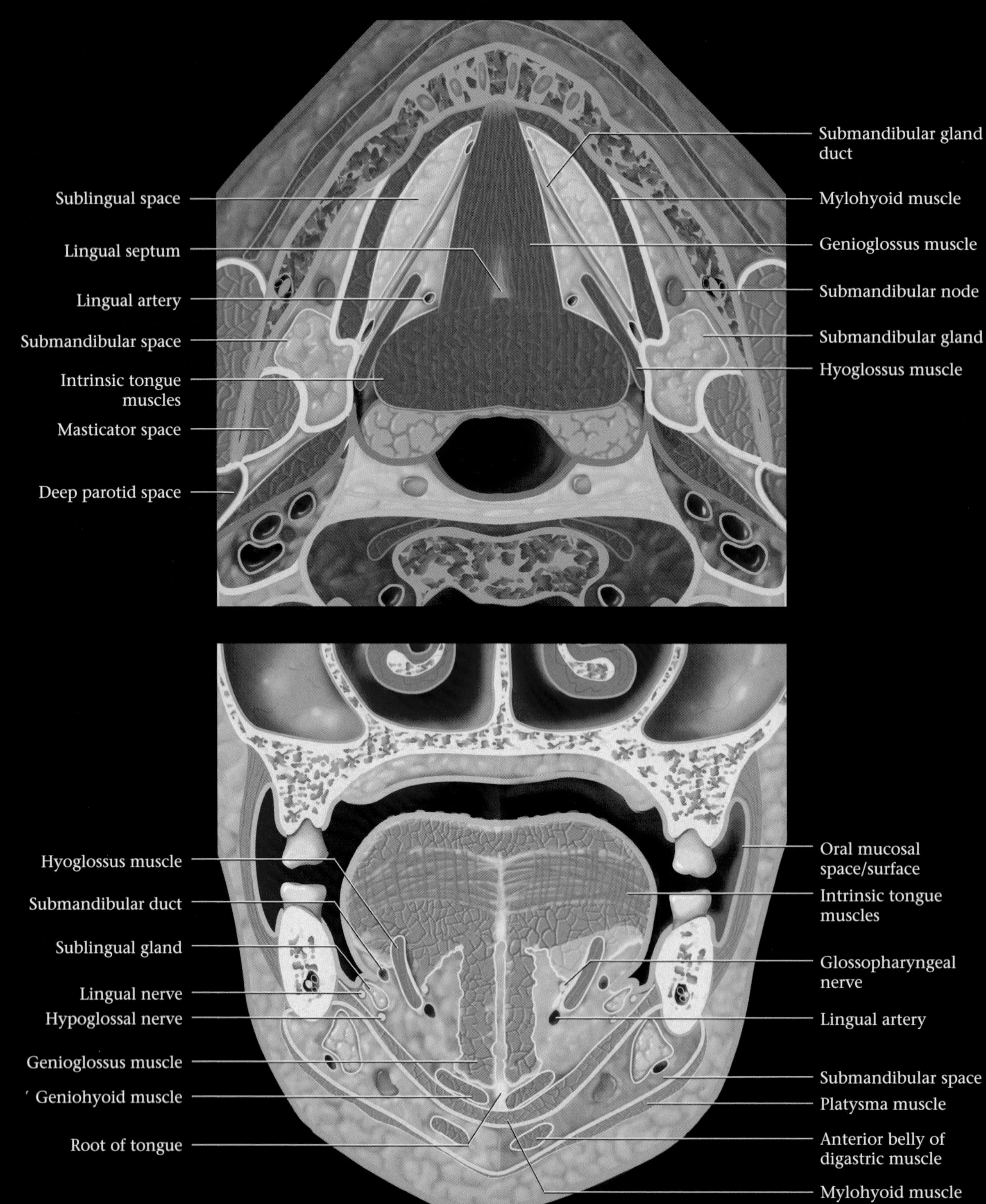
Submandibular gland duct
Sublingual space
Mylohyoid muscle
Lingual septum
Genioglossus muscle
Lingual artery
Submandibular node
Submandibular space
Submandibular gland
Intrinsic tongue muscles
Hyoglossus muscle
Masticator space
Deep parotid space
Hyoglossus muscle
Oral mucosal space/surface
Submandibular duct
Intrinsic tongue muscles
Sublingual gland
Glossopharyngeal nerve
Lingual nerve
Hypoglossal nerve
Lingual artery
Genioglossus muscle
Submandibular space
Geniohyoid muscle
Platysma muscle
Root of tongue
Anterior belly of digastric muscle
Mylohyoid muscle

(Top) Axial graphic through oral cavity shows superficial layer of deep cervical fascia (yellow line) circumscribing masticator and parotid spaces posteriorly and defining deep margin of SMS anteriorly colored in blue. Notice principal occupants of SMS are submandibular gland and nodes. Green sublingual space has many structures within it including the sublingual gland, submandibular duct, anterior margin of hyoglossus to name a few. **(Bottom)** In this coronal graphic through oral cavity the mylohyoid muscle is seen stretched from side to side from the mylohyoid ridges. This muscle separates sublingual space (green) from submandibular space (blue). Sublingual space contains the lingual nerve and artery, submandibular duct, CN9 and CN12 and sublingual gland. Genioglossus and geniohyoid complex with lower lingual septum forms the root of the tongue.

AXIAL CECT

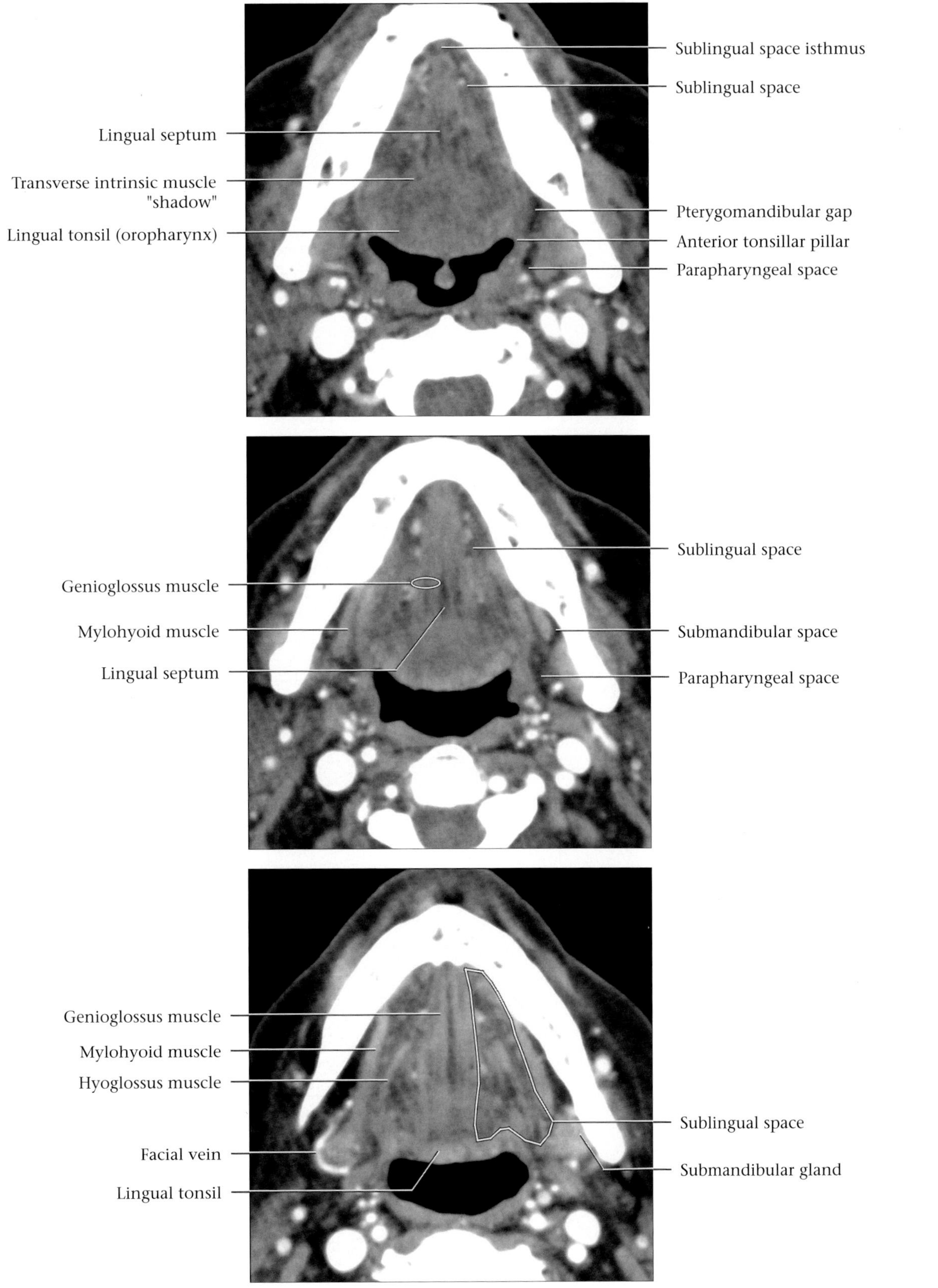
Sublingual space isthmus
Sublingual space
Lingual septum
Transverse intrinsic muscle "shadow"
Lingual tonsil (oropharynx)
Pterygomandibular gap
Anterior tonsillar pillar
Parapharyngeal space
Sublingual space
Genioglossus muscle
Mylohyoid muscle
Lingual septum
Submandibular space
Parapharyngeal space
Genioglossus muscle
Mylohyoid muscle
Hyoglossus muscle
Facial vein
Lingual tonsil
Sublingual space
Submandibular gland

(Top) First of six axial CECT images of oral cavity are presented from superior to inferior. On the most cephalad image the parapharyngeal space can be seen emptying anteriorly into the submandibular space via the pterygomandibular gap. **(Middle)** The large paired genioglossus muscles are seen on either side of the lingual septum. The cephalad submandibular space fat is just coming into view. **(Bottom)** The sublingual space is lateral to the genioglossus muscle, superomedial to the mylohyoid muscle and anterior to the lingual tonsil. On the patient's right the facial vein curves around the lateral margin of the submandibular gland.

ORAL CAVITY OVERVIEW

AXIAL CECT

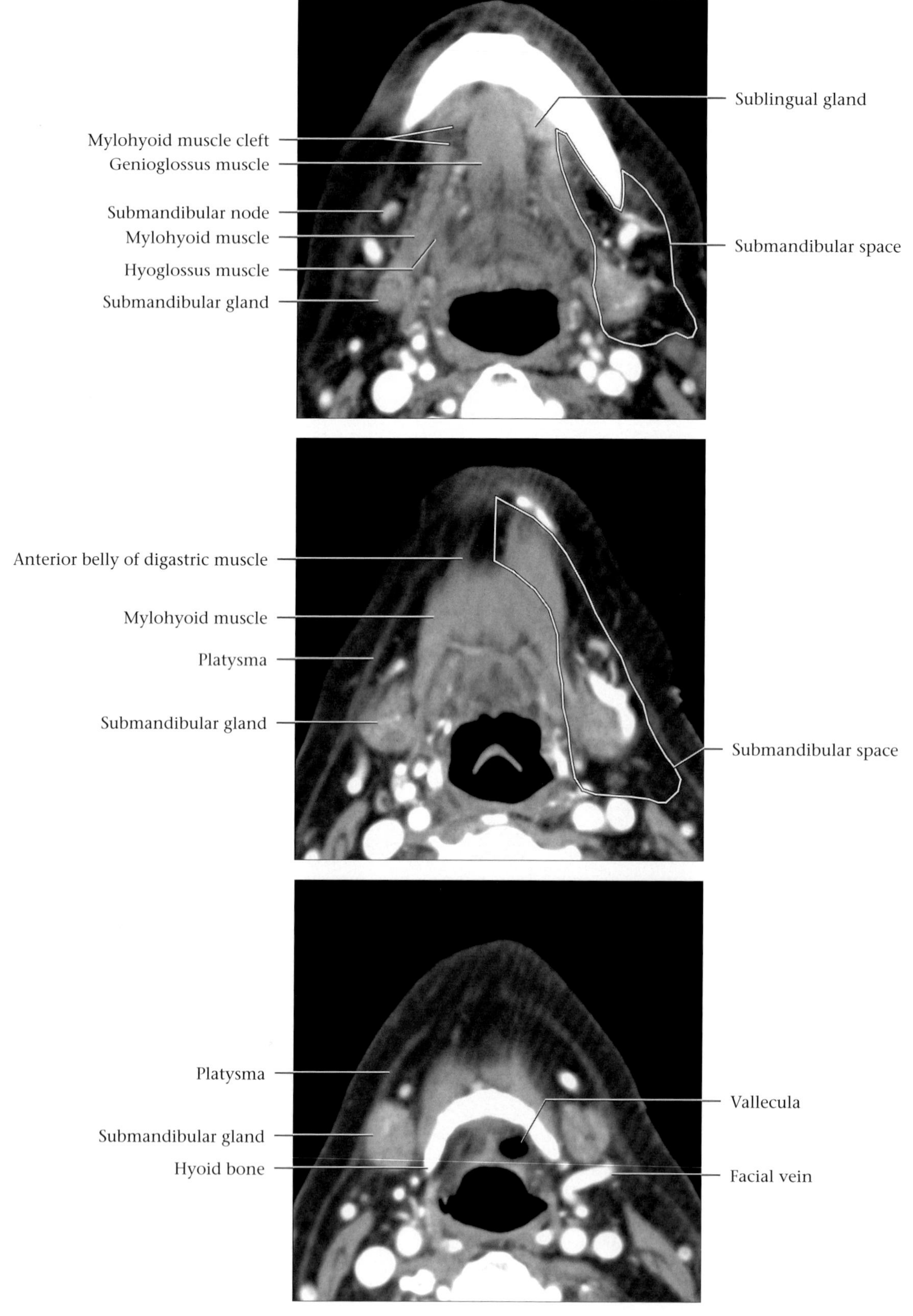
Mylohyoid muscle cleft
Genioglossus muscle
Submandibular node
Mylohyoid muscle
Hyoglossus muscle
Submandibular gland
Sublingual gland
Submandibular space
Anterior belly of digastric muscle
Mylohyoid muscle
Platysma
Submandibular gland
Submandibular space
Platysma
Submandibular gland
Hyoid bone
Vallecula
Facial vein

(Top) The complex shape of the submandibular space is outlined on the patient's left. Notice the mylohyoid muscle gap anteriorly on the right. This is a normal variant and can be large and fat-filled as in this image. **(Middle)** The left half of the more inferior submandibular space is outlined. The submandibular gland and anterior belly of the digastric muscles are seen as normal occupants of the this space. Remember there is no vertical fascia dividing the two sides of the submandibular space. **(Bottom)** The platysma muscle represents the superficial border of the submandibular space. The anterior cervical space connects to the submandibular space in the infrahyoid neck.

AXIAL T2 MR

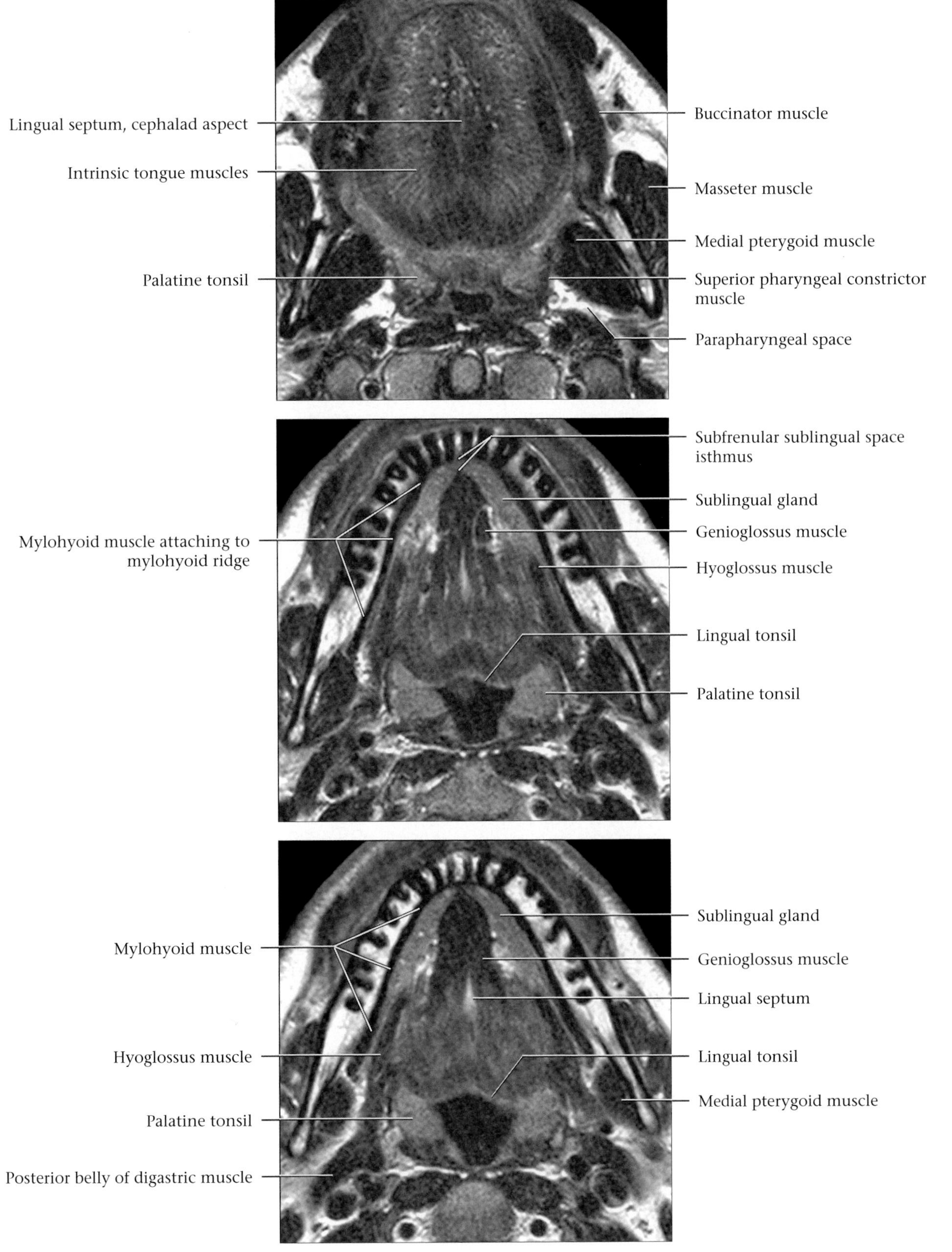
Lingual septum, cephalad aspect
Intrinsic tongue muscles
Palatine tonsil
Buccinator muscle
Masseter muscle
Medial pterygoid muscle
Superior pharyngeal constrictor muscle
Parapharyngeal space
Mylohyoid muscle attaching to mylohyoid ridge
Subfrenular sublingual space isthmus
Sublingual gland
Genioglossus muscle
Hyoglossus muscle
Lingual tonsil
Palatine tonsil
Mylohyoid muscle
Hyoglossus muscle
Palatine tonsil
Posterior belly of digastric muscle
Sublingual gland
Genioglossus muscle
Lingual septum
Lingual tonsil
Medial pterygoid muscle

(Top) First of six axial T2 MR images through the oral cavity presented from superior to inferior. This first image reveals the cephalad surface of the oral tongue. **(Middle)** In this image the mylohyoid muscle can be seen attaching to the mylohyoid ridge bilaterally. The sublingual space communicates anteriorly in the subfrenular isthmus. **(Bottom)** In this image the hyoglossus muscle is seen projecting into the posterior aspect of the sublingual space.

ORAL CAVITY OVERVIEW

AXIAL T2 MR

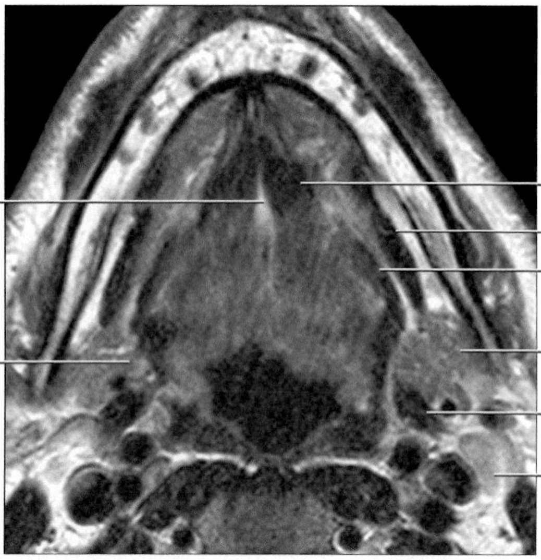

Lingual septum
Genioglossus muscle
Mylohyoid muscle
Hyoglossus muscle
Deep portion of submandibular gland in posterior sublingual space
Superficial portion of submandibular gland
Posterior belly of digastric muscle
Jugulodigastric node

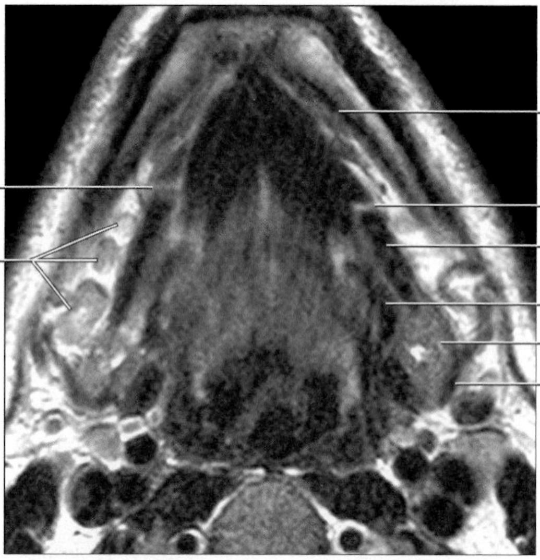

Inner cortical table of mandible
Mylohyoid cleft
Mylohyoid cleft
Submandibular nodes
Mylohyoid muscle
Hyoglossus muscle
Submandibular gland
Facial vein

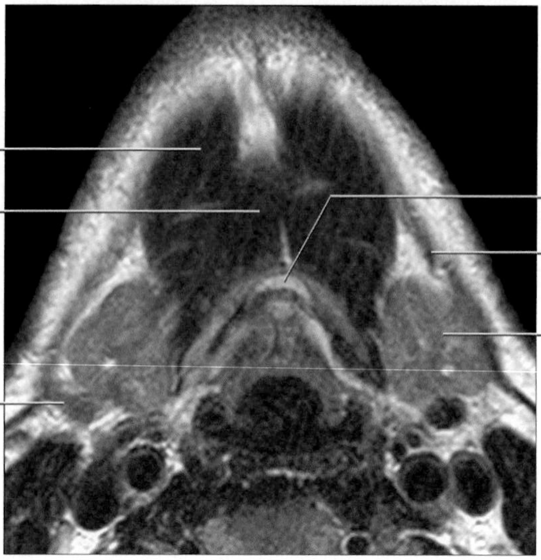

Anterior belly of digastric muscle
Mylohyoid muscle
Hyoid bone
Platysma muscle
Submandibular gland
Submandibular node

(Top) In lower oral cavity the submandibular gland becomes visible. Notice the deep portion "plugs" the back of the sublingual space (visible on left). The larger superficial submandibular gland is in the submandibular space proper. **(Middle)** At the level of the inferior body of mandible the fatty gap in the mylohyoid muscle is visible. Also notice the multiple reactive submandibular nodes on the left. **(Bottom)** At the level of the hyoid bone the bulk of the anterior bellies of the digastric muscles are visible. The platysma is seen as the superficial margin of the submandibular space.

CORONAL T1 MR

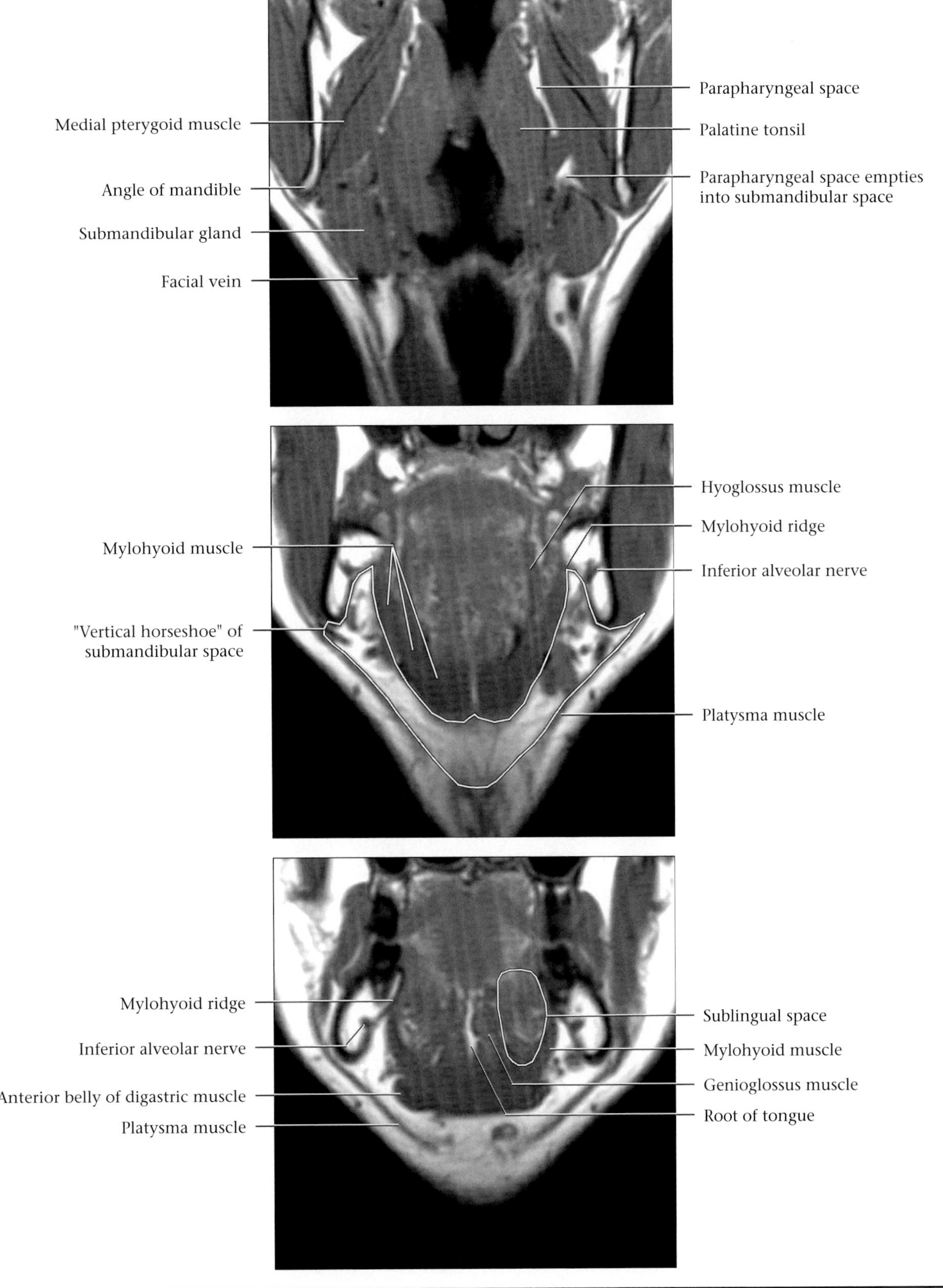
Medial pterygoid muscle
Angle of mandible
Submandibular gland
Facial vein
Parapharyngeal space
Palatine tonsil
Parapharyngeal space empties into submandibular space
Mylohyoid muscle
"Vertical horseshoe" of submandibular space
Hyoglossus muscle
Mylohyoid ridge
Inferior alveolar nerve
Platysma muscle
Mylohyoid ridge
Inferior alveolar nerve
Anterior belly of digastric muscle
Platysma muscle
Sublingual space
Mylohyoid muscle
Genioglossus muscle
Root of tongue

(Top) First of three coronal T1 MR images through oral cavity presented from posterior to anterior. In this most posterior image the parapharyngeal space can be seen "emptying" inferiorly into the posterior submandibular space on the right. **(Middle)** This more anterior view delineates the "vertical horseshoe" of the submandibular space bounded superficially by the platysma and superomedially by the mylohyoid muscle. **(Bottom)** The sublingual space becomes more obvious in the anterior oral cavity. Notice it is a potential space drawn in on the right lateral to the genioglossus muscle and superomedial to the mylohyoid muscle.

ORAL MUCOSAL SPACE

Terminology

Abbreviations

- Oral mucosal space/surface (OMS)
- Oral cavity (OC)

Definitions

- OMS: Mucosal surface of oral cavity extending from skin-vermilion junction of lips to junction of hard and soft palate above and to line of circumvallate papillae below

Imaging Anatomy

Overview

- OMS is constructed to complete radiologist's thinking regarding OC locations where specific lesions primarily occur
- Since OMS describes mucosal surface of entire oral cavity, it represents continuous sheet of mucosa where squamous cell carcinoma (SCCa) may originate

Extent

- Anterior extent of OMS: Skin-vermilion junction of upper and lower lips
- Posterior extent of OMS
  - Posterosuperior extent: Junction of hard and soft palate
  - Posteroinferior extent: Junction of anterior 2/3 of tongue and posterior 1/3 of tongue at circumvallate papillae
    - Anterior 2/3 of tongue is **oral tongue**
    - Posterior 1/3 of tongue is **lingual tonsil**; part of **oropharynx**

Anatomy Relationships

- OMS represents continuous mucosal surface of OC which sits anterior to mucosal surface of oropharynx
- Superior OMS overlies hard palate
  - Floor of nose and maxillary sinuses (palatine process of maxillary palatine bones) lie deep to this mucosa
- Inferior OMS overlies sublingual spaces and mylohyoid muscles

Internal Structures-Critical Contents

- Oral mucosal space/surface is divided into eight specific areas
  - **Mucosal lip**
    - Lip begins at vermilion border junction with skin
    - Includes only vermilion surface or portion of lip that makes contact with opposing lip
  - **Upper alveolar ridge mucosal surface**
    - Refers to mucosa overlying alveolar process of maxilla
    - Extends from line of attachment of mucosa in upper gingival buccal gutter to junction of hard palate
    - Posterior margin is upper end of pterygopalatine arch
  - **Lower alveolar ridge mucosal surface**
    - Refers to mucosa overlying alveolar process of mandible
    - Extends from line of attachment of mucosa in buccal gutter to line of free mucosa of floor of mouth
    - Posteriorly extends to ascending ramus of mandible
  - **Retromolar trigone** mucosal surface
    - Attached mucosa overlying ascending ramus of mandible
    - Extends from level of posterior surface of last molar tooth to apex superiorly, adjacent to tuberosity of maxilla
  - **Buccal mucosa**
    - Includes all membranes that line inner surface of cheeks and lips
    - Extends from line of contact of opposing lips to line of attachment of mucosa of alveolar ridge (upper and lower) and pterygomandibular raphe
  - **Floor of mouth, mucosal surface**
    - Semilunar mucosal surface overlying mylohyoid and hyoglossus muscles
    - Extends from inner surface of lower alveolar ridge to undersurface of tongue
    - Posterior boundary is base of anterior pillar of tonsil
    - Divided into two sides by tongue **frenulum**
    - Contains ostia of submandibular and sublingual salivary glands
  - **Hard palate mucosal surface**
    - Semilunar mucosal area between upper alveolar ridge and mucous membrane covering palatine process of maxillary palatine bones
    - Extends from inner surface of superior alveolar ridge to posterior edge of palatine bone
  - **Anterior 2/3 of tongue (oral tongue) mucosal surface**
    - Mucosal surface overlying oral tongue
    - Extends anteriorly from line of circumvallate papillae (anterior edge of lingual tonsil) to undersurface of tongue at junction of mucosal surface of floor of mouth
    - Composed of 4 areas including tongue tip, lateral borders, dorsum and undersurface (nonvillous oral tongue ventral surface)
- Contents of OMS
  - Mucosal surface of OC
  - **Minor salivary glands** (MSG)
    - Lie within submucosa of OC, paranasal sinuses, pharynx, larynx, trachea, and bronchi
    - Particularly concentrated in buccal, palatal and lingual submucosal regions
    - Mucinous or seromucinous in nature

Fascia

- **No** fascia exists to define OMS

Clinical Implications

Clinical Importance

- Primary malignancies arising from OMS include SCCa and MSG malignancy
- Vast majority of malignancies of OMS are SCCa while MSG malignancy is relatively rare

ORAL MUCOSAL SPACE

GRAPHICS

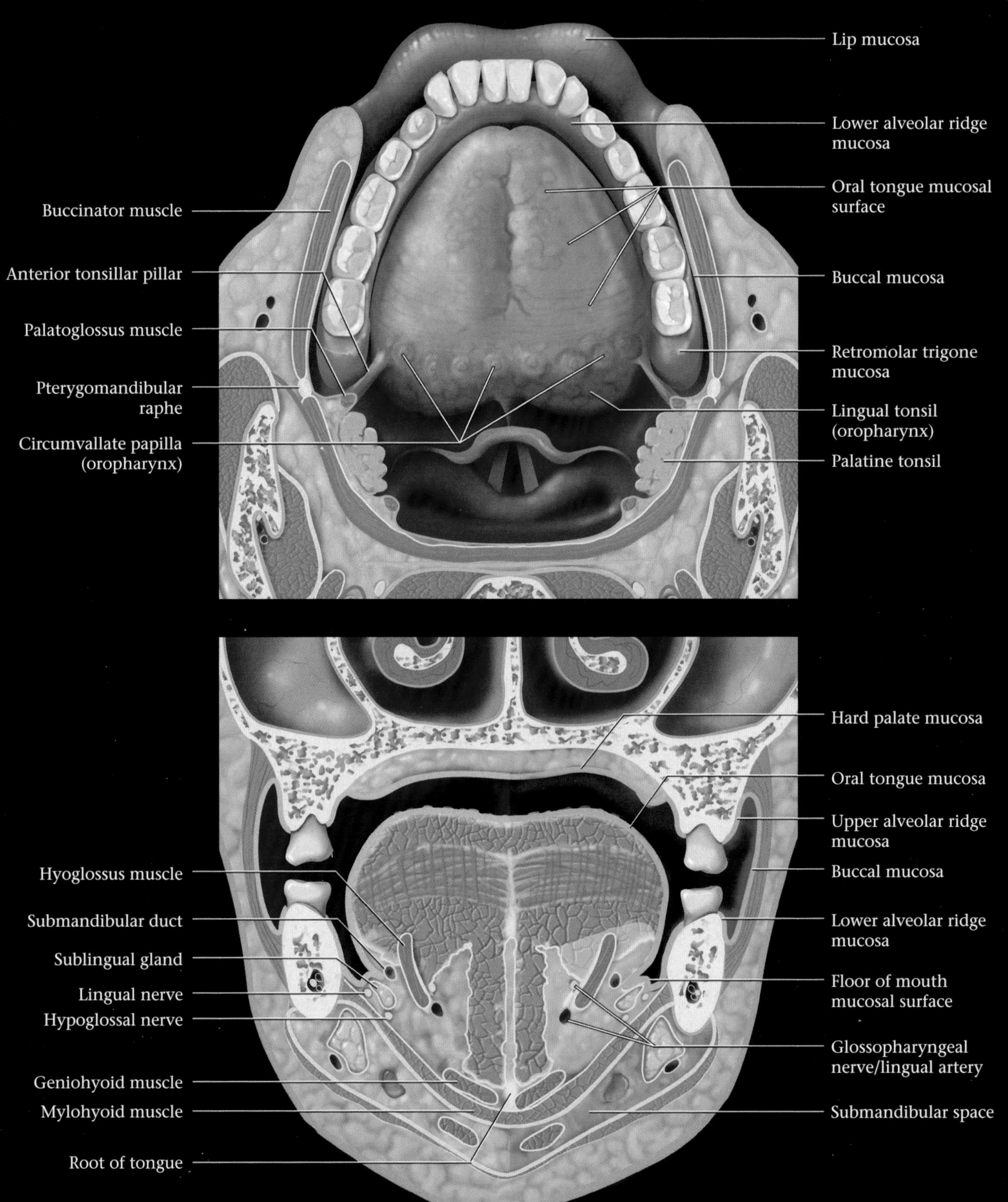
Lip mucosa
Lower alveolar ridge mucosa
Oral tongue mucosal surface
Buccinator muscle
Anterior tonsillar pillar
Buccal mucosa
Palatoglossus muscle
Retromolar trigone mucosa
Pterygomandibular raphe
Lingual tonsil (oropharynx)
Circumvallate papilla (oropharynx)
Palatine tonsil
Hard palate mucosa
Oral tongue mucosa
Upper alveolar ridge mucosa
Hyoglossus muscle
Buccal mucosa
Submandibular duct
Lower alveolar ridge mucosa
Sublingual gland
Floor of mouth mucosal surface
Lingual nerve
Hypoglossal nerve
Glossopharyngeal nerve/lingual artery
Geniohyoid muscle
Mylohyoid muscle
Submandibular space
Root of tongue

(Top) Axial graphic through the oral cavity and oropharynx. The area in blue delineates the oral mucosal space/surface. Notice the posterior oropharynx contains the lingual and palatine tonsils. The circumvallate papilla are a superficial line of taste buds that separate the anterior oral cavity from the posterior oropharynx. **(Bottom)** In this coronal graphic through the oral cavity the oral mucosal space/surface is again highlighted in blue. In this image the hard palate, oral tongue, upper and lower alveolar ridge, buccal and floor of mouth mucosal surfaces are seen. Also notice the four main areas of the oral cavity are all present: 1. Oral mucosal space/surface (blue), 2. Sublingual space (green), 3. Submandibular space (light blue) and 4. Root of tongue.

SUBLINGUAL SPACE

Terminology

Abbreviations

- Sublingual space (SLS)
- Submandibular space (SMS)
- Oral mucosal space/surface (OMS)

Definitions

- SLS: Paired non-fascial lined spaces of oral cavity in deep oral tongue above floor of mouth superomedial to mylohyoid muscle

Imaging Anatomy

Overview

- SLS contains key neurovascular structures of oral cavity
  - Includes glossopharyngeal nerve (CN9), hypoglossal nerve (CN12), lingual nerve (branch of V3), lingual artery and vein
- When a lesion involves both SLSs across anterior isthmus, it appears as a "**horizontal horseshoe**" parallel to line of inferior mandibular surface

Anatomy Relationships

- Sublingual space relationships
  - SLS in deep oral tongue **superomedial to mylohyoid muscle** and lateral to genioglossus-geniohyoid muscles
  - Communication between sublingual spaces occurs in midline anteriorly as a narrow **isthmus** beneath frenulum
  - SLS communicates with SMS and inferior parapharyngeal space (PPS) at posterior margin of mylohyoid muscle
    - There is **no fascia** dividing posterior SLS from adjacent SMS
    - Therefore there is direct communication with SMS and PPS in this location

Internal Structures-Critical Contents

- Posterior aspect of SLS is divided into medial and lateral compartments by hypoglossal muscle
- Lateral compartment contents
  - **Hypoglossal nerve**: Motor to intrinsic and extrinsic muscles of tongue
    - Intrinsic muscles of tongue include inferior lingual, vertical and transverse muscles
    - Extrinsic muscles of tongue include genioglossus, hyoglossus, styloglossus & palatoglossus muscles
  - **Lingual nerve**: Branch of mandibular division of trigeminal nerve (CNV3) combined with chorda tympani branch of facial nerve
    - Lingual nerve branch of CNV3: Sensation to anterior 2/3 of oral tongue
    - Chorda tympani branch of facial nerve: Anterior 2/3 of tongue taste and parasympathetic secreto-motor fibers to submandibular ganglion/gland
  - **Sublingual glands and ducts**
    - Lie in anterior SLS bilaterally
    - About 5 small ducts open under oral tongue into oral cavity
    - With age sublingual glands atrophy, becoming difficult to see on imaging
  - **Submandibular gland deep portion and submandibular duct**
    - Submandibular gland deep margin extends into posterior opening of SLS
    - Enlarging lesions of SLS in effect push this deep margin of submandibular gland out of the way as they emerge from SLS into SMS
    - Submandibular duct runs anteriorly to papillae in anteromedial subfrenular mucosa
- Medial compartment contents
  - **Glossopharyngeal nerve** (CN9)
    - Provides sensation to posterior 1/3 of tongue
    - Carries taste input from posterior 1/3 of tongue
    - Located more cephalad in medial compartment compared to lingual artery and vein
  - **Lingual artery and vein**
    - Vascular supply to oral tongue
    - Seen running just lateral to genioglossus muscle

Fascia

- SLS is **not fascia-lined** space but instead is **potential space** only

Anatomy-Based Imaging Issues

Key Concepts or Questions

- What defines a mass as primary to SLS?
  - Center of lesion is superomedial to mylohyoid muscle and lateral to genioglossus muscle
- Besides spilling out back of SLS into posterior SMS, how can a lesion of SLS access SMS?
  - **Mylohyoid** muscle has a variably sized **cleft** between its anterior 1/3 and posterior 2/3 area
  - Lesions may "escape" SLS into SMS through this cleft
  - When this occurs, lesion is found in anterior SMS **in front of** submandibular gland

Imaging Recommendations

- CECT or T1 C+ MR with fat-saturation are both excellent imaging tools to evaluate SLS lesions
- MR better in cooperative patient
  - MR less affected by dental amalgam artifact compared to CT
  - MR permits direct coronal imaging to assess relationship of lesion to mylohyoid muscle

Imaging Pitfalls

- Extension of oral cavity squamous cell carcinoma (SCCa) into floor of mouth or root of tongue can be obscured by dental amalgam on CECT

Clinical Implications

Clinical Importance

- Since neurovascular bundle to tongue travels in SLS, oral cavity SCCa involving posterior SLS is challenging to treat
- If SCCa crosses lingual septum to contralateral SLS, lesion becomes unresectable for cure

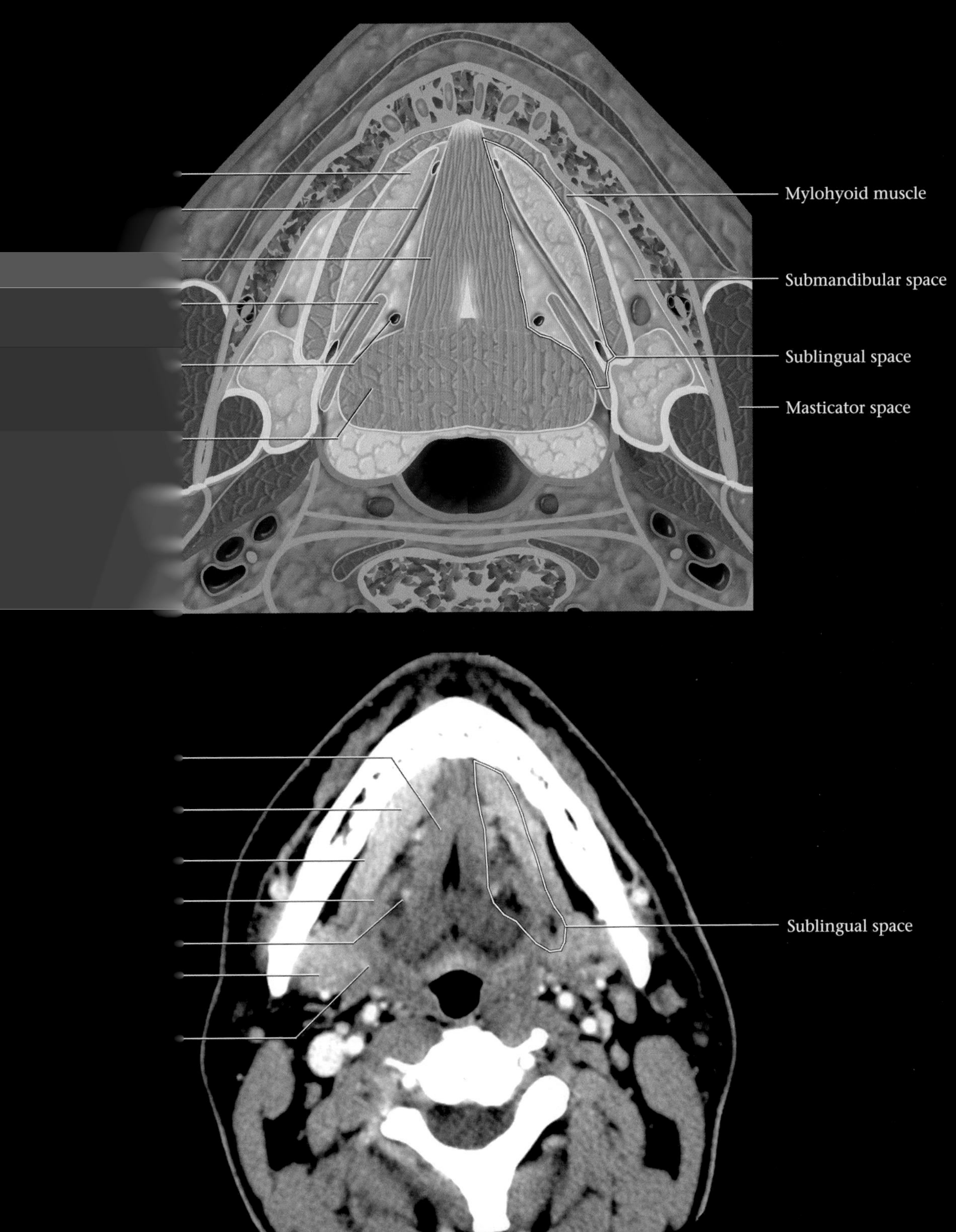
Mylohyoid muscle
Submandibular space
Sublingual space
Masticator space
Sublingual space

gh the body of the mandible shows the sublingual space (on patient's left shaded in green) the mylohyoid muscle and lateral to the genioglossus muscle. Notice the absence of fascia al space. The yellow line represents the superficial layer of deep cervical fascia. **(Bottom)** blingual space outlined on the patient's left. Notice the difficulty on enhanced CT in muscle from the sublingual gland. The deep portion of the submandibular gland projects

SUBLINGUAL SPACE

GRAPHIC & CORONAL T1 MR

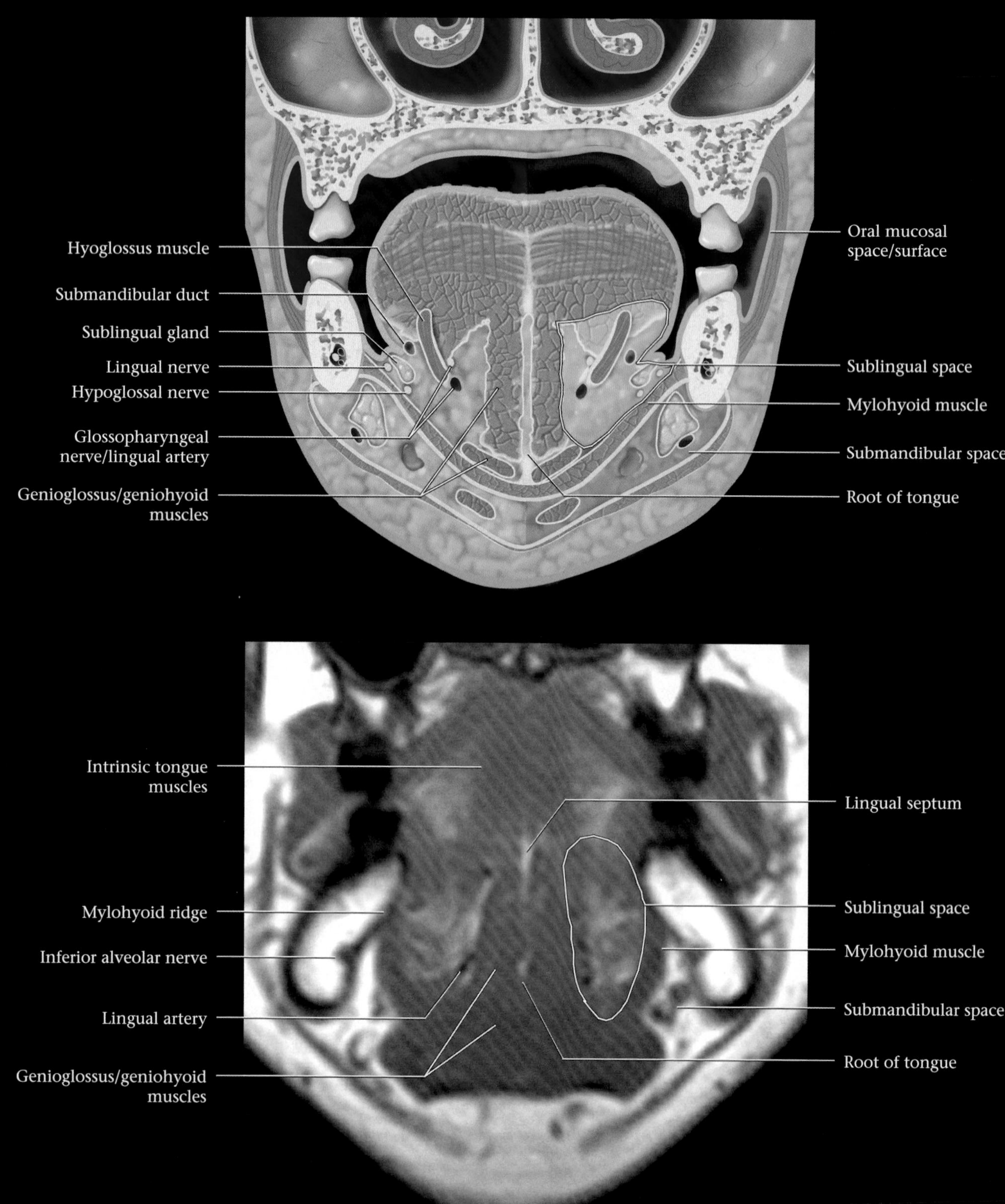
Hyoglossus muscle
Submandibular duct
Sublingual gland
Lingual nerve
Hypoglossal nerve
Glossopharyngeal nerve/lingual artery
Genioglossus/geniohyoid muscles
Oral mucosal space/surface
Sublingual space
Mylohyoid muscle
Submandibular space
Root of tongue
Intrinsic tongue muscles
Mylohyoid ridge
Inferior alveolar nerve
Lingual artery
Genioglossus/geniohyoid muscles
Lingual septum
Sublingual space
Mylohyoid muscle
Submandibular space
Root of tongue

(Top) In this coronal graphic through the oral cavity the SLS is shaded in green. The SLS medial compartment contents include the glossopharyngeal nerve (CN9) and lingual artery/vein. Lateral SLS compartment contents include the submandibular duct, sublingual gland, lingual nerve and hypoglossal nerve (CN12). The fascia-lined (yellow line) submandibular space is inferolateral to the mylohyoid muscle. **(Bottom)** In this coronal T1 MR image the "potential" SLS is superomedial to the mylohyoid muscle and lateral to the genioglossus muscle. It is difficult to identify the margins of the genioglossus muscles.

AXIAL CECT

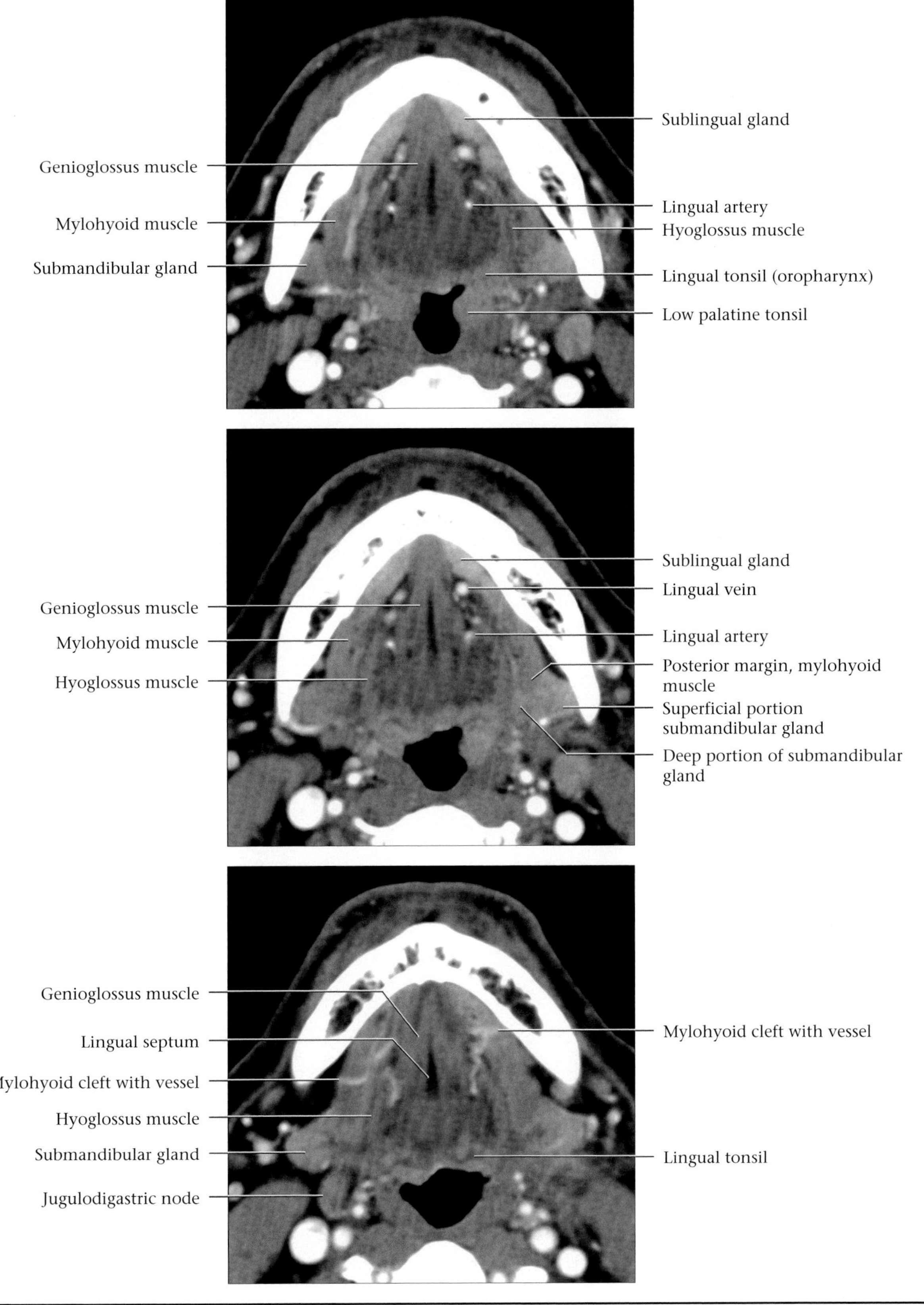

Sublingual gland
Genioglossus muscle
Lingual artery
Mylohyoid muscle
Hyoglossus muscle
Submandibular gland
Lingual tonsil (oropharynx)
Low palatine tonsil
Sublingual gland
Lingual vein
Genioglossus muscle
Mylohyoid muscle
Lingual artery
Hyoglossus muscle
Posterior margin, mylohyoid muscle
Superficial portion submandibular gland
Deep portion of submandibular gland
Genioglossus muscle
Mylohyoid cleft with vessel
Lingual septum
Mylohyoid cleft with vessel
Hyoglossus muscle
Submandibular gland
Lingual tonsil
Jugulodigastric node

(Top) First of three axial CECT images of the sublingual space within the oral cavity. This most superior image shows the medial border of the sublingual space is the genioglossus muscle. The hyoglossus muscles are seen projecting into the posterior sublingual spaces. **(Middle)** More inferiorly a larger portion of the mylohyoid muscle can be seen forming the inferolateral border of the sublingual space. Notice the submandibular gland wrapping around the posterior margin of this muscle on the patient's left. The deep portion of the submandibular gland is found in the posterior sublingual space. **(Bottom)** Inferiorly the sublingual spaces becomes smaller with the hyoglossus muscle filling most of this space. Both mylohyoid muscles demonstrate small clefts with a vessel present bilaterally.

SUBLINGUAL SPACE

AXIAL T2 FS MR

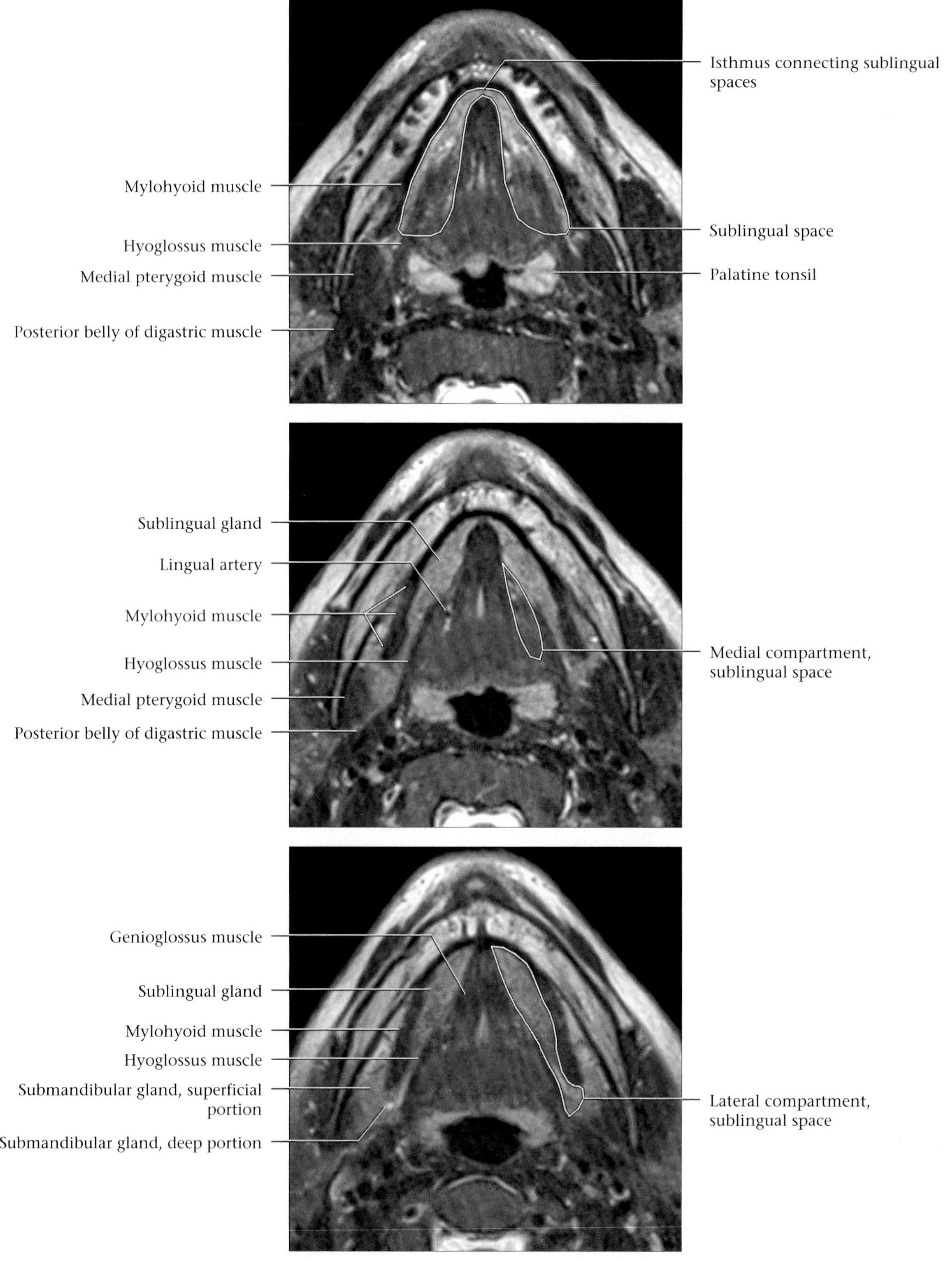

Isthmus connecting sublingual spaces
Mylohyoid muscle
Sublingual space
Hyoglossus muscle
Medial pterygoid muscle
Palatine tonsil
Posterior belly of digastric muscle
Sublingual gland
Lingual artery
Mylohyoid muscle
Medial compartment, sublingual space
Hyoglossus muscle
Medial pterygoid muscle
Posterior belly of digastric muscle
Genioglossus muscle
Sublingual gland
Mylohyoid muscle
Hyoglossus muscle
Submandibular gland, superficial portion
Lateral compartment, sublingual space
Submandibular gland, deep portion

(Top) First of three axial T2 FS MR images are presented from superior to inferior through the oral cavity. In this most superior image the two sublingual spaces are outlined to highlight the anterior connecting isthmus that is present under the frenulum of the oral tongue. **(Middle)** Slightly inferior the medial compartment of the SLS is outlined on the patient's left. The medial compartment is defined as the SLS area medial to the hyoglossus muscle containing the lingual artery and vein as well as the glossopharyngeal nerve (CN9). **(Bottom)** Continuing inferiorly the submandibular gland deep portion is seen projecting into posterior margin of sublingual space. The lateral compartment of SLS is outlined. It is defined as SLS component lateral to hyoglossus muscle. It contains the sublingual gland, lingual nerve, hypoglossal nerve and submandibular gland duct.

CORONAL T1 MR

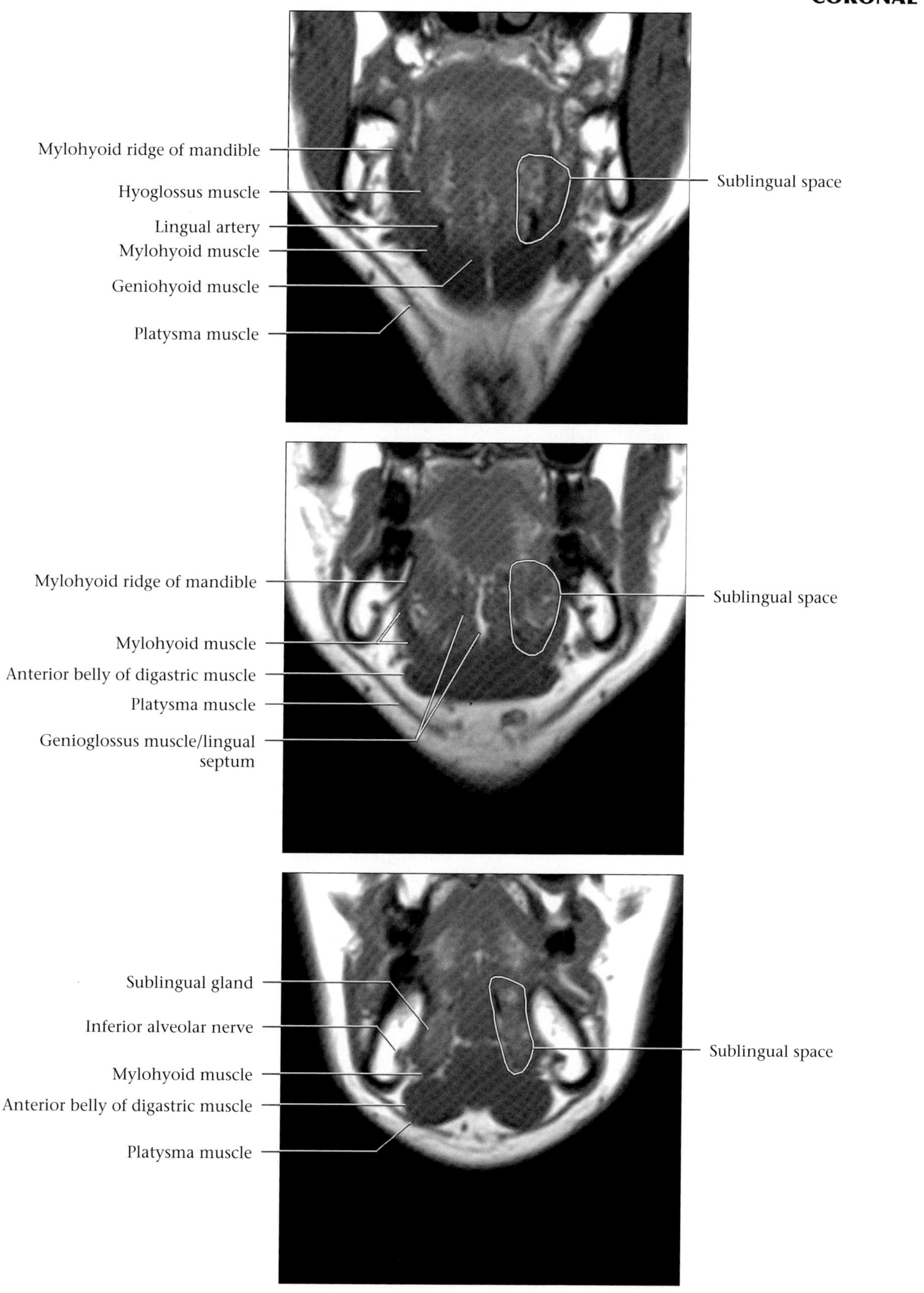
Mylohyoid ridge of mandible
Hyoglossus muscle
Lingual artery
Mylohyoid muscle
Geniohyoid muscle
Platysma muscle
Sublingual space
Mylohyoid ridge of mandible
Mylohyoid muscle
Anterior belly of digastric muscle
Platysma muscle
Genioglossus muscle/lingual septum
Sublingual space
Sublingual gland
Inferior alveolar nerve
Mylohyoid muscle
Anterior belly of digastric muscle
Platysma muscle
Sublingual space

(Top) First of three coronal T1 MR images of normal oral cavity/sublingual space presented from posterior to anterior. In this most posterior image the mylohyoid sling is slung from side to side between mylohyoid ridges of inner mandibular cortex. The sublingual space is superomedial to mylohyoid muscle & lateral to genioglossus & geniohyoid muscles. **(Middle)** Anteriorly in oral cavity the true size of sublingual space is visible as delineated on patient's left. Although it is possible to see the low signal lingual artery, the remaining normal sublingual space structures are blended into the fibrofatty space itself. **(Bottom)** In the very anterior floor of mouth the anterior belly of digastric muscles are the most prominent occupants of the submandibular space. The sublingual gland is mostly found within the anterior sublingual space where it takes up much of the space's volume.

SUBMANDIBULAR SPACE

Terminology

Abbreviations

- Submandibular space (SMS)

Synonyms

- Term submaxillary space used by surgeons

Definitions

- SMS: Fascial-lined space inferolateral to mylohyoid muscle containing submandibular gland, nodes and anterior belly of digastric muscles

Imaging Anatomy

Overview

- SMS is one of four distinct locations within oral cavity (OC) that may be used to develop location specific differential diagnoses
  - Other 3 locations include oral mucosal space/surface, sublingual space and root of tongue

Extent

- SMS is defined as a superficial space above hyoid bone deep to platysma and superficial to mylohyoid sling

Anatomy Relationships

- **Inferolateral to mylohyoid muscle** of floor of mouth
- Deep to platysma muscle
- Cephalad to hyoid bone
- "**Vertical horseshoe-shaped**" space between hyoid bone below and mylohyoid sling above
- Communicates posteriorly with sublingual space and inferior parapharyngeal space at posterior margin of mylohyoid muscle
- Continues inferiorly into infrahyoid neck as anterior cervical space

Internal Structures-Critical Contents

- **Submandibular gland**
  - Superficial portion is larger and in SMS itself
    - Superficial layer, deep cervical fascia (SL-DCF) forms submandibular gland capsule
    - Crossed by facial vein and cervical branches of facial nerve (marginal mandibular branch)
  - Smaller deep portion often called deep "process"
    - Deep process is tongue-like extension of gland
    - Wraps around posterior margin of mylohyoid muscle
    - Projects into posterior aspect of sublingual space
    - Submandibular duct projects off deep process into sublingual space
  - Submandibular gland innervation
    - Parasympathetic secretomotor supply from chorda tympani branch of facial nerve
    - Comes via lingual branch of cranial nerve V3
- **Submental (level IA) and submandibular (level IB) nodal groups**
  - Receives lymph drainage from anterior facial region
    - Including oral cavity, anterior sinonasal and orbital areas
- Facial vein and artery pass through SMS
- **Caudal loop of CN12** passes through SMS on way before looping anteriorly and cephalad into tongue muscles
- **Anterior belly of digastric muscles**
- Tail of parotid may "hang down" into posterior submandibular space

Fascia

- **SMS is lined by SL-DCF**
  - Superficial surface of mylohyoid muscle is covered by SL-DCF
  - Deep surface of platysma covered by SL-DCF
- There is **no midline fascia** separating two sides of SMS
  - Consequently lesion growth from side to side in SMS is unobstructed

Anatomy-Based Imaging Issues

Key Concepts or Questions

- Major clinical-imaging question when mass present in SMS: Is lesion nodal or submandibular gland in origin?
  - Fatty cleavage plane between mass & submandibular gland identifies lesion as nodal in origin
    - If facial vein separates lesion from submandibular gland, then lesion is from a node
  - "Beaking" of submandibular gland tissue around lesion margin identifies lesion as submandibular gland in origin
- What are major diagnoses in the SMS differential diagnoses list?
  - Congenital: Epidermoid, cystic hygroma
  - Inflammatory: Submandibular gland sialoadenitis with ductal calculus; diving ranula; reactive or suppurative adenopathy
  - Benign tumor: Benign mixed tumor of submandibular gland, lipoma
  - Malignant tumor: Salivary gland carcinomas; nodal squamous cell carcinoma and non-Hodgkin lymphoma

Imaging Recommendations

- CECT or T1 C+ fat-saturated MR both effective in SMS
- Ultrasound with needle aspiration of lesion also used

Imaging Pitfalls

- Do not mistake obstructed, enlarged submandibular gland for malignant node in setting of anterior floor of mouth primary squamous cell carcinoma

Clinical Implications

Clinical Importance

- Majority of lesion of SMS are either from submandibular gland or nodes
  - Sorting lesions into these two categories helps work through imaging differential diagnosis
- Remember clinicians can see and feel area of SMS
  - Fine needle cytopathology may have already been done at time of imaging
- Lesions of parotid tail may appear in posterior submandibular space clinically

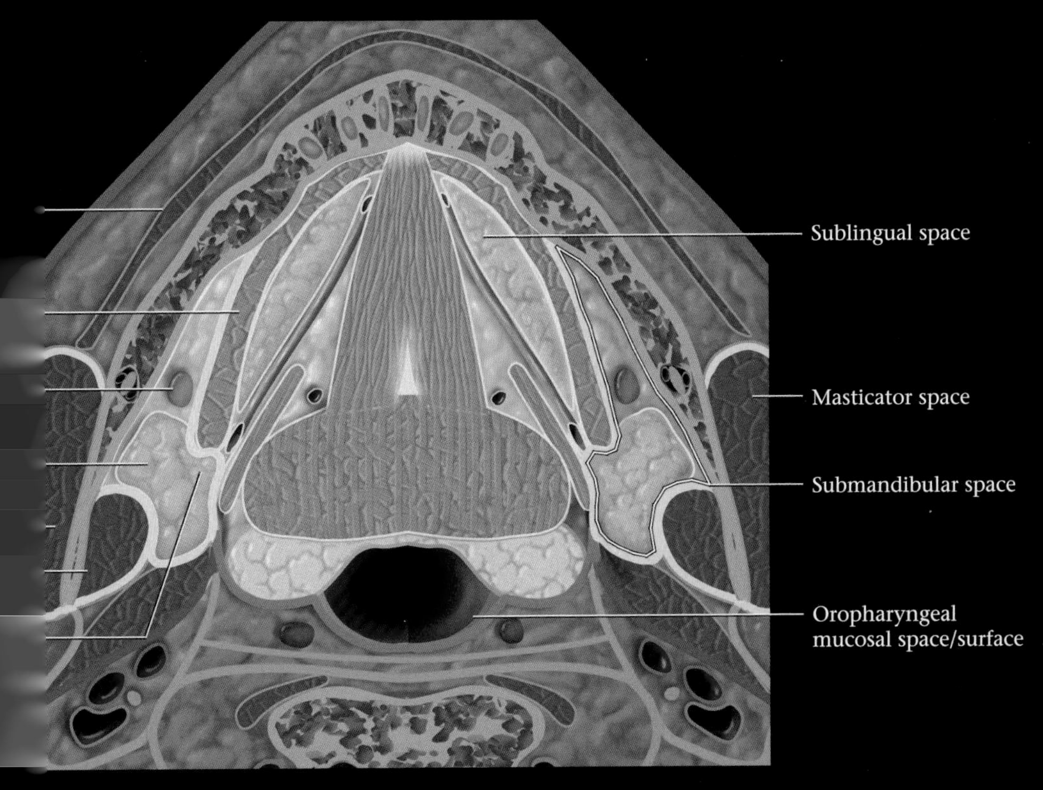
Sublingual space
Masticator space
Submandibular space
Oropharyngeal
mucosal space/surface

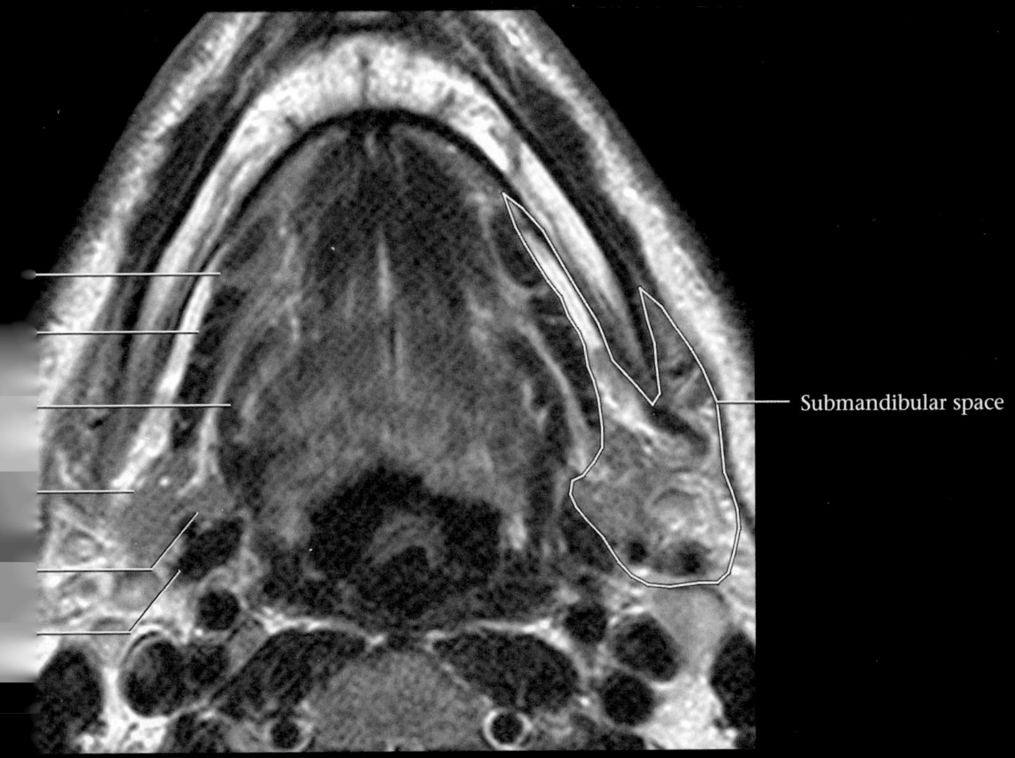
Submandibular space

l cavity with emphasis on the SMS shaded in light blue on patient's left. The ferolateral to the mylohyoid muscle. Note the principal occupants of the SMS are the nodes. **(Bottom)** Axial T2 MR image demonstrates the axial appearance of the ined on the patient's left. The principal occupant of the submandibular space are the nodes. Consequently the differential diagnosis of lesions of this space includes gland

SUBMANDIBULAR SPACE

GRAPHIC & CORONAL T1 MR

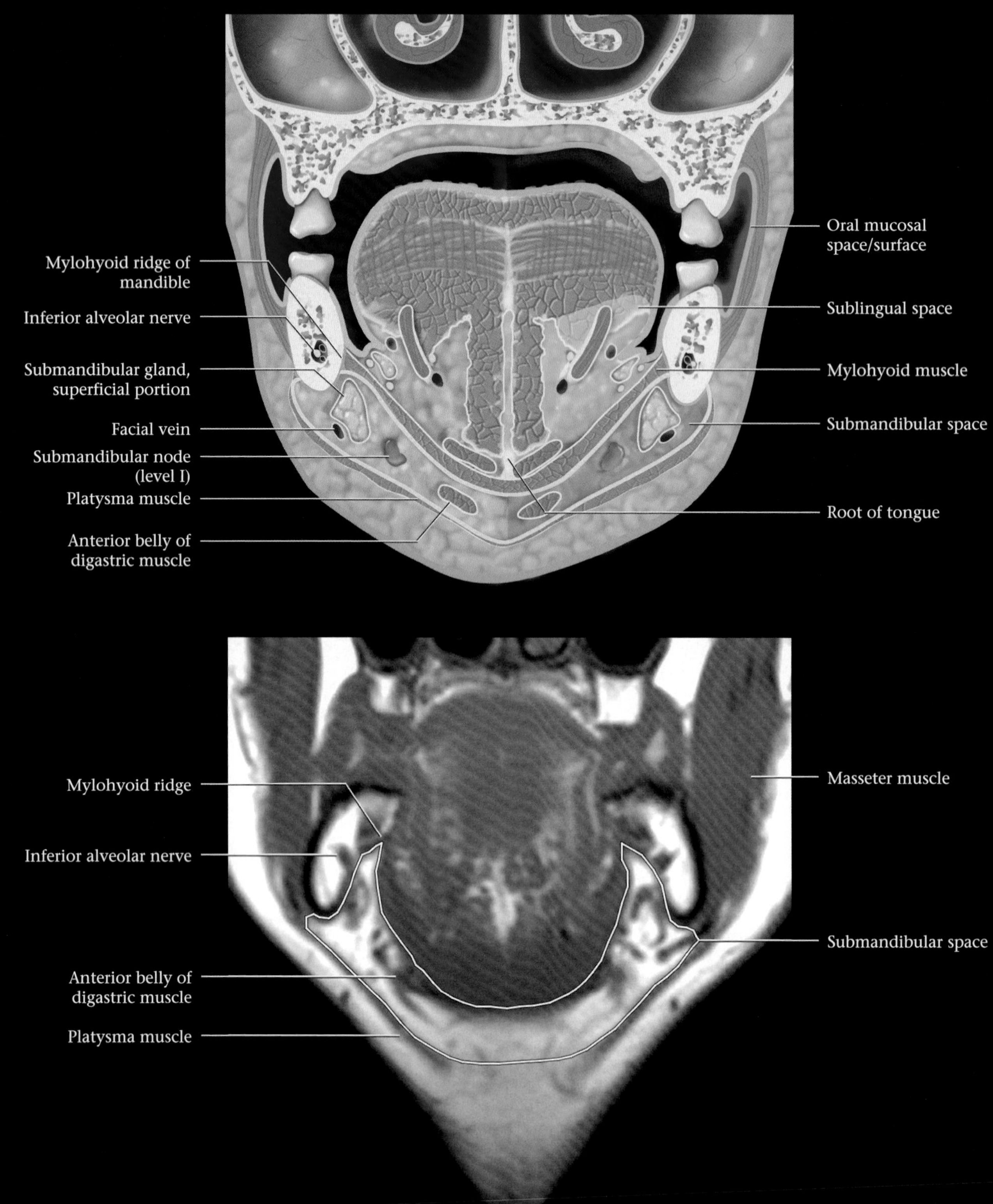
Mylohyoid ridge of mandible
Inferior alveolar nerve
Submandibular gland, superficial portion
Facial vein
Submandibular node (level I)
Platysma muscle
Anterior belly of digastric muscle
Oral mucosal space/surface
Sublingual space
Mylohyoid muscle
Submandibular space
Root of tongue
Mylohyoid ridge
Inferior alveolar nerve
Anterior belly of digastric muscle
Platysma muscle
Masseter muscle
Submandibular space

(Top) In this coronal graphic through the oral cavity the submandibular space is shaded in light blue. The superficial layer of deep cervical fascia (yellow line) is seen lining the "vertical horseshoe-shaped" SMS inferolateral to the mylohyoid muscle. Contents of SMS are the anterior belly of digastric muscle, submandibular nodes, submandibular gland and facial vein. Notice the platysma forms the superficial margin of the SMS. **(Bottom)** Coronal T1 MR shows the "horseshoe-shaped" submandibular space extending from side-to-side inferior and inferolateral to the mylohyoid muscle and deep to the platysma muscle. Notice the lack of vertical fascia or septation. Consequently lesions of the submandibular space spread readily across the midline.

AXIAL CECT

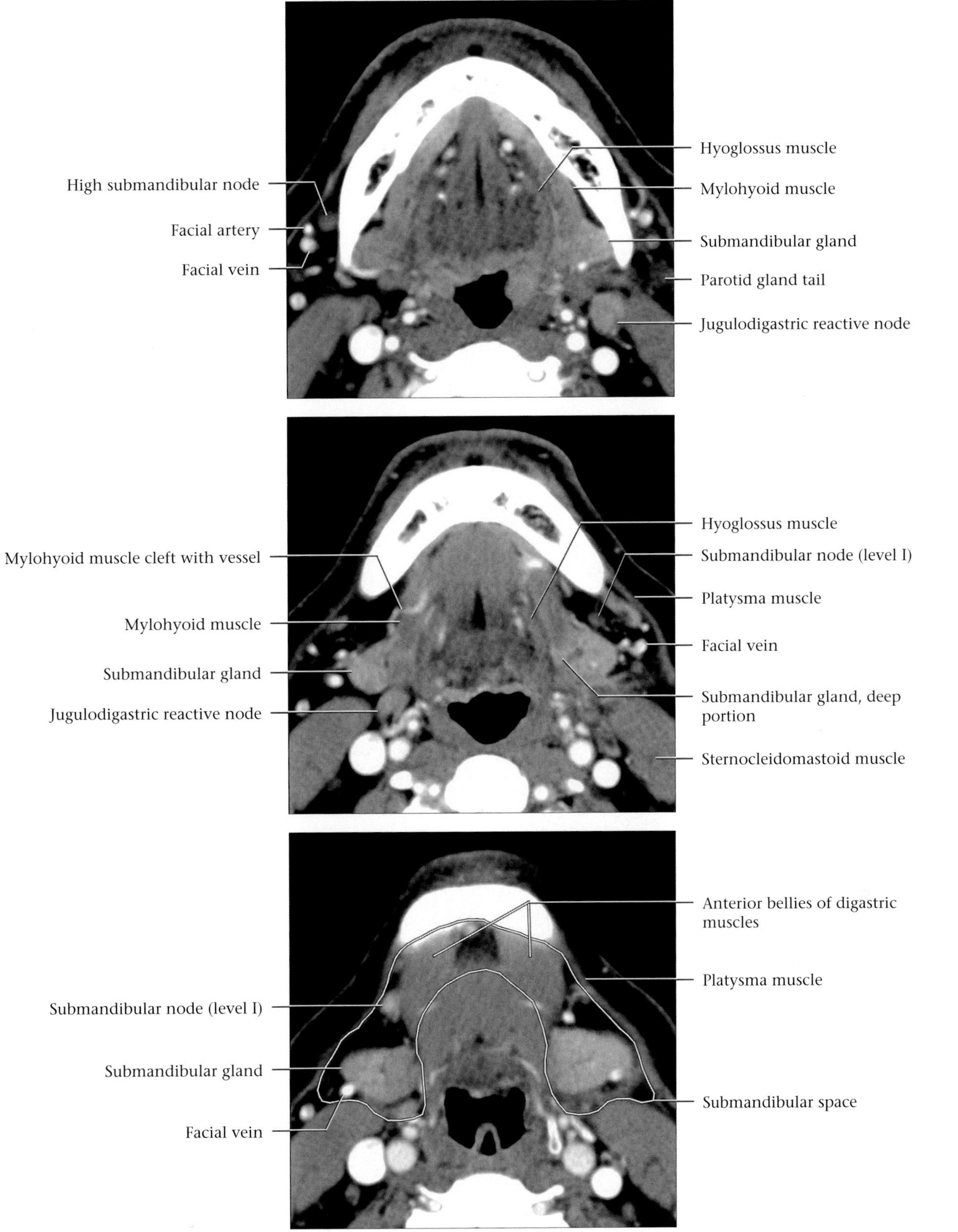

Hyoglossus muscle
High submandibular node
Mylohyoid muscle
Facial artery
Submandibular gland
Facial vein
Parotid gland tail
Jugulodigastric reactive node
Hyoglossus muscle
Mylohyoid muscle cleft with vessel
Submandibular node (level I)
Platysma muscle
Mylohyoid muscle
Facial vein
Submandibular gland
Submandibular gland, deep portion
Jugulodigastric reactive node
Sternocleidomastoid muscle
Anterior bellies of digastric muscles
Platysma muscle
Submandibular node (level I)
Submandibular gland
Submandibular space
Facial vein

(Top) First of three axial CECT images presented from superior to inferior. This most superior image reveals the upper most portion of the SMS. Notice the parotid gland tail projecting into the posterior SMS on the patient's left. **(Middle)** More inferiorly this image shows the enlarging SMS filled with the submandibular gland, nodes and facial vein. The submandibular gland deep portion extends to fill the posterior margin of the sublingual space on the patient's left. **(Bottom)** Low SMS axial CECT image highlights the full extent of these spaces. Notice how large the submandibular glands become inferiorly. Also note that the anterior bellies of the digastric muscles fill the anteromedial SMS.

AXIAL T2 MR

Mental foramen
Inferior alveolar nerve
Sublingual gland
Mylohyoid muscle
Submandibular duct
Hyoglossus muscle
Submandibular gland, superficial portion
Medial pterygoid muscle
Submandibular gland, deep portion
Posterior belly of digastric muscle

Mylohyoid cleft
Genioglossus muscles
Mylohyoid muscle
Hyoglossus muscle
Submandibular gland hilum
Facial vein
Posterior belly of digastric muscle
Jugulodigastric node

Anterior bellies of digastric muscles
Platysma
Facial vein
Submandibular gland
Submandibular space

(Top) First of three axial T2 MR images of the oral cavity presented from superior to inferior. In this most superior image the upper SMS is evident, filled with fat and the upper submandibular glands. Notice the high signal submandibular ducts entering the posterior sublingual spaces bilaterally. **(Middle)** Moving inferiorly more fat is seen in the SMS bilaterally surrounding the submandibular glands. Both submandibular glands can be seen wrapping around the posterior margins of the mylohyoid muscles. Remember that the neurovascular pedicle to each side of the tongue enters closely approximated to the hyoglossus muscles. **(Bottom)** Low in the SMS the full extend of both SMSs is visible. Notice that the anterior bellies of the digastric muscles fill the anteromedial SMS. Remember there is no midline fascia so diseases can move across midline from side-to-side.

CORONAL T1 MR

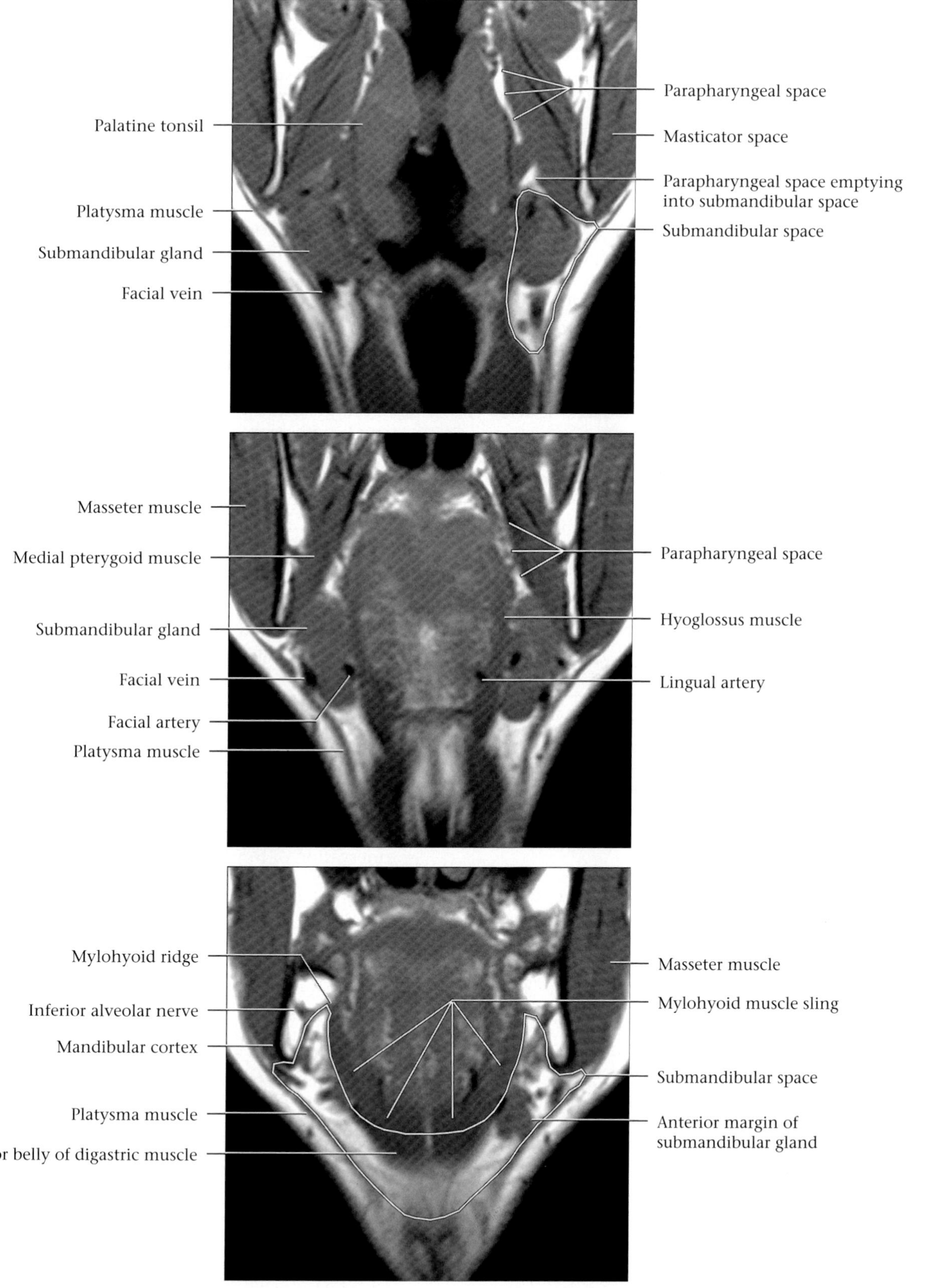

Palatine tonsil
Platysma muscle
Submandibular gland
Facial vein
Parapharyngeal space
Masticator space
Parapharyngeal space emptying into submandibular space
Submandibular space
Masseter muscle
Medial pterygoid muscle
Submandibular gland
Facial vein
Facial artery
Platysma muscle
Parapharyngeal space
Hyoglossus muscle
Lingual artery
Mylohyoid ridge
Inferior alveolar nerve
Mandibular cortex
Platysma muscle
Anterior belly of digastric muscle
Masseter muscle
Mylohyoid muscle sling
Submandibular space
Anterior margin of submandibular gland

(Top) First of three coronal T1 MR images are presented from posterior to anterior. This most posterior image shows the area of the submandibular space (SMS) outlined on the patient's left. Notice the parapharyngeal space empties inferiorly into the posterior SMS. **(Middle)** More anteriorly the connection between the parapharyngeal space and the SMS is still visible. The facial vein is visible snaking along the inferolateral margin of the submandibular gland. Remember that if the facial vein is seen between a mass and the gland, it is most likely nodal in origin. **(Bottom)** In this image through the mid-oral cavity the full extent of the SMS is clearly visible from side-to-side. The location of the superficial layer of deep cervical fascia is outlined. The mylohyoid sling forms the superomedial border of the SMS. The superficial margin of the SMS is the platysma muscle.

TONGUE

Terminology

Abbreviations

- Oral mucosal space/surface (OMS)
- Root of tongue (ROT)
- Floor of mouth (FOM)
- For muscles: Origin (O), insertion (I), function (F), innervation (N)

Definitions

- **Oral tongue**: Anterior 2/3 of tongue not including tongue base
  - By imaging includes freely mobile portion of tongue that is anterior to the lingual tonsil
- **Root of tongue**: Undersurface of oral tongue at its junction with anterior floor of mouth and mandible
  - By imaging includes lingual septum, inferior portion of genioglossus muscles and geniohyoid muscles
- **Floor of mouth**: Crescent-shaped region of mucosa overlying mylohyoid and hyoglossus muscles, extending from inner aspect of lower alveolar ridge to undersurface of anterior oral tongue
  - By imaging includes mylohyoid muscle as it hangs from side-to-side from medial mandible (mylohyoid ridge) to medial mandible and hyoglossus muscle
- **Base of tongue**: Posterior 1/3 of tongue in oropharynx
  - By imaging includes lingual tonsil

Imaging Anatomy

Overview

- Oral tongue sits centrally within oral cavity
  - Mucosal covering of oral tongue part of OMS
  - SLS is non-fascia lined space within oral tongue
- Surfaces of oral tongue is covered with mucosa

Anatomy Relationships

- **Sublingual space**
  - Part of oral tongue between mylohyoid muscle inferolaterally and genioglossus medially
  - Communicates with contralateral SLS beneath **frenulum** anteriorly
  - Empties posteriorly into posterosuperior aspect of submandibular space (SMS) and inferior parapharyngeal space (PPS)
- **Root of tongue**
  - Inferiorly ROT ends at mylohyoid sling
  - Superiorly ends at intrinsic tongue muscles
  - Anteriorly ends at mandibular symphysis

Internal Structures-Critical Contents

- Oral tongue consists of four anatomic regions
  - Tip of oral tongue
  - Lateral borders of oral tongue
  - Dorsum of oral tongue
  - Undersurface (nonvillous surface) of oral tongue
- Sublingual space
  - Anterior hyoglossus muscle
  - Lingual nerve; CN9 and 12
  - Lingual artery and vein
  - Sublingual glands and ducts
  - Submandibular gland duct
- **Extrinsic tongue muscles**: Move tongue body and alter its shape
  - **Genioglossus**: Large, fan-shaped muscle lying parallel to median plane in sagittal plane
    - O: Upper genial tubercle and internal surface of symphysis menti of mandible
    - I: Along entire length of under surface of tongue
    - F: Protrudes tongue
    - N: CN12
  - **Hyoglossus**: Thin and quadrilateral-shaped muscle; "arms reaching up from posteroinferior floor of mouth into posterior sublingual space"
    - O: Body and greater cornu of hyoid bone
    - I: Passes vertically upward to insert into side of tongue
    - F: Depresses tongue
    - N: CN12
  - **Styloglossus**
    - O: Arises from styloid process and stylomandibular ligament
    - I: Passes anteroinferiorly between internal and external carotid arteries to insert into side of tongue, merging with hyoglossus muscle
    - F: Retracts tongue upward and backward
    - N: CN12
  - **Palatoglossus**
    - O: Undersurface of palatine aponeurosis
    - I: Side and dorsum of tongue
    - F: Forms palatoglossal arch (anterior tonsillar pillar)
    - N: CN10, pharyngeal plexus branch
- **Intrinsic tongue muscles**: Alters shape of tongue during deglutition and speech
  - Complicated bundles of interlacing fibers innervated by CN12
  - Superior and inferior longitudinal
  - Transverse and vertical
- Innervation of tongue
  - Sensory supply (touch, pain, temperature and **taste**)
    - Anterior 2/3: Lingual nerve (taste fibers are from chorda tympani branch of CN7)
    - Posterior 1/3: CN9
  - **Hypoglossal nerve** (CN12)
    - Emerges from nasopharyngeal carotid space
    - Receives fibers from 1st and 2nd cervical nerves
    - Loops inferiorly to level of hyoid bone
    - Rises anteriorly to enter posterior sublingual space just lateral to hyoglossus muscle
    - Runs in sublingual space on lateral surface of genioglossus muscle
    - Innervates extrinsic and intrinsic tongue muscles
- Vasculature of tongue
  - Lingual artery: 2nd branch of external carotid artery
    - Divides in sublingual space into sublingual and deep lingual branches
  - Lingual vein: Parallels lingual artery; drains into internal jugular or facial veins
- Oral tongue lymph vessels
  - Two systems: Superficial mucosa and deep collecting
  - Superficial system: Crossing vessels in anterior FOM drain bilaterally into anterior submandibular nodes
  - Deep collecting system: Drain into ipsilateral anterior submandibular nodal chain only

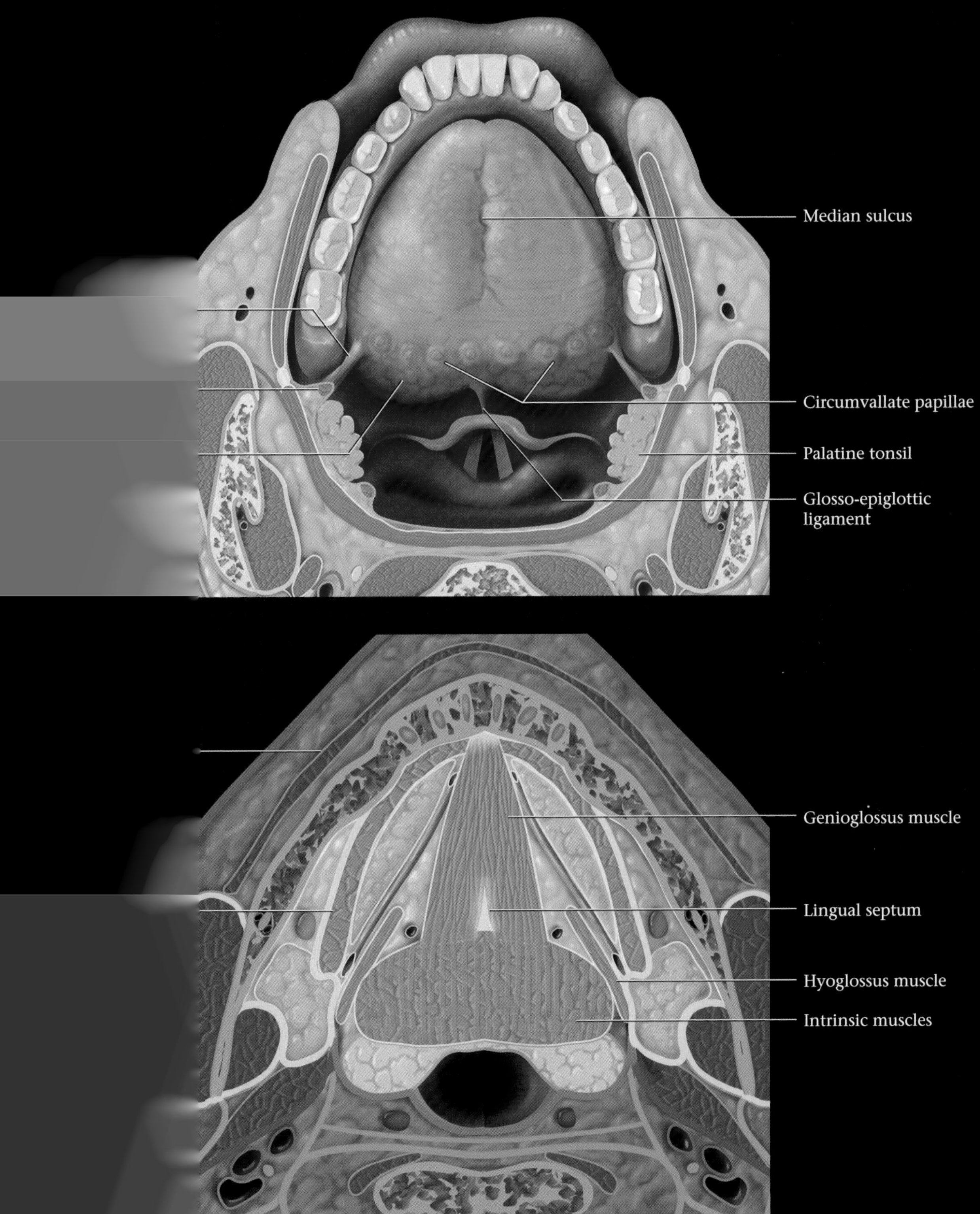
Median sulcus
Circumvallate papillae
Palatine tonsil
Glosso-epiglottic ligament
Genioglossus muscle
Lingual septum
Hyoglossus muscle
Intrinsic muscles

surface of the oral tongue. The oral tongue sits anterior to the oropharyngeal lingual umvallate papillae delineates the mucosal surface transition to the more anterior oral xial graphic through the deep portion of the oral tongue it is possible to see the large, oglossus muscles bordering the midline lingual septum. The genioglossus muscles rise to tangle of intrinsic tongue muscles. The hyoglossus muscles are also seen rising from the

GRAPHICS

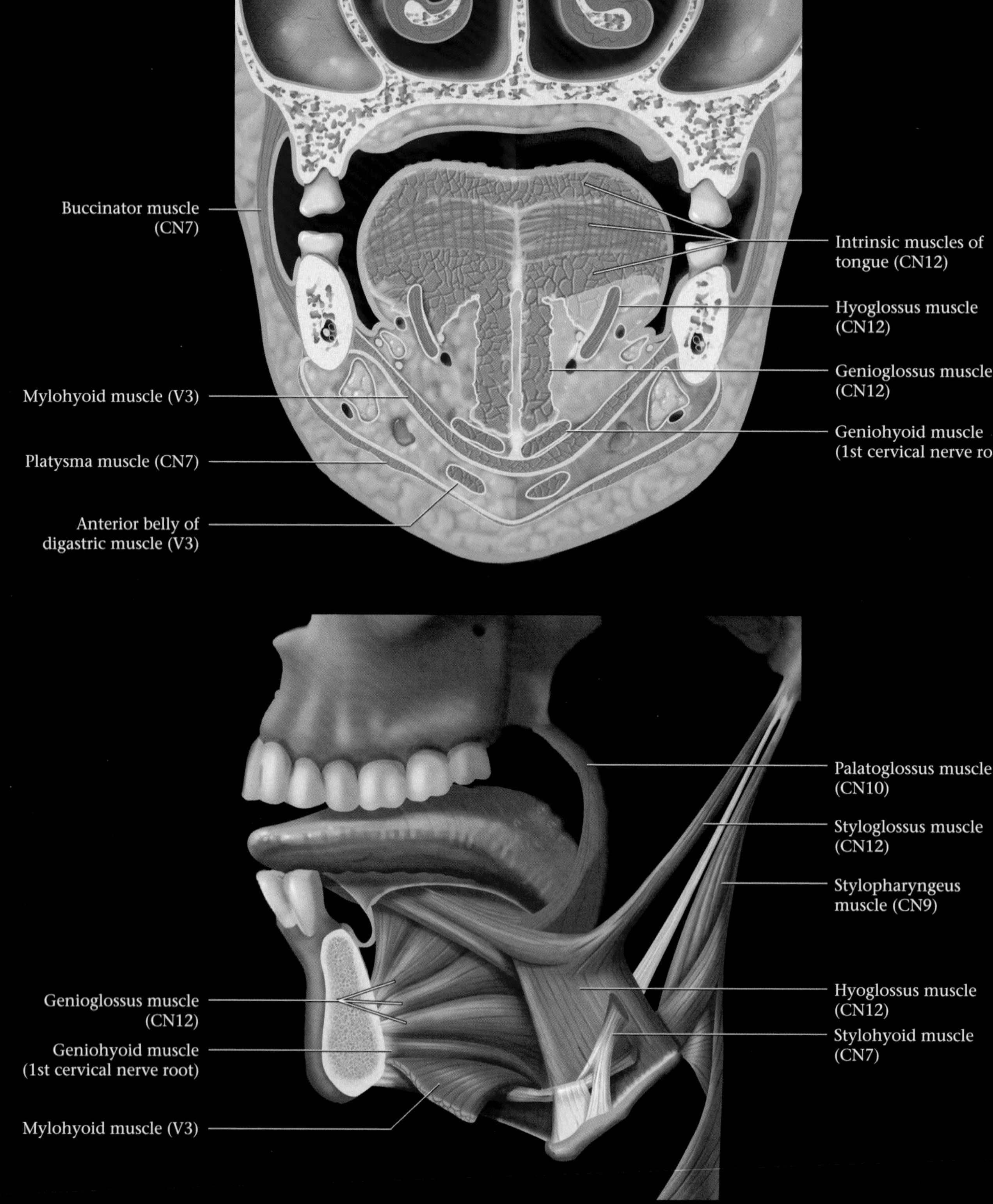

Buccinator muscle (CN7)
Intrinsic muscles of tongue (CN12)
Hyoglossus muscle (CN12)
Genioglossus muscle (CN12)
Mylohyoid muscle (V3)
Geniohyoid muscle (1st cervical nerve root)
Platysma muscle (CN7)
Anterior belly of digastric muscle (V3)
Palatoglossus muscle (CN10)
Styloglossus muscle (CN12)
Stylopharyngeus muscle (CN9)
Genioglossus muscle (CN12)
Hyoglossus muscle (CN12)
Geniohyoid muscle (1st cervical nerve root)
Stylohyoid muscle (CN7)
Mylohyoid muscle (V3)

(Top) Coronal graphic through oral cavity highlights all major muscles with their innervations indicated in parentheses. Note all intrinsic & extrinsic (genioglossus, hyoglossus, styloglossus, palatoglossus) tongue muscles are innervated by CN12 except palatoglossus. The buccinator & platysma, both muscles of facial expression, are innervated by CN7. **(Bottom)** Sagittal graphic of muscles of tongue area. Each muscle is labeled with its innervating nerve in parentheses. Pay attention to fan-shaped genioglossus which represents much of oral tongue extrinsic musculature. Note hyoglossus muscle projecting upward from hyoid bone like two big arms into oral tongues posterior sublingual space. Geniohyoid muscle is not considered part of the extrinsic muscles of the tongue but instead is suprahyoid neck muscle innervated by the CN12 branch with 1st cervical nerve root in it.

SAGITTAL & CORONAL T1 MR

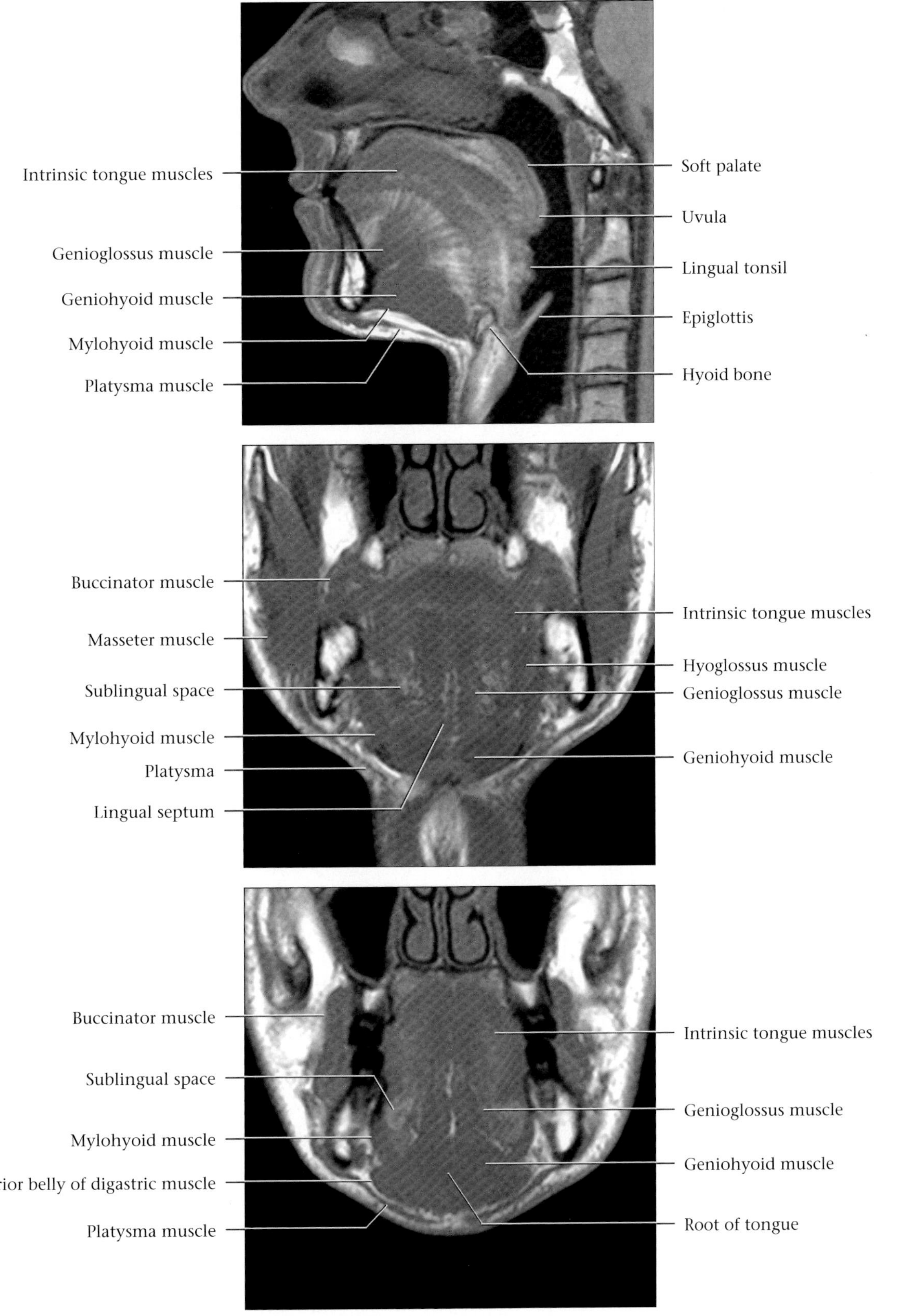

Intrinsic tongue muscles
Genioglossus muscle
Geniohyoid muscle
Mylohyoid muscle
Platysma muscle
Soft palate
Uvula
Lingual tonsil
Epiglottis
Hyoid bone
Buccinator muscle
Masseter muscle
Sublingual space
Mylohyoid muscle
Platysma
Lingual septum
Intrinsic tongue muscles
Hyoglossus muscle
Genioglossus muscle
Geniohyoid muscle
Buccinator muscle
Sublingual space
Mylohyoid muscle
Anterior belly of digastric muscle
Platysma muscle
Intrinsic tongue muscles
Genioglossus muscle
Geniohyoid muscle
Root of tongue

(Top) In this sagittal T1 MR image the full extent of the genioglossus muscle can be seen extending cephalad in a fan shape from its attachment to the posteroinferior mandible. Notice that it is difficult to distinguish the mylohyoid, geniohyoid and inferior genioglossus muscles. **(Middle)** More posterior coronal T1 MR reveals the oral tongue superomedial to mylohyoid muscle. Again the 3 stacked muscles (mylohyoid, geniohyoid and genioglossus) are difficult to distinguish. Remember that the sublingual spaces lie lateral to the genioglossus muscles and superolateral to the mylohyoid muscle. **(Bottom)** In this more anterior coronal T1 MR image, 4 muscles can be identified from inferior to superior, namely the anterior belly of digastric, mylohyoid, geniohyoid and genioglossus muscles. Notice also the root of tongue area.

AXIAL T2 MR

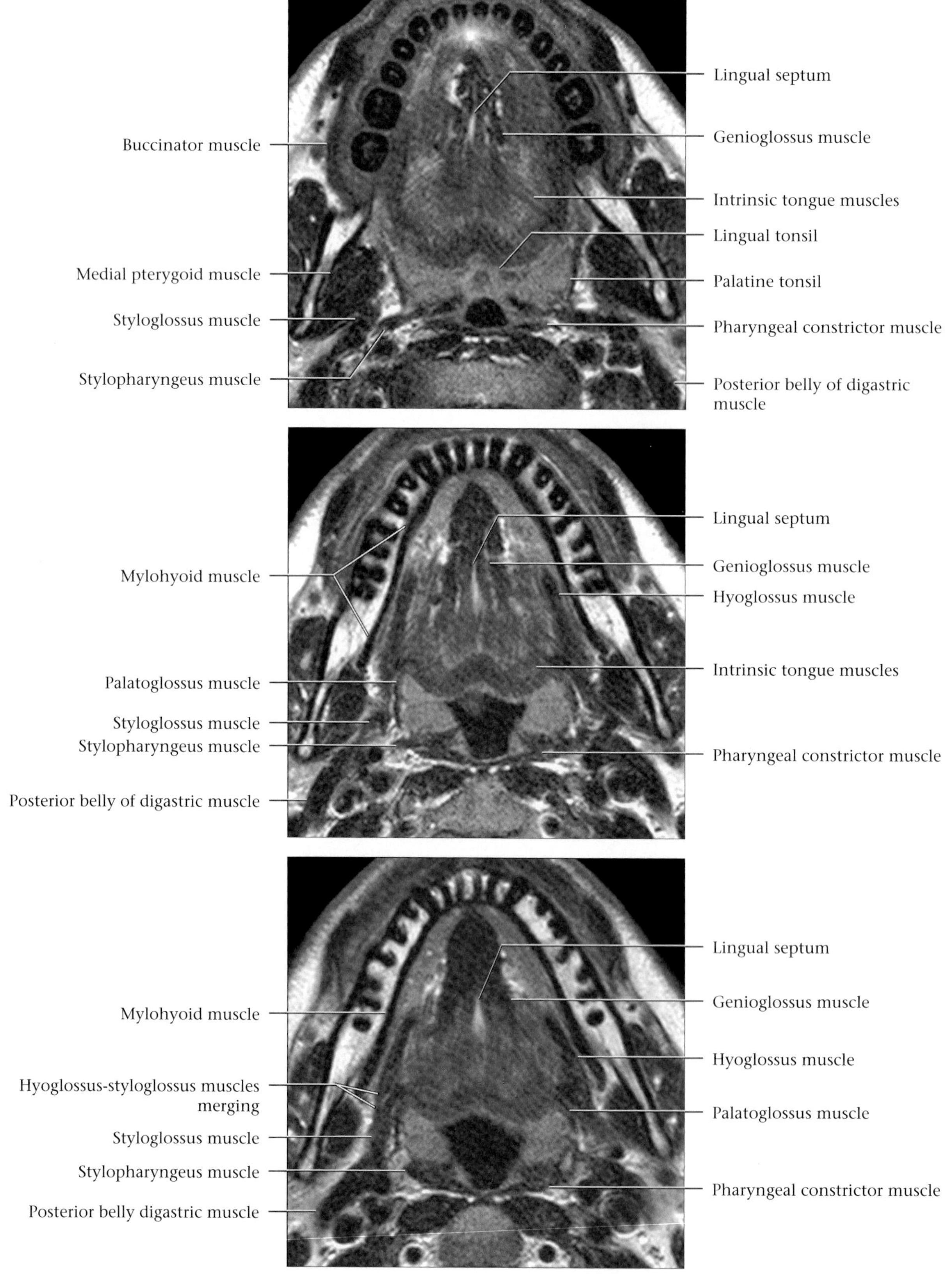
Lingual septum
Genioglossus muscle
Buccinator muscle
Intrinsic tongue muscles
Lingual tonsil
Medial pterygoid muscle
Palatine tonsil
Styloglossus muscle
Pharyngeal constrictor muscle
Stylopharyngeus muscle
Posterior belly of digastric muscle
Lingual septum
Genioglossus muscle
Mylohyoid muscle
Hyoglossus muscle
Intrinsic tongue muscles
Palatoglossus muscle
Styloglossus muscle
Stylopharyngeus muscle
Pharyngeal constrictor muscle
Posterior belly of digastric muscle
Lingual septum
Genioglossus muscle
Mylohyoid muscle
Hyoglossus muscle
Hyoglossus-styloglossus muscles merging
Palatoglossus muscle
Styloglossus muscle
Stylopharyngeus muscle
Pharyngeal constrictor muscle
Posterior belly digastric muscle

(Top) First of six axial T2 MR images of the oral tongue are presented from superior to inferior. In this first most superior MR image the superior aspect of the oral tongue is seen. The intrinsic muscles, especially the transverse group is well seen with just the top of the genioglossus muscle visible. The stylopharyngeus muscle is seen in its expected location just medial to the medial pterygoid muscle. The styloglossus is identified melding with the pharyngeal constrictor muscle. **(Middle)** On this inferior image the hyoglossus upper margin is seen rising into the posterior sublingual space. The genioglossus is now readily apparent on either side of the fibrofatty lingual septum. **(Bottom)** In this image the styloglossus can be seen merging with the hyoglossus (labeled on patient's right). The palatoglossus is now visible along anterior margin of palatine tonsil.

TONGUE

AXIAL T2 MR

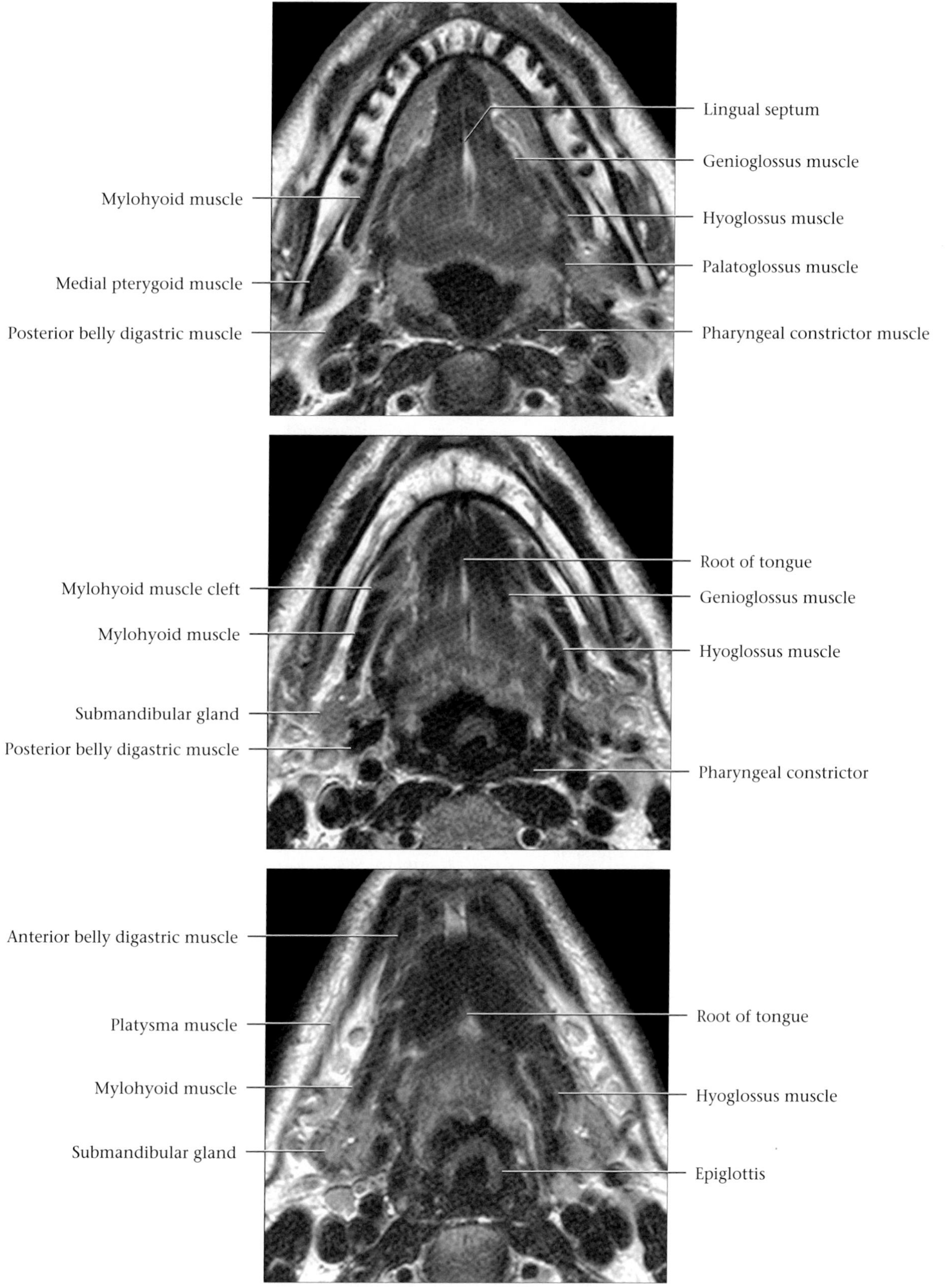
Lingual septum
Genioglossus muscle
Mylohyoid muscle
Hyoglossus muscle
Palatoglossus muscle
Medial pterygoid muscle
Posterior belly digastric muscle
Pharyngeal constrictor muscle
Root of tongue
Mylohyoid muscle cleft
Genioglossus muscle
Mylohyoid muscle
Hyoglossus muscle
Submandibular gland
Posterior belly digastric muscle
Pharyngeal constrictor
Anterior belly digastric muscle
Root of tongue
Platysma muscle
Mylohyoid muscle
Hyoglossus muscle
Submandibular gland
Epiglottis

(Top) At the level of the mandibular teeth roots the posterior belly of the digastric muscle is seen passing deep to the most inferior aspect of the medial pterygoid muscle on the patient's right. The posterior belly of digastric muscle is larger and more inferior than the styloglossus muscle. **(Middle)** In this image the mylohyoid muscle has left the mylohyoid ridge of the mandible. A prominent mylohyoid muscle cleft is present on the patient's right. The area of the root of tongue is labeled. **(Bottom)** This most inferior image shows the convergence of the anteroinferior genioglossus muscle with the geniohyoid muscle to form the area of the root of the tongue. The origins of the hyoglossus muscles are also seen rising off the hyoid bone. The free margin of the epiglottis is visible within the pharyngeal airway.

RETROMOLAR TRIGONE

Terminology

Abbreviations

- Retromolar trigone (RMT)
- Pterygomandibular raphe (PMR)
- Oral mucosal space/surface (OMS)

Definitions

- RMT: Triangle-shaped area of mucosa posterior to last mandibular molar that covers anterior surface of lower ascending ramus of mandible
- PMR: Thick fascial band that extends between posterior border of mandibular mylohyoid ridge and hamulus of medial pterygoid plate
  - Fascial band represents thickening of middle layer of deep cervical fascia condensed between posterior margin of buccinator muscle and anterior margin of superior constrictor muscle

Imaging Anatomy

Overview

- Pterygomandibular raphe lies beneath mucosa of retromolar trigone
- If retromolar trigone is affected by squamous cell carcinoma (SCCa), PMR is involved early
- PMR provides both inferior and superior routes of spread for SCCa

Extent

- RMT extent
  - Cephalad tip is at level of base of pterygoid plate
  - Base of mucosal triangle is posterior margin of last mandibular molar tooth
- PMR extent
  - Fascial band extends from **posterior border of mylohyoid ridge of mandible** to hamulus of medial pterygoid plate

Anatomy Relationships

- Retromolar trigone relationships
  - Deep to RMT mucosa & posterior mandibular body
  - Also covers anterior surface of inferior mandibular ramus
- PMR can be located at line of junction between buccinator (posterior margin) muscle and superior constrictor muscle (anterior margin)

Internal Structures-Critical Contents

- **Retromolar trigone**
  - Paired triangle-shaped mucosal surface in posterolateral oral cavity
- **Pterygomandibular raphe**
  - PMR forms line of attachment for buccinator and superior constrictor muscles
  - Represents junction of oropharynx posteriorly and oral cavity anteriorly
  - Lies between anterior tonsillar pillar & retromolar trigone

Fascia

- PMR: **Thick fascial band formed at junction of buccinator and superior constrictor muscles**
  - Fascia made up of focally thickened middle layer of deep cervical fascia
  - Middle layer of deep cervical fascia runs along superficial margin of buccinator muscle and along deep and lateral margins of superior constrictor muscle

Anatomy-Based Imaging Issues

Key Concepts or Questions

- Retromolar trigone SCCa can spread in multiple directions
  - Posterior spread of SCCa: May involve mandibular ramus, masticator space and perineural CNV3
  - Anterior spread of SCCa: Along alveolar ridge
  - Inferior spread of SCCa
    - If directly into mandible may extend anteriorly via perineural spread along inferior alveolar nerve
    - If along caudal spread along PMR, reaches posterior mylohyoid line of mandible and thereby posterior margin of mylohyoid muscle
  - Superior spread of SCCa: Cephalad spread along PMR to inferior margin of medial pterygoid plate at hamulus

Imaging Recommendations

- CECT provides both soft tissue and bone information
  - May be severely degraded by dental amalgam artifact
- MR less affected by dental amalgam artifact in most cases
  - Reserve for invasive retromolar trigone SCCa
  - Axial T2 and T1 fat-saturated enhanced MR sequences best for evaluation of cephalad PMR

Imaging Pitfalls

- Dental amalgam artifact on CECT may obscure RMT primary SCCa primary site ± spread along PMR in cephalad direction
  - Key CT observation
    - Always check **above CT artifact** in oral cavity in area of cephalad PMR (inferior margin of pterygoid plate) for evidence of tumor spread if primary RMT SCCa is known to be present

Clinical Implications

Clinical Importance

- SCCa of RMT may spread along PMR
  - Cephalad spread along PMR takes tumor up to inferolateral pterygoid plate-anteromedial masticator space
    - Tumor is seen at level of inferior pterygoid plate involving posterior buccinator muscle and anterior superior constrictor muscle
    - Enlarging tumor involves maxillary sinus, buccal and masticator spaces
  - Caudal spread along PMR takes tumor inferiorly to posterior margin of mylohyoid muscle
    - Enlarging tumor in this location involves floor of mouth of oral cavity

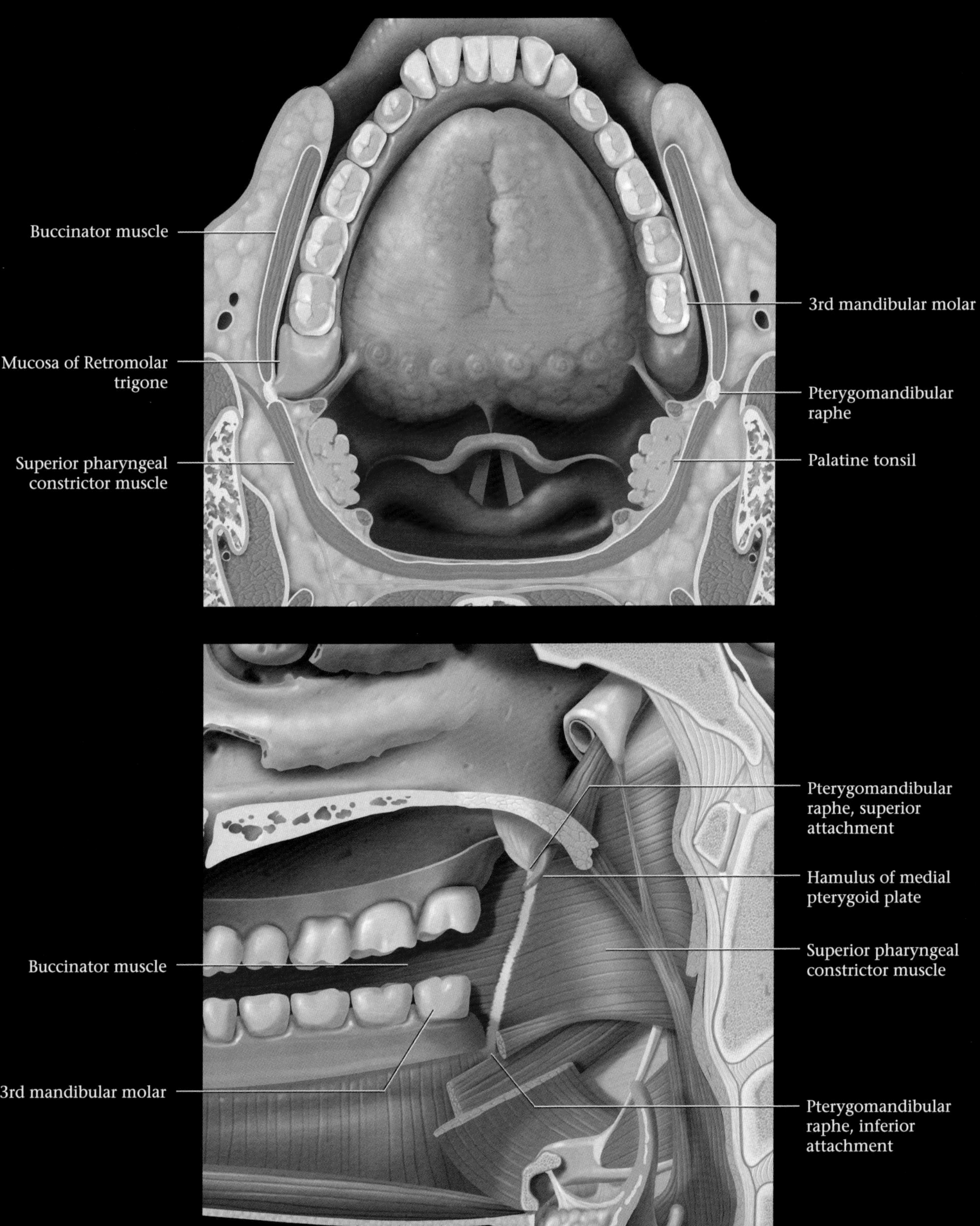
Buccinator muscle
Mucosa of Retromolar trigone
Superior pharyngeal constrictor muscle
3rd mandibular molar
Pterygomandibular raphe
Palatine tonsil
Pterygomandibular raphe, superior attachment
Hamulus of medial pterygoid plate
Buccinator muscle
Superior pharyngeal constrictor muscle
3rd mandibular molar
Pterygomandibular raphe, inferior attachment

(Top) Axial graphic highlighting the retromolar trigone (shaded in blue on patient's right) and the pterygomandibular raphe. Notice that the mucosal surface of the retromolar trigone is found directly behind the mandibular 3rd molar. Its proximity to the pterygomandibular raphe (fascial band connecting buccinator and superior pharyngeal constrictor muscles) is important when squamous cell carcinoma occurs here because of this tumors propensity for spreading cephalad on this fascia. **(Bottom)** Sagittal graphic viewed from inside the mouth delineating the full extent of the PMR. Note the cephalad PMR attachment to the hamulus of the medial pterygoid plate & its inferior attachment to the posterior aspect of the mylohyoid ridge on the inner mandibular cortex. The PMR "connects" the buccinator muscle to the superior pharyngeal constrictor muscle.

RETROMOLAR TRIGONE

AXIAL T2 MR

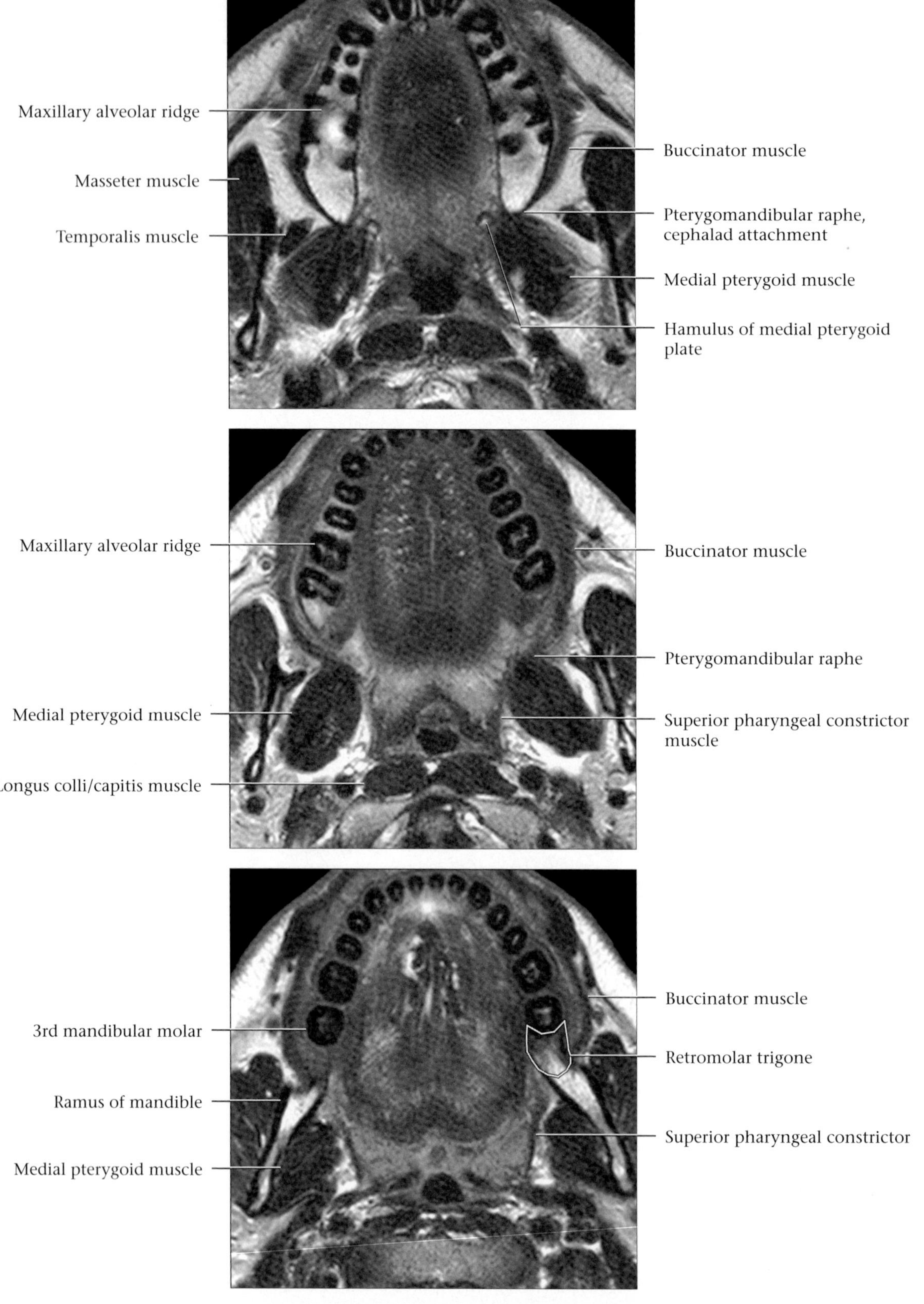
Maxillary alveolar ridge
Masseter muscle
Temporalis muscle
Buccinator muscle
Pterygomandibular raphe, cephalad attachment
Medial pterygoid muscle
Hamulus of medial pterygoid plate
Maxillary alveolar ridge
Medial pterygoid muscle
Longus colli/capitis muscle
Buccinator muscle
Pterygomandibular raphe
Superior pharyngeal constrictor muscle
3rd mandibular molar
Ramus of mandible
Medial pterygoid muscle
Buccinator muscle
Retromolar trigone
Superior pharyngeal constrictor

(Top) First of three axial T2 MR images presented from superior to inferior. This most superior image shows the point of attachment of the pterygomandibular raphe to the hamulus of the medial pterygoid plate. **(Middle)** On this more inferior image the buccinator can be seen meeting the superior pharyngeal constrictor muscle at the pterygomandibular raphe. The raphe itself is difficult to visualize. **(Bottom)** At the level of the mandibular alveolar ridge the area of the retromolar trigone can be outlined. Notice it is found directly behind the mandibular 3rd molar tooth. The buccinator is seen along its lateral margin while the superior pharyngeal constrictor can be seen approaching its medial margin. Just above this slice these two muscles meet at the pterygomandibular raphe. Squamous cell carcinoma of the retromolar trigone often spread cephalad along this raphe.

AXIAL T1 MR

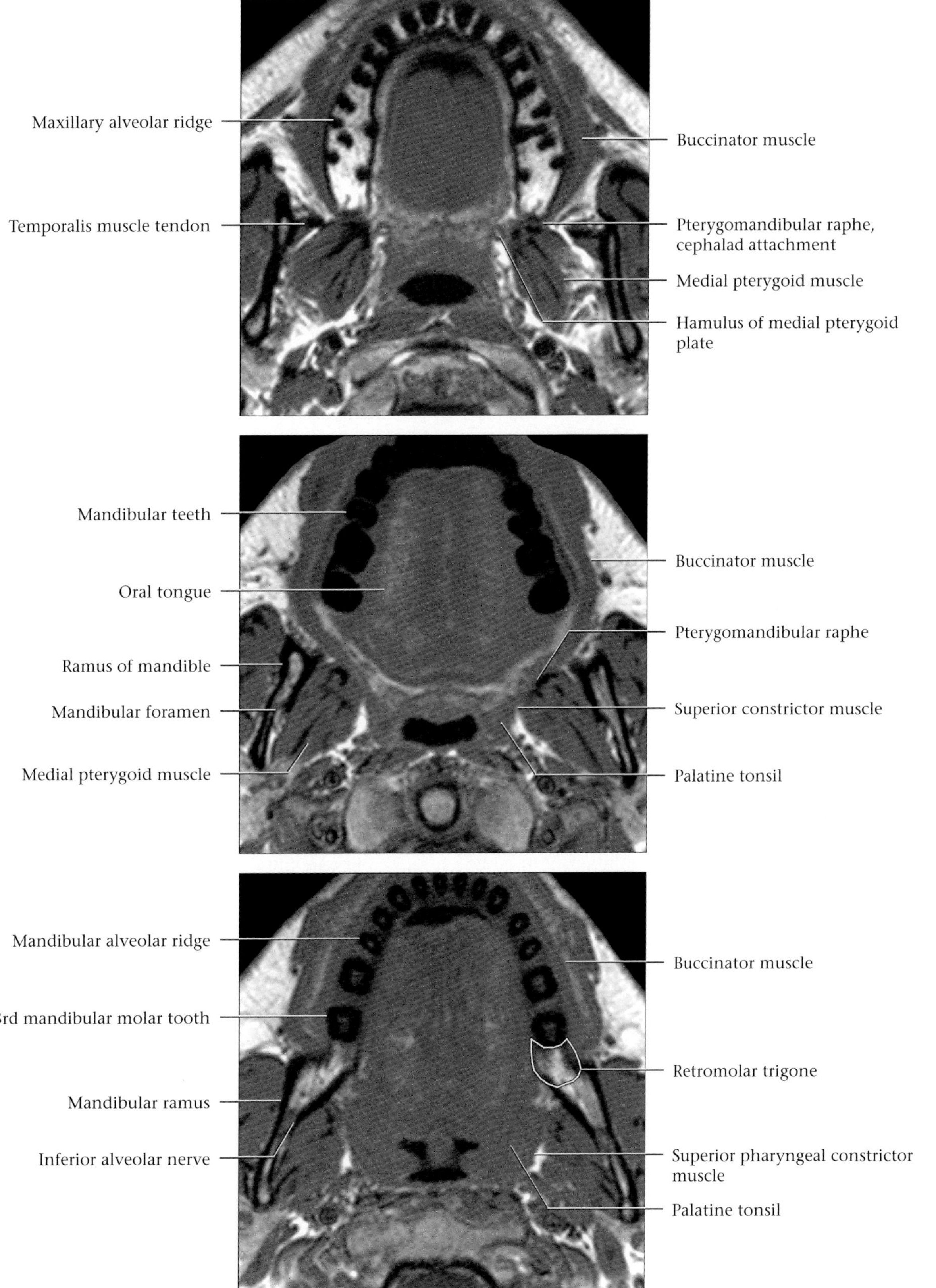
Maxillary alveolar ridge
Temporalis muscle tendon
Buccinator muscle
Pterygomandibular raphe, cephalad attachment
Medial pterygoid muscle
Hamulus of medial pterygoid plate
Mandibular teeth
Oral tongue
Ramus of mandible
Mandibular foramen
Medial pterygoid muscle
Buccinator muscle
Pterygomandibular raphe
Superior constrictor muscle
Palatine tonsil
Mandibular alveolar ridge
3rd mandibular molar tooth
Mandibular ramus
Inferior alveolar nerve
Buccinator muscle
Retromolar trigone
Superior pharyngeal constrictor muscle
Palatine tonsil

(Top) First of three axial T1 MR images through oropharynx-oral cavity presented from superior to inferior. On this most superior image the buccinator can be seen inserting at the inferolateral margin of the pterygoid plate with the most superior aspect of the pterygomandibular raphe. **(Middle)** Inferiorly at the level of the mandibular teeth the buccinator and the superior constrictor muscle meet at the pterygomandibular raphe. The superior constrictor muscle cannot be differentiated from the palatine tonsil on T1 images. **(Bottom)** On this most inferior image at the level of the mandibular alveolar ridge the area of the retromolar trigone is outlined on the patient's left. Note that the retromolar trigone is found directly behind the 3rd mandibular molar tooth. Squamous cell carcinoma can spread up the pterygomandibular raphe from this location.

MANDIBLE AND MAXILLA

Terminology

Abbreviations

- Mandible (Md)
- Maxilla (Mx)

Definitions

- Angle of mandible: Obtuse angle of Md where inferior segment of ramus becomes contiguous with posterior mandibular body

Imaging Anatomy

Internal Structures-Critical Contents

- Mandible anatomy: Bony
  - 2 vertical rami attached to horizontal, horseshoe-shaped body
  - Each ramus has 2 upwardly directed processes
    - **Condylar process**: Condylar head and neck contains articular surface of TMJ
    - **Coronoid process**: Temporalis muscle inserts here
    - Mandibular notch separates these 2 processes
    - Mandibular ramus divides masticator space into lateral and medial compartments
  - **Mandibular foramen**
    - Location: Center, medial surface of Md ramus
    - Nerve transmitted: Inferior alveolar nerve
    - Lingula: Small, osseous lip extending from anterior aspect of mandibular foramen
  - Mandibular body
    - U-shaped, horizontal body composed of 2 halves; fuses in anterior midline at **symphysis menti**
    - Alveolar process consists of external buccal & internal lingual plates, covered by periosteum
    - **Mental foramen**: Paired external openings of mandibular canal that transmits mental nerve
    - **Mylohyoid ridge**: Bony ridge on lingual Md body; site of attachment of mylohyoid muscle
  - Mandibular canal
    - Lies within distal ramus and proximal body of Md
    - Extends from mandibular to mental foramen
    - Contains inferior alveolar nerve and vessels
- Mandible anatomy: Nerves
  - **Inferior alveolar nerve**
    - Extends from mandibular foramen, through mandibular canal to mental foramen
    - Innervates ipsilateral premolars and molars
    - Divides into mental and incisive branches
  - **Mental nerve**
    - Exits mental foramen
    - Provides sensory innervation to skin and mucosa of lower lip and labial gingiva
  - **Incisive nerve**
    - Innervates ipsilateral canine and incisors
- Maxillary alveolar and palatine processes: Bony
  - Represents inferior aspect of maxillary bone
  - Maxillary alveolar ridge (arch)
    - Adult version contains 16 teeth
  - **Premaxilla**: Anterior hard palate and alveolar ridge
    - Contains **incisive foramen** (nasopalatine nerve)
    - Paired nasopalatine canals terminates as single incisive foramen
  - Palatine process of maxillary bone
    - Forms anterior 2/3 of hard palate
  - Posterior 1/3 hard palate formed by horizontal plate of palatine bone
- Maxillary alveolar and palatine processes: Nerves
  - **Nasopalatine nerve** (V2 sensory branch) travels through incisive foramen
    - Supplies sensory fibers to anterior hard palate
  - **Greater palatine nerve** comes down greater palatine canal in palatine bone
    - Supplies sensation to posterior 2/3 of hard palate
    - Exits greater palatine foramen anteriorly to hard palate mucosa
  - **Lesser palatine nerve** also comes down lesser palatine canal in palatine bone
    - Exits lesser palatine foramen posterior to greater palatine foramen
    - Supplies sensory fibers to palatine tonsil
- Dental anatomy, mandible and maxilla
  - 32 total permanent teeth in Md (16) and Mx (16)
    - Each tooth has crown, root and pulp
  - 16 adult teeth in each "dental arch"
    - Each arch consists of 2 quadrants
    - Each quadrant contains 3 molars, 2 premolars, 1 canine, 1 lateral incisor, and 1 medial incisor
  - **Teeth numbering convention**
    - Maxillary alveolar ridge: Begin with right 3rd molar, 1-16 across to left 3rd molar
    - Mandibular alveolar ridge: Begin with left 3rd molar, 17-32 across to right 3rd molar
  - Each tooth crown has 3 rings: Outer enamel surrounding dentin; pulp in center
    - **Enamel**: Densest material in body
    - **Dentin**: Encases pulp
    - **Pulp**: Nourishes the dentin
  - Tooth root covered by cementum
    - Cementum acts as a medium for attaching fibers of periodontal ligament to tooth
    - Periodontal ligament located in periodontal space
    - Periodontal space is radiolucency surrounding tooth root

Anatomy-Based Imaging Issues

Key Concepts or Questions

- V2 perineural malignant tumor
  - If malignancy affects skin of upper lip, **hard palate**, soft palate, check for V2 perineural tumor (PNT)
  - Major locations to identify V2 PNT extend from incisive canal-greater palatine foramen to root entry zone of V in lateral pons
  - If imaging for V2 PNT, check incisive canal, greater and lesser palatine foramen, pterygopalatine canal and fossa, foramen rotundum, Meckel cave, preganglionic segment of CN5, and root entry zone
- V3 perineural malignant tumor
  - If malignant tumor of skin of chin, mandibular alveolar ridge or masticator space, check for V3 PNT
  - If imaging for V3 PNT check entire length of V3 to root entry zone
    - Pay special attention to inferior alveolar canal, mandibular foramen, masticator space

Mandibular nerve
(CNV3)
Lingual nerve
Coronoid process
Inferior alveolar nerve
Mental nerve
Angle of mandible
Mental foramen
Incisive nerve

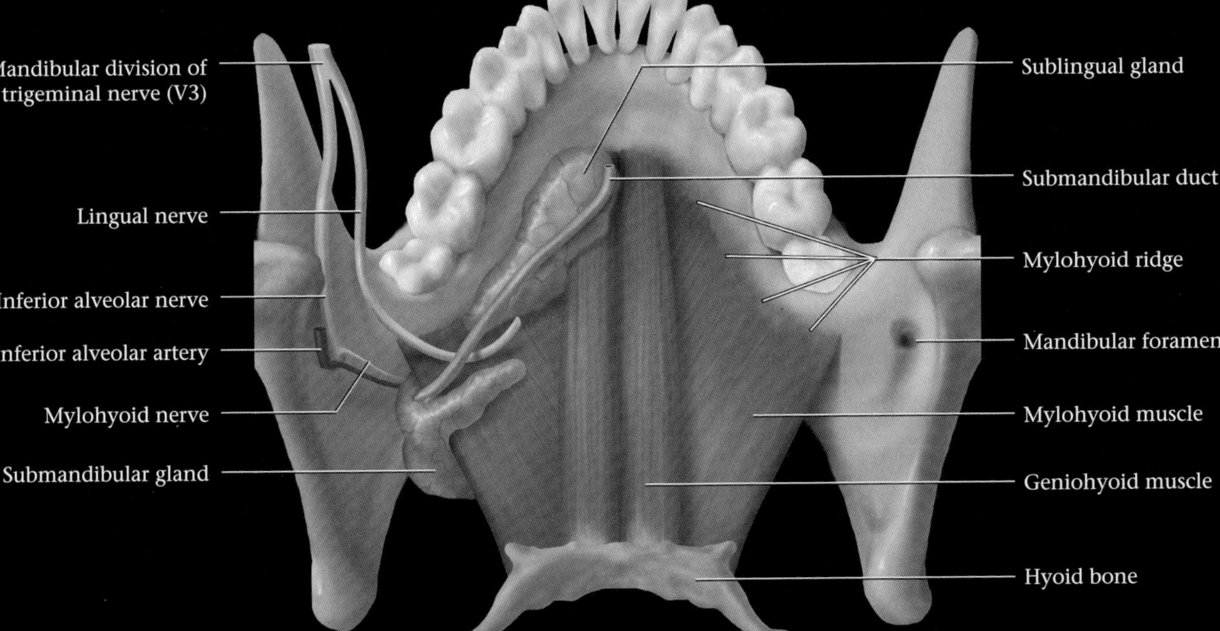
landibular division of
trigeminal nerve (V3)
Sublingual gland
Submandibular duct
Lingual nerve
Mylohyoid ridge
nferior alveolar nerve
Mandibular foramen
nferior alveolar artery
Mylohyoid nerve
Mylohyoid muscle
Submandibular gland
Geniohyoid muscle
Hyoid bone

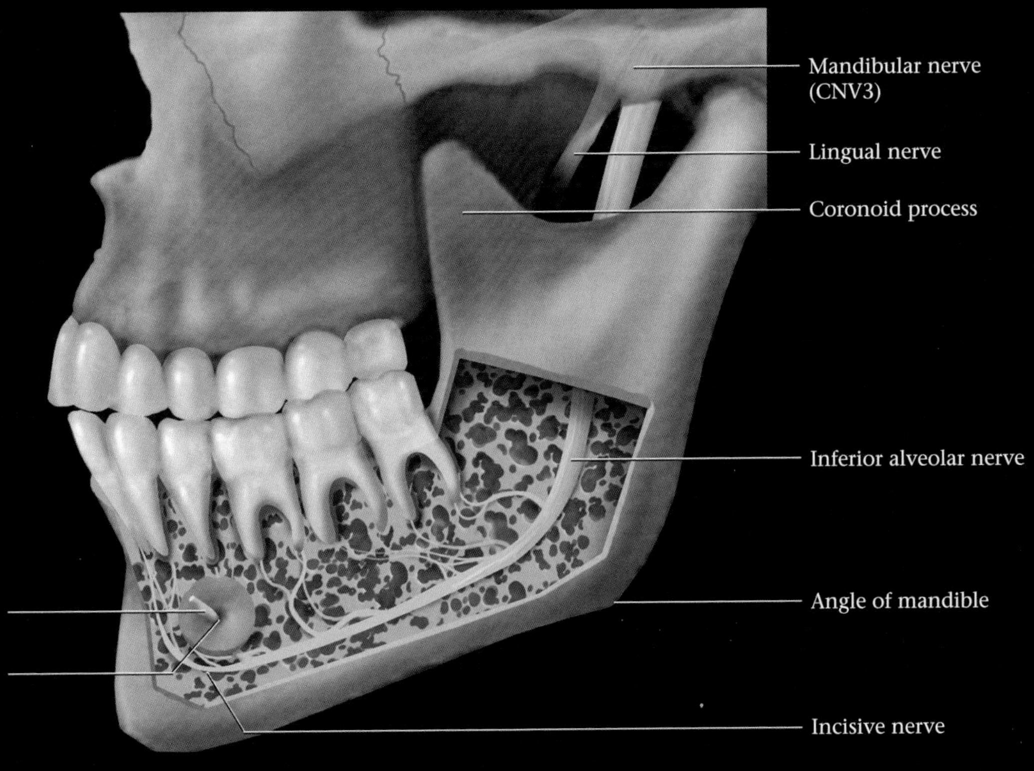

Top) Lateral drawing of mandible with its lateral cortex removed reveals the mandibular nerve divides into lingual nd inferior alveolar nerves. The inferior alveolar nerve divides distally into mental and incisive branches. The hental nerve branch reaches the superficial chin through the mental foramen. **(Bottom)** Drawing of posterior view f floor of mouth and mandible shows the S-shaped mylohyoid ridge where the mylohyoid muscle attaches to the nandible. Also note the mandibular division of the trigeminal nerve bifurcates into the lingual nerve and the nferior alveolar nerve. Just prior to entering the mandibular foramen the inferior alveolar nerve gives off the nylohyoid motor branch that innervates the mylohyoid and anterior belly of the digastric muscles.

MANDIBLE AND MAXILLA

GRAPHICS

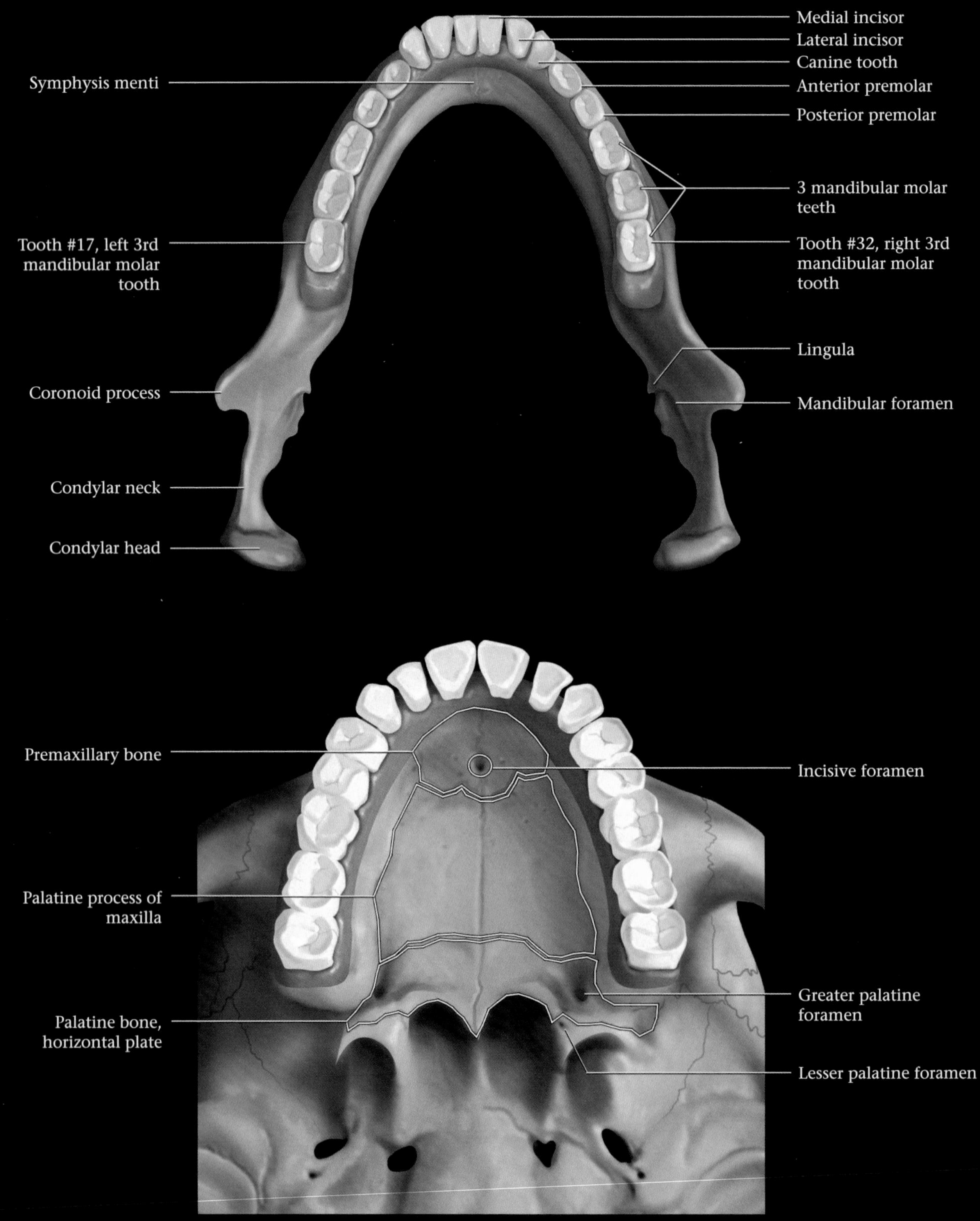
Medial incisor
Lateral incisor
Canine tooth
Anterior premolar
Posterior premolar
Symphysis menti
3 mandibular molar teeth
Tooth #17, left 3rd mandibular molar tooth
Tooth #32, right 3rd mandibular molar tooth
Lingula
Coronoid process
Mandibular foramen
Condylar neck
Condylar head
Premaxillary bone
Incisive foramen
Palatine process of maxilla
Greater palatine foramen
Palatine bone, horizontal plate
Lesser palatine foramen

(Top) Axial graphic of mandible seen from above demonstrates the cephalad condylar head and neck leading to the more inferior ramus. The mandibular foramen is seen on the inner surface of the mandibular ramus. The cephalad projecting coronoid processes attach to the temporalis muscle tendons. The U-shaped mandibular bodies fuse in the midline at the symphysis menti. Notice there are 16 adult teeth, numbered beginning at the left 3rd molar from 17 to 32 (right 3rd molar tooth). **(Bottom)** Axial graphic of hard palate and maxillary alveolar ridge viewed from below shows the anterior premaxillary bone and the larger more posterior palatine process of the maxillary bone. The horizontal plate of the palatine bone completes the hard palate picture. Notice the anterior midline incisive canal and the posterolateral greater and lesser palatine foramina.

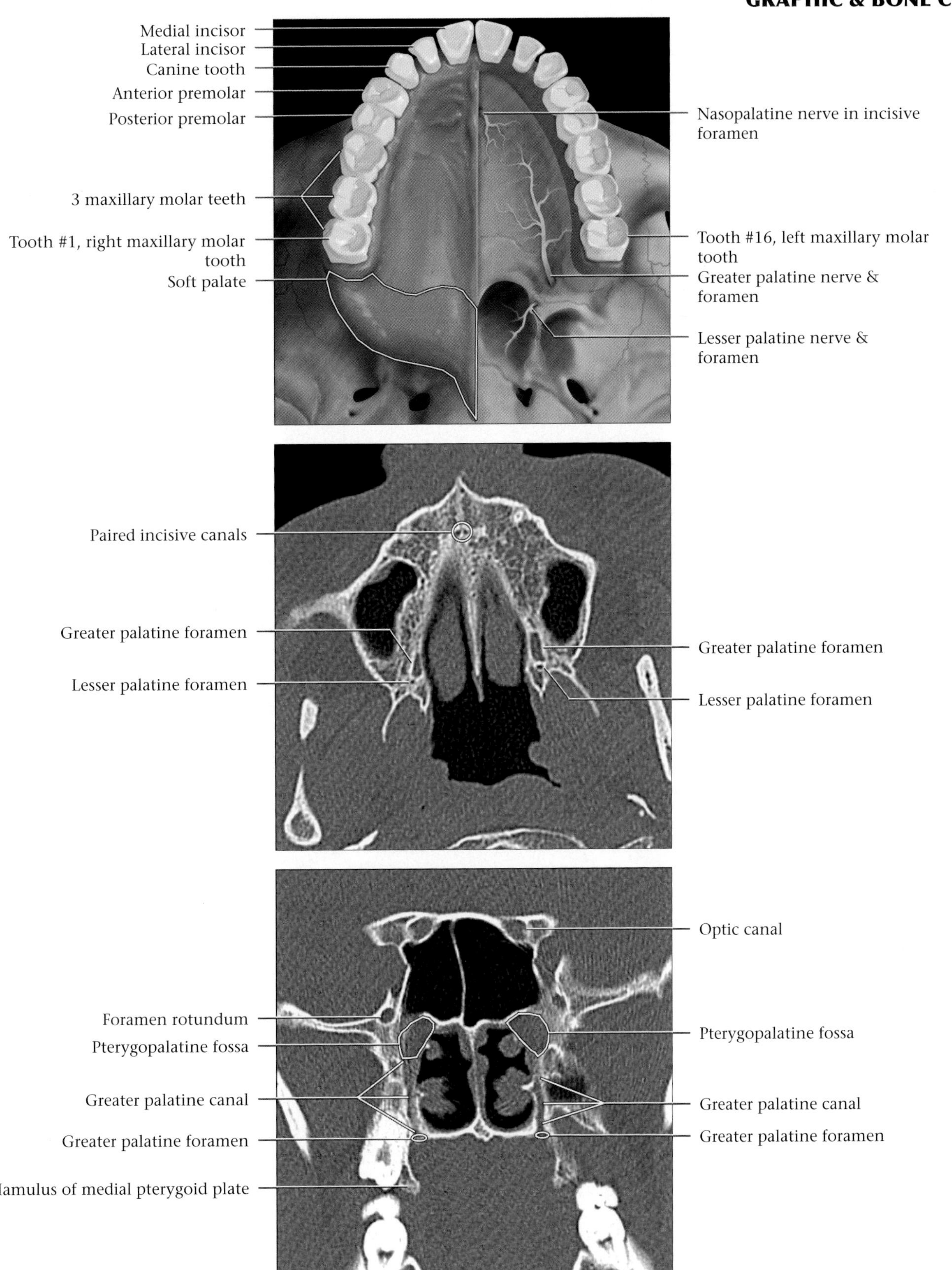

Medial incisor
Lateral incisor
Canine tooth
Anterior premolar
Posterior premolar
3 maxillary molar teeth
Tooth #1, right maxillary molar tooth
Soft palate
Nasopalatine nerve in incisive foramen
Tooth #16, left maxillary molar tooth
Greater palatine nerve & foramen
Lesser palatine nerve & foramen
Paired incisive canals
Greater palatine foramen
Lesser palatine foramen
Greater palatine foramen
Lesser palatine foramen
Optic canal
Foramen rotundum
Pterygopalatine fossa
Greater palatine canal
Greater palatine foramen
Hamulus of medial pterygoid plate
Pterygopalatine fossa
Greater palatine canal
Greater palatine foramen

(Top) Axial graphic of hard palate viewed from below with mucosa removed on right side of drawing. Hard palate sensory innervation is shown on right with anterior 1/3 of hard palate supplied by the nasopalatine nerve, the posterior 2/3 of the hard palate supplied by the greater palatine nerve. Notice there are 16 adult teeth, numbered beginning at the right 3rd molar from 1 to 16. **(Middle)** Axial bone CT image depicts foramina carrying nerves to hard palate. Anterior paired incisive canals lead to more inferior incisive foramen (not seen). Greater & lesser palatine foramina transmit greater & lesser palatine nerves respectively. **(Bottom)** Coronal bone CT through vertical aspect of greater palatine canal shows this canal connecting pterygopalatine fossa above with greater palatine foramen below. Greater palatine nerve uses the greater palatine canal to access the palate.

MANDIBLE AND MAXILLA

AXIAL BONE CT

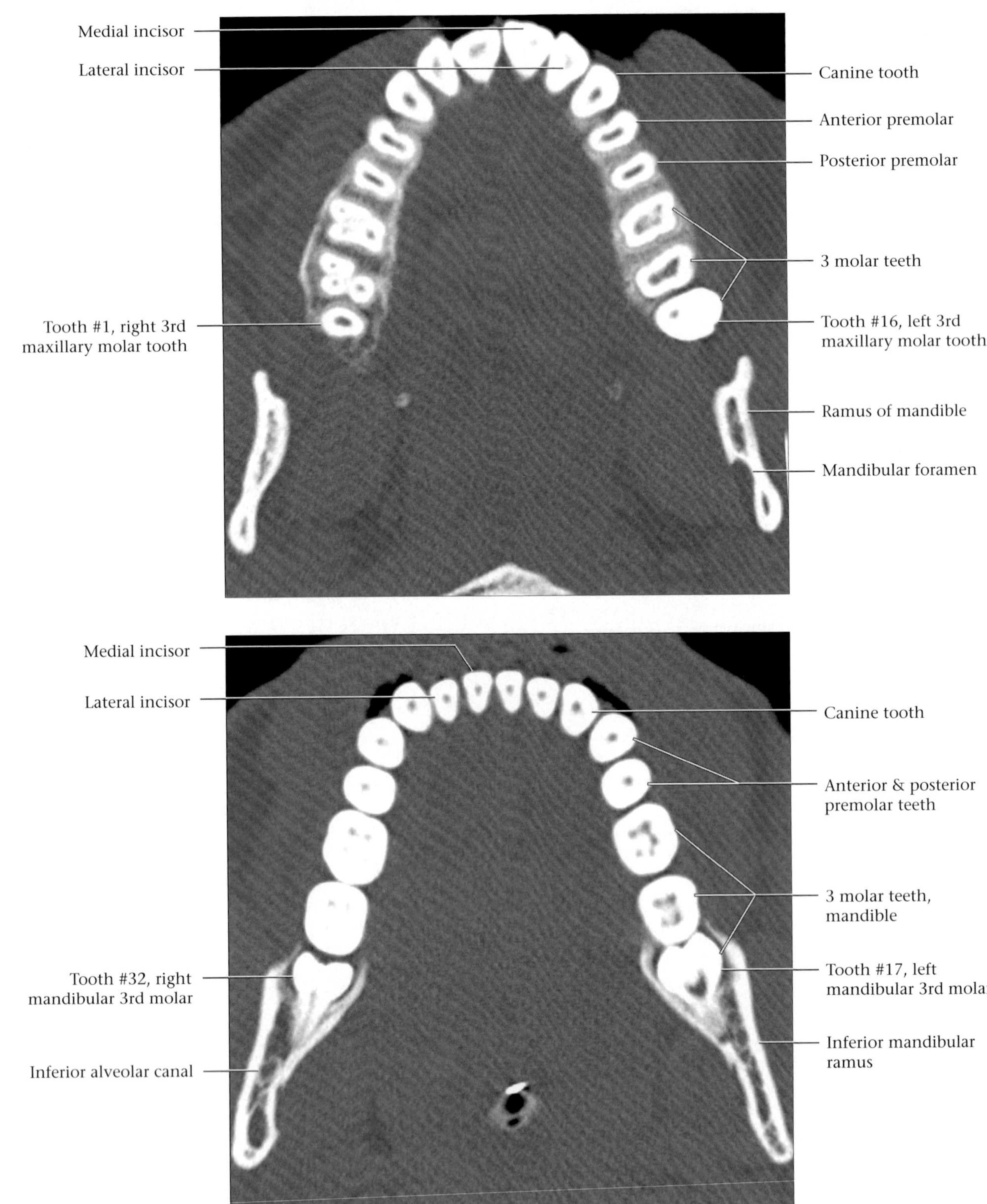
Medial incisor
Lateral incisor
Canine tooth
Anterior premolar
Posterior premolar
3 molar teeth
Tooth #1, right 3rd maxillary molar tooth
Tooth #16, left 3rd maxillary molar tooth
Ramus of mandible
Mandibular foramen
Medial incisor
Lateral incisor
Canine tooth
Anterior & posterior premolar teeth
3 molar teeth, mandible
Tooth #32, right mandibular 3rd molar
Tooth #17, left mandibular 3rd molar
Inferior alveolar canal
Inferior mandibular ramus

(Top) Axial bone CT at the level of the maxillary ridge delineates the 16 upper teeth. Numbering convention begins with tooth #1 (upper posterior right molar tooth) extending from there across to the opposite left posterior maxillary molar which is designated tooth #16. Note there are two each of medial and lateral incisors, canine, anterior and posterior premolars and three molar teeth. **(Bottom)** Axial bone CT of the 16 mandibular teeth is shown. Continuing the numbering convention for the mandibular teeth, the left 3rd molar is considered tooth #17 with numbering moving across to the opposite right 3rd mandibular molar designated tooth #32. Note again there are paired medial and lateral incisors, canines, anterior and posterior premolars and three molar teeth in the mandible.

3D CT OF MANDIBLE

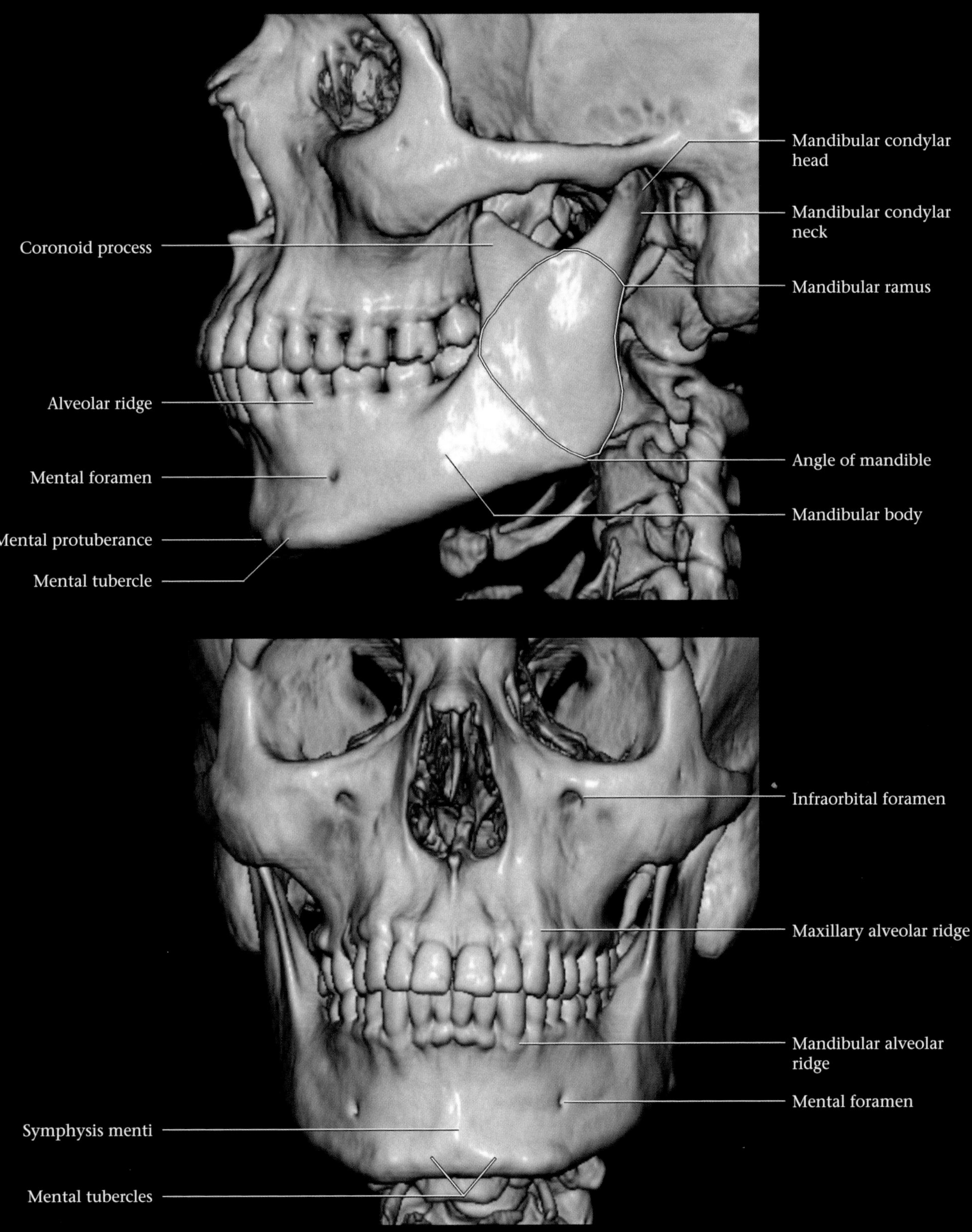
Mandibular condylar head
Mandibular condylar neck
Coronoid process
Mandibular ramus
Alveolar ridge
Angle of mandible
Mental foramen
Mandibular body
Mental protuberance
Mental tubercle
Infraorbital foramen
Maxillary alveolar ridge
Mandibular alveolar ridge
Mental foramen
Symphysis menti
Mental tubercles

(Top) Lateral view of 3D reconstruction of facial bones. The mandible can be divided into condyle, neck, ramus, coronoid process, body and alveolar ridge. The mental foramen is seen in the anterior body and transmits the mental nerve, a sensory nerve to the chin. **(Bottom)** Frontal view of 3D reconstruction of facial bones. The mandible anterior body is best delineated with the paired mental foramina evident. The infraorbital nerves are transmitted via the paired infraorbital foramina.

PART III

Spine

Vertebral Column, Discs & Paraspinal Muscle

Cord, Meninges and Spaces

Vascular

Plexus

Peripheral Nerves

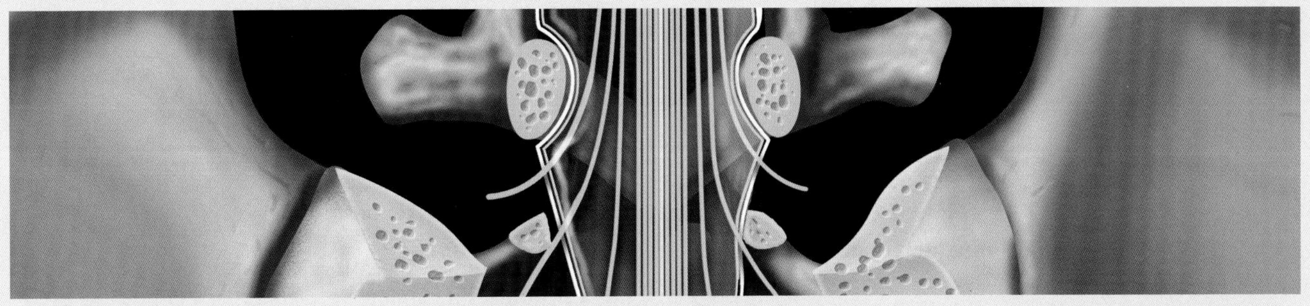

SECTION 1: Vertebral Column, Discs & Paraspinal Muscle

VERTEBRAL COLUMN OVERVIEW

Terminology

Abbreviations

- C1 (atlas), C2 (axis)
- Atlanto-occipital (AO)
- Anterior, posterior longitudinal ligaments (ALL, PLL)

Gross Anatomy

Overview

- Normally 33 spinal vertebrae (varies from 32-35)
  - 7 cervical (most constant); 12 thoracic; 5 lumbar
  - 5 sacral elements fuse → sacrum
  - 4-5 coccygeal elements → coccyx (most variable)
- Classic anatomic division into anterior (vertebral body), posterior elements (neural arch)
- "**Three columns**" concept (used by spine surgeons)
  - **Anterior column**
    - Anterior half of vertebral body/disc/annulus
    - ALL
  - **Middle column**
    - Posterior half of vertebral body/disc/annulus
    - PLL
  - **Posterior column**
    - Posterior elements (pedicles, facet joints, laminae, spinous processes)
    - Ligamentum flavum
    - Interconnecting ligaments (interspinous, etc.)

Components

- **Bones**
  - **Body**: Cylindrical ventral bone mass
  - **Arch**: Composed of 2 pedicles, 2 laminae, 7 processes (1 spinous, 2 transverse, 4 articular)
    - Pedicles: Extend from dorsolateral body to unite with pair of arched, flat laminae
    - Laminae: Arch over canal, join at midline to dorsal projection (spinous process)
    - Transverse processes: Arise from sides of arch
    - Articular processes: Each has superior process (with facet directed dorsally), inferior process (facet directed ventrally), pars interarticularis (between facets)
- **Intervertebral disc**
  - Composed of inner nucleus pulposus, outer annulus fibrosus
  - Adhere to hyaline cartilage of vertebral endplates
  - Avascular (except in young children and peripheral annular fibers in adults)
- **Ligaments**
  - ALL
    - Fibrous band along entire ventral surface of spine
    - Skull to sacrum
  - PLL
    - Dorsal surface of vertebral bodies
    - Skull to sacrum
  - Craniocervical ligaments
  - Interspinous ligaments
- **Nerves** (31 pairs)
  - 8 cervical, 12 thoracic
  - 5 lumbar (exit above disc, below pedicle)
  - 5 sacral, 1 coccygeal
- **Meninges**
  - Single (meningeal) layer of dura
  - Arachnoid (continuous with cranial arachnoid, loosely adherent to dura)
  - Pia (covers spinal cord, nerves)
- **Vasculature**
  - Arteries: Segmental arteries arise as dorsal rami from vertebral, subclavian, intercostal arteries
  - Veins: Y-shaped basivertebral veins connect with valveless epidural venous plexus; extensive anastomoses with cavae, azygos/hemiazygos systems

Imaging Anatomy

Overview

- MR
  - Body: Signal intensity of marrow varies with age
    - Hemopoietic ("red") marrow is hypointense on T1WI, becomes hyperintense with conversion from red → yellow (age 8-12 years)
    - End-plate, reactive marrow changes normally with aging (can be fibrovascular, fatty, or sclerotic)
  - Intervertebral disc: Signal intensity varies with age
    - Hyperintense on T2WI in children, young adults; progressive ↓ water → hypointense on T2WI
    - Disc degeneration, dessication, shape change (bulge) normal after second decade
  - Ligaments: Hypointense on both T1 & T2WI
  - Nerves: No enhancement until reach dorsal root ganglia, where they loose blood-nerve barrier
  - Meninges: Dura, basi-/epidural veins enhance

Anatomy-Based Imaging Issues

Imaging Recommendations

- CT: Use both bone, soft tissue algorithms; sagittal, coronal reconstructions helpful
- MR: Use STIR, fat-sat T1 C+ scans for marrow disorders
  - Standard planes = axial/sagittal but coronal useful in elderly, scoliotic patients
  - Obtain axial scans through discs using coronal localizer for scoliotic patients

Imaging Pitfalls

- Classic number (7-12-5-5-4) found in only 20%
- Foci of T1 hyperintensity (focal fatty marrow deposits, incidental hemangiomas) are common & normal
- Vertebral marrow in middle-aged, elderly patients may appear very inhomogeneous

Embryology

Embryologic Events

- Cranial half of C1, occipital sclerotomes combine → occiput
  - C1 exits below occiput, above C1 ring
- Lower half of upper, upper half of lower sclerotomes combine → vertebral bodies
  - C8 exits below lowest cervical vertebra (C7)
  - All thoracic and lumbar nerves arise below their respective pedicles

VERTEBRAL COLUMN OVERVIEW

GRAPHICS

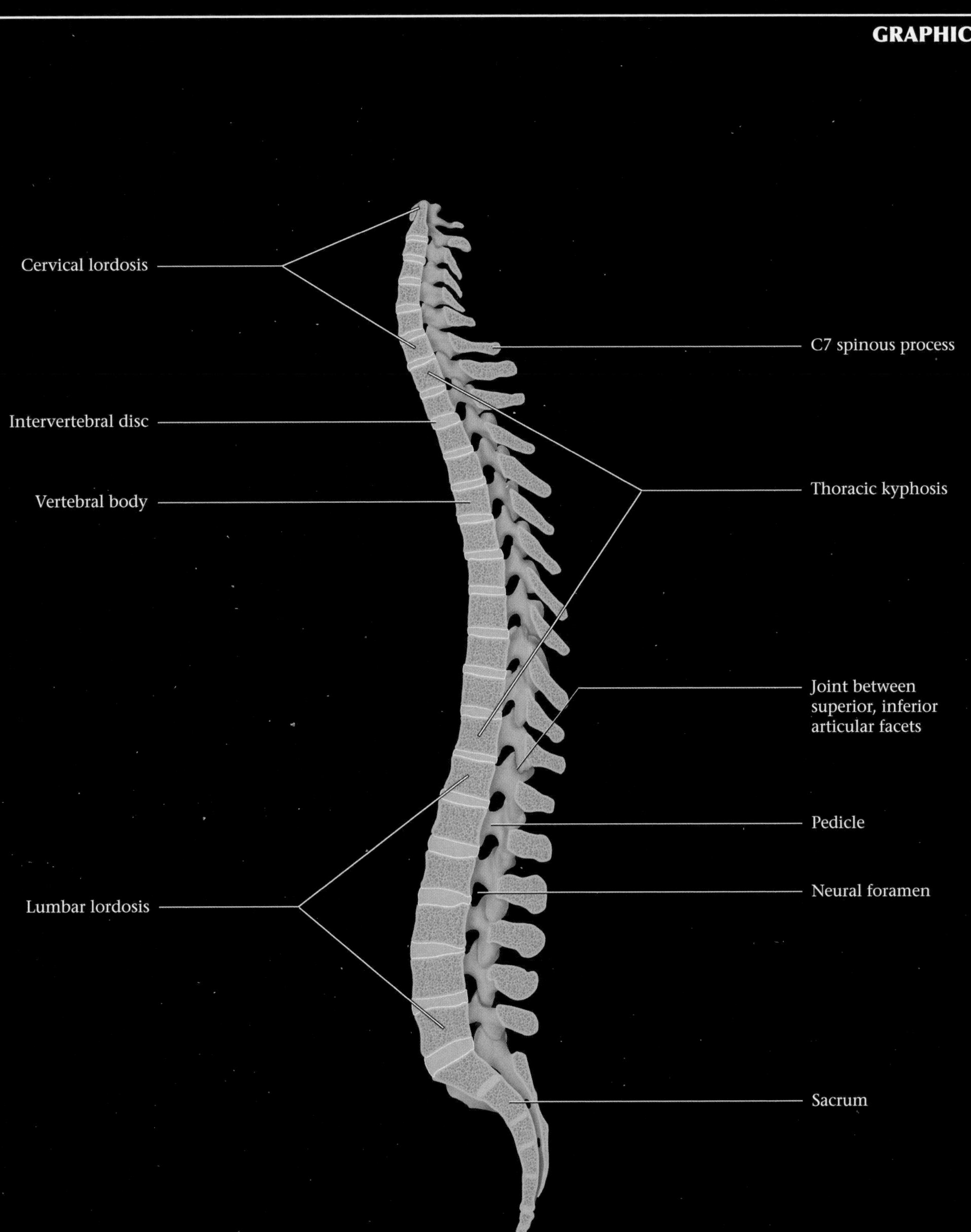
Cervical lordosis
C7 spinous process
Intervertebral disc
Vertebral body
Thoracic kyphosis
Joint between superior, inferior articular facets
Pedicle
Neural foramen
Lumbar lordosis
Sacrum

Sagittal midline graphic of the adult spine with soft tissues removed provides a nice overview of vertebral column. Note three curvatures: Cervical (lordosis) is the least marked. Thoracic curve is a kyphosis. The lumbar lordosis extends from T12 to the lumbosacral junction, with the most convexity in its caudal three segments. Most vertebrae, except for the specialized C1, C2, and sacrococcygeal segments, have a larger ventral body and thinner posterior neural arch. Generally the vertebral bodies increase in width from C2-L3, reflecting their increased load-bearing function. Pedicles attach the neural arches to the vertebral bodies. The vertebral canal extends from the foramen magnum to the sacrum, varying in diameter with the largest dimension generally at the thoracolumbar junction. Note spinous process in thoracic area overlap like shingles on a roof.

VERTEBRAL COLUMN OVERVIEW

GRAPHICS

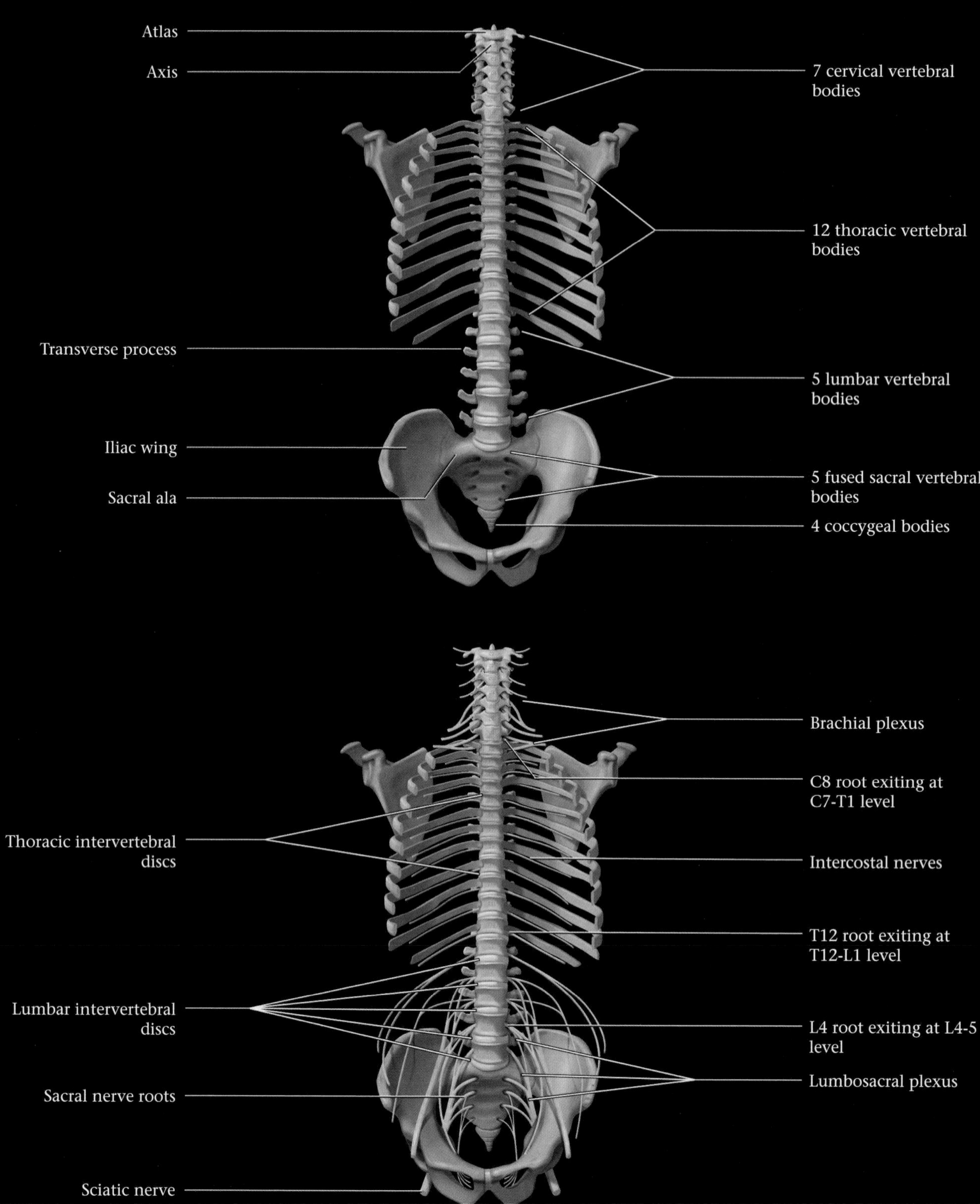

Atlas
Axis
7 cervical vertebral bodies
12 thoracic vertebral bodies
Transverse process
5 lumbar vertebral bodies
Iliac wing
Sacral ala
5 fused sacral vertebral bodies
4 coccygeal bodies
Brachial plexus
C8 root exiting at C7-T1 level
Thoracic intervertebral discs
Intercostal nerves
T12 root exiting at T12-L1 level
Lumbar intervertebral discs
L4 root exiting at L4-5 level
Sacral nerve roots
Lumbosacral plexus
Sciatic nerve

(Top) Coronal graphic of the spinal column as a whole shows relationship of the 7 cervical, 12 thoracic, 5 lumbar, 5 fused sacral and 4 coccygeal bodies. Note cervical bodies are smaller with neural foramina oriented at 45° and capped by the unique C1 and C2 morphology. Thoracic bodies are heart-shaped with thinner intervertebral discs, and are stabilized by the rib cage. Lumbar bodies are more massive, with prominent transverse processes and thick intervertebral discs. Sacrum shows a unique morphology with fusion of multiple segments forming a triangular bone mass. **(Bottom)** Coronal graphic demonstrates exiting spinal nerve roots as they exit above the intervertebral disc spaces, just under the pedicles. C1 exits between the occiput and C1 while the C8 root exits at the C7-T1 level. Thoracic and lumbar roots exiting below their respective pedicles.

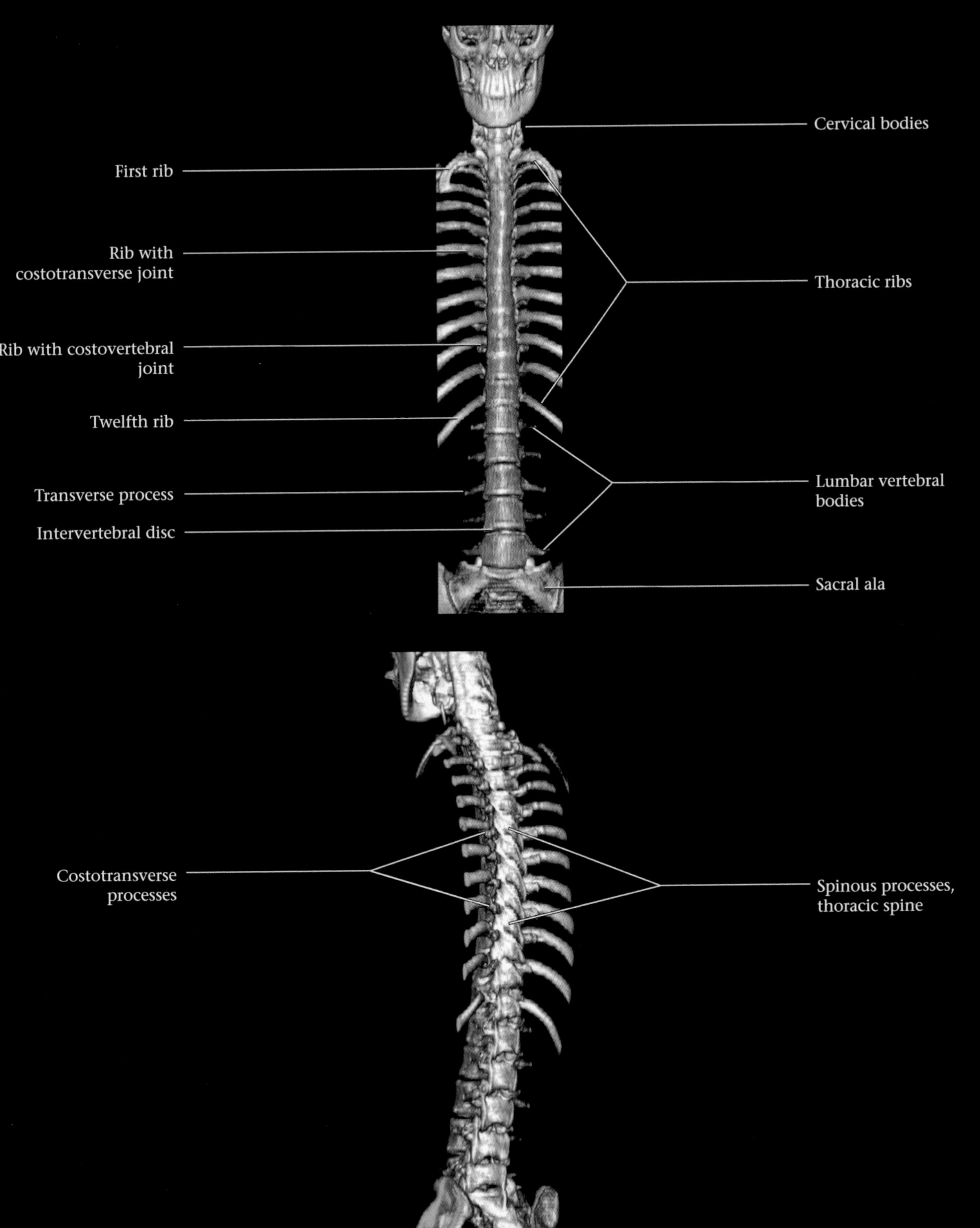
Cervical bodies
First rib
Rib with costotransverse joint
Thoracic ribs
Rib with costovertebral joint
Twelfth rib
Transverse process
Lumbar vertebral bodies
Intervertebral disc
Sacral ala
Costotransverse processes
Spinous processes, thoracic spine

(Top) Anterior 3D-VRT NECT scan of the spine shows the relationships of the cervicothoracic junction, thoracic, lumbar and sacral spine. The strong costotransverse and costovertebral joints provide stabilization for the long thoracic column, and limit rotation. The lumbar intervertebral discs are thick and separately defined on this reconstruction. The thinner thoracic intervertebral discs are poorly defined on this reconstruction. **(Bottom)** Oblique view of a 3D-VRT NECT seen from behind and slightly to the left, demonstrates relationship of the ribs to the transverse processes especially well. Thoracic transverse processes project laterally from the pediculolaminar junctions. Note that thoracic spinous processes overlap each other, especially from T5-8.

VERTEBRAL COLUMN OVERVIEW

3D-VRT NECT & SAGITTAL CT

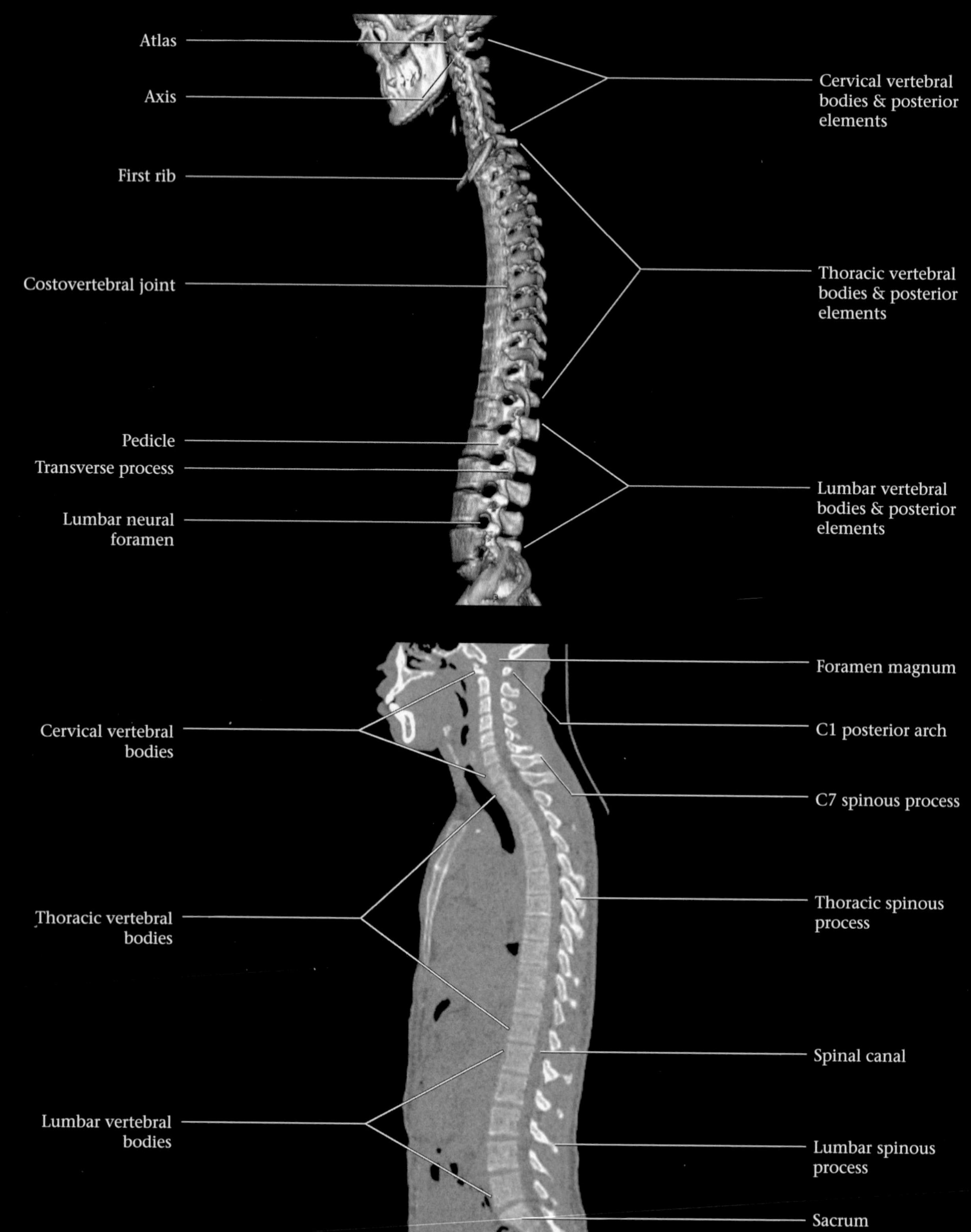
Atlas
Axis
First rib
Costovertebral joint
Pedicle
Transverse process
Lumbar neural foramen
Cervical vertebral bodies & posterior elements
Thoracic vertebral bodies & posterior elements
Lumbar vertebral bodies & posterior elements
Cervical vertebral bodies
Thoracic vertebral bodies
Lumbar vertebral bodies
Foramen magnum
C1 posterior arch
C7 spinous process
Thoracic spinous process
Spinal canal
Lumbar spinous process
Sacrum

(Top) Sagittal 3D-VRT NECT examination shows the balancing set of 4 spinal curves. The 2 primary flexed segments present at birth are the thoracic and sacral, with the secondarily developing lordotic curves occurring in the cervical and lumbar spinal segments. **(Bottom)** Sagittal reformat of CT examination shows overall vertebral body, spinal canal morphology. The cranium rests upon the lordotic curves of the cervical spine, with their smaller bodies and prominent spinous processes. Note the flexed posture of the thoracic spine with characteristic long, oblique inferiorly directed spinous processes extending over the body level below. The lumbar lordosis with large bodies and posterior elements provides a platform for large muscle attachment.

CORONAL NECT

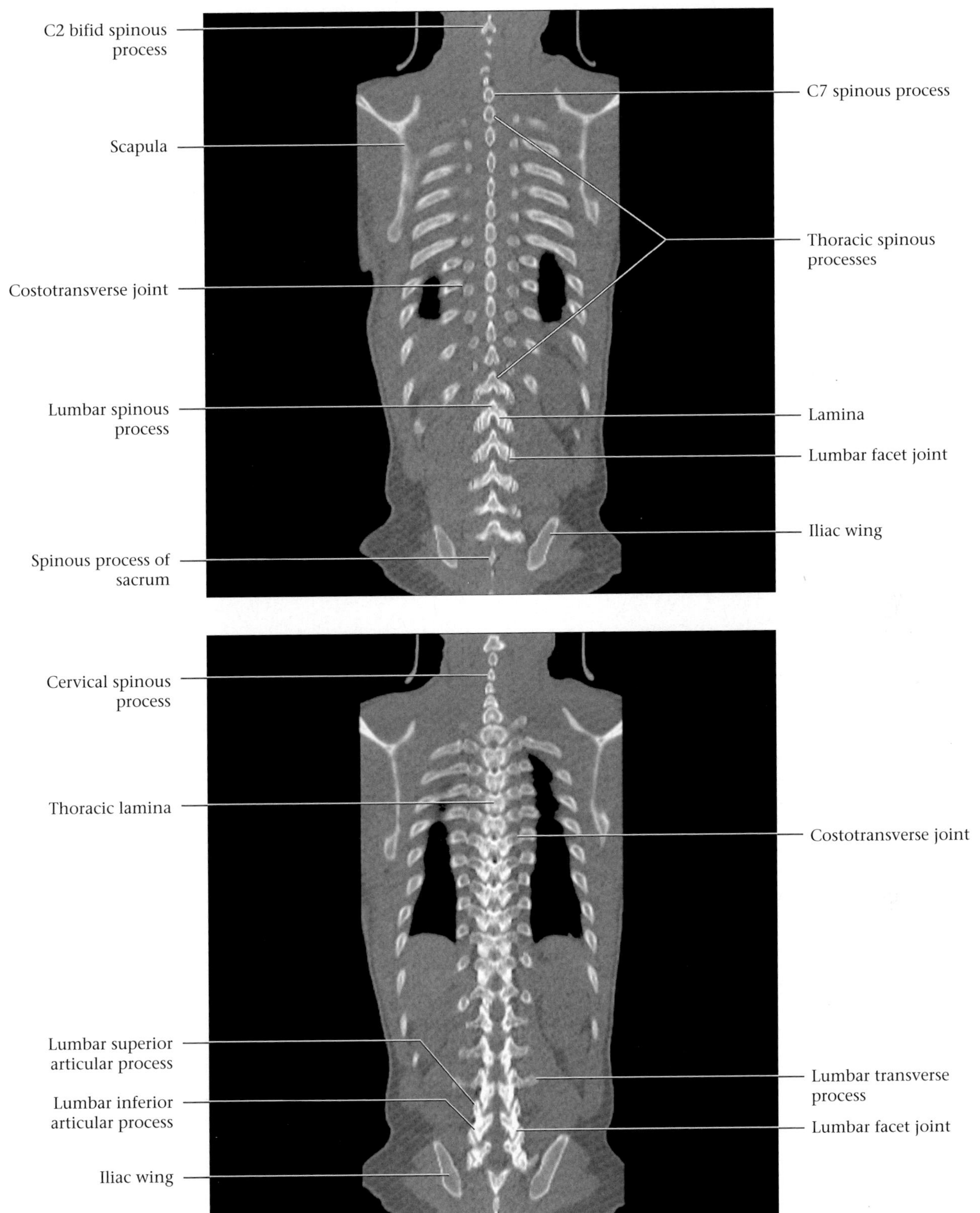

C2 bifid spinous process
C7 spinous process
Scapula
Thoracic spinous processes
Costotransverse joint
Lumbar spinous process
Lamina
Lumbar facet joint
Iliac wing
Spinous process of sacrum
Cervical spinous process
Thoracic lamina
Costotransverse joint
Lumbar superior articular process
Lumbar transverse process
Lumbar inferior articular process
Lumbar facet joint
Iliac wing

(Top) First of four coronal reformatted CT images shows the dorsal aspects of the spinal column. Spinous processes are seen as ovoid bony corticated densities, with the symmetrical costovertebral joints surrounding each posterior element. The more anterior section through the lumbar regions shows the junction of the spinous process with the lamina, and the lumbar facet joints. **(Bottom)** Section more anteriorly shows the appearance of the laminae and costotransverse joints that lie superolateral to the laminae. Inferiorly the lumbar region demonstrates the facet joints and the opposed superior and inferior articular processes.

VERTEBRAL COLUMN OVERVIEW

CORONAL NECT

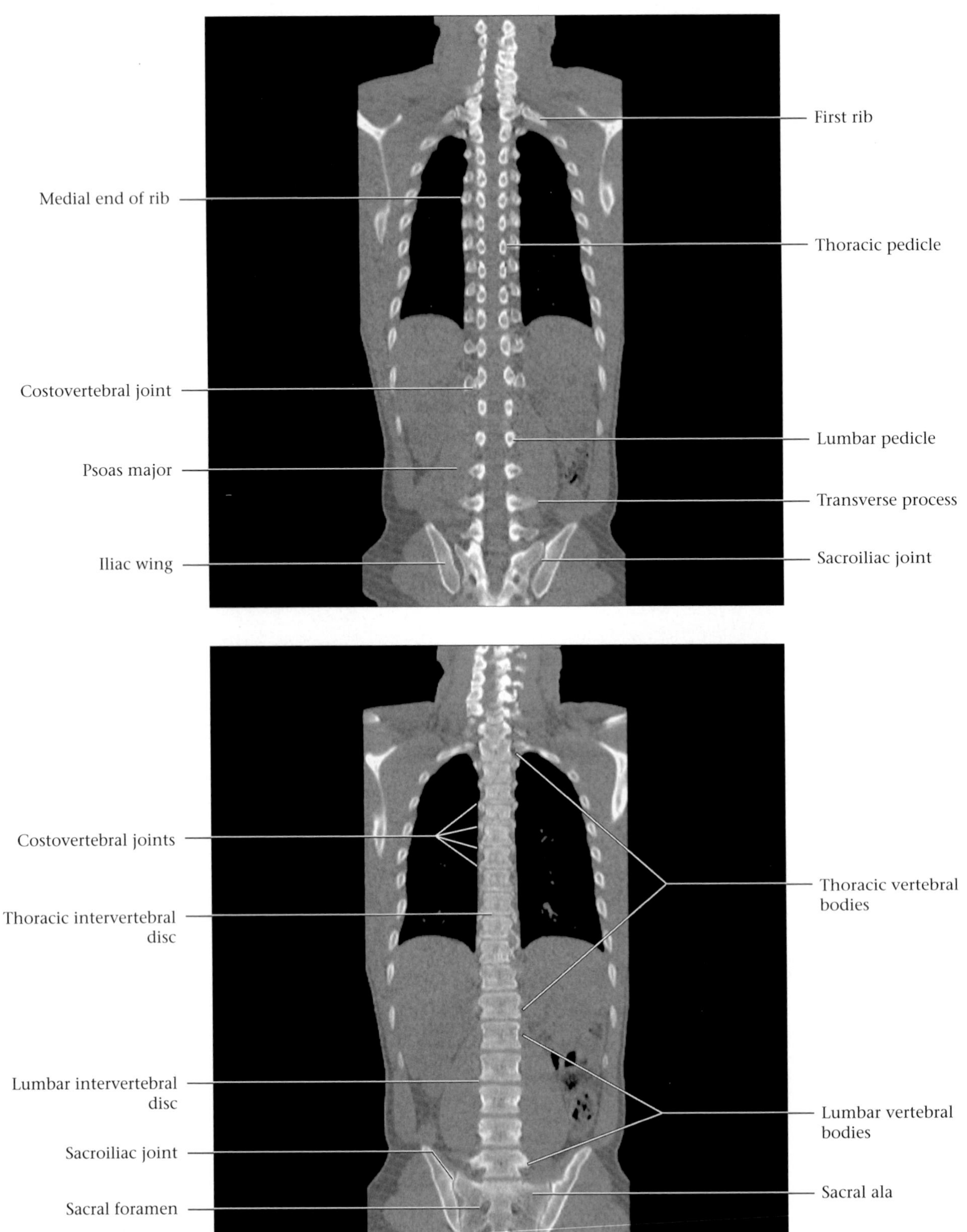
First rib
Medial end of rib
Thoracic pedicle
Costovertebral joint
Lumbar pedicle
Psoas major
Transverse process
Iliac wing
Sacroiliac joint
Costovertebral joints
Thoracic vertebral bodies
Thoracic intervertebral disc
Lumbar intervertebral disc
Lumbar vertebral bodies
Sacroiliac joint
Sacral ala
Sacral foramen

(Top) Image through the pedicles shows the width of the bony spinal canal in the thoracic and lumbar segments. The medial rib heads and pedicles are seen as paired ovoid bony densities on either side of midline. The transition to the lumbar spine is defined by the lack of medial rib component, and a large horizontally directed transverse process. **(Bottom)** Image through the mid-vertebral body level shows the rectangular shaped bodies of the thoracic and lumbar segments. The costovertebral joints are present in the thoracic spine centered at the disc levels since they attach to two adjacent vertebral bodies with demifacets. The thick and stout lumbar bodies are seen atop the triangular shaped sacrum with the ventral directed sacral neural foramina.

SAGITTAL T2 MR & CT MYELOGRAM

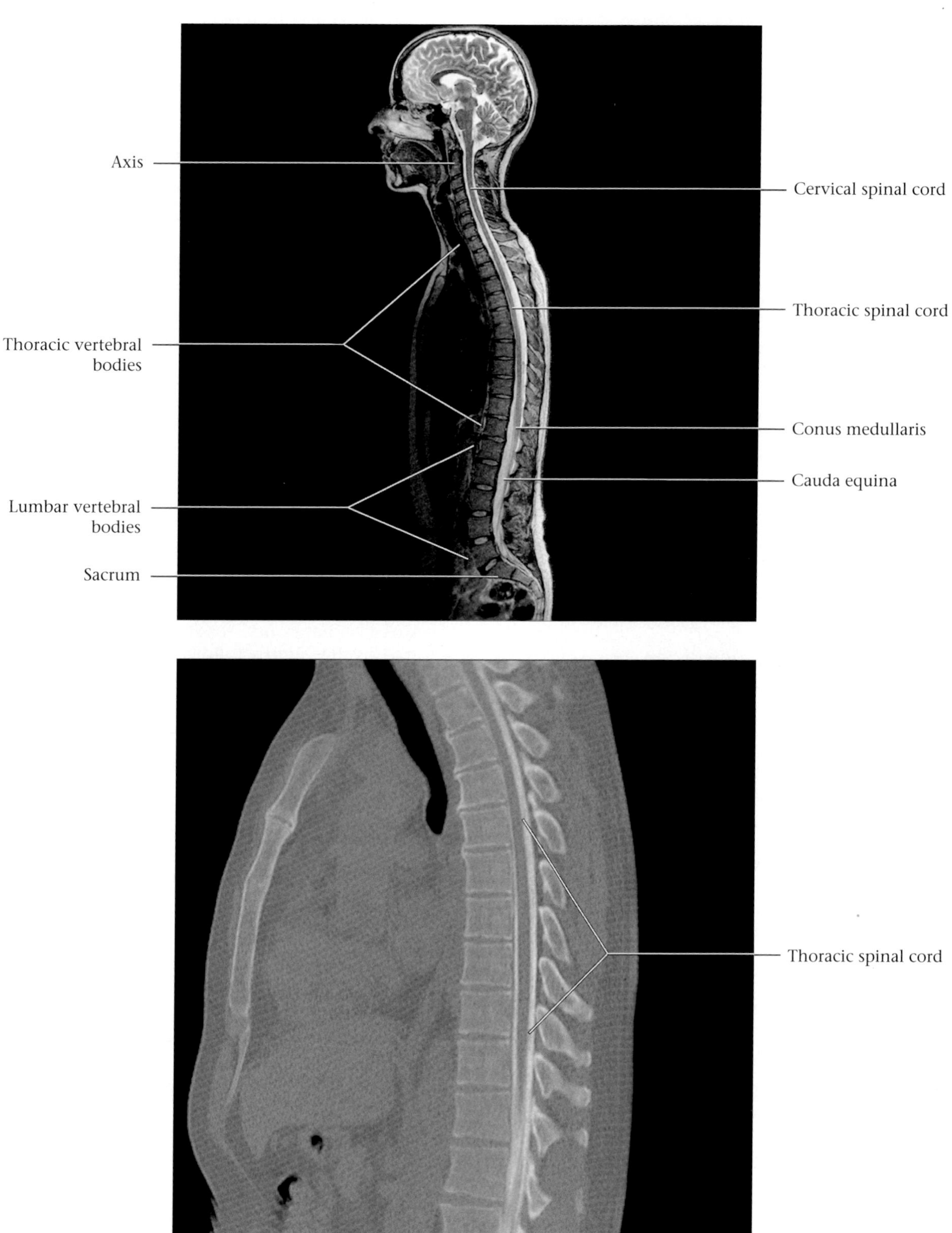
Axis
Cervical spinal cord
Thoracic spinal cord
Thoracic vertebral bodies
Conus medullaris
Cauda equina
Lumbar vertebral bodies
Sacrum
Thoracic spinal cord

(Top) Sagittal T2 MR image of the entire spine shows the general morphology of the spinal canal and spinal cord. The cord follows the gentle undulating course of the two upper spinal curves to end at the conus medullaris around the L1 level. The multiple roots of the cauda equina descend from the distal cord to their exiting foramen in the lumbar and sacral spines. **(Bottom)** Sagittal midline CT myelogram is shown for comparison with the overview T2 MR "myelogram". Both provide excellent visualization of the spinal cord and subarachnoid space. Normal filling defects seen on myelography are typically due to denticulate ligaments and septum posticum whereas on MR they are artifacts caused by inhomogeneous cerebrospinal fluid flow and spin dephasing.

OSSIFICATION

Gross Anatomy

Overview

- **Primary (1°) ossification center**
  - Primary focus of spinal ossification
  - At site of blood vessel invasion of future vertebrae cartilaginous model
  - Present at birth
- **Secondary (2°) ossification center**
  - Secondary focus of spinal ossification
  - Appears around puberty
- **Ring (annular) apophysis**
  - 2° ossification of superior/inferior centrum edges
  - Separated from remainder of vertebral body by thin hyaline cartilage rim
  - Appears between 6-8 years (girls) to 7-9 years (boys)
  - Coalesces by ≈ 21 years into single ring
  - Fusion with vertebral body (age 14-21 years) → longitudinal growth stops
- **Synchondrosis**
  - Cartilaginous junction between nonmobile vertebral articulating surfaces
  - Neurocentral suture = synchondrosis between vertebral centrum, neural arches

Imaging Anatomy

Overview

- **General ossification patterns**
  - Centrum ossification
    - Starts at lower thoracic/upper lumbar spine of fetus
    - Moves in both cranial, caudal directions
  - Neural arch ossification
    - Begins at cervicothoracic level → upper cervical → thoracolumbar
  - At birth most vertebrae have three 1° and five 2° ossification centers connected by hyaline synchondroses
  - Exceptions to typical ossification occur at C1, C2, C7, lumbar vertebra, sacrum, coccyx
- **Atlas (C1)**
  - Two to five (3 most common) 1° ossification centers
    - Anterior arch (1), posterior arch (1) + lateral masses (2)
  - No 2° ossification centers
- **Axis (C2)**
  - Five 1° ossification centers
    - Centrum (1), posterior vertebral neural arch (2), odontoid process (2)
    - Dens separated from C2 centrum by remnant of embryonic C1-2 disc
  - Two 2° ossification centers
    - Inferior annular epiphysis, apex of odontoid
- **C3-6**
  - Three 1° ossification centers per each vertebra
    - Centrum (1), posterior vertebral neural arch (2)
  - Five 2° ossification centers per each vertebra
    - Spinous process apex (1), transverse process apex (2), annular epiphysis (2)
- **C7**
  - Same 1°/2° ossification centers as C3-6
    - Plus 1° ossification centers for two costal processes
    - These appear by 6 months of age
    - Fuse with transverse process, vertebral body by 5-6 years
    - If remain unfused → cervical ribs (1%)
- **Thoracic (T1-12)**
  - Three 1° ossification centers per vertebra
    - Centrum (1), posterior vertebral neural arch (2)
  - Five 2° ossification centers per vertebra
    - Spinous process apex (1), transverse process apex (2), annular epiphysis (2)
- **Lumbar (L1-5)**
  - Three 1° ossification centers per vertebra
    - Centrum (1), posterior vertebral neural arch (2)
  - Seven 2° ossification centers per vertebra,
    - Spinous process apex (1), transverse process apex (2), annular epiphysis (2), base of mamillary processes (2)
- **Sacrum (S1-5)**
  - Five 1° ossification centers per vertebra
    - Centrum (1), posterior neural arch (2), costal element remnants (2)
  - Four 2° ossification centers
    - Sacroiliac (SI) joint epiphyseal plates (fuse ≈ 25 years)
- **Coccyx (Co1-Co4)**
  - Co1 has three 1° ossification centers: Centrum (1), cornua (2)
  - Co2-Co4 have one 1° ossification center each
  - Co1 ossifies shortly following birth; remaining coccygeal vertebra ossify into 3rd decade
  - No 2° ossification centers

Anatomy-Based Imaging Issues

Key Concepts or Questions

- Centrum smaller than adult vertebral body
  - Centrum → central vertebral body
  - Anterior extent of neural arch → posterolateral vertebral body
- Progression of synchondrosis closure important for imaging interpretation
  - C1
    - Anterior C1 arch: 8-12 months
    - Posterior C1 arch: 1-7 years
    - C1 lateral masses: 7-9 years
  - C2
    - Odontoid: C2 body: 3-7 years
    - Superior odontoid center appears ≈ 2-6 years, fuses ≈ 11-12 years
    - Posterior C2 synchondrosis: 4-7 years
  - Below C2
    - Neurocentral synchondrosis closes ≈ 3-7 years, posterior synchondrosis ≈ 4-7 years

Imaging Pitfalls

- Symmetry, location, corticated margins, patient age help distinguish open synchondrosis from fracture
- Cervical vs. thoracic ribs: Transverse processes oriented inferiorly in cervical, superiorly in thoracic spine

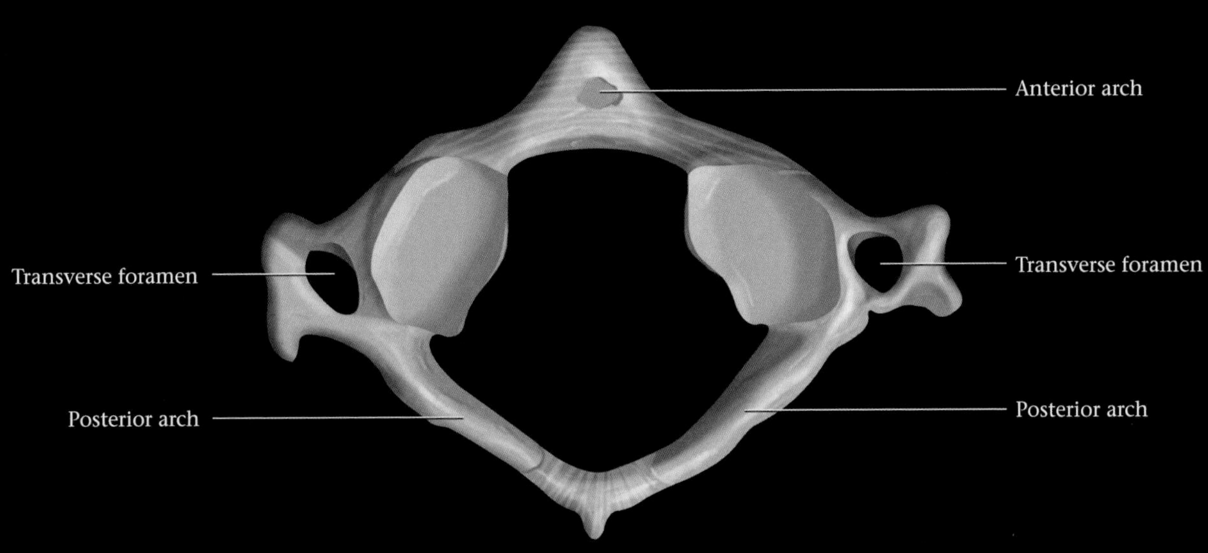
Anterior arch
Transverse foramen
Transverse foramen
Posterior arch
Posterior arch

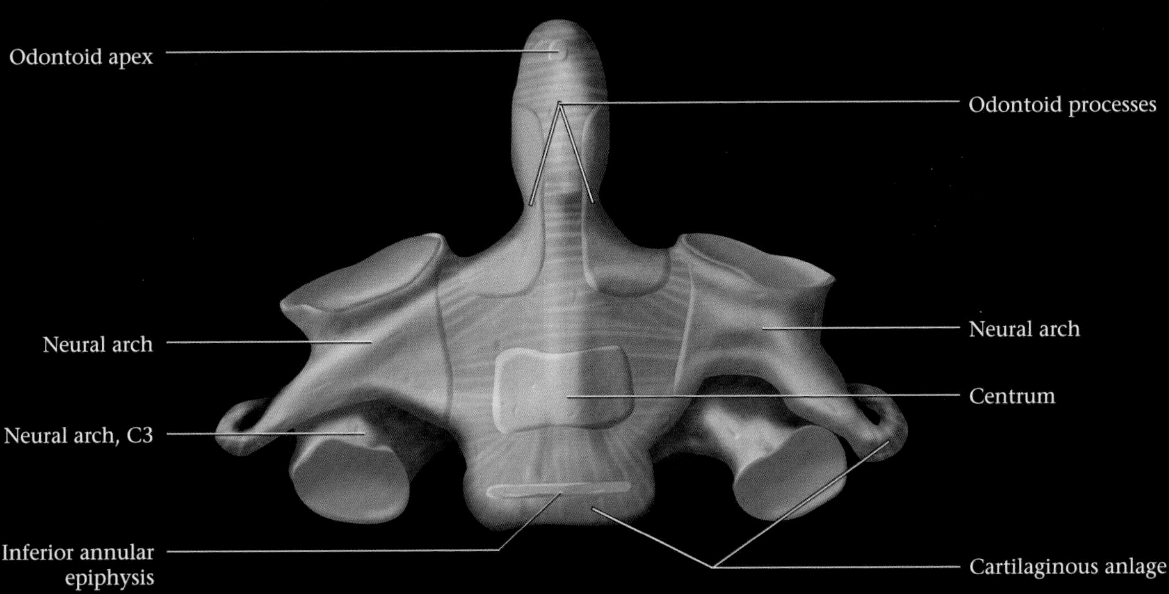
Odontoid apex
Odontoid processes
Neural arch
Neural arch
Centrum
Neural arch, C3
Inferior annular epiphysis
Cartilaginous anlage

(Top) Axial graphic of the atlas (C1) in a skeletally immature child, seen from above, depicts the most common configuration of anterior and posterior arch primary ossification centers, joined by cartilaginous synchondroses (shown in blue). The transverse foramen contains the vertebral artery and vertebral veins. **(Bottom)** Coronal graphic of the axis (C2) in a skeletally immature child, viewed from in front, depicts the five 1° ossification centers (centrum, neural arches, odontoid processes) and two 2° ossification centers (odontoid tip, inferior annular epiphysis) arising within the cartilaginous model (shown in blue).

OSSIFICATION

GRAPHICS

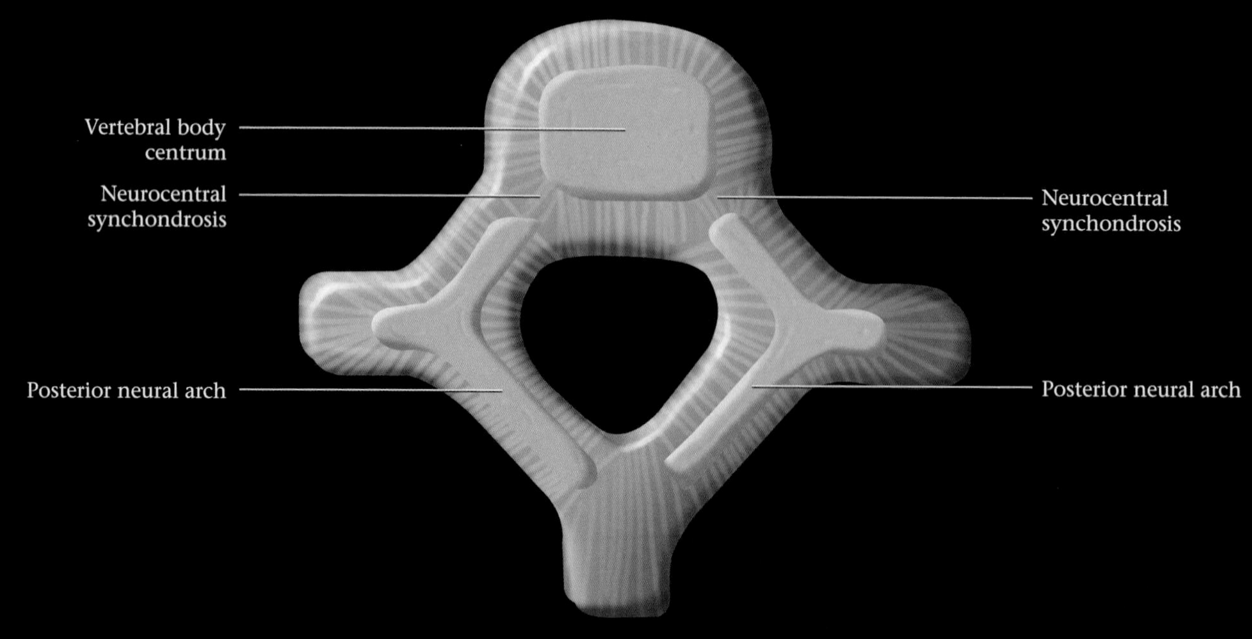
Vertebral body centrum
Neurocentral synchondrosis
Neurocentral synchondrosis
Posterior neural arch
Posterior neural arch

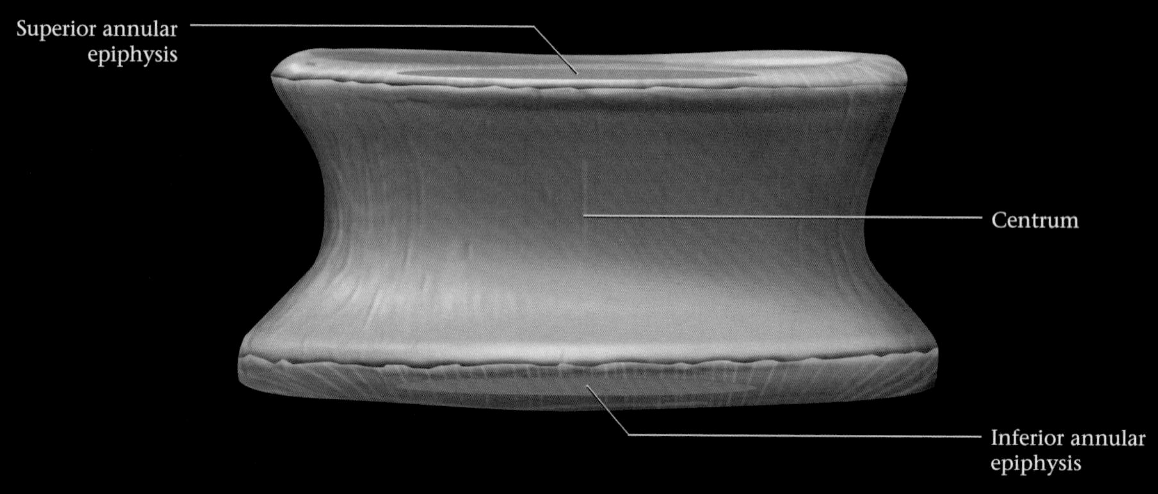
Superior annular epiphysis
Centrum
Inferior annular epiphysis

(Top) Axial graphic of a skeletally immature child, shown from above, depicts a stylized typical lumbar vertebra with three primary ossification centers (including the centrum) and two posterior neural arches separated by cartilaginous synchondroses. **(Bottom)** Graphic representation of a typical lumbar vertebral body, depicting the relationship of the centrum to the cartilaginous (shown in blue) endplate and annular (ring) apophyses. The superior and inferior annular epiphyses are 2° ossification centers (fuse at puberty).

OSSIFICATION

GRAPHICS

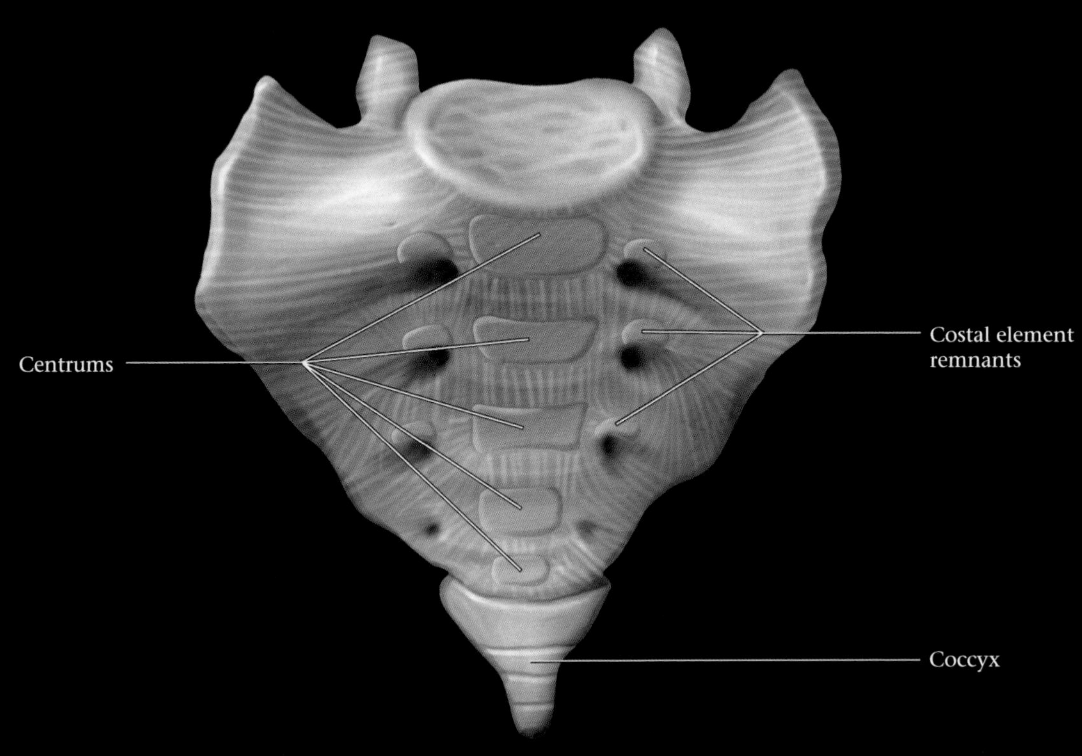
Centrums
Costal element remnants
Coccyx

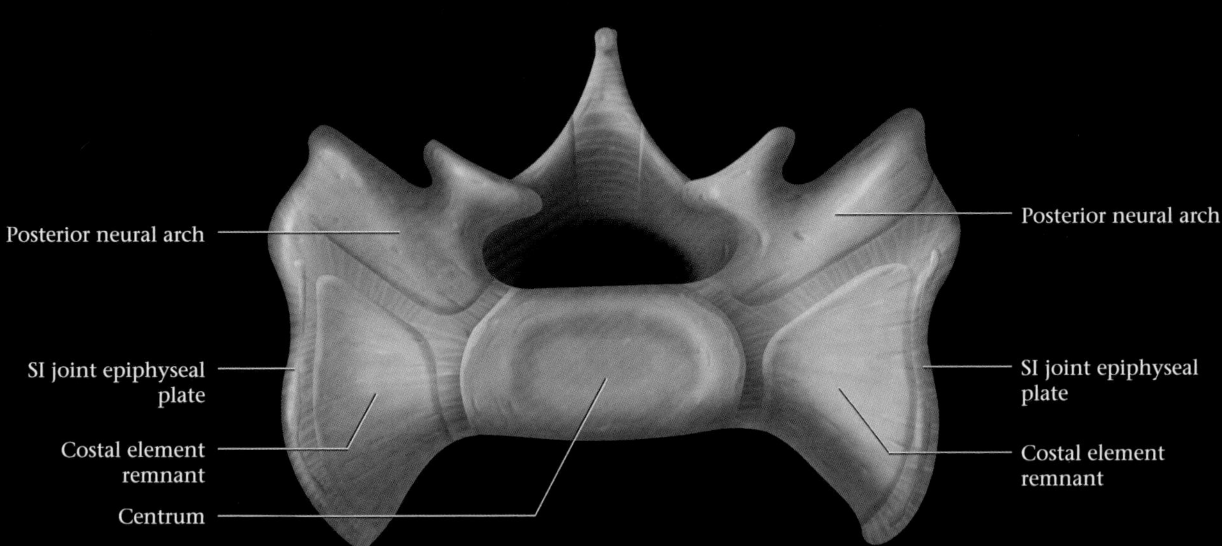
Posterior neural arch
Posterior neural arch
SI joint epiphyseal plate
SI joint epiphyseal plate
Costal element remnant
Costal element remnant
Centrum

(Top) Coronal graphic of the infant sacrum, seen from in front, depicts ossification in the sacral centrum and lateral costal element remnant 1° ossification centers. The majority of the sacrum and entire coccyx is cartilaginous (shown in blue) at this stage in development. **(Bottom)** Axial graphic representation of the sacrum in an older child, seen from above, depicts the five 1° ossification centers (centrum, 2 posterior arches, 2 costal elements remnants) connected by cartilaginous synchondroses (shown in blue). The sacral sacroiliac (SI) joint epiphyseal plates (2° ossification centers) fuse at approximately 25 years.

AXIAL BONE CT, ATLAS (C1) VERTEBRA

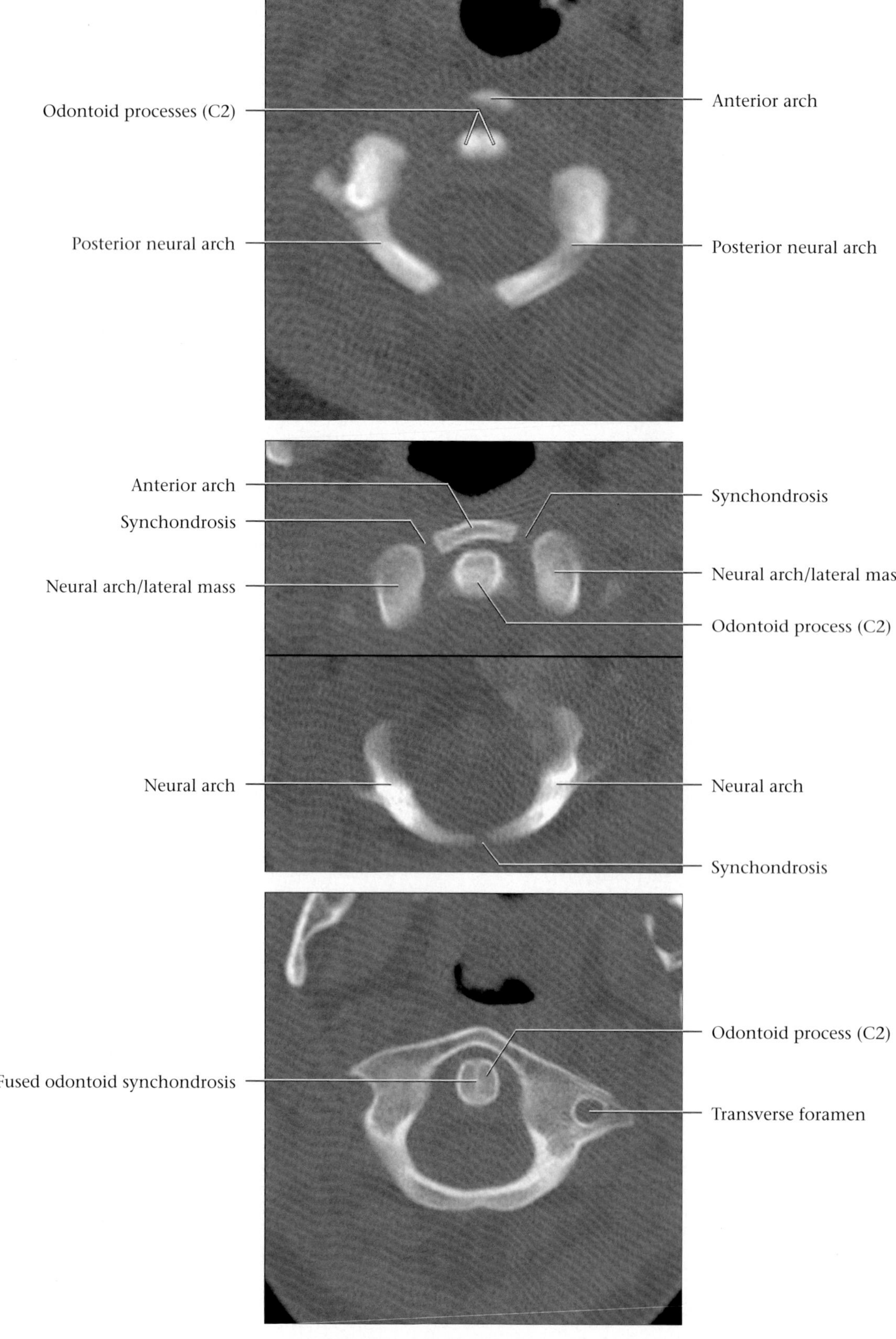
Odontoid processes (C2)
Anterior arch
Posterior neural arch
Posterior neural arch
Anterior arch
Synchondrosis
Synchondrosis
Neural arch/lateral mass
Neural arch/lateral mass
Odontoid process (C2)
Neural arch
Neural arch
Synchondrosis
Odontoid process (C2)
Fused odontoid synchondrosis
Transverse foramen

(Top) Axial bone CT of a 2 week old female demonstrates the three atlas 1° ossification centers. Much of the atlas is unossified cartilage at this age. The odontoid process ossification centers (C2) are identified posterior to the C1 anterior arch. **(Middle)** Composite image from two contiguous axial bone CT images of C1 of a 14 month old male shows further development of the three 1° ossification centers. The synchondroses between the centrum and posterior neural arches are smaller. **(Bottom)** Axial bone CT of the atlas of a 6 year old female shows fusion of the anterior and posterior neural arch 1° ossification centers to form a complete C1 ring. Note that the two C2 odontoid process 1° ossification centers show residual sclerotic line at the synchondrosis.

AXIAL BONE CT, AXIS (C2) VERTEBRA

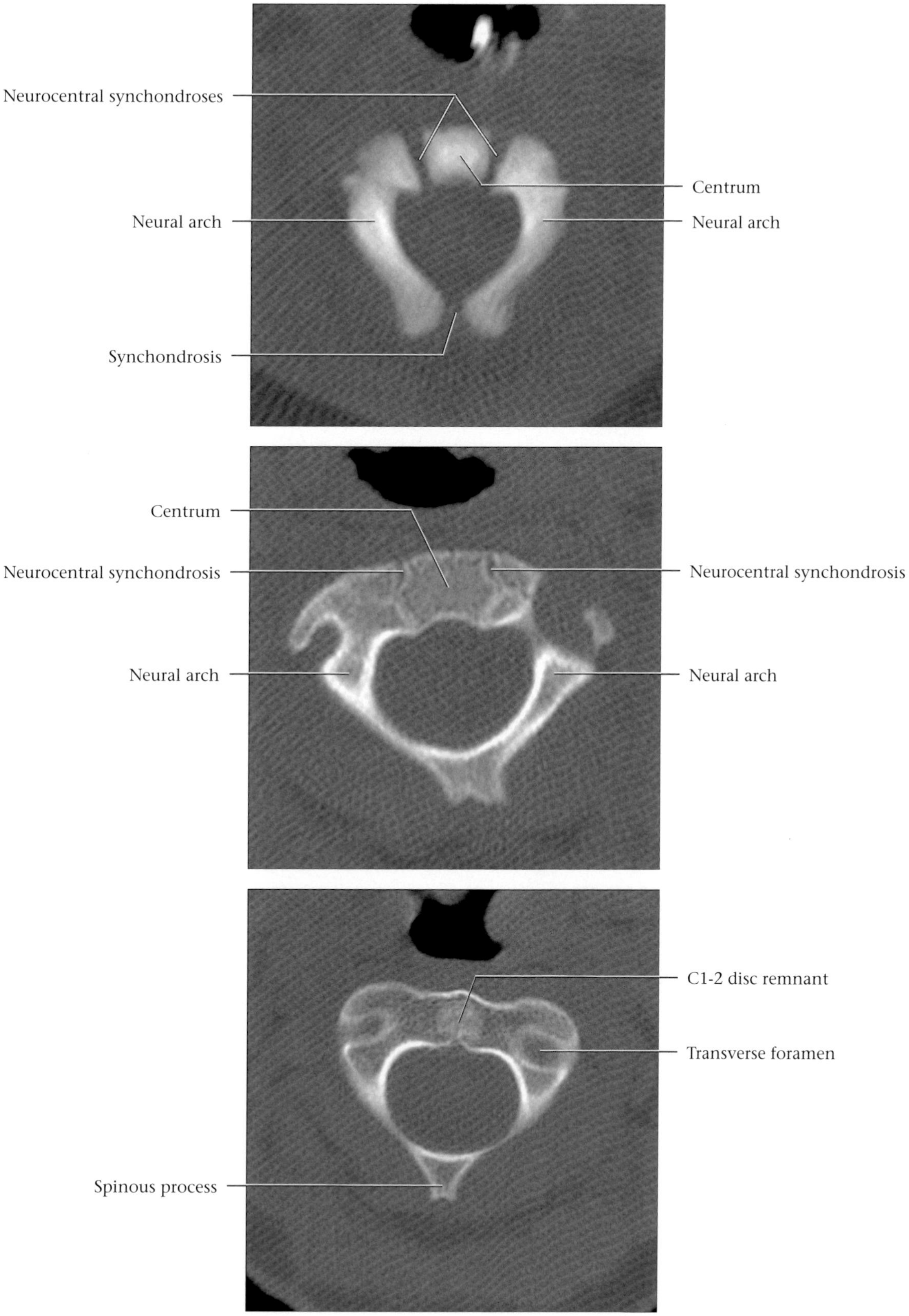

Neurocentral synchondroses
Centrum
Neural arch
Neural arch
Synchondrosis

Centrum
Neurocentral synchondrosis
Neurocentral synchondrosis
Neural arch
Neural arch

C1-2 disc remnant
Transverse foramen
Spinous process

(Top) Axial bone CT of a 2 week old female demonstrates the three axis 1° ossification centers separated by synchondroses. **(Middle)** Axial bone CT of a 4 year old male demonstrates progressive ossification of the three axis 1° ossification centers. Note that the centrum comprises only the central vertebral body, while the anterior portion of the neural arches form the lateral vertebral body. The posterior arch synchondrosis is fused. **(Bottom)** Axial bone CT of a 10 year old male shows fusion of the 1° ossification centers by closure of the neurocentral synchondroses. Sclerosis at the dens base indicates ossification within the rudimentary C1-2 intervertebral disc remnant joining the odontoid process to the C2 centrum.

CORONAL BONE CT, AXIS (C2) VERTEBRA

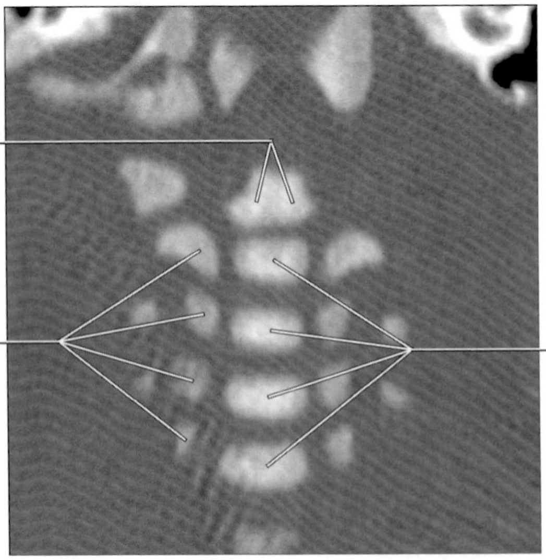

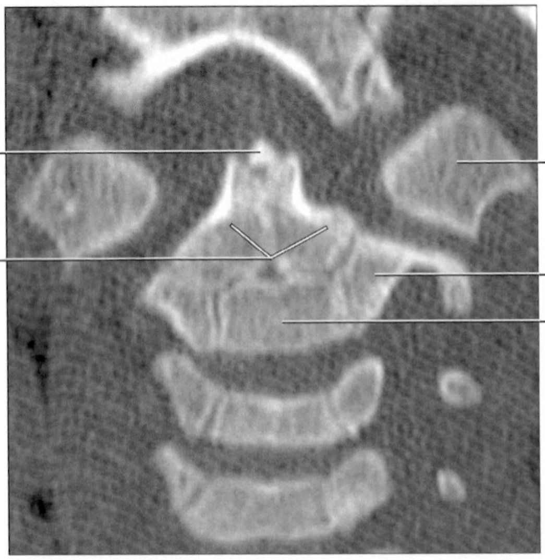

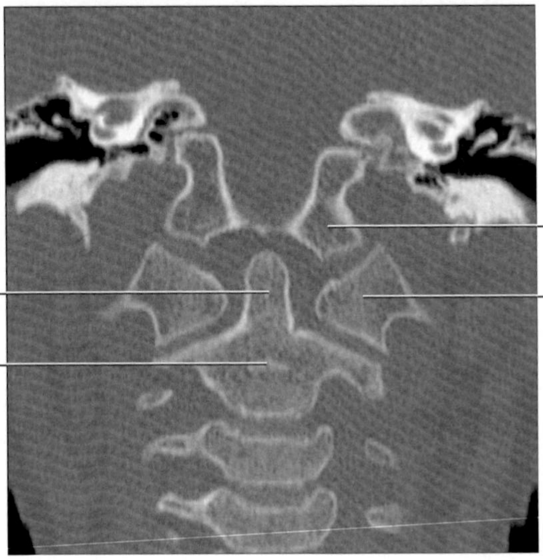

Odontoid 1° ossification centers
Neural arch 1° ossification centers
Centrum 1° ossification centers

Dens tip 2° ossification center
C1 lateral mass
Odontoid 1° ossification centers
Neural arch
Centrum

Occipital condyle
Odontoid process
C1 lateral mass
C1-2 intervertebral disc remnant

(Top) Coronal bone CT of the upper cervical spine of a 2 week old female shows the three cervical vertebra 1° ossification centers and two 1° odontoid ossification centers. The dens tip is cartilaginous at this developmental stage. **(Middle)** Coronal bone CT of the cervical spine of a 4 year old male shows progressive ossification of the centrum and neural arches connected by thin synchondroses. The characteristic location, symmetry, and well corticated margins of the synchondroses helps distinguish them from fracture. Note that the ossified odontoid tip 2° ossification center is now visible. **(Bottom)** Coronal bone CT of a 10 year old male shows fusion of the synchondroses. The C1-2 intervertebral disc remnant separating the dens from the C2 centrum remains visible as a sclerotic line.

OSSIFICATION

AXIAL & SAGITTAL BONE CT, CERVICAL (C3-6) VERTEBRA

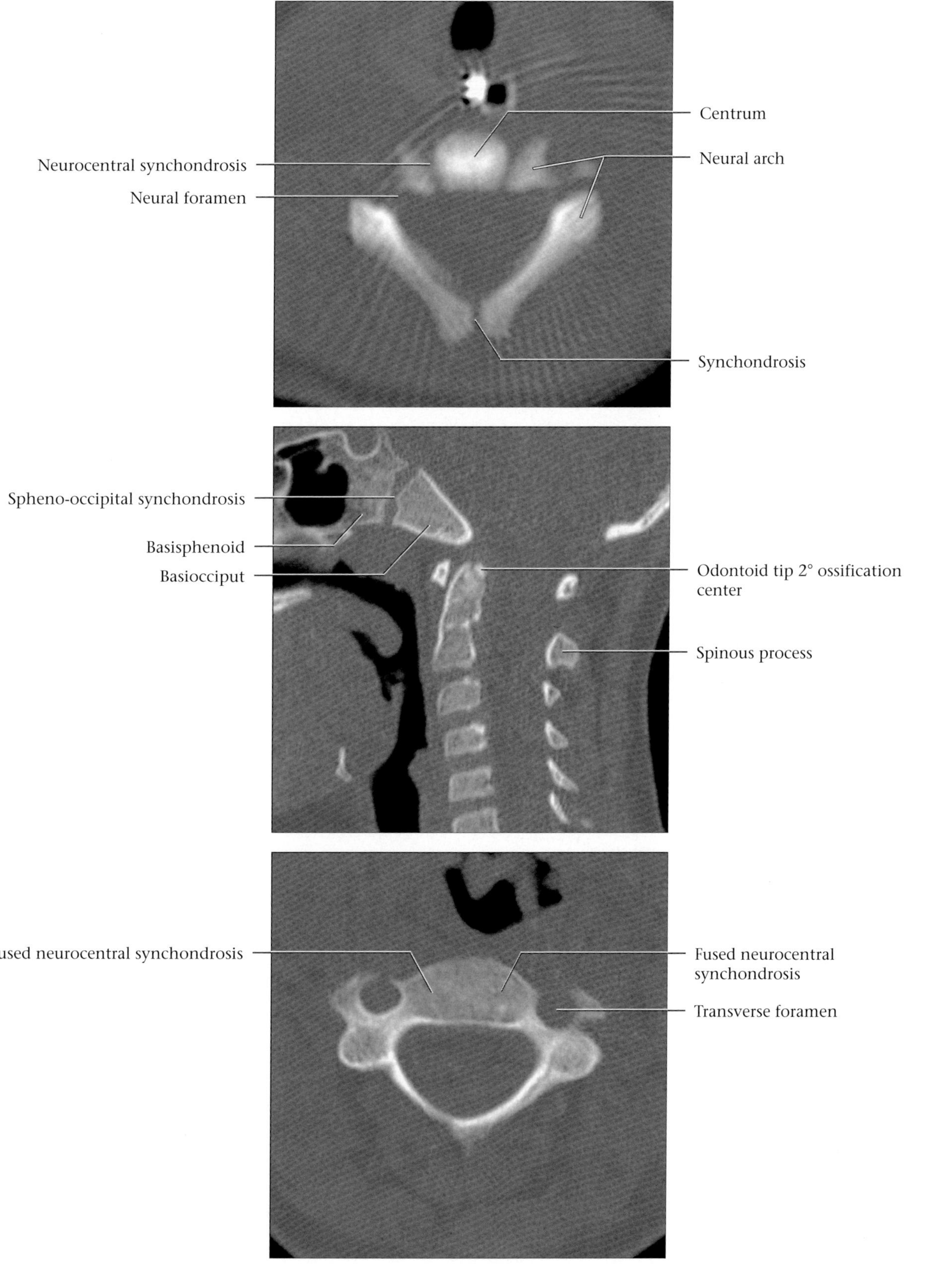

Centrum
Neurocentral synchondrosis
Neural arch
Neural foramen
Synchondrosis
Spheno-occipital synchondrosis
Basisphenoid
Basiocciput
Odontoid tip 2° ossification center
Spinous process
Fused neurocentral synchondrosis
Fused neurocentral synchondrosis
Transverse foramen

(Top) Axial bone CT of C5 of a 2 week old female demonstrates neurocentral synchondroses and synchondrosis junction of the neural arches. Note that the lateral vertebral body arises from the neural arches. **(Middle)** Sagittal bone CT of a 6 year old male demonstrates the normal appearance of the mid-cervical vertebra. The wide intervertebral distance between the ossified centrums represents the intervertebral discs and nonossified annular epiphysis 2° ossification centers. There is normal sclerosis at the fusion of the odontoid process to the C2 centrum. The odontoid tip persists as a separate 2° ossification center. **(Bottom)** Axial bone CT of a mid-cervical vertebra of a 6 year old female shows complete synchondrosis fusion, with only a faint sclerotic line visible at the site of the fused neurocentral synchondroses.

AXIAL BONE CT, C7 VERTEBRA

Neurocentral synchondrosis
Posterior neural arch
Centrum
Transverse process

Neurocentral synchondrosis
Neurocentral synchondrosis
Neural foramen
Transverse process 2° ossification center

Transverse process 2° ossification center

(Top) Axial bone CT of a 7 week old female demonstrates the normal appearance of C7. The transverse processes are characteristically longer than the other cervical vertebra, assisting identification of C7. **(Middle)** Axial bone CT of a 4 year old male demonstrates posterior fusion of the neural arches. The neurocentral synchondrosis is faintly apparent. The transverse process tip 2° ossification centers are visible. **(Bottom)** Axial bone CT of a 6 year old female shows synchondrosis fusion between the centrum and posterior neural arches. The synchondrosis between the transverse process tip 2° ossification center and neural arch transverse process remains open (normally closes at puberty).

AXIAL BONE CT, THORACIC VERTEBRA

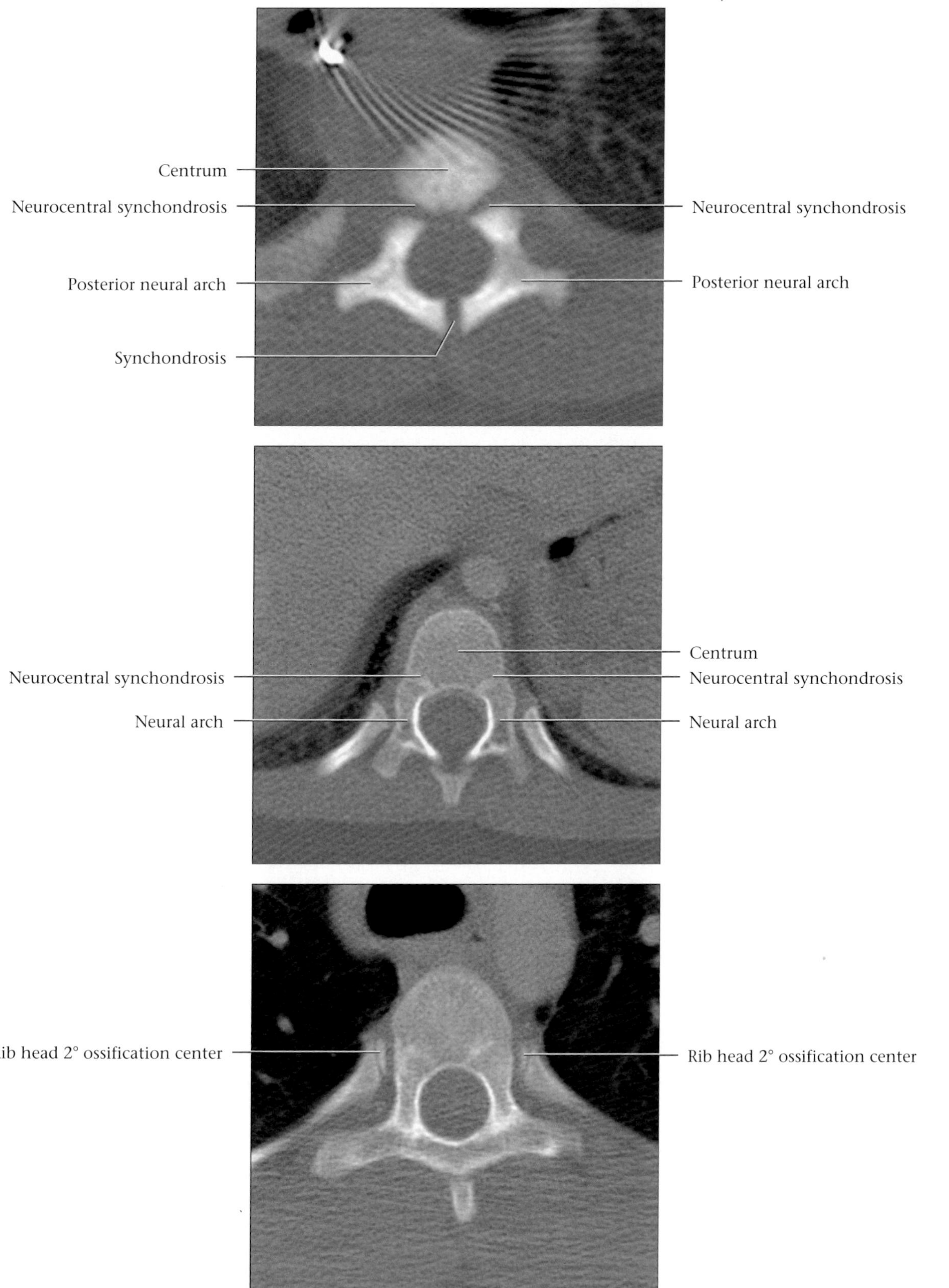
Centrum
Neurocentral synchondrosis
Neurocentral synchondrosis
Posterior neural arch
Posterior neural arch
Synchondrosis
Centrum
Neurocentral synchondrosis
Neurocentral synchondrosis
Neural arch
Neural arch
Rib head 2° ossification center
Rib head 2° ossification center

(Top) Axial bone CT of a 3 day old male demonstrates the three 1° ossification centers + synchondroses seen in a typical thoracic vertebra. **(Middle)** Axial bone CT of a 2 year old female shows narrowing of the neurocentral synchondroses and enlargement of the ossified centrum. The rib 2° ossification centers have not yet appeared. **(Bottom)** Axial bone CT of a 13 year old male shows fusion of the neurocentral and transverse process 2° ossification center synchondroses. The rib head 2° ossification centers are now ossified.

AXIAL BONE CT, LUMBAR VERTEBRA

Centrum
Neurocentral synchondrosis
Neurocentral synchondrosis
Neural arch
Neural arch
Synchondrosis

Centrum
Neurocentral synchondrosis
Neurocentral synchondrosis
Posterior neural arch
Posterior neural arch

Transverse process
Transverse process
Transverse process 2° ossification center
Transverse process 2° ossification center

(Top) Axial bone CT of a 4 day old male demonstrates the three 1° vertebral ossification centers and synchondroses in a typical lumbar vertebra. **(Middle)** Axial bone CT of L1 of a 2 year old male shows maturational development of the 1° ossification centers and neurocentral synchondroses. The transverse process 2° centers are not yet ossified. **(Bottom)** Axial bone CT of L2 of a 13 year old male shows completed fusion of the 1° synchondroses. The transverse process 2° ossification centers are ossified but not yet fused to the transverse processes.

AXIAL BONE CT, SACRUM

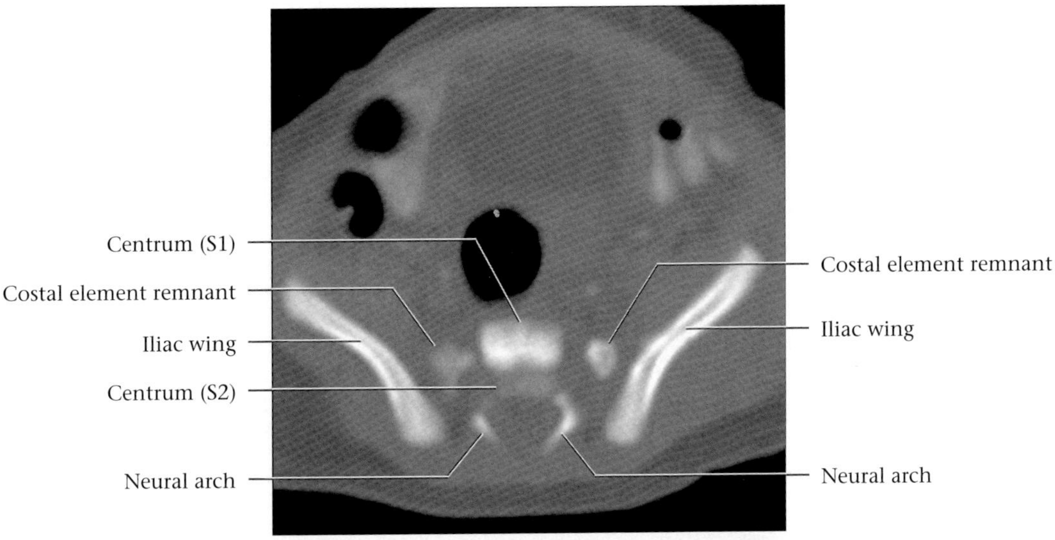

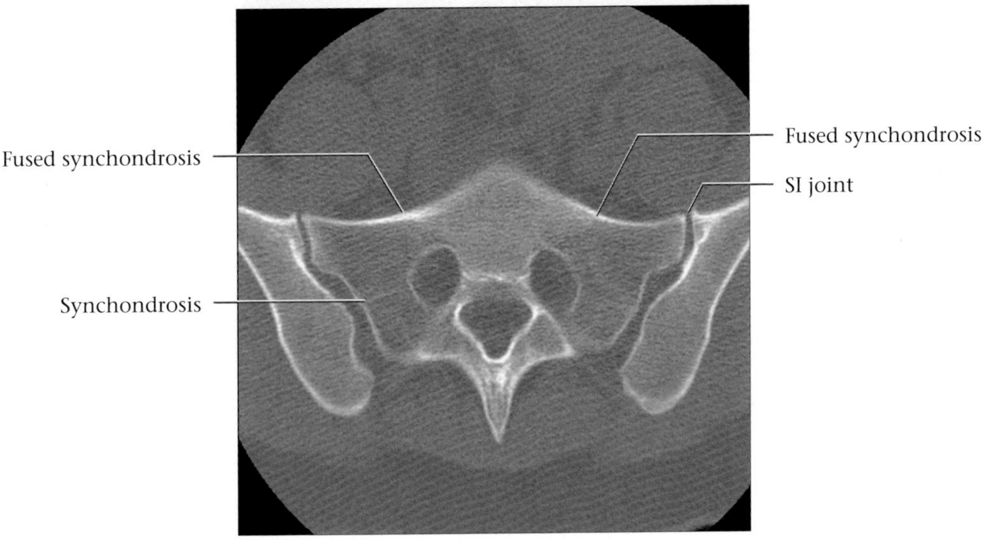

Centrum (S1)
Costal element remnant
Iliac wing
Centrum (S2)
Neural arch
Costal element remnant
Iliac wing
Neural arch

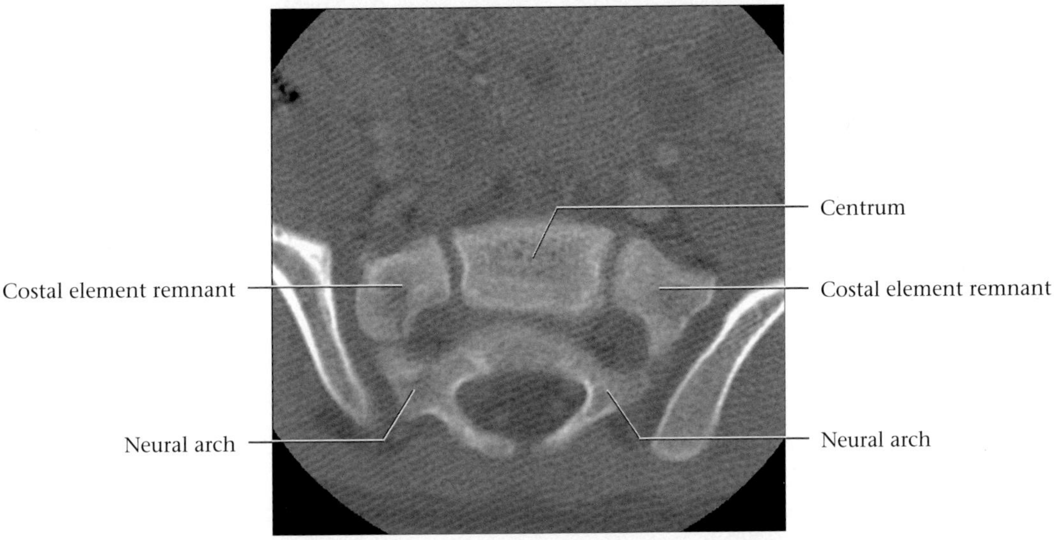

Centrum
Costal element remnant
Costal element remnant
Neural arch
Neural arch

Fused synchondrosis
Synchondrosis
Fused synchondrosis
SI joint

(Top) Axial bone CT of S2 of a 3 day old female shows the five 1° ossification centers (centrum, costal element remnants, neural arches) present at birth, separated by synchondroses. Both the S1 and S2 centrums are visible in this single slice because of the oblique angulation of the sacrum relative to the axial CT slice. **(Middle)** Axial bone CT of the sacrum of a 2 year old male shows typical configuration of the five 1° sacral ossification centers. The SI joints appear widened because the SI joint epiphyseal plates are not yet ossified. **(Bottom)** Axial bone CT of the sacrum of a 16 year old female demonstrates closure of the synchondroses and completed ossification of the 1° and 2° ossification centers. The site of the synchondroses persist as faint sclerotic lines.

SAGITTAL BONE CT, COCCYX

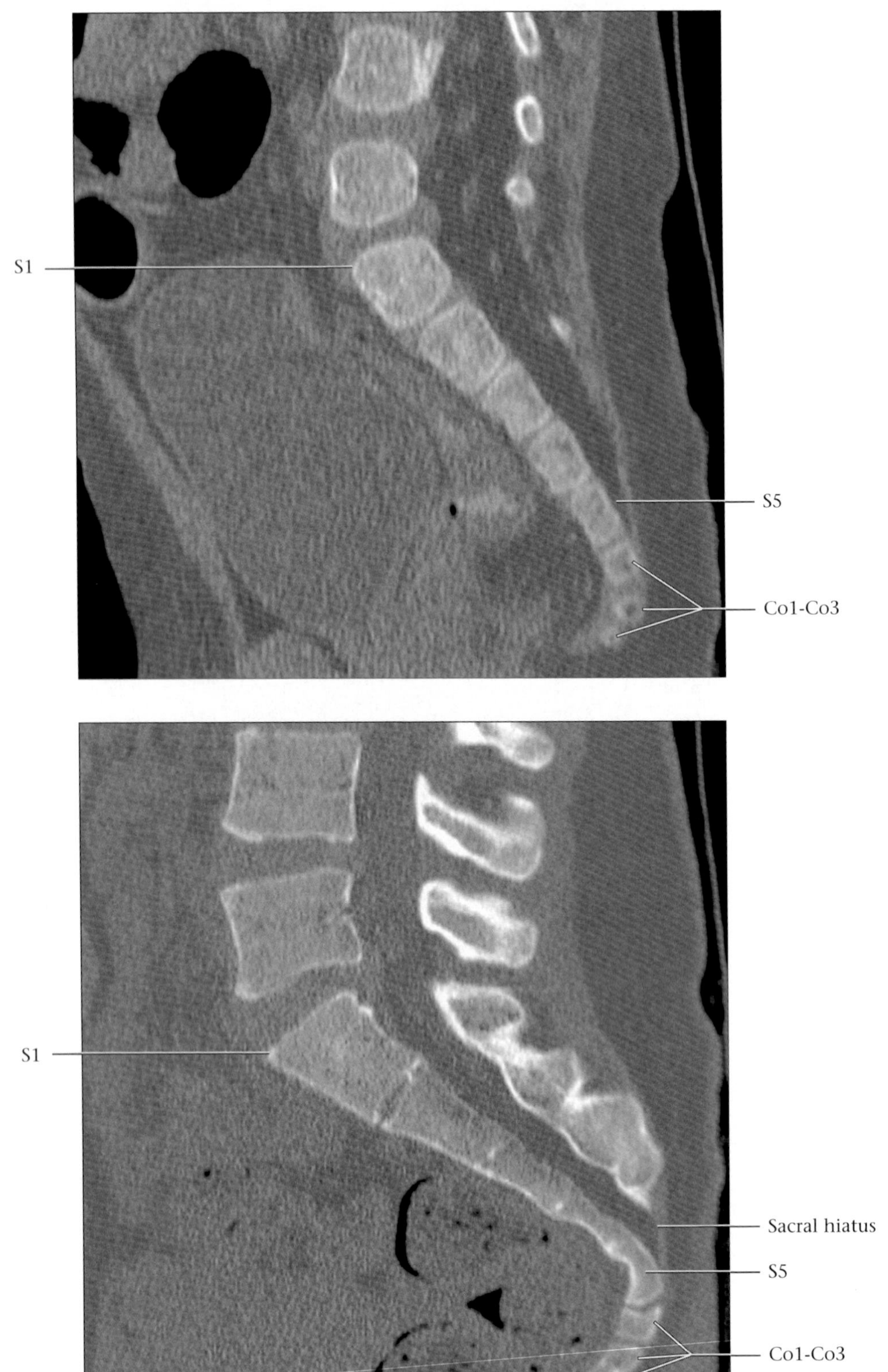
S1
S5
Co1-Co3
S1
Sacral hiatus
S5
Co1-Co3

(Top) Sagittal bone CT of the sacrum and coccyx of a 24 month old female demonstrates ossification of the five sacral vertebra. The first three coccygeal vertebra show ossification in the primary ossification centers only. The underlying cartilaginous model is visible as soft tissue density containing the ossified centrums. **(Bottom)** Sagittal bone CT of the sacrum and coccyx of a 16 year old female. Note the more mature appearance of the five sacral vertebra and first three coccygeal vertebra.

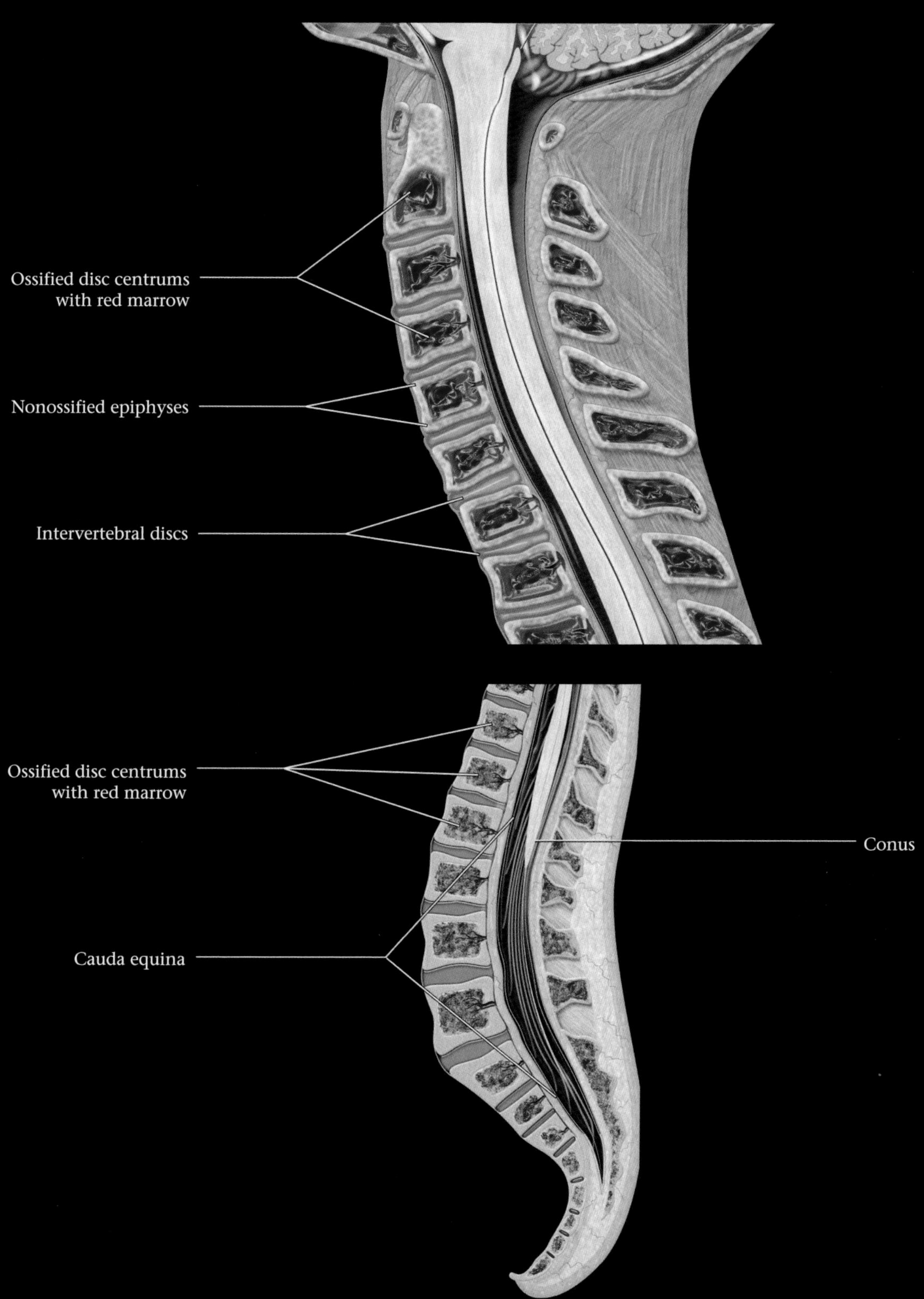
Ossified disc centrums with red marrow
Nonossified epiphyses
Intervertebral discs
Ossified disc centrums with red marrow
Conus
Cauda equina

(Top) Sagittal graphic depicts cervical vertebral bodies and intervertebral discs of a 6 year old male. Centrums of the disc are ossified at this age and contain hemopoietic ("red") marrow. Nonossified annular epiphyses surround the bodies and spinous processes. The nonossified epiphyses plus the intervertebral discs account for the wide intervertebral distance between the ossified centrums seen on imaging studies at this age. The odontoid tip persists as a separate 2° ossification center. **(Bottom)** Sagittal midline graphic depicts lumbar vertebral bodies, intervertebral discs, and sacrum of a 6 year old male. As in the cervical spine, the centers of the vertebral bodies and spinous processes are ossified at this age and contain hemopoietic ("red") marrow. The intervertebral distances between the ossified centra are even more prominent in the lumbar spine.

OSSIFICATION

SAGITTAL T1 MR

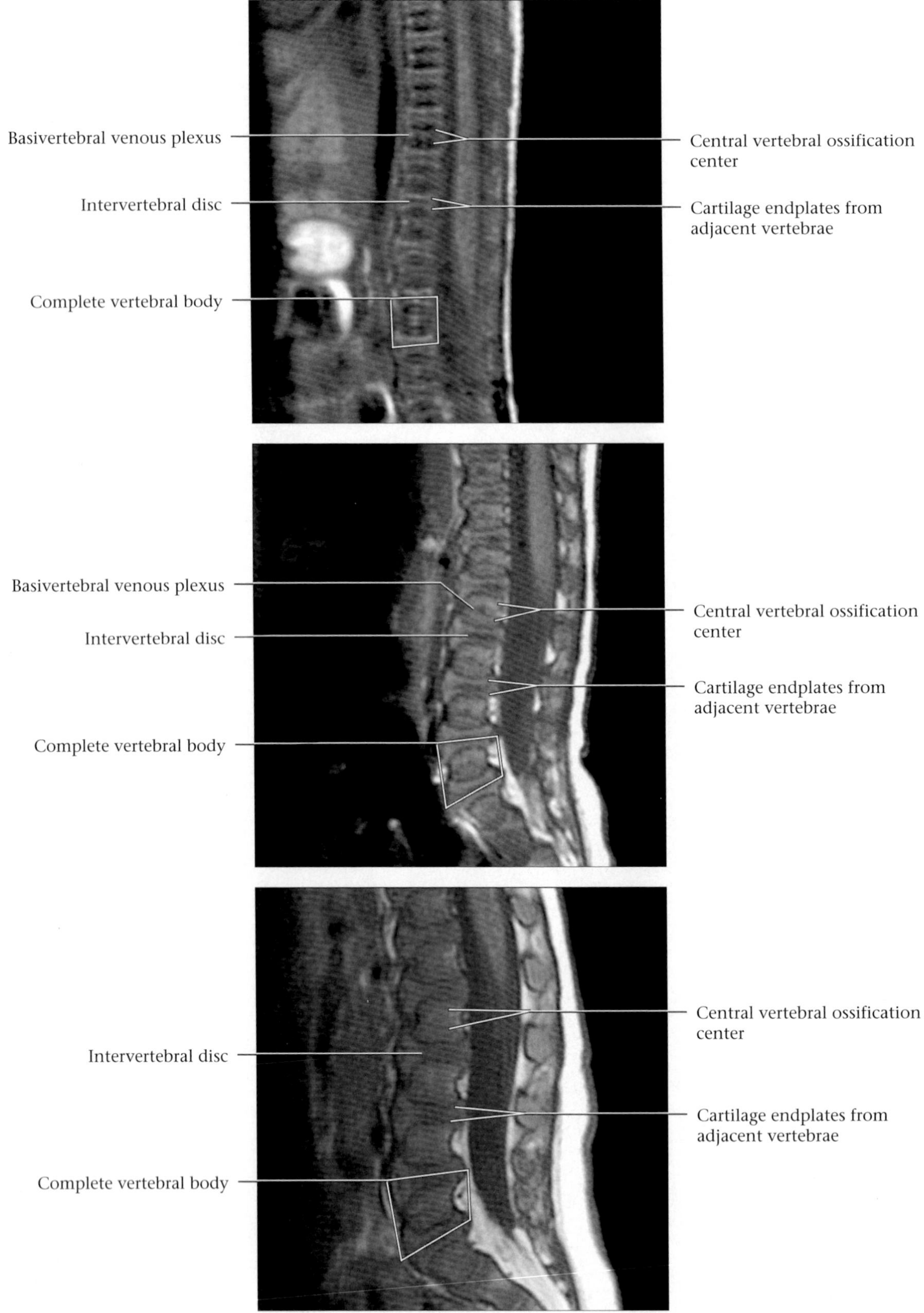
Basivertebral venous plexus
Intervertebral disc
Complete vertebral body
Central vertebral ossification center
Cartilage endplates from adjacent vertebrae
Basivertebral venous plexus
Intervertebral disc
Complete vertebral body
Central vertebral ossification center
Cartilage endplates from adjacent vertebrae
Intervertebral disc
Complete vertebral body
Central vertebral ossification center
Cartilage endplates from adjacent vertebrae

(Top) Sagittal T1 MR in 4 day old infant shows characteristic appearance of vertebrae & intervening disc. The central vertebral ossification center is markedly hypointense & contains a linear horizontal hyperintense cleft from the developing basivertebral venous plexus. The very prominent cartilaginous endplates are hyperintense & separated by hypointense disc. **(Middle)** Sagittal T1 MR in 5 month old infant showing gradual increasing signal within the ovoid vertebral ossification center, and decreasing prominence of the hyperintense cartilage endplates. **(Bottom)** Sagittal T1 MR in 1 year old infant shows continued increasing signal within the vertebral ossification center which now has a more rectangular shape. The cartilage endplates are less prominent & have continued decreased signal relative to the vertebral ossification center.

SAGITTAL T2 MR

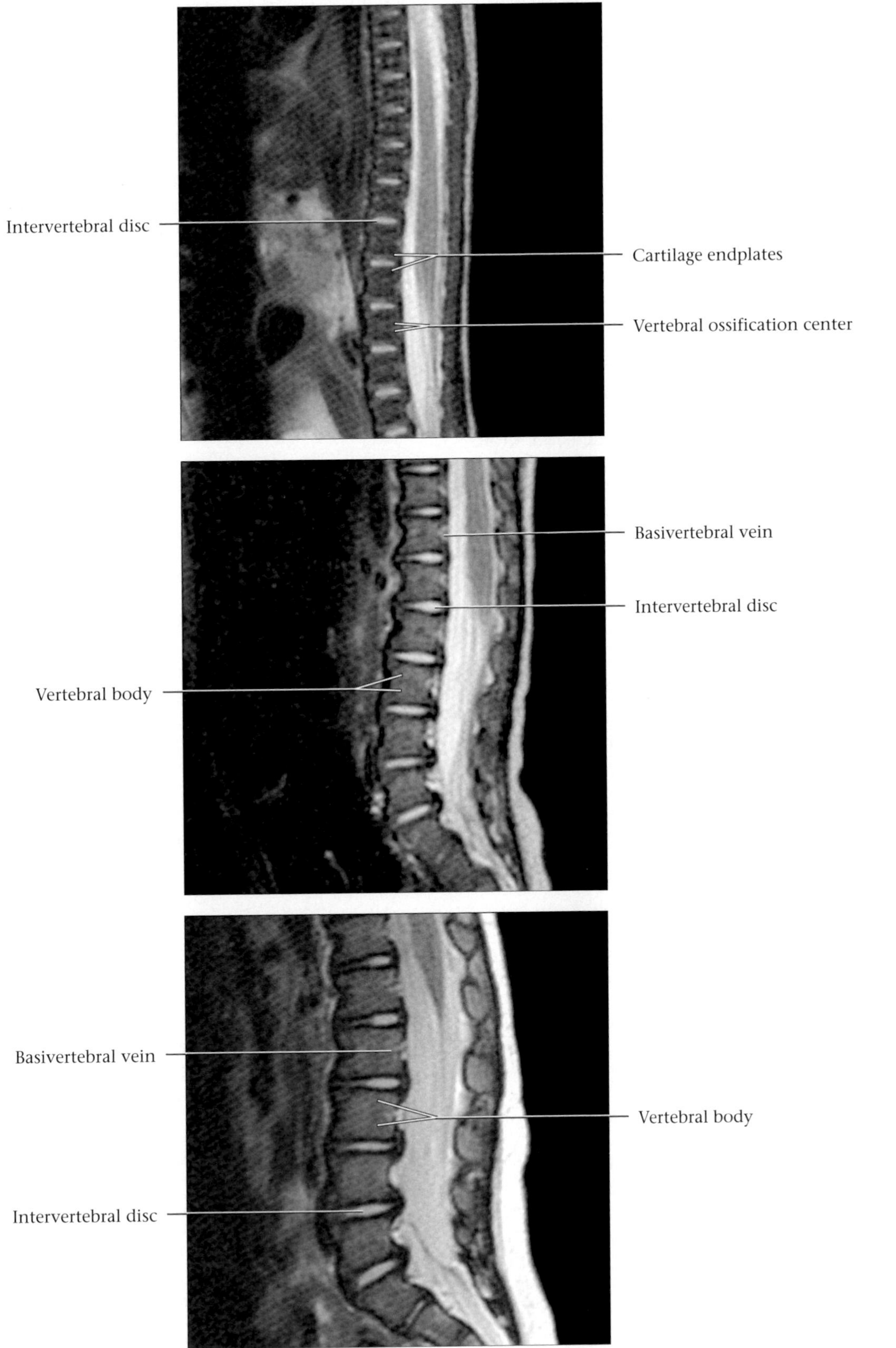
Intervertebral disc
Cartilage endplates
Vertebral ossification center
Basivertebral vein
Intervertebral disc
Vertebral body
Basivertebral vein
Vertebral body
Intervertebral disc

(Top) Corresponding sagittal T2 MR in same 4 day old infant shows very hypointense central ossification centers, mildly hyperintense cartilage endplates & hyperintense intervertebral discs. **(Middle)** Corresponding sagittal T2 MR in same 5 month old infant shows increasing signal within the central vertebral body which are now isointense with the endplates. **(Bottom)** Corresponding sagittal T2 MR in same 1 year old infant shows similar increasing signal within the central vertebral body with corticated hypointense margins. The intervertebral disc remains hyperintense.

VERTEBRAL BODY AND LIGAMENTS

Terminology

Abbreviations

- Anterior, posterior longitudinal ligaments (ALL, PLL)

Gross Anatomy

Overview

- **Vertebral body**
  - Varies in size, shape depending on region
  - Generally ↑ size from cervical to lumbar, then ↓ from sacrum to coccyx
- **Cervical:** Upper 7 vertebrae
  - **C1 (atlas)**: No body, spinous process; circular shape
    - Anterior, posterior arches; 2 lateral masses; transverse processes
  - **C2 (axis)**: Body with bony peg (dens/odontoid process)
    - Large, flat ovoid articular facets
    - Broad pedicles, thick laminae
    - Transverse processes contain L-shaped foramina for vertebral artery
  - **C3-6** similar in size, shape
    - Bodies small, thin relative to size of arch
    - Transverse diameter > AP; triangular central canal
    - Lateral edges of superior surface turn upward, form uncinate processes
    - Pedicles short, small, directed posterolaterally
    - Lateral masses rhomboid-shaped with slanted superior/inferior articular surfaces
    - Transverse processes contain transverse foramina for VAs
    - C3-5 spinous processes usually short, bifid
  - **C7** marked by longest spinous process
- **Thoracic**
  - Bodies heart-shaped, central canal round
  - Pedicles short, directed posteriorly
  - Laminae broad/thick
  - Spinous processes point caudally, dorsally
  - Superior articular processes vertical, flat, face posteriorly
  - T12 resembles upper lumbar bodies with inferior facet directed more laterally
  - Costal articular facets on body/transverse processes
    - Articulate with heads of ribs
    - T1 has complete facet for first rib, inferior demifacet for second rib
- **Lumbar**
  - Body large, wide, thick
  - Pedicles strong, thick, directed posteriorly
  - Laminae strong, broad
  - Superior articular processes face dorsomedial
  - Inferior articular processes face anterolateral
- **Sacrum:** Fusion of 5 segments
  - Large triangular shaped bone with base, apex, 3 surfaces (pelvic, dorsal, lateral), 2 alae
  - Base: Round/ovoid; articulates with L5
  - Pelvic surface
    - Anterior sacral foramina at lateral ends of ridges
    - Concave, crossed by 4 transverse ridges
  - Posterior surface
    - Median sacral crest in midline
    - Sacral groove on either side of crest
    - Intermediate crest lateral to sacral groove
    - Posterior sacral foramina lateral to crest
    - Lateral crest is lateral to sacral foramina
  - Lateral surface: Formed by costal, transverse processes
    - Alae on sides articulate with iliac bone
  - Apex: Inferior aspect of S5, articulates with coccyx
- **Coccyx:** Fusion of 3-5 segments
  - Anterior surface concave with transverse ridges
  - Posterior surface convex with transverse ridges
  - Apex round, directed caudally, may be bifid
- **Ligaments**
  - **ALL**: Fibrous band on ventral surface of spine from skull to sacrum
    - Firmly attached at ends of each vertebral body
    - Loosely attached at midsection of disc
    - 3 sets of fibers: Deep span 1 disc; intermediate 2-3 discs; superficial 4-5 levels
  - **PLL**: Dorsal surface of bodies from skull to sacrum
    - Attached at discs, margins of vertebral bodies
    - Cervical/thoracic: Broad, uniform
    - Lumbar: Narrow at body, broad at disc level
  - **Ligamentum flavum**
    - Largest elastic ligament in body
    - Connects adjacent lamina from C2 to lumbosacral junction
    - Extends from capsule of apophyseal joint to junction of lamina with spinous process
    - Thin, broad in cervical region, thicker in lumbar
  - **Intertransverse ligaments**: Extend between transverse processes
    - Cervical: Sparse or absent
    - Thoracic: Stronger associated with muscles
  - **Interspinous ligaments**: Connect adjoining spinous processes
    - Between ligamentum flavum, supraspinous ligaments
    - Strongest in lumbar spine
  - **Supraspinous ligaments**: Extend from tips of spinous processes from C7 to sacrum
    - Fused with dorsal margin of interspinous ligament
    - Broader, thicker in lumbar spine
    - Merges with ligamentum nuchae in cervical spine
    - Ligamentum nuchae extends from external occipital protuberance to C7

Imaging Anatomy

Overview

- Transitional lumbosacral bodies (up to 25% in normal)
  - Sacralization of lumbar body: Spectrum extending from expanded transverse processes of L5 articulating with top of sacrum to incorporation of L5 into sacrum
  - Lumbarization of sacrum: Elevation of S1 above sacral fusion mass assuming lumbar body shape
  - Sacralization and lumbarization may be similar in appearance, requiring evaluation of entire spinal axis to define anatomy and correct level nomenclature

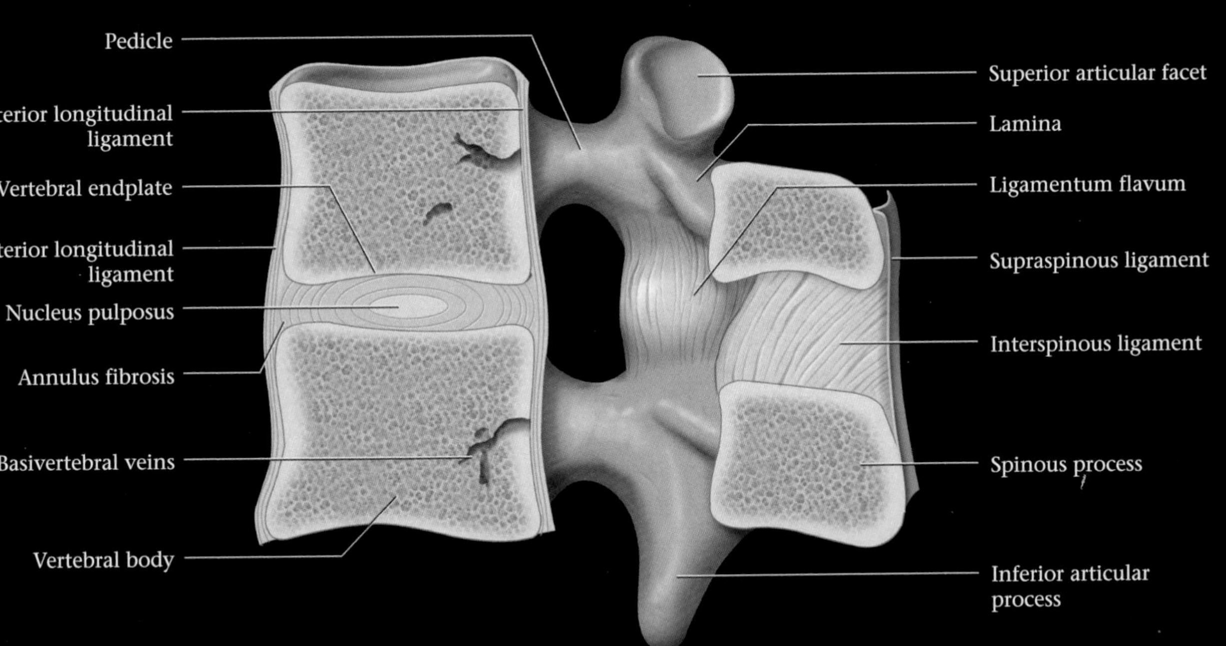
Pedicle
erior longitudinal ligament
Vertebral endplate
erior longitudinal ligament
Nucleus pulposus
Annulus fibrosis
Basivertebral veins
Vertebral body
Superior articular facet
Lamina
Ligamentum flavum
Supraspinous ligament
Interspinous ligament
Spinous process
Inferior articular process

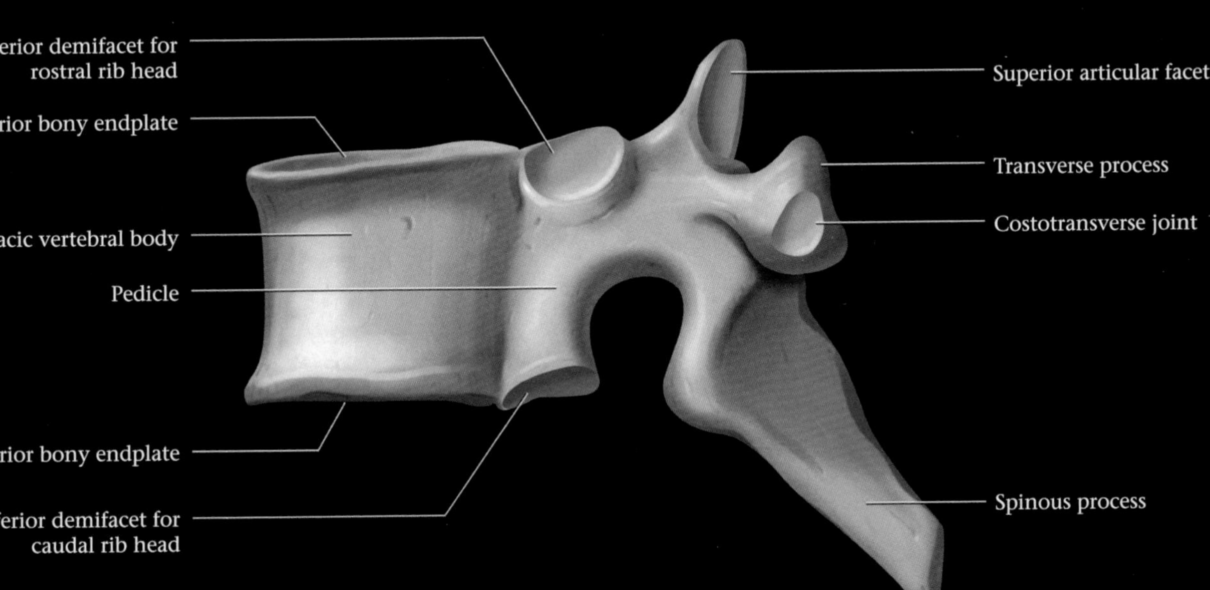
erior demifacet for rostral rib head
rior bony endplate
acic vertebral body
Pedicle
rior bony endplate
erior demifacet for caudal rib head
Superior articular facet
Transverse process
Costotransverse joint
Spinous process

) Sagittal cut away graphic through lumbar vertebral bodies as viewed from the left demonstrates major ctures of the discovertebral unit. The vertebral bodies are joined by the intervertebral disc and the anterior and erior longitudinal ligaments. The posterior elements consist of the paired pedicles, transverse processes, articular s, lamina and terminates in the dorsally directed spinous process. The paired ligamentum flavum and rspinous ligaments join adjacent posterior elements, capped by the single midline supraspinous ligament. **tom)** Lateral view of thoracic vertebral body shows the characteristic features of this spinal segment. The unique erior and inferior demifacets form a concavity spanning the intervening disc to house the rib head and form the overtebral joint. The spinous process is typically long and oblique.

GRAPHICS

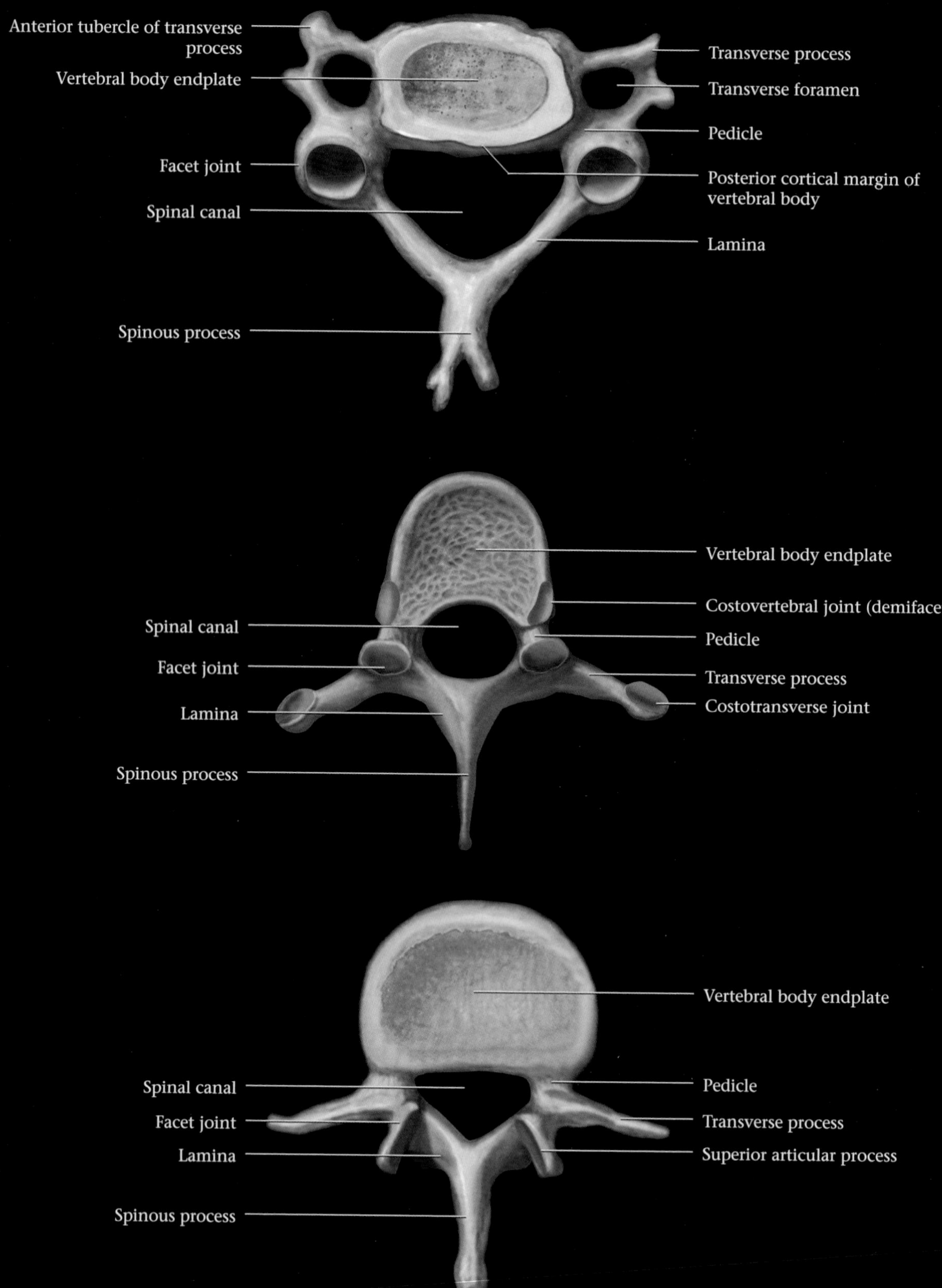
Anterior tubercle of transverse process
Vertebral body endplate
Facet joint
Spinal canal
Spinous process
Transverse process
Transverse foramen
Pedicle
Posterior cortical margin of vertebral body
Lamina
Vertebral body endplate
Costovertebral joint (demifacet)
Pedicle
Transverse process
Costotransverse joint
Spinal canal
Facet joint
Lamina
Spinous process
Vertebral body endplate
Pedicle
Transverse process
Superior articular process
Spinal canal
Facet joint
Lamina
Spinous process

(Top) Graphic of cervical vertebral body, viewed from above. The lateral margins of the vertebral bodies are dominated by the facet joints, with their articulating superior and inferior processes, and the transverse processes with their characteristic transverse foramen which transmits the vertebral artery. **(Middle)** Graphic of thoracic vertebral body, viewed from above. The thoracic bodies are characterized by long spinous processes and transverse processes. The complex rib articulation includes both costotransverse joints, and costovertebral joints. **(Bottom)** Graphic of lumbar vertebral body, viewed from above. The large sturdy lumbar vertebral bodies connect to thick pedicles and transversely directed transverse processes. The facets maintain an oblique orientation favoring flexion/extension motion.

VERTEBRAL BODY AND LIGAMENTS

CERVICAL RADIOGRAPHY

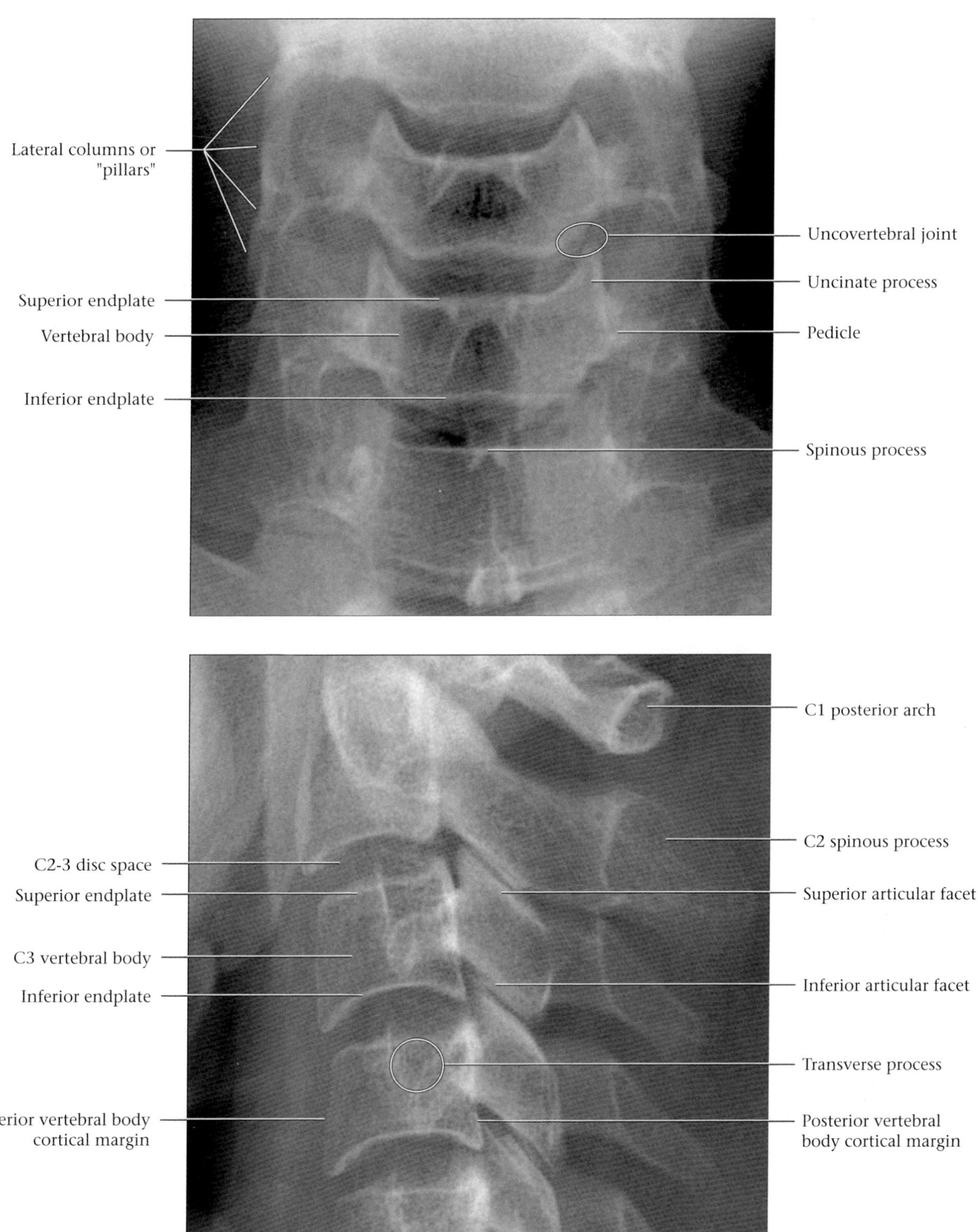
Lateral columns or "pillars"
Uncovertebral joint
Uncinate process
Superior endplate
Vertebral body
Pedicle
Inferior endplate
Spinous process
C1 posterior arch
C2 spinous process
C2-3 disc space
Superior endplate
Superior articular facet
C3 vertebral body
Inferior endplate
Inferior articular facet
Transverse process
Anterior vertebral body cortical margin
Posterior vertebral body cortical margin

(Top) AP view of the cervical spine. The vertebral bodies show a distinctive shape with their curved lateral margins with uncinate processes forming the uncovertebral ("Luschka") joints. The pedicles are poorly seen due to their obliquity to the plane, as are the facet joints. The lateral masses assume a flowing or undulating contour to the lateral aspects of the spine. The superior and inferior endplates are well-defined. The bifid spinous processes project through the vertebra body. **(Bottom)** Lateral view of cervical spine. The superior and inferior vertebral endplates are well-defined in this projection. The pedicles are poorly seen due to obliquity. The transverse processes overlap the vertebra bodies and are not well-defined. With proper positioning, the facet joints of each side overlap to merge into what appears to be one joint with a well-defined joint space.

THORACIC RADIOGRAPHY

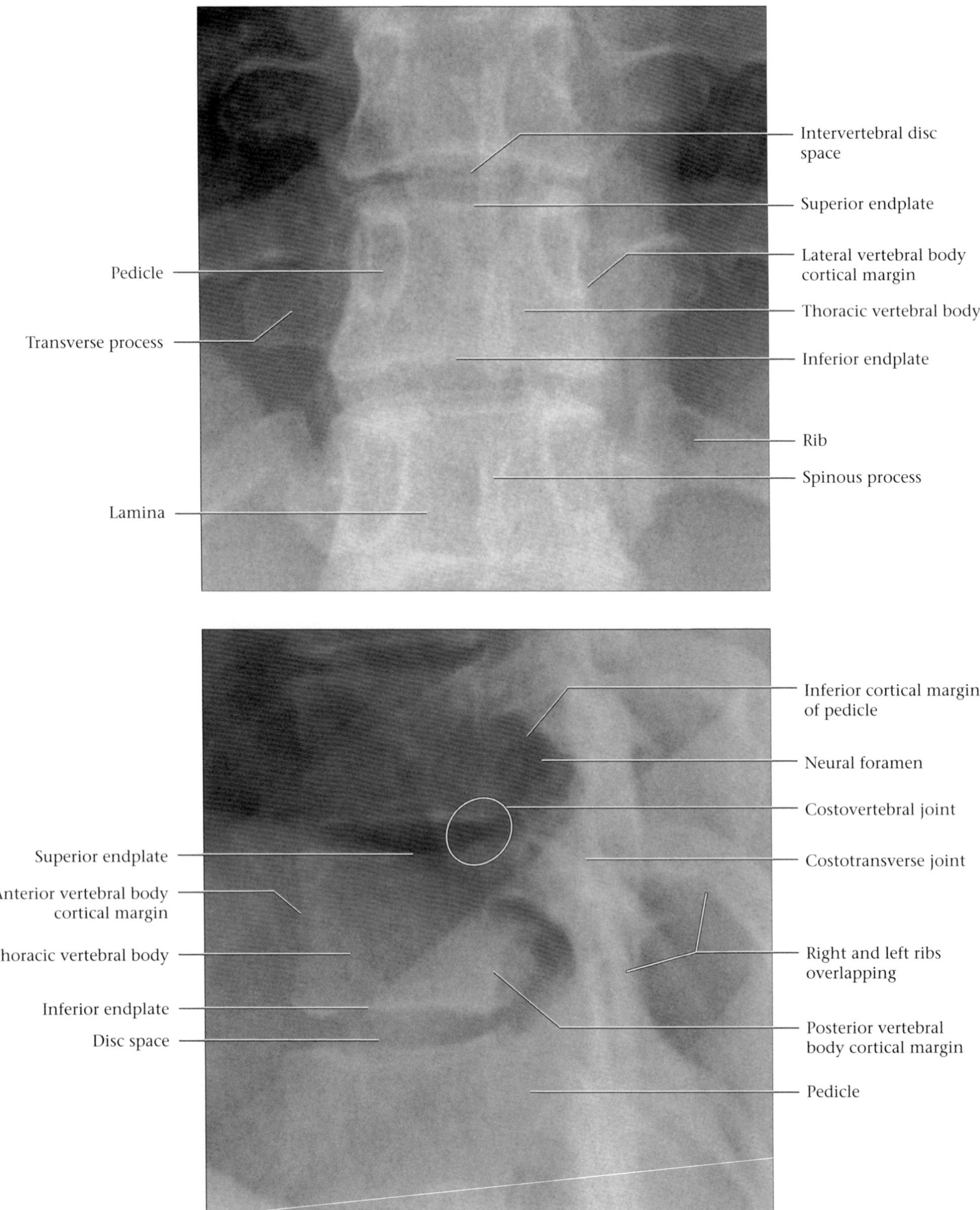

Intervertebral disc space
Superior endplate
Lateral vertebral body cortical margin
Pedicle
Thoracic vertebral body
Transverse process
Inferior endplate
Rib
Spinous process
Lamina
Inferior cortical margin of pedicle
Neural foramen
Costovertebral joint
Superior endplate
Costotransverse joint
Anterior vertebral body cortical margin
Thoracic vertebral body
Right and left ribs overlapping
Inferior endplate
Disc space
Posterior vertebral body cortical margin
Pedicle

(Top) AP view of the thoracic spine. The vertebral bodies are square with well-defined cortical margins. The intervertebral disc spaces are small relative to the lumbar region. The pedicles are visible end on with an oval configuration. The spinous process are long and obliquely oriented and extend caudally, overlapping the more inferior vertebral body on this view. **(Bottom)** Lateral view of the thoracic spine. The anterior and posterior thoracic body cortical margins are well-defined and maintain a smooth alignment in the vertical direction. The bony endplates are well-defined, separating the thin intervertebral discs. The region of the costovertebral joints is poorly-defined, just anterior to the inferior margin of the neural foramen. The costotransverse joints are seen end on.

VERTEBRAL BODY AND LIGAMENTS

LUMBAR RADIOGRAPHY

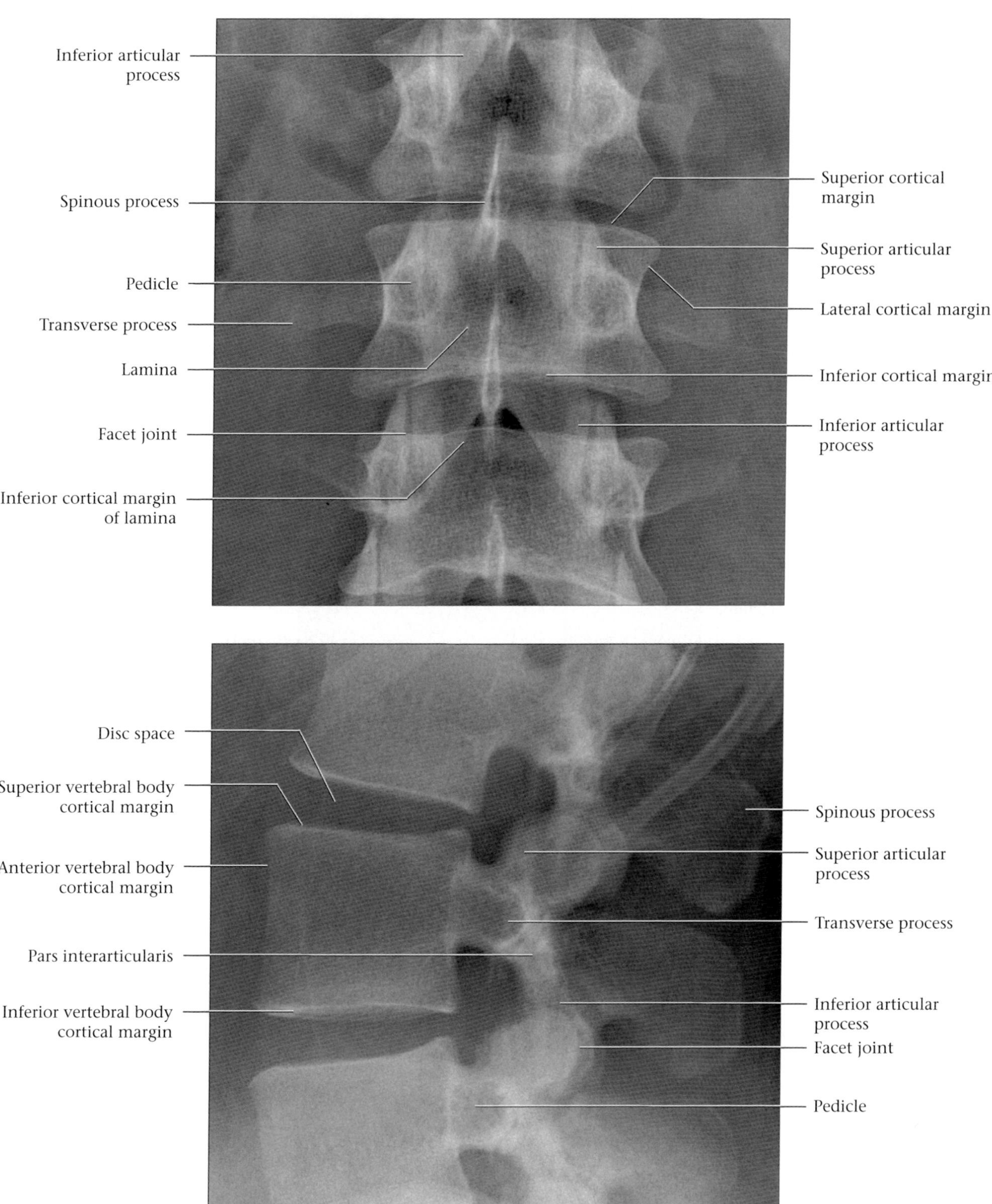
Inferior articular process
Spinous process
Pedicle
Transverse process
Lamina
Facet joint
Inferior cortical margin of lamina
Superior cortical margin
Superior articular process
Lateral cortical margin
Inferior cortical margin
Inferior articular process
Disc space
Superior vertebral body cortical margin
Anterior vertebral body cortical margin
Pars interarticularis
Inferior vertebral body cortical margin
Spinous process
Superior articular process
Transverse process
Inferior articular process
Facet joint
Pedicle

(Top) AP view of the lumbar spine. The vertebral bodies assume a more rectangular appearance in this view, with strong, large ovoid pedicles seen end on. A portion of the facet joints are visualized, being relatively oriented in the sagittal plane and allowing flexion and extension. The posterior elements forming the "H" pattern are well-defined with their superior and inferior articular processes and broad lamina. The spinous process is midline, pointing slightly inferior. **(Bottom)** Lateral view of the lumbar spine. The broad and square shaped bodies in this view separate the large intervertebral disc spaces. The anterior and posterior vertebral body cortical margins line up, allowing a gentle lordotic curvature. The pedicles and neural foramina are well visualized in this plane, with bony overlap obscuring the facet joint space.

VERTEBRAL BODY AND LIGAMENTS

AXIAL NECT

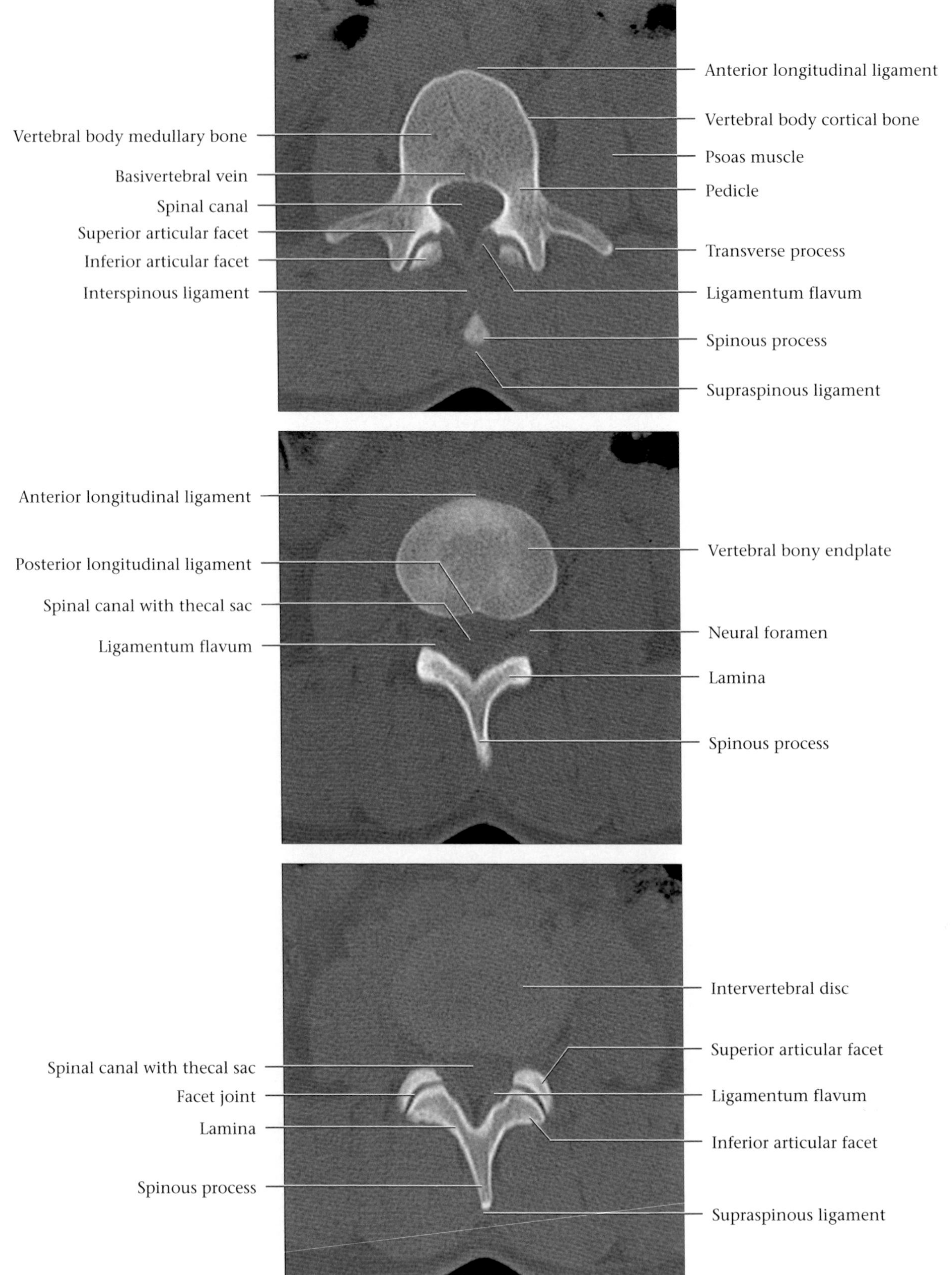

Anterior longitudinal ligament
Vertebral body cortical bone
Vertebral body medullary bone
Psoas muscle
Basivertebral vein
Pedicle
Spinal canal
Superior articular facet
Transverse process
Inferior articular facet
Interspinous ligament
Ligamentum flavum
Spinous process
Supraspinous ligament
Anterior longitudinal ligament
Vertebral bony endplate
Posterior longitudinal ligament
Spinal canal with thecal sac
Neural foramen
Ligamentum flavum
Lamina
Spinous process
Intervertebral disc
Superior articular facet
Spinal canal with thecal sac
Facet joint
Ligamentum flavum
Lamina
Inferior articular facet
Spinous process
Supraspinous ligament

(Top) Axial NECT image through mid-pedicle level of lumbar vertebra shows the thick pedicles extending into the superior articular process with the obliquely angled facet (zygapophyseal) joint. The ligamentum flavum extends to the midline as a paired structure and laterally along the lamina and facet joint margins. The basivertebral veins are seen as paired lucencies in the midline of the posterior portion of the vertebral body. **(Middle)** Axial CT image though the endplate shows the triangular shaped junction of the lamina with the dorsally directed spinous process. The neural foramina are large and directed laterally. **(Bottom)** Axial CT image through the intervertebral disc level. The ligamentum flavum is well-defined and does not cross the midline, extending laterally towards the facet joints.

VERTEBRAL BODY AND LIGAMENTS

LUMBAR CORONAL NECT

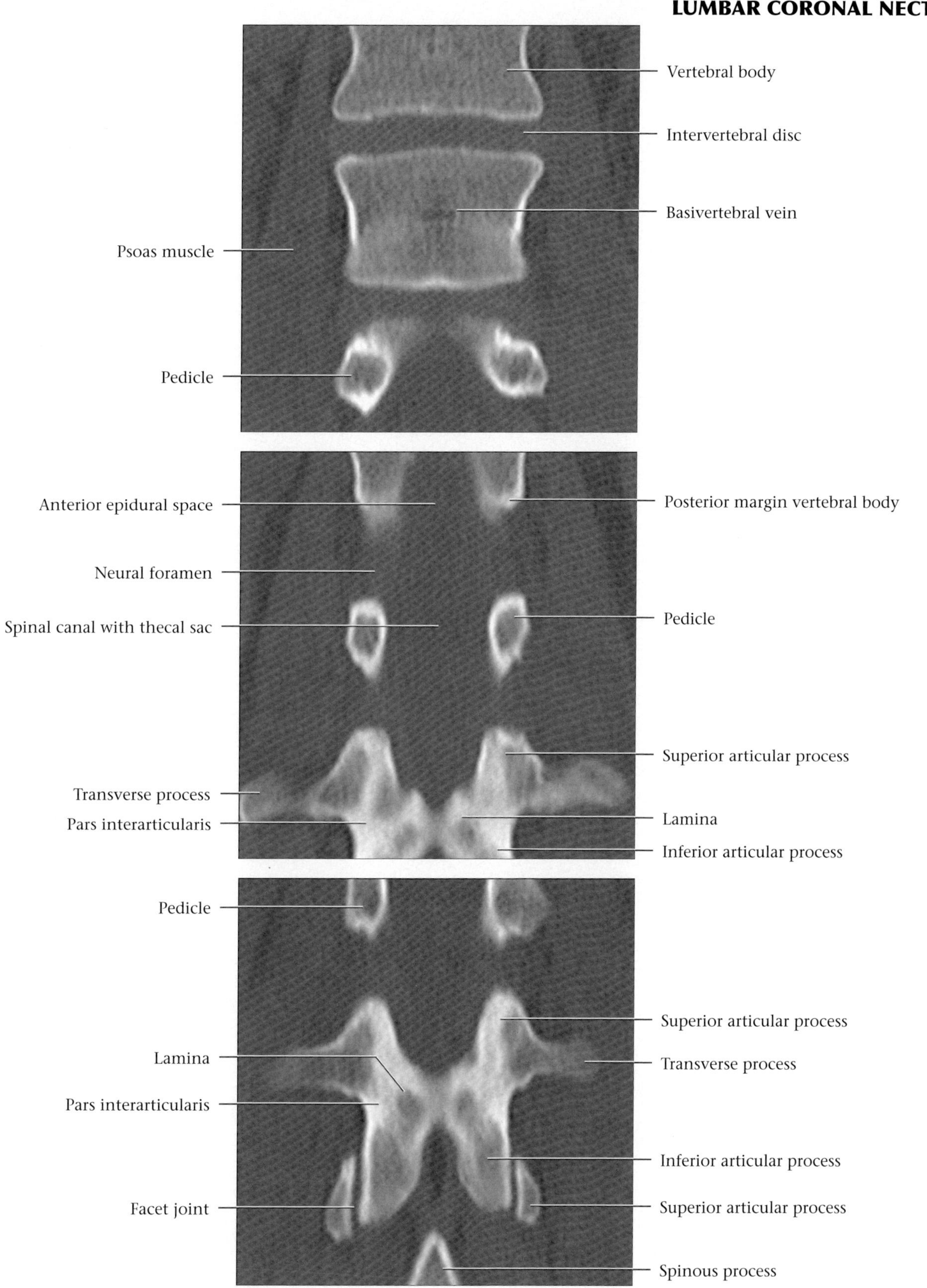

Vertebral body
Intervertebral disc
Basivertebral vein
Psoas muscle
Pedicle
Anterior epidural space
Posterior margin vertebral body
Neural foramen
Spinal canal with thecal sac
Pedicle
Superior articular process
Transverse process
Pars interarticularis
Lamina
Inferior articular process
Pedicle
Superior articular process
Lamina
Transverse process
Pars interarticularis
Inferior articular process
Facet joint
Superior articular process
Spinous process

(Top) First of three coronal NECT reformats of lumbar spine presented from anterior to posterior shows the rectangular-shaped vertebral bodies. The posterior margin of the body is pierced by the basivertebral veins. The pedicles arise dorsally from the vertebral bodies and are seen in transverse section. **(Middle)** Section more posteriorly extending through three levels of the spinal canal. The slightly oblique coronal section extends from the posterior vertebral body at top, through the pedicles in the middle, to the lamina at the bottom. The neural foramina are large and bounded superiorly by the pedicles. **(Bottom)** Section more posteriorly through the articular processes. The posterior elements in this plane assume a typical "H" configuration with the superior and inferior articular processes forming the vertical components and the lamina forming the central bar.

VERTEBRAL BODY AND LIGAMENTS

CERVICAL 3D-VRT NECT

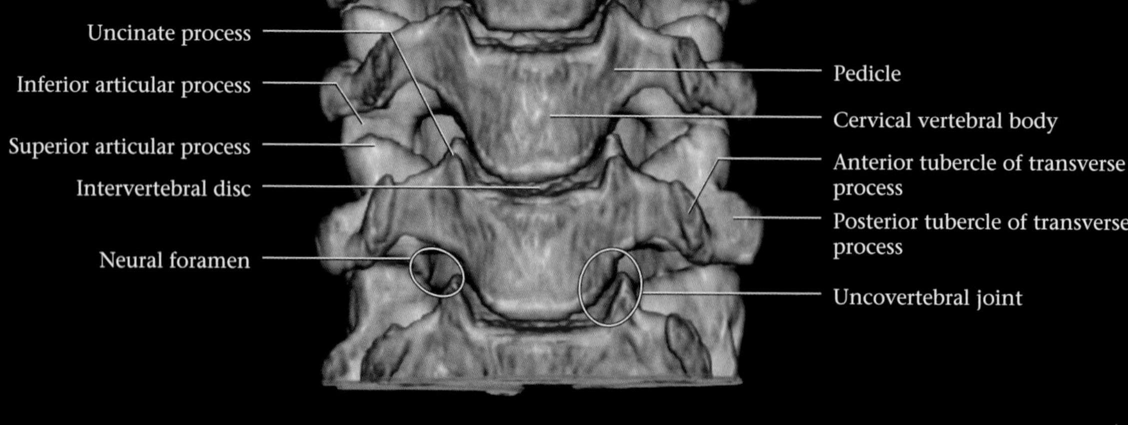
Uncinate process
Inferior articular process
Superior articular process
Intervertebral disc
Neural foramen
Pedicle
Cervical vertebral body
Anterior tubercle of transverse process
Posterior tubercle of transverse process
Uncovertebral joint

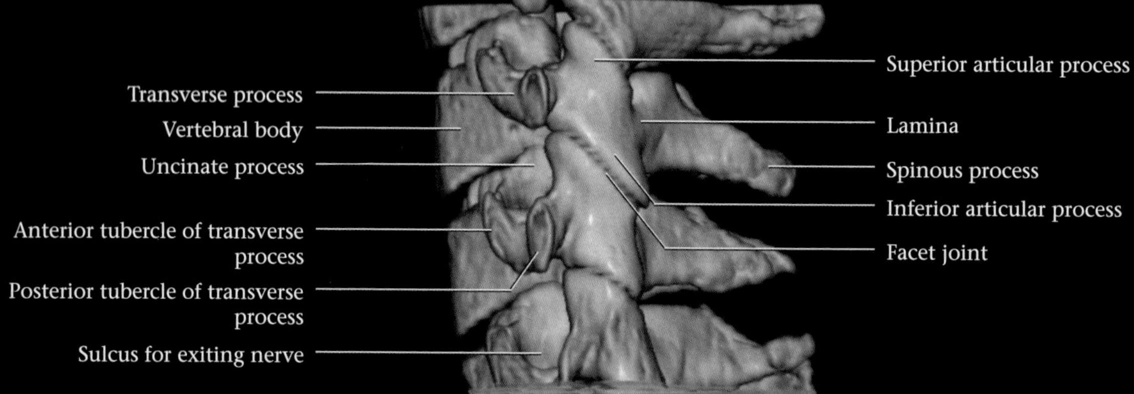
Transverse process
Vertebral body
Uncinate process
Anterior tubercle of transverse process
Posterior tubercle of transverse process
Sulcus for exiting nerve
Superior articular process
Lamina
Spinous process
Inferior articular process
Facet joint

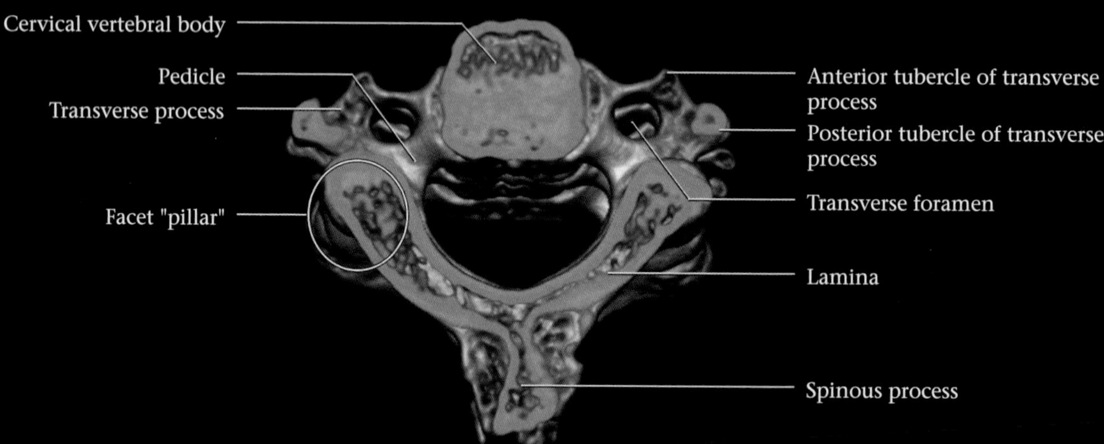
Cervical vertebral body
Pedicle
Transverse process
Facet "pillar"
Anterior tubercle of transverse process
Posterior tubercle of transverse process
Transverse foramen
Lamina
Spinous process

(Top) Anterior view of 3D-VRT NECT examination of the cervical spine. Cervical vertebral bodies are defined by the unique paired uncinate processes forming the margin of the uncovertebral joint (joints of Luschka). The pedicles are small, with large and complex transverse processes with anterior and posterior tubercles for muscle attachment, and the transverse foramen for the vertebral artery. **(Middle)** Lateral view of a 3D-VRT NECT study of the cervical spine. The posterior columns or "pillars" of the cervical spine are well-defined in this view comprised of the lateral masses with their superior and inferior articular processes. **(Bottom)** Axial 3D-VRT NECT viewed from below shows the large transverse foramen for passage of the vertebral arteries. The spinal canal is large relative to the pedicle and vertebral body. Note 45° anterior angulation of neural foramina.

THORACIC 3D-VRT NECT

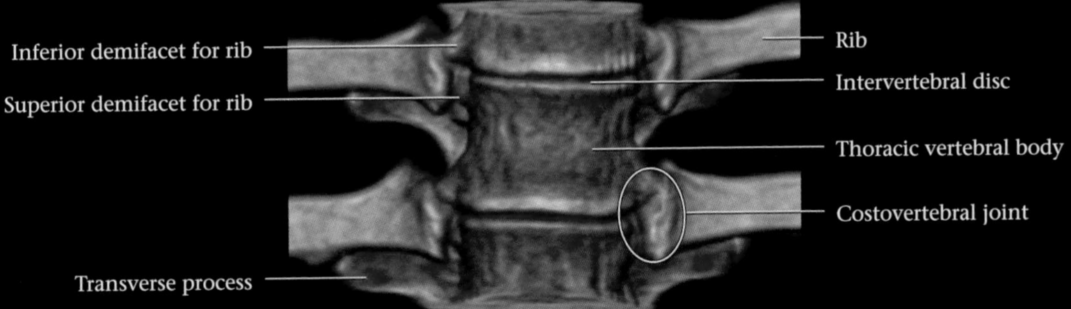
Inferior demifacet for rib
Superior demifacet for rib
Transverse process
Rib
Intervertebral disc
Thoracic vertebral body
Costovertebral joint

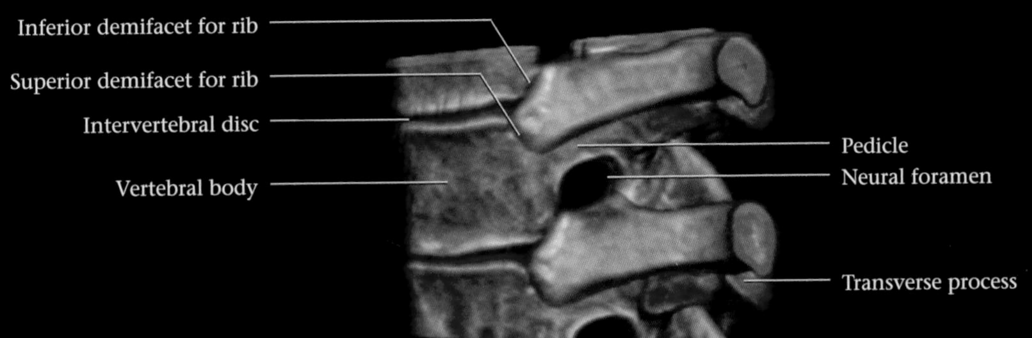
Inferior demifacet for rib
Superior demifacet for rib
Intervertebral disc
Vertebral body
Pedicle
Neural foramen
Transverse process

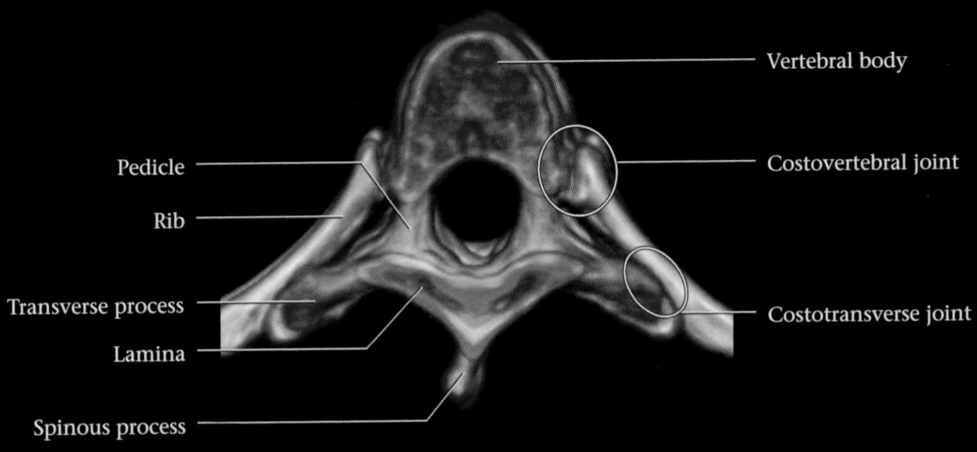
Vertebral body
Pedicle
Rib
Transverse process
Lamina
Spinous process
Costovertebral joint
Costotransverse joint

(Top) Anterior view of a 3D-VRT NECT examination of thoracic spine. The intervertebral discs are relatively small in the thoracic spine relative to cervical and lumbar segments. The bodies are held rigidly in place by the strong costotransverse and costovertebral joints for the ribs. The costovertebral joint crosses the disc with an inferior demifacet on the superior positioned vertebrae, and superior demifacet on the inferior positioned vertebrae. **(Middle)** Lateral view of a 3D-VRT NECT study of thoracic spine. The relationship of the neural foramen is well-defined on this view relative to the rib positions. **(Bottom)** Axial 3D-VRT examination of the thoracic spine viewed from below. The rib articulates at two points, the costotransverse joint laterally, and costovertebral joint medially. The vertebral bodies are heart-shaped, and the bony spinal canal is small.

VERTEBRAL BODY AND LIGAMENTS

LUMBAR 3D-VRT NECT

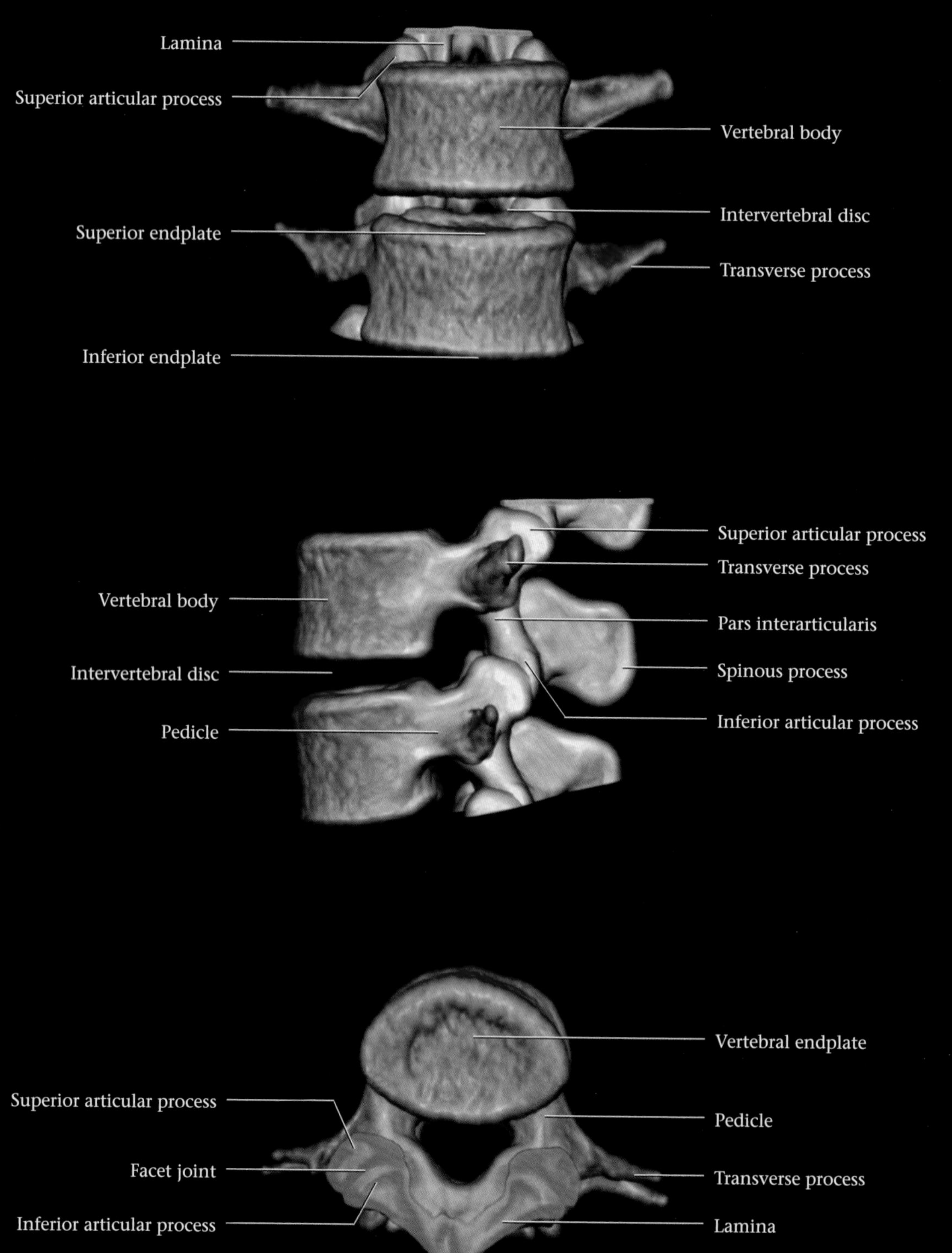
Lamina
Superior articular process
Vertebral body
Intervertebral disc
Superior endplate
Transverse process
Inferior endplate
Superior articular process
Transverse process
Vertebral body
Pars interarticularis
Spinous process
Intervertebral disc
Inferior articular process
Pedicle
Vertebral endplate
Superior articular process
Pedicle
Facet joint
Transverse process
Inferior articular process
Lamina
Spinous process

(Top) Anterior view of a 3D-VRT examination of the lumbar spine. The vertebral bodies are massive, with prominent lateral transverse processes. The intervertebral discs are large and thick. **(Middle)** Lateral view of a 3D-VRT examination of the lumbar spine. The large vertebral bodies are offset by the thick and sturdy posterior elements with their superior and inferior articular processes which are angled in a sagittal plane. Flexion/extension is permitted, but lateral rotation is limited. The transverse processes jut out laterally for muscle attachments. The pars interarticularis forms the junction between the superior and inferior articular processes. **(Bottom)** Axial view of a 3D-VRT NECT examination of the lumbar spine. The spinal canal assumes a more triangular shape, with thick pedicles and the obliquely oriented facets.

VERTEBRAL BODY AND LIGAMENTS

CERVICAL SAGITTAL T2 MR

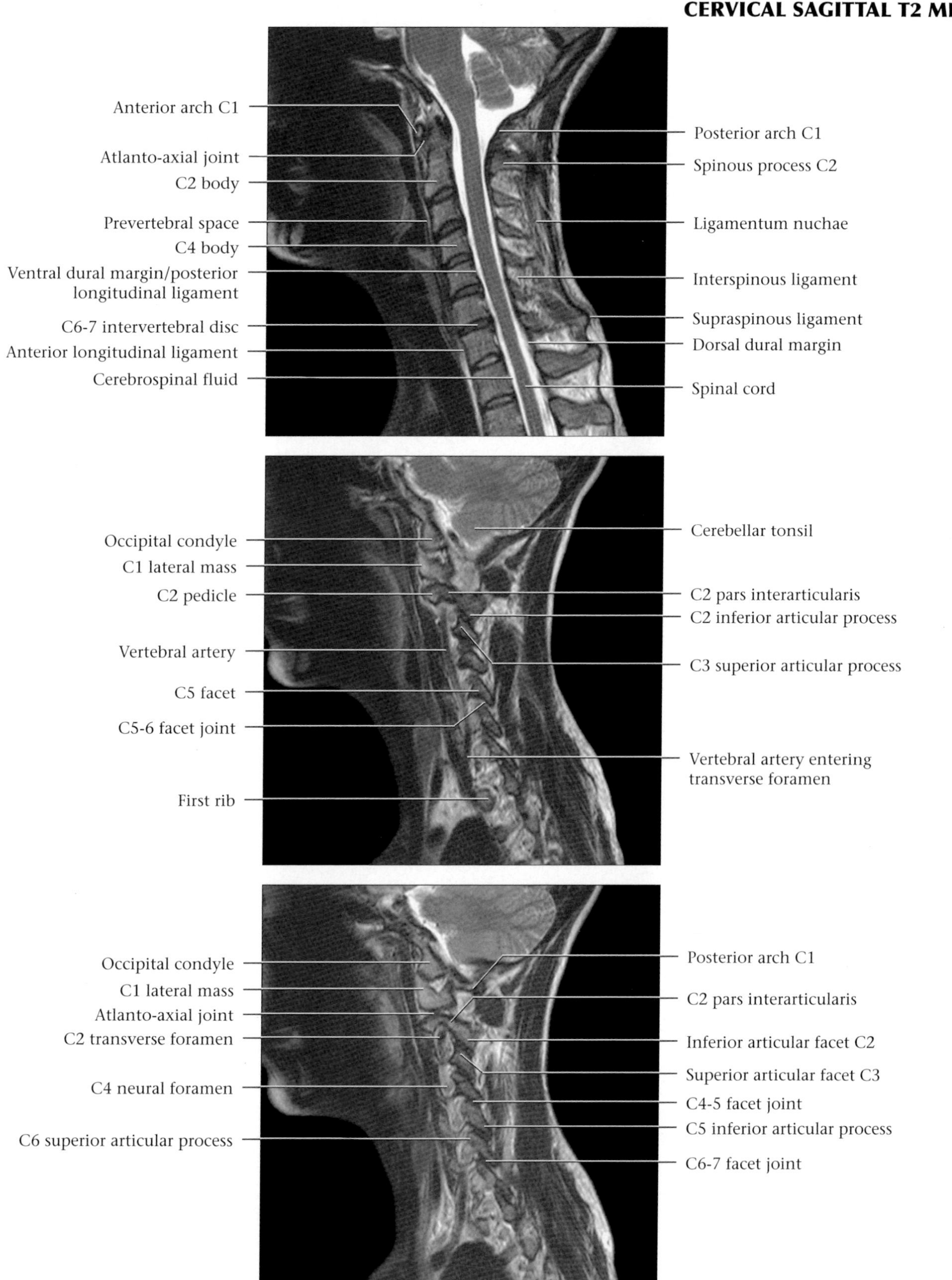
Anterior arch C1
Atlanto-axial joint
C2 body
Prevertebral space
C4 body
Ventral dural margin/posterior longitudinal ligament
C6-7 intervertebral disc
Anterior longitudinal ligament
Cerebrospinal fluid
Posterior arch C1
Spinous process C2
Ligamentum nuchae
Interspinous ligament
Supraspinous ligament
Dorsal dural margin
Spinal cord
Occipital condyle
C1 lateral mass
C2 pedicle
Vertebral artery
C5 facet
C5-6 facet joint
First rib
Cerebellar tonsil
C2 pars interarticularis
C2 inferior articular process
C3 superior articular process
Vertebral artery entering transverse foramen
Occipital condyle
C1 lateral mass
Atlanto-axial joint
C2 transverse foramen
C4 neural foramen
C6 superior articular process
Posterior arch C1
C2 pars interarticularis
Inferior articular facet C2
Superior articular facet C3
C4-5 facet joint
C5 inferior articular process
C6-7 facet joint

(Top) Midline sagittal T2 MR image shows the relationship of the cervical cord, vertebral bodies and spinous processes with smooth straight margins and alignment. The posterior dural margin merges with the ligamentum flavum and spinous process cortex low signal. The anterior dural margin merges with the posterior body cortex and posterior longitudinal ligament. **(Middle)** Paramedian T2 MR image shows the lateral facets at each level, and the flow void of the vertebral artery within the transverse foramen. **(Bottom)** Paramedian sagittal T2 MR image shows normal alignment of the lateral cervical bodies and facet joints. The rhomboidal configuration of the cervical facets is noted, with their complementary superior and inferior articular facets.

VERTEBRAL BODY AND LIGAMENTS

THORACIC SAGITTAL T2 MR

Intervertebral disc
Posterior longitudinal ligament
Superior endplate
Thoracic vertebral body
Inferior endplate
Anterior longitudinal ligament
Basivertebral veins
Thoracic cord
Ligamentum flavum
Spinous process
Interspinous ligament
Supraspinous ligament
Cerebrospinal fluid

Intervertebral disc
Lateral aspect thoracic vertebral body
Superior endplate
Inferior endplate
Segmental artery and vein
Superior articular process
Inferior articular process
Facet joint
Pedicle
Thoracic segmental nerve within foramen
Neural foramen

Costovertebral joint
Inferior demifacet for rib
Superior demifacet for rib
Segmental artery and vein
Intervertebral disc
Lateral margin thoracic vertebral body
Lateral aspect neural foramen
Segmental nerve within foramen

(Top) First of three sagittal midline T2 MR images of the thoracic spine presented from medial to lateral. The interspinous and supraspinous ligaments show typical normal low signal, attaching the adjacent spinous processes with their well-defined cortical margins and intermediate signal fatty marrow. The anterior longitudinal ligament low signal merges with the low signal of the anterior cortex of the vertebral body. The posterior longitudinal ligament is not separately defined from the anterior dural margin. **(Middle)** More lateral image of the thoracic spine. The lateral body marrow signal extends into the broad pedicle with the well-defined superior and inferior articular processes. The neural foramina are oval with rostral segmental vessels and nerves **(Bottom)** More lateral image of thoracic spine show the costovertebral joints spanning the posterior intervertebral discs.

VERTEBRAL BODY AND LIGAMENTS

LUMBAR SAGITTAL T2 MR

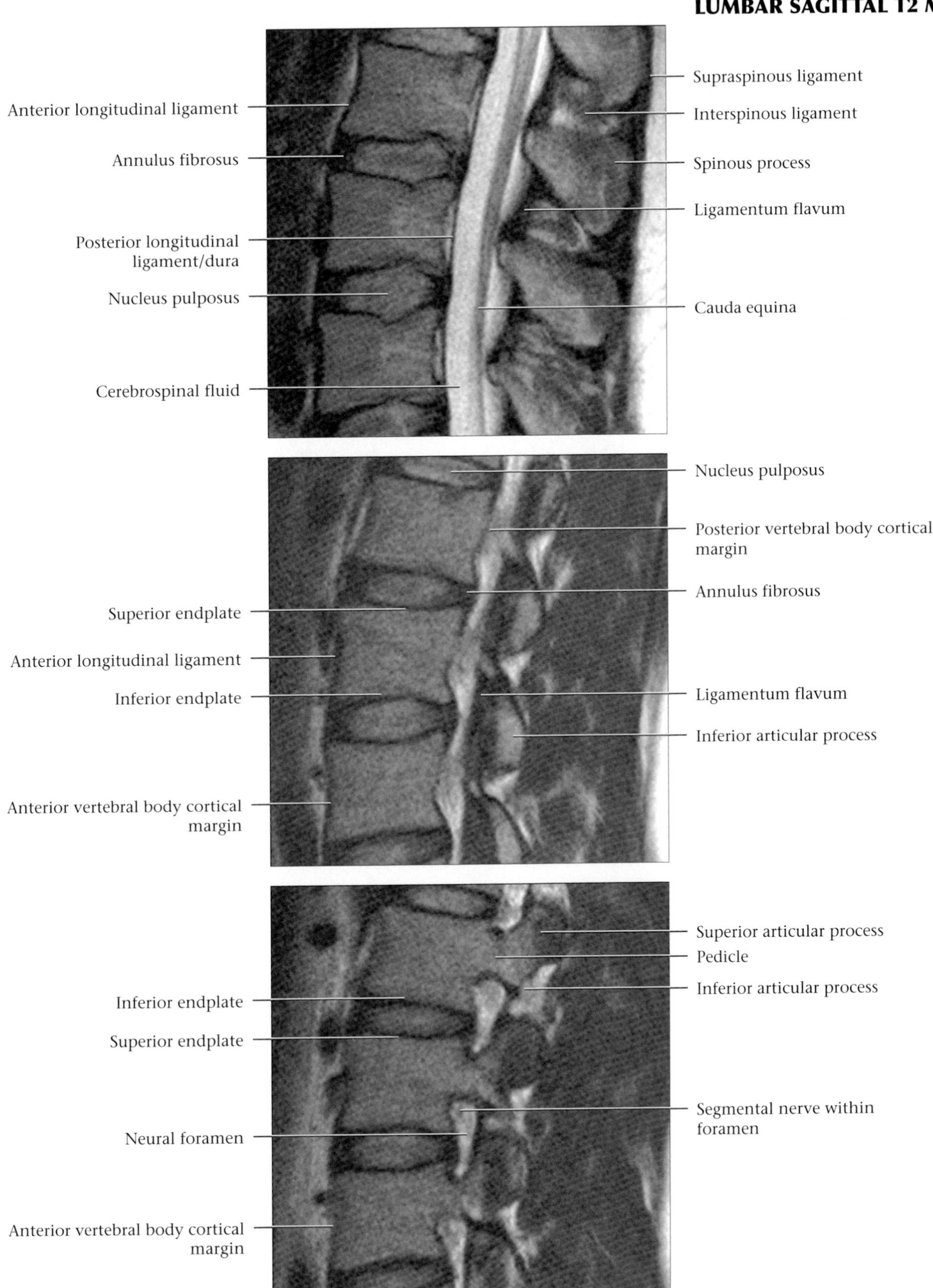

Anterior longitudinal ligament
Annulus fibrosus
Posterior longitudinal ligament/dura
Nucleus pulposus
Cerebrospinal fluid
Supraspinous ligament
Interspinous ligament
Spinous process
Ligamentum flavum
Cauda equina
Nucleus pulposus
Posterior vertebral body cortical margin
Annulus fibrosus
Superior endplate
Anterior longitudinal ligament
Inferior endplate
Ligamentum flavum
Inferior articular process
Anterior vertebral body cortical margin
Superior articular process
Pedicle
Inferior articular process
Inferior endplate
Superior endplate
Neural foramen
Segmental nerve within foramen
Anterior vertebral body cortical margin

(Top) First of three sagittal midline T2 MR images of the lumbar spine presented from medial to lateral. The medial portion of the ligamentum flavum is seen as a linear low signal posterior to the dural margin. The PLL and dura are seen as prominent linear low signal line spanning the discs and vertebral bodies. The ALL is seen as a smooth linear low signal along the anterior cortical margin of the vertebra body. **(Middle)** More lateral view of the lumbar spine. The articular processes are seen as oval bone masses posterior to the high signal cerebrospinal fluid of the thecal sac. The ligamentum flavum is more prominent as low signal along the ventral margin of the posterior elements. **(Bottom)** More lateral view of the lumbar spine. The neural foramina are key hole shaped, with larger superior portion bounded superiorly by the inferior margin of the pedicle.

VERTEBRAL BODY AND LIGAMENTS

THORACIC AXIAL T2 MR

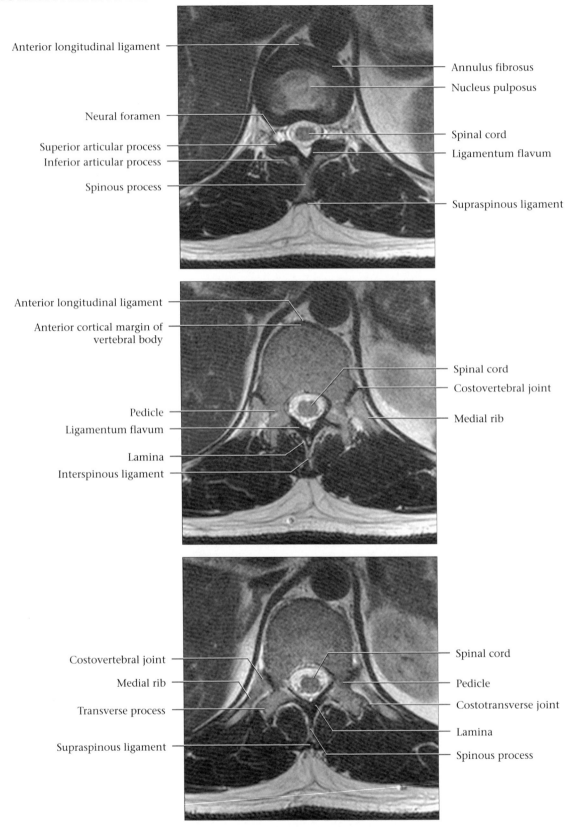

Anterior longitudinal ligament
Annulus fibrosus
Nucleus pulposus
Neural foramen
Spinal cord
Superior articular process
Inferior articular process
Ligamentum flavum
Spinous process
Supraspinous ligament

Anterior longitudinal ligament
Anterior cortical margin of vertebral body
Spinal cord
Costovertebral joint
Pedicle
Medial rib
Ligamentum flavum
Lamina
Interspinous ligament

Costovertebral joint
Spinal cord
Medial rib
Pedicle
Transverse process
Costotransverse joint
Lamina
Supraspinous ligament
Spinous process

(Top) First of three axial T2 MR images of the thoracic spine through the intervertebral disc presented from superior to inferior. The thoracic spine shows coronal orientation of the facet joints with a less distinct ligamentum flavum. The low signal outer component of the annulus fibrosus merges with the low signal of the anterior longitudinal ligament. The posterior longitudinal ligament is not visualized. **(Middle)** More inferior view of the thoracic spine through the vertebral body level. The costovertebral joint is well-defined, with the costotransverse joint out of plane of imaging. The pedicles at this level are short, encompassing the small central bony canal. **(Bottom)** More inferior image of the thoracic spine. The costovertebral and costotransverse joints are both visualized on this section, with rectangular shaped transverse processes.

Anterior longitudinal ligament
Anterior cortex of vertebral body
Ligamentum flavum
Superior articular process
Inferior articular process
Thecal sac
Pedicle
Transverse process
Facet joint
Interspinous ligament
Spinous process

Anterior longitudinal ligament
Anterior cortex of vertebral body
Thecal sac
Neural foramen
Ligamentum flavum
Segmental ganglion
Lamina
Spinous process
Supraspinous ligament

Intervertebral disc
Thecal sac
Neural foramen
Ligamentum flavum
Inferior articular process
Supraspinous ligament
Superior articular process
Facet joint
Lamina
Spinous process

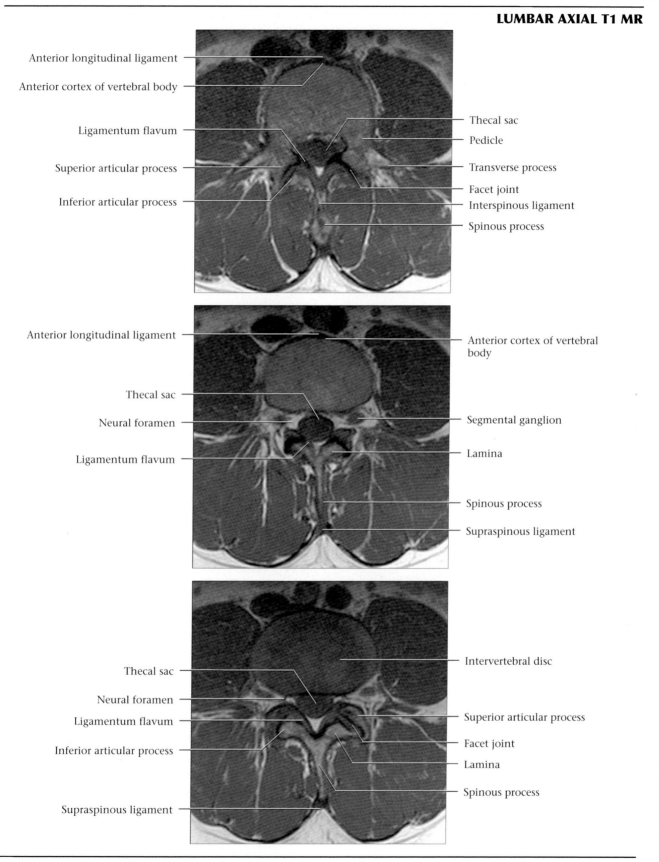

(Top) First of three axial T1 MR images of the lumbar spine through the vertebral body presented from superior to inferior. The low signal anterior longitudinal ligament merges with the low signal of the anterior cortical margin. The ligamentum flavum is seen along its medial portion, extending laterally towards the facet joint. The facet joint is obliquely oriented around 45 degrees, with a well-defined joint space. **(Middle)** More inferior axial T1 weighted image of the lumbar spine. The neural foramina are outlined by the high signal foraminal fat, with the centrally situated ganglion. The lamina and spinous process form a "Y" shaped structure projecting dorsally. **(Bottom)** More inferior axial T1 weighted image of the lumbar spine through the intervertebral disc. The facet or zygapophyseal joints are well visualized with the facet joint space, and ventral margin bounded by the ligamentum flavum.

INTERVERTEBRAL DISC & FACET JOINTS

Terminology

Synonyms

- Facet joint; apophyseal joint; zygapophyseal joint

Gross Anatomy

Overview

- C2 → S1 vertebrae articulate in 3 joint complex
  - Secondary cartilaginous joints (symphyses) between vertebral bodies
  - Synovial joints between articular processes (zygapophyses)
- Other articulations
  - Fibrous (between laminae, transverse/spinous processes)
  - Uncinate processes (C3-7)

Intervertebral Discs

- **Overview**
  - Lie between thin horizontal hyaline/fibrocartilage end-plates on superior, inferior surfaces of vertebrae
  - With ALL/PLL, link vertebrae from C2 → sacrum
  - Comprise 1/3 of spinal column height
    - Thickness varies (thinnest in upper T, thickest in lower L)
    - Lumbar discs 7-10 mm thick, 4 cm diameter
  - Components
    - Central nucleus pulposus
    - Peripheral annulus fibrosus
  - Major function is mechanical
    - Transmit, distribute load from weight/activity
    - Allow flexion/extension, lateral bending, torsion
    - Discs loaded preferentially in flexion
- **Annulus fibrosus**
  - Concentric series of 15-25 fibrous lamellae
    - Surround, constrain nucleus pulposus
    - Collagen fibers lie parallel within each lamina
    - Fibers oriented 60° to vertical
    - Type I collagen predominates in outer annulus
    - Type II predominates in inner annulus
  - Inner annulus blends gradually with nucleus
  - Outer annulus attaches to ALL, PLL and to fused epiphyseal ring of vertebral bodies by Sharpey fibers
  - Innervation: Branch of ventral primary ramus
  - Vasculature: Outer annulus supplied by capillaries from spinal branches of dorsal rami
- **Nucleus pulposus**
  - Origin: Remnant of notochord
  - Eccentric position within annulus
    - More dorsal compared to center of vertebral body
  - Components
    - 85-95% water
    - Loose fibrous strands of collagen, elastin with gelatinous matrix
    - Scattered chondrocytes
    - Major macromolecular component = proteoglycans
    - Proteoglycans = protein core + attached glycosaminoglycan chains
    - Glycosaminoglycan chains have negatively charged sulphate, carboxyl groups
    - Cations attract anions → high osmotic pressure enables disc to absorb water
  - Except for outer annulus, disc relies on nutrient diffusion from endplate vessels
    - Steep metabolic gradient between vessels, disc centrum
    - Centrum has ↓ glucose + oxygen, ↑ lactic acid
    - Carbohydrate utilization dominated by glycolysis

Facet Joints

- **Articular processes** (zygapophyses)
  - Paired posterior lateral joints
    - Superior facet surface directed dorsally
    - Inferior facet surface directed ventrally
    - Facets joined by pars interarticularis
  - True synovial joint
    - Hyaline cartilage surfaces, synovial membrane, fibrous capsule
  - Orientation
    - Obliquely sagittal in lumbar spine (protects disc from axial rotation)
    - Coronal in cervical and thoracic spine (protects against shear)
  - Innervation: Nociceptive fibers from medial branch of dorsal ramus
  - Function: Load bearing in extension, rotation
- **Pars interarticularis**
  - Lies between subatlantal superior/inferior articular facets
  - C2 unique
    - Anterior relation of superior to posterior placed inferior facet
    - C2 pars interarticularis unusually elongated

Imaging Anatomy

Overview

- Signal on MR related to water content
  - Nucleus, inner annulus high signal on T2WI
  - Outer annulus hypointense on T1 & T2WI
  - ↑ Collagen/proteoglycan cross-linking with age → decreased water binding, ↓ T2 signal
- Disc "bulge"
  - Normal age-related change (begins as early as mid-teens)
  - Posterior margin convex
  - Disc extends circumferentially beyond end plates
- Concentric annular tear in posterior disc common
  - High signal on T2WI
  - Vascularized granulation tissue enhances on T1 C+

Anatomy-Based Imaging Issues

Key Concepts or Questions

- Spondylolysis
  - Pars interarticularis fracture
  - Superior facets displace ventrally
  - Inferior facets remain attached to dorsal arch
- Spondylolisthesis
  - Slip of one vertebrae relative to adjacent level
  - Many etiologies (congenital dysplasia of articular processes, trauma, degenerative instability, etc.)

INTERVERTEBRAL DISC & FACET JOINTS

GRAPHICS

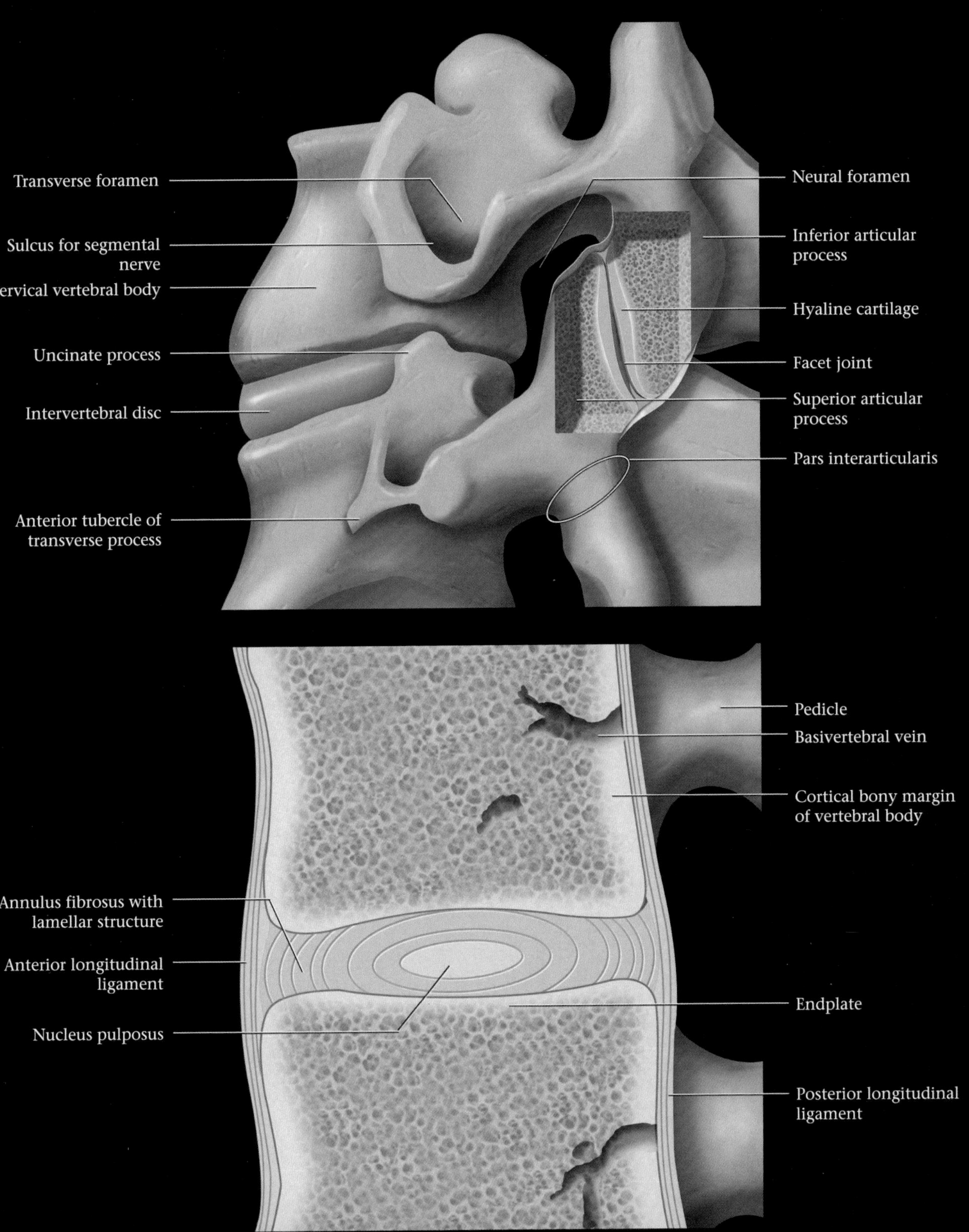

Transverse foramen
Sulcus for segmental nerve
Cervical vertebral body
Uncinate process
Intervertebral disc
Anterior tubercle of transverse process
Neural foramen
Inferior articular process
Hyaline cartilage
Facet joint
Superior articular process
Pars interarticularis
Pedicle
Basivertebral vein
Cortical bony margin of vertebral body
Annulus fibrosus with lamellar structure
Anterior longitudinal ligament
Nucleus pulposus
Endplate
Posterior longitudinal ligament

(Top) Posterior oblique graphic view of the cervical spine. The facet joint is highlighted with a cut away view, showing the opposed cartilaginous articular facets of the superior and inferior articular processes. The uncovertebral joint, or joint of Luschka is along the posterior lateral margin of the vertebral body and the anterior margin of the neural foramen. **(Bottom)** Sagittal midline graphic through the lumbar disc. The discovertebral unit is composed of the anterior and posterior longitudinal ligaments, the annulus fibrosus, the nucleus pulposus and the bony and cartilaginous endplates. The annulus fibrosus is composed of multiple layers, similar to an onion skin in appearance. The inner annulus merges into the central more gelatinous nucleus pulposus. The endplate maintains nutrition to the disc via diffusion of solutes.

INTERVERTEBRAL DISC & FACET JOINTS

3D-VRT NECT

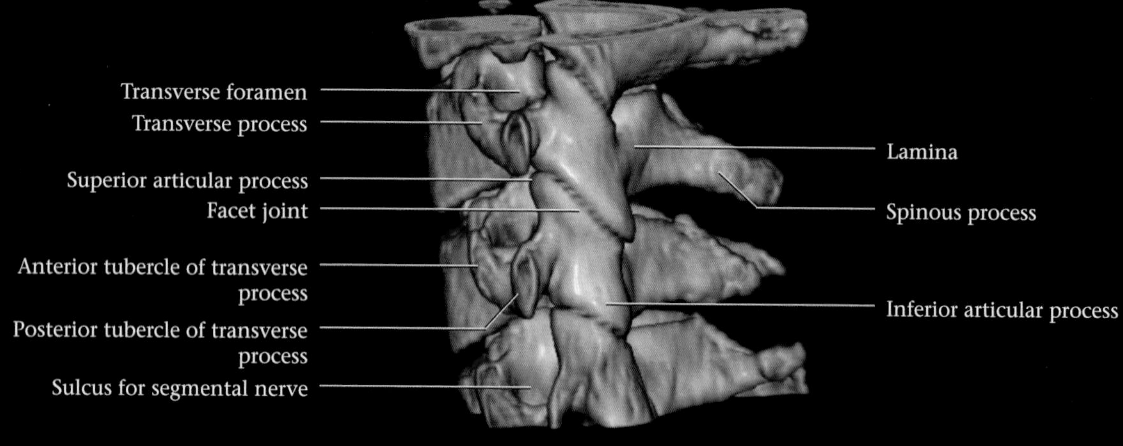
Transverse foramen
Transverse process
Superior articular process
Facet joint
Anterior tubercle of transverse process
Posterior tubercle of transverse process
Sulcus for segmental nerve
Lamina
Spinous process
Inferior articular process

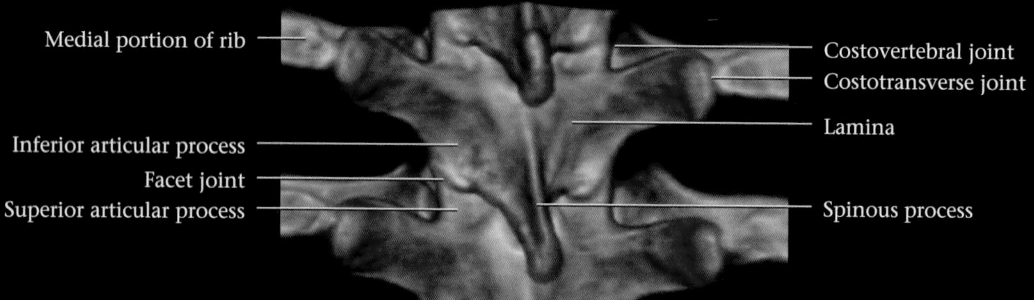
Medial portion of rib
Inferior articular process
Facet joint
Superior articular process
Costovertebral joint
Costotransverse joint
Lamina
Spinous process

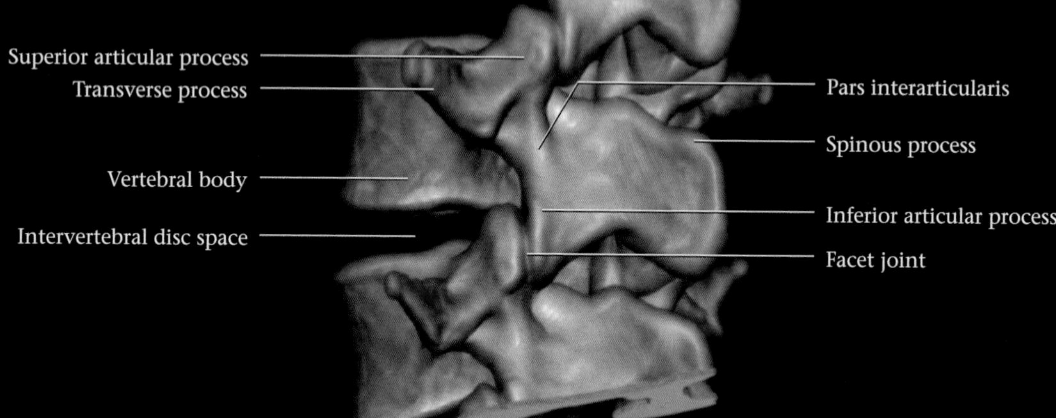
Superior articular process
Transverse process
Vertebral body
Intervertebral disc space
Pars interarticularis
Spinous process
Inferior articular process
Facet joint

(Top) Lateral oblique view of a 3D-VRT NECT examination of the cervical spine. The facet joints in the cervical spine form paired vertical columns or "pillars", which together with the discovertebral unit provide the three pronged structural support for the cervical segment. The obliquity of the facet joints allow degrees of both flexion/extension and rotation. **(Middle)** Posterior view of a 3D-VRT NECT examination of the thoracic spine. The coronally oriented facet joints are viewed from their posterior margins, with the interlocking superior and inferior processes. Structural stability is provided by the tough costovertebral and costotransverse joints and their accompanying ligaments. **(Bottom)** Oblique view of a 3D-VRT NECT examination of the lumbar spine shows the "Scotty dog" appearance of the transverse process, articular processes and pars interarticularis.

INTERVERTEBRAL DISC & FACET JOINTS

CERVICAL AXIAL & SAGITTAL NECT

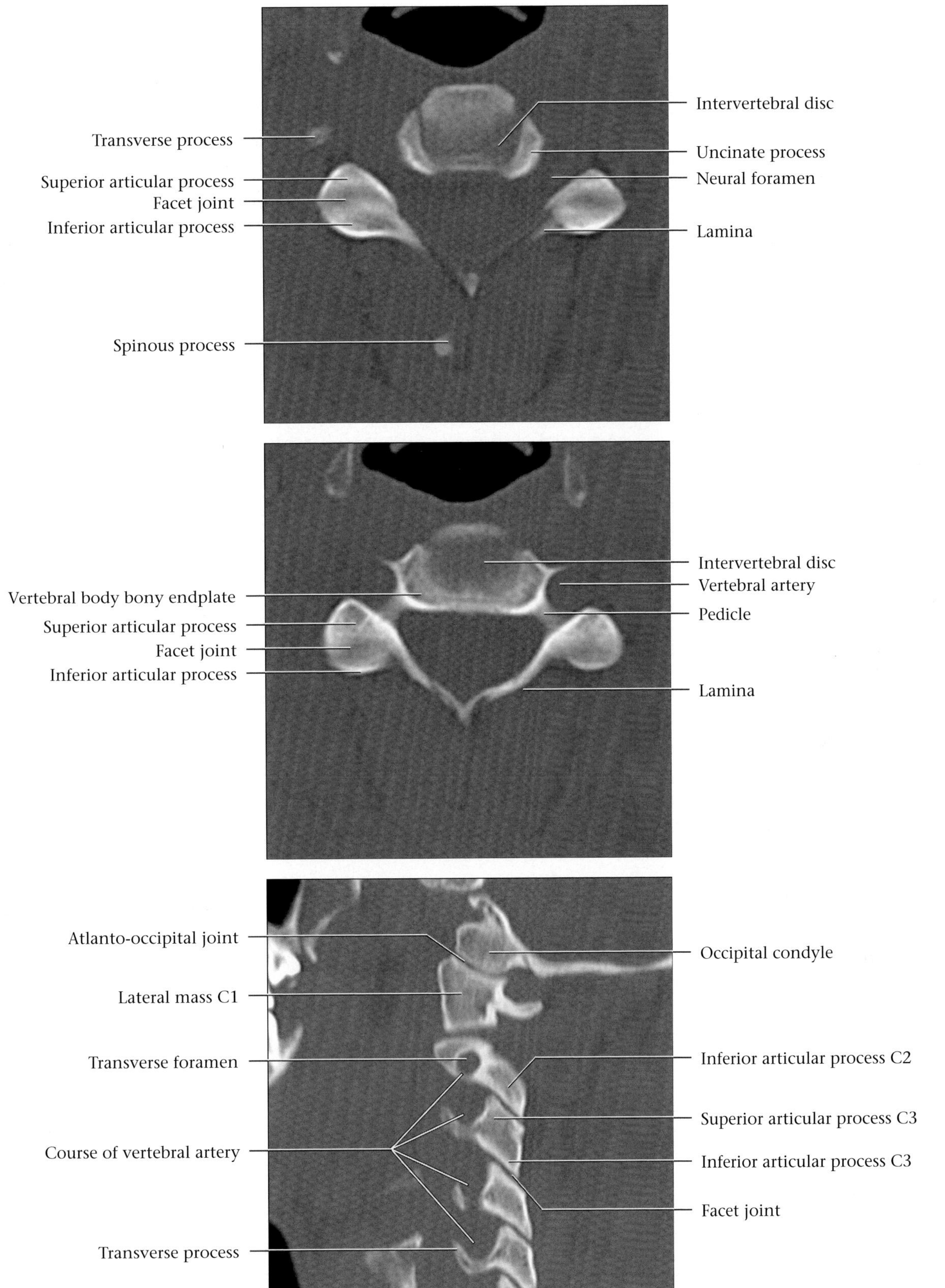
Transverse process
Superior articular process
Facet joint
Inferior articular process
Spinous process
Intervertebral disc
Uncinate process
Neural foramen
Lamina
Vertebral body bony endplate
Superior articular process
Facet joint
Inferior articular process
Intervertebral disc
Vertebral artery
Pedicle
Lamina
Atlanto-occipital joint
Lateral mass C1
Transverse foramen
Course of vertebral artery
Transverse process
Occipital condyle
Inferior articular process C2
Superior articular process C3
Inferior articular process C3
Facet joint

(Top) Axial NECT image of the cervical spine. The facet joint is viewed obliquely, with the superior to inferior articular process forming the oval-shaped facet mass. The intervertebral disc is cup-shaped, bounded along the posterior aspect by the upturned bony uncinate process. The anterior border of the neural foramen is shielded from the intervertebral disc by the uncinate process. **(Middle)** More inferior axial NECT view of the cervical spine. The cup shape of the intervertebral disc is also apparent on this section, with upturned bone of the posterior and lateral endplates. The facet joint is again viewed in oblique section forming an oval facet mass. **(Bottom)** Sagittal NECT reformat of cervical spine better defines the margins of the facet joints with their oblique inferior course. Just ventral to the facets is the long course of the vertebral artery.

THORACIC AXIAL & SAGITTAL NECT

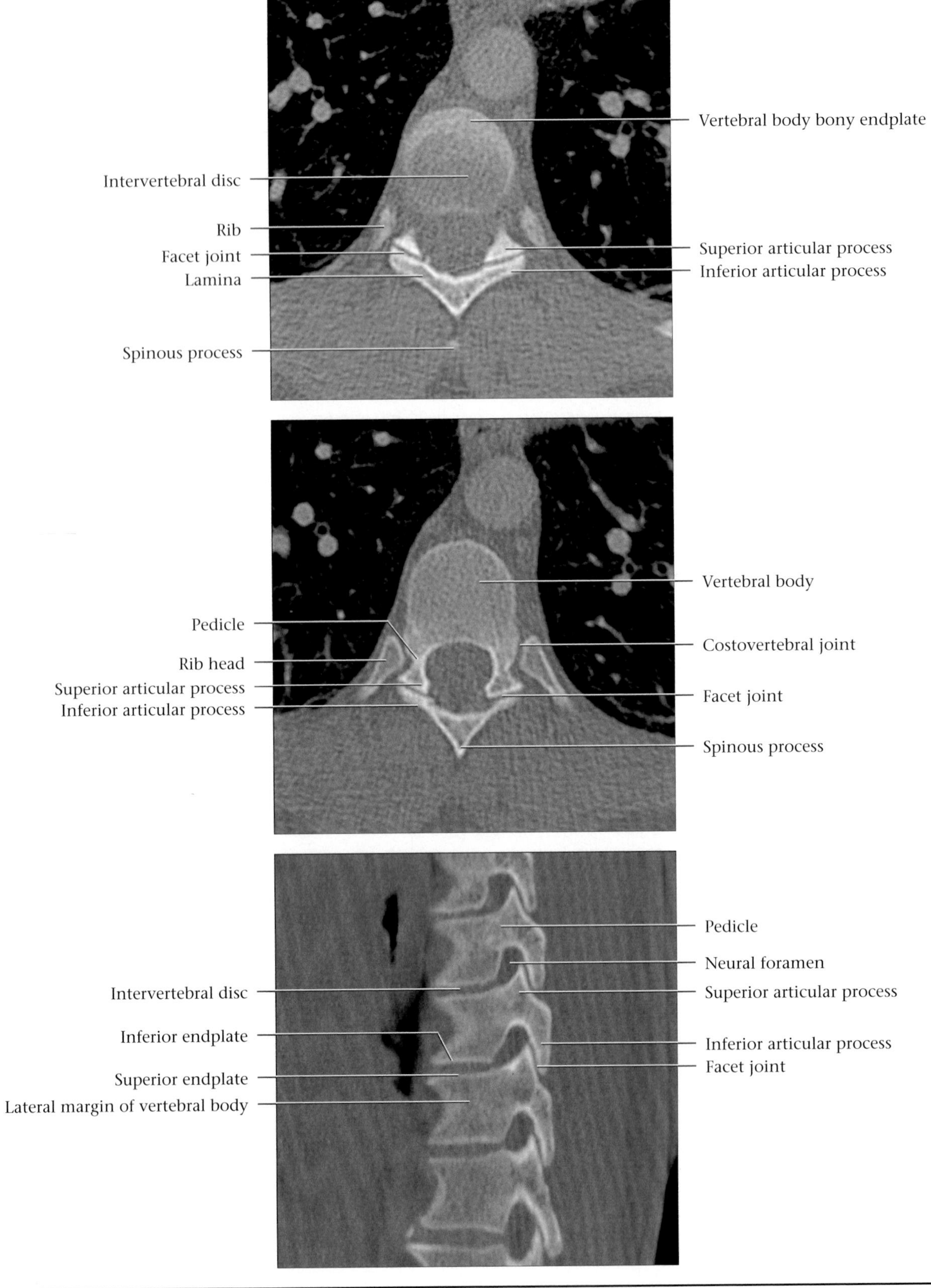
Vertebral body bony endplate
Intervertebral disc
Rib
Facet joint
Lamina
Superior articular process
Inferior articular process
Spinous process
Vertebral body
Pedicle
Costovertebral joint
Rib head
Superior articular process
Inferior articular process
Facet joint
Spinous process
Pedicle
Neural foramen
Intervertebral disc
Superior articular process
Inferior endplate
Inferior articular process
Facet joint
Superior endplate
Lateral margin of vertebral body

(Top) Axial NECT image through the thoracic spine. The facet joints show a more coronal orientation, relative to the oblique coronal (or horizontal) cervical joint orientation, and the oblique sagittal orientation of the lumbar joints. The bony spinal canal containing the thoracic cord is relatively small with respect to the body and posterior elements. **(Middle)** More inferior axial NECT view of the thoracic spine. The coronal oriented facet joints are again visualized, merging into the lamina and inferiorly directed spinous process. The costovertebral joint laterally provides additional stabilization. **(Bottom)** Sagittal reformat of thoracic spine NECT. The facet joint orientation is well-defined in this view, showing the articulation of the adjacent vertebral bodies with their superior and inferior articular processes.

INTERVERTEBRAL DISC & FACET JOINTS

LUMBAR AXIAL & SAGITTAL NECT

Vertebral bony endplate
Intervertebral disc
Neural foramen
Superior articular process
Facet joint
Inferior articular process
Lamina
Spinous process

Anterior cortical margin of vertebral body
Pedicle
Transverse process
Superior articular process
Facet joint
Inferior articular process
Ligamentum flavum
Spinous process

Inferior endplate
Neural foramen
Superior endplate
Superior articular process
Anterior cortical margin of vertebral body
Pars interarticularis
Intervertebral disc
Inferior articular process
Facet joint
Pedicle

(Top) Axial NECT of the lumbar spine. The oblique sagittal orientation of the facet joint is evident in this section, with the well-defined articular processes, forming the posterolateral margin of the spinal canal. The ventral margin of the facet forms the posterior aspect of the neural foramen. **(Middle)** More inferior axial NECT section of the lumbar spine through the pedicles. The oblique sagittal orientation of the facets is maintained. **(Bottom)** Sagittal reformat of NECT examination of the lumbar spine. The facet joints are well-defined with their large, robust superior and inferior articular processes. The ventral facet joint forms the posterior margin of the neural foramen. The anterior margin of the neural foramen is composed of cortical margin of two vertebral bodies, and the intervening intervertebral disc.

INTERVERTEBRAL DISC & FACET JOINTS

SAGITTAL T2 INTERVERTEBRAL DISC

Anterior arch C1
Cerebrospinal fluid
C2-3 intervertebral disc
Annulus fibrosus/anterior longitudinal ligament complex
Inferior endplate C6
Cerebellar tonsil
Foramen magnum
Spinal cord
Annulus fibrosus/posterior longitudinal ligament complex
Superior endplate C7
Intervertebral disc
Nucleus pulposus

Annulus fibrosus/anterior longitudinal ligament complex
Inferior endplate T6
Thoracic intervertebral disc
Annulus fibrosus/posterior longitudinal ligament complex
Superior endplate T7
T8 vertebral body
Thoracic spinal cord
Basivertebral vein

Superior endplate L3
Inferior endplate L3
Nucleus pulposus
Intranuclear cleft
Cerebrospinal fluid
Annulus fibrosus/anterior longitudinal ligament complex
Conus medullaris
Cauda equina
Annulus fibrosus
Posterior longitudinal ligament

(Top) Sagittal midline T2 MR image through the cervical spine. The intervertebral discs are relatively small, with thin low signal outer annular fibers and a predominate high signal central nucleus pulposus. The intranuclear cleft is not usually visible. **(Middle)** Sagittal T2 MR of the thoracic spine. The vertebral bodies are square in morphology, with slightly more pronounced intervertebral discs. The intranuclear cleft is not usually visible in the mid and upper thoracic region, but becomes progressively more pronounced at the thoracolumbar junction. **(Bottom)** Sagittal T2 MR image of the lumbar spine. The intervertebral discs are large, with pronounced low signal annulus fibrosus. The intranuclear cleft is a typical feature of the adult lumbar disc on T2 MR images.

SAGITTAL T2 FACET JOINTS

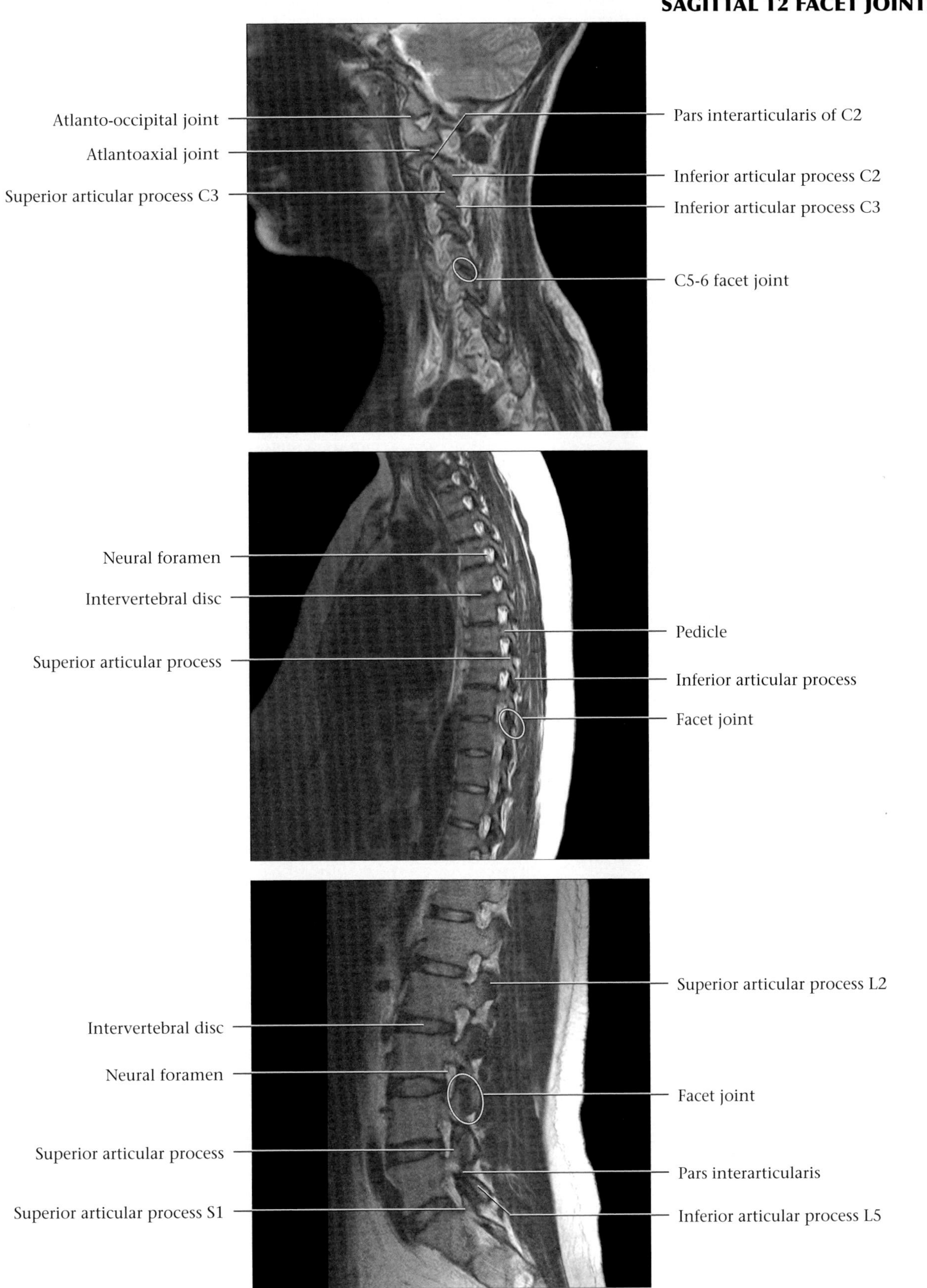
Atlanto-occipital joint
Atlantoaxial joint
Superior articular process C3
Pars interarticularis of C2
Inferior articular process C2
Inferior articular process C3
C5-6 facet joint
Neural foramen
Intervertebral disc
Superior articular process
Pedicle
Inferior articular process
Facet joint
Superior articular process L2
Intervertebral disc
Neural foramen
Facet joint
Superior articular process
Pars interarticularis
Superior articular process S1
Inferior articular process L5

(Top) Sagittal T2 MR image through the cervical spine. The cervical pillars are readily visible, composed of the adjacent superior and inferior articular processes and the intervening joint. The C2 body is transitional with the inferior articular process forming the rostral part of the pillar. The superior process of C2 is more ventral, and articulates with the inferior articular facet of C1. **(Middle)** Sagittal T2 MR image of the thoracic spine. The orientation of the thoracic facets allows good visualization of the facet joints, as well as the neural foramen. **(Bottom)** Sagittal T2 MR image of the lumbar spine. The facet joints are more obliquely oriented, allowing flexion and extension. The superior articular process forms the dorsal margin of the neural foramen.

PARASPINAL MUSCLES

Terminology

Abbreviations

- Origin (O), insertion (I), innervation (N), function (F)
- Ligamentum nuchae (LN)
- Spinous, transverse processes (SP, TP)

Gross Anatomy

Overview

- Musculature of back arranged in layers
  - Superficial (extrinsic or "immigrant") muscles
    - Innervated by anterior rami of spinal nerves
    - Run between upper limb, axial skeleton
  - Deep (intrinsic or "true") muscles
    - Innervated by spinal nerve dorsal rami
    - Lie deep to thoracolumbar fascia
- Muscles of back enclosed by fascia
  - Fascia attaches medially to LN, SP, supraspinous ligaments, medial crest of sacrum
  - Cervical (deep cervical fascia)
    - Prevertebral layer covers anterior vertebral muscles
  - Thoracic: Thin, transparent; joins ribs
  - Thoracolumbar fascia
    - Dense; continuous with abdominal aponeurosis

Imaging Anatomy

Superficial Muscles

- **Trapezius**
  - O: EOP, LN, SP C7-T12
  - I: Clavicle, acromion, scapular spine
  - F: Rotation, adduction, raising, lowering scapula
  - N: CN11, C3, C4
- **Latissimus dorsi**
  - O: Lumbar aponeurosis to T6-12 SP, iliac crest, lower 4 ribs
  - I: Intertubercular groove of humerus
  - F: Extends, adducts, rotates arm medially
  - N: Thoracodorsal
- **Levator scapulae**
  - O: Posterior tubercles + TP C1-4
  - I: Medial border scapula
  - F: Elevate and rotate scapula
  - N: C3-5
- **Rhomboid minor**
  - O: LN, SP C7-T1
  - I: Medial border scapula
  - F: Scapula medially
  - N: Dorsal scapular
- **Rhomboid major**
  - O: SP T2-5
  - I: Medial border scapula, below spine
  - F: Scapula medially
  - N: Dorsal scapular

Deep Muscles

- **C/T/L general musculature**
  - F: All extend vertebral column
  - N: All by posterior divisions of spinal nerves
  - **Splenius capitis**
    - O: LN, SP C7-T3
    - I: Occipital bone, mastoid
    - F: Draws head back, bends head laterally
  - **Splenius cervicis**
    - O: SP T3-6
    - I: TP C1-3
  - **Erector spinae** (iliocostalis, longissimus, spinalis)
    - O: SP T1-L5, lower 6 ribs, iliac crest, TP T1-5
    - I: Upper border ribs 1-6, TP C2-7, lumbar and thoracic TP
  - **Semispinalis** (capitis, cervical, thoracic)
    - O: TP C7-T10
    - I: SP C2-T4, occipital bone
    - F: Rotate head/column to opposite side
  - **Multifidus**
    - O: C4-7 articular processes, thoracic TP, lumbar superior articular facets
    - I: Crosses 1-4 vertebrae to reach SP C2-L5
    - F: Rotate column to opposite side
  - **Rotatores**
    - O: TP
    - I: SP adjacent vertebrae
    - F: Rotate column to opposite side
  - **Interspinalis**
    - Connect apices of adjoining SP C2-L5
  - **Intertransverse**
    - Connect adjacent TP
- **Suboccipital**
  - **Rectus capitis**
    - O: SP C2, posterior arch C1
    - I: Occipital bone
    - F: Extend, rotate head
  - **Oblique capitis superior**
    - O: TP C1
    - I: Occipital bone
    - F: Extend, bend head same side
  - **Oblique capitis inferior**
    - O: Spine of C2
    - I: TP C1
    - F: Turn head same side
- **Prevertebral**
  - **Rectus capitis**
    - O: TP C1
    - I: Occipital bone
    - F: Flexes head
    - N: C1-2
  - **Longus colli**
    - O: TP C3-5, vertebral bodies C5-T3
    - I: Anterior arch C1, vertebral bodies C2-4
    - F: Flexes, rotates neck
    - N: C2-7
  - **Longus capitis**
    - O: TP C3-6
    - I: Occipital bone
    - F: Flexes head
    - N: C1-3
  - **Scalene** (anterior, middle, posterior)
    - O: TP, vertebrae C2-7
    - I: Ribs 1, 2
    - F: Lateral bending, flexing neck
    - N: C5-8
  - **Psoas** (major, minor) functionally part of iliac region, thigh flexors

PARASPINAL MUSCLES

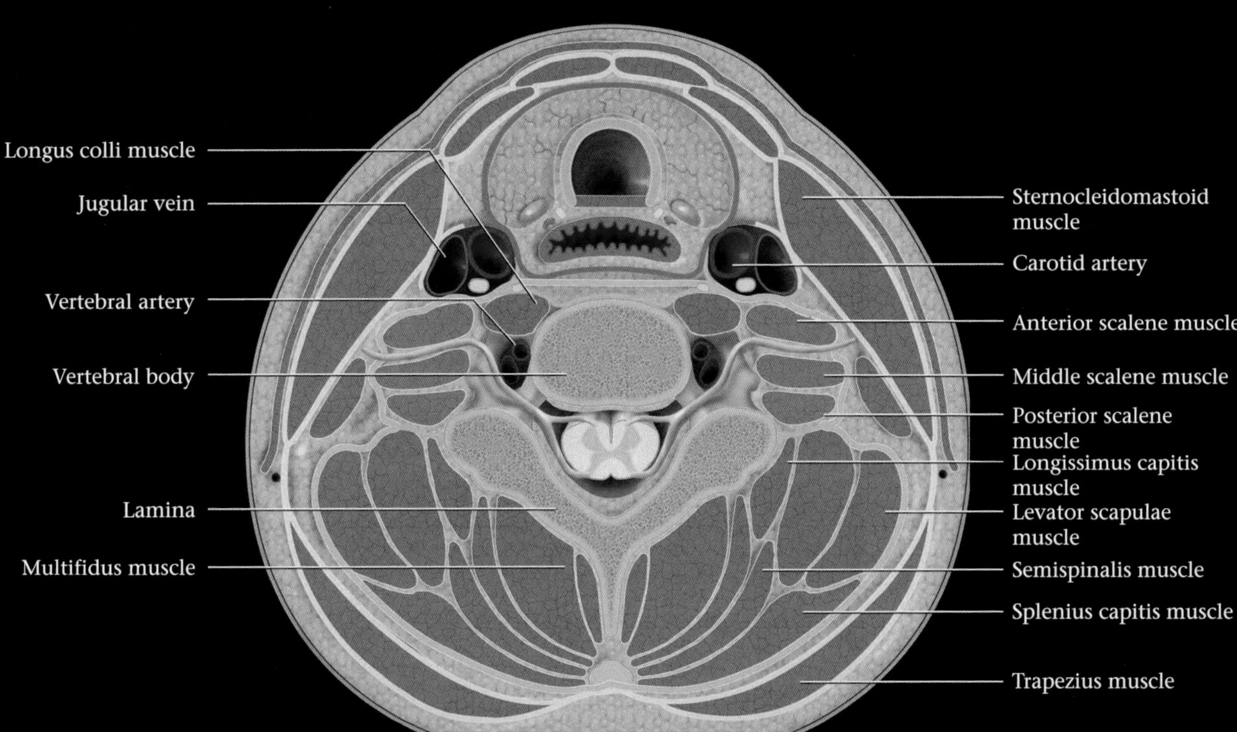
Longus colli muscle
Jugular vein
Vertebral artery
Vertebral body
Lamina
Multifidus muscle
Sternocleidomastoid muscle
Carotid artery
Anterior scalene muscle
Middle scalene muscle
Posterior scalene muscle
Longissimus capitis muscle
Levator scapulae muscle
Semispinalis muscle
Splenius capitis muscle
Trapezius muscle

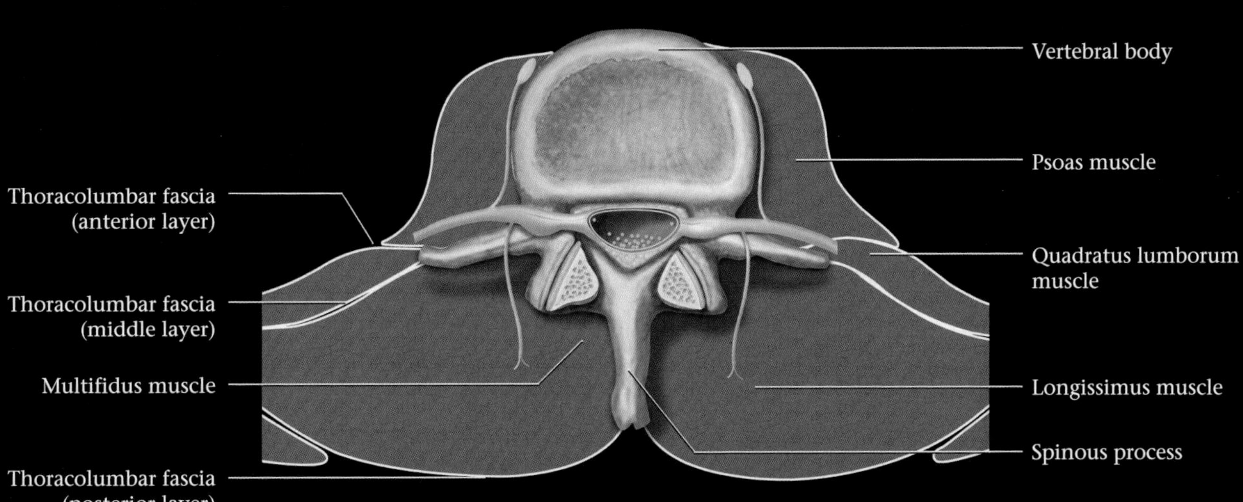
Vertebral body
Psoas muscle
Thoracolumbar fascia (anterior layer)
Quadratus lumborum muscle
Thoracolumbar fascia (middle layer)
Multifidus muscle
Longissimus muscle
Spinous process
Thoracolumbar fascia (posterior layer)

(Top) Axial graphic of cervical muscles. The superficial neck muscles are dominated by the anterior sternocleidomastoid muscles, and the posterior trapezius muscles. The anterolateral deep neck shows the scalene muscles, with the brachial plexus passing between the anterior and middle scalene muscles. The dorsal neck muscles are a complex of semispinalis, longus capitis, and splenius capitis muscles. **(Bottom)** Axial graphic of lumbar muscles. The dorsal muscle complex contains the longissimus and multifidus muscles. The quadratus lumborum muscle defines the planes between middle and anterior layers of the thoracolumbar fascia. The large psoas muscles define the lateral paravertebral regions.

AXIAL CECT CERVICAL

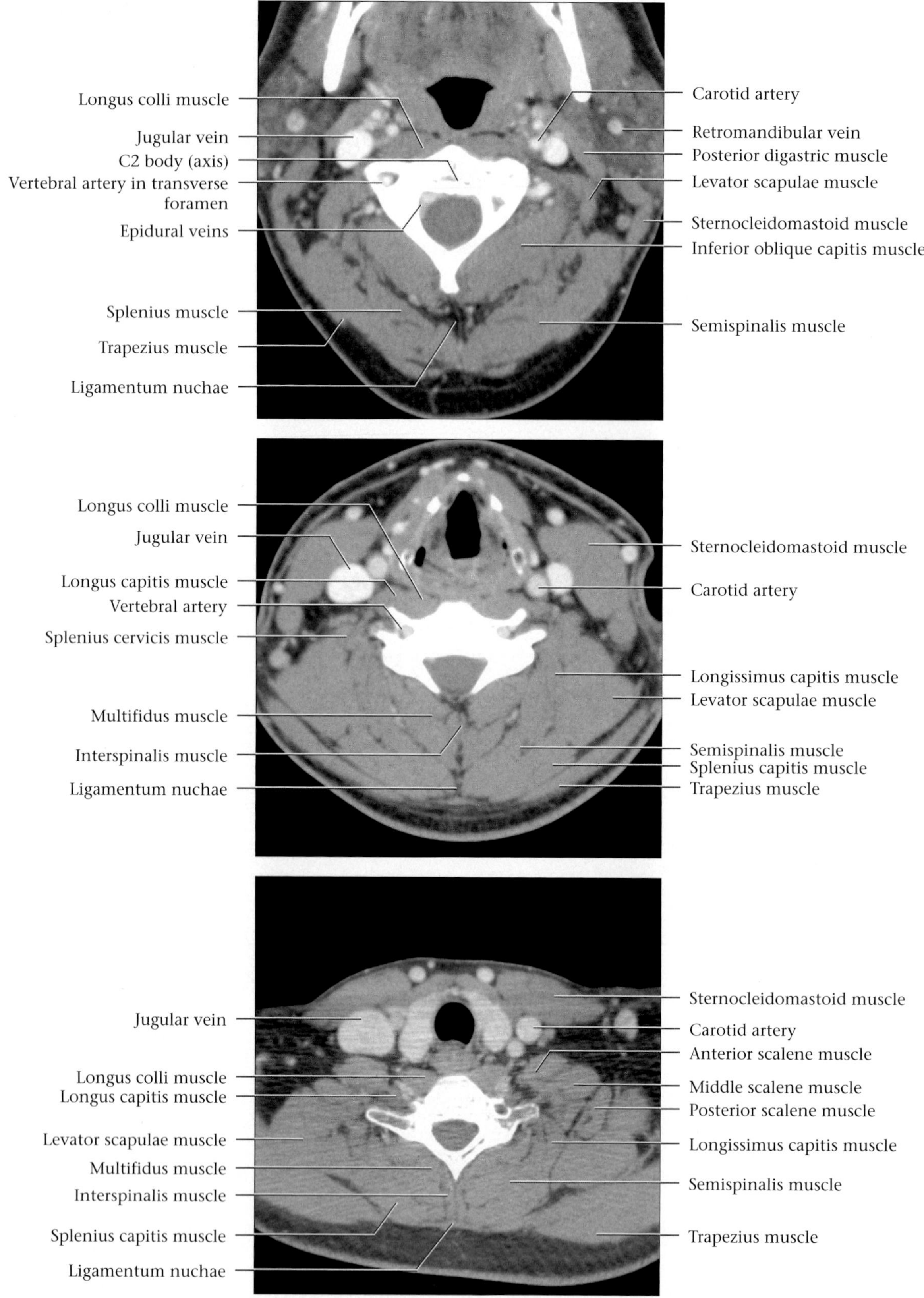

Longus colli muscle
Jugular vein
C2 body (axis)
Vertebral artery in transverse foramen
Epidural veins
Splenius muscle
Trapezius muscle
Ligamentum nuchae
Carotid artery
Retromandibular vein
Posterior digastric muscle
Levator scapulae muscle
Sternocleidomastoid muscle
Inferior oblique capitis muscle
Semispinalis muscle
Longus colli muscle
Jugular vein
Longus capitis muscle
Vertebral artery
Splenius cervicis muscle
Multifidus muscle
Interspinalis muscle
Ligamentum nuchae
Sternocleidomastoid muscle
Carotid artery
Longissimus capitis muscle
Levator scapulae muscle
Semispinalis muscle
Splenius capitis muscle
Trapezius muscle
Jugular vein
Longus colli muscle
Longus capitis muscle
Levator scapulae muscle
Multifidus muscle
Interspinalis muscle
Splenius capitis muscle
Ligamentum nuchae
Sternocleidomastoid muscle
Carotid artery
Anterior scalene muscle
Middle scalene muscle
Posterior scalene muscle
Longissimus capitis muscle
Semispinalis muscle
Trapezius muscle

(Top) First of three axial CECT image of the cervical spine presented from superior to inferior. The ligamentum nuchae and many of the deep neck extensor muscles are attached to the spinous processes within the cervical spine, such as the semispinalis (thoracic and cervical components), multifidus and interspinalis muscles. The vertical segment of the longus colli is located within the shallow depression along the anterior margins of the vertebral bodies. **(Middle)** Image through mid-cervical spine. The paired deep cervical musculature is identified in this view, including the multifidus, semispinalis and splenius capitis muscles. The longus colli attaches to the anterior tubercle, while the longus capitis is slightly more lateral. **(Bottom)** View of lower cervical spine. The anterior and middle scalene muscles insert on the first rib, with the posterior scalene inserting on the second rib.

AXIAL CECT THORACIC

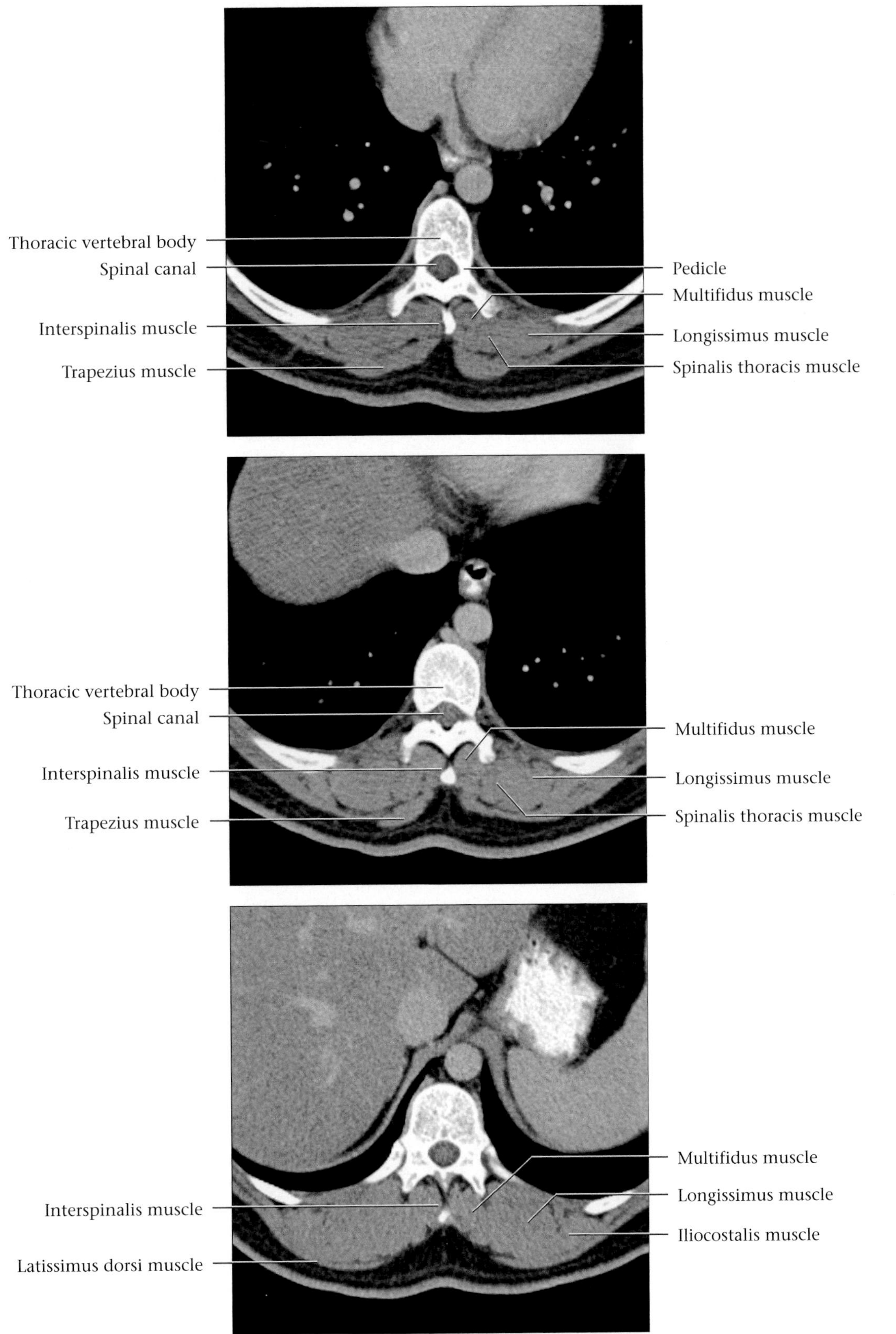

Thoracic vertebral body
Spinal canal
Interspinalis muscle
Trapezius muscle
Pedicle
Multifidus muscle
Longissimus muscle
Spinalis thoracis muscle
Thoracic vertebral body
Spinal canal
Interspinalis muscle
Trapezius muscle
Multifidus muscle
Longissimus muscle
Spinalis thoracis muscle
Interspinalis muscle
Latissimus dorsi muscle
Multifidus muscle
Longissimus muscle
Iliocostalis muscle

(Top) First of three axial CECT images of the thoracic spine presented from superior to inferior. The posterior margins of the transverse processes provide attachment for the deep thoracic muscles. The erector spinae muscle group includes the medial spinalis thoracis, longissimus, and laterally positioned iliocostalis muscles. The spinous processes provide attachment for multiple muscle groups, such as the more superficial trapezius, rhomboids, latissimus dorsi, serratus posterior, as well as the deep muscles groups. **(Middle)** View of mid-thoracic spine. Many small muscle groups are attached to the posterior elements. The transversospinalis group includes the interspinalis, rotatores, multifidus and semispinalis muscles. **(Bottom)** Image at thoracolumbar junction. The erector spinae group (e.g., medial multifidus and the lateral iliocostalis muscles) are well-defined here.

AXIAL CECT LUMBAR

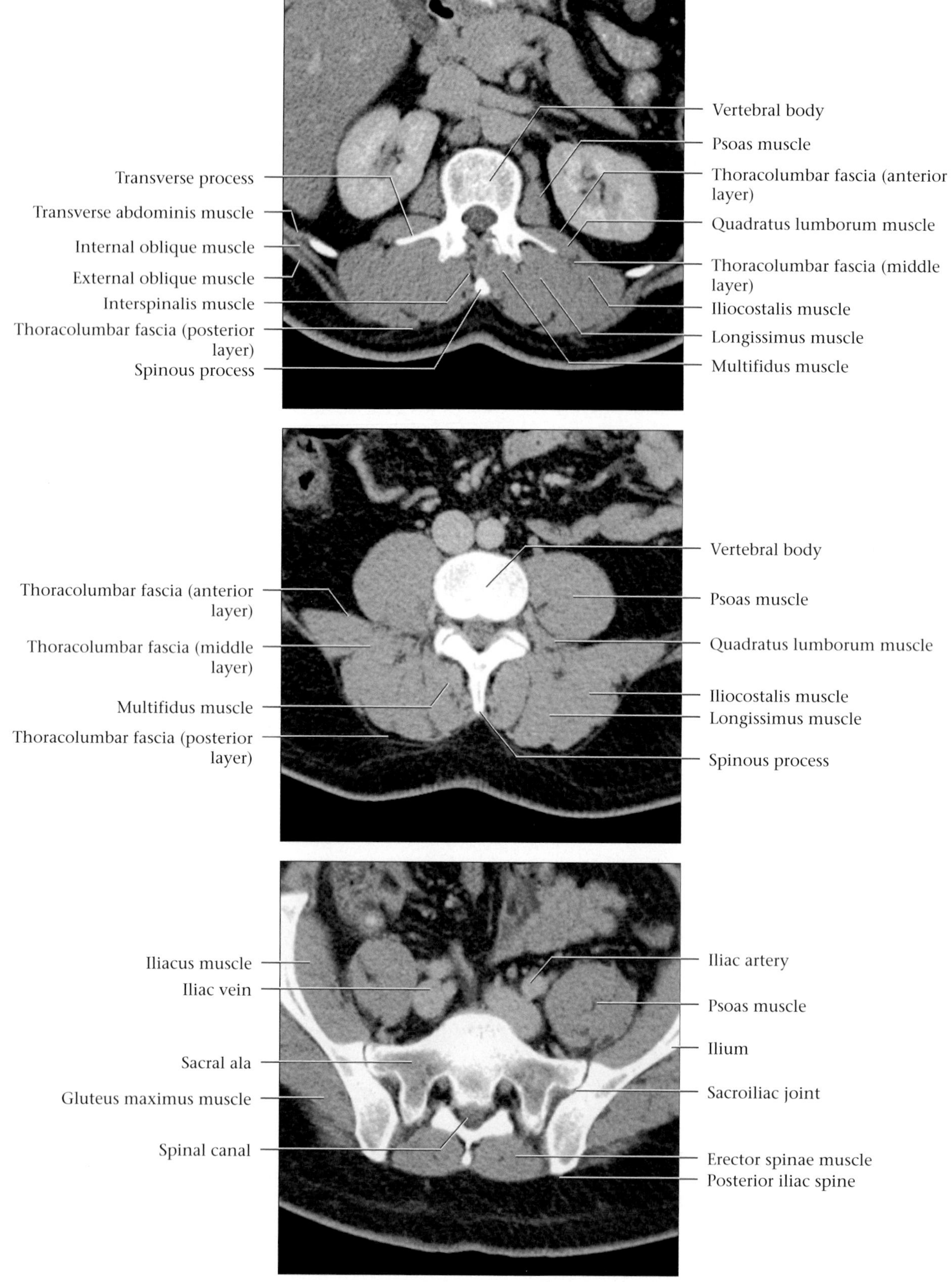

Transverse process
Transverse abdominis muscle
Internal oblique muscle
External oblique muscle
Interspinalis muscle
Thoracolumbar fascia (posterior layer)
Spinous process
Vertebral body
Psoas muscle
Thoracolumbar fascia (anterior layer)
Quadratus lumborum muscle
Thoracolumbar fascia (middle layer)
Iliocostalis muscle
Longissimus muscle
Multifidus muscle
Thoracolumbar fascia (anterior layer)
Thoracolumbar fascia (middle layer)
Multifidus muscle
Thoracolumbar fascia (posterior layer)
Vertebral body
Psoas muscle
Quadratus lumborum muscle
Iliocostalis muscle
Longissimus muscle
Spinous process
Iliacus muscle
Iliac vein
Sacral ala
Gluteus maximus muscle
Spinal canal
Iliac artery
Psoas muscle
Ilium
Sacroiliac joint
Erector spinae muscle
Posterior iliac spine

(Top) First of three axial CECT images through the lumbar spine presented from superior to inferior. The posterior layer of thoracolumbar fascia is adjacent to the erector spinae muscle group. The quadratus lumborum muscle provides the landmark for the middle and anterior layers; the anterior margin of the muscle is the anterior fascial layer, while the posterior margin of the muscle defines the middle layer. **(Middle)** Image through the mid-lumbar spine. The psoas muscles are prominent on either side of the vertebral body. The psoas muscles attach to the superior and inferior margins of all the lumbar vertebral bodies. The posterior layer of the thoracolumbar fascia is the boundary of the dorsal spinal muscles. **(Bottom)** Image through the S1 level. This level is defined by the ventral psoas and iliacus muscles, the dorsolateral gluteus maximus and the dorsomedial erector spinae group.

CORONAL CECT THORACOLUMBAR

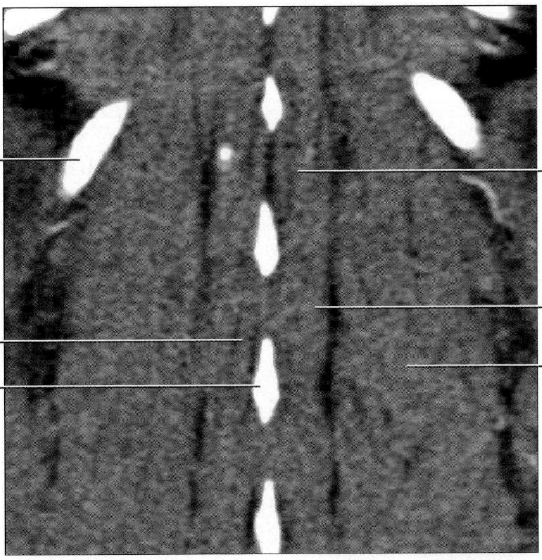

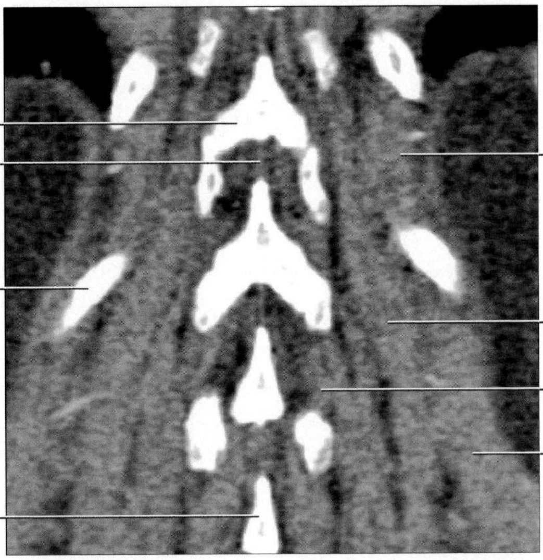

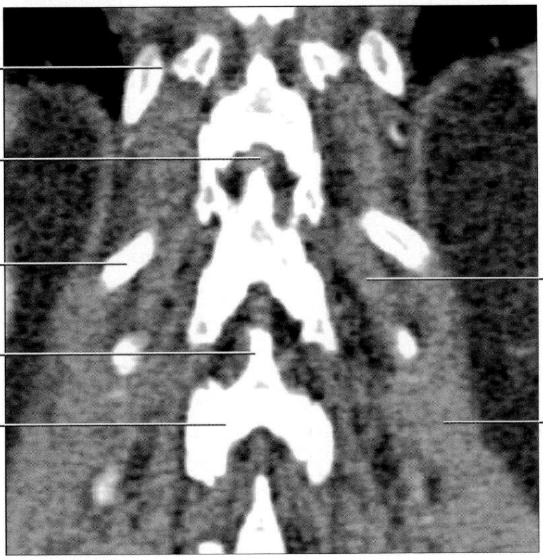

Rib
Spinalis thoracis muscle
Semispinalis thoracis muscle
Multifidus muscle
Longissimus thoracis muscle
Spinous process

Lamina
Interspinous ligament
Intercostal muscle
Rib
Spinalis thoracis muscle
Rotatores muscle
Longissimus thoracis muscle
Spinous process

Costotransverse joint
Interspinous ligament
Rib
Multifidus muscle
Spinous process
Lamina
Longissimus thoracis muscle

(Top) First of three coronal CECT images of the thoracolumbar junction dorsal musculature presented from posterior to anterior. The longissimus thoracis bend the spinal column to one side, and can depress the ribs. The semispinalis thoracis rotate the spinal column to one side, while the multifidus muscles and the small rotatores muscles rotate the column to the opposite side. **(Middle)** Image of the thoracolumbar junction dorsal musculature, just ventral to superior image. The multiple, paired small slips of erector muscles are demonstrated, with the rotatores and spinalis thoracis shown. **(Bottom)** Image of the thoracolumbar junction dorsal musculature, just ventral to upper image. The oblique angled multifidus muscles are shown, extending from transverse processes towards the spinous processes.

CRANIOCERVICAL JUNCTION

Terminology

Definitions

- Craniocervical junction (CCJ) = C1, C2 and articulation with skull base

Gross Anatomy

Overview

- Craniocervical junction comprises occiput, atlas, axis, their articulations, ligaments

Components of Craniocervical Junction

- **Bones**
  - **Occipital bone**
    - Occipital condyles are paired, oval-shaped, inferior prominences of lateral exoccipital portion of occipital bone
    - Articular facet projects laterally
  - **C1 (atlas)**
    - Composed of anterior and posterior arches, no body
    - Paired lateral masses with their superior and inferior articular facets
    - Large transverse processes with transverse foramen
  - **C2 (axis)**
    - Large body and superiorly projecting odontoid process
    - Superior articulating facet surface is convex & directed laterally
    - Inferior articular process + facet surface is typical of lower cervical vertebrae
    - Superior facet is positioned relatively anteriorly, inferior facet is posterior with elongated pars interarticularis
- **Joints**
  - **Atlanto-occipital joints**
    - Inferior articular facet of occipital condyle: Oval, convex surface, projects laterally
    - Superior articular facet of C1: Oval, concave anteroposteriorly, projects medially
  - **Median atlanto-axial joints**
    - Pivot type joint between dens + ring formed by anterior arch + transverse ligament of C1
    - Synovial cavities between transverse ligament/odontoid & atlas/odontoid articulations
  - **Lateral atlanto-axial joints**
    - Inferior articular facet of C1: Concave mediolaterally, projects medially in coronal plane
    - Superior articular facet of C2: Convex surface, projects laterally
- **Ligaments** (from anterior to posterior)
  - **Anterior atlanto-occipital membrane**: Connects anterior arch C1 with anterior margin foramen magnum
  - **Odontoid ligaments**
    - Apical ligament: Small fibrous band extending from dens tip to basion
    - Alar ligaments: Thick, horizontally directed ligaments extending from lateral surface of dens tip to anteromedial occipital condyles
  - **Cruciate ligament**
    - Transverse ligament: Strong horizontal component between lateral masses of C1, passes behind dens
    - Craniocaudal component: Fibrous band running from transverse ligament superiorly to foramen magnum and inferiorly to C2
  - **Tectorial membrane**: Continuation of posterior longitudinal ligament; attaches to anterior rim foramen magnum (posterior clivus)
  - **Posterior atlanto-occipital membrane**
    - Posterior arch C1 to margin of foramen magnum
    - Deficit laterally where vertebral artery enters on superior surface of C1
- **Biomechanics**
  - Atlanto-occipital joint: 50% cervical flexion/extension and limited lateral motion
  - Atlanto-axial joint: 50% cervical rotation

Imaging Anatomy

Overview

- **Lateral assessment of CCJ**
  - **C1-2 interspinous space**: ≤ 10 mm
  - **Atlanto-dental interval (ADI)**
    - Adults < 3 mm, children < 5 mm in flexion
  - **Pseudosubluxation**
    - Physiologic anterior displacement seen in 40% at C2-3 level and 14% at C3-4 level to age 8
    - Anterior displacement of C2 on C3 up to 4 mm
  - **Posterior cervical line**: Line is drawn from anterior aspect of C1-3 spinous processes ⇒ anterior C2 spinous process should be within 2 mm of this line
  - **Wackenheim line**
    - Posterior surface of clivus ⇒ posterior odontoid tip should lie immediately inferior
    - Relationship does not change in flexion/extension
  - **Welcher basal angle**
    - Angle between lines drawn along plane of sphenoid bone and posterior clivus
    - Normal < 140°, average 132°
  - **Chamberlain line**
    - Between hard palate and opisthion
    - Odontoid tip ≥ 5 mm above line abnormal
  - **McGregor line**
    - Between hard palate to base of occipital bone
    - Odontoid tip ≥ 7 mm above line abnormal
  - **Clivus canal angle**
    - Junction of Wackenheim line and posterior vertebral body line
    - 180° extension, 150° flexion, < 150° abnormal
  - **McRae line**
    - Drawn between basion and opisthion
    - Normal 35 mm diameter
- **Frontal assessment of CCJ**
  - Lateral masses of C1 and C2 should align
    - Overlapping lateral masses can be a normal variant in children
  - **Atlanto-occipital joint angle**
    - Angle formed at junction of lines traversing joints
    - 125-130° normal, < 124° may reflect condyle hypoplasia

GRAPHICS

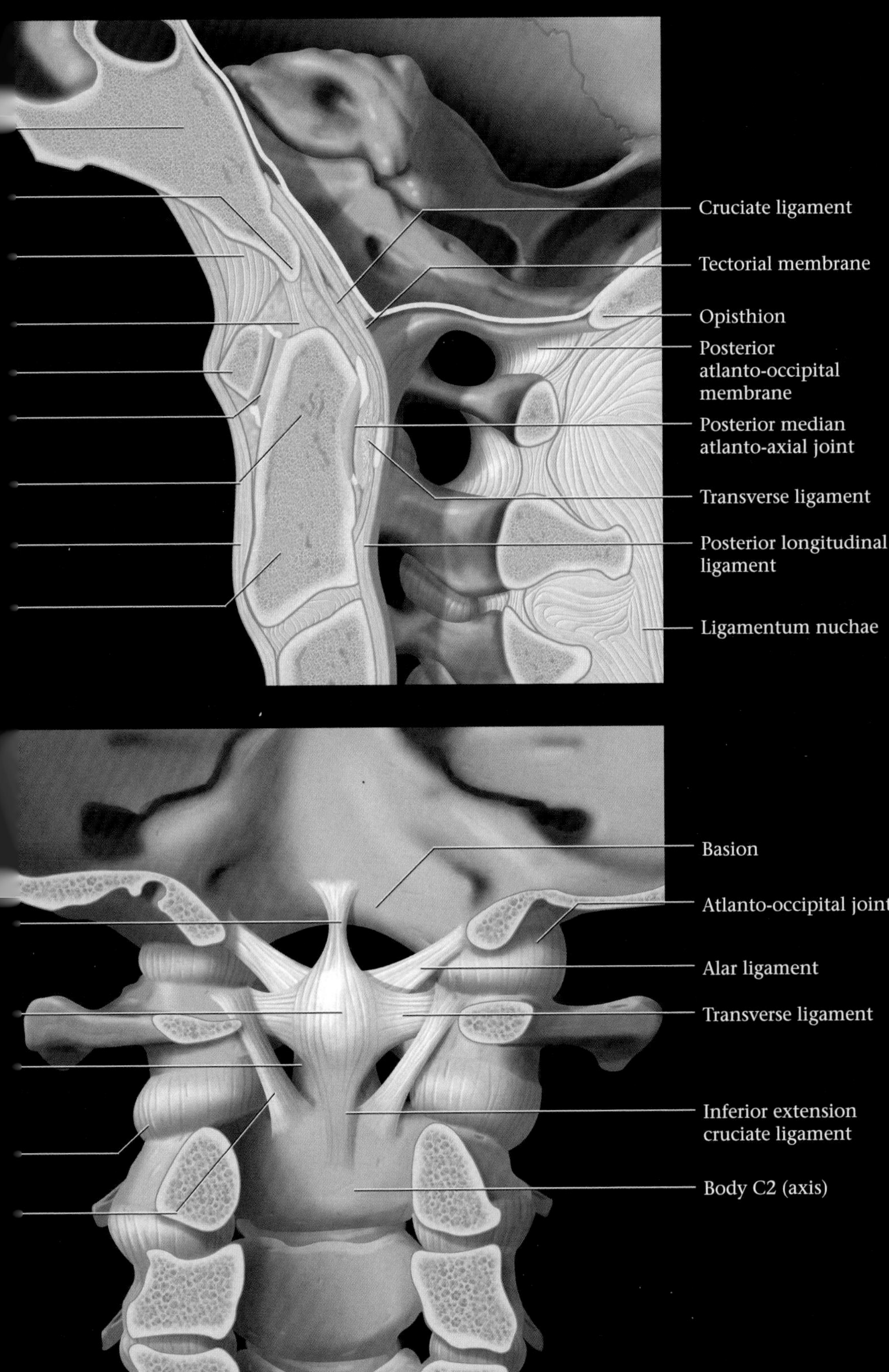
Cruciate ligament
Tectorial membrane
Opisthion
Posterior atlanto-occipital membrane
Posterior median atlanto-axial joint
Transverse ligament
Posterior longitudinal ligament
Ligamentum nuchae
Basion
Atlanto-occipital joint
Alar ligament
Transverse ligament
Inferior extension cruciate ligament
Body C2 (axis)

phic of the craniocervical junction. The complex articulations and ligamentous
ed. The midline atlanto-axial articulations consist of anterior & posterior median
nterior joint is between the posterior aspect of the anterior C1 arch and the ventral aspect
posterior joint is between the dorsal aspect of the odontoid process and the cruciate
w shows a series of ligamentous connection to the skull base including the anterior
ne, apical ligament, superior component of cruciate ligament, tectorial membrane &
membrane. **(Bottom)** Posterior view of craniocervical junction with posterior elements cut
nents of the cruciate ligament & alar ligaments

CRANIOCERVICAL JUNCTION

C1 GRAPHICS

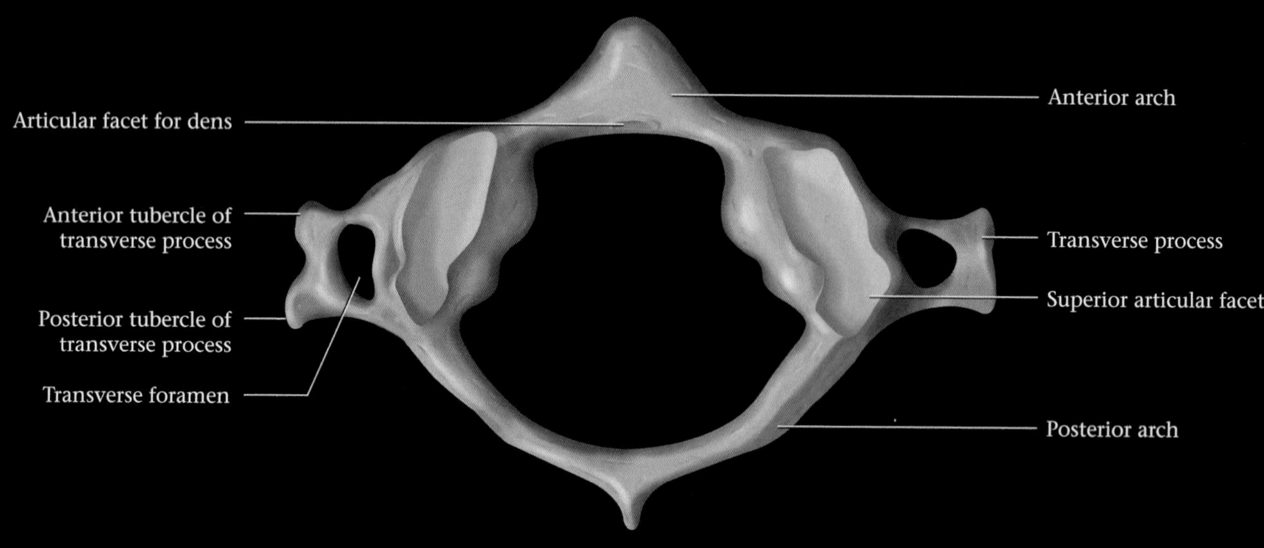
Articular facet for dens
Anterior tubercle of transverse process
Posterior tubercle of transverse process
Transverse foramen
Anterior arch
Transverse process
Superior articular facet
Posterior arch

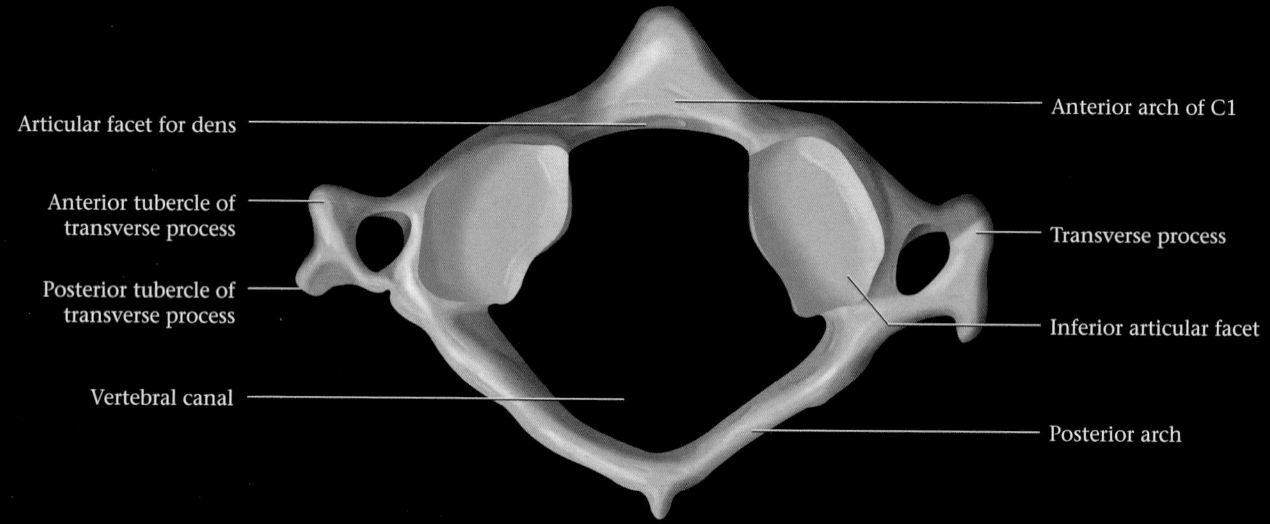
Articular facet for dens
Anterior tubercle of transverse process
Posterior tubercle of transverse process
Vertebral canal
Anterior arch of C1
Transverse process
Inferior articular facet
Posterior arch

(Top) Axial graphic view of atlas viewed from above. The characteristic ring shape is shown, composed of anterior & posterior arches & paired large lateral masses. The superior articular facet is concave anteroposteriorly & projects medially for articulation with the convex surface of the occipital condyle at the atlanto-occipital joint. The anterior arch articulates with the odontoid process at the anterior median atlanto-axial joint. **(Bottom)** Atlas viewed from below. The large inferior facet surface is concave mediolaterally & projects medially for articulation with the convex surface of the superior articular facet of C2. The canal of the atlas ± 3 cm in AP diameter: Spinal cord, odontoid process & free space for cord are each about 1 cm in diameter. The size of the anterior midline tubercle of the anterior arch, and spinous process of posterior arch are quite variable.

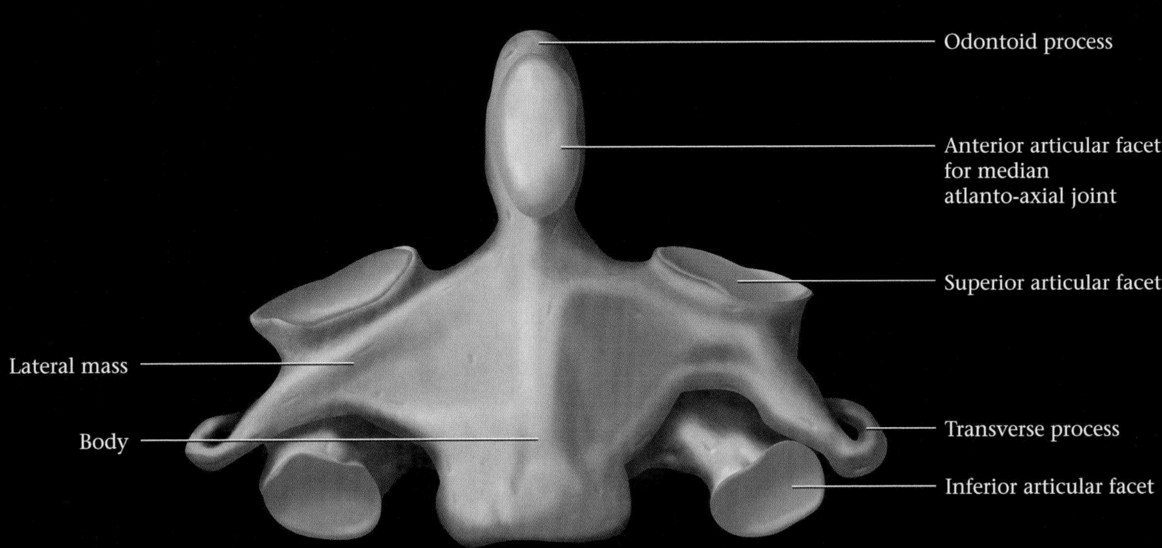
Odontoid process
Anterior articular facet for median atlanto-axial joint
Superior articular facet
Lateral mass
Body
Transverse process
Inferior articular facet

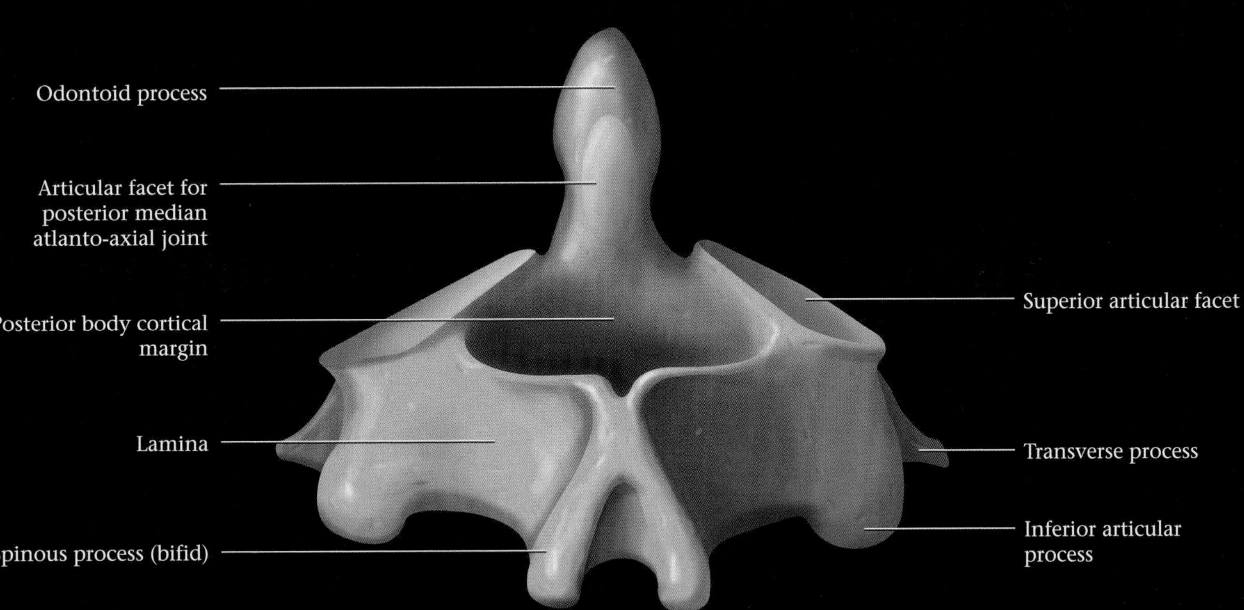
Odontoid process
Articular facet for posterior median atlanto-axial joint
Superior articular facet
Posterior body cortical margin
Lamina
Transverse process
Inferior articular process
Spinous process (bifid)

(Top) Atlas viewed from anterior perspective. The odontoid process is the "purloined" embryologic centrum of C1 which is incorporated into C2, giving C2 its unique morphology. The C2 body laterally is defined by large lateral masses for articulation with the inferior facet of C1. The elongated pars interarticularis of C2 ends with the inferior articular process for articulation with the superior articular facet of C3. **(Bottom)** Atlas viewed from posterior perspective. The odontoid process has anterior and posterior joints for articulation with C1. The anterior median joint articulates with the C1 arch, while the posterior median joint (shown here) involves the transverse ligament.

CRANIOMETRY GRAPHICS

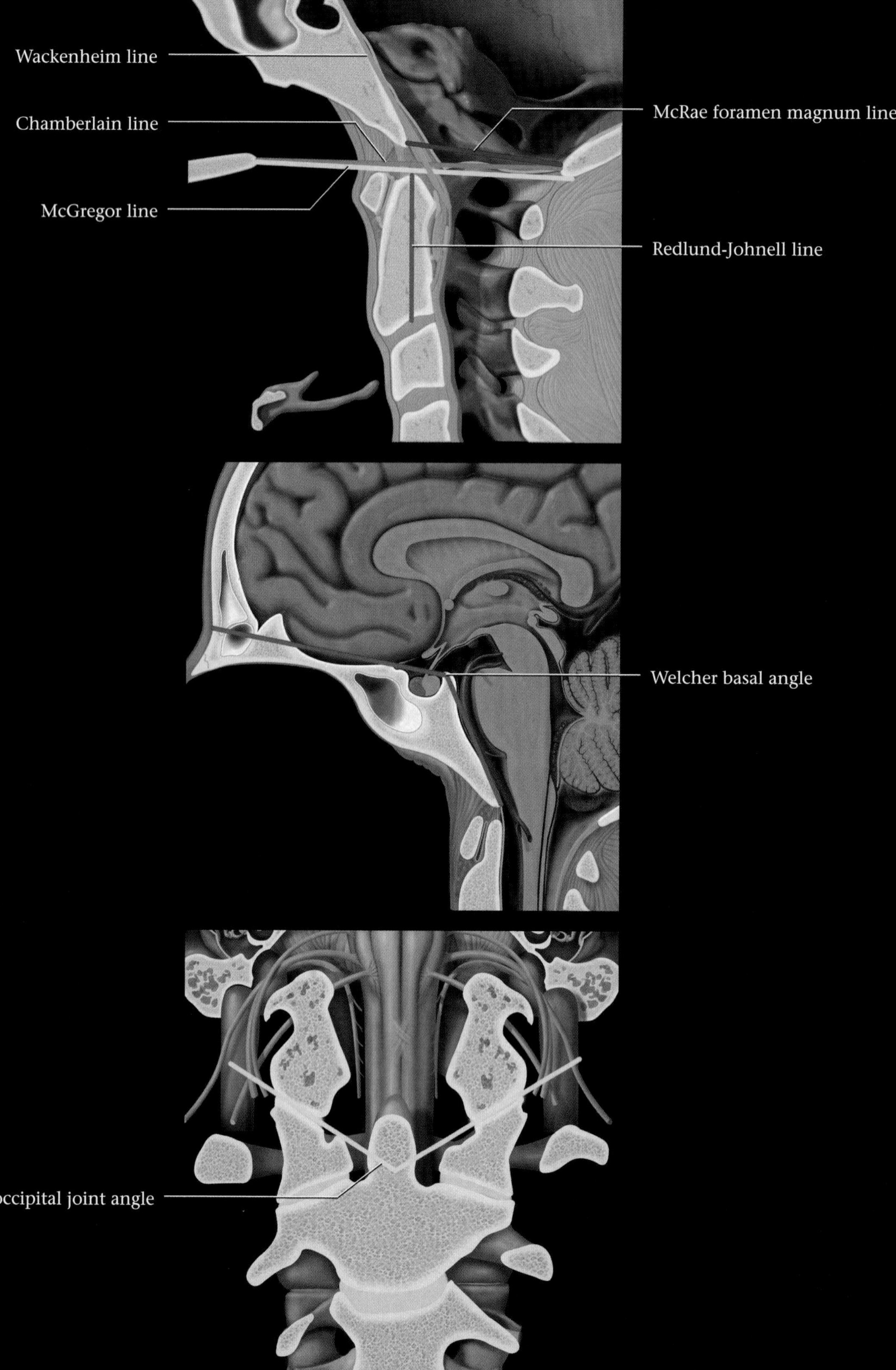
Wackenheim line
Chamberlain line
McGregor line
McRae foramen magnum line
Redlund-Johnell line
Welcher basal angle
Atlanto-occipital joint angle

(Top) Sagittal graphic shows important skull base craniometry. Orange: Chamberlain line - drawn between hard palate & opisthion. Yellow: McGregor line - drawn between hard palate to caudal point of occipital bone (base of occipital bone). Green: Wackenheim line - drawn along posterior surface of clivus. Blue: McRae foramen magnum line - drawn between basion & opisthion. Red: Redlund-Johnell line - drawn from base of C2 to McGregor line. **(Middle)** Sagittal midline graphic of Welcher basal angle - defined by angle between lines drawn along plane of sphenoid bone & along clivus (nasion to sella, sella along posterior clivus to basion). Normal < 140°, platybasia if > 140°. **(Bottom)** Coronal graphic of craniocervical junction showing lines drawn along atlanto-occipital joints to measure atlanto-occipital joint angle. Normal 125-130°, < 124° may reflect condyle hypoplasia.

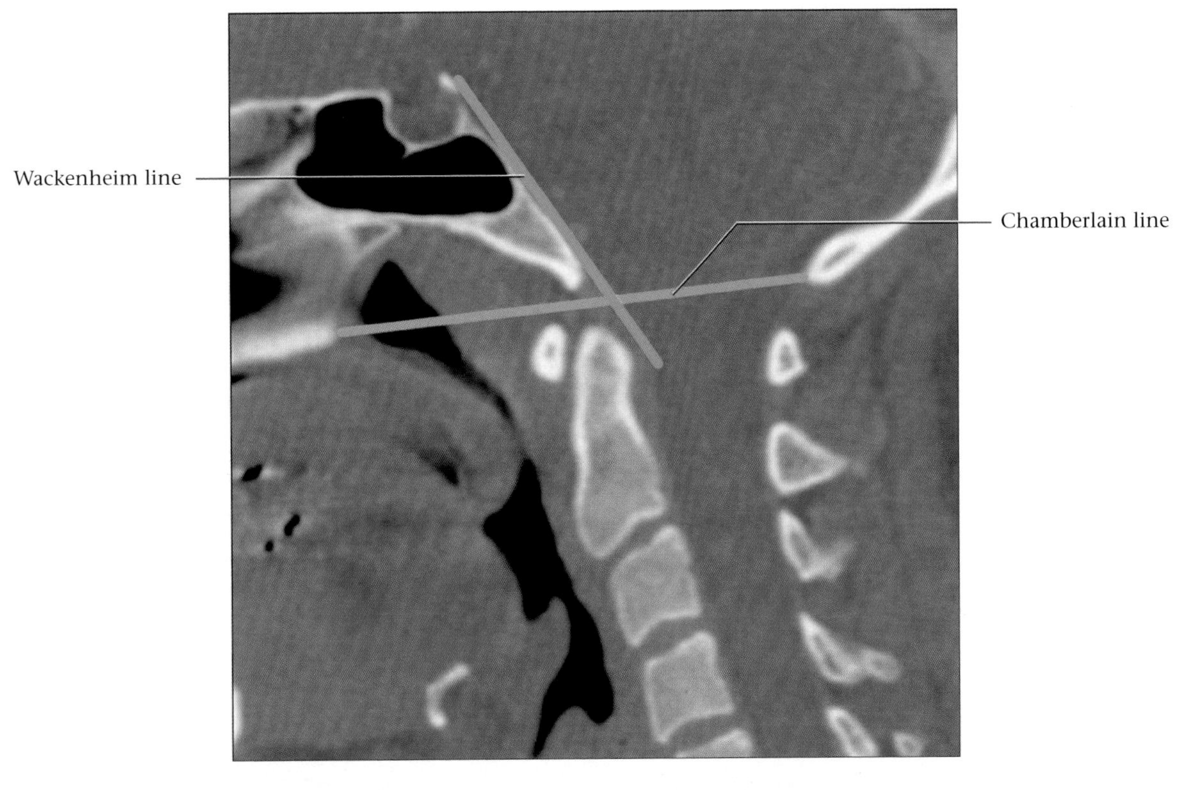
Wackenheim line
Chamberlain line

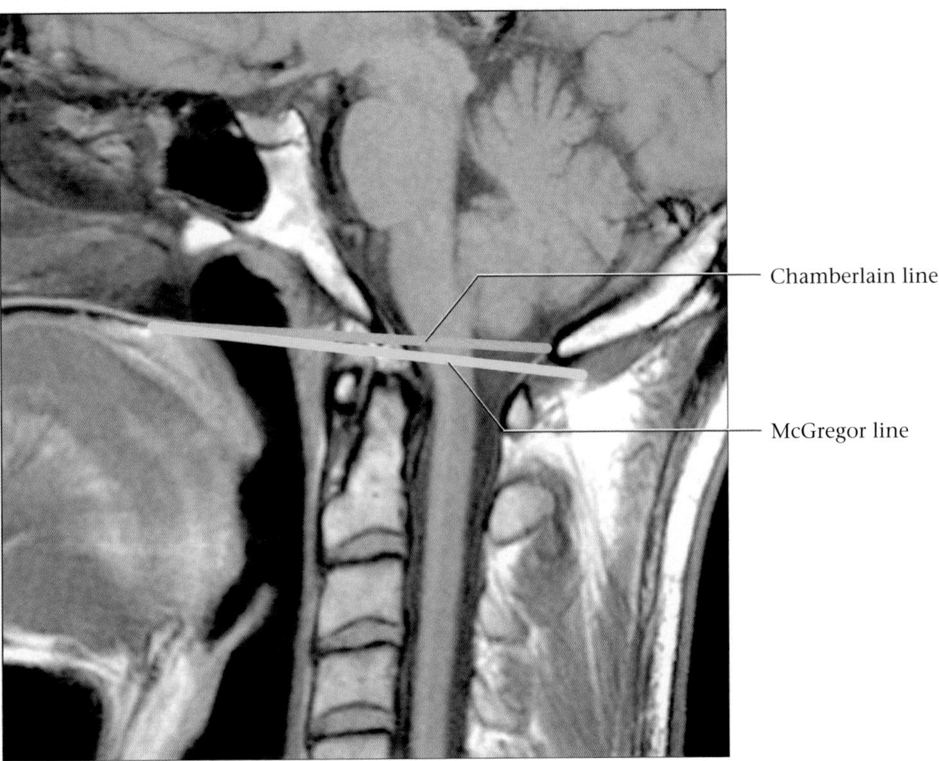
Chamberlain line
McGregor line

(Top) Sagittal CT reformat in the midline. Chamberlain line is shown in orange extending from hard palate to opisthion. Projection of up to 1/3 of dens (5 mm) above this line normal. Wackenheim line is shown in green along the clivus. The dens should lie immediately inferior to line, & any intersection is considered abnormal. **(Bottom)** Sagittal T1 MR with Chamberlain line shown in orange. Odontoid tip 5 mm or more above line defines basilar impression. McGregor line shown in yellow. This line has the same significance as Chamberlain line, with the odontoid tip 7 mm or more above line defining basilar impression.

CRANIOCERVICAL JUNCTION

LATERAL RADIOGRAPH CRANIOMETRY

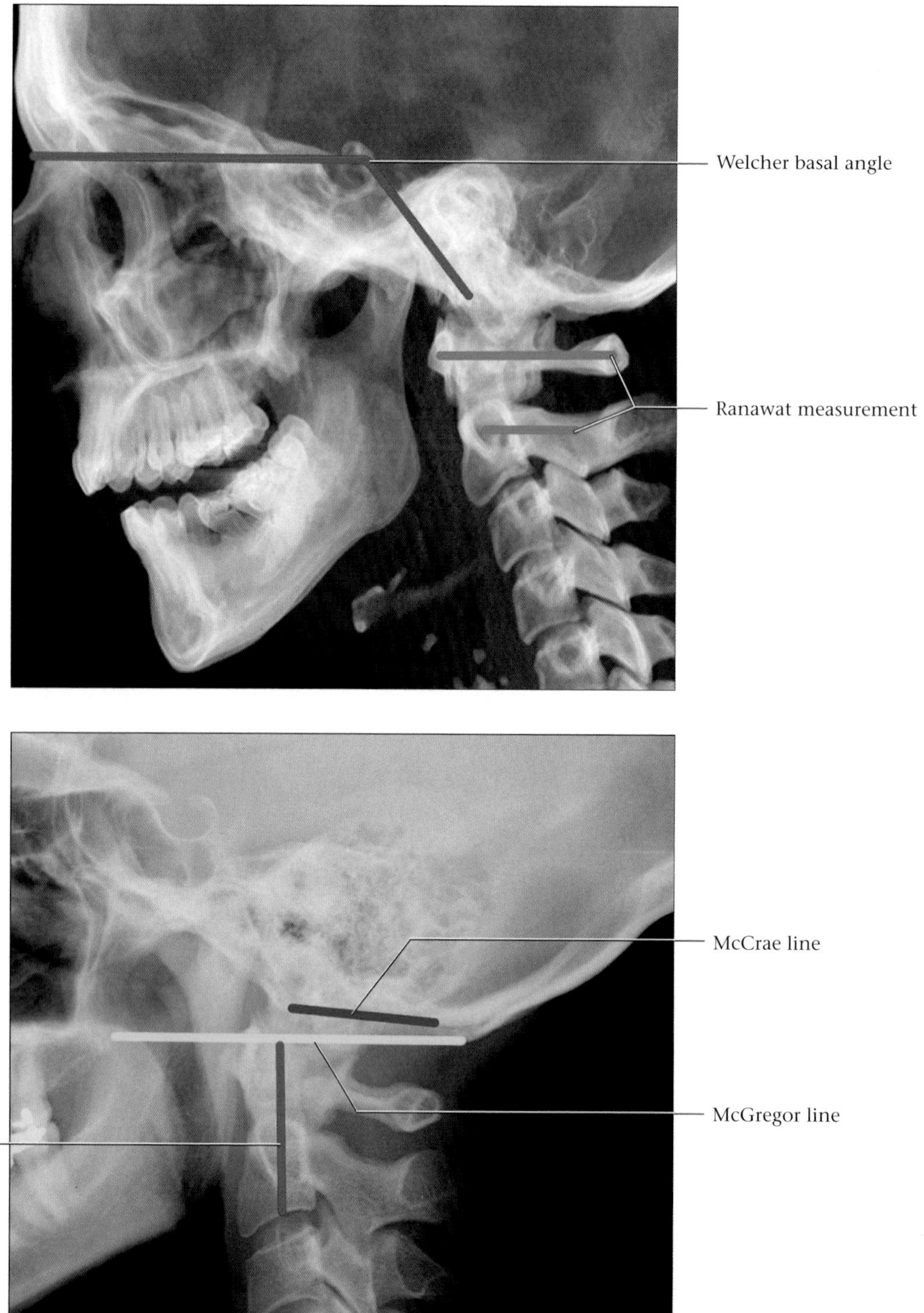
Welcher basal angle
Ranawat measurement
McCrae line
McGregor line
Redlund-Johnell measurement

(Top) In this lateral plain film the Welcher basal angle is shown in red. Platybasia exists if angle > 140° (normal < 140°). Ranawat measurement shown in blue - used to assess collapse at the C1-2 articulation. Measurement taken from center of C2 pedicle to line connecting anterior & posterior arch of C1. Normal ≥ 14 mm in men & ≥ 13 mm in women. < 13 mm is consistent with impaction. **(Bottom)** In this lateral plain film, McCrae line is shown in blue. Normal ≈ 35 mm diameter. The normal odontoid process does not extend above this line. Redlund-Johnell measurement shown in red. This measurement is from the base of C2 body to McGregor line (shown in yellow). Normal ≥ 34 mm in men, ≥ 28 mm for women.

CRANIOCERVICAL JUNCTION

LATERAL RADIOGRAPH

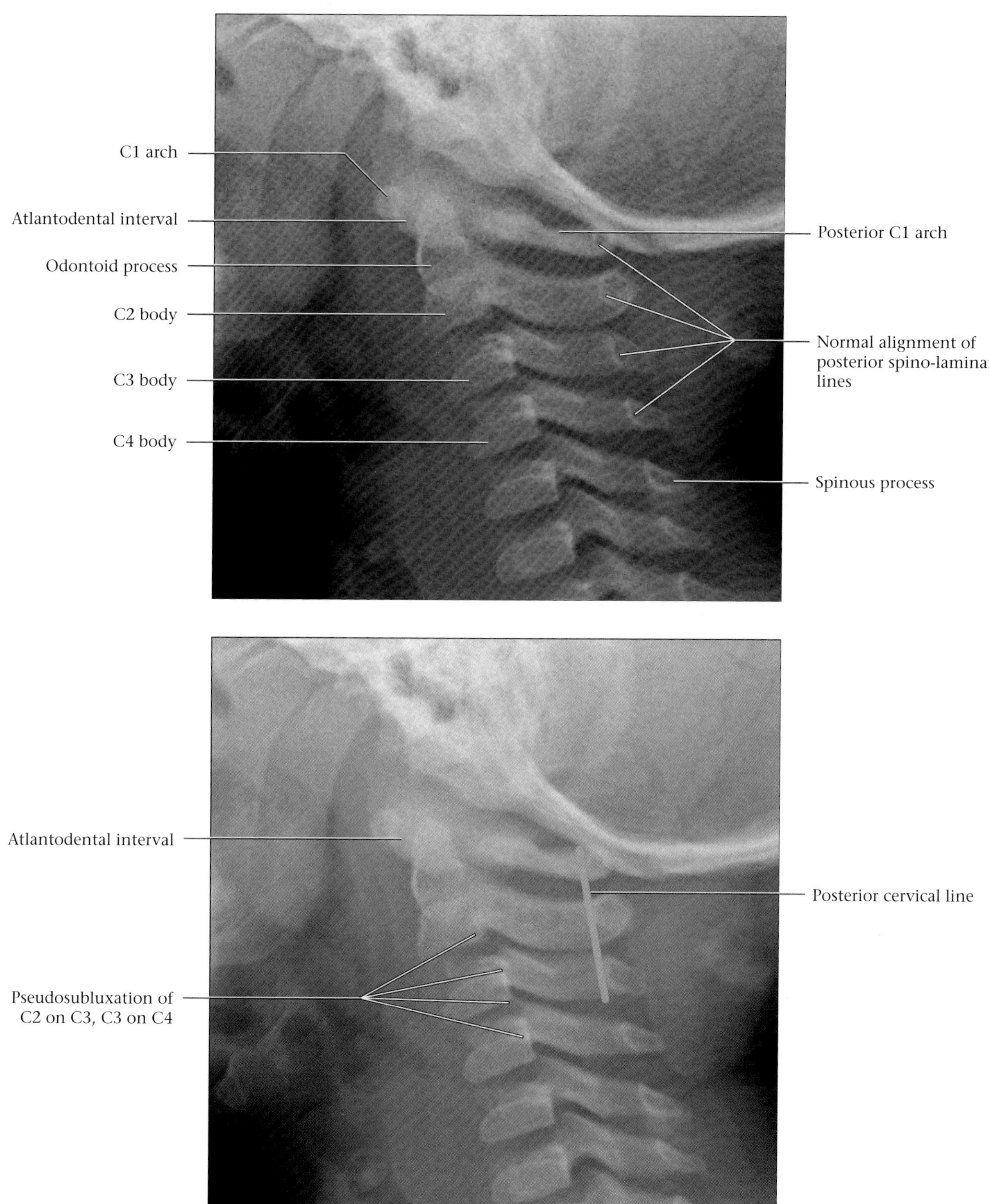

C1 arch
Atlantodental interval
Odontoid process
C2 body
C3 body
C4 body
Posterior C1 arch
Normal alignment of posterior spino-laminar lines
Spinous process
Atlantodental interval
Posterior cervical line
Pseudosubluxation of C2 on C3, C3 on C4

(Top) Lateral plain film of the cervical spine in a child shows physiologic anterior displacement of C2 with respect to C3, and C3 with respect to C4, the so-called pseudosubluxation. Physiologic subluxation is differentiated from pathologic anterior displacement by the absence of prevertebral soft tissue swelling, reduction on extension & assessment of the posterior cervical line as described below. **(Bottom)** Posterior cervical line is drawn along anterior aspect of C1-3 spinous processes. The anterior C2 spinous process should be within 2 mm of this line in flexion & extension. Atlantodental interval < 3.5 mm in children (< 3 mm in adults).

RADIOGRAPHY

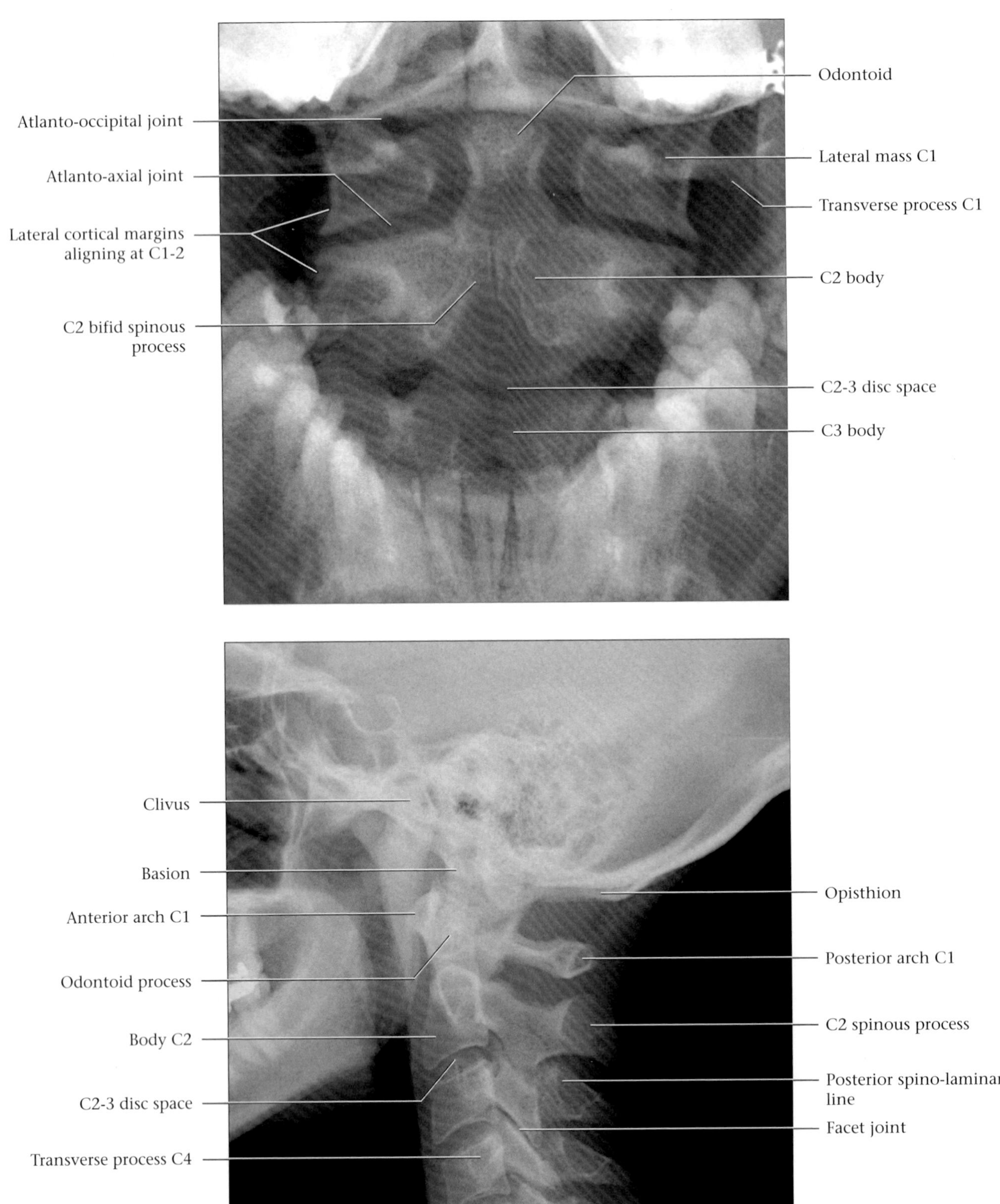

Odontoid
Atlanto-occipital joint
Lateral mass C1
Atlanto-axial joint
Transverse process C1
Lateral cortical margins aligning at C1-2
C2 body
C2 bifid spinous process
C2-3 disc space
C3 body
Clivus
Basion
Opisthion
Anterior arch C1
Posterior arch C1
Odontoid process
C2 spinous process
Body C2
Posterior spino-laminar line
C2-3 disc space
Facet joint
Transverse process C4

(Top) AP open mouth view of odontoid process. With proper positioning, the odontoid process is visualized in the midline with symmetrically placed lateral C1 masses on either side. The medial space between odontoid and C1 lateral masses should be symmetric as well. The lateral cortical margins of the C1 & C2 lateral masses should align. The atlanto-occipital and atlanto-axial joints are visible bilaterally, with smooth cortical margins. The bifid C2 process should not be confused for fracture. **(Bottom)** Lateral radiograph of craniocervical junction. There is smooth anatomic alignment of the posterior vertebral body margins, and the posterior spino-laminar line of the posterior elements. The anterior arch of C1 should assume a well-defined oval appearance, with sharp margination between the anterior C1 arch and the odontoid process.

CORONAL BONE CT

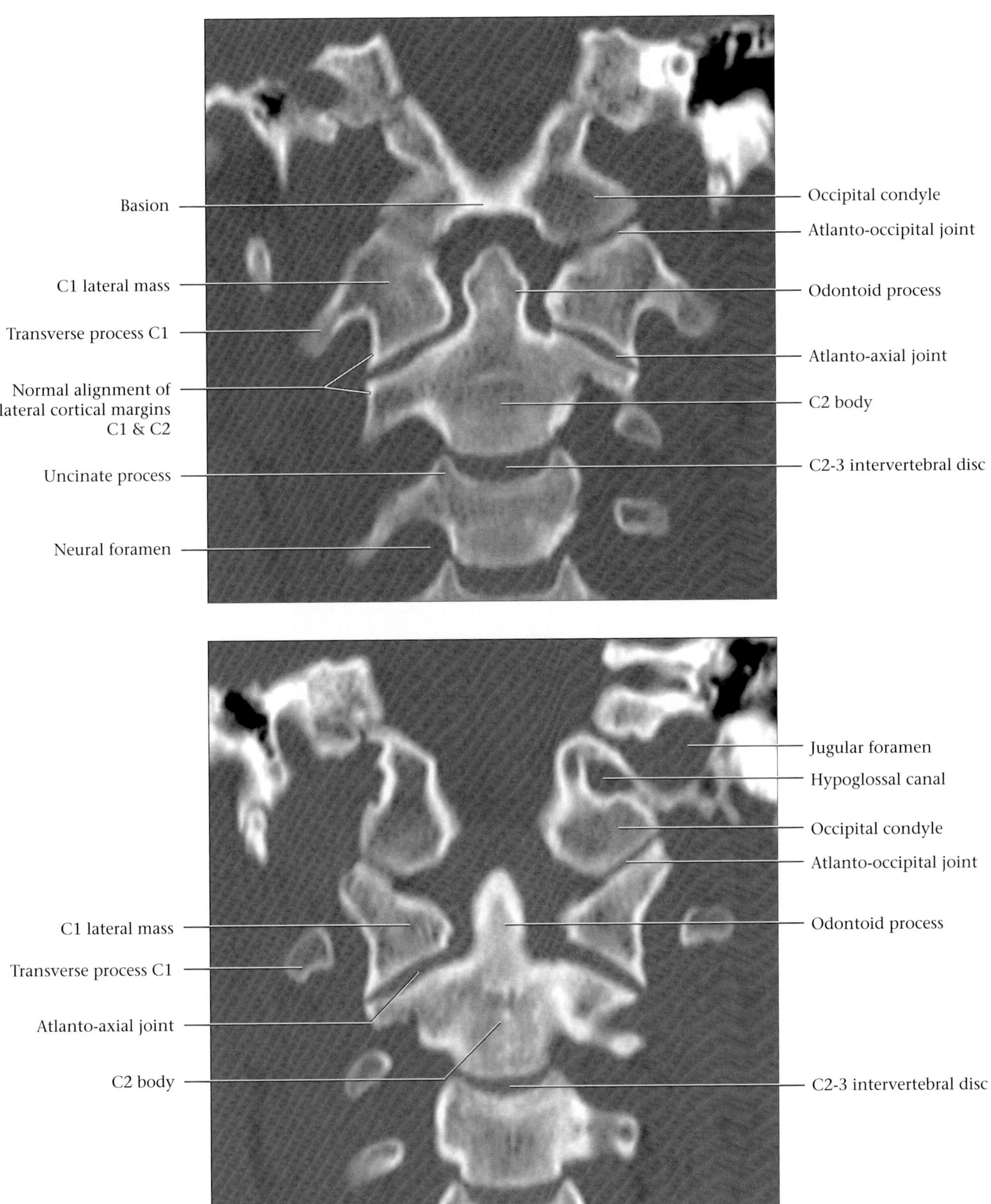
Basion
C1 lateral mass
Transverse process C1
Normal alignment of lateral cortical margins C1 & C2
Uncinate process
Neural foramen
Occipital condyle
Atlanto-occipital joint
Odontoid process
Atlanto-axial joint
C2 body
C2-3 intervertebral disc
C1 lateral mass
Transverse process C1
Atlanto-axial joint
C2 body
Jugular foramen
Hypoglossal canal
Occipital condyle
Atlanto-occipital joint
Odontoid process
C2-3 intervertebral disc

(Top) First of two coronal bone CT reconstructions of the craniocervical junction are presented from anterior to posterior. The odontoid process is visualized in the midline as a sharply corticated bony peg with symmetrically placed lateral C1 masses on either side. The lateral cortical margins of the C1 lateral masses, and the C2 lateral masses should align. The atlanto-occipital and atlanto-axial joints are visible bilaterally, with even joint margins, and sharp cortical margins. **(Bottom)** More posterior view of the craniocervical junction. Both atlanto-occipital joints are now well-defined with smooth cortical margins, sloping superolateral to inferomedial. The atlanto-axial joints are smoothly sloping inferolateral to superomedial.

CRANIOCERVICAL JUNCTION

AXIAL BONE CT

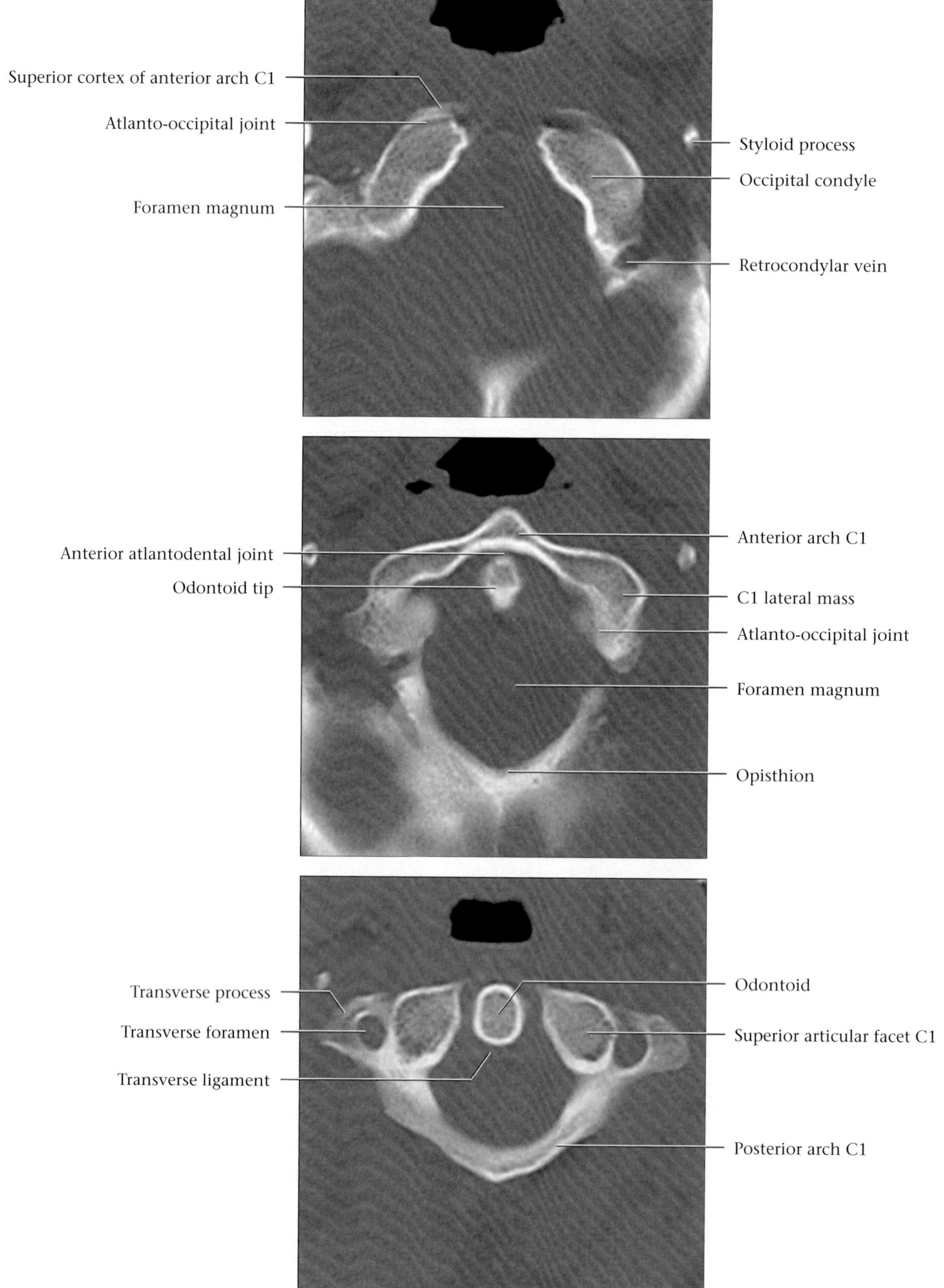
Superior cortex of anterior arch C1
Atlanto-occipital joint
Foramen magnum
Styloid process
Occipital condyle
Retrocondylar vein
Anterior atlantodental joint
Odontoid tip
Anterior arch C1
C1 lateral mass
Atlanto-occipital joint
Foramen magnum
Opisthion
Transverse process
Transverse foramen
Transverse ligament
Odontoid
Superior articular facet C1
Posterior arch C1

(Top) First of six axial bone CT images through the craniocervical junction are presented from superior to inferior. The anterolateral margin of the foramen magnum is formed by the prominent occipital condyles which articulate with the superior articular facets of the C1 lateral masses. **(Middle)** More inferior image of craniocervical junction. The anterior arch of C1 is now well-defined, with the odontoid process of C2 coming into plane. The atlanto-occipital joint is seen in oblique section and therefore has poorly-defined margins. The odontoid is tightly applied to the posterior margin of the C1 arch, held in place by the strong transverse component of the cruciate ligament. **(Bottom)** Image at level of atlas. The unique morphology of the C1 body is defined with its large transverse process with transverse foramen and ring shape.

AXIAL BONE CT

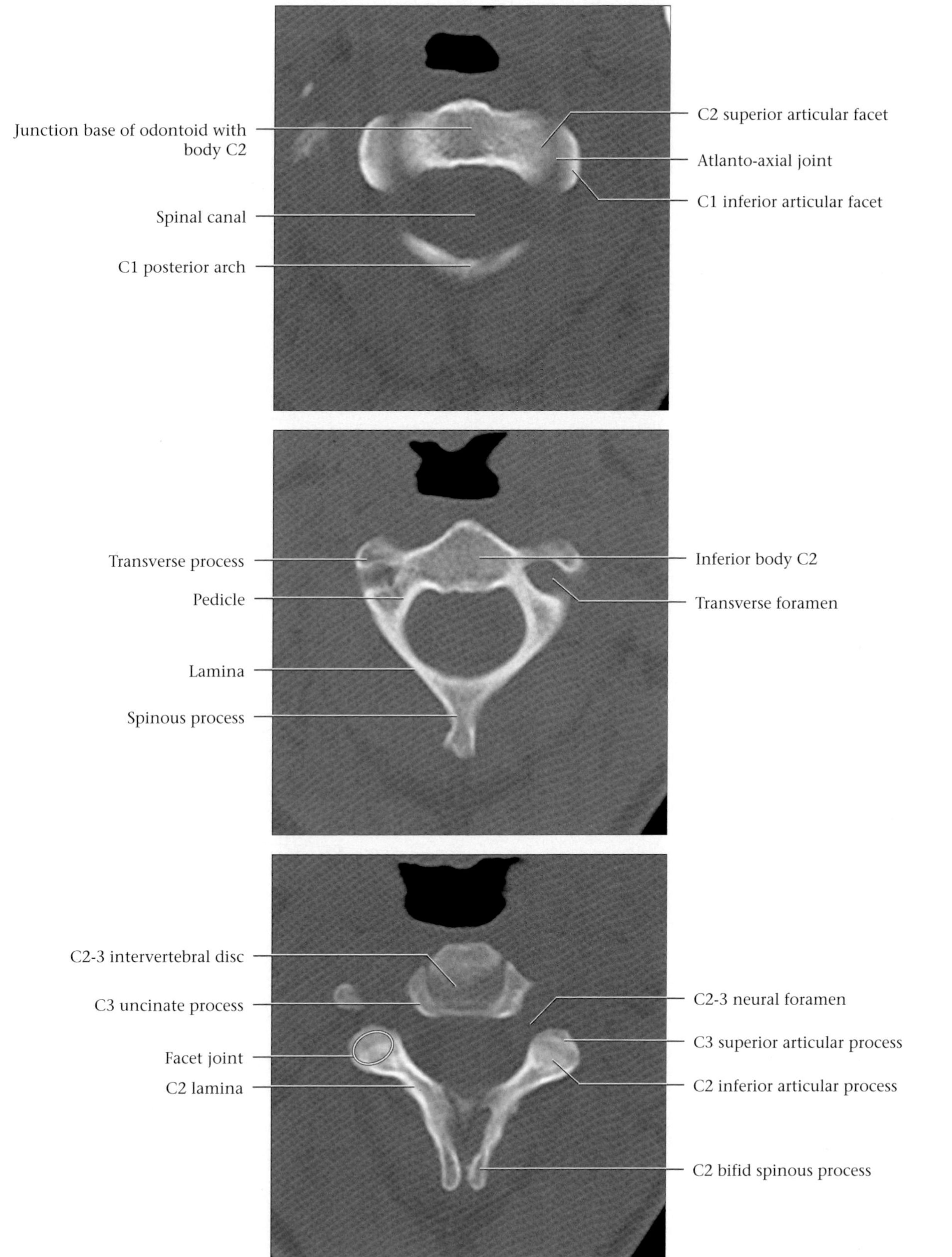
Junction base of odontoid with body C2
Spinal canal
C1 posterior arch
C2 superior articular facet
Atlanto-axial joint
C1 inferior articular facet
Transverse process
Pedicle
Lamina
Spinous process
Inferior body C2
Transverse foramen
C2-3 intervertebral disc
C3 uncinate process
Facet joint
C2 lamina
C2-3 neural foramen
C3 superior articular process
C2 inferior articular process
C2 bifid spinous process

(Top) Image through lateral atlanto-axial joints. This section defines the junction of the odontoid process with the body of C2. The obliquely oriented atlanto-axial joints are partially seen, with the C1 component lateral to the joint space, and the C2 component medial. **(Middle)** Image through inferior C2 body level showing large C2 vertebral body & vertebral arch formed by gracile pedicles & laminae. **(Bottom)** Image through C2-3 intervertebral disc level. The C2-3 neural foramen is well-defined, with the posterior margin formed by the superior articular process of C3. The spinous process of C2 is large and typically bifid. The C2-3 disc assumes the characteristic cervical cup-shaped morphology bounded by uncinate processes.

CRANIOCERVICAL JUNCTION

3D-VRT NECT

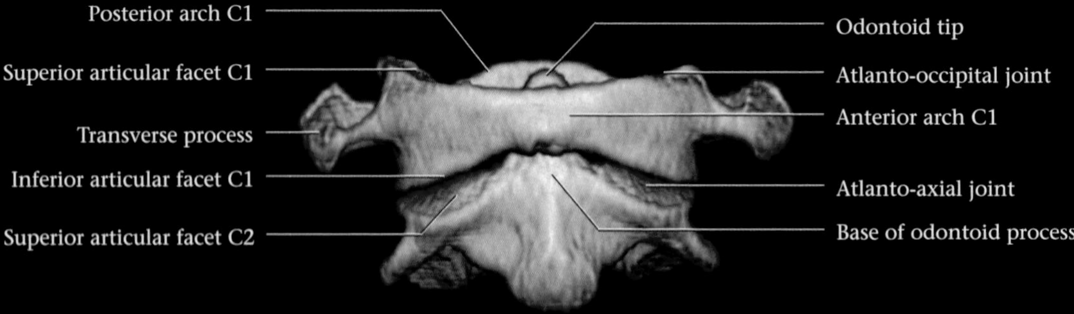
Posterior arch C1
Superior articular facet C1
Transverse process
Inferior articular facet C1
Superior articular facet C2
Odontoid tip
Atlanto-occipital joint
Anterior arch C1
Atlanto-axial joint
Base of odontoid process

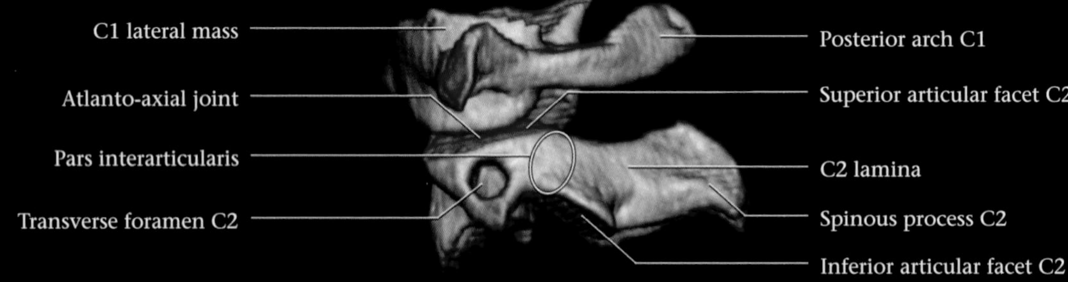
C1 lateral mass
Atlanto-axial joint
Pars interarticularis
Transverse foramen C2
Posterior arch C1
Superior articular facet C2
C2 lamina
Spinous process C2
Inferior articular facet C2

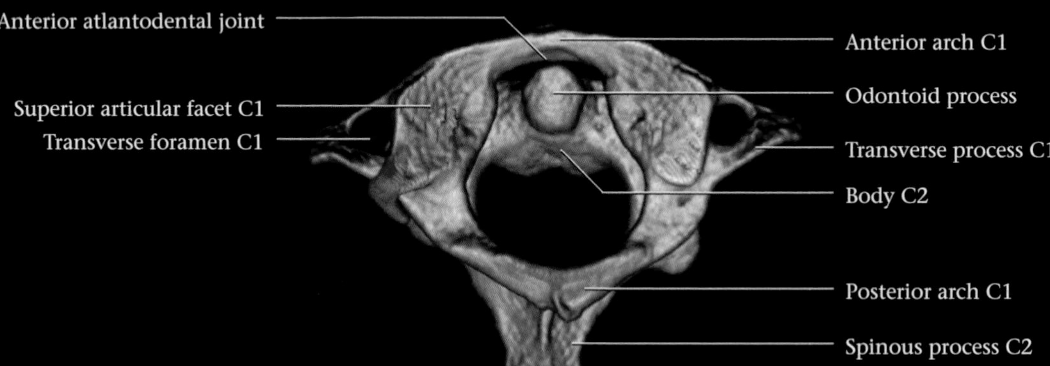
Anterior atlantodental joint
Superior articular facet C1
Transverse foramen C1
Anterior arch C1
Odontoid process
Transverse process C1
Body C2
Posterior arch C1
Spinous process C2

(Top) Anterior view of a 3D-VRT NECT examination. The unique ability of the C1-2 articulation to provide rotation is apparent in this projection, with the bony peg of the odontoid process forming the pivot point for the C1 ring. **(Middle)** Lateral view of a 3D-VRT NECT examination. The complex lateral components of C1 and C2 bodies are highlighted in this projection. The superior facet of C2 is anteriorly positioned to articulate with the inferior articular facet of C1 while the inferior articular facet of C2 is more posterior, and forms the top of the cervical articular "pillar". The articular facets are separated by the elongated pars interarticularis. **(Bottom)** Superior view of a 3D-VRT NECT examination shows relationship of C1 ring with underlying C2 odontoid and lateral masses.

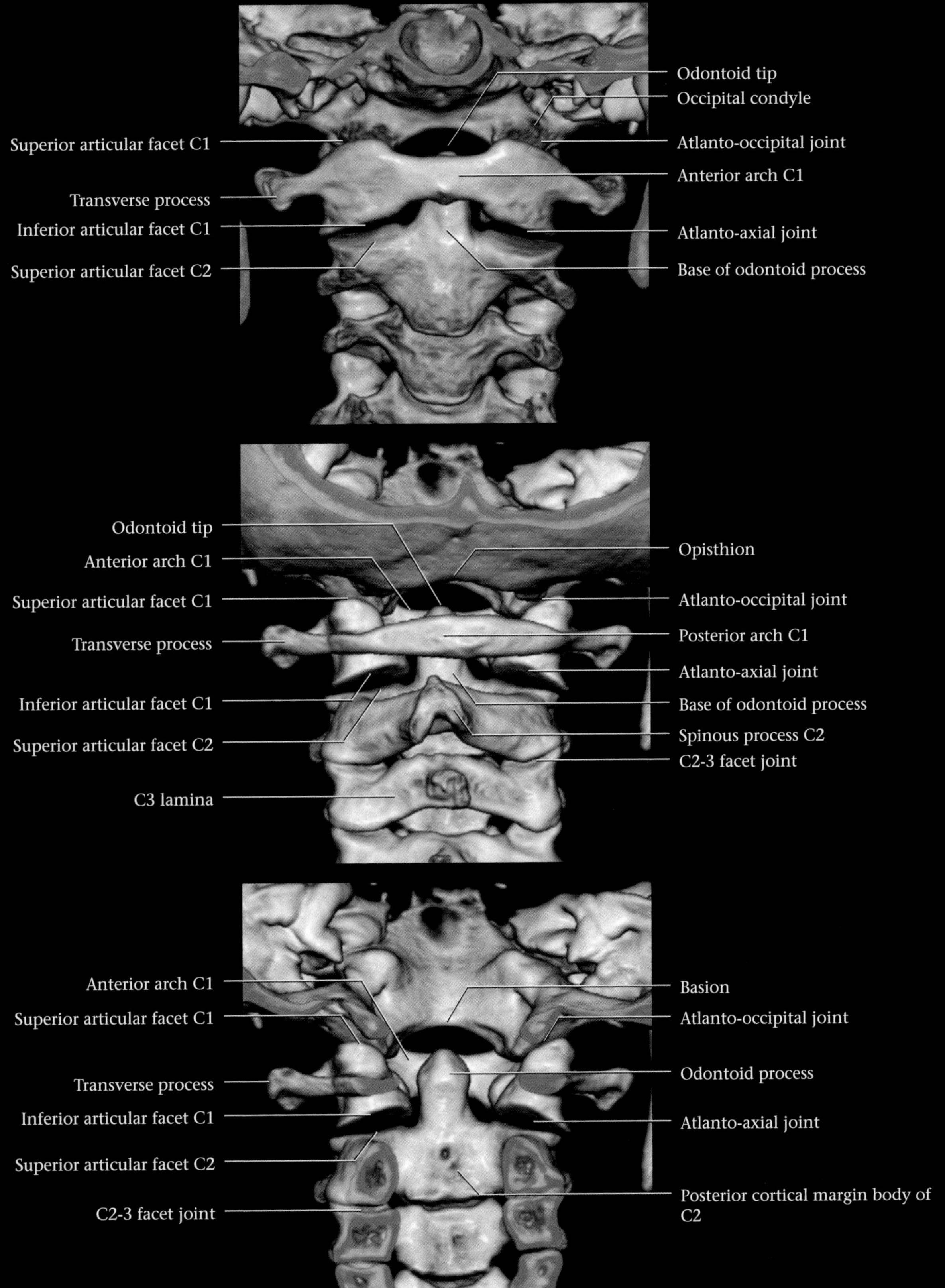
Odontoid tip
Occipital condyle
Superior articular facet C1
Atlanto-occipital joint
Anterior arch C1
Transverse process
Inferior articular facet C1
Atlanto-axial joint
Superior articular facet C2
Base of odontoid process
Odontoid tip
Anterior arch C1
Opisthion
Superior articular facet C1
Atlanto-occipital joint
Transverse process
Posterior arch C1
Atlanto-axial joint
Inferior articular facet C1
Base of odontoid process
Superior articular facet C2
Spinous process C2
C2-3 facet joint
C3 lamina
Anterior arch C1
Basion
Superior articular facet C1
Atlanto-occipital joint
Transverse process
Odontoid process
Inferior articular facet C1
Atlanto-axial joint
Superior articular facet C2
C2-3 facet joint
Posterior cortical margin body of C2

(Top) Anterior view of a 3D-VRT NECT examination of craniocervical junction. The relationship of the atlanto-axial complex with the skull base is highlighted in this projection. The basion forms the anterior margin of the foramen magnum, with the tip of the odontoid process below that level. **(Middle)** Posterior view of a 3D-VRT NECT examination of cervical spine. The opisthion forms the posterior margin of the foramen magnum. The sloping nature of both the C0-1 and C1-2 articulation is evident. The posterior elements form broad attachments for muscles, with prominent spinous processes. **(Bottom)** Posterior view of a 3D-VRT NECT examination of craniocervical junction with removal of posterior elements shows the orientation of atlanto-occipital & atlanto-axial joints well. The proximity of the basion to the odontoid tip is evident.

CRANIOCERVICAL JUNCTION

3D-VRT NECT

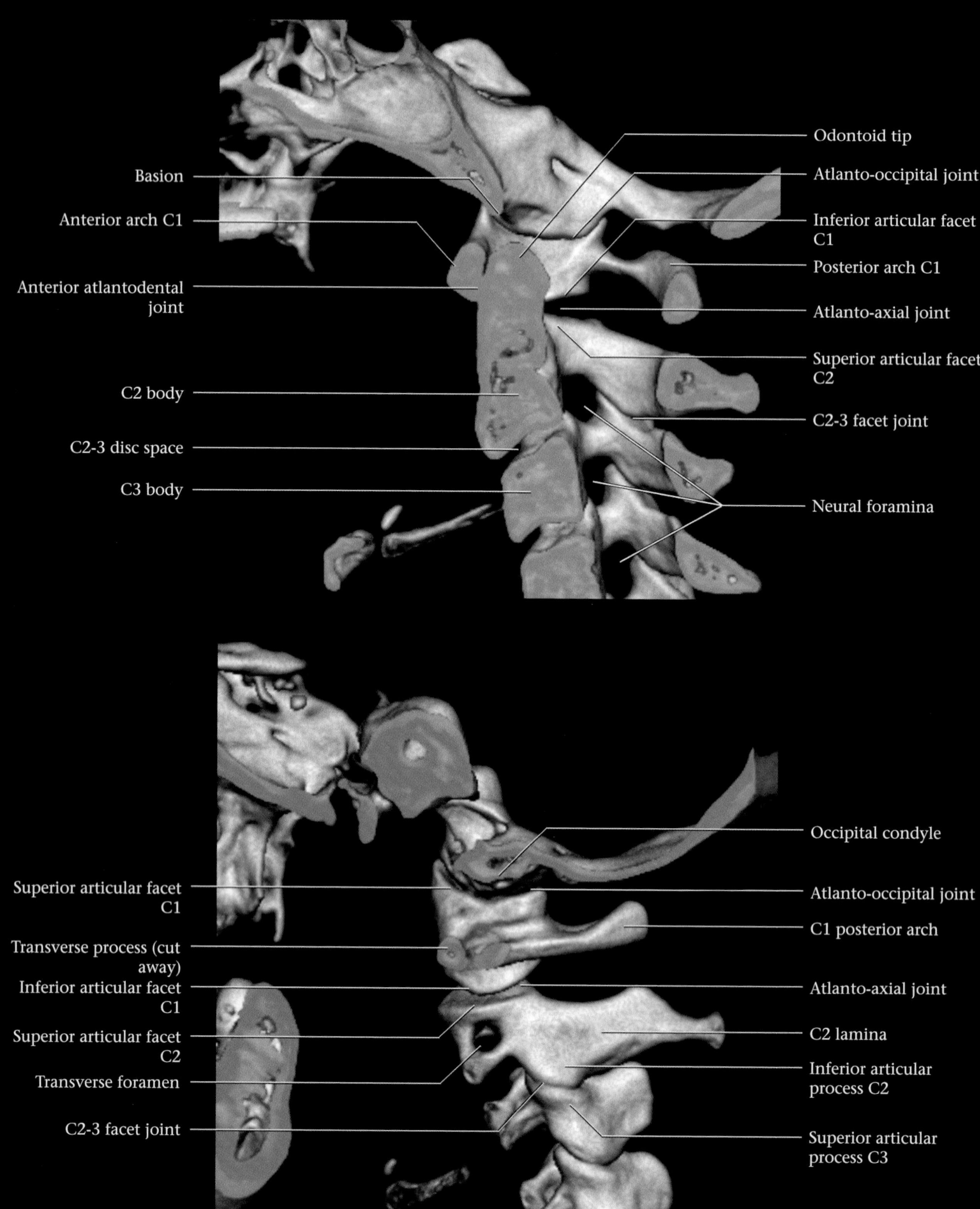

Basion
Anterior arch C1
Anterior atlantodental joint
C2 body
C2-3 disc space
C3 body
Odontoid tip
Atlanto-occipital joint
Inferior articular facet C1
Posterior arch C1
Atlanto-axial joint
Superior articular facet C2
C2-3 facet joint
Neural foramina
Superior articular facet C1
Transverse process (cut away)
Inferior articular facet C1
Superior articular facet C2
Transverse foramen
C2-3 facet joint
Occipital condyle
Atlanto-occipital joint
C1 posterior arch
Atlanto-axial joint
C2 lamina
Inferior articular process C2
Superior articular process C3

(Top) Midline sagittal view of a 3D-VRT NECT examination of cervical spine shows the right half of the craniocervical junction. Note the anterior position of the atlanto-occipital & atlanto-axial joints relative to the facet joints of the sub-axial cervical spine. The midline relationship of the basion, anterior C1 arch, and odontoid tip are well shown. **(Bottom)** Sagittal view of a 3D-VRT NECT examination of cervical spine with attention to the lateral elements. The midline structures have been cut away, showing the posterior "pillar" of the left side of the cervical spine starting with the inferior articular process of C2 and extending caudally. The atlanto-axial and atlanto-occipital joints form a more anterior column. The convex inferior shape of the occipital condyles allows for flexion and extension.

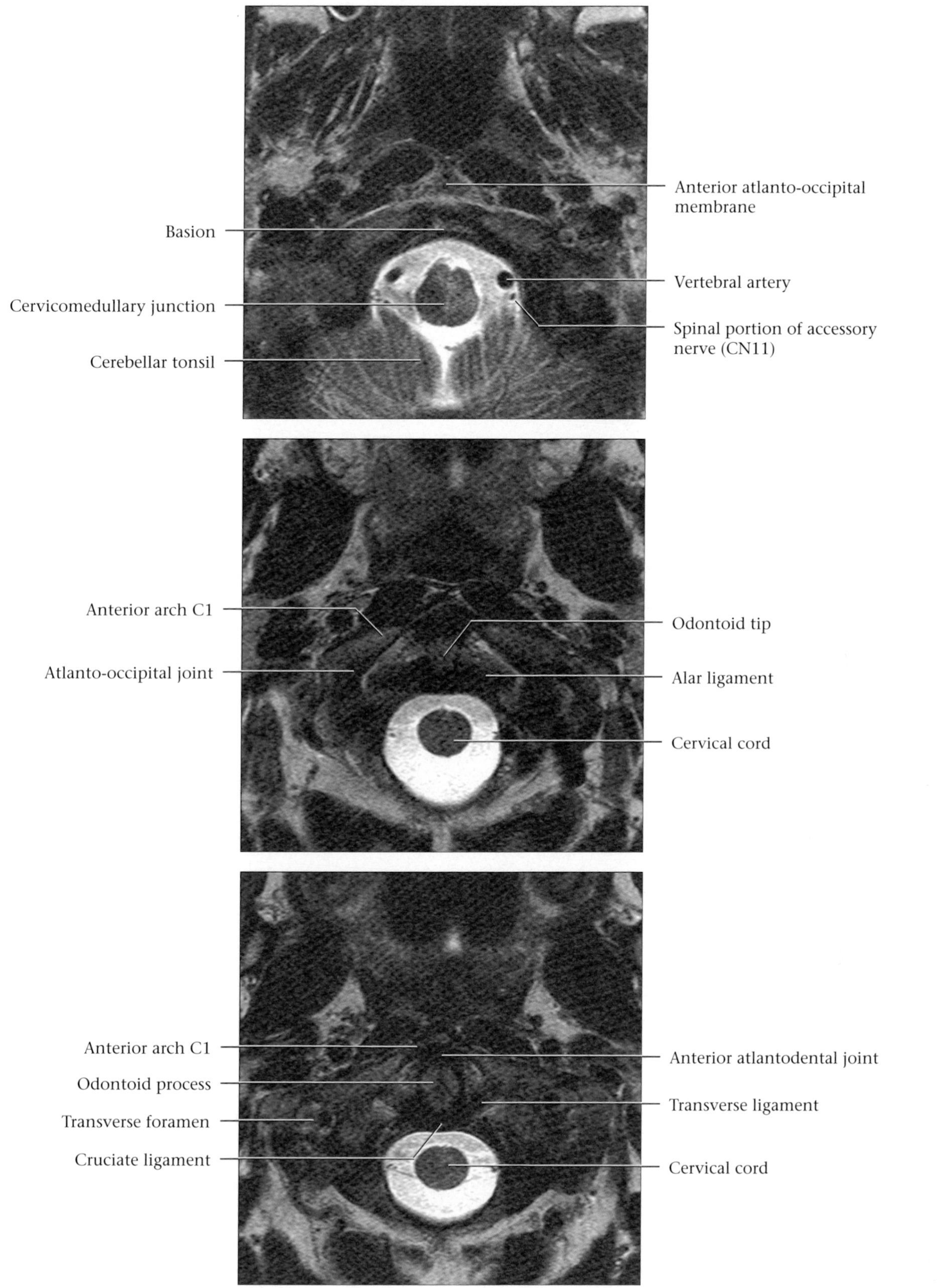

Anterior atlanto-occipital membrane
Basion
Vertebral artery
Cervicomedullary junction
Spinal portion of accessory nerve (CN11)
Cerebellar tonsil
Anterior arch C1
Odontoid tip
Atlanto-occipital joint
Alar ligament
Cervical cord
Anterior arch C1
Anterior atlantodental joint
Odontoid process
Transverse ligament
Transverse foramen
Cruciate ligament
Cervical cord

(Top) First of three axial T2 MR images through the craniocervical junction from superior to inferior shows the anterior margin of the foramen magnum, the cervicomedullary junction and adjacent vertebral artery flow voids. **(Middle)** Image at level of C1 anterior arch. The odontoid tip is seen as rounded intermediate signal in the midline, ventral to the cervical cord. The anterior arch of C1 is visible, with its well-defined cortical margins. The alar ligaments are identified as low signal intensity bands extending laterally from the lateral margins of the odontoid process towards the occipital condyles. **(Bottom)** More inferior image through atlantodental joint. The anterior atlantodental joint is seen along ventral margin of odontoid process. The cruciate ligament (transverse component) is seen as low signal bands curving over dorsal margin of odontoid.

CRANIOCERVICAL JUNCTION

SAGITTAL CT & MR

Anterior atlanto-occipital membrane
Apical ligament
Anterior arch C1
Anterior atlantodental joint
Base of odontoid process
C2-3 intervertebral disc
Basion
Tectorial membrane
Odontoid tip
Cruciate ligament
Opisthion
C1 posterior arch
C2 spinous process

Anterior atlanto-occipital membrane
Anterior arch C1
Anterior atlantodental joint
Anterior longitudinal ligament
Base of odontoid process
C2-3 intervertebral disc
Basion
Apical ligament
Tectorial membrane
Opisthion
Cruciate ligament
C1 posterior arch
C2 spinous process

Anterior atlanto-occipital membrane
Apical ligament
Anterior arch C1
Anterior longitudinal ligament
Base of odontoid process
C2-3 intervertebral disc
Basion
Superior extension of cruciate ligament
Tectorial membrane
Odontoid tip
Cruciate ligament
C1 posterior arch
Posterior longitudinal ligament

(Top) Sagittal midline CT reformat shows the ligamentous structures visible at the craniocervical junction. The apical ligament is visible as a linear band between odontoid tip and clivus. The tectorial membrane is the superior extension of the posterior longitudinal ligament. The anterior atlanto-occipital membrane is the extension of the anterior longitudinal ligament. **(Middle)** Sagittal T1 MR midline image of craniocervical junction. The atlantodental interval is well-defined by the adjacent low signal cortical margins of C1 anterior arch and the odontoid process. The cruciate ligament is a low signal band dorsal to the odontoid. **(Bottom)** Sagittal T2 MR image of the craniocervical junction. The tectorial membrane, superior extension of cruciate ligament, apical ligament & anterior atlanto-occipital membranes are evident.

SAGITTAL T1 MR

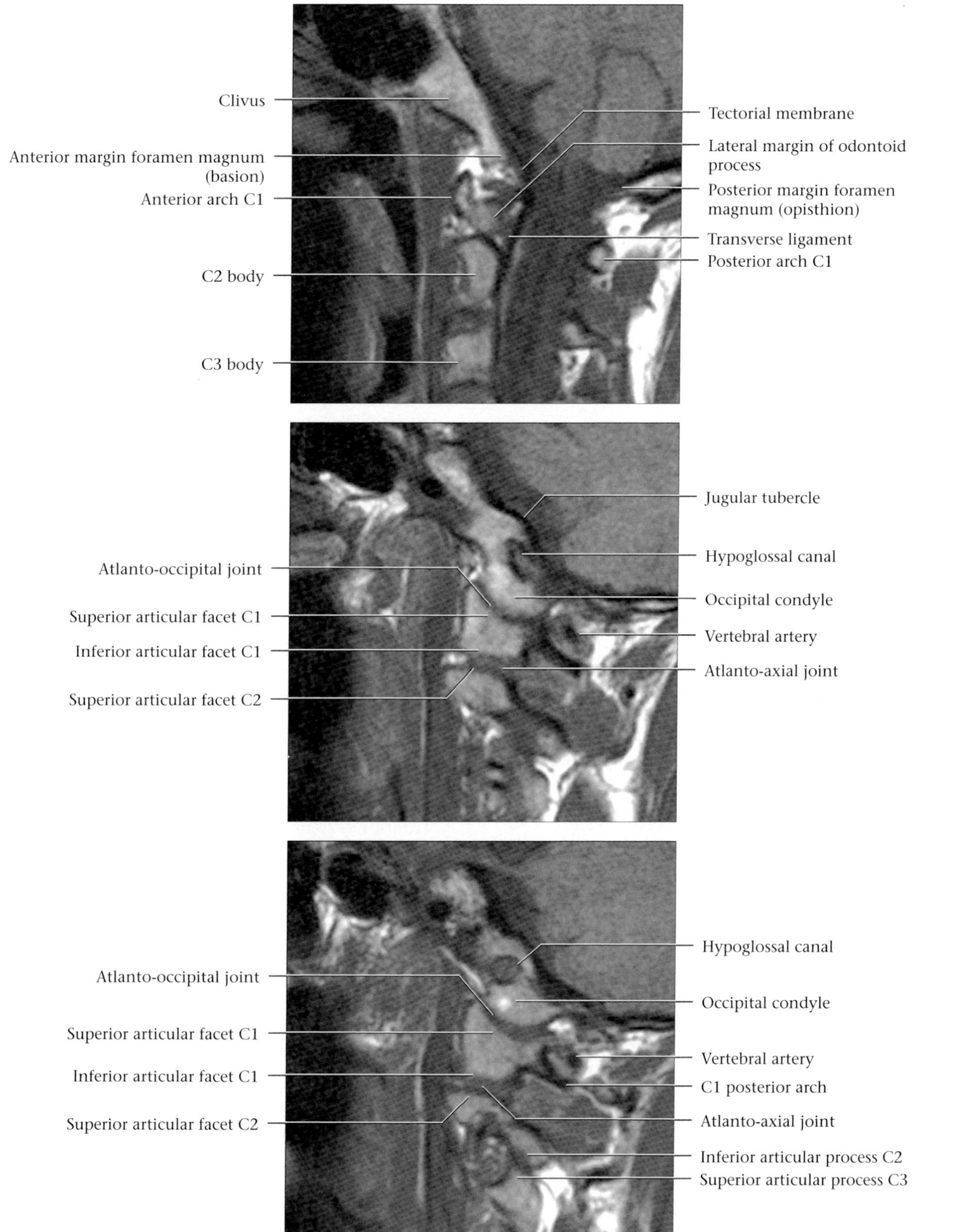
Clivus
Anterior margin foramen magnum (basion)
Anterior arch C1
C2 body
C3 body
Tectorial membrane
Lateral margin of odontoid process
Posterior margin foramen magnum (opisthion)
Transverse ligament
Posterior arch C1
Atlanto-occipital joint
Superior articular facet C1
Inferior articular facet C1
Superior articular facet C2
Jugular tubercle
Hypoglossal canal
Occipital condyle
Vertebral artery
Atlanto-axial joint
Atlanto-occipital joint
Superior articular facet C1
Inferior articular facet C1
Superior articular facet C2
Hypoglossal canal
Occipital condyle
Vertebral artery
C1 posterior arch
Atlanto-axial joint
Inferior articular process C2
Superior articular process C3

(Top) First of three parasagittal T1 MR images shown from medial to lateral through atlanto-occipital joint. This image extends through the lateral cortical margin of the odontoid, which is incompletely visualized. The anterior arch of C1 is obliquely visualized as it curves posterolaterally. The lateral extension of the cruciate ligament, the transverse ligament is prominent. **(Middle)** The relationship of the occipital condyle, C1 lateral mass + atlanto-axial joint is highlighted in this image. The articular surface of occipital condyle is convex & the superior facet of C1 is concave allowing for flexion/extension. **(Bottom)** More lateral image of craniocervical junction. The atlanto-occipital joint and atlanto-axial joints are visible with sharp, smooth cortical margins.

CERVICAL SPINE

Terminology

Synonyms

- Uncovertebral joint (joint of Luschka)
- C1 (atlas); C2 (axis)

Definitions

- Sub-axial cervical spine = C3-C7

Gross Anatomy

Overview

- Consists of 7 vertebrae (C1-C7)
  - **Craniocervical junction (CCJ)**: C1, C2 & articulation with skull base constitutes craniocervical junction
  - **Sub-axial spine**: C3-C7
    - C3-C6 typical cervical vertebrae
    - C7 has features that differ slightly from C3-C6

Components of Sub-Axial Cervical Spine

- **Bones C3-C7**
  - **Body**
    - Small, broader transversely than in AP dimension
    - Posterolateral edges of superior surface are turned upward = uncinate process
  - **Vertebral arch**
    - Pedicle: Delicate, project posterolaterally
    - Lamina: Thin and narrow
    - Vertebral foramen: Large, triangular-shaped
  - **Transverse process**
    - Project laterally and contain foramen for vertebral artery
    - Anterior and posterior tubercles are separated by a superior groove for exiting spinal nerve
  - **Articular processes**
    - Superior and inferior articular processes with articular facets oriented approximately 45° superiorly from transverse plain
    - Form paired osseous shafts posterolateral to vertebral bodies = articular pillars
  - Spinous process: Short and bifid
  - **C7 unique features**
    - Spinous process: Long, prominent
    - Transverse process: Short and project inferolaterally compare with T1 spinous processes which are long & project superolaterally
- **Intervertebral foramen**
  - Oriented anterolaterally below pedicles at approximately 45° to sagittal plane
- **Joints**
  - Intervertebral disc
    - Narrowest in cervical region
    - Thinner posteriorly than anteriorly
    - Do not extend to lateral margins of vertebral bodies in cervical spine ⇒ joints of Luschka
  - **Uncovertebral joint** (joints of Luschka)
    - Oblique, cleft-like cavities between superior surfaces of uncinate processes & lateral lips of inferior articular surface of next superior vertebrae
    - Lined by cartilaginous endplate of vertebral body
    - No true synovial lining present; contains serum, simulating synovial fluid
    - Uncinate process develops during childhood with uncovertebral joint forming by fibrillation and fissuring in fibers of annulus fibrosus
  - **Facet (zygapophyseal) joints**
    - Facet joints oriented approximately 45° superiorly from transverse plane in upper cervical spine; assume more vertical orientation towards C7
    - Formed by articulation between superior & inferior articular processes = articular pillars
    - Forms two sides of a flexible tripod of bone (vertebral bodies, right and left articular pillars) for support of cranium
- **Ligaments**
  - Anterior & posterior longitudinal, ligamentum flavum, interspinous & supraspinous ligaments
  - Additional ligaments of CCJ include apical, alar and cruciate ligaments
- **Biomechanics**
  - Sub-axial cervical spine shows free motion range relative to remainder of presacral spine
    - Cervical extension checked by anterior longitudinal ligament & musculature
    - Cervical flexion checked by articular pillars & intertransverse ligaments

Imaging Anatomy

Lateral Assessment of Sub-Axial Spine

- Principals apply equally to radiography, CT or MR
- **Prevertebral soft tissues**: Distance between air column and anterior aspect of vertebral body
  - Adults: < 7 mm at C2 & < 22 mm at C6
  - Child: < 14 mm at C6
- Bony alignment
  - **Anterior vertebral line**: Smooth curve paralleling anterior vertebral cortex
    - Less important than posterior cortical line
  - **Posterior vertebral line**: Smooth curve paralleling posterior vertebral cortex
    - Translation > 3.5 mm is abnormal
    - Flexion and extension allow physiological offset < 3 mm of posterior cortical margin of successive vertebral bodies
  - **Spino-laminar line**: Smooth curve from opisthion to C7 formed by junction of laminae with spinous processes
  - **Spinous process angulation**: Cervical spinous processes should converge towards a common point posteriorly
    - Widening is present when distance is > 1.5x interspinous distance of adjacent spinal segments

Frontal Assessment of Sub-Axial Spine

- Lateral masses: Bilateral smooth undulating margins
- Spinous processes: Midline
  - Lateral rotation of one spinous process with respect to others is abnormal
- Interspinous distance: Symmetric throughout
  - Interspinous distance 1.5x distance of level above or below is abnormal

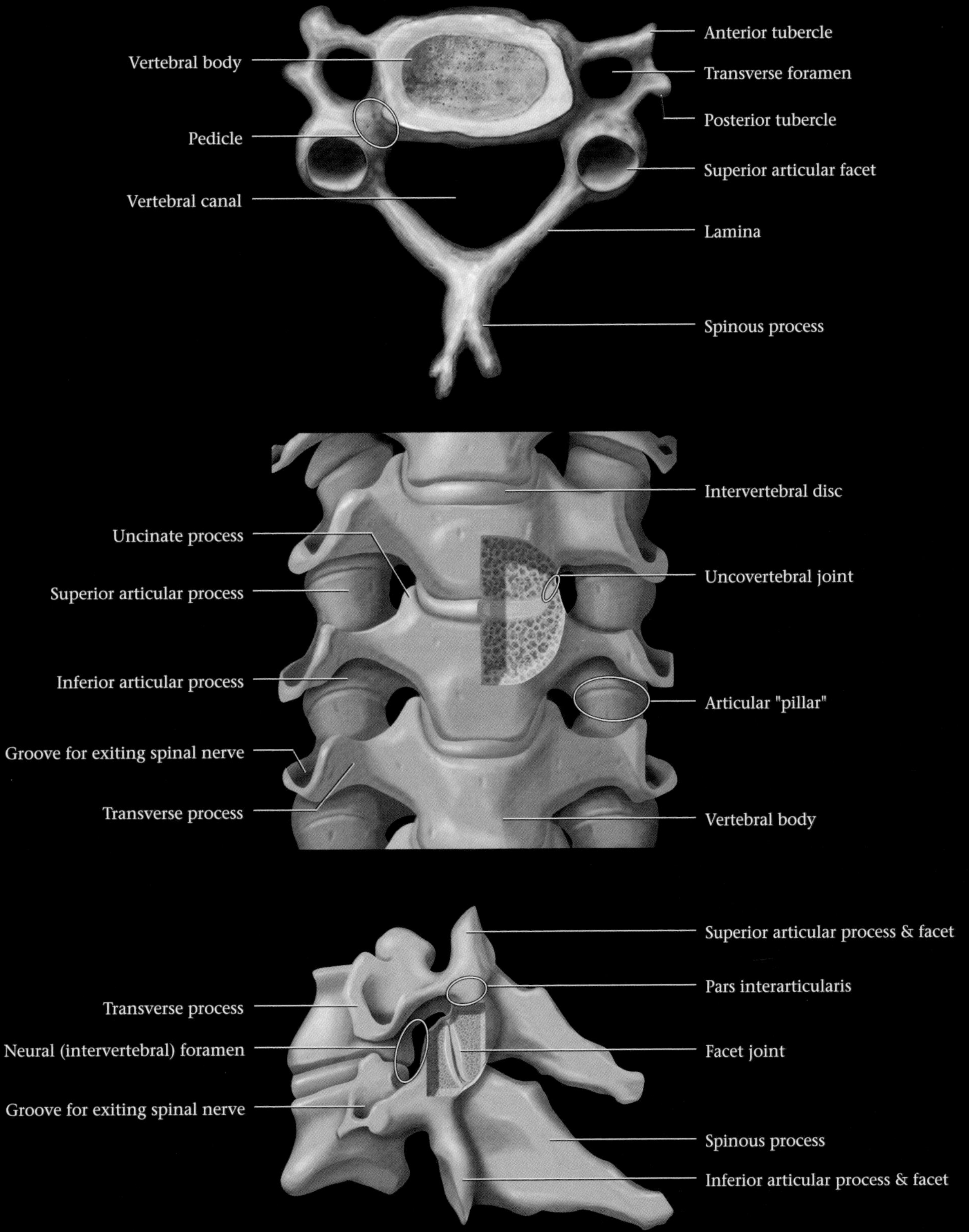
Vertebral body
Pedicle
Vertebral canal
Anterior tubercle
Transverse foramen
Posterior tubercle
Superior articular facet
Lamina
Spinous process
Intervertebral disc
Uncinate process
Superior articular process
Inferior articular process
Groove for exiting spinal nerve
Transverse process
Uncovertebral joint
Articular "pillar"
Vertebral body
Superior articular process & facet
Pars interarticularis
Transverse process
Neural (intervertebral) foramen
Facet joint
Groove for exiting spinal nerve
Spinous process
Inferior articular process & facet

(Top) Graphic of a typical cervical vertebra viewed from above demonstrates important morphology. Vertebral body is broader transversely than in AP dimension, central vertebral canal is large & triangular in shape, pedicles are directed posterolaterally, laminae are delicate & give rise to a spinous process with a bifid tip. Lateral masses contain the vertebral foramen for passage of vertebral artery & veins. **(Middle)** Frontal graphic of sub-axial cervical spine with cutout showing intervertebral disc & uncovertebral joints. Paired lateral articular "pillars" are formed by articulation between superior & inferior articular processes. **(Bottom)** Lateral graphic of two consecutive typical cervical vertebrae with cutout showing facet (zygapophyseal) joint detail. Note also the prominent groove on superior surface of transverse process for exiting spinal nerves.

CERVICAL SPINE

GRAPHICS

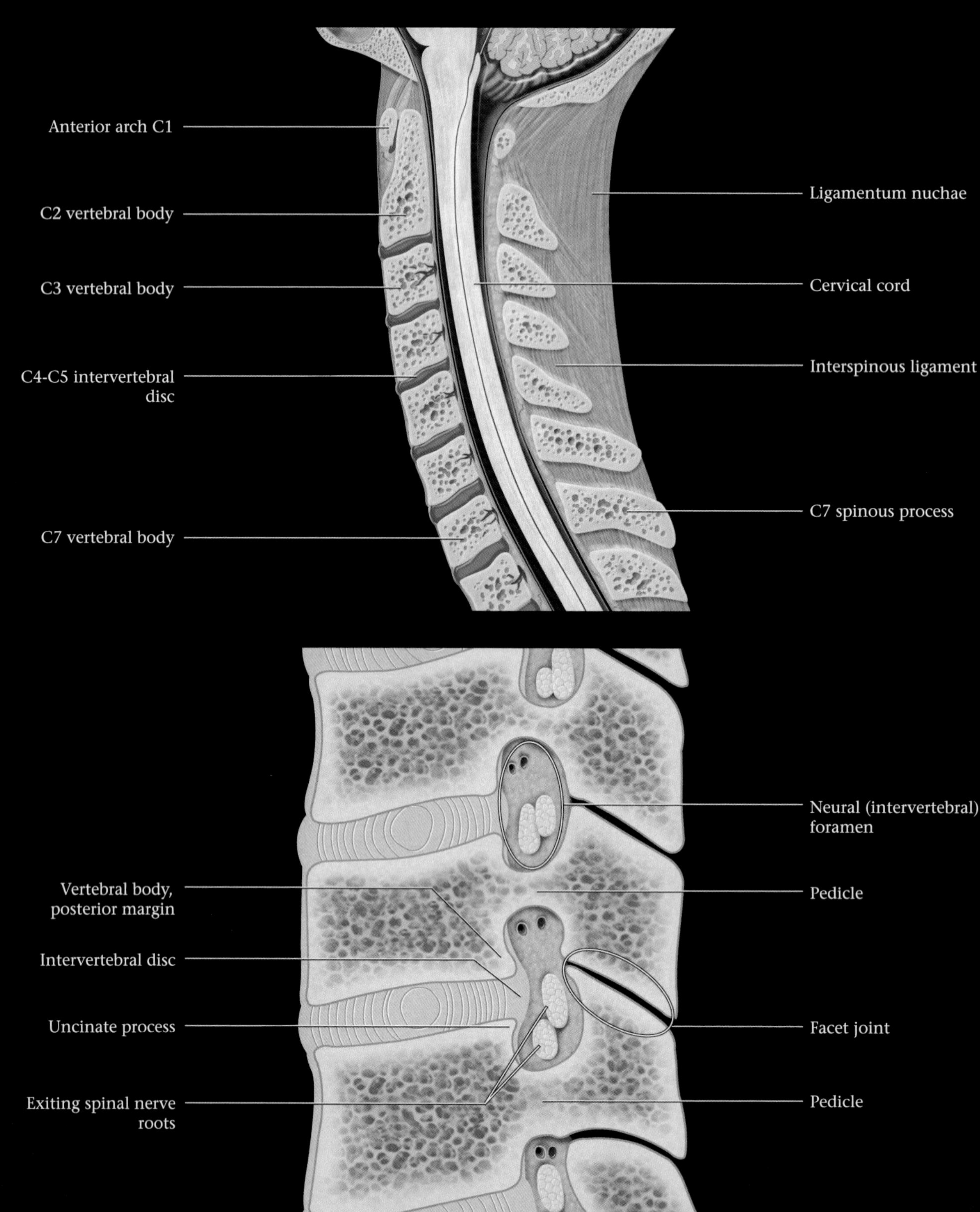
Anterior arch C1
C2 vertebral body
C3 vertebral body
C4-C5 intervertebral disc
C7 vertebral body
Ligamentum nuchae
Cervical cord
Interspinous ligament
C7 spinous process
Neural (intervertebral) foramen
Pedicle
Vertebral body, posterior margin
Intervertebral disc
Uncinate process
Exiting spinal nerve roots
Facet joint
Pedicle

(Top) Sagittal midline graphic of cervical spine & cord showing gentle lordotic curve & smooth alignment of adjacent vertebrae. C1, C2 & their articulation with the skull base constitutes the craniocervical junction. C3-C7 constitutes the sub-axial cervical spine. C3-C6 are regarded as typical cervical vertebrae, whereas C7 has features that differ slightly from C3-C6 including a long, prominent spinous process. **(Bottom)** Sagittal graphic through cervical neural foramen showing position of exiting spinal nerves within lower part of neural foramen. Neural foramina are oriented anterolaterally (compare with thoracic & lumbar regions). Anterior boundary of neural foramen include uncinate process, intervertebral disc & vertebral body from inferior to superior. Pedicles form superior & inferior boundaries. Posterior boundary is the facet joint complex.

GRAPHIC & 3D-VRT NECT

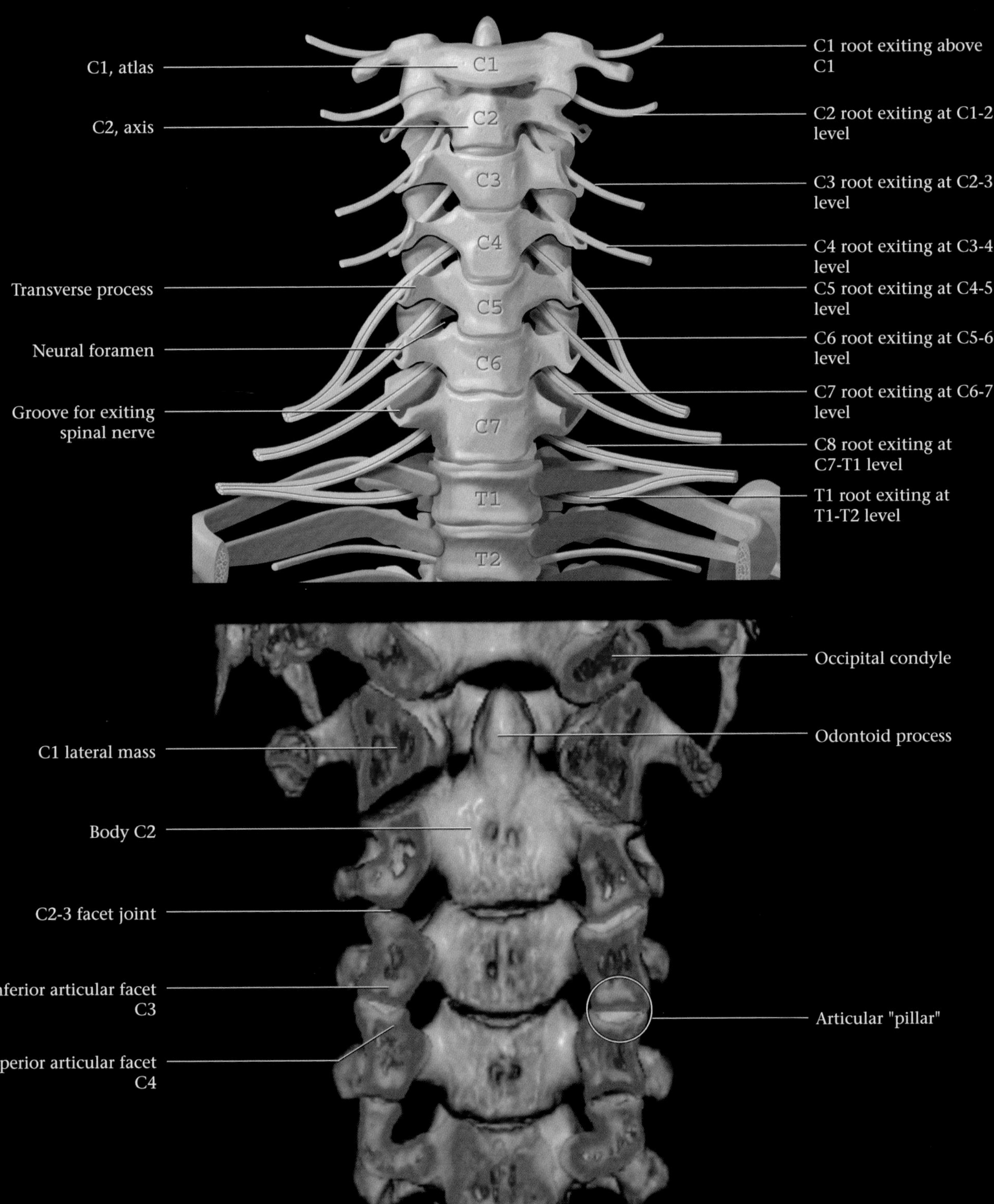
C1, atlas
C2, axis
Transverse process
Neural foramen
Groove for exiting spinal nerve
C1
C2
C3
C4
C5
C6
C7
T1
T2
C1 root exiting above C1
C2 root exiting at C1-2 level
C3 root exiting at C2-3 level
C4 root exiting at C3-4 level
C5 root exiting at C4-5 level
C6 root exiting at C5-6 level
C7 root exiting at C6-7 level
C8 root exiting at C7-T1 level
T1 root exiting at T1-T2 level
C1 lateral mass
Body C2
C2-3 facet joint
Inferior articular facet C3
Superior articular facet C4
Occipital condyle
Odontoid process
Articular "pillar"

(Top) Coronal graphic of the cervical spine showing vertebrae & corresponding cervical nerves. The vertebra are numbered & are shown with their exiting nerves. There are 8 cervical nerves, with C1 nerve exiting above the C1 body & C2 nerve exiting at the C1-2 level. The C8 nerve exits at C7-T1. Below this level, the thoracic roots exit below their respective numbered vertebra. The roots exit inferiorly within the neural foramen, along the bony groove in the transverse process. **(Bottom)** Coronal 3D-VRT examination of the cervical spine, viewed posteriorly with the dorsal elements partially removed to show the dorsal vertebral body surface. The concept of the cervical articular pillars is well shown in this view with the facets forming paired columns of bone with superior & inferior articulating facets.

CERVICAL SPINE

GRAPHIC & LATERAL RADIOGRAPH

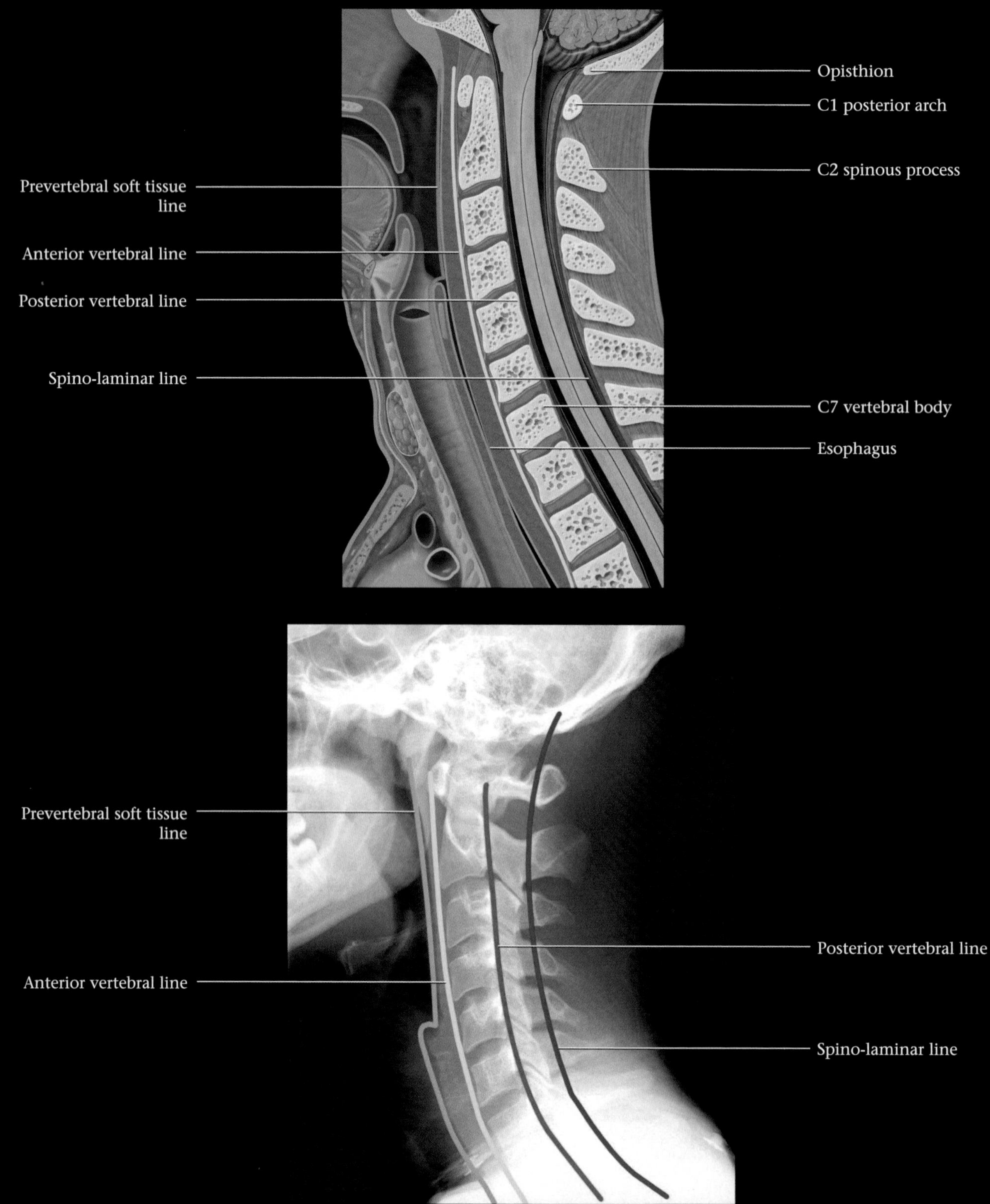

Opisthion
C1 posterior arch
C2 spinous process
Prevertebral soft tissue line
Anterior vertebral line
Posterior vertebral line
Spino-laminar line
C7 vertebral body
Esophagus
Prevertebral soft tissue line
Posterior vertebral line
Anterior vertebral line
Spino-laminar line

(Top) Sagittal midline graphic of the cervical spine. The normal cervical spine shows a smooth lordotic curve, with smooth alignment of a series of lines going from ventral to dorsal including prevertebral soft tissues (orange), anterior vertebral body cortical margins (yellow), posterior vertebral body margins (green), & posterior spino-laminar line (blue). In adults, the prevertebral soft tissues measure < 7 mm at C2 & < 22 mm at C6. In children they measure < 14 mm at C6. **(Bottom)** Lateral radiograph of the cervical spine showing normal alignment. A series of gently curving lines make up the normal cervical curvature, extending from prevertebral soft tissues to the posterior spino-laminar line. In addition, the cervical spinous processes should all converge towards a common point posteriorly.

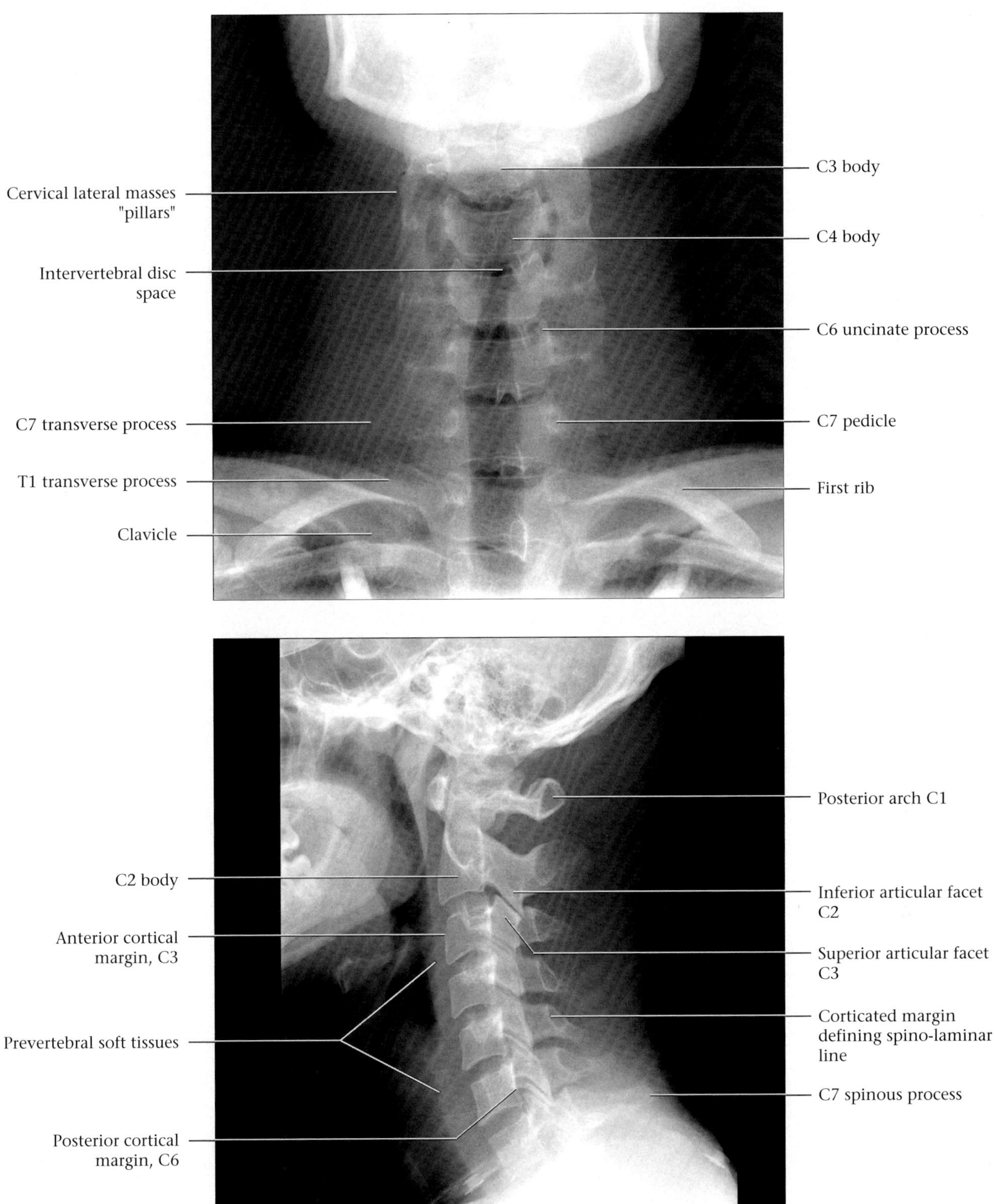

Cervical lateral masses "pillars"
Intervertebral disc space
C7 transverse process
T1 transverse process
Clavicle
C3 body
C4 body
C6 uncinate process
C7 pedicle
First rib
C2 body
Anterior cortical margin, C3
Prevertebral soft tissues
Posterior cortical margin, C6
Posterior arch C1
Inferior articular facet C2
Superior articular facet C3
Corticated margin defining spino-laminar line
C7 spinous process

(Top) AP plain film view of the cervical spine. The articular facets are viewed obliquely in this projection & therefore not defined, giving the appearance of smoothly undulating lateral columns of bone. The superior & inferior vertebral endplate margins are sharp, with regular spacing of the intervertebral discs. The spinous processes are midline. C7 transverse process is directed inferolaterally compared with T1 which is directed superolaterally. **(Bottom)** Lateral radiograph of cervical spine. The prevertebral soft tissues should form a defined, abrupt "shelf" at approximately C4/5 where the hypopharynx/esophagus begins, hence thickening the prevertebral soft tissues. The bony cervical spine is aligned from anteriorly to posteriorly with the anterior vertebral body margins, the posterior vertebral body margins & ventral margins of the spinous processes (spino-laminar line).

RADIOGRAPHY & 3D-VRT NECT

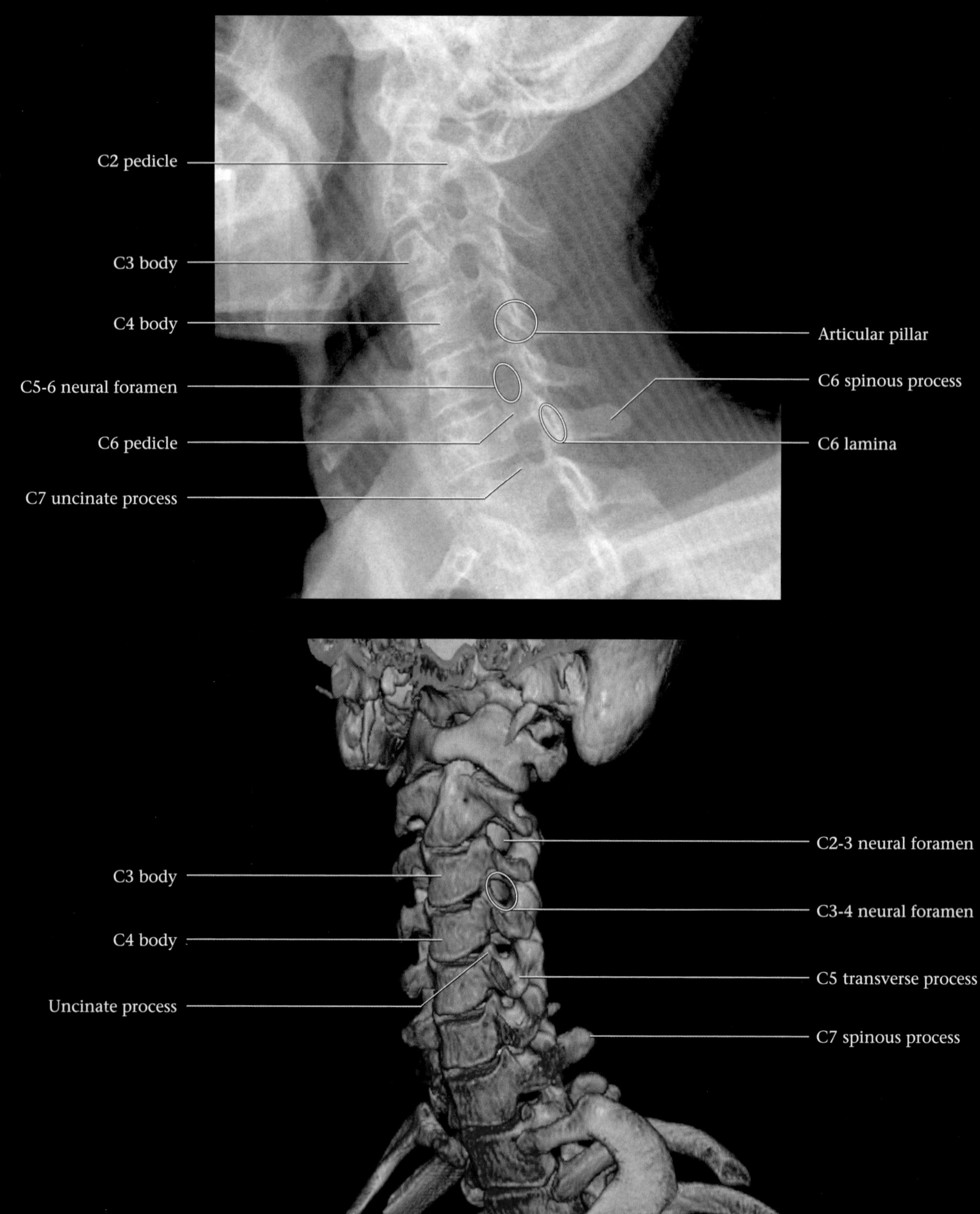
C2 pedicle
C3 body
C4 body
C5-6 neural foramen
C6 pedicle
C7 uncinate process
Articular pillar
C6 spinous process
C6 lamina
C3 body
C4 body
Uncinate process
C2-3 neural foramen
C3-4 neural foramen
C5 transverse process
C7 spinous process

(Top) Oblique radiograph of the cervical spine best demonstrates the neural foramina, as these are oriented obliquely at approximately 45° from sagittal plane. With the patient rotated to the left, the radiograph demonstrates the right-sided foramina. The anterior boundary of the neural foramina includes the uncinate process, intervertebral disc & vertebral body. The posterior boundary is the facet joint complex. The articular pillar facet joints are viewed obliquely and are hence not well-defined. The lamina are seen end-on & hence sharply corticated. **(Bottom)** Oblique 3D-VRT examination of the cervical spine showing the neural foramina end-on. The groove on the superior surface of the transverse processes for the exiting spinal nerves is well shown.

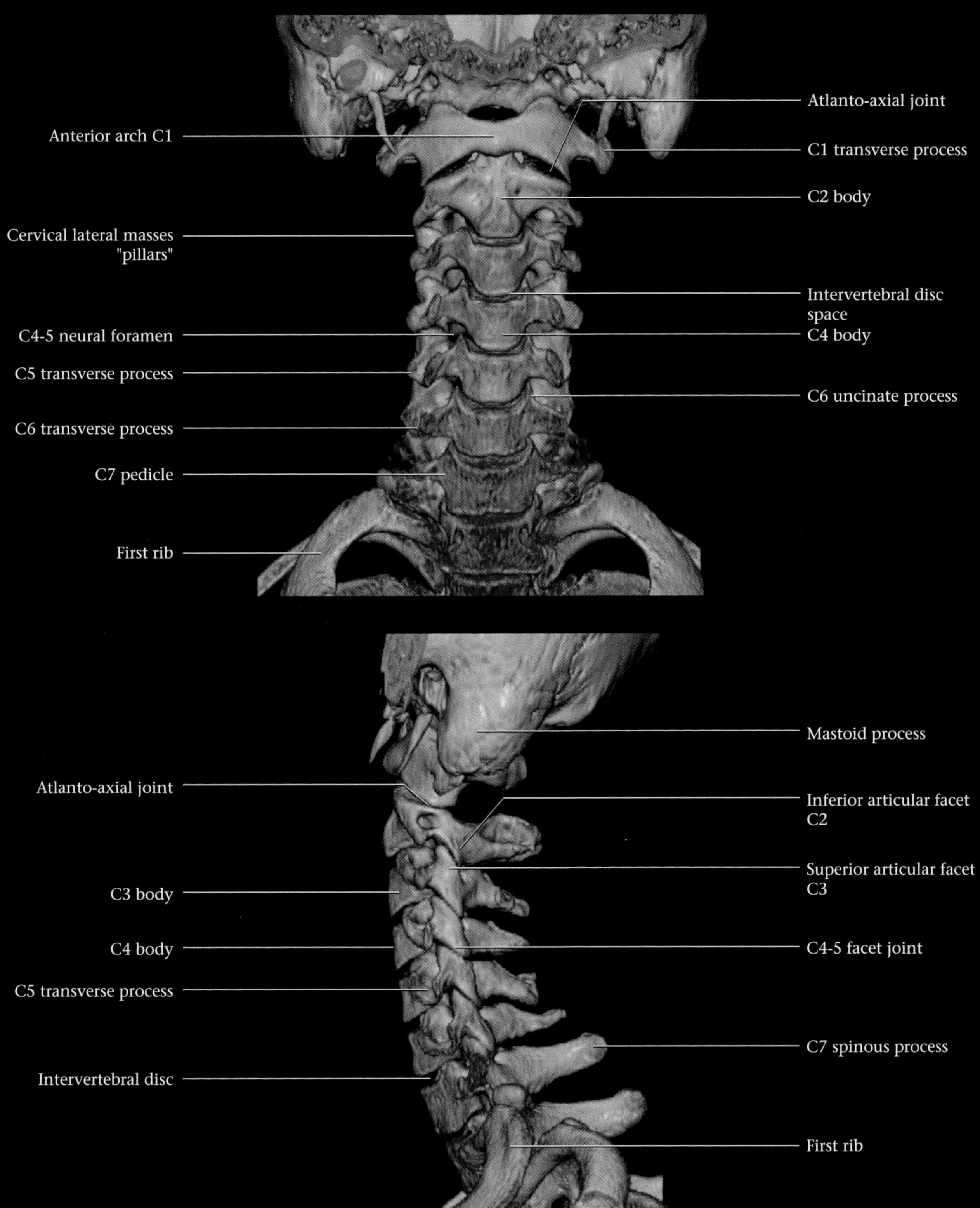
Anterior arch C1
Cervical lateral masses "pillars"
C4-5 neural foramen
C5 transverse process
C6 transverse process
C7 pedicle
First rib
Atlanto-axial joint
C1 transverse process
C2 body
Intervertebral disc space
C4 body
C6 uncinate process
Atlanto-axial joint
C3 body
C4 body
C5 transverse process
Intervertebral disc
Mastoid process
Inferior articular facet C2
Superior articular facet C3
C4-5 facet joint
C7 spinous process
First rib

(Top) Anterior view of 3D-VRT NECT examination of the cervical spine. The wide neural foramina, with the groove or sulcus on the superior surface of the transverse processes for the exiting nerves are well seen. The transverse processes with the tubercles for muscle attachments are well identified from C3-7 levels. The uncinate processes are acquired, superior bony projections along the posterolateral margins of the vertebral bodies & form the uncovertebral joints with the adjacent superior vertebral body. **(Bottom)** Lateral view of 3D-VRT NECT examination of the cervical spine. The facet joints are seen in profile angled approximately 45° superiorly from the transverse plain. They align in a smooth interlocking fashion, with the superior articular facets directed posteriorly & the inferior articular facets directed anteriorly.

AXIAL BONE CT

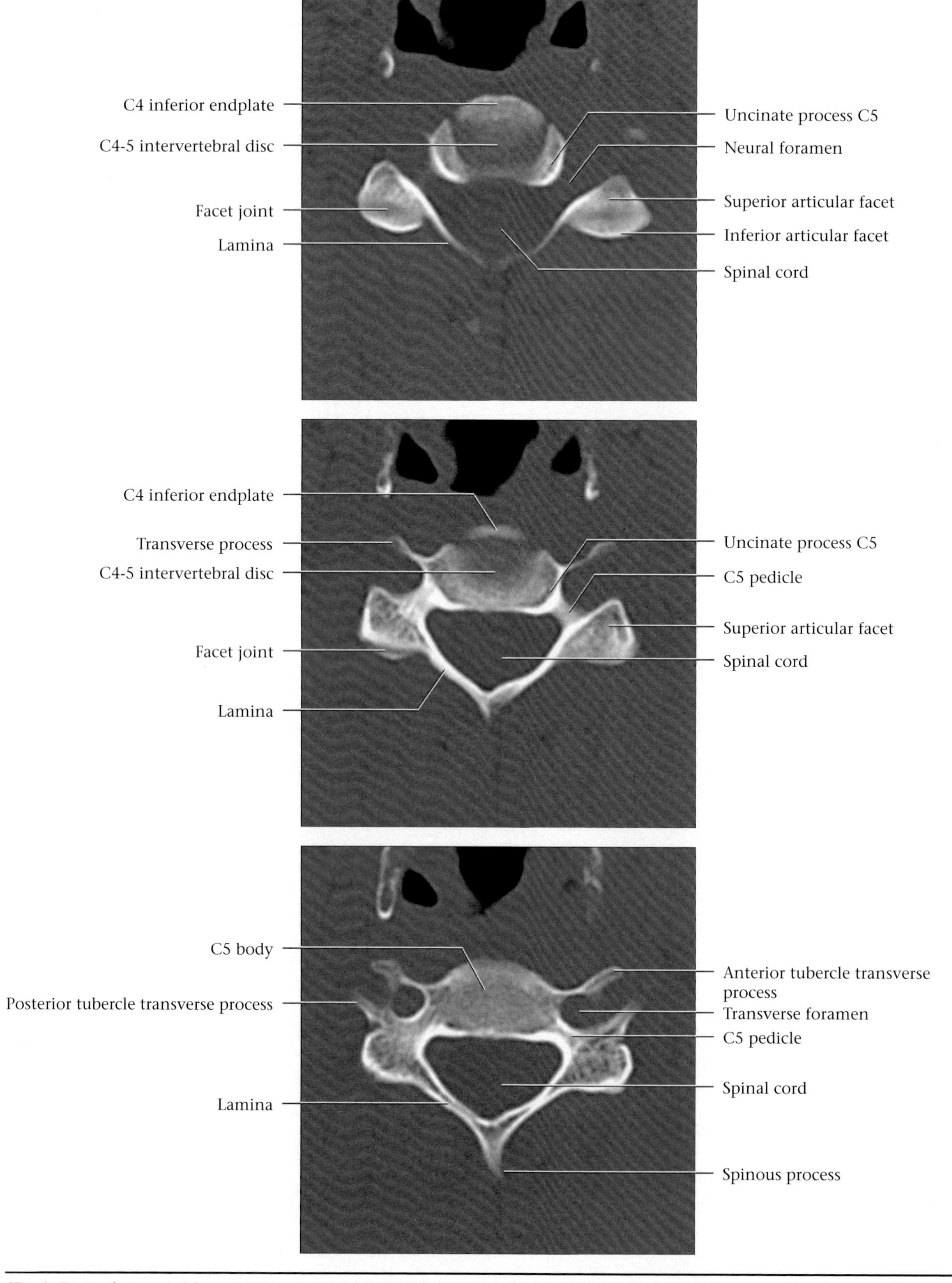
C4 inferior endplate
C4-5 intervertebral disc
Facet joint
Lamina
Uncinate process C5
Neural foramen
Superior articular facet
Inferior articular facet
Spinal cord
C4 inferior endplate
Transverse process
C4-5 intervertebral disc
Facet joint
Lamina
Uncinate process C5
C5 pedicle
Superior articular facet
Spinal cord
C5 body
Posterior tubercle transverse process
Lamina
Anterior tubercle transverse process
Transverse foramen
C5 pedicle
Spinal cord
Spinous process

(Top) First of six axial bone CT images presented from superior to inferior through the cervical spine starting at the C4-5 level. The cup-shaped intervertebral disc of the cervical region is seen centrally, bounded along the posterolateral margin by the uncinate processes. The uncinate process defines the joint of Luschka between adjacent vertebral segments. The neural foramina exit at around 45° in an anterolateral direction, bounded posteriorly by the superior articular process. **(Middle)** Image through inferior margin of intervertebral disc. The gracile pedicles arise obliquely from the posterolateral margins of the vertebral bodies. The bony canal is large relative to the posterior elements, & assumes a triangular configuration. **(Bottom)** Image through C5 body level. The transverse process contains the transverse foramen for the vertebral artery.

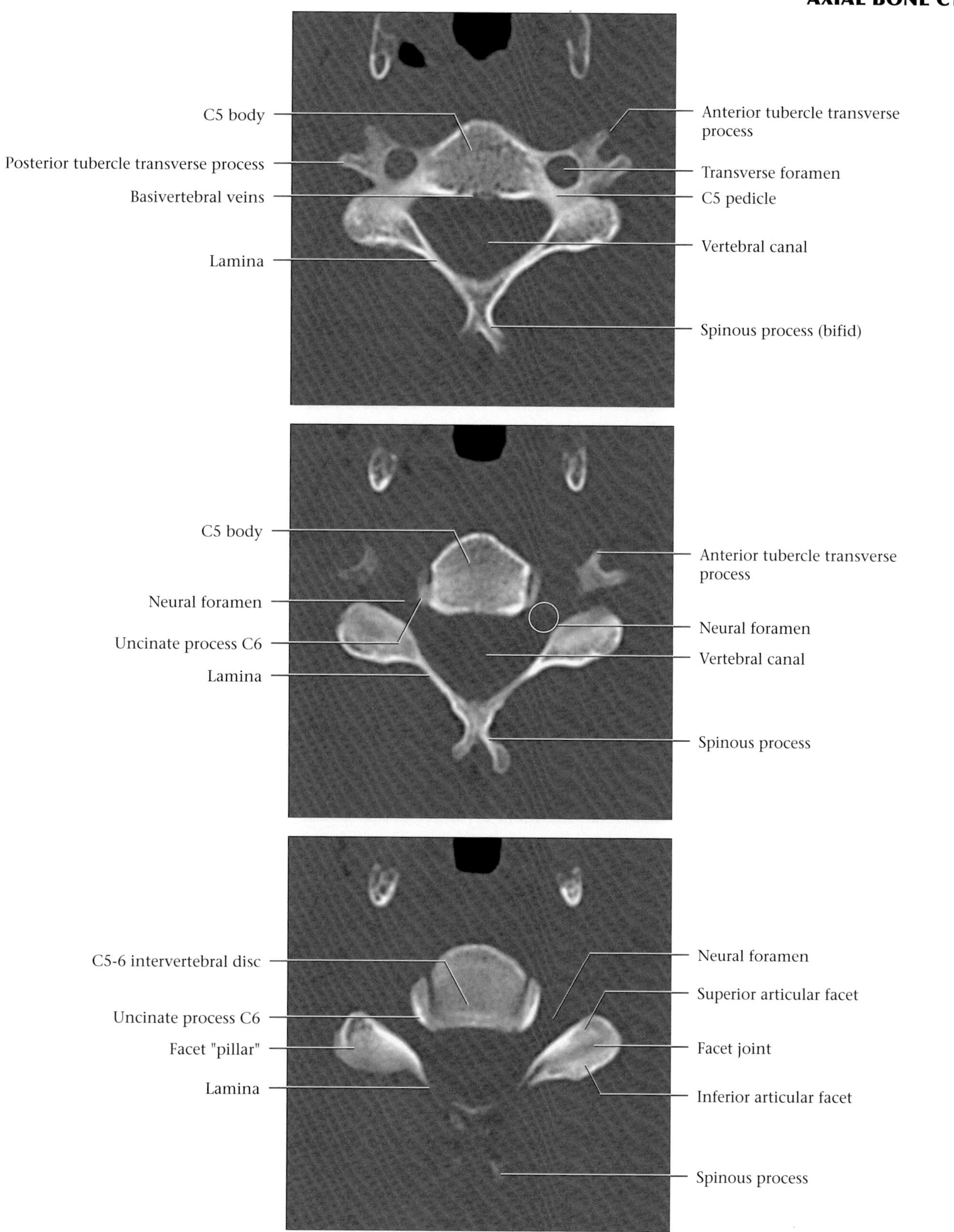
C5 body
Posterior tubercle transverse process
Basivertebral veins
Lamina
Anterior tubercle transverse process
Transverse foramen
C5 pedicle
Vertebral canal
Spinous process (bifid)
C5 body
Neural foramen
Uncinate process C6
Lamina
Anterior tubercle transverse process
Neural foramen
Vertebral canal
Spinous process
C5-6 intervertebral disc
Uncinate process C6
Facet "pillar"
Lamina
Neural foramen
Superior articular facet
Facet joint
Inferior articular facet
Spinous process

(Top) Image through mid C5 body at the pedicle level. The transverse foramina are prominent at this level, with the round, sharply marginated transverse foramen encompassing the vertical course of the vertebral artery. The anterior & posterior tubercles give rise to muscle attachments in the neck. The vertebral body is interrupted along the posterior cortical margin for the passage of the basivertebral venous complex. **(Middle)** Image at the inferior C5 body level. The uncinate process arising off of the next inferior vertebral body is coming into view. The inferior margins of the transverse processes are incompletely visualized. The spinous process is well seen joining with the thin lamina. **(Bottom)** View at C5-6 level shows the next neural foraminal level bounded by uncovertebral joint anteriorly, & facet posteriorly.

CERVICAL SPINE

CORONAL CT MYELOGRAM

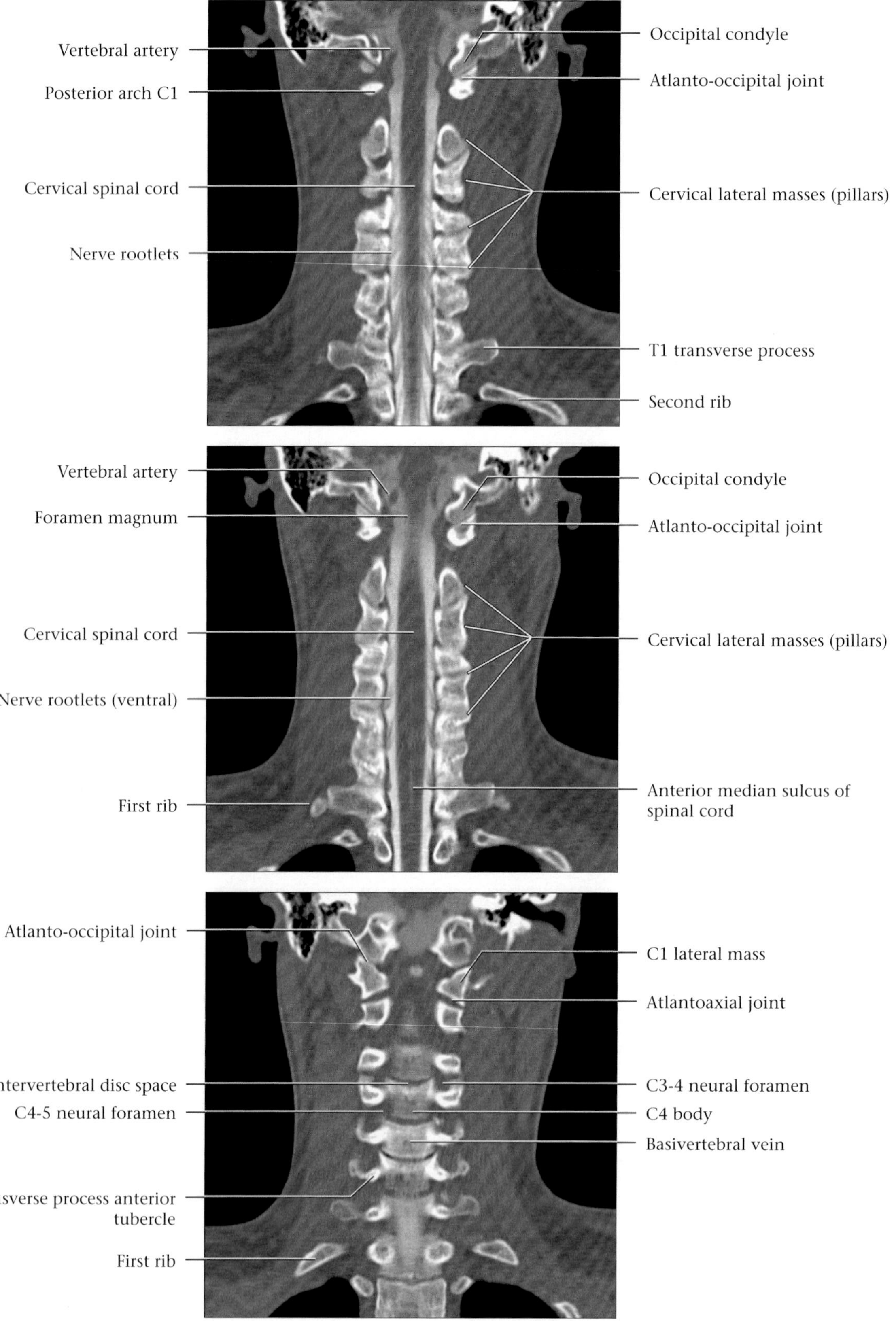

Vertebral artery
Posterior arch C1
Cervical spinal cord
Nerve rootlets
Occipital condyle
Atlanto-occipital joint
Cervical lateral masses (pillars)
T1 transverse process
Second rib
Vertebral artery
Foramen magnum
Cervical spinal cord
Nerve rootlets (ventral)
First rib
Occipital condyle
Atlanto-occipital joint
Cervical lateral masses (pillars)
Anterior median sulcus of spinal cord
Atlanto-occipital joint
Intervertebral disc space
C4-5 neural foramen
C6 transverse process anterior tubercle
First rib
C1 lateral mass
Atlantoaxial joint
C3-4 neural foramen
C4 body
Basivertebral vein

(Top) First of three coronal reformatted images from a CT myelogram displayed from posterior to anterior. Most posterior view shows the spinal cord with exiting nerve rootlets at each segmental level traversing in a craniocaudal direction within the thecal sac. T1 transverse process is prominent & directed superolaterally. **(Middle)** More anterior view shows the ventral margin of the cervical spinal cord with the anterior median sulcus, which would contain the anterior spinal artery. The ventral nerve rootlets are also visible. The articular pillars of the facet joints are well shown, giving a view similar to an AP radiograph of the undulating lateral margin of the cervical pillars. **(Bottom)** More anterior view shows transverse processes with adjacent neural foramina. The posterior margins of the vertebral bodies show the midline basivertebral veins.

SAGITTAL CT MYELOGRAM

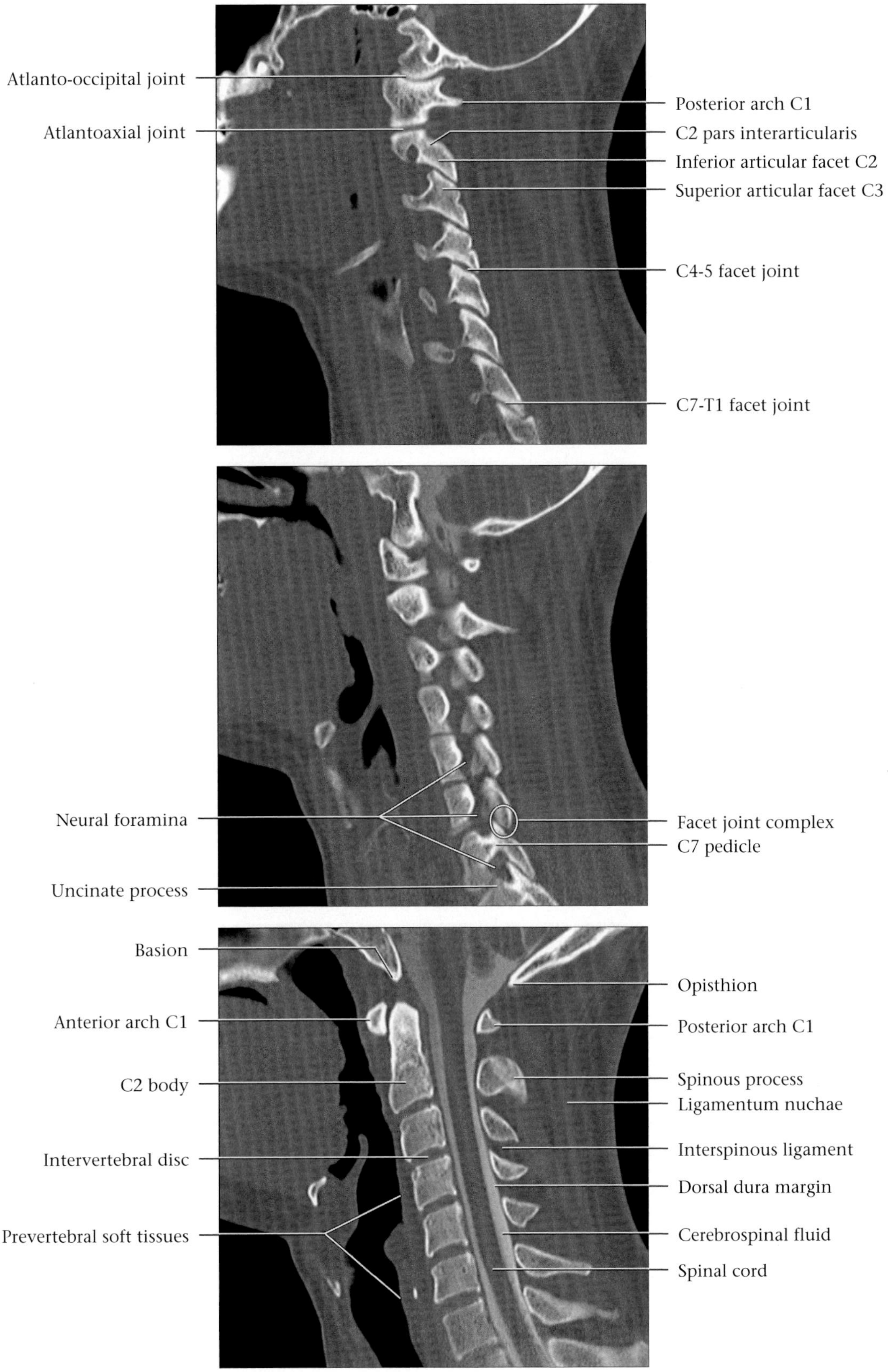

Atlanto-occipital joint
Atlantoaxial joint
Posterior arch C1
C2 pars interarticularis
Inferior articular facet C2
Superior articular facet C3
C4-5 facet joint
C7-T1 facet joint

Neural foramina
Uncinate process
Facet joint complex
C7 pedicle

Basion
Anterior arch C1
C2 body
Intervertebral disc
Prevertebral soft tissues
Opisthion
Posterior arch C1
Spinous process
Ligamentum nuchae
Interspinous ligament
Dorsal dura margin
Cerebrospinal fluid
Spinal cord

(Top) First of three sagittal reformatted images from CT myelogram. Paramedian sagittal section through the articular pillar showing the facet joints in profile. Superior articular facets are directed posteriorly while inferior facets are directed anteriorly. The curvilinear shape of the atlanto-occipital joint is visible, allowing for flexion/extension. **(Middle)** More medial section through obliquely oriented neural foramina which are bounded above & below by pedicles, anteriorly by uncovertebral joint, disc & vertebral body, & posteriorly by facet joint complex. **(Bottom)** Midline section shows the spinal cord outlined by the high attenuation of the contrast within the cerebrospinal fluid. Vertebral alignment is normal & prevertebral soft tissues demonstrate an abrupt "shelf" at approximately C4-5 level where esophagus begins.

SAGITTAL T1 MR

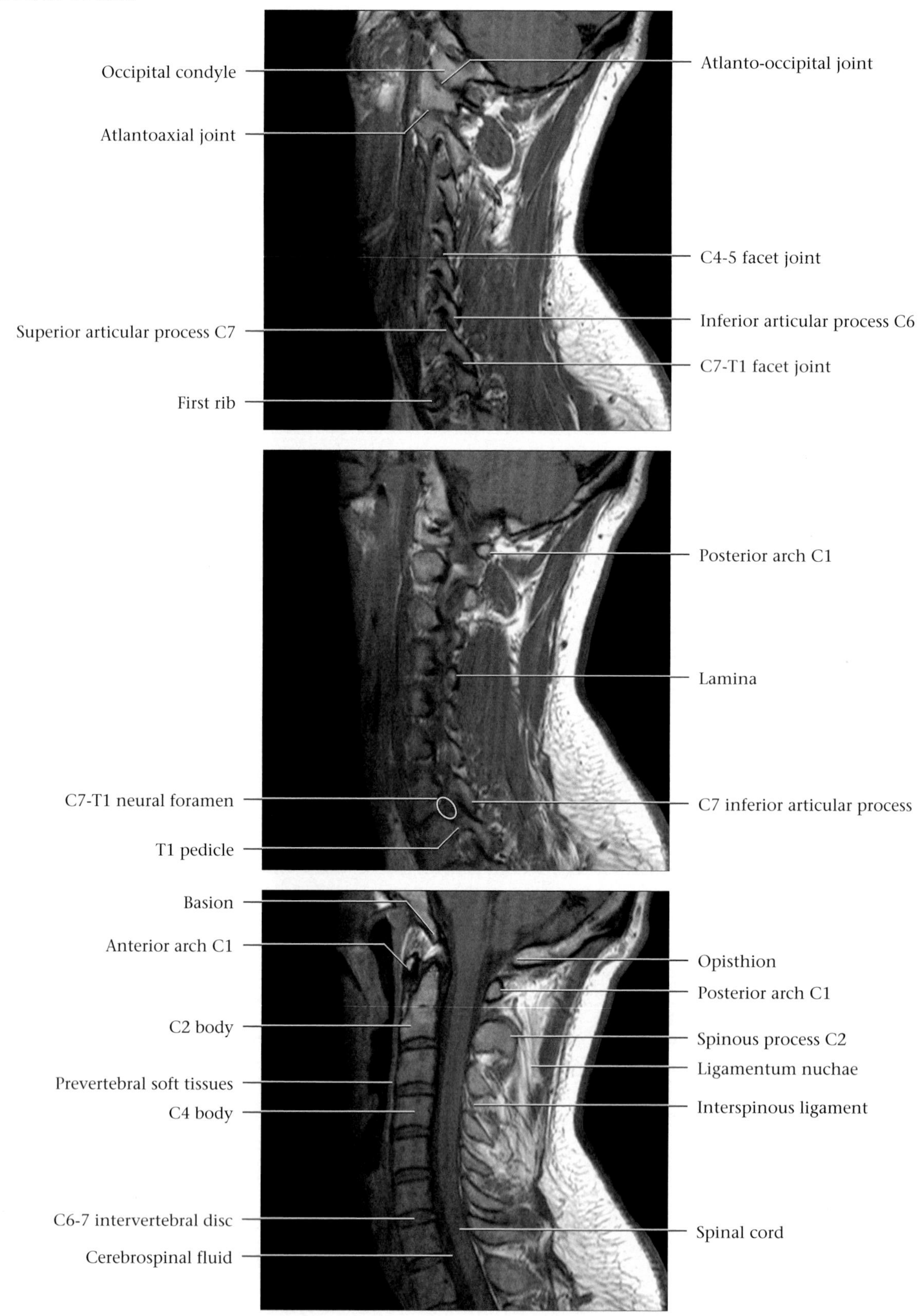
Occipital condyle
Atlantoaxial joint
Superior articular process C7
First rib
Atlanto-occipital joint
C4-5 facet joint
Inferior articular process C6
C7-T1 facet joint
Posterior arch C1
Lamina
C7-T1 neural foramen
T1 pedicle
C7 inferior articular process
Basion
Anterior arch C1
C2 body
Prevertebral soft tissues
C4 body
C6-7 intervertebral disc
Cerebrospinal fluid
Opisthion
Posterior arch C1
Spinous process C2
Ligamentum nuchae
Interspinous ligament
Spinal cord

(Top) First of three sagittal T1 MR images viewed from lateral to medial. View through the articular pillar showing the facet joints in profile. Margins of the facet joints are well corticated & seen as thin hypointense lines. **(Middle)** More medial section through obliquely oriented neural foramina. **(Bottom)** Midline image shows the well-defined low signal cortical margins of the vertebral bodies, which merge along their anterior & posterior margins with the hypointense anterior & posterior longitudinal ligaments respectively. Vertebral marrow signal is hyperintense relative to intervening discs on T1 MR. Cerebrospinal fluid is hypointense.

SAGITTAL T2 MR

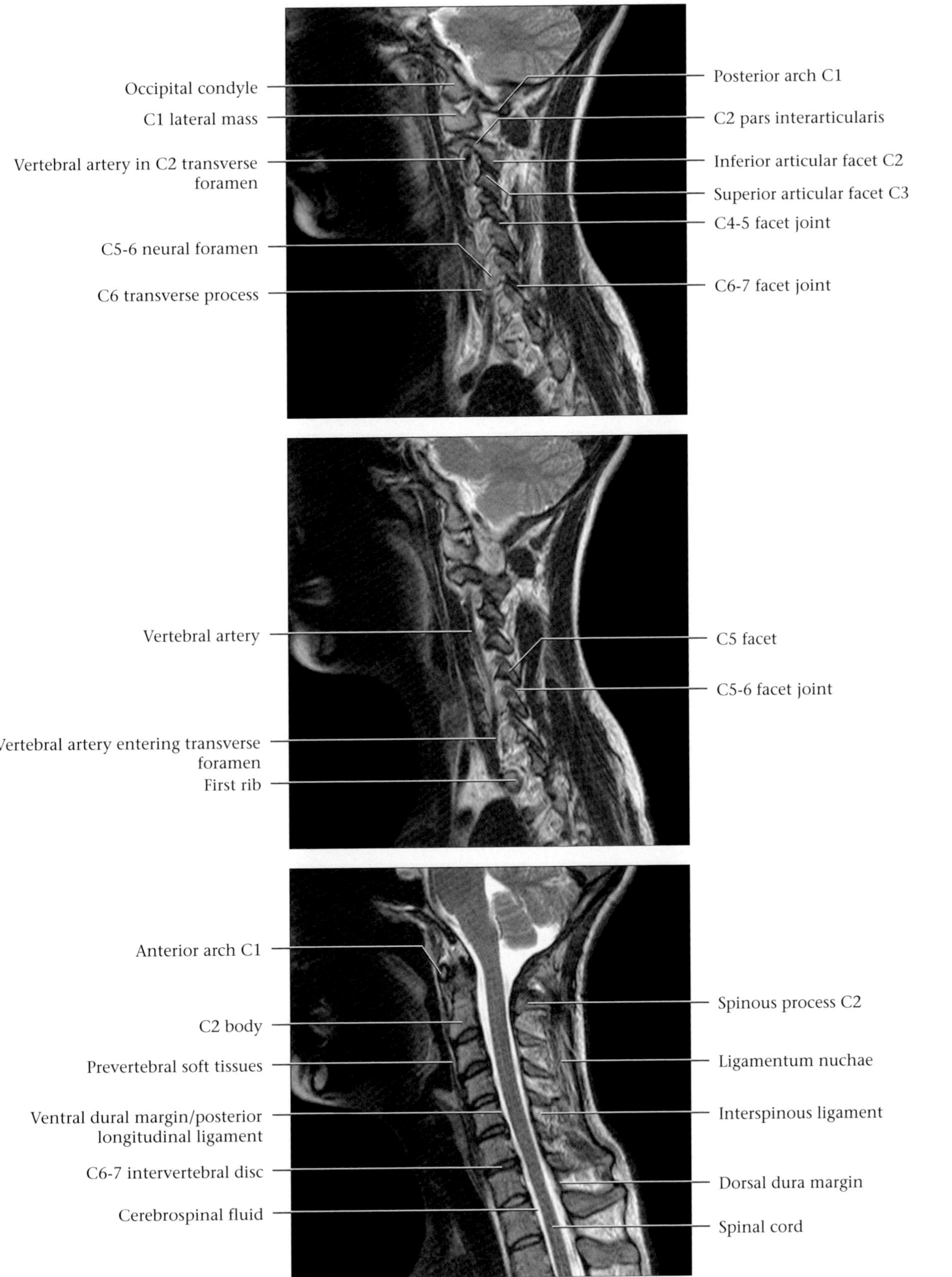
Occipital condyle
C1 lateral mass
Vertebral artery in C2 transverse foramen
C5-6 neural foramen
C6 transverse process
Posterior arch C1
C2 pars interarticularis
Inferior articular facet C2
Superior articular facet C3
C4-5 facet joint
C6-7 facet joint
Vertebral artery
Vertebral artery entering transverse foramen
First rib
C5 facet
C5-6 facet joint
Anterior arch C1
C2 body
Prevertebral soft tissues
Ventral dural margin/posterior longitudinal ligament
C6-7 intervertebral disc
Cerebrospinal fluid
Spinous process C2
Ligamentum nuchae
Interspinous ligament
Dorsal dura margin
Spinal cord

(Top) First of three sagittal T2 MR images viewed from lateral to medial. View through the articular pillars show normal alignment of the facet joints. The rhomboidal configuration of the cervical facets is noted, with their complementary superior & inferior articular facets. The exiting spinal nerves run in the groove along the superior aspect of transverse processes. **(Middle)** More medial section shows the overlapping facets at each level, & the flow void of the vertebral artery within the transverse foramen. **(Bottom)** Midline image shows the relationship of the cervical cord, vertebral bodies & spinous processes with smooth straight margins & alignment. The posterior dural margin merges with the ligamentum flavum & spinous process cortex low signal. The anterior dural margin merges with the posterior body cortex & posterior longitudinal ligament.

AXIAL GRE MR

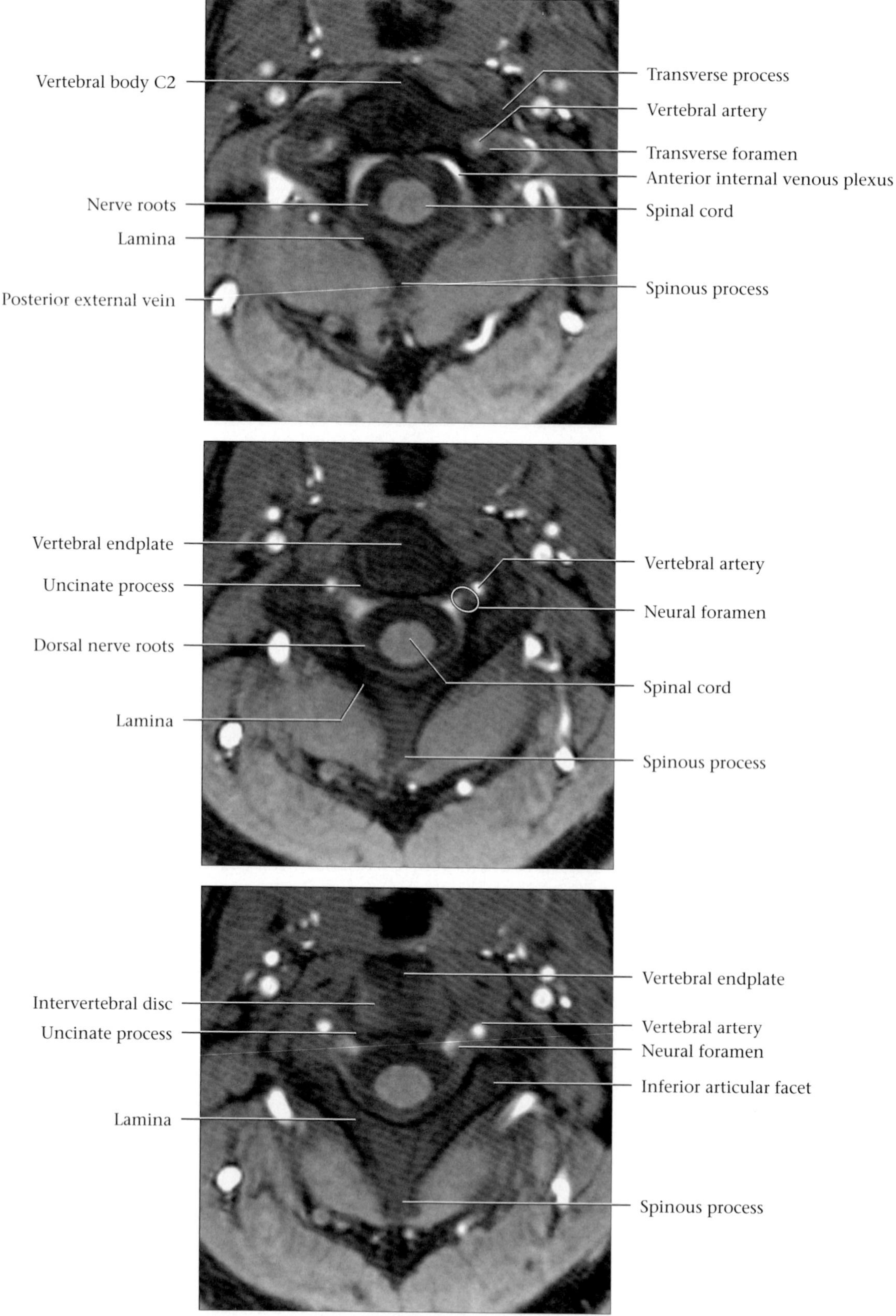
Vertebral body C2
Nerve roots
Lamina
Posterior external vein
Transverse process
Vertebral artery
Transverse foramen
Anterior internal venous plexus
Spinal cord
Spinous process
Vertebral endplate
Uncinate process
Dorsal nerve roots
Lamina
Vertebral artery
Neural foramen
Spinal cord
Spinous process
Intervertebral disc
Uncinate process
Lamina
Vertebral endplate
Vertebral artery
Neural foramen
Inferior articular facet
Spinous process

(Top) First of six axial gradient echo MR images with large flip angle (giving dark CSF signal) shown from superior to inferior beginning at the inferior C2 body level. The prominent transverse foramen with the vertebral artery is apparent. Flow related enhancement is also visible in the cervical dorsal veins, as well as the epidural veins (anterior internal venous plexus). **(Middle)** Image at the inferior endplate of C2. The neural foramina are directed at 45° anterolaterally & show flow related enhancement in epidural/foraminal venous plexus, & the ascending vertebral arteries. The spinal cord & dural margins are well-defined & smooth. The dorsal nerve rootlets are barely visible within the dorsal thecal sac. **(Bottom)** Image at the C2-3 disc level. The inferior articular facet of C2 & the prominent C2 spinous process are visible.

AXIAL GRE MR

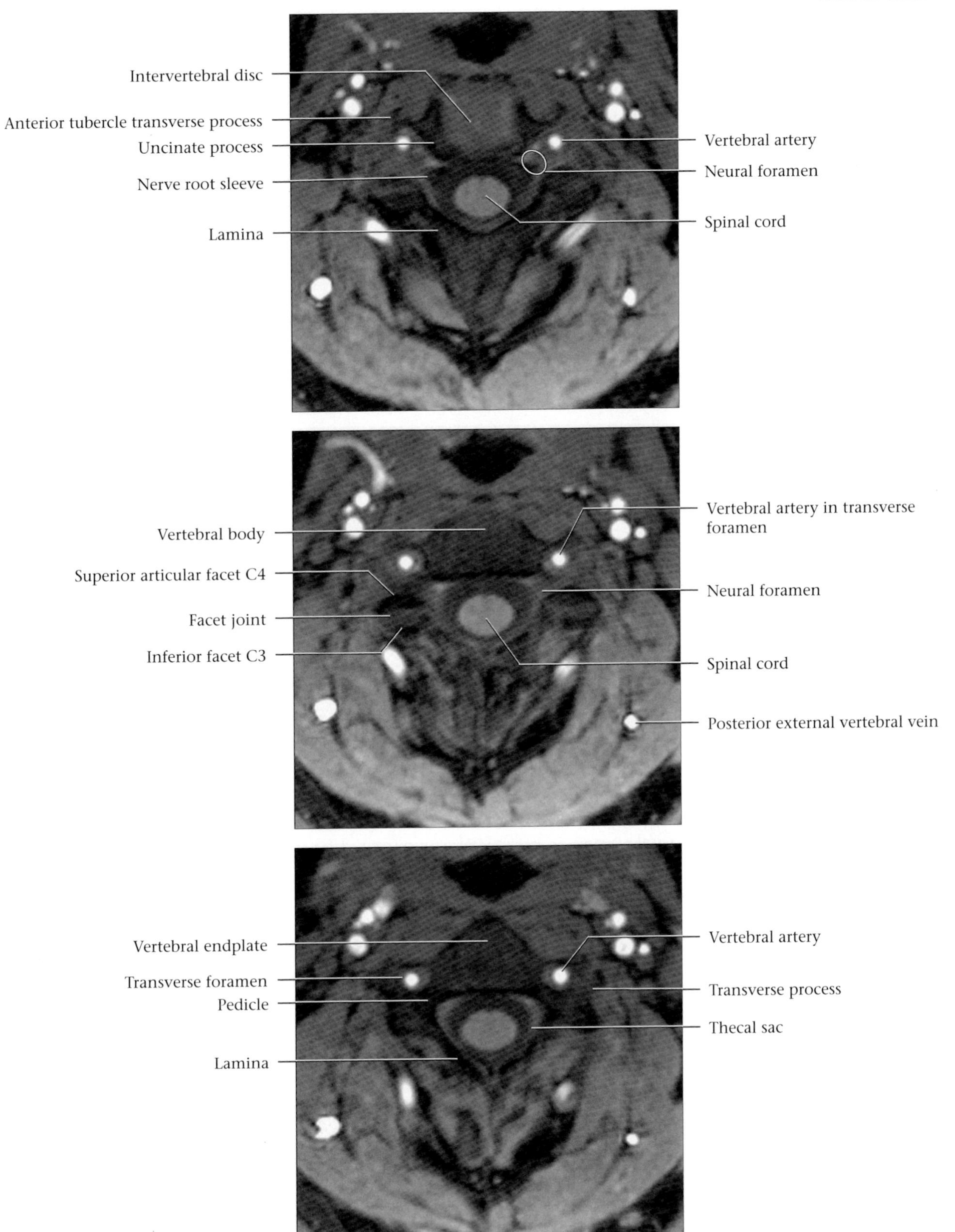
Intervertebral disc
Anterior tubercle transverse process
Uncinate process
Nerve root sleeve
Lamina
Vertebral artery
Neural foramen
Spinal cord
Vertebral body
Superior articular facet C4
Facet joint
Inferior facet C3
Vertebral artery in transverse foramen
Neural foramen
Spinal cord
Posterior external vertebral vein
Vertebral endplate
Transverse foramen
Pedicle
Lamina
Vertebral artery
Transverse process
Thecal sac

(Top) Image through C2-3 intervertebral disc. The intermediate signal, square shaped intervertebral disc is evident, with the bounding lower signal uncinate processes. The low signal, CSF containing, triangular shaped root sleeves are seen extending anterolaterally into the neural foramina. **(Middle)** Image through superior C3 vertebral body shows the C3-4 facet joint with the anterior low signal superior facet of C4, the intermediate signal linear joint space, & the dorsal positioned low signal inferior facet of C3. **(Bottom)** Image through C3 pedicles which project posterolaterally from the vertebral body. The delicate laminae complete the triangular shaped vertebral foramen containing the thecal sac & contents. The transverse foramina containing the vertebral arteries are prominent within the transverse processes.

AXIAL T2 MR

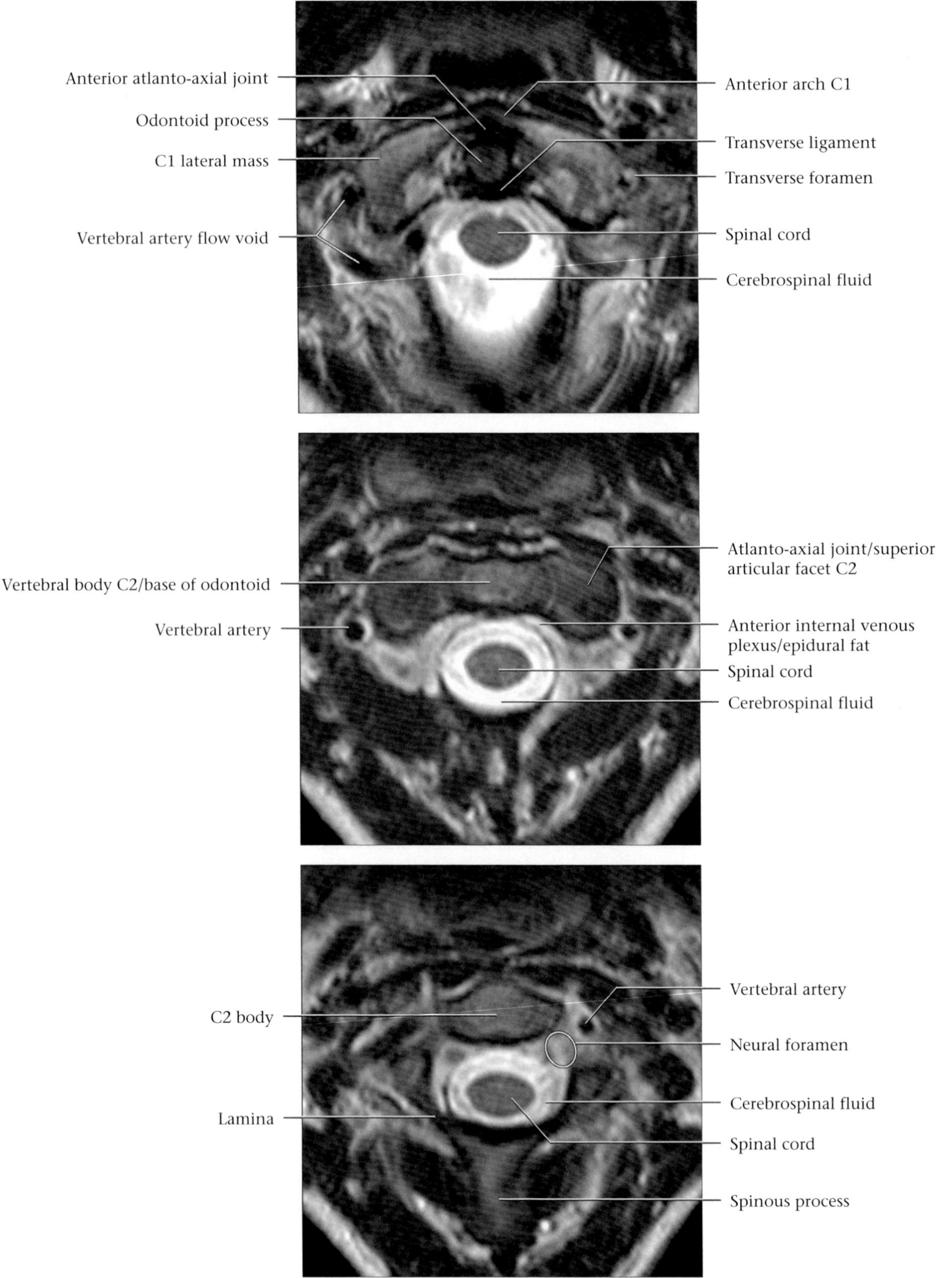
Anterior atlanto-axial joint
Odontoid process
C1 lateral mass
Vertebral artery flow void
Anterior arch C1
Transverse ligament
Transverse foramen
Spinal cord
Cerebrospinal fluid
Vertebral body C2/base of odontoid
Vertebral artery
Atlanto-axial joint/superior articular facet C2
Anterior internal venous plexus/epidural fat
Spinal cord
Cerebrospinal fluid
C2 body
Lamina
Vertebral artery
Neural foramen
Cerebrospinal fluid
Spinal cord
Spinous process

(Top) First of six axial T2 MR images shown from superior to inferior beginning at the level of the anterior arch of C1. The anterior atlantodental joint is well-identified, bounded by the low signal cortical margins of the anterior odontoid & anterior arch of C1. Posterior to the odontoid is the low signal transverse ligament complex. **(Middle)** Image at odontoid/C2 body level. The base of the odontoid is at the level of the lateral atlanto-axial articulation. This joint is sloped, being more superior at the medial margin. The vertebral arteries are identified by their flow voids, located just lateral to the lateral masses, passing superiorly toward the C1 transverse foramen. **(Bottom)** Image at C2 body level. The relationship of the vertically oriented vertebral artery to the neural foramen is highlighted in this section.

AXIAL T2 MR

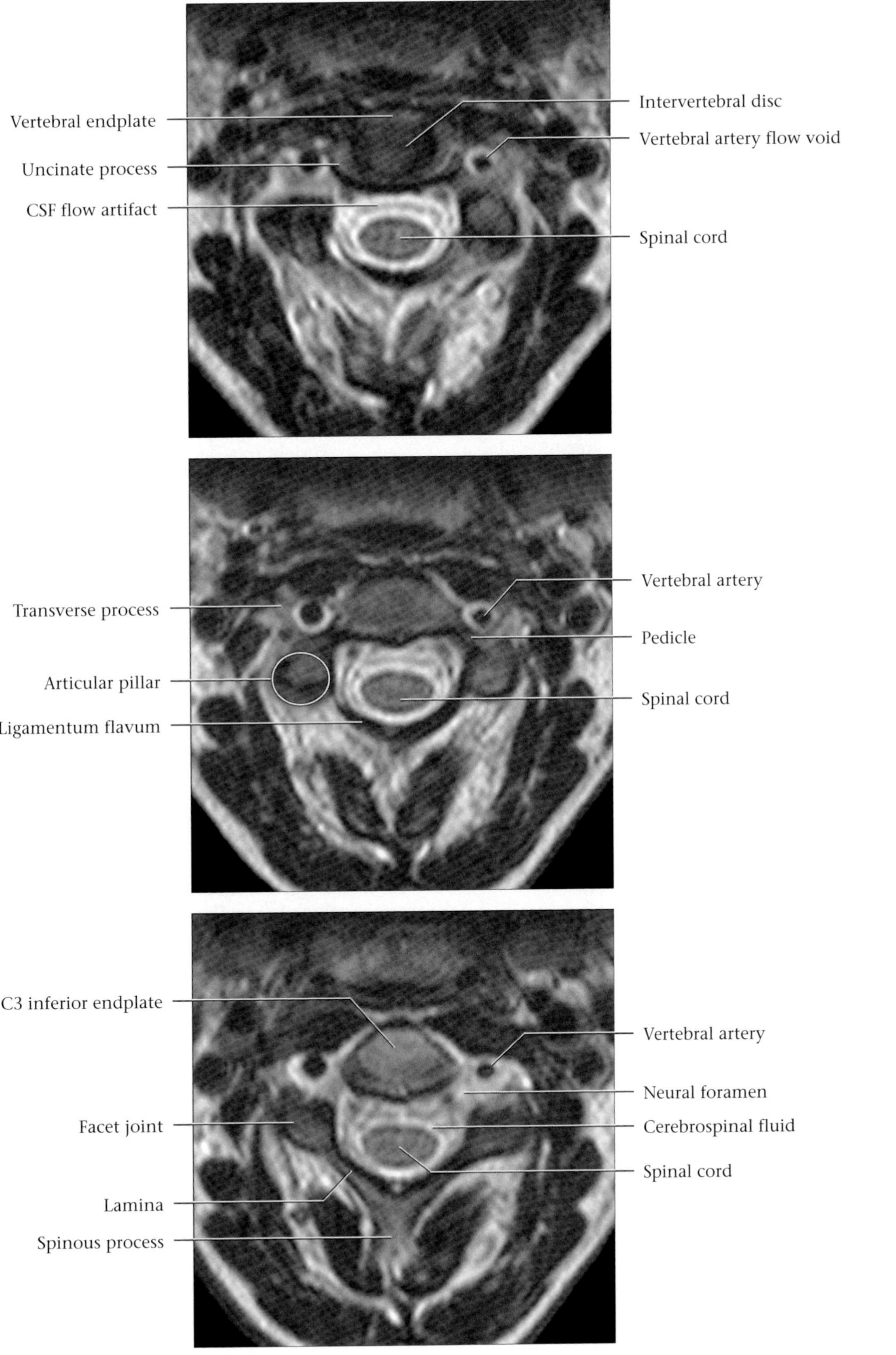
Vertebral endplate
Uncinate process
CSF flow artifact
Intervertebral disc
Vertebral artery flow void
Spinal cord
Transverse process
Articular pillar
Ligamentum flavum
Vertebral artery
Pedicle
Spinal cord
C3 inferior endplate
Facet joint
Lamina
Spinous process
Vertebral artery
Neural foramen
Cerebrospinal fluid
Spinal cord

(Top) Image at C2-3 disc level. The intervertebral disc is fully visualized as low signal, with the bounding posterior lateral uncovertebral joints. **(Middle)** Image through pedicles of C3. Pedicles are delicate & are directed posterolaterally from the vertebral body. The articular pillars are formed by the superior & inferior articular processes & intervening facet joints. Prominent vertebral artery flow voids are seen within the transverse foramina of the transverse processes. **(Bottom)** Image through the neural foramina of C3 which are oriented approximately 45° anterolaterally. The posterior margin of the neural foramen is the facet joint & the ventral margin the disc & uncinate process.

THORACIC SPINE

Terminology

Abbreviations

- Costovertebral (CV)

Synonyms

- Costal facet = demifacet

Gross Anatomy

Overview

- Consists of 12 vertebrae (T1-12)
- **Thoracic kyphosis**
  - One of two primary spinal curves (thoracic & sacral) present at birth, maintained throughout life
  - Cervical & lumbar lordoses are secondary curves, more flexible & result of development
    - Considerable variability in amount of kyphosis (20-45°)
    - Each body contributes 3.8° of kyphosis via wedge-shaped angulation
    - Apex at T7
    - Increases with age
    - M < F
- **Thoracolumbar junction**
  - Transition from rigid thoracic spine to more mobile lumbar spine
  - T11, T12 ribs provide less rigidity compared to rest of thoracic spine
  - No connection to sternum (free floating)
  - Only single rib articulation on vertebral bodies
- **Thoracic spine unique features**
  - Articulation with rib cage
  - Coronal facet orientation
  - Small spinal canal relative to posterior element size

Components

- **Bones**
  - Thoracic vertebrae increase in size from T1 ⇒ T12
  - **Body**
    - Typical body contains two costal demifacets laterally
    - T1 has complete facet superiorly and demifacet inferiorly, T10 has superior demifacet only, T11 and 12 have complete facet
  - **Arch**
    - Pedicle: Projects directly posteriorly
    - Transverse process: T1 transverse process projects superolaterally; T1-10 transverse process costal facet articulates with costal tubercle
    - Articular processes: Superior & inferior articular process with coronally oriented facet joint
    - Lamina
    - Spinous process: T1-9 project inferiorly; T10-12 project more horizontally
- **Intervertebral foramen**
  - Oriented laterally below pedicle
- **Joints**
  - Intervertebral disc
  - Facet (zygapophyseal) joints
    - Facets oriented near vertical in coronal plane
    - Limit flexion & extension
  - **Rib articulations**
    - **Costovertebral joint:** Rib head articulates with two costal demifacets; superior costal facet of same number vertebrae as rib & inferior costal facet of next vertebral body
    - **Costotransverse joint:** Transverse process of vertebral body T1-10
- **Muscles**
  - Superficial muscles include trapezius, rhomboid, latissimus dorsi & serratus inferior & superior
  - Deep muscles include erector spinae (sacrospinalis), iliocostalis, longissimus, spinalis & semispinalis thoracis, multifidus, rotatores & interspinalis
- **Ligaments**
  - Anterior & posterior longitudinal, interspinous, supraspinous ligaments & ligamentum flavum
  - Costovertebral ligaments
    - Radiate ligament connects head of rib & adjacent vertebral bodies
    - Costotransverse ligaments (lateral & superior) connect neck of rib with transverse process
- **Biomechanics**
  - Intact rib cage increases axial load resistance 4x
  - Rib cage & facets limit rotation

Imaging Anatomy

Radiography

- Short C7 transverse process projects inferolaterally; long T1 transverse process projects superolaterally

MRI

- Body: Signal intensity of marrow varies with age
  - Hemopoietic ("red") marrow is hypointense on T1WI, becomes hyperintense with conversion from red → yellow (age 8-12 years)
  - End-plate, reactive marrow changes normally with aging (can be fibrovascular, fatty, or sclerotic)
- Intervertebral disc: Signal intensity varies with age
  - Hyperintense on T2WI in children, young adults; progressive ↓ water → hypointense on T2WI
  - Disc degeneration, dessication, shape change (bulge) normal after second decade
- Ligaments: Hypointense on both T1 & T2WI

Anatomy-Based Imaging Issues

Key Concepts or Questions

- Thoracic spinal cord is protected & shielded from injury by paraspinal muscles & rib cage
- Narrow spinal canal of thoracic spine allows for easy cord compression with malalignment or trauma
- Normal kyphotic posture increases risk of fracture
- Thoracolumbar junction at more traumatic risk due to lack of rib cage stabilization

Imaging Pitfalls

- **Cervicothoracic junction**
  - Cervical ribs arising from C7 found in 0.5% population
  - Short C7 transverse process projects inferolaterally
  - Long T1 transverse process projects superolaterally

THORACIC SPINE

GRAPHICS

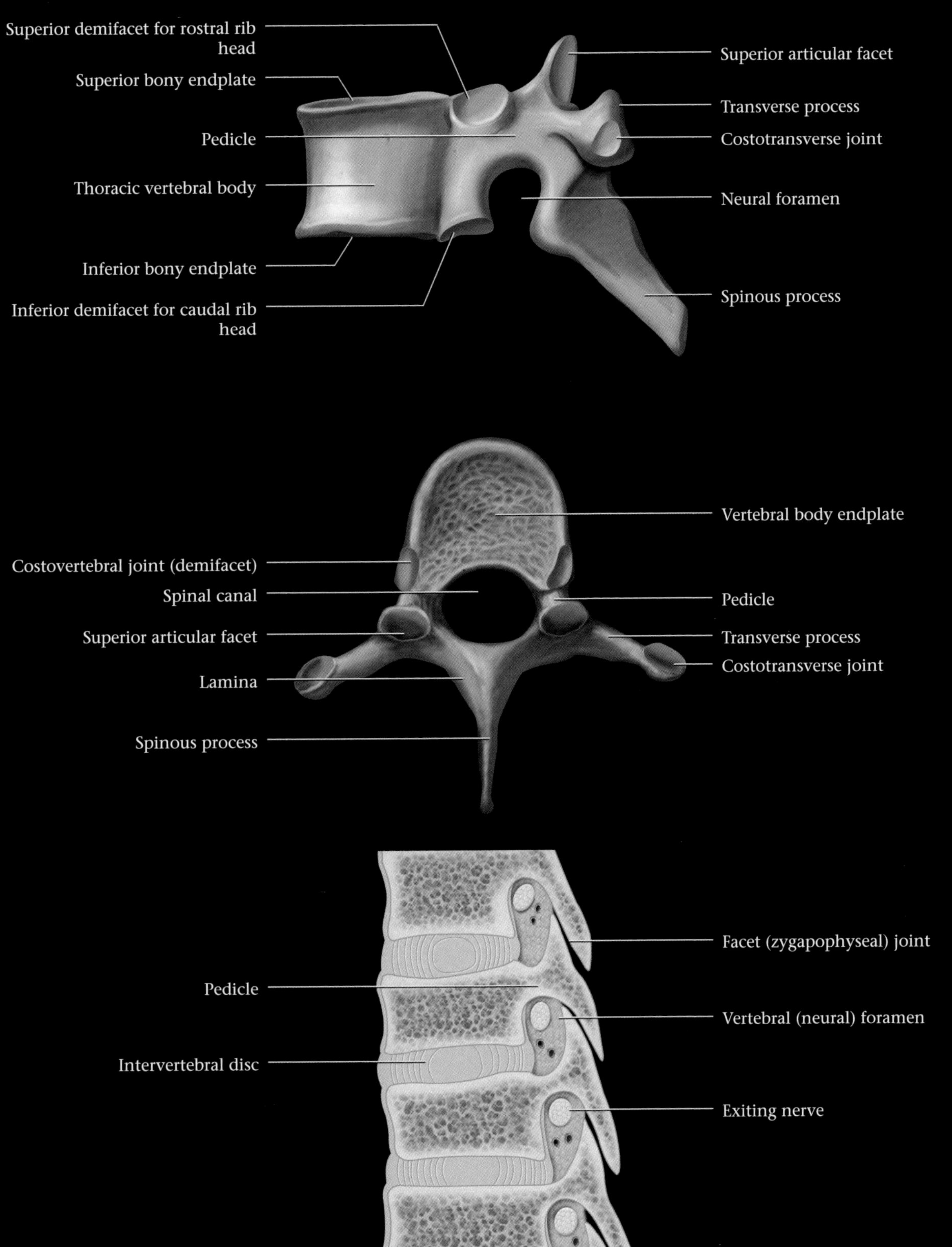
Superior demifacet for rostral rib head
Superior bony endplate
Pedicle
Thoracic vertebral body
Inferior bony endplate
Inferior demifacet for caudal rib head
Superior articular facet
Transverse process
Costotransverse joint
Neural foramen
Spinous process
Vertebral body endplate
Costovertebral joint (demifacet)
Spinal canal
Superior articular facet
Lamina
Spinous process
Pedicle
Transverse process
Costotransverse joint
Facet (zygapophyseal) joint
Pedicle
Vertebral (neural) foramen
Intervertebral disc
Exiting nerve

(Top) Lateral view of thoracic vertebral body shows the characteristic features of this spinal segment. The unique superior & inferior demifacets form a concavity spanning the intervening disc to house the rib head & form the costovertebral joint. The spinous process is typically long & oblique. **(Middle)** Graphic of thoracic vertebral body, viewed from above. The thoracic bodies are characterized by long spinous processes & transverse processes. The complex rib articulation includes both costotransverse joints, & costovertebral joints. The facet joints are oriented in a coronal direction. **(Bottom)** Sagittal graphic through thoracic vertebral foramen. The exiting nerve is positioned superiorly bounded by the vertebral body anteriorly, pedicle above & facet joint posteriorly. Facet joints are oriented in near coronal plane in thoracic spine.

RADIOGRAPHY

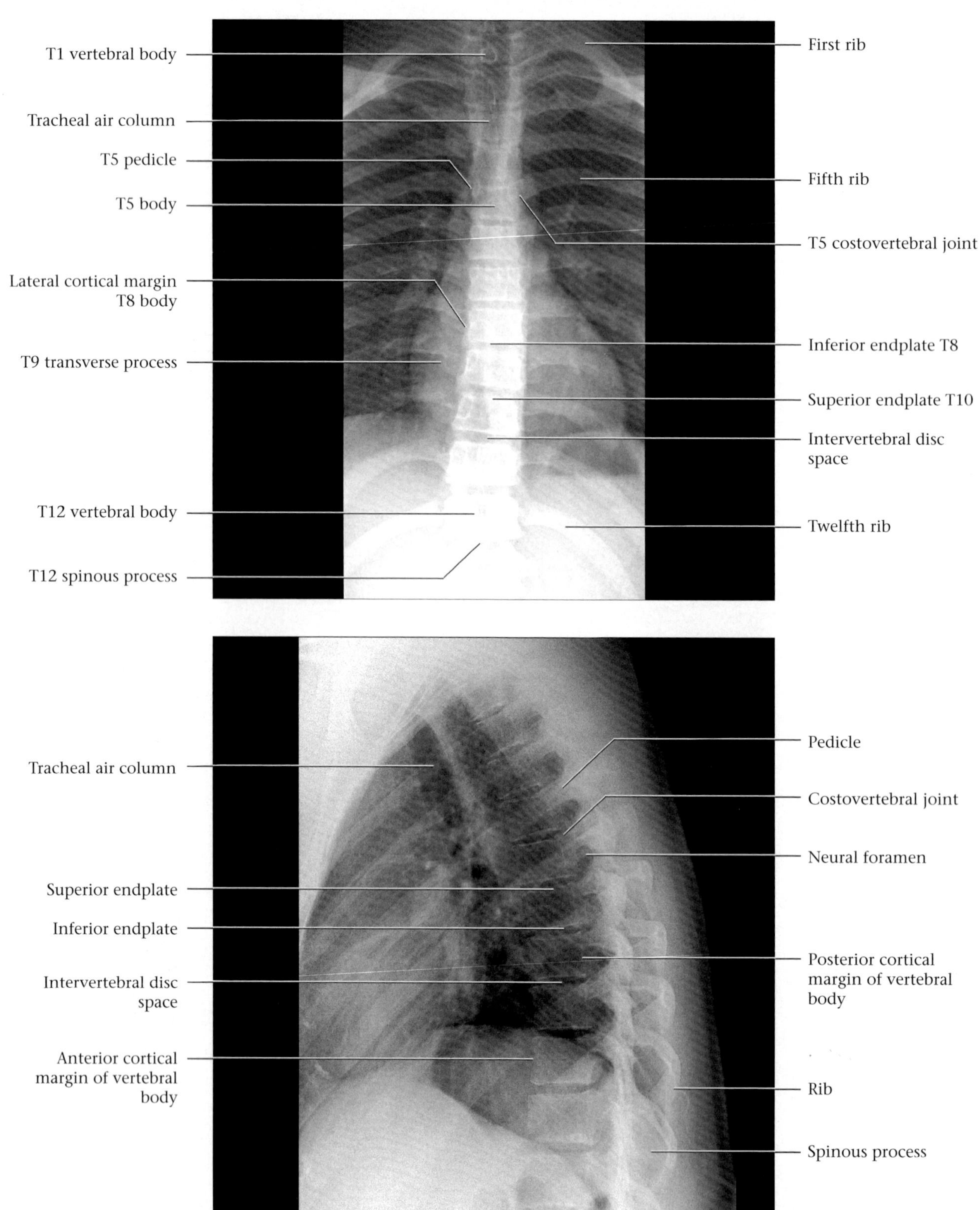
T1 vertebral body
Tracheal air column
T5 pedicle
T5 body
Lateral cortical margin T8 body
T9 transverse process
T12 vertebral body
T12 spinous process
First rib
Fifth rib
T5 costovertebral joint
Inferior endplate T8
Superior endplate T10
Intervertebral disc space
Twelfth rib
Tracheal air column
Superior endplate
Inferior endplate
Intervertebral disc space
Anterior cortical margin of vertebral body
Pedicle
Costovertebral joint
Neural foramen
Posterior cortical margin of vertebral body
Rib
Spinous process

(Top) AP view of the thoracic spine. The square thoracic vertebral bodies are aligned in the midline, with symmetrical paired & sharp corticated ovals of the pedicles. The endplates are well-defined with smooth intervertebral discs. The spinous processes also align in the midline, with the tips extending to the next inferior level. The rib heads articulate with the two adjacent vertebra (T5 rib articulates with T4 & T5 bodies). **(Bottom)** Lateral view of the thoracic spine. The vertebral bodies are identified with sharp cortical margins on all four sides, well-defined intervertebral disc spaces, & a gentle thoracic kyphotic curvature. The neural foramina are well identified on this projection. The posterior elements are ill-defined, due to considerable overlap of the right & left-sided ribs.

CORONAL CT MYELOGRAM

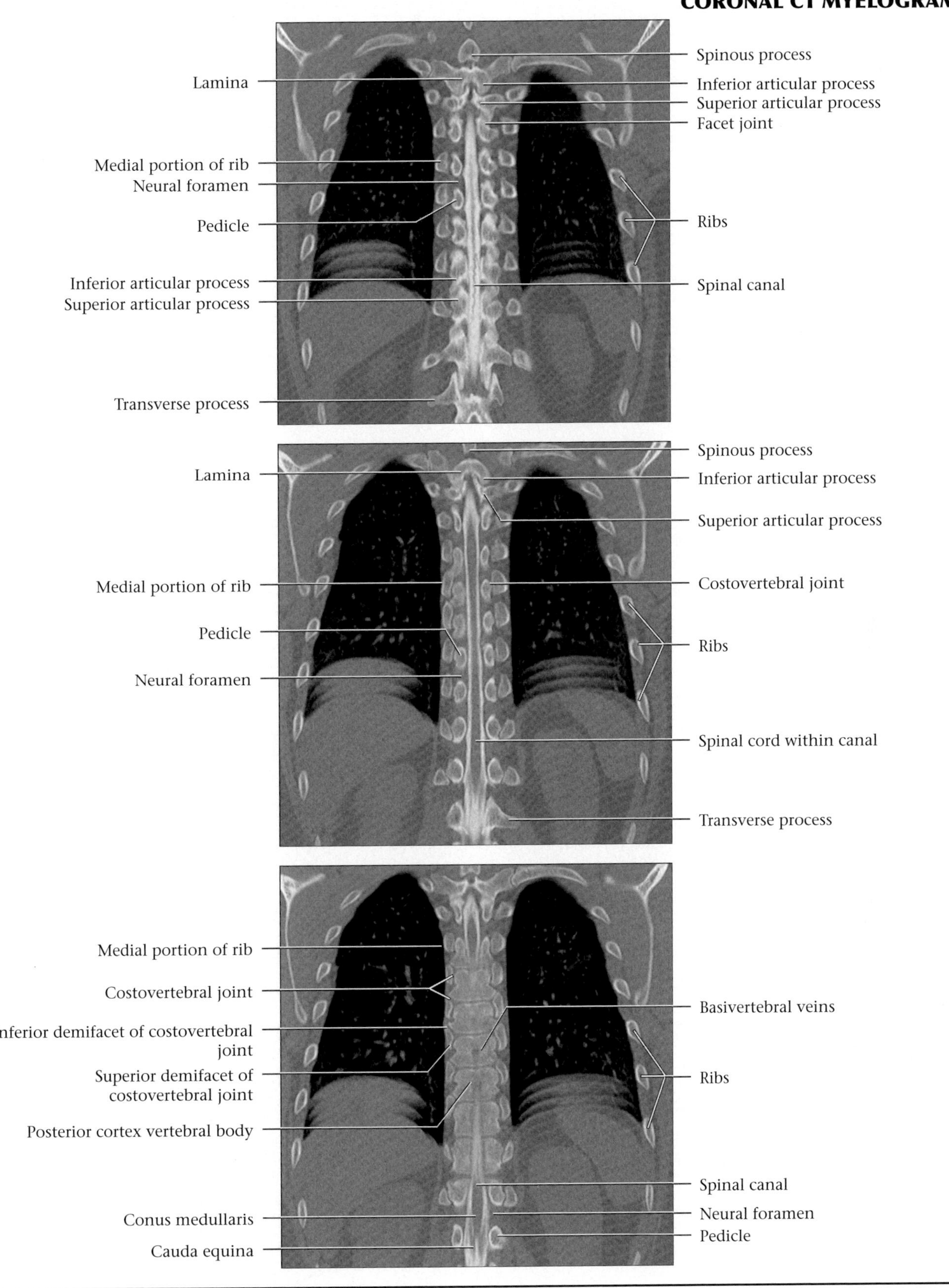
Lamina
Medial portion of rib
Neural foramen
Pedicle
Inferior articular process
Superior articular process
Transverse process
Spinous process
Inferior articular process
Superior articular process
Facet joint
Ribs
Spinal canal
Lamina
Medial portion of rib
Pedicle
Neural foramen
Spinous process
Inferior articular process
Superior articular process
Costovertebral joint
Ribs
Spinal cord within canal
Transverse process
Medial portion of rib
Costovertebral joint
Inferior demifacet of costovertebral joint
Superior demifacet of costovertebral joint
Posterior cortex vertebral body
Conus medullaris
Cauda equina
Basivertebral veins
Ribs
Spinal canal
Neural foramen
Pedicle

(Top) First of three coronal reformat images from CT myelogram through the thoracic spine presented from posterior to anterior. The posterior spinal canal is identified with the intrathecal contrast, bounded laterally by the pairs of medial ribs/pedicles seen as well-defined corticated oval bony densities. With the normal thoracic kyphosis, the superior & inferior thoracic spine is seen in more anterior section than the mid portion. **(Middle)** More anterior image through mid canal level. The relationship of the neural foramen, pedicle & adjacent medial rib is identified. **(Bottom)** More anterior image through the posterior vertebral body level. The costovertebral joint articulations are particularly well identified in this view. Note the superior & inferior costal facets (demifacets) with the rib head at disc level.

3D-VRT NECT

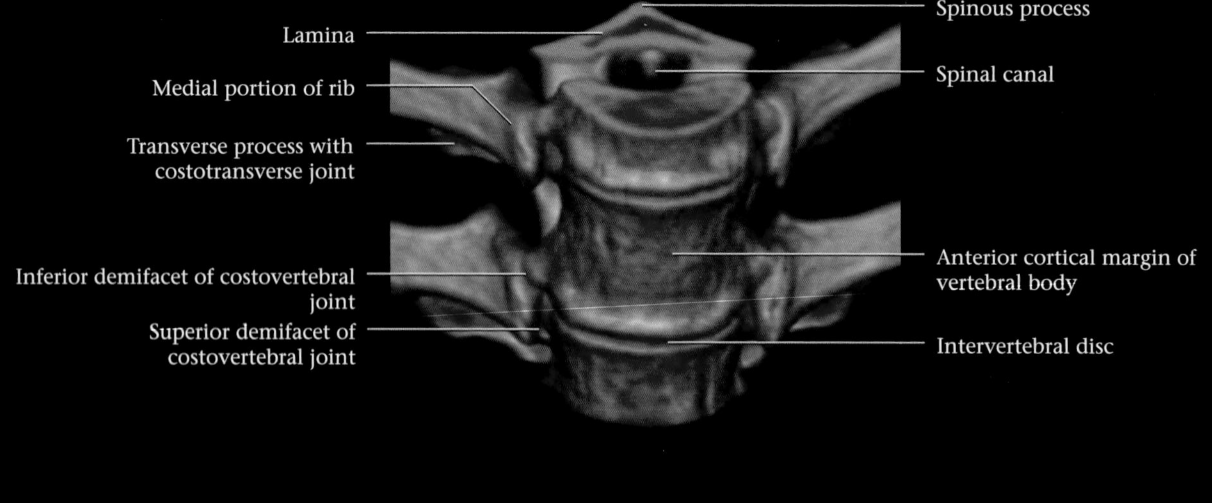
Lamina
Medial portion of rib
Transverse process with costotransverse joint
Inferior demifacet of costovertebral joint
Superior demifacet of costovertebral joint
Spinous process
Spinal canal
Anterior cortical margin of vertebral body
Intervertebral disc

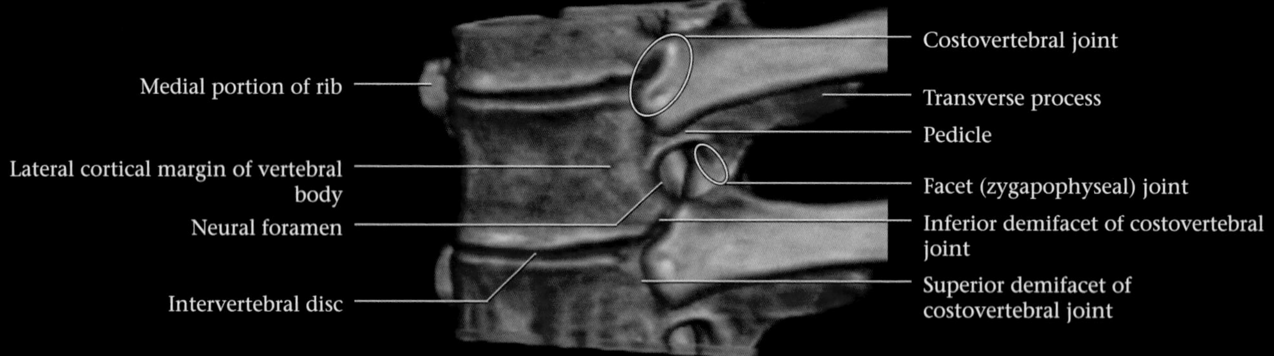
Medial portion of rib
Lateral cortical margin of vertebral body
Neural foramen
Intervertebral disc
Costovertebral joint
Transverse process
Pedicle
Facet (zygapophyseal) joint
Inferior demifacet of costovertebral joint
Superior demifacet of costovertebral joint

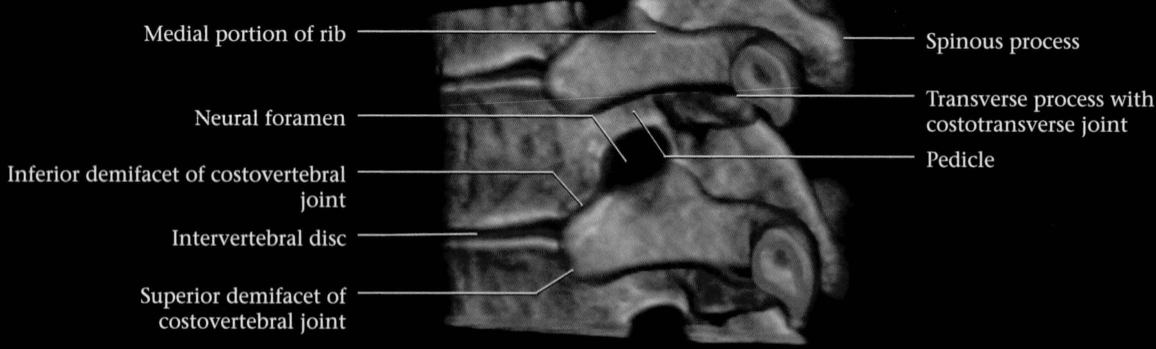
Medial portion of rib
Neural foramen
Inferior demifacet of costovertebral joint
Intervertebral disc
Superior demifacet of costovertebral joint
Spinous process
Transverse process with costotransverse joint
Pedicle

(Top) Oblique anterior 3D-VRT examination of the thoracic spine. The complex costovertebral & costotransverse joints are highlighted in the projection. The superior & inferior demifacets are identified, with the joint proper crossing the intervertebral disc space. **(Middle)** Lateral oblique 3D-VRT examination of the thoracic spine. The relationship of the neural foramen & the posterior elements & costal joints is visualized in this projection. The foramen is bounded posteriorly by the facet joint, superiorly by the pedicle, & ventrally by the posterior margin of the vertebral body. **(Bottom)** Lateral 3D-VRT examination of the thoracic spine. The neural foramina are oriented laterally & therefore viewed en face in this projection bounded by vertebral body anteriorly, pedicle superiorly & facet joint posteriorly.

3D-VRT NECT

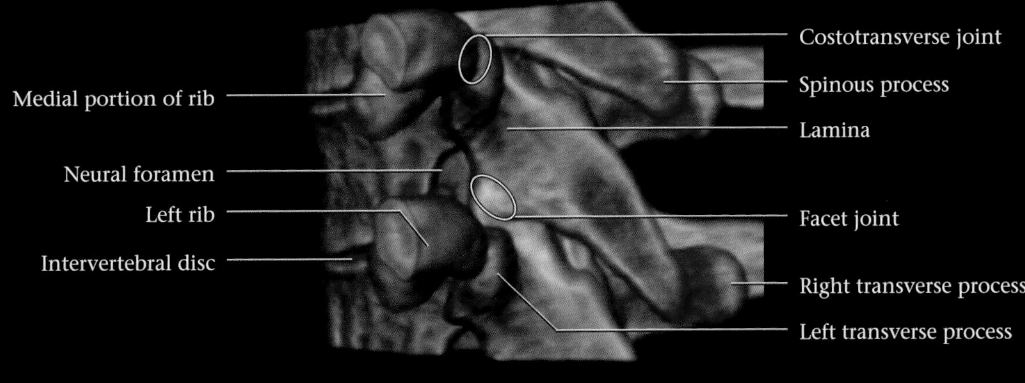

Medial portion of rib
Neural foramen
Left rib
Intervertebral disc
Costotransverse joint
Spinous process
Lamina
Facet joint
Right transverse process
Left transverse process

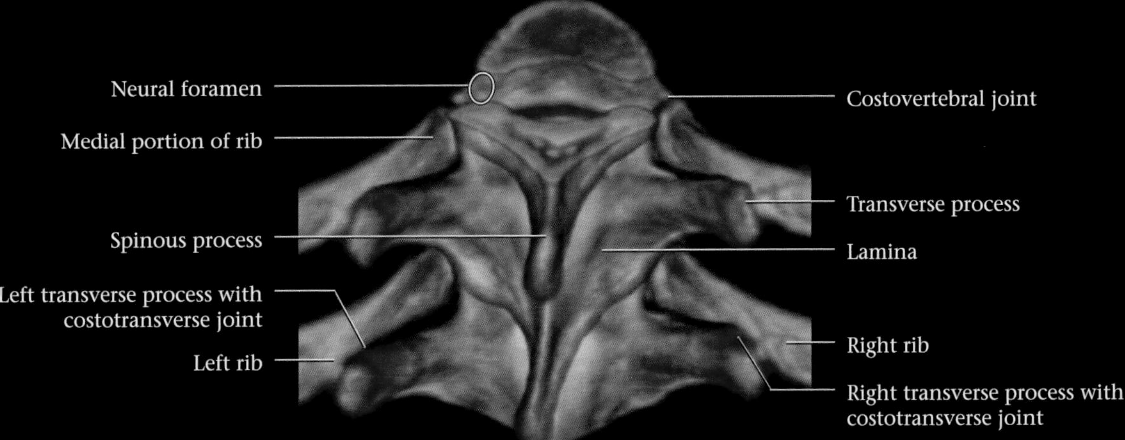

Neural foramen
Medial portion of rib
Spinous process
Left transverse process with costotransverse joint
Left rib
Costovertebral joint
Transverse process
Lamina
Right rib
Right transverse process with costotransverse joint

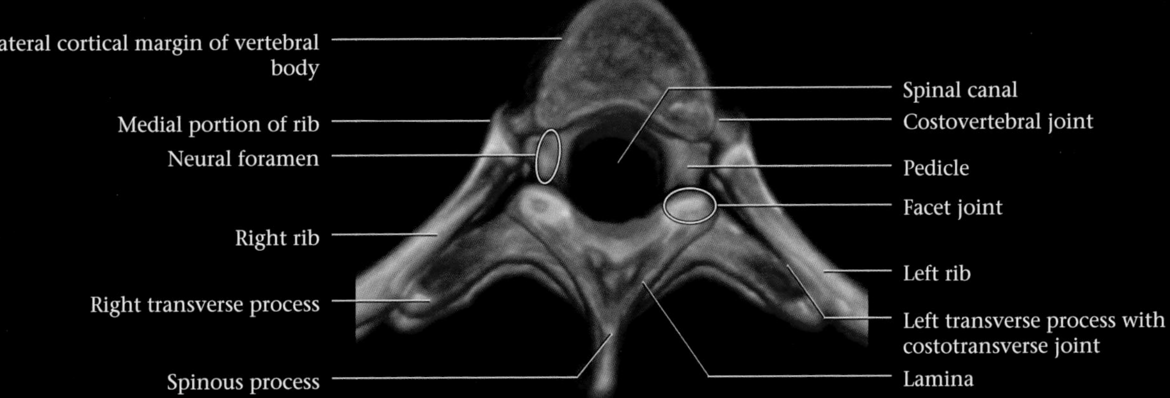

Lateral cortical margin of vertebral body
Medial portion of rib
Neural foramen
Right rib
Right transverse process
Spinous process
Spinal canal
Costovertebral joint
Pedicle
Facet joint
Left rib
Left transverse process with costotransverse joint
Lamina

(Top) Oblique anterior 3D-VRT examination of the thoracic spine. The facet joints are partially seen in this projection, primarily obscured by the posterior surface of the inferior articular facet, which overlaps the dorsal surface of the superior articular facet from the next caudal vertebra. The thoracic spinous processes are long & directed inferiorly, overlapping the next vertebral body level. **(Middle)** Posterior 3D-VRT examination of the thoracic spine. The posterior bony projections of the thoracic spine are highlighted in this projection, including the spinous processes, transverse processes & the costotransverse articulations. **(Bottom)** Axial 3D-VRT examination of the thoracic spine. The 2 costal articulations are viewed in this projection. The neural foramen are immediately adjacent to the costovertebral articulations.

AXIAL BONE CT

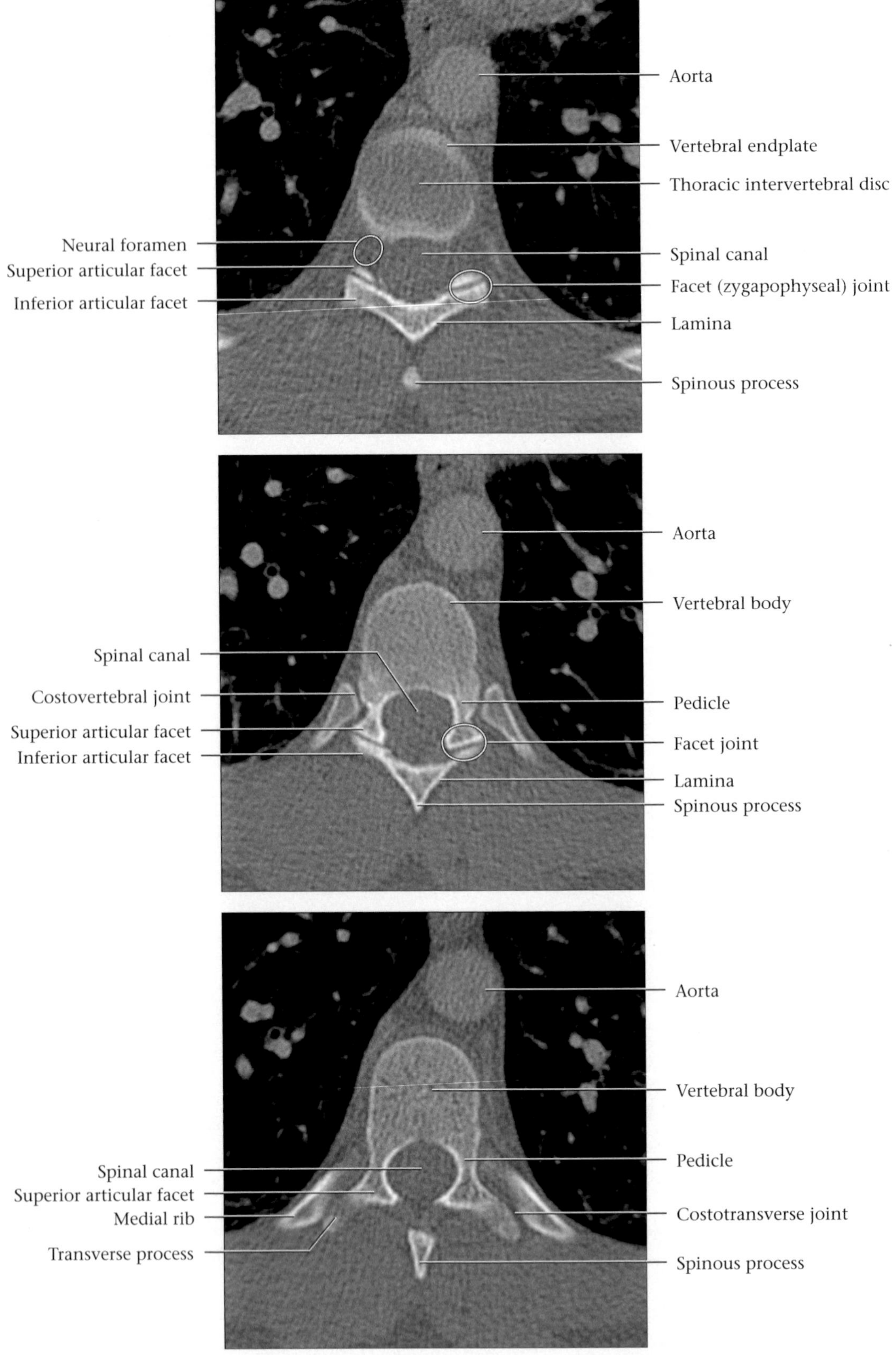
Aorta
Vertebral endplate
Thoracic intervertebral disc
Neural foramen
Superior articular facet
Inferior articular facet
Spinal canal
Facet (zygapophyseal) joint
Lamina
Spinous process
Aorta
Vertebral body
Spinal canal
Costovertebral joint
Superior articular facet
Inferior articular facet
Pedicle
Facet joint
Lamina
Spinous process
Aorta
Vertebral body
Pedicle
Spinal canal
Superior articular facet
Medial rib
Transverse process
Costotransverse joint
Spinous process

(Top) First of six axial bone CT images presented from superior to inferior at intervertebral disc level. Neural foramina are directed laterally & bounded anteriorly by the posterior vertebral body margin & dorsally by facet joint (superior articular facet). The facet joints are oriented in a coronal plane & strongly resist rotation combined with the costovertebral joints. **(Middle)** Image through the pedicle level of the thoracic spine. The coronal orientation of the facet joints are well identified in this section. The pedicles are relatively thin & gracile, with the adjacent rib articulations. **(Bottom)** Image through vertebral body level. The posterior bony projections are highlighted in this view, including spinous process, transverse processes & medial ribs.

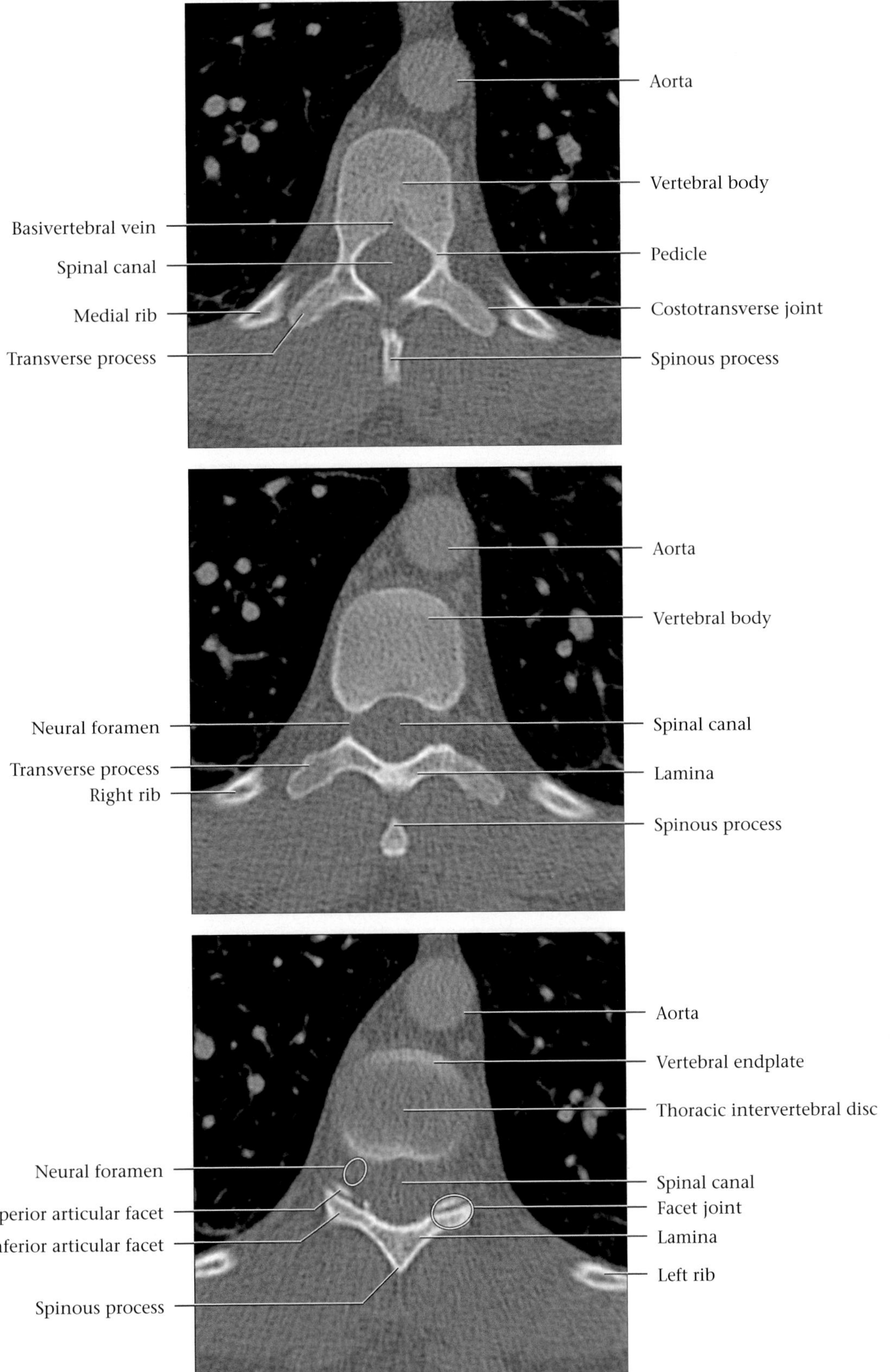

Aorta
Vertebral body
Basivertebral vein
Pedicle
Spinal canal
Costotransverse joint
Medial rib
Transverse process
Spinous process
Aorta
Vertebral body
Neural foramen
Spinal canal
Transverse process
Lamina
Right rib
Spinous process
Aorta
Vertebral endplate
Thoracic intervertebral disc
Neural foramen
Spinal canal
Superior articular facet
Facet joint
Inferior articular facet
Lamina
Left rib
Spinous process

(Top) Image through mid vertebral body level. The posterior vertebral body is pierced by the basivertebral veins in the midline. The thoracic pedicles are gracile, leading to large obliquely oriented transverse processes supporting the costotransverse joints for the ribs. **(Middle)** Image through the neural foraminal level of the thoracic spine. The large neural foramina are directed laterally. The orientation of the transverse processes is posterior & laterally as shown. **(Bottom)** Image at intervertebral disc level. Neural foramina are directed laterally, & bounded anteriorly by the posterior vertebral body margin, & dorsally by the facet joint (superior articular facet). The facet joints are oriented in a coronal plane, & strongly resist rotation combined with the costovertebral joints.

SAGITTAL CT MYELOGRAM

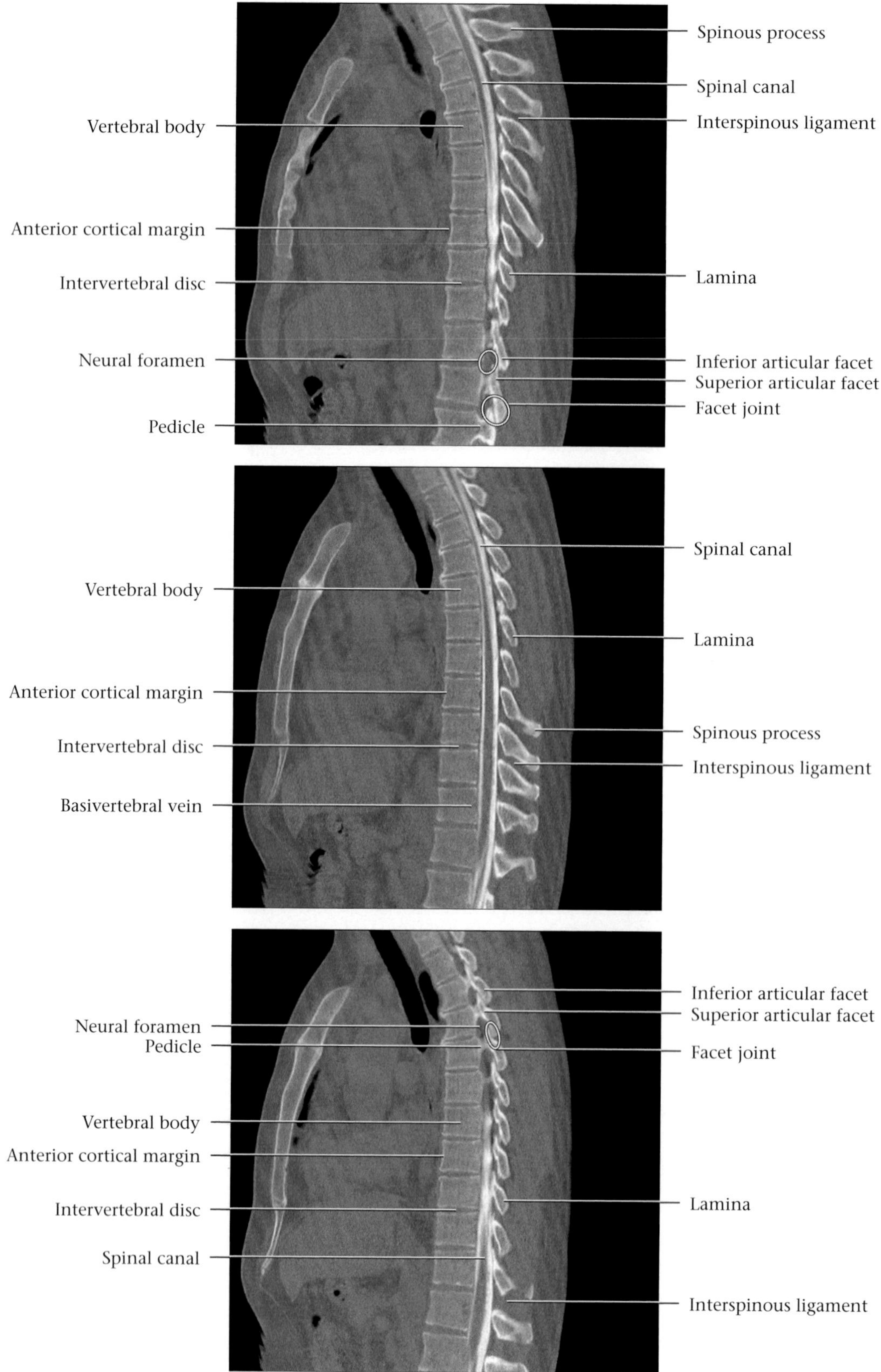
Spinous process
Spinal canal
Interspinous ligament
Vertebral body
Anterior cortical margin
Intervertebral disc
Lamina
Neural foramen
Inferior articular facet
Superior articular facet
Facet joint
Pedicle
Spinal canal
Vertebral body
Lamina
Anterior cortical margin
Spinous process
Intervertebral disc
Interspinous ligament
Basivertebral vein
Inferior articular facet
Superior articular facet
Neural foramen
Pedicle
Facet joint
Vertebral body
Anterior cortical margin
Intervertebral disc
Lamina
Spinal canal
Interspinous ligament

(Top) First of three sagittal reformat images from CT myelogram presented from medial to lateral. The slight off midline alignment allows for visualization of the midline spinous processes of the superior thoracic spine, & the more lateral lamina & facet joints of the inferior thoracic spine. **(Middle)** The oblique alignment again allows for visualization of the lamina of the upper thoracic spine, with the midline spinous processes visible in the lower thoracic segment. The vertebral bodies are square, with well-defined cortical margins, & relatively thin intervertebral discs. **(Bottom)** The upper thoracic segment demonstrates the pedicles extending into the superior & inferior articular facets. The laterally directed neural foramen, bounded by vertebral body, pedicle & facet are evident.

SAGITTAL T1 MR

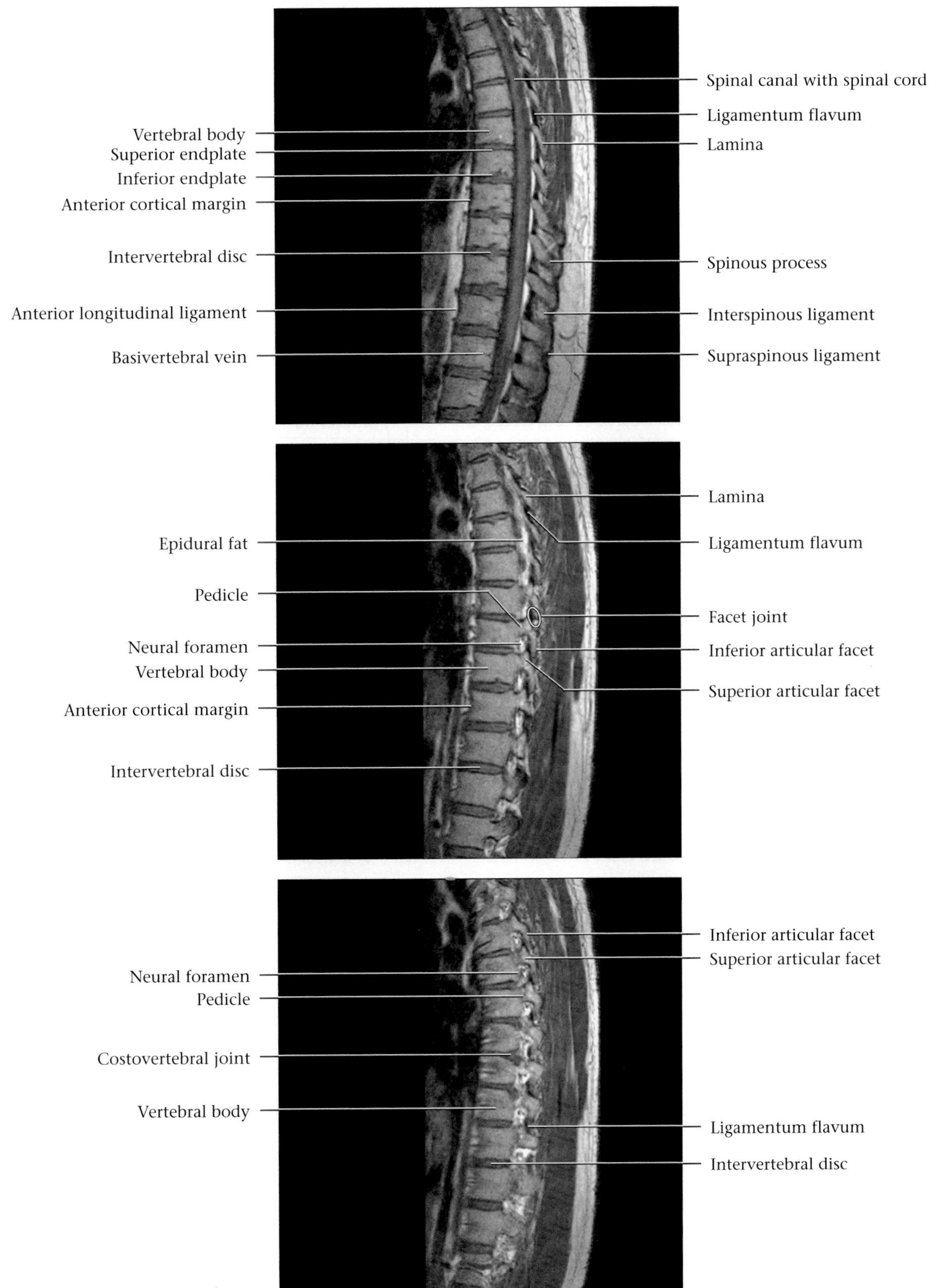
Spinal canal with spinal cord
Ligamentum flavum
Lamina
Vertebral body
Superior endplate
Inferior endplate
Anterior cortical margin
Intervertebral disc
Spinous process
Anterior longitudinal ligament
Interspinous ligament
Basivertebral vein
Supraspinous ligament
Lamina
Epidural fat
Ligamentum flavum
Pedicle
Facet joint
Neural foramen
Inferior articular facet
Vertebral body
Superior articular facet
Anterior cortical margin
Intervertebral disc
Inferior articular facet
Superior articular facet
Neural foramen
Pedicle
Costovertebral joint
Vertebral body
Ligamentum flavum
Intervertebral disc

(Top) First of three sagittal T1 MR images of the thoracic spine presented from medial to lateral. The posterior supporting ligamentous structures are identified on this view, including the interspinous ligaments, ligamentum flavum, & supraspinous ligament. The anterior & posterior longitudinal ligaments are not separately identified, rather they merged into the low signal of the anterior & posterior vertebral body cortical margins, respectively. **(Middle)** The neural foramina are highlighted by high signal foraminal fat content. The posterior, coronally oriented facet joints are evident. **(Bottom)** The costovertebral joint articulations are viewed as triangular shaped areas of intermediate signal along the posterior disc margins.

THORACIC SPINE

SAGITTAL T2 MR

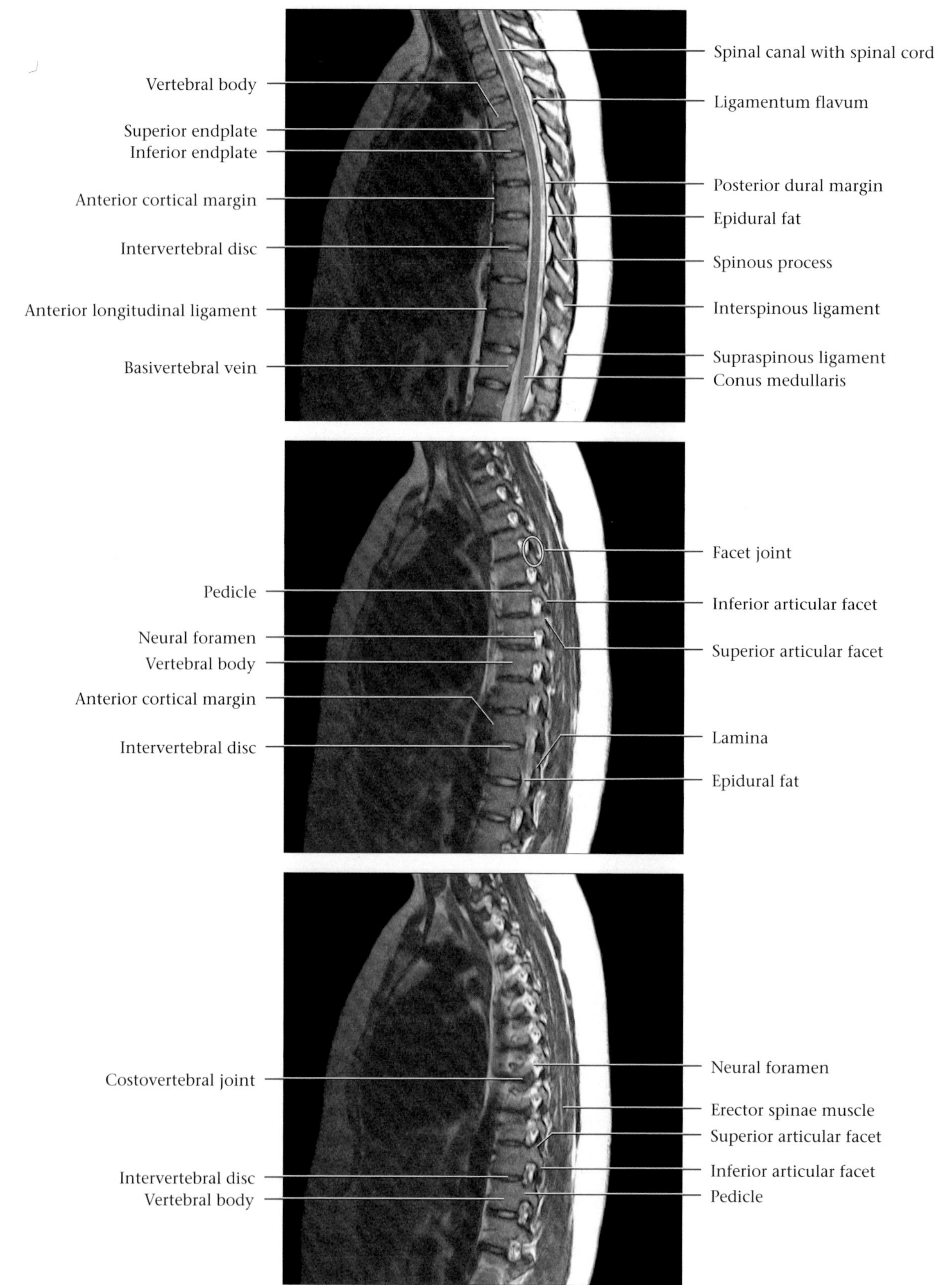
Vertebral body
Superior endplate
Inferior endplate
Anterior cortical margin
Intervertebral disc
Anterior longitudinal ligament
Basivertebral vein
Spinal canal with spinal cord
Ligamentum flavum
Posterior dural margin
Epidural fat
Spinous process
Interspinous ligament
Supraspinous ligament
Conus medullaris
Pedicle
Neural foramen
Vertebral body
Anterior cortical margin
Intervertebral disc
Facet joint
Inferior articular facet
Superior articular facet
Lamina
Epidural fat
Costovertebral joint
Intervertebral disc
Vertebral body
Neural foramen
Erector spinae muscle
Superior articular facet
Inferior articular facet
Pedicle

(Top) First of three sagittal T2 MR images of the thoracic spine presented from medial to lateral. The square thoracic vertebral bodies with the small intervening intervertebral discs are identified in this midline view. The spinous processes are large & dominate the dorsal soft tissues. The thoracic cord is seen in its entirety, with its smoothly tapering conus medullaris. **(Middle)** The facet joints are identified on this sagittal image, with the coronal oriented joints seen in lateral view. The superior & inferior articular processes & neural foramen are easily viewed in this plane. **(Bottom)** The more lateral margin of the neural foramen are identified on this section, as well as the costovertebral joints at the disc levels.

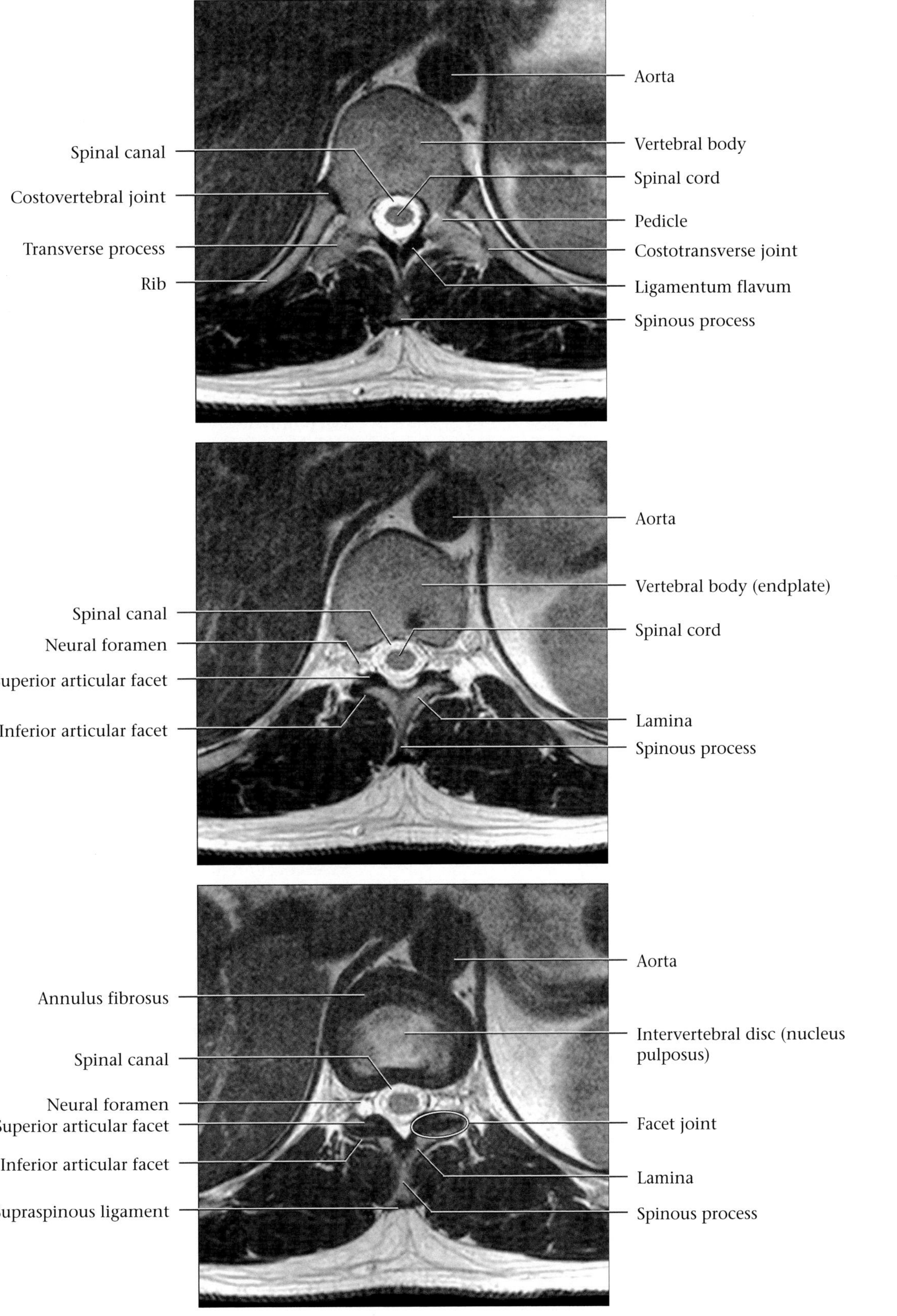

Aorta
Spinal canal
Vertebral body
Costovertebral joint
Spinal cord
Pedicle
Transverse process
Costotransverse joint
Rib
Ligamentum flavum
Spinous process
Aorta
Vertebral body (endplate)
Spinal canal
Spinal cord
Neural foramen
Superior articular facet
Lamina
Inferior articular facet
Spinous process
Aorta
Annulus fibrosus
Intervertebral disc (nucleus pulposus)
Spinal canal
Neural foramen
Superior articular facet
Facet joint
Inferior articular facet
Lamina
Supraspinous ligament
Spinous process

(Top) First of three axial T2 MR images of the thoracic spine. The relationship of the medial rib forming the strong costotransverse & costovertebral joints is highlighted. The transverse processes extend out dorsally, & laterally to articulate with the medial ribs. The spinous process is large, & directed caudally. **(Middle)** Image through the foraminal level of the thoracic spine. The neural foramina are directed laterally, with their posterior margin formed by the facet joints, & anterior margin by the vertebral body & disc. **(Bottom)** Image through the disc level. The coronal orientation of the facet joints are identified in this section, forming the posterior boundary of the neural foramen. The components of the intervertebral disc are shown in this section, with well-defined nucleus pulposus & annulus fibrosus.

LUMBAR SPINE

Terminology

Abbreviations

- Anterior longitudinal ligament (ALL)
- Posterior longitudinal ligament (PLL)

Synonyms

- Articular processes = facets = zygapophyses

Gross Anatomy

Overview

- 5 discovertebral units (L1-5)

Components

- **Bones**
  - **Body**
    - Large oval cancellous ventral mass
    - Larger in transverse width than AP diameter
  - **Endplates**
    - Formed by superior & inferior surfaces of vertebral bodies
    - Consist of concave surfaces of 1 mm thick cortical bone & hyaline cartilage plates
    - Endplates are transitional between fibrocartilage disc & vertebral body
    - Nutrients to disc diffuse via endplates
  - **Arch**
    - Pedicle: Project directly posteriorly
    - Transverse process: Extend out laterally, long and flat on L1-4, small at L5
    - Articular process: Superior and inferior articular processes with pars interarticularis between; facet joints oriented obliquely
    - Lamina: Broad, thick, overlap minimally
    - Spinous process
- **Intervertebral foramen**
  - Aperture giving exit to segmental spinal nerves and entrance to vessels
  - Oriented laterally below pedicle
  - Boundaries
    - Superior & inferior pedicles of adjacent vertebrae
    - Ventral boundary is dorsal aspect vertebral body above and intervertebral disc below
    - Dorsal boundary is joint capsule of facets and ligamentum flavum
  - Vertical elliptical shape in lumbar region
    - Vertical diameter 12-19 mm
    - Transverse diameter from disc to ligamentum flavum ≈ 7 mm, thus little room for pathologic narrowing
- **Joints**
  - **Intervertebral disc**
    - Outer annulus fibrosus (alternating layers of collagen fibers)
    - Inner annulus fibrosus (fibrocartilaginous component)
    - Transitional region
    - Central nucleus pulposus (elastic mucoprotein gel with high water content)
  - **Facet (zygapophyseal) joints**
    - Facet joints oriented obliquely
    - Superior facet: Concave, faces dorsomedially to meet inferior facet from above
    - Inferior facet: Faces ventrolaterally to meet superior facet from body below
- **Ligaments**
  - Anterior and posterior longitudinal ligaments, interspinous and supraspinous ligaments
  - **Ligamentum flavum**
    - Thick in lumbar region
    - Connects adjacent lamina
    - Extends from capsule of facet joint to junction of lamina with spinous process, discontinuous in midline
- **Muscles**
  - Erector spinae: Poorly differentiated muscle mass composed of iliocostalis, longissimus, spinalis
  - Multifidi (best developed in lumbar spine)
  - Deep muscles: Interspinalis, intertransversarius
  - Quadratus lumborum & psoas muscles
- **Biomechanics**
  - Lumbar articulations permit ventral flexion, lateral flexion, extension
  - Facets prevent rotation
  - Lumbosacral junction motion checked by strong iliolumbar ligaments

Imaging Anatomy

Radiography

- **"Scotty dog"** demonstrated on oblique view
  - Nose = transverse process, eye = pedicle, ear = superior articular process, neck = pars interarticularis, front leg = inferior articular process

Cross-Sectional Imaging

- **Facet joint orientation**
  - Facet joint angle is measured relative to coronal plane
  - Normal facet joint angle ≈ 40°
  - More sagittally oriented facet joints (> 45°) at L4 & L5 levels ↑ incidence of disc herniation & degenerative spondylolisthesis

Anatomy-Based Imaging Issues

Imaging Pitfalls

- **Lumbosacral junction**
  - Transitional lumbosacral vertebrae
    - Congenital malformation of vertebrae, usually last lumbar or first sacral vertebra
    - Bony characteristics of both lumbar vertebrae and sacrum
  - Vertebral facet asymmetry (**tropism**)
    - Asymmetry between left & right vertebral facet (zygapophyseal) joint angles
    - Tropism defined as mild (6-10°), moderate (10-16°), or severe (> 16°)
    - Variable relationship between facet joint tropism & disc herniation at L4 and L5 level

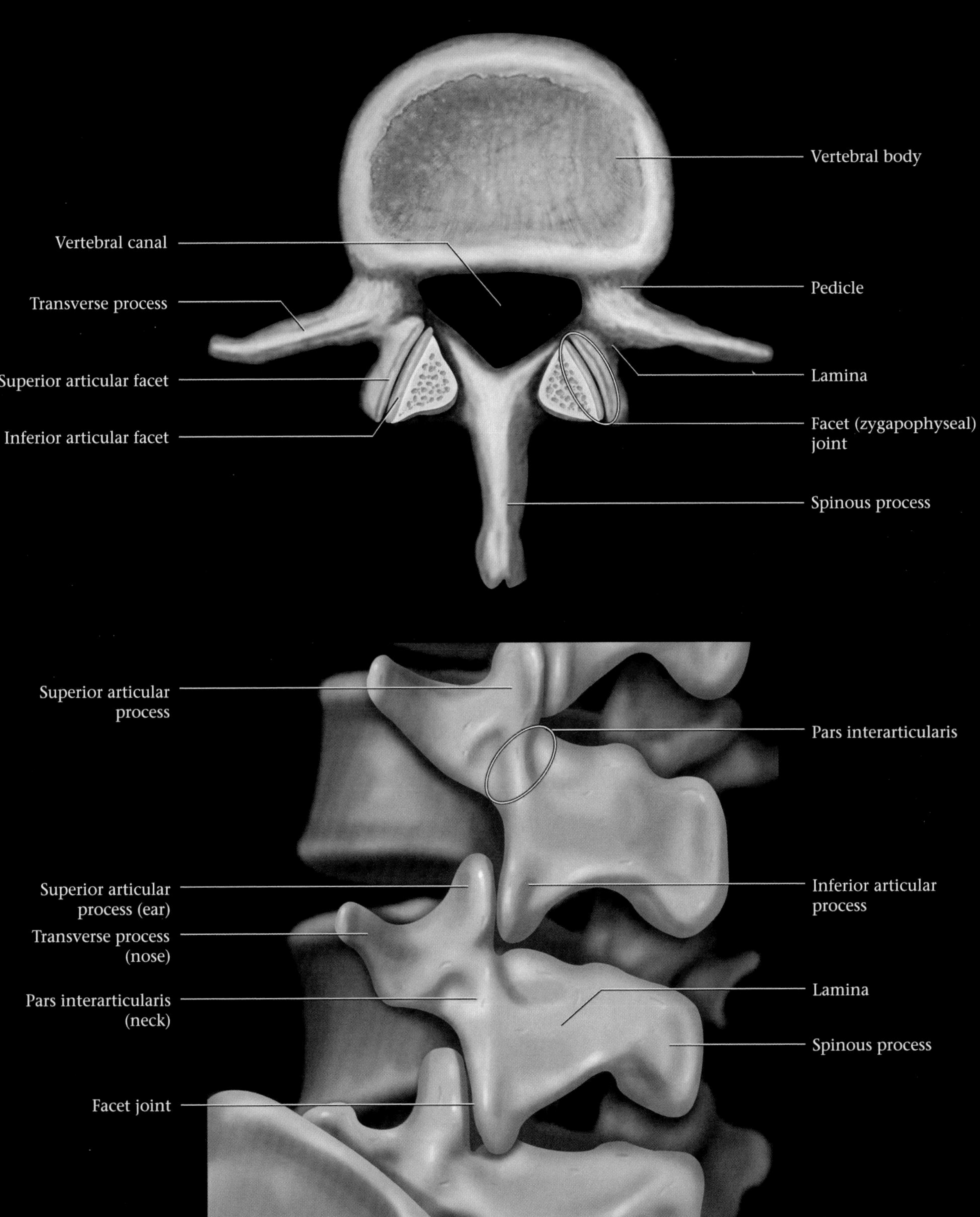
Vertebral body
Vertebral canal
Pedicle
Transverse process
Lamina
Superior articular facet
Facet (zygapophyseal) joint
Inferior articular facet
Spinous process
Superior articular process
Pars interarticularis
Superior articular process (ear)
Inferior articular process
Transverse process (nose)
Lamina
Pars interarticularis (neck)
Spinous process
Facet joint

(Top) Graphic of lumbar vertebral body from above with section passing through facet (zygapophyseal) joints. The large lumbar vertebral body is wider from side to side than in the AP dimension. The pedicles are strong & project directly posteriorly from the upper part of the body. The central vertebral canal is triangular (cervical > lumbar > thoracic). The spinous process is thick & broad & projects backward. The superior articular facets are concave, & face posteromedially; the inferior articular facets are convex, & face anterolaterally. **(Bottom)** Oblique graphic shows the characteristic "Scotty dog" appearance of the superior (ear) & inferior (front leg) articular facets, with the intervening pars interarticularis (neck). The well-defined superior & inferior articular processes project respectively upward & downward from the junctions of pedicles & laminae.

GRAPHICS

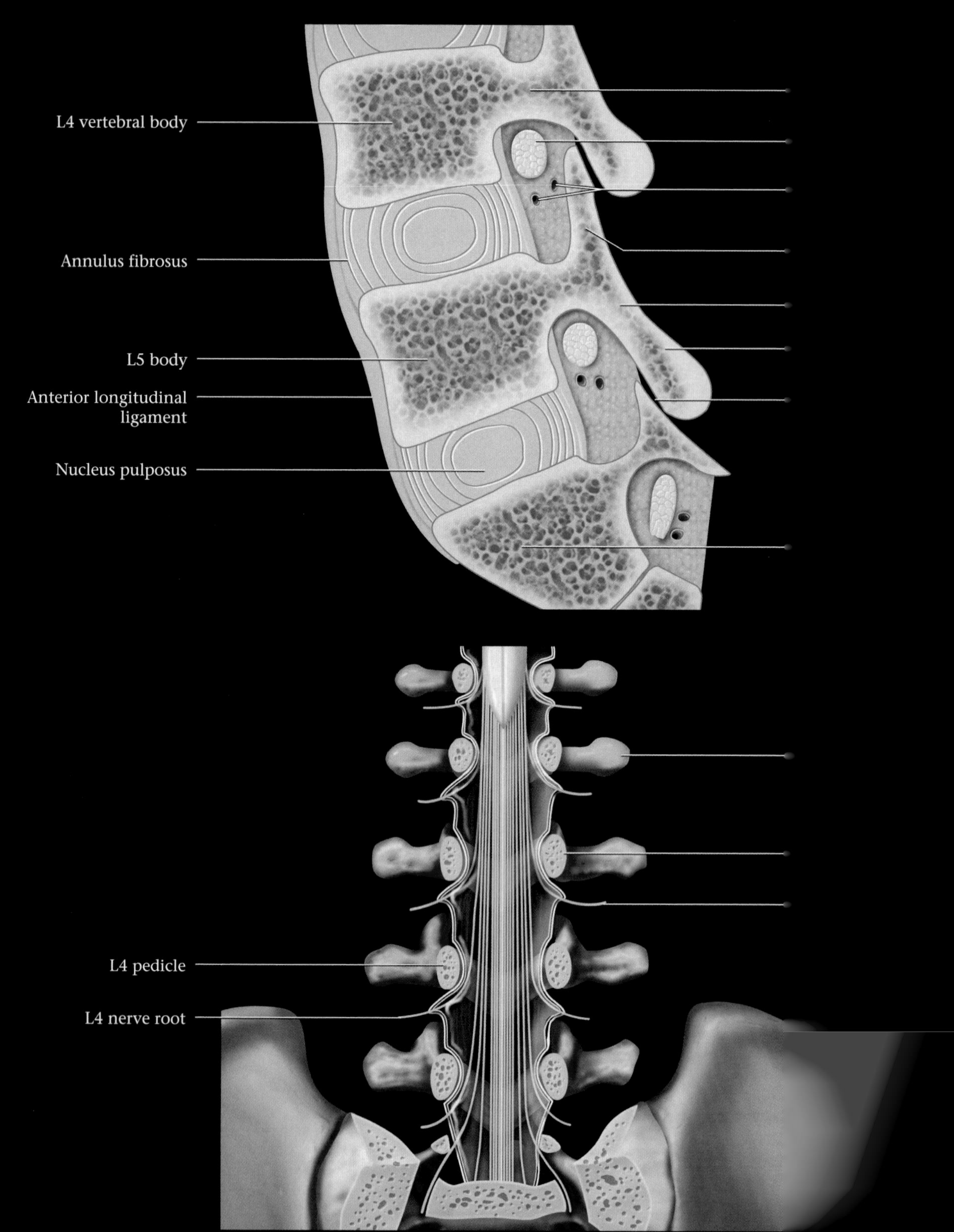
L4 vertebral body
Annulus fibrosus
L5 body
Anterior longitudinal ligament
Nucleus pulposus
L4 pedicle
L4 nerve root

(Top) Sagittal graphic of lumbar spine through neural foramen shows position of exiting ne
aspect of the neural foramen. The segmental vessels are located inferior to the exiting nerve
bounded anteriorly by dorsal vertebral body above & intervertebral disc below, pedicle abov
ligamentum flavum posteriorly. The lumbar vertebral bodies are large, with a large interveni
The pedicles are directed posteriorly, giving rise to large superior & inferior articular facets. (
through pedicles of lumbar spine shows exiting nerve roots passing below their respective p

LUMBAR SPINE

RADIOGRAPHY

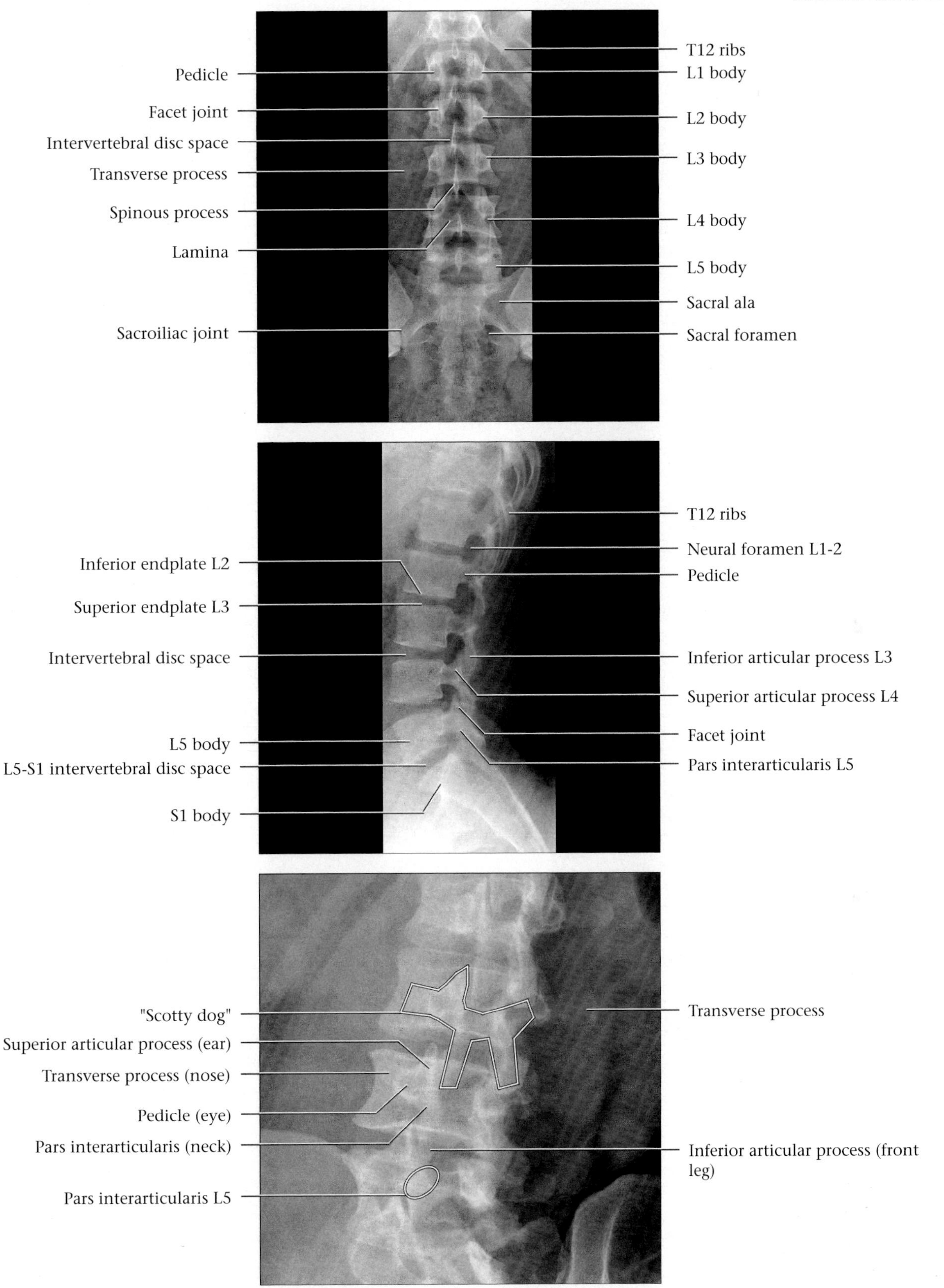
Pedicle
Facet joint
Intervertebral disc space
Transverse process
Spinous process
Lamina
Sacroiliac joint
T12 ribs
L1 body
L2 body
L3 body
L4 body
L5 body
Sacral ala
Sacral foramen
Inferior endplate L2
Superior endplate L3
Intervertebral disc space
L5 body
L5-S1 intervertebral disc space
S1 body
T12 ribs
Neural foramen L1-2
Pedicle
Inferior articular process L3
Superior articular process L4
Facet joint
Pars interarticularis L5
"Scotty dog"
Superior articular process (ear)
Transverse process (nose)
Pedicle (eye)
Pars interarticularis (neck)
Pars interarticularis L5
Transverse process
Inferior articular process (front leg)

(Top) AP view of the lumbar spine. The lumbar bodies are large & rectangular in shape, with relatively thick intervertebral disc spaces. The pedicles are viewed en face, with the adjacent facet joints incompletely visualized due to their obliquity. The large horizontal transverse processes are easily identified, at the pedicle levels. **(Middle)** Lateral view of the lumbar spine. The large, strong lumbar bodies join with the stout lumbar pedicles & posterior elements. The neural foramina are large & directed laterally. The boundary of the neural foramen includes posterior vertebral body, inferior & superior pedicle cortex, & superior articular process. **(Bottom)** Oblique view of the lumbar spine. The typical "Scotty dog" appearance of the posterior elements is visible. The neck of the dog is the pars interarticularis.

LUMBAR SPINE

3D-VRT NECT

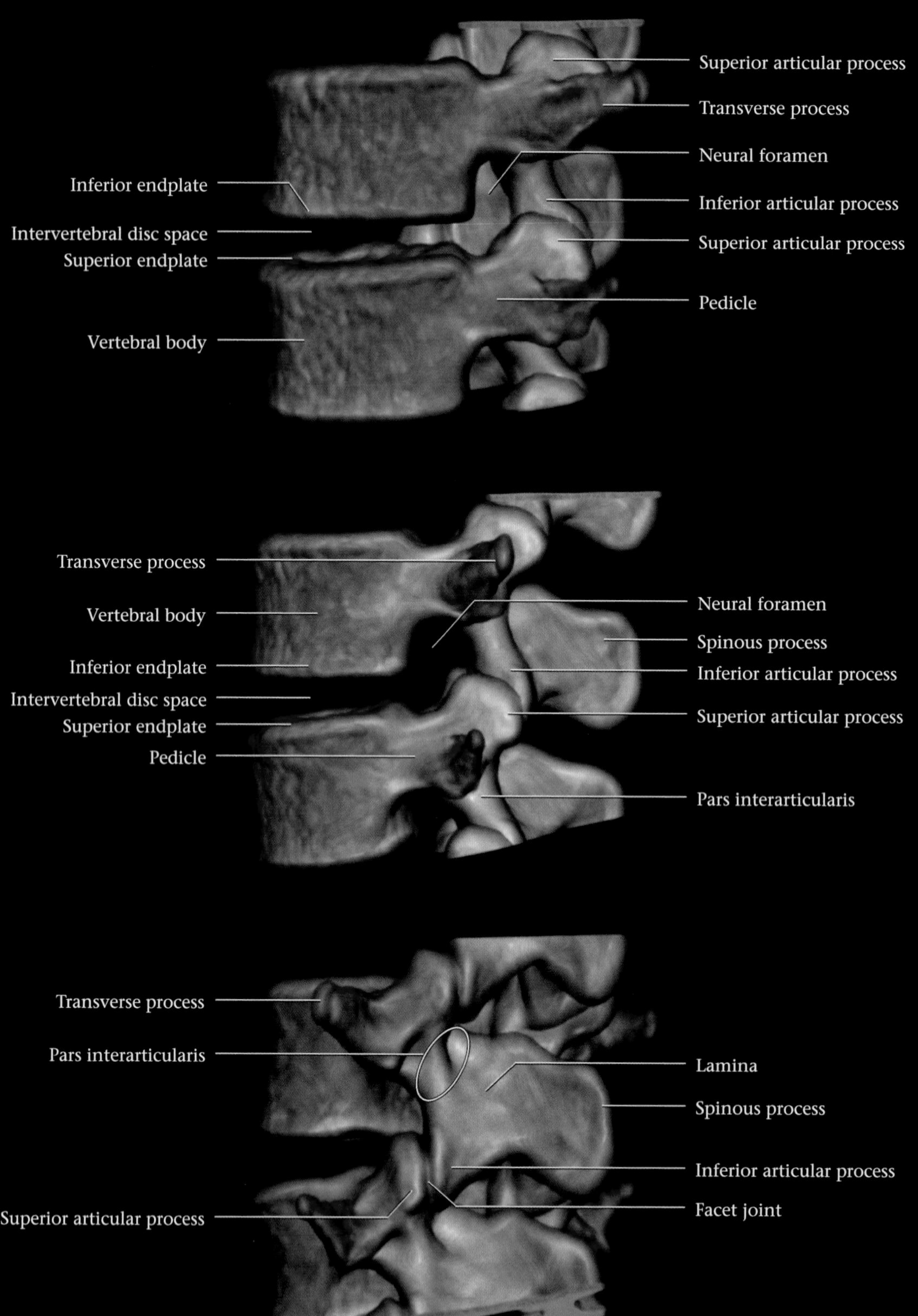
Superior articular process
Transverse process
Neural foramen
Inferior articular process
Superior articular process
Pedicle
Inferior endplate
Intervertebral disc space
Superior endplate
Vertebral body
Transverse process
Vertebral body
Inferior endplate
Intervertebral disc space
Superior endplate
Pedicle
Neural foramen
Spinous process
Inferior articular process
Superior articular process
Pars interarticularis
Transverse process
Pars interarticularis
Superior articular process
Lamina
Spinous process
Inferior articular process
Facet joint

(Top) Left anterior oblique 3D-VRT NECT examination of the lumbar spine. The broad, stout pedicle/vertebral body junction is highlighted in this projection, with the superior facet arising as the dorsal extension. **(Middle)** Left lateral 3D-VRT NECT examination of the lumbar spine shows the neural foramen seen en face as it projects laterally. **(Bottom)** Left posterior oblique 3D-VRT NECT examination of the lumbar spine. This view shows the surface anatomy inherent in the "Scotty dog". The transverse process (nose), superior articular process (ear), inferior articular process (front leg) & intervening pars interarticularis (neck) are well-defined. The pedicle which forms the "eye" on oblique radiographs is obscured. The oblique sagittal orientation of the facet joints is evident in this view, restricting lumbar rotation, & allowing flexion/extension.

LUMBAR SPINE

3D-VRT NECT

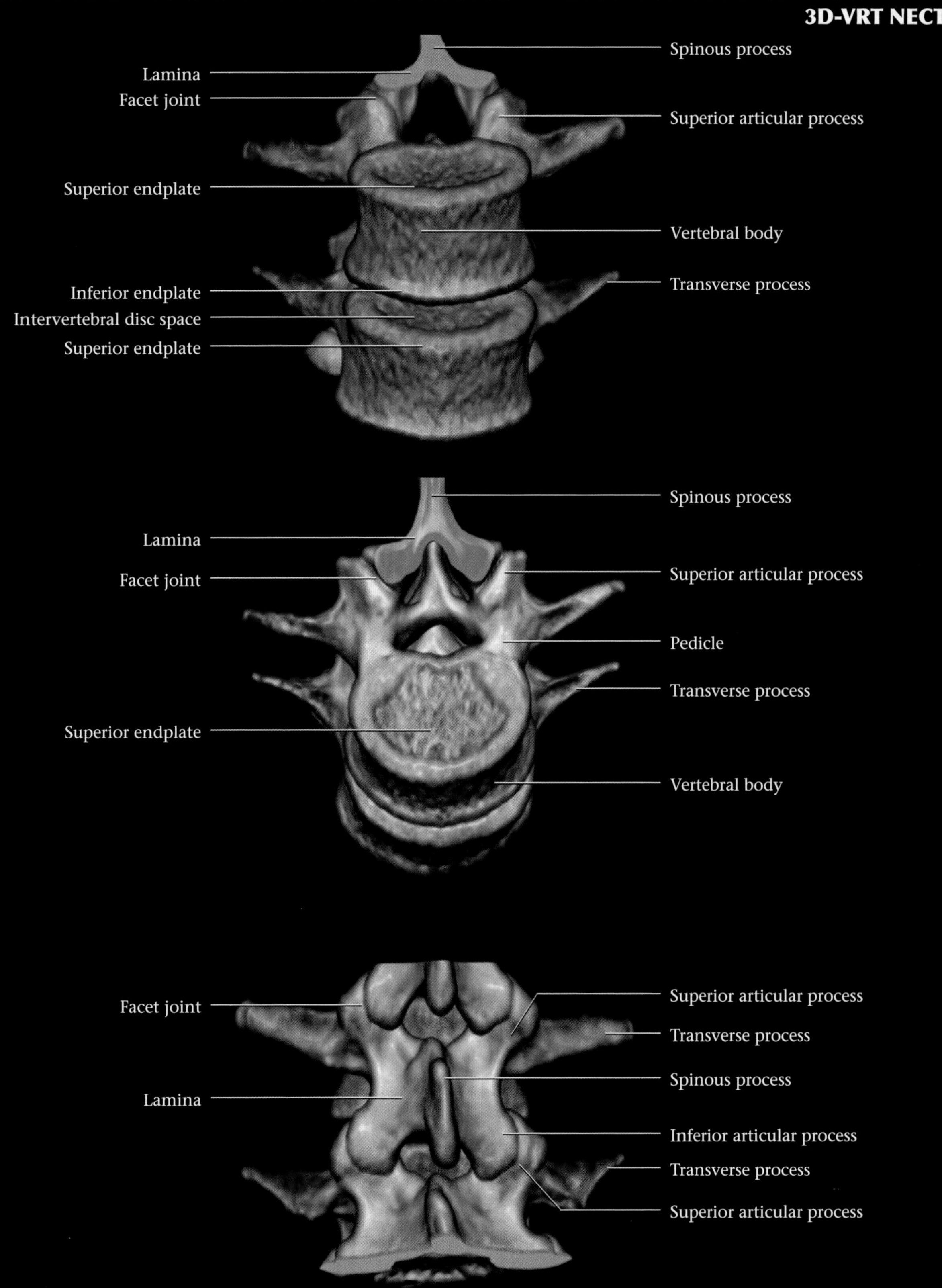
Spinous process
Lamina
Facet joint
Superior articular process
Superior endplate
Vertebral body
Transverse process
Inferior endplate
Intervertebral disc space
Superior endplate
Spinous process
Lamina
Facet joint
Superior articular process
Pedicle
Transverse process
Superior endplate
Vertebral body
Superior articular process
Facet joint
Transverse process
Spinous process
Lamina
Inferior articular process
Transverse process
Superior articular process

(Top) Anterior 3D-VRT NECT examination of the lumbar spine, with superior angulation. The large intervertebral disc space is identified, in contrast to the cervical or thoracic segments. **(Middle)** Superior view of 3D-VRT NECT examination of the lumbar spine. The large surface area of the posterior elements with their dorsal projections is evident, allowing broad muscle attachments. **(Bottom)** Posterior view of 3D-VRT NECT examination of the lumbar spine. The "H" shape of the dorsal elements is apparent in this projection. The superior arms of the "H" are formed by the superior articular processes. The horizontal bar reflects the lamina & spinous process. The inferior arms of the "H" are the inferior articular processes.

AXIAL BONE CT

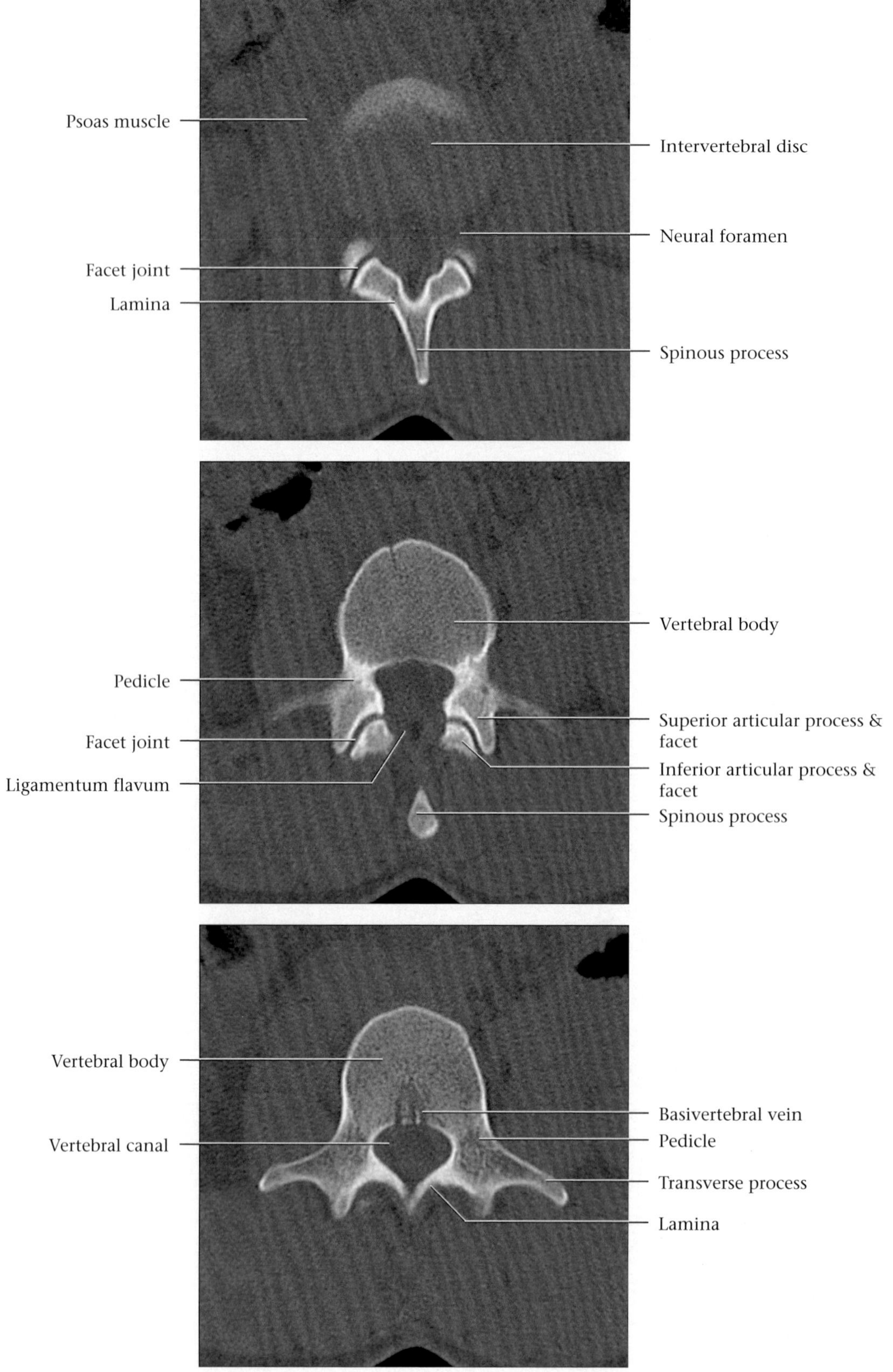
Psoas muscle
Intervertebral disc
Neural foramen
Facet joint
Lamina
Spinous process
Vertebral body
Pedicle
Superior articular process & facet
Facet joint
Inferior articular process & facet
Ligamentum flavum
Spinous process
Vertebral body
Basivertebral vein
Pedicle
Vertebral canal
Transverse process
Lamina

(Top) First of six axial bone CT images through the lumbar spine presented from superior to inferior. Image at intervertebral disc & lower neural foraminal level. Posterior intervertebral disc forms the lower anterior border of neural foramen which contains primarily fat. Exiting nerves are in upper neural foramen. **(Middle)** Image through facet joints. Facet joint shows typical lumbar morphology, with superior facet showing a concave posterior surface & inferior facet showing the complementary convex anterior surface. Facet joints are oriented approximately 40° from coronal plane. An angle of > 45° from coronal plane increases incidence of disc herniation & degenerative spondylolisthesis at L4 & L5 levels. **(Bottom)** Image showing triangular central vertebral canal & posteriorly oriented pedicles. Basivertebral veins enter vertebral body through posterior cortex.

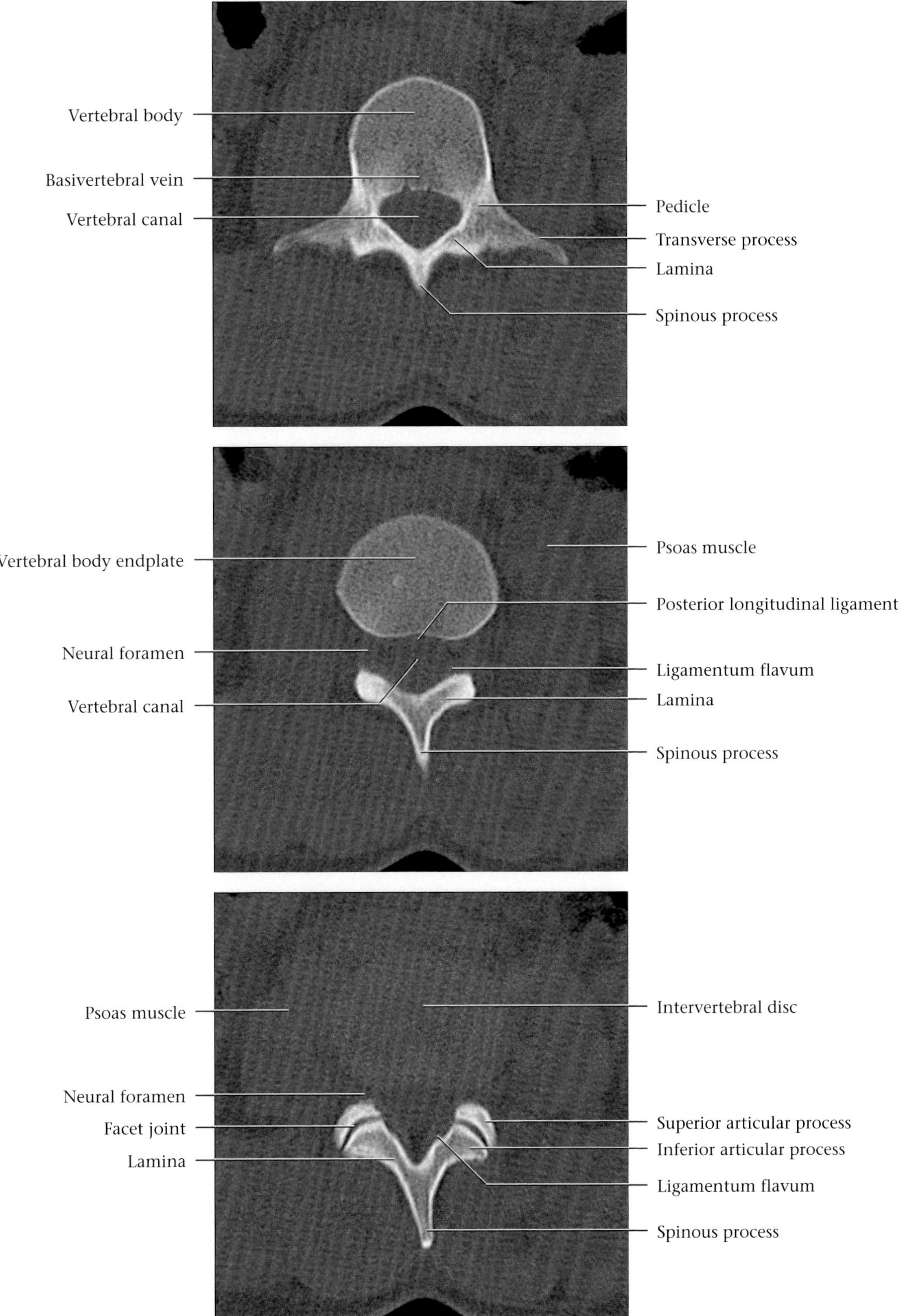

Vertebral body
Basivertebral vein
Vertebral canal
Pedicle
Transverse process
Lamina
Spinous process
Vertebral body endplate
Neural foramen
Vertebral canal
Psoas muscle
Posterior longitudinal ligament
Ligamentum flavum
Lamina
Spinous process
Psoas muscle
Neural foramen
Facet joint
Lamina
Intervertebral disc
Superior articular process
Inferior articular process
Ligamentum flavum
Spinous process

(Top) Image at mid vertebral body level showing thick cortical vertebral body margin & midline posterior basivertebral veins. The pedicles are strong, thick & directed posteriorly. Large transverse processes project from the lateral margins. **(Middle)** Image at endplate level. The neural foramen are identified, opening laterally. The posterior elements have a "T" pattern with the large posteriorly directed spinous process. **(Bottom)** Image through the intervertebral disc level again demonstrates lower neural foramen bounded anteriorly by intervertebral disc & posteriorly by the superior articular process & facet joint. Oblique coronal orientation of facet joints is again appreciated. Asymmetry between left & right vertebral facet joint angles, with one joint having a more sagittal orientation than the other is termed "tropism".

SAGITTAL T1 MR

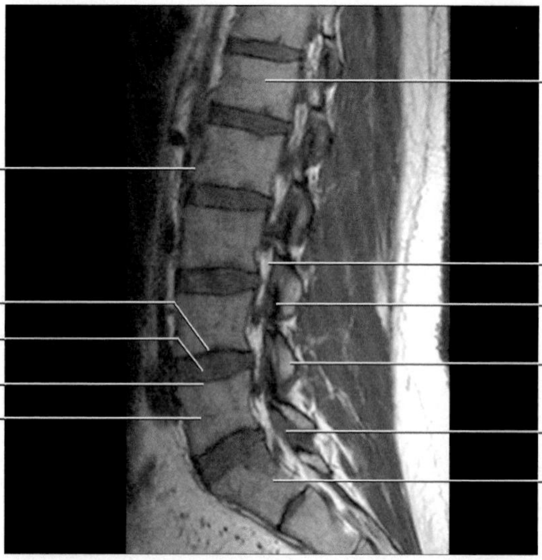

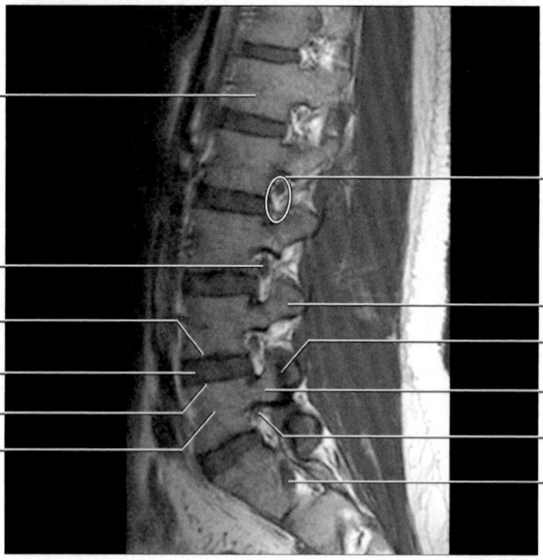

Conus medullaris
Basivertebral vein
Spinous process
Supraspinous ligament
Anterior longitudinal ligament
Interspinous ligament
Epidural fat
Inferior endplate L4
Dorsal dural margin
Intervertebral disc
Lumbar cerebrospinal fluid
Superior endplate L5
L5 body
S1 body
L1 vertebral body
Anterior longitudinal ligament
Epidural fat
Inferior endplate L4
Facet joint
Intervertebral disc
Inferior articular process L4
Superior endplate L5
L5 body
Ligamentum flavum
S1 body
L1 vertebral body
Neural foramen
L3 nerve root
Superior articular process L4
Inferior endplate L4
Facet joint
Intervertebral disc
Pedicle L5
Superior endplate L5
Nerve root L5
L5 body
S1 nerve root

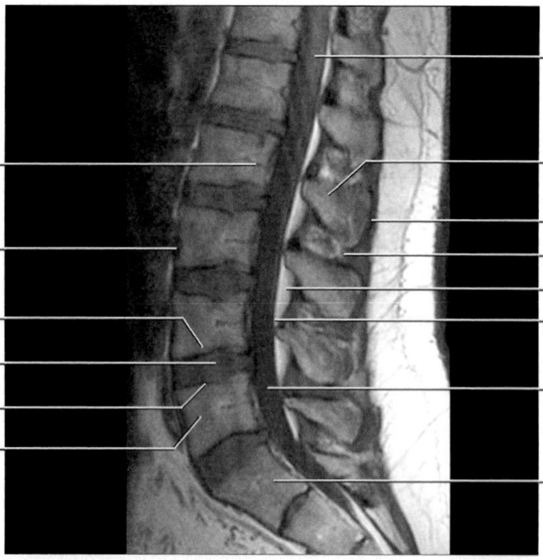

(Top) First of three sagittal T1 MR images of the lumbar spine presented from medial to lateral. The normal marrow signal on T1 images is of increased signal compared to the adjacent intervertebral discs in the adult, due to fatty marrow content. The basivertebral veins are seen as signal voids in the midline of the posterior vertebral bodies, often with surrounding high signal fatty marrow. The intervertebral disc morphology is poorly identified on this sequence, with little differentiation of annulus or nucleus. **(Middle)** In this image the lateral vertebral bodies are evident, with the pronounced oblong shaped inferior articular facets dominating the posterior aspect. **(Bottom)** In this image the anterior boundaries of the neural foramina are evident, as is the relationship of the disc to the exiting nerve.

AXIAL T1 MR

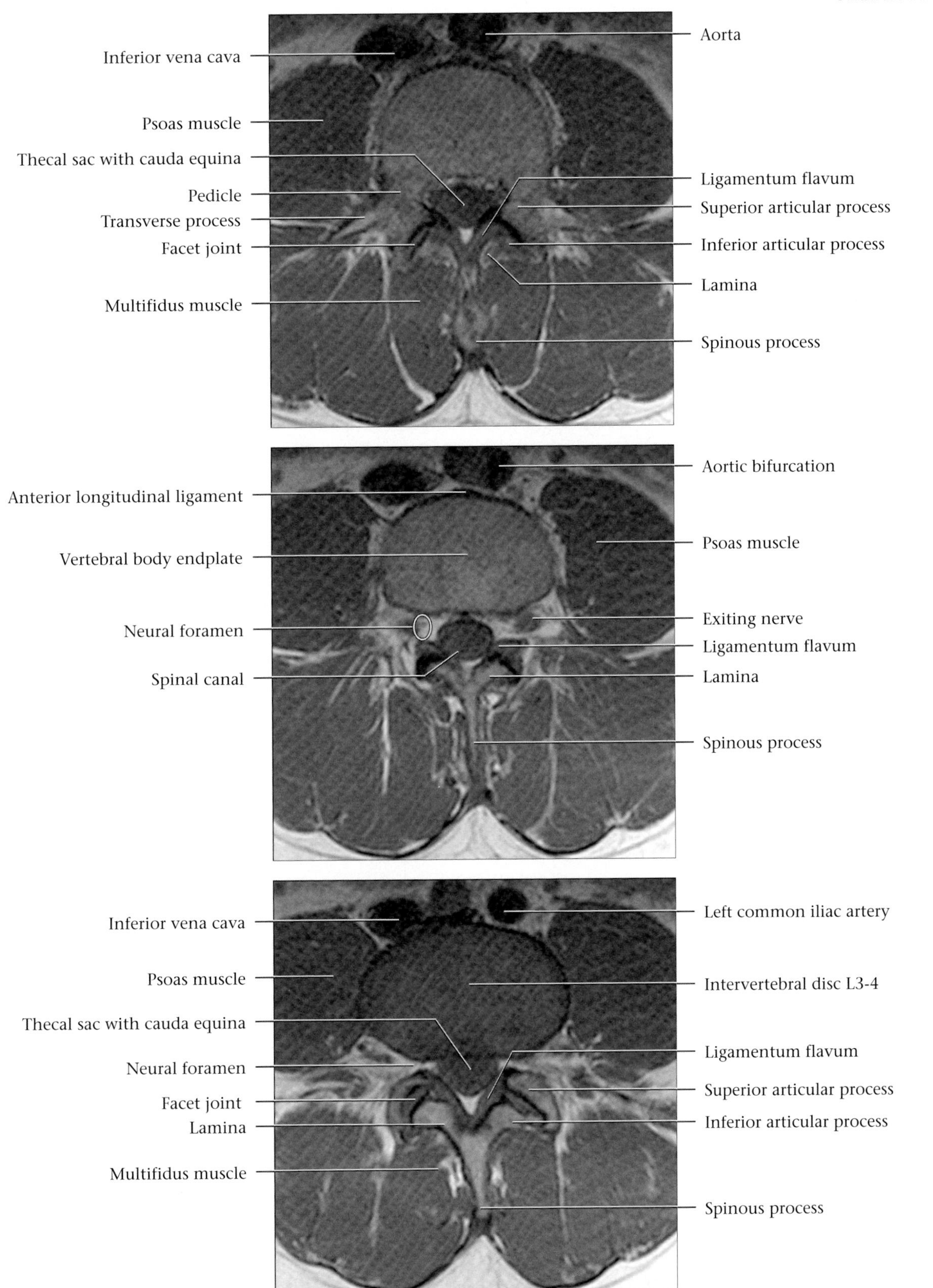
Inferior vena cava
Psoas muscle
Thecal sac with cauda equina
Pedicle
Transverse process
Facet joint
Multifidus muscle
Aorta
Ligamentum flavum
Superior articular process
Inferior articular process
Lamina
Spinous process
Anterior longitudinal ligament
Vertebral body endplate
Neural foramen
Spinal canal
Aortic bifurcation
Psoas muscle
Exiting nerve
Ligamentum flavum
Lamina
Spinous process
Inferior vena cava
Psoas muscle
Thecal sac with cauda equina
Neural foramen
Facet joint
Lamina
Multifidus muscle
Left common iliac artery
Intervertebral disc L3-4
Ligamentum flavum
Superior articular process
Inferior articular process
Spinous process

(Top) First of three axial T1 MR images of the lumbar spine presented from superior to inferior. This superior view shows the thick broad pedicles extending into the posterior elements. The transverse processes are large, providing surface area for muscle attachment. **(Middle)** Image though the upper neural foraminal level. The neural foramina are directed laterally, bounded anteriorly by the posterior vertebral body & intervertebral disc & posteriorly by the facet complex. Exiting peripheral nerves are surrounded by hyperintense fat within neural foramen. **(Bottom)** Image at intervertebral disc & lower neural foramen level. The facet joints are well-defined in this plane, & are oriented approximately 40° from coronal plane. The spinal canal assumes a triangular configuration with the ventral disc margin, & the dorsal ligamentum flavum.

CORONAL T1 MR

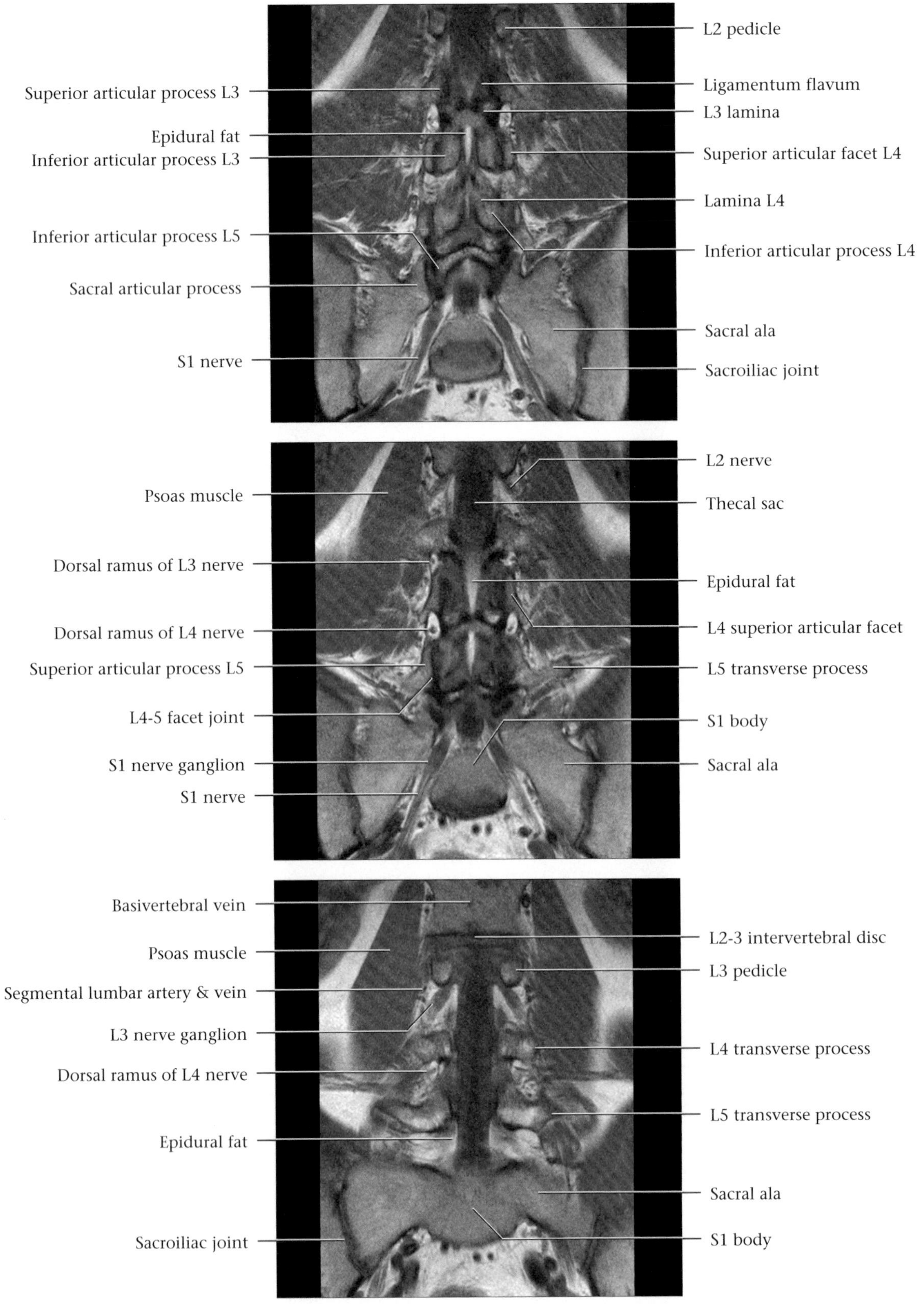

L2 pedicle
Superior articular process L3
Ligamentum flavum
L3 lamina
Epidural fat
Inferior articular process L3
Superior articular facet L4
Lamina L4
Inferior articular process L5
Inferior articular process L4
Sacral articular process
Sacral ala
S1 nerve
Sacroiliac joint
L2 nerve
Psoas muscle
Thecal sac
Dorsal ramus of L3 nerve
Epidural fat
L4 superior articular facet
Dorsal ramus of L4 nerve
Superior articular process L5
L5 transverse process
L4-5 facet joint
S1 body
S1 nerve ganglion
Sacral ala
S1 nerve
Basivertebral vein
L2-3 intervertebral disc
Psoas muscle
L3 pedicle
Segmental lumbar artery & vein
L3 nerve ganglion
L4 transverse process
Dorsal ramus of L4 nerve
L5 transverse process
Epidural fat
Sacral ala
Sacroiliac joint
S1 body

(Top) First of six coronal T1 MR images through the lumbar spine presented from posterior to anterior. The posterior elements are visualized in this section, with the lateral margins of the facet joints in view. **(Middle)** More anterior image of the lumbar spine. Dorsal (posterior) ramus of L4 nerve is demonstrated surrounded by fat passing posteriorly following its exit through the neural foramen. Midline epidural fat is seen as a linear band separating the paired ligamentum flavum. **(Bottom)** More anterior image of the lumbar spine. The L3 nerve is seen extending underneath the L3 pedicle. The spinal nerve ganglia are surrounded by fat within the neural foramen. Distal to the ganglion, the spinal nerve divides into anterior & posterior branches. Posterior branches supply motor innervation to deep muscles of the back & sensation to skin of the back.

CORONAL T1 MR

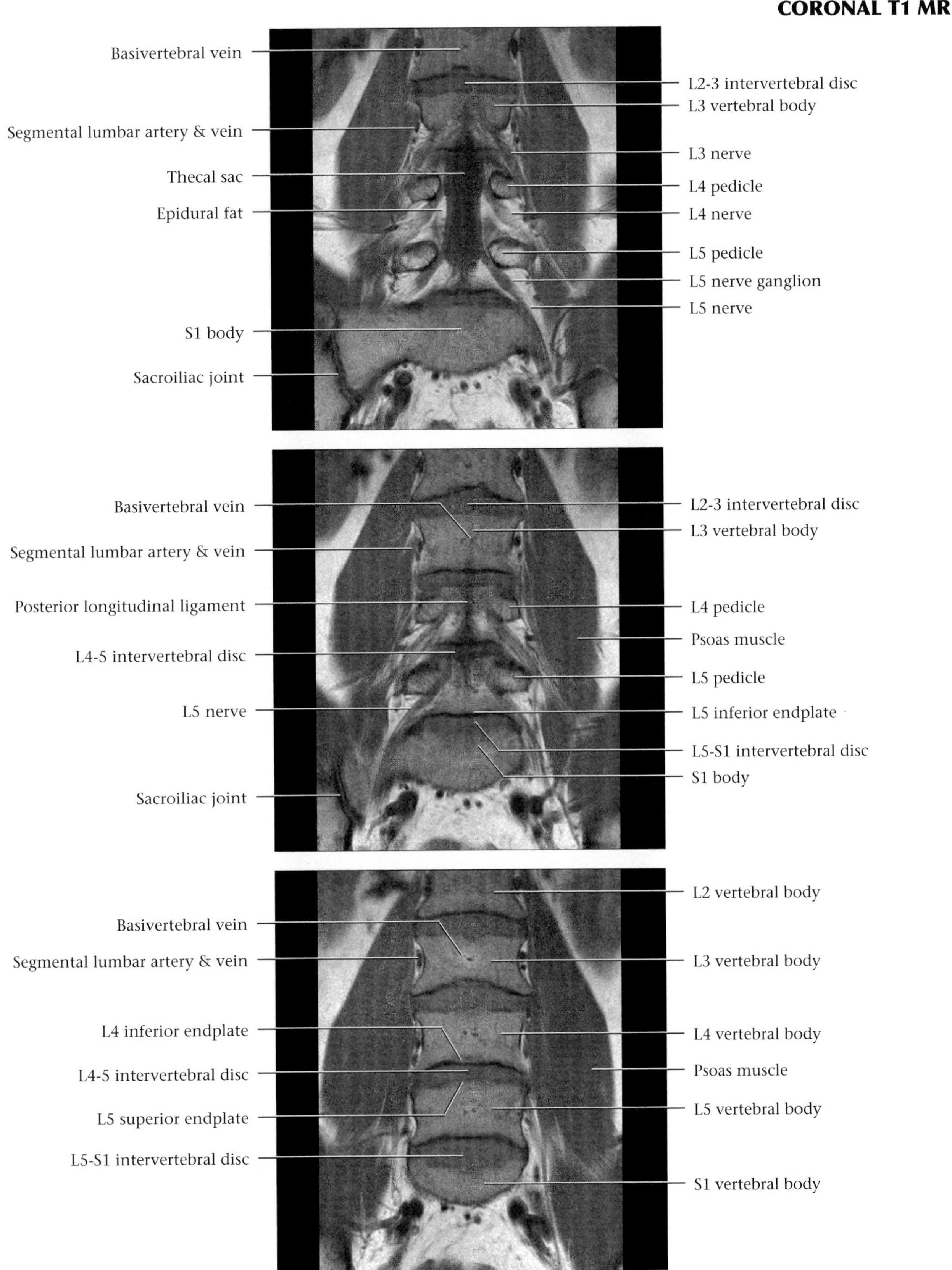
Basivertebral vein
Segmental lumbar artery & vein
Thecal sac
Epidural fat
S1 body
Sacroiliac joint
L2-3 intervertebral disc
L3 vertebral body
L3 nerve
L4 pedicle
L4 nerve
L5 pedicle
L5 nerve ganglion
L5 nerve
Basivertebral vein
Segmental lumbar artery & vein
Posterior longitudinal ligament
L4-5 intervertebral disc
L5 nerve
Sacroiliac joint
L2-3 intervertebral disc
L3 vertebral body
L4 pedicle
Psoas muscle
L5 pedicle
L5 inferior endplate
L5-S1 intervertebral disc
S1 body
Basivertebral vein
Segmental lumbar artery & vein
L4 inferior endplate
L4-5 intervertebral disc
L5 superior endplate
L5-S1 intervertebral disc
L2 vertebral body
L3 vertebral body
L4 vertebral body
Psoas muscle
L5 vertebral body
S1 vertebral body

(Top) More anterior image of the lumbar spine showing relationship of exiting nerves to the pedicles. Nerves exit the foramina in an inferior lateral direction at the same numbered pedicle level (i.e., L5 root exits below L5 pedicle). **(Middle)** The junction of the vertebral bodies with the ventral epidural space is highlighted in this view. The posterior longitudinal ligament is seen as a dark vertically oriented band in the midline. The adjacent epidural fat shows high signal. The vertebral bodies are defined by the superior & inferior endplates. **(Bottom)** Most anterior image of the lumbar spine. The vertebral body endplates are visualized for each segment, with the intervening thick intervertebral disc.

AXIAL T2 MR

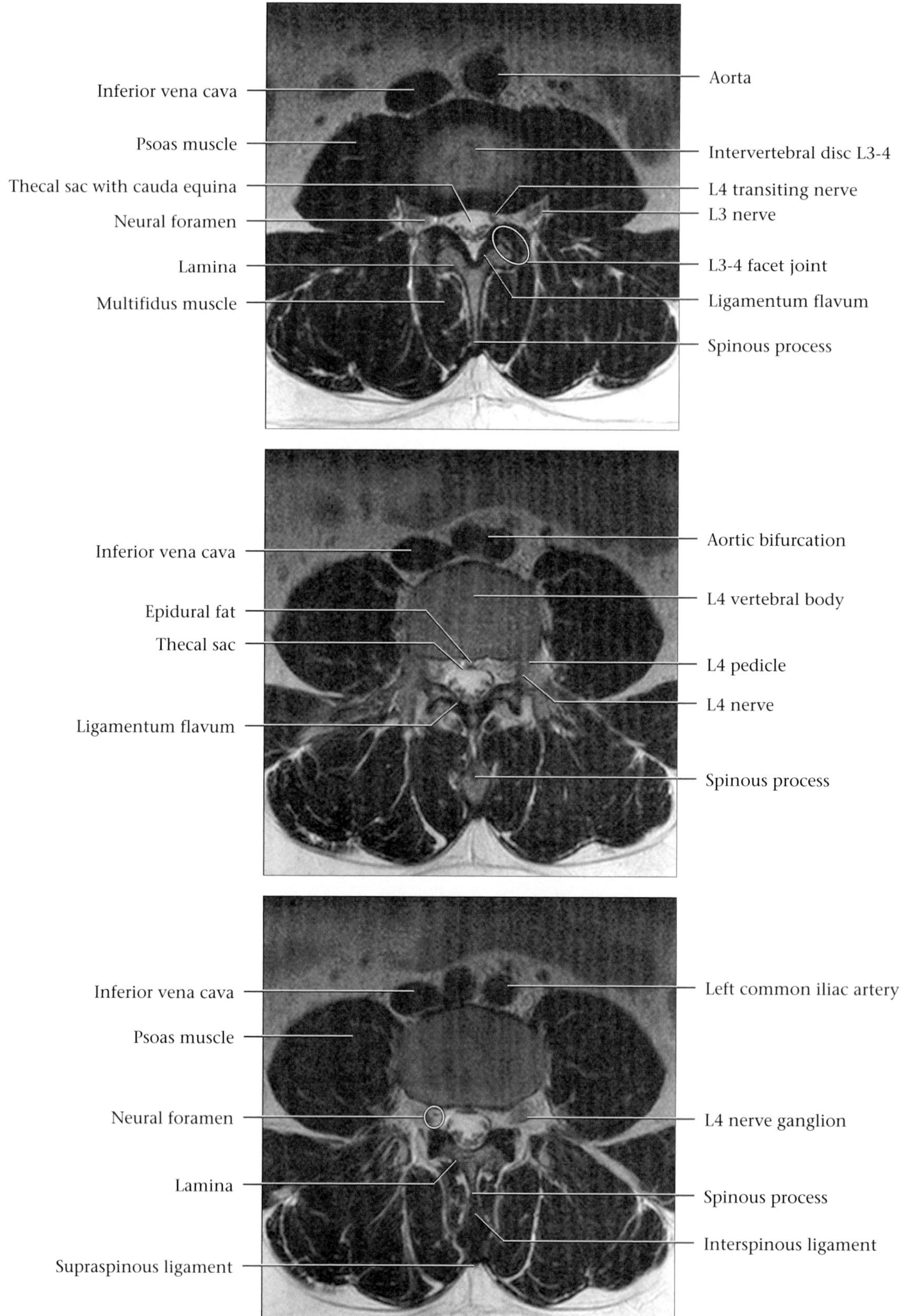
Inferior vena cava
Psoas muscle
Thecal sac with cauda equina
Neural foramen
Lamina
Multifidus muscle
Aorta
Intervertebral disc L3-4
L4 transiting nerve
L3 nerve
L3-4 facet joint
Ligamentum flavum
Spinous process
Inferior vena cava
Epidural fat
Thecal sac
Ligamentum flavum
Aortic bifurcation
L4 vertebral body
L4 pedicle
L4 nerve
Spinous process
Inferior vena cava
Psoas muscle
Neural foramen
Lamina
Supraspinous ligament
Left common iliac artery
L4 nerve ganglion
Spinous process
Interspinous ligament

(Top) First of six axial T2 MR images of lumber spine presented from superior to inferior. This view through the intervertebral disc shows increased disc signal within the central nucleus pulposus due to its high water content, & low signal within the peripheral annulus fibrosus. The margin with the thecal sac is sharp, with the cauda equina seen as punctate nerves within the high signal cerebrospinal fluid. L3 nerve is extraforaminal in location, L4 nerve is transiting in lateral recess. **(Middle)** Image just below L4 pedicle shows exiting L4 nerve passing just below pedicle within the upper neural foramen. **(Bottom)** This image shows L4 nerve ganglion & surrounding fat within mid neural foramen. Posterior margin of neural foramen at this level is facet joint complex, & anterior margin is posterior vertebral body

AXIAL T2 MR

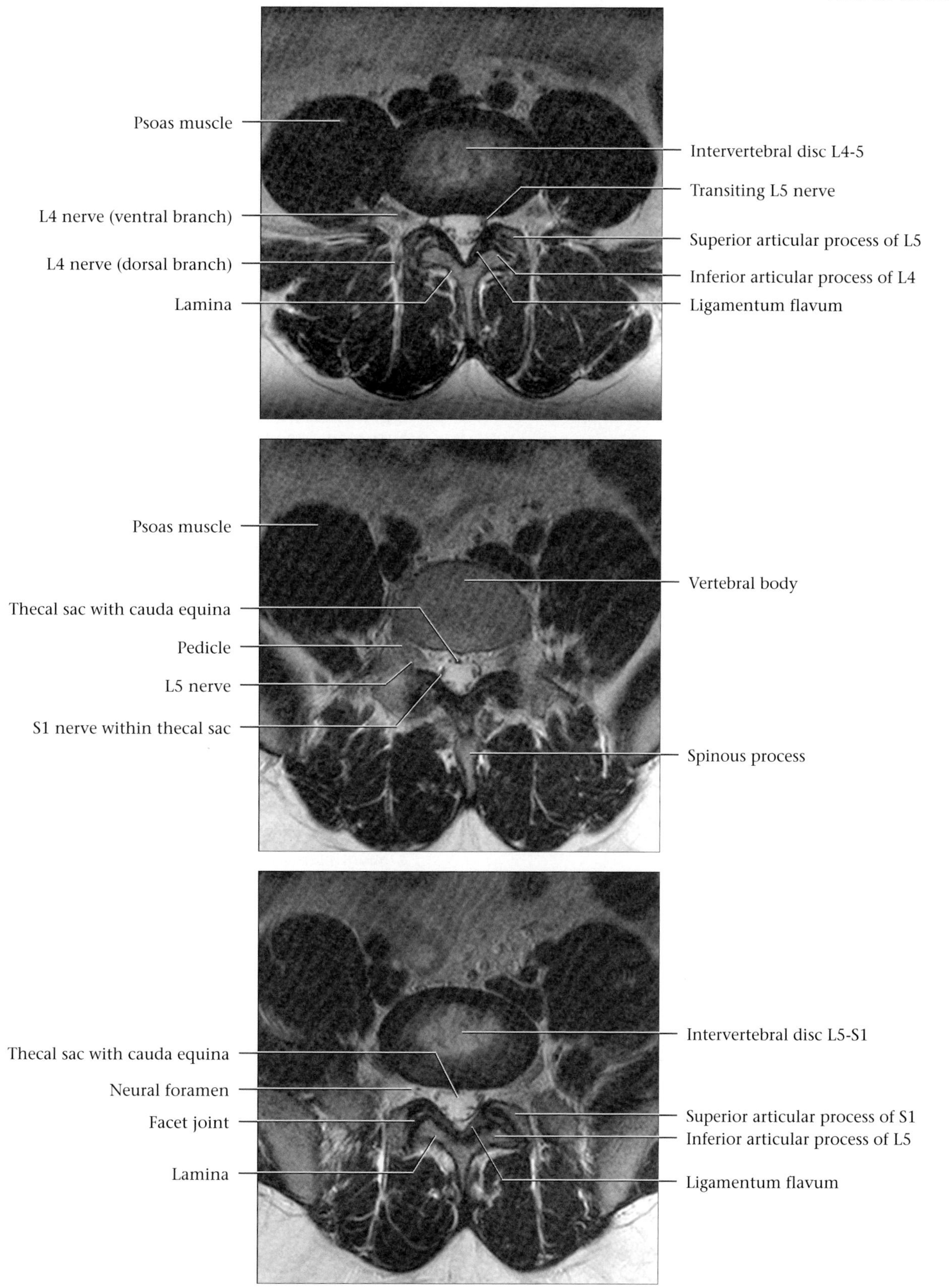

Psoas muscle
Intervertebral disc L4-5
Transiting L5 nerve
L4 nerve (ventral branch)
Superior articular process of L5
L4 nerve (dorsal branch)
Inferior articular process of L4
Lamina
Ligamentum flavum
Psoas muscle
Vertebral body
Thecal sac with cauda equina
Pedicle
L5 nerve
S1 nerve within thecal sac
Spinous process
Intervertebral disc L5-S1
Thecal sac with cauda equina
Neural foramen
Facet joint
Superior articular process of S1
Inferior articular process of L5
Lamina
Ligamentum flavum

(Top) Image through lower neural foramen bordered anteriorly by posterior margin of intervertebral disc & posteriorly by facet joint. L4 nerve has divided into anterior & posterior branches. **(Middle)** Image through upper L5 neural foramina show exiting L5 nerves just below the pedicles. **(Bottom)** Image through L5-S1 intervertebral disc. The typical facet morphology is again identified. The superior articular facet is seen as a convex anterior bony mass with low signal cortical margin. The joint space is seen as a linear focus of high signal due to joint fluid & cartilage. The inferior articular facet is typically convex anteriorly, although can be seen as a more straight margin or even slightly concave (as is seen on the left). Facet joints are oriented approximately 40° from coronal plane.

SACRUM AND COCCYX

Terminology

Definitions

- Sacrum is a large triangular bone formed from 5 fused vertebrae at base of vertebral column

Gross Anatomy

Overview

- **Sacrum**
  - Consists of 5 fused vertebrae (S1-5)
  - Large, triangular shape, forms dorsal aspect of pelvis
  - 3 surfaces: Pelvic, dorsal & lateral
  - Base: Articulates superiorly with L5
  - Apex: Articulates inferiorly with coccyx
- **Coccyx**
  - Consists of 3-5 rudimentary fused segments

Components of Sacrum

- **Bones**
  - Central body, lateral sacral ala, posterior triangular shaped sacral canal
  - 4 paired ventral & dorsal sacral foramina extend laterally from sacral canal to pelvic & dorsal surfaces respectively
  - **Pelvic surface**
    - Concave, forms dorsal aspect of pelvis
    - 4 paired anterior sacral foramina
    - 4 transverse ridges between anterior sacral foramina
  - **Dorsal surface**
    - Convex
    - **Median sacral crest** in midline ≈ fused spinous processes
    - Sacral groove on either side of crest
    - **Intermediate sacral crest** lateral to groove ≈ fused remnants of articular processes
    - 4 paired posterior sacral foramina are lateral to intermediate crest
    - **Lateral sacral crest** lateral to foramina ≈ remnants of transverse processes
    - **Sacral hiatus**: Dorsal bony opening below termination of median sacral crest
  - Lateral surface
    - Broad upper part, tapers inferiorly
    - Ventral articular surface for sacroiliac joint & dorsal roughened area for ligamentous attachment
- **Joints**
  - **Lumbosacral junction**
    - Joins with 5th lumbar vertebra by L5-S1 disc & facet joints
    - Superior base articulates with L5
    - Superior articular processes of S1 faces dorsally
  - **Sacrococcygeal joint**
    - Apex of sacrum & base of coccyx
    - Contains fibrocartilaginous disc
  - **Sacroiliac joints**
    - Ventral synovial joint: Between hyaline covered articular surface of sacrum & fibrocartilage covered surface of iliac bone
    - Dorsal syndesmosis: Interosseous sacroiliac ligament
- **Soft tissues**
  - **Thecal sac**
    - Thecal sac terminates at S2 level
    - Extradural component of filum terminale continues from S2 to attach at 1st coccygeal segment
  - **Nerves**
    - Sacral canal contains sacral & coccygeal nerve roots
    - Nerves emerge via ventral & dorsal sacral foramina
  - **Muscles**
    - **Piriformis**: Arises from ventral sacrum, passes laterally through greater sciatic foramen to insert on greater trochanter; nerves of sacral plexus pass along anterior surface of piriformis muscle
    - Gluteus maximus, erector spinae & multifidis arise from dorsal sacrum
  - **Ligaments**
    - Anterior longitudinal ligament passes over sacral promontory
    - Posterior longitudinal ligament on dorsal surface of lumbosacral disc forming ventral margin of bony canal
    - Sacroiliac joint secured by broad anterior, interosseous & posterior sacroiliac ligaments
    - Sacrospinous ligament bridges lateral sacrum to ischial spine
    - Sacrotuberous ligament bridges lateral sacrum to ischial tuberosity

Imaging Anatomy

Overview

- Lumbosacral junction
  - **Transitional vertebrae**
    - 25% of normal cases
    - **Sacralization** of lumbar body: Spectrum from expanded transverse processes of L5 articulating with top of sacrum to incorporation of L5 into sacrum
    - **Lumbarization** of sacrum: Elevation of S1 above sacral fusion mass assuming lumbar body shape
  - Sacrum lies at 40° incline from horizontal at lumbosacral junction
    - Axial load result in rotational forces at LS junction
    - Rotation forces checked by sacrotuberous, sacrospinous ligaments

Anatomy-Based Imaging Issues

Imaging Pitfalls

- Lumbarization & sacralization may appear similar, require counting from C2 caudally to precisely define anatomy

GRAPHICS

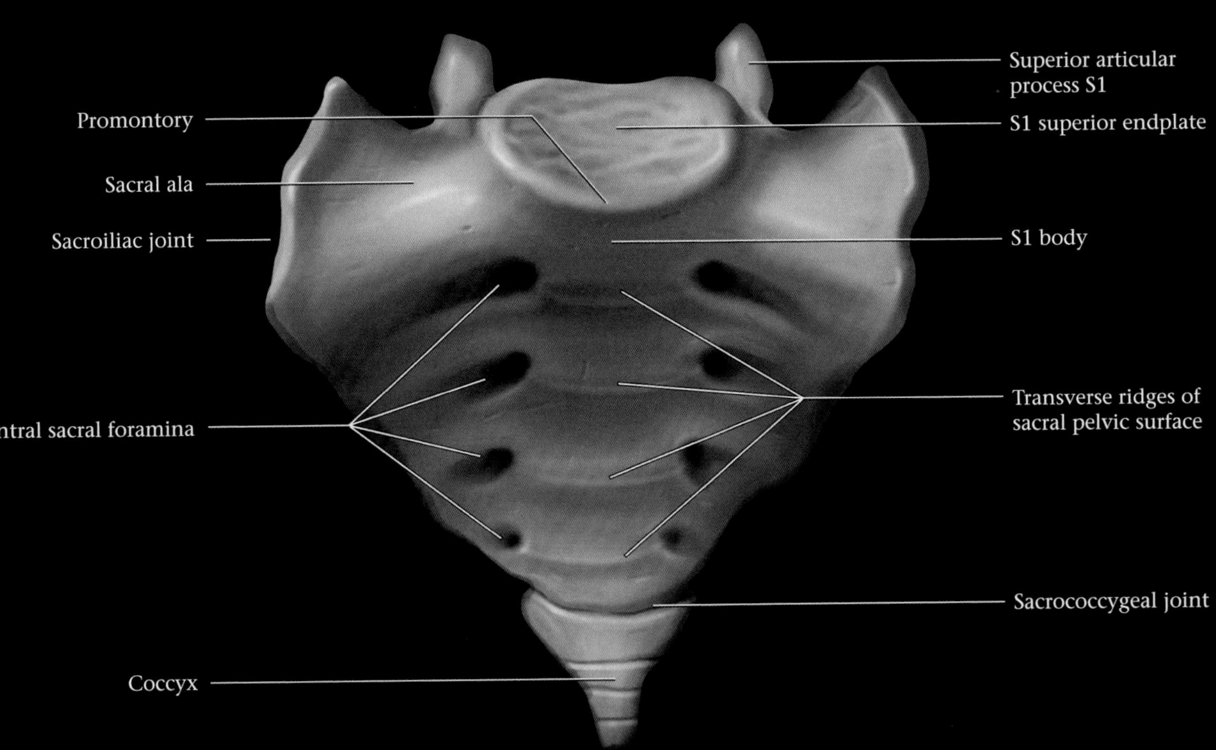
Superior articular process S1
Promontory
S1 superior endplate
Sacral ala
Sacroiliac joint
S1 body
Ventral sacral foramina
Transverse ridges of sacral pelvic surface
Sacrococcygeal joint
Coccyx

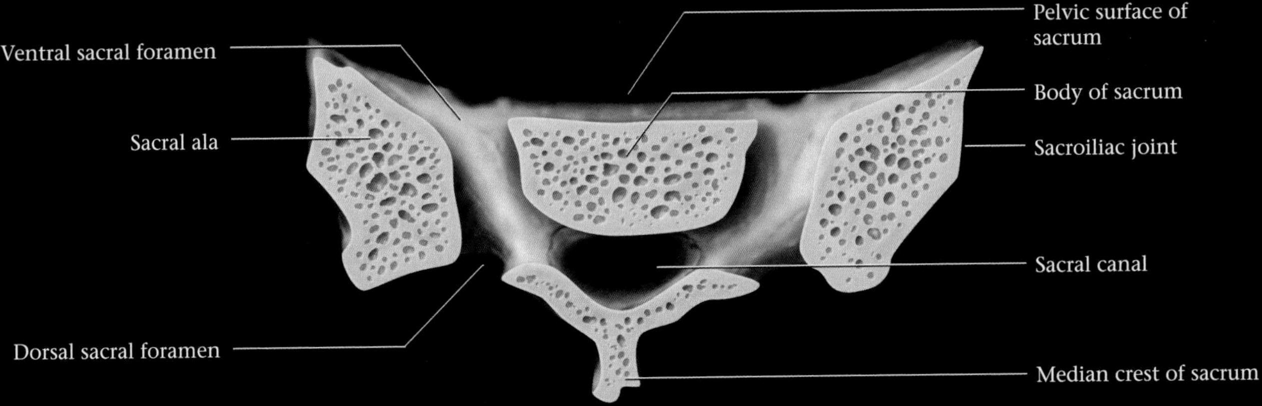
Pelvic surface of sacrum
Ventral sacral foramen
Body of sacrum
Sacral ala
Sacroiliac joint
Sacral canal
Dorsal sacral foramen
Median crest of sacrum

(Top) Anterior graphic view of the sacrum. The sacrum is a large fused bony mass of 5 vertebra, forming the posterior aspect of the pelvis. The superior articular facets arise off of the sacrum & articulate with the inferior articular processes of L5 to form the lumbosacral junction. **(Bottom)** Axial graphic through the sacrum. The sacrum is highlighted as three bony masses, with the central body & lateral sacral ala. The ventral & dorsal sacral foramina are visible arising from the central sacral canal, extending to the pelvic & dorsal surfaces respectively.

GRAPHICS

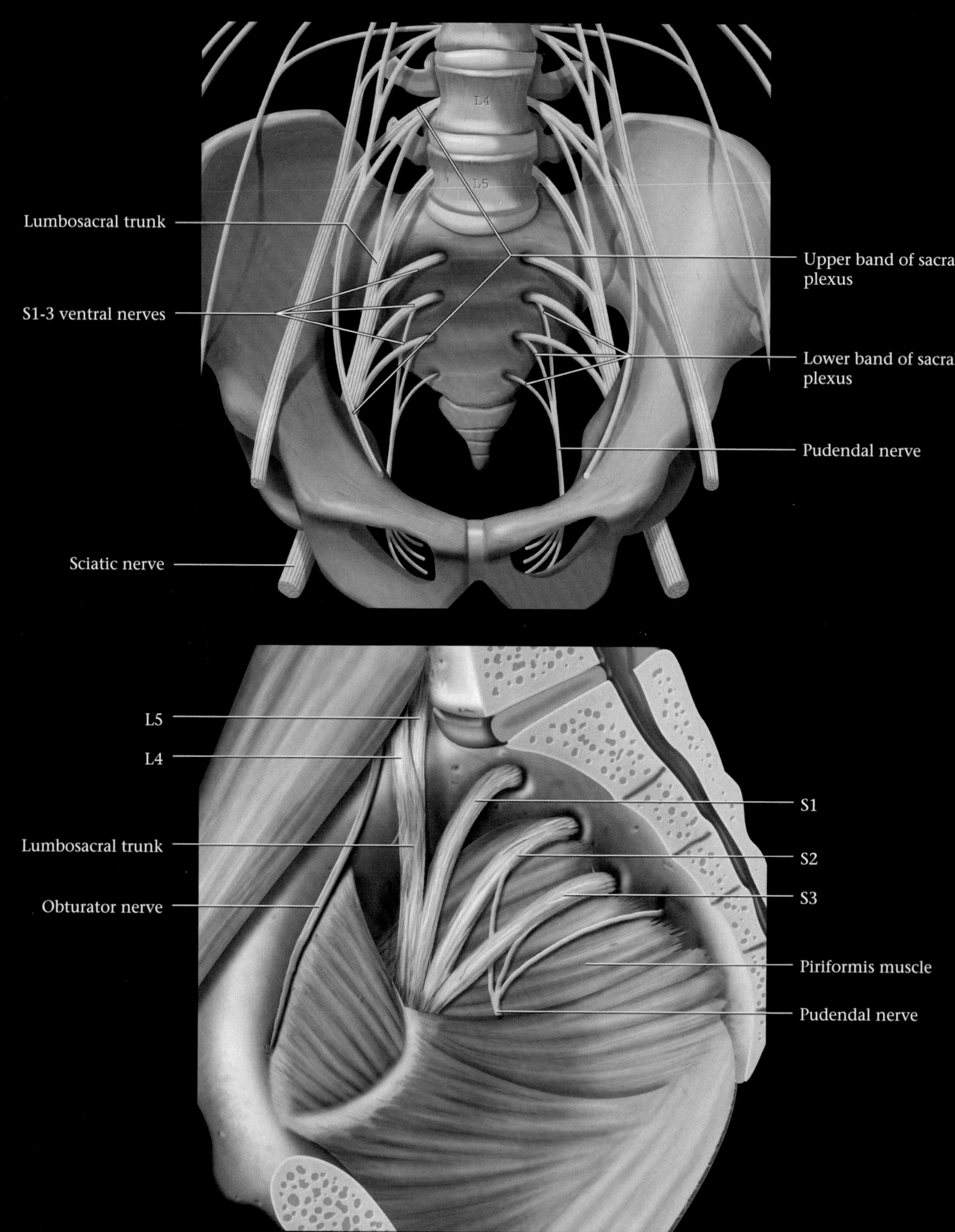

L4
L5
Lumbosacral trunk
S1-3 ventral nerves
Sciatic nerve
Upper band of sacral plexus
Lower band of sacral plexus
Pudendal nerve
L5
L4
Lumbosacral trunk
Obturator nerve
S1
S2
S3
Piriformis muscle
Pudendal nerve

(Top) Coronal graphic showing relationship of sacrum to sacral nerve plexus. Graphic depicts upper & lower sacral bands of sacral plexus. The primary terminal branch of the upper sacral band is the sciatic nerve, which consists of the lumbosacral trunk & the first 3 ventral sacral nerves. The lower sacral band forms the pudendal nerve to the perineum. **(Bottom)** Sagittal graphic depicts upper & lower bands of sacral plexus in anatomic relationship to musculature of pelvic bowl. The upper sacral bands coalesce into the sciatic nerve on the ventral surface of the piriformis muscle.

3D-VRT NECT

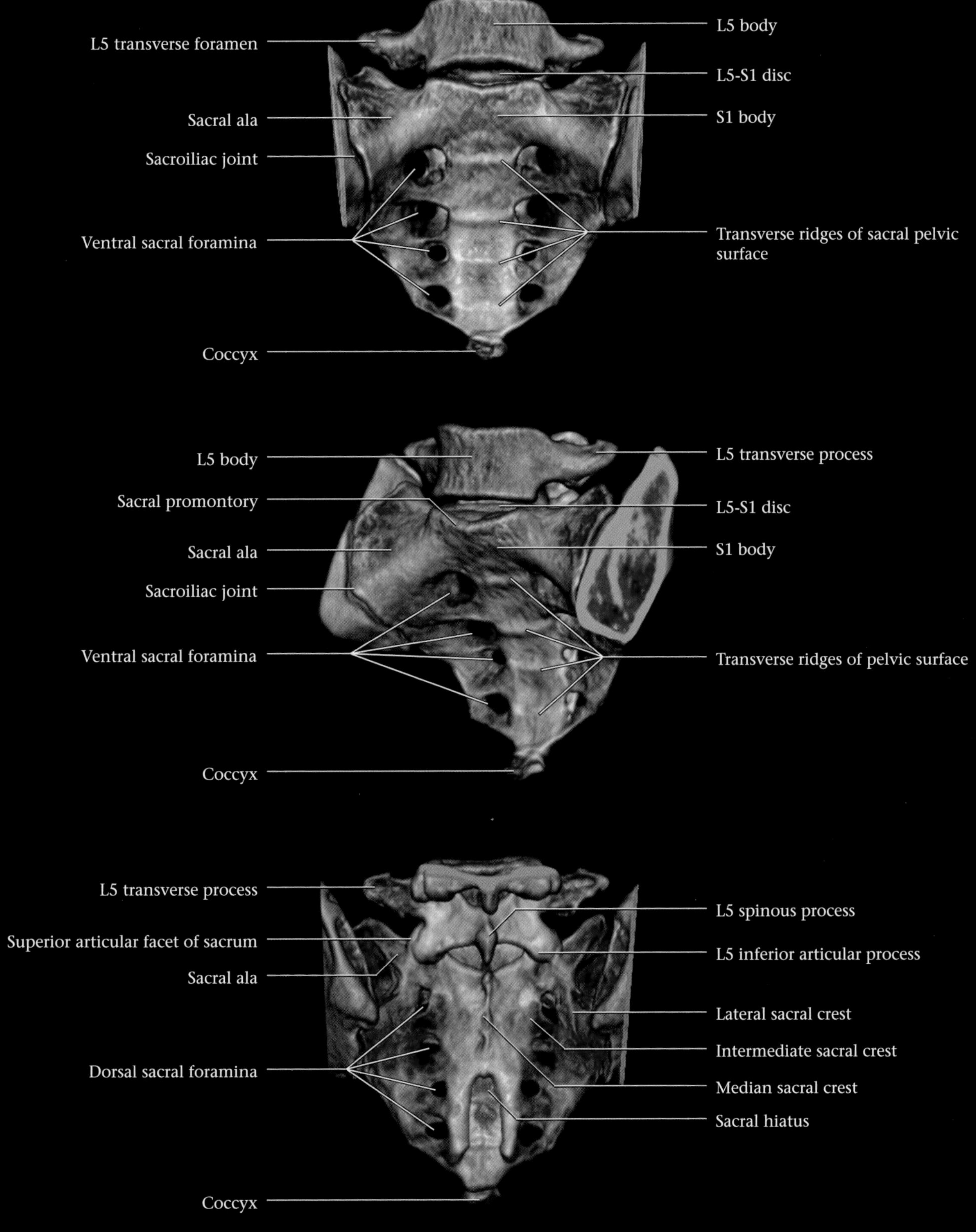
L5 transverse foramen
L5 body
L5-S1 disc
Sacral ala
S1 body
Sacroiliac joint
Ventral sacral foramina
Transverse ridges of sacral pelvic surface
Coccyx
L5 body
L5 transverse process
Sacral promontory
L5-S1 disc
Sacral ala
S1 body
Sacroiliac joint
Ventral sacral foramina
Transverse ridges of pelvic surface
Coccyx
L5 transverse process
L5 spinous process
Superior articular facet of sacrum
L5 inferior articular process
Sacral ala
Lateral sacral crest
Intermediate sacral crest
Dorsal sacral foramina
Median sacral crest
Sacral hiatus
Coccyx

(Top) Anterior view of a 3D-VRT NECT examination of the sacrum. The sacrum is seen as a large fused bony mass of 5 vertebra, forming the posterior aspect of the pelvis. The multiple sacral roots exit via the 4 paired sacral foramen. The superior aspect of the sacrum articulates with the inferior endplate of L5. **(Middle)** Anterior oblique view of a 3D-VRT NECT examination of the sacrum. The superior aspect of the sacrum, with the broad sacral ala & the sacral promontory are highlighted in this projection. **(Bottom)** Posterior view of a 3D-VRT NECT examination of the sacrum. The dorsal sacrum has vertically oriented ridges which are homologous to the more cephalad spinal column. The median sacral crest is homologous to the spinous processes. The intermediate sacral crest is analogous to the facets. The lateral sacral crest is analogous to the transverse process.

SACRUM AND COCCYX

AXIAL T2 MR

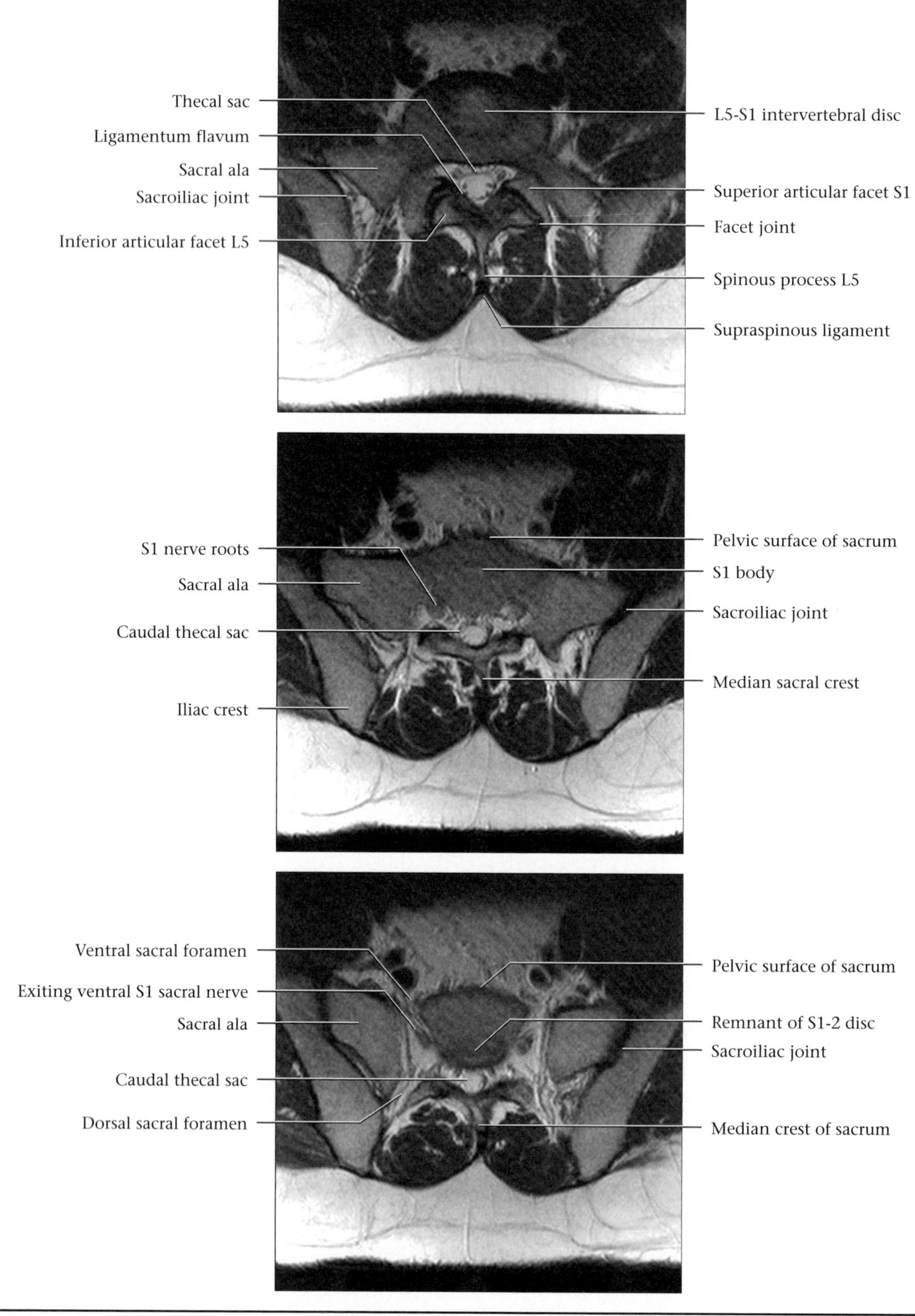
Thecal sac
Ligamentum flavum
Sacral ala
Sacroiliac joint
Inferior articular facet L5
L5-S1 intervertebral disc
Superior articular facet S1
Facet joint
Spinous process L5
Supraspinous ligament
S1 nerve roots
Sacral ala
Caudal thecal sac
Iliac crest
Pelvic surface of sacrum
S1 body
Sacroiliac joint
Median sacral crest
Ventral sacral foramen
Exiting ventral S1 sacral nerve
Sacral ala
Caudal thecal sac
Dorsal sacral foramen
Pelvic surface of sacrum
Remnant of S1-2 disc
Sacroiliac joint
Median crest of sacrum

(Top) First of six axial T2 MR images of the sacrum presented from superior to inferior. The lumbosacral facet articulations are visible between the functioning anterior positioned superior articular process of S1 (which faces medially & dorsally) articulating with the posterior positioned inferior articular facet of L5. **(Middle)** Image through S1 body. At this level, the sacral body & sacral ala are seen as one large bony mass extending between the lateral sacroiliac joints. Posteriorly, the median crest of the sacrum is prominent. **(Bottom)** Image more inferiorly through the S1/S2 junction. The exiting ventral & dorsal S1 nerves are seen passing through the ventral & dorsal foramina respectively.

AXIAL T2 MR

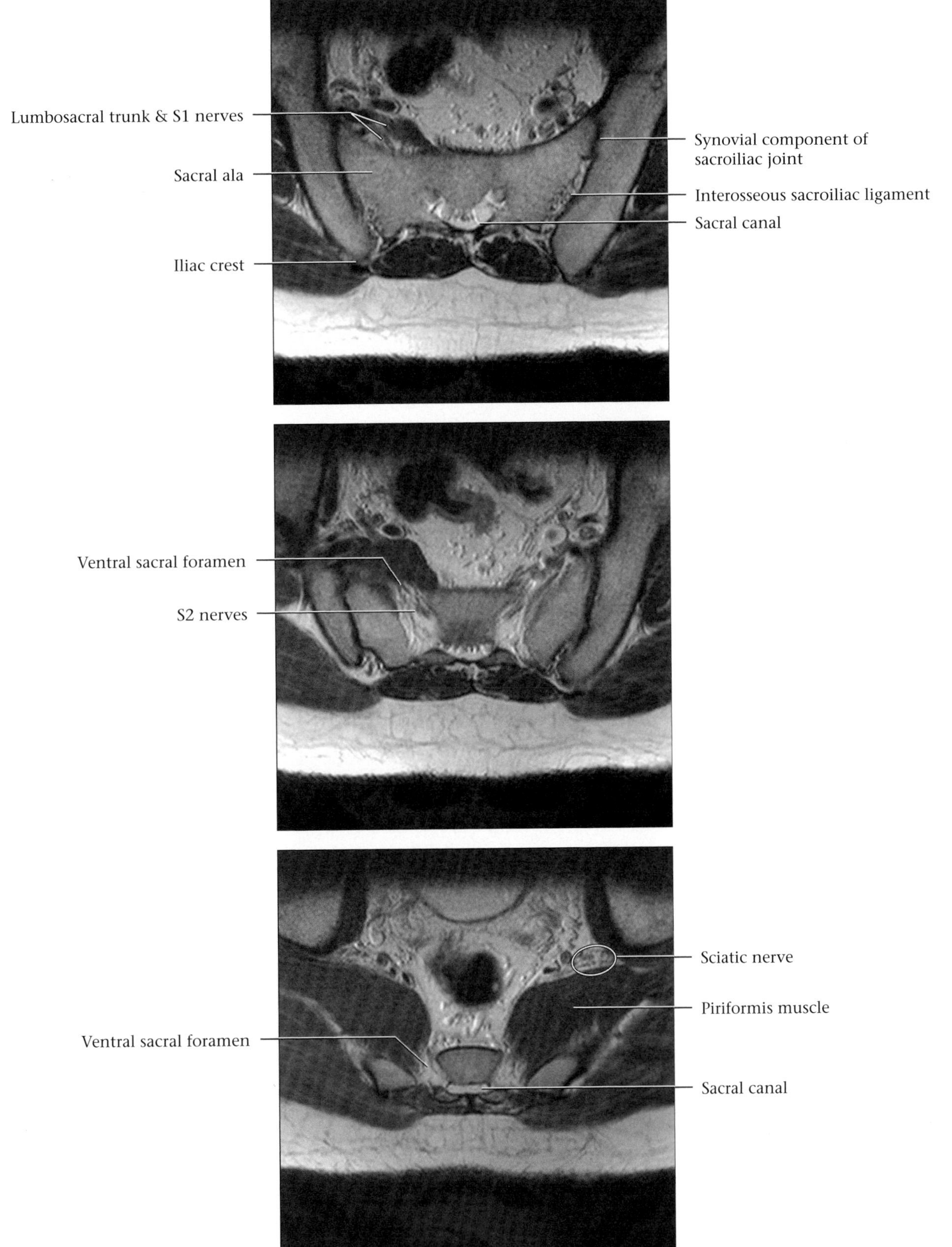

Lumbosacral trunk & S1 nerves
Sacral ala
Iliac crest
Synovial component of sacroiliac joint
Interosseous sacroiliac ligament
Sacral canal
Ventral sacral foramen
S2 nerves
Sciatic nerve
Piriformis muscle
Ventral sacral foramen
Sacral canal

(Top) Image through S2 body (incidental spina bifida is seen on this and the lower two images). At this level, the sacral body & sacral ala are again seen as one large bony mass extending between the lateral sacroiliac joints. The sacroiliac joints consist of a ventral synovial joint & a dorsal syndesmosis bridged by the interosseous sacroiliac ligament. The thecal sac has terminated at this level (S2) & the sacral canal now only contains peripheral lower sacral & coccygeal nerves, fat & extradural portion of filum terminale. **(Middle)** Ventral S2 nerves are seen exiting anteriorly. **(Bottom)** Section through lower sacrum demonstrates piriformis muscle arising from lateral sacrum & extending laterally through greater sciatic foramen. Note the large sciatic nerve on the anterior surface of the piriformis muscle.

AXIAL NECT

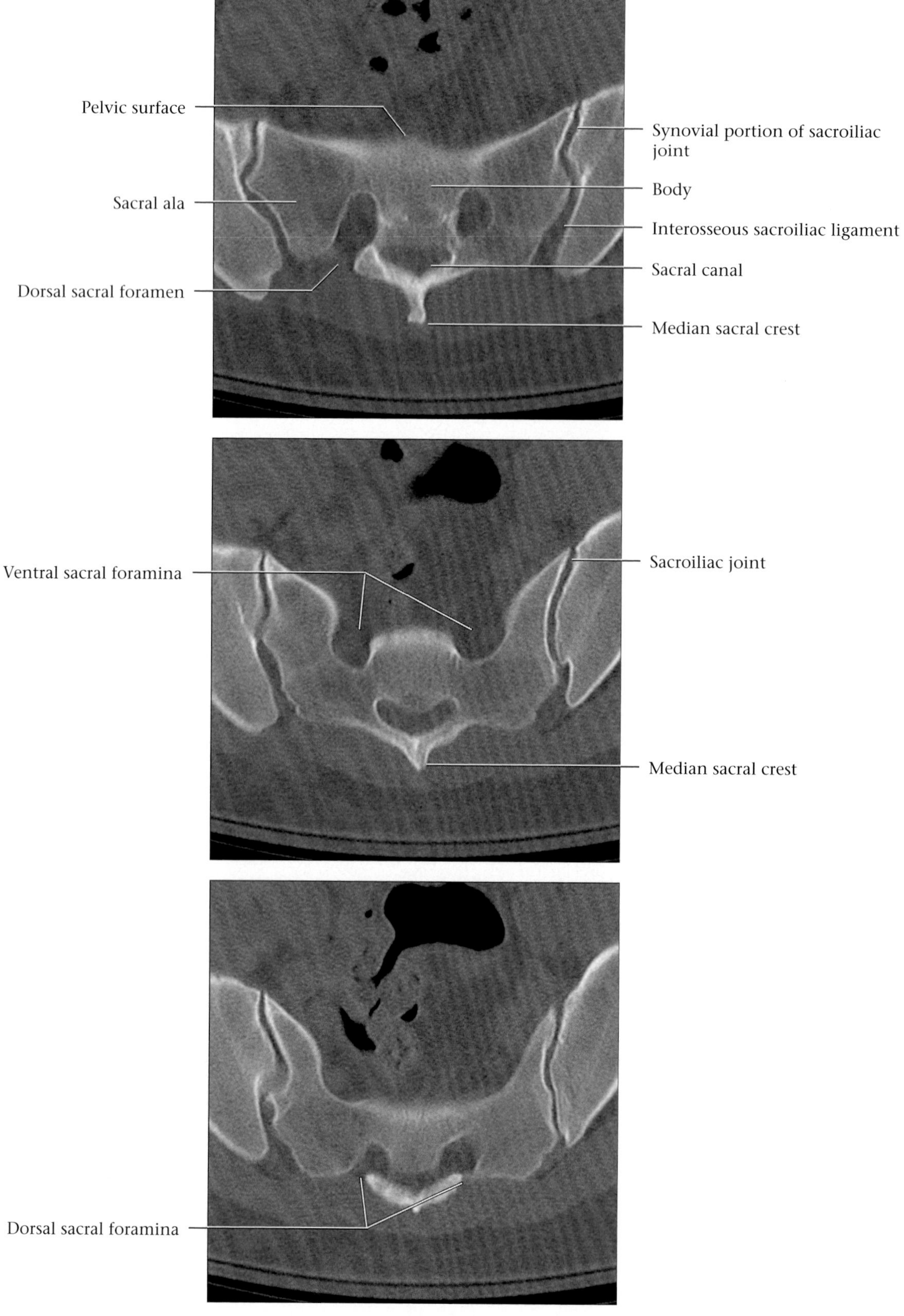

Pelvic surface
Sacral ala
Dorsal sacral foramen
Synovial portion of sacroiliac joint
Body
Interosseous sacroiliac ligament
Sacral canal
Median sacral crest
Ventral sacral foramina
Sacroiliac joint
Median sacral crest
Dorsal sacral foramina

(Top) First of three axial NECT images through sacrum presented from superior to inferior. Bony components of sacrum include central body, paired lateral ala & dorsal sacral canal. The different components of the sacroiliac joints are seen. The ventral synovial & dorsal syndesmosis are evident. **(Middle)** More inferior image through sacrum showing one of the 4 paired ventral sacral foramina where the S1-S4 ventral sacral nerves exit into the pelvis. **(Bottom)** Image through mid-sacrum showing one of the paired dorsal sacral foramina.

ANTERIOR RADIOGRAPH & CORONAL NECT

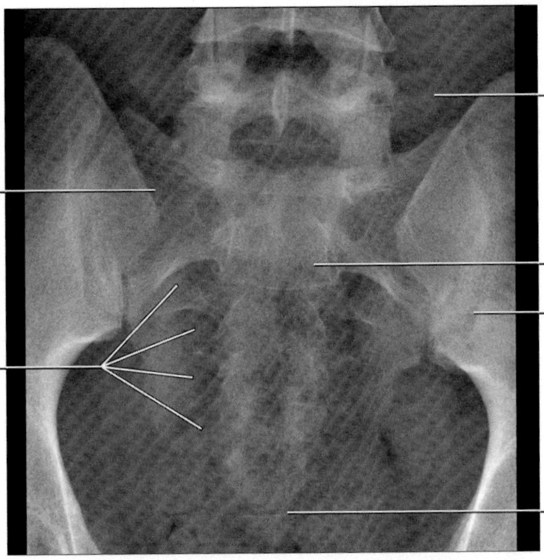

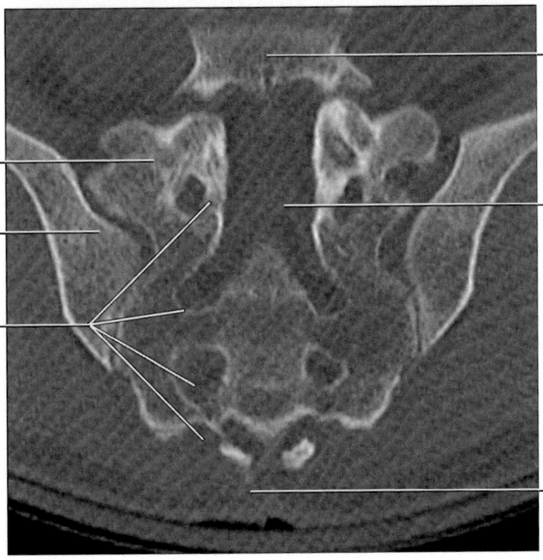

L5 transverse process
Sacral ala
Body
Sacroiliac joint
4 ventral sacral foramina
Sacrococcygeal joint

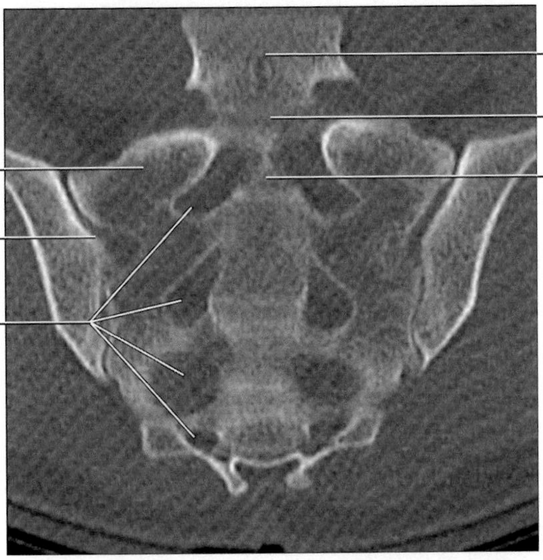

L5 body
L5-S1 disc
Sacral ala
S1 body
Sacroiliac joint
Ventral sacral foramina

L5 body
Sacral ala
S1 body
Sacroiliac joint
Ventral sacral foramen
Coccyx

(Top) Anterior radiograph of sacrum showing paired sacroiliac joints on either side of the triangular sacrum, composed of 5 fused sacral vertebrae. The ventral sacral foramina are clearly outlined by a corticated superomedial margin & an indistinct inferior margin. **(Middle)** Coronal CT image through the sacrum. The paired ventral sacral foramina are evident. The broad sacroiliac joint is identified. The fused 5 sacral segments are visible in the midline. **(Bottom)** More posterior image through the sacrum. The ventral sacral foramina are seen at various degrees of obliquity, giving a variety of appearances from circular to rectangular.

CORONAL T1 MR

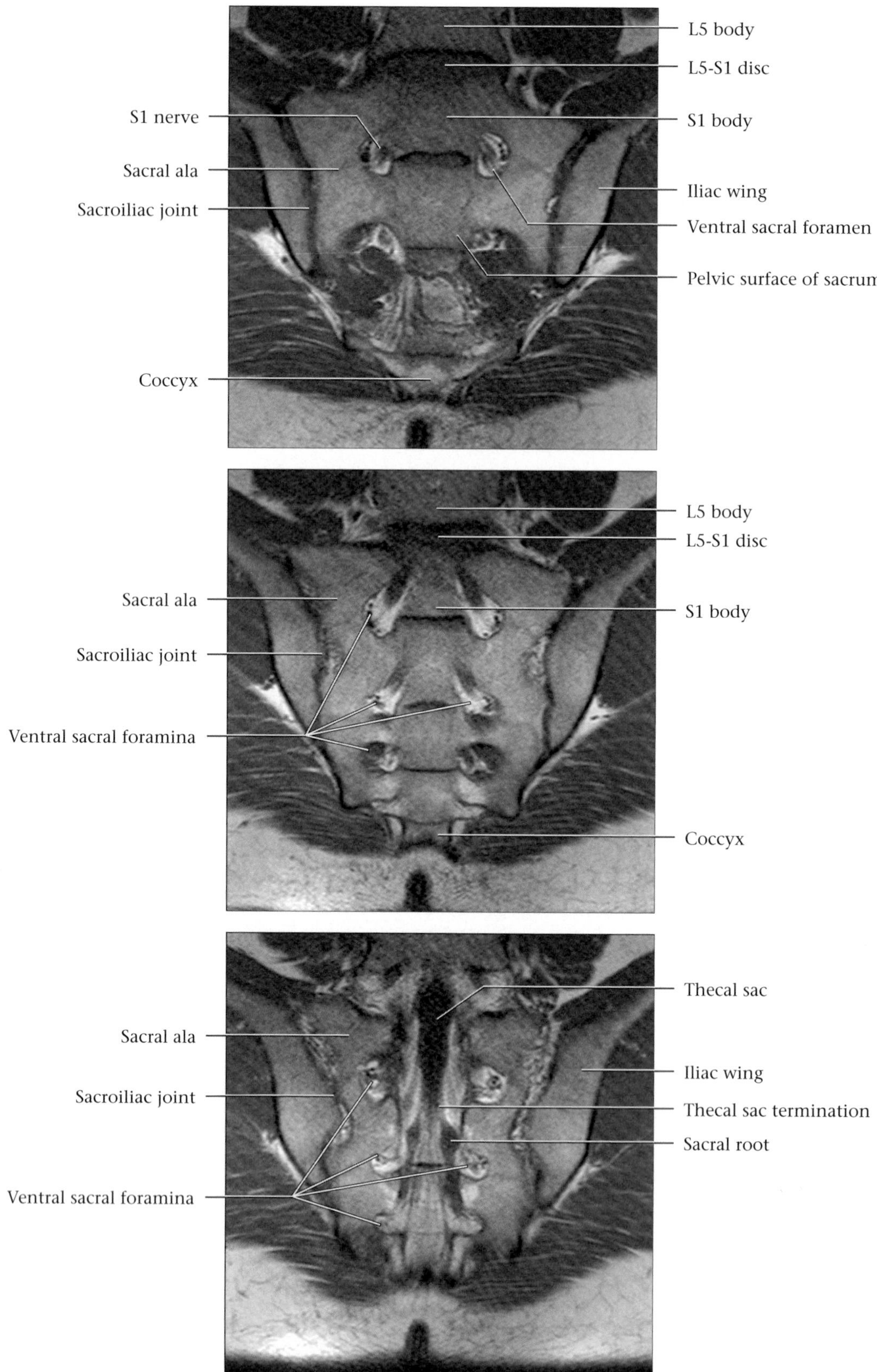
L5 body
L5-S1 disc
S1 nerve
S1 body
Sacral ala
Iliac wing
Sacroiliac joint
Ventral sacral foramen
Pelvic surface of sacrum
Coccyx
L5 body
L5-S1 disc
Sacral ala
S1 body
Sacroiliac joint
Ventral sacral foramina
Coccyx
Thecal sac
Sacral ala
Iliac wing
Sacroiliac joint
Thecal sac termination
Sacral root
Ventral sacral foramina

(Top) First of three coronal T1 MR images through the sacrum presented from anterior to posterior. The ventral sacral foramina are readily identified by the target appearance of cortical bone, foraminal fat & central nerve. The sacrum & coccyx are partially identified due to the sacral & coccygeal curvature. **(Middle)** Image through the mid-sacrum. The paired ventral sacral foramina are evident with their rounded foci of high signal fat with central low signal exiting roots. The broad sacroiliac joint is identified as low signal separating the ala from iliac wings. The fused 5 sacral segments are visible in the midline. **(Bottom)** In this image the distal thecal sac is evident terminating at S2 level.

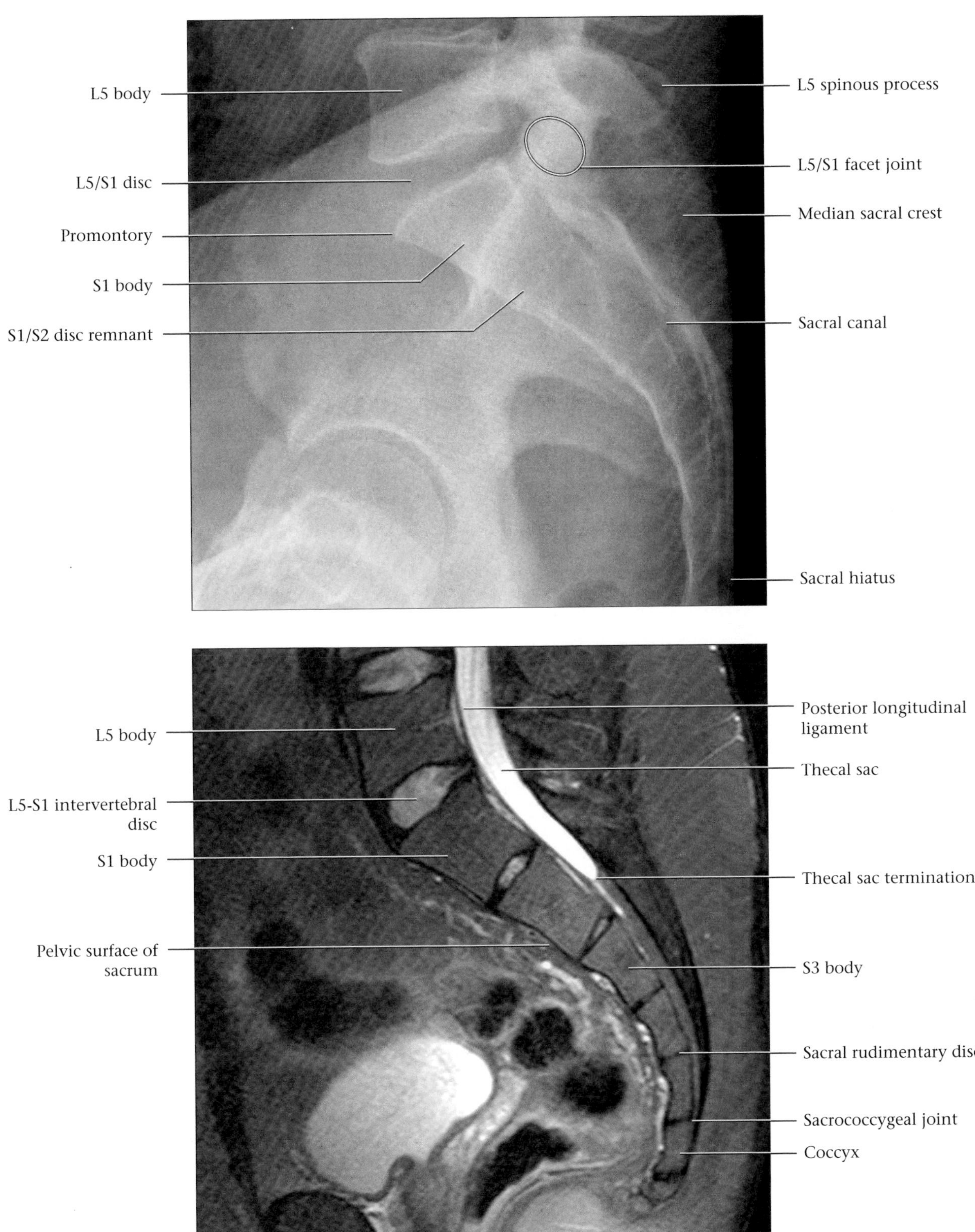

L5 body
L5/S1 disc
Promontory
S1 body
S1/S2 disc remnant
L5 spinous process
L5/S1 facet joint
Median sacral crest
Sacral canal
Sacral hiatus
L5 body
L5-S1 intervertebral disc
S1 body
Pelvic surface of sacrum
Posterior longitudinal ligament
Thecal sac
Thecal sac termination
S3 body
Sacral rudimentary disc
Sacrococcygeal joint
Coccyx

(Top) Lateral radiograph of sacrum & lumbosacral junction. Sacrum consists of 5 fused vertebrae with pelvic, dorsal & lateral surfaces. It articulates at its base with L5, at its apex with the coccyx & laterally with the iliac bones bilaterally. The anterior margin of S1 body is termed the promontory & forms the posterior margin of the pelvic inlet. **(Bottom)** Sagittal midline T2 weighted image of the sacrum. The typical lumbosacral junction morphology is present, with well-defined L5-S1 intervertebral disc, square shape of L5, & trapezoidal shape of S1. Rudimentary sacral intervertebral discs are seen as linear low signal. Note the thecal sac termination at the S2 level.

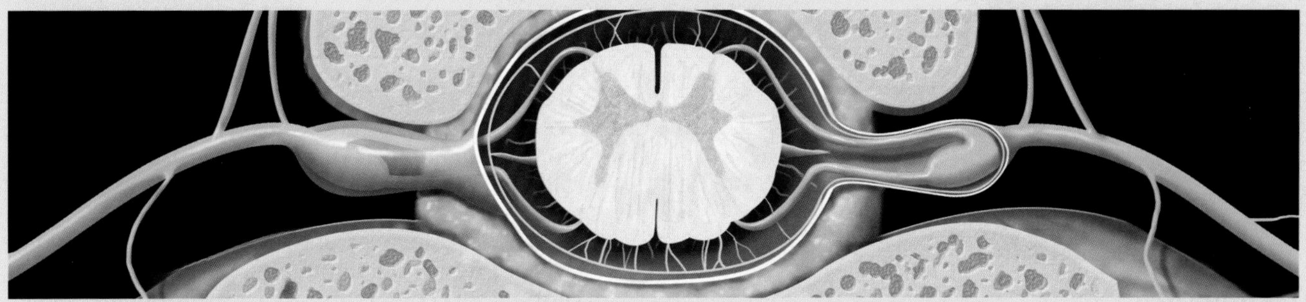

SECTION 2: Cord, Meninges and Spaces

SPINAL CORD AND CAUDA EQUINA

Terminology

Abbreviations

- Spinal cord (SC); cauda equina (CE)
- Cerebrospinal fluid (CSF); subarachnoid space (SAS)
- Dorsal root ganglion (DRG)

Definitions

- Tract: Nerve fibers with shared origin, destination or function
- Root: Coalescence of rootlets into dorsal (sensory), ventral (motor) roots
- Nerve: Union of dorsal, ventral roots
- Ganglion: Aggregation of cell bodies, nerve fibers

Gross Anatomy

Overview

- **Spinal cord**
  - Suspended within thecal sac
  - Anchored to dura by denticulate ligaments
  - Long tapered cylindrical conduit between medulla, peripheral nervous system
  - Two enlargements
    - Cervical enlargement (C3-T2) with maximum diameter at C6
    - Lumbar enlargement at T9-12
  - Cord tapers to diamond-shaped point (conus medullaris)
  - Conus normally ends between T12 to L2-3 interspace (T12-L1 most common level)
  - External landmarks
    - Deep ventral (anterior) median fissure extends along entire ventral surface
    - Dorsal (posterior) median sulcus is more shallow
    - Posterolateral sulcus (dorsal rootlets enter cord here)
    - Ventral rootlets emerge from ventrolateral sulci
  - Internal landmarks
    - In contrast to brain, gray matter is on inside with white matter on periphery of cord
    - Central gray matter formed by columns ("horns") of neuronal cell bodies, is roughly "H"-shaped
    - Anterior, posterior gray commissures connect two near-vertical arms of "H"
    - Ventral (anterior) horn of "H" is shorter, thicker, contains multipolar motor neurons
    - Dorsal (posterior) horn is longer, more narrow, receives sensory axons from DRGs
    - Small lateral horn only found between T2, L1 cord segments
    - Ependymal-lined central canal
    - Three white matter columns (funiculi): Dorsal, ventral, lateral
    - Descending motor, ascending sensory tracts mostly in lateral, ventral funiculi
    - Fibers for position, discriminative touch in dorsal funiculi
- **Filum terminale**
  - Strand of connective tissue extending inferiorly from conus
  - Fuses distally into dura, attaches to dorsal coccyx
- **Spinal nerve roots**
  - 8 cervical (first exits between skull base, C1), 12 thoracic, 5 lumbar, 5 sacral, 1 coccygeal
  - Paired dorsal, ventral roots exit from their respective hemicords
  - Descend separately across SAS, dura, then unite in/near intervertebral foramina
  - Ventral roots contain mostly efferent somatic, some sympathetic fibers
  - Dorsal roots mostly contain afferent axons (both somatic, visceral)
  - Lose pia at dorsal root ganglia level
- **Cauda equina**
  - "Horse's tail" of lumbar, sacral, coccygeal nerve roots below conus

Imaging Anatomy

Overview

- **Spinal cord**
  - "H"-shaped central gray matter hypointense compared to myelinated (hyperintense) white matter
  - Maximal cord diameter in axial section varies with location
    - Up to 75% at cervical enlargement
    - Generally 50% or less in thoracic region except for slight ↑ at thoracic enlargement
  - Filum terminale
    - Normally 2 mm or less in diameter
    - Has distal branch of anterior spinal artery, which normally enhances
- **Spinal nerve roots**
  - Course becomes longer, more oblique at caudal levels
  - Intrathecal nerve roots have blood-nerve barrier, do not normally enhance
  - DRG has no blood-nerve barrier, enhances normally
- **Cauda equina**
  - On axial T2WI, normally lie in a "U"-shaped configuration within thecal sac

Anatomy-Based Imaging Issues

Key Concepts or Questions

- Somatotopic cord organization predicates clinical findings, pathology
- Central gray matter = cord "watershed" zone
- Conus is at normal "adult" level at birth

Imaging Recommendations

- Multiplanar T2WI best demonstrates cord, roots
- T2 FSE or CISS sequence for "MR myelogram" effect

Imaging Pitfalls

- Sagittal plane less reliable than axial for determining conus position
- Pulsatile CSF flow, spin dephasing often causes "flow voids" and should not be mistaken for vascular malformation

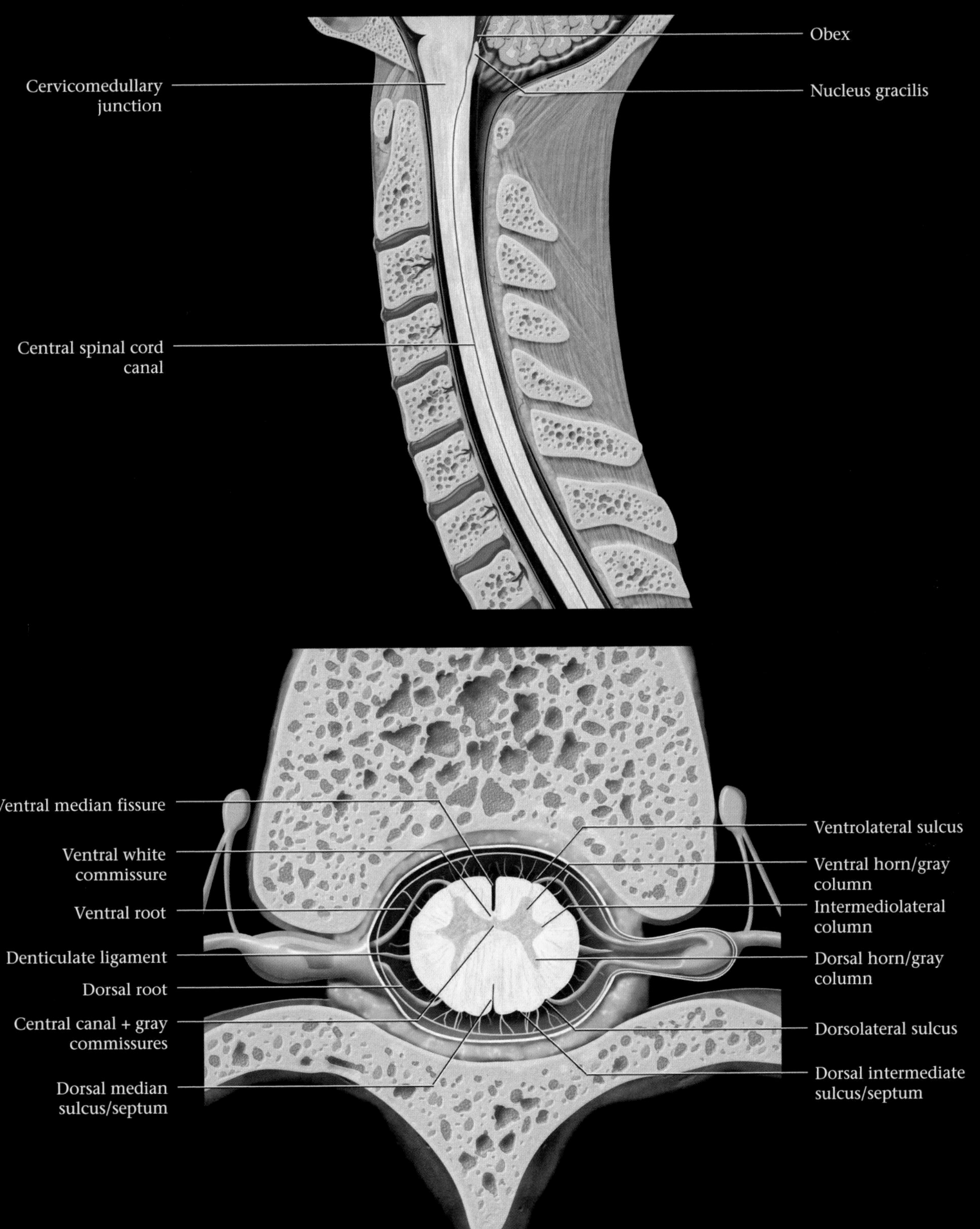

Obex
Cervicomedullary junction
Nucleus gracilis
Central spinal cord canal
Ventral median fissure
Ventrolateral sulcus
Ventral white commissure
Ventral horn/gray column
Ventral root
Intermediolateral column
Denticulate ligament
Dorsal horn/gray column
Dorsal root
Central canal + gray commissures
Dorsolateral sulcus
Dorsal median sulcus/septum
Dorsal intermediate sulcus/septum

(Top) Sagittal graphic of the cervical spinal cord. The central spinal cord canal is contiguous with the obex, the inferior point of the fourth ventricle. The transition from obex to central canal of the spinal cord is marked by the dorsal "bump" of the nucleus gracilis, which is easily seen on sagittal T2 MR scans through the craniocervical junction. **(Bottom)** Axial graphic depicts internal anatomy of the distal thoracic spinal cord. The deep ventral median fissure divides the ventral hemicords, while the smaller dorsal median sulcus/septum divides the dorsal hemicords. The dorsal intermediate sulcus separates the dorsal funiculus into gracile and cuneate tracts. The dorsal and ventral nerve roots arise from the dorsolateral and ventrolateral sulci respectively.

SPINAL CORD AND CAUDA EQUINA

GRAPHICS

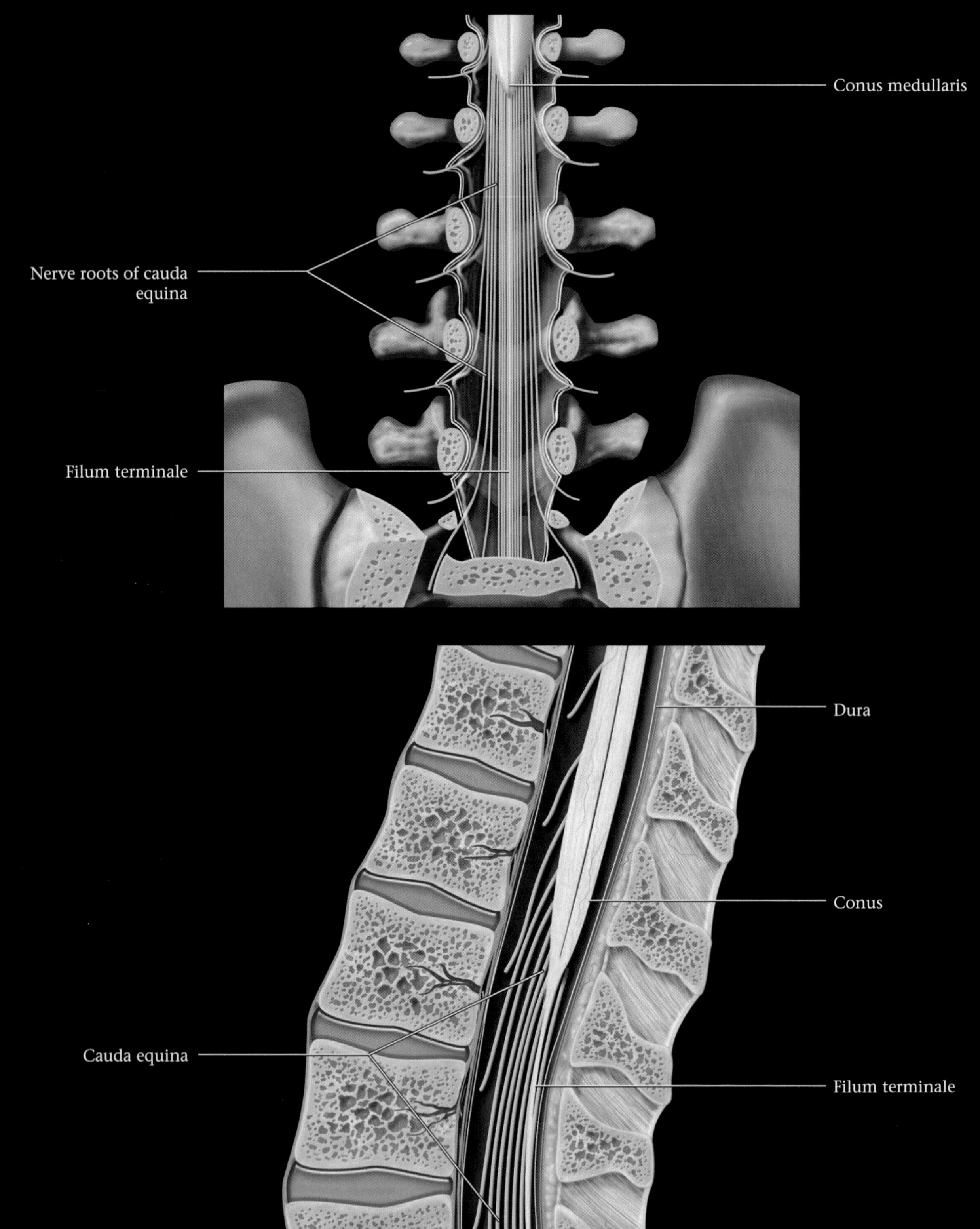
Conus medullaris
Nerve roots of cauda equina
Filum terminale
Dura
Conus
Cauda equina
Filum terminale

(Top) Coronal graphic through the middle of the spinal canal shows the distal thoracic spinal cord and nerve roots of the cauda equina. Note the cord ends in a diamond-shaped point, the conus medullaris. Lumbar nerve roots exit the thecal sac just under the pedicles of their same-numbered vertebral segments. The filum terminale is a strand of connective tissue that extends inferiorly from the conus to the dorsal coccyx. It typically contains no functional neural tissue and no fat. **(Bottom)** Sagittal graphic of the thoracolumbar junction demonstrates normal conus and cauda equina anatomy. The filum terminale lies among the cauda equina roots and affixes the conus to the terminal thecal sac.

CORONAL CT MYELOGRAM

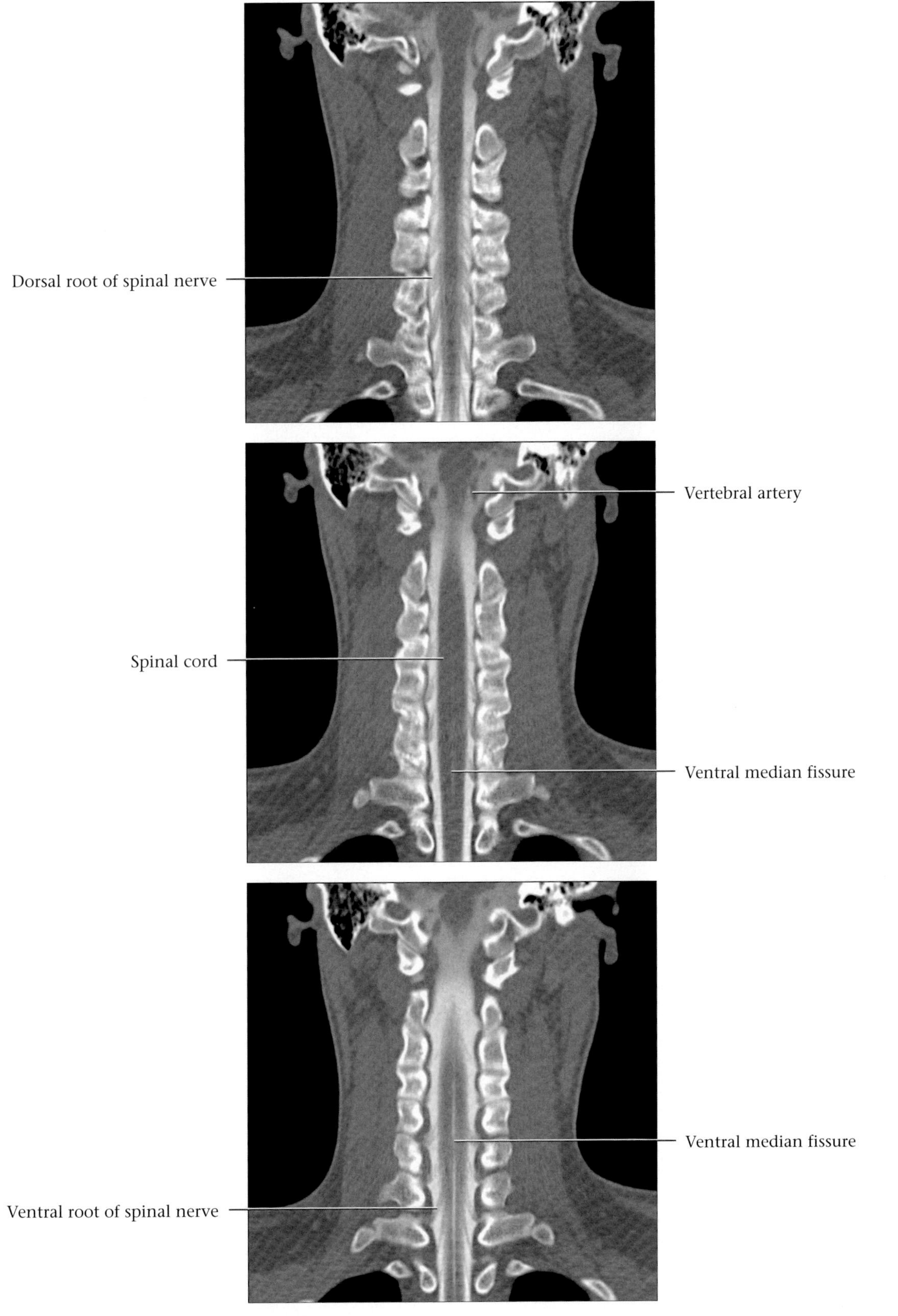
Dorsal root of spinal nerve
Vertebral artery
Spinal cord
Ventral median fissure
Ventral median fissure
Ventral root of spinal nerve

(Top) First of three coronal CT myelograms presented from posterior to anterior demonstrates the dorsal (sensory) roots surrounded by dense CSF. **(Middle)** This image depicts the spinal cord within the thecal sac. The central spinal cord canal may imbibe myelographic contrast in some cases (especially on delayed scans), although in this case the high density in the central cord represents partial volume averaging with the ventral median fissure. Note that CT provides little information regarding the internal cord structure due to its limited contrast resolution. **(Bottom)** This image shows the ventral spinal cord and ventral (motor) nerve roots and dense contrast opacified CSF within the ventral median fissure.

SPINAL CORD AND CAUDA EQUINA

CORONAL CT MYELOGRAM

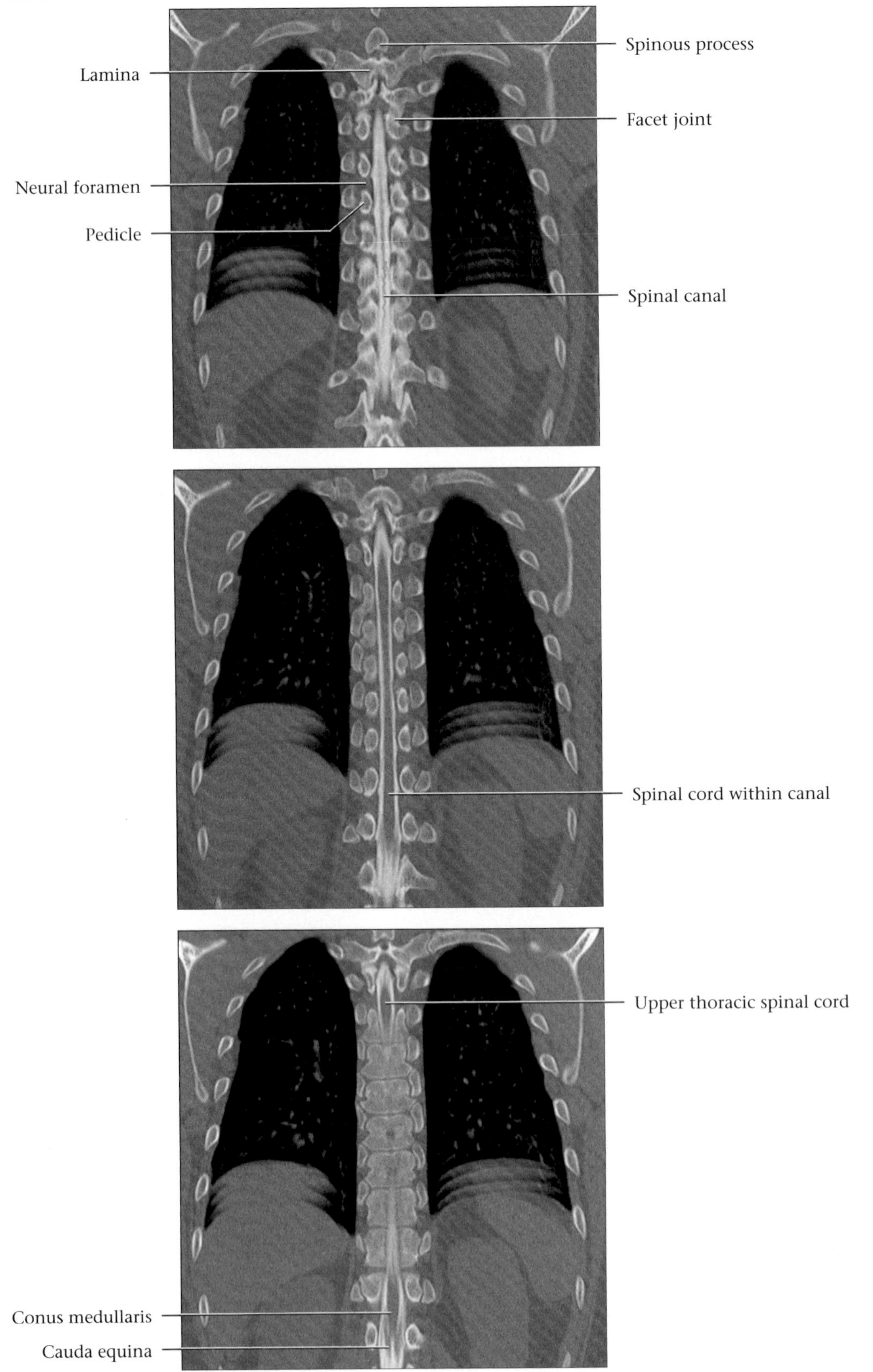
Lamina
Spinous process
Facet joint
Neural foramen
Pedicle
Spinal canal
Spinal cord within canal
Upper thoracic spinal cord
Conus medullaris
Cauda equina

(Top) First of three coronal reformatted images from CT myelogram through the thoracic spine presented from posterior to anterior. The posterior spinal canal is identified with the intrathecal contrast, bounded laterally by the pairs of medial rib/pedicles seen as well-defined corticated oval bony densities. With the normal thoracic kyphosis, the superior & inferior thoracic spine is seen in more anterior section than the mid portion. **(Middle)** More anterior image through mid-canal level. In the thoracic spine, the cord typically occupies approximately 50% of the subarachnoid space. **(Bottom)** Image through the posterior vertebral body level. The conus medullaris is well seen here. There is a slight expansion of the distal thoracic spinal cord before it tapers into its diamond-shaped point, the conus.

SPINAL CORD AND CAUDA EQUINA

SAGITTAL T2 & CORONAL STIR MR

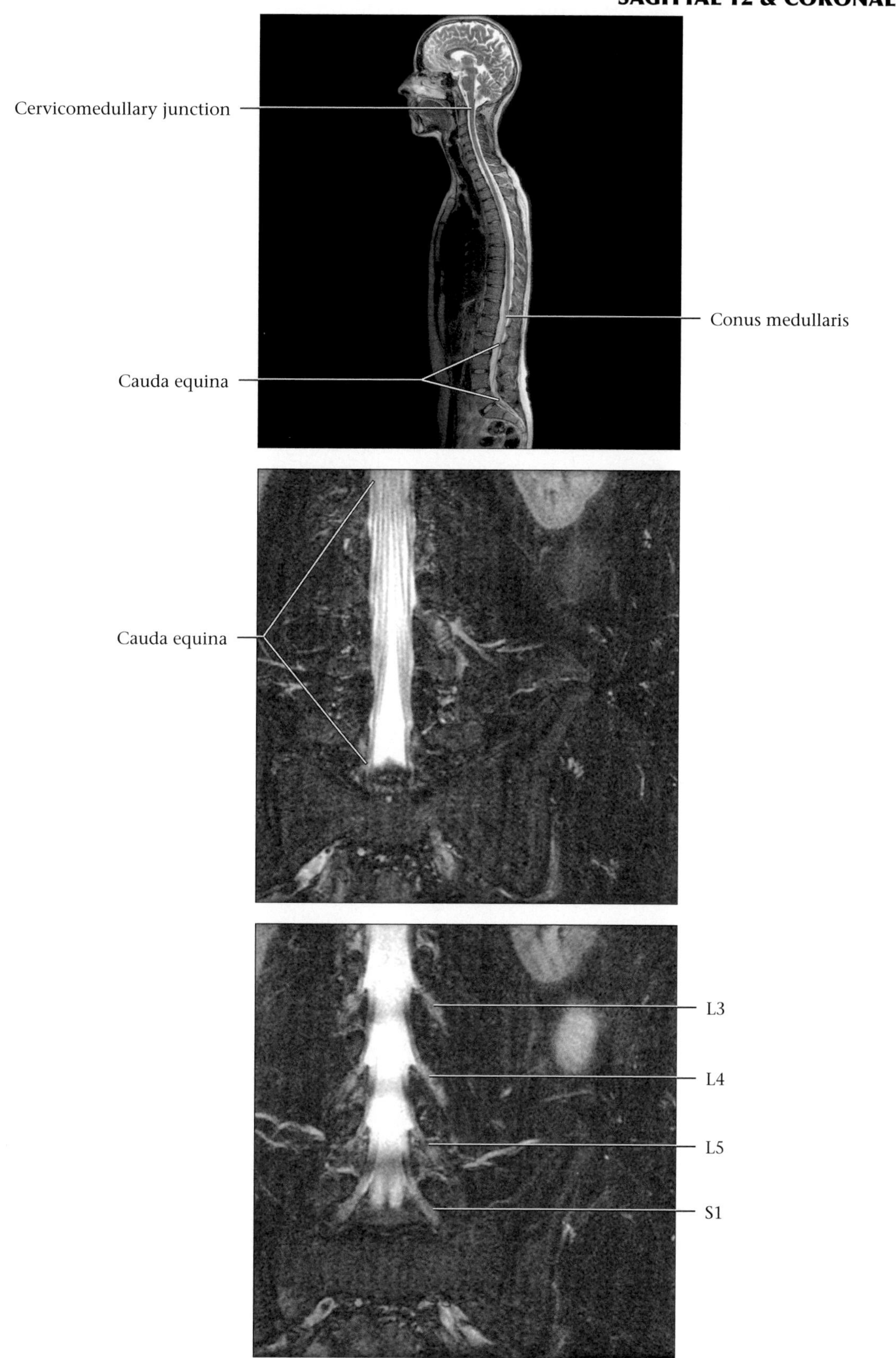
Cervicomedullary junction
Conus medullaris
Cauda equina
Cauda equina
L3
L4
L5
S1

(Top) Sagittal T2 MR demonstrates the entire spinal cord from the cervicomedullary junction to the conus. The cauda equina is draped dependently within the caudal thecal sac. Although the patient is imaged supine, it is typical for the normal thoracic spinal cord to be anteriorly positioned and conus posteriorly positioned in the thecal sac because of the normal kyphotic thoracic and lordotic lumbar curvature. **(Middle)** First of two coronal STIR MR images demonstrates the cauda equina roots somatotopically organized within the caudal thecal sac. The nerve roots are arranged with more rostral (lumbar) levels laterally and caudal (sacral, coccygeal) levels medially. **(Bottom)** A more ventral image shows the lumbosacral spinal nerves exiting through their named neural foramina.

AXIAL CISS & T2 MR

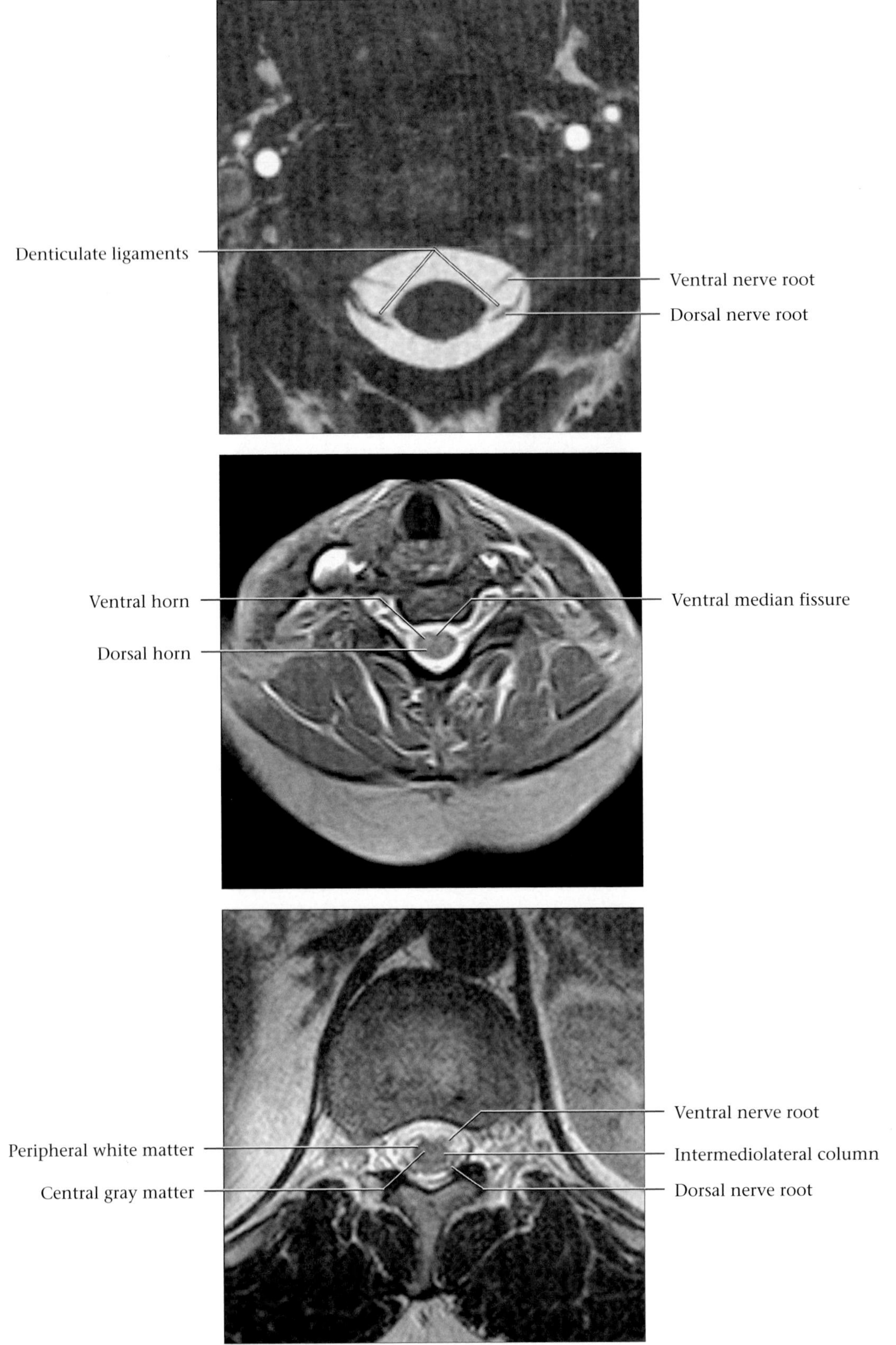

Denticulate ligaments
Ventral nerve root
Dorsal nerve root
Ventral horn
Dorsal horn
Ventral median fissure
Peripheral white matter
Central gray matter
Ventral nerve root
Intermediolateral column
Dorsal nerve root

(Top) Axial CISS sequence provides bright, homogeneous CSF signal intensity. The hypointense bilateral denticulate ligaments anchor the spinal cord to the dura. The dorsal and ventral roots are resolved as separate structures within the thecal sac, and join at the neural foramen to produce the proper spinal nerve. **(Middle)** First of two axial T2 MR images shows the normal cervical spinal cord gray and white matter clearly delineated. The intermediolateral gray matter column representing the cell bodies of the sympathetic nervous system is only present in the thoracolumbar spinal cord and not seen at the cervical level. **(Bottom)** Image of the conus demonstrates normal conus anatomy. The peripheral white matter and central gray matter are easily distinguished. Note the characteristic bump of the intermediolateral column of the sympathetic nervous system.

SPINAL CORD AND CAUDA EQUINA

AXIAL T2 MR

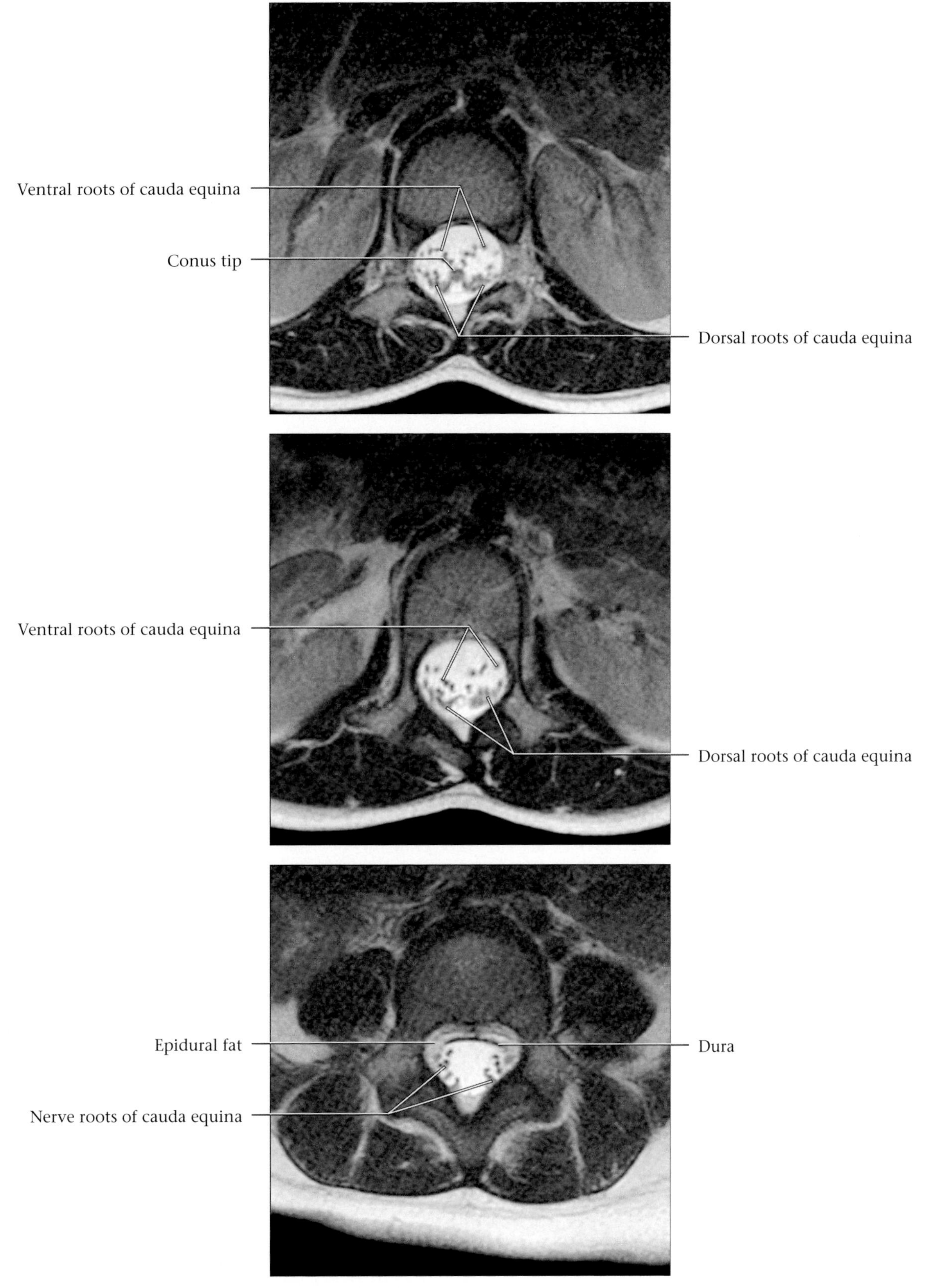
Ventral roots of cauda equina
Conus tip
Dorsal roots of cauda equina
Ventral roots of cauda equina
Dorsal roots of cauda equina
Epidural fat
Dura
Nerve roots of cauda equina

(Top) First of three axial T2 MR images at the L1 foraminal level shows the conus tip and cauda equina. At this level, the ventral and dorsal nerve roots of the cauda equina are separately positioned ventrally and dorsally respectively within the thecal sac. **(Middle)** This image at the mid L2 level reveals the cauda equina nerve roots moving laterally in preparation to form the spinal nerve proper and exit through the appropriate neural foramen. Note that the ventral roots remain ventral and dorsal roots dorsal. **(Bottom)** This image at the L4 level shows the nerve roots losing their ventral/dorsal orientation in order to congregate near the lateral thecal sac in preparation to form the appropriate spinal nerves. At this and lower levels the roots assume a "U" shaped configuration around the margins of the thecal sac.

SPINAL CORD AND CAUDA EQUINA

LONGITUDINAL ULTRASOUND

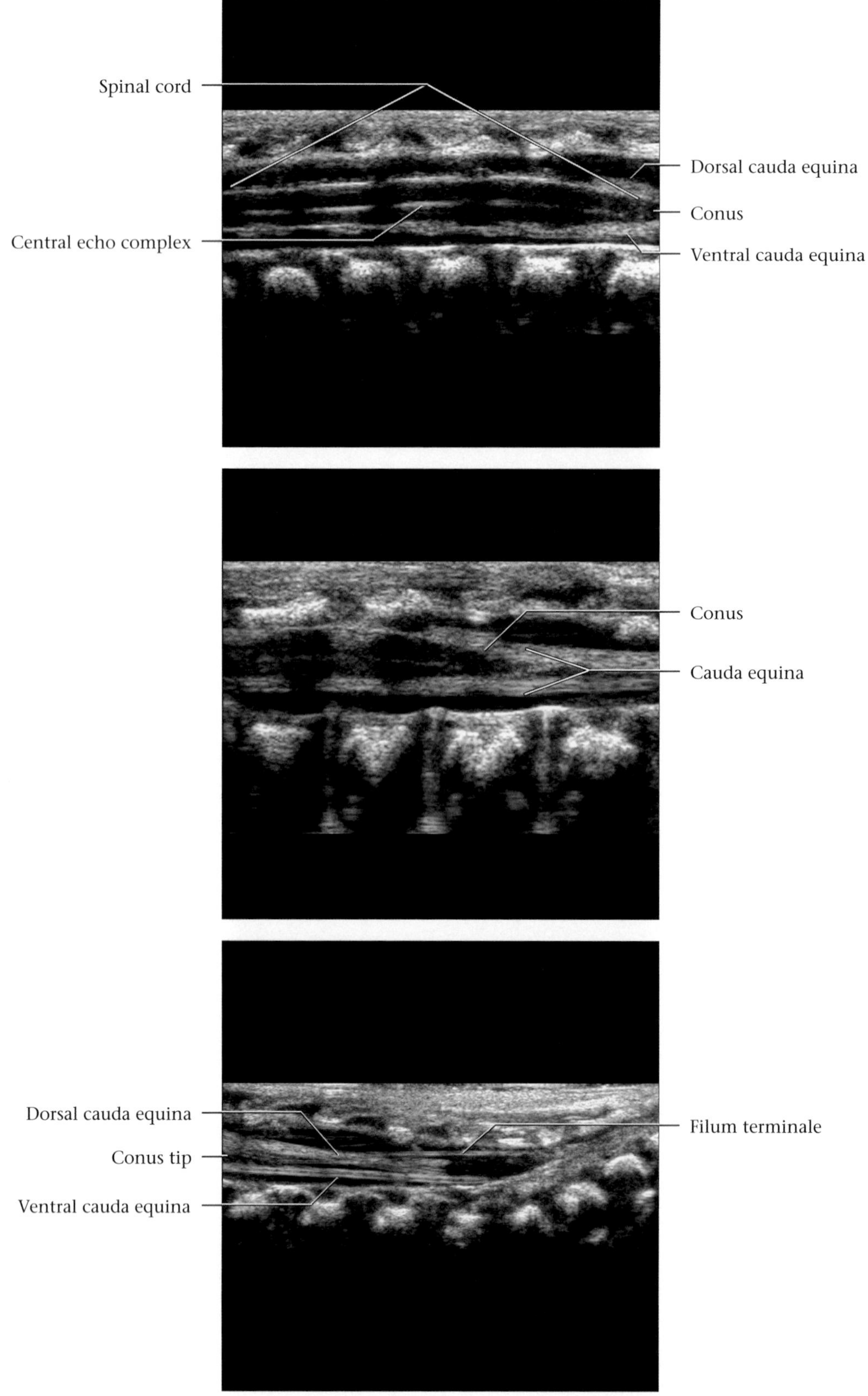
Spinal cord
Central echo complex
Dorsal cauda equina
Conus
Ventral cauda equina
Conus
Cauda equina
Dorsal cauda equina
Conus tip
Ventral cauda equina
Filum terminale

(Top) First of three longitudinal ultrasound images shows the normal hypoechoic spinal cord with hyperechoic central echo complex. Contrary to popular misunderstanding, this central echo complex is a reflection of echoes from the interface between the ventral white commissure and CSF within the ventral median fissure rather than from the central canal. **(Middle)** Image centered more caudally best demonstrates the hypoechoic spinal cord terminating as the conus. The hyperechoic cauda equina drapes around the conus and undulates with each CSF pulsation during real-time observation. **(Bottom)** This image demonstrates the mildly hyperechoic filum terminale anchoring the spinal cord to the terminal thecal sac. The cauda equina nerve roots drape dependently within the thecal sac.

TRANSVERSE ULTRASOUND

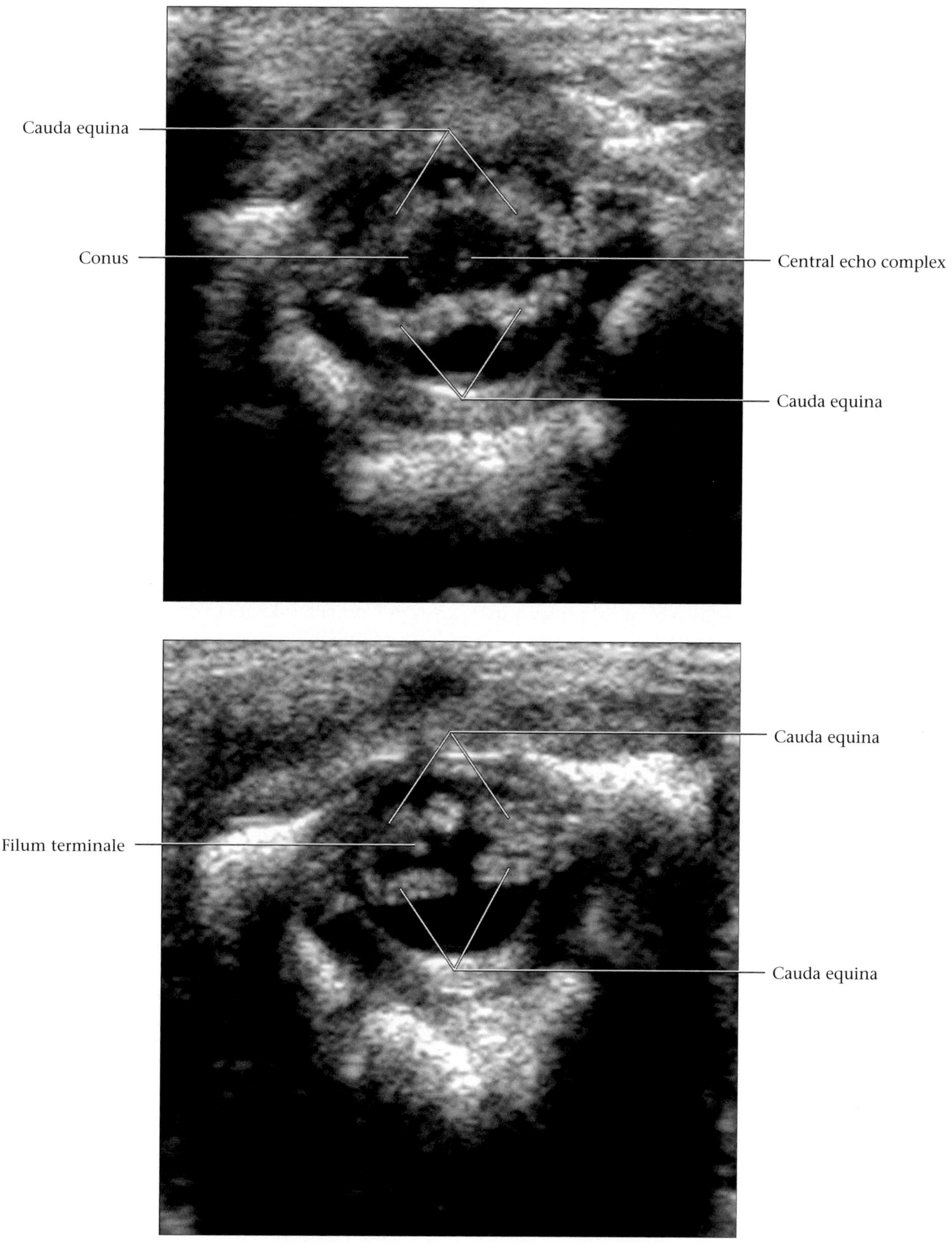
Cauda equina
Conus
Central echo complex
Cauda equina
Cauda equina
Filum terminale
Cauda equina

(Top) First of two transverse ultrasound images demonstrates the hypoechoic conus surrounded by hyperechoic cauda equina nerve roots. The central echo complex is well visualized. **(Bottom)** A more caudal image shows the hypoechoic cauda equina suspended within cerebrospinal fluid. The filum is positioned centrally within the cauda equina.

MENINGES AND COMPARTMENTS

Terminology

Abbreviations

- Dorsal root ganglia (DRG)

Definitions

- Meninges = collective term for dura, arachnoid, pia
  - Pachy ("thick") meninges = dura
  - Lepto ("thin") meninges = arachnoid, pia
- Spaces = real or potential spaces between meningeal layers or adjacent structures
- Ligaments = suspend cord within thecal sac
- Compartments = anatomic construct for location-based imaging differential diagnoses

Gross Anatomy

Overview

- **Meninges**
  - **Dura**
    - Dense, tough outermost layer of connective tissue
    - Only one dural layer in spine
    - Attached by fibrous bands to posterior longitudinal ligament
    - Tubular prolongations of dura/arachnoid extend around roots/nerves through intervertebral foramina, terminate near DRG
    - Dura fuses with epineurium of spinal nerves distal to DRG
  - **Arachnoid**
    - Thin, delicate, continuous with cranial arachnoid
    - Two layers: Outer (loosely attached to dura), intermediate (attached to pia)
  - **Pia**
    - Delicate, innermost layer of meninges
    - Closely applied to cord, spinal nerves
- **Ligaments**
  - **Denticulate ligaments**
    - Flat, fibrous, serrated sheets that support spinal cord
    - Collagenous core is continuous with pia
    - Extend laterally from pia along each side of cord, between ventral/dorsal roots
    - Insert into dura mater
  - **Dorsal, dorsolateral, ventral spinal cord ligaments**
    - Thin irregular, fenestrated; extend from cord to arachnoid
  - **Septum posticum**
    - Incomplete longitudinal midline membrane
    - Connects pia/cord dorsally to dura
    - Partially divides subarachnoid space (SAS), creating "pseudocompartments"
- **Spaces**
  - **Epidural** space (extradural compartment)
    - Between dura & surrounding vertebral canal
    - Extends from foramen magnum to posterior sacrococcygeal ligament
    - Contains fat, loose connective tissue, small arteries, veins, lymphatics
  - **Subdural** space
    - Potential space between dura, outer surface of arachnoid
  - **Subarachnoid** space (SAS)
    - Between inner surface of arachnoid, pia
    - Contains CSF, vessels, spinal cord ligaments, nerves, filum terminale
    - Continuous with intracranial SAS
  - **Subpial** space (potential space only)
- **Compartments**
  - **Extradural** compartment
    - Epidural space
    - Vertebral bodies, neural arches, intervertebral discs, paraspinous muscles
  - **Intradural extramedullary** compartment
    - SAS
    - Spinal cord ligaments, nerve roots, cauda equina, filum terminale
  - **Intramedullary** compartment
    - Spinal cord, pia

Imaging Anatomy

Overview

- **Meninges**
  - Dura
    - Thin black line on T2WI
    - Vessels lack endothelial tight junctions so dura enhances strongly, uniformly
  - Arachnoid
    - Normally adheres to dura; not visualized separately
- **Ligaments**
  - Seen as thin, linear "filling defects" on T2WI
- **Spaces**
  - Spinal CSF isointense with intracranial CSF

Anatomy-Based Imaging Issues

Key Concepts or Questions

- Localization of a lesion to specific anatomic compartment greatly assists differential diagnosis
- Position of spinal needle for lumbar puncture, myelography should be in SAS
  - Spinal needles are beveled, may "tent" arachnoid as they are pushed through dura
  - May result in "split" injection (mixed subarachnoid, subdural contrast)
  - Subdural injection usually localized
  - Epidural injection results in "epidurogram" with contrast spreading freely in epidural space, along nerve roots

Imaging Recommendations

- T2 weighted, CISS sequences best for "MR myelogram"
- Nicely demonstrate spinal meninges, ligaments, outline cord/roots

Imaging Pitfalls

- Denticulate ligaments, septum posticum create "pseudocompartments" where CSF may flow at different rates, directions
- Spin dephasing → "flow voids" in CSF, should not be mistaken for vascular malformation!

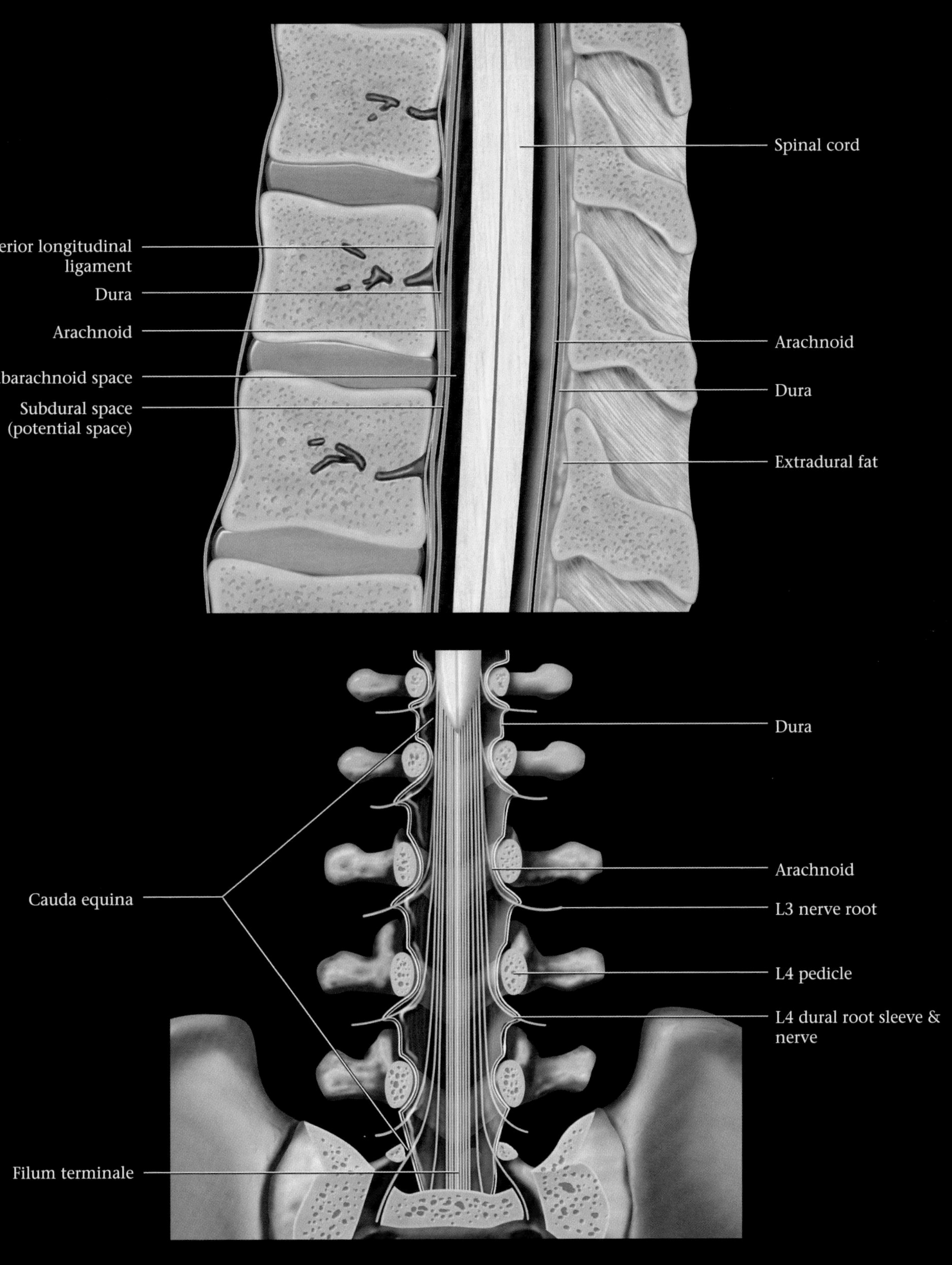

terior longitudinal ligament
Dura
Arachnoid
ubarachnoid space
Subdural space (potential space)
Spinal cord
Arachnoid
Dura
Extradural fat
Dura
Cauda equina
Arachnoid
L3 nerve root
L4 pedicle
L4 dural root sleeve & nerve
Filum terminale

) Sagittal graphic of thoracic level showing relationship of central cord and surrounding meninges within ebral canal. The thick dura defines the intra- & extradural compartments. Extradural compartment contains arily fat and veins. Arachnoid is closely adherent to inner dura creating the potential subdural space. rachnoid space contains CSF which surrounds the spinal cord, and is continuous with intracranial subarachnoid cisterns. Pia mater is closely adherent to the surface of the cord. **(Bottom)** Coronal cutaway graphic onstrates relationship between dura, nerve roots. Note nerve root/sleeve exit spinal canal just under the pedicle e same numbered level.

GRAPHICS

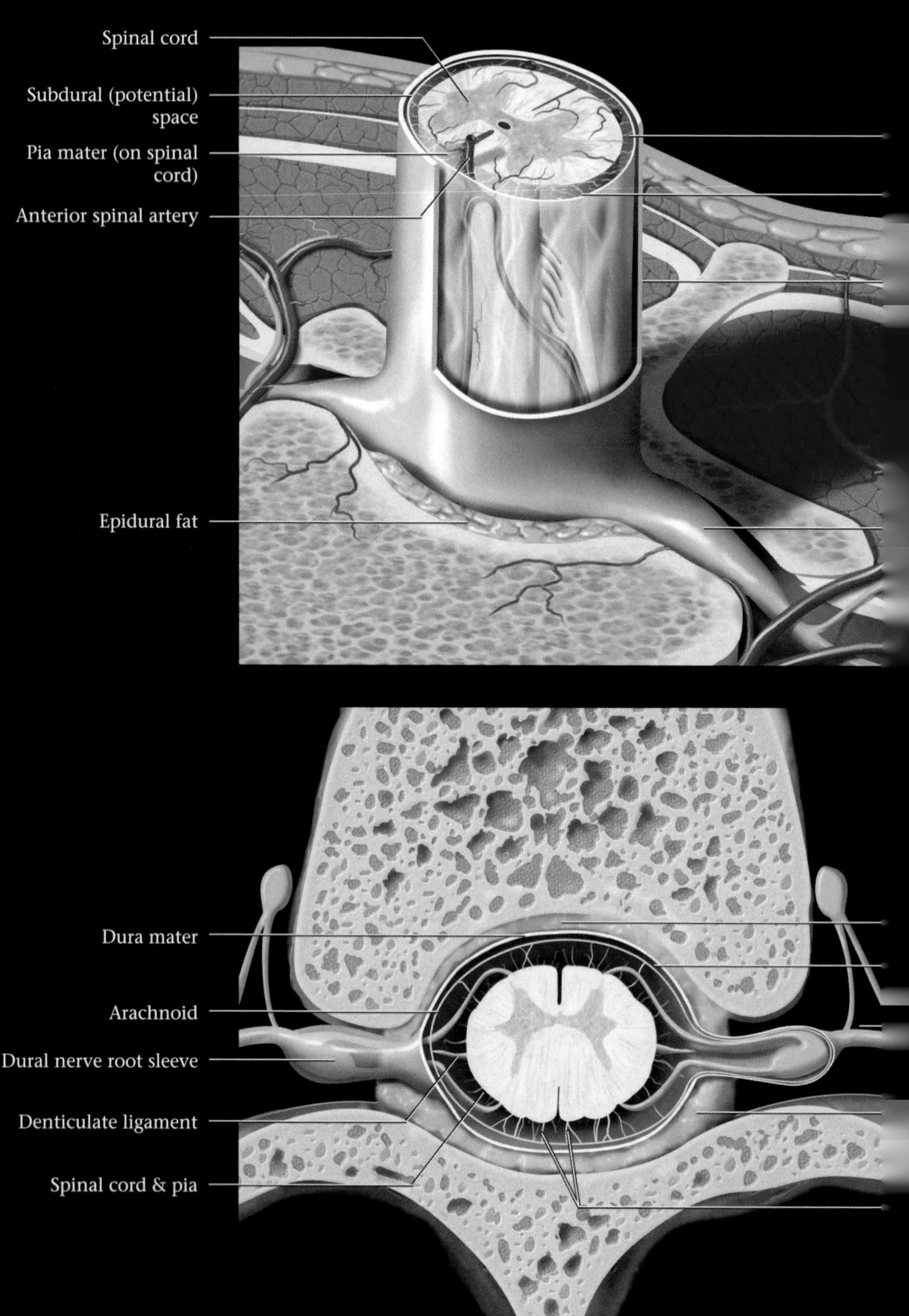
Spinal cord
Subdural (potential) space
Pia mater (on spinal cord)
Anterior spinal artery
Epidural fat
Dura mater
Arachnoid
Dural nerve root sleeve
Denticulate ligament
Spinal cord & pia

(Top) Cut-away graphic of the spinal cord and its coverings demonstrates the meningeal lay to adjacent regional structures. **(Bottom)** Axial graphic demonstrates cross sectional anatom meningeal layers. Nerve root sleeves are directly contiguous with the dura mater which join epineurium lateral to the neural foramen. Arachnoid lines root sleeves. The web-like tissue v space represents the inner trabecular portion of the arachnoid mater. The denticulate ligame dorsal and ventral spinal nerve roots and anchor the spinal cord laterally to the dura mater

AXIAL CT MYELOGRAM

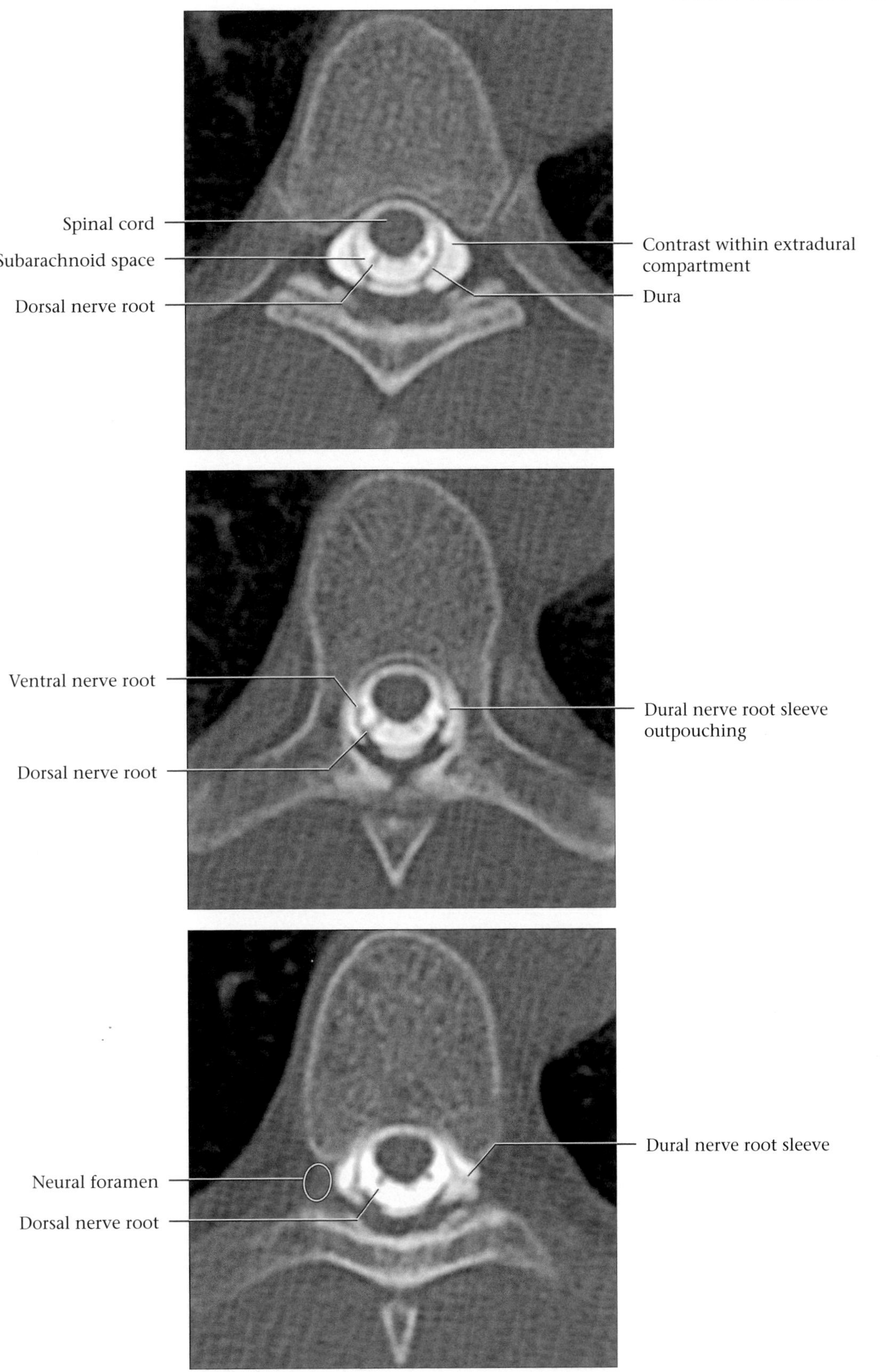
Spinal cord
Subarachnoid space
Dorsal nerve root
Contrast within extradural compartment
Dura
Ventral nerve root
Dorsal nerve root
Dural nerve root sleeve outpouching
Neural foramen
Dorsal nerve root
Dural nerve root sleeve

(Top) First of three axial CT myelogram images through thoracic spine presented from superior to inferior in a patient with a CSF leak. Contrast injected into the subarachnoid space has leaked into the extradural compartment and as a result beautifully demonstrates the dura surrounded on both sides by contrast material. **(Middle)** The ventral and dorsal nerve roots are seen traversing the subarachnoid space toward the dural nerve root sleeve, which is an outpouching of dura and arachnoid. **(Bottom)** Here the dural nerve root sleeve containing the exiting nerve is seen extending laterally towards the neural foramen surrounded by CSF in the extradural compartment. Dura of nerve root sleeve is directly contiguous with the peripheral nerve epineurium lateral to the neural foramen. The dorsal nerve root exiting at the next level down is seen within the subarachnoid space.

LONGITUDINAL & TRANSVERSE ULTRASOUND

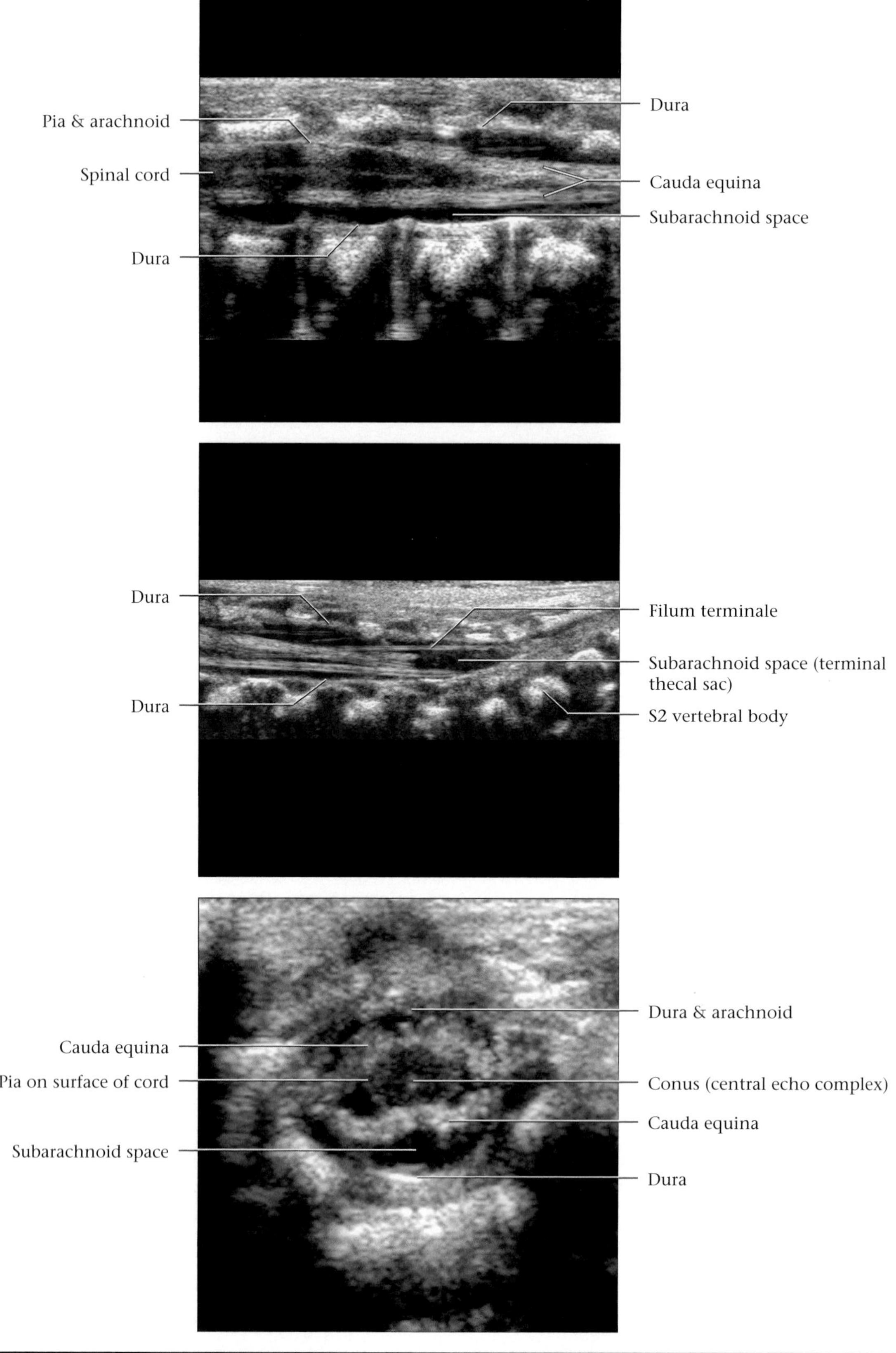
Pia & arachnoid
Spinal cord
Dura
Dura
Cauda equina
Subarachnoid space
Dura
Dura
Filum terminale
Subarachnoid space (terminal thecal sac)
S2 vertebral body
Cauda equina
Pia on surface of cord
Subarachnoid space
Dura & arachnoid
Conus (central echo complex)
Cauda equina
Dura

(Top) First of two longitudinal ultrasound images in a normal infant demonstrates the hypoechoic conus medullaris surrounded by hyperechoic cauda equina nerve roots. The hyperechoic dura defines the margins of the thecal sac filled with anechoic CSF. The arachnoid-dura mater complex of the thecal sac corresponds to the echogenic border of the spinal canal dorsal and ventral to the subarachnoid space. **(Middle)** This image demonstrates the mildly hyperechoic filum terminale anchoring the spinal cord to the terminal thecal sac at the S2 level. The cauda equina nerve roots drape dependently within the thecal sac. **(Bottom)** Transverse ultrasound image shows the normal conus and its coverings suspended within the CSF filled thecal sac.

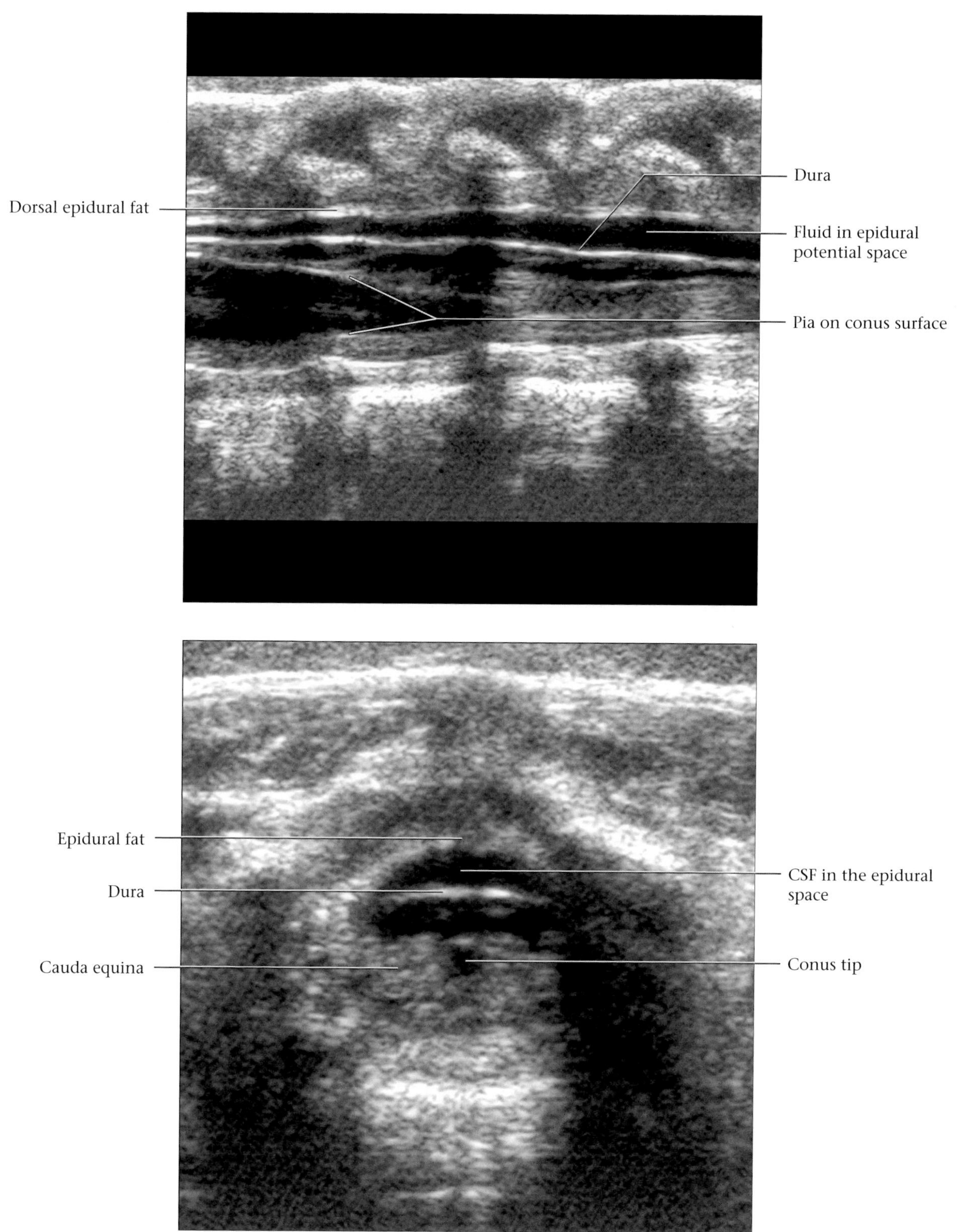
Dorsal epidural fat
Dura
Fluid in epidural potential space
Pia on conus surface
Epidural fat
Dura
Cauda equina
CSF in the epidural space
Conus tip

(Top) Longitudinal ultrasound image demonstrates anechoic CSF within the extradural (epidural) potential space. The extradural effusion developed following lumbar puncture with CSF leak. The extradural fluid separates the hyperechoic dura from normally adjacent hyperechoic dorsal extradural fat. **(Bottom)** Transverse ultrasound image demonstrates CSF within the dorsal extradural (epidural) potential space. The extradural effusion developed following lumbar puncture with CSF leak.

SAGITTAL & AXIAL CT MYELOGRAM

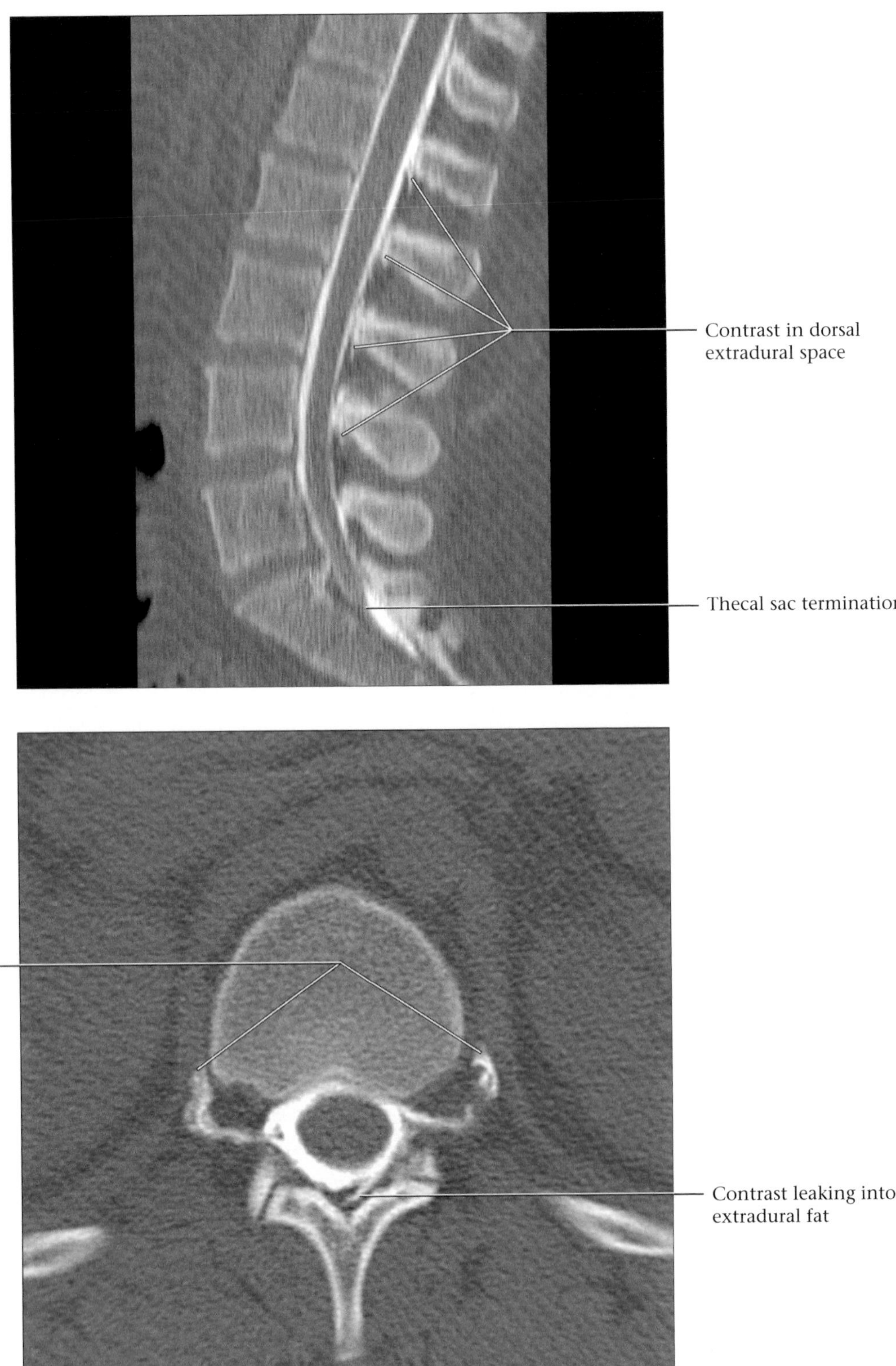
Contrast in dorsal extradural space
Thecal sac termination
Extradural contrast leaking around nerve sheathes
Contrast leaking into extradural fat

(Top) Sagittal CT reformat following myelography with unintentional administration of the entire contrast bolus into the extradural space. The thecal sac terminates at around S2 in normal position. Contrast is leaking around the dorsal extradural fat confirming its localization in the extradural space. A small L5/S1 disc protrusion is incidentally noted. **(Bottom)** Axial CT image following inadvertent extradural administration of contrast demonstrates the extradural space. Contrast surrounds the unopacified thecal sac and dural nerve root sleeves and leaks out through the neural foramina along the nerve root sleeve. A similar appearance would be intentionally produced following contrast injection during therapeutic extradural nerve root injection. The extradural contrast also invaginates into the dorsal extradural fat confirming injection into the extradural space.

SAGITTAL & AXIAL CT MYELOGRAM

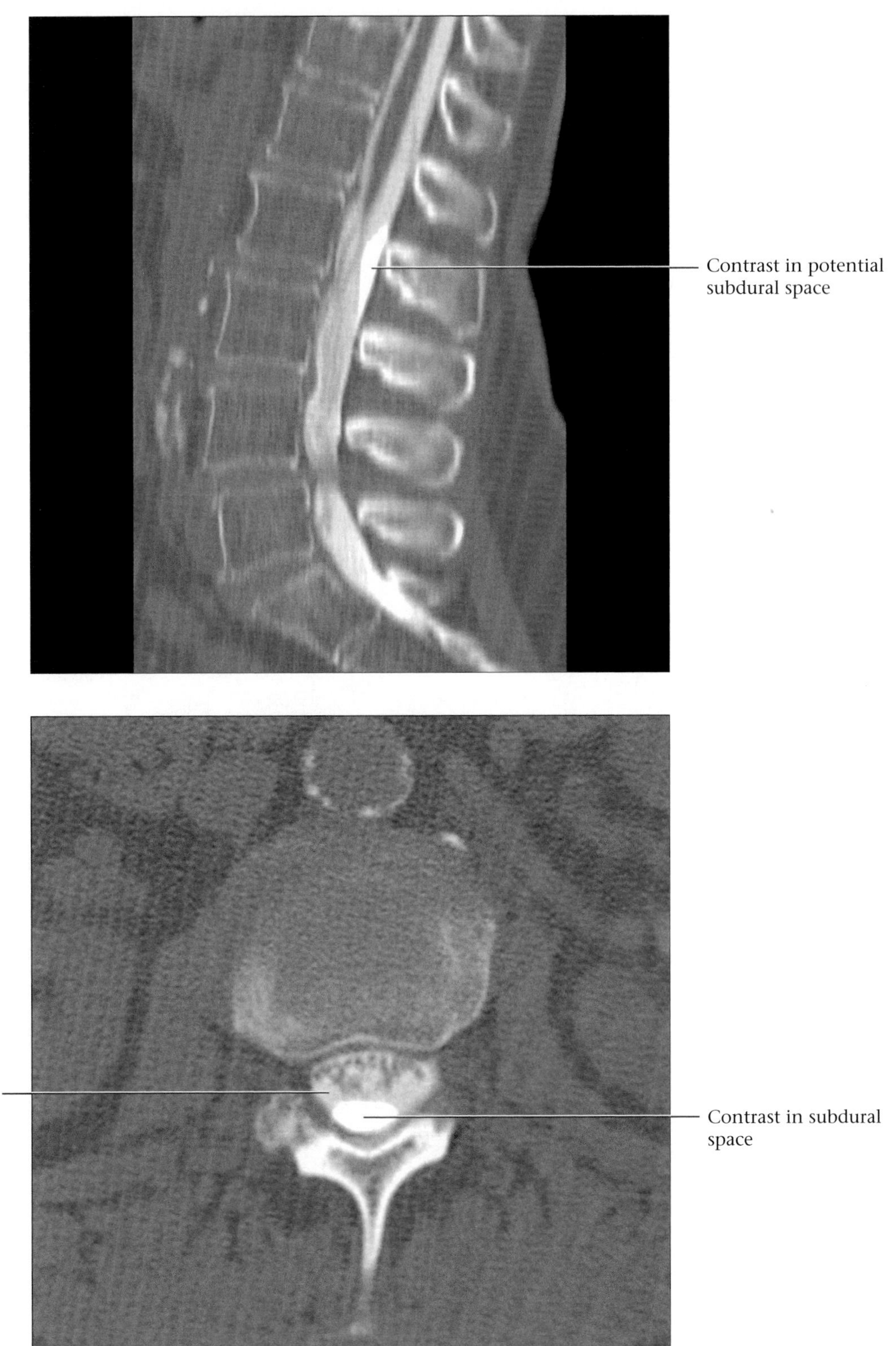
Contrast in potential subdural space
Subarachnoid space
Contrast in subdural space

(Top) Sagittal CT reformat following myelography demonstrates the subdural potential space, permitted by inadvertent administration of intrathecal contrast into the subdural space. There is ventral displacement of the arachnoid without disruption of the dura. **(Bottom)** Axial CT following myelography demonstrates the subdural potential space, seen here because of a "split" injection of intrathecal contrast into the subdural and subarachnoid spaces. There is slight ventral displacement of the arachnoid without disruption of the dura. The acute margins within the thecal sac and lack of mixing with the subarachnoid contrast confirms split injection partly into the subdural space.

AXIAL T2 MR

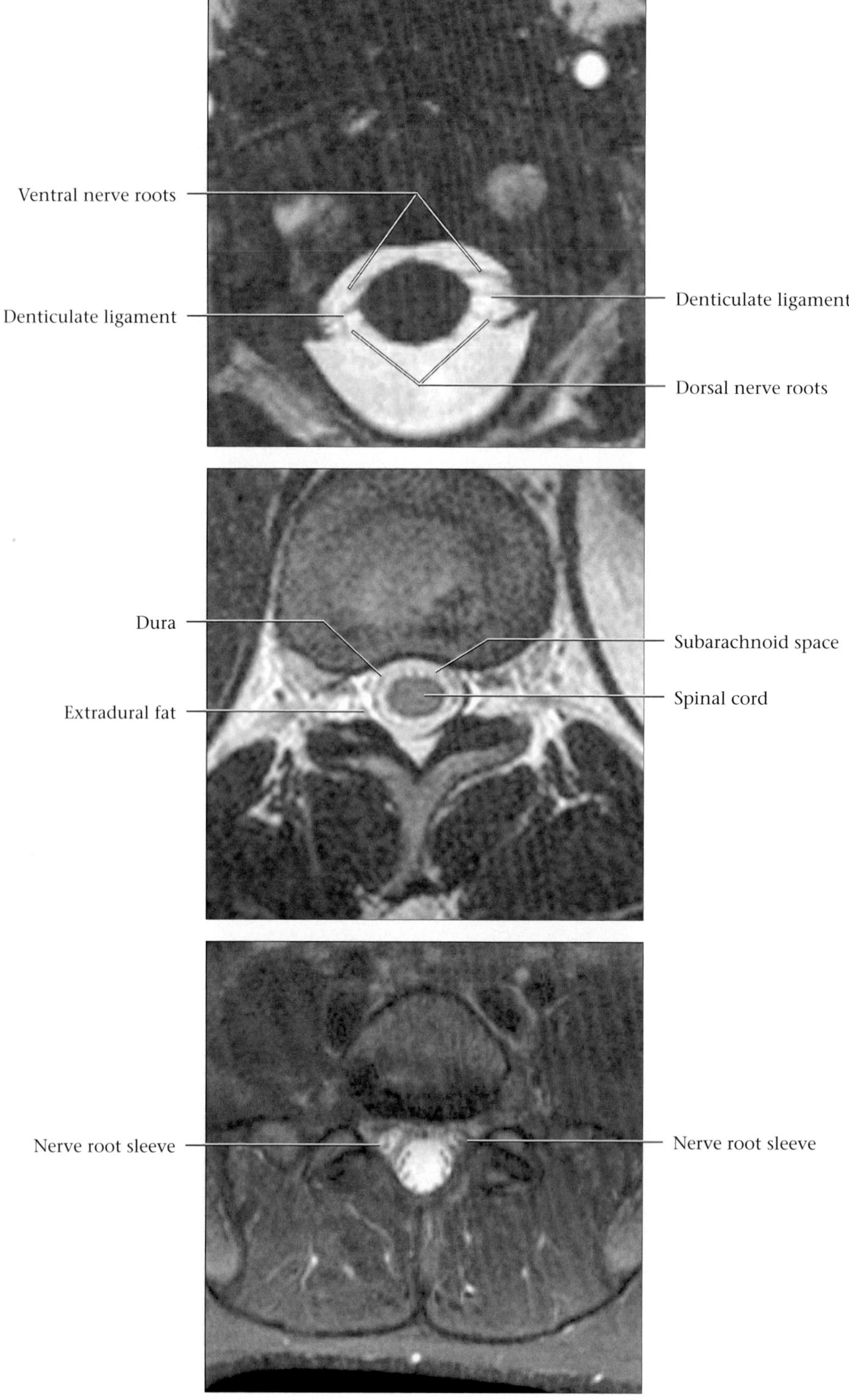
Ventral nerve roots
Denticulate ligament
Denticulate ligament
Dorsal nerve roots
Dura
Subarachnoid space
Spinal cord
Extradural fat
Nerve root sleeve
Nerve root sleeve

(Top) Axial steady state free precession (CISS) MR image of the upper cervical spine shows the normal denticulate ligaments anchoring the spinal cord laterally to the dura within the subarachnoid space. The denticulate ligaments are found between the ventral and dorsal nerve roots, and are a surgical landmark. **(Middle)** Axial T2 MR of the lower thoracic spine demonstrates hypointense dura delineating the thecal sac and its bright (CSF) contents. On T2 FSE MR, the CSF appears similar in signal intensity to extradural fat. **(Bottom)** Axial fat-saturated T2 FSE MR mostly negates fat signal permitting visualization of the distal thecal sac (lumbar cistern) and cauda equina. The CSF-filled, arachnoid-lined dural root sleeves are noted adjacent to the thecal sac preparing to exit through the neural foramina.

AXIAL T1 C+, AXIAL & CORONAL T1 MR

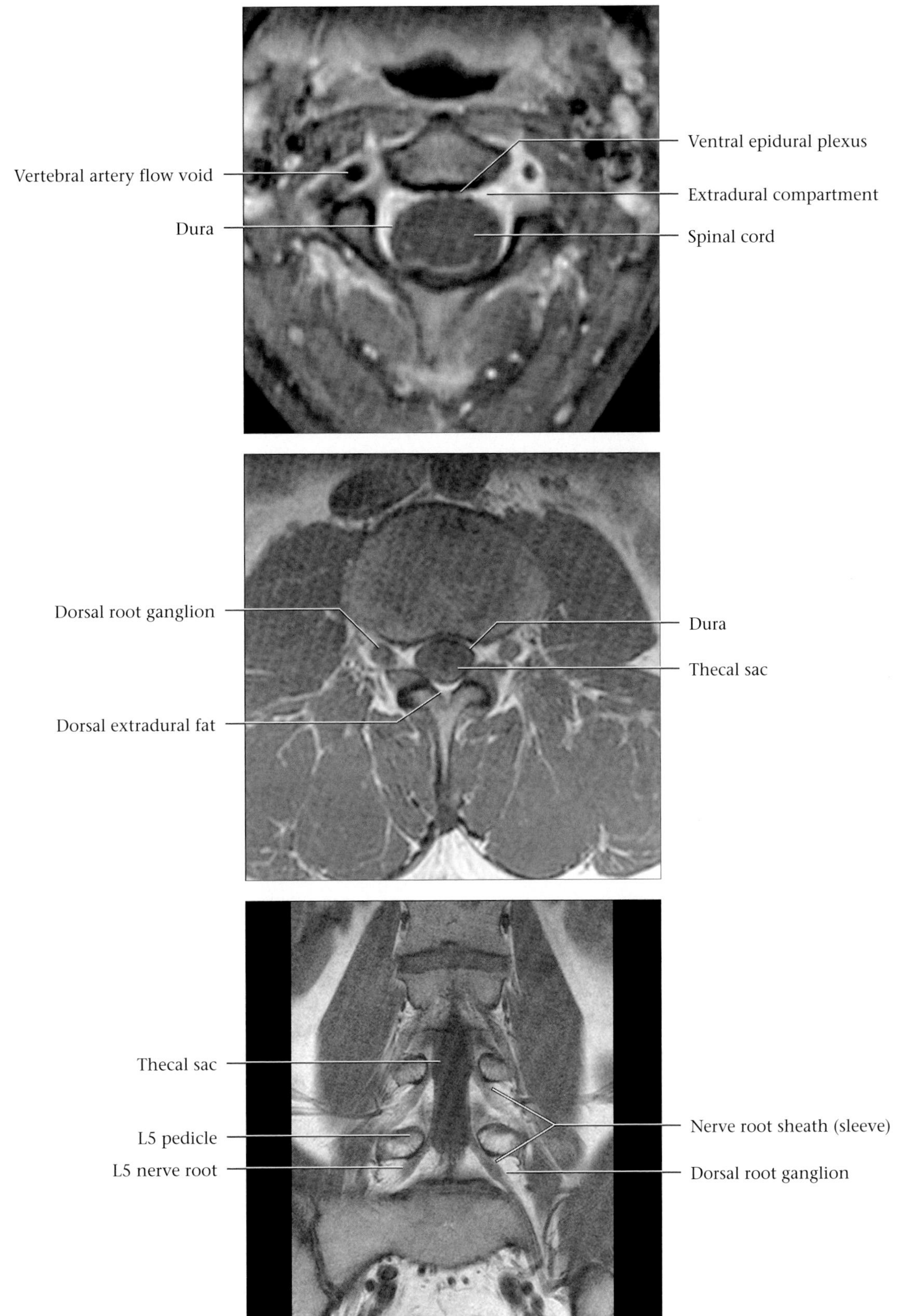
Vertebral artery flow void
Dura
Ventral epidural plexus
Extradural compartment
Spinal cord
Dorsal root ganglion
Dorsal extradural fat
Dura
Thecal sac
Thecal sac
L5 pedicle
L5 nerve root
Nerve root sheath (sleeve)
Dorsal root ganglion

(Top) Axial T1 C+ fat-saturated MR of the cervical spine shows intense, but normal enhancement of venous plexus within extradural compartment outlining the isointense dura & hypointense CSF. Extradural compartment contains primarily fat and veins. **(Middle)** Axial T1 MR at L1 level shows the hypointense dura delineating the CSF-filled thecal sac surrounded by hyperintense fat within extradural compartment. Also note fat surrounding the dorsal root ganglion within the neural foramina bilaterally. **(Bottom)** Coronal T1 MR shows the hypointense nerve root sheaths (sleeve) which represent dural outpouchings (nerve root sheath or sleeve) exiting via the neural foramina. The nerve roots descend in the thecal sac as the cauda equina and exit under the pedicle at their named levels. Bright signal intensity fat defines the extradural space.

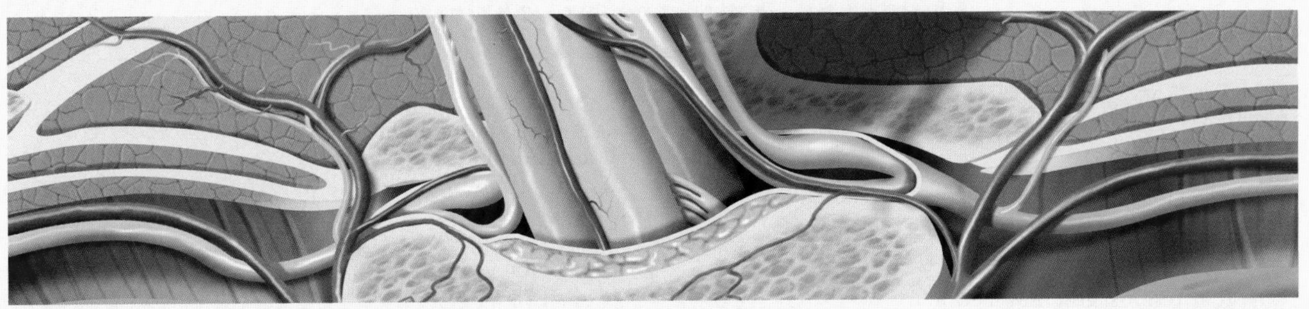

SECTION 3: Vascular

SPINAL ARTERIAL SUPPLY

Terminology

Abbreviations

- Anterior, posterior spinal arteries (ASA, PSA)
- Vertebral artery (VA), basilar artery (BA)

Synonyms

- Great anterior segmental medullary artery = artery of Adamkiewicz

Gross Anatomy

Vertebral Column, Epidural Soft Tissues

- Segmental arrangement
  - Arteries numbered for segments from which they arise
  - Numerous transverse, longitudinal anastomoses extend over several segments
  - **Cervical**
    - VAs (dorsal intersegmental anastomoses)
    - Thyrocervical trunk (ventral intersegmental anastomoses)
  - **Thoracic**
    - Arise from paired intercostal arteries
    - Pre-, postcentral branches to vertebral bodies
    - Pre-, postlaminar, spinal branches to canal, neural arch
  - **Lumbar**
    - Arise from paired lumbar segmental arteries

Dura, Cord, Roots, Nerves

- **Spinal cord circulation** derived from
  - VAs (ASA, PSA)
  - Segmental vessels at multiple levels
    - Ascending cervical, deep cervical, intercostal, lumbar, sacral
- **Anterior spinal artery**
  - Arises at junction of intradural segment of VAs
  - Lies in midline on ventral cord surface (in anterior median fissure)
  - Courses inferiorly from foramen magnum to filum terminale
  - Supplies anterior 2/3 of cord
    - Anterior horns, spinothalamic/corticospinal tracts
    - Penetrating (central) branches have few collaterals
  - Augmented by segmental feeders
- **Posterior spinal arteries**
  - Arise from PICA or posterior rami of VA
  - Paired longitudinal channels on dorsal cord medial to dorsal roots
  - Numerous plexiform anastomoses between PSAs
  - Supply posterior 1/3 of cord
    - Posterior columns, some corticospinal tracts (variable)
  - Augmented by medullary feeders from posterior radicular arteries
- **Segmental arteries**
  - Dorsal rami of segmental arteries arising from vertebral, subclavian, thoracic intercostal, lumbar intercostal arteries
  - Enter canal through foramen, penetrate dura
  - Divide into dural, radiculomedullary branches
    - Dural arteries supply dura, nerve root sleeves
    - Radiculomedullary branches supply roots, cord
- **Radiculomedullary arteries**
  - Arise from dorsal segmental arteries, penetrate SAS
  - Radicular branches supply anterior/posterior roots
  - Medullary branches anastomose with ASA/PSA, provide variable supply to cord
- **Cervical**
  - Major radicular feeders between C5-7 level
  - 2-3 anterior cervical cord feeders
  - 3-4 posterior cervical cord feeders
- **Thoracic**
  - Anterior thoracic cord feeders ≈ 2-3
    - Usually left sided
    - Small ventral feeders may also be present
    - Inverse relationship between number, caliber of ventral radicular vessels
    - "Pauci-segmental" fewer vessels (< 5) with larger caliber
    - "Pluri-segmental" more vessels with smaller caliber
  - Dominant thoracic anterior radicular = **artery of Adamkiewicz**
    - Left side origin (73%)
    - T9-12 origin (62%)
    - Lumbar origin (26%)
    - T6-8 (12%)
  - Posterior thoracic cord feeders ≈ 9-12 (average 8)
    - No right-left lateralization preference
    - Vessel caliber 150-400 μ
    - Variable reporting of "great posterior radicular artery"
- **Lumbosacral and pelvic**
  - 0-1 major cord feeders
  - ASA ends at conus, gives communicating branches ("rami cruciantes") to PSAs
  - Posterior division of iliac artery ⇒ inferior & superior lateral sacral branches ⇒ spinal arteries via anterior sacral foramina
  - Anterior division iliac artery ⇒ inferior gluteal artery ⇒ supplies sciatic nerve
  - Posterior division internal iliac artery ⇒ iliolumbar artery supplies femoral nerve at iliac wing level
- **Cord nutrient vessels**
  - Central and peripheral systems
  - Central ⇒ ASA and flow centrifugal
  - Peripheral ⇒ PSA, pial plexus &and flow centripetal
  - Dense capillary network in gray matter of cord

Imaging Anatomy

Overview

- Artery of Adamkiewicz has characteristic "hairpin" turn on DSA
- Vascular "watershed" of cord = central gray matter
  - Hypotensive infarcts affect central gray
  - ASA infarct affects anterior 2/3 of cord
- Evaluation of vascular malformations requires visualization of entire spinal vasculature
  - VAs to iliac arteries

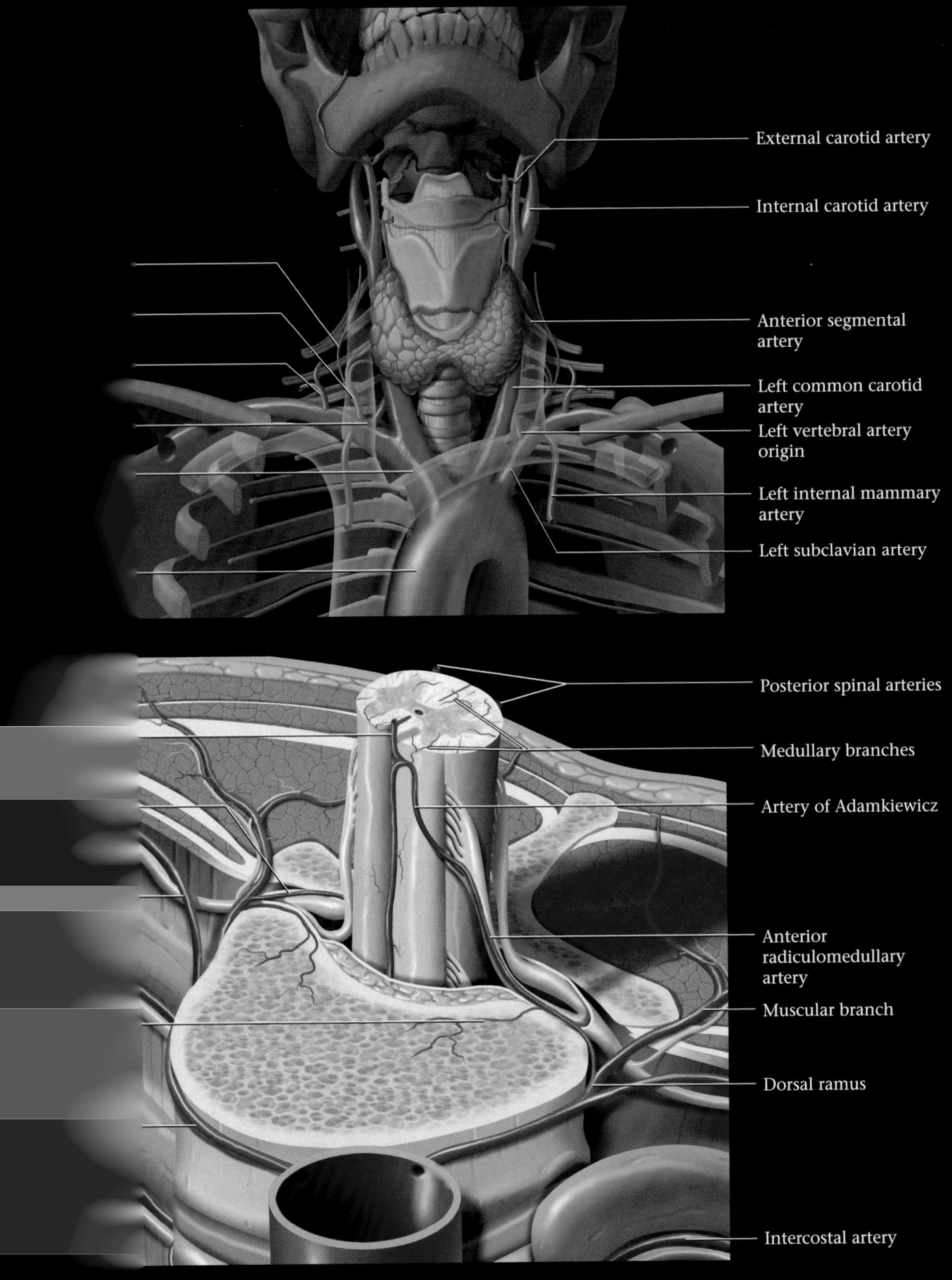
External carotid artery
Internal carotid artery
Anterior segmental artery
Left common carotid artery
Left vertebral artery origin
Left internal mammary artery
Left subclavian artery
Posterior spinal arteries
Medullary branches
Artery of Adamkiewicz
Anterior radiculomedullary artery
Muscular branch
Dorsal ramus
Intercostal artery

ne aortic arch and arterial great vessels in red. The vertebral arteries give rise to the anterior es. The ascending cervical arteries, branches of the thyrocervical trunks, give off anterior nedullary arteries that anastomose with the ASA and PSA on the cord surface. Complete les evaluation of all these vessels. **(Bottom)** Oblique axial graphic rendering of T10 depicts ries arising from the lower thoracic aorta. The artery of Adamkiewicz is the dominant o the thoracic cord, supplying the anterior aspect of the cord via the anterior spinal artery. rpin" turn on the cord surface as it first courses superiorly, then turns inferiorly.

SPINAL ARTERIAL SUPPLY

GRAPHICS

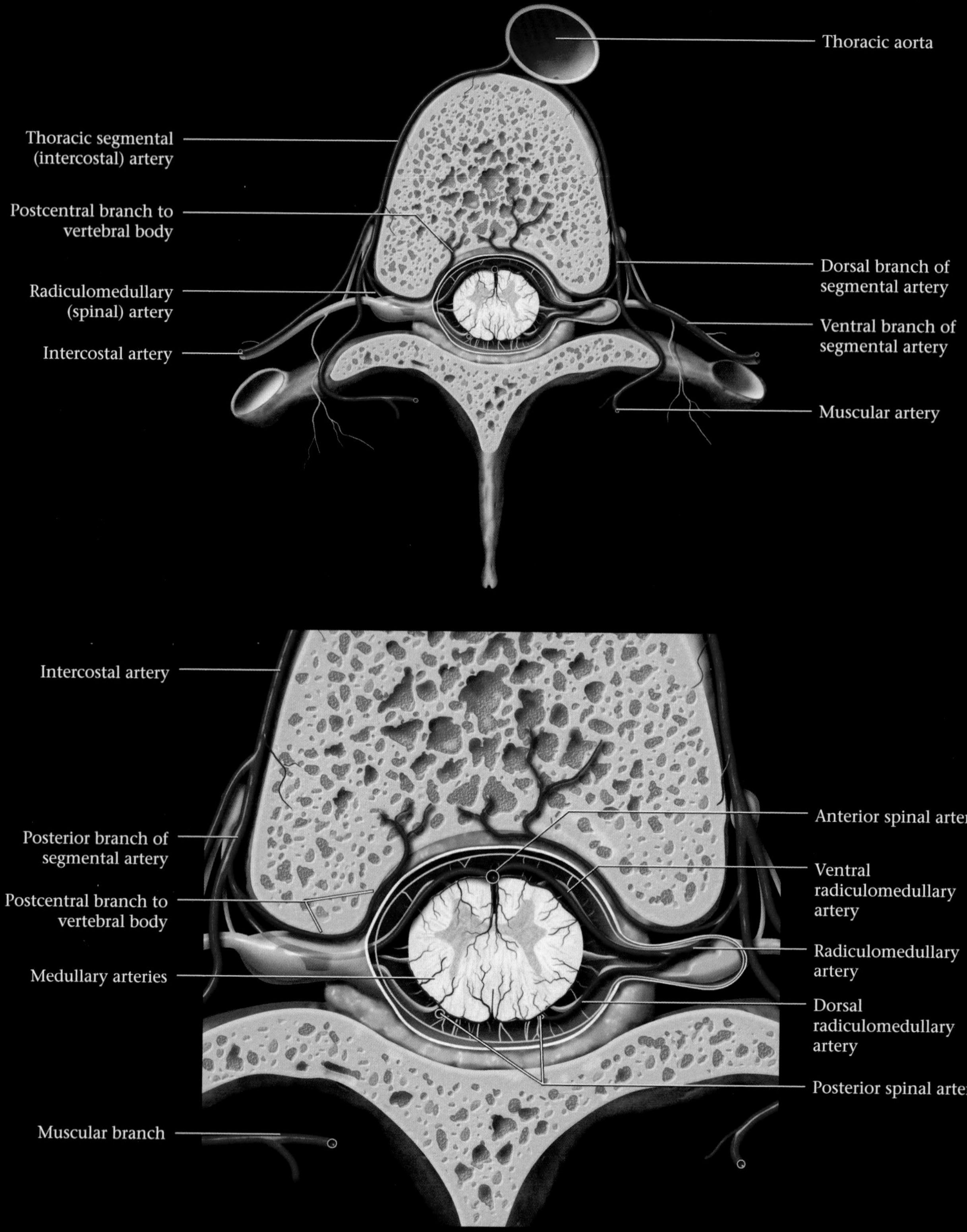
Thoracic aorta
Thoracic segmental (intercostal) artery
Postcentral branch to vertebral body
Radiculomedullary (spinal) artery
Intercostal artery
Dorsal branch of segmental artery
Ventral branch of segmental artery
Muscular artery
Intercostal artery
Posterior branch of segmental artery
Postcentral branch to vertebral body
Medullary arteries
Muscular branch
Anterior spinal arte
Ventral radiculomedullary artery
Radiculomedullary artery
Dorsal radiculomedullary artery
Posterior spinal arte

(Top) Axial graphic shows overview of the arterial supply to the vertebral column & its contents, depicted here in lower thoracic spine. A series of paired segmental arteries (cervical region arise from the vertebral & thyrocervical arteries, thoracic region are intercostal arteries & lumbar region are lumbar arteries) divide into anterior & posterio branches. The posterior branch gives rise to a muscular branch, a branch to the vertebral body, and the radiculomedullary artery. The radiculomedullary artery enters the vertebral canal via neural foramen. **(Bottom)** Anterior & posterior radiculomedullary arteries anastomose with the anterior & posterior spinal arteries. Penetratin medullary arteries in the cord are largely end-arteries with few collaterals. The cord "watershed" zone is at the centr gray matter.

3D-VRT CECT

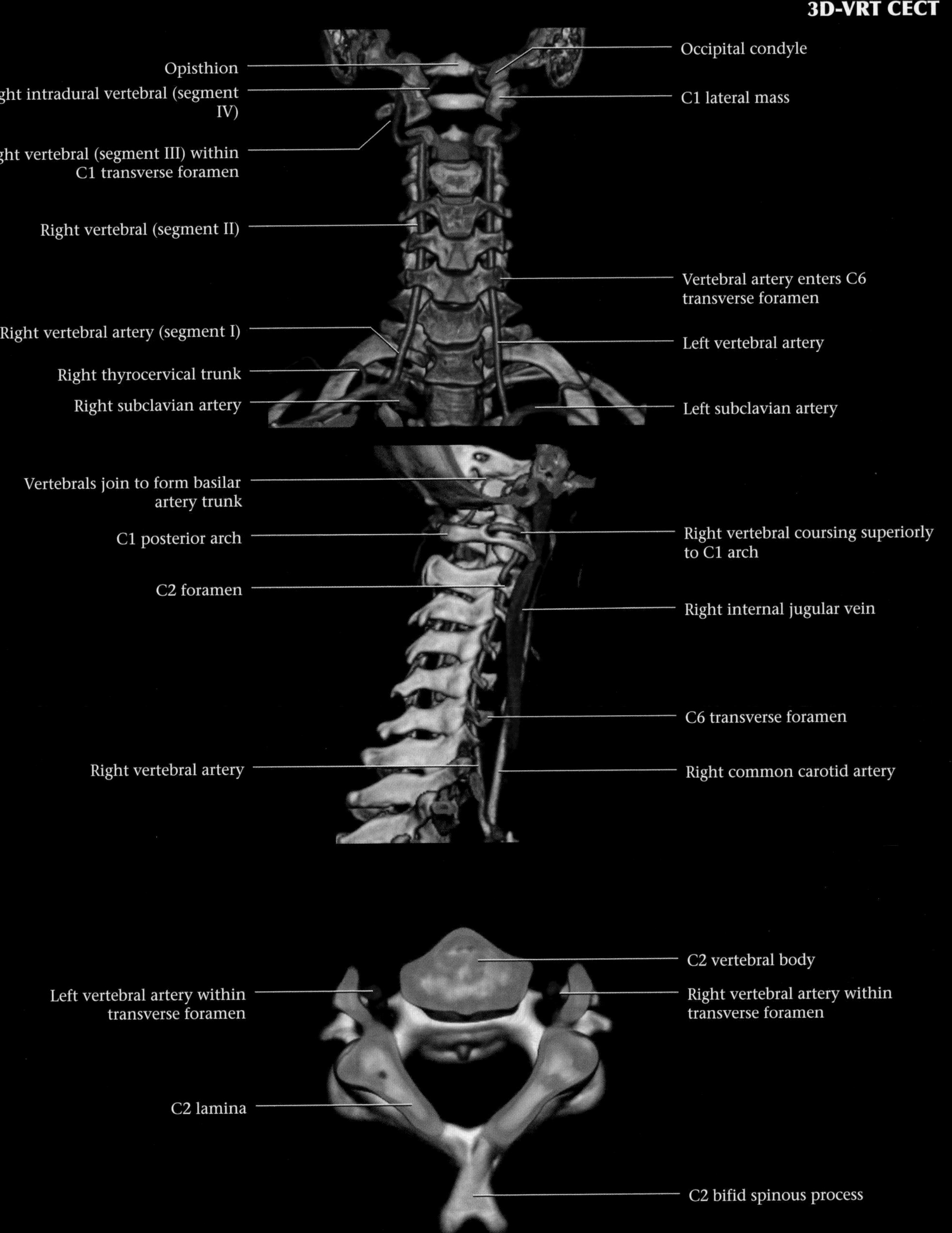
Opisthion
Right intradural vertebral (segment IV)
Right vertebral (segment III) within C1 transverse foramen
Right vertebral (segment II)
Right vertebral artery (segment I)
Right thyrocervical trunk
Right subclavian artery
Occipital condyle
C1 lateral mass
Vertebral artery enters C6 transverse foramen
Left vertebral artery
Left subclavian artery
Vertebrals join to form basilar artery trunk
C1 posterior arch
C2 foramen
Right vertebral artery
Right vertebral coursing superiorly to C1 arch
Right internal jugular vein
C6 transverse foramen
Right common carotid artery
Left vertebral artery within transverse foramen
C2 lamina
C2 vertebral body
Right vertebral artery within transverse foramen
C2 bifid spinous process

(Top) First of six 3D-VRT angiographic images. AP volume rendered image of CTA shows the course of the vertebral arteries, entering the transverse foramen and ascending to the foramen magnum. Both vertebral arteries in this patient enter the C6 level, but this can show wide normal variation. **(Middle)** Lateral oblique volume rendered CTA image of the cervical spine shows the course of the vertebral artery within the transverse processes. Note the ventral to dorsal course of the artery as it ascends towards the C6 transverse foramen. The distal vertebral makes a lateral course from the C2 foramen, then ascends through the C1 foramen where it turns posteriorly to pass over the posterior arch of C1 to enter the foramen magnum. **(Bottom)** Axial oblique image of cervical CTA at the C2 level shows the relationship of the vertebral artery to the transverse foramen.

SPINAL ARTERIAL SUPPLY

3D-VRT CECT

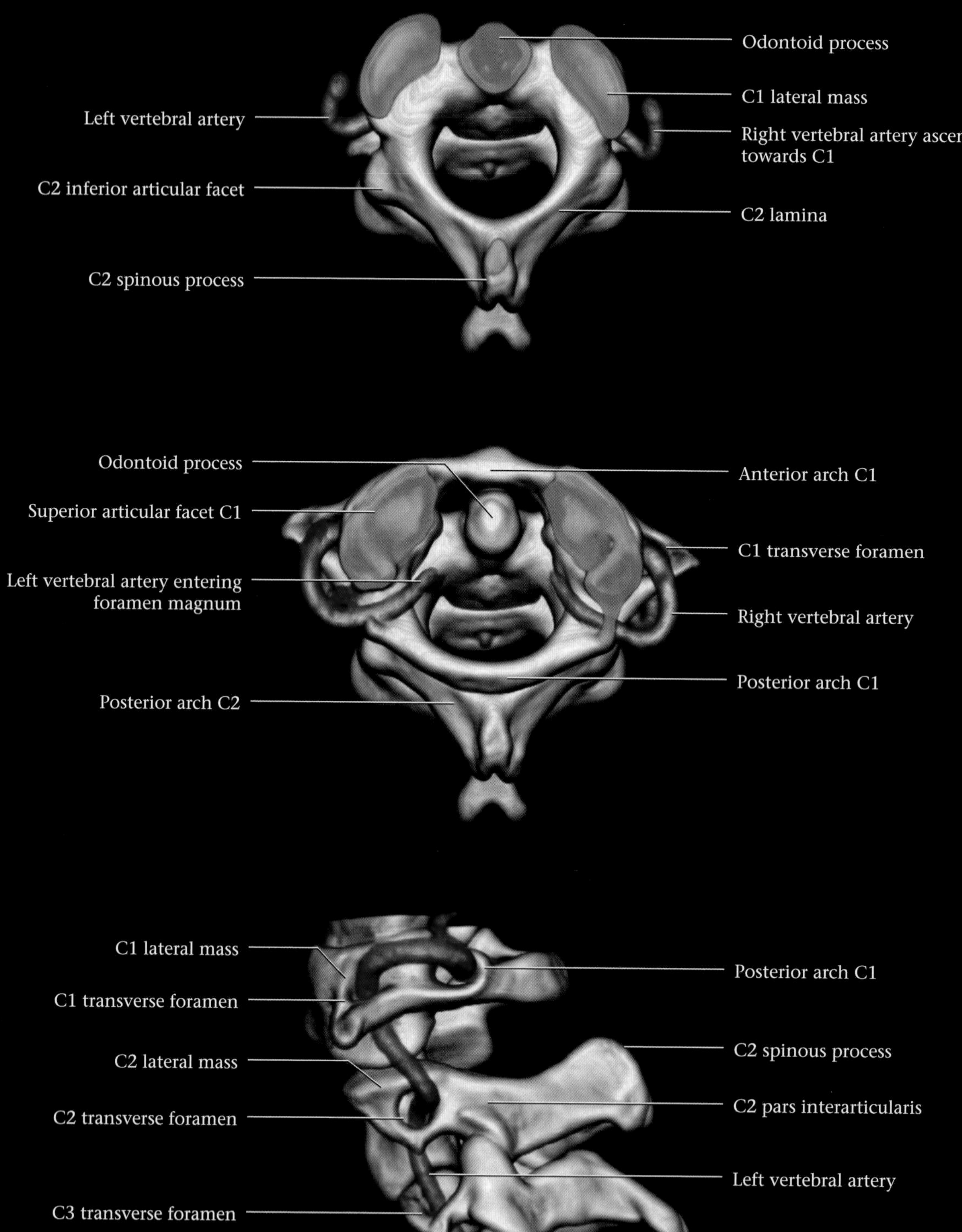
Odontoid process
C1 lateral mass
Left vertebral artery
Right vertebral artery ascending towards C1
C2 inferior articular facet
C2 lamina
C2 spinous process
Odontoid process
Anterior arch C1
Superior articular facet C1
C1 transverse foramen
Left vertebral artery entering foramen magnum
Right vertebral artery
Posterior arch C1
Posterior arch C2
C1 lateral mass
Posterior arch C1
C1 transverse foramen
C2 lateral mass
C2 spinous process
C2 transverse foramen
C2 pars interarticularis
Left vertebral artery
C3 transverse foramen

(Top) Cranial oblique view of volume rendered CTA images shows the vertebral arteries leaving the C2 transverse foramen and coursing lateral to the lateral masses as they ascend towards the transverse foramen of C1. The cut plane extends superiorly through the lateral masses of C1 and odontoid process of C2. **(Middle)** Cranial oblique view of CTA examination with cut plane superior to the C1 arch. The image demonstrates the course of the distal vertebral arteries as they exit the C1 transverse foramen and turn medial to extend over the posterior C1 arch to then ascend through the foramen magnum. **(Bottom)** Lateral volume rendered CTA shows the course of the distal left vertebral artery passing through C1 and horizontally oriented C2 transverse foramen.

AP DSA

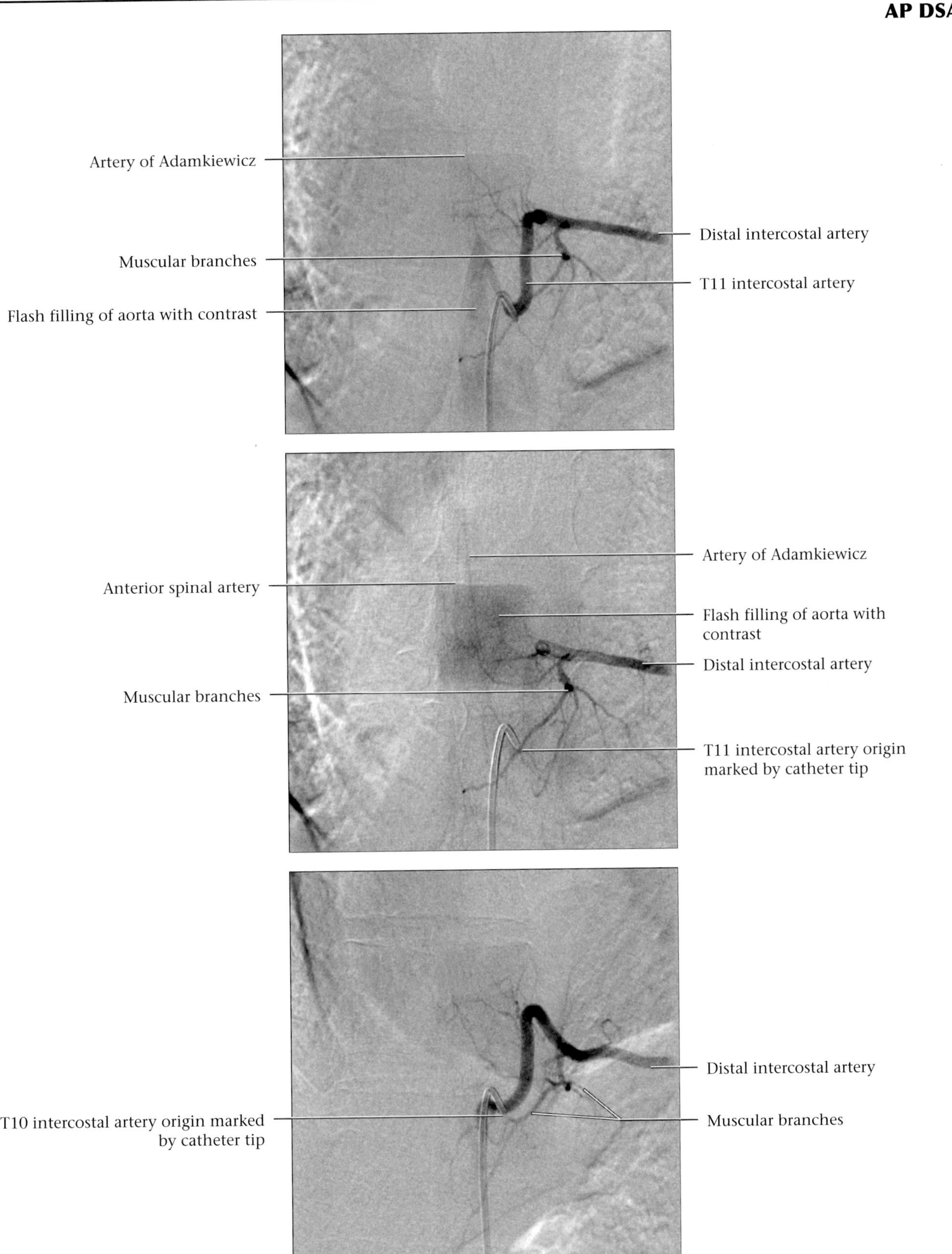

Artery of Adamkiewicz
Muscular branches
Flash filling of aorta with contrast
Distal intercostal artery
T11 intercostal artery
Artery of Adamkiewicz
Anterior spinal artery
Flash filling of aorta with contrast
Distal intercostal artery
Muscular branches
T11 intercostal artery origin marked by catheter tip
Distal intercostal artery
T10 intercostal artery origin marked by catheter tip
Muscular branches

(Top) AP IA-DSA image from left T11 injection. The T11 intercostal artery gives rise to the major segmental feeding vessel of the thoracic cord (artery of Adamkiewicz). The artery of Adamkiewicz shows a characteristic sharp hairpin turn as it joins the anterior spinal artery. **(Middle)** AP IA-DSA later arterial phase T11 intercostal injection shows the typical hairpin turn of the artery of Adamkiewicz. The anterior spinal artery is present in the midline as vertical arteries both superior and inferior to the junction with Adamkiewicz. **(Bottom)** T10 intercostal injection shows the intercostal and muscular branches with no major feeding segmental vessel extending to the cord at this level.

SPINAL ARTERIAL SUPPLY

DSA & CTA

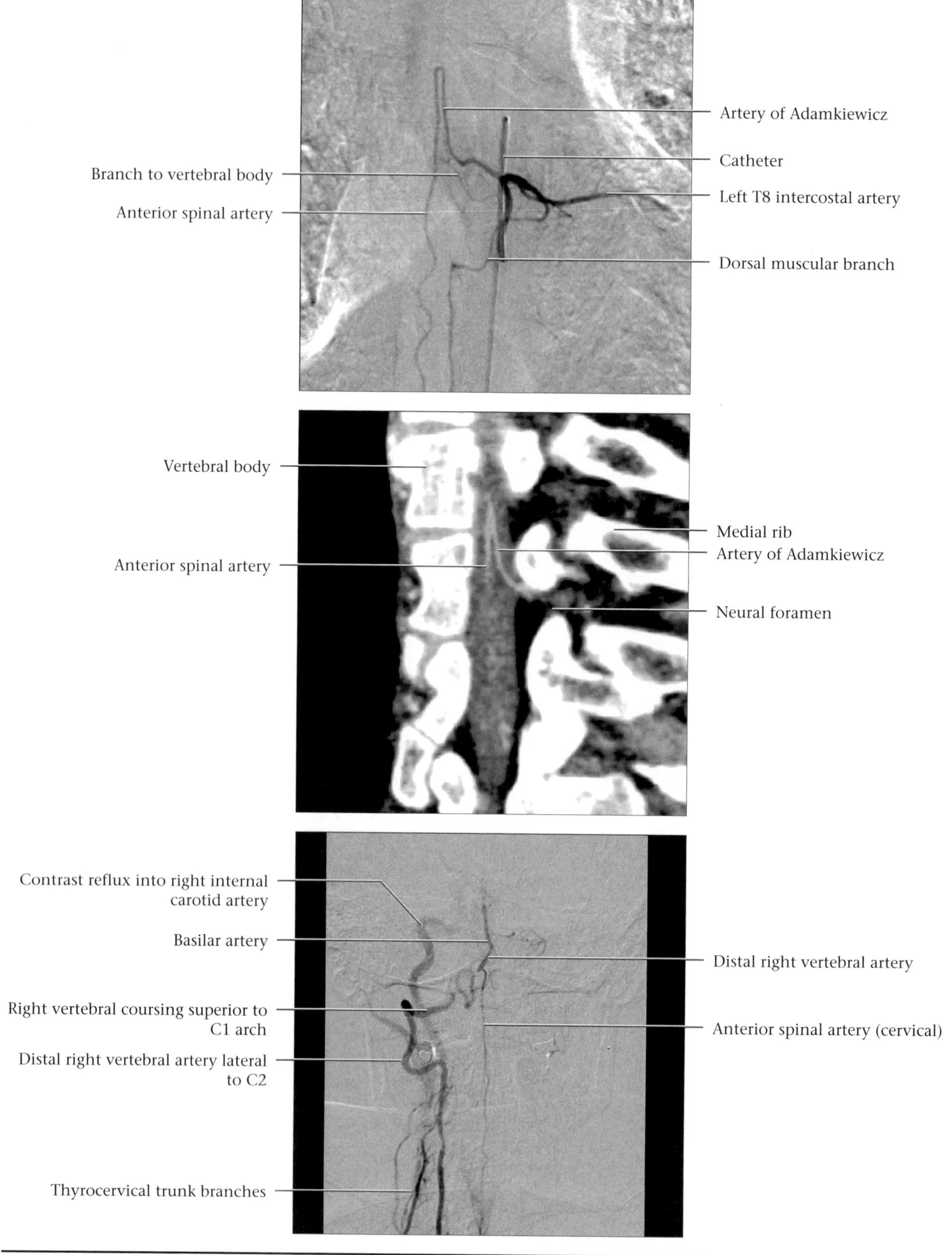
Artery of Adamkiewicz
Catheter
Branch to vertebral body
Left T8 intercostal artery
Anterior spinal artery
Dorsal muscular branch
Vertebral body
Medial rib
Artery of Adamkiewicz
Anterior spinal artery
Neural foramen
Contrast reflux into right internal carotid artery
Basilar artery
Distal right vertebral artery
Right vertebral coursing superior to C1 arch
Anterior spinal artery (cervical)
Distal right vertebral artery lateral to C2
Thyrocervical trunk branches

(Top) AP view of a left T8 intercostal injection gives rise to the characteristic hairpin turn of the major segmental feeding vessel to the thoracic cord, the artery of Adamkiewicz. Extending inferiorly from the top of the hairpin turn is the anterior spinal artery, which supplies the anterior 2/3 of the cord. **(Middle)** Sagittal CTA shows the left T8 intercostal segmental artery gives rise to the characteristic hairpin turn of the major segmental feeding vessel to the thoracic cord, the artery of Adamkiewicz. Extending inferiorly from the top of the hairpin turn is the anterior spinal artery, supplying the anterior 2/3 of the cord. **(Bottom)** AP view of right vertebral injection shows the anterior spinal artery extending inferiorly from the right distal vertebral artery. The anterior spinal artery is well seen due to occlusion of the distal right vertebral with collateral reconstitution of the basilar.

AP DSA

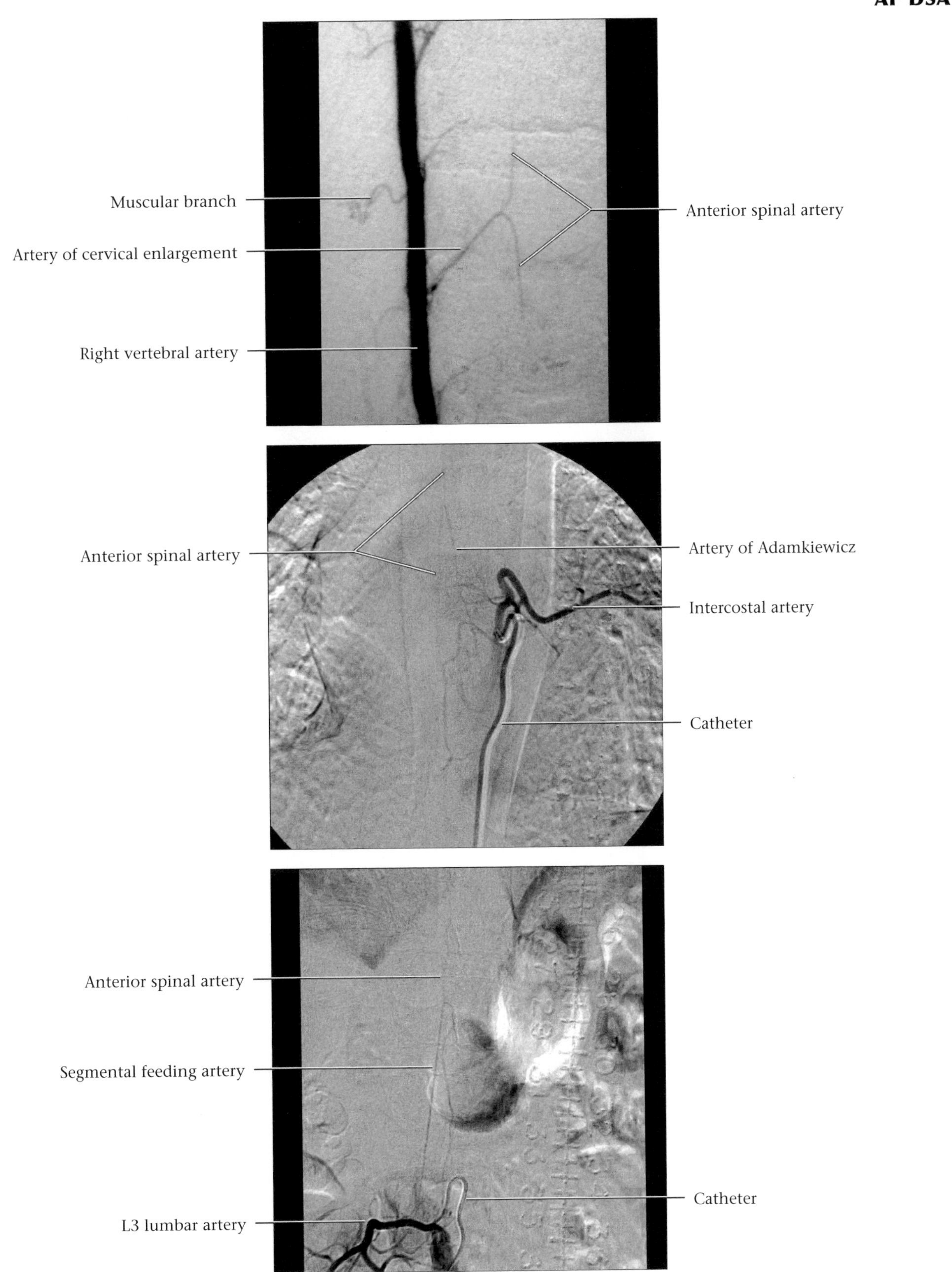
Muscular branch
Artery of cervical enlargement
Right vertebral artery
Anterior spinal artery
Anterior spinal artery
Artery of Adamkiewicz
Intercostal artery
Catheter
Anterior spinal artery
Segmental feeding artery
L3 lumbar artery
Catheter

(Top) AP view of right vertebral injection shows a dominant segmental branch (artery of cervical enlargement) supplying the cervical anterior spinal artery and arising off of the mid cervical vertebral artery. **(Middle)** AP thoracic view of left intercostal injection shows the artery of Adamkiewicz with a hairpin turn configuration, and supplying the anterior spinal artery. **(Bottom)** AP view of L3 lumbar artery injection shows a dominant segmental feeding vessel extending to L1 level.

AXIAL CT ANGIOGRAM

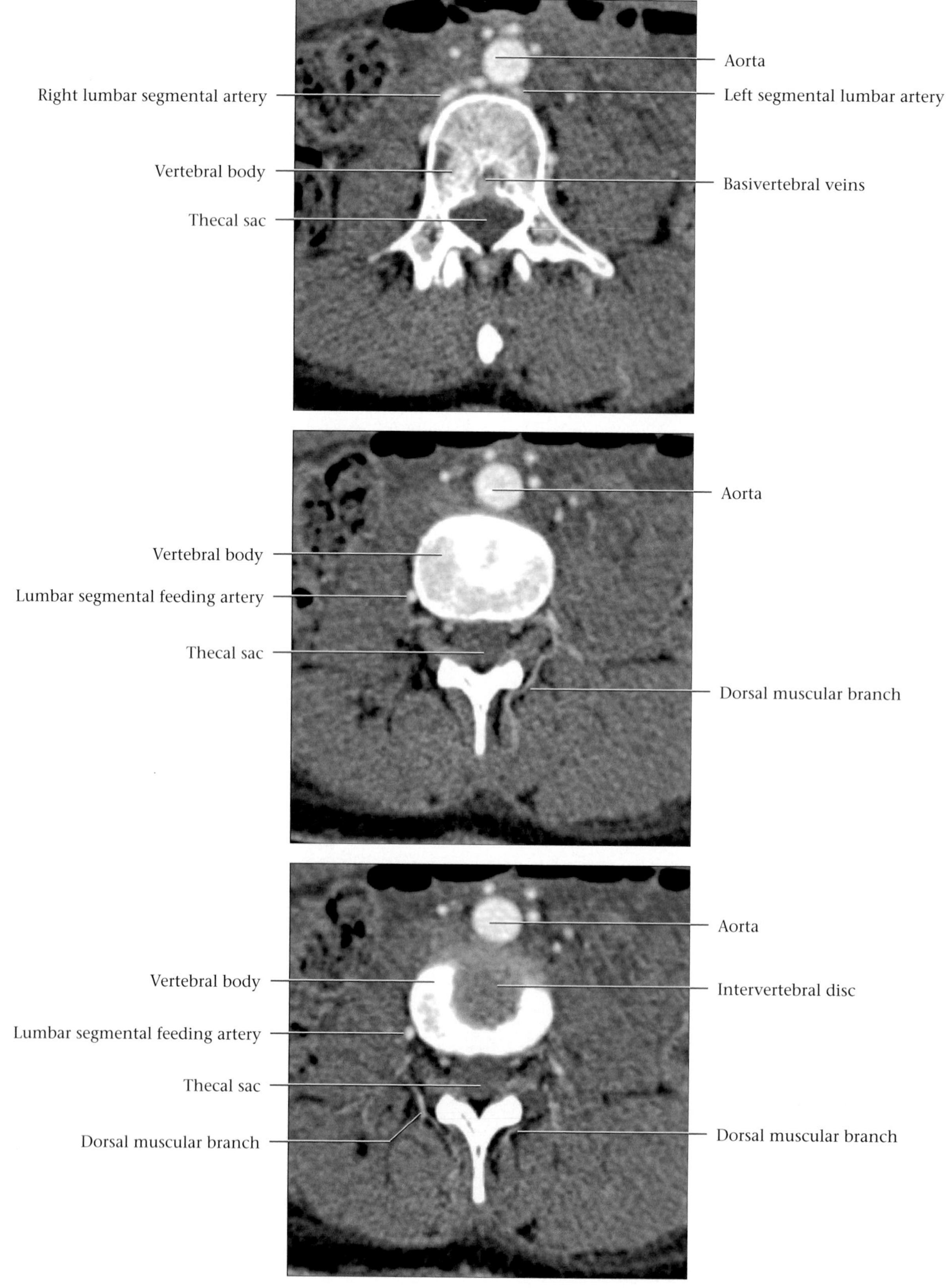

Aorta
Right lumbar segmental artery
Left segmental lumbar artery
Vertebral body
Basivertebral veins
Thecal sac
Aorta
Vertebral body
Lumbar segmental feeding artery
Thecal sac
Dorsal muscular branch
Aorta
Vertebral body
Intervertebral disc
Lumbar segmental feeding artery
Thecal sac
Dorsal muscular branch
Dorsal muscular branch

(Top) First of three axial CTA source images show the arterial supply to the spine via lumbar segmental arteries. Upper section through the vertebral body and transverse processes shows both right and left segmental arteries. Note basivertebral vein, seen here as a funnel-shaped area of contrast in the middle of the vertebral body, connecting posteriorly to the epidural venous plexus. **(Middle)** Scan through the middle of the vertebral body shows segmental vessels with a dorsal muscular branch seen especially well. **(Bottom)** Scan at level of the intervertebral disc space shows two dorsal muscular branches supplying the paraspinous muscles adjacent to the lamina and posterior spinous processes.

CT ANGIOGRAPHY

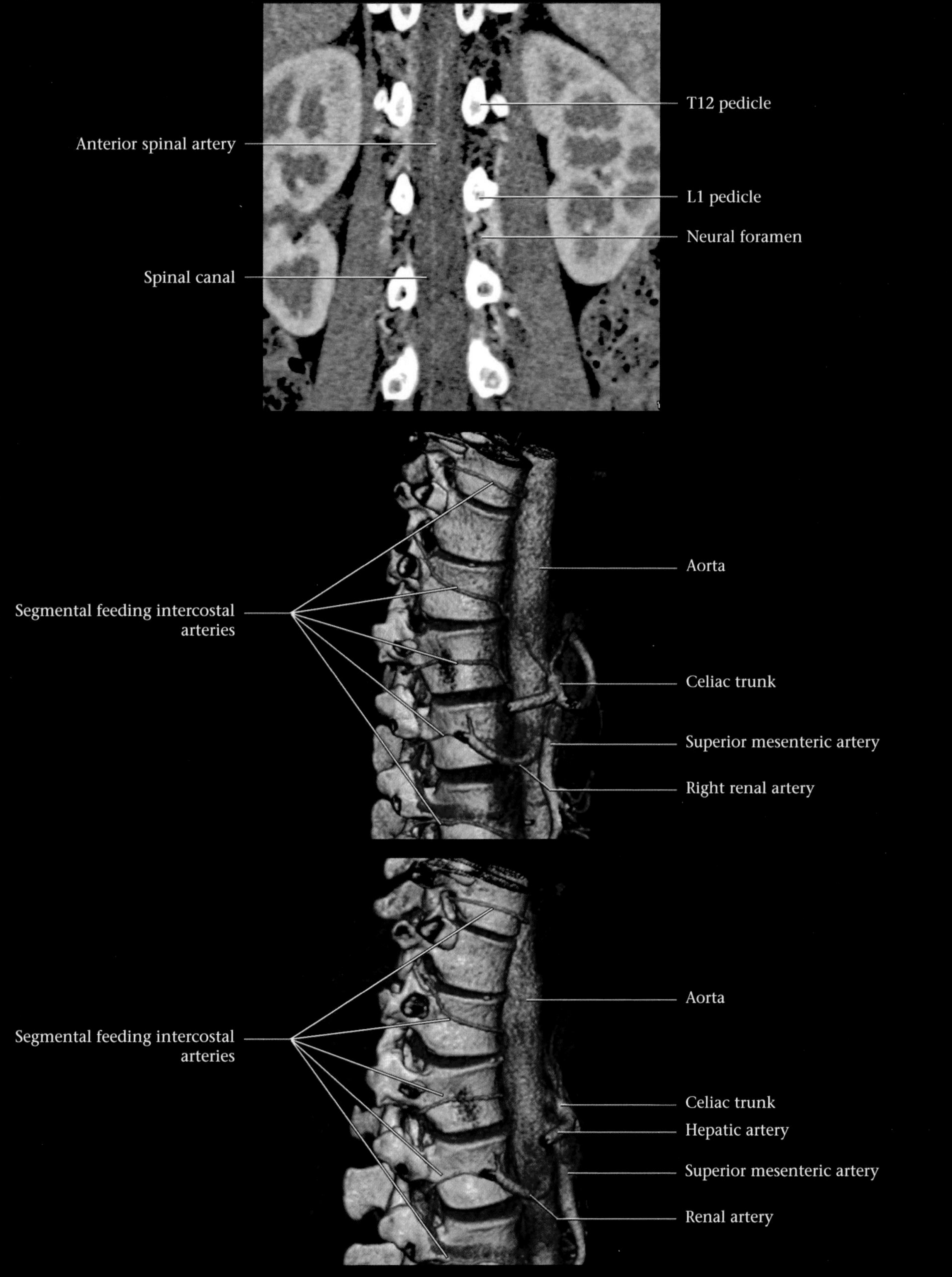

T12 pedicle
Anterior spinal artery
L1 pedicle
Neural foramen
Spinal canal
Aorta
Segmental feeding intercostal arteries
Celiac trunk
Superior mesenteric artery
Right renal artery
Aorta
Segmental feeding intercostal arteries
Celiac trunk
Hepatic artery
Superior mesenteric artery
Renal artery

(Top) Coronal spinal CTA multiplanar reformat shows the anterior spinal artery as a linear contrast-enhancement along the conus and proximal filum. **(Middle)** Right anterior oblique CTA volume rendered image shows the distal aorta giving rise to multiple segmental feeding vessels extending around the right lateral margin of the vertebral bodies towards the neural foramen. **(Bottom)** Lateral volume rendered image of spinal CTA shows the close relationship of the segmental feeding vessels extending posteriorly towards the neural foramen of the thoracic spine and their intimate relationship with the vertebral bodies.

SPINAL VEINS AND VENOUS PLEXUS

Terminology

Abbreviations

- Vertebral venous system/plexus (VVS, VVP)
- Superior, inferior vena cava (SVC, IVC)
- Internal jugular vein (IJV)

Synonyms

- Epidural plexus = Batson plexus

Gross Anatomy

Overview

- **Vertebral venous system**
  - Large valveless network in/around vertebral column
  - Part of extradural neural axis compartment (EDNAC)
  - Extent: Sacral hiatus to foramen magnum
    - Ends in clival plexus, suboccipital sinus
  - Extensive collaterals, anastomoses
    - Unites superior and inferior vena cava (like azygos system)
    - Three major external complexes: Internal VVP, basivertebral veins, external VVP
    - Smaller intradural veins
  - Function
    - Blood flows either direction, varies with thoracic/abdominal pressure
    - Large volume relative to arterial supply (20x greater)
- **Internal vertebral venous plexus**
  - Epidural venous network surrounds thecal sac
    - Series of irregular, thin-walled valveless sinuses
    - Arranged in ladder-like series of cross-connected expansions up vertebral column
    - Embedded in epidural fat
    - Tributaries: Radicular veins, veins along posterior elements
  - Anterior/posterior epidural regions
    - Anterior more prominent
    - Formed from two continuous channels along posterior surface of vertebral bodies between pedicles
    - Channels expand to cross anastomose with each other, receive basivertebral veins
    - Largest at central dorsal region of vertebral body
    - Thinnest at disc level
- **Basivertebral veins**
  - Paired valveless intravertebral veins
  - Extend horizontally through anterior, posterior vertebral bodies
  - Collect numerous small venous channels within vertebral bodies
  - Drain into anterior internal VVP
  - Drain anteriorly into external VVP
- **External vertebral venous plexus**
  - Anterior, posterior components in paravertebral region
  - Surround vertebral column
  - Connect with: Internal VVP; azygos, lumbar veins ⇒ IVC, SVC
  - Posterior veins form paired system, lie in vertebrocostal grooves
  - Cross anastomoses lie between spinous processes
  - Extensive in posterior nuchal region, drain into deep cervical veins, IJV
- **Intradural veins**
  - Parallel spinal arteries
  - Symmetric pattern of venous drainage (compared with highly asymmetric arterial supply)
    - Minimal anterior-posterior, right-left, segmental variations
  - Central, peripheral groups of radial veins drain into anastomoses on cord surface
  - Central group provides return for anterior horns, surrounding white matter
    - ⇒ Drain into central veins in anterior median fissure
    - ⇒ Form anterior median vein
  - Peripheral dorsal, lateral cord drainage via small valveless radial vein plexus
    - ⇒ Coronal venous plexus on cord surface
    - ⇒ Epidural venous plexus of Batson
    - Epidural plexus connects with SVC, IVC, azygos/hemiazygos systems, intracranial dural sinuses
  - 30-70 medullary radicular veins
    - No anterior or posterior dominance
    - Anterior median vein continues caudally along filum terminale to end of dural sac
  - Coronal, median veins drain ⇒ medullary veins
    - No intradural valves but medullary veins have functional valve-like mechanism at dural margin
    - Prevents epidural reflux into intradural space
    - Medullary veins leave intradural space at root sleeve ⇒ epidural plexus

Imaging Anatomy

Overview

- CT
  - Normal funnel-shaped discontinuity in cortex of posterior vertebral bodies
  - Represents site at which basivertebral veins drain into anterior internal VVP
- Spinal veins, plexi enhance strongly on T1 C+ MR
  - External, internal VVPs surround vertebral column, thecal sac
  - Basivertebral vein enhances in "Y" configuration
  - Thin, linear enhancement on cord surface normal, caused by venous anastomoses
  - Faint filum terminale enhancement normal

Anatomy-Based Imaging Issues

Key Concepts or Questions

- Retrograde flow from pelvis → epidural plexus
  - Provides natural route of spread from pelvic neoplasms, infection to vertebral bodies
- Pharyngovertebral veins penetrate anterior atlanto-occipital membrane ⇒ surround atlantoaxial joint
  - Permits inflammatory relaxation/subluxation (Grisel syndrome)

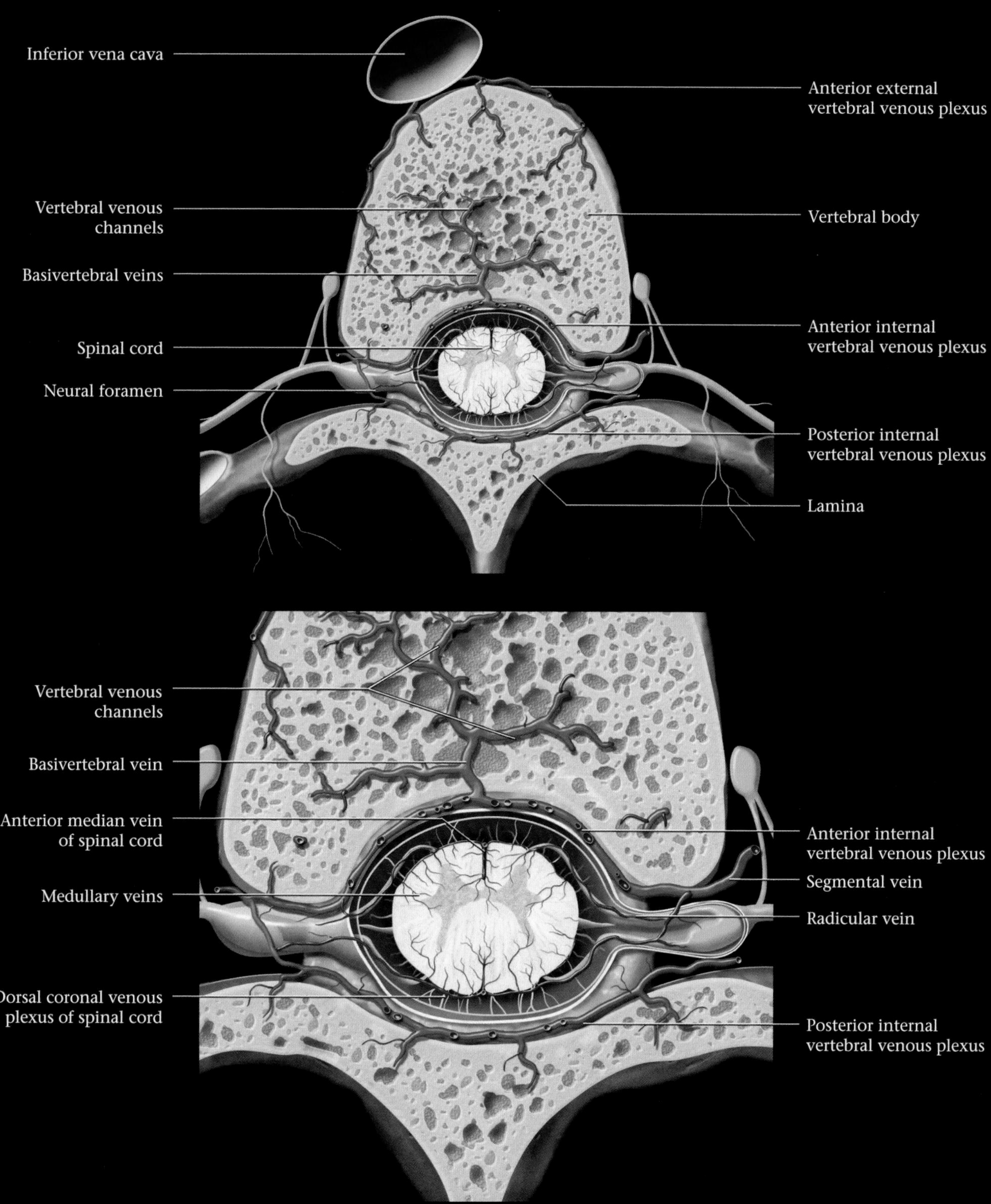

Inferior vena cava
Anterior external vertebral venous plexus
Vertebral venous channels
Vertebral body
Basivertebral veins
Anterior internal vertebral venous plexus
Spinal cord
Neural foramen
Posterior internal vertebral venous plexus
Lamina
Vertebral venous channels
Basivertebral vein
Anterior median vein of spinal cord
Anterior internal vertebral venous plexus
Segmental vein
Medullary veins
Radicular vein
Dorsal coronal venous plexus of spinal cord
Posterior internal vertebral venous plexus

(Top) Axial graphic of thoracic vertebral bodies and venous anatomy. The vertebral bodies are drained by anterior perforating veins, as well as via the basivertebral venous plexus. The anterior perforating veins are part of the anterior external plexus, while the basivertebral veins are part of the anterior internal plexus. The spinal central canal contains the anterior and posterior internal vertebral venous plexi. **(Bottom)** Magnified graphic of the internal vertebral venous plexus. The radicular veins course along the dorsal and ventral rami, eventually draining into components of the anterior or posterior internal plexus, and subsequently the segmental veins, which will drain into the superior or inferior vena cava.

SPINAL VEINS AND VENOUS PLEXUS

AXIAL T1 C+ MR

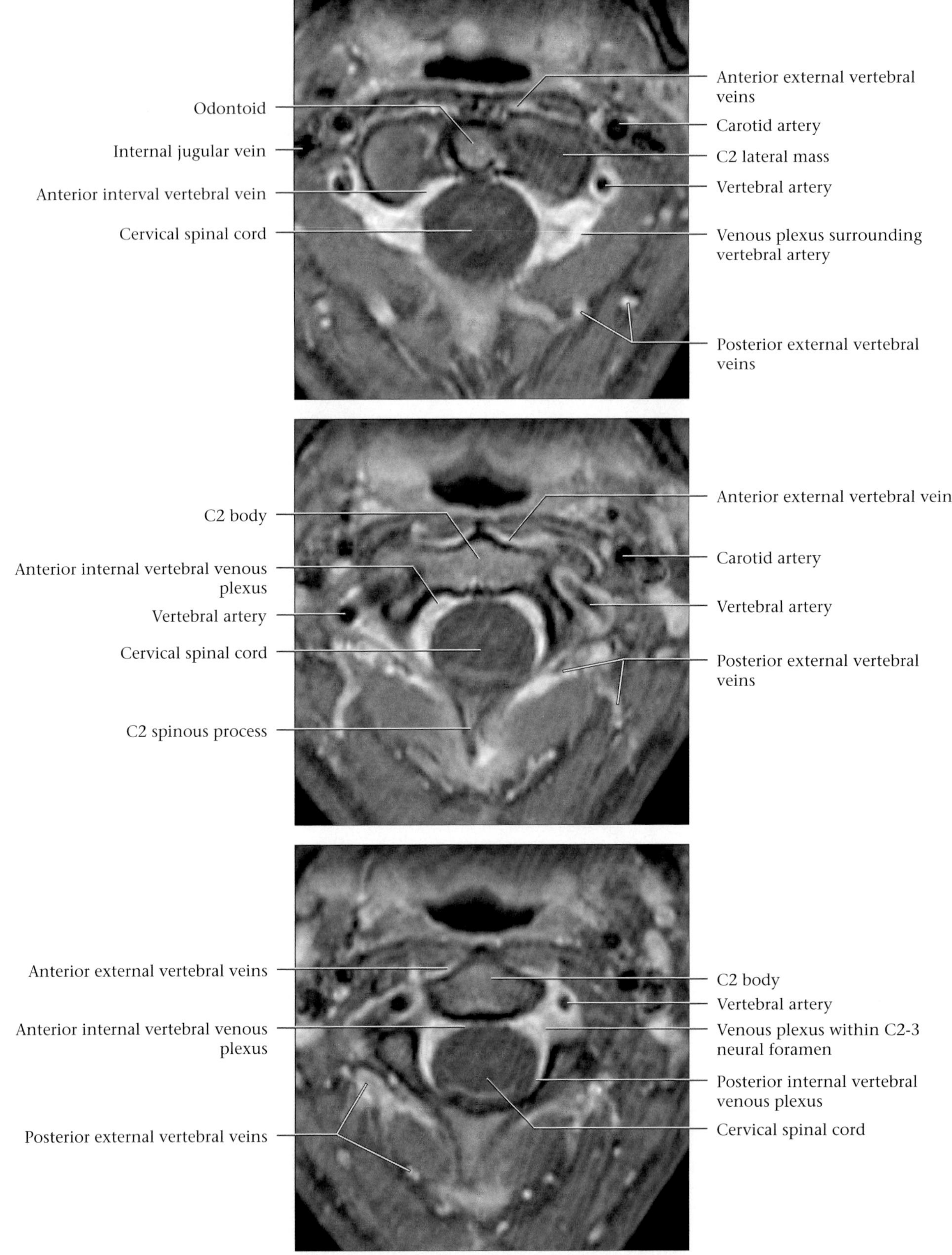
Odontoid
Internal jugular vein
Anterior interval vertebral vein
Cervical spinal cord
Anterior external vertebral veins
Carotid artery
C2 lateral mass
Vertebral artery
Venous plexus surrounding vertebral artery
Posterior external vertebral veins
C2 body
Anterior internal vertebral venous plexus
Vertebral artery
Cervical spinal cord
C2 spinous process
Anterior external vertebral vein
Carotid artery
Vertebral artery
Posterior external vertebral veins
Anterior external vertebral veins
Anterior internal vertebral venous plexus
Posterior external vertebral veins
C2 body
Vertebral artery
Venous plexus within C2-3 neural foramen
Posterior internal vertebral venous plexus
Cervical spinal cord

(Top) First of six axial fat suppressed T1 C+ MR images through cervical spine presented from superior to inferior shows the distribution of cervical venous plexus surrounding the vertebral arteries, and joining with the anterior and posterior internal vertebral venous plexus. The posterior external plexus forms two parallel columns of veins to either side of the spinous processes. **(Middle)** Image through C2 body shows the anastomoses between the different venous components such as anterior internal plexus and posterior external plexus dorsal to lamina, and surrounding vertebral arteries. **(Bottom)** Image through the C2-3 neural foramen shows the prominent venous plexus surrounding vertically oriented vertebral artery flow void, and anastomosing with the internal venous plexus circumferentially surrounding the thecal sac.

SPINAL VEINS AND VENOUS PLEXUS

AXIAL T1 C+ MR

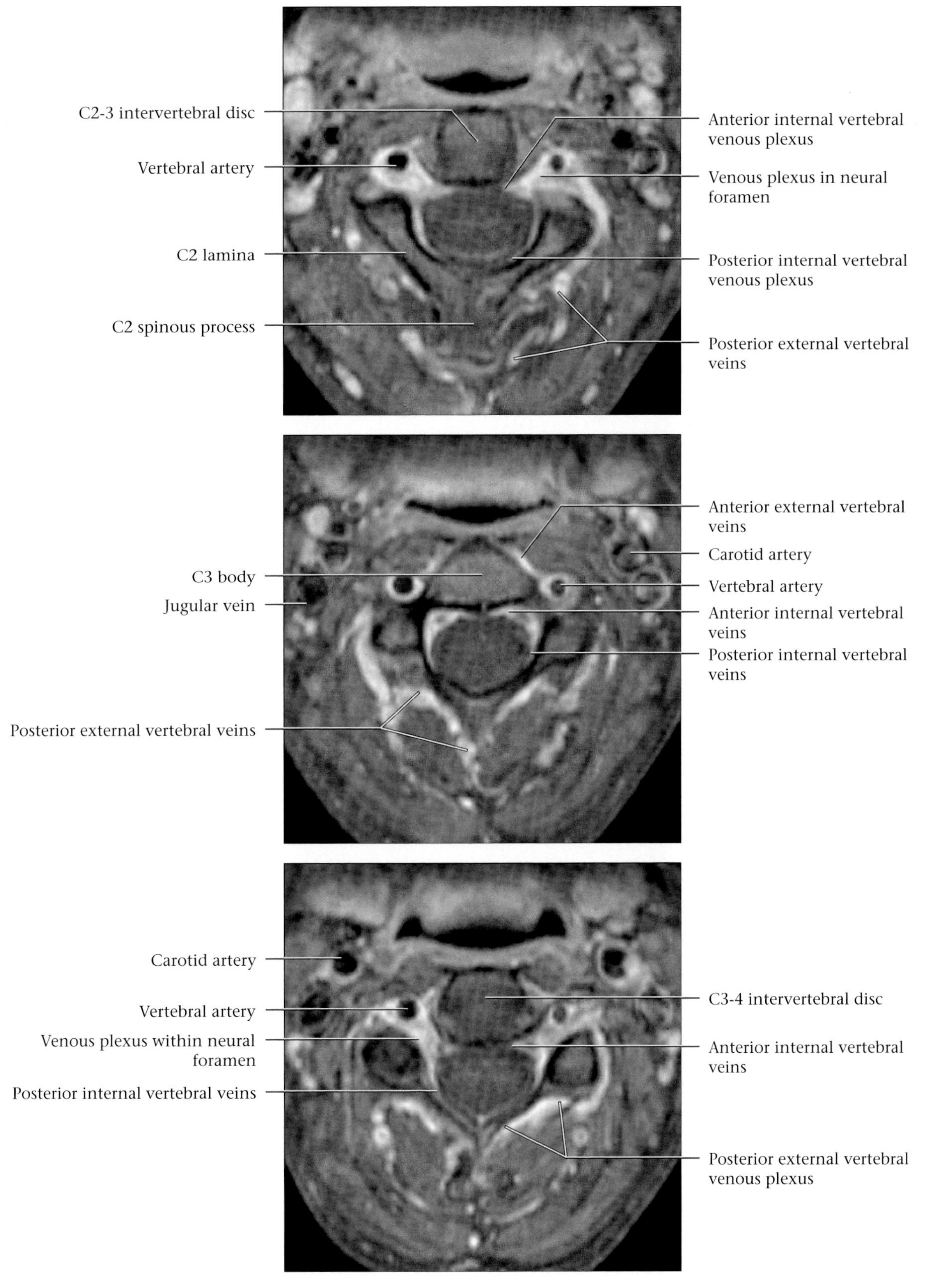
C2-3 intervertebral disc
Vertebral artery
C2 lamina
C2 spinous process
Anterior internal vertebral venous plexus
Venous plexus in neural foramen
Posterior internal vertebral venous plexus
Posterior external vertebral veins
C3 body
Jugular vein
Posterior external vertebral veins
Anterior external vertebral veins
Carotid artery
Vertebral artery
Anterior internal vertebral veins
Posterior internal vertebral veins
Carotid artery
Vertebral artery
Venous plexus within neural foramen
Posterior internal vertebral veins
C3-4 intervertebral disc
Anterior internal vertebral veins
Posterior external vertebral venous plexus

(Top) Image through more inferior aspect of the C2-3 neural foramen shows the prominent venous plexus surrounding vertically oriented vertebral artery flow void, and anastomosing with thin crescentic internal venous plexus circumferentially surrounding the thecal sac. The communication between the posterior external vertebral veins and the more anterior foraminal plexus are pronounced. **(Middle)** Image at C3 body level shows typical pattern of epidural enhancement due to anterior internal venous plexus, most prominent along lateral margins of anterior canal, and thinning in the midline. The anastomoses of the plexus surrounding the vertebral artery and the more ventral anterior external plexus are shown. **(Bottom)** Image through C3-4 level shows the marked enhancement of the foraminal plexus, merging with the external plexus lateral to the facets.

SPINAL VEINS AND VENOUS PLEXUS

CORONAL T1 C+ MR

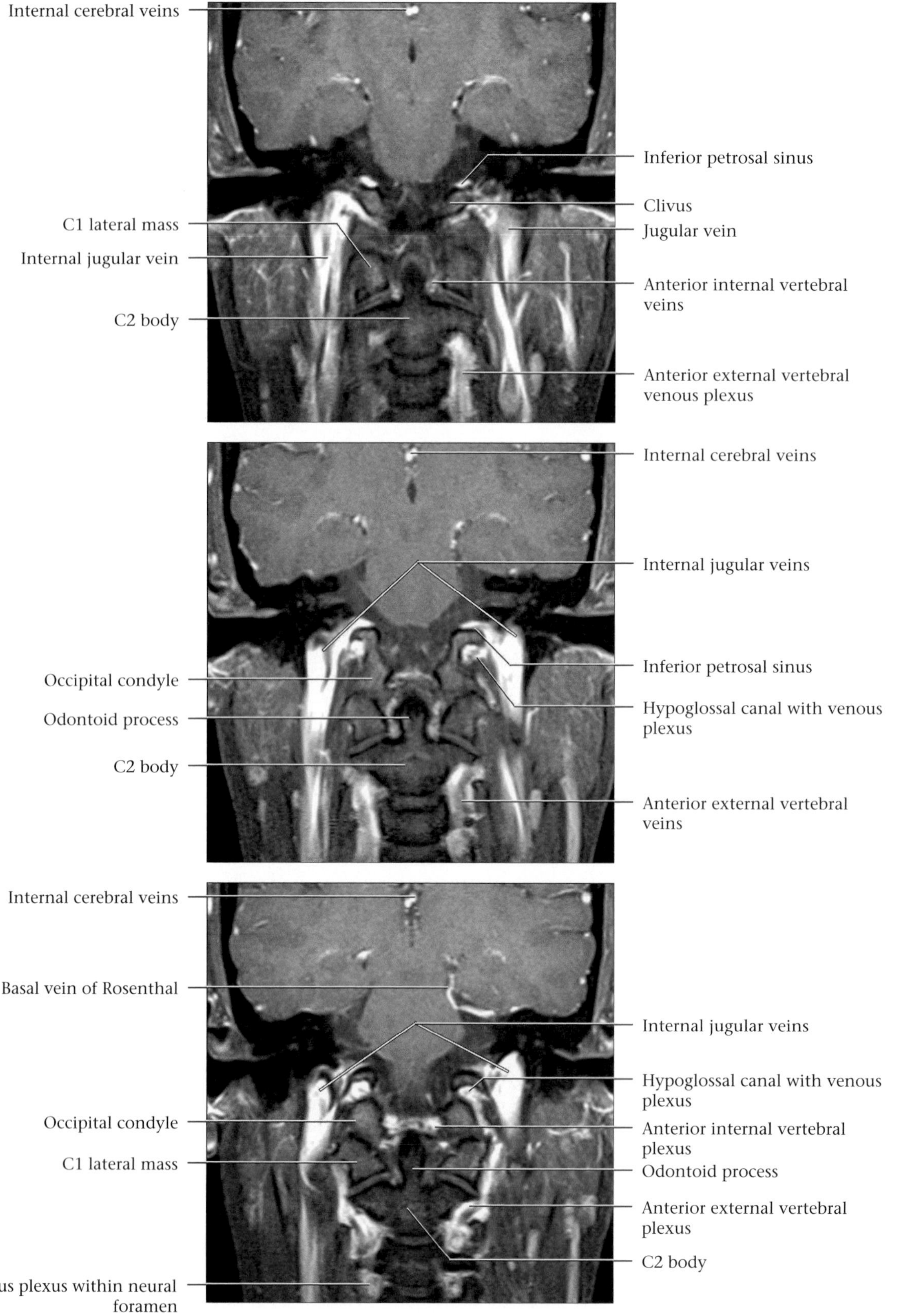
Internal cerebral veins
Inferior petrosal sinus
Clivus
C1 lateral mass
Jugular vein
Internal jugular vein
Anterior internal vertebral veins
C2 body
Anterior external vertebral venous plexus
Internal cerebral veins
Internal jugular veins
Inferior petrosal sinus
Occipital condyle
Hypoglossal canal with venous plexus
Odontoid process
C2 body
Anterior external vertebral veins
Internal cerebral veins
Basal vein of Rosenthal
Internal jugular veins
Hypoglossal canal with venous plexus
Occipital condyle
Anterior internal vertebral plexus
C1 lateral mass
Odontoid process
Anterior external vertebral plexus
C2 body
Venous plexus within neural foramen

(Top) First of six coronal fat suppressed T1 C+ MR images are presented from anterior to posterior. The course of the internal jugular veins from the jugular bulb inferiorly are shown bilaterally, and their relationship to the inferior petrosal sinus and basisphenoid. **(Middle)** Image though mid-odontoid level shows inferior petrosal sinus draining into jugular vein, and adjacent hypoglossal canal with venous plexus. Anterior external venous plexus of upper cervical spine is defined by diffuse enhancement along course of neural foramina. **(Bottom)** Section towards posterior margin of odontoid process continues to define relationship of prominent left jugular bulb with hypoglossal canal, and inferior anterior external vertebral venous plexus.

SPINAL VEINS AND VENOUS PLEXUS

CORONAL T1 C+ MR

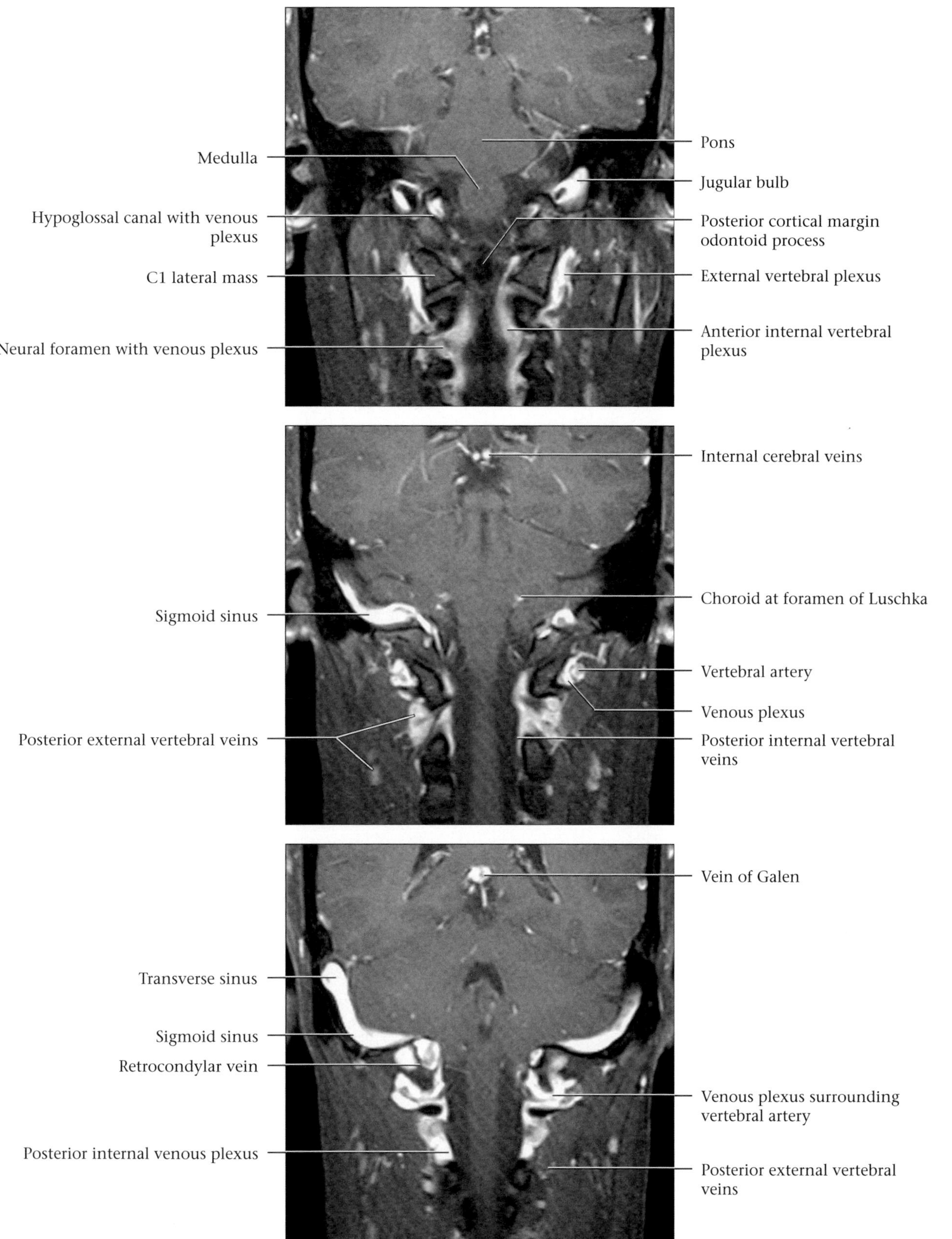

Medulla
Hypoglossal canal with venous plexus
C1 lateral mass
Neural foramen with venous plexus
Pons
Jugular bulb
Posterior cortical margin odontoid process
External vertebral plexus
Anterior internal vertebral plexus
Internal cerebral veins
Choroid at foramen of Luschka
Sigmoid sinus
Vertebral artery
Venous plexus
Posterior external vertebral veins
Posterior internal vertebral veins
Vein of Galen
Transverse sinus
Sigmoid sinus
Retrocondylar vein
Venous plexus surrounding vertebral artery
Posterior internal venous plexus
Posterior external vertebral veins

(Top) Section through posterior margin of odontoid process shows posterior margin of the jugular bulbs and hypoglossal canals. The anterior internal vertebral venous plexus (anterior epidural plexus) is now prominent and merges with the plexus within each neural foramen. **(Middle)** Section through midportion of upper cervical canal shows cerebral venous drainage extending to the skull base with a prominent right sigmoid sinus. The venous plexus surrounding the vertebral artery is present cephalad to the enhancement of the internal venous plexus at C1-2. **(Bottom)** Section through midportion of upper cervical canal shows the cerebral venous drainage at skull base with transverse and sigmoid sinuses curving along occipital bone. The retrocondylar venous system is also present, merging with the upper cervical external plexus.

SPINAL VEINS AND VENOUS PLEXUS

AXIAL, SAGITTAL & CORONAL CECT MIP

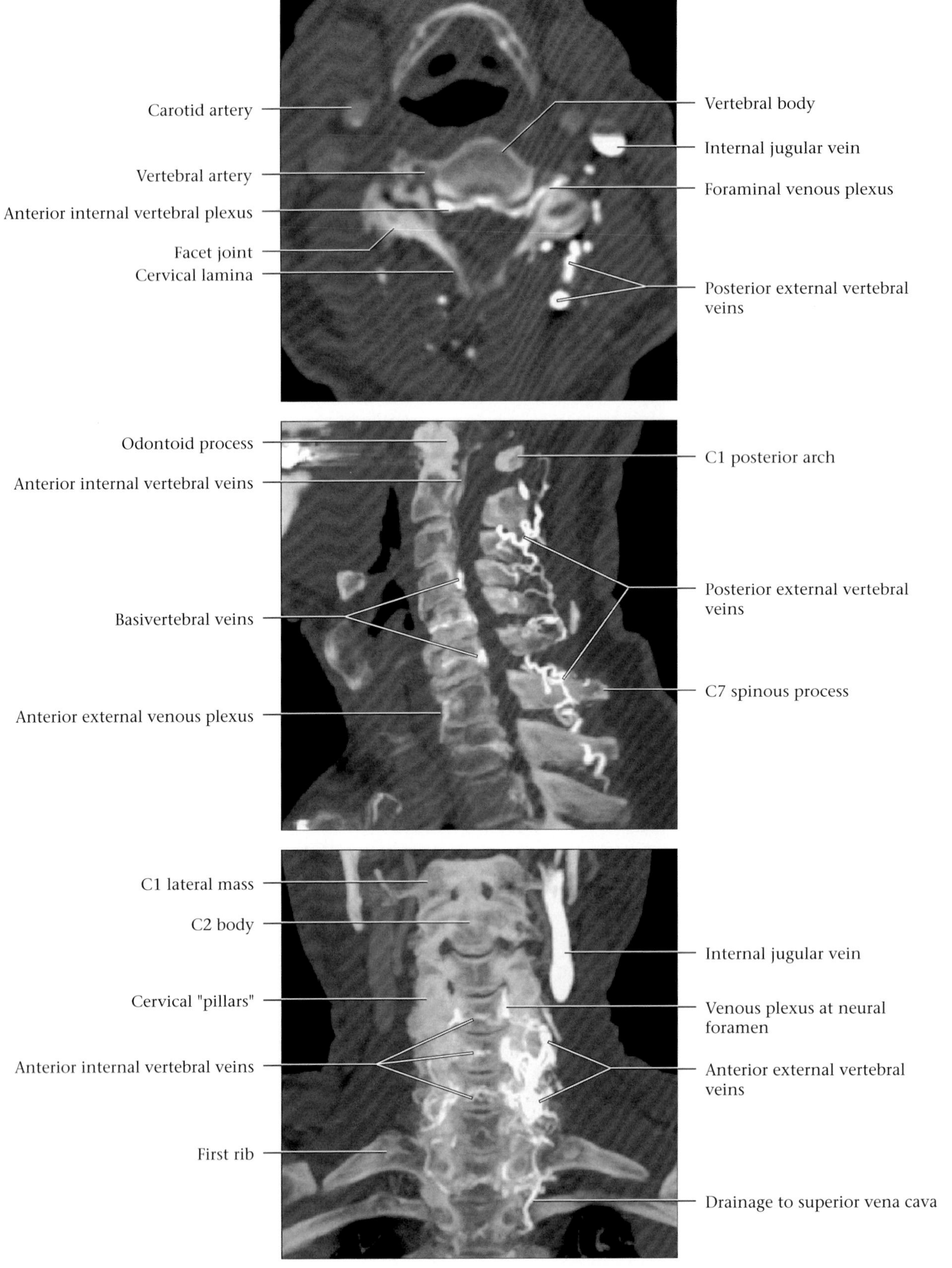

Carotid artery
Vertebral artery
Anterior internal vertebral plexus
Facet joint
Cervical lamina
Vertebral body
Internal jugular vein
Foraminal venous plexus
Posterior external vertebral veins
Odontoid process
Anterior internal vertebral veins
Basivertebral veins
Anterior external venous plexus
C1 posterior arch
Posterior external vertebral veins
C7 spinous process
C1 lateral mass
C2 body
Cervical "pillars"
Anterior internal vertebral veins
First rib
Internal jugular vein
Venous plexus at neural foramen
Anterior external vertebral veins
Drainage to superior vena cava

(Top) Axial CECT MIP image shows reflux of contrast into both external and internal venous plexus, with opacification of left internal jugular vein. **(Middle)** Sagittal CECT MIP of cervical spine shows reflux opacification of venous system, including basivertebral veins, and posterior external venous drainage surrounding spinous processes. **(Bottom)** Coronal CECT MIP projection shows reflux of contrast into anterior external and internal venous systems. The anterior internal venous plexus assumes the typical "step ladder" pattern crossing the midline at the mid vertebral body level.

SPINAL VEINS AND VENOUS PLEXUS

AXIAL & SAGITTAL CECT MIP

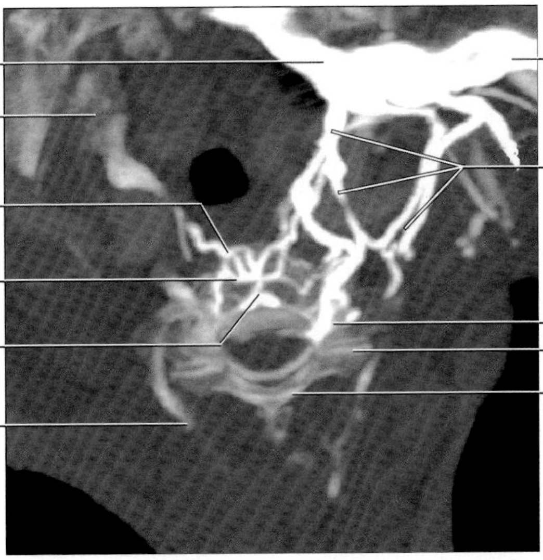

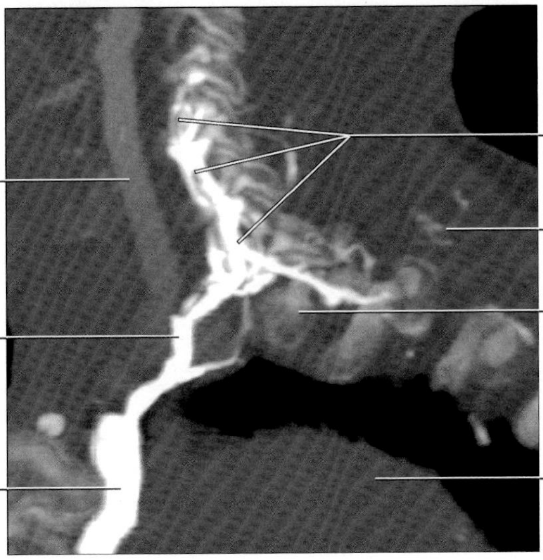

Innominate vein
Right subclavian vein
Anterior external vertebral venous plexus
Intravertebral venous sinuses
Basivertebral veins
Posterior external vertebral veins
Left subclavian vein
Cervical veins draining towards superior vena cava
Foraminal plexus
Facet joint
Cervical lamina

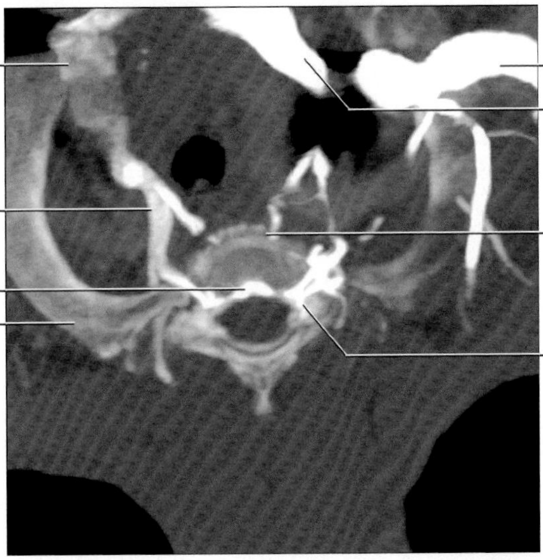

Right subclavian vein
Cervical veins draining toward superior vena cava
Basivertebral vein
First rib
Left subclavian vein
Innominate vein
Anterior external vertebral venous plexus
Foraminal venous plexus

Carotid artery
Cervical vein draining towards superior vena cava
Innominate vein
Anterior external vertebral venous and foraminal venous plexus
Posterior external vertebral veins
First rib
Aortic arch

(Top) Series of CECT MIP projections of neck CT following intravenous contrast administration through left arm vein. The first axial MIP image at cervicothoracic junction shows reflux of contrast retrograde into the cervical vertebral veins outlining both external and internal vertebral venous plexus anatomy. The foraminal component of the external plexus drain through multiple cervical muscular veins into the subclavian system. **(Middle)** Axial CECT MIP image at the T1 level shows the anterior internal vertebral veins crossing midline with the central basivertebral veins. The drainage of the cervical veins towards both left and right subclavian systems is demonstrated. **(Bottom)** Sagittal CECT MIP image through the left cervical facet level shows the confluence of the external plexus along the neural foramen, and the drainage towards the innominate vein.

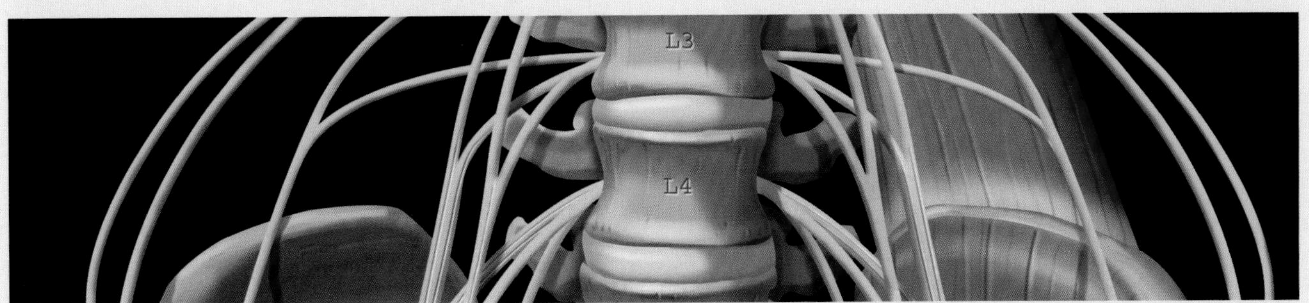
L3
L4

SECTION 4: Plexus

BRACHIAL PLEXUS

Gross Anatomy

Overview

- **Cervical plexus**
  - Formed from ventral rami of C1-4 +/- minor branch of C5
  - Has ascending superficial, descending superficial, deep branches
  - Supplies nuchal muscles, diaphragm, cutaneous head/neck tissues
- **Brachial plexus (BP)**
  - Formed from ventral rami of C5-T1 +/- minor branches from C4, T2
  - Has some proximal branches originating above BP proper
    - Dorsal scapular nerve; long thoracic nerve; nerves to scalene/longus colli muscles; branch to phrenic nerve
  - Remaining minor, all major peripheral branches arise from BP proper
  - BP divided into roots/rami, trunks, divisions, cords, terminal branches
  - **Roots/rami**
    - Originate from spinal cord levels C5 to T1
  - **Trunks**
    - Superior (C5-6), middle (C7), inferior (C8, T1)
    - Minor nerves arising directly from trunks: Suprascapular nerve, nerve to subclavius muscle
  - **Divisions**
    - Anterior divisions innervate anterior (flexor) muscles
    - Posterior divisions innervate posterior (extensor) muscles
    - No named minor nerves arising directly from divisions
  - **Cords**
    - Lateral cord (anterior divisions of superior, middle trunks) innervates anterior (flexor) muscles
    - Medial cord (anterior division of inferior trunk) innervates anterior (flexor) muscles
    - Posterior cord (posterior divisions of all 3 trunks) innervates posterior (extensor) muscles
  - **Branches (terminal)**
    - Musculocutaneous nerve (C5-6) arises from lateral cord
    - Ulnar nerve (C8-T1) arises from medial cord
    - Axillary nerve (C5-6), radial nerve (C5-T1), thoracodorsal nerve (C6-8), upper (C6-7) and lower (C5-6) subscapular nerves all arise from posterior cord

Anatomy Relationships

- Cervical/thoracic
  - BP enters thorax between anterior, middle scalene muscles (scalene triangle)
  - Close anatomic proximity to subclavian artery, lymphatics
  - Subclavian vein courses anterior to anterior scalene muscle, not in direct proximity to brachial plexus
- Axilla
  - Cords surround axillary artery
  - In lower axilla cords divide into nerves to upper limb

Imaging Anatomy

Overview

- Surrounding perineural fat provides excellent visualization of nerves, and allows them to be distinguished from adjacent soft tissues
- Characteristics of normal nerve
  - Well defined oval structure
  - Discrete fascicles are uniform size, shape
    - Distinct fascicular pattern distinguishes peripheral nerves schwannoma or ganglion cyst, which also have high intrinsic T2 signal intensity
  - Isointense to adjacent muscle tissue on T1WI
  - Slightly hyperintense to adjacent muscle on fat-saturated T2WI, STIR

Anatomy-Based Imaging Issues

Key Concepts or Questions

- Essential to assess for anatomic integrity of plexus and search for signs of edema or injury
- Knowledge of normal brachial plexus anatomy critical for evaluating clinical abnormalities

Imaging Recommendations

- Multiplanar high-resolution MR peripheral nerve imaging using surface coil

Imaging Approaches

- Preferred coil: Multipurpose flexible phase array surface coil
- Alternative coil: Neurovascular phase array coil
- Best imaging planes: Coronal and oblique sagittal planes from C3 (rostral) through T2 (caudal), nerve roots (medial) through axilla (lateral)
- Best imaging sequences: Coronal T1, coronal STIR, oblique sagittal T1, and oblique sagittal STIR
- Optional sequences: Oblique sagittal and coronal contrast-enhanced fat-saturated T1WI (for cases of known or suspected neoplasm, scar, or infection)

Imaging Pitfalls

- Too large field of view reduces spatial resolution, compromises visualization of internal BP architecture
- Technically simpler to evaluate the supraclavicular plexus than infraclavicular plexus
- STIR provides more reliable fat suppression than chemical fat-saturated T2WI

Clinical Implications

Clinical Importance

- Complex BP anatomy predisposes to characteristic clinical syndromes
  - Erb palsy - avulsion of upper plexus elements
  - Klumpke palsy - avulsion of lower plexus elements
  - Thoracic outlet syndrome - neural compression at the scalene triangle

BRACHIAL PLEXUS

GRAPHICS

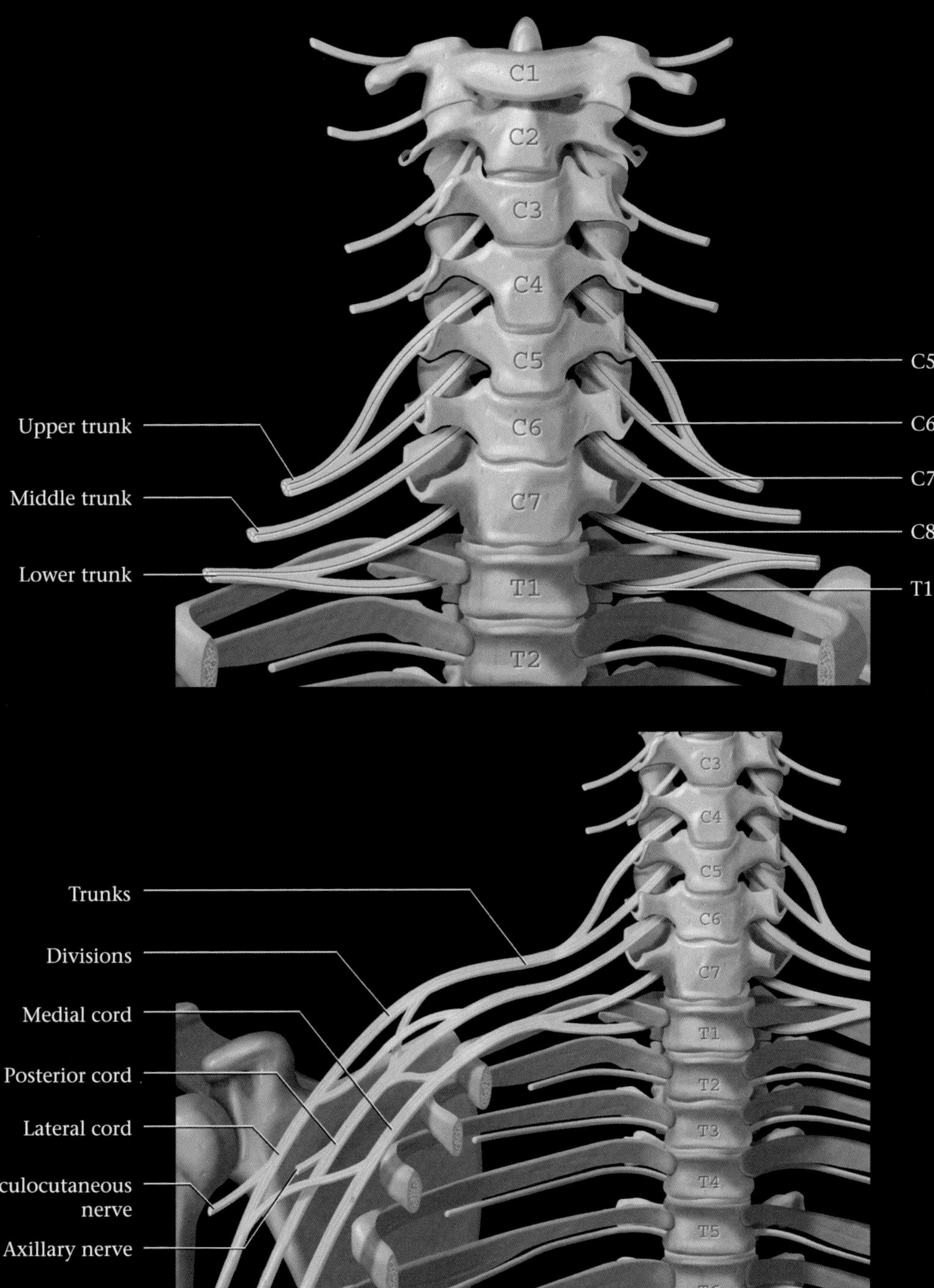
C1
C2
C3
C4
C5
C6
C7
T1
T2
Upper trunk
Middle trunk
Lower trunk
C5
C6
C7
C8
T1
C3
C4
C5
C6
C7
T1
T2
T3
T4
T5
T6
T7
T8
Trunks
Divisions
Medial cord
Posterior cord
Lateral cord
Musculocutaneous nerve
Axillary nerve
Median nerve
Radial nerve
Ulnar nerve

(Top) Coronal graphic of the cervical spine and supraclavicular brachial plexus demonstrates the cervical ventral primary rami combining to form the brachial plexus. The C1-7 roots exit above the same numbered pedicle, C8 exits above the T1 pedicle, and more caudal roots exit below their numbered pedicle. **(Bottom)** Coronal graphic of the brachial plexus demonstrates the more distal plexus elements extending into the axilla. The trunks recombine into posterior and anterior divisions that form the cords. The posterior cord forms the radial and axillary nerves. The medial cord forms the ulnar nerve, while the lateral cord forms the musculocutaneous nerve. The median nerve is formed from branches of both the lateral and medial cords.

CORONAL STIR MR

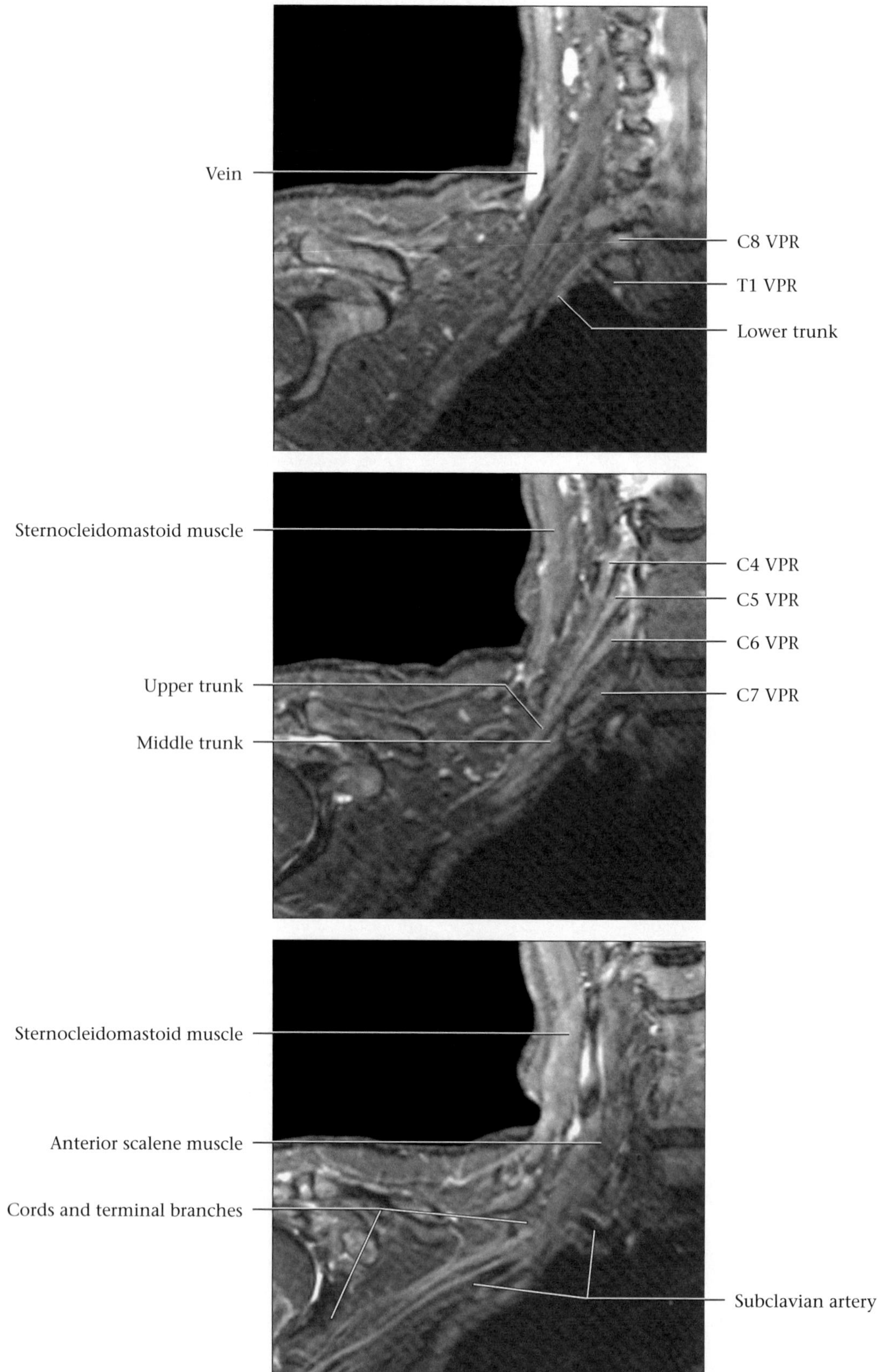
Vein
C8 VPR
T1 VPR
Lower trunk
Sternocleidomastoid muscle
C4 VPR
C5 VPR
C6 VPR
C7 VPR
Upper trunk
Middle trunk
Sternocleidomastoid muscle
Anterior scalene muscle
Cords and terminal branches
Subclavian artery

(Top) First of three coronal STIR MR images presented from posterior to anterior demonstrates the lower cervical roots and ventral primary rami (VPR) (C8, T1) combining into the lower trunk. **(Middle)** This image shows the proximal cervical roots/VPR combining to form the upper and middle trunks of the brachial plexus. Normal nerve is slightly hyperintense to muscle on STIR and fat-saturated T2 MR imaging. **(Bottom)** The distal cords and terminal branches of the brachial plexus are depicted emerging from behind the anterior scalene muscle. The brachial plexus normally exits the neck between the anterior and middle scalene muscles with the subclavian artery, while the subclavian vein travels anterior to the anterior scalene muscle.

CORONAL T1 MR

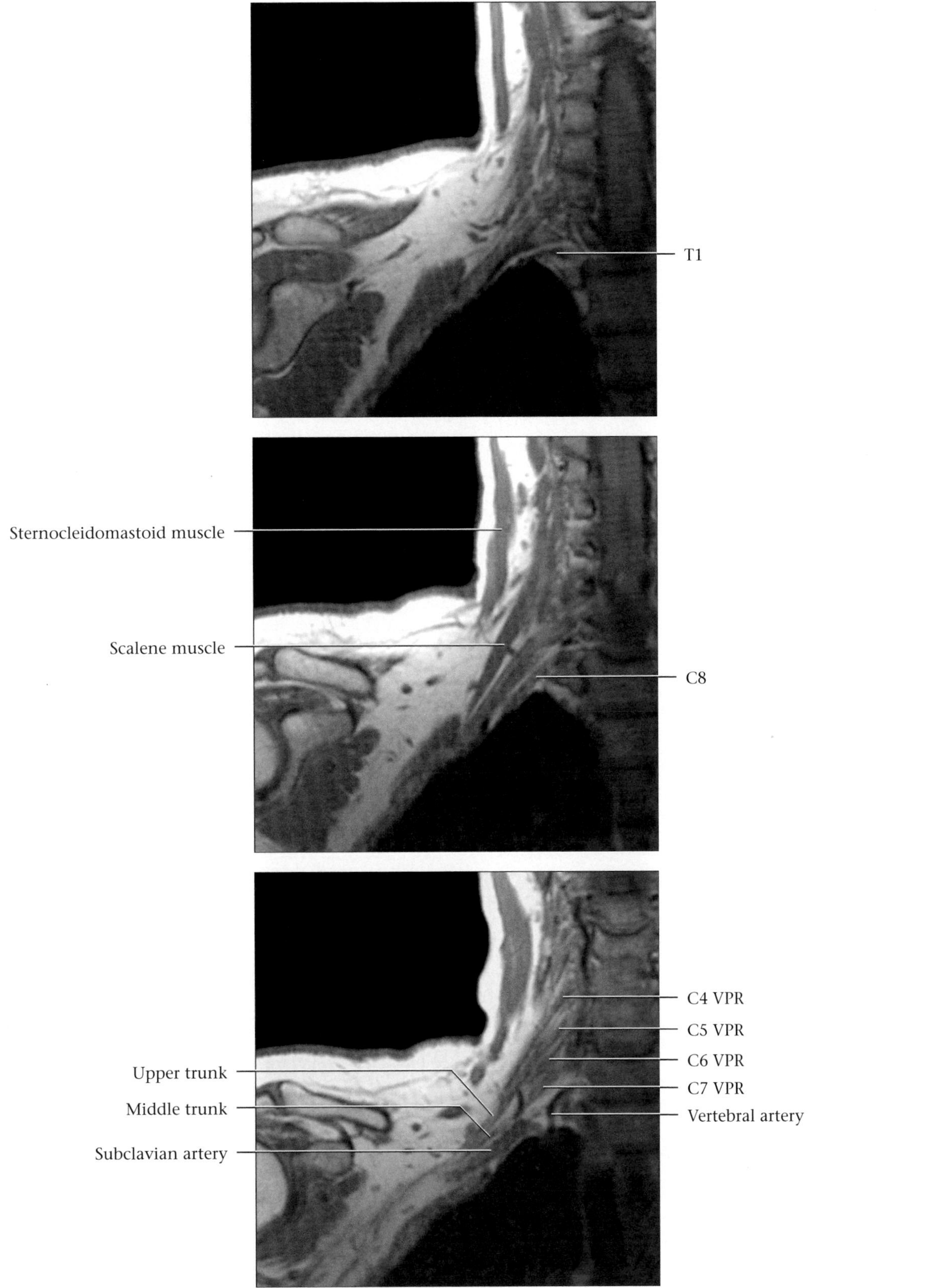

T1
Sternocleidomastoid muscle
Scalene muscle
C8
Upper trunk
Middle trunk
Subclavian artery
C4 VPR
C5 VPR
C6 VPR
C7 VPR
Vertebral artery

(Top) First of three coronal T1 MR images presented from posterior to anterior demonstrates the T1 root/VPR exiting at T1/2 and traversing over the lung apex. **(Middle)** The C8 root/VPR descends over the lung apex. The T1 root, which is out of plane and not seen on this image, will combine with C8 to form the lower trunk. Note that C8 exits from the C7/T1 interspace. Since the nerves are isointense to muscle on T1 MR, it can be sometimes difficult to distinguish nerve from slips of scalene muscle. **(Bottom)** Slightly more anterior image demonstrates the proximal cervical roots/VPR combining to form the upper and middle trunks of the brachial plexus. Normal nerve is slightly isointense to muscle on T1 MR imaging. Note the close anatomic proximity of the brachial plexus elements to the subclavian artery.

OBLIQUE SAGITTAL STIR MR

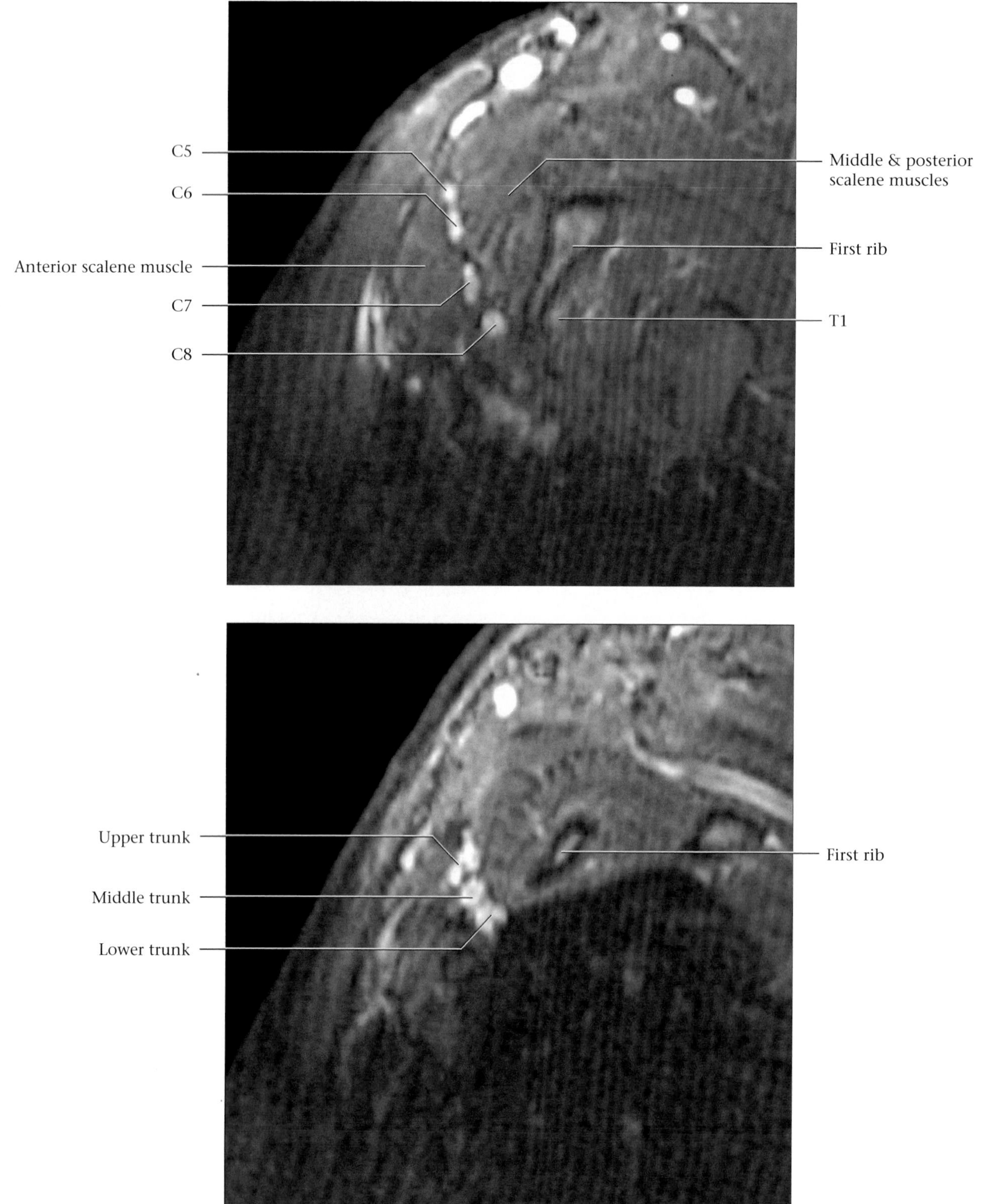
C5
C6
Anterior scalene muscle
C7
C8
Middle & posterior scalene muscles
First rib
T1
Upper trunk
Middle trunk
Lower trunk
First rib

(Top) First of four oblique sagittal STIR MR images presented from medial to lateral demonstrates the ventral primary rami of C5 through T1 proximal to the trunks. C8 exits above the first rib, while T1 exits below. The BP is normally sandwiched between the anterior and middle scalene muscles. **(Bottom)** Slightly more lateral slice demonstrates the formation of the upper, middle, and lower trunks arranged in a vertical line between the scalene muscles. The C5 and C6 VPR can be still resolved as distinct elements within the upper trunk at this level.

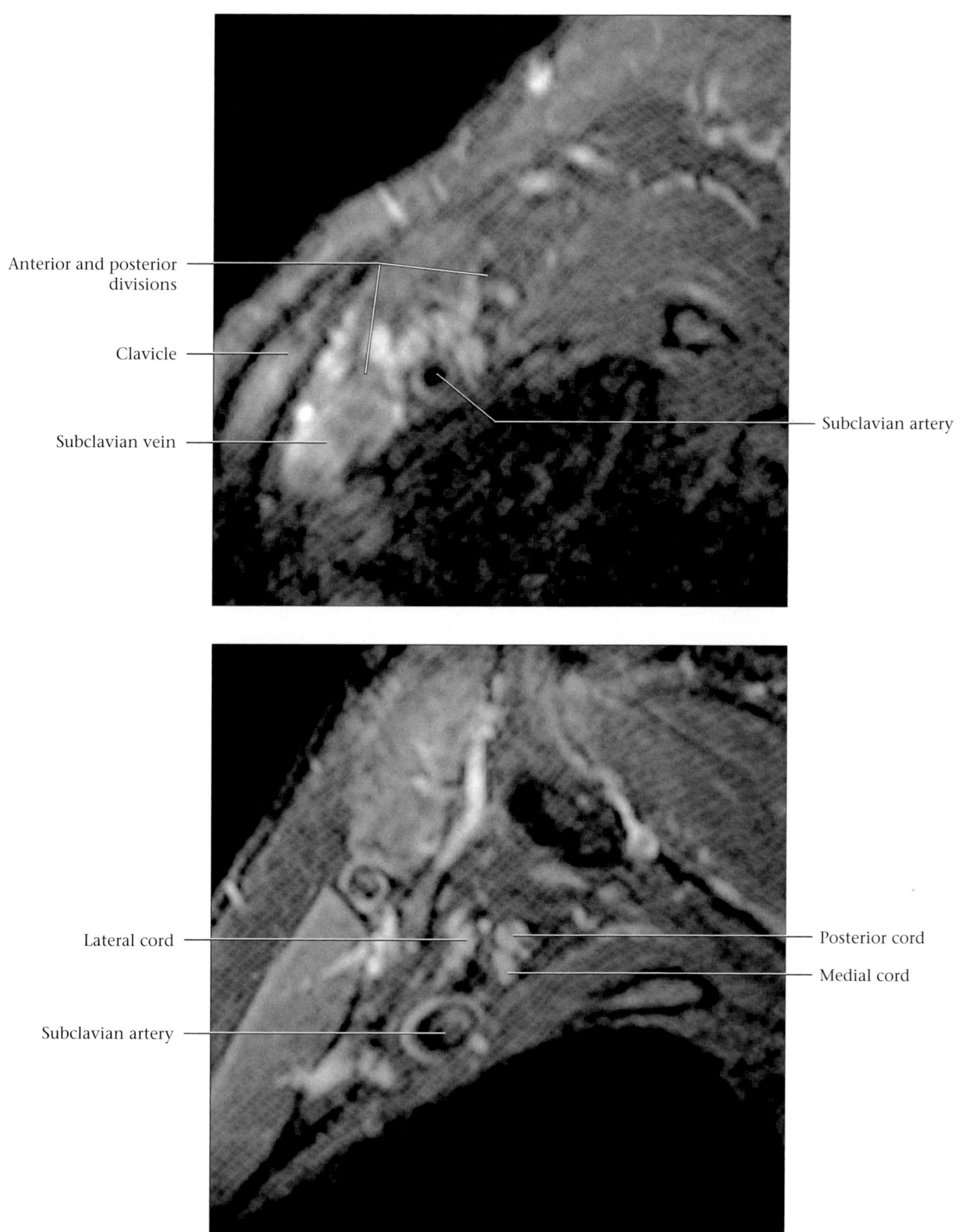
Anterior and posterior divisions
Clavicle
Subclavian vein
Subclavian artery
Lateral cord
Subclavian artery
Posterior cord
Medial cord

(Top) Image at the division level shows mixing and matching of the trunks into anterior and posterior divisions. Note that the divisions are retroclavicular. The posterior divisions will form the posterior cord and the anterior divisions will form the lateral and medial cords. It is generally not possible to follow individual branches of the divisions from trunk to cord. **(Bottom)** Image demonstrates the formation of the three cords (lateral, medial, and posterior). The most important terminal branch of the lateral cord is the musculocutaneous nerve. The posterior cord forms the axillary and radial nerve terminal branches. The medial cord terminates as the ulnar nerve.

AXIAL STIR MR

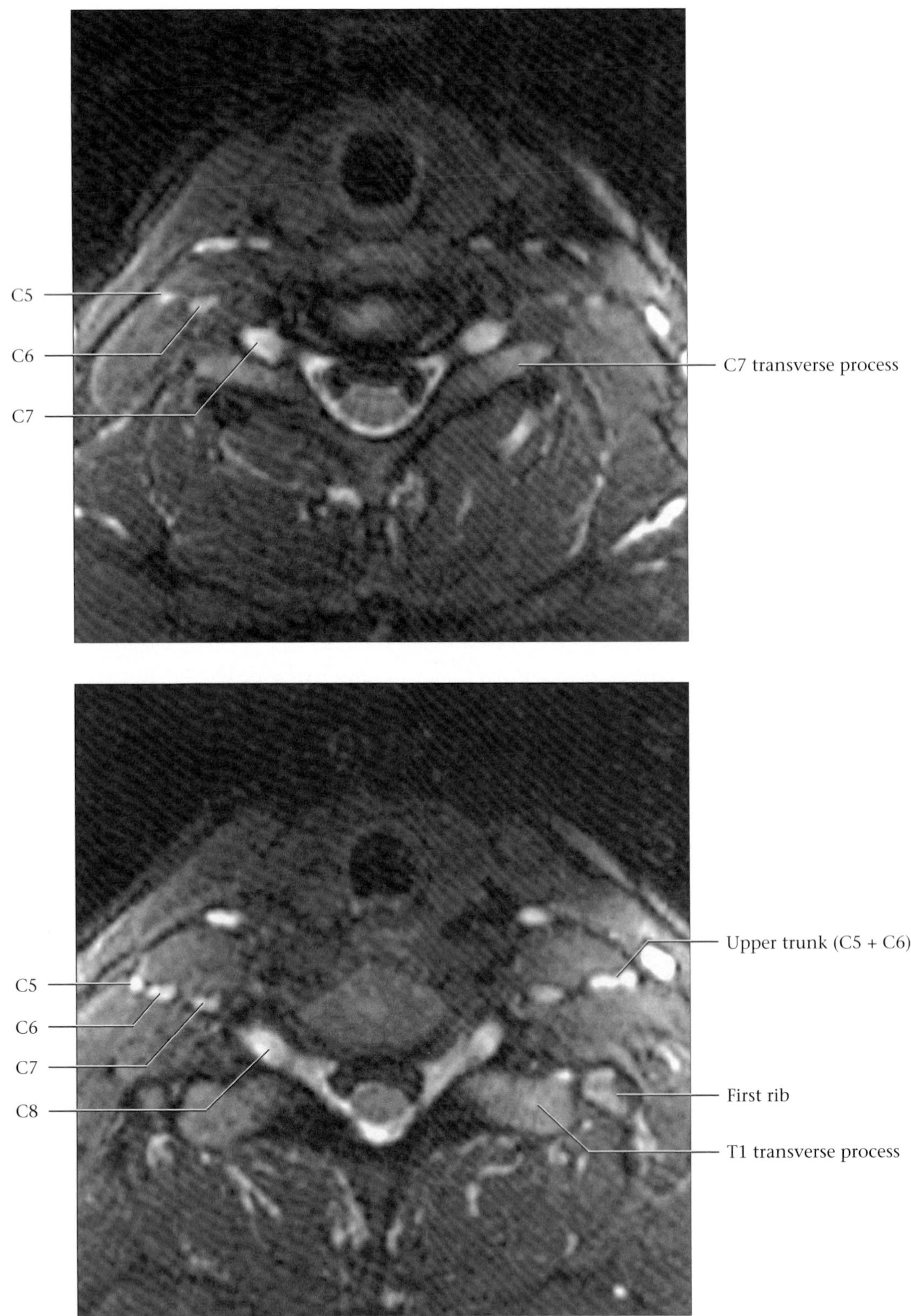
C5
C6
C7
C7 transverse process
C5
C6
C7
C8
Upper trunk (C5 + C6)
First rib
T1 transverse process

(Top) First of four axial STIR MR images presented from rostral to caudal shows the upper brachial plexus elements (C5-7 VPR) traveling between the anterior and middle scalene muscles in preparation to form the brachial plexus. **(Bottom)** Image at the C7/T1 level depicts the linear alignment of the C5 through C8 VPR. C5 and C6 are closely approximated and forming the left upper trunk.

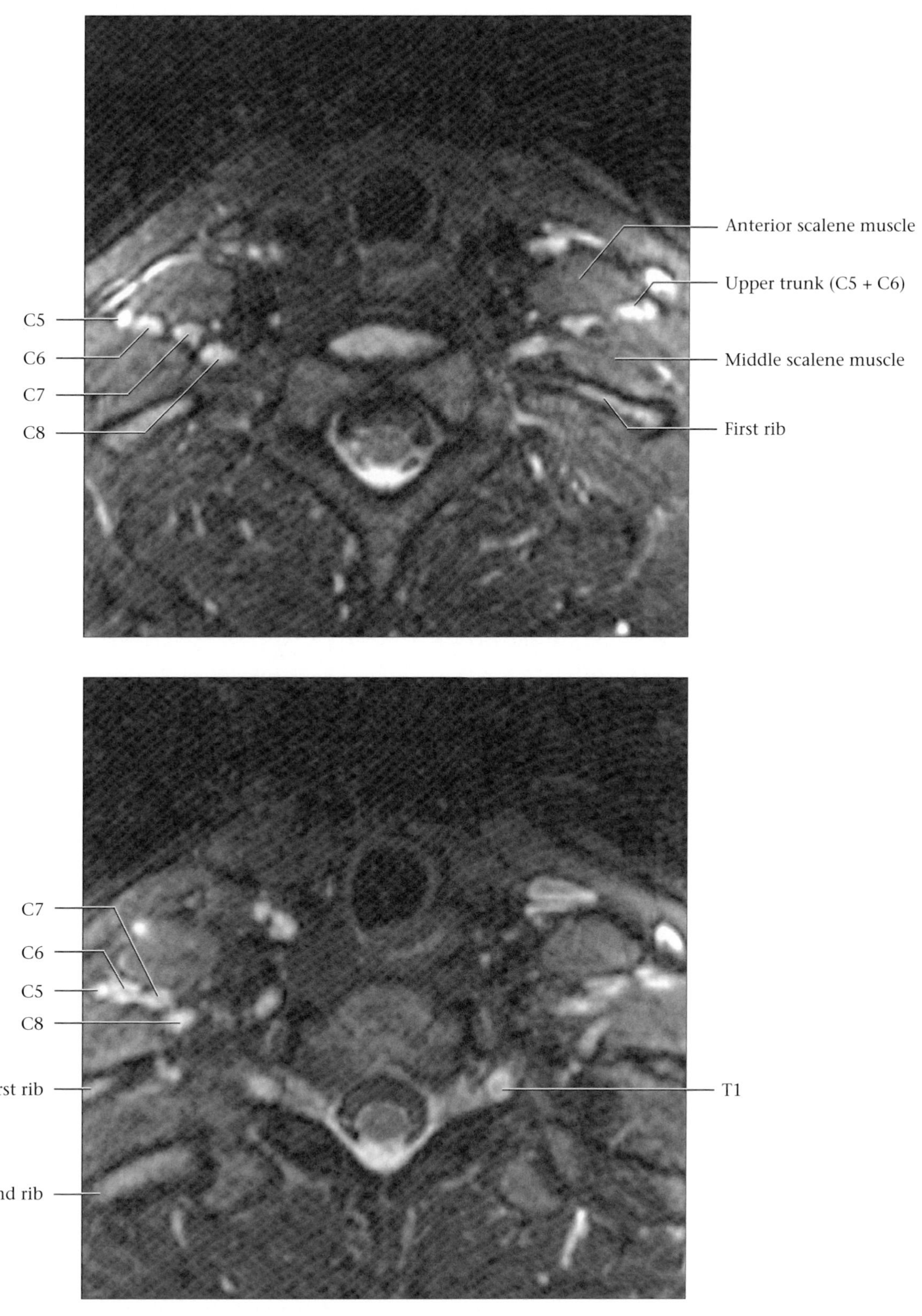
Anterior scalene muscle
Upper trunk (C5 + C6)
Middle scalene muscle
First rib
C5
C6
C7
C8
C7
C6
C5
C8
First rib
Second rib
T1

(Top) Imaging more caudal at C7/T1 level depicts the upper trunk on the left. Note that the brachial plexus elements exit the neck between the anterior and middle scalene muscles. **(Bottom)** Image at the T1/2 level reveals the 5 roots/ventral primary rami and their relationship to the scalene muscles and ribs. They are arranged linearly on axial imaging, and are always most easily located by finding the scalene muscles and following the roots out from the spinal cord laterally as they exit the neck into the thorax.

LUMBAR PLEXUS

Terminology

Abbreviations

- Lumbar plexus (LP)
- Lumbosacral plexus, trunk (LSP, LST)

Gross Anatomy

Overview

- **Lumbar plexus**
  - Formed by
    - L2-4 ventral rami
    - Minor branches of L1, T12
  - Two major branches
    - **Femoral nerve** (posterior divisions, L2-4)
    - **Obturator nerve** (anterior divisions, L2-4)
  - Minor branches, constituent rami
    - Iliohypogastric (L1)
    - Ilioinguinal (L1)
    - Genitofemoral (L1, L2)
    - Lateral femoral cutaneous (L2, L3)
    - Superior gluteal nerves (L4-S1)
- **Lumbosacral trunk**
  - Formed by
    - L5
    - L4 ventral rami (minor branch)
- **Lumbosacral plexus**
  - Formed by
    - LST (L5, minor branch of L4)
    - S1-4

Anatomy Relationships

- **Lumbar plexus**
  - Lies in posterior aspect of psoas major
  - Anterior to lumbar vertebral transverse processes
  - Courses medial to psoas, ventral to quadratus lumborum
- **Femoral nerve**
  - Largest and major terminal branch of LP
  - Arises from L2-4
  - Courses inferiorly, medial to psoas major
  - Emerges between psoas, iliacus
  - Passes behind inguinal ligament into thigh
  - Splits into anterior, posterior divisions
  - Sensory, motor fibers mixed in peripheral nerves
  - Femoral artery lies medially

Imaging Anatomy

Overview

- General concepts
  - Perineural fat surrounds, provides excellent visualization of LP
  - Normal nerve fascicles are uniform size, shape
- MR
  - Intrafascicular signal intensity determined by
    - Endoneurial fluid
    - Axoplasmic water
  - Interfascicular signal intensity
    - Mostly fibrofatty connective tissue
    - Susceptible to fat suppression

Anatomy-Based Imaging Issues

Key Concepts or Questions

- MR
  - T1WI + fat-saturated T2WI/STIR sequences complementary
  - T1WI
    - Normal LP is well-defined ovoid structure
    - Discrete fascicles isointense to adjacent muscle
  - Fat-saturated T2WI/STIR
    - LP slightly hyperintense to adjacent muscle
    - Hypointense to regional vessels
    - Discrete fascicles clearly-defined, separated by lower intensity connective tissue

Imaging Recommendations

- Coils
  - Torso wrap-around or pelvis phase array preferred
  - Spine phase array alternative coil
    - Provides inferior signal to noise ratio (SNR)
    - Especially notable in lateral aspects of posterior abdomen, pelvis
  - Body coil
    - Good spatial coverage
    - Poor SNR severely limits utility
- Planes
  - Coronal, oblique sagittal
  - From L3 superiorly through ischial tuberosity inferiorly
  - From spine medially through greater trochanter laterally
- Sequences
  - Coronal T1WI
  - Coronal STIR or fat-saturated T2WI
  - Direct axial or oblique axial T1WI
  - Direct axial or oblique axial fat-saturated T2WI/STIR
  - Optional: T1 C+ (if known/suspected neoplasm, scar, infection)
- Specific recommendations
  - For neural foramina, proximal L4-5 ventral rami, LST, sciatic nerve: Direct coronal, axial planes preferred
  - For optimal visualization of LP internal architecture: Oblique axial plane preferred

Imaging Pitfalls

- Nerves, vessels may be difficult to differentiate
  - Nerves
    - Round/ovoid linear structures
    - No "flow voids"
    - Branch at relatively acute angles
    - Enhance minimally
    - Show distinctive "fascicular" architecture (on axial)
  - Vessels
    - Round/ovoid, linear
    - Have internal "flow voids"
    - Branch at large angles
    - Enhance intensely
- Normal peripheral nerves, lesions (e.g., schwannoma) both have high T2 signal
  - Nerves have distinct fascicular pattern

LUMBAR PLEXUS

GRAPHICS

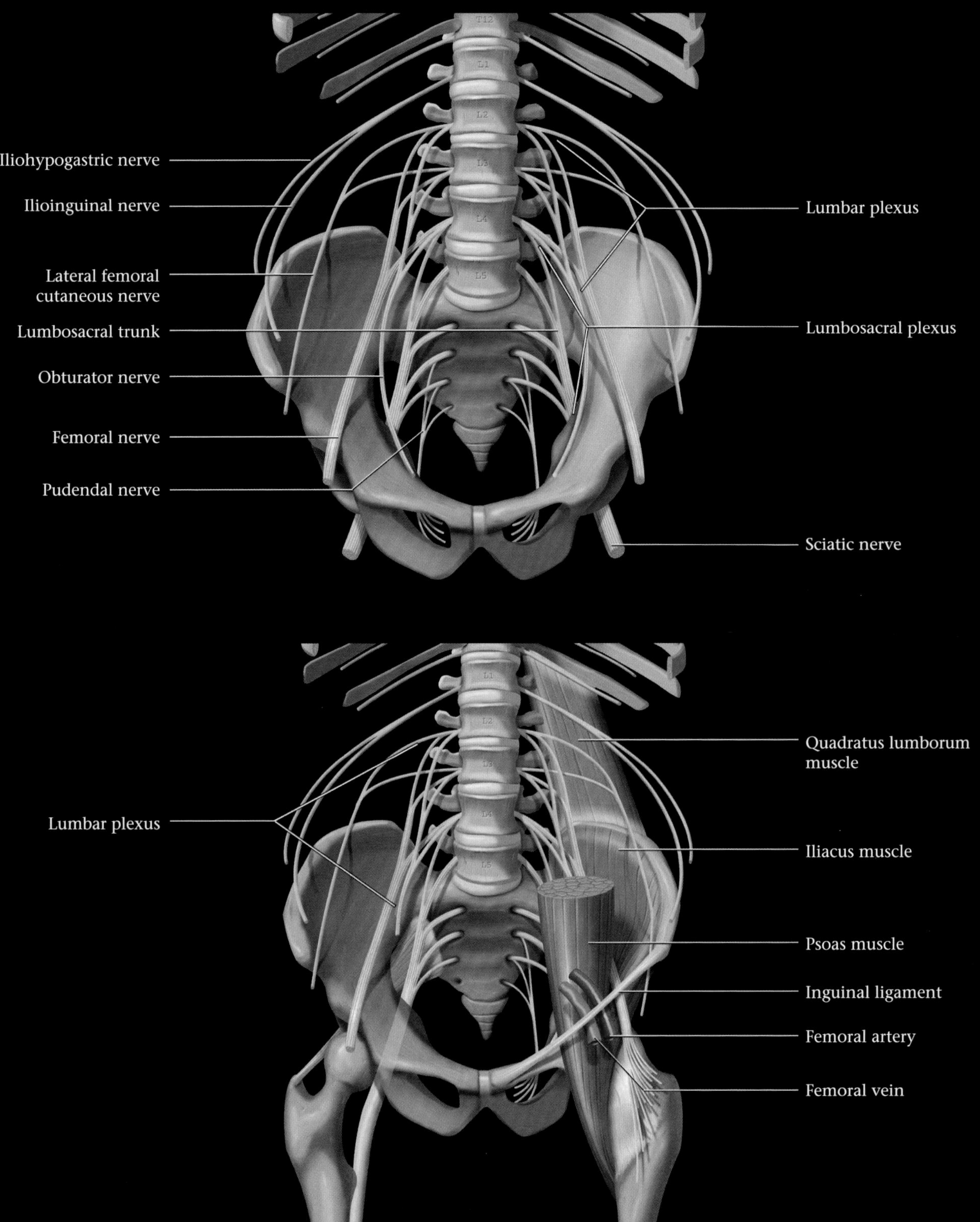

T12
L1
L2
L3
L4
L5
Iliohypogastric nerve
Ilioinguinal nerve
Lateral femoral cutaneous nerve
Lumbosacral trunk
Obturator nerve
Femoral nerve
Pudendal nerve
Lumbar plexus
Lumbosacral plexus
Sciatic nerve
Lumbar plexus
Quadratus lumborum muscle
Iliacus muscle
Psoas muscle
Inguinal ligament
Femoral artery
Femoral vein

(Top) Coronal graphic shows the lumbosacral spine, pelvis, coccyx, and nerves. The lumbar plexus is composed of ventral primary rami of L2-L4. The plexus splits into a larger posterior division which forms femoral nerve and a smaller anterior division forming obturator nerve. **(Bottom)** Coronal graphic demonstrates relationship of plexi to pelvic musculature and soft tissues. The lumbar plexus runs ventral to quadratus lumborum and iliacus muscles and medial to the psoas muscle. The femoral nerve, the major terminal branch of the lumbar plexus, travels in the groove between iliacus and psoas muscles and passes under the inguinal ligament to exit pelvis at the femoral canal. The femoral artery and vein lie medial to the femoral nerve.

LUMBAR PLEXUS

CORONAL T1 MR

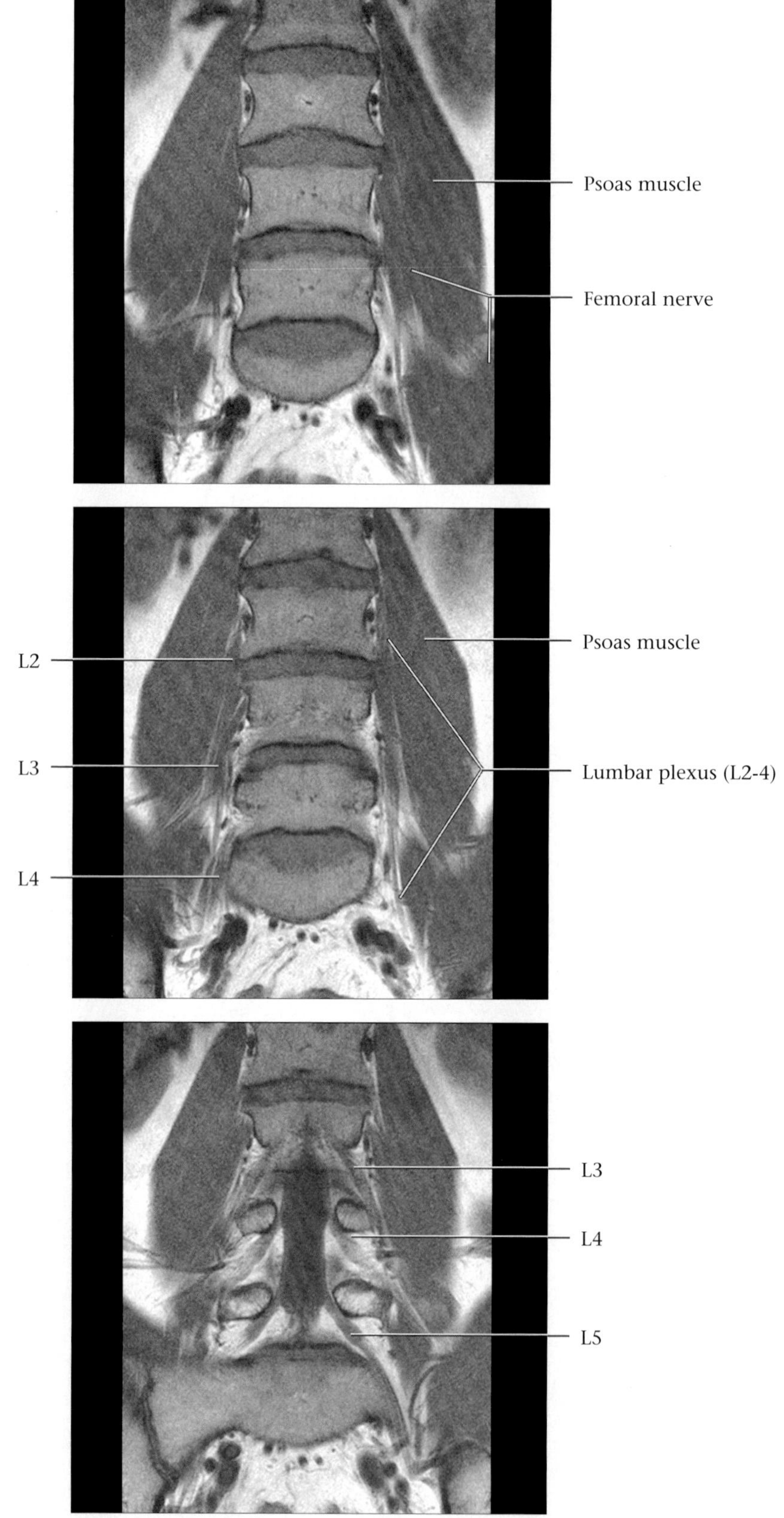
Psoas muscle
Femoral nerve
Psoas muscle
L2
L3
L4
Lumbar plexus (L2-4)
L3
L4
L5

(Top) First of three coronal T1 MR images presented from anterior to posterior demonstrates the lumbar plexus and ipsilateral femoral nerve traveling along the medial aspect of the psoas muscle. **(Middle)** This image demonstrates the normal lumbar plexus arising from its primary neural inputs (L2-L4). Normal nerve is isointense to normal muscle. The lumbar plexus is easily identified by locating the medial border of the psoas muscle. **(Bottom)** Image more posteriorly shows the normal proximal L3, L4, and L5 roots and rami exiting under the vertebral pedicle. L3 and L4 will join L2 to form the lumbar plexus and subsequently divide into anterior and posterior divisions respectively to form the obturator and femoral nerves. L5 will join a minor branch of L4 to form the lumbosacral trunk, a primary component of the sacral plexus.

CORONAL T2 FS MR

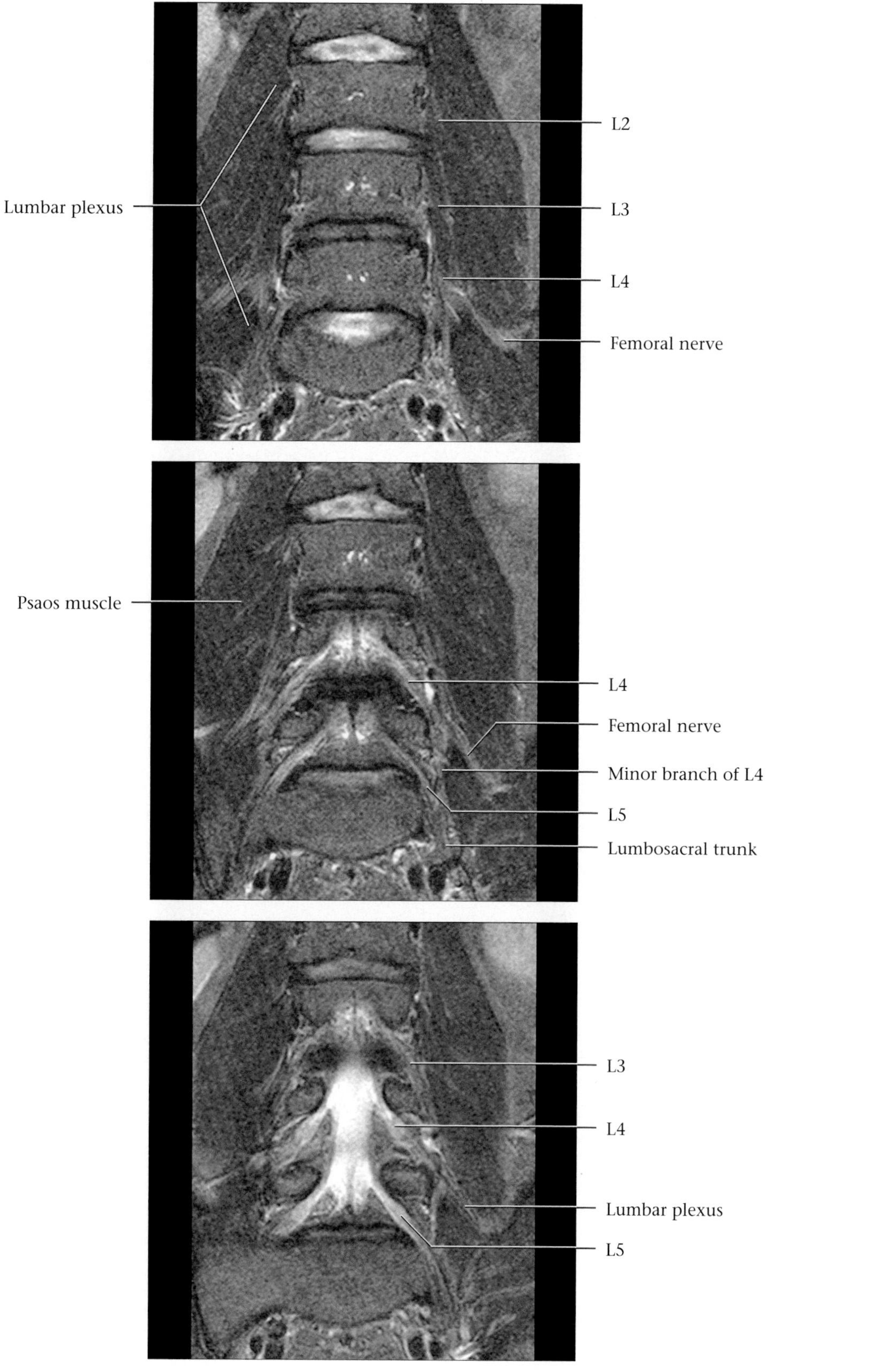

L2
Lumbar plexus
L3
L4
Femoral nerve
Psaos muscle
L4
Femoral nerve
Minor branch of L4
L5
Lumbosacral trunk
L3
L4
Lumbar plexus
L5

(Top) First of three coronal fat-saturated T2 MR images presented from anterior to posterior demonstrates the lumbar plexus and its component L2-L4 roots/rami. Also seen is the proximal femoral nerve transiting along the medial ipsilateral psoas muscle into the iliopsoas groove. Normal nerve is mildly hyperintense to muscle on fat saturated T2 or STIR MR imaging. **(Middle)** This image better demonstrates the L4 contribution to the lumbar plexus as well as the proximal lumbosacral trunk, which will contribute to the sacral plexus. **(Bottom)** More posterior image shows the proximal L3 and L4 roots and rami exiting under the vertebral pedicles to form the lumbar plexus along the medial psoas border.

AXIAL T1 MR

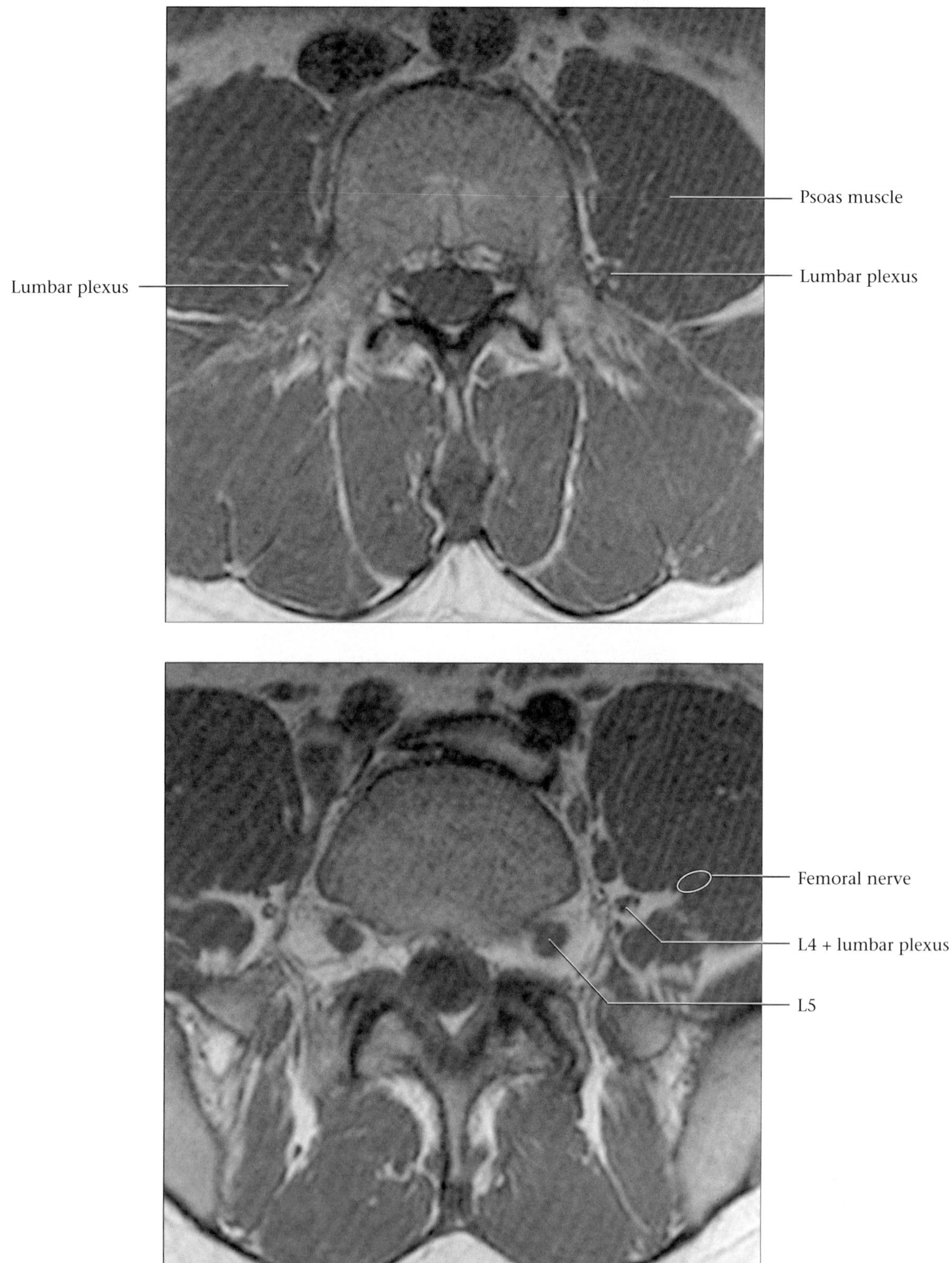
Psoas muscle
Lumbar plexus
Lumbar plexus
Femoral nerve
L4 + lumbar plexus
L5

(Top) First of two axial T1 MR images presented from superior to inferior depicts the lumbar plexus (composed of L2 and L3 at this level) traveling adjacent to the medial psoas muscle. A faint fascicular architecture is apparent. Surrounding bright fat helps identification of the plexus. **(Bottom)** More caudal image shows the femoral nerve along the medial psoas muscle. It is hard to identify the femoral nerve at this level on T1 MR imaging because of its isointensity to the muscle. L4 has joined the remainder of the lumbar plexus at this level, and contributes to both the LP and the lumbosacral trunk.

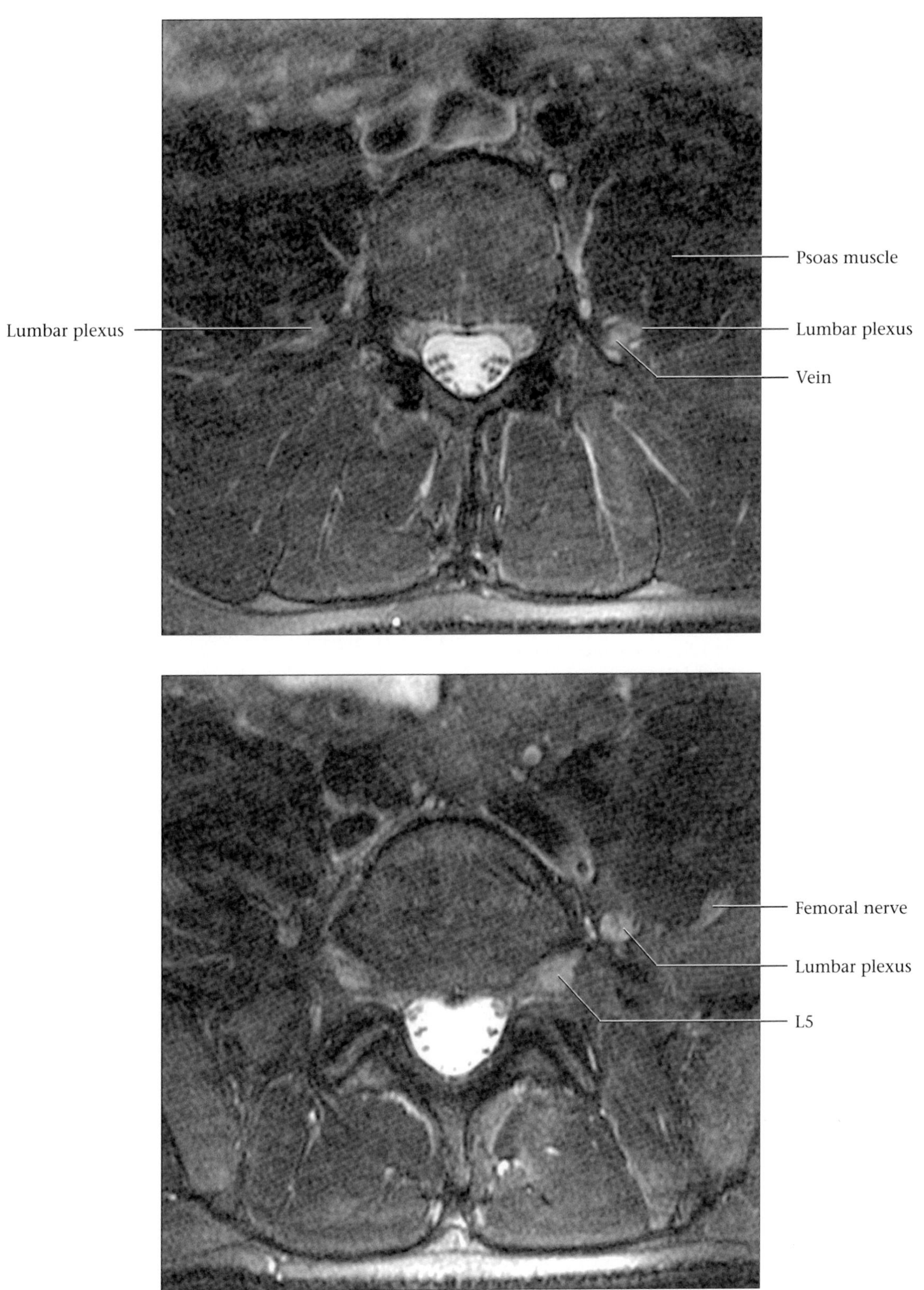
Psoas muscle
Lumbar plexus
Lumbar plexus
Vein
Femoral nerve
Lumbar plexus
L5

(Top) First of two axial fat-saturated T2 MR images from superior to inferior demonstrates the lumbar plexus in its normal location medial to the ipsilateral psoas muscle. At this level it is composed of L2 and L3, with the L4 contribution joining caudal to this slice. **(Bottom)** Imaging more inferiorly demonstrates the more caudal lumbar plexus after the L4 contribution. The femoral nerve has branched off and is tracking in the iliopsoas groove in expected location.

SACRAL PLEXUS AND SCIATIC NERVE

Terminology

Abbreviations

- Lumbosacral trunk, plexus (LST, LSP)
- Sacroiliac (SI), sciatic nerve (SN)

Gross Anatomy

Overview

- **Lumbosacral trunk**
  - Formed by L4 (minor branch), L5
  - Nerve supply to pelvis, lower limb; autonomic to pelvic viscera
  - Lumbar part
    - Appears at medial margin of psoas major
    - Courses inferiorly over pelvic rim anterior to SI joint
    - Joins S1
  - Sacral part
    - S2-3 converge on LST in greater sciatic foramen → **sciatic nerve**
- **Sacral plexus**
  - Formed by
    - LST
    - Ventral rami, S1-3
    - Minor branch of S4
  - Two "bands"
    - Upper band: LST (L4, L5) + S1-3 → **sciatic nerve**
    - Lower band: S2-4 → **pudendal nerve**
- **Sciatic nerve**
  - Major branch of sacral plexus
  - Coalesces from sacral plexus on ventral piriformis muscle surface
  - Innervates
    - Capsule of hip joint
    - Posterior thigh (biceps femoris, semitendinosus, semimembranosus, adductor magnus)
    - All leg muscles (via common peroneal, tibial nerves)
- **Pudendal nerve**
  - Formed by S2-4 ventral rami
  - Exits pelvis via greater sciatic foramen between piriformis/ischiococcygeus
  - Innervates
    - Inferior rectal nerve
    - Perineal nerve
    - Penis or clitoris
- **Coccygeal plexus**
  - Formed by
    - Minor branch of S4 (forms anococcygeal nerve)
    - S5 ventral rami
    - Coccygeal ventral rami

Anatomy Relationships

- **Sacral plexus**
  - Lies against posterior pelvic wall, behind presacral fascia
    - Anterior to piriformis
    - Posterior to ureter
    - Posterior to internal iliac vessels
    - Behind sigmoid colon
  - Iliolumbar artery accompanies L5 nerve
  - Lateral sacral artery branches accompany sacral nerves
  - Superior gluteal artery passes backward between L5/S1 nerves
  - Inferior gluteal vessels lie between S1/S2 or S2/S3
- **Sciatic nerve**
  - Thickest nerve in body
  - Exits pelvis
    - Via greater sciatic foramen
    - Below piriformis muscle
  - Descends between greater trochanter of femur, ischial tuberosity
  - Descends along posterior thigh
  - Divides (usually near apex of popliteal fossa) into two branches
    - Tibial nerve
    - Common peroneal nerves
- **Pudendal nerve**
  - Courses through greater sciatic foramen between piriformis, ischiococcygeus
  - Lies medial to internal pudendal vessels on spine
  - Accompanies internal pudendal artery through lesser sciatic foramen into pudendal canal

Anatomy-Based Imaging Issues

Imaging Approaches

- **Sciatic nerve**
  - Coils
    - Torso wrap-around phase array coil preferred
    - Flexible extremity surface coil alternative
  - Planes: Coronal, oblique or direct axial
  - Sequences
    - Coronal T1WI, coronal STIR or fat-saturated T2WI
    - Direct axial or oblique axial T1WI
    - Direct axial or oblique axial fat-saturated T2WI or STIR
    - Optional: Coronal/direct or oblique axial fat-saturated T1 C+

Clinical Implications

Clinical Importance

- Compression syndromes
  - Piriformis
    - Sciatic neuropathy
    - Trapped/irritated at piriformis muscle (controversial)
  - Ischial tunnel
    - Sciatic neuropathy
    - Compressed between obturator internus/gluteus maximus
    - At level of ischium
  - Sacral plexus
    - Dense presacral fascia protects sacral plexus
    - Sacral plexus rarely directly involved in malignant pelvic tumors
    - Sacral plexus can be compressed indirectly

SACRAL PLEXUS AND SCIATIC NERVE

GRAPHICS

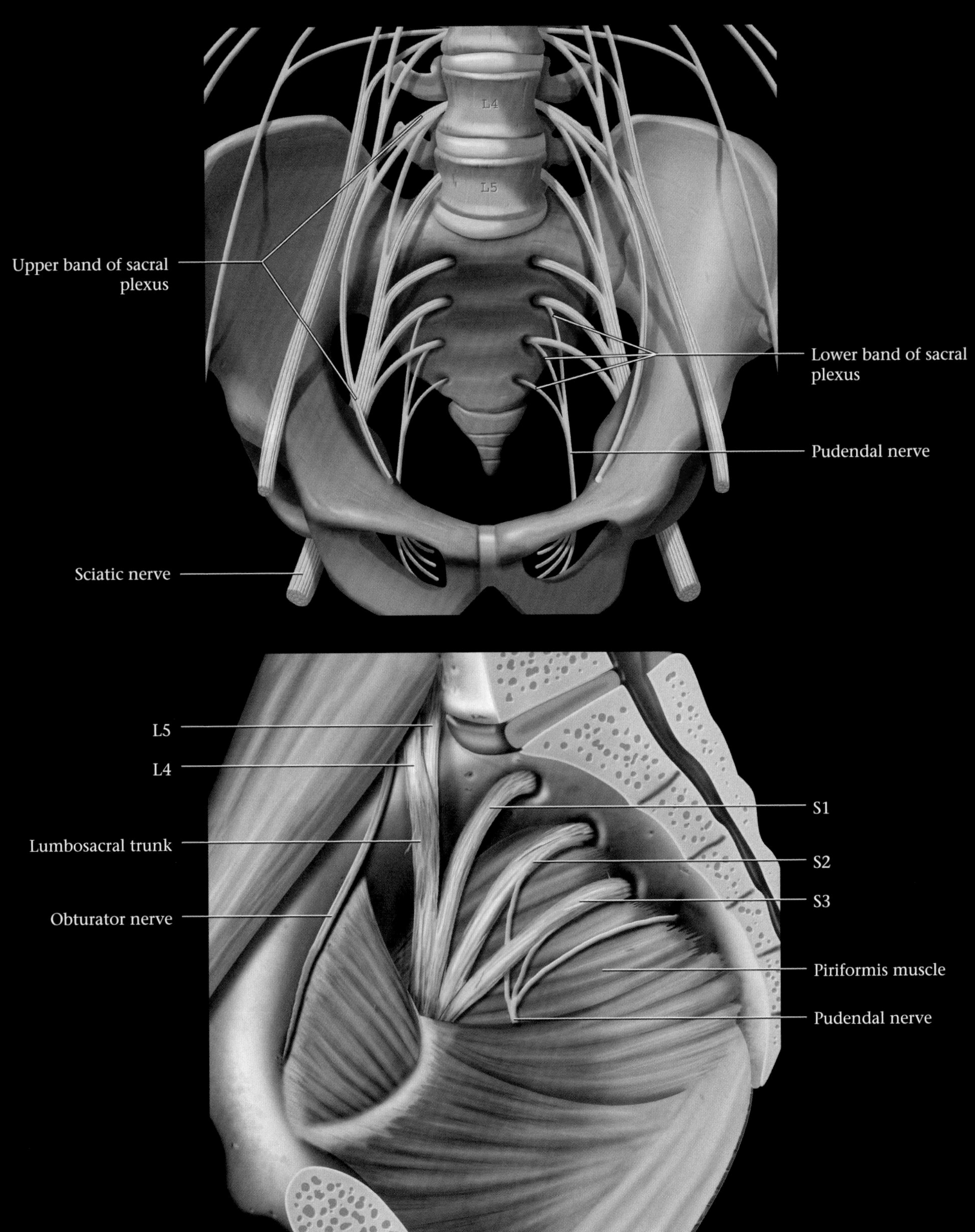
L4
L5
Upper band of sacral plexus
Lower band of sacral plexus
Pudendal nerve
Sciatic nerve
L5
L4
Lumbosacral trunk
Obturator nerve
S1
S2
S3
Piriformis muscle
Pudendal nerve

(Top) Coronal graphic depicts upper and lower sacral bands of sacral plexus. The primary terminal branch of the upper sacral band is the sciatic nerve, which supplies many thigh and all leg muscles (via the tibial and common peroneal nerves). The lower sacral band forms the pudendal nerve to the perineum. **(Bottom)** Sagittal graphic depicts upper and lower bands of sacral plexus in anatomic relationship to musculature of pelvic bowl. The upper sacral bands coalesce into the sciatic nerve on the ventral surface of the piriformis muscle.

SACRAL PLEXUS AND SCIATIC NERVE

CORONAL T1 MR

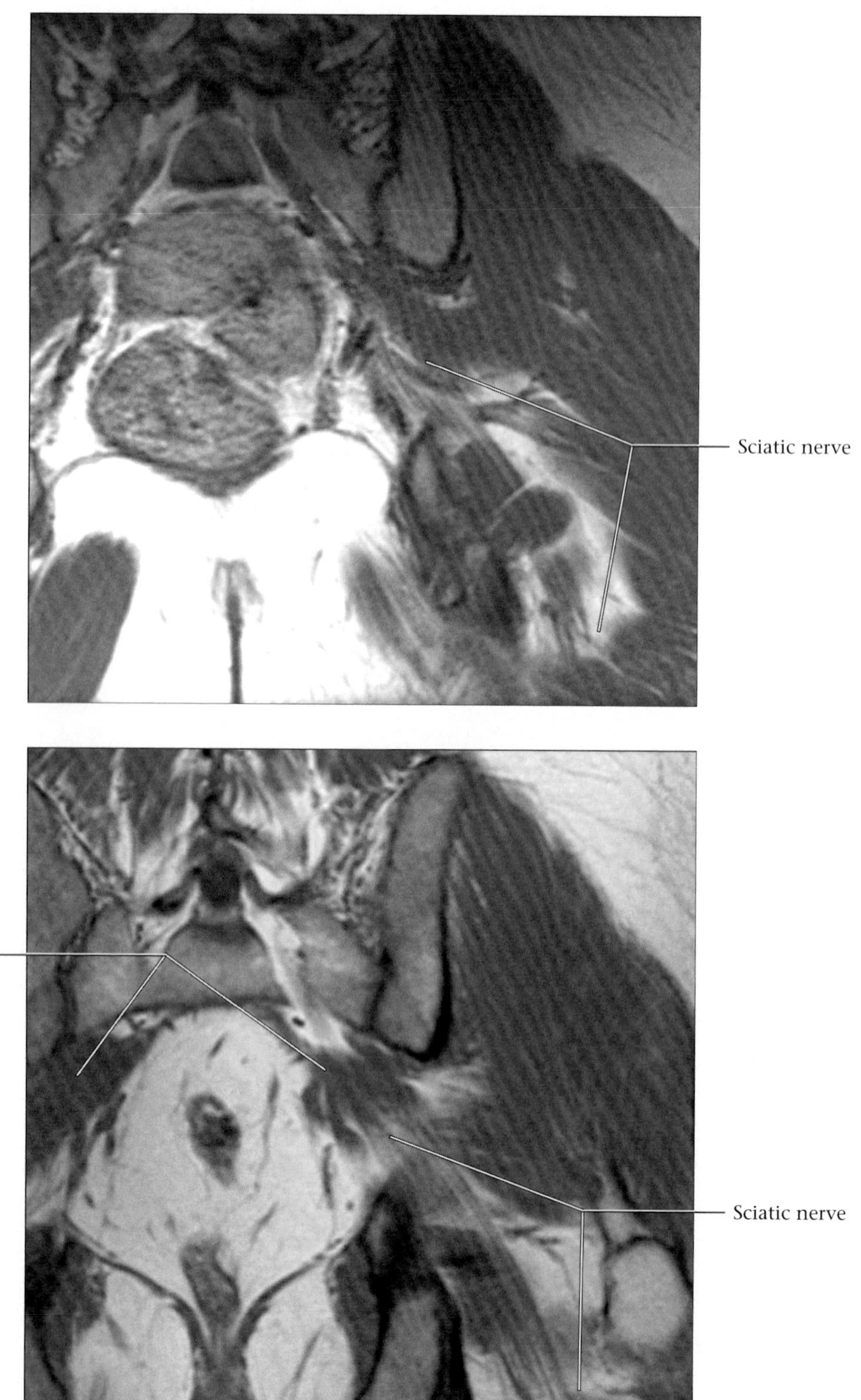
Sciatic nerve
Piriformis muscles
Sciatic nerve

(Top) First of two coronal T1 MR images through the pelvis presented from posterior to anterior demonstrates the S2 nerve contributing to the sacral plexus and sciatic nerve. **(Bottom)** Image obtained more anterior in the pelvis demonstrates the sacral plexus coalescing into the sciatic nerve on the ventral surface of the piriformis muscle.

OBLIQUE AXIAL T1 MR & FS T2 MR

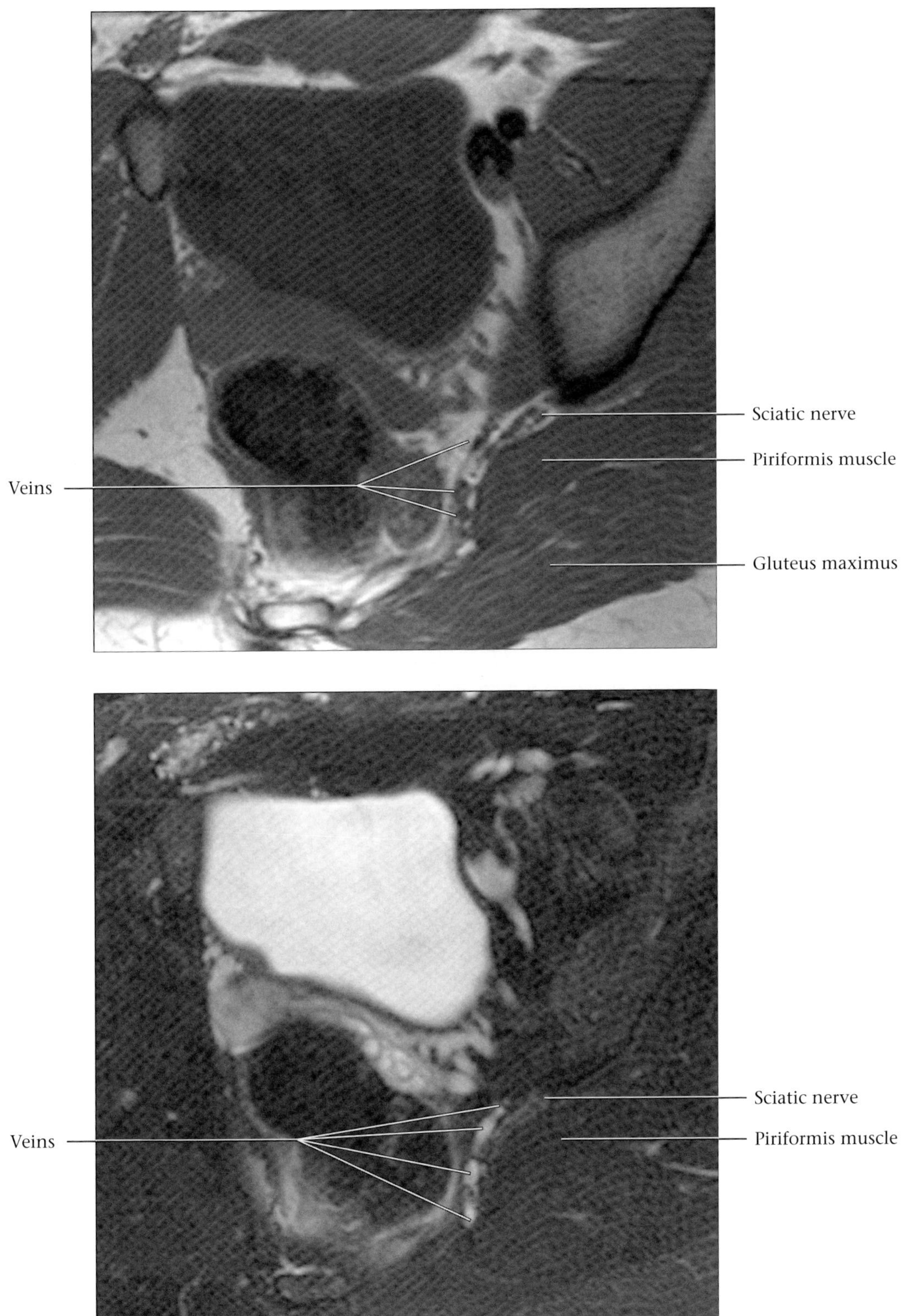

Sciatic nerve
Piriformis muscle
Veins
Gluteus maximus
Sciatic nerve
Piriformis muscle
Veins

(Top) The sciatic nerve coalesces from the sacral plexus on the ventral surface of the piriformis muscle. On T1 MR images, the fascicles are isointense to muscle separated by bright fibrofatty connective tissue. The fascicular architecture permits ready distinction from vessels. **(Bottom)** The sciatic nerve coalesces from the sacral plexus on the ventral surface of the piriformis muscle. On FS T2 MR images, the fascicles are mildly hyperintense to muscle separated by dark (fat suppressed) fibrofatty connective tissue. The fascicular architecture permits ready distinction from vessels.

OBLIQUE AXIAL T1 MR & FS T2 MR

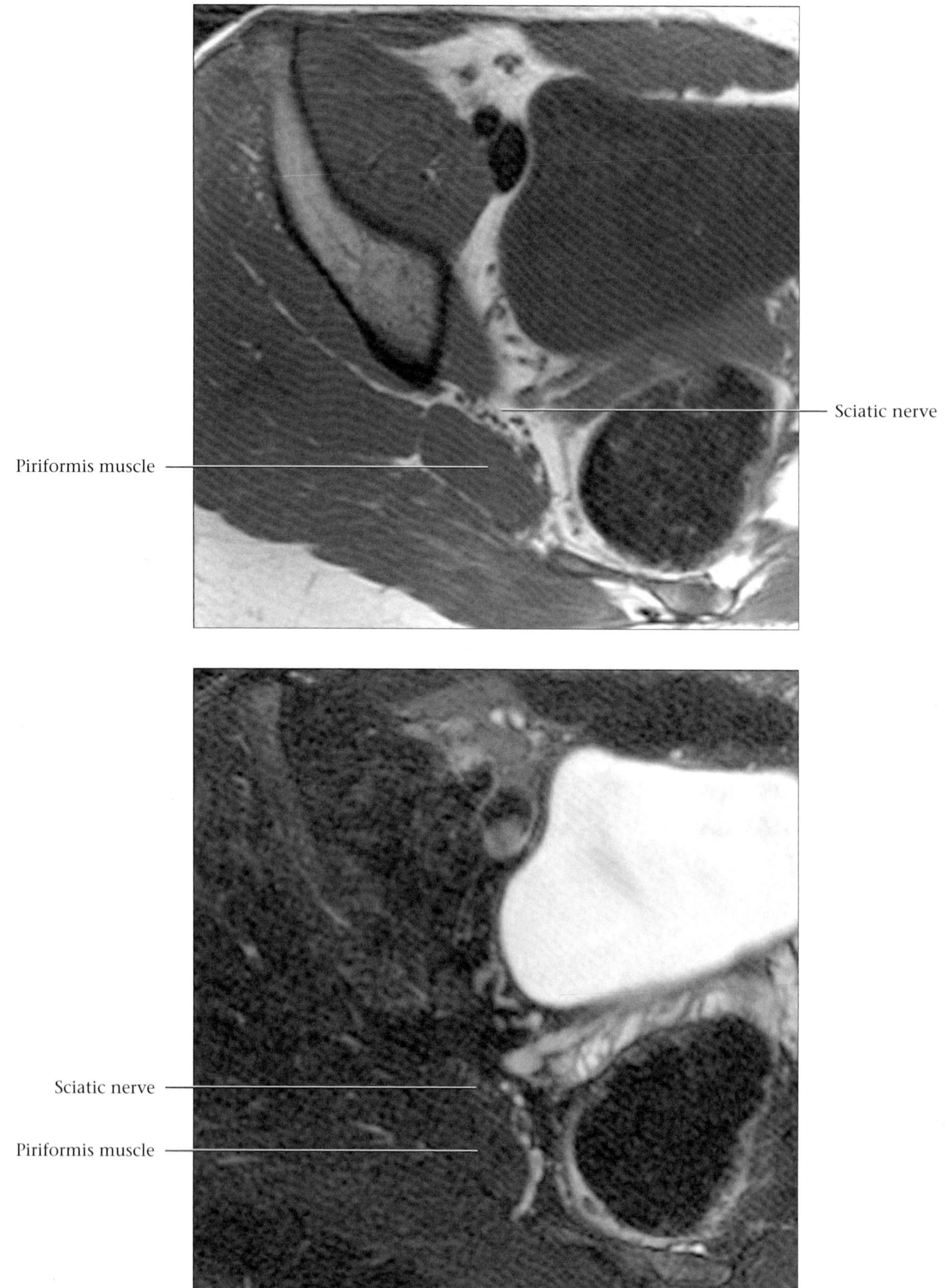
Sciatic nerve
Piriformis muscle
Sciatic nerve
Piriformis muscle

(Top) Oblique axial T1 MR image shows the sciatic nerve on the ventral piriformis muscle. Although the nerve (largest single nerve in the body) is enveloped by epineurium, the abundant fibrofatty epineurium gives the impression that the individual fascicles are free in pelvic fat. **(Bottom)** The sciatic nerve is a more discrete structure on fat-saturated T2 or STIR MR, with distinctive mildly hyperintense fascicles separated by interspersed dark (fat suppressed) fibrofatty connective tissue.

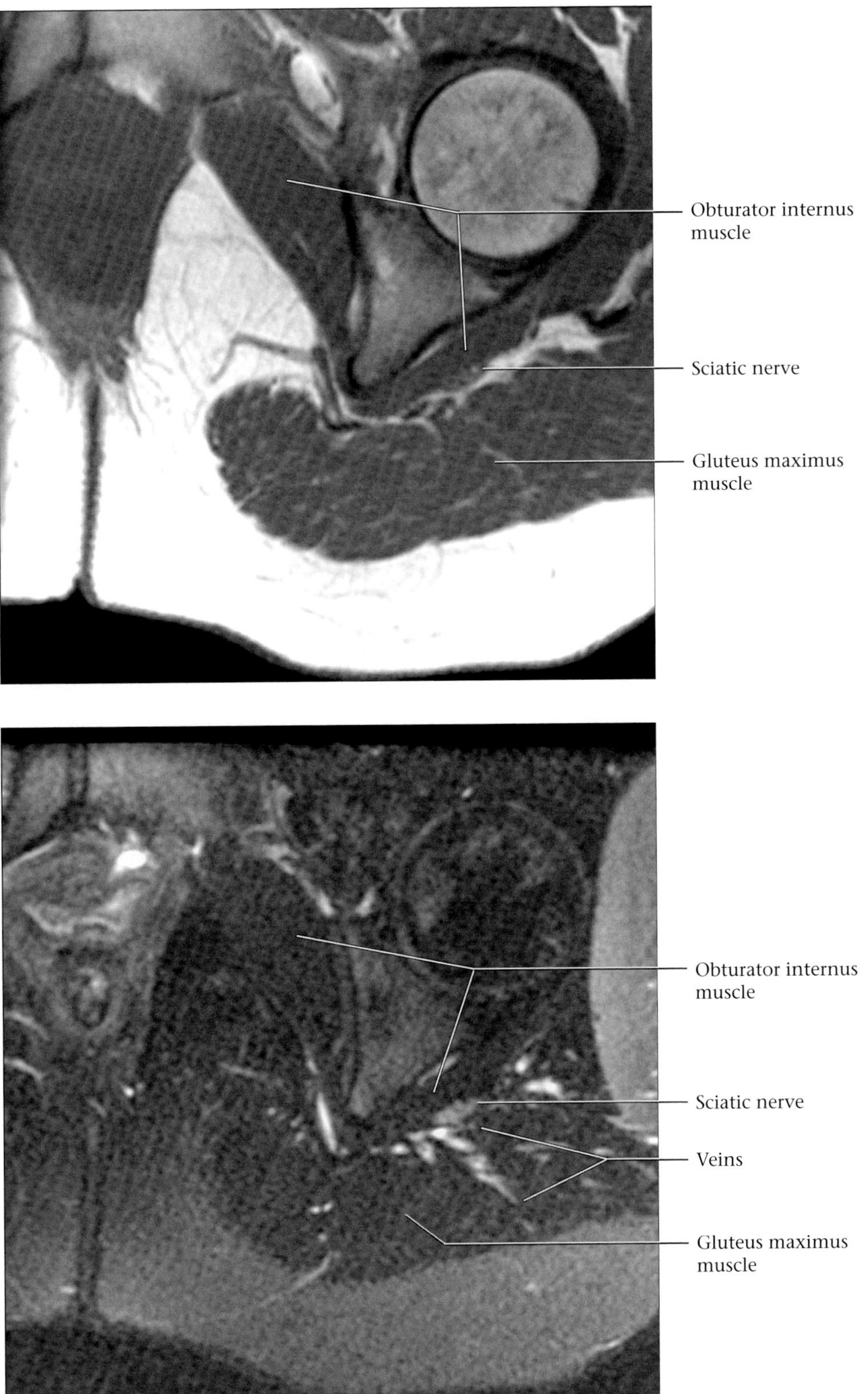
Obturator internus muscle
Sciatic nerve
Gluteus maximus muscle
Obturator internus muscle
Sciatic nerve
Veins
Gluteus maximus muscle

(Top) Axial T1 MR of the sciatic nerve at the obturator internus level is readily identified between the obturator internus and gluteus maximus muscles. The normal sciatic nerve is smaller and flatter appearing at this level than at the piriformis level. **(Bottom)** Axial T2 MR of the sciatic nerve at the obturator internus level is readily identified between the obturator internus and gluteus maximus muscles. The normal fascicular architecture is distinctive and permits discrimination from adjacent veins.

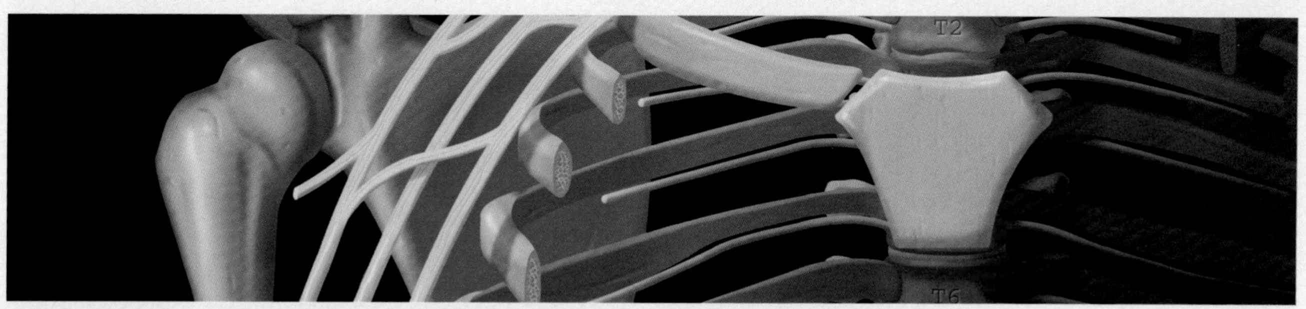
T2
T6

SECTION 5: Peripheral Nerves

PERIPHERAL NERVE OVERVIEW

Terminology

Abbreviations

- Peripheral nervous system (PNS)
- Ventral, dorsal primary ramus (VPR, DPR)
- Dorsal root ganglion (DRG)

Gross Anatomy

General Concepts

- **Ramus**
  - First branch(es) of spinal nerve proper
    - VPR (larger branch) → ventral musculature, facet
    - DPR (smaller branch) → paraspinal muscles, facet
- **Nerve**
  - 4-10 or more fascicles surrounded by epineurium
- **Fascicle**
  - Nerve fibers (hundreds) surrounded by connective tissue
- **Connective tissue** (covers nerve fibers)
  - **Epineurium**
    - Outer layer of connective tissue
    - Longitudinally oriented
    - Continuous with surrounding connective tissues
    - Groups fascicles into nerves, limits stretching
  - **Perineurium**
    - Intermediate layer of connective tissue
    - Multilayered sheath that invest fascicles
    - Extends from nerve roots to nerve ends
    - Functions as blood-nerve barrier
  - **Endoneurium**
    - Innermost layer of connective tissue
    - Intrafascicular, surrounds individual nerve fibers
- **Peripheral nerve**
  - Combination of one or more rami
  - +/- Schwann cell myelin sheath
  - Sensory, motor fibers usually mixed
    - Some PNS branches purely sensory
- **Plexus**
  - Network of anastomosing nerves

Overview

- **Brachial plexus**
  - Composed of
    - C5-T1 VPRs
    - +/- Minor C4, T2
  - Major branches
    - Radial nerve
    - Median nerve
    - Ulnar nerve
    - Musculocutaneous nerve
    - Axillary nerve
- **Lumbar plexus**
  - Composed of
    - L2-4 VPRs
    - Minor T12, L1 branches
  - Major branches
    - Obturator nerve
    - Femoral nerve
- **Lumbosacral trunk (LST)**
  - Composed of
    - L5 + L4 VPR (minor)
  - Functionally part of sacral plexus
- **Sacral plexus**
  - Composed of
    - LST + S1-3 VPRs
    - Minor branch of S4
  - Major branches
    - Sciatic nerve
    - Common peroneal nerve
    - Tibial nerve

Anatomy Relationships

- Nerves usually accompanied by similarly-named arteries, veins
  - Supply similar target tissues
  - Form "neurovascular 'bundle'"

Imaging Anatomy

Normal

- MR findings
  - Nerves appear round/ovoid
  - Well-defined internal fascicular architecture
  - No abrupt change in caliber, course
  - STIR/fat suppressed T2WI
    - Fascicles appear mildly hyperintense
    - Interspersed with hypointense fibrofatty connective tissue

Abnormal

- Abnormal size (usually enlarged)
- +/- Loss of normal fascicular architecture
- Abrupt change in caliber or course
- STIR/fat suppressed T2WI
  - Hyperintense; approach signal of vessels

Imaging Recommendations

- High-resolution MR
  - T1WI MR (relationship to adjacent structures)
  - STIR/fat suppressed T2WI (fascicular anatomy)
  - Fat-saturated T1 C+ (neuritis vs. tumor, etc.)

Imaging Pitfalls

- Nerves, vessels sometimes difficult to differentiate
  - Nerves
    - Round/ovoid, linear
    - No "flow void"
    - Branch at relatively acute angles
    - Enhance minimally
    - Distinctive axial fascicular architecture
  - Vessels
    - Also round/ovoid, linear
    - Have internal "flow voids"
    - Branch at large angles
    - Enhance intensely

Clinical Implications

Clinical Importance

- Neuropathy syndromes specific to abnormal nerve(s)
- Imaging complimentary to clinical exam, electrodiagnostic testing

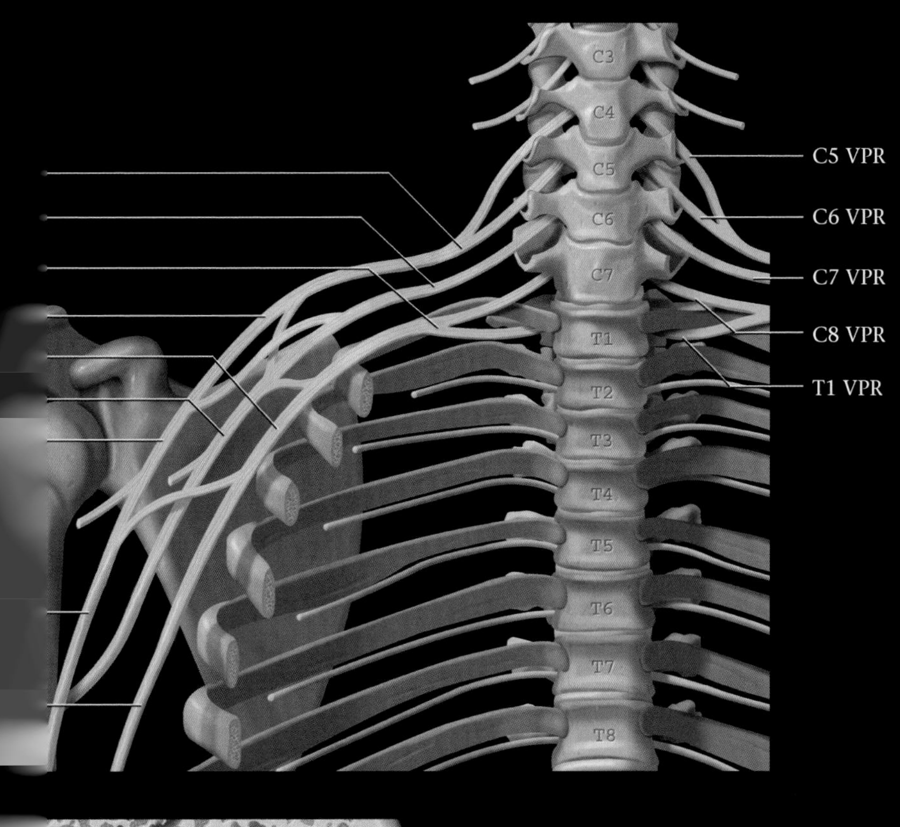
C3
C4
C5
C6
C7
T1
T2
T3
T4
T5
T6
T7
T8
C5 VPR
C6 VPR
C7 VPR
C8 VPR
T1 VPR

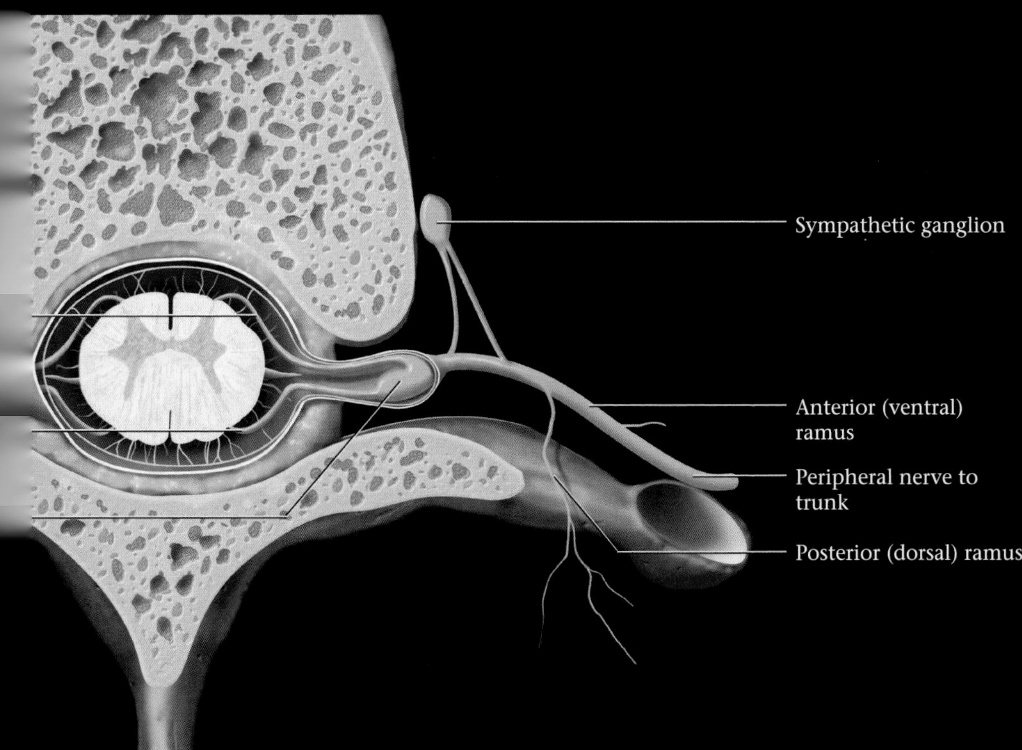
Sympathetic ganglion
Anterior (ventral) ramus
Peripheral nerve to trunk
Posterior (dorsal) ramus

f the lower cervical and upper thoracic spinal nerves as seen from the front shows the
ntral primary rami (VPRs) form plexi and peripheral nerves. Upper four cervical ventral
s; lower four plus contributions from the first thoracic ventral ramus form the brachial
). The VPRs form trunks, which then form divisions and cords. Peripheral nerves arise from
houlder and upper limb, seen here on right. **(Bottom)** Close-up axial graphic shows how a
ned and then gives rise to ventral and dorsal primary rami. A lower thoracic vertebral
ventral branch supplies ventral musculature while the dorsal branch is smaller and supplies

PERIPHERAL NERVE OVERVIEW

GRAPHIC

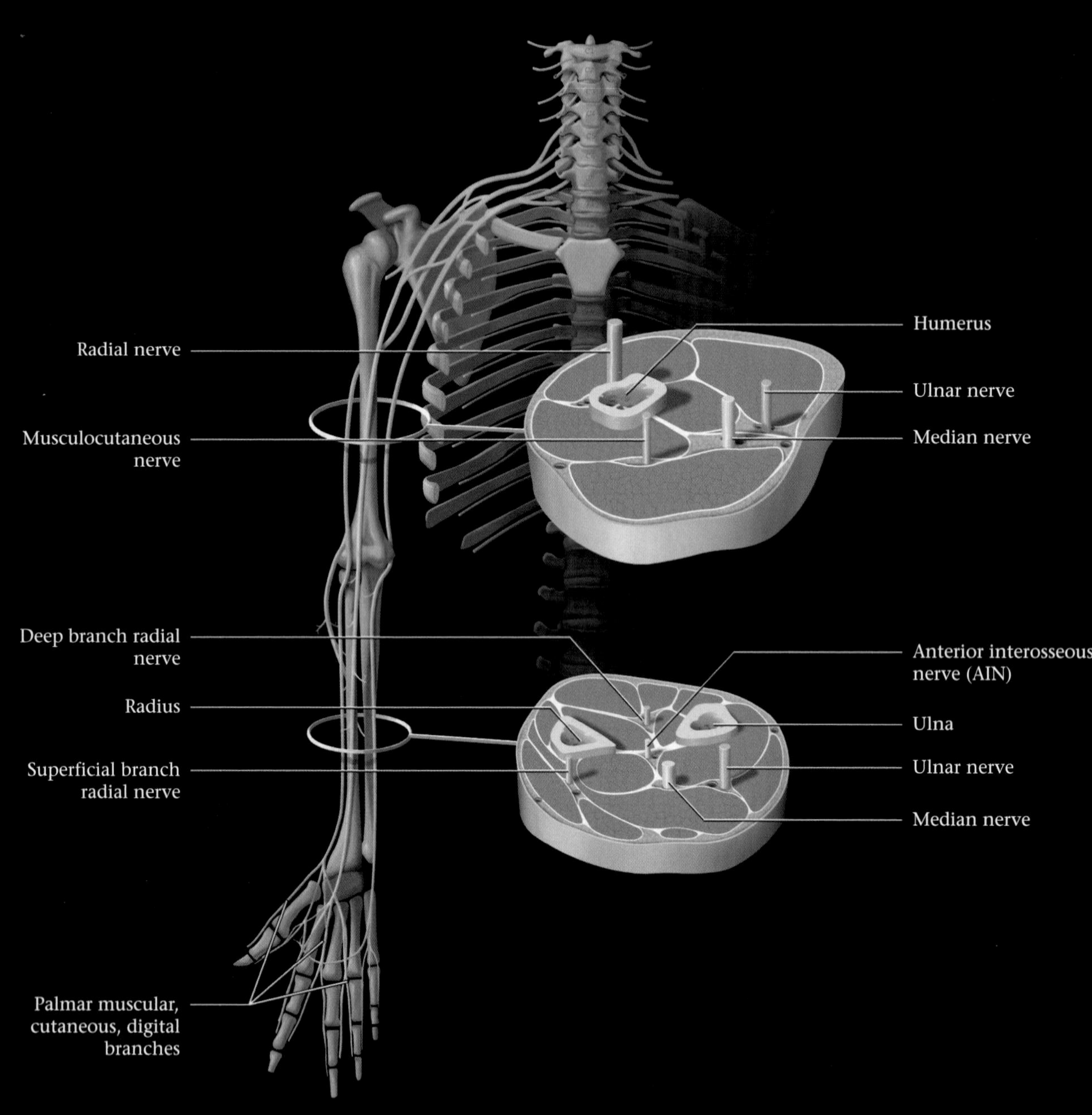
Radial nerve
Musculocutaneous nerve
Deep branch radial nerve
Radius
Superficial branch radial nerve
Palmar muscular, cutaneous, digital branches
Humerus
Ulnar nerve
Median nerve
Anterior interosseous nerve (AIN)
Ulna
Ulnar nerve
Median nerve

Graphic depicts formation of a prominent peripheral nerve to the arm, the median nerve. The median nerve arises from branches of both the lateral and medial brachial plexus cords, and passes directly through the arm [median nerve has no branches in axilla or arm, and serves no brachial (arm) muscles]. At the elbow, median nerve gives off the anterior interosseous nerve branch and continues as the median nerve proper into the hand under the flexor retinaculum.

PERIPHERAL NERVE OVERVIEW

GRAPHIC

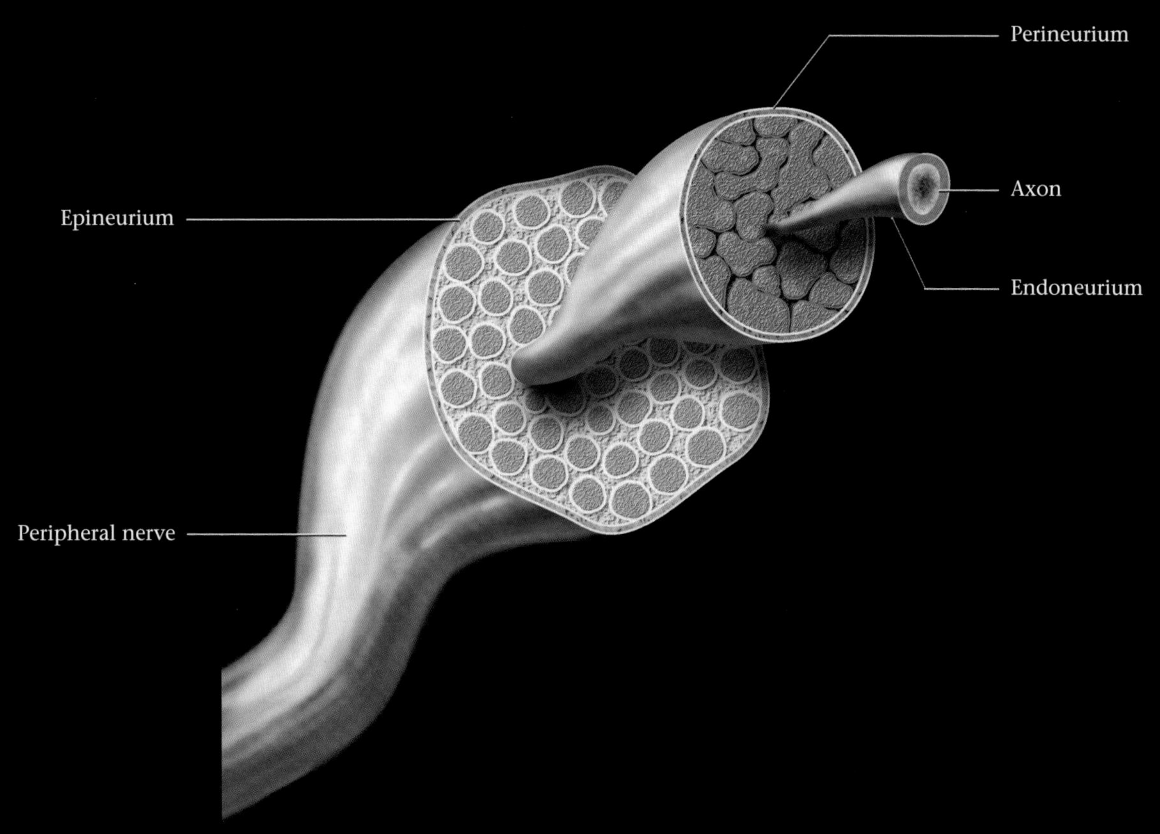
Perineurium
Epineurium
Axon
Endoneurium
Peripheral nerve

Graphic cutaway of a typical peripheral nerve illustrates the characteristic internal architecture that permits imaging distinction from vessels. Each axon has a connective tissue covering, the endoneurium. Axons are bundled together to form fascicles that are bounded externally by perineurium. Fascicles are bundled together to form a peripheral nerve, surrounded by the tough epineurium. This general pattern is followed for all peripheral nerves of both extremities and the trunk.

CORONAL T1 & STIR MR

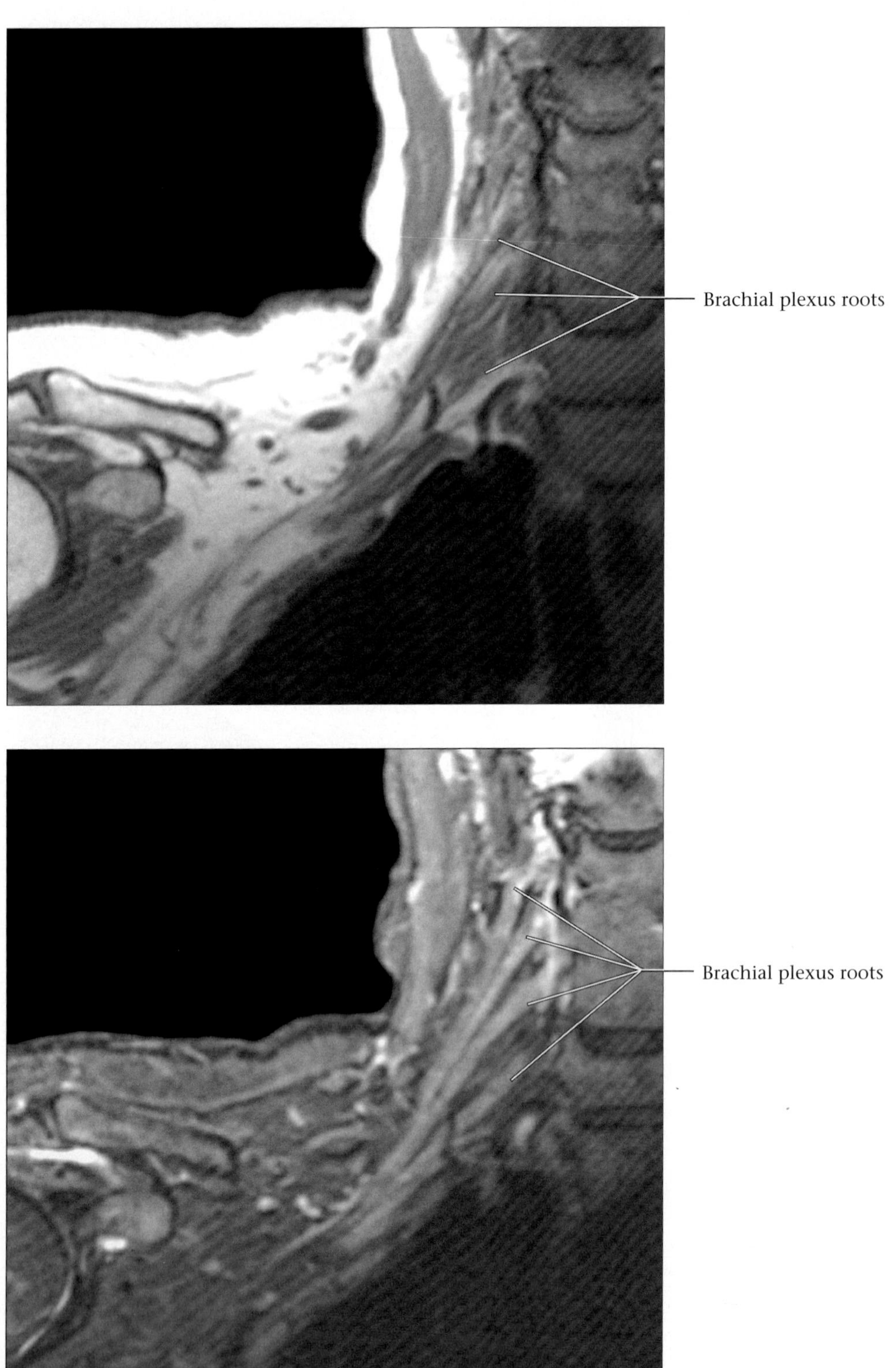
Brachial plexus roots
Brachial plexus roots

(Top) Coronal T1 MR of the right brachial plexus and its roots shows the normal longitudinal T1 appearance of peripheral nerves. Peripheral nerves are isointense to normal muscle on T1 MR images. **(Bottom)** Coronal STIR MR of the right brachial plexus shows the normal longitudinal T2 appearance of peripheral nerves. Peripheral nerves are mildly hyperintense to normal muscle on fat-saturated T2 or STIR MR images. Note that the fascicular architecture is not always apparent on longitudinal imaging.

AXIAL T1 AND FS T2 MR

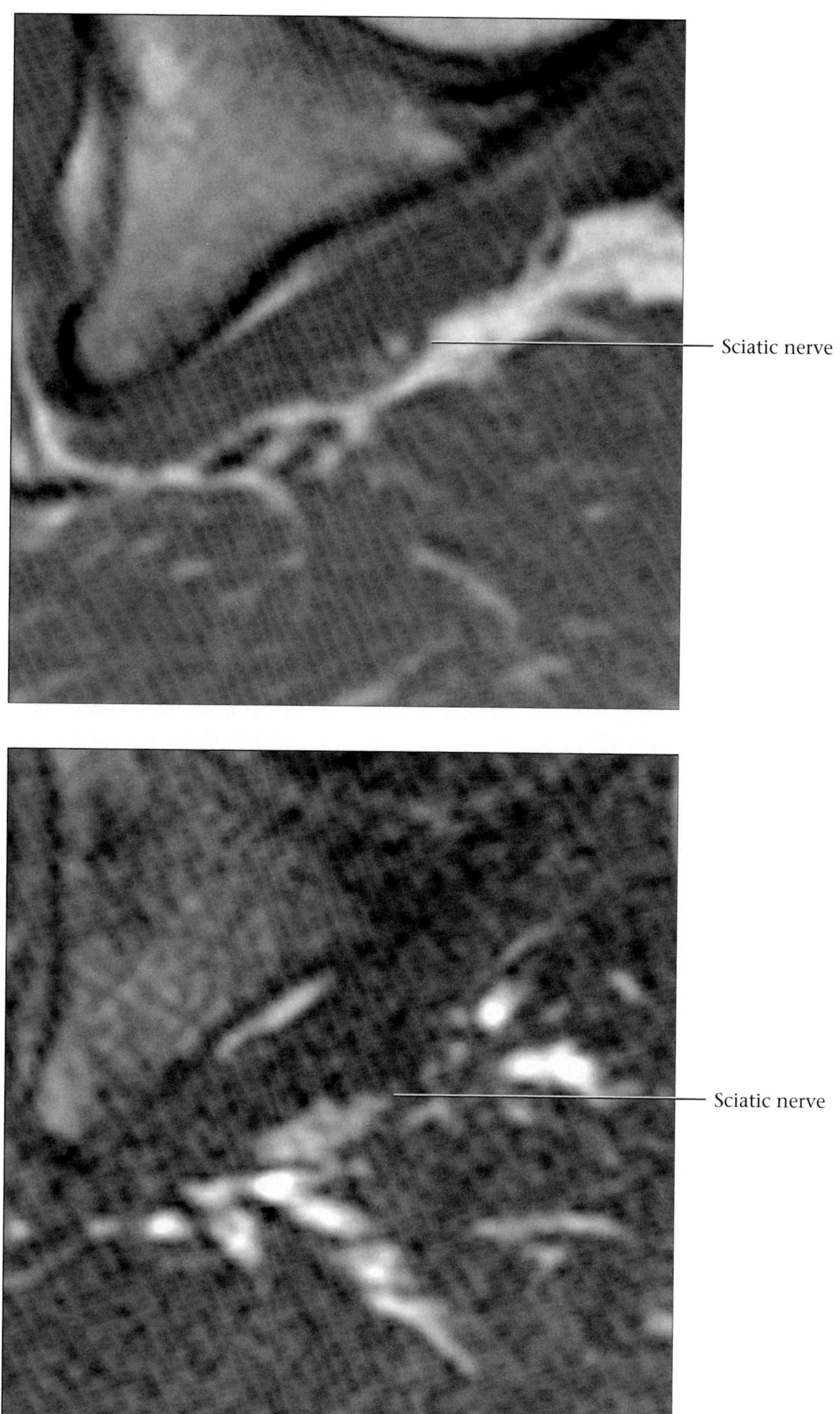
Sciatic nerve
Sciatic nerve

(Top) Direct axial T1 MR of the sciatic nerve is coned and magnified to show characteristic transverse fascicular appearance of peripheral nerves. The sciatic nerve is the largest single nerve in the body, and is well suited for learning to recognize normal nerve internal architecture. The nerve fascicles are isointense to muscle and are surrounded by higher signal intensity fibrofatty tissue. As in this instance, peripheral nerves are frequently marginated by bright fat which assists delineation from surrounding soft tissues. **(Bottom)** Axial fat-saturated T2 MR image of the left sciatic nerve reveals the normal T2 appearance of peripheral nerve. The individual fascicles are distinct and slightly hyperintense to adjacent muscle. Low signal fibrofatty connective tissue (fat is suppressed by fat-saturation or STIR MR imaging) accentuates conspicuity of the individual fascicles.

RADIAL NERVE

Terminology

Abbreviations

- Brachial plexus (BP)
- Radial nerve (RN)
- Posterior interosseous nerve (PIN)
- Radial tunnel syndrome (RTS)
- Metacarpal phalangeal joints (MCPs)

Gross Anatomy

Overview

- RN is largest branch of BP
- Continuation of posterior cord of BP
- Primary nerve of forearm posterior (extensor) compartment
- Innervates extensor muscles of arm, forearm
- Does NOT innervate hand muscles
- RN divided anatomically into five segments
  - Shoulder/axilla
  - Upper arm
  - Elbow
  - Forearm
  - Wrist/hand
- **Radial nerve in shoulder/axilla**
  - Arises from BP posterior cord (C5-T1)
  - Descends behind third part of axillary, upper part of brachial arteries
  - Passes dorsally between long/medial heads of triceps
- **Radial nerve in upper arm**
  - Lies in spiral groove of humerus
  - Accompanies profunda brachii artery, veins
  - Enters posterior (extensor) compartment
    - Muscular branches innervate triceps, brachioradialis, etc.
    - Cutaneous branches supply skin along posterior surface of upper arm
  - Pierces lateral intermuscular septum to re-enter anterior compartment
- **Radial nerve at elbow**
  - Lies anterior to lateral epicondyle
  - Gives off articular branches
  - Divides into superficial, deep branches
- **Radial nerve in forearm**
  - **Superficial branch of RN**
    - Direct continuation of RN
    - Smaller of the two terminal RN branches
    - Descends lateral to radial artery
    - Curves around lateral aspect of radius
    - Pierces deep fascia
    - Entirely sensory
  - **Deep branch of RN**
    - Larger of two terminal RN branches
    - Largest branch is **posterior interosseous nerve**
    - PIN is entirely muscular, articular
    - Enters radial tunnel proximal to radiocapitellar joint
    - Passes between heads of supinator
    - Curves around lateral side of radius
    - Enters posterior fascial compartment of forearm
    - Terminates on dorsum of wrist
    - Does not pass into hand
    - Supplies extensor forearm muscles, brachioradialis
- **Radial nerve at wrist, hand**
  - Superficial branch of RN curves around wrist
  - Passes deep to brachioradialis tendon
  - Reaches hand
  - Divides into dorsal digital cutaneous nerves
  - Supplies skin over dorsum of wrist, thumb/index/middle/radial half of ring fingers
  - Communicates with posterior, lateral cutaneous nerves of forearm (ulnar nerve)

Anatomy-Based Imaging Issues

Imaging Recommendations

- Coils
  - Preferred: Multipurpose flexible phase array surface coil
  - Alternative: Flexible extremity surface coil
- Best planes
  - Direct axial
- Best sequences
  - T1WI
  - STIR/fat suppressed T2WI
  - Optional: Fat-saturated T1 C+

Imaging Pitfalls

- Easy to image RN along spiral groove of humerus
- Difficult to image distal RN after it bifurcates into superficial, deep branches

Clinical Implications

Clinical Importance

- RN most vulnerable to injury in humeral groove
- **RN palsy**
  - Following fracture of mid-numerous
    - Nerve laceration
    - Entrapment by bone fragments
  - "Saturday night palsy"
    - Prolonged pressure compressing RN in spiral groove of humerus
- **RN sensory branch entrapment**
  - Injury to superficial RN branch as it emerges below brachioradialis tendon
  - Pain, paresthesias over radial side of dorsum of wrist/hand
- **Radial tunnel syndrome (RTS)**
  - Symptoms
    - Pain over extensors just distal to elbow
    - No sensory disturbance, motor loss
  - Entrapment neuropathy
  - Near elbow can be compressed by
    - Fibrous bands
    - Tendinous border of extensor carpi radialis brevis
    - Supinator aponeurosis
- **Posterior interosseous nerve palsy**
  - Symptoms
    - Pain like RTS
    - Weakness, paralysis
    - Inability to extend MCP joints of thumbs, fingers
    - Radial deviation of wrist with extension
  - Entrapment at same anatomic sites as RTS

RADIAL NERVE

GRAPHIC

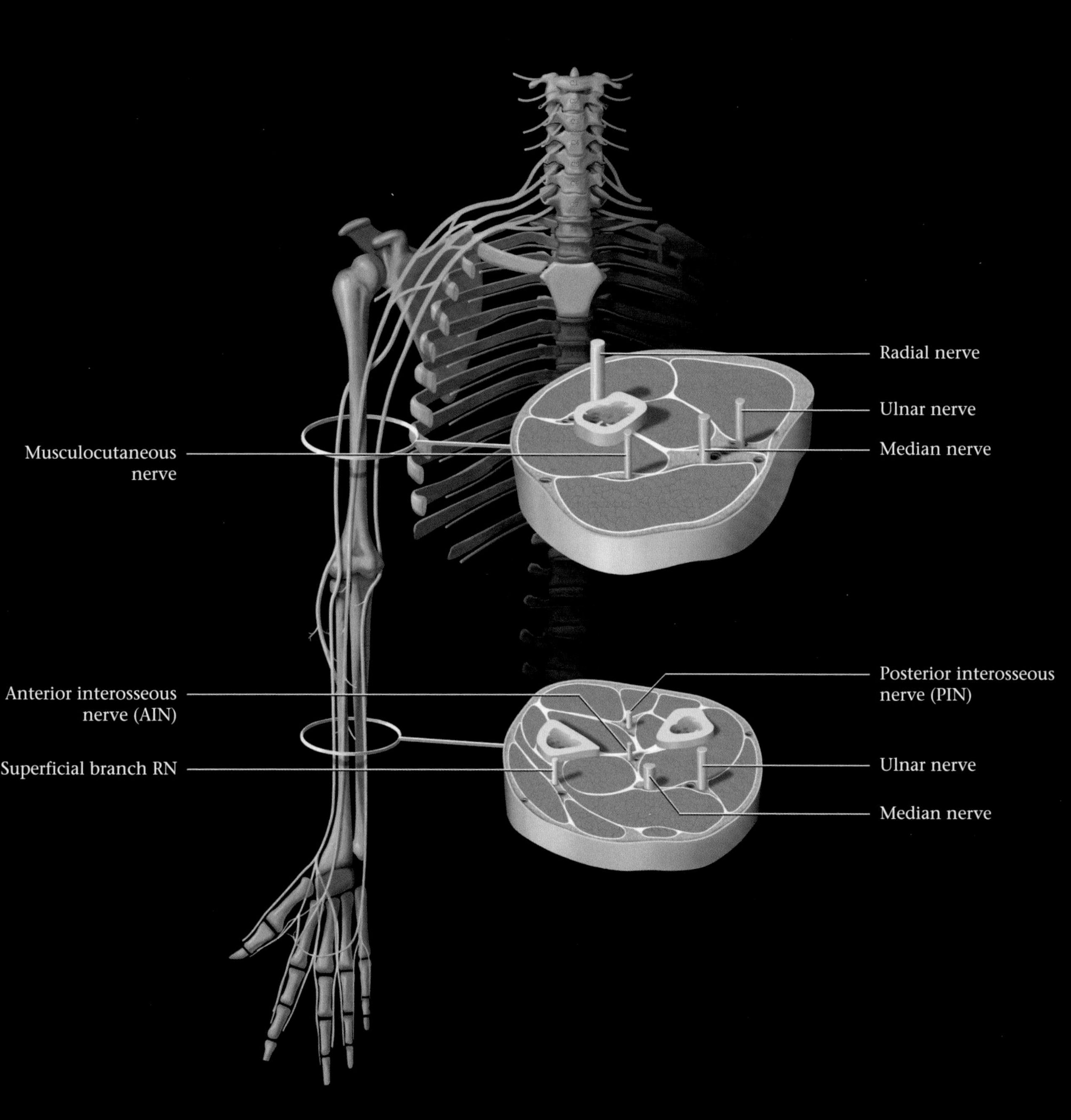
Radial nerve
Ulnar nerve
Musculocutaneous nerve
Median nerve
Posterior interosseous nerve (PIN)
Anterior interosseous nerve (AIN)
Superficial branch RN
Ulnar nerve
Median nerve

Graphic depicts radial nerve in arm and forearm. Radial nerve arises as the terminal branch of posterior brachial plexus cord and enters posterior arm, wrapping around the midhumeral shaft and into the lateral arm. At the elbow, radial nerve divides into a deep motor and articular branch (posterior interosseous nerve) and superficial sensory branch.

RADIAL NERVE

AXIAL T1 MR

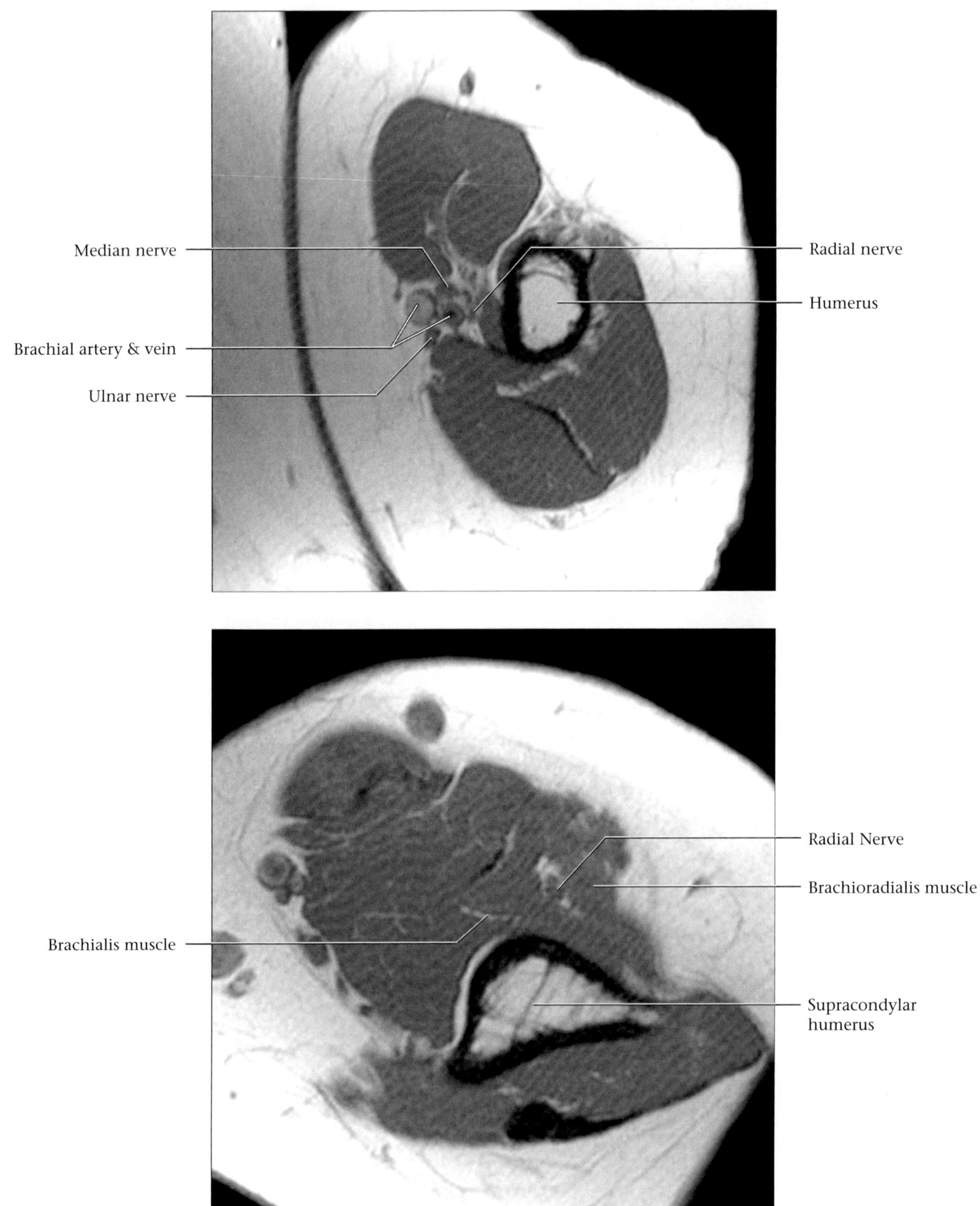
Median nerve
Radial nerve
Humerus
Brachial artery & vein
Ulnar nerve
Radial Nerve
Brachioradialis muscle
Brachialis muscle
Supracondylar humerus

(Top) First of two axial T1 MR images in the arm presented from superior to inferior demonstrates the radial nerve traveling in close anatomic proximity to the ulnar nerve and median nerve and brachial vessels. The nerve will move posteriorly around the midhumeral shaft as it descends distally. It is difficult to follow the radial nerve around the humeral shaft on T1 MR. **(Bottom)** Slice at the level of supracondylar humerus, the radial nerve has previously transited around the humeral shaft and now descends anterolaterally between the brachialis and brachioradialis muscles towards the cubital fossa.

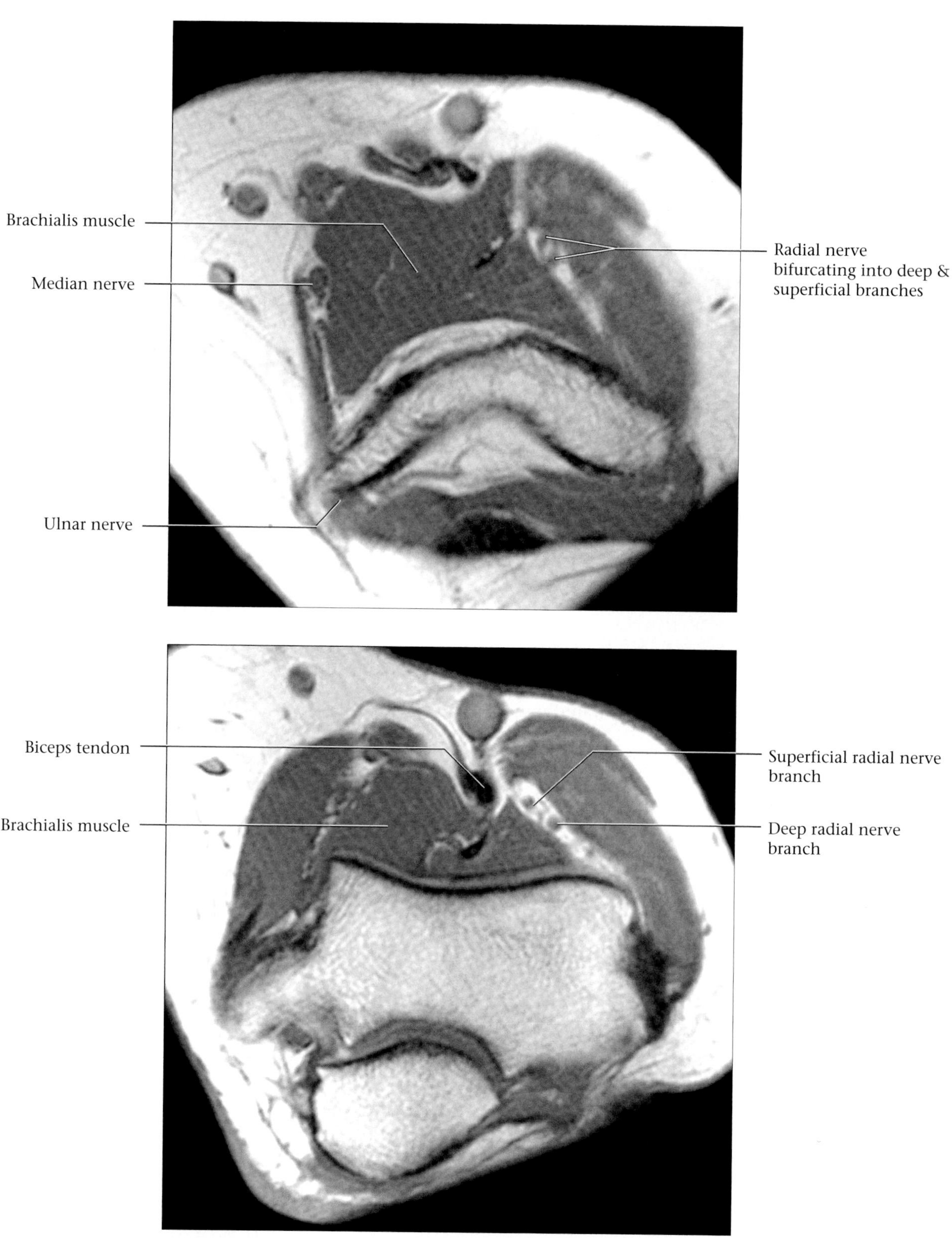
Brachialis muscle
Median nerve
Ulnar nerve
Radial nerve bifurcating into deep & superficial branches
Biceps tendon
Brachialis muscle
Superficial radial nerve branch
Deep radial nerve branch

(Top) First of two axial T1 MR images obtained just proximal to the elbow presented from superior to inferior shows the radial nerve bifurcation into the deep and superficial branches. **(Bottom)** Image obtained more distal within the cubital fossa clearly depicts the separate superficial and deep radial nerve branches moving apart. The deep branch forms the posterior interosseous nerve which will travel deep within the posterior compartment and provide motor and articular innervation to the forearm, and the superficial branch which is entirely sensory and supplies sensory fibers to dorsum of wrist, hand, and radial (lateral)1.5 fingers.

ULNAR NERVE

Terminology

Abbreviations

- Brachial plexus (BP), ulnar nerve (UN)

Gross Anatomy

Overview of Ulnar Nerve

- UN is major terminal branch of BP
  - Formed from C8, T1
  - Gives off no branches in arm
- Has both motor, sensory functions
- Motor: To forearm flexors, intrinsic hand muscles
  - Flexor carpi ulnaris (FCU)
  - Flexor digitorum profundus III/IV
  - Adductor pollicis, flexor pollicis brevis
  - Hypothenar muscles
  - First palmar, dorsal interosseous muscles
  - Third, fourth lumbricals
- Sensory: Articular, cutaneous innervation
  - Articular branches: Elbow, wrist, intercarpal, carpometacarpal, intermetacarpal joints
  - Cutaneous branches: Ulnar aspect of hand, 5th finger, ulnar half of 4th finger

Anatomy Relationships

- **Axilla**
  - Courses between axillary artery, vein
- **Arm**
  - Runs in anterior compartment along medial intermuscular septum
  - Pierces medial intermuscular septum at midhumerus
  - Enters posterior compartment
  - Descends anterior to medial head of triceps
  - Lies between medial epicondyle, olecranon process of humerus
  - Passes into cubital tunnel at elbow posterior to medial epicondyle between two heads of FCU
    - Cubital tunnel borders: Medial epicondyle (anterior), olecranon (lateral), Osborne fascia (posterior)
  - UN, radial, median nerves in close approximation
- **Forearm**
  - UN enters forearm
  - Descends on medial forearm, lying on flexor digitorum profundus
  - Ulnar nerve/artery/veins travel together
  - Becomes superficial in distal forearm (covered by skin, fascia)
  - Transits under medial flexor retinaculum (Guyon canal) at wrist
  - Divides into superficial, deep branches
  - Deep branch is muscular and articular
    - Muscular branches: Supply hypothenar muscles, medial two lumbricales
    - Articular branches: Supply wrist, intercarpal, carpometacarpal, intermetacarpal joints
  - Superficial branch is entirely sensory
    - Cutaneous fibers: Supply anterior palmar surfaces of medial 1.5 fingers

Internal Structures-Critical Contents

- Three layers of connective tissue surround nerve
  - From outside to inside: Epi-, peri-, endoneurium
  - Extrinsic arterioles/venules/capillaries lie in epi-, perineurium
  - Fascicular microvessels in endoneurium

Imaging Anatomy

Overview

- MR
  - T1WI
    - UN appears as well-defined oval
    - Discrete fascicles
    - Isointense to adjacent muscle tissue
  - Fat-saturated T2WI/STIR
    - UN slightly hyperintense to adjacent muscle
    - Hypointense compared to adjacent vessels
    - Clearly defined fascicles separated by interposed lower signal intensity connective tissue

Anatomy-Based Imaging Issues

Key Concepts or Questions

- Predict where lesion resides (elbow, wrist) to place coil

Imaging Recommendations

- Preferred coil: Multipurpose flexible phase array surface coil
  - May need to use sequential stations to achieve desired coverage
- Alternative coil: Flexible extremity surface coil
- Best plane: Direct axial
- Best sequences: T1WI, STIR/fat-saturated T2WI
- Optional sequence: Fat-saturated T1 C+

Imaging Pitfalls

- Nerves, vessels occasionally difficult to differentiate
  - Nerve
    - Round/ovoid linear structure
    - No flow voids, minimal enhancement
    - Branches at relatively acute angles
    - Distinct fascicular architecture on axial scans
  - Vessel
    - Internal flow void
    - Branches at large angles
    - Enhances intensely

Clinical Implications

Clinical Importance

- Clinical syndromes (compressive neuropathies)
  - Cubital tunnel syndrome
    - Transient paresthesias in ring, little fingers
    - +/- Clawing of digits
    - Hypothenar atrophy
  - Guyon tunnel syndrome
    - Hand weakness
    - Dorsoulnar hand sensory deficit
    - Positive Tinel over medial wrist

ULNAR NERVE

GRAPHIC

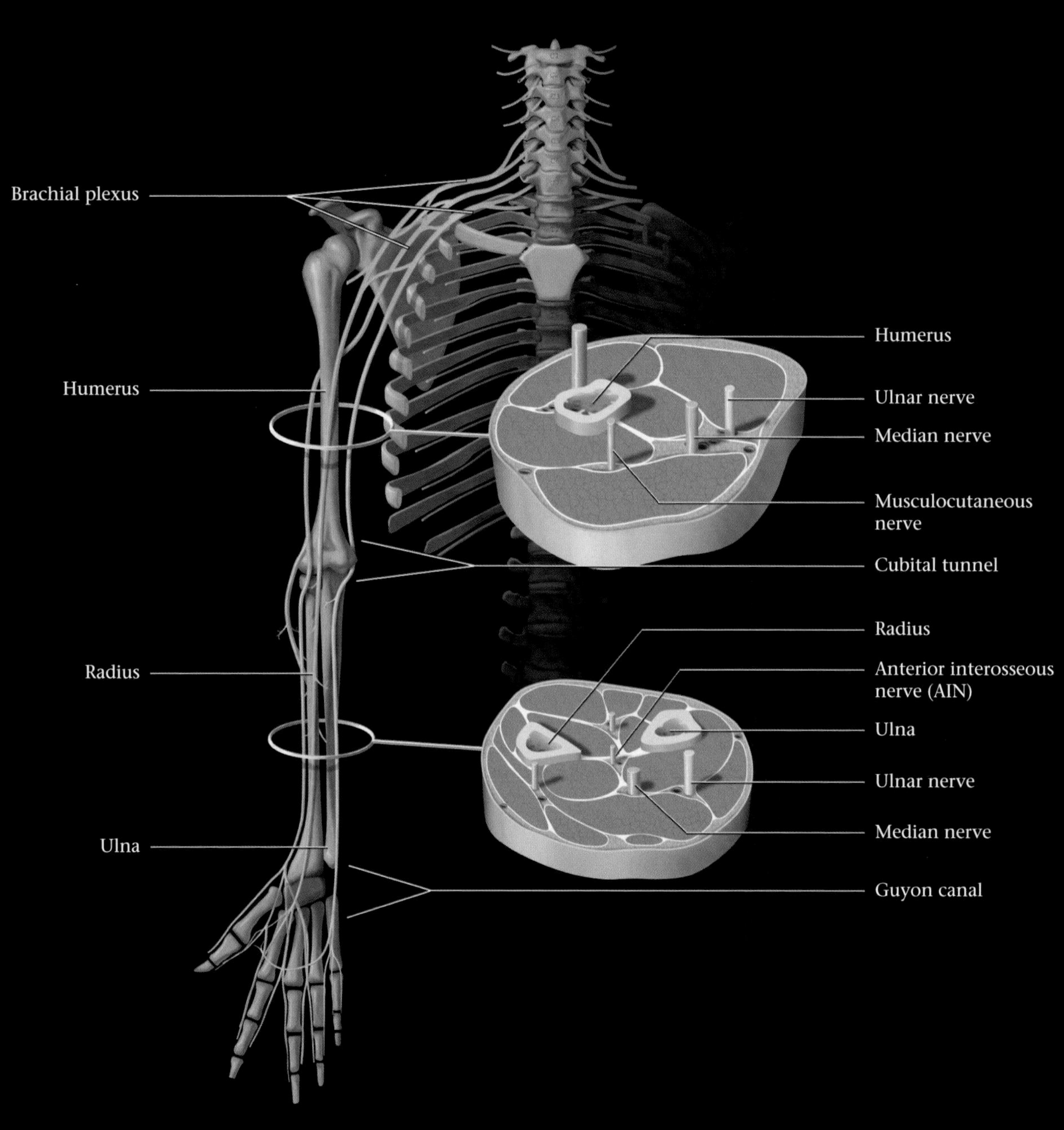
Brachial plexus
Humerus
Radius
Ulna
Humerus
Ulnar nerve
Median nerve
Musculocutaneous nerve
Cubital tunnel
Radius
Anterior interosseous nerve (AIN)
Ulna
Ulnar nerve
Median nerve
Guyon canal

Graphic seen from anterior perspective with three-dimensional rendered axial cuts through the middle of the upper arm and forearm. The normal course of the ulnar nerve (yellow) is shown as it courses from the brachial plexus all the way down into the hand. The ulnar nerve arises from the inferior brachial plexus trunk (C8, T1) and anterior division of the medial cord. The ulnar nerve has no branches in the arm, providing innervation to the forearm and hand only.

ULNAR NERVE

AXIAL T1 MR

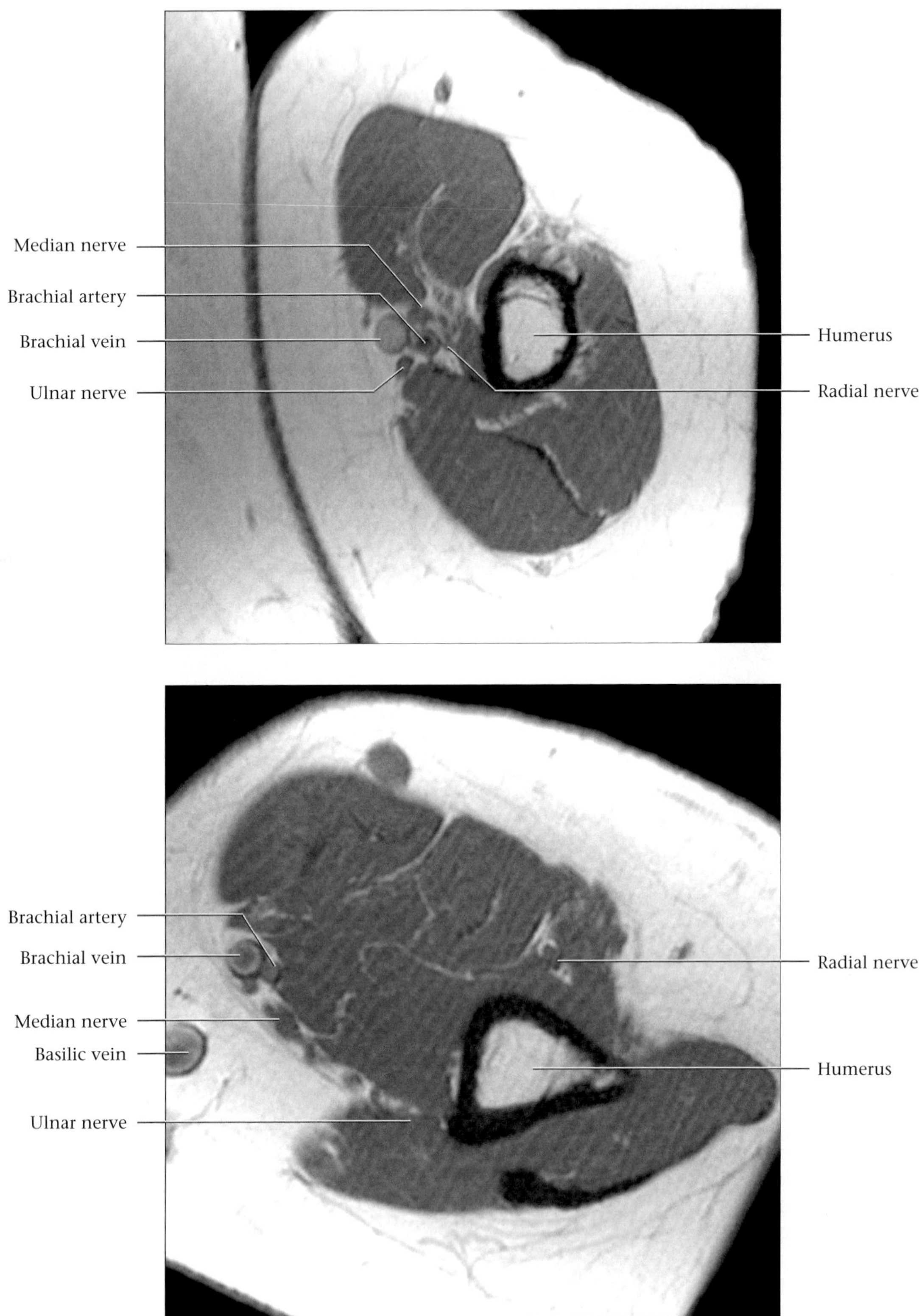
Median nerve
Brachial artery
Brachial vein
Ulnar nerve
Humerus
Radial nerve
Brachial artery
Brachial vein
Median nerve
Basilic vein
Ulnar nerve
Radial nerve
Humerus

(Top) First of two axial T1 MR images presented from superior to inferior through the upper left arm demonstrates the ulnar nerve traveling with the radial and median nerves and brachial artery and vein. **(Bottom)** Image obtained more distally in the arm above the supracondylar humerus demonstrates the ulnar nerve moving medially in preparation to travel under the medial epicondyle. Note the separate courses of the ulnar, radial, and median nerves in the distal arm.

AXIAL T1 MR

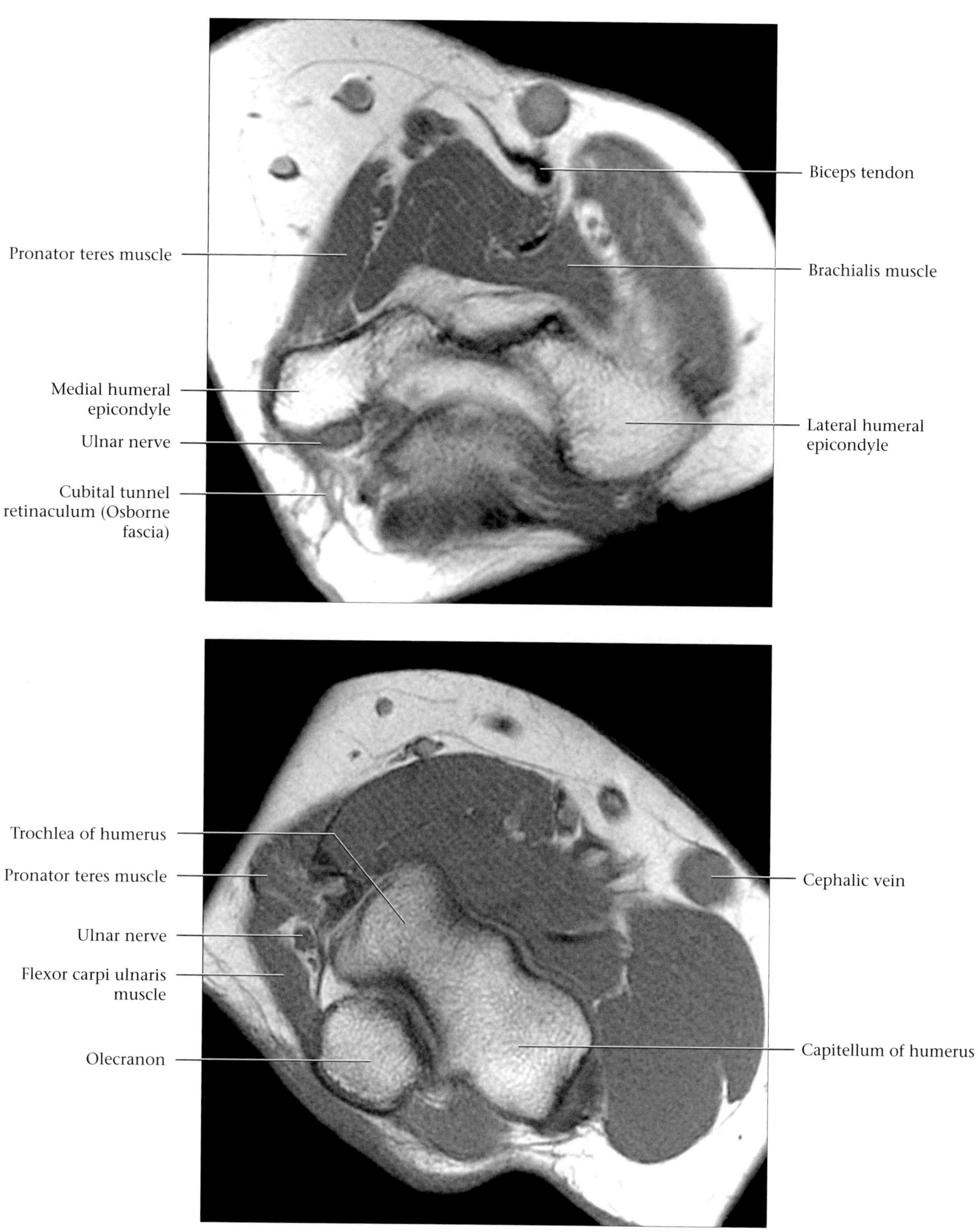

Biceps tendon
Pronator teres muscle
Brachialis muscle
Medial humeral epicondyle
Ulnar nerve
Lateral humeral epicondyle
Cubital tunnel retinaculum (Osborne fascia)
Trochlea of humerus
Pronator teres muscle
Cephalic vein
Ulnar nerve
Flexor carpi ulnaris muscle
Olecranon
Capitellum of humerus

(Top) First of two axial T1 MR images centered at the left elbow presented from superior to inferior depicts the ulnar nerve transiting under the medial epicondyle of the humerus. The characteristic fascicular neural architecture is distinctive, with nerve fascicles isointense to muscle and the intervening fibrofatty tissue slightly hyperintense. The ulnar nerve normally is plumper and more conspicuous at the cubital tunnel. **(Bottom)** Imaging at the left elbow distal to the medial epicondyle demonstrates the ulnar nerve entering the medial forearm. Note that the nerve caliber is normally smaller than at the level of the medial epicondyle (cubital tunnel).

ULNAR NERVE

AXIAL T1 MR

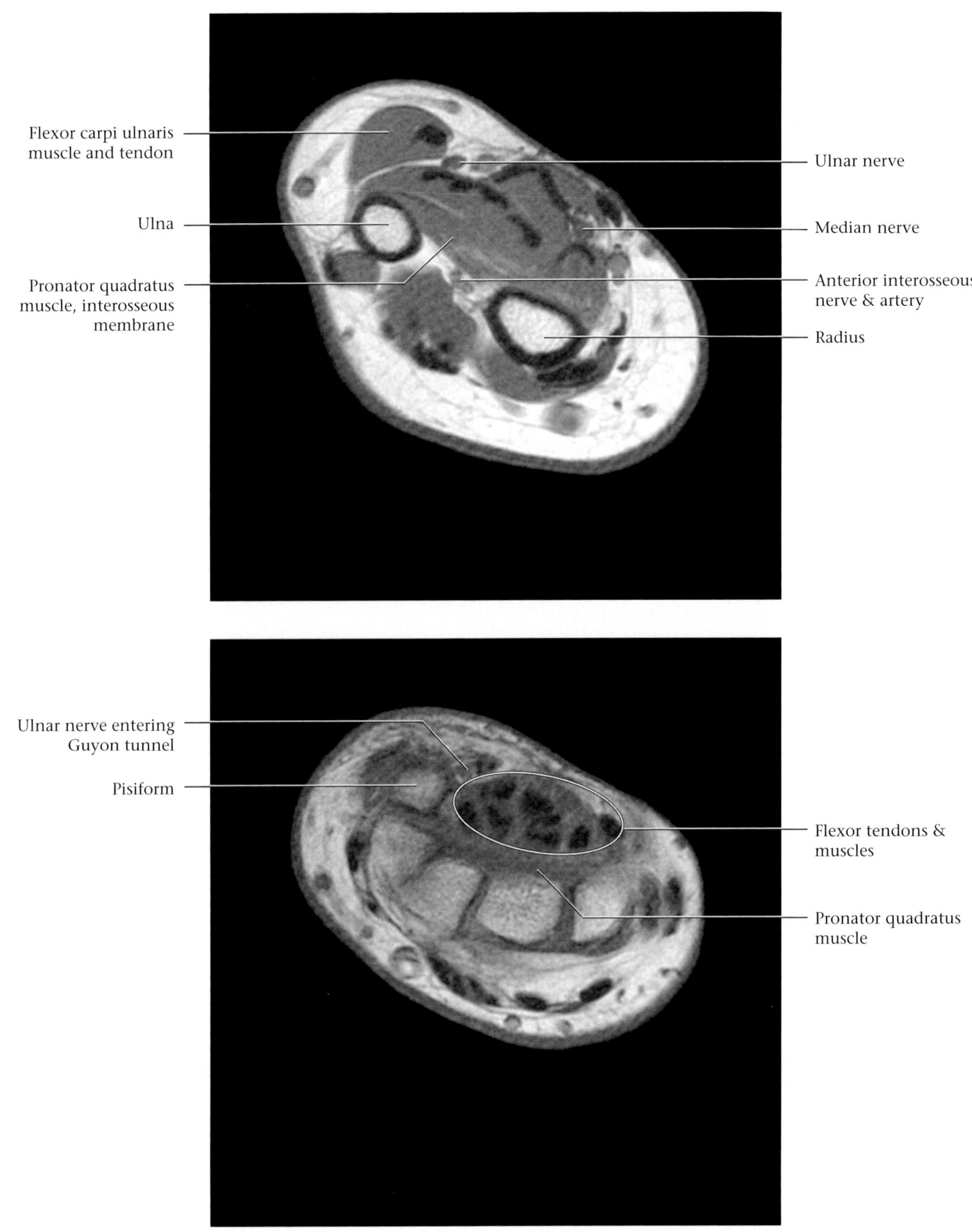

Flexor carpi ulnaris muscle and tendon
Ulna
Pronator quadratus muscle, interosseous membrane
Ulnar nerve
Median nerve
Anterior interosseous nerve & artery
Radius
Ulnar nerve entering Guyon tunnel
Pisiform
Flexor tendons & muscles
Pronator quadratus muscle

(Top) First of two axial T1 MR images of the left forearm presented from superior to inferior shows the ulnar nerve in the medial forearm coursing lateral to the flexor carpi ulnaris muscle. The anterior interosseous nerve branch travels with the interosseous artery adjacent to the interosseous membrane. **(Bottom)** Imaging of the left forearm shows the ulnar nerve in the medial forearm entering the medial (Guyon) tunnel at the wrist. This is a less common point of nerve entrapment than the cubital tunnel at the elbow.

AXIAL PD FS MR

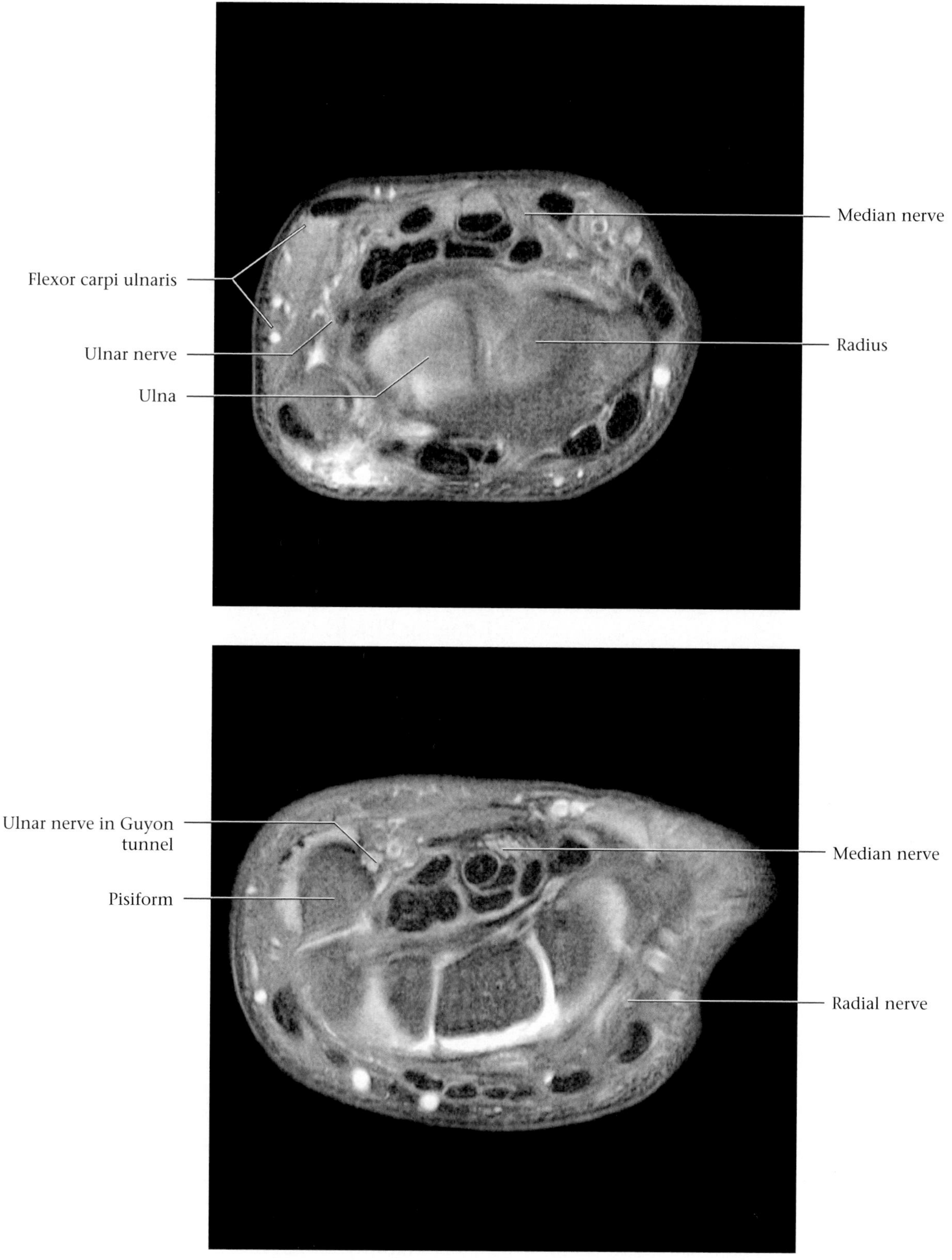

Median nerve
Flexor carpi ulnaris
Ulnar nerve
Radius
Ulna
Ulnar nerve in Guyon tunnel
Median nerve
Pisiform
Radial nerve

(Top) First of two axial fat-saturated proton density images of the forearm and wrist presented from superior to inferior demonstrates the ulnar nerve as mildly hyperintense to muscle with distinctive fascicular architecture that permits distinction from adjacent tendons and vessels. **(Bottom)** This image depicts the ulnar nerve in Guyon tunnel adjacent to the pisiform carpal bone. The median nerve is also distinctive with its characteristic fascicular architecture.

MEDIAN NERVE

Terminology

Abbreviations

- Brachial plexus (BP)
- Median nerve (MN)
- Anterior interosseous nerve (AIN)

Gross Anatomy

Overview

- MN = principle nerve of anterior forearm fascial compartment
- MN passes through (but has no branches in) axilla or upper arm
- MN anatomically divided into six segments
  - Shoulder/axilla
  - Upper arm
  - Cubital fossa
  - Forearm
  - Wrist
  - Palm
- **Median nerve (shoulder/axilla)**
  - Infraclavicular branch of BP
  - Two roots
    - Lateral root from lateral cord of BP (C5-7)
    - Medial root from medial cord of BP (C8, T1)
  - Roots surround, unite in front of axillary artery
  - MN exits lower axilla
- **Median nerve (upper arm)**
  - Enters upper arm lateral to brachial artery
  - In mid-arm
    - MN crosses brachial artery
    - Descends medially, between biceps/triceps
    - MN, musculocutaneous, medial cutaneous, radial, ulnar nerves all lie relatively superficially
    - MN, other nerves surround/lie adjacent to brachial artery, basilic vein
- **Median nerve in cubital fossa (elbow)**
  - MN lies medial to brachial artery, deep to bicipital aponeurosis, anterior to brachioradialis
  - Courses deep to median cubital vein
  - Gives off articular, muscular branches to most superficial flexor muscles
- **Median nerve in forearm**
  - MN travels with ulnar artery, veins
  - Courses into deep forearm between heads of pronator teres
  - Gives off anterior interosseous nerve
  - Descends posterior to flexor digitorum superficialis
- **Median nerve at wrist**
  - MN larger, flatter at wrist than other levels
  - Becomes superficial as nears wrist
  - Enters palm deep to flexor retinaculum
- **Median nerve in palm**
  - Palmar cutaneous branch
    - Arises just proximal to flexor retinaculum
    - Therefore is spared in carpal tunnel syndrome
  - Muscular branch to thenar muscles
  - Palmar digital branches
- **Anterior interosseous nerve**
  - Arises from MN between heads of pronator teres
  - Proximal to point at which MN passes under tendinous arch of flexor digitorum superficialis
  - Descends on interosseous membrane with anterior interosseous artery (branch of ulnar artery)
  - Between flexor digitorum profundus, flexor pollicis longus muscles
  - Enters palm through osseofibrous carpal tunnel
  - Close to deep surface of flexor retinaculum (transverse carpal ligament)
    - AIN can become entrapped by flexor retinaculum at wrist

Anatomy-Based Imaging Issues

Imaging Recommendations

- Coils
  - Preferred: Multipurpose flexible phase array surface coil (dedicated wrist coil for CTS)
  - Alternative: Flexible extremity surface coil
  - Coverage: Sequential stations needed to cover MN course fully
- Best planes
  - Direct axial
- Best sequences
  - T1WI
  - STIR/fat-saturated T2WI
  - Optional: T1 C+

Imaging Pitfalls

- Must extend axial imaging into palm for complete MN, AIN delineation

Clinical Implications

Clinical Importance

- MN can be injured during deep median cubital vein puncture
- MN vulnerable to wrist lacerations
- Three major neural compression syndromes
  - **Carpal tunnel syndrome** (CTS)
    - Most common entrapment mononeuropathy
    - Caused by MN compression at wrist as it passes through fibro-osseous tunnel under flexor retinaculum
    - Intermittent pain, paresthesias, numbness in thumb, index/middle/medial ring fingers
    - +/- Thenar atrophy, weakness
    - Loss of palmar hand sensation
  - **Anterior interosseous nerve syndrome**
    - Weakness of "pinch grip"
    - Flexor pollicis longus/digitorum profundus (index finger), pronator quadratus
    - No sensory symptoms (distinguishes from pronator syndrome)
  - **Pronator syndrome**
    - Caused by MN entrapment at elbow
    - Uncommon
    - Pain in proximal anterior forearm aggravated by flexing elbow or pronating forearm against resistance
    - Intermittent paresthesias

MEDIAN NERVE

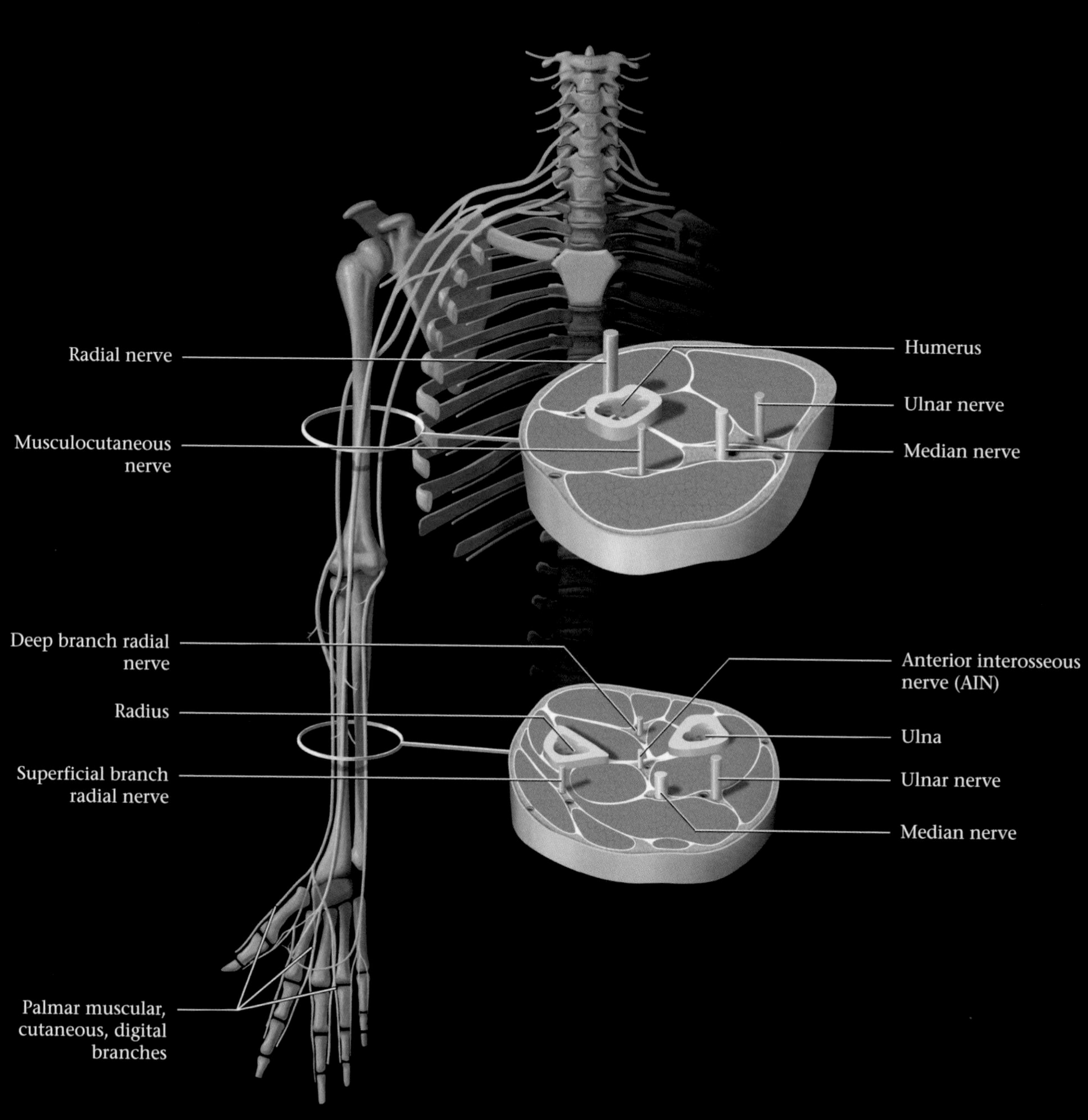
Radial nerve
Musculocutaneous nerve
Deep branch radial nerve
Radius
Superficial branch radial nerve
Palmar muscular, cutaneous, digital branches
Humerus
Ulnar nerve
Median nerve
Anterior interosseous nerve (AIN)
Ulna
Ulnar nerve
Median nerve

Graphic image demonstrates the normal course of the median nerve. Median nerve arises from branches of both the lateral and medial brachial plexus cords, and passes directly through the arm [median nerve has no branches in axilla or arm, and serves no brachial (arm) muscles]. At the elbow, MN gives off the anterior interosseous nerve branch and continues as the median nerve proper into the hand under the flexor retinaculum.

AXIAL T1 MR

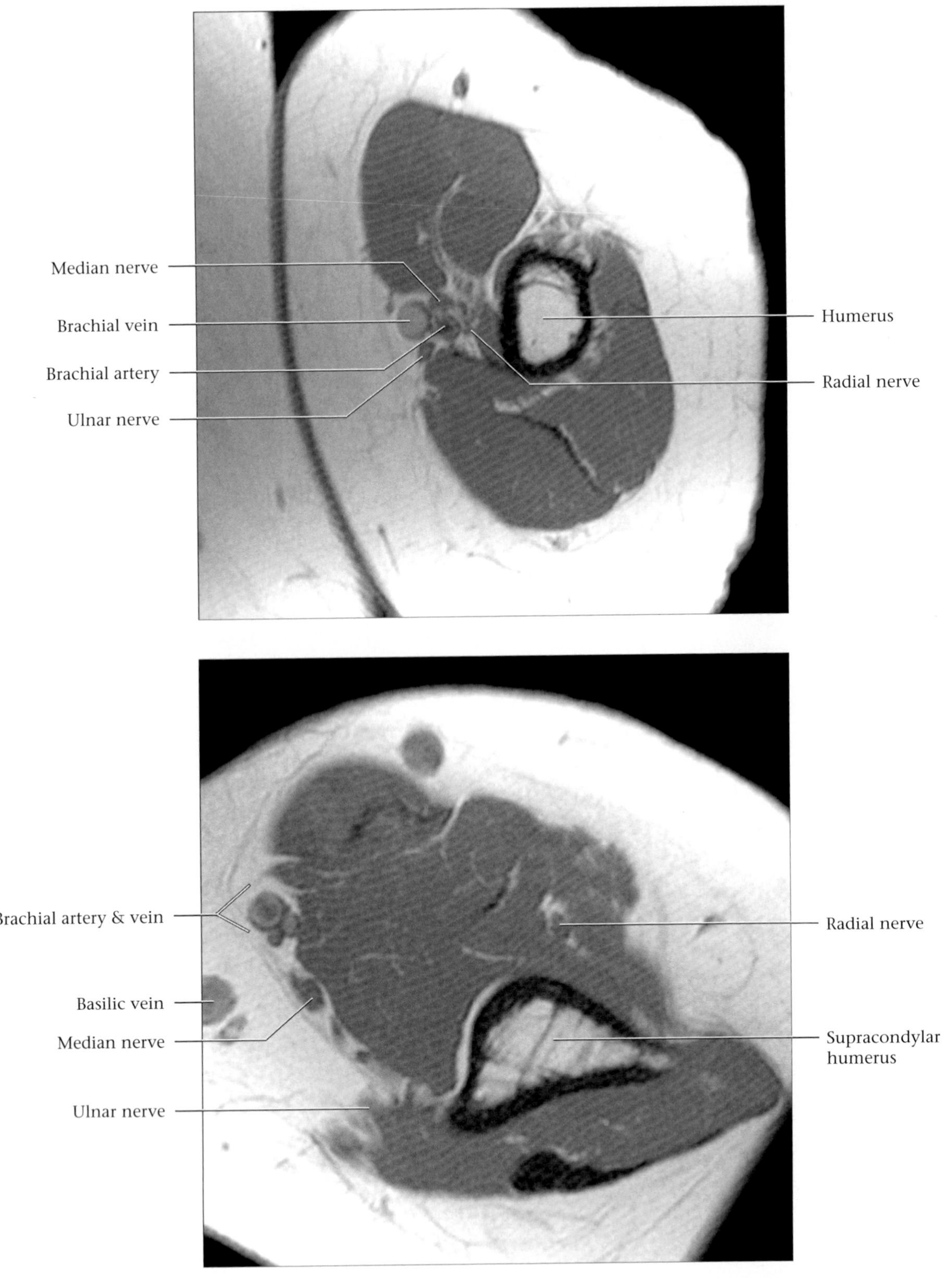
Median nerve
Brachial vein
Brachial artery
Ulnar nerve
Humerus
Radial nerve
Brachial artery & vein
Basilic vein
Median nerve
Ulnar nerve
Radial nerve
Supracondylar humerus

(Top) First of two axial T1 MR images presented from superior to inferior demonstrates median nerve traveling with the radial and ulnar nerves in the arm. The neurovascular complex also includes the brachial artery and brachial vein. **(Bottom)** Image lower in arm at the supracondylar humerus level depicts median nerve traveling separately from the radial and ulnar nerves and the brachial vessels.

AXIAL T1 MR

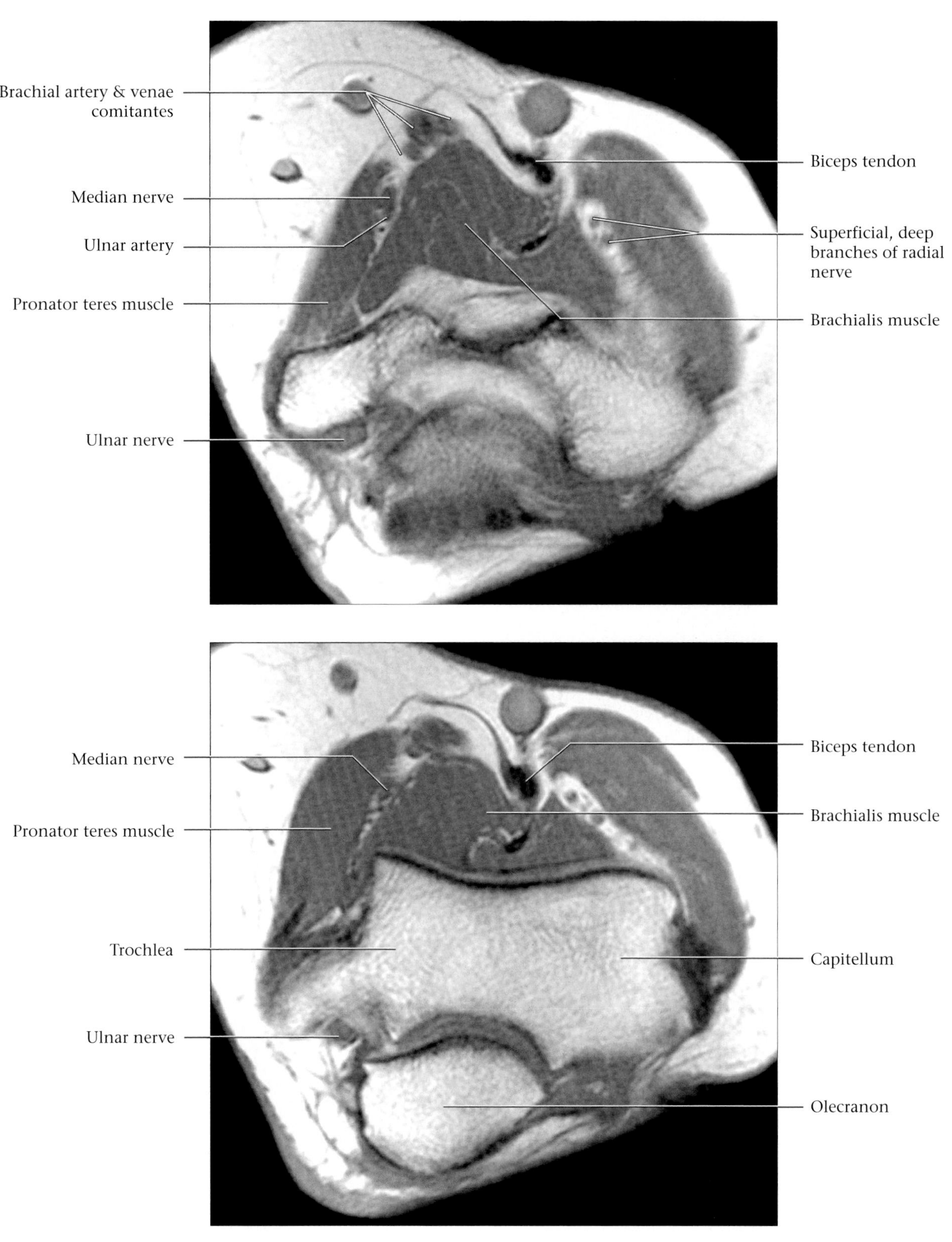
Brachial artery & venae comitantes
Median nerve
Ulnar artery
Pronator teres muscle
Ulnar nerve
Biceps tendon
Superficial, deep branches of radial nerve
Brachialis muscle
Median nerve
Pronator teres muscle
Trochlea
Ulnar nerve
Biceps tendon
Brachialis muscle
Capitellum
Olecranon

(Top) First of two axial T1 MR images at the left elbow presented from superior to inferior demonstrates median nerve traveling with the ulnar artery between the pronator teres and brachialis muscles in the medial volar forearm. At this level, the caliber of median nerve is smaller than the ulnar nerve. **(Bottom)** Image lower in the left elbow at the level of the humeral condyles shows median nerve within the volar medial forearm. The median nerve travels between the pronator teres and brachialis muscles at the elbow.

AXIAL T1 MR

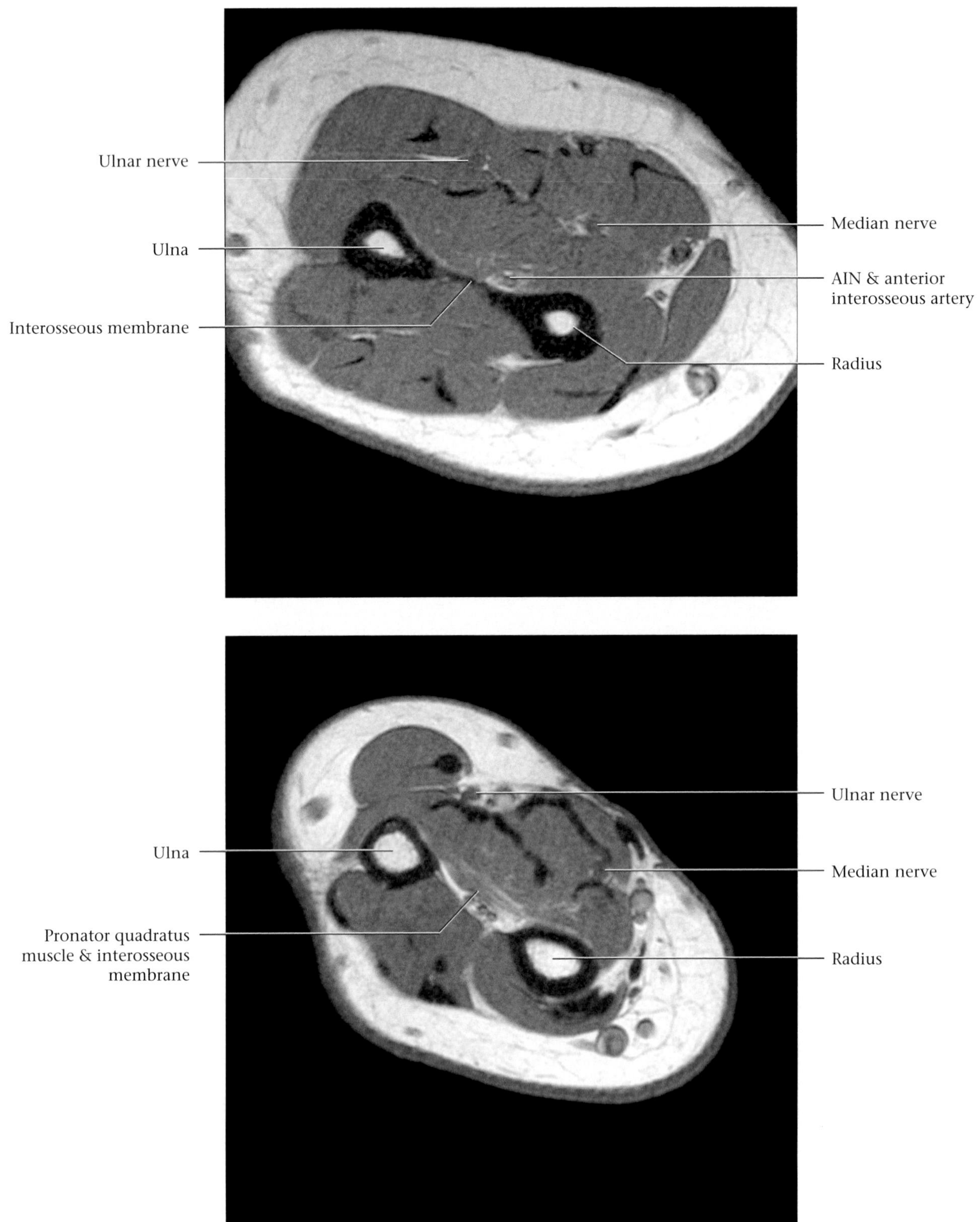
Ulnar nerve
Ulna
Interosseous membrane
Median nerve
AIN & anterior interosseous artery
Radius
Ulnar nerve
Ulna
Median nerve
Pronator quadratus muscle & interosseous membrane
Radius

(Top) First of two axial T1 MR images of the forearm presented from superior to inferior depicts median nerve relative to other important regional structures. Note that median nerve has divided into the AIN, which travels deep along the volar surface of the interosseous membrane with the anterior interosseous artery, and the main median nerve which continues into the wrist through the carpal tunnel. **(Bottom)** Image more distal in the forearm demonstrates the normal course of AIN and median nerve proper in the distal forearm. At this level, the median nerve is fairly superficial but readily identifiable.

AXIAL PD FS MR

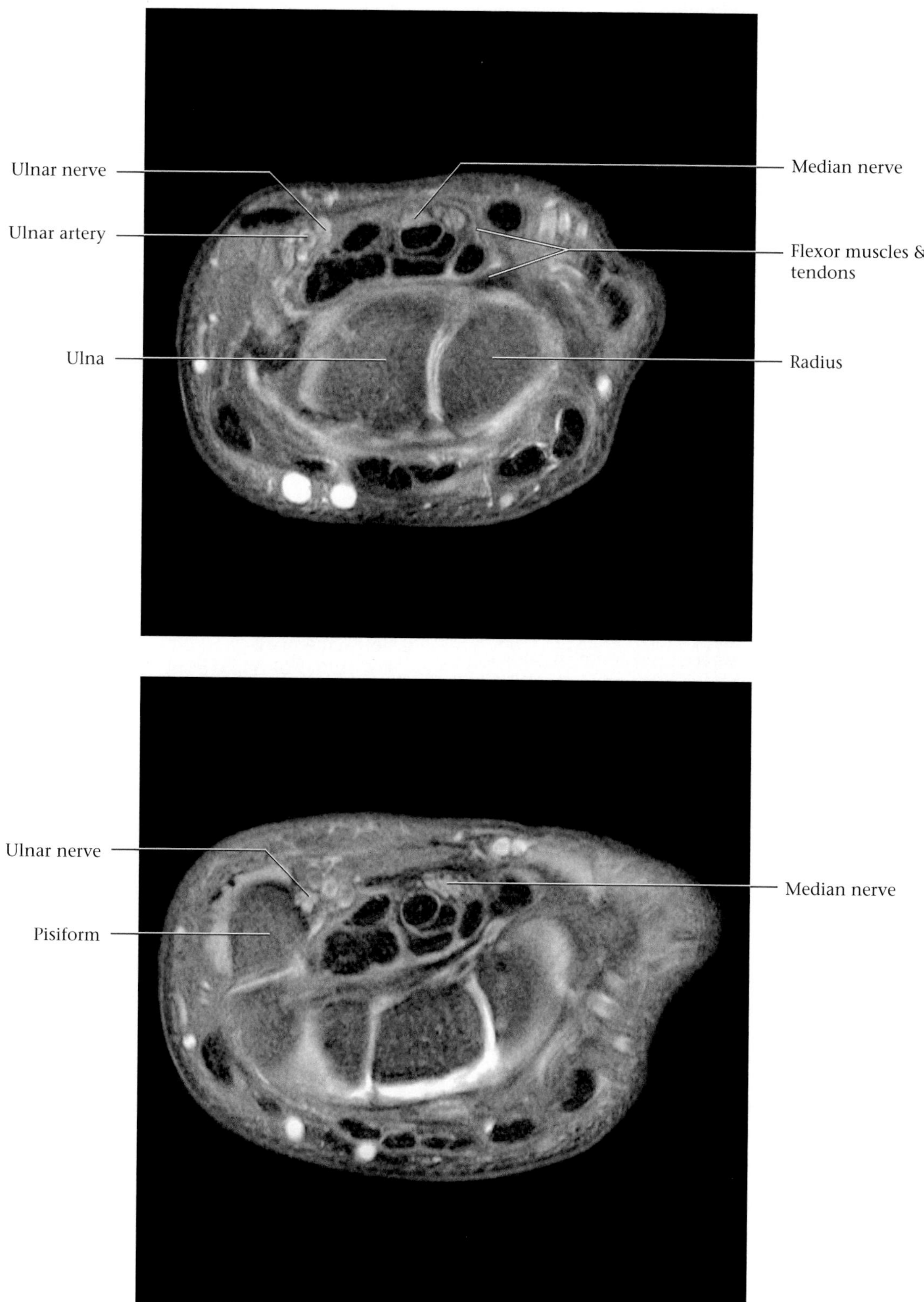
Ulnar nerve
Ulnar artery
Ulna
Median nerve
Flexor muscles & tendons
Radius
Ulnar nerve
Pisiform
Median nerve

(Top) First of two axial fat-saturated PD MR images through the wrist presented from superior to inferior shows the median nerve well relative to adjacent important regional structures. Median nerve travels superficial to the flexor muscles and tendons and lateral (radial) to the ulnar nerve. **(Bottom)** Image at the level of the Guyon and carpal tunnels shows the normal median nerve appearance, with mildly hyperintense (to muscle) fascicles. The nerve is normally a bit larger and flatter at the wrist than other levels, which must be remembered when imaging for clinically suspected carpal tunnel entrapment syndrome.

FEMORAL NERVE

Terminology

Abbreviations

- Femoral nerve (FN)
- Lumbar plexus (LP)
- Ventral primary ramus (VPR)

Gross Anatomy

Overview

- **Lumbar plexus**
  - Paraspinal nerve plexus
  - Lies in posterior part of psoas major
  - Formed by L2-4 VPRs
  - Branches
    - Ventral branches of L2-4 VPRs form **obturator nerve**
    - Smaller dorsal branches of L2, L3 VPRs unite to form **lateral femoral cutaneous nerve**
    - Larger dorsal branches of L2-4 VPRs form **femoral nerve**
- **Femoral nerve**
  - Largest branch of LP
  - Composed of
    - Dorsal branches of L2-4 VPRs
    - Abdominal branches supply iliacus, pectineus muscles
  - In thigh, FN splits into anterior, posterior divisions
  - Anterior division branches
    - **Intermediate femoral cutaneous nerve**
    - **Medial femoral cutaneous nerve**
    - Branches to sartorius muscle
  - Posterior division
    - **Saphenous nerve** (largest femoral cutaneous branch)
    - **Muscular branches** to quadriceps, rectus femoris, vastus muscles

Anatomy Relationships

- FN descends through psoas major
- Runs caudally in iliopsoas groove, deep to iliac fascia
- Exits pelvis by passing behind inguinal ligament
- Runs inferiorly in close proximity to femoral artery/vein
- Courses lateral to femoral artery/vein within femoral canal
  - Acronym for femoral canal contents from lateral to medial = NAVL (nerve, artery, vein, lymphatics)
- FN splits into anterior, posterior divisions
- Anterior division branches
  - **Intermediate femoral cutaneous nerve**
    - Pierces fascia lata
    - Descends on front of thigh
    - Supplies skin to knee
  - **Medial femoral cutaneous nerve**
    - Lateral, then anterior to femoral artery at apex of femoral triangle
    - Anterior branch descends on sartorius, supplies skin as low as medial aspect of knee
    - Posterior branch anastomoses with saphenous, obturator nerve branches; supplies medial leg
- Posterior division branches
  - **Saphenous nerve**
    - Descends in adductor canal
    - First lateral, then medial to femoral artery
    - Descends on medial side of leg
    - Supplies skin of medial thigh, knee, leg

Imaging Anatomy

Overview

- MR of normal FN
  - T1WI: Round/ovoid shape
  - STIR/fat suppressed T2WI
    - Well-defined internal fascicular architecture
    - Uniformly mildly hyperintense fascicles + interspersed hypointense fibrofatty connective tissue

Anatomy-Based Imaging Issues

Imaging Recommendations

- MR
  - Best coils
    - Preferred: Torso wrap-around phase array coil
    - Alternative: Flexible extremity surface coil
  - Best planes
    - Direct coronal, axial
  - Best sequences
    - Coronal T1WI, STIR or fat-saturated T2WI
    - Axial T1WI, STIR or fat-saturated T2WI
    - Optional: Coronal, axial fat-saturated T1 C+
  - Area to cover: Similar to sciatic nerve imaging in thigh
    - Extend scan from sacrum (posterior) to skin of groin (anterior)
    - Visualizes FN under inguinal ligament

Clinical Implications

Clinical Importance

- FN neuropathy characterized by
  - Quadriceps wasting/weakness
  - Pain/paresthesias anteromedial thigh, medial leg
- FN especially vulnerable to injuries at two points
  - Within iliopsoas groove
  - At groin
- FN generally not subject to entrapment but may be compressed
- Compressive FN neuropathy
  - Secondary to pelvic tumor such as
    - Lymphoma
    - Sarcoma
  - Secondary to psoas hematoma
    - Trauma
    - Coagulopathy
    - Hemophilia
- Noncompressive FN neuropathy
  - Diabetes
  - Surgical (e.g., inadvertent ligation during herniorrhaphy)

FEMORAL NERVE

GRAPHIC

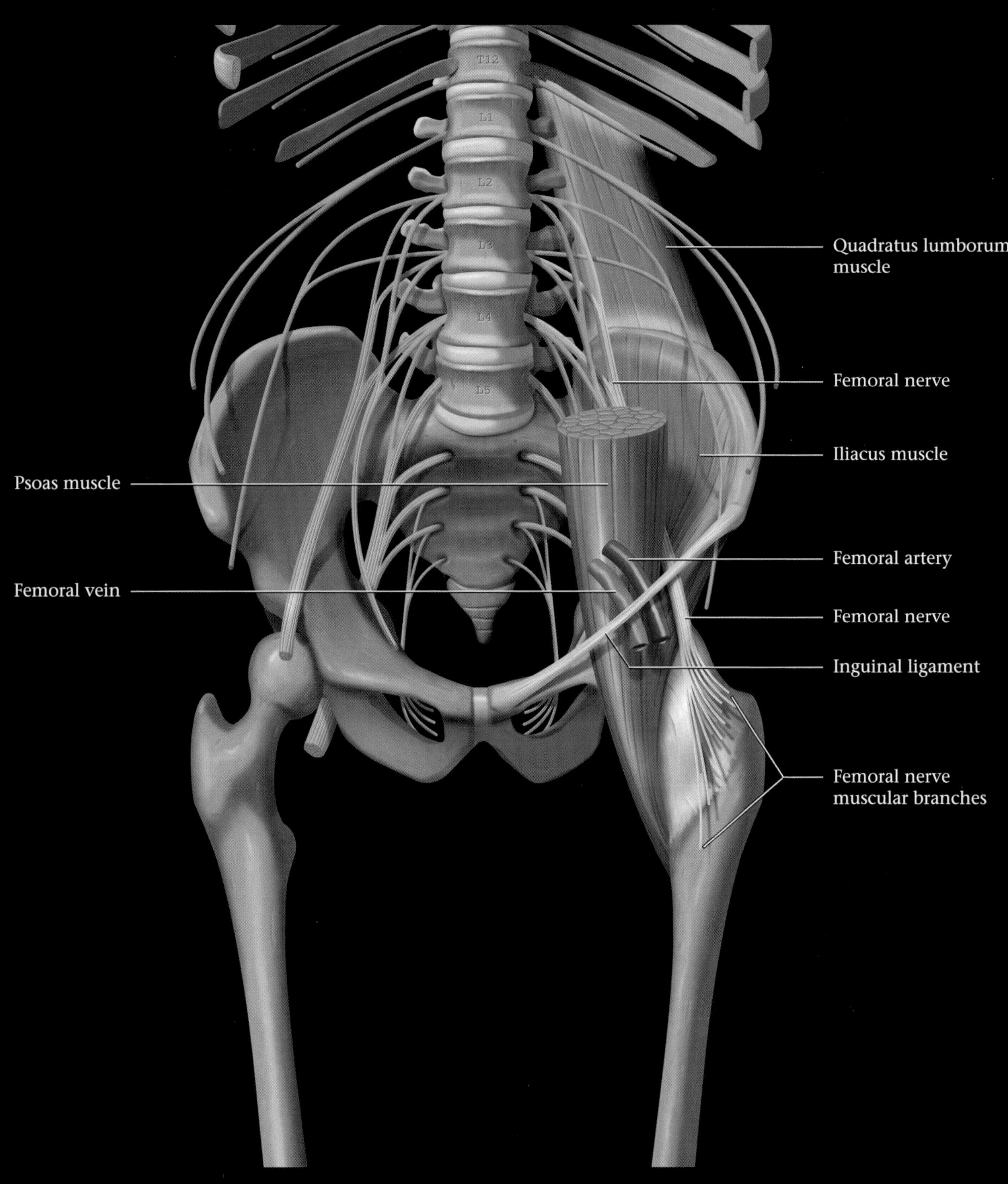
T12
L1
L2
L3
L4
L5
Quadratus lumborum muscle
Femoral nerve
Iliacus muscle
Psoas muscle
Femoral artery
Femoral vein
Femoral nerve
Inguinal ligament
Femoral nerve muscular branches

Graphic shows the femoral nerve arising from L2, L3, and L4 nerve roots (ventral primary rami) and traveling in groove created by iliacus and psoas muscles (iliopsoas groove). FN travels with the femoral artery and vein under the inguinal ligament to provide innervation to quadriceps muscles in thigh. The well known acronym "NAVL" (nerve, artery, vein, lymphatics) describes the order of femoral canal contents from lateral to medial.

CORONAL T1 MR

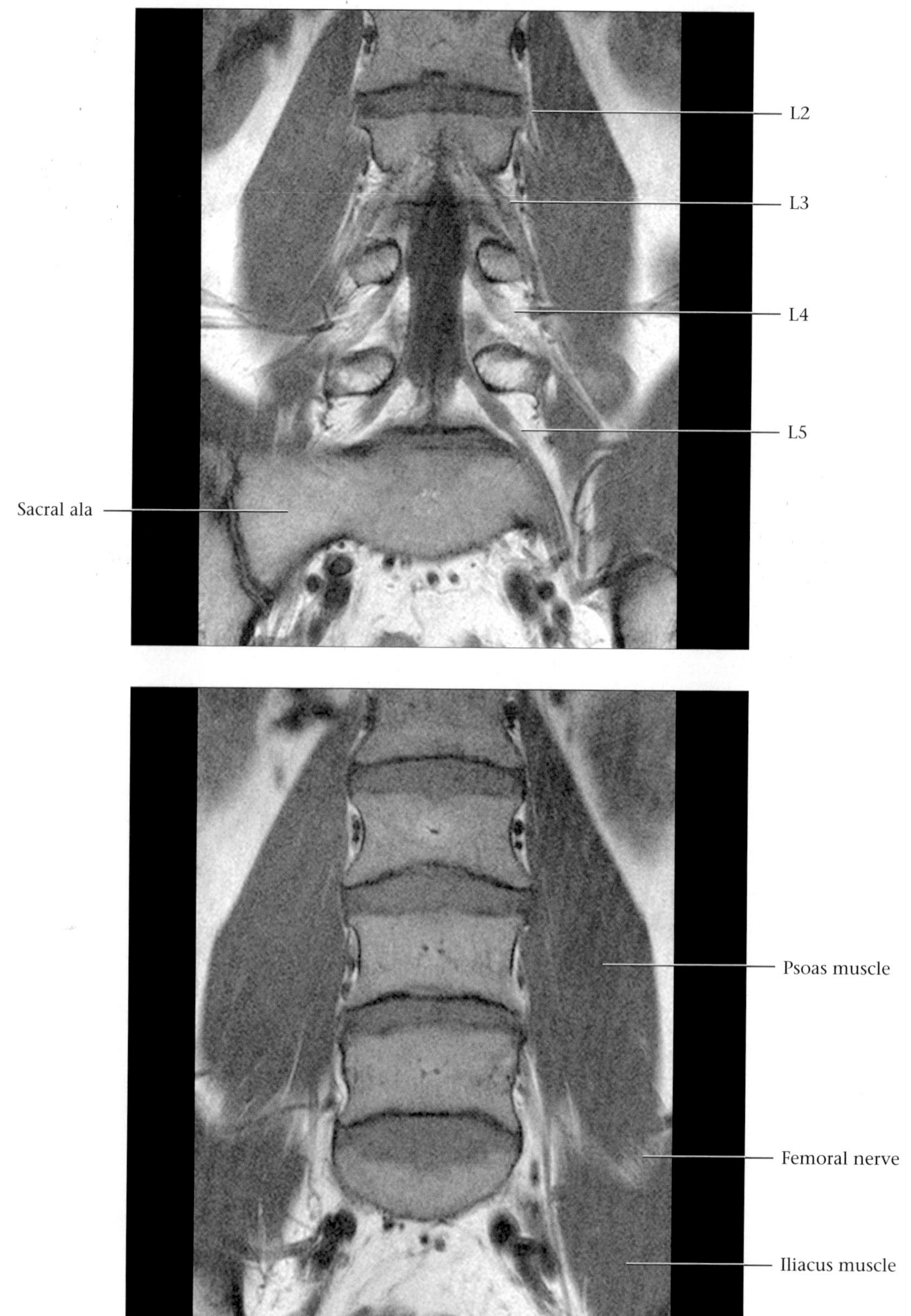
L2
L3
L4
L5
Sacral ala
Psoas muscle
Femoral nerve
Iliacus muscle

(Top) First of two coronal T1 MR images presented from posterior to anterior demonstrates the ventral primary rami (L2-4) which will form the lumbar plexus. L5 will combine with a minor branch of L4 to form the lumbosacral trunk. **(Bottom)** Image more anteriorly after formation of the lumbar plexus shows the femoral nerve in the iliopsoas groove. The lumbar plexus is isointense to muscle signal, and often difficult to identify on coronal T1 MR images.

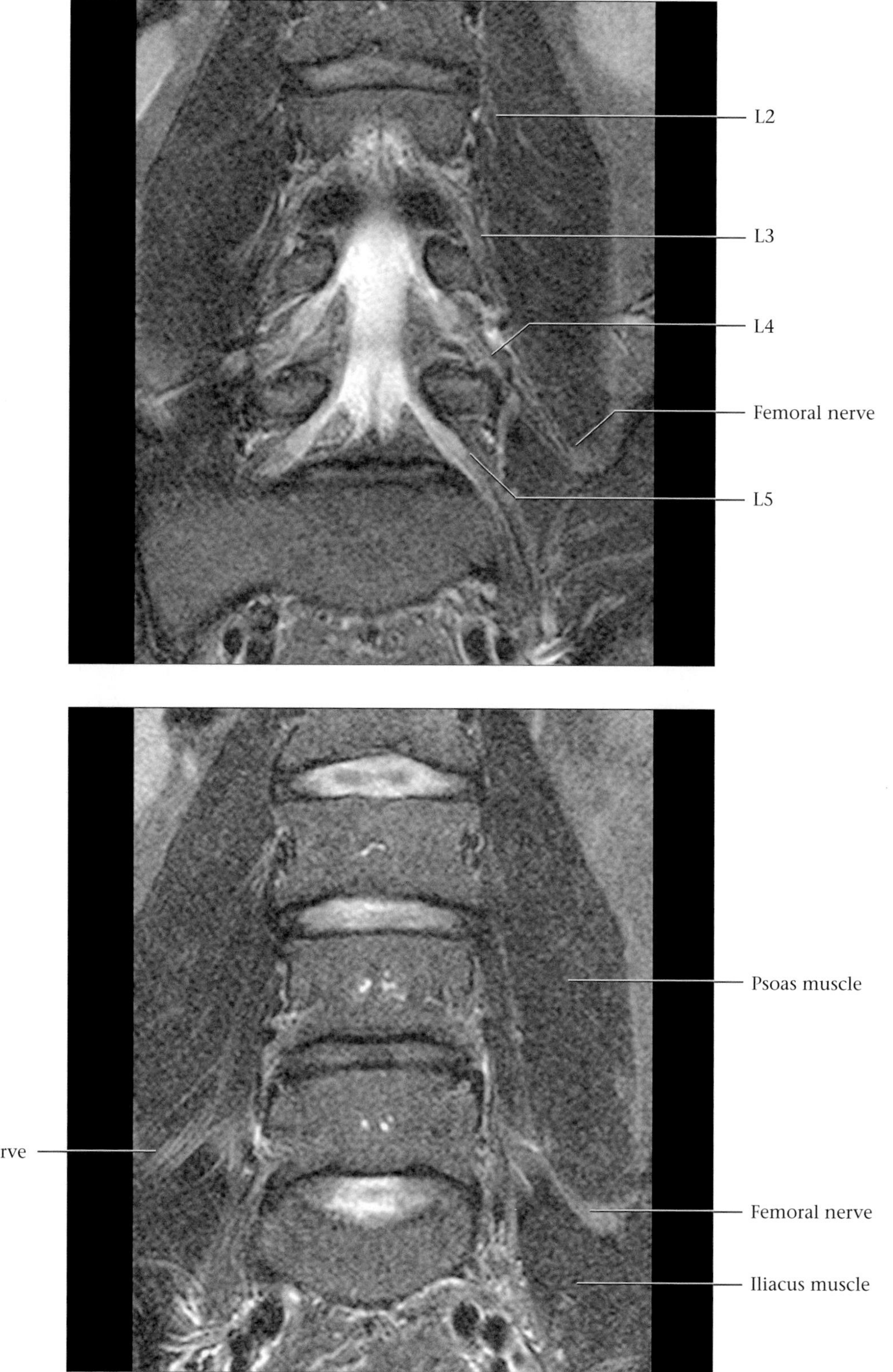
L2
L3
L4
Femoral nerve
L5
Psoas muscle
Femoral nerve
Femoral nerve
Iliacus muscle

(Top) First of two coronal STIR MR images depicts the proximal rami contributions to the lumbar plexus. The proximal femoral nerve travels in the iliopsoas groove, and is easily identifiable by its fascicular nature and mild hyperintensity (to adjacent muscle). **(Bottom)** Image more anteriorly located shows the bilateral femoral nerves traveling in the iliopsoas grooves. The distinct fascicular pattern is unique to normal nerves and readily permits their distinction from vessels.

CORONAL & AXIAL STIR MR

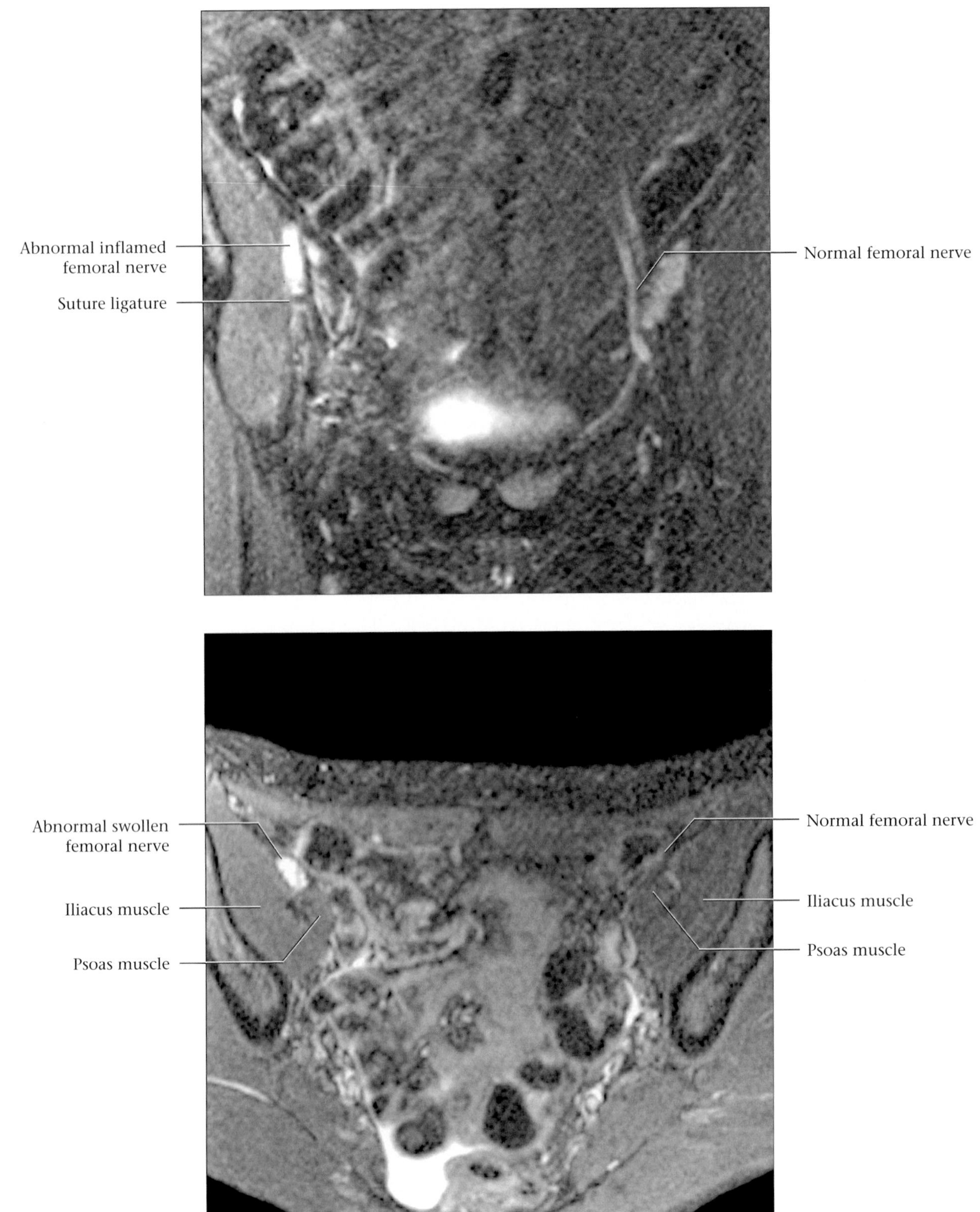

Abnormal inflamed femoral nerve
Suture ligature
Normal femoral nerve
Abnormal swollen femoral nerve
Iliacus muscle
Psoas muscle
Normal femoral nerve
Iliacus muscle
Psoas muscle

(Top) Coronal STIR MR shows the femoral nerves as they descend out of the pelvis into the femoral canal. The normal left femoral nerve is mildly hyperintense to muscle. The right femoral nerve is swollen and abnormally hyperintense to the level of a suture inadvertently ligating the femoral nerve during a herniorrhaphy. This image reinforces the importance of continuing coronal slices anteriorly to groin skin to avoid missing lesions within the femoral canal. **(Bottom)** Axial STIR MR image obtained in the pelvis contrasts the normal left femoral nerve within the iliopsoas groove to the abnormally swollen hyperintense right femoral nerve proximal to an inadvertent surgical ligature during herniorrhaphy. Note that both nerves clearly demonstrate the distinctive fascicular architecture of nerves. At this level, the iliacus and psoas muscles functionally form the iliopsoas muscle.

FEMORAL NERVE

AXIAL T1 MR

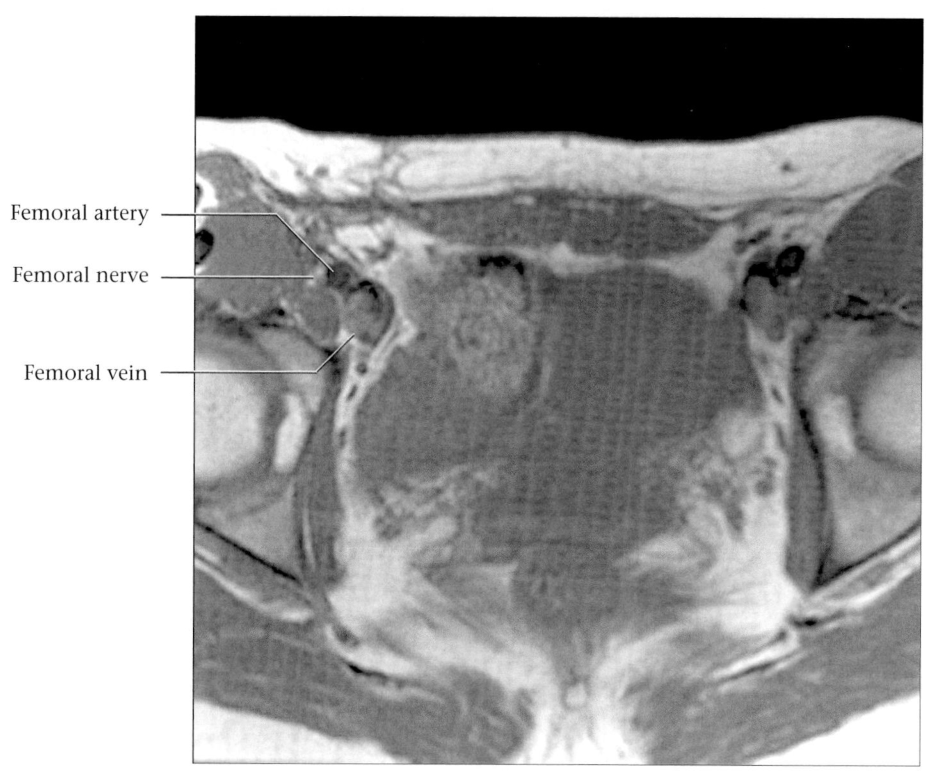
Femoral artery
Femoral nerve
Femoral vein

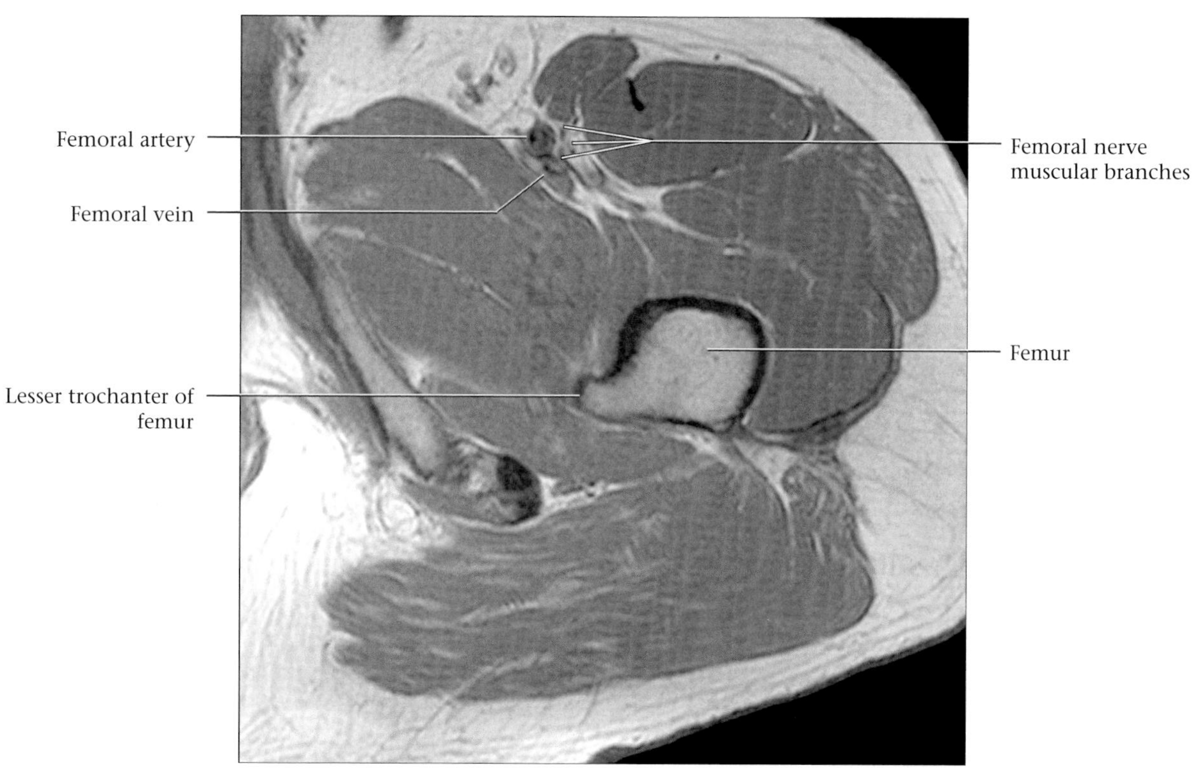
Femoral artery
Femoral vein
Lesser trochanter of femur
Femoral nerve muscular branches
Femur

(Top) Axial T1 MR image obtained at the level of the femoral canal demonstrates the right femoral nerve lateral to the femoral artery, veins, and lymphatics (not seen). The acronym "NAVL" helps to remember the order of structures within the femoral canal from lateral to medial. The left femoral nerve is not seen well. The femoral nerve is small at this level and often difficult to identify as a discrete structure unless abnormally swollen. **(Bottom)** Axial T1 MR image through the proximal thigh shows the femoral nerve branching into muscular branches that will supply the anterior thigh quadriceps muscles. It is difficult to image femoral nerve distal to these proximal branches because of their small size and similar signal intensity to muscles.

COMMON PERONEAL/TIBIAL NERVES

Terminology

Abbreviations

- Sciatic nerve (SN)
- Common peroneal nerve (CPN)
- Tibial nerve (TN)

Gross Anatomy

Overview

- **Sciatic nerve**
  - Major continuation of sacral plexus
  - Passes behind, below piriformis muscle
    - Common variation: Passes through piriformis
  - Exits pelvis through greater sciatic foramen
  - Passes between greater trochanter, ischial tuberosity
  - Descends along posterior thigh
  - Proximal to knee, divides into two major terminal branches
    - Common peroneal (fibular) nerve
    - Tibial nerve
    - CPN, TN divisions discrete entities within SN prior to division
    - TN usually larger, more medially located than CPN
  - Supplies knee flexors + all muscles below knee
- **Tibial nerve**
  - Larger terminal branch of SN
  - VPR of L4-5, S1-3
  - Descends along back of thigh, popliteal fossa
  - Sends articular branches to knee
  - Branches to posterior leg muscles
    - Gastrocnemius
    - Plantaris
    - Soleus
    - Popliteus
    - Tibialis posterior
    - Flexor digitorum longus
    - Flexor hallucis longus
  - Sural nerve (posterior/lateral skin of distal third of leg, lateral foot)
  - Medial calcanean branches (skin of heel, medial plantar surface)
  - Medial plantar nerve (main termination of tibial nerve to medial sole of foot, plantar muscles)
  - Lateral plantar nerve
    - Lateral sole of foot
    - Most deep muscles of foot
- **Common peroneal nerve**
  - Smaller terminal branch of SN
  - Descends obliquely along lateral popliteal fossa to fibula
  - Traverses lateral aspect of head of fibula
    - Especially vulnerable to injury at this point
  - Two major terminal branches
    - Superficial peroneal nerve (SPN)
    - Deep peroneal nerve (DPN)
  - DPN supplies anterior compartment leg muscles
    - Tibialis anterior
    - Peroneus
    - Extensor hallucis longus, brevis
    - Skin on lateral aspect of ankle, dorsal foot
  - SPN supplies
    - Peroneus longus, brevis
    - Skin of lower leg

Anatomy-Based Imaging Issues

Imaging Recommendations

- **Tibial nerve**
  - Coils
    - Preferred: Torso wrap-around phase array coil
    - Alternative: Flexible extremity surface coil
  - Best plane: Direct axial
  - Best sequences
    - T1WI, STIR/fat-saturated T2WI
    - Optional: Fat-saturated T1 C+
- **Common peroneal nerve**
  - Coils
    - Preferred: Torso wrap-around phase array coil
    - Alternative: Knee coil (excellent images but limited coverage) or flexible extremity surface coil
  - Best plane: Direct axial
  - Best sequences
    - T1WI, STIR/fat-saturated T2WI
    - Optional: Fat-saturated T1 C+

Imaging Approaches

- Torso coil preferred for most suspected TN, CPN lesions
  - Excellent signal-to-noise (SNR)
  - Large coverage distance
  - Wrap coil around both legs
  - Image one leg at a time ⇒ maximizes spatial resolution
  - Imaging both legs simultaneously ⇒ ↑ FOV, ↓ SNR
- Knee coil
  - Optimal if specifically imaging CPN at fibular head

Clinical Implications

Clinical Importance

- Lesions of SN, branches (CPN, TN) can occur at numerous locations
- Sciatic nerve
  - Compression as components leave lumbosacral spine
  - Compression as SN leaves pelvis
  - Piriformis syndrome (common anatomic variant but entrapment rare)
- CPN neuropathy
  - Paresis/weakness of ankle/toe dorsiflexion (foot drop)
  - Most common cause = CPN compression at fibular head
  - Less common: After total knee arthroplasty, proximal tibial osteotomy
- TN neuropathy
  - Pain, paresthesias, paresis of plantar flexion at ankle
  - TN can be entrapped as traverses tarsal tunnel

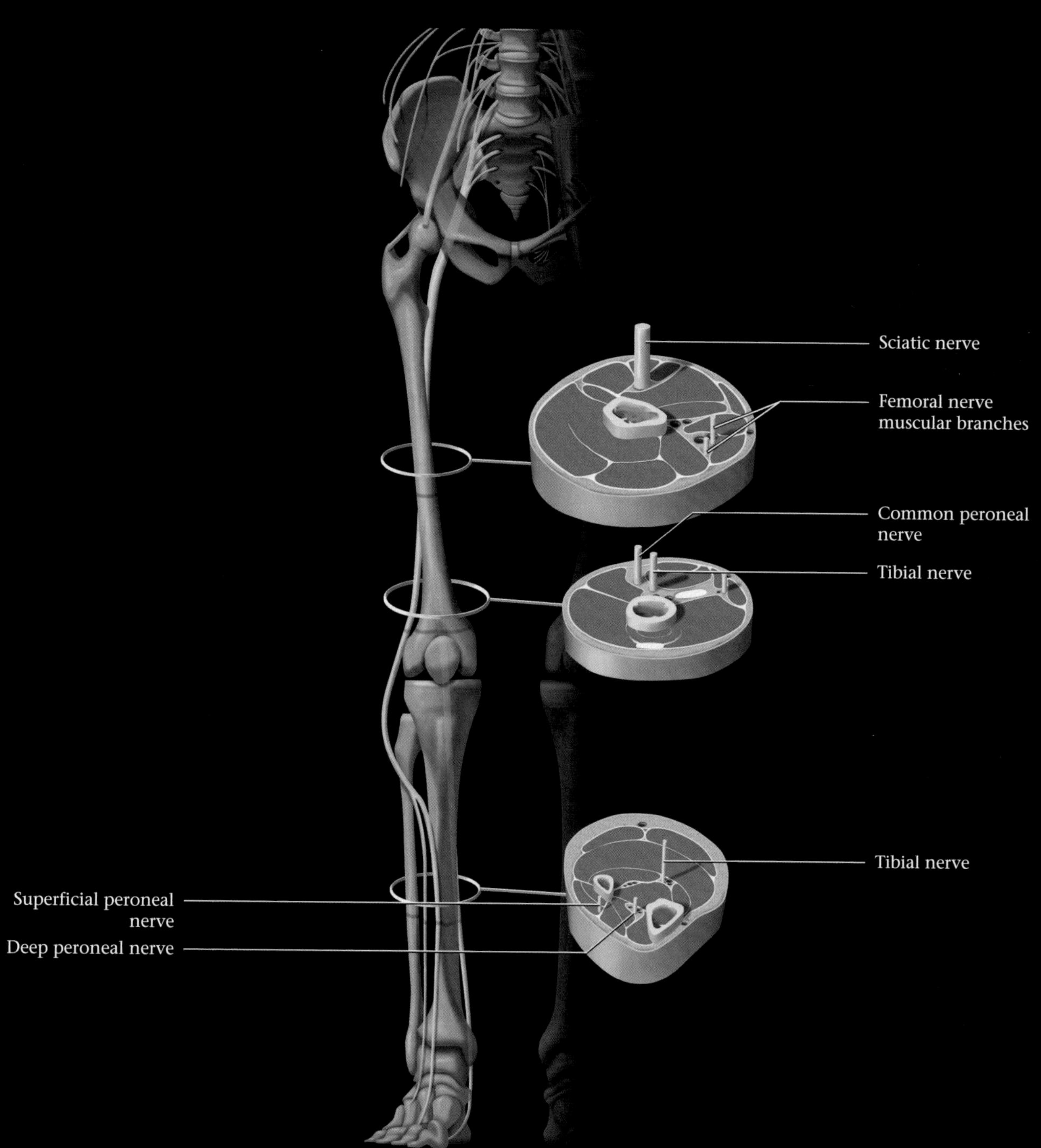

Sciatic nerve
Femoral nerve muscular branches
Common peroneal nerve
Tibial nerve
Tibial nerve
Superficial peroneal nerve
Deep peroneal nerve

Graphic of the right leg, seen from anterior perspective, demonstrates the normal course of the sciatic nerve and its terminal tibial nerve and common peroneal nerve branches. The tibial nerve remains in the posterior compartment where it supplies the muscles of the posterior leg, while the common peroneal nerve moves laterally around the fibular head (where it is vulnerable to injury) and descends in the anterolateral leg to supply the anterior leg muscles. Common peroneal nerve divides into superficial and deep terminal branches. The superficial peroneal nerve supplies the peroneus muscles and extensor digitorum brevis muscle, while the deep peroneal nerve supplies the tibialis anterior, extensor digitorum longus, and extensor hallucis longus muscles.

COMMON PERONEAL/TIBIAL NERVES

AXIAL T1 MR

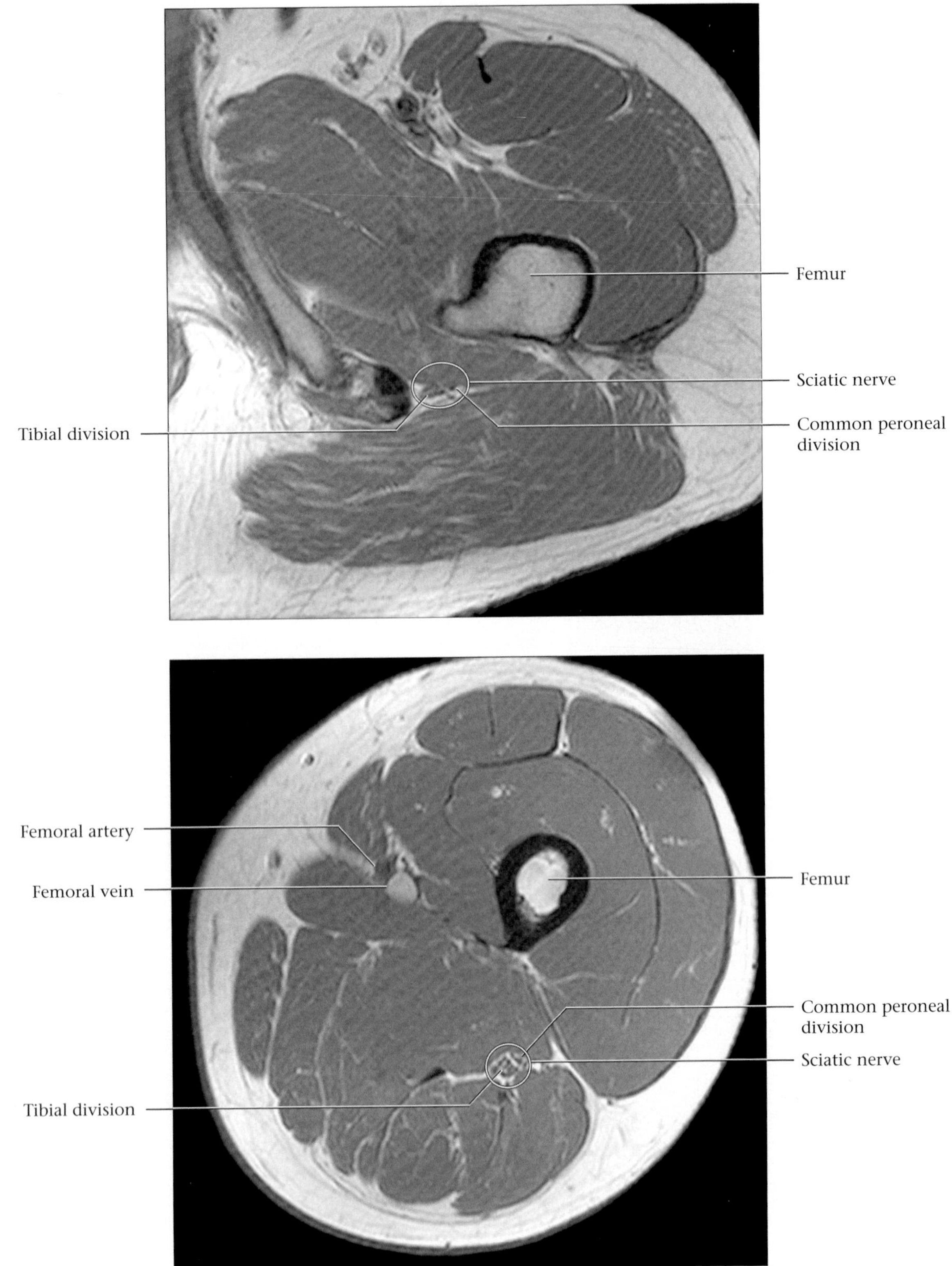
Femur
Sciatic nerve
Common peroneal division
Tibial division
Femoral artery
Femoral vein
Femur
Common peroneal division
Sciatic nerve
Tibial division

(Top) First of two axial T1 MR images through the left thigh presented from superior to inferior demonstrates the left sciatic nerve residing between the obturator internus and gluteus maximus muscles. Even at this level, the common peroneal division and tibial division fibers are anatomically distinguishable even though the sciatic nerve proper contains both divisions within a single epineurium layer. **(Bottom)** Image obtained more distally through the left thigh shows clear separation of the common peroneal nerve and tibial nerve fibers within the sciatic nerve. This somatotopic distribution of nerve fibers explains why some patients with sciatic nerve lesions may clinically demonstrate either a common peroneal or tibial neuropathy only.

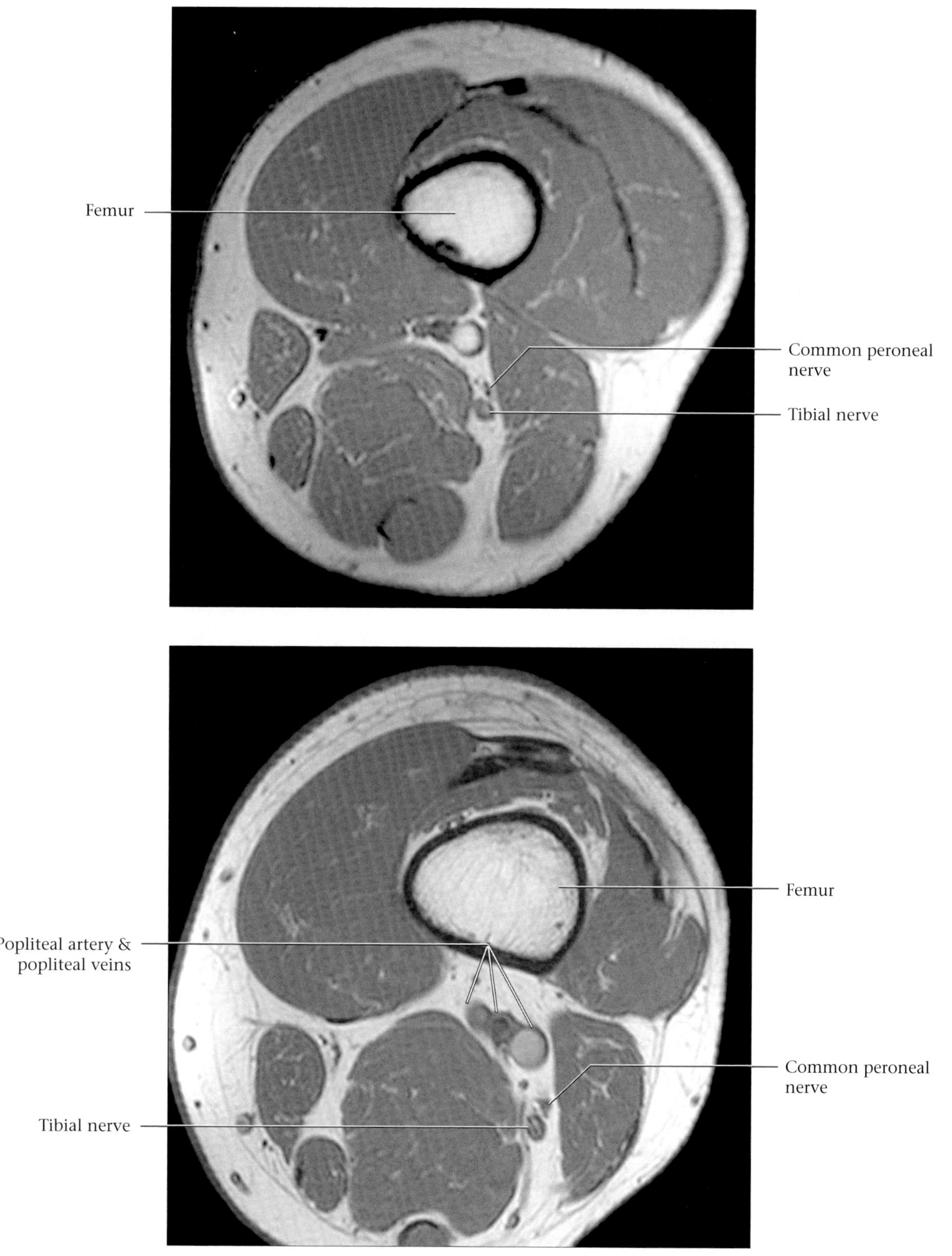

Femur
Common peroneal nerve
Tibial nerve
Femur
Popliteal artery & popliteal veins
Common peroneal nerve
Tibial nerve

(Top) First of two axial T1 MR images through the left mid-thigh depicts the proximal bifurcation of the sciatic nerve into common peroneal and tibial nerve branches. The tibial nerve is normally larger than the common peroneal nerve. **(Bottom)** Image more distal in the left thigh depicts the common peroneal and tibial nerves as separate nerves with separate epineurium, but traveling adjacent to each other in the posterior thigh.

AXIAL T1 MR

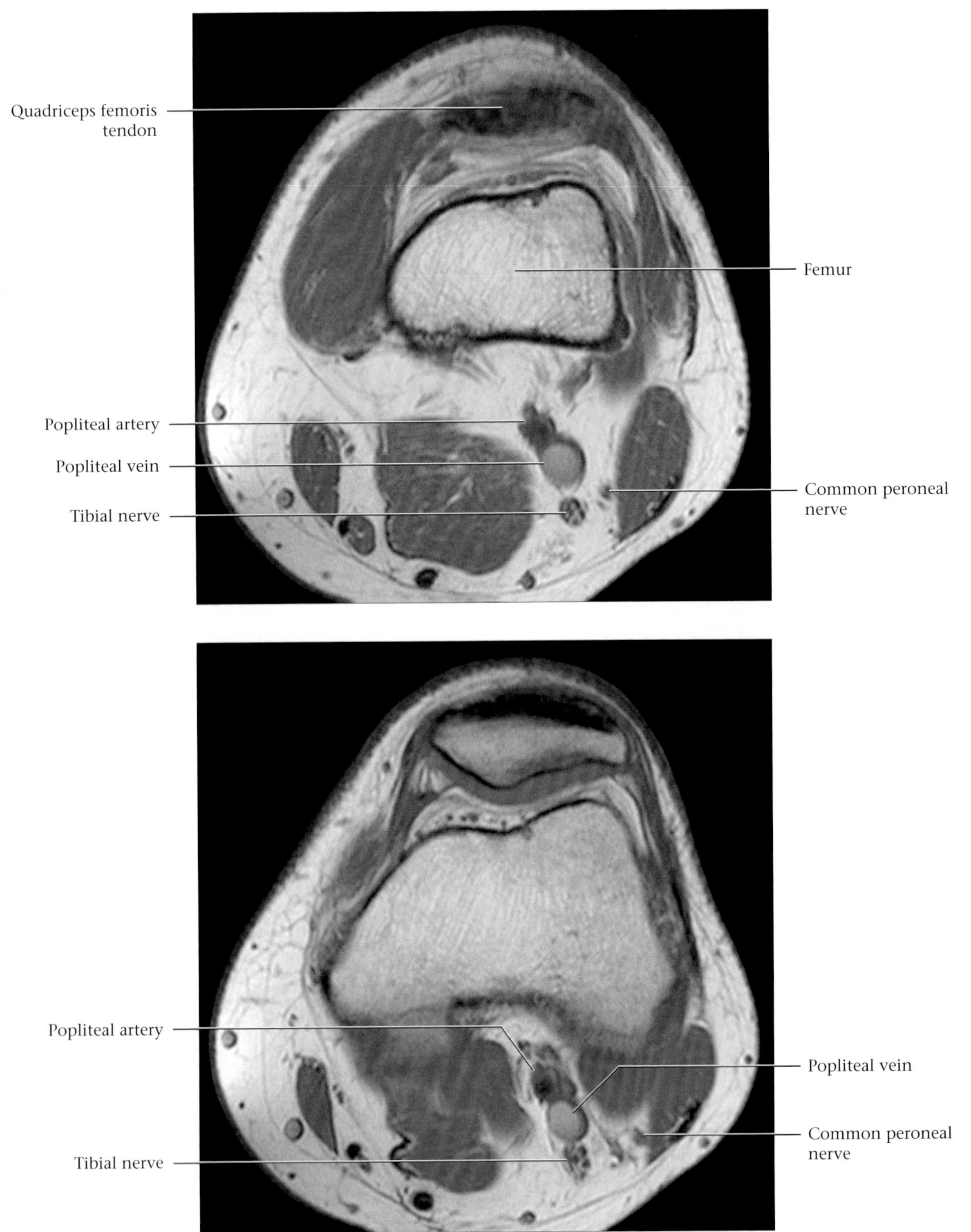
Quadriceps femoris tendon
Femur
Popliteal artery
Popliteal vein
Tibial nerve
Common peroneal nerve
Popliteal artery
Popliteal vein
Common peroneal nerve
Tibial nerve

(Top) First of two axial T1 MR images through the distal thigh presented from superior to inferior depicts the larger tibial nerve continuing straight distally and the smaller common peroneal nerve moving laterally in preparation to transit around the fibular head. **(Bottom)** Image obtained more distally in the left thigh at the level of the supracondylar femur clearly depicts the isointense (to muscle) tibial nerve fascicles separated by bright fibrofatty connective tissue. The smaller common peroneal nerve is laterally positioned.

AXIAL T1 MR

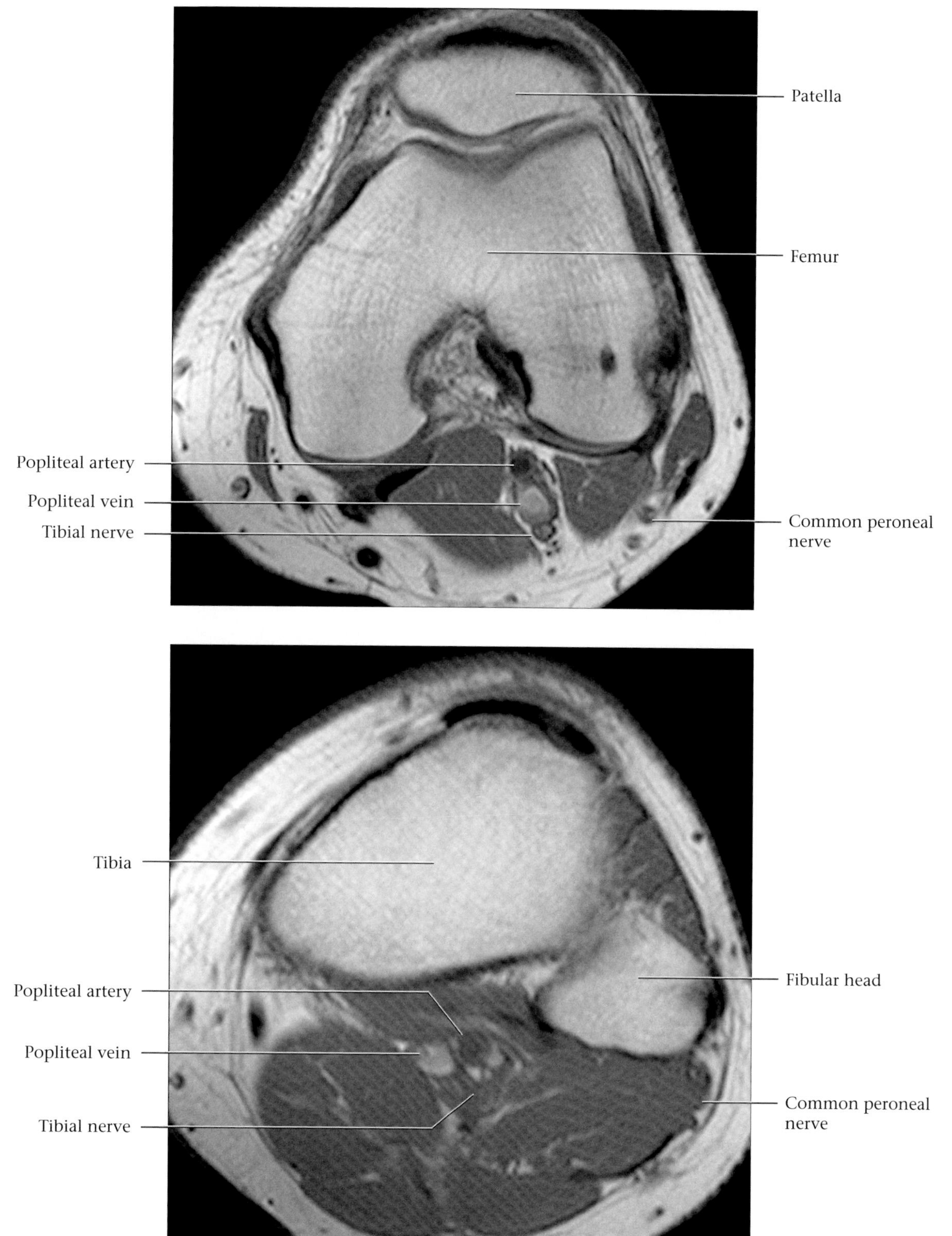

Patella
Femur
Popliteal artery
Popliteal vein
Tibial nerve
Common peroneal nerve
Tibia
Fibular head
Popliteal artery
Popliteal vein
Tibial nerve
Common peroneal nerve

(Top) Axial T1 MR image obtained at the femoral condyle level confirms little change in location of the tibial nerve as it moves distally towards the knee joint. Conversely, the common peroneal nerve is moving progressively laterally. **(Bottom)** Axial T1 MR image obtained below the knee joint at the level of the proximal tibia and fibula reveals the lateral superficial position of the common peroneal nerve at the fibular head. Because of this superficial anatomical position adjacent to the hard fibular head, the common peroneal nerve is commonly injured in this location.

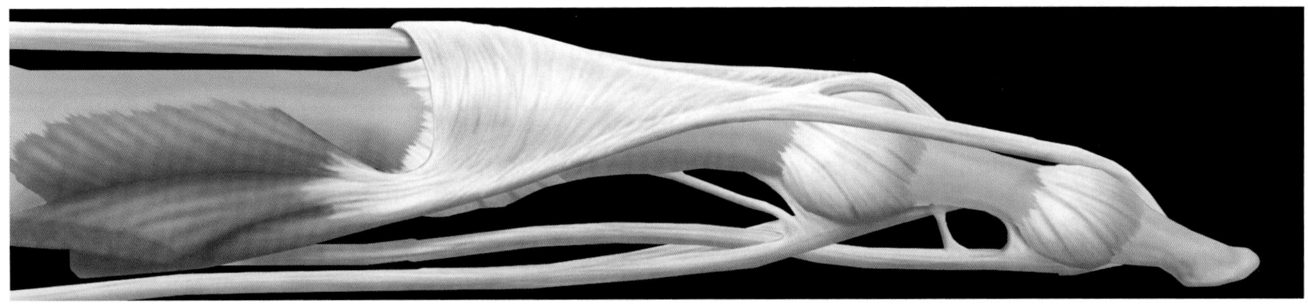

INDEX

A

INDEX

INDEX

B

INDEX

C

INDEX

INDEX

INDEX

INDEX

INDEX

INDEX

INDEX

INDEX

INDEX

F

INDEX

INDEX

G

H

INDEX

I

INDEX

INDEX

INDEX

J

INDEX

INDEX

INDEX

M

INDEX

INDEX

N

INDEX

O

INDEX

INDEX

P

INDEX

INDEX

INDEX

INDEX

INDEX

INDEX

INDEX

INDEX

INDEX

INDEX

INDEX

U

V

INDEX

INDEX

W

Z